Every Decker book is accompanied by a CD-ROM.

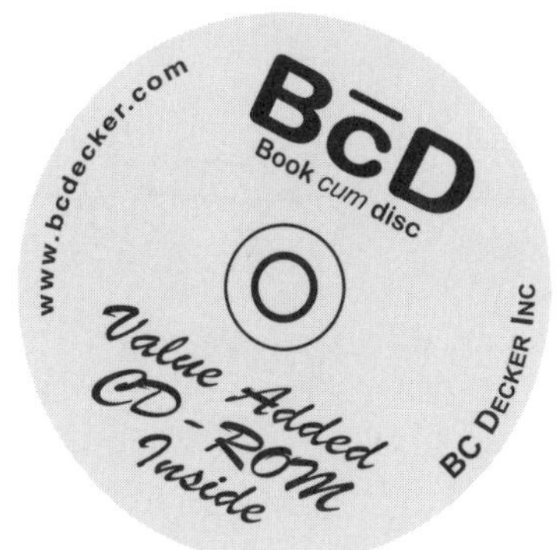

The disc appears in the front of each copy, in its own sealed jacket. Affixed to the front of the book will be a distinctive Bc̄D sticker "Book *cum* disc."

The disc contains the complete text and illustrations of the book, in fully searchable PDF files. The book and disc are sold *only* as a package; neither is available independently, and no prices are available for the items individually.

BC Decker Inc is committed to providing high-quality electronic publications that complement traditional information and learning methods.

We trust you will find the book/CD package invaluable and invite your comments and suggestions.

Brian C. Decker
CEO and Publisher

ENDODONTICS

Fifth Edition

ENDODONTICS

Fifth Edition

JOHN I. INGLE, DDS, MSD
Lecturer, Department of Endodontics
Loma Linda University School of Dentistry
Loma Linda, California

Formerly Dean and Professor of Endodontics and Periodontics
School of Dentistry
University of Southern California
Los Angeles, California

Formerly Professor and Chairman of Endodontics and Periodontics
School of Dentistry, University of Washington
Seattle, Washington
Diplomate, American Board of Endodontics and American Board of Periodontology

LEIF K. BAKLAND, DDS
Professor and Chairman, Department of Endodontics
Associate Dean, Advanced Education
Loma Linda University School of Dentistry
Loma Linda, California
Diplomate, American Board of Endodontics

2002
BC Decker Inc
Hamilton • London

BC Decker Inc
P.O. Box 620, L.C.D. 1
Hamilton, Ontario L8N 3K7
Tel: 905-522-7017; 800-568-7281
Fax: 905-522-7839; 888-311-4987
E-mail: info@bcdecker.com
www.bcdecker.com

BC Decker

Fourth edition 1994

05 06 07 08/WPC/9 8 7 6 5 4 3 2

ISBN 1-55009-188-3
Printed in the United States of America

Sales and Distribution

United States
BC Decker Inc
P.O. Box 785
Lewiston, NY 14092-0785
Tel: 905-522-7017; 800-568-7281
Fax: 905-522-7839; 888-311-4987
E-mail: info@bcdecker.com
www.bcdecker.com

Canada
BC Decker Inc
20 Hughson Street South
P.O. Box 620, LCD 1
Hamilton, Ontario L8N 3K7
Tel: 905-522-7017; 800-568-7281
Fax: 905-522-7839; 888-311-4987
E-mail: info@bcdecker.com
www.bcdecker.com

Foreign Rights
John Scott & Company
International Publishers' Agency
P.O. Box 878
Kimberton, PA 19442
Tel: 610-827-1640
Fax: 610-827-1671
E-mail: jsco@voicenet.com

Japan
Igaku-Shoin Ltd.
Foreign Publications Department
3-24-17 Hongo
Bunkyo-ku, Tokyo, Japan 113-8719
Tel: 3 3817 5680
Fax: 3 3815 6776
E-mail: fd@igaku-shoin.co.jp

UK, Europe, Scandinavia, Middle East
Elsevier Science
Customer Service Department
Foots Cray High Street
Sidcup, Kent
DA14 5HP, UK
Tel: 44 (0) 208 308 5760
Fax: 44 (0) 181 308 5702
E-mail: cservice@harcourt.com

Singapore, Malaysia,Thailand, Philippines, Indonesia, Vietnam, Pacific Rim, Korea
Elsevier Science Asia
583 Orchard Road
#09/01, Forum
Singapore 238884
Tel: 65-737-3593
Fax: 65-753-2145

Australia, New Zealand
Elsevier Science Australia
Customer Service Department
STM Division
Locked Bag 16
St. Peters, New South Wales, 2044
Australia
Tel: 61 02 9517-8999
Fax: 61 02 9517-2249
E-mail: stmp@harcourt.com.au
www.harcourt.com.au

Mexico and Central America
ETM SA de CV
Calle de Tula 59
Colonia Condesa
06140 Mexico DF, Mexico
Tel: 52-5-5553-6657
Fax: 52-5-5211-8468
E-mail: editoresdetextosmex@prodigy.net.mx

Brazil
Tecmedd Importadora E Distribuidora
De Livros Ltda.
Avenida Maurílio Biagi, 2850
City Ribeirão, Ribeirão Preto – SP – Brasil
CEP: 14021-000
Tel: 0800 992236
Fax: (16) 3993-9000
E-mail: tecmedd@tecmedd.com.br

India, Bangladesh, Pakistan, Sri Lanka
Elsevier Health Sciences Division
Customer Service Department
17A/1, Main Ring Road
Lajpat Nagar IV
New Delhi – 110024, India
Tel: 91 11 2644 7160-64
Fax: 91 11 2644 7156
E-mail: esindia@vsnl.net

Dedicated to the Memory of my Father,
John James Ingle, Jr., DDS–1892-1954

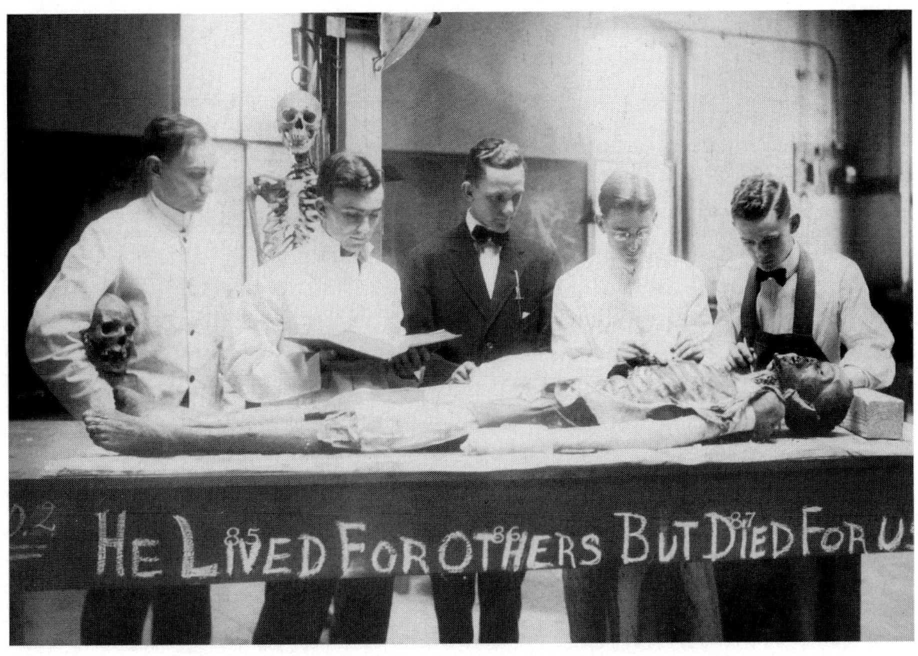

Vanderbilt University Dental School, circa 1912.
Dr. Ingle is on the far right.

Dr. Ingle graduated from Northwestern University Dental School in 1914, the last class under G.V. Black.

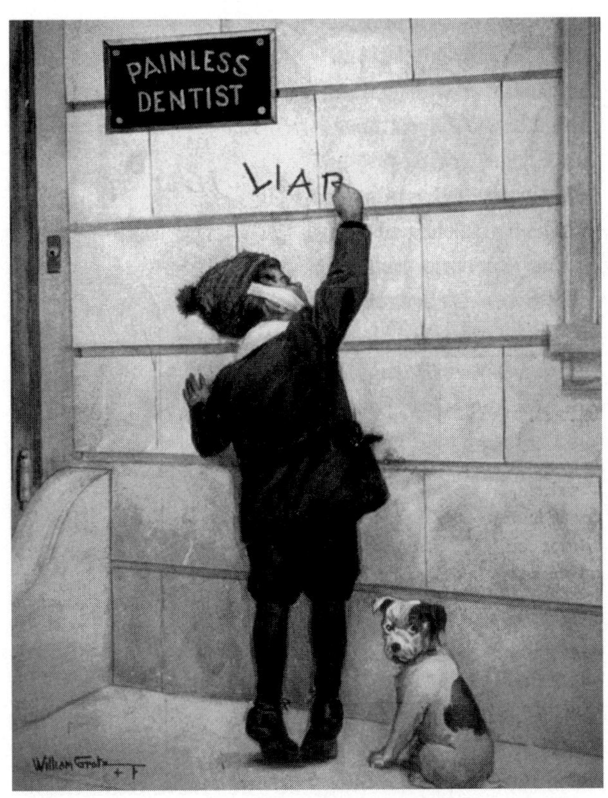

"TESTIMONIAL", cover of the old Life Magazine, 73:(1890), January 16, 1919.

These two pictures hung in my father's dental laboratory for 35 years.

ACKNOWLEDGMENTS

A number of years ago, I (JII) served on a committee to select a new dean for a school of medicine. The committee was made up mostly of physicians. I was the only dentist. The meeting started in the traditional way - each participant stating their name and specialty. When it came to my turn, I gave my specialty as endodontics.

"Endodontics," said the neurosurgeon, "What in the world is endodontics?" "Endodontics," I explained, "deals with the diagnosis and treatment of diseases of the dental pulp." "You mean inside the tooth?" he inquired. "I guess you could say that." I answered. He uttered an expletive and declared that endodontics had to be the ultimate in limited specialties.

Over the years I've thought many times of this encounter. How could one write 900 pages about the inside of the tooth? And yet, we have. Because it deserves it!

We have realized for a long time that one person could not be an expert in all phases of this limited, yet demanding discipline. For that reason we have mustered an assembly of world experts, each enjoying an international reputation in their particular area of expertise, be it microanatomy, pathology, pharmacology, microbiology, radiography, anesthesiology, pain management, canal preparation and obturation, trauma, surgery, bleaching, pediatric endodontics, whatever.

We are very proud of our contributing authors, and to them we owe an endearing debt of gratitude. And you~ the reader should as well, for they bring you the finest, stated honestly and unsparingly!

Once again, I (JII) acknowledge the genuine assistance and loving care I have received from my wife of 62 years - Joyce Ingle. How fortunate I have been. And likewise, I (LKB) thank my wife. Grete, for her understanding when I spent numerous hours reading and writing.

At Loma Linda University, we wish to express our gratitude to the individuals who helped with the graphics: Richard Tinker and Richard Cross. and the secretaries who so carefully worked on the text: Luci Denger, Dawn Pellerin, and Marjorie Sweet. Without their care and dedication, this book would still be just a dream.

At the University of Southern California, we gratefully acknowledge the expertise of Frank Mason, Associate Professor and Director of the School of Dentistry library and his associates.

Special thanks to Ron and Mary Prottsman for their wonderful indexes.

In addition, we are indebted to Brian Decker, Peggy Dalling and the entire team at BC Decker Inc for their hard work involved in the preparation of this material.

PREFACE TO THE FIRST EDITION

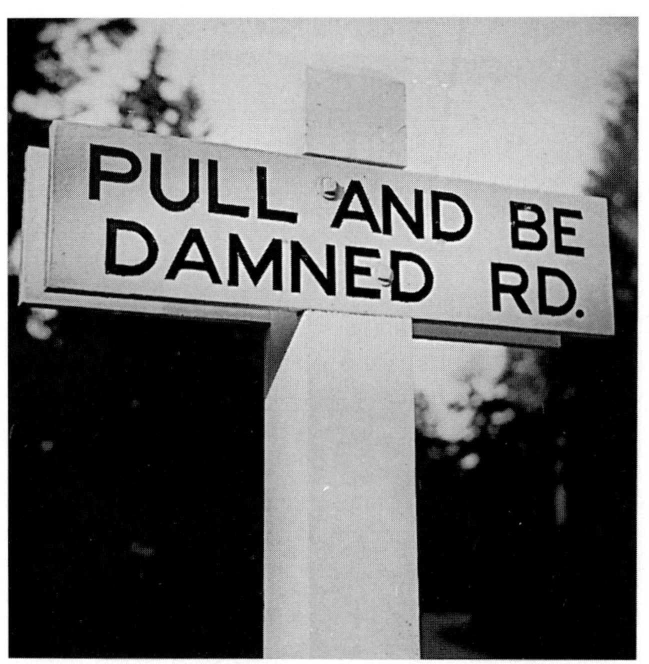

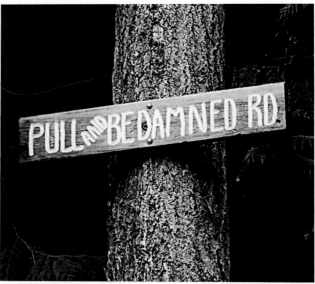

The original sign for Pull and Be Damned Road has been pilfered so many times the authorities have had to place a new sign over 20 feet above ground. (Courtesy of Dr. James Stephens.)

This book was begun at Snee-oosh Beach, a quiet retreat overlooking Puget Sound and the San Juan Islands. At Snee-oosh it is possible to escape from complex civilization, and to concentrate upon the job at hand—writing a text.

Hard by Snee-oosh is an old Indian trail called PULL AND BE DAMNED ROAD. One can hardly imagine a more fitting location while writing a text on the pulpless tooth than nearby PULL AND BE DAMNED ROAD, for "Pull and be damned" could well be the motto of the dental profession from its inception.

PULL AND BE DAMNED ROAD goes down to the shores of Skagit Bay an inside passage of the gentle Pacific leading ominously to DECEPTION PASS. This delusive inlet which so easily deceived the early explorers reminds us how our profession has practiced self-deception over the years. Unfortunately, many pass into the "pull and be damned"' deceptive phase of dental practice, never to return.

Inside DECEPTION PASS, however, lies HOPE ISLAND, a symbol of the future. HOPE we must have, coupled with resolve. HOPE that the future of dentistry will noticeably improve. HOPE that an enlightened profession will be guided by the concept of retention and rehabilitation of the dental apparatus. HOPE for the rejection of "oral amputation."

To say that the ideas contained within this text are ours or are original is ridiculous. Nothing really is new under the dental sun. We have liberally borrowed from our contemporaries as well as from the past. We only hope we give credit where credit is due. The student who chooses this text for an encyclopedia will be disappointed. In this age of "do it yourself" this is a "how to do it" book. We have attempted to discuss and illustrate in great detail the operative aspects of endodontic therapy, for we estimate that in treating a pulpless tooth the dentist will spend at least 75 percent of treatment time in endodontic cavity preparation, canal debridement, and filling. Operative endodontics is therefore presented first in the text, and a correspondingly significant section deals with these matters.

We leave to other authors the detailed discussion of anti-infectives, local anesthesia, or oral microbiology. Although these subjects are dealt with in this text, we have tried to keep the material in proper context; brief, and to the point. We have spent, however, an unusual amount of space and time in developing the chapter on DIFFERENTIAL DIAGNOSIS OF ORAL AND PERIORAL PAIN.

Diagnosis of pain is an area of dental practice that more frequently is falling into the province of Endodontics. It has often been said that any well-trained person can practice the mechanics of dentistry, but that proper diagnosis is the discipline that separates the really competent dentist from the merely mechanical; hence the extensive coverage of the subject.

A great deal of thought and talent was put into developing the four chapters on the normal and pathologic pulp and periapical tissues. This discussion builds the background for diagnosis of endodontic problems and sets the stage for a better understanding of oral and perioral pain.

Snee-oosh Beach is no Walden Pond, nor we Thoreau for that matter. But we may learn a lesson from Walden. "Simplify, simplify!" was Thoreau's text, and simplification is one text we may well take to heart. There has been far too much complicated mumbo-jumbo in endodontic treatment, a significant factor in discouraging the profession from including endodontic therapy in their practices.

We will attempt to present the subject not only in a simplified form, but in a systemic manner; for the simplified systematic practice of endodontics will lead to successful results achieved with pleasure and profit. We have attempted to remove the mystery and retain the basic core of the subject. We only hope we succeed in bringing some order out of the present chaos.

Finally, we would like to eulogize Dr. Balint J. Orban to whom the first edition is dedicated. Dr. Orban's death was a great loss to the profession and an even greater loss to those of us fortunate enough to have known him well. His ability to clarify and delineate a problem is apparent in the Classification of Pulpal and Periapical Pain which we discussed just prior to his death. The profession is forever in the debt of Balint Orban; not the least for his matchless descriptions of pulpal histopathology. We are proud to be the recipients of this priceless collection of microscopic material. We are more proud to have been his friends and disciples.

JOHN INGLE
Seattle, Washington
1964

PREFACE

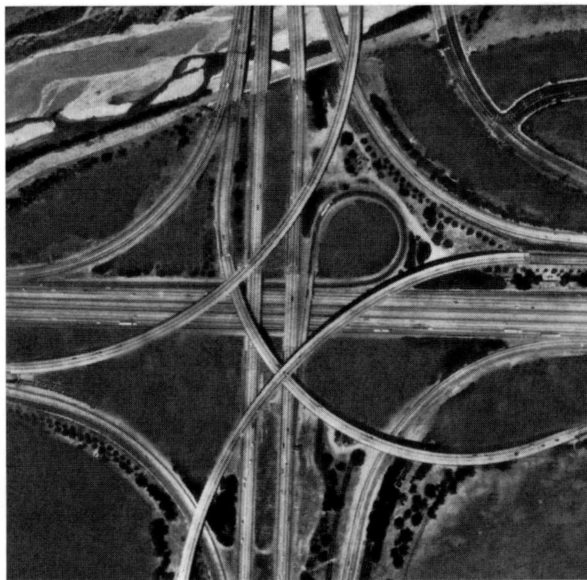

California Crossroads. The interchange between highways I-10 and I-215, near Loma Linda, California, February 2000. (Courtesy of the California Department of Transportation [Caltrans].

Thirty-six years ago, this text was started at "PULL AND BE DAMNED ROAD". And now, after a third of a century, we have reached another road—a crossroads, as it turns out.

In our fast moving world, the publishing business is approaching a major intersection. What future directions will be taken: hard copy printing, CD-ROM, Internet, or a combination of all three? This is not a simple fork in the road. This is a freeway interchange, with more to come for sure.

The authors and publishers of this text were faced with a dilemma, a tectonic shift in storage and retrieval, so to speak. Should we just abandon the textbook altogether? Should we grossly reduce the contents and make it a paperback? Should we create a CD-ROM or a combination of text and CD-ROM? Or should we update the 4th edition to produce a 5th edition?

We decided on the latter option! BC Decker Inc, our publisher, stated that the text had become a classic – respected worldwide – and should continue as the pace-setter, the landmark, the milestone against which other texts are compared. The endodontic "Bible", if you will.

This text will continue to provide eager students of the discipline with the latest and most complete information available–unvarnished, impartial, and reliable.

The discipline of endodontics is also reaching a crossroads, brought about by two elements—nickel and titanium (NiTi). More and more, root canal therapy today is done with the aid of mechanical means. As new instruments and materials are added, endodontics will be more precise and less time consuming. But, in this rush to mechanize, let us not forget our major concerns, namely bacteria and pain. We feel that this new edition of *Endodontics* addresses well all of these aspects of the discipline.

CONTRIBUTORS

James K. Bahcall, DMD, MS
Assistant Professor and Chair
Department of Surgical Sciences
Director, Postgraduate Endodontic Education
School of Dentistry, Marquette University
Formerly Assistant Professor and Chairman
Department of Endodontics
Northwestern University Dental School
Diplomate, American Board of Endodontics

Leif K. Bakland, DDS
Professor and Chairman, Department of Endodontics
Associate Dean, Advanced Education
Loma Linda University School of Dentistry
Diplomate, American Board of Endodontics

Joseph T. Barss, DDS, MS
Assistant Professor and Ph.D. Fellow
Department of Cell and Molecular Biology
Northwestern University Medical School
Formerly Clinical Assistant Professor
Department of Endodontics
Northwestern University Dental School

J. Craig Baumgartner, BS, DDS, MS, PhD
Professor and Chairman
Department of Endodontology
Oregon Health Sciences University
Formerly Chief of Microbiology
U.S. Army Institute of Dental Research
Chief of Endodontics
Walter Reed Army Medical Center, Washington DC
Diplomate, American Board of Endodontics

Edward E. Beveridge, DDS, MSD (deceased)
Formerly Professor and Chairman
Department of Endodontics
School of Dentistry
University of Southern California

Patrick Bogaerts, LSD
Private Endodontic Practice
Brussels, Belgium

L. Stephen Buchanan, BA, DDS
Founder, Dental Education Laboratories
Adjunct Clinical Professor
Department of Endodontics
University of the Pacific
Diplomate, American Board of Endodontics

Joe H. Camp, AB, DDS, MSD
Adjunct Associate Professor of Endodontics
University of North Carolina School of Dentistry

Silvia C. M. Cecchini, DDS, MSc, MS, PhD
Clinical Assistant Professor, School of Dentistry
University of California San Francisco
Formerly Assistant Professor
Department of Endodontics
Loma Linda University School of Dentistry
Formerly Assistant Professor
Department of Restorative Dentistry
Paulista University School of Dentistry, Brazil

Jeffrey M. Coil, DMD, MSD, PhD
Assistant Professor and Chairman
Division of Endodontics
Department of Oral Biological and Medical Sciences
University of British Columbia, Canada
Diplomate, American Board of Endodontics and The Royal College of Dentists of Canada

Clifton O. Dummett Jr., DDS, MSD, MEd
Professor and Coordinator
Postgraduate Pediatric Dentistry
Louisiana State University School of Dentistry
Formerly Staff Instructor and Coordinator of Dental Research
Children's Medical Center, Dayton, Ohio
Formerly Director of Pediatric Dentistry
Charles R. Drew Neighborhood Health Center,
Dayton, Ohio
Diplomate, American Board of Pediatric Dentistry

Paul D. Eleazer, DDS, MS
Professor and Chairman
Department of Endodontics and Pulp Biology
University of Alabama
Formerly Associate Professor and Director
Post Graduate Endodontics
Interim Chair, Department of Periodontics, Endodontics, and Dental Hygiene
University of Louisville
Formerly Director, Pharmacology for Dental Hygienists
Darton College
Diplomate, American Board of Endodontics

Alfred L. Frank, BS, DDS
Guest Consultant, Department of Endodontics
School of Dentistry
University of California, Los Angeles
Formerly Adjunct Professor of Endodontics
University of Southern California
Formerly Adjunct Professor of Endodontics
Loma Linda University School of Dentistry
Diplomate, American Board of Endodontics

Robert J. Frank, BS, DDS
Associate Professor of Endodontics
Loma Linda University School of Dentistry
Formerly Director, Endodontic Clinic
Loma Linda University School of Dentistry
Diplomate, American Board of Endodontics

Cyril Gaum, DDS
Professor Emeritus, Endodontics
Tufts University School of Dental Medicine
Formerly Clinical Professor and Chairman of Endodontics
Tufts University
Diplomate, American Board of Endodontics

Dudley H. Glick, BS, DDS
Director of Endodontics, Dental Residency Program
Surgery Department, Cedar Sinai Medical Center
Lecturer, Department of Endodontics
School of Dentistry, University of California, Los Angeles
Formerly Clinical Professor of Endodontics
School of Dentistry
University of Southern California
Diplomate, American Board of Endodontics

Gerald N. Glickman, DDS, MS, MBA, JD
Professor and Chairman, Department of Endodontics
Director, Graduate Program in Endodontics
School of Dentistry, University of Washington

Albert C. Goerig, BS, DDS, MS
Private practice of endodontics
Olympia, Washington
Diplomate, American Board of Endodontics

Charles J. Goodacre, DDS, MSD
Dean, School of Dentistry
Professor, Department of Restorative Dentistry
Loma Linda University School of Dentistry
Formerly Professor and Chairman
Department of Prosthodontics
Director, Undergraduate Fixed and Removable Prosthodontics
Indiana University School of Dentistry
Diplomate, American Board of Prosthodontics

James L. Gutmann, DDS
Formerly Professor and Chairman, Department of Endodontics
Program Director, Graduate Endodontics
Baylor College of Dentistry
Formerly Professor and Chairman
Department of Endodontics
Baltimore College of Dental Services
Diplomate, American Board of Endodontics

Gary R. Hartwell, DDS, MS
Chair, Department of Endodontics
Director, Advanced Education Program in Endodontics
Virginia Commonwealth University School of Dentistry
Formerly Director, Advanced Education Program in Endodontics
U.S. Army Dental Activity, Fort Gordon, Georgia
Formerly Director, Advanced Program in Endodontics
Madigan Army Medical Center, Fort Lewis, Washington
Diplomate, American Board of Endodontics

Carl E. Hawrish, BA, DDS, MSc (deceased)
Formerly Professor and Chairman
Department of Oral Diagnosis and Oral Surgery
Faculty of Dentistry, University of Alberta, Canada

Geoffrey S. Heithersay, BDS, MDS, FDSCRCS, FRACDS
Clinical Associate Professor
University of Adelaide, Australia
Formerly Lecturer in Endodontics
Supervisor of undergraduate and graduate endodontic studies
University of Adelaide, Australia

Van T. Himel, BS, DDS
Professor and Chair
Department of Biologic and Diagnostic Sciences
University of Tennessee
Formerly Director of Postgraduate Endodontics
Louisiana State University
Formerly Director, Division of Endodontics
University of Tennessee
Diplomate, American Board of Endodontics

Anthony E. Hoskinson, BDS, MSc
Private practice limited to endodontics
Prestwood, England
Senior Clinical Lecturer, Conservation Department
Eastman Dental Institute, United Kingdom

John I. Ingle, DDS, MSD
Lecturer, Department of Endodontics
Loma Linda University School of Dentistry
Formerly Dean and Professor of Endodontics and Periodontics
School of Dentistry
University of Southern California
Formerly Professor and Chairman of Endodontics and Periodontics
School of Dentistry, University of Washington
Diplomate, American Board of Endodontics and American Board of Periodontology

Bernadette Jaeger, DDS
Adjunct Associate Professor, Section of Orofacial Pain
School of Dentistry
University of California, Los Angeles
Diplomate, American Board of Oraofacial Pain

Frederick H. Kahn, DDS
Clinical Professor of Endodontics
Advanced Education Faculty
New York University College of Dentistry

Joseph Y. K. Kan, DDS
Assistant Professor
Department of Restorative Dentistry
Loma Linda University School of Dentistry
Formerly Clinical Director and Assistant Professor
Center for Prosthodontics and Implant Dentistry
Loma Linda University School of Dentistry

John A. Khademi, DDS
Private practice of endodontics
Durango, Colorado

Hugh M. Kopel, DDS, MS
Professor Emeritus, School of Dentistry
University of Southern California
Lecturer, Pediatric Dentistry
University of California, Los Angeles
Lecturer, Rancho Las Amigos Hospital
National Rehabilitation Center
Formerly Senior Attending and Acting Head
Dental Division, Children's Hospital of Los Angeles
Diplomate, American Board of Pediatric Dentistry

Barry H. Korzen, DDS
Associate Professor, Department of Endodontics
Faculty of Dentistry University of Toronto, Canada
Active Staff, Section of Endodontics
Department of Dentistry
Mount Sinai Hospital, Canada
Formerly Associate Professor and Head
Department of Endodontics
Faculty of Dentistry, University of Toronto, Canada
Formerly Head, Section of Endodontics
Department of Dentistry
Mount Sinai Hospital, Canada

Robert M. Krasny, DDS, MSD, MA
Professor Emeritus, Endodontics
School of Dentistry
University of California, Los Angeles
Formerly Professor and Chairman
Section of Endodontics
School of Dentistry
University of California, Los Angeles

Pierre Machtou, DDS, MS, PhD
Professor, Department of Endodontics
Faculte de Chirurgie Dentaire
Universite Par Denis Diderot, France

Stanley F. Malamed, DDS
Professor, Division of Surgical, Therapeutic and Bioengineering Sciences
School of Dentistry
University of Southern California
Diplomate, American Board of Dental Anesthesiology

F. James Marshall, DMD, MS
Professor and Chairman Emeritus
Oregon Health Sciences University
Diplomate, American Board of Endodontics

Howard Martin, DMD
Private practice of endodontics
Rockville, Maryland
Formerly Professorial Lecturer
Georgetown University School of Dentistry
Formerly Clinical Research Endodontist
Dental Department
V.A. Medical Center, Washington DC
Diplomate, American Board of Endodontics

Steven G. Morrow, DDS, MS
Associate Professor, Department of Endodontics
Loma Linda University School of Dentistry
Diplomate, American Board of Endodontics

Carl W. Newton, DDS, MSD
Professor, Department of Restorative Dentistry
Indiana University School of Dentistry
Formerly Chairman, Department of Endodontics
Indiana University School of Dentistry
Diplomate, American Board of Endodontics

David H. Pashley, BS, DMD, PhD
Regents Professor of Oral Biology
School of Dentistry, Medical College of Georgia
Honorary member, American Association of Endodontists

James B. Roane, BS, DDS, MS
Professor and Co-Chair, Department of Endodontics
College of Dentistry, University of Oklahoma
Diplomate, American Board of Endodontics

Paul A. Rosenberg, DDS
Professor and Chairman, Department of Endodontics
Director, Post Graduate Endodontics
New York University College of Dentistry
Diplomate, American Board of Endodontics

Ilan Rotstein, CD
Associate Professor and Chair
Division of Surgical, Therapeutic and Bioengineering Sciences
School of Dentistry
University of Southern California
Formerly Associate Professor, Acting Chair and Director, Graduate Endodontics
Hebrew University
Hadassah Faculty of Dental Medicine, Israel
Diplomate, Israel Board of Endodontics

Richard A. Rubinstein, DDS, MS
Adjunct Assistant Professor
Department of Endodontics
School of Dental Medicine
University of Pennsylvania

Clifford J. Ruddle, DDS
Lecturer, Department of Endodontics
Loma Linda University School of Dentistry
Adjunct Assistant Professor of Endodontics
University of the Pacific School of Dentistry

Thomas P. Serene, BS, DDS, MSD
Emeritus Chairman and Professor
Section of Endodontics
School of Dentistry
University of California, Los Angeles
Formerly Chairman and Professor
Department of Endodontics
School of Dentistry
Medical University of South Carolina
Formerly Chairman and Professor
Department of Endodontics
School of Dentistry, Emory University
Diplomate, American Board of Endodontics

Barnet B. Shulman, DDS
Attending and Senior Lecturer
Manhattan Veterans Administration Hospital
Clinical Associate Professor of Endodontics
Advanced Education Faculty
New York University College of Dentistry
Formerly Attending
Bellevue Hospital, New York, New York
Formerly Instructor, Dental Auxiliary Utilization
New York University College of Dentistry

James H. Simon, AB, DDS
Professor and Director
Advanced Endodontics Program
University of Southern California
Professor of Endodontics
Loma Linda University School of Dentistry
Formerly Director, Endodontic Residency Program
Veterans Administration Medical Center, Long Beach, California
Diplomate, American Board of Endodontics

Harold C. Slavkin, DDS
Dean, School of Dentistry
University of Southern California
Formerly Director
National Institute of Dental and Craniofacial Research
National Institute of Health, Bethesda, Maryland

Harold R. Stanley, BS, DDS, MS (deceased)
Formerly Professor Emeritus
Department of Oral and Maxillofacial Surgery and Diagnostic Sciences
Division of Oral and Maxillofacial Pathology and Oncology
Formerly Clinic Director, National Institute of Dental Research
Formerly Director of Pulp Registry

Eugene I. Sugita, DDS, MPH
Private practice of Endodontics
El Cajon, California
Diplomate, American Board of Endodontics

Mahmoud Torabinejad, DMD, MSD, PhD
Professor of Endodontics
Director, Graduate Endodontics
Loma Linda University School of Dentistry
Diplomate, American Board of Endodontics

Richard E. Walton, DMD, MS
Professor of Endodontics
Director, Junior Endodontic Clerkship
University of Iowa College of Dentistry
Formerly Chair, Department of Endodontics
University of Iowa College of Dentistry
Formerly Chair, Department of Endodontics
Medical College of Georgia
Diplomate, American Board of Endodontics

John D. West, DDS, MSD
Clinical Associate Professor, Graduate Endodontics
Department of Endodontics
University of Washington School of Dentistry
Clinical Instructor, Boston University Goldman School of Dental Medicine
Guest Faculty, Pacific Endodontic Research Foundation
Founder and Director, Center for Endodontics
Tacoma, Washington

CONTENTS

Chapter 1

MODERN ENDODONTIC THERAPY

John I. Ingle, Leif K. Bakland, Edward E. Beveridge, Dudley H. Glick, and Anthony E. Hoskinson

"Because I'll have you know, Sancho, that a mouth without teeth is like a mill without its stone, and you must value a tooth more than a diamond."

– Miguel de Cervantes, ***Don Quixote***

The newspaper headline read, "Ancient Root Canal Filling Found." Datelined Jerusalem, the article went on to state that "a green tooth containing the oldest known root canal filling was discovered in the skull of a Nabatean warrior who was buried in a mass grave **2,200 years ago.**"

Joseph Zias, curator of the State of Israel Department of Antiquities, later reported on this historic archeologic finding in the *Journal of the American Dental Association.*[1] The tooth in question—a maxillary right lateral incisor—dated from the Hellenistic period (200 BC). Radiographic examination of the ancient skull "disclosed a 2.5 mm bronze wire that had been implanted in the root canal—the earliest known archeologic example of a tooth filled with a metal object" (Figure 1-1). Professor Zias went on to explain the probable reason for the primitive "endodontics": "The accepted cause of tooth disease in the Mediterranean—a worm burrowing inside the tooth—may give a clue as to why this tooth was filled with a metal wire. It is possible that the wire was implanted into the tooth canal to close the passage and prevent 'toothworms' from burrowing into the tooth and causing further dental pain." The first mention of the "toothworm" theory is found in the Anastasia Papyrus of the thirteenth century BC.[1]

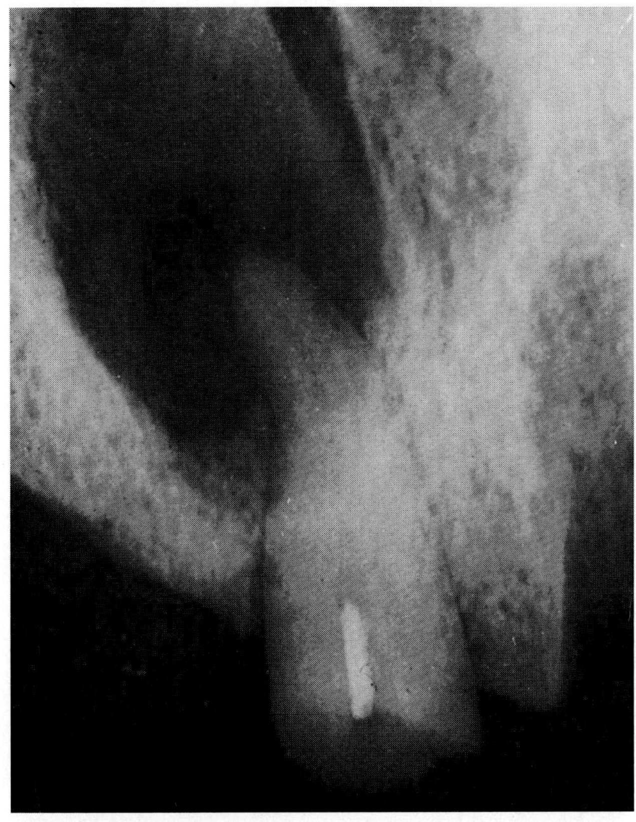

Figure 1-1 Oldest known root canal filling. Radiograph of skeletal remains showing maxillary incisor with bronze wire implanted in the root canal of a Nabatean warrior buried in the Negev desert 2,200 years ago (200 BC). Reproduced with permission from Dr. Joseph Zias, State of Israel Department of Antiquities, and J Am Dent Assoc 1987;114:665.

Somewhat earlier in China, the ancient Chinese subscribed to the "toothworm" theory of dental caries as well. According to Tsai-Fang, "The oracle bone inscription, excavated from the ruins of the Ying Dynasty (fourteenth century BC), clearly shows a character meaning 'caries.'"[2] Since the cause of tooth decay was thought to be an invasion of "worms" into teeth, the Chinese language character for "caries" was composed of a worm on top of a tooth[2] (Figure 1-2).

Fifteen hundred years later, by the year 200 AD, the Chinese were using arsenicals to treat pulpitis, preceding Spooner, who was the first to do so in Europe, by

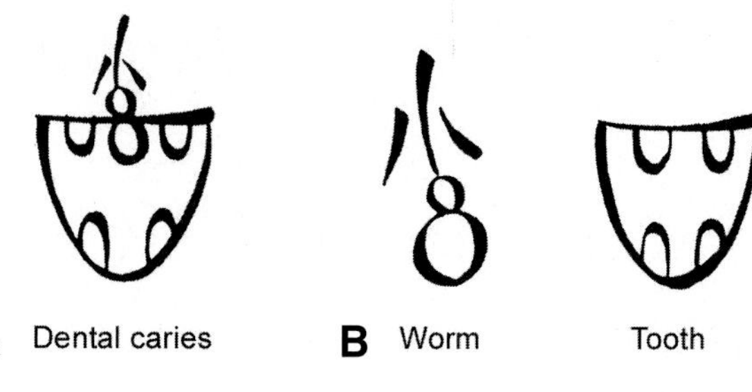

Figure 1-2 A, A piece of "oracle bone" inscribed with Chinese character meaning "caries" (fourteenth century BC). **B**, Chinese characters for "worm" and "tooth" combined to form the word "caries." Reproduced with permission from Dr. Tsai-fang Tsao, Faculty of Stomatology, Peking Medical College; Int Endodont J 1984;17:163; and L.F. Zhens. Diseases of the mouth and teeth. 4th ed. Beijing (PRC): People's Health Publishing House; 1957. p. 2–5.

1,600 years.[2] The Chinese also used amalgam to fill cavities in the teeth as early as 659 AD.[2]

This ancient history, preceding dentistry in North America and even Europe by thousands of years, was a harbinger of things to come.

Jumping ahead to more modern times, Dr. Louis I. Grossman (Figure 1-3), dean of endodontists in America, if not the world, pointed out that, by 1750, "Pierre Fauchard, the noted French dentist (1678-1761), had dispelled the 'toothworm' legend and was recommending the removal of diseased pulps as well."[3] Dr. Grossman also chronicled the historical events impacting on root canal therapy since the American Revolution.[4]

In his usual orderly manner, Dr. Grossman divided the 200 years between 1776 and 1976 into four 50-year periods.[4] During the first period, 1776 to 1826, he noted that treatment was crude—abscessed teeth were treated with leeches or toasted fig poultices, and pulps were cauterized with red-hot wires. Nevertheless, it was during this same period that root canals were being filled from apex to crown with gold foil.

The second half-century, 1826 to 1876, was marked by the founding of the first dental journal and the first dental school, the introduction of general anesthesia, rubber dam, gutta-percha root canal points, and the barbed broach, as well as three- and four-sided tapering broaches for cleaning and enlarging root canals, intracanal antiseptics, and oxyphosphate of zinc cement. At the same time, however, pulps were still being removed by driving wooden pegs into the canal, and crowns of the teeth were also being "snipped" off at the gingival level to cure toothache. Arsenicals were still being used to devitalize pulps.

The third half-century, 1876 to 1926, was highlighted by the discovery and development of the x-ray, the advent of local anesthetics, and the acceptance of antisepsis as a part of endodontic therapy. In 1891, for example, Otto Walkhoff introduced camphorated monoclorophenol (CMCP) as an intracanal medicament. It was this same Dr. Walkhoff who took the first dental radiograph in 1895.[3]

Beginning about 1912, dentistry in general and endodontics in particular were set back by the wide acceptance of the theory of **focal infection**. Wholesale extraction of both vital and pulpless teeth took place. The professions were not to recover their senses until well after World War II.

The final 50-year period, 1926 to 1976, saw improvements in radiographs, anesthetics, and procedures as well as the introduction of new methods and agents. Calcium hydroxide made its appearance, as did ethylenediaminetetraacetic acid (EDTA) for chelation. Many root canal medications appeared, and arsenic finally disappeared from the dental pharmacopeia. This same period saw the publication of the first major text devoted to endodontics, Dr. Grossman's **Root Canal Therapy**, as well as the introduction of standardized instruments and cavity preparation.[5–7] The period also witnessed the rise and decline of the silver root canal

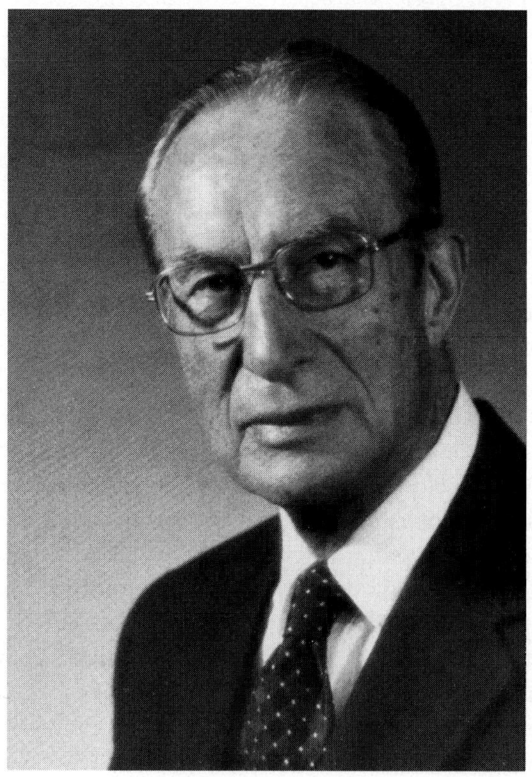

Figure 1-3 The late Louis I. Grossman, DDS, Dr. med. dent., dean of American endodontists. His substantial contributions over more than half of the twentieth century enormously improved the practice, science, and standing of endodontics.

point. A more sensible attitude toward endodontic surgery developed.

During this period, the American Association of Endodontists (AAE) was formed, followed by the American Board of Endodontics. Continuing education in endodontics widely disseminated information, skills, and techniques to an eager profession. The prevention of pulp disease began to play a more important role in dental practice. In part because of fluoridation, there was a decline in dental caries. Research into the causes and biology of dental trauma led to improved awareness and treatment of dental injuries. Antibiotics greatly improved the profession's ability to control infection, while new anesthetics and injection techniques increased control over pain. The high-speed air rotor handpiece added to patient comfort and the speed and ease of operation, as did prepackaged sterilized supplies. The mandatory use of masks, gloves, and better sterilizing methods rapidly emerged with the spread of human immunodeficiency virus/acquired immune deficiency syndrome (HIV/AIDS) and hepatitis. The widespread use of auxiliaries expanded dental services.

It is now more than two decades since Grossman's historic report, a period in which new instruments and techniques for cleaning and shaping as well as filling root canals have been introduced. Some of them are still in the development stage. All in all, the new decade, if not the new millennium, should prove exciting and profitable for the profession and patients alike.

RECENT ATTITUDES TOWARD DENTISTRY AND ENDODONTIC THERAPY

Increasingly, the term "root canal" has become fashionable and generally known. In conversation, people proudly proclaim that they have had a "root canal." The stigma of fear and pain is fast disappearing.

Another impressive factor in the acceptance of endodontics is television. Countless advertisements emphasize a beautiful smile—not just toothpaste advertisements, but commercials in every field, from Buicks to beer. At the same time, the constant barrage of denture adhesive and cleanser advertisements produces a chilling effect. The public sees the problems that develop from the loss of teeth. Obvious missing teeth are anathema.

There is no question that the public's acceptance of endodontic treatment is on the rise. In 1969, for example, the American Dental Association (ADA) estimated that 6 million root canal fillings were done each year. By 1990, their estimate had risen to 13,870,000. One might add that the ADA also estimated that another 690,000 "endodontic surgeries and root amputations" were done in 1990.[8] By the year 2000, it was estimated that 30 million teeth were root-filled annually.[9]

This upward trend was also documented by the Public Affairs Committee of the AAE. Reporting on surveys of the general public made by the Opinion Research Institute in 1984 and 1986, the Committee noted that **28%** of 1,000 telephone respondents reported that they had had root canal therapy by 1986, an increase of 5% over 23% in 1984.[10] Also, in 1986, 62% said they would choose root canal therapy over extraction, an increase of 10% over 52% in 1984. More than half the respondents (53%) believed that an endodontically treated tooth would last a lifetime.[10]

On the other hand, the perceptions of younger people (under 25 years) in this survey were disappointing in that 70% described root canal therapy as "painful" and 58% thought it would be less expensive to extract the tooth and place a bridge.[10] Clearly, the profession has a mission in educating this age group to reverse their image of endodontics and the value of a treated pulpless tooth.

A rate of use of endodontic services similar to the rate in the United States (28%) was also reported from Norway, where 27% of an older age group (66 to 75 years) had had root canal therapy, as had 12% of a younger age group (26 to 35 years). Incidentally, 100% of the root-filled teeth in the younger group were still present 10 to 17 years later, a remarkable achievement.[11]

The growth in endodontic services is also reflected in the sale of endodontic equipment, supplies, and instruments. In 1984, endodontics was a $20 million market, growing at a rate of 4% a year.[12] By 1997, 13 years later, the endodontic market, through dental dealer retail stores alone, was $72 million, up from $65.6 million in 1996, a growth of nearly 10%. One must add to these sales another 10% to account for mail-order/telephone sales, a grand total in 1997 of nearly $80 million. Worldwide sales are probably double this figure![13]

There is no question that the greatest share of endodontic procedures is carried out by America's general practitioners. On the other hand, the specialty of endodontics is growing as well. In 1986, for example, only 5% of those patients who had root canal therapy were treated by a specialist.[10] By 1990, this percentage had grown to 28.5%.[8] In 1989, there were 2,500 endodontic specialists in the United States.[9] By 2,000, the figure was around 3,300 endodontists,[14] and these endodontists were completing 39% of all of the root canal therapy and endodontic surgery in the United States.[8]

In spite of these encouraging figures for the **immediate** future of endodontics, one has to question what the **distant** future will bring. The rate of dental caries is declining precipitously.

In two separate reports, the US National Institute of Dental Research (NIDR) proudly announced in 1988 that half of all children in the United States aged 5 to 17 years had no decay in their permanent teeth. None![15] In contrast, in the early 1970s, only 28% of the permanent teeth of American children were caries free. By 1980, this figure had risen to 36.6%, and by 1986–1987, 49.9% were caries free. Furthermore, there was a 50% improvement in 17 year olds, a most encouraging sign for dentists, who were once faced with repairing the ravaged mouths of adolescents in the 1950s through the 1970s. The national decayed-missing-filled surfaces (DMFS) rate had dropped to 3.1 for all US schoolchildren and, even more importantly, "82 percent of the DMF surfaces are **filled,** about 13% decayed and 4% are missing."[15]

A comparable radiographic survey in 1980 on 1,059 US Air Force basic trainees 18 to 20 years old found that 10% had "no restorations, no decay and no missing teeth." Moreover, another 10% had at least one root canal filling.[16] A comparison between these 1980 recruits and Navy recruits in 1956 proved that **missing** teeth per recruit had dropped from 2.4 to 0.75 in 24 years, a reduction of 31%.[16]

As far as older adults are concerned, the NIDR reported a remarkable decline in edentulism as well, particularly in the middle-aged, a group in which "total tooth loss has been practically eliminated."[17] The elderly (age 65 and older), however, "are still in serious trouble," root caries and periodontal disease being the primary offenders.[17]

All of these encouraging figures suggest greater preventive measures and higher use of dental services by the public. Part of the improvement can be credited to a healthier economy and lifestyle, part to the national water supply and dentifrice fluoridation programs, part to the dental profession's efforts, and part to dental insurance. Bailit et al. have shown that third-party payment has increased dental use and improved oral health.[18] By 1995, the ADA estimated that 63% of all US citizens were covered by a private insurance program and another 5.3% by public assistance. A remaining 31.4% were not covered by any insurance program.[19]

In providing these burgeoning services, the dental profession has fared well financially. Over the past 30 years, the net income of dentists has more than doubled in constant 1967 dollars.[20] Moreover, between 1986 and 1995, the net income of dentists rose 30.7%, from $102,953 to $134,590.[19]

Dental expenditures by the public have increased as well, from $3.4 billion in 1967 to $10 billion in 1977, to $25.3 billion in 1987 and $47.5 billion in 1996.[21] In 1996, the average person spent $172.70 for dental services, up from $108 (adjusted to 1996 dollars) in 1967. This amounts to a 60% increase in outlay for dental care in 30 years.[21]

After all of this expenditure and care, one is hard-pressed to explain why 15.1 million workdays are lost annually because of dental pain.[22]

ENDODONTIC CASE PRESENTATION

All of these improvements notwithstanding, many patients still must be convinced that root canal therapy is an intelligent, practical solution to an age-old problem—the loss of teeth. The "case for endodontic treatment" must be presented to the patient in a straightforward manner. The patient with the correct "oral image" will be anxious to proceed with therapy.

"Is this tooth worth saving, doctor?" This sentiment is voiced more often than not by the patient who has been informed that his or her tooth will require endodontic therapy. Superficially, this appears to be a simple question that requires a direct, uncomplicated answer. It should not be interpreted as hostile or as a challenge to the treatment recommendations presented for the retention of the tooth. Psychologically, however, this initial question is a prelude to a Pandora's box of additional queries that disclose doubts, fears, apprehensions, and economic considerations: for example, "Is it painful?" "Will this tooth have to be extracted later?" "How long will this tooth last?" "Is it a dead tooth?" "Will it turn black?" and "How much will it cost?"

Following the first question, the dentist should anticipate such a series of questions. These may be avoided, however, by including the answers to anticipated questions in the presentation. In turn, the dentist will gain a decided psychological advantage. By this apparent insight into his or her problems, the patient is assured that the dentist is cognizant of the very questions the patient was about to raise or possibly was too reticent to ask. Most of the patient's fear and doubts can be allayed by giving a concise answer to each question. The dentist should be able to explain procedures intelligently as ideas are exchanged with the patient.

To do this, one must be endodontically oriented. That is, one must believe in the value of endodontic therapy. By believing in such treatment, one cannot help but influence the patient favorably. The dentist will soon gain the confidence of the patient who realizes that professional recommendations emanate from an honest desire to preserve the mouth's functional efficiency.[23]

To answer patients' questions, the ADA produced an inexpensive pamphlet entitled "**Your Teeth Can be Saved...by Endodontic.**"[24] The AAE also publishes a number of pamphlets[25] for patients: the "**Your Guide To**"* series: "**Endodontic Treatment, Cracked Teeth, Endodontic Retreatment, and Endodontic Surgery.**"* Dr. Joel Burns has beautifully illustrated a booklet entitled **Why Root Canal Therapy?**[26] Although this approach is a little impersonal, it is a tangible reference, particularly when the patient returns home and tries to explain to an interested spouse what endodontic therapy involves.

Based on previous experiences in the office, the average patient has sufficient confidence in the dentist's ability to help. He or she is ready to accept the professional knowledge and advice offered but likes to have some part in evaluating the reasonableness of treatment. The professional person and the staff must spend the time and thought necessary to understand the patient's initial resistance, which is often based on false assumptions and beliefs in matters dealing with pulpless teeth. However, once the patient is secure in the thought that this is the correct treatment, most of the fears and apprehensions related to unfamiliarity with endodontic therapy will be dissipated.

A dental appointment is still associated with fear in the minds of many people[27–29] (Figure 1-4). The mere thought of treating the "nerve" of a tooth implies pain. Patients require reassurance, supported by all available psychological and therapeutic methods of relaxation and pain control. The patient must be reassured that endodontic therapy need not be painful and usually requires no more than a local anesthetic.

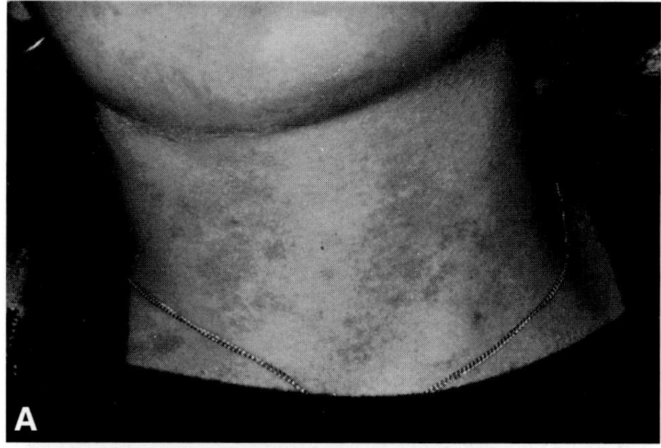

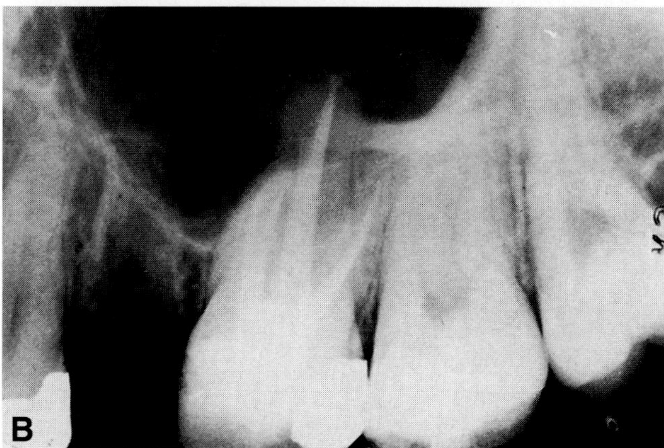

Figure 1-4 **A**, Rash occurred in this terrified patient, who was merely sitting in the dental chair. **B**, The patient's apprehension was allayed by sympathetic management, allowing successful completion of endodontic therapy in a four-canal molar. (Courtesy of Dr. Norbert Hertl.)

All too often, we hear negative remarks about root canal therapy: "Trying to do anything positive in Tacoma is akin to getting a **root canal** without Novocain." Or "Whew! What you just heard was a collective sigh of relief following 7 months of agonizing **root canal**"—remarks made following President Clinton's "confession" on television. In contrast to these commonly heard excoriations, LeClaire et al. reported that 43.9% of endodontic patients reported a decrease in fearfulness **after** having root canal therapy. Furthermore, 96.3% said that "they would have root canal therapy again to save a tooth."[29]

It should be explained to the concerned patient that root canal therapy is a specialized form of dental procedure designed to retain a tooth safely and comfortably. The tooth, when properly treated and restored, can be retained as long as any other tooth. It is not a "dead tooth" as long as the roots of the tooth are embedded in healthy surrounding tissues. Although teeth do not turn "black" following root canal therapy, a slight change in color owing to reduced translucency may occur. Discoloration associated with pulp necrosis and leakage around restorations can be managed successfully (see Chapter 16). Most often, retention of the tooth and bleaching, veneering, or crowning (Figure 1-5) are preferable to extraction and replacement with a prosthetic appliance.[10]

There is little doubt that economic considerations play an important role (and for some a supreme role) in the final decision. Some patients "think financially," and even though they are able to afford treatment, they allow financial considerations to govern decisions that should logically be made on a physiologic basis only. It

*Available from the American Association of Endodontists Information Services, 211 East Chicago Ave., Suite 1100, Chicago, IL 60611-2691.

is necessary to point out to these people the **financial advantage** of retaining a tooth by endodontic therapy rather than by extraction and prosthetic replacement. The properly informed patient is quick to recognize that the fee for a bridge is more than that for root canal therapy and proper restoration.[10] In addition, it should be mentioned in all honesty that any vital tooth prepared for a crown could become a possible candidate for future endodontic therapy. Also, the patient who says "Pull it out"' should be informed of the problems that arise if a space is left unfilled (ie, tilting, reduced masticatory efficiency, future periodontal problems, and cosmetic effects).

Another commonly heard statement by the patient is, "It's only a back tooth, anyway," or "If it were a front tooth I would save it, but no one sees it in back." This patient thinks cosmetically. The disadvantages of the loss of any tooth, let alone a posterior one so essential for mastication, must be explained.

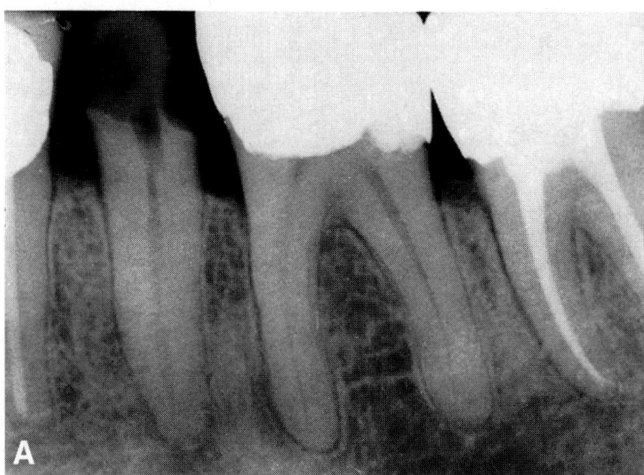

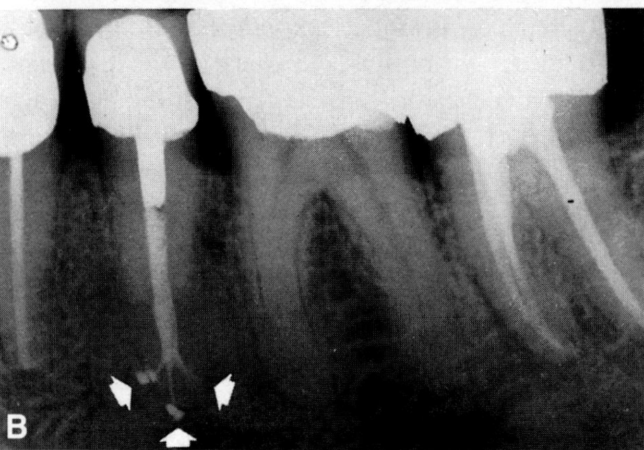

Figure 1-5 Fractured premolar restored by endodontics and post-and-core crown. **A**, Tooth immediately following fracture. **B**, Restoration and periradicular healing at 3-year recall. Note the spectacular fill of arborization (**arrows**) at the apex. (Courtesy of Dr. Clifford J. Ruddle.)

Fortunately, today's patient is becoming more sophisticated, too "tooth conscious" to permit indiscriminate extraction without asking whether there is an alternative. Extraction contributes to a crippling aberration from the normal dentition. There is no doubt that a normally functioning, endodontically treated, and well-restored tooth is vastly superior to the best prosthetic or implant replacement.

INDICATIONS

The indications for endodontic therapy are legion. Every tooth, from central incisor to third molar, is a potential candidate for treatment. Far too often, the expedient measure of extracting a pulpless tooth is a short-sighted attempt at solving a dental problem. Endodontic therapy, on the other hand, extends to the dentist and the patient the opportunity to save teeth.

The concept of retaining every possible tooth, and even the healthy roots of periodontally involved teeth, is based on the even distribution of the forces of mastication. The final success of any extensive restorative procedure depends on the root-surface area attached through the periodontal ligaments to the alveolar bone. Like the proverbial horseshoe nail, root-filled teeth may often be the salvation of an otherwise hopeless case.

To carry this concept one step further, recognized today is the importance of retaining even endodontically treated **roots**, over which may be constructed a full denture, the so-called **overdenture**.[30] On some occasions, attachments may be added to these roots to provide additional retention for the denture above. At other times, the treated roots are merely left in place on the assumption that the alveolar process will be retained around roots, and there will not be the usual ridge resorption so commonly seen under full or even partial dentures.

Most dentists would agree that the retained and restored individual tooth is better than a bridge replacement and that a bridge is better than a removable partial denture, which, in turn, is superior to a full denture. Although recent success with dental implants is impressive, the long-term outcome is not known, and, functionally, the patient's own tooth is superior. Treatment in every case should adhere to the standards set by the dentist for himself or herself and his or her family.

Modern dentistry incorporates endodontics as an integral part of restorative and prosthetic treatment. Most any tooth with pulpal involvement, provided that it has adequate periodontal support, can be a candidate for root canal treatment. Severely broken down teeth, and potential and actual abutment teeth, can be candidates for the tooth-saving procedures of endodontics.

One of the greatest services rendered by the profession is the retention of the first permanent molar (Figure 1-6). In contrast, the long-range consequences of breaking the continuity of either arch are also well known (Figure 1-7). Root canal therapy often provides the only opportunity for saving first molars with pulp involvement.

In addition to saving molars for children, saving posterior teeth for adults is also highly desirable. Retaining a root-filled terminal molar, for example, means saving two teeth—the molar's opposite tooth as well (Figure 1-8, A). Moreover, root canal treatment may save an abutment tooth of an existing fixed prosthesis. The gain is doubled if the salvaged abutment is also the terminal posterior tooth in the arch and has a viable opponent (Figure 1-8, B).

Another candidate for endodontic therapy is the adolescent who arrives in the office with a grossly damaged dentition and is faced with multiple extractions and dentures (Figure 1-9). Many of these children are mortified by their appearance. It is gratifying to see the blossoming personality when an esthetic improvement has been achieved. The end result in these cases would not be possible without root canal therapy (Figure 1-10).

Intentional Endodontics

Occasionally, intentional endodontics of teeth with perfectly vital pulps may be necessary. Examples of situations requiring intentional endodontics include hypererupted teeth or drifted teeth that must be reduced so drastically that the pulp is certain to be involved.[31] On other occasions, a pulp is intentionally removed and the canal filled so that a post and core may be placed for increased crown retention. In these cases, the endodontic treatment may be completed before tooth reduction is started.

Over and above these quite obvious indications for intentional endodontics, it has been recommended that pulpectomy and root canal filling be done for vital teeth badly discolored by tetracycline ingestion.

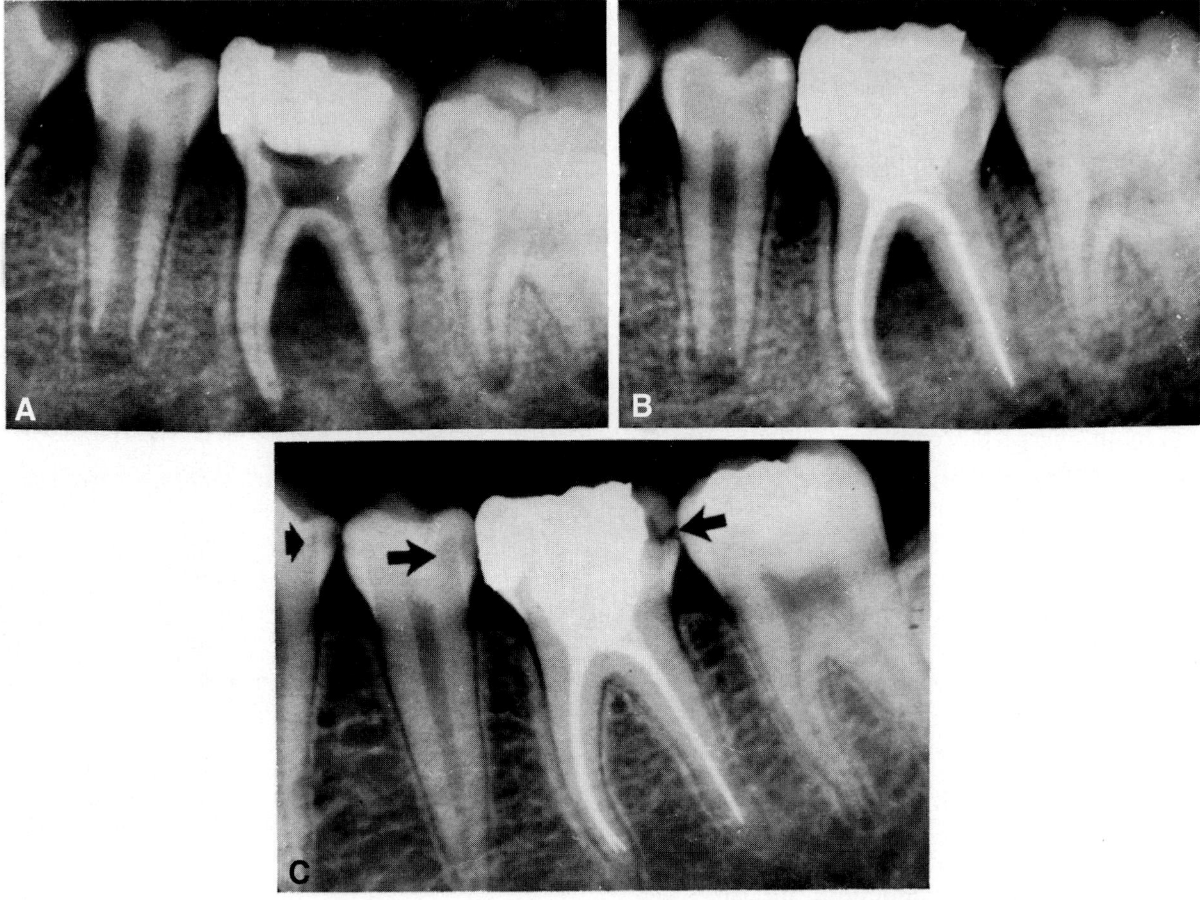

Figure 1-6 A, Pulpless first molar following failure of pulpotomy. Note two periradicular lesions and complete loss of intraradicular bone. Draining sinus tract opposite furca is also present. **B**, Completion of endodontic therapy without surgery. **C**, Two-year recall radiograph. Complete healing was evident in 6 months. New carious lesions (**arrows**) now involve each interproximal surface.

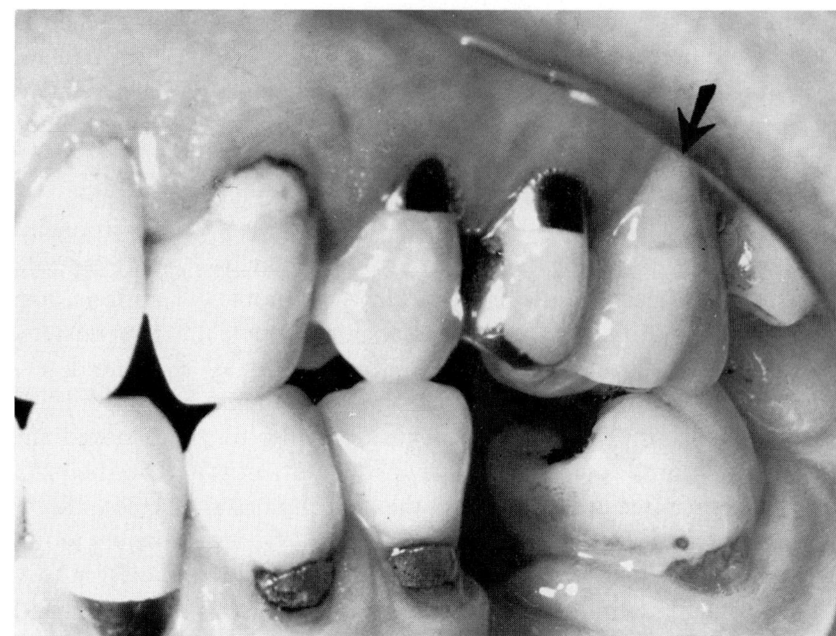

Figure 1-7 Extrusion, recession (**arrow**) tipping, malocclusion, rotation, and gingival cemental caries are only a few of the long-range consequences following early extraction of a permanent first molar.

Following root canal therapy, internal bleaching may be carried out.[32]

Considerations Prior to Endodontic Therapy

Although it is true that root canal treatment can be performed on virtually any tooth in the mouth, there are some important considerations that must be evaluated prior to recommending root canal treatment. Some of these were delineated by Beveridge (personal communication, June 1971):

1. Is the tooth needed or important? Does it have an opponent? Could it some day serve as an abutment for prosthesis?
2. Is the tooth salvageable, or is it so badly destroyed that it cannot be restored?
3. Is the entire dentition so completely broken down that it would be virtually impossible to restore?
4. Is the tooth serving esthetically, or would the patient be better served by its extraction and a more cosmetic replacement?
5. Is the tooth so severely involved periodontally that it would be lost soon for this reason?
6. Is the practitioner capable of performing the needed endodontic procedures?

In regard to the last point, today in the United States and many other countries, endodontic specialists are available to whom patients may be referred. A decision to refer is preferable **before** a mishap, such as perforation of the root canal, occurs. If a mishap does occur

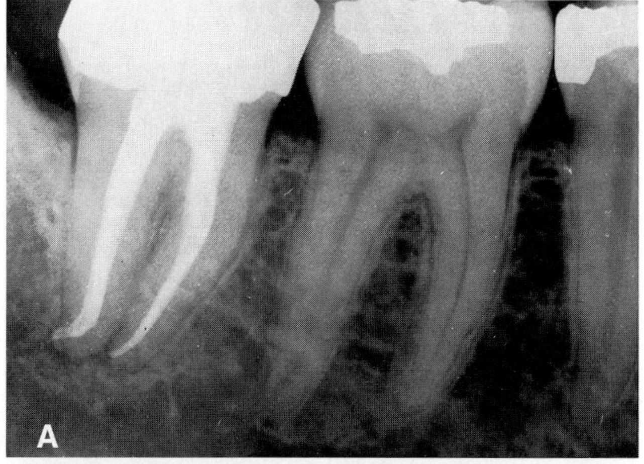

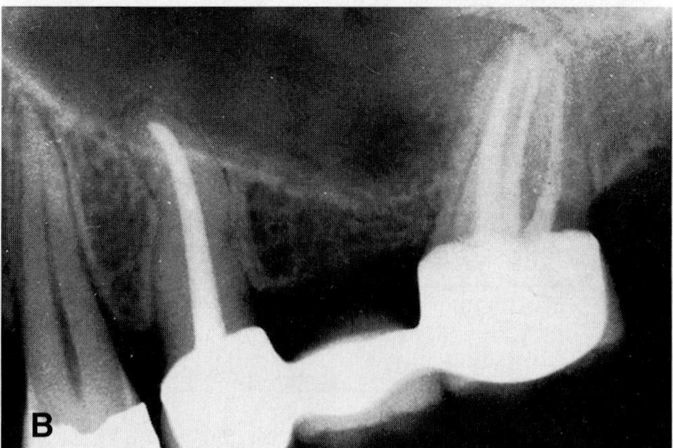

Figure 1-8 A, Terminal molar retained by endodontic therapy saves opposing molar as well. (Courtesy of Dr. L. Stephen Buchanan.) **B**, Fixed partial denture possible only because abutment teeth are retained by root canal therapy. (Courtesy of Dr. Norbert Hertl.)

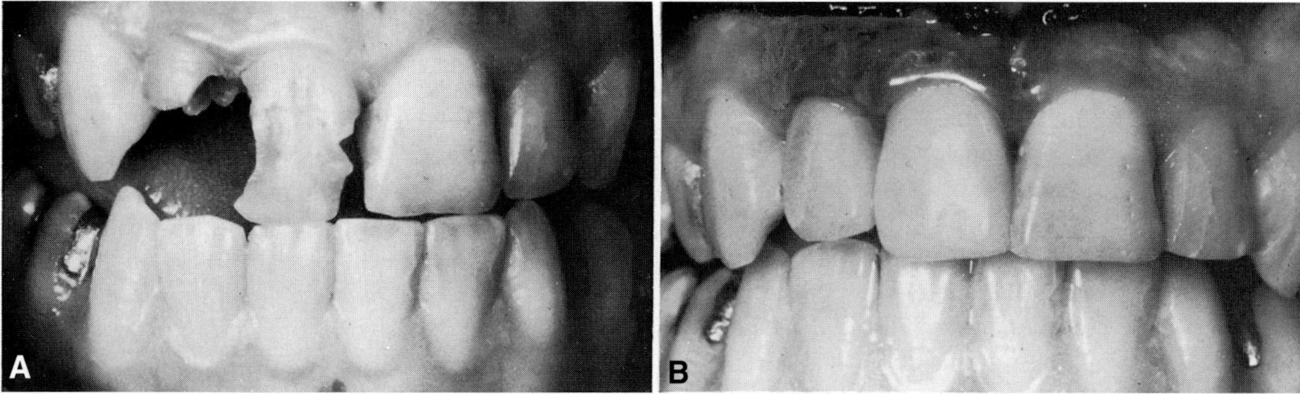

Figure 1-9 **A**, Caries-decimated dentition in a 14-year-old girl. Personality problems had developed in this youngster related to her feeling embarrassed about her appearance. **B**, Provisional restoration following endodontic therapy has restored the cosmetic appearance and confidence so necessary for the adolescent.

during treatment, the patient must be given the option of seeing a specialist before the decision to extract the tooth is made.

The well-trained dentist should have no fear of the pulpally involved tooth. If a carious exposure is noted during cavity preparation, the patient is informed of the problem and the recommended treatment, and, if consented to, the endodontic therapy is started while the tooth is anesthetized. The prepared dentist can begin pulpectomy immediately, using sterile instruments packaged and stored for just such an emergency.

Age and Health as Considerations

Age need not be a determinant in endodontic therapy. Simple and complex dental procedures are routinely performed on deciduous teeth in young children and

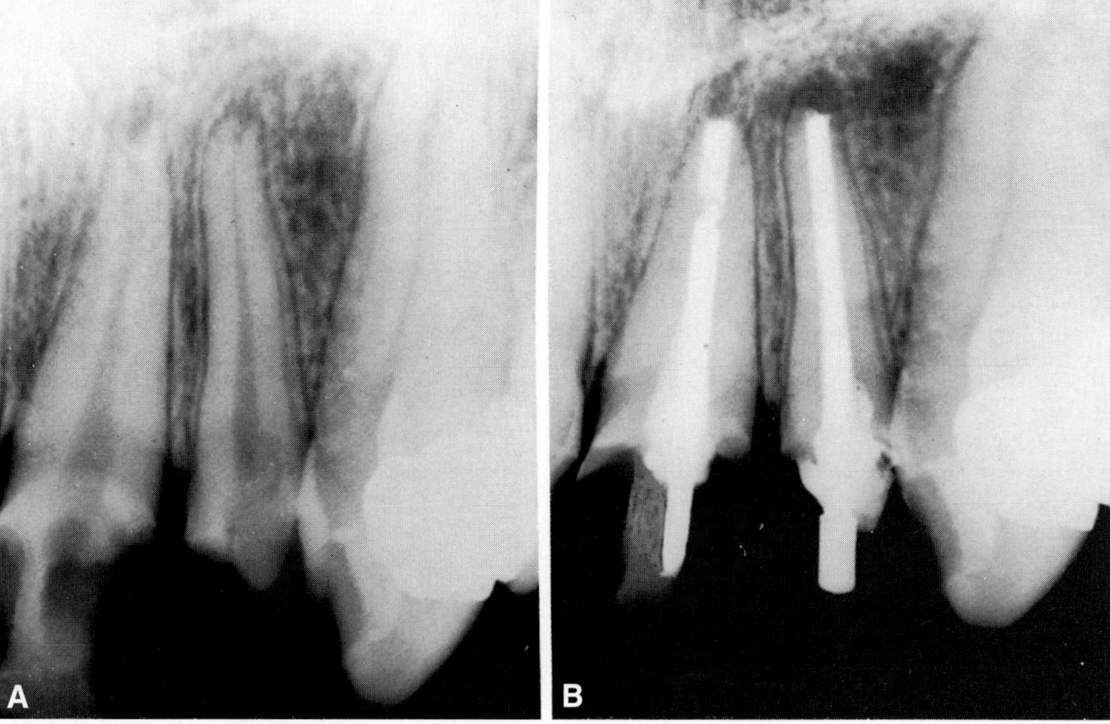

Figure 1-10 **A**, Obvious pulp involvement of incisors shown in Figure 1-9. **B**, Root canal treatment of these incisors makes possible dowel restoration followed by cosmetic provisional plastic crowns.

on permanent teeth in patients well into their nineties. The same holds true for endodontic procedures. It should be noted, however, that complete removal of the pulp in young immature teeth should be avoided if possible. Procedures for pulp preservation are more desirable and are fully discussed in chapter 15.

Health consideration must be evaluated for endodontics as it would for any other dental procedure. Most often, root canal therapy will be preferable to extraction. In severe cases of heart disease, diabetes, or radiation necrosis,[33] for example, root canal treatment is far less traumatic than extraction. Even for terminal cases of cancer, leukemia, or AIDS, endodontics is preferred over extraction. Pregnancy, particularly in the second trimester, is usually a safe time for treatment. In all of these situations, however, endodontic surgery is likely to be as traumatic as extraction.

Status of the Oral Condition

Pulpally involved teeth may simultaneously have periodontal lesions and be associated with other dental problems such as rampant decay, orthodontic malalignment, root resorption, and/or a history of traumatic injuries. Often the treatment of such teeth requires a team effort of dental specialists along with the patient's general dentist.

The presence of **periodontal lesions** must be evaluated with respect to the correct diagnosis: Is the lesion of periodontal or endodontic origin, or is it a combined situation? The answer to that question will determine the treatment approach and the outcome; generally, lesions of endodontic origin will respond satisfactorily to endodontic treatment alone[34] (Figure 1-11), whereas those of periodontal origin will not be affected simply by endodontic procedures (Figure 1-12). Combined

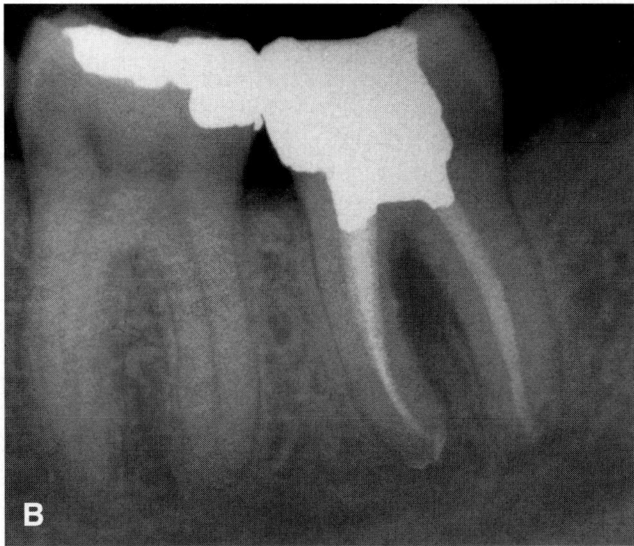

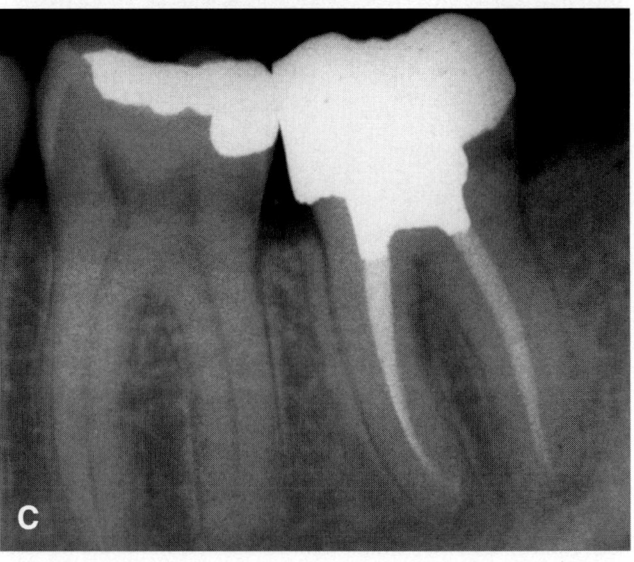

Figure 1-11 **A**, Mandibular molar with furcal bone loss (**arrow**) owing to endodontic infection and no periodontal disease. **B**, Root canal treatment completed without any periodontal intervention. **C**, One-year control shows recovery of furcal lesion by endodontic treatment alone.

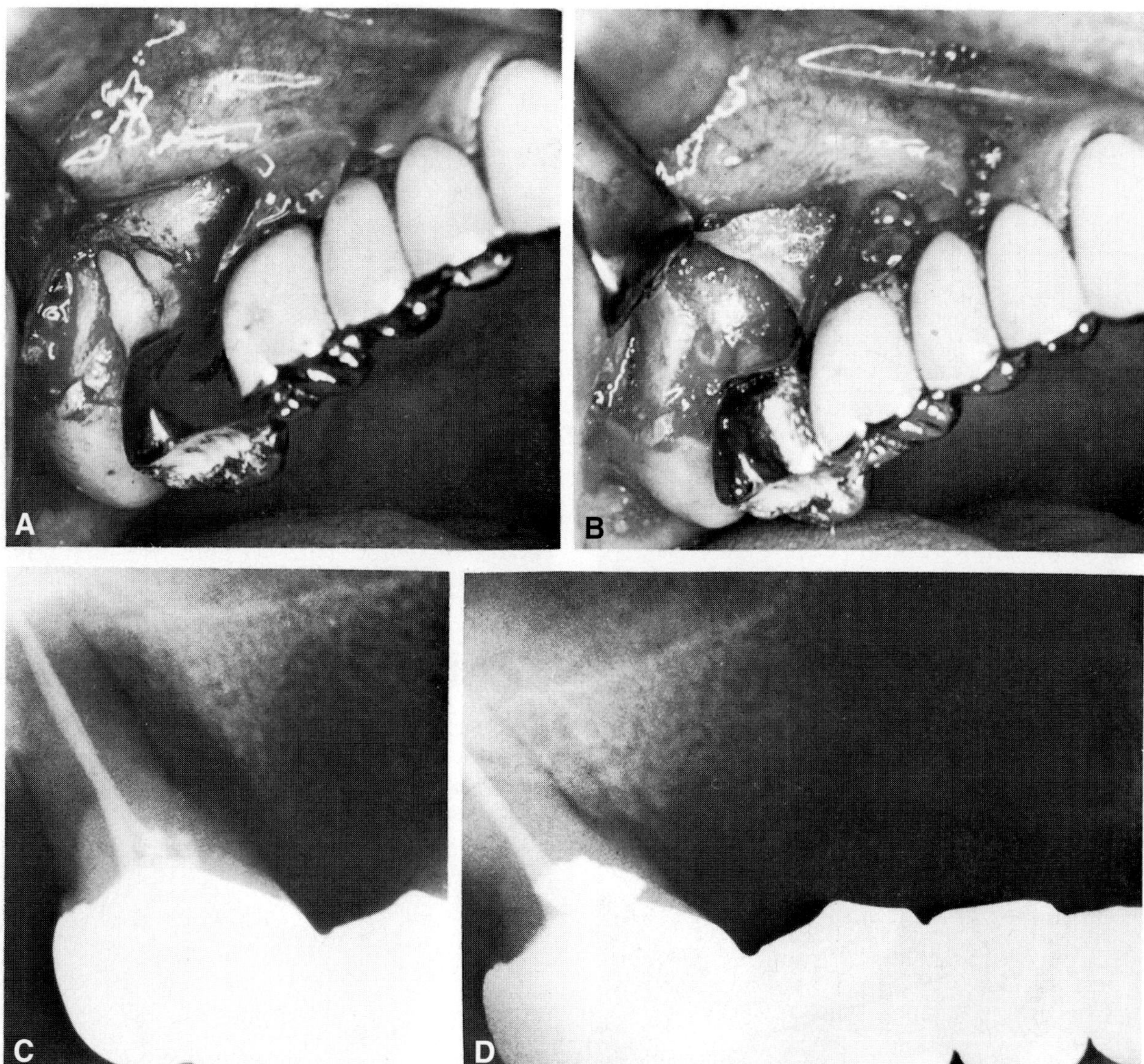

Figure 1-12 **A**, Retraction of surgical flap reveals the extent of periodontal lesion completely involving buccal roots of second molar abutment of full-arch periodontal prosthesis. Root canal therapy of a healthy, palatal root is completed before surgery. **B**, Total amputation of buccal roots reveals extent of cavernous periodontal lesion. **C**, Extensive bone loss, seen in *A* and *B*, is apparent in a radiograph taken at the time of treatment (the root outline was retouched for clarity). **D**, Osseous repair, 1 year following buccal root amputation. A solidly supported palatal root serves as an adequate terminal abutment for a full-arch prosthesis. Endodontic therapy was completed in 1959 and has remained successful. (Courtesy of Dr. Dudley H. Glick.)

lesions—those that develop as a result of both pulpal infection and periodontal disease—respond to a combined treatment approach in which endodontic intervention precedes, or is done simultaneously with, periodontal treatment[35] (Figure 1-13). Even teeth with apparently hopeless root support can be saved by endodontic treatment and root amputation (Figure 1-14).

Today, many pulpless teeth, once condemned to extraction, are saved by root canal therapy: teeth with large periradicular lesions or apical cysts[36–39] (Figure 1-15), teeth with perforations or internal or external resorption (Figure 1-16), teeth badly broken down by caries or horizontal fracture (Figure 1-17), pulpless teeth with tortuous or apparently obstructed canals or broken instruments within,[40] teeth with flaring open apices (Figure 1-18), teeth that are hopelessly discolored (Figure 1-19), and even teeth that are wholly or partially luxated.

All of these conditions can usually be overcome by endodontic, orthodontic, periodontic, or surgical procedures. In some cases, the prognosis may be somewhat guarded. But in the majority of cases, the patient and dentist are pleased with the outcome, especially if the final result is an arch fully restored.

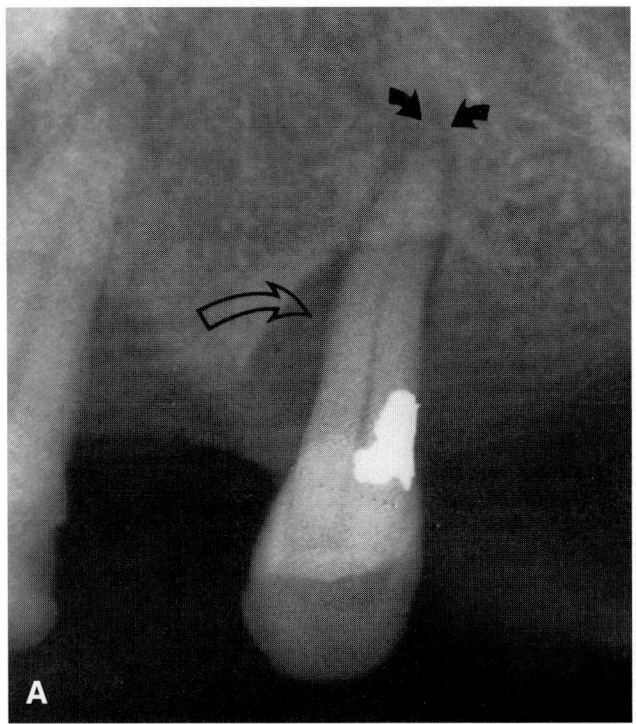

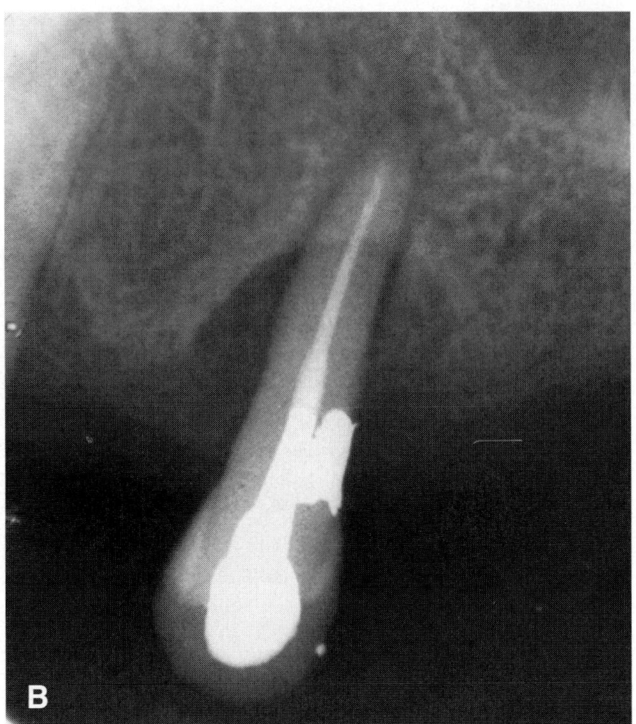

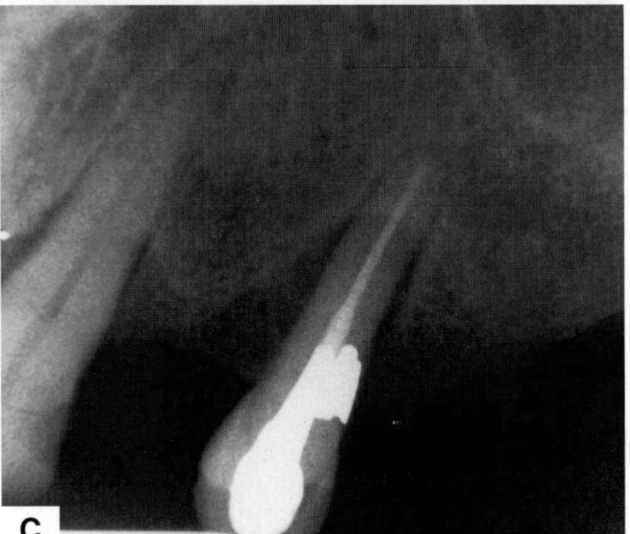

Figure 1-13 A, Maxillary premolar with both periodontal bone loss (**open arrow**) and an apical lesion (**small closed arrows**) from pulpal infection. **B**, Root canal treatment was done along with periodontal pocket maintenance. **C**, One-year control shows apical bony response to the endodontic procedure; the periodontal condition is unchanged.

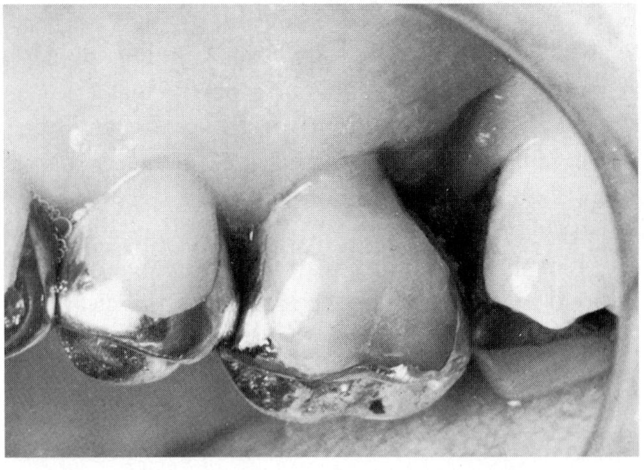

Figure 1-14 Amputation of periodontally involved distobuccal root allows retention of well-restored maxillary first molar. Root canal therapy of two remaining roots is necessary. Buccal-lingual narrowing of the occlusal table reduces the forces of mastication on these roots. The vulva-like soft tissue defect should be corrected with gingivoplasty.

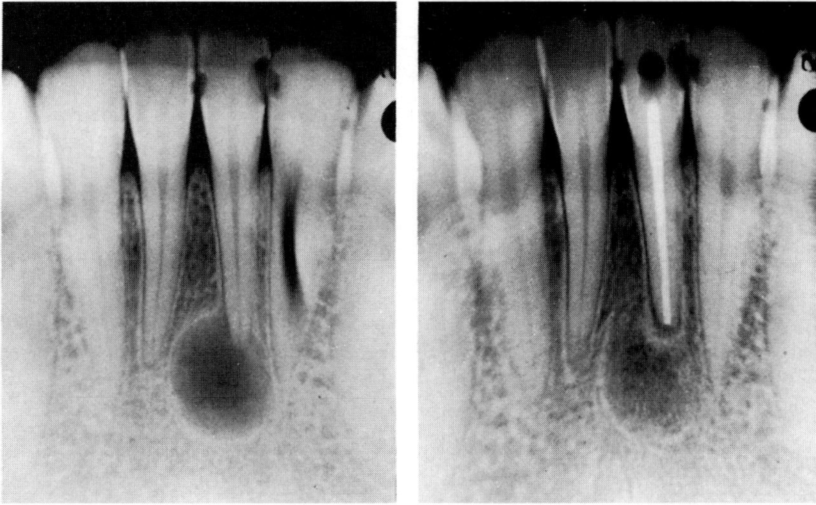

Figure 1-15 Classic apical cyst (**left**) apparent in pretreatment radiograph. Total repair of cystic cavity in 6-month recall film is signaled by complete lamina dura that has developed periradicularly. Biopsy confirmed the initial diagnosis of an apical cyst.

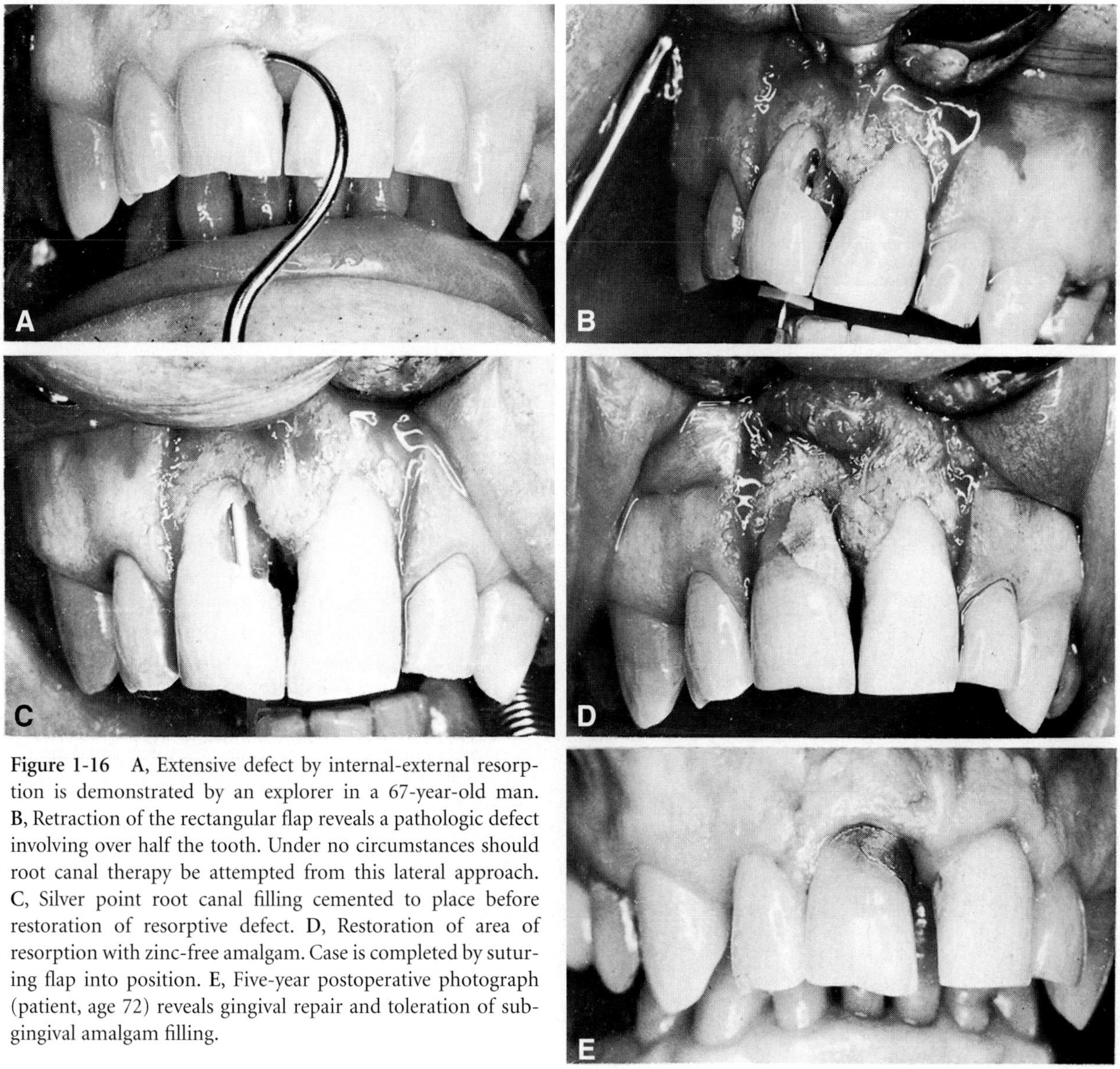

Figure 1-16 **A,** Extensive defect by internal-external resorption is demonstrated by an explorer in a 67-year-old man. **B,** Retraction of the rectangular flap reveals a pathologic defect involving over half the tooth. Under no circumstances should root canal therapy be attempted from this lateral approach. **C,** Silver point root canal filling cemented to place before restoration of resorptive defect. **D,** Restoration of area of resorption with zinc-free amalgam. Case is completed by suturing flap into position. **E,** Five-year postoperative photograph (patient, age 72) reveals gingival repair and toleration of subgingival amalgam filling.

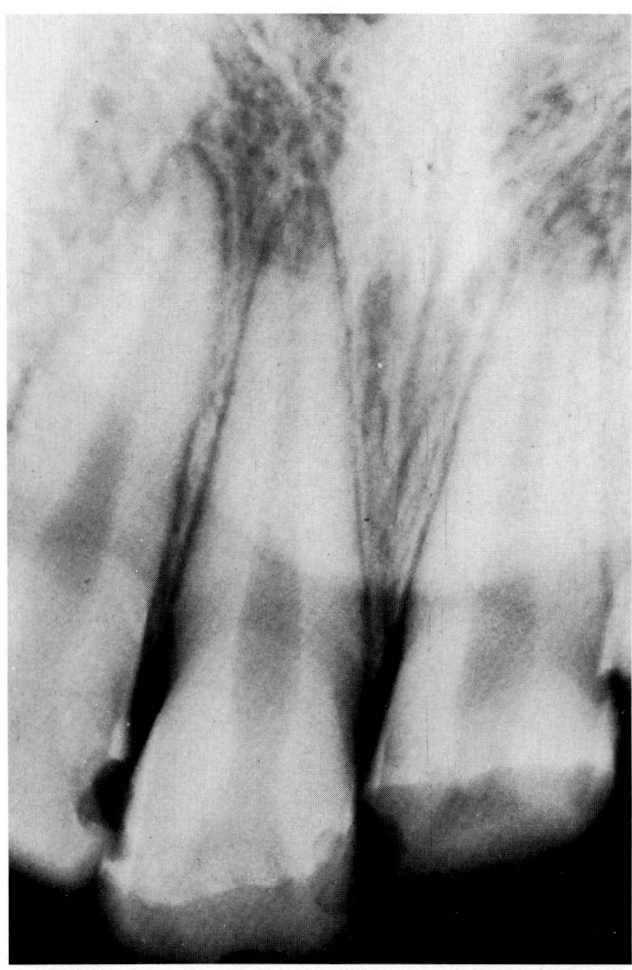

Figure 1-17 Four maxillary incisors with coronal fractures into pulp. Radiograph is necessary to determine whether root fracture has occurred and the stage of root development and apical closure. Immediate pulpectomy and root canal filling are indicated for all four incisors.

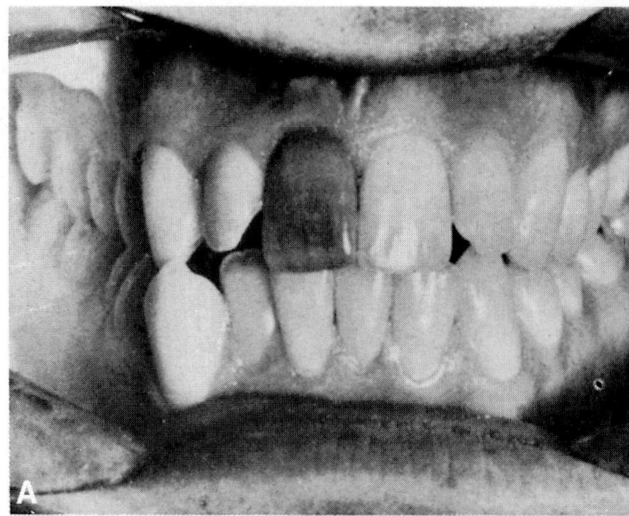

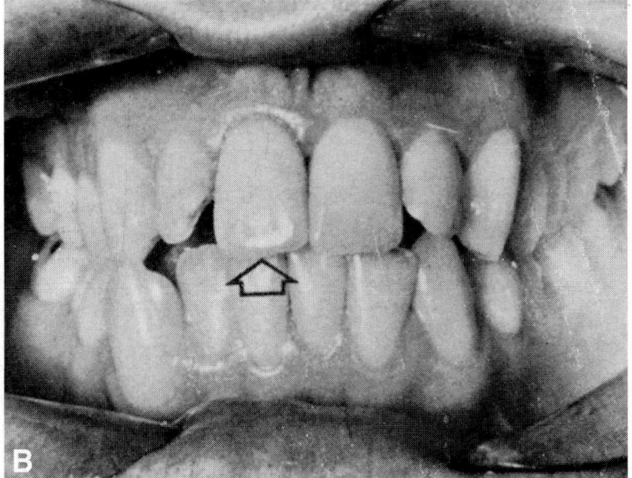

Figure 1-19 **A,** Intense discoloration of a pulpless maxillary central incisor. **B,** Successful bleaching with Superoxol (30% H_2O_2). The incisor has been restored to its normal color.

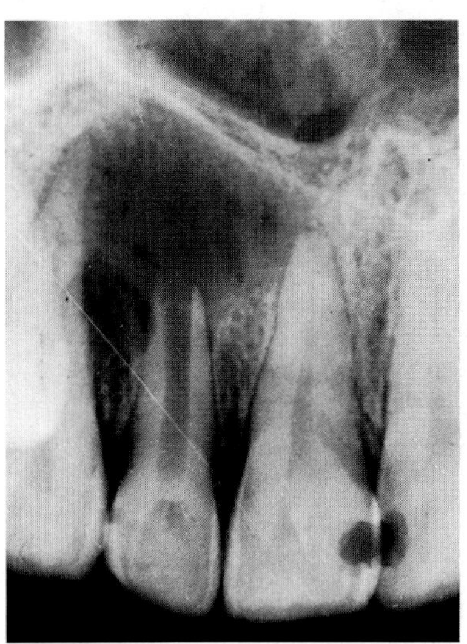

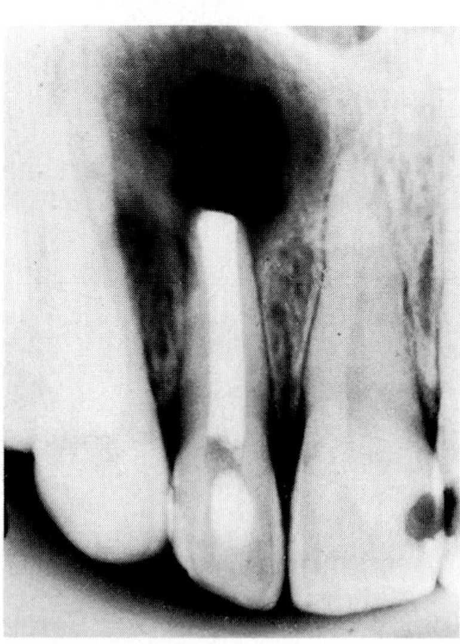

Figure 1-18 **Left,** Flaring apex of incompletely formed root follows pulpal death caused by impact injury at early age. **Right,** Obturation of the "blunderbuss" canal is accomplished by retrofilling from surgical approach. Reproduced with permission from Ingle JI. Dent Digest 1956;62:410.

ONE-APPOINTMENT THERAPY

Single-appointment root canal therapy has become a common practice. When questioned, however, most dentists reply that they reserve one-appointment treatment for vital pulp and immediate periradicular surgery cases. In 1982, only 12.8% of dentists queried thought that necrotic teeth would be successfully treated in one appointment.[41] Endodontists have been treating patients in one-appointment visits for some time. At one time, 86% of the directors of postgraduate endodontic programs, when surveyed, reported that nonsurgical one-visit treatment was part of their program.[42]

What are the advantages and disadvantages of single-visit endodontics?

Advantages:

1. Immediate familiarity with the internal anatomy, canal shape, and contour facilitates obturation
2. No risk of bacterial leakage beyond a temporary coronal seal between appointments
3. Reduction of clinic time
4. Patient convenience—no additional appointment
5. Less cost

Perceived Disadvantages:

1. No easy access to the apical canal if there is a flare-up
2. Clinician fatigue with extended one-appointment operating time
3. Patient fatigue and discomfort with extended operating time
4. **No opportunity to place an intracanal disinfectant** (other than allowing NaOCl to disinfect during treatment)

What has held back one-appointment endodontics? The major consideration has been concern about postoperative pain and failure.

Postoperative Pain

The fear that patients will probably develop postoperative pain and that the canal has been irretrievably sealed has probably been the greatest deterrent to single-visit therapy. Yet the literature shows no real difference in pain experienced by patients treated with multiple appointments.[41–57] In spite of this evidence, however, 40% of the endodontic course directors surveyed were of the opinion that necrotic cases treated in one visit have more flare-ups.[41] Galberry did not find this to be true in Louisiana,[49] nor did Nakamuta and Nagasawa in Japan, who had only a 7.5% pain incidence after treating 106 infected cases in single appointments.[50] Moreover, the symptoms the patients experienced were mild and needed no drugs or emergency treatment.

Oliet reported that only 3% of his sample of 264 patients receiving single-appointment treatment had severe pain, compared with 2.4% of the 123 patients treated in two visits.[48] Wolch's records of over 2,000 cases treated at a single appointment showed that less than 1% of patients indicated any severe reaction.[44] Pekruhn reported no statistically significant difference between his two groups.[47] Mulhern et al. reported no significant difference in the incidence of pain between 30 single-rooted teeth with necrotic pulps treated in one appointment and 30 similar teeth treated in three appointments.[51] At the University of Oklahoma, however, Roane and his associates found a "two to one higher frequency of pain following treatment completed in multiple visits when compared to those completed in one visit."[52] More recent reports from Brazil and Fava from the Netherlands found no difference in the incidence of pain between one- and two-visit cases,[53–56] and Trope reported **no flare-ups** in one-appointment cases **with no apical lesions.**[57] Re-treatment of failed cases with apical periodontitis made the difference, however. These cases suffered a 13.6% flare-up rate.[57] One might expect pain from any case, as reported by Harrison et al. from Baylor University.[58] Of 229 patients **treated twice,** 55.5% had no interappointment pain, 28.8% had slight pain, and 15.7% had moderate to severe pain. Eleazer and Eleazer compared the flare-up rate between one and two appointments in treating necrotic canal molars. In the two-visit cohort, there was a 16% flare-up rate, whereas in the **one-visit group**, there was only a **3% flare-up** experience, which proved to be significant.[59] In 1996, Ørstavik et al. also reported fewer flare-ups following single-appointment therapy.[60]

In light of these studies, **pain does not appear to be a valid reason** to avoid single-appointment root canal therapy.

Success versus Failure

If pain is not a deterrent, how about fear of failure? Pekruhn has published a definitive evaluation of **single-visit endodontics.**[61] From the clinics of the Arabian-American Oil Company, he reported a 1-year recall of 925 root-filled teeth of 1,140 possible cases. His failure rate was 5.2%, very comparable to many multiple-visit studies. Pekruhn was surprised to learn that his rate of failure was higher (15.3%) in teeth with periradicular lesions that had had **no prior access opening.** If this type of case had been previously opened, the incidence of failure dropped to 6.5%. The highest failure rate (16.6%) was in endodontic re-treatment cases. Symptomatic cases were twice as likely to fail as were asymptomatic cases (10.6% versus 5.0%).

A Japanese study followed one-visit cases for as long as 40 months and reported an 86% success rate.[50] Oliet again found no statistical significance between his two groups.[48] The majority of the postgraduate directors of endodontics felt that the chance of successful healing was equal for either type of therapy.[42] The original investigators in this field, Fox et al.,[43] Wolch,[44] Soltanoff,[45] and Ether et al.,[46] were convinced that single-visit root canal therapy could be just as successful as multiple-visit therapy. **None, however, treated the acutely infected or abscess case with a single visit.**

In more recent times, and in marked contrast to these positive reports, Sjögren and his associates in Sweden sounded **a word of caution.**[62] At **a single appointment**, they cleaned and obturated 55 single-rooted teeth with apical periodontitis. All of the teeth were initially infected. After cleaning and irrigating with sodium hypochlorite and just before obturation, they cultured the canals. Using advanced **anaerobic** bacteriologic techniques, they found that 22 (40%) of the 55 canals tested positive and the other 33 (60%) tested negative.

Periapical healing was then followed for **5 years.** Complete periapical healing occurred in **94%** of the 33 cases that yielded **negative** cultures! But in those 22 cases in which the canals tested **positive** prior to root canal filling, "the success rate of healing had **fallen to just 68%**," a statistically significant difference.[62] In other words, if a canal is still infected before filling at a single dental appointment, there may be a **26%** greater chance of failure than if the canal is free of bacteria. Their conclusions emphasized the importance of eliminating bacteria from the canal system before obturation and that this objective could not be achieved reliably without an effective intracanal medicament. This is one limited study, but it was done carefully and provides the recent evidence correlating the presence of bacteria to longer-term outcomes.

Ørstavik et al. faced up to this problem and studied 23 teeth with apical periodontitis, all but one infected initially. At the end of each sitting, apical dentin samples were cultured anaerobically. No chemical irrigants were used during cleaning and shaping, and at the end of the first appointment, 14 of the 23 canals were still infected.[63] At an earlier time, Ingle and Zeldow, using aerobic culturing, found much the same.[64,65] Ørstavik et al. then sealed calcium hydroxide in the canal. In 1 week, at the start of the second appointment, only one root canal had sufficient numbers of bacteria "for quantification"—the calcium hydroxide was that effective! They also found "a tendency for teeth causing symptoms to harbour more bacteria than symptomless teeth."[63]

In a follow-up study, Trope et al. treated teeth with apical periodontitis, with and without calcium hydroxide, in one or two visits. They reached a number of conclusions: (1) "[C]alcium hydroxide disinfection after chemomechanical cleaning will result in negative cultures in most cases"; (2) "[I]nstrumentation and irrigation alone decrease the number of bacteria in the canal 1000-fold, however the canals cannot be rendered free of bacteria by this method alone"; and (3) "[T]he additional disinfecting action of calcium hydroxide before obturation resulted in a **10% increase in healing rates.** This difference should be considered clinically important."[66]

In another 52-week comparative study in North Carolina, of the "periapical healing of infected roots [in dogs] obturated **in one step** or with prior calcium hydroxide disinfection," the researchers concluded that "$Ca(OH)_2$ disinfection before obturation of infected root canals results in significantly less periapical inflammation than obturation alone."[67]

One has to ask, therefore, wouldn't it be better to extend one more appointment, properly medicate the canal between appointments, and improve the patient's chances of filling a bacteria-free canal? Unfortunately, there is a widely held but anecdotal opinion that current chemomechanical cleaning techniques are superior, predictably removing the entire bacterial flora. If this is so, single-visit treatment of necrotic pulp cases would definitely be indicated. However, the research has yet to be published to corroborate these opinions. Until then, it may be more prudent to use an intracanal medicament such as calcium hydroxide, within a multiple-visit regimen, for cases in which a mature bacterial flora is present within the canal system prior to treatment. Although single appointments would be very appropriate in **cases with vital pulps**, on the other hand, for teeth with necrotic pulps and periapical periodontitis, and for failed cases requiring retreatment, there may be a risk of lower success rates in the long term. To date, the evidence for recommending either one- or multiple-visit endodontics is not consistent. The prudent practitioner needs to make decisions carefully as new evidence becomes available.

Wolch said it best: "In the treatment of any disease, a cure can only be effected if the cause is removed. Since endodontic diseases originate from an infected or affected pulp, it is axiomatic that the root canal must be thoroughly and carefully debrided and obturated" (personal communication, 1983).

"ENDODONTICS AND THE LAW"[68]

If today's patients are becoming more sophisticated about their dental wants, they are also becoming more sophisticated about their legal rights. As Milgrom and Ingle have noted, the dentist can no longer consider himself immune to malpractice litigation by hiding behind a doctrine of "local community standards."[69]

Local community standards today are those standards set by the specialists in the community, in this case the board-certified endodontists, not the general practitioner. More and more often, specialists are willing to testify in court, supporting patients who, in their view, have been treated below the standard of care. Along with authors who have alluded to the subject,[70–72] the AAE has issued guidelines that could well establish a **national standard of care.** Titled "**Appropriateness of Care and Quality Assurance Guidelines,**" it is now in its third edition and may be obtained from the AAE.[73]

Cohen and Schwartz have pointed out that a meritorious claim by a patient is "**any departure** from the minimum quality of endodontic care that reasonably prudent practitioners would perform under the same or similar circumstances."[68] "**Any** departure"' is rather broad and includes failure to properly diagnose; failure to perform comprehensive diagnostic tests; failure to properly document and record all findings and treatment; treatment of the wrong tooth; use of paraformaldehyde/steroid pastes such as N2, RC2B, Endomethazone, and SPAD; root perforations; failure to receive informed consent; failure of yet-to-be-approved endodontic implants; failure because of instruments broken in the canal; and failure to use a rubber dam.[74] From this list, "failure to use a rubber dam" is unconscionable and may result in the most disastrous consequences, namely the swallowing or inhalation of an endodontic instrument (Figure 1-20).

Instrument breakage or, as it is euphemistically referred to, "instrument separation" is a "disquieting event." One must ask, "Did the file break because of overzealous use... or was it defectively manufactured?"[74] The unbroken end of the file should be saved in a coin envelope and placed in the patient's treatment record. If defective manufacturing can be proved, liability shifts to the manufacturer. In either event, **the patient must be promptly informed.**[74]

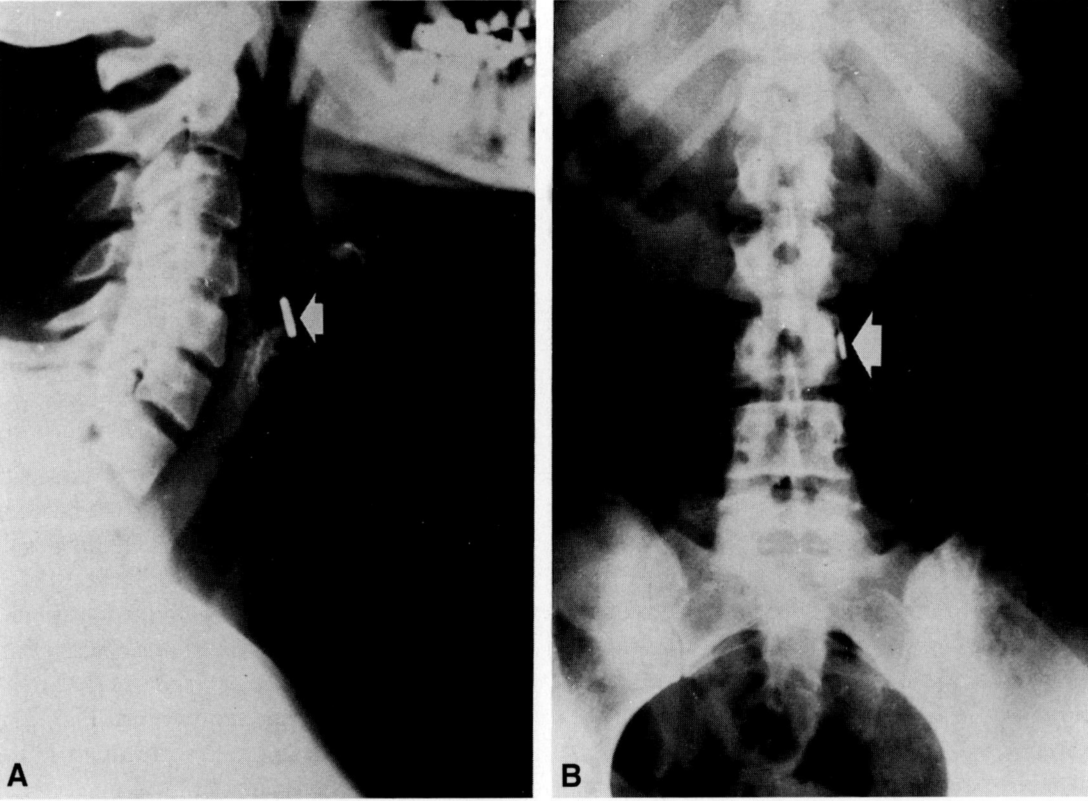

Figure 1-20 Two examples of swallowed endodontic instruments because the rubber dam was not used. **A**, Radiograph taken 15 minutes after an endodontic broach (**arrow**) was swallowed. Reproduced with permission from Heling B, Heling I. Oral Surg 1977;43:464. **B**, Abdominal radiograph showing a broach in the duodenum (**arrow**). The broach was surgically removed 1 month later. Reproduced with permission from Goultschin J, Heling B. Oral Surg 1971;32:621.

A major standard of care controversy has also erupted over the issue of overfilling or overextending the root canal filling versus filling "short." One would be hard-pressed in court to defend gross overfilling, sometimes even to the point of filling the mandibular canal (Figure 1-21). On the other hand, a "puff" of cement from the apical constriction has become acceptable.

Filling just short of the radiographic apex, at the apical constriction, 0.5 to 1.0 mm, is backed by a host of positive reports. By the same token, an inadequate root canal filling is hardly defensible as rising to the standard of care, even though the filling might appear to extend to the apex.

Grossly underfilled canals, 3.0 to 6.0 mm short, are also hard to defend, particularly if an associated periradicular lesion is radiographically apparent. One must realize, however, that some root canals are so thoroughly calcified (obliterated) that penetration to the apex is virtually impossible.

Facing this problem, Swedish scientists analyzed 70 cases of "obliterated" canals over a recall period of 2 to 12 years.[75] The overall success rate for the partially filled canals was 89%. If in the initial radiograph there was an intact periradicular contour, the success rate was an amazing 97.9%. If a preoperative periradicular radiolucency was present, however, the success rate dropped to a disappointing 62.5%.[75]

In the incompletely filled failure cases, it was theorized that canals were present but so narrow that they could not be negotiated by the smallest instruments, but were still large enough for the passage of bacteria and their toxins.[75] Buchanan has shown that with care and persistence, many so-called obliterated canals can be negotiated (personal communication, 1989).

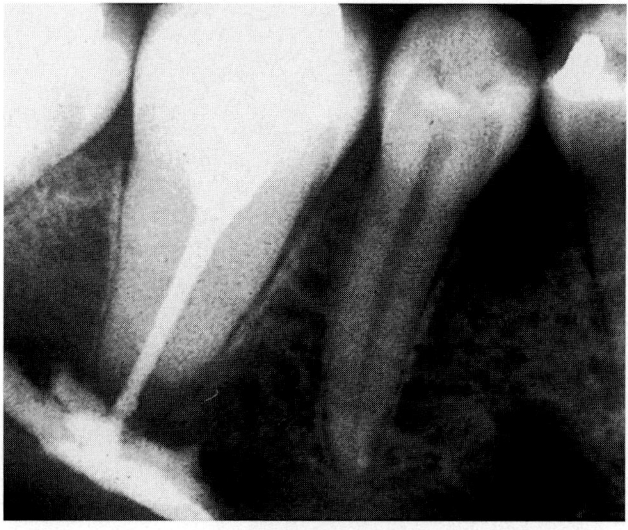

Figure 1-21 Massive overextension of RC2B into the inferior alveolar canal. The patient suffered permanent paresthesia. A lawsuit was settled out of court against the dentist and in favor of the 26-year-old female secretary in Pennsylvania. (Courtesy of Edwin J. Zinman, DDS, JD.)

In the light of the low success rate (62.5%) of unfilled "obliterated" canals with apical radiolucencies, the dentist must seriously consider a surgical approach and retrofillings. This would be well within the standard of care if done expertly.

Paresthesia is another patient complaint following endodontic treatment. Lip numbness ("the injection didn't wear off")[76] is usually caused by gross overfilling, nearly always when root canal sealers or cements impinge on the inferior alveolar nerve. This is particularly true when neurotoxic filling materials are used (eg, N2, RC2B, Endomethazone, SPAD).

Ørstavik et al. surveyed the literature for reported cases of paresthesia related to endodontic treatment.[76] They found 24 published cases; 86% of patients were female, and usually a paste-type filling had been used. Although 5 cases "healed in four months to two years, 14 showed no indication of the paraesthesia healing...from 3 months up to 18 years." The remaining cases were resolved by surgical removal of the offending material. Ørstavik et al. reported the twenty-fifth case, paresthesia following overfilling with Endomethazone. The condition still persisted 3 years later and "the possibility of regeneration of the nerve must be considered negligible."[76] Others have reported the same or similar causes of nerve damage and paresthesia.[77–80]

In California, endodontics became number one in terms of the frequency of malpractice claims filed.[68] Nationally, "endodontic claims are the second most frequent producer of claims and dollar losses with oral surgery being number one."[72] There is obviously "an increase in the number of malpractice claims involving endodontics, primarily against general dentists."[73] Many of these tragedies, for dentist and patient alike, could have been avoided had the patient been referred to a dentist more skilled in endodontics. "When in doubt, refer it out."[74]

Just such a tragic case—a failure to timely or properly refer a patient—involved five dentists enmeshed in a recent malpractice suit: one general dentist, three endodontists, and a prosthodontist. None of the four specialists was board certified, although all were educationally qualified. The patient was first seen by the general dentist, who took full-mouth radiographs, did an oral examination, and established a treatment plan that said nothing about an unusual bony lesion in the left mandible. The patient was not satisfied with the generalist, asked for her radiographs, and transferred to a prosthodontist, who also used the original films for his examination. He established that a number of crowns and a bridge should be done and that he would start on tooth #19, which had had root canal therapy that failed. So, quite properly, he referred the patient to an endodontist, who, for some unexplained reason, retreated only two of the three canals. Up to this time, all three dentists had failed to notice the unusual bone trabeculation and apparent lesion that extended from the mesial of #19 and around the roots of #20 and #21 to the distal of #22, nor had they noted the buccal swelling in the region! If they had done so, they should have referred the patient to an oral surgeon, a competent radiologist, or an oral pathologist.

The prosthodontist continued treatment, and, finally, when the patient complained, noted the swelling in the vestibule opposite the radiographic lesion. So he sent her back to the endodontist, who was not in his office, so his associate saw her. The associate stated that the patient had an abscess and that root canal therapy would have to be done on both teeth, #20 and #21. She was very displeased with this second endodontist and so went to a third, who stated that she had an abscess and proceeded to do root canal therapy on tooth #21, right in the middle of the lesion, which, by this time, had grown almost to the midline. The patient was very concerned about the swelling, but the endodontist assured her that it was an abscess that was about to "fistulate," even though there were no other signs of inflammation—no redness, no pain, no loss of function—only swelling. He did not suggest that she be referred to an oral surgeon, nor did he aspirate the buccal swelling for exudate. He stated that they should "watch and wait" to see if the root canal therapy improved the situation. When it did not and the buccal swelling increased, the patient finally went to an oral surgeon. The case was diagnosed as an ameloblastoma, and the mandible had to be amputated from first molar to first molar. The case against the five dentists was settled out of court for nearly one million dollars.

This case is a sad example of dentists so eager to treat the patient that they did not thoroughly examine the evidence that was present, ignored the signs and symptoms, and neglected to refer the patient to someone better trained or more competent.

REFERRALS

Just when should an endodontic patient be referred? Dietz has listed four general categories in which referral should be considered[81]:

1. The **complex case** involving multiple, dilacerated, obstructed, or curved canals; malpositioned and malformed teeth; and complex root morphology. To this one might add unusual radiographic lesions that do not appear to be "standard" periradicular lesions.
2. **Emergencies** in which a patient needs immediate treatment for toothaches, broken crowns, clinical exposures, infection, or traumatically injured teeth.
3. **Medically compromised patients** with cardiovascular conditions, diabetes, and blood disorders.
4. **Mentally compromised patients**, those with a true mental disorder and those who have problems with dentistry.

Then there is "the dentist who is too busy to perform the procedures..."[81]

To this list, Harman has added, "If the general dentist believes that a good and proper diagnosis goes beyond his or her abilities, then the dentist should refer the patient."[82] Nash has estimated that 85 to 90% of all endodontic referrals come from other dentists.[83] The remainder are self-referrals, walk-ins, and patient or physician referrals.

The endodontist would much rather receive the patient at the beginning of treatment than become a "retreat-odontist," retrieving his fellow dentist's "chestnuts from the fire."

INFORMED CONSENT

Weichman has pointed out the importance of the **doctrine of informed consent**, as well as other steps that must be taken by the dentist to maintain good patient relations.[84] According to the doctrine of informed consent, a dentist must (1) describe the proposed treatment so that it is fully understood by the patient, (2) explain all of the risks attendant to such treatment, and (3) discuss alternative procedures or treatments that might apply to the patient's particular problem.[85] To this should be added (4) the risks associated with doing nothing!

The courts have decided that a patient can give a valid or an informed consent for treatment only after receiving all of this information. If a dentist does not obtain an informed consent, he or she is guilty of professional negligence and is liable for any injury resulting from so-called unauthorized treatment. One way of handling this is to list the options in the patient's chart and **have the patient sign**. "Inform before you perform."[68]

Weichman points out that, at a minimum, the dentist must tell the patient what he or she intends to accomplish and what any follow-up treatment, such as final restoration, might entail; the dentist must list other ways of treating the condition, as well as their advantages and disadvantages, such as extraction versus root canal therapy, and, above all, must discuss possible complications—what might go wrong or the fact that the treatment could lose its effectiveness after a few months.[84]

In spite of this detailed recitation, just informing the patient is not enough, as a famous court decision has made quite clear: "The test for determining whether a potential peril must be divulged to the patient is its materiality to the patient's decision." For the patient to give informed consent, he or she must understand what the dentist is stating. In other words, technical terms are to be avoided. For example, use "numbness" rather than "paresthesia." Also, the explanation must be in the language the patient understands (eg, Spanish rather than English). It should be pointed out that in some states, "guaranteeing" the outcome of professional services is against the law.

Another type of informed consent is **parental consent**. A minor should never be treated without the written consent of a parent. Again, "age of consent" varies by state. One may also encounter the "emancipated minor," who may give consent. The definition of "emancipated minor" also varies by state.

Weichman goes on to list the other aspect of practicing defensive dentistry, maintaining good patient relations. He recommends showing concern for the patient's welfare by (1) establishing good anesthesia, (2) anticipating problems such as unavoidable pain and forewarning the patient, (3) telephoning patients after treatment to inquire about their comfort, (4) placing high priority on emergencies, (5) consulting with other professionals to provide the best possible care for each patient, and (6) providing competent "coverage" in the event that the dentist is unavailable.[84] Selbst has added another caveat. He shows "data suggesting an increased incidence of complications associated with retreatment cases, particularly the retreatment of paste fills." He recommends that special care be taken to advise the re-treatment patient of this increased jeopardy.[85]

Patient Records

The importance of maintaining good patient records, not just financial ones, is also emphasized by Weichman.[84] These records should consist, at a minimum, of good, well-processed radiographs; a health history signed by the patient; the patient's complaints, from "chief complaint" to any variance at subsequent appointments; any objective findings made during treatment, such as the state of the pulp's vitality found on opening the chamber, as well as the results of all testing before treatment; any possible complications foreseen or encountered, such as curved roots, obliterated canals, postoperative problems, and associated periodontal problems; a list of allergies and illnesses; any prescription written or medications given, including anesthetics injected; and full disclosure of any procedural accidents occurring during treatment, such as broken instruments or fractured roots.[84]

Hourigan emphasized that, at the very least, records should show the following:

- Diagnosis (Dx)
- Treatment (Tx) (eg, "carpules"—what, how many)
- Medications (Rx) (what, how much; write out)
- Follow-up (Fx)
- Complications (Cx) (broken instruments, perforations, patient's reaction to anesthetic, etc)[86]

When records are filled out, abbreviations may be used, but the dentist must know what they stand for. If someone other than the dentist writes on the patient's record, the writer must initial the writing. An office record of initials and the names they stand for should be kept for possible future use.

The AAE has suggested an informed consent form that will cover most situations (Figure 1-22). However, the Association has stated that "a written consent form cannot be used as a substitute for the doctor's discussion with each individual patient."[87]

Sample Statement Of Consent For Endodontic Treatment

1. I hereby authorize Dr. ________________, and any other agents or employees of ________________ and such assistants as may be selected by any of them to treat the condition(s) described below:

____

____

2. The procedure(s) necessary to treat the condition(s) have been explained to me and I understand the nature of the procedure to be:

____

____

3. I have been informed of possible alternative methods of treatment including no treatment at all.
4. The doctor has explained to me that there are certain inherent and potential risks in any treatment plan or procedure.
5. It has been explained to me and I understand that a perfect result is not guaranteed or warranted and cannot be guaranteed or warranted.
6. I have been given the opportunity to question the doctor concerning the nature of the treatment, the inherent risks of the treatment, and the alternatives to this treatment.
7. This consent form does not encompass the entire discussion I had with the doctor regarding the proposed treatment.

____

Patient's signature

Figure 1-22 Informed consent form for endodontic procedures recommended by the American Association of Endodontists (may be copied and enlarged).

Others have written extensively about informed consent.[88–92] Bailey and Curley have both noted that informed consent was an outgrowth of assault and battery law—the unauthorized "offensive touching without consent."[88,89] In 1960, Kansas was the first state to formalize informed consent applied to dentists. The practitioner must bear in mind that informed consent is the "**rule of law rather than just a standard of practice.**"[89]

Bailey has pointed out the wide variance among states in applying or interpreting the law. In Alaska and Washington state, for example, informed consent is not mandatory in severe emergencies.[88]

The Council on Insurance of the ADA made note of the fact that the issue of informed consent will be tried in court as a civil action and that guilt will be based on the "**preponderance of evidence**," which is easier to prove than "**beyond a reasonable doubt**," used in criminal cases.[90]

Paladino et al. have warned of the indefensibility of using the Sargenti endodontic technique (N2 or RC2B), informed consent or no informed consent: "A general dentist who performs a Sargenti root canal is going to have as an expert witness testifying against him virtually every endodontist in town."[91] Further, "any patient who comes to [a lawyer] with a Sargenti treated tooth has a *prima facie* case of negligence" against the dentist. "There is no way that... a dentist can justify performing that procedure."[91]

Weichman has stated that the statute of limitations does not begin **until the patient discovers** (or should have discovered) such problems as a broken instrument or a poorly filled canal.[84] He also points out the futility of adding to or changing records at a later date, noting the dishonesty of the procedure and the dentist's culpability when proved a fraud in court.

A serious problem in patient management that has developed in this age of specialization revolves around responsibility. Who among the many professionals caring for the patient shall assume responsibility? "Who should be captain of the ship?" asked Beveridge. "Let it become a mutual objective that no patient shall move from one practitioner to another without someone in command. Every patient deserves to have a clearly understood, readily identified, 'captain of his dental ship,'" he stated. Ideally, the dentist most responsible should be the general practitioner who has referred the patient to the endodontist, periodontist, or oral surgeon. His office should be the "clearinghouse" for central records and coordination of treatment. Howard has also emphasized the importance of the general dentist being the "captain of the ship."[92]

It would be easy to become discouraged about providing medical and dental care after reviewing the number of malpractice suits in recent decades. The fact of the matter is that heightened patient awareness of their rights, and the standard of care to be expected, forces the health care provider to be prudent and careful in caring for patients and makes the patient take more responsibility for his or her medical and dental health.

REFERENCES

1. Zias J, Numeroff K. Operative dentistry in the second century BCE. J Am Dent Assoc 1987;114:665.
2. Tsai-Fang T. Endodontic treatment in China. Int Endodont J 1984;17:163.
3. Grossman LI. Pioneers in endodontics. JOE 1987;13:409.
4. Grossman LI. Endodontics 1776-1976: a bicentennial history against the background of general dentistry. J Am Dent Assoc 1976;93:78.
5. Pucci FM. Conductos radiculares. Vol. II. Buenos Aires: Editorial Medico-Quirurgica; 1945.
6. Ingle JI, Levine M. The need for uniformity of endodontic instruments, equipment, and filling materials. In: Grossman LI, editor. Transactions of the Second International Congress on Endodontics. Philadelphia: 1958. p. 133–45.
7. Ingle JI. A standardized endodontic technique utilizing newly designed instruments and filling materials. Oral Surg 1961;14:83.
8. American Dental Association. 1990 Services rendered report (estimates).
9. American Association of Endodontists recertification document, 1989.
10. Burns R. Surveys document more people choosing root canal therapy over extractions. Report of the Public Affairs Committee of the American Association of Endodontists. Public education report. April 1987.
11. Molven O, et al. Prevalence and distribution of root-filled teeth in former dental school patients: follow-up after 10-17 years. Int Endodont J 1985;18:247.
12. Torrey Report. American Dental Trade Association, 1984.
13. Dental products marketing strategic survey-1997: Strategic Dental Marketing.
14. AAE Internet report, 1999.
15. National Institute of Dental Research. Dental caries continues downward trend in children. J Am Dent Assoc 1988;117:625.
16. Burgess JO. A panoramic radiographic analysis of Air Force basic trainees. Oral Surg 1985;60:113.
17. National Institute of Dental Research. Survey of adult dental health. J Am Dent Assoc 1987;114:829.
18. Bailit H, et al. Does more generous dental insurance coverage improve oral health? J Am Dent Assoc 1985;110:701.
19. ADA 1996 Survey of dental practice.
20. Waldman BH. A favorable prognosis for dentistry. Dent Econom 1984;74:51.
21. U.S. Health Care Financing Administration and the Bureau of Labor Statistics, 1997.
22. Louis Harris Associates. Nuprin pain report. Newsweek 1985;Dec 2.
23. Gale EN, et al. Effect of dentist's behavior on patient's attitudes. J Am Dent Assoc 1984;109:444.

24. What is root canal treatment? American Dental Association pamphlet No. W-117.
25. American Association of Endodontists, survey. ADA News 1985; Apr 15;7.
26. Burns JM. Why root canal therapy? Chicago: Quintessence; 1986.
27. Milgrom P, et al. The prevalence and practice management consequences of dental fear in a major U.S. city. J Am Dent Assoc 1988;116:641.
28. Gatchel RJ. The prevalence of dental fear and avoidance: expanded adult and recent adolescent surveys. J Am Dent Assoc 1989;118:591.
29. LeClaire AJ, et al. Endodontic fear survey. JOE 1988;14:560.
30. Lord J, Teel S. The overdenture: patient selection, use of copings. J Prosthet Dent 1974;32:41.
31. Bohannan HM, Abrams L. Intentional vital extirpation in periodontal prosthesis. J Prosthet Dent 1961;11:781.
32. Abou-Rass M. The elimination of tetracycline discoloration by intentional endodontics and internal bleaching. JOE 1982;8:101.
33. Hayward JR, Kerr DA, Jesse RH, Ingle JI. The management of teeth related to the treatment of oral cancer. CA Cancer J Clin 1969;19:98.
34. Hiatt WH. Regeneration of the periodontium after endodontic therapy and flap operation. Oral Surg 1959;12:1471.
35. Prichard J. The intrabony technique as a predictable procedure. J Periodontol 1957;28:202.
36. Sommer RF, Ostrander FD, Crowley MC. Clinical endodontics. 2nd ed. Philadelphia: WB Saunders; 1961.
37. Grossman LI, Rossman SR. Correlation of clinical diagnosis and histopathologic findings in 101 pulpless teeth with areas of rarefaction [abstract]. J Dent Res 1955;34:692.
38. Priebe WA, Lazansky JP, Wuehrmann AH. The value of roentgenographic film in the differential diagnosis of periradicular lesions. Oral Surg 1954;7:979.
39. Bhaskar SN. Synopsis of oral pathology. 7th ed. St. Louis: CV Mosby; 1986.
40. Crump MC, Natkin E. Relationship of broken root canal instruments to endodontic case prognosis: a clinical investigation. J Am Dent Assoc 1970;80:1341.
41. Calhoun RL, Landers RR. One-appointment endodontic therapy: a nationwide survey of endodontists. JOE 1982;8:35.
42. Landers RR, Calhoun RL. One-appointment endodontic therapy: an opinion survey. JOE 1980;6:799.
43. Fox JL, Atkinson JS, Dinin PA. Incidence of pain following one-visit endodontic treatment. Oral Surg 1970;30:123.
44. Wolch I. The one-appointment endodontic technique. J Can Dent Assoc 1975;41:613.
45. Soltanoff W. Comparative study of the single visit and multiple visit endodontic procedure. JOE 1978;4:278.
46. Ether S, et al. A comparison of one and two visit endodontics. J Farmacia Odontol New Orleans, Louisiana State University 1978;8:215.
47. Pekruhn RB. Single-visit endodontic therapy: a preliminary clinical study. J Am Dent Assoc 1981;103:875.
48. Oliet S. Single-visit endodontic therapy: a preliminary clinical study. J Am Dent Assoc 1981;103:873.
49. Galberry JH. Incidence of post-operative pain in one appointment and multi-appointment endodontic treatment: a pilot study [thesis]. Louisiana State University; 1983.
50. Nakamuta H, Nagasawa H. Study on endodontic treatment of infected root canals in one visit. Personal communication, 1983.
51. Mulhern JM, Patterson SS, Newton CW, Ringel AM. Incidence of postoperative pain after one appointment endodontic treatment of asymptomatic pulpal necrosis in single-rooted teeth. JOE 1982;8:370.
52. Roane JB, Dryden JA, Grimes EW. Incidence of post-operative pain after single- and multiple-visit endodontic procedures. Oral Surg 1983;55:68.
53. Genet J. Factors determining the incidence of post-operative pain in endodontic therapy. JOE 1986;12:126.
54. Fava L. A comparison of one versus two appointment endodontic therapy in teeth with non-vital pulps. Int Endodont J 1979;22:179.
55. Fava L. One appointment root canal treatment: incidence of post-operative pain using a modified double flared technique. Int Endodont J 1991;24:258.
56. Fava L. A clinical evaluation of one and two-appointment root canal therapy using calcium hydroxide. Int Endodont J 1994;27.
57. Trope M. Flare-up rate of single-visit endodontics. Int J Endodont 1991;24:24.
58. Harrison JW, Baumgartner JC, Svec TA. Incidence of pain associated with clinical factors during and after root canal therapy. Part I. Interappointment pain. JOE 1983;9:384.
59. Eleazer PD, Eleazer KR. Flare-up rate in pulpally necrotic molars in one-visit versus two-visit endodontic treatment. JOE 1998;24:614.
60. Ørstavik O, et al. Sensory and affective characteristics of pain following treatment of chronic apical periodontitis [abstract]. J Dent Res 1996;75:373.
61. Pekruhn R. The incidence in failure following single-visit endodontic therapy. JOE 1986;12:68.
62. Sjogren U, et al. Influence of infection at the time of root filling on the outcome of the endodontic treatment of teeth with apical periodontitis. Int Endodont J 1997;30:297.
63 Ørstavik D, et al. Effects of apical reaming and calcium hydroxide dressing on bacterial infection during treatment of apical periodontitis. Int Endodont J 1991;24:1.
64. Ingle JI, Zeldow BJ. An evaluation of mechanical instrumentation and the negative culture in endodontic therapy. J Am Dent Assoc 1958;57:471.
65. Zeldow BJ, Ingle JI. Correlation of the positive culture to the prognosis of endodontically treated teeth. J Am Dent Assoc 1963;66:23.
66. Trope M, Delano EO, Orstavik D. Endodontic treatment of teeth with apical periodontitis: single vs. multivisit treatment. JOE 1999;25:345.
67. Katebzadeh N, Hupp J, Trope M. Histological periapical repair after obturation of infected canals in dogs. JOE 1999;25:364.
68 Cohen S, Schwartz S. Endodontics and the law. Calif Dent Assoc J 1985;13:97.
69. Milgrom P, Ingle JI. Consent procedures as a quality control. J Oral Surg 1975;33:115.
70. Association reports. Code on dental procedures and nomenclature. J Am Dent Assoc 1989;118:369.
71. Quality assurance guidelines. Chicago: American Association of Endodontists; 1988.
72. Harman B. A roundtable on referrals. Dent Econ 1987;77:44.
73. Appropriateness of care and quality assurance guidelines. 3rd ed. Chicago: American Association of Endodontics; 1998.
74. Cohen S, Schwartz S. Endodontic complications and the law. JOE 1987;13:191.

75. Åkerblom A, Hasselgren G. The prognosis for endodontic treatment of obliterated root canals. JOE 1988;14:565.
76. Ørstavik D, et al. Paraesthesia following endodontic treatment: survey of the literature and report of a case. Int Endodont J 1983;16:167.
77. Rowe AHR. Damage to the inferior alveolar nerve during or following endodontic treatment. Br Dent J 1983;153:306.
78. Cohenca C, Rotstein I. Mental nerve paresthesia associated with a non vital tooth. Endod Dent Traumatol 1996;12:298.
79. Reeh ES. Messer HH. Long term paresthesia following inadvertent forcing sodium hypochlorite through perforation in incisor. Endod Dent Traumatol 1989;5:200.
80. Joffe E. Complications during root canal therapy following accidental extrusion of sodium hypochlorite through the apical foramen. Gen Dent 1991;39:460.
81. Dietz G. A roundtable on referrals. Dent Econ 1987;77:51.
82. Harman B. Op cit, p. 72.
83. Nash K. Endodontic referrals. Calif Dent Assoc J 1987;15:47.
84. Weichman JA. Malpractice prevention and defense. Calif Dent Assoc J 1975;3:58.
85. Selbst AG. Understanding informed consent and its relationship to the incidence of adverse treatment events in conventional endodontic therapy. JOE 1990;16:387.
86. Hourigan MJ. Oral surgery for the general practitioner. Palm Springs Seminars, Mar., 1989.
87. American Association of Endodontists. Informed consent. Communique 1986;3:4.
88. Bailey B. Informed consent in dentistry. J Am Dent Assoc 1985;110:709.
89. Curley A. Informed consent, past, present and future [bulletin]. Sacramento (CA): The Dentists Insurance Co.; 1989. p. 3.
90. Association Reports, Council on Insurance. Informed consent: a risk management view. J Am Dent Assoc 1987;115:630.
91. Paladino T, Linoff K, Zinman E. Informed consent and record keeping. AGD Impact 1986;14:1.
92. Howard W. A roundtable on referrals. Dent Econ 1987;77:50.

Chapter 2

HISTOLOGY AND PHYSIOLOGY OF THE DENTAL PULP

David H. Pashley, Richard E. Walton, and Harold C. Slavkin

As the principal source of pain within the mouth and as the major site of attention in endodontic treatment, the pulp warrants direct inspection. By its very location deep within the tooth, it defies visualization, other than its appearance as radiolucent lines on radiographs. Occasionally, when required to deal with an accidentally fractured cusp, the dentist is afforded a glimpse of the normal pulp. A pink, coherent soft tissue is noted, obviously dependent on its normal hard dentin shell for protection and hence, once exposed, extremely sensitive to contact and to temperature changes.

When pulp tissue is removed *en masse* from a tooth in the course of, say, vital pulpectomy, the dentist gains a new perspective of the pulp. Here is connective tissue obviously rich in fluid and highly vascular. After exposure to air, the appearance and volume of the tissue change as the fluid evaporates. Another dimension of the physical characteristics of pulp tissue can be demonstrated by grasping a freshly extirpated vital pulp between thumb and forefinger in both hands and attempting to pull the pulp apart. Surprisingly, this tiny strand has much the feel of dental floss: it is tough, fibrous, and inelastic. This is a reflection of an important structural component of the pulp, namely collagen.

FUNCTION

The pulp lives for the dentin and the dentin lives by the grace of the pulp. Few marriages in nature are marked by a greater interrelationship. Thus it is with the pulp and the four functions that it serves: namely, the formation and the nutrition of dentin and the innervation and defense of the tooth.[1]

Formation of the dentin is the primary task of the pulp in both sequence and importance. From the mesodermal aggregation known as the dental papilla arises the specialized cell layer of odontoblasts adjacent and internal to the inner layer of the ectodermal enamel organ. Ectoderm interacts with mesoderm, and the odontoblasts initiate the process of dentin formation.[2] Once under way, dentin production continues rapidly until the main form of the tooth crown and root is created. Then the process slows, eventually to a complete halt.

Nutrition of the dentin is a function of the odontoblast cells and the underlying blood vessels. Nutrients exchange across the capillaries into the pulp interstitial fluid, which, in turn, travels into the dentin through the network of tubules created by the odontoblasts to contain their processes.

Innervation of the pulp and dentin is linked by the fluid and by its movement between the dentinal tubules and peripheral receptors, and thus to the sensory nerves of the pulp proper.[3]

Defense of the tooth and the pulp itself has been speculated to occur by the creation of new dentin in the face of irritants. The pulp may provide this defense by intent or by accident; the fact is that formation of layers of dentin may indeed decrease ingress of irritants or may prevent or delay carious penetration. The pulp galvanizes odontoblasts into action or produces new odontoblasts to form needed hard tissue.

The defense of the pulp has several characteristics. First, dentin formation is localized. Dentin is produced at a rate faster than that seen at sites of nonstimulated primary or secondary dentin formation. Microscopically, this dentin is often different from secondary dentin and has earned several designations: irritation dentin, reparative dentin, irregular secondary dentin, osteodentin, and tertiary dentin.

The type and amount of dentin created during the defensive response appear to depend on numerous factors. How damaging is the assault? Is it chemical, ther-

---

*Supported, in part, by grant DE 06427 from the National Institute of Dental and Craniofacial Research.

mal, or bacterial? How long has the irritant been applied? How deep was the lesion? How much surface area was involved? What is the status of the pulp at the time of response? A second defensive reaction, inflammation within the pulp at the site of injury, should not be ignored. This phenomenon will be explored in more detail in chapter 4.

INDUCTION AND DEVELOPMENT OF DENTIN AND CEMENTUM

Human tooth development spans an extremely long period of time, starting with the induction of the primary dentition during the second month of embryogenesis until completion of the permanent dentition toward the end of adolescence. The primary dentition is induced during the fifth week of gestation, and biomineralization begins during the fourteenth week of gestation. In tandem, the first permanent teeth have reached the bud stage, and they begin biomineralization just prior to birth. The **first primary teeth** begin to erupt in children at 6 months of age, and the **first permanent teeth** erupt at 5 to 6 years of age. The third molars are the last teeth to be formed, and their crown development is completed between 12 and 16 years of age. Therefore, the induction and development of the human dentition persists during embryonic, fetal, neonatal, and postnatal childhood stages of development. Detailed descriptions of the histology and timing of human tooth development can be readily found in a number of excellent textbooks.[4]

Inductive tissue interactions, specifically epithelium-mesenchyme interactions, have been extensively investigated and characterized throughout the various stages of tooth crown and root morphogenesis.[5–8] The developing tooth system has become a well-characterized model for defining the molecular mechanisms required for reciprocal signaling during epithelium-mesenchyme interactions in crown and root morphogenesis and cytodifferentiation.[9–13]

It is now evident that the initial inductive signals for tooth formation are synthesized and secreted from specific sites defined as odontogenic placodes within the oral ectoderm that cover the maxillary and mandibular processes.[13] The oral ectodermally derived inductive signals are received by multiple cognate receptors located on the cell surfaces of a specific subpopulation of cranial neural crest–derived ectomesenchymal cells during the initial induction process and the subsequent dental lamina, bud, and stages of tooth development[8–13] (Figure 2-1).

During the transition from bud to cap stages, the ectomesenchyme provides several cell lineages, including one that becomes dental papilla mesenchyme and others that become progenitor cells for the subsequent development of the periodontium.[8,14,15] At this time, multiple and reciprocal signals are secreted by the dental papilla mesenchyme, and these signals bind to the extracellular matrix and transmembrane cell receptors along the adjacent enamel organ epithelium. A discrete structure within the enamel organ, termed the "enamel knot," synthesizes and secretes a number of additional signals that also participate in the determination for the patterns of morphogenesis within the maxillary and mandibular dentitions: incisiform, caninform, and molariform.[12,13]

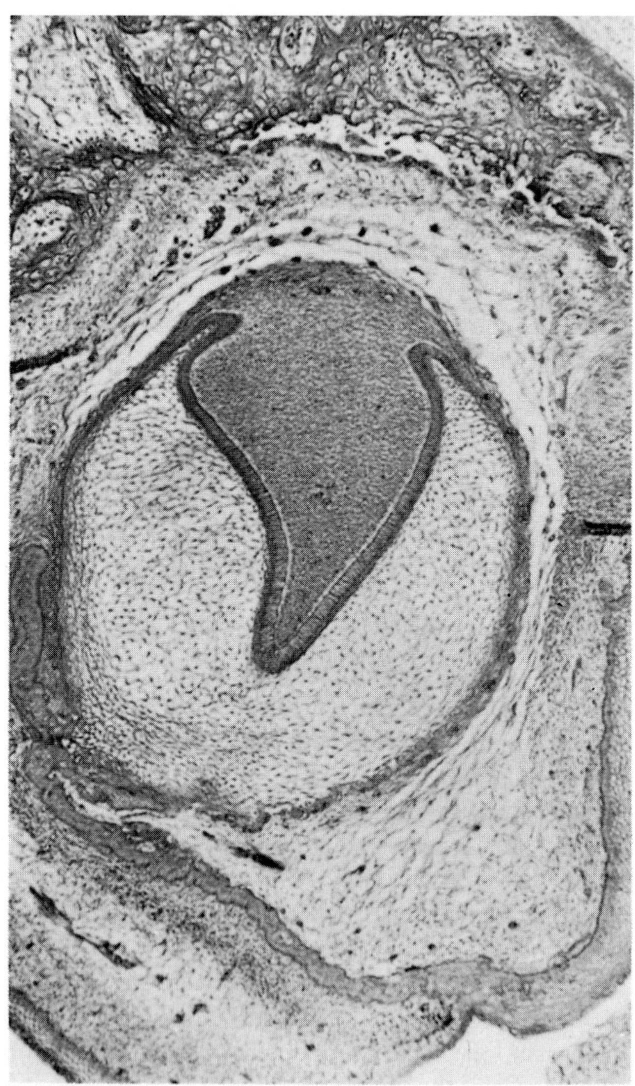

Figure 2-1 Early dental pulp, or dental papilla, exhibiting a cellular mass at the center of this tooth bud in the early bell stage. Nerve fiber bundles are evident in cross-section as dark bodies apical to dental papilla yet are absent in the papilla itself. Human fetus, 19 weeks. Palmgren nerve stain. Reproduced with permission from Arwil T, Häggströms I. Innervation of the teeth. Transactions Royal School of Dentistry (Stockholm), 3:1958.

The human genome was basically completed by the year 2000[16]; essentially all of the 100,000 regulatory and structural genes within the human lexicon have been identified, sequenced, and mapped to specific chromosomal locations. Further, combinations of genes encoded within the human genomic deoxyribonucleic acid (DNA) are now known to be expressed during development that controls morphogenesis. A number of these genes have been identified and characterized as being expressed in the odontogenic placode, dental lamina, and the bud, cap, bell, and crown stages of tooth development in either the epithelial or mesenchymal cells or both. Significantly, these genes are expressed in various combinations during induction processes associated with many developing epidermal organ systems including the salivary gland, sebaceous glands, mammary glands, tooth, hair, and skin morphogenesis.[5]

The specificity of induction reflects the particular combinations of signaling molecules, their cognate cell surface receptors, various intracellular signal pathways, and a large number of transcriptional factors that regulate gene expression. These combinations further are modified according to temporal and spatial information during development; the combination used to induce the dental lamina is different than that required for cap stage development and subsequent odontoblast cytodifferentiation. The hierarchy of these molecular mechanisms associated with the initiation and subsequent early stages of tooth development is shown in Figure 2-2.

Specific mutations or alternations in one or more of these molecules result in clinical phenotypes including cleft lip and/or palate and a range of dental abnormalities with enamel, dentin, cementum, periodontal ligament, or alveolar bone disorders; for example, hypodontia or missing teeth as seen in X-linked anhydrotic ectodermal dysplasia, which is caused by a mutation in the gene *EDA*; familial tooth agenesis, which is caused by a mutation in the gene *MSX1*; and X-linked amelogenesis imperfecta, which is caused by a mutation in the gene amelogenin.[17,18] Recently, a mutation in the gene *CBF-alpha1*, a transcription factor, was found to cause cleidocranial dysplasia with hyperdontia.[19]

The development of dentin is intriguing for several reasons. First, signals within the inner enamel epithelia of the enamel organ induce adjacent cranial neural crest–derived ectomesenchymal cells to become progenitor odontoblasts. Mutations in either the signaling molecules, cognate receptors, intracellular signal pathways, transcription factors, or extracellular matrix molecules can result in severe dental anomalies including

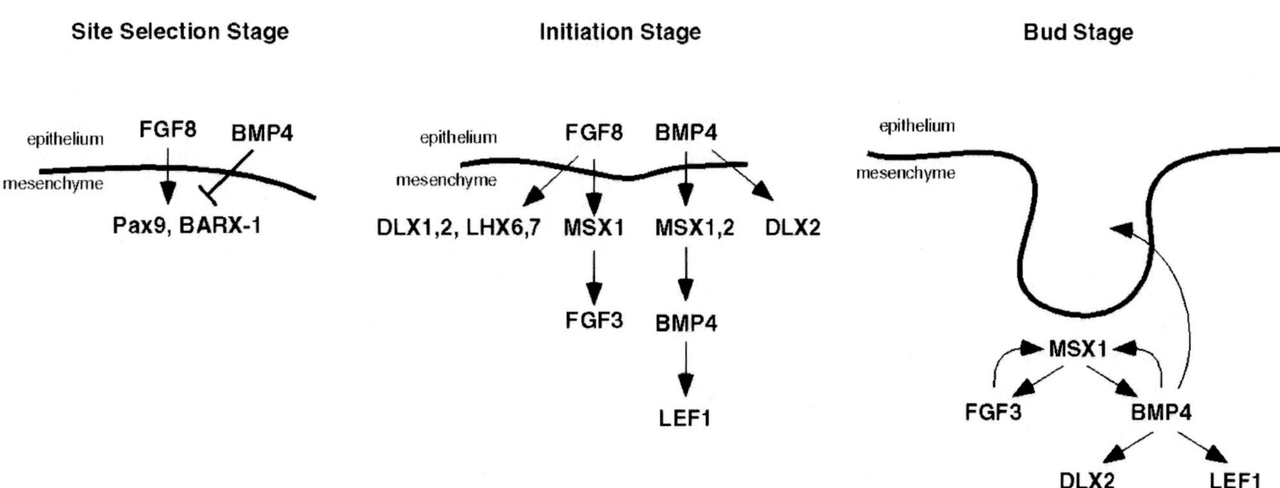

Figure 2-2 Molecular controls for the initiation and early stages of tooth morphogenesis. The initiation or site selection for tooth development is controlled by oral ectoderm-derived epithelial fibroblast growth factor (**FGF**) and bone morphogenetic protein (**BMP**) through their signaling pathways. The actions of these signaling pathways or circuits are dependent on the stage and position of development and the combination of transcription factors that are either induced (→) or repressed (_). This establishes the odontogenic placode. Thereafter, epithelium regulates the adjacent mesenchyme during the bud stage and the mesenchyme then promotes differentiation and influences the adjacent inner enamel epithelium through feedback loops in the cap, bell, and crown stages of tooth development. The reader is encouraged to see the following references for detailed analyses of these morphoregulatory molecules.[2,7–10,14,16]

tooth *agenesis*, *hypodontia*, and *oligodontia* and defects in dentin deposition or biomineralization, termed *dentinogenesis imperfecta.* Several dentin extracellular matrix proteins—dentin sialoprotein, dentin matrix protein, and dentin phosphoprotein—are produced by alternative splicing from one single gene product. Mutations in any one of these encoded sequences, or in type I collagen, result in *dentinogenesis imperfecta.* Mutations that are limited to type I collagen produce *osteogenesis imperfecta* with a form of *dentinogenesis imperfecta.*

Following crown morphogenesis, cells from the cervical loop give rise to Hertwig's epithelial root sheath (HERS) cells, which, in turn, induce adjacent dental papilla mesenchymal cells to engage in root formation.[6–8] Progressive cell proliferation and migrations eventually outline the shape and size of the forming roots. In this developmental process, two interpretations are currently being considered. First, evidence is available to support the hypothesis that HERS cells transdifferentiate into cementoblasts and secrete acellular cementum matrix.[8] Second, evidence is also available to support the hypothesis that peripheral ectomesenchymal cells penetrate through the HERS and become cementoblasts and secrete acellular cementum.[6,7] Of course, both processes may take place at different times and positions of cementogenesis.

The understanding of the induction and development of cementum has also progressed in recent years. Hertwig's epithelial root sheath cells provide signals that induce the differentiation of odontoblasts and the formation of the first peripheral layer of dentin. It has been known for almost 100 years that a small percentage of the human population expresses enamel pearls along the root surfaces of permanent teeth. These enamel-like aberrations in cementogenesis are intriguing and could offer new insights and strategies to regenerate acellular cementum.

Recent advances have indicated that molecules presumed to be uniquely restricted to inner enamel epithelium and ameloblasts associated with enamel formation are also expressed in HERS.[6–8] Specifically, ameloblastin has recently been identified in both ameloblasts and HERS.[20] This association between enamel and cementum has been previously discussed with respect to coronal cementum.[21] These and other studies have suggested that enamel matrix contains molecular constitutents, presumably with growth factor bioactivities, that can induce acellular regeneration when active on denuded human dentin root surfaces. Recently, an enamel matrix preparation has been demonstrated to induce acellular cementum regeneration on root surfaces associated with advanced periodontitis.[22] The available evidence strongly supports the hypothesis that enamel organ epithelium-derived cell phenotypes control coronal enamel deposition and the initiation of acellular cementum formation.[23,24]

ANATOMY

The living pulp, as we have seen, creates and shapes its own locale in the center of the tooth. The pulp, under normal conditions, tends to form dentin evenly, faciolingually and mesiodistally.[25] The pulp therefore tends to lie in the center of the tooth and shapes itself to a miniaturization of the tooth. This residence of the pulp is called the pulp cavity, and one speaks of its two main parts as the **pulp chamber** and the **root canal.** The clinical implications of pulp form and variation are extensively covered in chapter 10. Indeed, the key word in understanding the gross anatomy of the pulp is "variation." Equally evident in any study of the pulp is the reduction in size of the chamber and canals with age. Such reduction in size thus becomes a new variation.

In addition to changes in pulp size and shape with aging, external stimuli also exert an effect. Caries, attrition, abrasion, erosion, impact trauma, and clinical procedures are some of the major irritants that may cause formation of irritation dentin. The clinician must appreciate the resultant alterations in internal anatomy that accompany disease and damage of the pulp and dentin.

Pulp Chamber

At the time of eruption, the pulp chamber of a tooth reflects the external form of the enamel.[1] Anatomy is less sharply defined, but the cusp form is present. Often the pulp suggests its original perimeter (and threatens its future) by leaving a filament of itself, the pulp horn, within the coronal dentin. A specific stimulus such as caries leads to the formation of irritation dentin on the roof or wall of the chamber adjacent to the stimulus. Of course, with time, the chamber undergoes steady reduction in size as secondary, and irritation dentin is produced on all surfaces (Figure 2-3).

Root Canal

An unbroken train of connective tissue passes from the periodontal ligament through the apical root canal(s) to the pulp chamber. Each root is served by at least one such pulp corridor. Actually, the root canal is subject to the same pulp-induced changes as the chamber. Its diameter becomes narrowed, rapidly at first as the foramen takes shape in the posteruptive months but with increasing slowness once the apex is defined. The canal diameter tends to decrease slightly with age; irritants such as periodontal disease may cause further constriction.

According to Orban, the shape of the canal, "to a large degree, conforms to the shape of the root. A few canals are round and tapering, but many are elliptical, broad and thin."[26] A curve at the end of the root means almost invariably that the canal follows this curve. Meyer stated that "roots that are round and cone-shaped usually contain only one canal, but roots that are elliptical and have flat or concave surfaces more frequently have more canals than one"[27] (Figure 2-4).

The foramen can change in shape and location because of functional influences on the tooth[28] (eg, tongue pressure, occlusal pressure, mesial drift). The pattern that develops is the reverse of the changes in the alveolar bone around the tooth. Cementum resorption occurs on the wall of the foramen farthest from the force and apposition on the wall nearest. The net result is a deviation of the foramen away from the true apex (Figure 2-5).

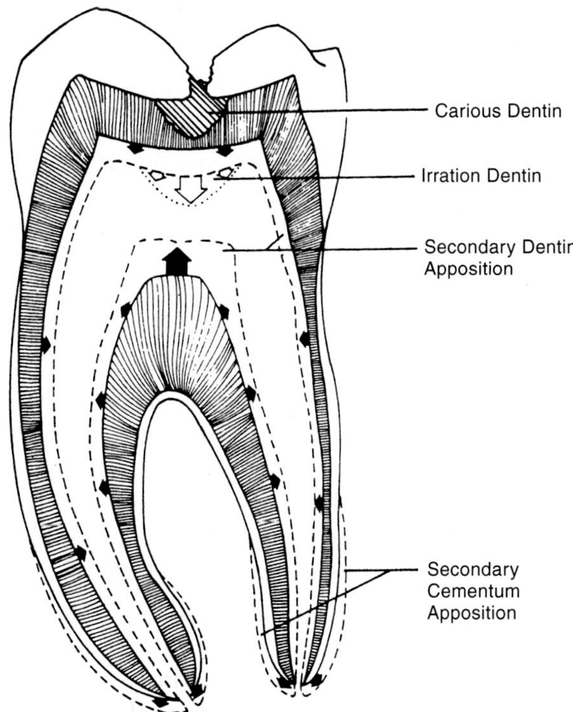

Figure 2-3 Schematic diagram of a mandibular molar showing hard tissue apposition with time and/or irritation. **Black arrows** indicate physiologic secondary cementum and dentin apposition; **white arrows** indicate formation of dentin in response to irritants. Pulp space undergoes continual reduction in size and volume. Note that the floor of the chamber is a region of maximum secondary dentin formation.

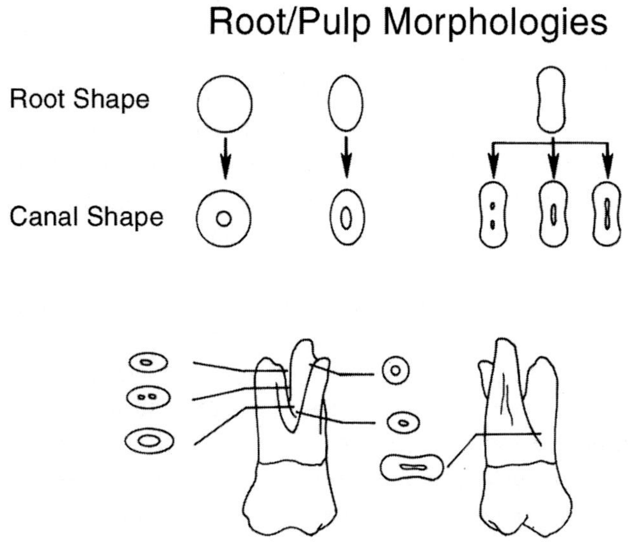

Root/Pulp Morphologies

Root Shape

Canal Shape

Figure 2-4 Canal size and shape are a reflection of the external root surface. The upper diagrams show the possible canal configurations within each shaped root. The maxillary molar root sections illustrate that all sizes and shapes of canals may be seen in a single tooth.

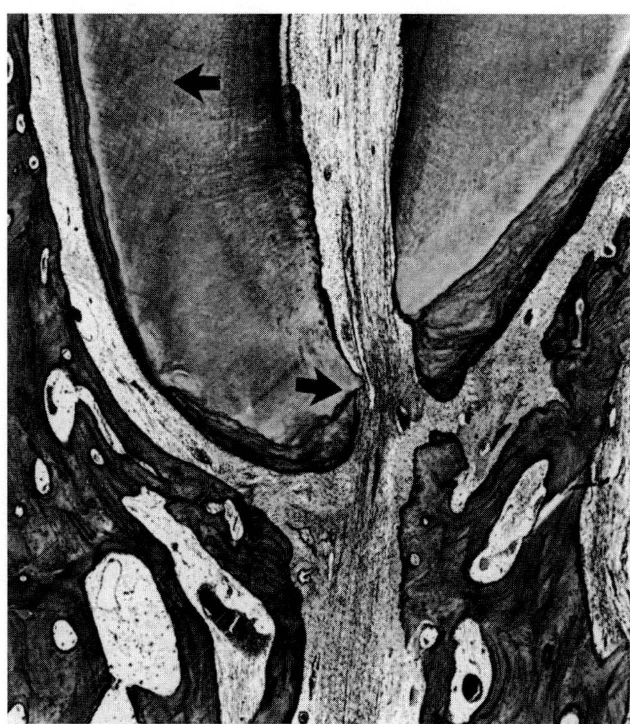

Figure 2-5 Features often noted in normal yet aging tooth: deviation of apical foramen as a result of mesial migration of the tooth (**top arrow**). Selective resorption and apposition of cementum have changed the position of the apex, causing narrowing of the apical third of the root canal by increments of secondary dentin and flaring of apical foramen from its smallest diameter at the dentinocemental junction (**bottom arrow**) to its greatest diameter at the cemental surface. Note the abundance of collagen fibers in the radicular pulp. Reproduced with permission from Matsumiya S. Atlas of oral pathology. Tokyo Dental College Press; 1955.

Foramina

The anatomy of the root apex is partially determined by the number and location of apical blood vessels present at the time of formation of the apex. When the tooth is young and just erupting, the foramen is open. Islands of dentin may appear within the mainstream of connective tissue when the root sheath has induced them, but these islands are widely separated. Progressively, the main channel narrows. The primary vessels and nerves, though never directly threatened with strangulation, have a restricted passage. Increments of cementum apposition contribute to this continuous modeling. The possibilities of vascular branching are so varied at the apex that prediction of the number of foramina in a given tooth becomes impossible (Figure 2-6).

It is known that the incidence of multiple foramina is high.[29,30] The majority of single-rooted teeth have a single canal that terminates in a single foramen. Less often, they possess an apical delta, which terminates in a major channel and one or more collateral exits. Occasionally, the delta has several channels of equal magnitude. Root canals of the multirooted teeth, on the other hand, tend to have a more complex apical anatomy. Multiple foramina are the rule rather than the exception. When accessory foramina are found in one root of a multirooted tooth, the other roots usually have a similar condition.[29] Moreover, because the individual roots of such teeth often contain two or even three canals, a new factor is introduced. These canals can merge, but they need not and often do not merge before making their exit. Indeed, **each may leave the root independently.** Branching of the emergent canals within the apical area is a common finding because the preexisting vessels are linked.[30]

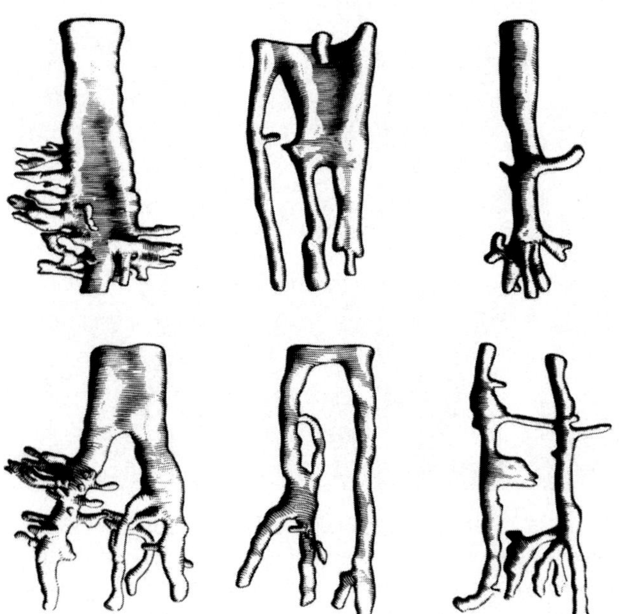

Figure 2-6 Diverse ramifications of apical pulp space anatomy. These models were made by drawing pulps from serial histologic sections and "stacking" the drawings. Many regions are obviously inaccessible to conventional débridement methods. Adapted with permission from Meyer W. Dtsch Zahnaerztl Z 1970;25:1064.

It is also important to recall that cementum forms in abundance at the root apex. Because of the apposition of new layers of cementum, in response to eruption, the foramen anatomy is by no means constant. As stated above, the center of the foramen tends to deviate increasingly from the apical center.[31] Also, many root canals have two apical diameters. The minor diameter at the level of the dentinocemental junction can be as small as one half that of the major diameter at the external surface of the root. Cementum deposition tends to produce an apical funnel of increasing divergence. Contributing to this is secondary dentin formation that narrows the dentinal orifices of the canal (see Figure 2-5).

Stereomicroscopic analysis of some 700 posterior root apices showed that at least half of the major foramina take eccentric positions that deviate as far as 2 mm from the apex.[29]Accessory foramina, on average, were found to be located twice the distance of the major foramina from the vertex (Figure 2-7).[29]

Accessory Canals

Communication of pulp and periodontal ligament is not limited to the apical region. Accessory canals are found at every level. Vascular perfusion studies have demonstrated vividly how numerous and persistent these tributaries are.[32] Many, in time, become sealed off by cementum and/or dentin; however, many remain viable. The majority appear to be encountered in the apical half of the root. These generally pass directly from the root canal to the periodontal ligament (Figure 2-8).

A common area in which accessory canals appear is the furcation area of molar teeth (Figure 2-9). Burch and Hulen[33] and Vertucci and Anthony[34] found that molars frequently presented openings in the furcation areas. However, the studies did not determine how many of these represented patent (continuous) accessory canals all the way from the pulp to the periodontal ligament. Morphologic and scanning electron microscopic studies consistently show the presence of patent accessory canals or depressions that were assumed to be the openings to such canals.[34–37] In other studies, dyes were injected or drawn by vacuum into the furcation of molars. Approximately one half of

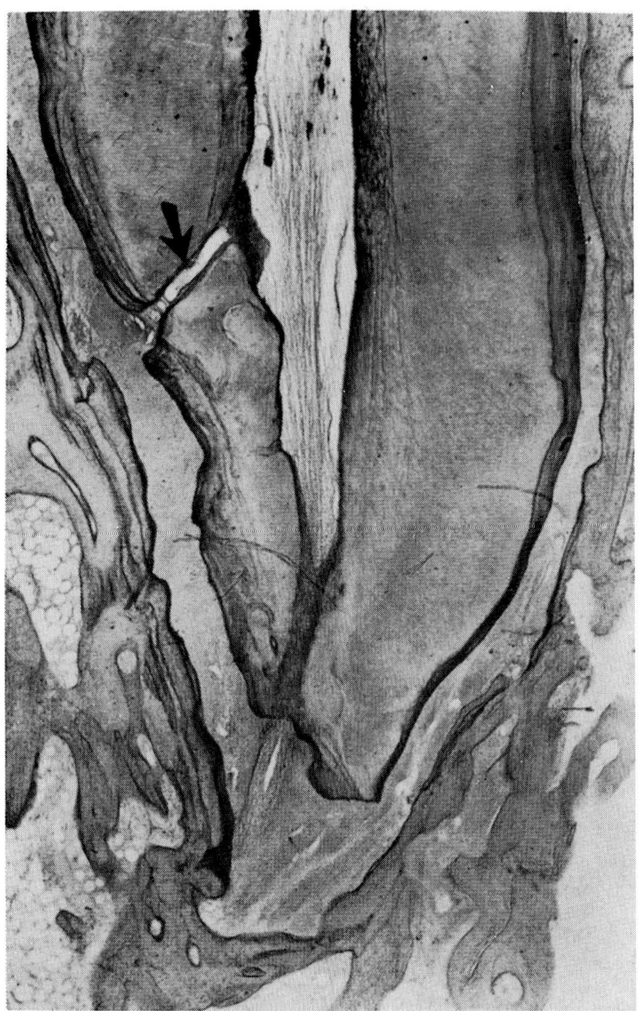

Figure 2-7 Accessory foramen (**arrow**) in mandibular anterior tooth. Accessory foramina are usually located within the apical 2 to 3 mm of root. (Orban collection.) Reproduced with permission from Sicher H. Oral histology and embryology. 5th ed. St. Louis: CV Mosby; 1962.

the teeth studied demonstrate patent accessory canals from pulp space to furcation.[38]

HISTOLOGY

Regions

Classically, the pulp is described as having two defined regions, central and peripheral.[39] Typically, however, studying sections of pulp under the microscope reveals that the classic description is not consistent; levels of activity dictate regional morphology. However, it is helpful to know the textbook description before studying the variations.

The pulp is in intimate contact with the dentin and survives only through the protection of its hard outer covering. As the price of this protection, the pulp contributes to a close symbiosis. The way in which the normal pulp relates to its immediate environment can be best explained by a review of its own morphology and that of the tissues with which it is confluent, namely, the dentin and the periodontal ligament. In general, the pulp demonstrates a homogeneity in its blend of cells, intercellular substance, fiber elements, vessels, and nerves.

Peripheral Pulp Zone. On the periphery of the pulp, adjacent to the calcified dentin, structural layers are apparent. These are usually evident in a medium-power photomicrograph (Figure 2-10). Next to the predentin lies the palisade of columnar odontoblast cells. Central to the odontoblasts is the subodontoblastic layer, termed the **cell-free zone of Weil.**[40]

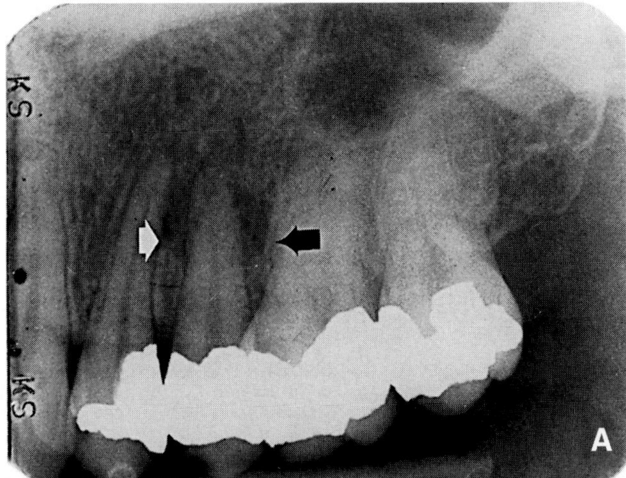

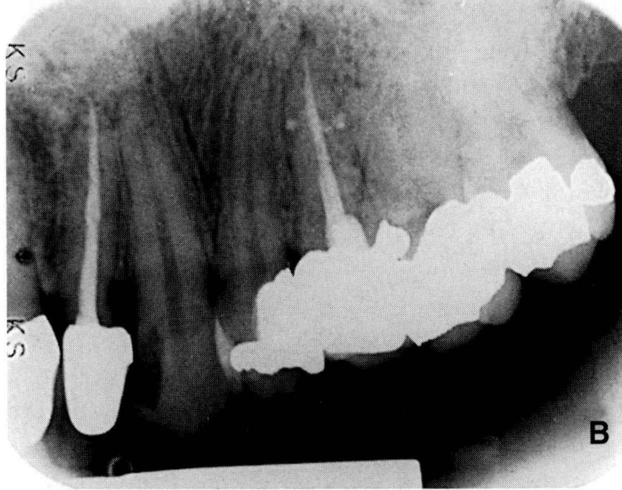

Figure 2-8 **A**, Necrotic pulp in maxillary second premolar in which irritants egress through lateral canals to the periodontium, creating inflammatory lesions (**arrows**). Although often invisible on pretreatment radiographs, the presence of lateral canals may be confirmed following obturation. **B**, Bony lesions healed several months following root canal treatment. Accessory canals are important, not so much for the irritants they contain but because of their communication to the PDL. (Courtesy of Dr. Manuel I. Weisman.)

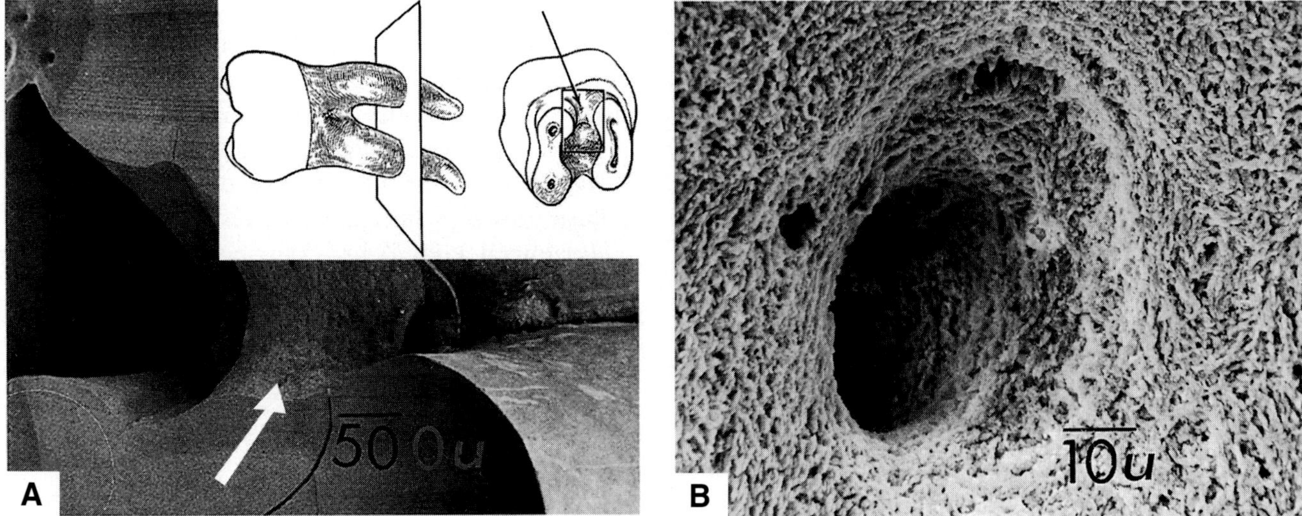

Figure 2-9 Inset demonstrates method of sectioning molars for viewing furcations. **A**, Foramina of accessory canal indicated by **arrow** (×20 original magnification). **B**, Foramen seen in **A**, magnified ×1,000. Canal is about 35 microns across, flaring to 60 microns at surface. Note two peripheral foramina on the rim. Reproduced with permission from Koenigs JG, Brilliant JD, Foreman DW. Oral Surg 1974;38:773.

Plexuses of capillaries and small nerve fibers ramify in this subodontoblastic layer. Deep to the odontoblastic layer is the **cell-rich zone**, which blends in turn with the dominant stroma of the pulp. The **cell-rich zone** contains fibroblasts and undifferentiated cells, which sustain the population of odontoblasts by proliferation and differentiation.[41]

These zones vary in their prominence from tooth to tooth and from area to area in the pulp of the same tooth. The cell-free and cell-rich zones are usually indistinct or absent in the embryonic pulp and usually appear when dentin formation is active. The zones tend to become increasingly prominent as the pulp ages. Both of these zones are less constant and less prominent near the root apex.

Central Pulp Zone. The main body of the pulp occupies the area circumscribed by cell-rich zones. It contains the principal support system for the peripheral pulp, which includes the large vessels and nerves (Figure 2-11) from which branches extend to supply the critical outer pulp layers. The principal cells are fibroblasts; the principal extracellular components are ground substance and collagen. The environment of the pulp is unique in that it is surrounded by an unyielding tissue and fed and drained by vessels that pass in and out at a distant site. However, it is classified as an areolar, fibrous connective tissue, containing cellular and extracellular elements that are found in other similar tissues. These elements will be discussed in more detail.

Structural Elements, Cellular

Reserve Cells. The pulp contains a pool of reserve cells, descendants of undifferentiated cells in the primitive dental papilla. These multipotential cells are likely a fibroblast type that retains the capability of dedifferentiating and then redifferentiating on demand into many of the mature cell types. Beneath the odontoblasts, in the cell-rich zone, are concentrations of such cells. However, Frank demonstrated by radioautography that these cells produce little collagen, which is circumstantial evidence that they are not mature fibroblasts.[42]

Baume has reviewed ultrastructural studies that suggest cytoplasmic connections between the odontoblasts and these subjacent mesenchymal cells.[43] Through such connections, on odontoblast injury or death, signals may be provided to these less differentiated cells that may cause them to divide and differentiate into odontoblasts or odontoblast-like cells, as required.[43]

Also important are the reserve cells scattered throughout the pulp, usually in juxtaposition to blood vessels. These retain the capacity, on stimulation, to divide and differentiate into other mature cell types. For example, mast cells and odontoclasts (tooth resorbers) arise in the presence of inflammation.

Significant are the unique cells that differentiate to form the calcified tissue that develops under a pulp cap or pulpotomy when calcium hydroxide is placed in direct contact with the pulp. These unique cells are also frequently observed along the calcified tissue forming at the base of tubules involved with caries, restorations, attrition, or abrasion. This calcified tissue is not a true

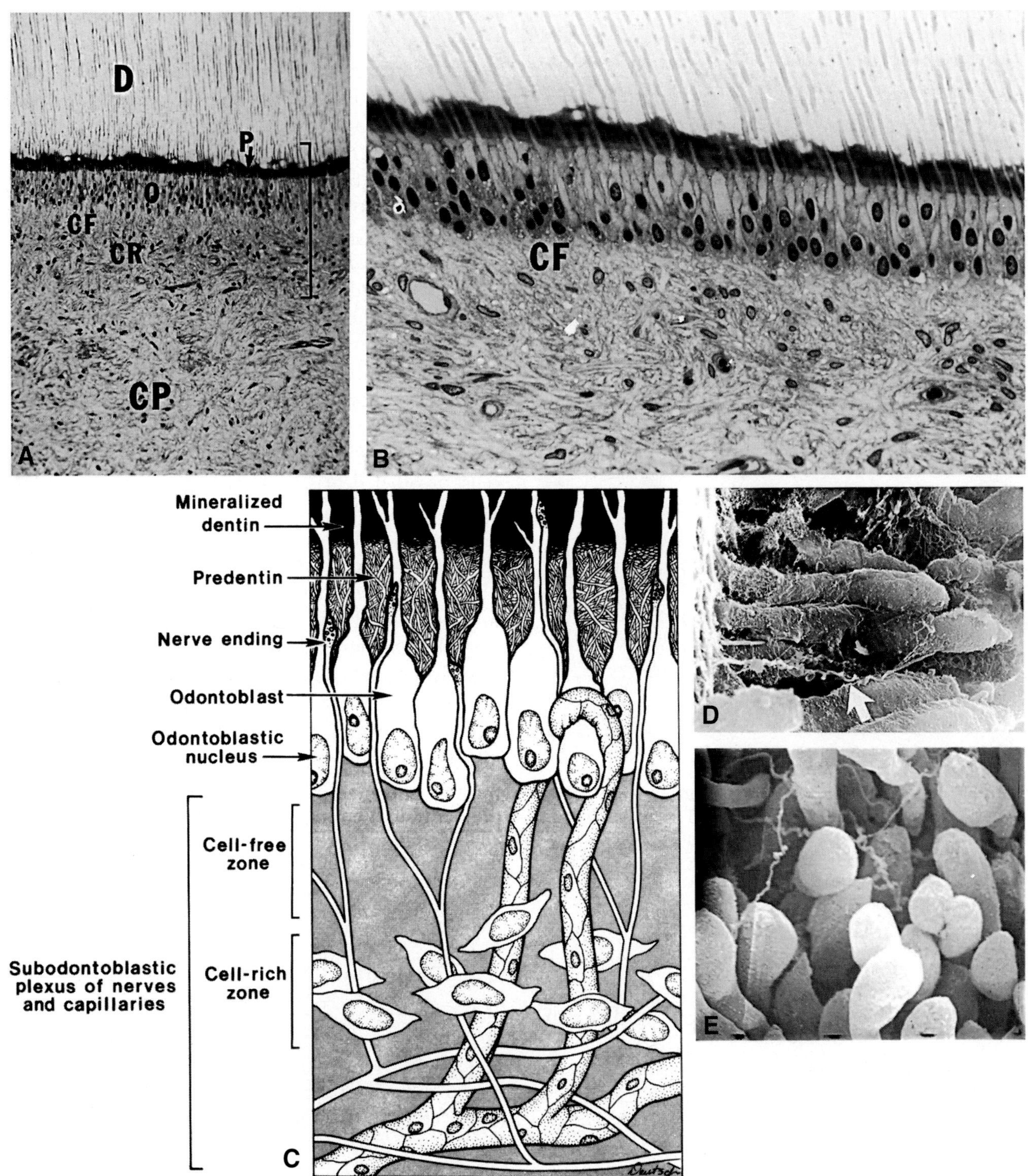

Figure 2-10 A, Medium-power photomicrograph from human pulp specimen showing dentin (D), predentin (P), odontoblast layer (O), cell-free zone (CF), cell-rich zone (CR), and central pulp (CP). **B**, Region similar to area bracketed in **A**. Cell-free zone contains large numbers of small nerves and capillaries not visible at this magnification. Underlying CR does not have high concentration of cells but contains more cells than does central pulp. (**A** and **B** courtesy of Drs. Dennis Weber and Michael Gaynor.) **C**, Diagram of peripheral pulp and its principal elements. **D**, Scanning electron micrograph of dentin-pulp junction. Note corkscrew fibers between odontoblasts (**arrow**). Reproduced with permission from Jean A, Kerebel JB, Kerebel LM. Oral Surg 1986;61:592. **E**, Scanning electron micrograph of pulpal surface of odontoblast layer. Thread-like structures are probably terminal raveling of nerves. (Courtesy of Drs. R. White and M. Goldman.)

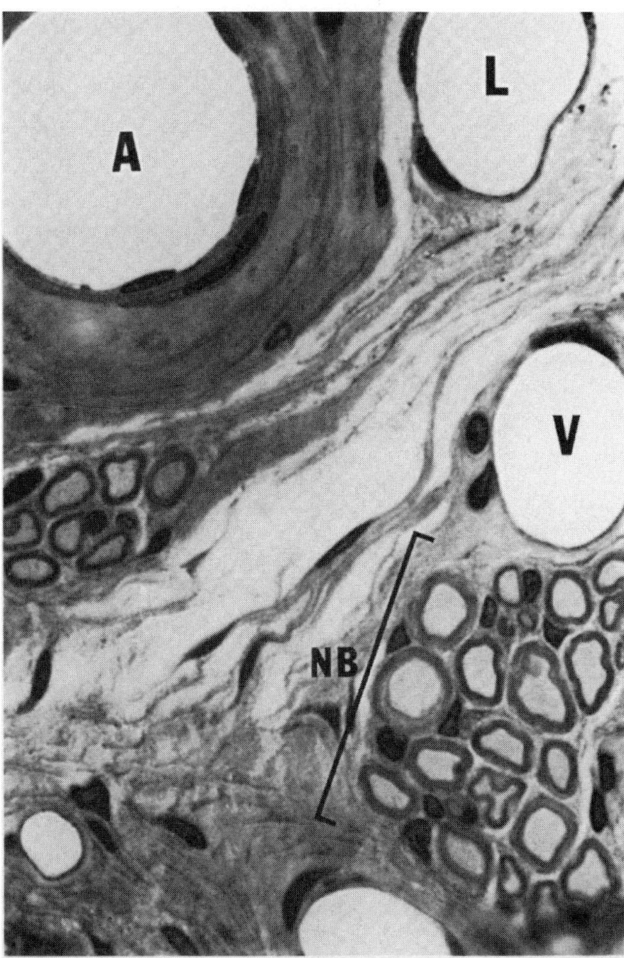

Figure 2-11 Cross-section from the central pulp showing major support systems, including arterioles (A) with a muscular wall, thin-walled lymphatics (L), venules (V), and nerve bundles (NB) containing myelinated and unmyelinated nerves. Reproduced with permission from Walton R, Leonard L, Sharawy M, Gangarosa L. Oral Surg 1979;48:545.

dentin, just as the cells that produce it are not true odontoblasts. However, like the odontoblast, these cells trace their origins to undifferentiated cells.

Fibroblasts. Most of the cells of the pulp are fibroblasts. These cells exhibit wide variation in their degree of differentiation.[44] Baume refers to them as mesenchymal cells, pulpoblasts, or pulpocytes in their progressive levels of maturation.[43] These distinctions are made, in part, because of the ability of these cells to form calcified tissues, something regular connective tissue fibroblasts apparently cannot accomplish.

Pulpal fibroblasts are spindle-shaped cells with ovoid nuclei (Figure 2-12). They synthesize and secrete the bulk of the extracellular components, that is, collagen and ground substance. The classic autoradiographic studies of Weinstock and Leblond, using ^{3}H-proline, demonstrated the process of collagen synthesis and secretion by the fibroblast.[45]

Not only are fibroblasts the principal producers of collagen, they also eliminate excess collagen or participate in collagen turnover in the pulp by resorption of collagen fibers. This has been demonstrated to occur intracellularly by the action of lysosomal enzymes, which literally digest the collagen components.[46]

Defense Cells.

Histiocytes and Macrophages. Undifferentiated mesenchymal cells (see Figure 2-12) around blood vessels (pericytes) can differentiate into fixed or wandering histiocytes under appropriate stimulation.[47] Wandering histiocytes (macrophages) may also arise from monocytes that have migrated from vessels. These cells are highly phagocytic and can remove bacteria, foreign bodies (endodontic paste, zinc oxide, etc), dead cells, or other debris.[48] Pulpal macrophages and dendritic cells thought to function like Langerhans' cells have been identified in normal rat pulp.[49] These cells seem to be associated with pulpal immunosurveillance.

Polymorphonuclear Leukocytes. The most common form of leukocyte in pulpal inflammation is the neutrophil, although eosinophils and basophils are occasionally detected. It is important to know that although neutrophils are not normally present in intact healthy pulps, with injury and cell death they rapidly migrate into the areas from nearby capillaries and venules.[50] They are the major cell type in microabscess formation and are very effective at destroying and phagocytizing bacteria or dead cells. Unfortunately, their participation often injures adjacent cells and may contribute to the development of wider zones of inflammation.

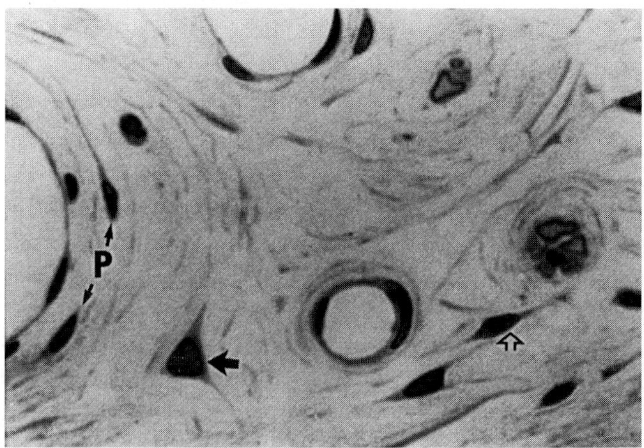

Figure 2-12 Pulpal fibroblasts showing spindle-shaped cytoplasm. Plump nuclei (**dark arrow**) usually indicate active collagen formation. Condensed nucleus is in a "quiet" cell, often termed a fibrocyte (**open arrow**). Pericytes (P) lie in close apposition to vessels and differentiate into other typical pulp cell types on demand.

Lymphocytes and Plasma Cells. These inflammatory cell types generally appear following invasion into the area of injury by neutrophils. These cells are not normally present in healthy pulp tissue but are associated with injury and resultant immune responses—attempts to destroy, damage, or neutralize foreign substance(s). Their presence would therefore indicate the presence of a persistent irritant.

Mast Cells. Interestingly, mast cells are seldom in large numbers in normal, healthy pulps[51] but are commonly found in inflamed pulps.[52,53] The granules of these cells contain histamine, a potent inflammatory mediator, and heparin. These cells release these granules or degranulate into the surrounding tissue fluid during inflammation.[52]

Since these cells are generally found near blood vessels, degranulation of mast cells releases histamine close to vascular smooth muscle, causing vasodilation. This increases vessel permeability, allowing fluids and leukocytes to escape.

Odontoblasts. The principal cell of the dentin-forming layer, the odontoblast, is the first cell type encountered as the pulp is approached from the dentin (Figure 2-13). These cells arise from peripheral mesenchymal cells of the dental papilla during tooth development (see Structural Elements) and differentiate by acquiring the characteristic morphology of glycoprotein synthesis and secretion[54] (Figure 2-14). Glycoprotein forms the predentin matrix, which is rendered mineralizable by the odontoblast, a unique cell producing a unique tissue, dentin. Synthesizing and secretory activities render the odontoblast highly polarized, with synthesis occurring in the cell body and secretion from the odontoblastic process.

The cell body contains organelles that represent different stages of secretion of collagen, glycoproteins, and calcium salts.[55] Matrix secretion precedes mineralization with these two events separated in time and space by the predentin. As happens in bone, the initial mineral seeding of predentin at the dentinoenamel junction is by formation of "matrix vesicles."[56,57] Classic studies by Weinstock and colleagues,[45,58,59] using an autoradiographic technique, have demonstrated the functional sequence of matrix production and secretion. This material has recently been reviewed by Holland.[60]

In histologic sections viewed under a light microscope, odontoblasts appear to vary from tall, pseudostratified columnar cells in the coronal pulp (see Figure 2-10) to a single row of cuboidal cells in radicular pulp to a flattened, almost squamous shape near the apex.[61,62] These squamous cells often form an irregular, atubular dentin.

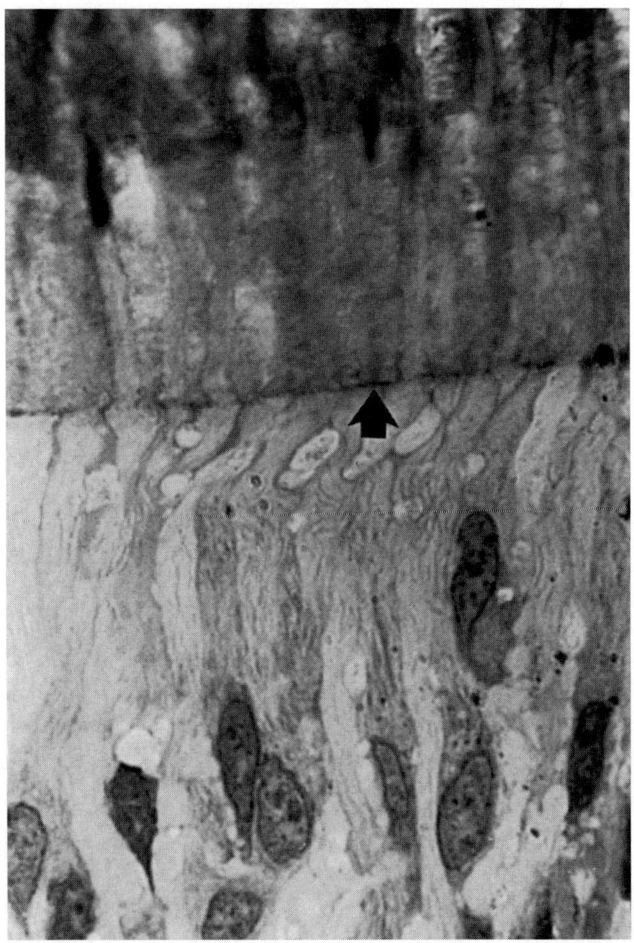

Figure 2-13 Pseudostratified appearance of odontoblasts. Dark horizontal line (**arrow**) delineates cell body from the odontoblastic processes and predentin and was once termed "pulpodentinal membrane." Ultrastructural examination has shown this to be a terminal cell web that forms a support and attachment area between adjoining cells. Reproduced with permission from Walton R, Leonard L, Sharawy M, Gangarosa L. Oral Surg 1979;48:545.

Scanning electron microscopy has provided a better view of the external morphology of the odontoblasts (see Figure 2-10, C and D). The large nucleus is located in the base of the cell, giving it a pear-shaped appearance.[63] From an exquisite scanning electron microscopic study, French dental scientists have demonstrated that odontoblast cell bodies "appear tightly packed in the pulp horn and successively pear shaped, spindle shaped, club shaped, or globular from the crown to the apex"[64] (Figure 2-15).

During dentin formation in the crown, the odontoblasts are pushed inward to form the periphery of a pulp chamber, the circumference of which is increasingly smaller than the original circumference at the dentinoenamel junction. This explains why the cells are packed and palisaded into a pseudostratified appear-

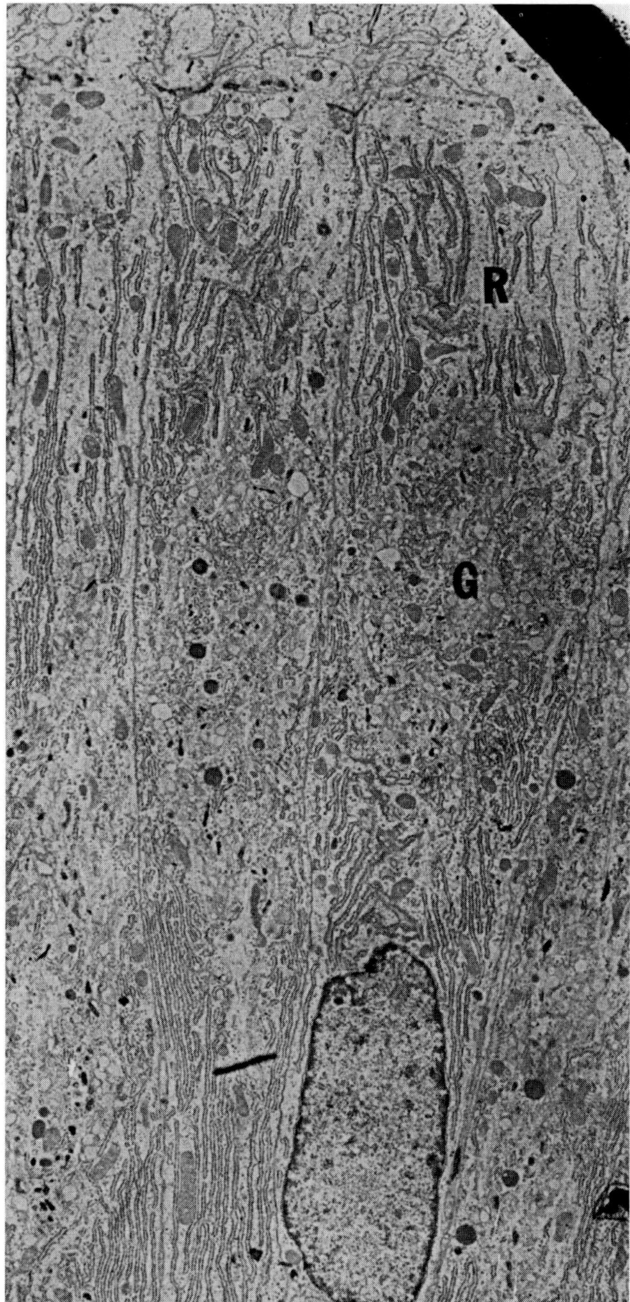

Figure 2-14 Odontoblasts, as viewed under the electron microscope, show organelles essential for protein synthesis, a plump nucleus filled with euchromatin, and cytoplasm rich with rough endoplasmic reticulum (R) and a well-developed Golgi apparatus (G). (Courtesy of Dr. Dale Eisenmann.)

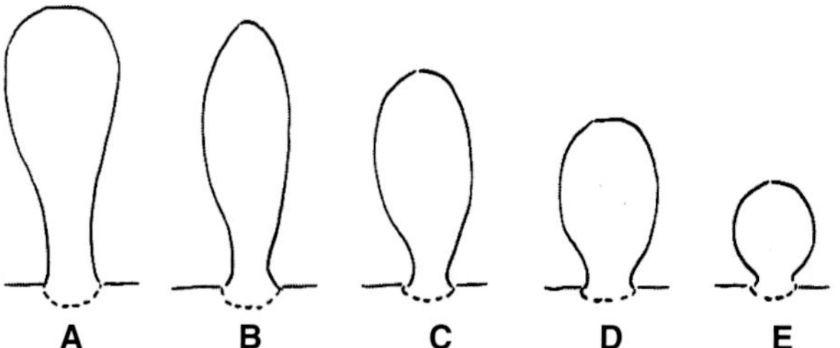

Figure 2-15 Diagram summarizing shape variation of odontoblast cell bodies. **A**, Pulp horn (pear shaped); **B**, coronal midpulp level (spindle shape); **C**, coronal midroot level (elongated club shape); **D**, mid-third of root (short club shape); **E**, apical third of root (globules). Reproduced with permission from Marion D, et al. Oral Surg 1991;72:473.

ance of coronal odontoblasts. Conversely, because the space is not so compressed in the radicular pulp, the odontoblasts maintain a columnar, cuboidal, or (in the apical region) squamous shape. Also, the resulting cell and tubule density is much higher in the pulp chamber than in the root pulp.[65] This increased tubule density in the chamber may explain the greater sensitivity and permeability of the dentin of the crown.

The cell body manufactures the matrix material; the material is transported to and secreted from the odontoblastic process. Classically, the odontoblastic process has been described as extending from the cell body to the dentinoenamel junction, a distance of 2 to 3 mm (ie, 2,000 to 3,000 μm). This concept was based on the observations of many light microscopists using a variety of special procedures and stains. [66] When dentin was examined by electron microscopy, the odontoblastic process was determined to be limited to the inner third of dentin, with the outer two-thirds of the tubule devoid of processes or of nerves but filled with extracellular fluid.[67–70] More recent investigations indicate that odontoblastic processes may indeed extend to the dentinoenamel junction.[71,72] However, tubular structures in dentinal tubules are not necessarily odontoblastic processes.[73,74] Unequivocal identification can be done only by identifying a trilaminar plasma membrane around the putative process using transmission electron microscopy.[75,76] The extent of the odontoblastic process remains controversial.[77]

Therefore, modern interpretations of pulpal injury following conservative cavity preparation may not be attributable to amputation of odontoblastic processes but to desiccation, heat, and osmotic effects. Further, dentin sensitivity may not be related to direct stimulation of either odontoblastic processes or nerves in peripheral dentin since the tubules may be devoid of such structures in the periphery of dentin.

After initial dentin formation, the odontoblast, via its process, can still modify dentin structure by producing peritubular dentin. This is a hypermineralized cuff with little organic matrix within the tubule, decreasing the diameter of the tubule.[78–80] When irritated, the odontoblast can accelerate peritubular dentin formation to the point of complete occlusion of the tubule (Figure 2-16).[81–83] When tubule occlusions extend over a large area, this is referred to as sclerotic dentin, commonly found in teeth with cervical erosion.[44]

Alternatively, irritated odontoblasts can secrete collagen,[84] amorphous material, or large crystals into the tubule lumen; these occlusions result in decreases in dentin permeability to irritating substances.[81–83] Although these secretions have been described as a defensive reaction by the odontoblast to protect itself and the underlying pulp, this "protection" has never been proved.

Extracellular. The dental pulp has most of its volume primarily composed of fibers and ground substance. These form the body and integrity of the pulp organ.

Fibers. The morphology of collagen fibers, a principal constituent in the pulp, has been described at the level of both light and electron microscopy. At the ultrastructural level, typical 640 angstrom banding or electron-dense periodicity provides positive proof of collagen fiber identity.[85] These fibers form a loose, reticular network to support other structural elements of the pulp. Collagen is synthesized and secreted by odontoblasts and fibroblasts. However, the type of collagen secreted by odontoblasts to subsequently mineralize differs from the collagen produced by pulpal fibroblasts, which normally does not calcify. They also differ not in basic structure but in the degree of cross-linking, and in slight variation in hydroxylysine content.[86]

Tropocollagen is immature collagen fibers that remain thin and stain black with silver nitrate, described in light microscopy as argyrophilic or reticular fibrils. If tropocollagen molecules aggregate into larger fibers, they no longer stain with silver and are generally termed "collagen fibers." If several collagen fibers aggregate (cross-link) and grow more dense, they are termed "collagen bundles." Collagen generally becomes more coarse (ie, develops more bundles) as the patient ages. Age also seems to permit ectopic calcification of pulp connective tissue, ranging from the development of random calcifications to diffuse calcifications[87] to denticle (pulp stone) formation. Elastin, the only other fibrous connective tissue protein, is found only in the walls of pulp arterioles.

Collagen has been described as having a unique arrangement in the peripheral pulp; these bundles of collagen are termed von Korff's fibers. Most textbooks describe von Korff's fibers as being corkscrew-like and originating between odontoblasts to pass into the dentin matrix (Figure 2-17). The tight packing of odontoblasts, predentin, capillaries, and nerves produces very narrow spaces between and around odontoblasts that can retain heavy metal stain (precipitates). Ten Cate's electron microscopic studies of the distribution of these precipitates demonstrated their presence in narrow intracellular tissue spaces.[88] He claimed that they represented artifactual "stains" that were not attached to collagen fibers.[88] However, more recent scanning electron microscopic studies (see Figure 2-10,

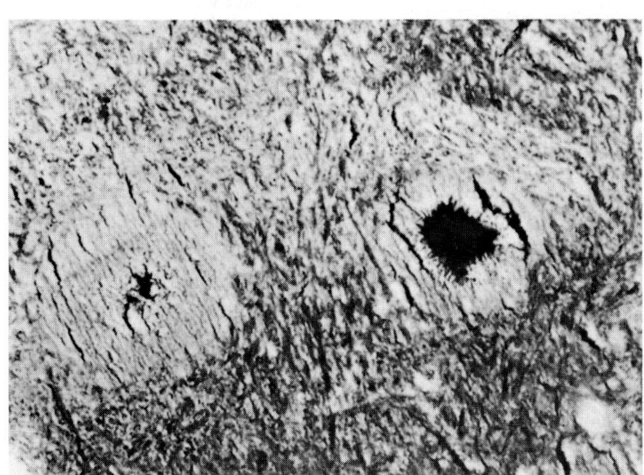

Figure 2-16 Mineralization of dentinal tubules in an aging human tooth. Electron micrograph of transparent root dentin from a 45-year-old person. The more densely mineralized peritubular dentin is white and the tubule itself is black. Two tubules are visible in cross-section. The tubule on the left is almost completely occluded. The progressive nature of mineralization is evident in the tubule on the right. (Courtesy of Dr. John Nalbandian.)

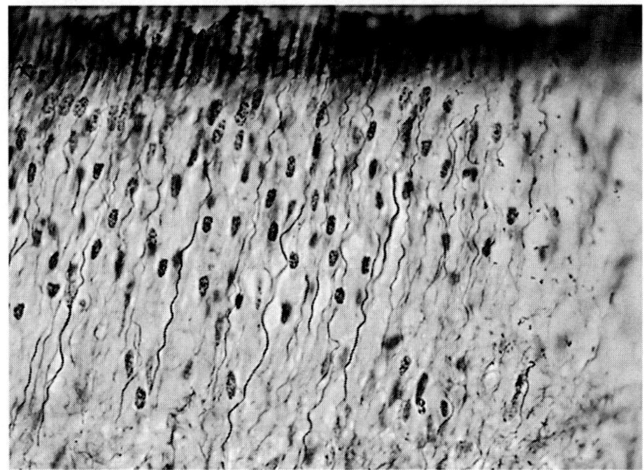

Figure 2-17 Peripheral pulp. The corkscrew-like structures (von Korff's fibers) reportedly are collagen fibers that originate in the pulp, pass between odontoblasts, and are incorporated into predentin. That these are collagen fibers is disputed. Reproduced with permission from Bernick S.[155]

D) of the predentin-pulpal border demonstrating screw-like fibrous material have stimulated new speculation that von Korff's fibers are real structures.[63]

Ground Substance. This structureless mass, gel-like in consistency, makes up the bulk of the pulp organ. It occupies the space between formed elements. The ground substance resembles that of other areolar, fibrous connective tissues, consisting primarily of complexes of proteins and carbohydrates and water. More specifically, these complexes are composed of combinations of glycosaminoglycans, that is, hyaluronic acid, chondroitin sulfate, and other glycoproteins.[89,90] The ground substance surrounds and supports structures and is the medium through which metabolites and waste products are transported to and from cells and vessels. Aging of the pulp alters the ground substance,[91] although there is no substantive proof that these alterations significantly inhibit pulp functions.

Supportive Elements.

Pulpal Blood Supply. Numerous investigators have described the blood supply of the dental pulp.[92–95] Because the pulp itself is small, pulp blood vessels do not reach a large size. At the apex and extending through the central pulp, one or more arterioles branch into smaller terminal arterioles or metarterioles that are directed peripherally (Figure 2-18, A). Before the arterioles break up into capillary beds, arteriovenous anastomoses often arise to connect the arteriole directly to a venule.[96] These arteriole-venule shunts are identified by the presence of irregularly oriented myoepithelium-like cells surrounding them and by the cuboidal nature of the cells lining their lumen.[97] The classic description of microcirculatory beds includes capillaries that branch off arterioles at right angles (Figure 2-18, B). Unfortunately, no such structures have been found in human pulps. Instead, arterioles branch into terminal arterioles, which, in turn, give rise to capillaries (Figure 2-19).

Capillary density is highest in the subodontoblastic region with loops passing between odontoblasts (Figure 2-20).[98–100] In the subodontoblastic region, capillaries with fenestrations occur frequently and regularly in both primary and permanent teeth (Figure 2-21). The fenestrae ("windows") are spanned by a thin diaphragm of plasma membrane. The frequency of fenestration falls off rapidly when examining central capillaries, being as low as 4% in the coronal pulp.[98,101]

Capillaries empty into small venules that connect with fewer and successively larger venules. At the apex, multiple venules exit the pulp. These venules connect with vessels that drain the periodontal ligament or adjacent alveolar bone. The vessels of the pulp have

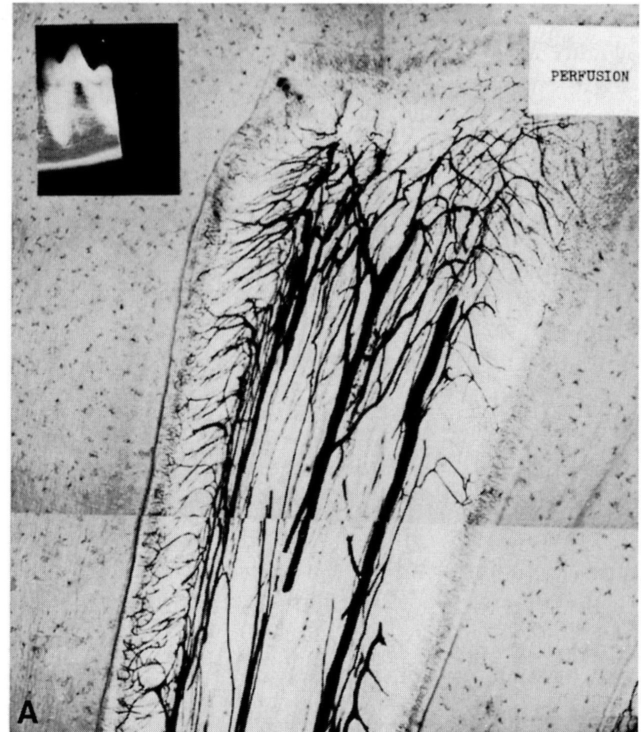

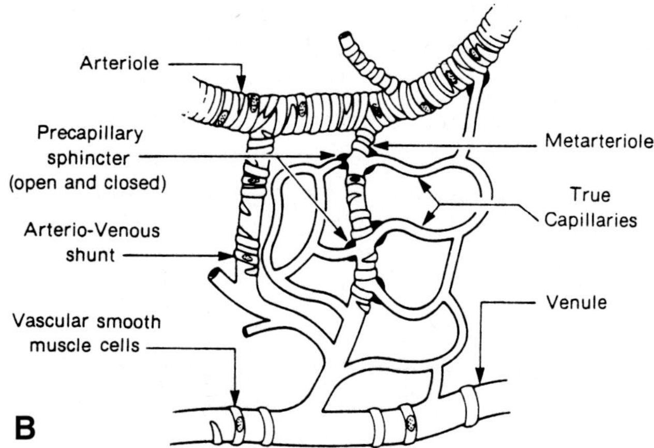

Figure 2-18 A, Perfused pulp of dog premolar showing the size and location of vessels. Larger central vessels are arterioles and venules. Peripherally directed are smaller metarterioles that branch into the rich network of looping capillaries of peripheral pulp. B, Schematic diagram of classic microcirculatory vascular bed that would represent a region of central and peripheral vessels as seen in A. Arterioles are invested by a continuous layer of smooth muscle cells. Metarterioles have discontinuous clusters of smooth muscle with capillaries branching directly off metarterioles. Precapillary smooth muscle sphincters are strategically located to control capillary blood flow. True capillaries lack smooth muscle. Arteriovenous shunts represent direct connections between arterioles and venules. Their muscles are innervated by sympathetic nerve fibers. A reproduced with permission from Seltzer S, Bender IB. The dental pulp. 2nd ed. Philadelphia: JB Lippincott; 1975. p. 106.

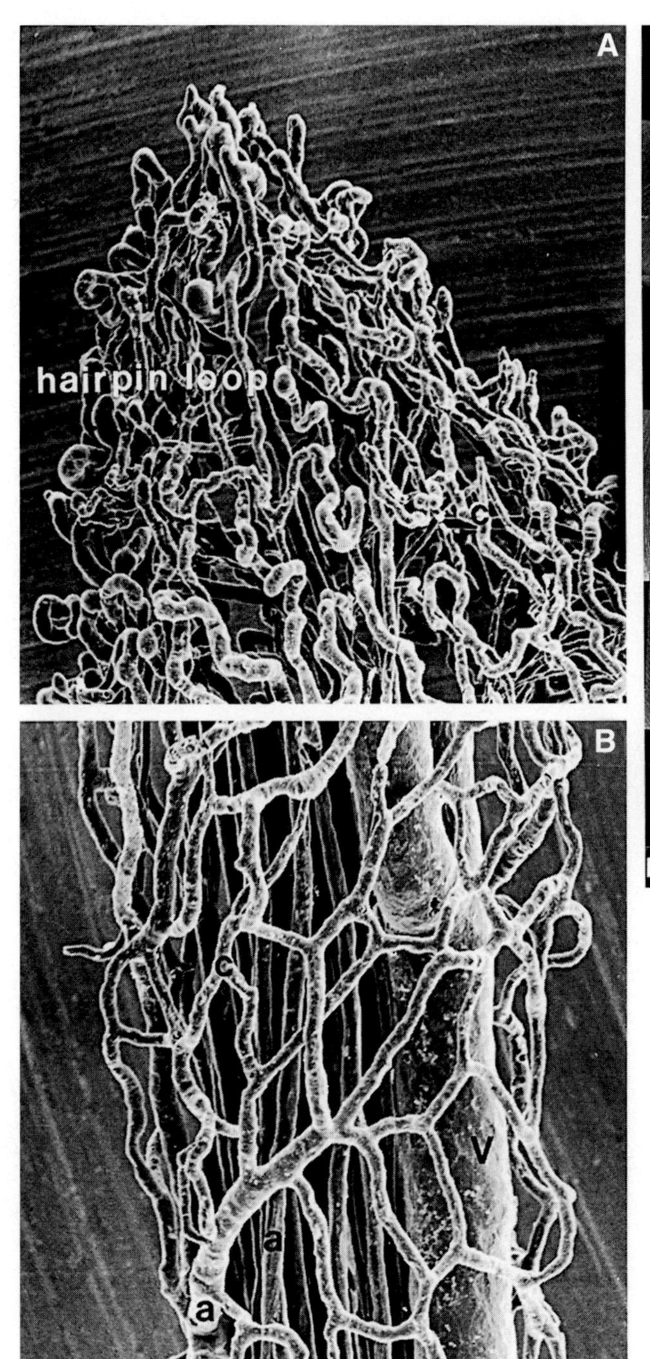

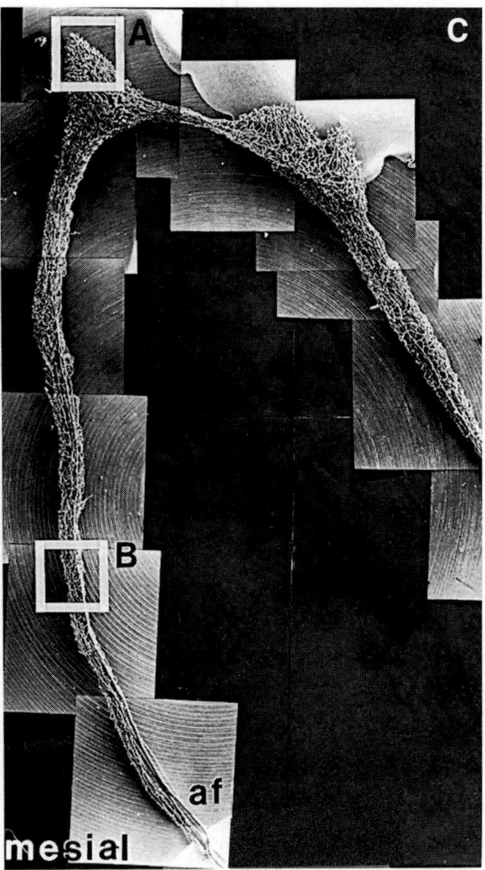

Figure 2-19 Corrosion resin casts of the pulp vessels of a dog premolar. **A**, Higher magnification of the region enclosed by the square labeled A in **C** demonstrates many hairpin capillary loops within the pulp horn (×300 original magnification). **B**, Higher magnification of the area enclosed by the square labeled B in **C**. Arterioles (a) arborize from artery to form a capillary (c) network on the surface of the radicular pulp. Venule (V) is about 50 micrometers in diameter. Arterioles are about 10 micrometers in diameter. Superficial capillary network demonstrates cross-fence shape. **C**, Montage of the entire pulp made from multiple, overlapping scanning electron micrographs (×50 original magnification). The three projections in the coronal region represent three pulp horns, apical foramen (af). (Courtesy of Drs. K. Takahashi, Y. Kishi, and S. Kim.)

thinner muscular walls (tunica media) than vessels of comparable diameter in other parts of the body. Undoubtedly, this is an adaptation to the surrounding protective and unyielding walls.[102] Kim and his associates have obtained evidence that suggests that most vasodilating agents induce only a transient, brief increase in pulpal blood flow followed by a decrease in blood flow owing to collapse of local venules.[103] Apparently, the vasodilation either directly impinges on venules or permits transudation of fluid across capillaries that indirectly compresses the thin-walled venules in the low-compliance system of the pulp chamber.

The above-described general vascular architecture is found in each tooth root. Alternate blood supply is available to multicanaled teeth, with the resulting rich anastomoses in the chamber. The occasional vessels that communicate via accessory canals have not been

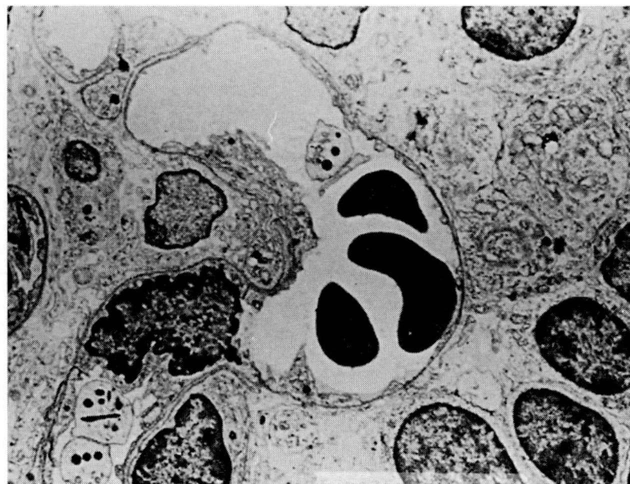

Figure 2-20 Electron micrograph of subodontoblastic capillary looping between odontoblasts. Portions of several red blood cells are seen within the lumen. Reproduced with permission from Avery J.[100]

demonstrated to contribute significantly as a source of collateral circulation.

Lymphatics. The presence of pulpal lymphatics is disputed.[104,105] However, lymphatics have been identified in the pulp at the ultrastructural[98] and histologic levels by the absence of red blood cells in their lumina, the lack of overlapping of endothelial margins, and the absence of a basal lamina.[87,98,106–108] They arise as lymphatic capillaries in the peripheral pulp zone (Figure 2-22) and join other lymph capillaries to form collecting vessels.[87] These vessels unite with progressively larger lymphatic channels that pass through the apex with the other vasculature. Numerous authors, using both histologic and functional methods, have described extensive anastomoses between lymph vessels of the pulp, periodontal ligament, and alveolar bone.[108–114]

Functional Implications. The presence of arteriovenous shunts[32,96] in the pulp provides the opportunity for blood to shunt[115,116] past capillary beds since these arteriole-venule connections are "upstream" from the capillaries. Alternatively, the arteriole-venule shunts could remain nearly closed (in a constricted state), and most of the blood would pass peripherally in the pulp to perfuse capillaries and the cells that they support.[115] It has been suggested that the distribution of blood flow might change during pulp inflammation.[117] Increased dilation of arteriole-venule shunts may produce "hyperemia," in which more blood vessels than normal are open and filled with blood cells; this may indicate more rapid blood flow or represent partial stasis. Further, this dilation of arteriole-venule shunts may "steal" blood from capillary beds, causing accumulation of waste products.

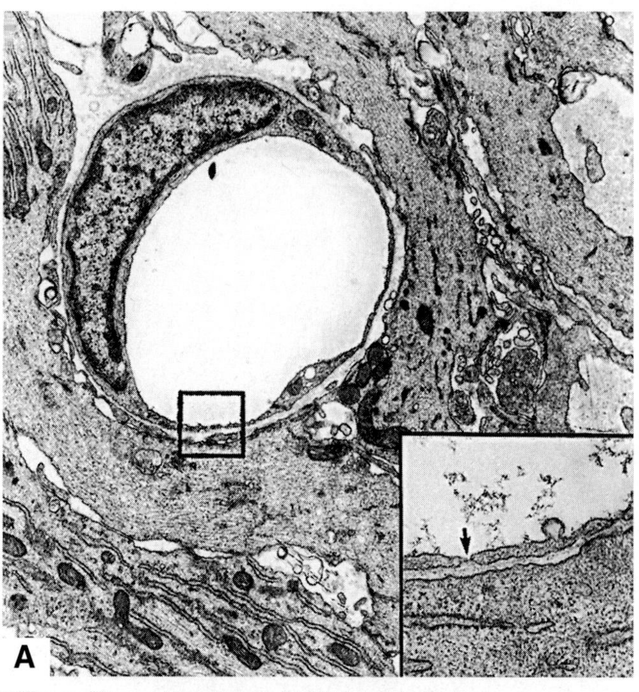

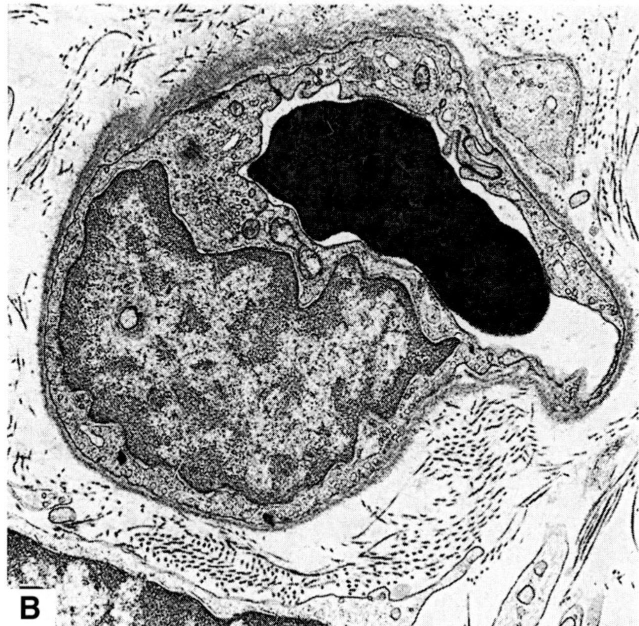

Figure 2-21 **A**, Electron micrograph of cross-section of the capillary loop passing between and closely surrounded by odontoblasts. Inset shows higher magnification of a portion of endothelial wall of the capillary demonstrating fenestrations (**arrow**). **B**, Subodontoblastic capillary with large nucleus of endothelial cell impinging on lumen. Plasticity of red blood cell (**black**) allows it to adapt to irregular contours of lumen. Prominent basement membrane encircles the periphery of the cell. (*A courtesy of Dr. K. Josephsen, Denmark; B courtesy of Dr. Robert Rapp.*)

Capillary fenestration may indicate that these capillaries are more permeable to large molecules or that they allow more rapid fluid movement across the endothelium.[118] However, studies on pulp capillaries

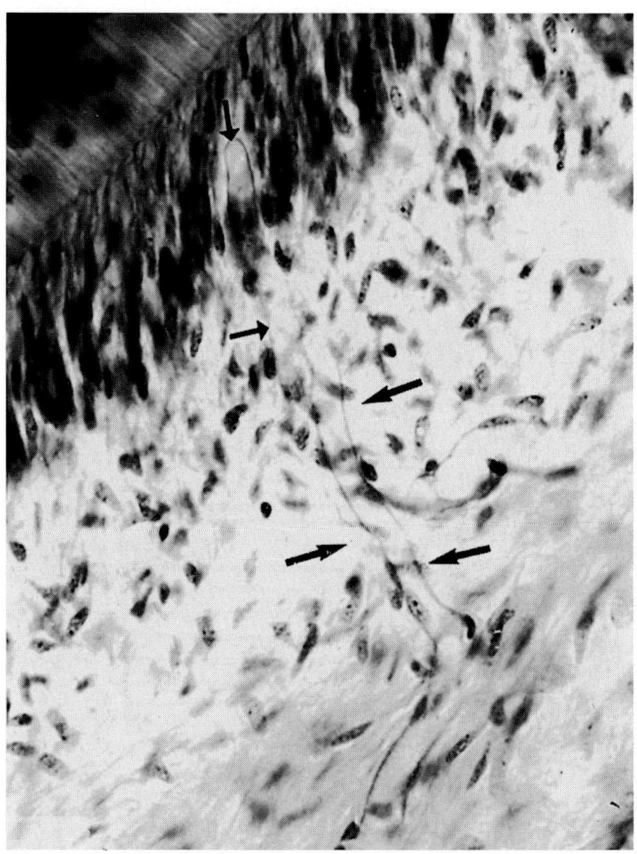

Figure 2-22 Lymphatic capillary arising and collecting from within the odontoblast-subodontoblast region of a human pulp. **Arrows** delineate margins of the vessel, draining toward the central pulp. Reproduced with permission from Bernick S.[87]

suggest a lower than normal permeability to large molecules. On the other hand, a higher rate of fluid movement has not been ruled out. Increased transudation of plasma and polymorphonuclear neutrophil leukocytes from the circulation occurs most often in venules[50] rather than capillaries.

The structural identification of lymph capillaries[87,98,107] complements the functional studies of Walton and Langeland,[108] who demonstrated that substances placed in the pulp chamber can be found in regional lymph nodes. The open endothelial margins and incomplete basal lamina permit entry of large molecules and even bacteria. The fact that materials placed on pulps can migrate to lymph nodes[119] indicates the possibility of immunologic reactions to substances that enter the pulp.[120] Bernick described the appearance of lymphatics in the inflamed pulp and surmised that their function is to remove the excess fluid and debris that accompanies inflammation.[87]

Unfortunately for the pulp, the lymphatics may collapse as pulp pressure rises, thus inhibiting removal of irritants and fluid. Clearly, more investigation is required before one can understand how lymphatic function is disturbed in pulp inflammatory conditions. The anastomoses of pulpal, periodontal, and alveolar lymphatics may be important routes for the spread of pulpal inflammation into adjacent tissues during the removal of irritants and fluid from the pulp. These structural interrelationships have not received the attention they deserve. Finally, the extent and degree of anastomoses of apical venules with those of the periodontal ligament and alveolar bone need investigation.[92] Vessels may provide a route for local anesthetic movement during intraosseous or periodontal ligament injections[121] rather than the fluid "dissecting" through perivascular tissue spaces.[122] These same pathways have been implicated as routes of spread of inflammation from pulp to periodontal ligament and/or bone and vice versa.

Nerves. Several nerve bundles, each containing numerous unmyelinated and myelinated nerves, pass into each root via the apical foramen. The majority are unmyelinated nerves,[123–125] most of which are part of the sympathetic division of the autonomic nervous system; these have been shown to cause reductions in pulp blood flow when stimulated.[126,127] The remaining nerves are myelinated sensory nerves of the trigeminal system (Figure 2-23).

The myelinated nerve fibers branch extensively beneath the cell-rich zone to form the so-called plexus of Raschkow (Figure 2-24). From here, many fibers lose their myelin sheath and pass through the cell-free zone to terminate as receptors or as free nerve endings near odontoblasts (Figure 2-25); others pass between odontoblasts to travel a short distance up the dentinal tubules adjacent to odontoblastic processes.[128] The nerve endings terminate far short of the dentinoenamel junction; rather, endings are found only in tubules of the inner dentin and predentin, on or between odontoblasts.[129] Byers has found that intradental nerves pass approximately 100 μm into the tubules, regardless of the dentin thickness, in a wide variety of animal species.[130] Perhaps nerve fibers cannot be nourished beyond a 100 μm diffusion distance. Some sensory axons exhibit terminal aborizations that innervate up to 100 dentinal tubules.[130] Significantly, sensory nerves of the pulp respond to noxious stimuli **with pain sensation only,** regardless of the stimulus. This pain is produced whether the stimulus is applied to dentin or the pulp.

Cavity preparation in the unanesthetized tooth is painful at any depth of dentin. How can this occur if there are no sensory nerves in the outer two-thirds of dentin? The answer probably lies in the hydrodynamic

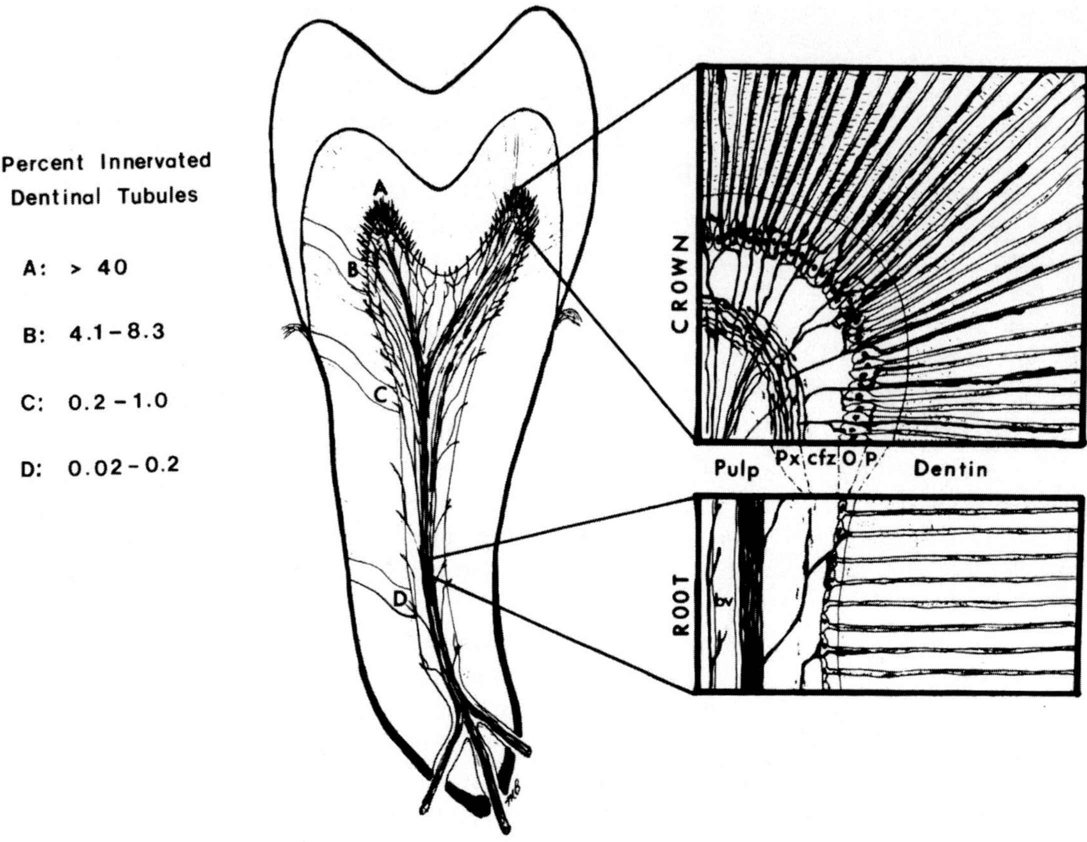

Figure 2-23 Schematic drawing showing sensory nerve location in pulp and dentin. Percentage of innervated tubules at regions A through D is indicated (**left**). Px = plexus of Raschkow; cfz = cell-free zone; O = odontoblasts; p = predentin. Reproduced with permission from Byers M.[144]

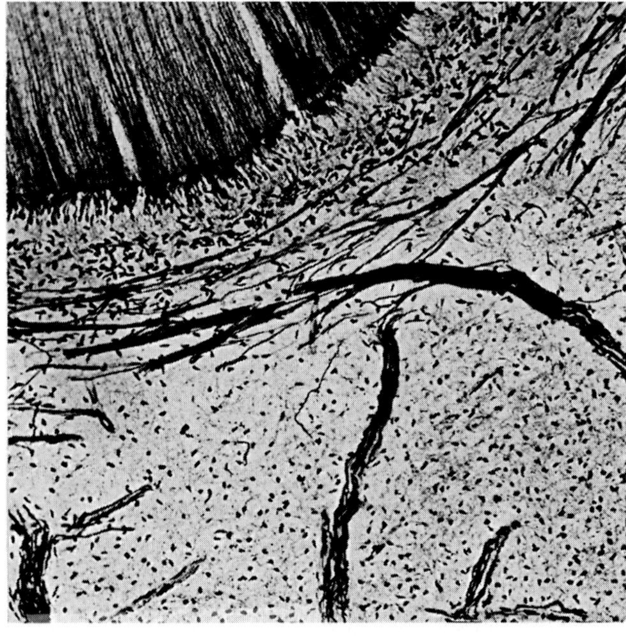

Figure 2-24 Branching of nerve bundles as they approach the subodontoblastic region (plexus of Raschkow). (Courtesy of Dr. James Avery.)

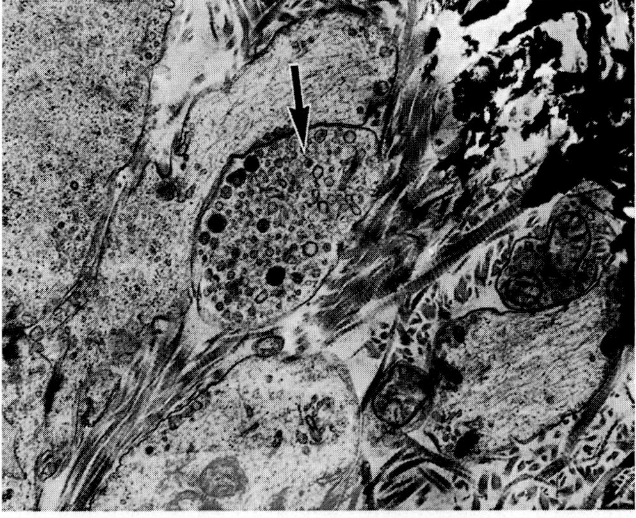

Figure 2-25 Nerve terminal (**arrow**) located between adjacent odontoblasts near calcifying dentin. Large number of vesicles is characteristic of nerve terminal. Terminal is closely applied to the adjacent odontoblastic process; this does not, however, represent a synapse. (Courtesy of Dr. James Avery.)

theory in which fluid movement within tubules stimulates distant sensory nerve endings (see Byers et al and Avery[128–131] for reviews).

Highly organized junctions have been demonstrated between some nerve fibers and odontoblasts.[132–136] Although they do not appear to be typical synaptic junctions, their existence must be functional. It is unclear whether the activity is sensory or motor.

An additional function of sympathetic nerves is the possible regulation of the rate of tooth eruption. Sympathetic nerve activity influences local blood flow and tissue pressure by opening or closing arteriovenous shunts as well as arteriolar blood flow; this may secondarily affect eruptive pressure.[137] Activation of sympathetic fibers not only reduces pulpal blood flow[138] but also decreases the excitability of intradental nerves.[139] Thus, there is a very intimate relationship between pulpal nerves and their excitability and local blood flow.[140]

Numbers and concentrations of nerves vary with the stage of tooth development and also with location. Fearnhead and others have reported that very few nerves appear in the human pulp prior to tooth eruption.[41,141,142] After eruption, the highest number of nerves is found in the pulp horns (about 40% of the tubules are "innervated"). The number of nerves per tubule drops off to about 4.8% in the more lateral parts of the coronal dentin to less than 1% in the cervical region (see Figure 2-23), with only an occasional nerve in radicular dentin.[143] Patterns of branching nerves seen with the light microscope would confirm numbers of nerves at different levels. There is little branching off the main nerve bundles until the coronal pulp. Regions of sensitivity also correlate in that coronal pulp and dentin are more painful to stimuli than are radicular pulp and dentin. The same stimuli applied to dentin were described as "sharp" when applied to coronal dentin but "dull" when applied to radicular dentin.[144] Restorative procedures in rat teeth cause sprouting of pulpal and intradental nerves that may modify both dentin sensitivity[145] and local inflammatory reactions.[146]

Interestingly, removal of the pulp by extraction of the tooth or by pulpectomy and, presumably, pulpotomy results in the successive degeneration of the cell bodies located in the spinal nucleus of the trigeminal nerve, the main sensory ganglion, and the peripheral nerve leading to the tooth in the socket.[147] Bernick observed the effects of caries and restorations on underlying nerves in the pulp.[148] He found a degeneration of the subodontoblastic plexus of nerves associated with the production of irritation dentin. He concluded that "the terminal nerves in the injured pulp are sensitive to the noxious products of caries and the restorative procedures. An apparent decrease in sensitivity results in restored teeth." The lack of sensitivity that accompanies the caries process may be attributable, at least partially, to degeneration of underlying nerves.

Calcifications. Basically, there are two distinct types of pulpal calcifications: formed structures commonly known as pulp stones (denticles) and tiny crystalline masses generally termed diffuse (linear) calcifications (Figure 2-26). Pulp stones seem to be found predominantly in the coronal pulp, whereas the calcifications found in radicular pulp seem to be of the diffuse variety.[149]

Calcifications are common in the dental pulp, with a tendency to increase with age and irritation. It has been speculated that these calcifications may aggravate or even incite inflammation of pulp or may elicit pain by pressing on structures; however, these speculations have not been proved and are improbable. Although these calcifications are not pathologic, their presence under certain conditions may be an aid in diagnosis of pulpal disease. Moreover, their bulk and position may interfere with endodontic treatment.

Pulp Stones. These discrete calcific masses appear with frequency in mature teeth.[150] Although there is increased incidence with age, they are not uncommon

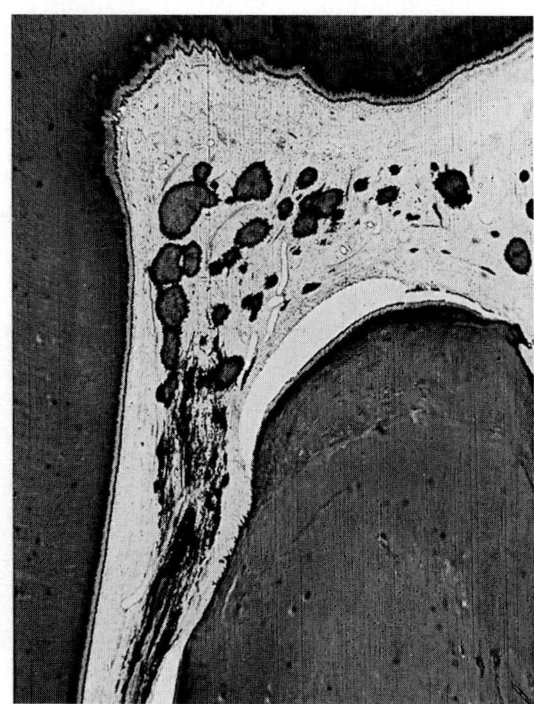

Figure 2-26 Uninflamed pulp. Typical pattern of calcifications. Larger pulp stones in the chamber blend into linear diffuse calcifications in the canal. Reproduced with permission from Bernick S.[155]

in young teeth. It has also been demonstrated that their occurrence and size often increase with external irritation.[151] Pulp stones also may arise spontaneously; their presence has been identified on radiographs (Figure 2-27) and, on histologic examination, even in impacted teeth.[152] Interestingly, there appears to be a predisposition for pulp stone formation in certain individuals, possibly a familial trait.

Pulp stones have been classified as two types, true or false. However, recent careful histologic examination has discounted the true pulp stone. Supposedly, true pulp stones are islands of dentin, demonstrating tubules and formative odontoblasts on their surface. However, serial sectioning has shown that these are not islands but peninsulas—extrusions from dentin walls.[152,153] Therefore, the term "denticle," which would imply dentin structure, is a misnomer. The term "pulp stone" is more correct, particularly because the "false" pulp stone so closely resembles gallstones and kidney or ureter stones.

Pulp stones, like other types of stones, are formed from clearly concentric or diffuse layers of calcified tissue on a matrix that seems to consist primarily of collagen.[154] Their structure may help explain their origin; it has been shown that potential nidi of pulp stones may occur in the sheaths associated with blood vessels (Figure 2-28) and nerves.[155] Other potential nidi are calcifications of thrombi in vessels or calcification of clumps of necrotic cells.[153] Whatever the nidus, growth is by incremental layering of a matrix that quickly acquires mineral salts.

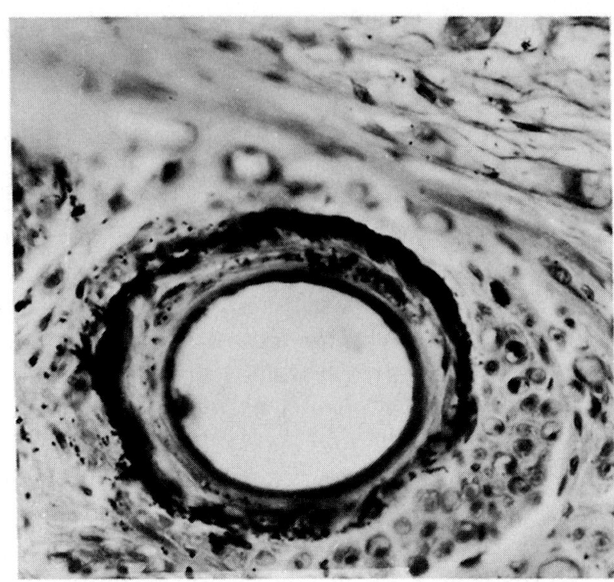

Figure 2-28 Calcification of the sheath surrounding this small vessel may form a nidus for growth of a larger calcified structure, a pulp stone. Reproduced with permission from Bernick S. J Dent Res 1967;46:544.

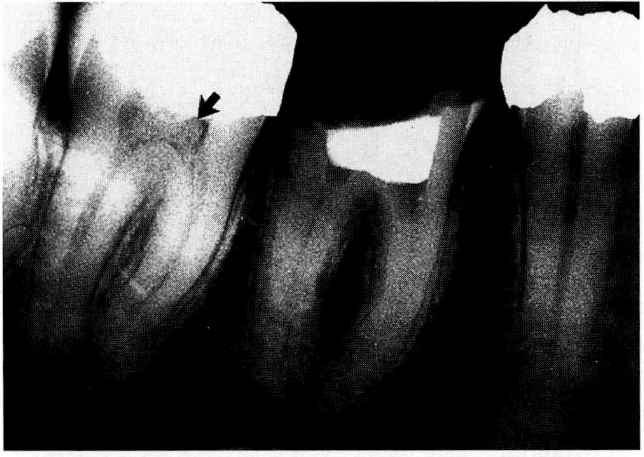

Figure 2-27 Second molar demonstrates chamber nearly filled with pulp stones (**arrow**). Stones may have arisen spontaneously, or their presence may indicate chronic irritation and inflammation from caries and/or deep restoration. (Courtesy of Dr. G. Norman Smith.)

Pulp stones are also classified according to location. "Free" stones are those that are islands, "attached" stones are free pulp stones that have become fused with the continuously growing dentin, and "embedded" stones are formerly attached stones that have now become surrounded by dentin.

Pulp stones may be important to the clinician who attempts access preparation or to negotiate canals. Either free or attached denticles may attain large size and occupy considerable volume of the coronal pulp (Figure 2-29). Their presence may alter the internal anatomy and confuse the operator by obscuring, but not totally blocking, the orifice of the canal. Attached denticles may deflect or engage the tip of exploring instruments in the canals, thus preventing their easy passage down the canal.[156]

Pulp stones of sufficient size are readily visible on radiographs, although the majority are too small to be seen except on histologic examination. The large, discrete masses, occasionally appearing to nearly fill the chamber (Figure 2-30), are likely to be those of natural occurrence. The chamber that appears to have a diffuse and obscure outline may represent a pulp that has been subjected to a persistent irritant and has responded by forming large numbers of irregular pulp stones. This finding is a diagnostic aid and indicates a pulp exposed to a persistent chronic irritant.

Diffuse Calcifications. Also known as linear calcifications because of their longitudinal orientation,

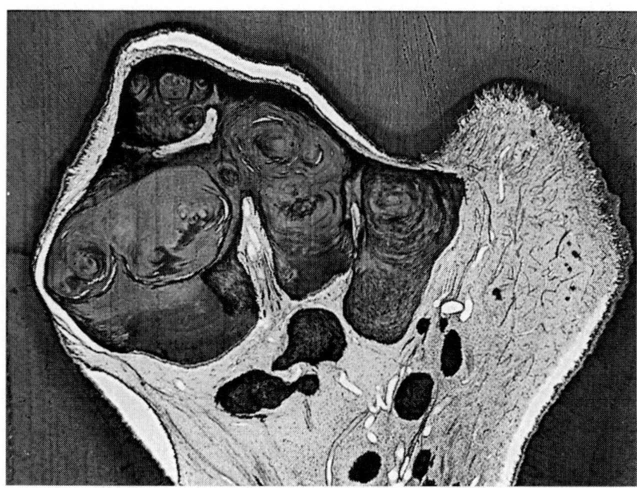

Figure 2-29 Large pulp stone may have been formed by growth and fusion of smaller stones such as those below it. Examination of other serial sections may show that this apparently "free" pulp stone is actually attached to dentin walls. Reproduced with permission from Bernick S.[155]

these are common pulp findings. They may appear in any area of the pulp but predominate in the radicular region.[157] Their form is that of tiny calcified spicules,[156] usually aligned close to blood vessels and nerves or to collagen bundles (see Figure 2-26). Because of their size and dispersion, they are not visible in radiographs and are seen only on histologic specimens. Like pulp stones, diffuse calcifications also tend to increase with age and with irritation but otherwise have no known clinical significance.

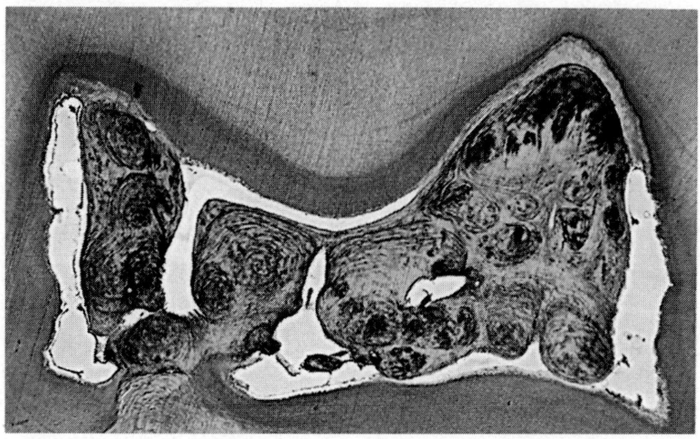

Figure 2-30 Large pulp stones may fill and nearly obscure the entire chamber. In some areas, the margins of the stone have fused with the dentin walls. Reproduced with permission from Bernick S.[155]

PULP CHANGES WITH AGE

Teeth age, not only with the passage of time but also under the stimulus of function and irritation. Therefore, age is a chronologic occurrence, but even more importantly, an "aged" tooth may represent a premature response to the abuses of caries, extensive restorative procedures, and inflicted trauma. Since the pulp reacts to its environment and is in intimate contact with dentin, it responds to abuses by altering the anatomy of its internal structures and surrounding hard tissue.

Dimensional

With time and/or injury, the pulp volume decreases by forming additional calcified tissues on the walls (see Figure 2-30). Ordinarily, with time, formation of dentin continues, with the greatest increase on the floor of the chamber of posterior teeth[158] (Figure 2-31) and on the incisal of anterior teeth. In such teeth, the location of the pulp chamber and/or root canals may be difficult. In anterior teeth, the clinician may have to search cervically to locate a remnant of the chamber. In molars, dentin formation may have rendered the chamber almost disk-like; while searching, it is easy to inadvertently pass a bur through the flattened chamber (Figure 2-32). If the preparation is continued, the next hemorrhage encountered will arise

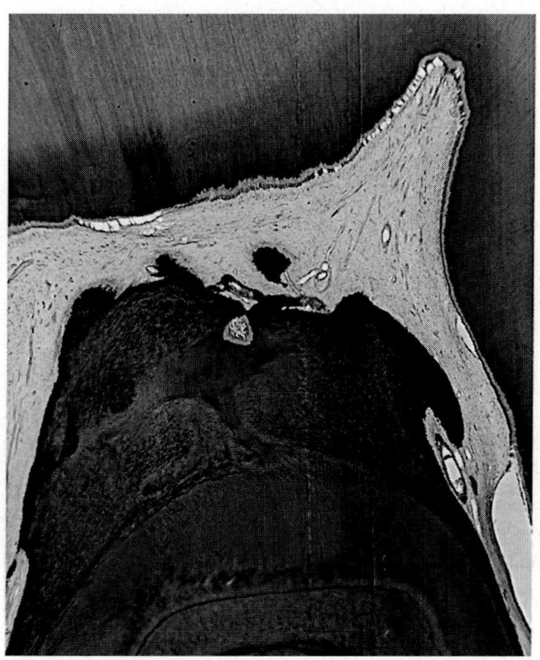

Figure 2-31 Pattern of dentin formation in "aged" posterior tooth from a 60-year-old patient. Typically irregular hard tissue apposition is greatest on the floor, decreasing chamber depth. (Courtesy of Dr. Sol Bernick.)

from the furcation, not from the chamber. Careful examination of radiographs to identify chamber size and location, followed by measurements of the occlusochamber distance, will prevent this mishap. Irritation dentin formation will also alter internal anatomy. Therefore, when the dentin has been violated by caries or by attrition, one should expect increased amounts of hard tissue in the underlying pulp. Irritation dentin may occasionally be extensive enough to obscure or fill large areas of the chamber.

Structural

Although exacting quantitative studies have not been published, there is agreement that the number of cells decreases and the fibrous component increases with aging of the pulp (Figure 2-33).[159] The increased fibrosis with time is not from continued formation of collagen but rather may be attributable to a persistence of connective tissue sheaths in an increasingly narrowed pulp space.[155,160]

Bernick observed a decrease in the number of blood vessels[155] and nerves[161] supplying the aging pulp, noting that many of the arteries demonstrated arteriosclerotic changes similar to those seen in other tissues[161] (Figure 2-34). These changes involve decreases in lumen size with intimal thickening and hyperplasia of elastic fibers in the media. Also common is calcification of arterioles and precapillaries.[161] Although these structural changes are described, it is not clear whether the vascular and neural changes alter the function of the older pulp.

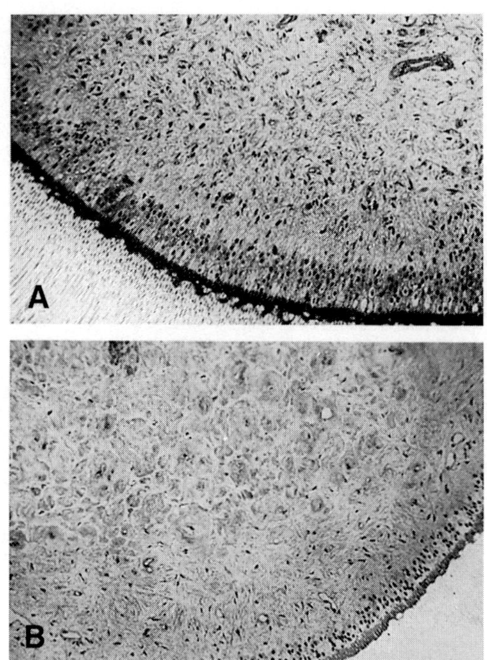

Figure 2-33 Age changes in cross-sections of human pulp. **A**, Young pulp with characteristic cellularity and relatively small scattered fibrous components of central pulp. **B**, Acellularity and large fiber bundles are common findings in mature pulps. (Courtesy of Dr. Dennis Weber.)

Not only do cells decrease in number, notably fibroblasts and odontoblasts, but the remaining cells are likely to appear relatively inactive. These ordinarily active cells demonstrate fewer organelles associated with synthesis and secretion.[1]

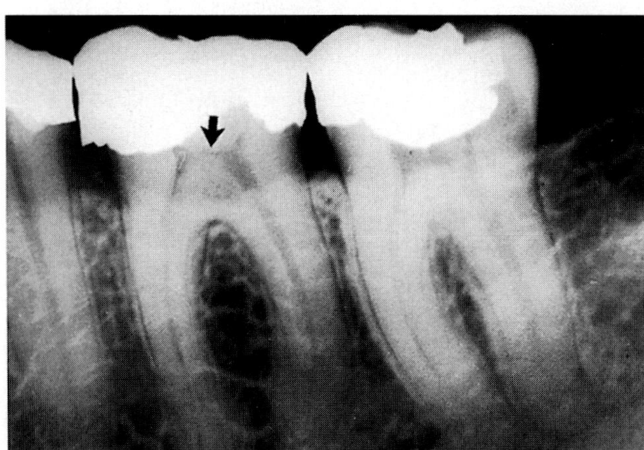

Figure 2-32 Disk-like chamber (**arrow**) is a result of hard tissue apposition on the floor and roof. The center of the chamber is difficult to locate. An access preparation should be started by locating the large orifice of the distal canal first. (Courtesy of Dr. G. Norman Smith.)

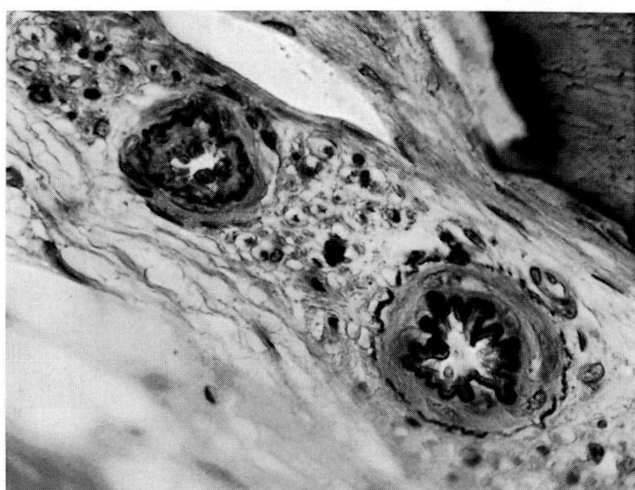

Figure 2-34 Cross-section of small arterioles in the apical third of pulp from an older person. The lumina are decreased in size, showing thickening of the tunica intima and hyperplasia of the tunica media—changes characteristic of arteriosclerosis. Reproduced with permission from Bernick S. J Dent Res 1967;46:544.

"Regressive" Changes

The term "regressive" is defined as a condition of decreased functional capability or of returning to a more primitive state. Older pulps have been described as regressive and as having a decreased ability to combat and recover from injury. This has been surmised because older pulps have fewer cells, a less extensive vasculature, and increased fibrous elements. In fact, there have never been experiments proving that aged pulps are more susceptible to irritants or less able to recover. Until these have been conclusively demonstrated, the term "regression" is not appropriate, and the dentist should not assume that pulps in older individuals are less likely to respond favorably than are younger pulps.

PULPAL RESPONSE TO INFLAMMATION

Pulp structures and functions are altered, often radically, by injury and resulting inflammation. As a part of the inflammatory response, neutrophilic leukocytes are chemotactically attracted to the site. Bacteria or dying pulp cells are phagocytosed, causing release of potent lysosomal enzymes. These enzymes may attack surrounding normal tissue, resulting in additional damage.

For instance, by-products of the hydrolysis of collagen and fibrin may act as kinins, producing vasodilation and increased vascular permeability.[162,163] Escaping fluid tends to accumulate in the pulp interstitial space, but because the space is confined, the pressure within the pulp chamber rises. This elevated tissue pressure produces profound, deleterious effects on the local microcirculation. When local tissue pressure exceeds local venous pressure, the local veins tend to collapse, increasing their resistance; hence blood will flow away from this area of high tissue pressure as it seeks areas of lower resistance. This process of blood diversion can be illustrated by applying slight pressure to the end of a fingernail. As the pressure increases, the nail bed blanches as blood is squeezed out of the local vessels, and new blood is prevented from flowing through this area of elevated tissue pressure. Persistent pressure continues to compromise circulation. The consequences of reduced local blood flow are minor in normal tissue but disastrous in inflamed tissue because the compromised circulation allows the accumulation of irritants such as injurious enzymes, chemotoxic factors, and bacterial toxins.

This event may lead to the development of the "compartment syndrome,"[164–166] a condition in which elevated tissue pressure in a confined space alters structure and severely depresses function of tissues within that space. Depressed function often leads to cell death, which, in turn, produces inflammation resulting in fluid escape and increased pressure within the compartment. The increased tissue pressure collapses veins, thereby increasing the resistance to blood flow through capillaries. Blood is then shunted from areas of high tissue pressure to more "normal" areas. Thus, a vicious cycle is produced in which inflamed regions tend to become more inflamed because they tend to limit their own local nutrient blood flow (Figure 2-35).

This is not to say that the pulp "strangulation" theory is valid. As shown by Van Hassel,[167] and more recently by Nahri[168] and Tönder and Kvinnsland,[169] pressures are not readily transmitted throughout the pulp. Therefore, inflammation and increased pressure in the coronal pulp will not collapse veins in the apical region. Pulps physiologically have multiple compartments throughout. It is as if small volumes of pulp tissue are enclosed in separate connective tissue sheaths, each of which can contain local elevations in tissue pressure. Although no histologic evidence exists to support this notion, these functional compartments may break down individually to become necrotic and may coalesce to form microabscesses.

The recent micropuncture work by Tönder and Kvinnsland demonstrated that there are highly localized elevations in interstitial tissue pressure in inflamed pulp.[169] This is thought by some to be caused by the release of vasoactive neuropeptides such as substance P and calcitonin gene–related peptide, both found in pulp nerve fibers.[170] During pulpal inflammation, there is an increase in the number of calcitonin gene–related peptide–containing nerves in areas previously devoid of nerves. The release of these peptides seems to promote and sustain inflammation, prompting some to call it neurogenic inflammation.[171]

PULPODENTINAL PHYSIOLOGY

As long as dentin is covered peripherally by enamel on coronal surfaces and cementum on radicular surfaces, the dental pulp will generally remain healthy for life, unless the apical blood supply is disrupted by excessive orthodontic forces or severe impact trauma. Most pathologic pulp conditions begin with the removal of one or both of these protective barriers via caries, fractures, or abrasion. The result is the communication of pulp soft tissue with the oral cavity via dentinal tubules, as has been demonstrated by dye penetration studies[172] and radioactive tracer experiments.[173]

It is apparent that substances easily permeate dentin, permitting thermal, osmotic, and chemical insults to act on the pulpal constituents. The initial stages involve stimulation or irritation of odontoblasts and may proceed to inflammation and often to tissue destruction.

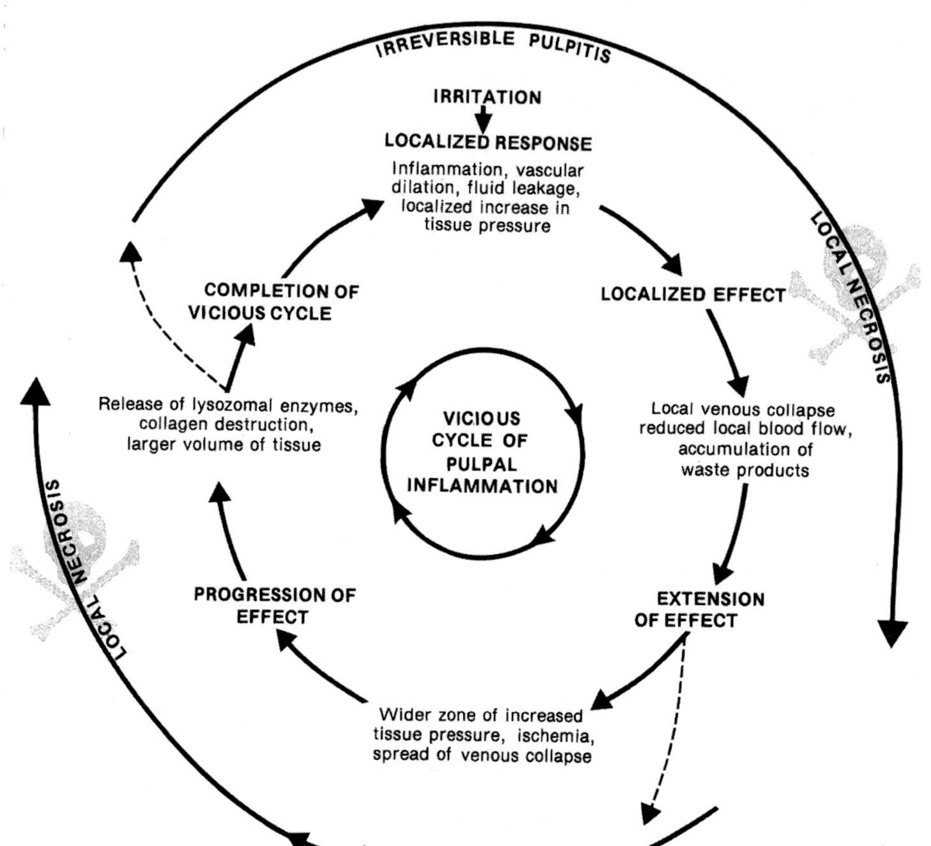

Figure 2-35 Vicious cycle of pulpal inflammation, which begins with irritation (**top**), leads to a localized response, and may progress to a lesion of increasing severity and eventual irreversible pulpitis.

To understand how these steps may lead to pulp damage, the pulpodentinal complex will be examined in its separate forms.

Dentin Structure

Dentin is a calcified connective tissue penetrated by millions of tubules; their density varies from 40,000 to 70,000 tubules per square mm.[174,175] Tubules are from 1 μm in diameter at the dentinoenamel junction to 3 μm at their pulpal surface and contain fluid that has a composition similar to extracellular fluid.[176] If the fluid becomes contaminated, for example, with carious bacterial endotoxins and exotoxins, then it develops a reservoir of injurious agents that can permeate through dentin to the pulp to initiate inflammation.[177] It is useful to understand the important variables that control dentin permeability.

Dentin Permeability. Dentinal tubules in the coronal dentin converge from the dentinoenamel junction to the pulp chamber.[178] This tends to concentrate or focus permeating substances into a smaller area at their terminus in the pulp. The surface area occupied by tubules at different levels indicates the effect of tubule density and diameter. One can calculate from Garberoglio and Brännström's[175] observations that the area of dentin occupied by tubules is only 1% at the dentinoenamel junction and increases to 45% at the pulp chamber. The clinical implications of this are enormous. As dentin becomes exposed to increasing depths by restorative procedures, attrition, or disease, the remaining dentin becomes increasingly permeable.[179,180] Thus, dentin removal, although necessary, renders the pulp more susceptible to chemical or bacterial irritation. This functional consequence of tubule area is also responsible for the decrease in dentin microhardness closer to the pulp[181,182]; as tubule density increases, the amount of calcified matrix between the tubules decreases. This relative softness of the dentin lining the pulp chamber somewhat facilitates canal enlargement during endodontic treatment.[183]

Overall dentin permeability is directly proportional to the total surface area of exposed dentin. Obviously, a leaking restoration over a full crown preparation provides more diffusional surface for bacterial products than would a small occlusal restoration.[184] Restorations requiring extensive and deep removal of dentin (ie, preparation for a full crown) would open more and larger tubules and increase the rate of injurious substances diffusing from the surface to the pulp—thus the importance of "remaining dentin thickness."[185,186] The

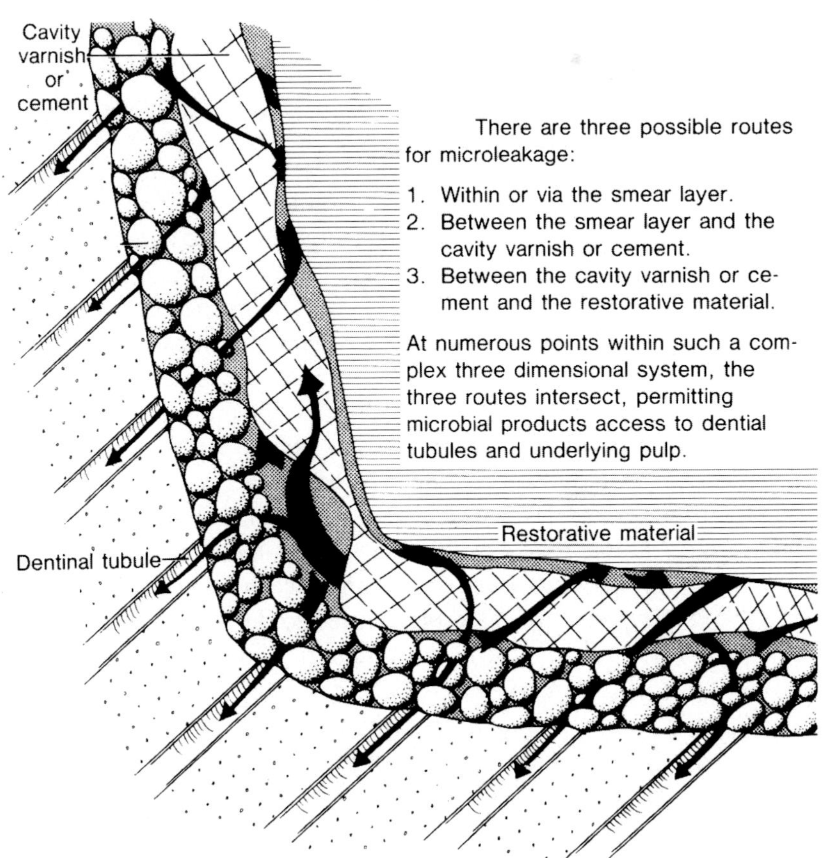

Cavity varnish or cement
There are three possible routes for microleakage:
1. Within or via the smear layer.
2. Between the smear layer and the cavity varnish or cement.
3. Between the cavity varnish or cement and the restorative material.
At numerous points within such a complex three dimensional system, the three routes intersect, permitting microbial products access to dential tubules and underlying pulp.
Restorative material
Dentinal tubule

Figure 2-36 Schematic representation of the interface of dentin and restorative material. The globular constituents of the smear layer have been exaggerated out of proportion for emphasis. Reproduced with permission from Pashley DH.[193] Oper Dent 1984;3:13.

permeability of the root is 10 to 20 times less than that of a similar thickness of coronal dentin.[187] This may account for the lack of pulpal reactions to periodontal therapy that removes cementum and exposes root dentin to the oral cavity.

Recent evidence indicates that dentin permeability is not constant after cavity preparation. In dogs, dentin permeability fell over 75% in the first 6 hours following cavity preparation.[188] Although there were no histologic correlates of the decreased permeability, dogs depleted of their plasma fibrinogen did not decrease their dentin permeability following cavity preparation.[189] The authors speculated that the irritation to pulpal blood vessels caused by cavity preparation increased the leakage of plasma proteins from pulpal vessels out into the dentinal tubules, where they absorb to the dentin, decreasing permeability. Future study of this phenomenon is required to determine if it occurs in humans.

The character of the dentin surface can also modify dentin permeability. Two extremes are possible: tubules that are completely open, as seen in freshly fractured[190] or acid-etched dentin,[191] and tubules that are closed either anatomically[66] or with microcrystalline debris.[192] This debris creates the "smear layer" (Figure 2-36), which forms on dentin surfaces whenever they are cut with either hand or rotary instruments.[193] The smear layer prevents bacterial penetration[194,195] but permits a wide range of molecules to readily permeate dentin. Small molecules permeate much faster than large molecules. Smear layers are often slowly dissolved over months to years as oral fluids percolate around microleakage channels between restorative materials and the tooth.[196] Removal of the "smear layer" by acid etching or chelation increases dentin permeability[197] because the microcrystalline debris no longer restricts diffusion of irritants and also permits bacteria to penetrate into dentin.[198] There is considerable debate as to whether smear layers created in the root canal during biomechanical preparation (Figure 2-37) should be removed.[199] Its removal may increase the quality of the seal between endodontic filling materials and root dentin. It may also increase the bond strength of resin posts.[200]

Pulp Metabolism. The rate at which pulpal cells are metabolizing can be quantitated by measuring their rate of oxygen consumption, CO_2 liberation, or lactic acid production.[201] Fisher and colleagues reported that zinc oxide–eugenol (ZOE) cement, eugenol, calcium hydroxide, silver amalgam, and procaine all depressed pulp oxygen consumption.[202] Shalla and Fisher demonstrated that lowering the medium pH of pulp

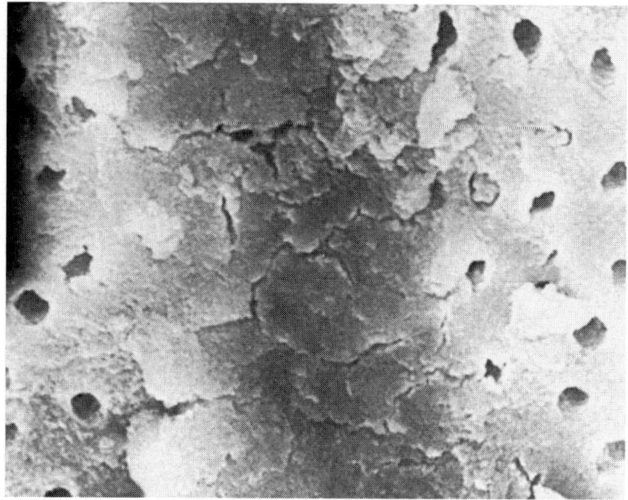

Figure 2-37 Scanning electron micrograph of root canal dentin treated with 5% NaOCl and 17% EDTA (ethylenediaminetetraacetic acid) to remove pulpal tissue and smear layer. A number 8 file drawn over the clean surface in the middle of the field creates a smear layer (×2,000 original magnification). Reproduced with permission from Goldman M et al.[199]

cells below 6.8 caused a progressive decrease in oxygen consumption.[203] This undoubtedly occurs during the development of pulp abscesses. Even though pulp respiration may decrease in an acid environment, Fisher and Walters have shown that bovine pulp has a very active ability to produce energy through anaerobic glycolysis.[204] Oxygen consumption has also been measured in dental pulp tissue using an oxygen electrode.[205]

A more sensitive technique has recently been applied to studying pulp respiration.[206–208] Pulp tissue was placed in ^{14}C-labeled substrates such as succinate and measured the rate of appearance of $^{14}CO_2$ from the reaction vessel. Using this technique, reduced pulp metabolism was demonstrated when ZOE cement, Dycal, Cavitec, and Sargenti's formula/N_2 were used.[206] It was also reported that the application of orthodontic force to human premolars for 3 days led to a 27% reduction in pulp respiration.[207] The depressant effects of eugenol on pulp respiration were reported as well.[208] Similar results were recently reported by Hume.[209,210] Pulpal irritation generally causes elevated tissue levels of cyclooxygenase products. Eugenol in ZOE cement has been shown to block this reaction.[211]

Pulp Reaction to Permeating Substances. What happens when permeating substances reach the pulp chamber? Although bacteria may not actually pass through dentin, their by-products[212,213] have been shown to cause severe pulp reaction.[177,212,214] The broad spectrum of pulp reaction, from no inflammation to abscess formation, may be related to the concentration of these injurious substances in the pulp. Although exposed dentin may permit substances to permeate, their concentrations may not reach levels high enough to trigger the cascade of events associated with inflammation. This would indicate that the interstitial fluid concentration of these substances can be maintained at vanishingly low concentrations. As long as the rate of pulp blood flow is normal, the microcirculation is very efficient at removing substances diffusing across dentin to the pulp chamber.[184] There is enough blood flowing through the pulp each minute to completely replace between 40 and 100% of the blood volume of the pulp.[215] Since blood is confined to the vasculature, which comprises only about 7% of the total pulpal volume,[215,216] the blood volume of the pulp is replaced 5 to 14 times each minute.

If pulpal blood flow is reduced,[217–230] there will be a resultant rise in the interstitial fluid concentration of substances that permeated across dentin.[184] The increased concentration of injurious agents may degranulate mast cells,[49,50] release histamine[231] or substance P,[232–236] produce bradykinin,[237] or activate plasma proteins.[238,239] All of these effects would initiate inflammation. The endogenous mediators of inflammation produce arteriolar vasodilation, elevated capillary hydrostatic pressure, increased leakage of plasma proteins into the pulp interstitium,[240] and increased pulp tissue pressure.[167,169,241] These events, by causing collapse of local venules, lead to a further reduction in pulp blood flow,[242] with an even higher interstitial concentration of irritants; thus, a vicious cycle[243] is created that may terminate in pulp death (see Figure 2-35).

Techniques for accurately measuring pulp tissue pressures were developed in the 1960s.[244–248] These methods all involve drilling carefully through the enamel and dentin to tap into the pulp chamber. Recently, several indirect methods of measuring pulp pressure through intact dentin have been devised. One group measured the pressure in a chamber cemented on cat dentin necessary to prevent outward movement of fluid as 15 cm H_2O.[249] Ciucchi et al, using the same technique in humans, reported a normal pulp pressure of 14 cm H_2O (10.4 mm Hg), far below systemic blood pressure but close to pulp capillary pressure (Figure 2-38).[250] Recent direct measurements of pulpal interstitial fluid pressures by micropuncture have given pressures of 6 to 10 mm Hg. However, they were done on pulps exposed to the atmosphere.[169]

Pulp blood flow has been measured by numerous authors using many different techniques.[251–254] Recently, Gazelius and his associates reported the use of a laser Doppler blood flowmeter that was sensitive enough to measure changes in pulpal blood flow in intact human teeth.[253] This method has begun to be used in pulp biology research.[138] Blood flow in the pulp falls in direct proportion to any increase in pulp tissue pressure. Van Hassel,[167] Stenvik and colleagues,[241] and Tönder and Kvinnsland[169] reported that pulp tissue pressure is elevated in pulpitis but that the elevation is localized within specific regions of the pulp, being normal in noninflamed areas. The localized reduction in pulp blood flow, however, allows the accumulation of mediators of inflammation, which, in turn, causes a spread in the elevation of tissue pressure, reducing pulp blood flow to a larger volume of pulp, etc.[167,243] The elevated pulp tissue pressure causes dull, aching, poorly localized pulp pain, a type of pain that differs from the brief, sharp, well-localized dentinal pain that is postulated to be caused by fluid movement within dentin.[3] Accordingly, when teeth with elevated pulp pressures are opened to the pulp, the pain generally subsides rapidly as tissue pressures rapidly fall.

Dentin Sensitivity. Clinicians recognize that dentin is exquisitely sensitive to certain stimuli.[255,256] It is unlikely that this sensitivity results from direct stimulation of nerves in dentin (Figure 2-39). As previously stated,

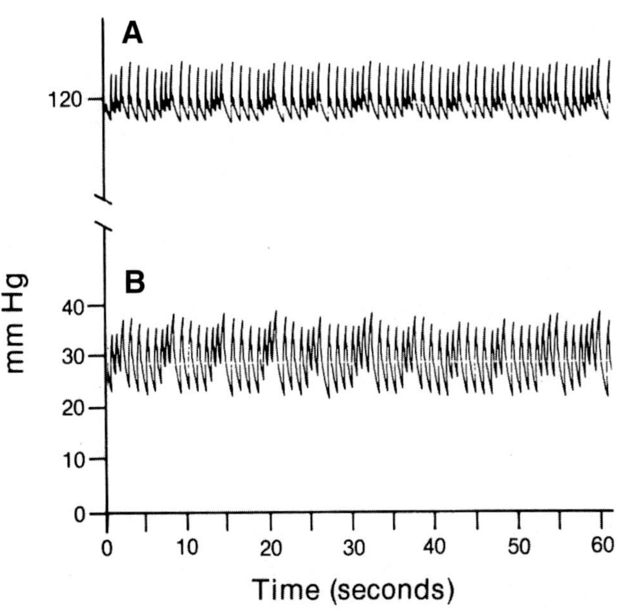

Figure 2-38 Comparison of pulp tissue pressure with systemic blood pressure in dog. **A**, Systemic blood pressure, shown on a different sensitivity and scale, demonstrates a mean value of about 120 mm Hg and a pulse pressure of about 60 mm Hg. **B**, Pulp tissue pressure taken simultaneously with systemic blood pressure and shown on different scale. Pulp tissue pressure demonstrates a mean value of about 30 mm Hg and a pulse pressure of about 10 mm Hg. (Courtesy of Dr. J. G. Weatherred.)

nerves cannot be shown in peripheral dentin.[143,144] Another speculation is that the odontoblastic process may serve as excitable "nerve endings" that would, in turn, excite nerve fibers shown to exist in deeper dentin, closer to the pulp.[143,144,257] The experiments of Anderson and colleagues[258] and Brännström[259] suggest that neither odontoblastic processes nor excitable nerves within dentin are responsible for dentin's sensitivity.

This led Brännström and colleagues to propose the "hydrodynamic theory" of dentin sensitivity, which sets forth that fluid movement through dentinal tubules, moving in either direction, stimulates sensory nerves in dentin or pulp.[259,260] Further support for the hydrodynamic theory came from electron microscopic examination of animal[67,261,262] and human dentin,[64,66,67] demonstrating that odontoblastic processes seldom extend more than one-third the distance of the dentinal tubules. Work by LaFleche and colleagues suggested that the process may retract from the periphery during extraction or processing.[77] Obviously, more investigation will be required before any definitive statement can be made regarding the distribution of the process. The tubules are filled with dentinal fluid that is similar in composition to interstitial fluid.[176]

The hydrodynamic theory satisfies numerous experimental observations. Although it cannot yet be regarded as fact, it has provided and will continue to provide a very useful perspective for the design of future experiments[263–265] (see Figure 2-39).

Effect of Posture on Pulpal Pain. Whenever an appendage is elevated above the heart, gravity acts on blood on the arterial side to reduce the effective pressure and, hence, appendage blood flow. This is why one's arm rapidly tires when working overhead. The reduced pressure effect occurs in structures in the head that, in normal upright posture, are well above the heart. When the patient lies down, however, the gravitational effect disappears, and there is a significant increase in pulp blood pressure and corresponding rise in tissue pressure over and above that caused by endogenous mediators of inflammation. In this position, an irritated and inflamed pulp becomes more sensitive to many stimuli and may spontaneously begin to fire a message of pain. This is why patients with pulpitis frequently call their dentists after lying down at night. In the supine position, a higher perfusion pressure and, presumably, a higher tissue pressure develop in the patient, which cause more pulp pain. Patients often discover that they are more comfortable if they attempt to sleep sitting up, which again emphasizes the effects of gravity on pulp blood flow.

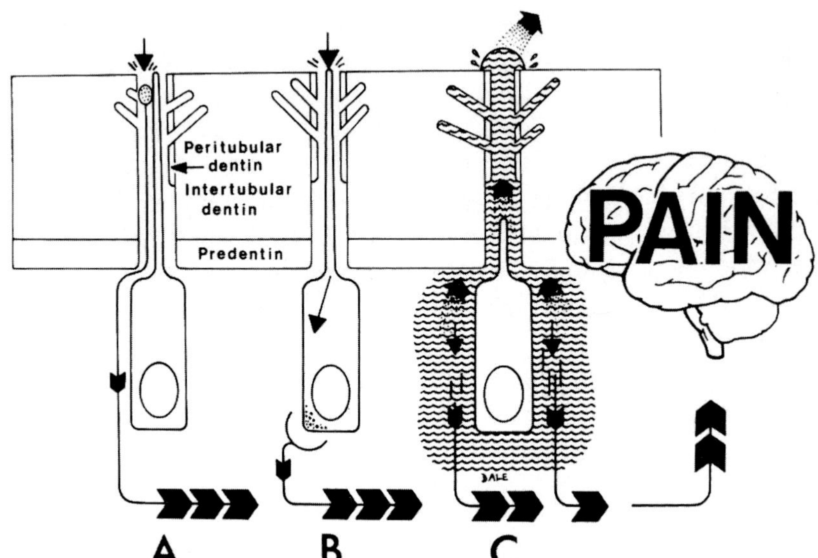

Figure 2-39 Schematic diagram of essentials of three theories of dentin sensitivity. **A,** Classical theory proposed that stimuli applied to dentin caused direct simulation of nerves in dentin. **B,** Modified theory proposed that stimuli applied to the odontoblastic process would be transmitted along the odontoblast and passed to the sensory nerves via some sort of synapse. **C,** Hydrodynamic theory proposed that fluid movement within tubules transmits peripheral stimuli to highly sensitive pulpal nerves. **C** more accurately represents the actual length of the odontoblastic process relative to the tubules. Nerves are seldom found more than one-third the distance from pulp to surface. Modified with permission from Torneck CD.[90]

Another factor contributing to elevated pulp pressure on reclining is the effect of posture on the activity of the sympathetic nervous system. When a person is upright, the baroreceptors (the so-called "carotid" sinus), located in the arch of the aorta and the bifurcation of the carotid arteries, maintain a relatively high degree of sympathetic stimulation to organs richly innervated by the sympathetic nervous system. Tönder demonstrated that canine pulps showed large reductions in blood flow when the baroreceptor system was manipulated.[226] If the human dental pulp is similar, it would result in slight pulpal vasoconstriction whenever a person is standing or sitting upright. Lying down would reverse the effect with an increase in blood flow and tissue pressure in the pulp. Lying down, then, increases pulp blood flow by removing both the effects of gravity and the effects of baroreceptor nerves, which decrease pulpal vasoconstriction. Thus, the increase in pain from inflamed pulps at night or the transformation of the pain from a dull to a throbbing ache has rational physiologic bases. The lack of documentation in the literature is owing to a lack of investigation.

Systemic Distribution of Substances from Dentin and Pulp. The rate of blood flow[115,230,266,267] in the pulp is moderately high and falls between that of organs of low perfusion, such as skeletal muscle, and highly perfused organs, such as the brain or kidney[267] (Figure 2-40). Since dentinal fluid (the fluid filling the tubules) is in communication with the vasculature of the pulp,[240] in theory, substances placed directly on pulp or dentin diffuse to the interstitial fluid and are quickly absorbed into the bloodstream or into the lymphatics. In vivo evidence indicates that both may occur. Numerous authors have demonstrated that substances placed onto dentin or into pulp chambers are absorbed systemically. These substances include radioactive labeled cortisone,[268] tetracycline,[269] lead,[270,271] formocresol,[272–275] glutaraldehyde,[276,277] and camphorated monochlorophenol.[278]

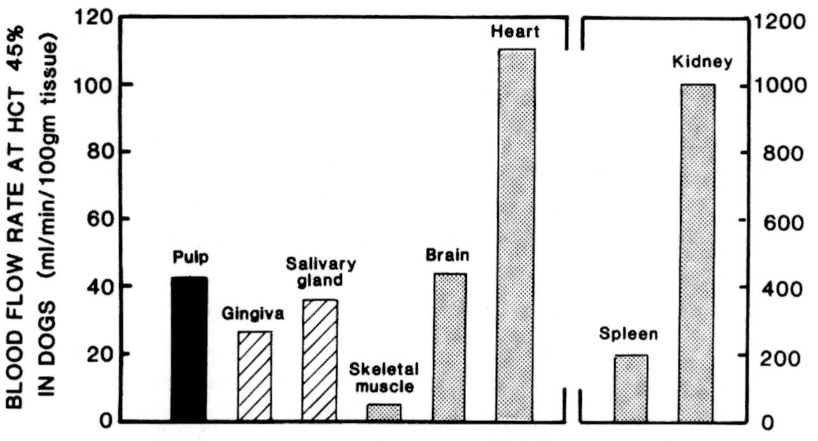

Figure 2-40 Comparison of blood flows among various tissues and organs, adjusted according to weight. **Pulpal** blood flow is intermediate between muscle and heart blood flow. Reproduced with permission from Kim S. J Dent Res 1985;64:590.

This direct communication of dentin to systemic circulation was proved by Pashley,[184] who demonstrated that radioactive iodide and albumin placed on dog dentin rapidly gave measurable blood levels of the substances. Systemic absorption of substances following pulp application was shown by Myers and colleagues, who measured the systemic appearance of ^{131}I from pulpotomy sites in monkeys both before and after treatment of the pulp stumps with formocresol.[276] Similar studies have recently been completed using ^{14}C-formaldehyde[274,275] and ^{14}C-glutaraldehyde.[276,277] Barnes and Langeland demonstrated that circulating antibodies were formed against bovine serum albumin and sheep erythrocytes placed on exposed pulps of monkeys.[120] Thus, the pulp provides an access route not only to the systemic circulation but also to the lymphatic system.[106]

Noyes and Ladd forced fluid into dog pulps and observed its collection in submaxillary lymph nodes.[279] Kraintz and coworkers placed radioactive colloidal gold on dog dentin and found that it appeared in the lymphatic drainage.[119] Walton and Langeland studied the distribution of zinc oxide and eugenol from pulpotomy sites in monkeys.[108] Within days, the particles were distributed throughout the pulp (Figure 2-41) and periodontium and appeared in the submandibular lymph nodes of the animals.

Feiglin and Reade deposited radioactive microspheres in rat pulps and found more microspheres in the submandibular lymph nodes in those rats whose pulps had been exposed for 5 days in comparison with those with acute pulp exposure.[280] This suggests enhanced lymphatic function during inflammation.

The relationship of teeth to the cardiovascular and lymphatic systems is intimate and absolute. Clinicians should remember this when performing dental procedures since their placement of materials on dentin or pulp may result in widespread distribution of that material or medicament.

HISTOLOGY OF THE PERIRADICULAR REGION

At the periapex, the connective tissues of root canal, foramen, and periradicular zone form a tissue continuum that is inseparable. This intimate relationship is confirmed by the frequency of disease in the pulp, inciting disease beyond the tooth. When both the pulp and periapex are jointly involved, immediate therapy must often focus on the periradicular region. More commonly, only pulp therapy is necessary. Healing of the periradicular tissue generally occurs spontaneously, demonstrating its capacity to repair. During preparation of the pulp space, the cardinal principles of instrumentation and obturation, aimed at confining everything to the canal space, indicate how necessary it is to respect the periradicular connective tissue.

The intimate communicative relationship of the structures at the periapex has been shown in experiments that traced substances placed in the coronal pulp to the periodontium. Markers migrated from the pulp and were observed in all areas of the periodontal ligament, the alveolar and medullary bone, and even in the marginal gingiva.[94,108]

The periapex is the apical continuation of the periodontal ligament. Actually, the tissue at the immediate apex of the tooth is more akin to the content of the root canal than to the periodontal ligament. The concentration of nerves and vessels coursing into the pulp is such, in fact, that attachment fibers and bone normally associated with the ligament space are generally excluded. The radiographic appearance of the interruption in bone to permit passage of the neurovascular bundle must not be confused with the bone resorption that accompanies periradicular inflammation (Figure 2-42).

The connective tissue sheaths of vessel and nerve groups lie close together. It is small wonder that inflammatory change is found concentrated at this zone of vessel egress; the spread of inflammation occurs via the connective tissue sheaths of vessels as a pathway of spread.[113,114]

Physiologically, as well as structurally, sharp contrasts set the periodontal ligament apparatus off from pulp tissue: (1) It is, for example, an organ of the finest tactile reception. The lightest contact on the tooth will stimulate its numerous pressor receptors. The pulp contains no such receptors. Proprioceptors of the periodontal ligament present the capability of spatial determination. It is for this reason that an inflamed periodontium can be more easily localized by the patient than can an inflamed pulp. (2) Collateral blood supply, so lacking within the pulp, is abundant in this area. This rich blood supply is undoubtedly a major factor in the periapex's ability to resolve inflammatory disease. In contrast, the pulp often succumbs to inflammation because it lacks collateral vessels. (3) The apical periodontium communicates with extensive medullary spaces of alveolar bone. The fluids of inflammation and resultant pressures apparently diffuse through this region more readily than is possible in the confined pulp space.

Histologically, the periapex demonstrates the major features of the remaining periodontium. Collagenous fibers anchor cementum to alveolar bundle bone. The arrangement of bone and fibers is discontinuous where the neurovascular bundle passes through to the pulp. A significant component of the periodontal ligament at all levels is the cords of ectodermal cells derived from the

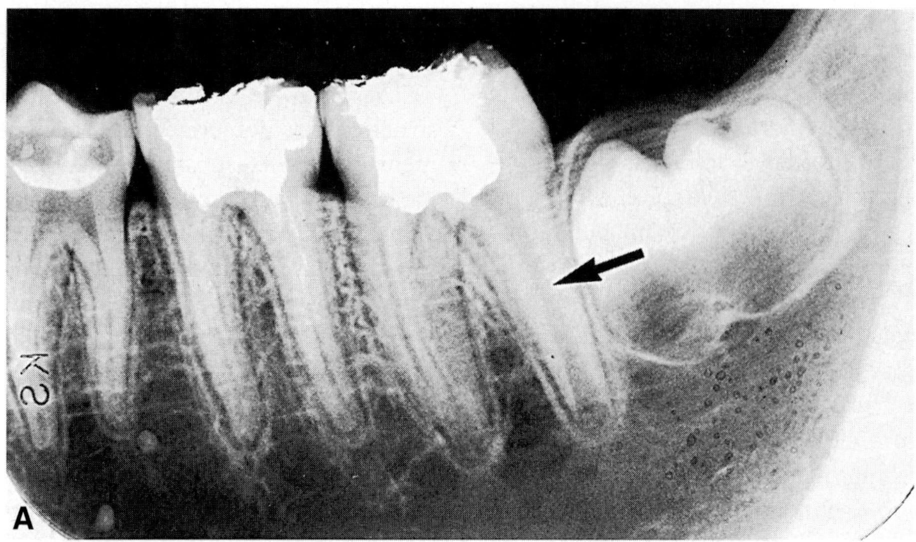

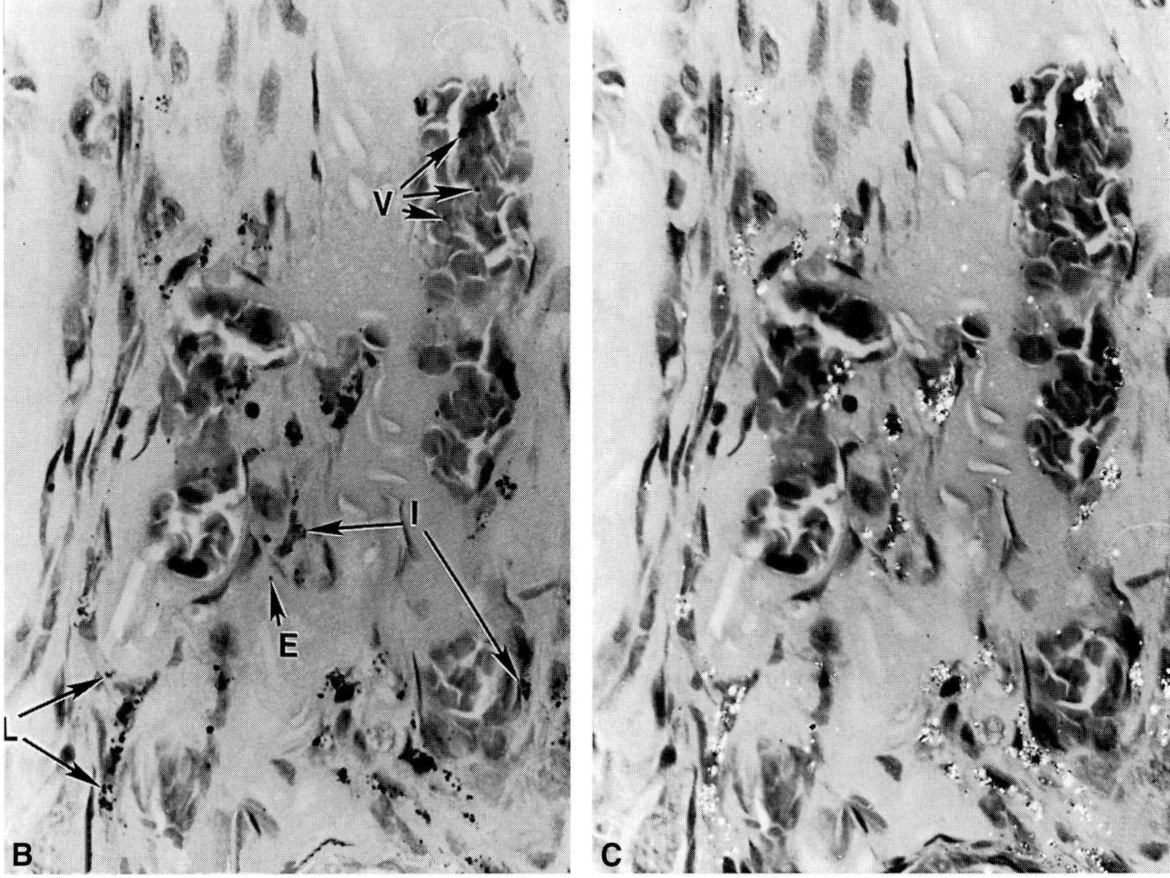

Figure 2-41 Experiment in monkeys showing time and spatial pattern of migration of material placed in contact with vital pulp. **A**, Human mandibular first and second molars after pulpotomy; application of a silver–zinc oxide–eugenol sealer and restoration with amalgam. **Arrow** indicates region shown histologically in **B** and **C**. **B**, Area of pulp canal indicated in **A**. Particles of silver and zinc oxide are visible in extracellular spaces (E) adjacent to vessels and intracellularly (I) within endothelial or perivascular cells. Material is also contained in venules (V) and in small vessels resembling capillaries, or in lymphatics (L). **C**, Same field as **B**; polarized light demonstrates particles seen in **B**, which are birefringent sealer particles. Reproduced with permission from Walton R and Langeland K.[108]

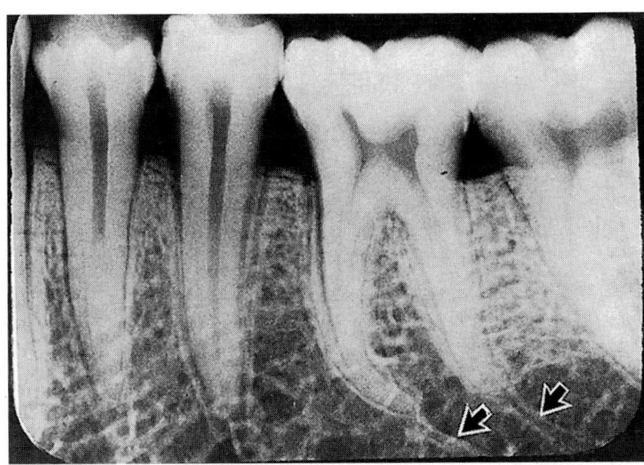

Figure 2-42 Radiographic appearance of bone surrounding apical neurovascular bundle (**arrows**). Because of configuration, these structures should not be confused with radiolucent apical lesion that is accompanied by loss of lamina dura and has a "hanging drop" appearance.

original root sheath, which form a tight network in this narrow zone between tooth and bone. These embryonic remnants, the epithelial rests of Malassez, may serve in a constructive capacity, and several such functions have been postulated.[281] However, interest has focused on their potential to undergo rapid hyperplasia when stimulated by periradicular inflammation. As will be seen in chapter 5, it is these cells that provide the epithelial "seed" for the lining sheet of the apical cysts.

Beyond the ligament is the alveolar bone with its associated marrow. The transition from ligament space to marrow is made through the myriad perforations of the alveolar bone proper. This bone, at the periapex as much as on the lateral walls of the socket, is truly a cribriform plate.[122] Interstitial connective tissue of the periodontal membrane passes through it, carrying vessels and nerves, to blend with the fatty marrow of the alveolar-supporting bone.

The potentials of this periradicular marrow are rich and significant. The reserve and other cells of the marrow contribute to nature's débridement and repair in the diseased periradicular zone following adequate pulp therapy.

REFERENCES

1. Bhaskar SN. Orban's oral histology and embryology. 9th ed. St. Louis; CV Mosby; 1980.
2. Slavkin HC. The nature and nurture of epithelial-mesenchymal interactions during tooth morphogenesis. J Biol Buccale 1978;6:189.
3. Brännström M, Astrom A. The hydrodynamics of the dentin: its possible relationship to dentinal pain. Int Dent J 1972;22:219.
4. Ten Cate AR. Oral histology, development, structure and function. St. Louis: CV Mosby Year Book; 1994.
5. Thesleff I. The teeth. In: Thorogood P, editor. Embryos, genes and birth defects. New York: John Wiley & Sons; 1997. p. 329.
6. MacNeil RI, Thomas HF. Development of the murine periodontium. I. Role of basement membrane in formation of a mineralized tissue on the developing root dentin surface. J Periodontol 1993;64:95.
7. MacNeil RI, Thomas HF. Development of the murine periodontium. II. Role of the epithelial root sheath in formation of the periodontal ligament. J Periodontol 1993;64:285.
8. Slavkin HC, Chai Y, Hu CC, et al. Intrinsic molecular determinants of tooth development from specification to root formation: a review. In: Davidovitch Z, editor. The biological mechanisms of tooth eruption, resorption and replacement by implants. Birmingham (AL): EBSCO Media; 1994. p. 263.
9. Slavkin HC, Diekwisch T. Evolution in tooth developmental biology of morphology and molecules. Anat Rec 1996;245:131.
10. Bei M, Maas R. FGFs and BMP4 induce both Msx1-independent and Msx1-dependent signaling pathways in early tooth development. Development 1998;125:4325.
11. Chen Y, Bei M, Woo I, et al. Msx1 controls inductive signaling in mammalian tooth morphogenesis. Development 1996;122:3035.
12. Neubuser A, Peters H, Balling R, Martin GR. Antagonistic interactions between FGF and BMP signaling pathways: a mechanism for positioning the sites of tooth formation. Cell 1997;90:247.
13. Tucker AS, Matthews KL, Sharpe PT. Transformation of tooth type induced by inhibition of BMP signaling. Science 1998;282:1136.
14. Lumsden AGS. Neural crest contribution to tooth development in the mammalian embryo. In: Maderson PFA, editor. Developmental and evolutionary aspects of the neural crest. New York: John Wiley and Sons; 1988. p. 261.
15. Thomas HF, MacNeil RL, Haydenblit R. The role of epithelium in the developing and adult murine periodontium. In: Davidovitch Z, editor. The biological mechanisms of tooth eruption, resorption and replacement by implants. Birmingham (AL): EBSCO Media; 1994. p. 317.
16. Collins F, Patrinos A, Jordan E, et al. New goals for the U.S. human genome project: 1998-2003. Science 1998;282:682.
17. Nuckolls GH, Shum L, Slavkin HC. Ectodermal dysplasia: a synthesis between evolutionary, developmental and molecular biology and human clinical genetics. In: Chuong CM, editor. Molecular basis of epithelial appendage morphogenesis. Georgetown (TX): RG Landes; 1998. p.15.
18. Bachman B. Inherited enamel defects. In: Chadwick DJ, Cardew G, editors. Dental enamel. London: John Wiley and Sons; 1997. p. 175.
19. Online Mendelian Inheritance of Man, OMIM™ [online]. Center for Medical Genetics, Johns Hopkins University (Baltimore, Maryland) and National Center for Biotechnology Information, National Library of Medicine (Bethesda, Maryland); 1998. http://www3.ncbi.nlm.nih.gov/omim/.
20. Fong CD, Slaby I, Hammarstrom L. Amelin, an enamel related protein transcribed in the epithelial root sheath of rat teeth. J Bone Miner Res 1996;11:892.
21. Schroeder HE. Development, structure and function of periodontal tissues. In: Oksche A, Vollrath L, editors. Handbook of microscopic anatomy. Berlin: Springer-Verlag; 1985. p. 23.

22. Hammarström L. The role of enamel matrix proteins in the development of cementum and periodontal tissues. In: Chadwick DJ, Cardew G, editors. Dental enamel. London: John Wiley and Sons; 1997. p. 246.
23. Slavkin HC, Bringas P, Bessem C. Hertwig's epithelial root sheath differentiation and initial cementum and bone formation during long term organ culture of mouse mandibular first molars using serumless, chemically-defined medium. J Periodontal Res 1988;23:28.
24. Slavkin HC. Towards a cellular and molecular understanding of periodontics: cementogenesis revisited. J Periodontol 1976;11:331.
25. Green D. Morphology of the pulp cavity of permanent teeth. Oral Surg 1955;8:743.
26. Coolidge E, Kesel RG. A textbook of endodontology. 2nd ed. Philadelphia: Lea & Febiger; 1956.
27. Meyer W. Ist das Foramen apicale stationar? Dtsch Monats F Zahnk 1927;45:1016.
28. Pucci FM, Reig R. Conductos radiculares. Vol 1. Montevideo (Uruguay): Casa A. Barreiro y Ramos S.A.; 1944.
29. Green D. Stereomicroscopic study of 700 root apices of maxillary and mandibular posterior teeth. Oral Surg 1960;13:728.
30. Green D. A stereomicroscopic study of the root apices of 400 maxillary and mandibular anterior teeth. Oral Surg 1956;9:1224.
31. Kuttler Y. Microscopic investigation of root apices. J Am Dent Assoc 1955;50:544.
32. Kramer IRH. The vascular architecture of the human dental pulp. Arch Oral Biol 1960;2:177.
33. Burch JG, Hulen S. A study of the presence of accessory foramina and the topography of molar furcations. Oral Surg 1974;38:451.
34. Vertucci FJ, Anthony R. A scanning electron microscopic investigation of accessory foramina in the furcation and pulp chamber floor of molar teeth. Oral Surg 1986;62:319.
35. Lowman JV, Burke RS, Pellen GV. Patent accessory canals: incidence in molar furcation region. Oral Surg 1973;36:580.
36. Perlich MA, Reader A, Foreman DW. A scanning electron microscopic investigation of accessory foramens on the pulpal floor of human molars. JOE 1981;7:402.
37. Vertucci FJ, Williams RG. Furcation canals in the human mandibular first molar. Oral Surg 1974;38:308.
38. Gutmann JL. Prevalence, location and patency of accessory canals in the furcation region of permanent molars. J Periodontol 1978;49:21.
39. Cappuccino CC, Sheehan RF. The biology of the dental pulp. In: Shaw JH, Sweeney EA, Cappuccino CC, Meller SM, editors. Textbook of oral biology. Philadelphia: WB Saunders; 1978.
40. Avery JK. Structural elements of the young and normal human pulp. Oral Surg 1971;32:113.
41. Zach I, Topal R, Cohen G. Pulpal repair following operative procedure: radioautographic demonstration with tritiated thymidine. Oral Surg 1969;28:587.
42. Frank RM. Etude autoradiographique de la dentinogenèse en microscopie électronique à l'aide de la proline tritiée chez le chat. Arch Oral Biol 1970;15:583.
43. Baume LJ. The biology of pulp and dentin. A historic, terminologicotaxonomic, histologic-biochemical, embryonic and clinical survey. Monographs in oral science. Myers HM, Karger S, editors. New York, 1980;8:69–123.
44. Han SS. The fine structure of cells and intercellular substance in the dental pulp. In: Finn SB, editor. Biology of the dental pulp organ. Birmingham (AL): University of Alabama Press; 1968.
45. Weinstock M, Leblond CP. Synthesis, migration and release of precursor collagen odontoblasts as visualized by radioautography after ^{3}H-proline administration. J Cell Biol 1974;60:92.
46. Torneck CD. Intracellular destruction of collagen in the human dental pulp. Arch Oral Biol 1978;23:745.
47. Stanley HR. The cells of the dental pulp. Oral Surg 1962; 15:839.
48. Watts A, Paterson RC. Migration of materials and microorganisms in the dental pulp of dogs and rats. JOE 1982;8:53.
49. Jontell M, Bergenholtz G, Scheynius A, Ambrose W. Dendritic cells and macrophages expressing class II antigens in the normal rat incisor pulp. J Dent Res 1988;67:1263.
50. Kogushi M, Nakamura S, Kishi Y, et al. A study of leukocyte extravasation in early inflammatory changes in the pulp. JOE 1988;14:475.
51. Miller GS, Sternberg RN, Pilrero SJ, Rosenberg PA. Histologic identification of mast cells in human dental pulp. Oral Surg 1978;46:559.
52. Zachrisson BU. Mast cells in human dental pulp. Arch Oral Biol 1971;16:555.
53. Farnoush A. Mast cells in human dental pulp. JOE 1984;10:250.
54. Gartner LP, Siebel W, Hiatt JL, Provenza DV. A fine structural analysis of mouse molar odontoblast maturation. Acta Anat 1979;103:16.
55. Garant PR. Microanatomy of the oral mineralized tissues. In: Shaw JH, Sweeney EA, Cappuccino CC, Meller SM, editors. Textbook of oral biology. Philadelphia: WB Saunders; 1968. p. 181.
56. Eisenmann DR, Glick PL. Ultrastructure of initial crystal formation in dentin. J Ultrastruc Res 1972;41:18.
57. Katchburian E. Membrane-bound bodies as initiators of mineralization of dentine. J Anat 1973;116:285.
58. Weinstock A. Matrix development in mineralizing tissues as shown by radioautography: formation of enamel and dentin. In: Slavkin HC, Bavetta LA, editors. Developmental aspects of oral biology. New York: Academic Press; 1972.
59. Weinstock M, Leblond CP. Radioautographic visualization of a phosphoprotein at the mineralization front in the rat incisor. J Cell Biol 1973;56:838.
60. Holland GR. The odontoblast process: form and function. J Dent Res 1985;64:499.
61. Grosdenovic-Selecki S, Qvist V, Hansen HP. Histologic variations in the pulp of intact premolars from young individuals. Scand J Dent Res 1973;81:433.
62. Seltzer S, Bender IB. The dental pulp: biologic considerations in dental procedures. 2nd ed. Philadelphia: JB Lippincott Co.; 1975. p. 48.
63. Jean A, Kerebel B, Kerebel L-M. Scanning electron microscope study of the predentin-pulpal border zone in human dentin. Oral Surg 1986;61:392.
64. Marion D, Jean A, Hamel H, et al. Scanning electron microscope study of odontoblasts and circum-pulpal dentin in a human tooth. Oral Surg 1991;72:473.
65. Forsell-Ahlberg K, Brännström M, Edwall L. The diameter and number of dentinal tubules in rat, cat, dog and monkey. A comparative scanning electron microscopic study. Acta Odontol Scand 1975;33:243.

66. Avery JK. In: Bhaskar SM, editor. Orban's oral histology and embryology. 9th ed. St. Louis: CV Mosby; 1980. p. 108.
67. Tsatsas BG, Frank RM. Ultrastructure of the dentinal tubular substances near the dentino-enamel junction. Calcif Tissue Res 1972;9:238.
68. Holland GR. The extent of odontoblastic process in the cat. J Anat 1976;121:133.
69. Brännström M, Garberoglio R. The dentinal tubules and the odontoblast processes. A scanning electron microscopic study. Acta Odontol Scand 1972;30:29.
70. Thomas HF. The extent of the odontoblastic process in human dentin. J Dent Res 1979;58:2207.
71. Maniatopoulos C, Smith DC. A scanning electron microscopic study of the odontoblastic process in human coronal dentine. Arch Oral Biol 1984;28:701.
72. Sigel MJ, Aubin JE, Ten Cate AR. An immunocyto-chemical study of the human odontoblast process using antibodies against tubulin, actin and vimentin. J Dent Res 1985; 64:1348.
73. Thomas HF, Payne RC. The ultrastructure of dentinal tubules from erupted human premolar teeth. J Dent Res 1983; 62:532.
74. Thomas HF, Carella P. Correlation of scanning and transmission electron microscopy of human dentinal tubules. Arch Oral Biol 1984;29:641.
75. Thomas HF. The dentin-predentin complex and its permeability: anatomic overview. J Dent Res 1985;64:607.
76. Weber DF, Zaki AE. Scanning and transmission electron microscopy of tubular structures presumed to be human odontoblast processes. J Dent Res 1986;65:982.
77. LaFleche RG, Frank RM, Steuer P. The extent of the human odontoblast process as determined by transmission electron microscopy: the hypothesis of a retractable suspensor system. J Biol Buccale 1985;13:293.
78. Nalbandian A, Gonzales F, Sognnaes RF. Sclerotic changes in root dentin of human teeth as observed by optical, electron and x-ray microscope. J Dent Res 1960;39:598.
79. Johansen E, Parks HF. Electron-microscopic observations on sound human dentine. Arch Oral Biol 1962;7:185.
80. Mjor IA. Dentin-predentin complex and its permeability: pathology and treatment overview. J Dent Res 1985;64:621.
81. Tronstad L. Scanning electron microscopy of attrited dentinal surfaces and subjacent dentin in human teeth. Scand J Dent Res 1973;81:112.
82. Mendis BRRM, Darling AI. A scanning electron microscopic and microradiographic study of human coronal dentinal tubules related to occlusal attrition and caries. Arch Oral Biol 1979;24:725.
83. Brännström M, Garberoglio R. Occlusion of dentinal tubules under superficial attrited dentin. Swed Dent J 1980;4:87.
84. Dai XF, Ten Cate AR, Limeback H. The extent and distribution of intratubular collagen fibers in human dentine. Arch Oral Biol 1991;36:775.
85. Griffin CJ, Harris R. Ultrastructure of collagen fibrils and fibroblasts of the developing human dental pulp. Arch Oral Biol 1966;11:656.
86. Barbanell RL, Lian JB, Keith DA. Structural proteins of the connective tissues. In: Shaw JH, Sweeney EA, Cappuccino CC, Meller SM, editors. Textbook of oral biology. Philadelphia: WB Saunders; 1978. p. 419.
87. Bernick S. Lymphatic vessels of the human dental pulp. J Dent Res 1977;56:70.
88. Ten Cate R. A fine structural study of coronal and root dentino-genesis in the mouse; observations on the so-called 'Von Korff fibers' and their contribution to mantle dentine. J Anat 1978;125:183.
89. Embery G. Glycosaminoglycans of human dental pulp. J Biol Buccale 1976;4:229.
90. Torneck CD. In: Ten Cate AR, editor. Dentin-pulp complex. Oral histology. Toronto: CV Mosby Co., 1980, p. 169.
91. Zerlotti E. Histochemical study of the connective tissue of the dental pulp. Arch Oral Biol 1964;9:149.
92. Boling LR. Blood vessels of the dental pulp. Anat Rec 1942;82:25.
93. Cutright DE, Bhaskar SN. A new method of demonstrating microvasculature. Oral Surg 1967;24:422.
94. Cutright DE, Bhaskar SN. Pulpal vasculature as demonstrated by a new method. Oral Surg 1969;27:678.
95. Takahashi K, Kishi V, Kim S. A scanning electron microscope study of the blood vessels of dog pulp using corrosion resin casts. JOE 1982;8:131.
96. Kim S, et al. Arteriovenous distribution of hemodynamic parameters in the rat dental pulp. Microvasc Res 1984;27:28.
97. Harris R, Griffin CJ. The ultrastructure of small blood vessels of the normal dental pulp. Aust Dent J 1971;16:220.
98. Dahl E, Mjor IA. The fine structure of the vessels in the human dental pulp. Acta Odontol Scand 1973;31:223.
99. Harris R, Griffin CJ. The fine structure of the mature odontoblasts and cell rich zone of the human dental pulp. Aust Dent J 1969;14:168.
100. Avery JK. Repair potential of the pulp. JOE 1981;7:205.
101. Rapp R, et al. Ultrastructure of fenestrated capillaries in human dental pulps. Arch Oral Biol 1977;22:317.
102. Ekblom A, Hansson P. A thin-section and freeze fracture study of the pulp blood vessels in feline and human teeth. Arch Oral Biol 1984;29:413.
103. Kim S, Dorscher-Kim J, Liu MT, Trowbridge HO. Biphasic pulp blood flow response in the dog as measured with a radiolabelled microsphere injection method. Arch Oral Biol 1988;33:305.
104. Isokava S. Uber das lymph System des Zahnes. Z Zellforsch 1960;52:140.
105. Kilhara T. Das extravaskulare Saftbahn system. Okajimas Folia Anat Jpn 1956;28:601.
106. Riedel H, et al. Elektronenmikroskopische Untersuchunger zur Frage der Kapillarmorphologie in der menschlichen Zahnpulpa. Arch Oral Biol 1966;11:1049.
107. Frank RM, Wiedermann P, Fellingeret E. Ultrastructure of lymphatic capillaries in the human dental pulp. Cell Tissue Res 1977;178:229.
108. Walton RE, Langeland K. Migration of materials in the dental pulp of monkeys. JOE 1978;4:167.
109. Stein JB. A study of the maxillae with regard to their blood and lymph supply. VI, Items of Interest (Dental) 1919;31:81.
110. Stein JB. A study of the maxillae with regard to their blood and lymph supply. VIII, Items of Interest (Dental) 1919;31:401.
111. MacGregor A. An experimental investigation of the lymphatic system of the teeth and jaws. Proc R Soc Med 1936;29:1237.
112. Dewey KW, Noyes FB. A study of the lymphatic vessels of the dental pulp. Dent Cosmos 1917;59:436.
113. Ruben MR, et al. Visualization of the lymphatic microcirculation of oral tissues: vital retrograde lymphography. J Periodontol 1971;42:774.

114. Levy BM, Bernick S. Studies on the biology of the periodontium of marmosets. Lymphatic vessels of the periodontal ligament. J Dent Res 1968;47:1166.
115. Path MG, Meyer M. Heterogeneity of blood flow in the canine tooth of the dog. Arch Oral Biol 1980;25:83.
116. Kim S, et al. Anatomical and functional heterogeneity of microcirculation in the dental pulp. Int J Microcir 1984;3:407.
117. Feiglin B, Reade PC. Arteriovenous shunts demonstrated in the apical circulation of rat incisor teeth by the use of radio-labeled microspheres. Oral Surg 1979;47:364.
118. Maul GG. Structure and formation of pores in fenestrated capillaries. J Ultrastruc Res 1971;36:768.
119. Kraintz L, et al. Lymphatic drainage of teeth in dogs demonstrated by radioactive colloid gold. J Dent Res 1959;38:198.
120. Barnes GW, Langeland K. Antibody formation in primates following introduction of antigens into the root canal. J Dent Res 1966;45:1111.
121. Smith GN, Walton RE. Periodontal ligament injection: distribution of the injected solutions. Oral Surg 1983;55:232.
122. Walton RE. Distribution of solutions with the periodontal ligament injection: clinical, anatomical and histological evidence. JOE 1986;12:492.
123. Johnsen D, Johns D. Quantitation of nerve fibers in the primary and permanent canine and incisor teeth in man. Arch Oral Biol 1978;23:825.
124. Johnson DC. Innervation of teeth: qualitative, quantitative and developmental assessment. J Dent Res 1985;64:555.
125. Hirvonen TJ. A quantitative electron microscopic analysis of the axons at the apex of the canine tooth pulp in the dog. Acta Anatomica 1987;128:134.
126. Edwall L, Kindlova M. The effect of sympathetic nerve stimulation on the rate of disappearance of tracers from various oral tissues. Acta Odont Scand 1971;29:387.
127. Tönder KH, Naess G. Nervous control of blood flow in the dental pulp in dogs. Acta Physiol Scand 1978;104:13.
128. Byers MR, Närhi MVO, Mecifi KB. Acute and chronic reactions of dental sensory nerve fibers to cavities and desiccation in rat molars. Anat Rec 1988;221:872.
129. Avery JK. Anatomic considerations in the mechanism of pain and sensitivity. In: Chasens AI, Kaslick RS, editors. The teeth and supporting structures. East Brunswick (NJ): Fairleigh Dickinson University; 1974. p. 16.
130. Byers MR. Terminal aborization of individual sensory axons in dentin and pulp of rat molars. Brain Res 1985;345:181.
131. Taylor PE, Byers MR, Redd PE. Sprouting of CGRP nerve fibers in response to dentin injury in rat molars. Brain Res 1988;461:371.
132. Arwill T. Studies on the ultrastructure of dental tissue. II. The predentin-pulp border zone. Odontol Rev 1967;18:191.
133. Frank RM. Attachment sites between the odontoblast, process and intradentinal nerve fibers. Arch Oral Biol 1968;13:833.
134. Arwill T, Edwall L, Lilja J, et al. Ultrastructure of nerves in the dentinal-pulp border zone after sensory and autonomic nerve transsection in the cat. Acta Odontol Scand 1973;31:273.
135. Dahl E, Mjor IA. The structure and distribution of nerves in the pulp-dentin organ. Acta Odontol Scand 1973;31:349.
136. Holland GR. The effect of nerve section on the incidence and distribution of gap junctions in the odontoblast layer of the cat. Anat Rec 1987;218:458.
137. Van Hassel HJ, McMinn RG. Pressure differential favouring tooth eruption in the dog. Arch Oral Biol 1972;17:183.
138. Edwall B, et al. Neuropeptide Y (NPY) and sympathetic control of blood flow in oral mucosa and dental pulp in the cat. Acta Physiol Scand 1985;125:253.
139. Olgart LM. The role of local factors in dentin and pulp in intradental pain mechanisms. J Dent Res 1985;64:572.
140. Kim S. Neurovascular interactions in the dental pulp in health and inflammation. JOE 1990;16:48.
141. Fearnhead RW. The neurohistology of human dentin. Proc R Soc Med 1961;54:877.
142. Bernick S. Differences in nerve distribution between erupted and non-erupted human teeth. J Dent Res 1964;43:406.
143. Byers MR. Development of sensory innervation in dentin. J Comp Neurol 1980;191:413.
144. Byers MR. Dental sensory receptors. Int Rev Neurobiol 1984;25:39.
145. Johnsen DC, Karlsson UL. Electron microscopic quantitations of feline primary and permanent incisor innervation. Arch Oral Biol 1974;19:671.
146. Lilja J. Sensory differences between crown and root dentin in human teeth. Acta Odontol Scand 1980;38:285.
147. Westrum LE, Canfield RB, Black RG. Transganglionic degeneration in the spinal trigeminal nucleus following removal of tooth pulps in adult cats. Brain Res 1976;101:137.
148. Bernick S. Vascular and nerve changes associated with healing of the human pulp. Oral Surg 1971;33:983.
149. Foreman PC. Micromorphology of mineralized deposits in the pulps of human teeth. Int Endodont J 1984;17:183.
150. Moss-Salentijn L, Hendricks-Klyvert M. Calcified structures in human dental pulps. JOE 1988;14:184.
151. Hall DC. Pulpal calcifications—a pathologic process? In: Symons NBB, editors. Dentine and pulp: their structure and function. Symposium at the Dental School, University of Dundee. Edinburgh-London: E. & S. Livingston; 1968. p. 269.
152. Langeland K. Tissue changes in the dental pulp. An experimental histological study. Odontol Rev 1957;65:239.
153. Johnson PL, Bevelander G. Histogenesis and histochemistry of pulp calcification. J Dent Res 1956;35:714.
154. Appleton J, Williams MJR. Ultrastructural observations on the calcification of human dental pulp. Calcif Tissue Res 1973;11:222.
155. Bernick S. Effects of aging on the human pulp. JOE 1975;1:88.
156. Langeland K. The histopathologic basis in endodontic treatment. Dent Clin North Am 1967;491.
157. Plackova A, Vah J. Ultrastructure of mineralizations in the human pulp. Caries Res 1974;8:172.
158. Tidmarsh BG. Micromorphology of molar pulp chambers [abstract]. J Dent Res 1979;59:1873.
159. Frohlich E. Altersveranderungen der Pulpa und des Parodontiums. Dtsch Zahnerztl Z 1970;25:175.
160. Stanley HR, Ranney RR. Age changes in the human dental pulp: the quantity of collagen. Oral Surg 1962;15:1396.
161. Bernick S. Effects of aging on the nerve supply to human teeth. J Dent Res 1967;46:694.
162. Buczko W, et al. Biological effects of degradation products of collagen by bacterial collagenase. Br J Pharmacol 1980;69:551.
163. Wisniewski K, et al. The effects of products of fibrinogen digestion by plasmin (P-FDP) on the central nervous system. Acta Neurobiol Exp 1975;35:275.

164. Matsen FA. Compartmental syndrome. Clin Orthop 1975;113:8.
165. Romanus EM, et al. Pressure-induced ischemia. Part I. An experimental model for intravital microscopic studies in hamster cheek pouch. Eur Surg Res 1977;9:444.
166. Reneman RS, et al. Muscle blood flow disturbances produced by simultaneously elevated venous and total muscle tissue pressure. Microvasc Res 1980;10:307.
167. Van Hassel HJ. Physiology of the human dental pulp. Oral Surg 1971;32:126.
168. Nahri M. Activation of dental pulp nerves of the cat and the dog with hydrostatic pressure. Proc Finn Dent Soc 1978; Suppl V:1.
169. Tönder K, Kvinnsland I. Micropuncture measurements of interstitial fluid pressure in normal and inflamed dental pulp in cat. JOE 1983;9:105.
170. Kimberly CL, Byers MR. Inflammation of rat molar pulp and periodontium causes increased calcitonin gene-related peptide and axonal sprouting. Anat Res 1988;222:289.
171. Khayat B, Byers MR, et al. Response of nerve fibers to pulpal inflammation and periapical lesions in rat molars demonstrated by CGRP immunocytochemistry. JOE 1988;14:577.
172. Fish EW. The physiology of dentine and its reaction to injury and disease. Br Dent J 1928;49:593.
173. Pashley DH, Kehl T, Pashley E, Palmer P. Comparison of *in vitro* and *in vivo* dog dentin permeability. J Dent Res 1981;60:763.
174. Ketterl W. Studie uber das Dentin der permanenten Zahne des Menschen. Stoma 1961;14:79.
175. Garberoglio R, Brännström M. Scanning electron microscopic investigation of human dentinal tubules. Arch Oral Biol 1976;21:355.
176. Coffey CT, Ingram MJ, Bjorndal A. Analysis of human dentinal fluid. Oral Surg 1970;30:835.
177. Bergenholtz, G.: Effect of bacterial products on inflammatory reactions in the dental pulp. Scand J Dent Res 1977;85:122.
178. Walton R, Outhwaite WC, Pashley DH. Magnification—an interesting optical property of dentin. J Dent Res 1976;55:639.
179. Outhwaite W, Livingston M, Pashley DH. Effects of changes in surface area, thickness, temperature and post-extraction time on dentine permeability. Arch Oral Biol 1976;21:599.
180. Reeder OW, Walton RE, Livingston MJ, Pashley DH. Dentin permeability: determinants of hydraulic conductance. J Dent Res 1978;57:187.
181. Craig RG, Gehring PE, Peyton FA. Relation of structure to the microhardness of human dentin. J Dent Res 1959;38:624.
182. Fusayama T, Okuse K, Hosoda H. Relationship between hardness, discoloration and microbial invasion of carious dentin. J Dent Res 1966;45:1033.
183. Pashley DH, Okabe A, Parham P. The relationship between dentin microhardness and tubule density. Endod Dent Traumatol 1985;1:176.
184. Pashley DH. The influence of dentin permeability and pulpal blood flow on pulpal solute concentration. JOE 1979;5:355.
185. Stanley HR. The factors of age and tooth size in human pulpal reactions. Oral Surg 1961;14:498.
186. Pashley DH. Dentin-predentin complex and its permeability: physiologic overview. J Dent Res 1985;64:613.
187. Fogel H, Marshall FJ, Pashley DH. Effect of distance from the pulp and thickness on the hydraulic conductance of human radicular dentin. J Dent Res 1988;67:1381.
188. Pashley DH, Kepler EE, Williams EC, O'Meara JA. The effect of dentine permeability of time following cavity preparation in dogs. Arch Oral Biol 1984;29:65.
189. Pashley DH, Galloway SE, Stewart FP. Effects of fibrinogen in vivo on dentine permeability in the dog. Arch Oral Biol 1984;29:725.
190. Johnson G, Brännström M. The sensivity of dentin: changes in relation to conditions at exposed tubules apertures. Acta Odontol Scand 1974;32:29.
191. Pashley DH, Livingston MJ, Reeder OW, Horner J. Effects of the degree of tubule occlusion on the permeability of human dentin, in vitro. Arch Oral Biol 1978;23:1127.
192. Pashley DH, Tao L, Boyd L, et al. Scanning electron microscopy of the substructure of smear layers in human dentine. Arch Oral Biol 1988;33:265.
193. Pashley DH. The smear layer: physiological considerations. Oper Dent 1984;Suppl 3:13.
194. Olgart L, Brännström M, Johnson G. Invasion of bacteria into dentinal tubules. Experiments in vivo and in vitro. Acta Odontol Scand 1974;32:61.
195. Michelich VJ, Schuster GS, Pashley DH. Bacterial penetration of human dentin, in vitro. J Dent Res 1980;59:1398.
196. Brännström M. Dentin and pulp in restorative dentistry. 1st ed. Nacka (Sweden): Dental Therapeutics AB; 1981.
197. Dippel HW, et al. Morphology and permeability of the dentinal smear layer. J Prosthet Dent 1984;52:657.
198. Pashley DH, Michelich V, Kehl T. Dentin permeability: effects of smear layer removal. J Prosthet Dent 1981;46:531.
199. Goldman LB, Goldman M, Kronman JH, Lin PS. The efficacy of several irrigating solutions for endodontics: a scanning electron microscopic study. Oral Surg 1981;52:197.
200. Goldman M, DeVitre R, Pier M. Effect of the dentin smeared layer on tensile strength of cemented posts. J Prosthet Dent 1984;52:485.
201. Biesterfeld RC, et al. The significance of alterations of pulpal respiration. A review of literature. J Oral Pathol 1979;8:129.
202. Fisher AK, et al. The effects of dental drugs and materials on the rate of oxygen consumption in bovine dental pulp. J Dent Res 1957;36:447.
203. Shalla CI, Fisher AK. Influence of hydrogen ion concentrations on oxygen consumption in bovine dental pulp. J Dent Res 1970;49:1154.
204. Fisher AK, Walters VE. Anaerobic glycolysis in bovine dental pulp. J Dent Res 1968;47:717.
205. Taintor JF, Shalla C. Comparison of respiration rates in different zones of rat incisor pulp. J Dent 1978;6:63.
206. Jones PA, et al. Comparative dental material cytotoxicity measured by depression of rat incisor pulp respiration. JOE 1979;5:48.
207. Hamersky PA, et al. The effect of orthodontic force application on the pulpal tissue respiration rate in the human premolar. Am J Orthod 1980;77:368.
208. Vallé GF, et al. The effect of varying liquid-to-powder in zinc oxide and eugenol of pulpal respiration. JOE 1980;6:400.
209. Hume WR. Effect of eugenol on respiration and division of human pulp, mouse fibroblasts and liver cells in vitro. J Dent Res 1984;63:1262.
210. Hume WR. The pharmacologic and toxicological properties of zinc oxide eugenol. J Am Dent Assoc 1986;113:789.

211. Hashimoto S, et al. In vivo and in vitro effects of zinc oxide-eugenol (ZOE) on biosynthesis of cyclo-oxygenase products in rat dental pulp. J Dent Res 1988;67:1092.
212. Mjor IA, Tronstad L. Experimentally induced pulpitis. Oral Surg 1972;34:102.
213. Bergenholtz G. Inflammatory response of the dental pulp to bacterial irritation. JOE 1981;7:100.
214. Warfringe J, Dahlen G, Bergenholtz G. Dental pulp response to bacterial cell wall material. J Dent Res 1985;64:1046.
215. Kraintz L, Conroy CW. Blood volume measurements of dog teeth. J Dent Res 1960;39:1033.
216. Kraintz L, et al. Blood volume determination of human dental pulp. J Dent Res 1980;59:544.
217. Pohto M, Scheinin A. Effects of local anesthetic solutions on the circulation of the pulp in rat incisor. Bibl Anat 1960;1:46.
218. Scheinin A. Flow characteristics of the pulpal vessels. J Dent Res 1963;438 Suppl 2:411.
219. Scott D, Scheinin A, Karjalainen S, Edwall L. Influence of sympathetic nerve stimulation on flow velocity in pulpal vessels. Acta Odontol Scand 1972;30:277.
220. Taylor AC. Microscopic observation of the living tooth pulp. Science 1950;111:40.
221. Meyer M, et al. Blood flow in the dental pulp. Proc Soc Exp Biol Med 1964;116:1038.
222. Ogilvie RW, et al. Physiologic evidence for the presence of vasoconstrictor fibers in the dental pulp. J Dent Res 1966;45:980.
223. Ogilvie RW. Direct observations of the cat dental pulp microvascular response to electrical and drug stimuli. Anat Rec 1967;157:379.
224. Edwall L, Kindlova M. The effect of sympathetic nerve stimulation on the rate of disappearance of tracers from various oral tissues. Acta Odontol Scand 1971;29:387.
225. Edwall L, Scott D. Influence of changes in microcirculation on the excitability of the sensory unit in the tooth of the cat. Acta Physiol Scand 1971;85:555.
226. Tönder KH. The effect of variations in arterial blood pressure and baroreceptor reflexes on pulpal blood flow in dogs. Arch Oral Biol 1975;20:345.
227. Ahlberg KF, Edwall L. Influence of local insults on sympathetic vasoconstrictor control in the feline dental pulp. Acta Odontol Scand 1977;35:103.
228. Olgart L, Gaelius B. Effects of adrenalin and elypressin (octapressin) on blood flow and sensory nerve activity in the tooth. Acta Odontol Scand 1977;35:69.
229. Tönder KH, Naess G. Nervous control of blood flow in the dental pulp in dogs. Acta Physiol Scand 1978;104:13.
230. Kim S. Microcirculation of the dental pulp in health and disease. JOE 1985;11:465.
231. DelBalso AM, et al. The effects of thermal and electrical injury on pulpal histamine levels. Oral Surg 1976;41:110.
232. Olgart L, Gazelius B, Brodin E, Nilsson G. Release of substance P-like immunoreactivity from the dental pulp. Acta Physiol Scand 1977;101:510.
233. Brodin E, Gazelius B, Lundberg JM, Olgart L. Substance P in trigeminal nerve endings: Occurrence and release. Acta Physiol Scand 1981;111:501.
234. Brodin E, Gazelius B, Panopoulos P, Olgart L. Morphine inhibits substance P release from peripheral sensory nerve endings. Acta Physiol Scand 1983;117:567.
235. Wakisaka S, et al. Immunohistochemical study on regeneration of substance P-like immunoreactivity in rat molar pulp and periodontal ligament following resection of the inferior alveolar nerve. Arch Oral Biol 1987;32:225.
236. Edwall L. Regulation of pulpal blood flow. JOE 1980;6:434.
237. Inoki R, et al. Elaboration of a bradykinin-like substance in dog's canine pulp during electrical stimulation and its inhibition by narcotic and non-narcotic analgesics. Naunyn Schmiedebergs' Arch Pharmacol 1973;279:387.
238. Okamura K, et al. Serum proteins and secretory component in human carious dentin. J Dent Res 1979;58:1127.
239. Okamura K, et al. Dentinal response against carious invasion: localization of antibodies in odontoblastic body and process. J Dent Res 1980;59:1368.
240. Pashley DH, Nelson R, Williams EC, Kepler EE. Use of dentine-fluid protein concentrations to measure pulp capillary reflection coefficients in dogs. Arch Oral Biol 1981;26:703.
241. Stenvik A, Iversion J, Mjor IA. Tissue pressure and histology of normal and inflamed tooth pulps in macaque monkeys. Arch Oral Biol 1972;17:1501.
242. Kim S, Trowbridge H, Kim B, Chien S. Effects of bradykinin on pulpal blood flow in dogs. J Dent Res 1982;61:1036.
243. Heyeraas KJ. Pulpal microvascular and tissue pressure. J Dent Res 1985;64:585.
244. Weatherred JG, Kroeger DC, Smith EL. Pressure response in dental pulp to inferior alveolar nerve stimulation. Fed Proc 1963;22:756.
245. Wynn W, et al. Pressure within the pulp chamber of the dog's tooth relative to arterial pressure. J Dent Res 1963;42:11.
246. Brown AC, Yankowitz D. Tooth pulp tissue pressure and hydraulic permeability. Circ Res 1964; 15:42.
247. Beveridge EE, Brown AC. The measurement of human dental intrapulpal pressure and its response to clinical variables. Oral Surg 1965;19:655.
248. Brown AC, Beveridge EE. The relationship between tooth pressure and systemic arterial pressure. Arch Oral Biol 1966;11:1181.
249. Christiansen RL, Meyer MW, Visscher MD. Tonometric measurement of dental pulpal and mandibular marrow blood pressures. J Dent Res 1977;56:635.
250. Ciucchi B, Bouillaguets S, Holz J, Pashley DH. In vivo estimation of pulp pressure in humans. J Dent Res 1993;72:1359.
251. Meyer MW, Path MG. Blood flow in the dental pulp in dogs determined by hydrogen polarography and radioactive microsphere methods. Arch Oral Biol 1979;24:601.
252. Meyer MW. Methodologies for studying pulpal hemodynamics. JOE 1980;6:466.
253. Gazelius B, Olgart L, Edwall B, Edwall L. Noninvasive recording of blood flow in human dental pulp. Endodont Dent Traumatol 1986;2:219.
254. Trope M, Jaggi J, Barnett F, Trontad L. Vitality testing of teeth with a radiation probe using ^{133}xenon radioisotope. Endodont Dent Traumatol 1986;2:215.
255. Rowe NH, editor. Hypersensitive dentin: origin and management. Ann Arbor (MI): University of Michigan; 1985.
256. Tronstad L, editor. Symposium on dentinal hypersensitivity. Endodont Dent Traumatol 1986;2:124.
257. Rapp R, Avery JK, Strachan D. The distribution of nerves in human primary teeth. Anat Rec 1967;159:89.
258. Anderson DJ, et al. Sensory mechanisms in mammalian teeth and their supporting structures. Physiol Rev 1970;50:171.

259. Brännström M. Sensitivity of dentin. Oral Surg 1966;21:517.
260. Brännström M, et al. The hydrodynamics of the dentinal tubule and of pulp fluid. A discussion of its significance in relation to dentinal sensitivity. Caries Res 1967;1:310.
261. Garant PR. The organization of microtubules within rat odontoblast processes revealed by perfusion fixation with glutaraldehyde. Arch Oral Biol 1972;17:1047.
262. Holland GR. The dentinal tubules and the odontoblast process in the cat. J Anat 1975;120:169.
263. Greenhill JD, Pashley DH. The effects of desensitizing agents on the hydraulic conductance of human dentin, in vitro. J Dent Res 1981;60:686.
264. Nahri MVO. Dentin sensitivity: a review. J Biol Buccale 1985;13:75.
265. Pashley DH. Dentine permeability, dentine sensitivity and treatment through tubule occlusion. JOE 1986;12:465.
266. Kim S, et al. Effects of change in systemic hemodynamic parameters on pulpal hemodynamics. JOE 1980;6:394.
267. Kim S. Regulation of pulpal blood flow. J Dent Res 1985;64:590.
268. deDeus QD, Hans SS. The fate of ^{3}H-cortisone applied on the exposed dental pulp. Oral Surg 1967;24:404.
269. Page PO, Trump GN, Schaeffer LD. Pulpal studies. I. Passage of ^{3}H-tetracycline into circulatory system through rat molar pulps. Oral Surg 1973;35:555.
270. Oswald RJ, Cohen SA. Systemic distribution of lead from root canal fillings. JOE 1975;1:59.
271 Chong R, Senzer J. Systemic distribution of ^{201}PbO from root canal fillings. JOE 1976;2:301.
272. Myers DR, Shoaf HK, Dirksen TR, et al. Distribution of ^{14}C-formaldehyde after pulpotomy with formocresol. J Am Dent Assoc 1978;96:805.
273. Pashley EL, Myers DR, Pashley DH, Whitford GM. Systemic distribution of ^{14}C-formaldehyde from formocresol-treated pulpotomy sites. J Dent Res 1980;59:603.
274. Ranley DM. Assessment of the systemic distribution and toxicity of formaldehyde following pulpotomy treatment: part one. J Dent Child 1985;52:431.
275. Ranley DM, Horn D. Assessment of the systemic distribution and toxicity of formaldehyde following pulpotomy treatment: part two. J Dent Child 1987;54:40.
276. Myers DR, Pashley DH, Lake FT, et al. Systemic absorption of ^{14}C-glutaraldehyde from glutaraldehyde-treated pulpotomy sites. Pediatr Dent 1986;8:134.
277. Ranley DM, Horn D, Hubbard JB. Assessment of the systemic distribution and toxicity of glutaraldehyde as a pulpotomy agent. J Pediatr Dent 1989;11:8.
278. Fager FK, Messer HH. Systemic distribution of camphorated monochlorophenol from cotton pellets sealed in pulp chambers. JOE 1986;12:225.
279. Noyes FB, Ladd RL. The lymphatics of the dental region. Dent Cosmos 1929;71:1041.
280. Feiglin B, Reade PC. The distribution of ^{14}C-leucine and ^{85}Sr microspheres from rat incisor root canals. Oral Surg 1979;47:277.
281. Lindskog S, Blomlöf L, Hammarström L. Evidence for a role of odontogenic epithelium in maintaining the periodontal space. J Clin Periodontol 1988;15:371.

Chapter 3

MICROBIOLOGY OF ENDODONTICS AND ASEPSIS IN ENDODONTIC PRACTICE

J. Craig Baumgartner, Leif K. Bakland, and Eugene I. Sugita

Microorganisms cause virtually all pathoses of the pulp and the periradicular tissues. To effectively treat endodontic infections, clinicians must recognize the cause and effect of microbial invasion of the dental pulp space and the surrounding periradicular tissues. Once bacterial invasion of pulp tissues has taken place, both nonspecific inflammation and specific immunologic response of the host have a profound effect on the progress of the disease. Knowledge of the microorganisms associated with endodontic disease is necessary to develop a basic understanding of the disease process and a sound rationale for effective management of patients with endodontic infections. Although the vast majority of our knowledge deals with bacteria, we are now aware of the potential for endodontic disease to be associated with fungi and viruses.[1–4] The topics of this chapter are directed toward the role of microorganisms in the pathogenesis of endodontic disease with recommendations for treatment of endodontic infections. Owing to much recent controversy over the "theory of focal infection," an update on this issue will be presented first.

THEORY OF FOCAL INFECTION REVISITED

In 1890, W. D. Miller associated the presence of bacteria with pulpal and periapical disease. In 1904, F. Billings described a "focus of infection" as a circumscribed area of tissue infected with pathogenic organisms. One of his students was E. C. Rosenow, who in 1909 described the "Theory of Focal Infection" as a **localized or generalized infection caused by bacteria traveling through the bloodstream from a distant focus of infection.** In 1910, a British physician, William Hunter, presented a lecture on the role of sepsis and antisepsis in medicine to the faculty of McGill University. He condemned the practice of dentistry in the United States, which emphasized restorations instead of tooth extraction. Hunter stated that the restorations were "a veritable mausoleum of gold over a mass of sepsis." He believed that this was the cause of Americans' many illnesses, including pale complexion, chronic dyspepsias, intestinal disorders, anemias, and nervous complaints.

Soon pulpless teeth (teeth with necrotic pulps) and endodontically treated teeth were also implicated. Weston Price began a 25-year study on pulpless and endodontically treated teeth and their association with focal infection. With expansion of the theory, many dentists and physicians became "100 Percenters," who recommended the extraction of all pulpless and endodontically treated teeth. The dental literature contained numerous testimonials reporting cures of illnesses following tooth extraction. These reports were empirical and without adequate follow-up. However, they wrongfully supported the continued extraction of teeth without scientific reason. In many cases, the diseases returned, and the patients had to face the additional difficulty of living with mutilated dentitions.

In the 1930s, editorials and research refuted the theory of focal infection and called for a return to constructive rather than destructive dental treatment rationale.[5,6] The studies by Rosenow and Price were flawed by inadequate controls, the use of massive doses of bacteria, and bacterial contamination of endodontically treated teeth during tooth extraction. In 1939, Fish recognized four zones of reaction formed in response to viable bacteria implanted in the jaws of guinea pigs.[7] He described the bacteria as being confined by polymorphonuclear neutrophil leukocytes to a zone of infection. Outside the zone of infection is the zone of contamination containing inflammatory cells but no bacteria. Next, the zone of irritation contained histocytes and osteoclasts. On the outside was a zone of stimulation with mostly fibroblasts, capillary buds, and osteoblasts. Fish theorized that removal of the nidus of infection would lead to resolution of the infection. This theory became the basis for successful root canal treatment

Today the medical and dental professions agree that there is no relationship between endodontically treated teeth and the degenerative diseases implicated in the theory of focal infection. However, a recent book entitled *Root Canal Cover-up Exposed* has resurrected the focal infection theory based on the poorly designed and outdated studies by Rosenow and Price.[8] This body of research has been evaluated and disproved. Unfortunately, uninformed patients may receive this outdated information and believe it to be credible new findings. To further confuse the issue, recent epidemiologic studies have found relationships between periodontal disease and coronary heart disease, strokes, and preterm low birth rate.[9,10] It must be kept in mind that epidemiologic research can identify relationships but not causation. Further research may show that periodontal disease constitutes an oral component of a systemic disorder or has etiologic features in common with medical diseases. They may occur at the same time without necessarily indicating a cause-effect relationship.

Endodontic infections can spread to other tissues. An abscess or cellulitis may develop if bacteria invade periradicular tissues and the patient's immune system is not able to stop the spread of bacteria and bacterial by-products. This type of infection/inflammation spreads directly from one anatomic space to an adjacent space. This is not an example of the theory of focal infection, whereby bacteria travel through the circulatory system and establish an infection at a distant site.

Practitioners are well aware of the relationship between bacteremias caused by dental procedures (especially tooth extraction) and infective endocarditis. This is an example of focal infection that is not related to the classic theory of focal infection. A bacteremia associated with a dental procedure introduces bacteria into the circulation. It does not arise because of the mere presence of an endodontically treated tooth. Studies have shown that the incidence and extent of a bacteremia are related to the amount of bleeding (trauma) produced by a dental procedure.[11–14] These studies have shown that nonsurgical endodontic procedures produce a relatively low incidence of bacteremia when compared to tooth extraction. Simple tooth extraction produces an extensive bacteremia 100% of the time.[12,15] Endodontic therapy should be the treatment of choice instead of tooth extraction for patients believed to be susceptible to infective endocarditis following a bacteremia.

A recent study found the frequency of bacteremia associated with **nonsurgical** root canal instrumentation to be from 31 to 54%.[16] If the endodontic instrument was confined to inside the root canal 1 mm short of the apical foramen, the incidence of bacteremia was 4 in 13 (31%). If the instruments (sizes 15, 20, and 25) were deliberately used to a level 2 mm beyond the apical foramen, the incidence of bacteremia was 7 in 13 (54%). Ribotyping with restriction enzymes showed identical characteristics for the clinical isolates from the root canals and for the bacteria isolated from the blood. This typing method suggests that the microorganisms recovered from the bloodstream during and after endodontic treatment had the root canal as their source. However, to show a causal relationship between an oral infection and systemic disease, it is not adequate to show only a potential relationship via a bacteremia. Hard evidence is needed to show that the organism in the nonoral site of infection actually came from the oral cavity. If possible, Koch's postulates should be fulfilled to establish a causal role of the microorganism from the oral cavity.

Successfully completed root canal therapy should not be confused with an untreated infected root canal system or a tooth with a periradicular abscess that may be a source of bacteremias. In addition, numerous bacteremias occur every day as a result of a patient's normal daily activities. Endodontics has survived the theory of focal infection because of recognition by the scientific community that successful root canal treatment is possible without endangering systemic health.

ENDODONTIC INFECTIONS

Colonization is the establishment of microbes in a host if appropriate biochemical and physical conditions are available for growth. Normal oral flora is the result of a permanent microbial colonization in a symbiotic relationship with the host. Although the microbes in the normal oral flora participate in many beneficial relationships, they are opportunistic pathogens if they gain access to a normally sterile area of the body such as the dental pulp or periradicular tissues and produce disease. The steps in the development of an endodontic infection include microbial invasion, multiplication, and pathogenic activity. Much of the pathogenic activity is associated with host response.

Pathogenicity is a term used to describe the capacity of a microbe to produce disease, whereas virulence describes the degree of pathogenicity. Bacteria have a number of virulence factors that may be associated with disease. They include pili (fimbriae), capsules, extracellular vesicles, lipopolysaccharides, enzymes, short-chain fatty acids, polyamines, and low-molecular-weight products such as ammonia and hydrogen sulfide. Pili may be important for attachment to surfaces and interaction with other bacteria in a polymicrobial infection. Bacteria including gram-negative black-pigmented bacteria (BPB) may have capsules that enable them to avoid or survive phagocytosis.[17]

Lipopolysaccharides are found on the surface of gram-negative bacteria and have numerous biologic effects when released from the cell in the form of **endotoxins.** The endotoxin content in canals of symptomatic teeth with apical rarefactions and exudate is higher than that of asymptomatic teeth.[18] Endotoxins have been associated with periapical inflammation and activation of complement.[19,20]

Enzymes are produced by bacteria that may be spreading factors for infections or proteases that neutralize immunoglobulins and complement components.[21–24] The enzymes in neutrophils that degenerate and lyse to form purulent exudate also have an adverse effect on the surrounding tissues.

Gram-negative bacteria produce **extracellular vesicles** (Figure 3-1). They are formed from the outer membrane and have a trilaminar structure similar to the outer membrane of the parent bacteria. These vesicles may contain enzymes or other toxic chemicals. It is believed that these vesicles are involved in hemagglutination, hemolysis, bacterial adhesion, and proteolytic activities.[25,26] Because these vesicles have the same antigenic determinants on their surface as their parent bacteria, they may protect the bacteria by combining with and neutralizing antibodies that would have reacted with the bacteria.

Anaerobic bacteria commonly produce short-chain fatty acids including propionic, butyric, and isobutyric acids. As virulence factors, these acids may affect neutrophil chemotaxis, degranulation, chemiluminescence, and phagocytosis. **Butyric acid** has been shown to have the greatest inhibition of T-cell blastogenesis and to stimulate the production of interleukin-1, which is associated with bone resorption.[27]

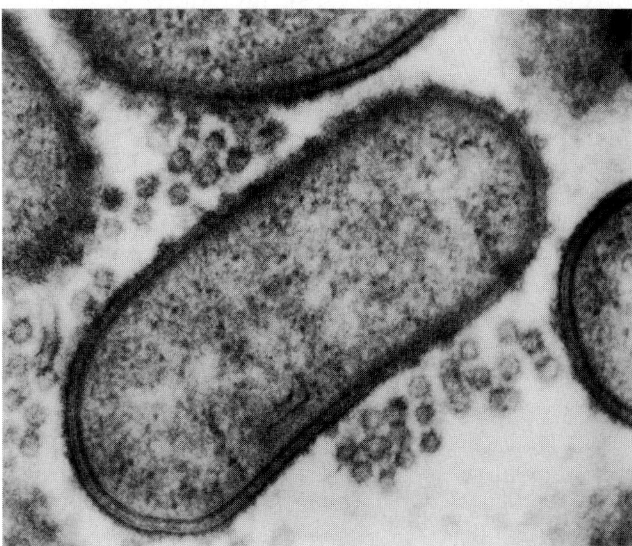

Figure 3-1 Extracellular vesicles are shown between *Prevotella intermedia* cells (×20,000 original magnification).

Polyamines are biologically active chemicals found in infected canals.[28] Bacteria and host cells contain polyamines. Putrescine, cadaverine, spermidine, and spermine are involved in the regulation of cell growth, regeneration of tissues, and modulation of inflammation. The amount of total polyamines and putrescine is higher in the necrotic pulps of teeth that are painful to percussion or with spontaneous pain.[28] When a sinus tract was present, a significantly greater amount of cadaverine was detected in the pulp space.[28] Although some correlations between some virulence factors and clinical signs and symptoms have been shown, an absolute cause and effect relationship has not been proven.

ASSOCIATION OF MICROBES WITH PULPAL DISEASE

Antony van Leewenhoek, the inventor of single-lens microscopes, was the first to observe oral flora.[29] His description of the "animalcules" observed with his microscopes included those from dental plaque and from an exposed pulp cavity. The father of oral microbiology is considered to be W. D. Miller. In 1890, he authored a book, *Microorganisms of the Human Mouth*, which became the basis for dental microbiology in this country. In 1894, Miller became the first researcher to associate the presence of bacteria with pulpal disease.[30]

The true significance of bacteria in endodontic disease was shown in the classic study by Kakehashi et al in 1965.[31] They found that no pathologic changes occurred in the exposed pulps or periradicular tissues in germ-free rats (Figure 3-2, A). In conventional animals, however pulp exposures led to pulpal necrosis and periradicular lesion formation (Figure 3-2, B). In contrast, the germ-free rats healed with dentinal bridging regardless of the severity of the pulpal exposure.[31] Thus, the presence or absence of microbial flora was the major determinant for the destruction or healing of exposed rodent pulps.

Invasion of the pulp cavity by bacteria is most often associated with dental caries. Bacteria invade and multiply within the dentinal tubules (Figure 3-3). **Dentinal tubules range in size from 1 to 4 μm in diameter,** whereas the majority of bacteria are less than 1 μm in diameter. If enamel or cementum is missing, microbes may invade the pulp through the exposed tubules. A

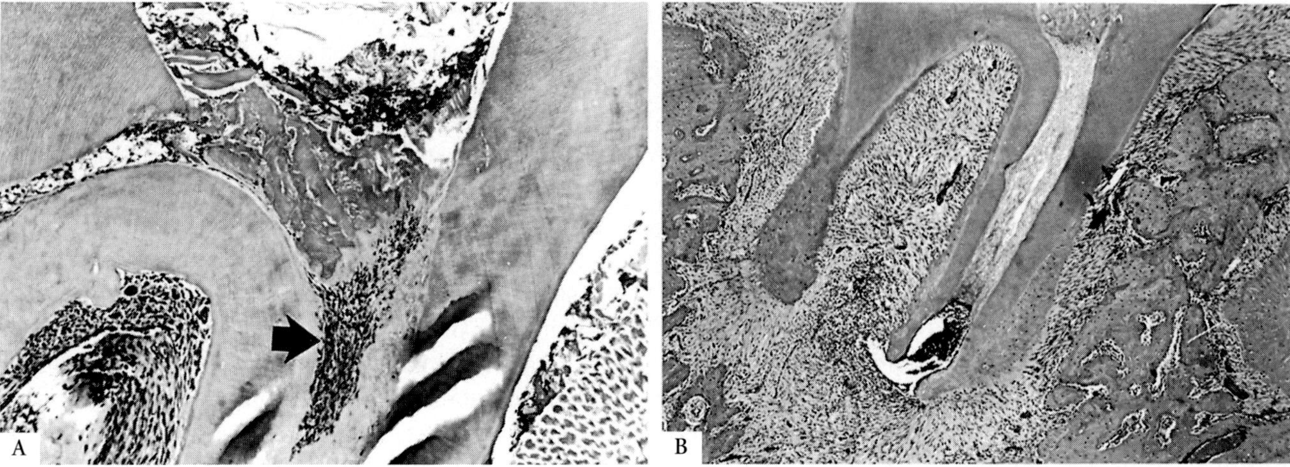

Figure 3-2 Role of bacteria in dentin repair following pulp exposure. **A**, Germ-free specimen obtained 14 days after surgery, with food and debris in the occlusal exposure. Nuclear detail of surviving pulp tissue (**arrow**) can be observed beneath the bridge consisting of dentin fragments united by a new matrix. **B**, Intentional exposure of first molar in control rat (with bacteria 28 days postoperatively). Complete pulp necrosis with apical abscess. **A** reproduced with permission from Kakehashi S, Stanley HR, Fitzgerald RJ. Oral Surg 1965;20:340. **B** reproduced with permission from Clark JW, Stanley HR. Clinical Dentistry. Hagerstown (MD): Harper & Row; 1976;4:10.

tooth with a vital pulp is resistant to microbial invasion. Movement of bacteria in dentinal tubules is restricted by viable odontoblastic processes, mineralized crystals, and various macromolecules within the tubules. Caries remains the most common portal of entry for bacteria and bacterial by-products into the pulpal space. However, bacteria and their **by-products** have been shown to have a direct effect on the dental pulp even without direct exposure.[32–34] These studies demonstrated inflammatory reactions opposite the exposed dentinal tubules. Although the inflammatory reactions could result in pulpal necrosis, the majority of pulps were able to undergo healing and repair.[32–34]

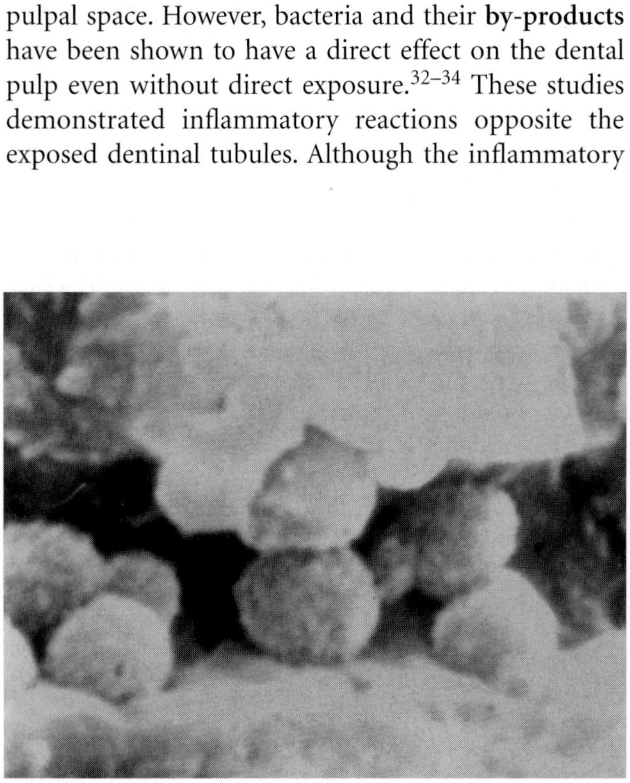

Figure 3-3 Coccal forms of bacteria seen in the cross-section of a fractured dentinal tubule (×15,000 original magnification).

Following trauma and **direct exposure** of the pulp, inflammation, necrosis, and bacterial penetration are no more than 2 mm into the pulp after 2 weeks.[35] In contrast, a necrotic pulp is rapidly invaded and colonized. Peritubular dentin and reparative dentin may impede the progress of the microorganisms. However, the "dead tracts" of empty dentinal tubules following dissolution of the odontoblastic processes may leave virtual highways for the microbes' passage to the pulp cavity. Microbes may reach the pulp via direct exposure of the pulp from restorative procedures or trauma injury and from pathways associated with anomalous tooth development.

It is believed that the egress of irritants from an infected root canal system through tubules, lateral or accessory canals, furcation canals, and the apical foramina may directly affect the surrounding attachment apparatus. However, it is debatable whether periodontal disease directly causes pulpal disease.[36–39] The presence of pulpitis and bacterial penetration into exposed dentinal tubules following root planing in humans has been demonstrated.[40] Langeland et al. found that changes in the pulp did occur when periodontal disease was present, but pulpal necrosis occurred only if the apical foramen was involved.[38] Recently, Kobayashi et al. compared the bacteria in root canals to those in periodontal pockets.[41] The authors believe that bacteria concurrent in both areas suggest that the sulcus or periodontal pocket is the source of the bacteria in root canal infections. To differentiate an abscess of periodontal origin from that of endodontic origin, the enumeration of spirochetes has been recommended.[42] Abscesses of periodontal origin contained 30 to 58% spirochetes, whereas those of endodontic origin were 0 to 10% spirochetes.

Anachoresis is a process by which microbes may be transported in the blood or lymph to an area of inflammation such as a tooth with pulpitis, where they may establish an infection. The phenomenon of anachoresis has been demonstrated in animal models both to nondental inflamed tissues and inflamed dental pulps.[43–45] However, the localization of bloodborne bacteria in instrumented but unfilled canals could not be demonstrated in an animal mode.[46,47] Infection of unfilled canals was possible only with overinstrumentation during the bacteremia to allow bleeding into the canals.[47] Anachoresis may be the mechanism through which traumatized teeth with intact crowns become infected.[48] The process of anachoresis has been especially associated with bacteremias and infective endocarditis.

Once the dental pulp becomes necrotic, the root canal system becomes a "privileged sanctuary" for clusters of bacteria, bacterial by-products, and degradation products of both the microorganisms and the pulpal tissue.[49–51]

PULPAL INFECTION

Polymicrobial interactions and nutritional requirements make the cultivation and identification of all organisms from endodontic infections very difficult. Prior to 1970, very few strains of strict anaerobes were isolated and identified because of inadequate anaerobic culturing methods. **The importance of anaerobic bacteria** in pulpal and periapical pathoses has been revealed with the development of anaerobic culturing methods and the use of both selective and nonselective culture media. However, even with the most sophisticated culturing methods, there are still many microorganisms that remain uncultivable. The bacteria in an infected root canal system are a restricted group compared to the oral flora.

Most of the bacteria in an endodontic infection are strict anaerobes. These bacteria grow only in the absence of oxygen but vary in their sensitivity to oxygen. They function at low oxidation-reduction potentials and generally lack the enzymes superoxide dismutase and catalase. Microaerophilic bacteria can grow in an environment with oxygen but predominantly derive their energy from anaerobic energy pathways. Facultative anaerobes grow in the presence or absence of oxygen and usually have the enzymes superoxide dismutase and catalase. Obligate aerobes require oxygen for growth and possess both superoxide dismutase and catalase.

Most species in endodontic infections have also been isolated from periodontal infections, but the root canal flora is not as complex.[41] Using modern techniques, five or more species of bacteria are usually isolated from root canals with contiguous apical rarefactions. The number of colony-forming units (CFUs) in an infected root canal is usually between 10^2 and 10^8. A positive correlation exists between an increase in size of the periapical radiolucency and both the number of bacteria species and CFUs present in the root canal.[52,53]

The dynamics of bacteria in infected root canals have been studied in monkeys.[51,54,55] After infecting the monkey root canals with indigenous oral bacteria, the canals were sealed and then sampled for up to 3 years. Initially, facultative bacteria predominated; however, with increasing time, the facultative bacteria were displaced by anaerobic bacteria.[51,54,55] The results indicate that a selective process takes place that allows anaerobic bacteria an increased capability of surviving and multiplying. After almost 3 years (1,080 days), 98% of the cultivable bacteria were strict anaerobes.

The root canal system is a selective habitat that allows the growth of certain species of bacteria in preference to others. Tissue fluid and the breakdown products of necrotic pulp provide nutrients rich with polypeptides and amino acids. These nutrients, low oxygen tension, and bacterial by-products determine which bacteria will predominate.

Antagonistic relationships between bacteria may occur. Some metabolites (eg, ammonia) may be either a nutrient or a toxin, depending on the concentration. In addition, bacteria may produce bacteriocins, which are antibiotic-like proteins produced by one species of bacteria to inhibit another species of bacteria. When Sundqvist et al. cultured intact root canals, 91% of the organisms were strict anaerobes.[56] When Baumgartner et al. cultured the apical 5 mm of root canals exposed by caries, 67% were found to be strict anaerobes.[57] **A polymicrobial ecosystem seems to be produced that selects for anaerobic bacteria over time.** Gomes et al.[58,59] and Sundqvist[50,60] used odds ratios to show that some bacteria tend to be associated in endodontic infections. This suggests a **symbiotic relationship** that may lead to an increase in virulence by the organisms in that ecosystem. Clinicians may consider chemomechanical cleaning and shaping of the root canal system as total disruption of that microbial ecosystem.

Although no absolute correlation has been made between any species of bacteria and severity of endodontic infections, several species have been implicated with some clinical signs and symptoms. Those species include BPB, *Peptostreptococcus*, *Peptococcus*, *Eubacterium*, *Fusobacterium*, and *Actinomyces*.[53,56,58,61–72] Table 3-1 shows the percentage of incidence of bacteria isolated from intact root canals from five combined studies.[53,56,73–75] Table 3-2 shows the taxonomic changes that have taken place with the bacteria formerly in the genus **Bacteroides.**

Studies of endodontically treated teeth requiring **retreatment** have shown a prevalence of facultative bacteria, especially **Streptococcus faecalis,** instead of strict anaerobes.[76–80] In addition, fungi have been shown to be associated with failed root canal treatment.[1,80,81] Infection at the time of refilling and the size of the periapical lesion were factors that had a negative influence on the prognosis for re-treatment.[80]

Black-pigmented bacteria have been associated with clinical signs and symptoms in several studies.[53,56,58,61,62,65–70,72] Unfortunately, taxonomic revision based on deoxyribonucleic acid (DNA) studies has made the interpretation of previous research results based on conventional identification of the bacteria at the very least confusing and in many cases impossible. Conventional identifications of microbes based on Gram stain, colonial morphology, growth characteristics, and biochemical tests are often inconclusive and yield presumptive identifications. Sundqvist described some of the taxonomic changes that have affected those species of bacteria often cultured from root canals.[82]

Previously, *Prevotella intermedia* was the species of BPB most commonly isolated from endodontic infections. In 1992, isolates previously thought to be *P. intermedia* were shown to be a closely related species now known as *P. nigrescens*.[83] Recent studies have demonstrated that *P. nigrescens* is actually the BPB

Table 3-1 Bacteria Cultured and Identified from the Root Canals of Teeth with Apical Radiolucencies

Bacteria	Incidence (%)
Fusobacterium nucleatum	48
Streptococcus sp	40
Bacteroides sp*	35
Prevotella intermedia	34
Peptostreptococcus micros	34
Eubacterium alactolyticum	34
Peptostreptococcus anaerobius	31
Lactobacillus sp	32
Eubacterium lentum	31
Fusobacterium sp	29
Campylobacter sp	25
Peptostreptococcus sp	15
Actinomyces sp	15
Eubacterium timidum	11
Capnocytophaga ochracea	11
Eubacterium brachy	9
Selenomonas sputigena	9
Veillonella parvula	9
Porphyromonas endodontalis	9
Prevotella buccae	9
Prevotella oralis	
Proprionibacterium propionicum	8
Prevotella denticola	6
Prevotella loescheii	6
Eubacterium nodatum	6

*Nonpigmenting species.

Other species isolated in low incidence included *Porphyromonas gingivalis, Bacteroides ureolyticus, Bacteroides gracilis, Lactobacillus minutus, Lactobacillus catenaforme, Enterococcus faecalis, Peptostreptococcus prevotii, Eienella corrodens,* and *Enterobacter agglomerans.*

Adapted from Sundqvist G.[82]

Table 3-2 Recent Taxonomic Changes for Previous Bacteroides Species

Porphyromonas—black-pigmented (asaccharolytic *Bacteroides* species)
- *Porphyromonas asaccharolyticas* (usually nonoral)
- *Porphyromonas gingivalis**
- *Porphyromonas endodontalis**

Prevotella—black-pigmented (saccharolytic *Bacteroides* species)
- *Prevotella melaninogenica*
- *Prevotella denticola*
- *Prevotella loescheii*
- *Prevotella intermedia**
- *Prevotella nigrescens*†
- *Prevotella corporis*
- *Prevotella tannerae*

Prevotella—nonpigmented (saccharolytic *Bacteroides* species)
- *Prevotella buccae**
- *Prevotella bivia*
- *Prevotella oralis*
- *Prevotella oris*

Prevotella oulorum

Prevotella ruminicola

*Studies have associated species with clinical signs and symptoms.

†Most commonly isolated species of black-pigmented bacteria from endodontic infections.

most commonly isolated from both root canals and periradicular abscesses of endodontic origin.[84–86] Another study associating BPB with endodontic infections found BPB in 55% of 40 intact teeth suffering necrotic pulps and apical periodontitis. Sixteen of the 22 teeth in the sample "were associated with purulent drainage or an associated sinus tract."[87] Future studies will likely use molecular methods to detect and identify the microbes using extracted DNA.

PULPAL PATHOGENESIS

Because of the polymicrobial nature of periodontal and endodontic disease, a modification of Koch's postulates has been recommended by Socransky.[88,89] This recommendation states that the humoral response to the organism should be suggestive of its role in the disease. Jontell et al. have demonstrated the presence of dendritic cells in the pulp that activate T lymphocytes, which, in turn, direct other immunocompetent cells to mount a local immune response.[90–92] Hahn and Falkler have shown the production by the pulp of immunoglobulin (Ig)G specific for bacteria in deep caries.[93] In addition, they found an increase in the ratio of T helper lymphocytes and B lymphocytes to T suppressor cells in response to approaching caries.[93] In general, the presence of a mononuclear cell infiltrate (lymphocytes, macrophages, and plasma cells) is indicative of an immune response. Bacterial antigens activate both T and B cells. This response may be stimulated by viable bacteria or soluble bacterial components. Lipopolysaccharides cause polyclonal stimulation of B cells and induce macrophage activation.

PERIRADICULAR INFECTIONS

Today we know that serious odontogenic infections, beyond the tooth socket, are much more common as a result of endodontic infections than as a result of periodontal disease.[94] The seriousness of an infection beyond the apex of a tooth depends on the number and virulence of the organisms, host resistance, and anatomic structures associated with the infection. Once the infection has spread beyond the tooth socket, it may localize or continue to spread through the bone and soft tissue as a diffuse abscess or cellulitis.

The terms abscess and cellulitis are often used interchangeably in common clinical use. An **abscess** is a cavity containing pus (purulent exudate) consisting of bacteria, bacterial by-products, inflammatory cells, numerous lysed cells, and the contents of those cells. **Cellulitis** is a diffuse, erythematous, mucosal, or cutaneous infection that may rapidly spread into deep facial spaces and become life threatening. As a diffuse cellulitis matures, it may contain foci of pus consistent with an abscess. The relationship of specific species of bacteria or aggregates of bacteria with the pathogenesis of endodontic abscesses/cellulitis has not been established. Endodontic infections occur when opportunistic pathogens gain access to the normally sterile dental pulp and produce disease. Infections of the root canal system may spread to the contiguous periradicular tissues. Endodontic abscesses are invariably polymicrobial, and several strains of bacteria are cultured from each infection.[66,70,95–100]

The microorganisms identified in periradicular infections (abscesses) of endodontic origin are similar to bacteria isolated and identified from within the root canal system.[53,56,58,61–72] Only a few strains of bacteria isolated from oral abscesses will produce an abscess in pure culture.[17,101–105] A recent study showed that *Fusobacterium nucleatum, Peptostreptococcus anaerobius,* and *Veillonella parvula*, but not any strains of BPB could produce abscesses in pure culture in a mouse model.[101] **In mixed culture** with *F. nucleatum,* the BPB *Prevotella intermedia* and ***Porphyromonas gingivalis*** were significantly more abscessogenic than *F. nucleatum* in pure culture.[101] This supports the concept of **synergistic relationships between bacteria in an endodontic infection.** *Porphyromonas gingivalis* has also been shown to express collagenase as a potential **virulence factor**. *Porphyromonas endododentalis,* however, does not appear to possess this same collagenase gene, *prtC*.[106]

Whether asymptomatic chronic apical periodontitis lesions (periapical granulomas) are sterile has been controversial since the beginning of the 1900s.[107–111] It was generally believed that bacteria usually stayed confined to the root canal system of an infected tooth except when associated with an abscess or cellulitis. It was believed that "a granuloma is not an area in which bacteria live, but in which they are destroyed.".[108] Since then, histologic studies have demonstrated intraradicular organisms, plaque-like material at the root apex, intracellular organisms in the body of the inflammatory lesions, and extracellular bacteria within the body of the lesions[1,112–114] (Figures 3-4 to 3-7).

In an elegant study by Nair using both light and electron microscopy, both intracellular and extracellular bacteria were observed within the body of four granulomas and one radicular cyst. Whereas these 5 teeth were **symptomatic** and clinically diagnosed as acute periapical inflammation, 25 other teeth that were **asymptomatic** did not have identifiable extracellular bacteria.[115]

Recently, several investigators have demonstrated the presence of bacteria by culturing lesions diagnosed

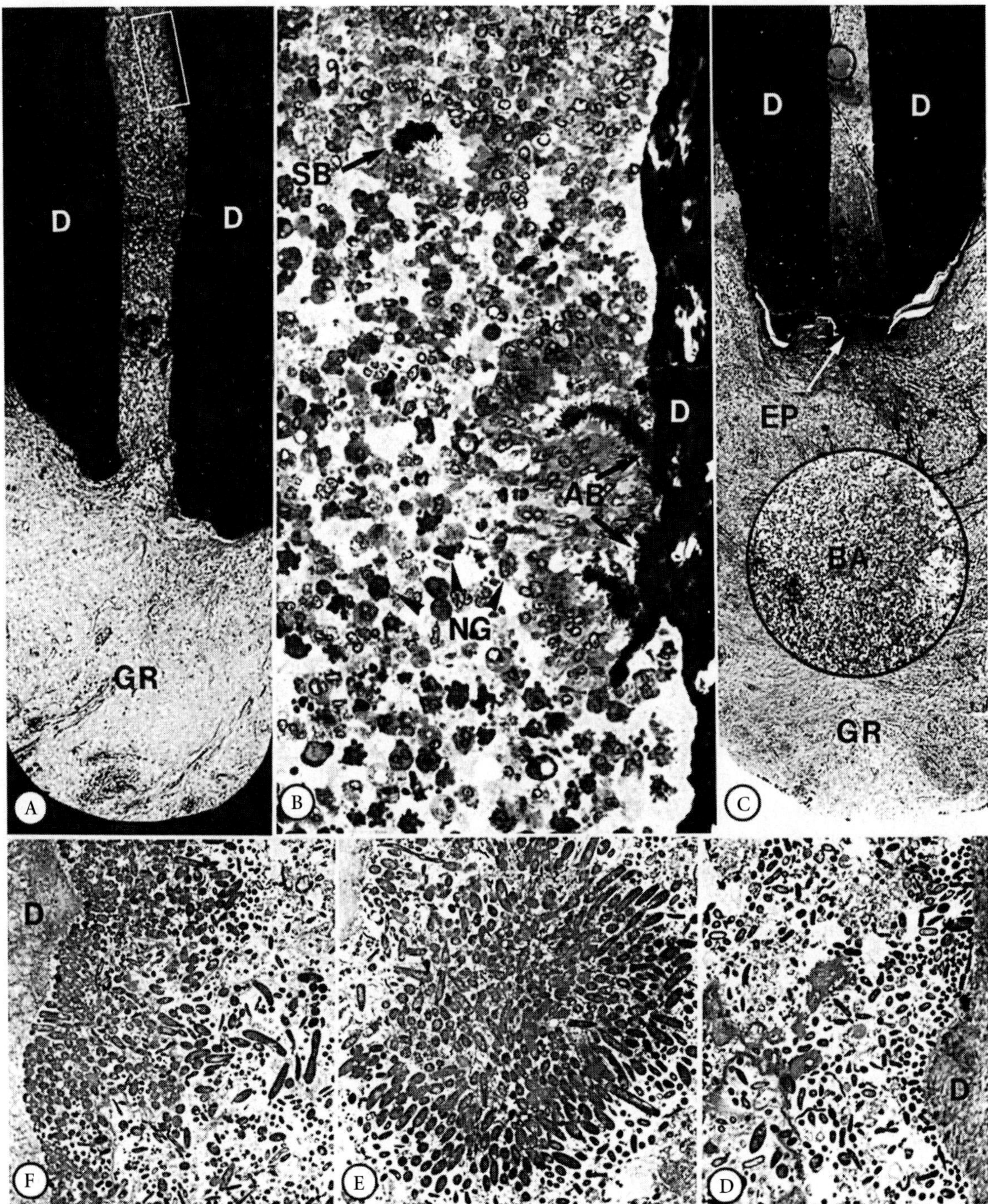

Figure 3-4 The endodontic flora in the radicular third of periradicularly affected human teeth. The flora appears to be blocked by a wall of neutrophils (NG in **B**) or by an epithelial plug (EP in **C**) in the apical foramen. Note the dense aggregates of bacteria sticking to the dentin wall (AB in **B**) and similar ones (SB in **B**) along with loose collections of bacteria (inset in **C**) remaining suspended in the root canal among neutrophils. A cluster of an apparently monobacterial colony is magnified in **D**. Electron micrographs show bacterial condensation on the surface of the dentin wall, forming thin (**E**)- or thick (**F**)-layered bacterial plaques. The rectangular demarcated portion in **A** and the circular one in **C** are magnified in **B** and the inset in **C**, respectively. GR = granuloma; D = dentin. Reproduced with permission from Nair PN.[115]

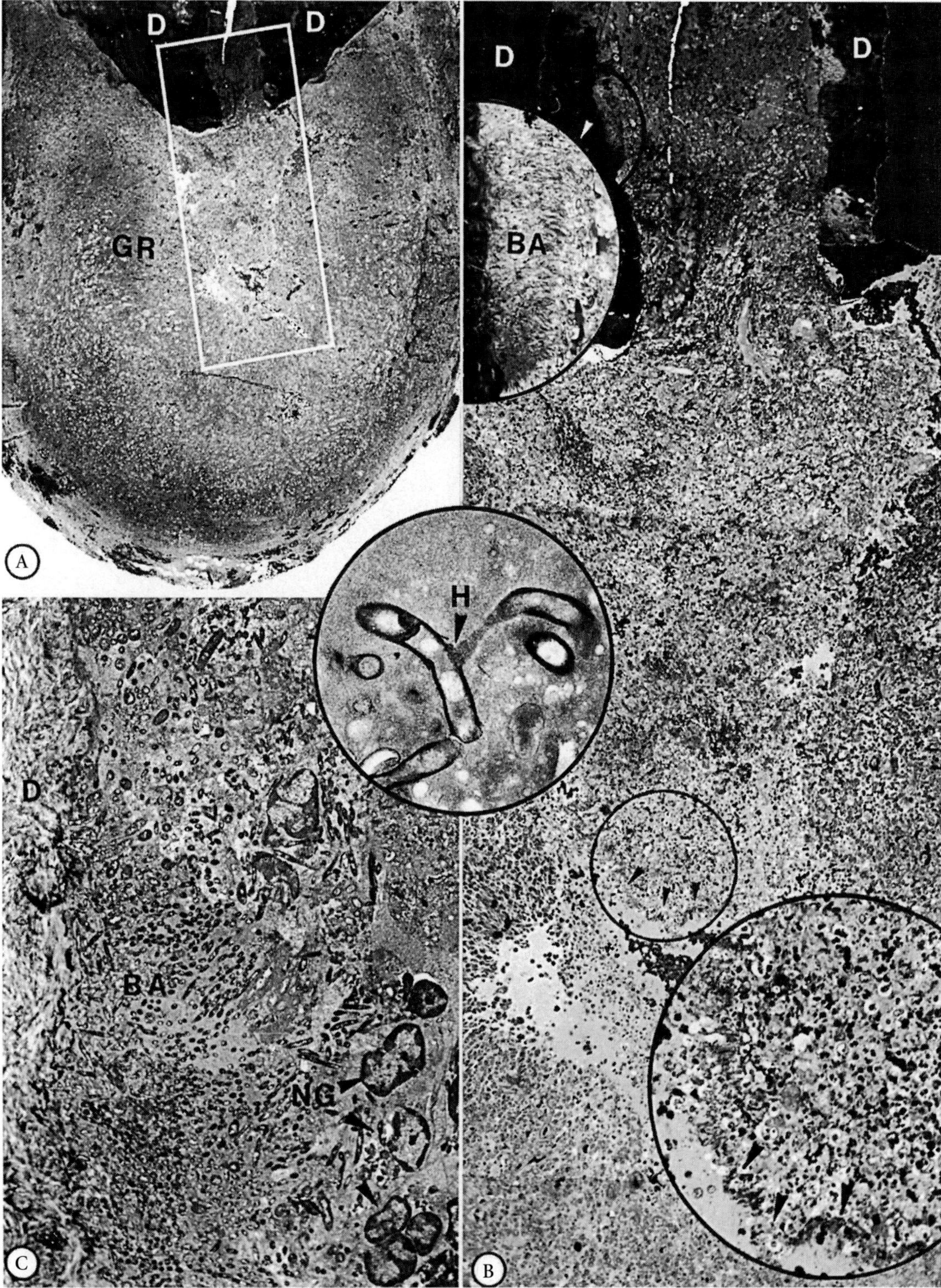

Figure 3-5 A radicular plaque invading a resting granuloma. (The rectangular demarcated area in **A** is magnified in **B**.) The well-encapsulated granuloma (GR in **A**) shows the bacterial front (**arrowheads** in **B** and lower inset) deep within the body of the lesion. Note the funnel-like area of tissue necrosis immediately in front of the apical foramen (**A** and **B**) and the plaque-like bacterial condensation (BA in **B** and upper inset) along the root dentin. This plaque is electron microscopically shown in **C**. The middle inset shows a high magnification of a branching or hyphal-like structure found among the plaque flora. D = dentin; NG = neutrophilic granulocytes. Reproduced with permission from Nair PN.[115]

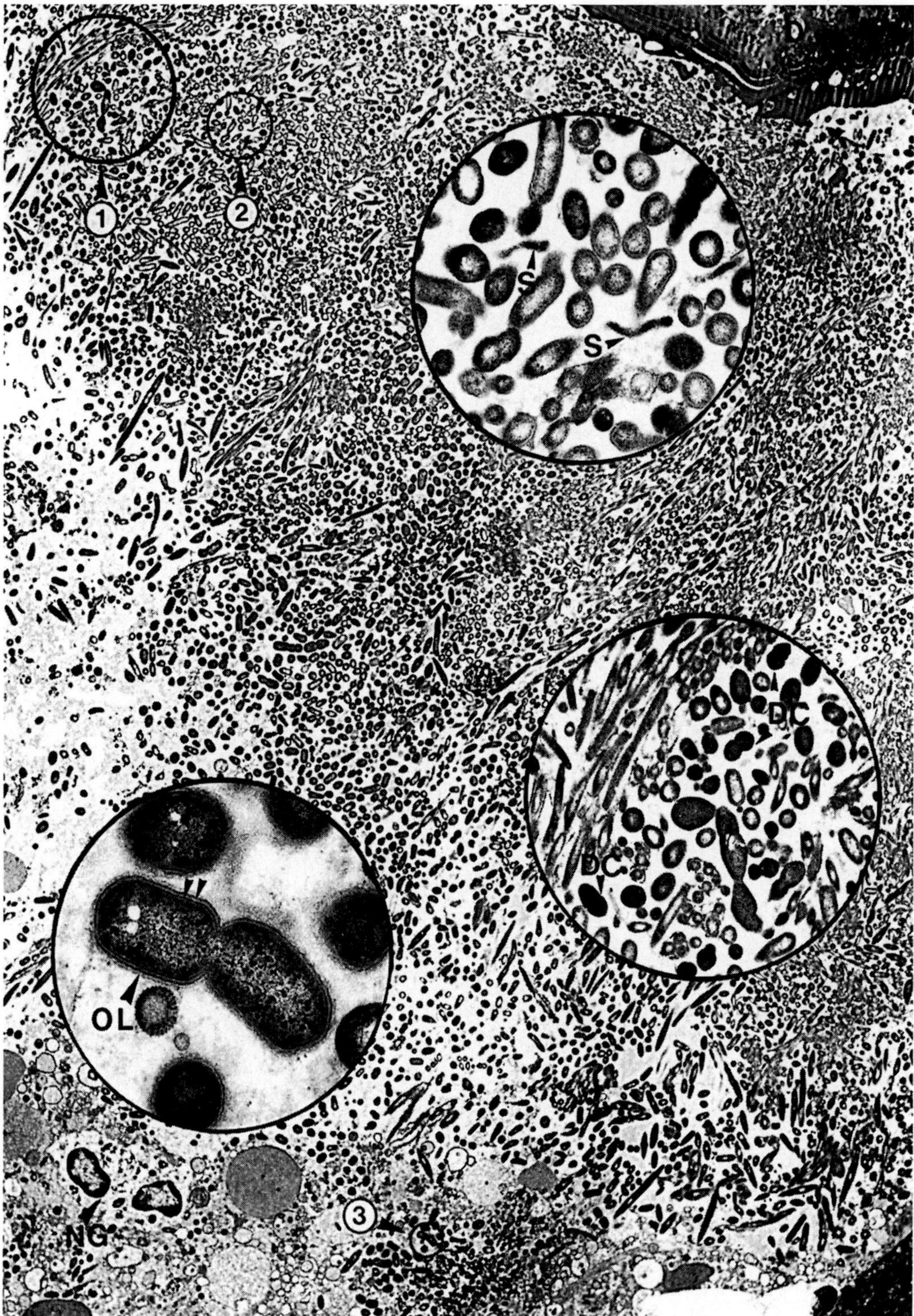

Figure 3-6 A massive periradicular plaque associated with an acute lesion. Note the mixed nature of the flora. Numerous dividing cocci (DC, middle inset), rods (lower inset), filamentous bacteria, and spirochetes (S, upper inset) can be seen. Rods often reveal a gram-negative cell wall (**double arrowhead**, lower inset), some of them showing a third outer layer (OL). The circular areas 1, 2, and 3 are magnified in the middle, upper, and lower insets, respectively. D = dentin; C = cementum; NG = neutrophils. Reproduced with permission from Nair PN.[115]

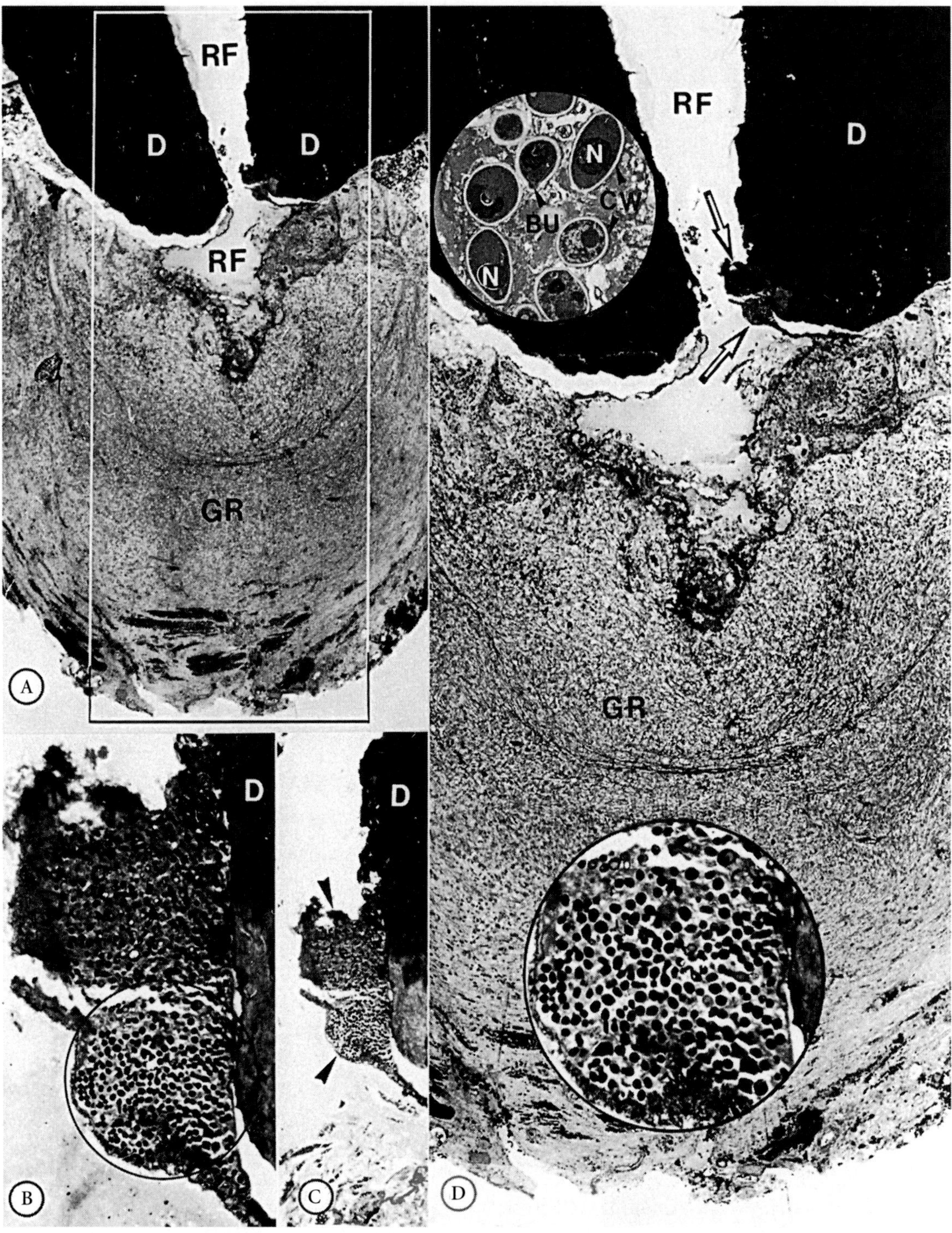

Figure 3-7 Presence of fungus in the root canal and apical foramen of a root-filled (RF in **A** and **D**) tooth with a therapy-resistant periradicular lesion (GR in **A** and **D**). The rectangular demarcated area in **A** is magnified in **D**. Note the two clusters of microorganisms located between the dentinal wall (D) and the root filling (**arrows** in **D**). Those microbial clusters are stepwise magnified in **C** and **B**. The circular demarcated area in **B** is further magnified in the lower inset in **D**. The upper inset is an electron microscopic view of the organisms. They are about 3 to 4 μm in diameter and reveal distinct cell wall (CW), nuclei (N), and budding forms (BU). Reproduced with permission from Nair PN.[1]

as chronic apical inflammation.[113,114,116,117] There is the possibility of microbial contamination from communication of the apical tissues with bacteria located in the apical foramen or the oral cavity or during a surgical procedure and collection of the microbial sample.

Depending on the host's resistance and the virulence of the bacteria, invasion of the periradicular tissues may occur from time to time. Perhaps asymptomatic periradicular inflammatory lesions (granulomas) may contain invading bacteria and even abscesses (microabscesses) not clinically detectable. If the opportunistic organism is successful in invading and establishing an infection, a clinically apparent abscess and possibly a cellulitis may develop (phoenix abscess). Further research is needed to clarify this aspect of endodontic infections.

PERIADICULAR PATHOGENESIS

Research has shown that periradicular inflammatory tissue is capable of an **immunologic response to bacteria.** Studies using an enzyme-linked immunosorbent assay (ELISA), radioimmunosorbent tests, and radial immunodiffusion assays have detected IgG, IgA, IgM, or IgE in fluids of explant (tissue) cultures of endodontic periapical lesions.[118–122] A DOT-ELISA was used to show that BPB (*P. intermedia, P. endodontalis,* and *P. gingivalis)* were the bacteria most reactive with IgG produced by explant cultures of periapical lesions.[120] An ELISA has also been used to show an increase in serum IgG reactive with *P. intermedia* in patients with periodontal disease or combined endodontic-periodontal disease.[123] Recently, exudates from root canals associated with symptomatic periapical lesions were shown to contain higher concentrations of β-glucuronidase and interleukin-1β.[124] Those with severe involvement had higher IgG, and those with a sinus tract or swelling contained higher concentrations of IgM.

Numerous studies have quantitatively analyzed the **lymphocytes** and their subsets in periapical lesions.[125–134] Periapical lesions associated with untreated teeth have a denser inflammatory cell infiltrate than periapical lesions associated with treated teeth.[135] No associations were seen between the histologic diagnosis, clinical signs and symptoms, or radiographic size of the lesions. Most studies have shown that the majority of **lymphocytes** in periapical lesions associated with untreated teeth are **T cells.** However, with treated teeth, Alavi et al. found that half of all inflammatory lesions associated with endodontically treated teeth had more B than T cells.[135] In a rat model, Stashenko and Wang showed that T helper cells outnumber T suppressor cells during lesion expansion up to 15 days.[136] After 15 days, the lesion expansion slows, and T suppressor cells outnumber T helper cells. They believe that T helper–mediated activities may involve bone destruction and lesion expansion. Others believe that lymphocyte proportion may shift in response to population shifts in microorganisms.[55,60,137]

The periapical inflammatory responses that occur following bacterial infection of the root canal system result in the formation of granulomas and cysts with the resorption of surrounding bone. **Interleukin-1** and **prostaglandins** have been especially associated with periapical bone resorption. Research is showing that these inflammatory responses are very complex and consist of several diverse elements.[138] Prostanoids, kinins, and neuropeptides are endogenous mediators responsible for intermediate-type responses that include vasodilatation, increased vascular permeability, and leukocyte extravasation. Bacteria and their byproducts produce nonspecific immune responses including neutrophil and monocyte migration/activation and cytokine production. Chronic apical periodontitis also involves specific T lymphocyte– and B lymphocyte–mediated antibacterial responses. Figure 3-8 shows some of the interactions believed to be associated with bone resorption.

TREATMENT OF ENDODONTIC ABSCESSES/CELLULITIS

The vast majority of infections of endodontic origin can be effectively managed without the use of antibiotics. Systemically administered antibiotics are not a substitute for proper endodontic treatment. Chemomechanical débridement of the infected root canal system with **drainage through the root canal** or by incision and drainage of soft tissue will decrease the bioburden so that a normal healthy patient can begin the healing process. Antibiotics are not recommended for healthy patients with a symptomatic pulpitis, symptomatic apical periodontitis, draining sinus tract, or localized swelling of endodontic origin or following endodontic surgery.[139,140]

An **antibiotic regimen** should be **prescribed** in conjunction with proper endodontic therapy when there are systemic signs and symptoms or a progressive/persistent spread of infection. The presence of a fever (>100°F), malaise, cellulitis, unexplained trismus, and progressive swelling are all signs and symptoms of systemic involvement and the spread of infection (Table 3-3). Under these circumstances, an antibiotic is indicated in addition to débridement of the root canal harboring the infection and drainage of any accumulated purulence.

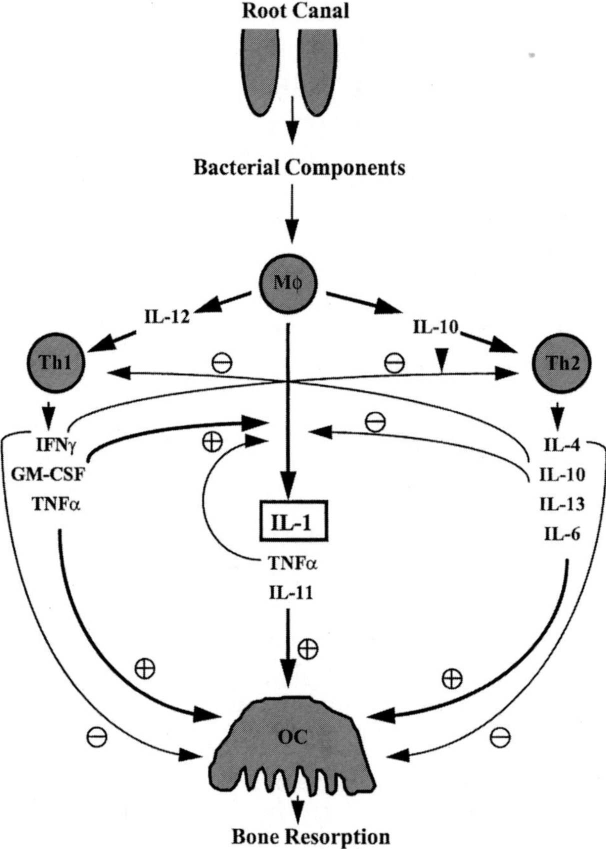

Figure 3-8 Regulation of periapical bone destruction by the cytokine network. GM-CSF = granulocyte-macrophage colony-stimulating factor; TNFa = tumor necrosis factor alpha; IL = interleukin; Th1, Th2 = T helper cell subsets; IFN = interferon; Mϕ = macrophage; OC = osteoclast. Heavy lines = stimulation; light lines = inhibition. Reproduced with permission from Stashenko P and Wang SM.[136]

Patients with serious endodontic infections should be closely followed on a daily basis. The patient's condition will usually rapidly improve once the source of the infection is removed. Because of the lack of circulation, systemically administered antibiotics are not effective against a reservoir of microorganisms within an infected root canal system. Likewise, a minimum inhibitory concentration of an antibiotic may not reach a space filled with pus because of poor circulation. The antibiotic moves via a diffusion gradient through the edematous fluid and purulent exudate that accumulates in an anatomic space. **Pus** contains mainly neutrophils with some other inflammatory cells, cellular debris, bacteria, bacterial by-products, enzymes, and edematous fluid. An **incision for drainage** will allow drainage of the purulent material and improve circulation to the area.

Empirical selection of an antibiotic (antimicrobial agent) must be based on one's knowledge of which bacteria are most commonly associated with endodontic infections and their antibiotic susceptibility.[139–143] The clinician must be thoroughly familiar with the antibiotic and inform the patient of the benefits, possible side effects, and possible sequelae of failing to take the proper dosage. The antibiotic should generally be continued for 2 to 3 days following resolution of the major clinical signs and symptoms of the infection. Following treatment of the source of the infection and adjunctive antibiotic therapy, significant improvement in the patient's status should be seen in 24 to 48 hours. A loading dose is important to provide an initial adequate therapeutic level of antibiotic. An adequate maintenance dose is recommended to prevent the selection of resistant bacteria.

Penicillin VK is the antibiotic of choice because of its effectiveness against both facultative and anaerobic microorganisms commonly found in polymicrobial endodontic infections.[141–144] However, up to 10% of the population may be allergic, so a careful history of drug hypersensitivity is important. **Amoxicillin** has an increased spectrum of activity that includes bacteria not routinely associated with infections of endodontic origin.

Erythromycin has traditionally remained the alternative choice for patients allergic to penicillin, but it is **not effective against anaerobes** associated with endodontic infections. **Clarithromycin** and **azithromycin** are macrolides like erythromycin, with some advantages over the latter. They have a spectrum of antimicrobial activity that includes facultative bacteria and some anaerobic bacteria associated with infections of endodontic origin. They also have less gastrointestinal upset than erythromycin.

Table 3-3 Indications for Adjunctive Antibiotics (Antimicrobial Therapy)

Systemic involvement
Fever > 100°F
Malaise
Lymphadenopathy
Trismus
Progressive infections
Increasing swelling
Cellulitis
Osteomyelitis
Persistent infections

For serious infections when the patient is allergic to penicillin, **clindamycin** is effective against both facultative and strict anaerobic bacteria associated with endodontic infections. It is well distributed throughout the body, especially to bone, where its concentration approaches that of plasma.

Metronidazole is a synthetic antimicrobial agent with **excellent activity against anaerobic bacteria**; however, it is ineffective against facultative bacteria. It is a valuable antimicrobial agent in combination with penicillin when penicillin alone has been ineffective.

When antibiotics are prescribed in conjunction with débridement of the root canal system and drainage of purulence, significant improvement should be seen within 24 to 48 hours. If the infection is not resolving, the diagnosis and initial treatment should be reviewed. If another source of the infection is not found or if additional attempts for drainage are unsuccessful, the **addition of metronidazole (250 mg every 6 hours) to penicillin is indicated.** Because metronidazole is effective only against anaerobic bacteria, penicillin should be continued to treat any facultative bacteria present.

For a more detailed discussion of the role of antibiotics in endodontics, the reader is referred to chapter 18.

PROPHYLACTIC ANTIBIOTICS FOR MEDICALLY COMPROMISED PATIENTS

Prophylactic antibiotic coverage may be indicated for medically compromised patients requiring endodontic treatment. The American Heart Association (AHA) has made major changes in their updated recommendations.[145] Their guidelines are meant to aid practitioners but are not intended as the standard of care or as a substitute for clinical judgment. The incidence of endocarditis following most procedures on patients with underlying cardiac disease is low. A reasonable approach for prescribing prophylactic antibiotics considers the degree to which the underlying disease creates a risk for endocarditis, the apparent risk for producing a bacteremia, adverse reactions to the prophylactic antibiotic, and the cost-benefit aspect of the regimen.[145]

The incidence of bacteremia has been shown to be low during root canal therapy; however, a transient bacteremia can result from the extrusion of the microorganisms infecting the root canal beyond the apex of the tooth.[11,12,14] In addition, care must be taken when positioning rubber dam clamps and accomplishing other dental procedures that may produce bleeding with an accompanying bacteremia. Medically compromised dental patients who are at risk of infection should receive a regimen of antibiotics that either follows the recommendations of the AHA or an alternate regimen determined in consultation with the patients' physicians.[145] Table 3-4 gives the antibiotic regimens recommended for dental procedures.[145] It is believed that the antibiotics **amoxicillin, ampicillin, and penicillin V are equally effective against alpha-hemolytic streptococci; however, amoxicillin is recommended** because it is better absorbed from the gastrointestinal tract and provides higher and more sustained serum levels.[145]

Table 3-4 Prophylactic Regimens for Dental Procedures

Situation	Agent	Regimen
Standard general prophylaxis	Amoxicillin	Adults: 2.0 g; children: 50 mg/kg orally 1 h before procedure
Unable to take oral medications	Ampicillin	Adults: 2.0 g IM, or IV; children: 50 mg/kg IM or IV 30 min before procedure
Allergic to penicillin	Clindamycin	Adults: 600 mg; children: 20 mg/kg orally 1 hr before procedure
	or cephalexin or cefadroxil	Adults: 2.0 g; children: 50 mg/kg orally 1 h before procedure
	Azithromycin or clarithromycin	Adults: 500 mg; children: 15 mg/kg orally 1 h before procedure
Allergic to penicillin and unable to take oral medications	Clindamycin	Adults: 600 mg; children 20 mg/kg IV within 30 min before procedure
	Cefazolin	Adults: 1.0 g; children: 25 mg/kg IM or IV within 30 min before procedure

From Dajani A et al.[145]

For more complete details concerning antibiotic prophylaxis, the reader is referred to chapter 18 and to the reports by Strom et al.[146] and Durack.[147]

COLLECTION OF A MICROBIAL SAMPLE

Adjunctive antibiotic therapy for endodontic infections is most often prescribed empirically based on our knowledge of the bacteria most often associated with endodontic infections. At times, culturing may provide valuable information to better select the appropriate antibiotic regimen. For example, an immunocompromised/immunosuppressed patient (not immunocompetent) or patients at high risk of developing an infection (eg, history of infective endocarditis) following a bacteremia require close monitoring. These patients may have an infection caused by bacteria usually not associated with the oral cavity. Other examples include a seemingly healthy patient who has persistent or progressive symptoms following surgical or nonsurgical endodontic treatment.

An aseptic microbial sample from a root canal is accomplished by first isolating the tooth with a rubber dam and disinfecting the tooth surface and rubber dam with sodium hypochlorite or other disinfectant. Sterile burs and instruments must be used to gain access to the root canal system. Antimicrobial solutions should not be used until after the microbial sample has been taken. If there is drainage from the canal, it may be sampled with a sterile paper point or aspirated into a syringe with a sterile 18- to 25-gauge needle. Any aspirated air should be vented from the syringe into a sterile gauze. The aspirate should either be taken immediately to a microbiology laboratory in the syringe or injected into pre-reduced transport media. To sample a dry root canal, a sterile syringe should be used to place some pre-reduced transport medium into the canal. A sterile endodontic instrument is then used to scrape the walls of the canal to suspend microorganisms in the medium.

To prevent contamination by "normal oral flora," a microbial sample from a soft tissue swelling should be obtained before making an incision for drainage. Once profound anesthesia is achieved, the surface of the mucosa should be dried and disinfected with an iodophor swab (The Purdue Frederick Company, Norwalk, Conn.). A sterile 16- to 20-gauge needle is then used to aspirate the exudate. The aspirate should then be handled as described above. If purulence cannot be aspirated, a sample can be collected on a swab after the incision for drainage has been made, but great care must be taken to prevent microbial contamination with normal oral flora. After collecting the specimen on a swab, it should be quickly placed in pre-reduced medium for transport to the laboratory.

Good communication with the laboratory personnel is important. The sample should be Gram-stained to demonstrate which types of microorganisms predominate. The culture results should show the prominent isolated microorganisms and not just be identified as "normal oral flora." Antibiotics can usually be chosen to treat endodontic infections based on the identification of the prominent microorganisms in the culture. With persistent infections, susceptibility testing can be undertaken to establish which antibiotics are the most effective against resistant microbial isolates. At present, it may take 1 to 2 weeks to identify anaerobes. In the future, molecular methods will be used to rapidly detect and identify known opportunistic bacteria.

ROOT CANAL DÉBRIDEMENT AND INTRACANAL MEDICATION

The goal of clinical treatment is to completely disrupt and destroy the bacteria involved in the endodontic infection. Endodontic disease will persist until the source of the irritation is removed. The microbial ecosystem in an infected root canal has been directly linked to both acute and chronic inflammation.[31,138]

Root Canal Débridement

Root canal débridement includes the removal of the microorganisms and their substrates required for growth. Chemomechanical cleaning and shaping of the root canal system remove a great deal of the irritants, but total débridement is impeded because of the complex root canal systems with accessory canals, fins, cul-de-sacs, and communications between the main canals. The last decade has seen the development and use of several innovative methods and materials to aid in root canal débridement. The ability of nickel-titanium instruments to remain centered in canals has facilitated the use of the step-down method of instrumentation without significant concern for ledge formation or canal transportation.[148,149] In addition, the step-down method removes debris as progress is made toward the apex, so irritating debris is not carried apically and extruded into the periapical tissues.[150] The step-down method also enlarges the coronal portions of the canal so that there is a larger reservoir for an irrigant. Numerous irrigants have been used and studied, but sodium hypochlorite (0.5 to 5.25%) remains the most popular irrigant in the United States. Sodium hypochlorite, in concentrations of 0.5 to 5.25%, has the ability to dissolve organic pulpal debris in areas not reached by endodontic instruments.[151–155] It is also an excellent antimicrobial.[73,75,156]

When sodium hypochlorite is alternated as an irrigant with 15% ethylenediaminetetraacetic acid (EDTA), both the instrumented and the noninstrumented surfaces of a root canal are chemically débrided.[157] Sodium hypochlorite reacts with organic tissue to facilitate cleaning; however, this reaction inactivates the agent and decreases its antibacterial capacity. Thus the **irrigant in the canal should be frequently replenished** to maintain the most optimum activity of sodium hypochlorite. Both 0.5% and 5% sodium hypochlorite have been shown to be effective antimicrobials in clinical studies.[158,159] However, **5% sodium hypochlorite is more effective than 0.5 sodium hypochlorite as a solvent of necrotic tissue.**[160] Research has shown that the combined use of 15% EDTA and 5.25% sodium hypochlorite was more efficient as an antimicrobial than 5.25% NaOCl by itself for irrigating infected root canals.[158] The irrigants must be passively introduced into the canal without wedging the needle and inadvertently infusing the irrigant into the periapical tissues, where they will produce pain and tissue injury.[161,162] Use of a needle with a slot at the tip or side opening helps to prevent wedging of the needle. Sonic and ultrasonic devices may be used to improve the efficacy of irrigation.[163–167]

Intracanal Antisepsis

Residual microorganisms left in the root canal system following cleaning and shaping or microbial contamination of a root canal system between appointments have been a concern. If root canal treatment is not completed in a single appointment, antimicrobial agents are recommended for intracanal antisepsis to prevent the growth of microorganisms between appointments. The access opening in the tooth must also be sealed with an effective interappointment filling to prevent microbial contamination by microleakage from the oral cavity. Despite the controversy over culturing root canals, most clinicians agree that healing is more likely in the absence of bacteria.[168–170]

A recent study used modern microbiologic techniques, with teeth root-filled at a single appointment and evaluated for clinical success.[76] Initially, all 55 single-rooted teeth were infected. After instrumentation and irrigation with 0.5% sodium hypochlorite, bacteria could still be cultivated from 22 of the 55 root canals. Periapical healing was followed for up to 5 years. Complete healing occurred in 94% of those teeth that had negative cultures but only 68% of those with positive cultures at the time of root canal obturation.[76] These findings suggest the importance of eliminating bacteria from the root canal system before obturation.

In the past, numerous antimicrobial agents have been used that were antigenic and cytotoxic and provided relatively short-term antisepsis.[171–175] These included traditional phenolic and fixative agents such as camphorated monochlorophenol, formocresol, eugenol, metacresylacetate, and halides (iodine-potassium iodide). A reliance on mechanical instrumentation and aversion to the use of cytotoxic chemicals have led to a lack of use of an intracanal dressing by many clinicians, a practice that allows remaining bacteria to multiply between appointments.

The current **intracanal dressing of choice is calcium hydroxide.** Although not characterized as an antiseptic, studies have shown calcium hydroxide to be an effective antimicrobial agent.[158,176–180] Other studies have shown it to be an effective interappointment dressing over several weeks.[181,182] When mixed into a paste with water, calcium hydroxide's solubility is less than 0.2%, with a pH of about 12.5. Some of its antibacterial activity may be related to the absorption of carbon dioxide that starves capnophilic bacteria in the root canal.[183] The Saunders group in Dundee was disappointed, however, in the lack of antibacterial activity of calcium hydroxide against the anaerobes *P. gingivalis* and *Peptostreptococcus micros*.[184]

On the other hand, calcium hydroxide has been shown to hydrolyze the lipid moiety of bacterial lipopolysaccharides, making them incapable of producing such biologic effects as toxicity, pyrogenicity, macrophage activation, and complement activation.[177] Lipopolysaccharides have been shown to be present in the dentinal tubules of infected root canals.[18,185] Obliterating the canal space with calcium hydroxide, during treatment, may minimize the ingress of tissue fluid used as a nutrient by microorganisms.[186] Removal of the smear layer facilitates the diffusion of calcium hydroxide into the dentinal tubules.[187] But smear layer or not, a Brazilian group was disappointed in the inability of calcium hydroxide to destroy bacteria in infected dentinal tubules,[188] whereas four root canal sealers appeared to be quite effective against tubuli bacteria, AH-26 being the best.[189] Moreover, zinc oxide–eugenol sealer was found to be more effective in inhibiting the growth of *Streptococcus anginosus* than three of the calcium hydroxide–containing sealers.[190]

Actinomyces israelii, a species of bacteria isolated from periapical tissues, has been reported to not respond to conventional endodontic therapy.[63,191,192] Recently, however, both sodium hypochlorite and calcium hydroxide have been shown to be highly effective in killing *A. israelii*.[193] The optimal treatment of **periapical actinomycosis** is endodontic surgery that removes the likely cause, enables microscopic confirmation, and has a high chance of success without prescribing antibiotics.[63,191,193] In classic forms of actinomycosis involving invasion and spread of *A. israelii* in the periradicular tissues, antibiotic treatment is justified. When actinomycosis cannot be controlled by surgery, **antibiotic therapy is justified** and optimized by prescribing for an extended period of 6 weeks with **amoxicillin or cephalexin.**[193]

Calcium hydroxide has been shown to have some efficacy in the dissolution of pulp tissue in vitro and may increase the ability of sodium hypochlorite to dissolve remaining organic tissue at subsequent appointments.[160,194] The tissue-dissolving property seems to work equally well in aerobic and anaerobic environments.[195] Some commercial preparations of calcium hydroxide come packaged in syringes, or the powder may be mixed with water or glycerin to form a thick paste. The paste is carried into the pulp chamber with a plastic instrument, amalgam carrier, or syringe and then carried down the canals using a lentulo, prefitted pluggers, or counterclockwise rotation of endodontic files. Calcium hydroxide is easily removed from the canal system at the next appointment using endodontic files and irrigation.

When exposed to carbon dioxide in an open container, some calcium hydroxide is slowly converted into inactive calcium carbonate. In a closed container, it is quite stable, with only 1 to 2% being converted after several months.[196] A good temporary filling that is several millimeters thick to prevent microleakage is important between appointments.[197–201] Calcium hydroxide has also been shown to decrease the amount of microbial contamination under temporary fillings.[202]

Another root canal medicament has more recently been introduced in Germany, a liquid medication known as camphorated chloroxylenol (ED84), which is claimed to be as effective as a "temporary root canal dressing for a duration of 2 days" and to be nontoxic to tissue.[203]

ASEPSIS IN ENDODONTIC PRACTICE

Endodontics has long emphasized the importance of aseptic techniques using sterilized instruments, disinfecting solutions such as sodium hypochlorite, and rubber dam barriers. In the past decade, numerous articles have been written regarding the exposure of dental personnel to infectious diseases.[204–209] In 1979, Crawford discussed guidelines for contamination control with respect to sterilization and disinfection in endodontic practice.[204] More recently, further recommendations have been made to prevent transmission of infectious diseases.[205–209] Interestingly, the basic tenets still apply today, but with many additions. The list of identified risks to health care professionals has increased tremendously. The Occupational Safety and Health Administration (OSHA) regulations have had a profound impact on the practice of dentistry.

Traditionally, hepatitis B has been the benchmark disease on which infection control has been based.[205] In an office that treats approximately 20 patients per day, the personnel can expect to encounter 1 active carrier of hepatitis B virus (HBV) every 7 working days. In addition, one can expect exposure to 2 patients with oral herpes and an unknown number of patients infected with human immunodeficiency virus (HIV). It is generally accepted that the potential for HBV transmission in the dental environment is greater than that for HIV.[210] Immediate exposure is one critical factor, but HBV and tubercle bacilli have been shown to survive on inanimate surfaces beyond 7 days, thus illustrating the longevity of the pathogens. Hepatitis B virus is also highly infectious, with as little as 0.00001 mL of contaminated blood capable of transmitting the disease. Human immunodeficiency virus has been recovered from 1 to 3 days after drying under certain conditions.[211]

Human immunodeficiency virus and HBV infections have raised the concern of the profession and the public alike. Health care workers worry about acquiring HIV from patients, and patients worry about being exposed to diseases in dental offices. Much attention has been aroused by the highly publicized case in Florida in which a dentist may have infected at least five of his patients before he himself died from acquired immune deficiency syndrome (AIDS).[212]

The transmission route of HIV/HBV in this two-way street is primarily through the exchange of blood. Percutaneous injury to dentists is the most direct patient-to-dentist transmission method. Infected dentists, in turn, can then unknowingly infect other patients.[213]

Percutaneous injuries to dentists are caused by burs (37%), syringe needles (30%), sharp instruments (21%), orthodontic wires (6%), suture needles (3%), scalpel blades (1%), and other objects (2%). In recent years, however, needlestick injuries have dropped dramatically.

Oral surgeons suffer the highest percutaneous injury rate and endodontists the lowest. The average dentist performs about 3,000 invasive procedures a year—37% of all procedures. The percutaneous injury rate ranges from 3.16 (general practice) to 3.43 (specialties) "sticks" per year, any one of which could be disastrous.[213] Proper sterilization and infection control procedures in dental offices have become important issues for the public, the dental profession, and government agencies such as OSHA.

INFECTION CONTROL

The basic theorems of asepsis in general dentistry apply to endodontics with little variance. Figure 3-9 illustrates the major aspects of infection control in the dental environment. Each of these areas is reviewed in this chapter.

Objectives

In the development of any program, including one for contamination control, certain goals should be formulated. The American Dental Association (ADA) Council on Dental Therapeutics has recommended the following[206]:

1. Decrease the number of pathogenic microbes to the level where normal body resistance mechanisms can prevent infection.
2. Break the cycle of infection from dentist, assistant, and patient and eliminate cross-contamination.
3. Treat all patients and instruments as though they could transmit an infectious disease.
4. Protect patients and personnel from infection and protect all dental personnel from the threat of malpractice.

Even though these are general objectives, they provide a framework for the development of a contamination control program.

Terminology

The following terms apply to the topic of infection control:

1. **Sterilization**: The process that **destroys** all types and forms of microorganisms, including viruses, bacteria, fungi, and bacterial endospores. Major methods of sterilization include steam autoclave, dry heat, chemical vapor under pressure, ethylene oxide gas, and immersion in liquid chemical disinfectants/ sterilizers.

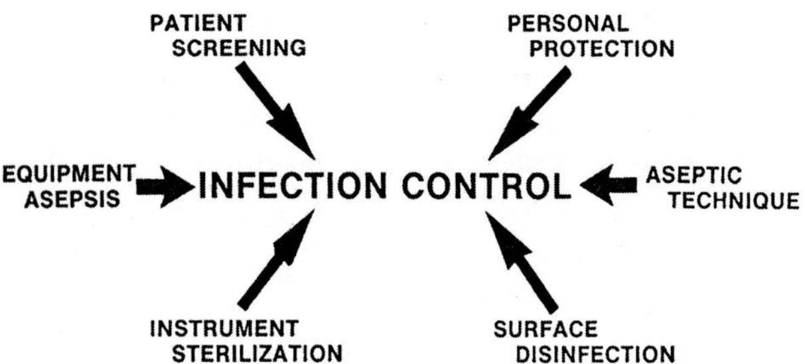

Figure 3-9 Major aspects of infection control in dentistry. (Courtesy of Dr. James A. Cottone, University of Texas Health Science Center at San Antonio, Texas.)

2. **Disinfection:** A process that is less lethal than sterilization. Three levels of disinfection are differentiated, depending on the type and form of microorganism destroyed.
   - **High-level disinfection:** A process that can kill some, but not necessarily all, bacterial spores. It is tuberculocidal, and if the disinfectant is capable of destroying bacterial spores, it is labeled sporicidal.
   - **Intermediate-level disinfection:** A process that is capable of killing *Mycobacterium tuberculosis,* HBV, and HIV. It may not be capable of killing bacterial spores.
   - **Low-level disinfection.** A process that kills most bacteria, some fungi, and some viruses. It does not kill *M. tuberculosis* or bacterial spores.
3. **Bactericidal:** A process or an agent that destroys (kills) bacteria.
4. **Bacteriostatic:** A process or an agent that inhibits growth or multiplication of bacteria.
5. **Contamination:** The introduction of an infectious agent into an area.
6. **Biomedical waste:** Generally any waste that is generated or has been used in the diagnosis, treatment, or immunization of human beings or animals, in research pertaining thereto, or in producing or testing a biologic agent, or that may contain infectious agents and may pose a substantial threat to health. This does not include hazardous waste.[214]
7. **Biohazardous waste:** Depending on regional regulations, this may include or exclude any of the following[214]:
   - **Laboratory waste**, including specimen cultures from medical and pathologic laboratories, culture dishes, and dishes and devices used to transfer, inoculate, and mix cultures or material that may contain infectious agents and may pose a substantial threat to health. All nonsterilized cultures are presumed biohazardous.
   - **Specimens** sent to a laboratory for microbiologic analysis are presumed biohazardous.
   - **Surgical specimens**, including human or animal parts or tissues removed surgically or by autopsy, are presumed biohazardous.
   - **Recognizable fluid and blood elements** and regulated body fluids and containers and articles contaminated with blood elements or regulated body fluids.
   - **Sharps**, including all objects or devices having acute rigid corners, edges, or protuberances capable of cutting or piercing and including, but not limited to, hypodermic needles, blades, and slides. [This would be likely to include endodontic instruments.]

8. **Medical solid waste:** Empty specimen containers, bandages or dressings containing nonliquid blood, surgical gloves, treated biohazardous waste, and other materials that are not biohazardous.[214]

PATIENT EVALUATION

The identification of patients with transmissible diseases and of those belonging to high-risk groups is essential before treatment begins.[205,207,208,215] The Ad Hoc Committee on Infectious Diseases of the American Association of Public Health Dentists has listed diseases of concern to dental personnel[207] (Table 3-5). Populations at high risk of contracting hepatitis B are listed in Table 3-6. According to the Centers for Disease Control and Prevention (CDC), however, because the medical history and examination cannot reliably identify all patients with bloodborne pathogens, blood and body fluid precautions should be consistently used for all patients.[210] The concept stresses that all patients should be assumed to be infectious for HIV and other bloodborne pathogens.[216] Unfortunately, the medical history is only an adjunct to the patient's background and cannot be considered a totally inclusive source of information.

In the daily practice of endodontics, one must **frequently re-evaluate** the patient's medical history, at least on a yearly basis. With the recent advances in the treatment of medically compromised patients, a greater number of patients will enter the office with immunocompromised conditions, cardiovascular susceptibilities, and a host of other physical limitations that may require special attention. Consultation with attending physicians is most important in proper care of such patients.

Table 3-5 Transmissible Diseases of Concern to Dental Providers

Hepatitis (types A, B, non-A/non-B) (hepatitis B virus)
Acquired immune deficiency syndrome (human immunodeficiency virus)
Syphilis
Gonorrhea
Influenzas
Acute pharyngitis (viral or streptococcal)
Pneumonias
Tuberculosis
Herpes
Chickenpox
Infectious mononucleosis
Rubella
Rubeola
Mumps

Reproduced with permission from the Ad Hoc Committee on Infectious Diseases.[207]

CLASSIFICATION OF INSTRUMENT STERILIZATION

Spaulding's classification for instruments has been cited as a methodology for instrument sterilization.[217] The categorization of instruments depends on the contact with different tissue types to determine whether sterilization or disinfection is required. The categories are as follows:

1. **Critical items:** Instruments that touch sterile areas of the body or enter the vascular system and those that penetrate the oral mucosa. Examples are scalpels, curettes, burs, and files. Because of their potential for harboring microorganisms, dental handpieces also must be sterilized.[218] Instruments in this category

Table 3-6 Groups at High Risk of Contracting Hepatitis B

Health care personnel
Selected patients and patient contacts
Patients and staff in hemodialysis units and hematology/oncology units
Patients requiring frequent or large-volume blood transfusions or clotting factors (ie, hemophiliac patients)
Residents and staff of institutions for the mentally handicapped
Household and sexual contacts of persons with persistent hepatitis B antigen
Newborns of hepatitis B surface antigen carrier mother
Populations with high incidence of the disease
Alaskan natives
Indo-Chinese refugees
Haitian refugees
Native Pacific Islanders
Sub-Saharan Africans
Morticians and embalmers
Blood bank and plasma fractionation workers
Persons at increased risk of disease because of sexual practices
Prisoners
Users of illicit injectable drugs
International travelers

Reproduced with permission from the Ad Hoc Committee on Infectious Diseases.[207]

must be sterilized and stored in appropriate packages. Single-use items must be properly discarded.

2. **Semicritical items:** Instruments that touch mucous membranes but do not penetrate tissues. This includes amalgam condensers and saliva ejectors. These items should be sterilized; however, if this is not feasible, high-level disinfection or disposal is required.
3. **Noncritical items:** Those items that do not come in contact with oral mucosa but are touched by saliva- or blood-contaminated hands while treating patients. Such items include light switches, countertops, and drawer pulls on cabinets. These areas should be properly disinfected.

STERILIZATION

A recent Minnesota study suggests that approximately one of every five efforts at instrument sterilization in dental offices fails. Errors made by the sterilizer operator were found to be the major cause of failure.[212]

Four elements essential to ensuring proper sterilization are recommended:

1. High-quality sterilization equipment and maintenance
2. Correct operation of sterilization equipment
3. Comprehensive operator training
4. Weekly use of biologic indicators (*Bacillus subtilis* strips) to monitor sterilization effectiveness.[212]

The four methods of sterilization that are generally accepted in dentistry include **steam** under pressure, **chemical vapor, dry heat** sterilization, and **glutaraldehyde** solutions.[208,219] Ethylene oxide gas, ultraviolet light, microwave, and other forms of radiation are effective but have limited use in dentistry at present.[217,220] Glutaraldehyde solutions are reviewed with disinfectants because of difficulties of attaining sterilization using the medium.

Steam Under Pressure—Autoclaving

The commonly accepted criteria for autoclaving are 121°C (249°F) at 15 psi for 15 to 40 minutes. The time depends on the items to be autoclaved, the size of the load, and the type of container used. Included in this method is the "flash" sterilization technique, for which shorter times with higher temperatures are used. There is, however, a greater chance for sterilization error to occur. The disadvantages of autoclaving include rusting, corroding, and dulling of instruments, especially those composed of carbon steel. Instruments removed from the chamber are wet, which increases the turnaround time of sterilization. Certain plastics and rubber are also sensitive to heat and moisture and cannot be placed in the autoclave.

Chemical Vapor Sterilization—Chemclave

This method is based on the factors of heat, water, and chemical synergism. The chemicals include alcohol, acetone, ketones, and formaldehyde. The water content is below the 15% level, above which rust, corrosion, and dullness of metal occur. The composition of heat and chemicals is much kinder to metal surfaces than are other techniques. The temperature requirements are 132°C (270°F) for 20 minutes. The main advantages are the fast turnaround time and the protection of carbon steel instruments. The main disadvantage is the odor that is released when the chemicals are heated. This method has become a popular mode of sterilization in endodontic offices.

Dry Heat Sterilization

This technique of sterilization requires a temperature of 160°C (320°F) for 2 hours. The primary disadvantage of this technique is the long sterilization time. Initial cost of the dry heat method is lower than that of the two previously described. During the loading process, instruments must be separated to prevent the creation of air pockets (stratification) leading to ineffective sterilization. Some units also have problems of uneven heating.

Recently, a Rapid Heat-Transfer Sterilizer was introduced as the Cox sterilizer (Alfa Medical Equipment Co.; Hempstead, N.Y.). Operated at 190°C, it will, by rapid airflow, sterilize unpackaged instruments in 6 minutes and packaged instruments in 12 minutes.

Preparation for Sterilization

Instruments and equipment intended for sterilization or disinfection procedures must first be carefully prepared. This precleaning is essential to remove blood, saliva, tissue, and other debris that can interfere with the sterilization process. The instruments should be cleaned thoroughly by scrubbing with soap and water or a detergent solution, or with a mechanical device (ultrasonic cleaner). The use of a covered ultrasonic cleaner is an effective method of increasing the efficiency of cleaning and reducing the handling of sharp instruments.

When it is not possible to clean and process instruments immediately after their use, they may be held in a "holding solution" to prevent organic material from drying on them, making them difficult to clean. Water, a detergent solution, or an intermediate-level disinfectant may be used for this purpose.

Verification

In a study of sterilizers in endodontic offices, 15% of those tested failed to adequately sterilize items.[221] Dry heat sterilizers were the most likely to have failures, although the most common problem was human error. Inadequate exposure time, equipment overloading, improper wrapping, and poor internal circulation were cited as only some of the problems encountered. Few failures were caused by the equipment.

Several sterilization monitors are available, including process indicators, control indicators, and biologic monitors.[219] Process indicators (ink compound on tape or paper) determine that certain conditions have been met but do not indicate sterility. Control or certified indicators better show that sterilization parameters have been achieved but still do not conclusively indicate sterility. Biologic monitoring is the only dependable method to verify sterility. These monitors are composed of strips of paper with live, resistant spores, which should be killed if properly sterilized. Biologic monitoring should be done weekly and the results recorded and stored.

DISINFECTION

All items that can be sterilized should be sterilized. Disinfection is added to the methods for preventing cross-contamination for instances in which sterilization is not possible. Disinfection is a compromise over sterilization; however, it does contribute substantially to the reduction of microorganisms. A disinfectant is deemed acceptable for dentistry if the solution is registered with the US Environmental Protection Agency (EPA) or approved/accepted by the ADA. Instrument and surface disinfectants suitable for dentistry are listed in the sections that follow.[222,223] These compounds have been accepted by the ADA as liquid disinfectants.

Glutaraldehyde Preparations

A plethora of glutaraldehyde preparations exists today. Disinfection occurs in 10 to 30 minutes, and various types of preparations are capable of sterilization:

- 2% acidic—60°C for 1 hour
- 2% alkaline—at room temperature for 10 hours
- 2% alkaline with phenolic buffer—at room temperature for 6.75 hours
- 2% neutral—at room temperature for 10 hours

Glutaraldehydes are generally not recommended for sterilization because of the instability of the activated solutions, problems of dilution, and the inability to monitor sterilization. Some glutaraldehyde solutions are ADA approved as disinfectants and sterilizers if used according to manufacturers' instructions. The solutions are registered with the EPA as immersion disinfectants only. They can be used on operatory surfaces and act in 3 to 30 minutes, depending on the amount of debris and types of viruses present. Glutaraldehydes have disadvantages as surface disinfectants, however, such as vapor toxicity, hand and eye irritation, and expense. They are therefore not recommended. A monitor strip to test the solution potency is available and recommended, rather than depending on the number of days the solution is used. A 1986 survey indicated that 71% of the dental practices participating were using glutaraldehyde solutions in some formulation.[224]

Chlorine Dioxide

The chlorine dioxide compounds disinfect instruments and operatory surfaces in 1 to 3 minutes when used correctly. The solution requires no rinsing and leaves no residue after use. There are no special handling or disposal requirements. Solutions can sterilize items in 6 hours at room temperature. This substance has been reported to be nontoxic, nonirritating, and nonsensitizing. The disadvantages are the corrosion of easily oxidized metals and the need for fresh new solutions for each sterilization/disinfection process.

Sodium Hypochlorite (Household Bleach)

Sodium hypochlorite is more suitable for surface **disinfection** than for instrument sterilization because of its highly corrosive action on metals. Dilutions of 1:5 to 1:1 are generally recommended. On surfaces, sodium hypochlorite is virucidal, bactericidal, and tuberculocidal. Disinfection can occur in 3 to 30 minutes, depending on the amount of debris present. It is the least expensive of the surface disinfectants. The major disadvantage, as previously mentioned, is the corrosion factor. The solution also tends to be unstable and should be prepared daily. As a surface disinfectant, there is a strong, unpleasant odor. Plastic chair covers have a tendency to crack under prolonged use.

Iodophors

Iodophor is a broad-spectrum disinfectant that is effective against a host of pathogens, including HBV, *M. tuberculosis,* poliovirus, and herpes simplex virus. One of the inherent advantages of the compound is the slow release of elemental iodine to enhance the bactericidal activity. A surfactant carrier keeps the surface moist to protect the iodophor during this release, and the action may continue even after the surface appears dry. The most effective dilution for hard-surface iodophors is 1 part iodophor concentrate to 213 parts of soft or distilled water. **Hard water inactivates the iodophor.** Biocidal activity occurs within 30 minutes.

Iodophors also have a built-in color indicator. When the solution is fresh, an amber color is present. With age, the solution changes to light yellow, indicating the loss of the iodophor molecules. A mixture of iodophor with alcohol was thought to enhance the activity, but research evidence is insufficient to support this claim.[222] The iodophor compound is to be used solely as a disinfectant. The sporicidal capabilities of the substance have not been shown.

Alcohols

Alcohols are not accepted by the ADA for disinfection of surfaces or instruments.

Quarternary Ammonium Compounds

This group of compounds, including benzalkonium chloride, is no longer recommended for instrument or surface disinfection. All quarternary ammonium compounds have been disapproved by the ADA for use in dentistry.

DISINFECTION TECHNIQUES

The following disinfection techniques are recommended by the ADA and The Center For Disease Control:

1. **Immersion disinfection:** Solutions must be fresh and changed according to manufacturers' recommendations. All instruments must be cleaned by thorough scrubbing with soap and water or with a mechanical cleaner, such as an ultrasonic unit. Heavy-duty rubber gloves should be worn during instrument decontamination. Instruments must be dried before being placed in the disinfectant to prevent dilution.
2. **Surface disinfection:** Countertops and surfaces that have become contaminated with blood, saliva, and debris must be wiped and/or scrubbed to remove organic material after being sprayed with an appropriate surface disinfectant. Once cleaned, the surface is again sprayed and left moist for the recommended period. Surface decontamination is approximately 80% effective in bacterial control.[205]
3. **Decontamination of dental units:** Dental units have come under scrutiny in the environment of infection control. Check-valves have been recommended to prevent aspiration of infective materials into handpieces and water lines.[208] A major implication would be if a patient were infected with HBV, HIV, or tuberculosis and these organisms were aspirated into the unit and allowed to colonize. They could later be discharged into the mouths of subsequent patients. A comparison of units with and without check-valves showed significant decreases in the amount of bacteria in the dental units with check valves.[225] Microorganisms, however, were still found even in units using the check-valve. Eliminating the fluid retraction valve was the most effective way to prevent fluid retraction, but then water continued to drip from the units. The CDC recommends that handpieces be flushed for 20 to 30 seconds between patients and for several minutes at the beginning of each day to reduce any overnight bacterial accumulation in the units. They also recommend that sterile saline or sterile water be used as a coolant/irrigant for any surgical procedures.[226]

BARRIER TECHNIQUES

Three factors determine whether disease develops in the host after exposure: virulence of the disease agent, resistance of the host, and the quantity of the disease agent.[227] Barrier techniques in infection control address the quantity factor in disease prevention. This may encompass protection of the body surfaces, protection of the environmental surfaces, or blockage of bacteria from the source.

Gloves

Gloves provide the patient with protection from contamination of microorganisms on the practitioner's hands and protect dental health care workers from contamination by the patient's blood and saliva.[227] Small cuts and abrasions on the hands can serve as portals of entry into the body. Gloves can provide a barrier between open wounds and bacteria from blood and saliva. In one research study, traces of blood were found beneath the fingernails of 44% of ungloved general dentists.[228]

One of the main concerns about the use of gloves has been the worry about possible loss of tactile sense, especially in the practice of endodontics. In a study focusing on tactile sense, no significant differences were found among gloved versus ungloved clinicians.[229] In a time test of endodontic performance, no differences were found between gloved and ungloved hands.[230] The difficulty lies in the fact that many clinicians were trained when gloves were not used. Studies have shown that learning periods of 1 to 2 months are necessary to become accustomed to wearing gloves.[231] Proper fit is important for tactile control and comfort. Gloves vary in size between manufacturers and even within the same brand, depending on the type of glove (ie, examination versus surgical).

The reuse of gloves has been reviewed by many authors.[208,231,232] Gobetti and associates have stated that washing a gloved hand removed significant amounts of bacteria.[233] If iodine scrub soap was used, the gloved hand would be free of bacteria. In a study of the evaluation of gloves, pinholes occurred randomly and were independent of the type or manufacturer.[231] Pinholes occurred in 1.7 to 9% of the gloves tested. Tear strength also varied. The investigators did not recommend reuse after conventional dental procedures because the clinician had no way to determine the integrity of the glove.

The ADA Council on Dental Therapeutics and the CDC recommend that gloves not be reused.[234] **Double gloves** may be indicated for patients with known infectious diseases, such as herpes, HBV, and HIV. Gloves that are known to have been contaminated with an infectious entity (ie, HBV, HIV) should be sterilized before being discarded.[234]

Hand Washing

Hands should be washed before gloves are placed and after gloves are removed because the integrity of the glove is not dependable.[208] Antimicrobial hand-washing solutions should be used.[209] If, during the course of treatment, a glove is torn, the glove should be removed and the hands washed and then regloved.

Face Masks

The face mask is an important barrier providing protection from inhalation of aerosols generated by high-speed handpieces and air-water syringes. The mask should remain dry to prevent transmission of organisms through moisture penetration. Masks may be composed of glass or synthetic fiber, paper, or gauze. The fiber-type mask is considered to be more efficient in filtering bacteria.[228] Masks should be worn by all treatment personnel and should be changed between patients because masks worn for prolonged periods may become a nidus of infection.

Eyeglasses

Protective eyewear is highly beneficial for dental care providers and for the patient. Herpes virus infection of the eye and infection from hepatitis B are possible consequences of viral contact with the eye.[227] Eyewear can prevent bacterial or viral contact with the eye by aerosol spray or droplet infection. Chin-length face shields are also effective in the prevention of splashing and splattering of blood and saliva; however, they do not provide protection from inhalation of aerosols.

Clothing

The general recommendations for clinic wear include reusable or disposable gowns and laboratory coats or uniforms with long sleeves. Head covers are also recommended during procedures that result in splashing blood or other body fluids. Gowns should be changed at least daily. Laundering can be effectively accomplished with a high-temperature (60 to 70°C) wash cycle with normal bleach, followed by machine drying (100°C or more). According to the CDC reports, this method, along with dry cleaning and steam pressing, is effective in killing the AIDS virus.[234] Shoes should be changed at the office or kept out of reach of small children at home because they are in constant contact with saliva and blood splatter that settle on the floor.

Procedural Barriers

The rubber dam has been shown to be an effective barrier to reduce the number of organisms contained in aerosols.[227] The number of infectious particles can be reduced by 99%. The rubber dam prevents aerosolization of saliva and should be used whenever possible. **Operating fields**, isolated by a rubber dam, however, showed bacterial contamination in 53% of the cases after 1 hour.[235] When silicone and adhesives were used to further seal around the dam, bacterial leakage was reduced to 20%.

Although high-speed evacuation is not a true form of barrier control, it should be used whenever possible. Evacuation decreases the amount of particles that become airborne.[208]

Disposable impervious-backed paper, plastic, or aluminum wrap can be used to cover surfaces and operatory equipment.[208,227] This aids in the prevention of surface contamination from blood or saliva. Plastic is more resistant to water penetration and can be molded into any shape more easily than can paper. Specially designed covers are commercially available to protect light handles, chairs, and bracket and instrument tables. Ash et al. developed a technique wherein radiographic film can be wrapped and sealed with a plastic to prevent contamination with saliva.[236] After the film has been exposed, the wrap is opened and the film handed to someone who is not contaminated and therefore can then develop the saliva-free film. Another method is to open the contaminated film packet in the darkroom or developing box using disposable gloves. The films should be dropped out of the packets without touching the films. Drop the contaminated packets in a paper cup. After all packets have thus been opened, the discarded packets and the gloves can be removed before processing the films. A recent study has demonstrated that bacterial contamination on radiographic films can survive the processing, thus pointing out the importance of preventing cross-contamination for this dental procedure.[237]

SHARP INSTRUMENTS

Needles, endodontic files, scalpels, and other sharp instruments must be handled with care to prevent percutaneous injury. After anesthetics or other injectables have been administered, the needle should be kept in a "sterile" area either uncapped or recapped, using the "scoop technique" (holding the cap in a hemostat or using a manufactured cap holder).

After needles or scalpel blades have been used, they should be removed with a hemostat to prevent injury. All sharps should be placed into puncture-resistant receptacles, which are then disposed of according to local regulations.

IMMUNIZATION

Hepatitis B is a major health hazard for dental health care personnel. Because of this risk, the ADA Council on Dental Therapeutics and the CDC have recommended that all dental personnel involved in patient care receive the hepatitis B vaccine if they do not already have immunity as a result of previous exposure to the virus.[206,238] Two types of vaccines are currently available: a plasma-derived HB vaccine and a recombinant DNA HB vaccine. Both are considered safe and effective in producing immunity to HBV. To date, no serious side effects have been reported from recipients of either vaccine.

Vaccines play an important role in the infection control process, but many bloodborne pathogens exist for which there is presently no vaccine, including HIV and non-A/non-B hepatitis. Proper infection control procedures are therefore important to prevent transmission of any pathogen.

ENDODONTIC INSTRUMENTS AND MATERIALS

Glass bead sterilizers have been commonly used in endodontic offices. Sterilization of clean endodontic files can be achieved with glass beads at 218°C (424.4°F) for 15 seconds or with salt at the same temperature for 10 seconds.[239] It is important to note that there is a wide variability among units in achieving operating temperatures. Preheating times ranged from 15 minutes to 3.5 hours, according to a test of sterilizers.[240] Larger instruments and more porous materials should be immersed in sterilizers for a minimum of 20 seconds. If larger-size instruments are being reused, the handles are not sterilized and require alternate methods of sterilization between patients.

Gutta-percha points are sterile in the manufacturer's package. Contaminated points can be sterilized with 5.25% sodium hypochlorite.[241] Researchers have found that gutta-percha can be sterilized after exposure to gram-positive, gram-negative, and spore-forming microorganisms within 1 minute after immersion in undiluted sodium hypochlorite (Clorox). No mention was made of viral forms. No changes were noted in the dimensional stability or integrity of the points immersed for up to 5 minutes in sodium hypochlorite versus points that were placed in water.[241]

Immersion in polyvinylpyrrolidone-iodine for 6 minutes is an alternate method for the disinfection of gutta-percha.[242] The reliability of this method against tuberculosis bacilli and some spore forms is questionable, however.

OCCUPATIONAL HEALTH AND SAFETY ADMINISTRATION

The OSHA requires employers, including dentists, to provide a safe working environment for their employees. Endodontists must obey guidelines developed by their specific state administrations and information set forth by the CDC and the ADA.[243] According to Miyasaki and associates, informing, educating, and providing for one's employees are ways to minimize the chance of an OSHA inspection.[244] Practitioners should inform their employees of the risks of exposure to hazardous materials and bloodborne diseases, educate employees on the prevention of the spread of disease, and provide protective equipment. All infection control procedures should be documented. Lastly, the endodontist can consult with an OSHA consultant regarding current regulations.

Chemical hazards are another area of regulation by OSHA. Again, depending on the location of practice, the endodontist must be aware of state and local regulations. Even though the endodontic office has fewer hazardous substances than does a general practice, items such as mercury, formaldehyde, and nitrous oxide may often be found. Generally, a complete list of hazardous substances in the office must be kept on file. This should be updated as materials are added to the office. Material safety data sheets from manufacturers must be available to employees. This documentation includes handling and use precautions, emergency and first-aid procedures, and control measures. Practitioners must also have a hazard communication program to disperse information to their employees.

CONCLUSION

A checklist recommended by the ADA is printed as Figure 3-10.[209] Practitioners should attempt to adhere to these recommendations to protect their patients, staff, and themselves from the risk of cross-contamina-

Infection control for the dental office: A checklist

Immunization

- Health care workers should have appropriate immunizations such as that for hepatitis B virus.

Before patient treatment

- Obtain a thorough medical history.
- Disinfect prostheses and appliances received from the laboratory.
- Place disposable coverings to prevent contamination of surfaces, or disinfect surfaces after treatment.

During patient treatment

- Treat all patients as potentially infectious.
- Use protective attire and barrier techniques when contact with body fluids or mucous membranes is anticipated.
  —Wear gloves.
  —Wear mask.
  —Wear protective eyewear.
  —Wear uniforms, laboratory coats, or gowns.
- Open intraorally contaminated X-ray film packets in the dark room with disposable gloves without touching the films.
- Minimize formation of droplets, spatters, and aerosols.
- Use a rubber dam to isolate the tooth and field when appropriate.
- Use high-volume vacuum evacuation.
- Protect hands.
  —Wash hands before gloving and after gloves are removed.
  —Change gloves between each patient.
  —Discard gloves that are torn, cut, or punctured.
  —Avoid hand injuries.
- Avoid injury with sharp instruments and needles.
  —Handle sharp items carefully.
  —Do not bend or break disposable needles.
  —If needles are not recapped, place in separate field. If recapping is necessary, use a method that protects hands from injury such as a holder for the cap.
  —Place sharp items in appropriate containers.

After patient treatment

- Wear heavy-duty rubber gloves.
- Clean instruments thoroughly.
- Sterilize instruments.
  —Sterilize instruments that penetrate soft tissue or bone.
  —Sterilize, whenever possible, all instruments that come in contact with oral mucous membranes, body fluids, or those that have been contaminated with secretions of patients. Otherwise, use appropriate disinfection.
  —Monitor the sterilizer with biological monitors.
- Clean handpieces, dental units, and ultrasonic scalers.
  —Flush handpieces, dental units, ultrasonic scalers, and air/water syringes between patients.
  —Clean and sterilize air/water syringes and ultrasonic scalers if possible; otherwise, disinfect them.
  —Clean and sterilize handpieces if possible; otherwise, disinfect them.
- Handle sharp instruments with caution.
  —Place disposable needles, scalpels, and other sharp items intact into puncture-resistant containers before disposal.
- Decontaminate environmental surfaces
  —Wipe work surfaces with absorbent toweling to remove debris, and dispose of this toweling appropriately.
  —Disinfect with suitable chemical disinfectant.
  —Change protective coverings on light handles, x-ray unit head, and other items.
- Decontaminate supplies and materials.
  —Rinse and disinfect impressions, bite registrations, and appliances to be sent to the laboratory.
- Communicate infection control program to dental laboratory.
- Dispense a small amount of pumice in a disposable container for individual use on each case and discard any excess.
- Remove contaminated wastes appropriately.
  —Pour blood, suctioned fluids, and other liquid waste into drain connected to a sanitary sewer system.
  —Place solid waste contaminated with blood or saliva in sealed, sturdy impervious bags; dispose according to local government regulations.
- Remove gloves and wash hands.

Figure 3-10 Infection control for the dental office: a checklist. (Report, Council on Dental Materials, ADA.[209])[may be copied]

tion. Recommendations from federal, state, and local authorities can change frequently; therefore, one must remain constantly updated on current information.

REFERENCES

1. Nair PNR, Sjogren U, Krey G et al. Intraradicular bacteria and fungi in root-filled, asymptomatic human teeth with therapy-resistant periapical lesions: a long-term light and electron microscopic follow-up study. JOE 1990;16:580.
2. Sen B, Safavi K, Spangberg L. Growth patterns of candida albicans in relation to radicular dentin. Oral Surg 1997;84:68.
3. Glick M, Trope M, Pliskin M. Detection of HIV in the dental pulp of a patient with AIDS. J Am Dent Assoc 1989; 119:649.
4. Glick M, Trope M, Pliskin E. Human immunodeficiency virus infection of fibroblasts of dental pulp in seropositive patients. Oral Surg 1991;71:733.
5. Easlick K. An evaluation of the effect of dental foci of infection on health. J Am Dent Assoc 1951;42:694.
6. Grossman LI. Focal infection: are oral foci of infection related to systemic disease? Dent Clin North Am 1960;4:749.
7. Fish EW. Bone infection. J Am Dent Assoc 1939;26:691.
8. Meinig G. Root canal cover-up exposed. Ojai (CA): Bion Publishing; 1993.
9. DeStefano F, Anda R, Kahn H, et al. Dental disease and risk of coronary heart disease and mortality. Br Dent J 1993;306:688.
10. Offenbacher S, Katz V, Fertik G, et al. Periodontal infection as a risk factor for preterm low birth weight. J Periodont 1996;67:1103.
11. Bender IB, Seltzer S, Yermish M. The incidence of bacteremia in endodontic manipulation. Oral Surg 1960;13:353.
12. Baumgartner JC, Heggers J, Harrison J. The incidence of bacteremias related to endodontic procedures. I. Nonsurgical endodontics. JOE 1976;2:135.
13. Baumgartner JC, Heggers JP, Harrison JW. Incidence of bacteremias related to endodontic procedures. II. Surgical endodontics. JOE 1977;3:399.
14. Debelian GF, Olsen I, Tronstad L. Bacteremia in conjunction with endodontic therapy. Endod Dent Traumatol 1995;11:142.
15. Heimdahl A, Hall G, Hedberg M, Sandberg H. Detection and quantitation by lysis-filtration of bacteremia after different oral surgical procedures. J Clin Microbiol 1990;28:2205.
16. Debelian GJ, Olsen I, Tronstad L. Bacteremia in conjunction with endodontic therapy. Endod Dent Traumatol 1995;11:142.
17. Sundqvist G, Bloom GD, Enberg K, Johansson E. Phagocytosis of *Bacteroides melaninogenicus* and *Bacteroides gingivalis* in vitro by human neutrophils. J Periodontal Res 1982;17:113.
18. Horiba N, Maekawa Y, Abe Y, et al. Correlations between endotoxin and clinical symptoms or radiolucent areas in infected root canals. Oral Surg 1991;71:492.
19. Horiba N, Maekawa Y, Yamauchi Y, et al. Complement activation by lipopolysaccharides purified from gram-negative bacteria isolated from infected root canals. Oral Surg 1992;74:648.
20. Dwyer TG, Torabinejad M. Radiographic and histologic evaluation of the effect of endotoxin on the periapical tissues of the cat. JOE 1981;7:31.
21. Sundqvist GK, Carlsson J, Herrmann B, et al. Degradation in vivo of the C3 protein of guinea-pig complement by a pathogenic strain of *Bacteroides gingivalis.* Scand J Dent Res 1984;92:14.
22. Sundqvist G, Carlsson J, Herrmann B, Tärnvik A. Degradation of human immunoglobulins G and M and complement factors C3 and C5 by black-pigmented *Bacteroides.* J Med Microbiol 1985;19:85.
23. Odell EL. Zinc as a growth factor for *Aspergillus sp.* and the antifungal effects of root canal sealants. Oral Surg 1995;79:82.
24. Sundqvist G, Carlsson J, Hånström L. Collagenolytic activity of black-pigmented *Bacteroides* species. J Periodontal Res 1987;22:300.
25. Shah HH. Biology of the species *Porphyromonas gingivalis.* Ann Arbor (MI): CRC Press; 1993.
26. Kinder SA, Holt SC. Characterization of coaggregation between *Bacteroides gingivalis* T22 and *Fusobacterium nucleatum* T18. Infect Immun 1989;57:3425.
27. Eftimiadi C, Stashenko P, Tonetti M, et al. Divergent effect of the anaerobic bacteria by-product butyric acid on the immune response: suppression of T-lymphocyte proliferation and stimulation of interleukin-1 beta production. Oral Microbiol Immunol 1991;6:17.
28. Maita E, Horiuchi H. Polyamine analysis of infected root canal contents related to clinical symptoms. Endod Dent Traumatol 1990;6:213.
29. Bibel D. The discovery of the oral flora: a 300-year retrospective. J Am Dent Assoc 1983;107:569.
30. Miller W.D. An introduction in the study of the bacteriopathology of the dental pulp. Dent Cosmos 1894;36:505.
31. Kakehashi S, Stanley HR, Fitzgerald RJ. The effects of surgical exposures of dental pulps in germ-free and conventional laboratory rats. Oral Surg 1965;20:340.
32. Langeland K. Tissue changes in the dental pulp. Odontol Tidskr 1957;65:239.
33. Bergenholtz G, Lindhe J. Effect of soluble plaque factors on inflammatory reactions in the dental pulp. Scand J Dent Res 1975;83:153.
34. Warfvinge J, Bergenholtz G. Healing capacity of human and monkey dental pulps following experimentally-induced pulpitis. Endod Dent Traumatol 1986;2:256.
35. Cvek M, Cleaton-Jones PE, Austin JC, Andreason JO. Pulp reactions to exposure after experimental crown fractures or grinding in adult monkeys. JOE 1982;8:391.
36. Torabinejad M, Kiger RD. A histologic evaluation of dental pulp tissue of a patient with periodontal disease. Oral Surg 1985;59:198.
37. Mazur B, Massler M. Influence of periodontal disease on the dental pulp. Oral Surg 1964;17:592.
38. Langeland K, Rodrigues H, Dowden W. Periodontal disease, bacteria, and pulpal histopathology. Oral Surg 1974;37:257.
39. Czarnecki RT, Schilder H. A histological evaluation of the human pulp in teeth with varying degrees of periodontal disease. JOE 1979;5:242.
40. Wong R, Hirsch RS, Clarke NG. Endodontic effects of root planing in humans. Endod Dent Traumatol 1989;5:193.
41. Kobayashi T, Hayashi A, Yoshikawa R, et al. The microbial flora from root canals and periodontal pockets of non-vital teeth associated with advanced periodontitis. Int Endod J 1990;23:100.
42. Trope M, Rosenberg E, Tronstad L. Darkfield microscopic spirochete count in the differentiation of endodontic and periodontal abscesses. JOE 1992;18:82.
43. Gier RE, Mitchell DF. Anachoretic effect of pulpitis. J Dent Res 1968;47:564.

44. Allard U, Nord CE, Sjoberg L, Stromberg T. Experimental infections with *Staphylococcus aureus*, *Streptococcus sanguis*, *Pseudomonas aeruginosa*, and *Bacteroides fragilis* in the jaws of dogs. Oral Surg 1979;48:454.
45. Robinson HB, Boling LR. The anachoretic effect in pulpitis. J Am Dent Assoc 1949;28:268.
46. Delivanis PD, Snowden RB, Doyle RJ. Localization of blood-borne bacteria in instrumented unfilled root canals. Oral Surg 1981;52:430.
47. Delivanis PD, Fan VSC. The localization of blood-borne bacteria in instrumented unfilled and overinstrumented canals. JOE 1984;10:521.
48. Grossman LI. Origin of microorganisms in traumatized pulpless sound teeth. JDR 1967;46:551.
49. Naidorf IJ. Inflammation and infection of pulp and periapical tissues. Oral Surg 1972;34: 486.
50. Sundqvist G. Ecology of the root canal flora. JOE 1992;18:427.
51. Moller AJR. Influence on periapical tissues of indigenous oral bacteria and necrotic pulp tissue in monkeys. Scand J Dent Res 1981;89:475.
52. Byström A, Happonen RP, Sjögren U, Sundqvist G. Healing of periapical lesions of pulpless teeth after endodontic treatment with controlled asepsis. Endod Dent Traumatol 1987;3:58.
53. Sundqvist GK. Bacteriological studies of necrotic dental pulps [dissertation]. Umea (Sweden): Univ. Umea; 1976.
54. Fabricius L, Dahlén G, Öhman AE, Möller ÅJR. Predominant indigenous oral bacteria isolated from infected root canals after varied times of closure. Scand J Dent Res 1982;90:134.
55. Fabricius L, Dahlén G, Holm SE, Möller ÅJR. Influence of combinations of oral bacteria on periapical tissues of monkeys. Scand J Dent Res 1982;90:200.
56. Sundqvist G, Johansson E, Sjögren U. Prevalence of black-pigmented *Bacteroides* species in root canal infections. JOE 1989;15:13.
57. Baumgartner JC, Falkler WA Jr. Bacteria in the apical 5 mm of infected root canals. JOE 1991;17:380.
58. Gomes B, Drucker D, Lilley J. Positive and negative associations between bacterial species in dental root canals. Microbios 1994;80:231.
59. Gomes BPFA, Drucker DB, Lilley JD. Association of specific bacteria with some endodontic signs and symptoms. Int Endod J 1994;27:291.
60. Sundqvist G. Associations between microbial species in dental root canal infections. Oral Microbiol Immunol 1992;7:257.
61. Griffee MB, Patterson SS, Miller CH, et al. The relationship of *Bacteroides melaninogenicus* to symptoms associated with pulpal necrosis. Oral Surg 1980;50:457.
62. Yoshida M, Fukushima H, Yamamoto K, et al. Correlation between clinical symptoms and microorganisms isolated from root canals of teeth with periapical pathosis. JOE 1987;13:24.
63. Happonen RP. Periapical actinomycosis: a follow-up study of 16 surgically treated cases. Endod Dent Traumatol 1986;2:205.
64. Heimdahl A, Von Konow L, Satoh T, Nord CE. Clinical appearance of orofacial infections of odontogenic origin in relation to microbiological findings. J Clin Microbiol 1985;22:299.
65. Hashioka K, Yamasaki M, Nakane A, et al. The relationship between clinical symptoms and anaerobic bacteria from infected root canals. JOE 1992;18:558.
66. Van Winkelhoff AJ, Carlee AW, de Graaff J. *Bacteroides endodontalis* and other black-pigmented *Bacteroides* species in odontogenic abscesses. Infect Immun 1985;49:494.
67. Drucker D, Lilley J, Tucker D, Gibbs C. The endodontic microflora revisited. Microbios 1992;71:225.
68. Gomes B, Lilley J, Drucker D. Clinical significance of dental root canal microflora. J Dent 1996;24:47.
69. Brook I, Frazier E. Clinical features and aerobic and anaerobic microbiological characteristics of cellulitis. Arch Surg 1995;130:786.
70. Brook I, Frazier E, Gher MJ. Microbiology of periapical abscesses and associated maxillary sinusitis. J Periodontol 1996;67:608.
71. Haapasalo M, Ranta H, Rantah K, Shah H. Black-pigmented *Bacteroides* spp. in human apical periodontitis. Infect Immun 1986;53:149.
72. Haapasalo M. *Bacteroides* spp. in dental root canal infections. Endod Dent Traumatol 1989;5:1.
73. Bystrom A, Sundqvist G. Bacteriologic evaluation of the efficacy of mechanical root canal instrumentation in endodontic therapy. Scand J Dent Res 1981;89:321.
74. Bystrom A, Sundqvist G. Bacteriologic evaluation of the effect of 0.5 percent sodium hypochlorite in endodontic therapy. Oral Surg 1983;55:307.
75. Bystrom A, Sundqvist G. The antibacterial action of sodium hypochlorite and EDTA in 60 cases of endodontic therapy. Int Endod J 1985;1:35.
76. Sjögren U, Figdor D, Persson S, Sundqvist G. Influence of infection at the time of root filling on the outcome of endodontic treatment of teeth with apical periodontitis. Int Endod J 1997;30:297.
77. Ranta H, Haapasalo M, Kontiainen S, et al. Bacteriology of odontogenic apical periodontitis and effect of penicillin treatment. Scand J Infect Dis 1988;20:187.
78. Molander A, Reit C, Dahlen G, Kvist T. Microbiological status of root-filled teeth with apical periodontitis. Int Endod J 1991;31:1.
79. Siren E, Haapasalo M, Ranta K, et al. Microbiological findings and clinical treatment procedures in endodontic cases selected for microbiological investigation. Int Endod J 1997;30:91.
80. Sundqvist G, Figdor D, Persson S, Sjögren U. Microbiologic analysis of teeth with failed endodontic treatment and the outcome of conservative re-treatment. Oral Surg 1998;85: 86.
81. Sen BH, Piskin B, Demirci T. Observation of bacteria and fungi in infected root canals and dentinal tubules by SEM. Endod Dent Traumatol 1995;11:6.
82. Sundqvist G. Taxonomy, ecology, and pathogenicity of the root canal flora. Oral Surg 1994;78:522.
83. Shah HN, Gharbia SE. Biochemical and chemical studies on strains designated *Prevotella intermedia* and proposal of a new pigmented species, *Prevotella nigrescens* sp. nov. Int J Syst Bacteriol 1992;42:542.
84. Bae K, Baumgartner JC, Xia T, David L. SDS-PAGE and PCR for differentation of *Prevotella intermedia* and *P. nigrescens*. JOE 1999;25:324.
85. Bae K, Baumgartner JC, Shearer T, David L. Occurence of *Prevotella nigrescens* and *Prevotella intermedia* in infections of endodontic origin. JOE 1997;23:620.
86. Dougherty W, Bae K, Watkins B, Baumgartner JC. Black-pigmented bacteria in coronal and apical segments of infected root canals. JOE 1998;24:356.

87. Baumgartner JC, Watkins BJ, Bae K-S, Xia T. Association of black-pigmented bacteria with endodontic infections. JOE 1999;25:413.
88. Socransky S. Criteria for the infectious agents in dental caries and periodontal disease. J Clin Periodontol 1979;6:16.
89. Slots J, Rams T. In: Slots J, Taubman M, editors. Contemporary oral microbiology and immunology. 1st ed. St. Louis: CV Mosby; p. 56.
90. Jontell M, Okiji T, Dahlgren U, Bergenholtz G. Immune defense mechanisms of the dental pulp. Crit Rev Oral Biol Med 1998;9:179.
91. Jontell M, Bergenholtz G, Scheynius A, Ambrose W. Dendritic cells and macrophages expressing Class II antigens in the normal rat incisor pulp. JDR 1988;67:1263.
92. Jontell M, Gunraj MN, Bergenholtz G. Immunocompetent cells in the normal dental pulp. JDR 1987;66:1149.
93. Hahn C, Falkler WAJ. Antibodies in normal and diseased pulps reactive with microorganisms isolated from deep caries. JOE 1992;18:28.
94. Topazian R, Goldberg M. Oral and maxillofacial infections. 3rd ed. Philadelphia: WB Saunders; 1994.
95. Sabiston CB Jr, Grigsby WR, Segerstrom N. Bacterial study of pyogenic infections of dental origin. Oral Surg 1976;41:430.
96. Lewis MAO, MacFarlane TW, McGowan DA. Quantitative bacteriology of acute dento-alveolar abscesses. J Med Microbiol 1986;21:101.
97. Brook I, Grimm S, Kielich RB. Bacteriology of acute periapical abscess in children. JOE 1981;7:378.
98. Brook I, Frazier EH, Gher ME. Aerobic and anaerobic microbiology of periapical abscess. Oral Microbiol Immunol 1991;6:123.
99. Williams BL. Bacteriology of dental abscesses of endodontic origin. J Clin Microbiol 1983;18:770.
100. Oguntebi B, Slee AM, Tanzer JM, Langeland K. Predominant microflora associated with human dental periapical abscesses. J Clin Microbiol 1982;15:964.
101. Baumgartner JC, Falkler WA. Experimentally induced infection by oral anaerobic microorganisms in a mouse model. Oral Microbiol Immunol 1992;7:253.
102. Odell LJ, Baumgartner JC, Xia T, Davids LL. Survey of collangenase gene prtC in *Porphyromonas gingivalis* and *Porphyromonas endodontalis* isolated from endodontic infections. JOE 1999;25:555.
103. Brook I, Walker RI. Infectivity of organisms recovered from polymicrobial abscesses. Infect Immun 1983;42:986.
104. Price SB, McCallum RE. Studies on bacterial synergism in mice infected with *Bacteroides intermedius* and *Fusobacterium necrophorum*. J Basic Microbiol 1987;27:377.
105. Sundqvist GK, Eckerbom MI, Larsson ÅP, Sjögren UT. Capacity of anaerobic bacteria from necrotic dental pulps to induce purulent infections. Infect Immun 1979;25:685.
106. Van Steenbergen TJM, Kastelein P, Touw JJA, De Graaff J. Virulence of black-pigmented *Bacteroides* strains from periodontal pockets and other sites in experimentally induced skin lesions in mice. J Periodontal Res 1982;17:41.
107. Henrici A, Hartzell T. The bacteriology of vital pulps. J Dent Res 1919;1:419.
108. Kronfeld R. Histopathology of the teeth and their surrounding structures. Philadelphia: Lea & Febiger; 1920.
109. Hedman WJ. An investigation into residual periapical infection after pulp canal therapy. Oral Surg 1951;4:1173.
110. Shindell E. A study of some periapical roentgenolucencies and their significance. Oral Surg 1961;14:1057.
111. Andreasen JO, Rud J. A histobacteriologic study of dental and periapical structures after endodontic surgery. Int J Oral Surg 1972;1:272.
112. Walton RE, Ardjmand K. Histological evaluation of the presence of bacteria in induced periapical lesions in monkeys. JOE 1992;18:216.
113. Tronstad L, Barnett F, Riso K, Slots J. Extraradicular endodontic infections. Endod Dent Traumatol 1987;3:86.
114. Wayman BE, Murata SM, Almeida RJ, Fowler CB. A bacteriological and histological evaluation of 58 periapical lesions. JOE 1992;18:152.
115. Nair PNR. Light and electron microscopic studies of root canal flora and periapical lesions. JOE 1987;13:29.
116. Iwu C, MacFarlane TW, MacKenzie D, Stenhouse D. The microbiology of periapical granulomas. Oral Surg 1990; 69:502.
117. Abou-Rass M, Bogen G. Microorganisms in closed periapical lesions. Int Endod J 1998;31:39.
118. Baumgartner JC. Microbiologic and pathologic aspects of endodontics. Curr Opin Dent 1991;1:737.
119. Baumgartner JC, Falkler WA Jr. Detection of immunoglobulins from explant cultures of periapical lesions. JOE 1991;17:105.
120. Baumgartner JC, Falkler WA Jr. Reactivity of IgG from explant cultures of periapical lesions with implicated microorganisms. JOE 1991;17:207.
121. Baumgartner JC, Falkler WA. Biosynthesis of IgG in periapical lesion explant cultures. JOE 1991;17:143.
122. Kettering JD, Torabinejad M, Jones SL. Specificity of antibodies present in human periapical lesions. JOE 1991; 17:213.
123. Baumgartner JC, Falkler WA. Serum IgG reactive with bacteria implicated in infections of endodontic origin. Oral Microbiol Immunol 1992;7:106.
124. Kuo M, Lamster I, Hasselgren G. Host mediators in endodontic exudates. JOE 1998;24: 598.
125. Bergenholtz G, Lekholm U, Liljenberg B, Lindhe J. Morphometric analysis of chronic inflammatory periapical lesions in root-filled teeth. Oral Surg 1983;55:295.
126. Babál P, Soler P, Brozman M, et al. In situ characterization of cells in periapical granuloma by monoclonal antibodies. Oral Surg 1987;64:348.
127. Piattelli A, Artese L, Rosini S, et al. Immune cells in periapical granuloma: morphological and immunohistochemical characterization. JOE 1991;17:26.
128. Stern MH, Dreizen S, Mackler BF, et al. Quantitative analysis of cellular composition of human periapical granuloma. JOE 1981;7:117.
129. Cymerman JJ, Cymerman DH, Walters J, Nevins AJ. Human T lymphocyte subpopulations in chronic periapical lesions. JOE 1984;10:9.
130. Nilson R, Johannessen AC, Skaug N, Matre R. In situ characterization of mononuclear cells in human dental periapical inflammatory lesions using monoclonal antibodies. Oral Surg 1984;58:160.
131. Torabinejad M, Kiger RD. Histological evaluation of a patient with periodontal disease. Oral Surg 1985;59:198.
132. Barkhordar RA, Desousa YG. Human T-lymphocyte subpopulations in periapical lesions. Oral Surg 1988;65:763.

133. Lukic A, Arsenijevic N, Vujanic G, Ramic Z. Quantitative analysis of the immunocompetent cells in periapical granuloma: correlation with the histological characteristics of the lesions. JOE 1990;16:119.
134. Alavi AM, Gulabivala K, Speight PM. Quantitative analysis of lymphocytes and their subsets in periapical lesions. Int Endod J 1998;31:233.
135. Alavi A, Gulabivala K, Speight, P. Quantitative analysis of lymphocytes and their subsets in periapical lesions. Int Endod J 1998;31:233.
136. Stashenko P, Wang SM. T-helper and T-suppressor cell reversal during the development of induced rat periapical lesions. JDR 1989;68:830.
137. Tani-Ishii N, Wang C-Y, Tanner A, Stashenko P. Changes in root canal microbiota during the development of rat periapical lesions. Oral Microbiol Immunol 1994;9:129.
138. Stashenko P, Teles R, D'Souza R. Periapical inflammatory responses and their modulation. Crit Rev Oral Biol Med 1998;9:498.
139. Fouad A, Rivera E, Walton R. Pencillin as a supplement in resolving the localized acute apical abscess. Oral Surg 1996;81:590.
140. Walton RE, Chiappinelli J. Prophylactic pencillin: effect on posttreatment symptoms following root canal treatment of asymptomatic periapical pathosis. JOE 1993;19:466.
141. Baker PT, Evans RT, Slots J, Genco RJ. Antibiotic susceptibility of anaerobic bacteria from the human oral cavity. JDR 1985;64:1233.
142. Ranta H. Bacteriology of odontogenic apical periodontitis and effect of penicillin treatment. Scand J Infect Dis 1988;20:187.
143. Vigil GV, Wayman BE, Dazey SE, et al. Identification and antibiotic sensitivity of bacteria isolated from periapical lesions. JOE 1997;23:110.
144. Yamamoto K, Fukushima H, Tsuchiya H, Sagawa H. Antimicrobial susceptibilities of *Eubacterium, Peptostreptococcus,* and *Bacteroides* isolated from root canals of teeth with periapical pathosis. JOE 1989;15:112.
145. Dajani A., et al. Prevention of bacterial endocarditis: recommendations by the American Heart Association. JAMA 1997;277:1794–801.
146. Strom B, Abrutyn E, Berlin J, et al. Dental and cardiac risk factors for infective endocarditis. A population-based, case-control study. Ann Intern Med 1998;129:761.
147. Durack D. Antibiotics for prevention of endocarditis during dentistry: time to scale back? Ann Intern Med 1998; 129:829.
148. Short JA, Morgan LA, Baumgartner J. A comparison of canal centering ability of four instrumentation techniques. JOE 1997;23:503.
149. Luiten D, Morgan L, Baumgartner J, Marshall J. A comparison of four instrumentation techniques on apical canal transportation. JOE 1995;21:26.
150. Reddy S, Hicks M. Apical extrusion of debris using two hand and two rotary instrumentation techniques. JOE 1998;24:180.
151. Baumgartner JC, Mader C. A scanning electron microscopic evaluation of four root canal irrigation regimens. JOE 1987;13:147.
152. Baumgartner JC, Cuenin PR. Efficacy of several concentrations of sodium hypochlorite for root canal irrigation. JOE 1992;18:605.
153. Senia ES, Marshall FJ, Rosen S. The solvent action of sodium hypochlorite on pulp tissue of extracted teeth. Oral Surg 1971;30:96.
154. Hand RE, Smith ML, Harrison JW. Analysis of the effect of dilution on the necrotic tissue dissolution property of sodium hypochlorite. JOE 1978;4:60.
155. Harrison JW, Hand RE. The effect of dilution and organic matter on the antibacterial property of 5.25% sodium hypochlorite. JOE 1981;7:128.
156. Shih M, Marshall FJ, Rosen S. The bactericidal efficiency of sodium hypochlorite as an endodontic irrigant. Oral Surg 1970;29:613.
157. Baumgartner JC, Mader CL. A scanning electron microscopic evaluation of four root canal irrigation regimens. JOE 1987;13:147.
158. Byström A, Sundqvist G. The antibacterial action of sodium hypochlorite and EDTA in 60 cases of endodontic therapy. Int Endod J 1985;18:35.
159. Cvek M, Nord C, Hollender L. Antimicrobial effect of root canal debridement in teeth with immature root. Odont Revy 1976;27:1.
160. Turkun M, Cengiz T. The effects of sodium hypochlorite and calcium hydroxide on tissue dissolution and root canal cleanliness. Int Endod J 1997;30:335.
161. Gatot A, Arbelle J, Leiberman A, Yanai-Inbar I. Effects of sodium hypochlorite on soft tissues after its inadvertent injection beyond the root apex. JOE 1991;17:573.
162. Reeh ES, Messer HH. Long-term paresthesia following inadvertent forcing of sodium hypochlorite through perforation in maxillary incisor. Endod Dent Traumatol 1989;5:200.
163. Metzler RS, Montgomery S. The effectiveness of ultrasonics and calcium hydroxide for the debridement of human mandibular molars. JOE 1989;15:373.
164. Sjögren U, Sundqvist G. Bacteriologic evaluation of ultrasonic root canal instrumentation. Oral Surg 1987;63:366.
165. Martin H. Ultrasonic disinfection of the root canal. Oral Surg 1976;42:92.
166. Martin H, Cunningham WT, Norris JP, Cotton WR. Ultrasonic versus hand filling of dentin: a quantitative study. Oral Surg 1980;49:79.
167. Huque J, Kota K, Yamaga M, et al. Bacterial eradication from root dentine by ultrasonic irrigation with sodium hypochlorite. Int Endod J 1998;31:242.
168. Engstrom B, Segerstad LHA, Ramstrom G, Frostell G. Correlation of positive cultures with the prognosis of root canal treatment. Odont Revy 1964;15:257.
169. Seltzer S, Vito A, Bender IB. A histologic evaluation of periapical repair following positive and negative root canal cultures. Oral Surg 1964;17:507.
170. Bender IB, Seltzer S, Turkenkopf S. To culture or not to culture. Oral Surg 1964;18:527.
171. Spångberg L, Rutberg M, Rydinge E. Biologic effects of endodontic antimicrobial agents. JOE 1979;5:166.
172. Spångberg L. Biologic effects of root canal filling materials. Oral Surg 1974;38:934.
173. Spångberg L, Engstrom G, Langeland K. Biologic effects of dental materials III. Toxicity and antimicrobial effect of endodontic antiseptics in vitro. Oral Surg 1973;36:856.
174. Thoden van, Velson S, Felt-kamp-Vroom T. Immunologic consequences of formaldehyde fixation of autologous tissue implants. JOE 1977;3:179.
175. Walton R. Intracanal medicaments. Dent Clin North Am 1984;28:783.

176. Stuart KG, Miller CH, Brown CE, Newton CW. The comparative antimicrobial effect of calcium hydroxide. Oral Surg 1991;72:101.
177. Safavi KE, Dowden WE, Introcasco JH, Langeland K. A comparison of antimicrobial effects of calcium hydroxide and iodine-potassium iodide. JOE 1985;11:454.
178. Estrela C, Pimenta F, Ito I, Bammann L. In vitro determination of direct antimicrobial effect of calcium hydroxide. JOE 1998;24:15.
179. Siqueira J, de Uzeda M. Intracanal medicaments: evaluation of the antibacterial effects of chlorhexidine, metronidazole, and calcium hydroxide associated with three vehicles. JOE 1997;23:167.
180. Barbosa CAM, Goncalves R, Siqueira J Jr, De Uzeda M. Evaluation of the antibacterial activities of calcium hydroxide, chlorhexidine and camphorated paramonochlorphenol as intracanal medicament. A clinical and laboratory study. JOE 1997;23:297.
181. Byström A, Claesson R, Sundqvist G. The antibacterial effect of camphorated paramonochlorophenol, camphorated phenol and calcium hydroxide in the treatment of infected root canals. Endod Dent Traumatol 1985;1:170.
182. Sjögren U, Figdor D, Spångberg L, Sundqvist G. The antimicrobial effect of calcium hydroxide as a short-term intracanal dressing. Int Endod J 1991;24:119.
183. Kontakiotis E, Nakou M, Georgopoulou M. In vitro study of the indirect action of calcium hydroxide on the anaerobic flora of the root canal. Int Endod J 1995;28:285.
184. Abdulkader A, Duguid R, Saunders EM. The antimicrobial activity of endodontic sealers to anaerobic bacteria. Int Endod J 1996;29:280.
185. Nissan R, Segal H, Pashley D, et al. Ability of bacterial endotoxin to diffuse through human dentin. JOE 1995;21:62.
186. Orstavik D, Haapasalo M. Disinfection by endodontic irrigants and dressings of experimentally infected dentinal tubules. Endod Dent Traumatol 1990;6:142.
187. Foster KH, Kulild JC, Weller RN. Effect of smear layer removal on the diffusion of calcium hydroxide through radicular dentin. JOE 1993;19:136.
188. Estrela C, Pimenta FC, Yoko I, Bammann L. Antimicrobial evaluation of calcium hydroxide in infected dentinal tubules. JOE 1999;25:416.
189. Heling I, Chandler NP. The antimicrobial effect within dentinal tubules of four root canal sealers. JOE 1996;22:257.
190. Mickel AK, Wright ER. Growth inhibition of *Streptococcus anginosa (milleri)* by three calcium hydroxide sealers and one zinc oxide-eugenol sealer. JOE 1999;25:34.
191. Sundqvist G, Reuterving CO. Isolation of *Actinomyces israelii* from periapical lesion. JOE 1980;6:602.
192. O'Grady JF, Reade PC. Periapical actinomycosis involving *Actinomyces israelii*. JOE 1988;14:147.
193. Barnard D, Davies J, Figdor D. Susceptibility of *Actinomyces israelii* to antibiotics, sodium hypochlorite and calcium hydroxide. Int Endod J 1996;29:320.
194. Hasselgren G, Olsson B, Cvek M. Effects of calcium hydroxide and sodium hypochlorite on the dissolution of necrotic porcine muscle tissue. JOE 1988;14:125.
195. Yang SF. Anaerobic tissue-dissolving abilities of calcium hydroxide and sodium hypochlorite. JOE 1995;21:613.
196. Cohen F, Lasfargues JJ. Quantitative chemical study of root canal preparations with calcium hydroxide. Endod Dent Traumatol 1988;4:108.
197. Webber R, del Rio C, Brady J, Segall R. Sealing quality of a temporary filling material. Oral Surg 1978;46:423.
198. Blaney TD, Peters DD, Setterstrom J, Bernier WE. Marginal sealing quality of IRM and cavit as assessed by microbial penetration. JOE 1981;7:453.
199. Bobotis HG, Anderson RW, Pashley DH, Pantera EA. A microleakage study of temporary restorative materials used in endodontics. JOE 1989;15:569.
200. Anderson RW, Powell BJ, Pashley DH. Microleakage of IRM® used to restore endodontic access preparations. Endod Dent Traumatol 1990;6:137.
201. Deveaux E, Hildelbert P, Neut C, et al. Bacterial microleakage of Cavit, IRM, and TERM. Oral Surg 1992;74:634.
202. Kontakiotis E, Wu M, Wesselink P. Effect of calcium hydroxide dressing on seal of permanent root filling. Endod Dent Traumatol 1997;13:281.
203. Schafer E, Bossmann K. Antimicrobial effect of camphorated chloroxylenol (ED 84) in the treatment of infected root canals. JOE 1999;25:547.
204. Crawford JJ. Office sterilization and asepsis procedures in endodontics. Dent Clin North Am 1979;23:717.
205. Crawford JJ. State-of-the-art: practical infection control in dentistry. J Am Dent Assoc 1985;110:629.
206. Council on Dental Therapeutics. Guidelines for infection control in the dental office and the commercial dental laboratory. J Am Dent Assoc 1985;110:968.
207. Ad Hoc Committee on Infectious Diseases: The control of transmissible disease in dental practice: a position paper on the American Association of Public Health Dentistry. J Public Health Dent 1986;46:13.
208. Centers for Disease Control and Prevention. Recommended infection-control practices for dentistry. Morb Mortal Wkly Rep 1986;35:237.
209. Council on Dental Materials, Instruments and Equipment, Council on Dental Practice, Council on Dental Therapeutics: Infection control recommendations for the dental office and the dental laboratory. J Am Dent Assoc 1988;116:241.
210. Centers for Disease Control and Prevention. Recommendations for prevention of HIV transmission in health-care settings. MMWR Morb Mortal Wkly Rep 1987;36:3.
211. Division of Scientific Affairs: Facts about AIDS for the dental team. J Am Dent Assoc 1991.
212. Hastreiter RJ, et al. Effectiveness of dental office instrument sterilization procedures. J Am Dent Assoc 1991;122:51.
213. Siew C, et al. Self-reported percutaneous injuries in dentists: implications for HBV, HIV, transmission risk. J Am Dent Assoc 1992;123:37.
214. County of San Diego, Department of Health Services. Document DHS: HM-9096, 1989.
215. Epstein JB, Mathias RG. Infection control in dental practice demands of the 1980's. J Can Dent Assoc 1986;8:695.
216. Centers for Disease Control and Prevention. Guidelines for prevention or transmission of human immunodeficiency virus and hepatitis B virus to health-care and public-safety workers. MMWR Morb Mortal Wkly Rep 1989;38:3.

217. Scarlett M. Emphasis: infection control in the dental office: a realistic approach. J Am Dent Assoc 1986;112:468.
218. ADA workshop on handpieces and other instruments in dentistry: sterilizing dental handpieces. J Am Dent Assoc 1992;123:44.
219. Runnells RR. Heat and heat/pressure sterilization. J Calif Dent Assoc 1985;13:46.
220. Rohrer MD, Bulard RA. Microwave sterilization. J Am Dent Assoc 1985;110:194.
221. Palenik CJ. A survey of sterilization practices in selected endodontic offices. JOE 1986;12:206.
222. Dental Products Report: Chemical disinfecting/sterilizing solutions—update '89. Irving Cloud; 1985: p. 17.
223. Mitchell E. Chemical disinfectant/sterilizing agents. J Calif Dent Assoc 1985;13:64.
224. Dental Products Report: disinfection/sterilizing solutions—update '86. Irving Cloud; 1986: p. 32.
225. Bagga BS, et al. Contamination of dental unit cooling water with oral microorganisms and its prevention. J Am Dent Assoc 1984;109:712.
226. Wirthlin MR. The performance of autoclaved high-speed dental handpieces. J Am Dent Assoc 1981;103:584.
227. Miller CH. Barrier techniques for infection control. J Calif Dent Assoc 1985;13:54.
228. Crawford JJ. Cross infection risks and their control in dentistry: an overview. J Calif Dent Assoc 1985;13:18.
229. Wilson MP, et al. Gloved versus ungloved dental hygiene clinicians, a comparison of tactile discrimination. Dent Hyg 1986;310.
230. Hardison JD, et al. Gloved and ungloved: performance time for two dental procedures. J Am Dent Assoc 1988;116:691.
231. Clinical Research Associates. Subject: gloves, disposable-operating. CRA Newsletter 1985;9:2.
232. Mitchell R, et al. The use of operating gloves in dental practice. Br Dent J 1983;154:372.
233. Gobetti JP, et al. Hand asepsis: the efficacy of different soaps in the removal of bacteria from sterile, gloved hands. J Am Dent Assoc 1986;113:219.
234. Council on Dental Therapeutics. Facts about AIDS for the dental team. Chicago: American Dental Association; 1985.
235. Fors UG, et al. Microbiological investigation of saliva leakage between the rubber dam and tooth during endodontic treatment. JOE 1986;17:396.
236. Ash JL, et al. The use of a sealed plastic bag of radiographic film to avoid cross-contamination. JOE 1984;10:512.
237. Bachman CE, et al. Bacterial adherence and contamination during radiographic processing. Oral Surg 1990;70:669.
238. Centers for Disease Control and Prevention. Protection against viral hepatitis. MMWR Morb Mortal Wkly Rep 1990;39:1.
239. Windeler AS, Walter RG. The sporicidal activity of glass bead sterilizers. JOE 1975;1:273.
240. Dayoub MB, Devin MJ. Endodontic dry-heat sterilizer effectiveness. JOE 1976;2:343.
241. Senia SE, Marraro RV. Rapid sterilization of gutta-percha cones with 5.25% sodium hypochlorite. JOE 1975;1:136.
242. Montgomery S. Chemical decontamination of gutta-percha cones with polyvinylpyrrolidone-iodine. Oral Surg 1971;31:258.
243. Controlling occupational exposure to blood-borne pathogens in dentistry. Washington (DC): US Government Printing Office; 1992. OSHA Bulletin 3129.
244. Miyasaki C, et al. Demystifying OSHA inspection guidelines. J Calif Dent Assoc 1989;17:28.

Chapter 4

PULPAL PATHOLOGY: ITS ETIOLOGY AND PREVENTION

John I. Ingle, James H. S. Simon, Richard E. Walton, David H. Pashley, Leif K. Bakland, Geoffrey S. Heithersay, and Harold R. Stanley

The noxious stimuli responsible for pulp inflammation, necrosis, and dystrophy are legion, ranging from bacterial invasion to hereditary dwarfism. Without question, bacterial invasion from a carious lesion is the most frequent initial cause of pulp inflammation. Paradoxically, an alarming amount of pulp involvement is induced by the very dental treatment designed to repair the carious lesion. An increase in automobile and cycle accidents, as well as accidents from body contact sports, has also brought about an increase in pulp death owing to trauma.

The causes of pulp inflammation, necrosis, and dystrophy are arranged below in logical sequence, beginning with the most frequent irritant, microorganisms:

I. Bacterial
  A. Coronal ingress
    1. Caries
    2. Fracture
      a. Complete
      b. Incomplete (cracks, infraction)
    3. Nonfracture trauma
    4. Anomalous tract
      a. Dens invaginatus (aka dens in dente)
      b. Dens evaginatus
      c. Radicular lingual groove (aka palatogingival groove)
  B. Radicular ingress
    1. Caries
    2. Retrogenic infection
      a. Periodontal pocket
      b. Periodontal abscess
    3. Hematogenic
II. Traumatic
  A. Acute
    1. Coronal fracture
    2. Radicular fracture
    3. Vascular stasis
    4. Luxation
    5. Avulsion
  B. Chronic
    1. Adolescent female bruxism
    2. Traumatism
    3. Attrition or abrasion
    4. Erosion
III. Iatral
  A. Cavity preparation
    1. Heat of preparation
    2. Depth of preparation
    3. Dehydration
    4. Pulp horn extensions
    5. Pulp hemorrhage
    6. Pulp exposure
    7. Pin insertion
    8. Impression taking
  B. Restoration
    1. Insertion
    2. Fracture
      a. Complete
      b. Incomplete
    3. Force of cementing
    4. Heat of polishing
  C. Intentional extirpation and root canal filling
  D. Orthodontic movement
  E. Periodontal curettage
  F. Electrosurgery
  G. Laser burn
  H. Periradicular curettage
  I. Rhinoplasty
  J. Osteotomy
  K. Intubation for general anesthesia
IV. Chemical
  A. Restorative materials
    1. Cements
    2. Plastics
    3. Etching agents

4. Cavity liners
5. Dentin bonding agents
6. Tubule blockage agents

B. Disinfectants
1. Silver nitrate
2. Phenol
3. Sodium fluoride

C. Desiccants
1. Alcohol
2. Ether
3. Others

V. Idiopathic
A. Aging
B. Internal resorption
C. External resorption
D. Hereditary hypophosphatemia
E. Sickle cell anemia
F. Herpes zoster infection
G. Human immunodeficiency virus (HIV) and acquired immune deficiency syndrome (AIDS)

BACTERIAL CAUSES

Coronal Ingress

Caries. Coronal caries is by far the most common means of ingress to the dental pulp for infecting bacteria and/or their toxins (Figure 4-1). Long before the bacteria reach the pulp to actually infect it, the pulp becomes inflamed from irritation by preceding bacterial toxins. Langeland reported pulp reactions he observed "with certainty" when superficial enamel fissure caries were found clinically[1] (Figure 4-2). Brännström and Lind observed inflammatory changes in the pulps of 50 of 74 premolars with initial enamel caries on proximal surfaces but with no radiographic evidence of penetration[2] (Figure 4-3).

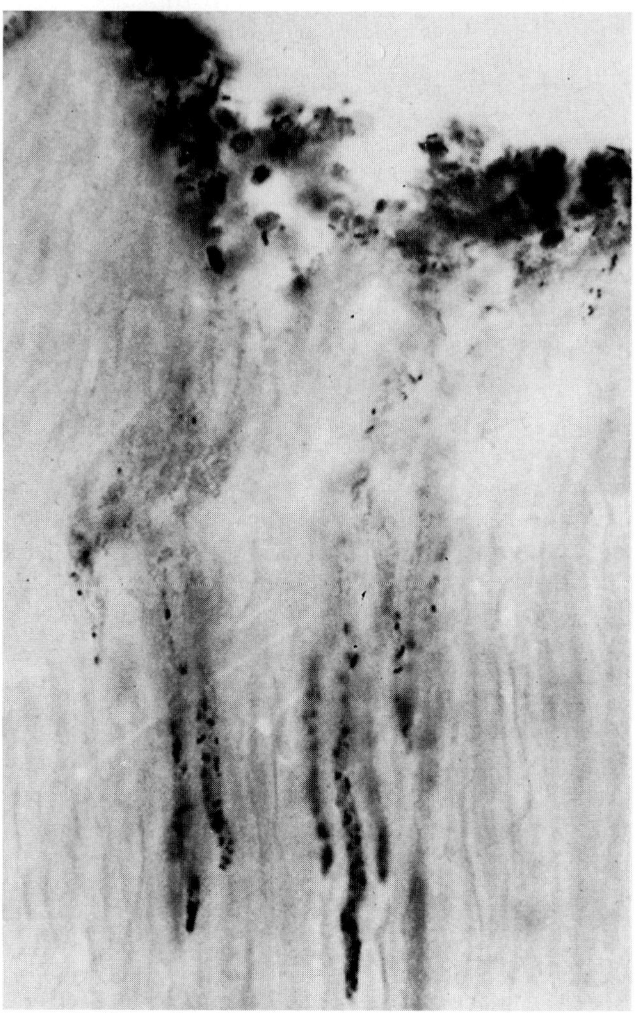

Figure 4-1 Bacteria penetrating through dentinal tubules from carious lesion (**top**). Pulp inflammation is already established from toxins that precede bacteria (Orban collection).

Brännström and his associates also demonstrated the alarming rapidity with which bacteria penetrate the enamel.[3] From incipient carious lesions, **without cavitation** on the enamel surface (Figure 4-4), microorganisms can reach the dentinoenamel junction. The ensuing gap between the enamel and dentin completely fills with microorganisms. The infection is then shown to spread not only laterally along the dentinoenamel junction but pulpally as well. It is quite conceivable that a degree of pulp inflammation could develop well before a visual or radiographic break in the enamel becomes apparent. To compound the problem, Douglass et al. have claimed that only 60% of dental caries lesions can be detected by radiographs alone.[4]

Seltzer et al. have described these pulp changes, from early irritation dentin formation under initial caries, through scattered macrophages and lymphocytes under moderately developed caries, to frank chronic inflammatory exudate under deep carious lesions.[5]

Skogedal and Tronstad remarked on how reasonable it is to expect pulp involvement subjacent to carious lesions in the dentin because of the intimate relationship between the dentin and the dental pulp.[6] They pointed out, however, the existing disagreement over attempts by some to correlate the **degree** of inflammation with the **depth** and "virulence" of the carious lesion. "It is conceivable," they surmised, "that the apparent discrepancies...are due to **variations** in the reaction known to occur in the dentin subjacent to carious lesions." This is discussed later in the chapter.

Most of the evidence to build and solve this enigma has been provided by Scandinavian researchers. Bergenholtz and Lindhe produced severe pulpitis with necrosis, **within hours,** merely by sealing an extract of

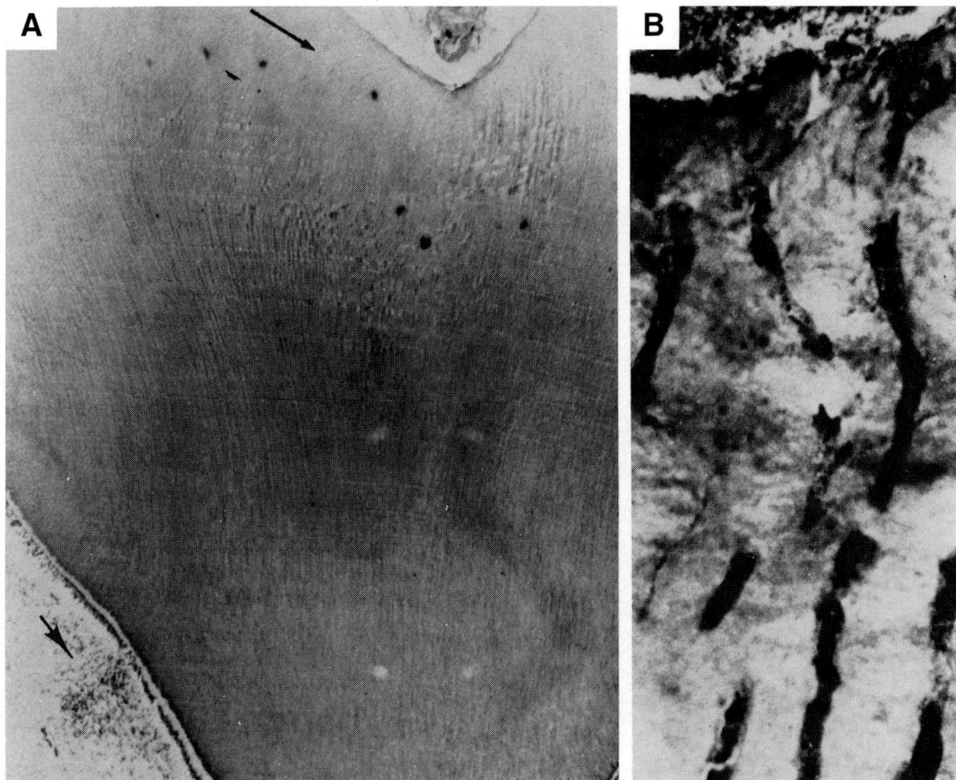

Figure 4-2 Enamel fissure caries leading to dentin and pulp involvement. **A,** At the top center, there is no break at the dentinoenamel junction, yet bacteria (**upper arrow**) have already penetrated dentin, and their toxins have caused pulp reaction (**lower left arrow**). Note break in the odontoblast layer and subjacent inflammatory cells. **B,** Bacteria in tubuli just below carious surface. (Courtesy of Dr. Karre Langeland.)

human dental plaque into deep class V cavity preparations[7] (Figure 4-5). Years before, Langeland achieved a similar result by sealing soft carious dentin into a prepared cavity.[8] Langeland's seminal research was confirmed by Mjör and Tronstad, who also compared the pulp reaction to carious dentin sealed into preparations in intact teeth against a control of gutta-percha temporaries[9] (Figure 4-6 to 4-8).

Dentin Permeability. One might assume from these studies that normal **primary** dentin is incapable of protecting the pulp from toxic agents or immune reactions triggered by the microorganisms of dental plaque or soft carious dentin. The **speed** with which pulp reactions take place is obviously related to the amount and degree of calcification of the remaining dentin. Reeves and Stanley found little inflammation if bacteria penetrated to within 1.1 mm (including irritation dentin) of the pulp.[10] Pathosis increased, however, when the lesion reached to within 0.5 mm of the pulp, and abscess formation developed when the irritation dentin barrier was breached.

For the remaining dentin to act as a barrier, it is important to consider both dentin thickness and the **degree of mineralization.** Trowbridge made the point that the rapidity and degree of flow of noxious stimuli toward the pulp are directly related to the absence or presence of a dense dentin barrier.[11] Thus, the most permeable would be dead tract dentin (empty tubules) followed by primary dentin (Figure 4-9). Irritation dentin, on the other hand, should be considerably less permeable (Figure 4-10).

The supposition can be made, therefore, that the **acuteness** or **chronicity** of caries as a disease serves to stimulate the production of an effective irritation dentin barrier. The highly acute lesion evidently overwhelms the pulp's calcific defense capability, whereas the chronic lesion allows time for an irritation and sclerotic dentin defense to develop. This could well explain the variance from normal pulp to advanced pulpitis under large carious lesions.

Reversible or Irreversible Pulpitis. Thus far in this chapter, nothing has been said about the pulp, which has been considered inflamed rather than infected. Here again, controversy develops: Does the inflamed and/or infected pulp represent reversible or irreversible pulpitis? What allows microorganisms to finally penetrate the dentin and invade and infect the pulp? Why is their movement relatively slow in the dentin yet

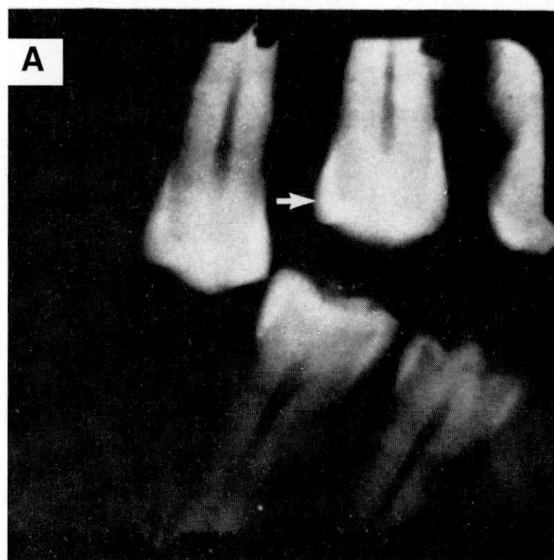

Figure 4-3 A, Radiograph does not reveal enamel or dentin caries, maxillary first premolar (**arrow**). B, Same tooth; brown discoloration on distal surface but no apparent break in enamel. C, No cavitation in distal enamel surface (**large arrow**), yet zone of altered dentin reaches to pulp (**arrows**). Reproduced with permission from Langeland K.[30]

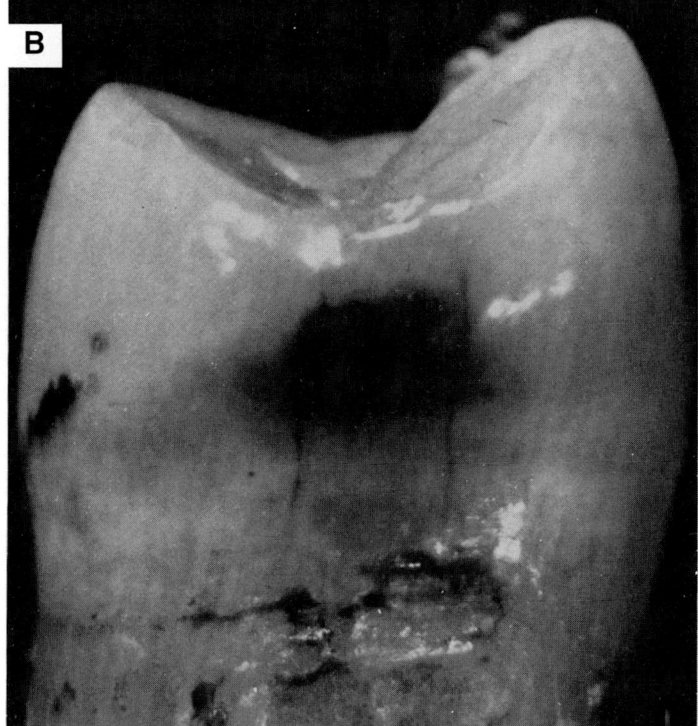

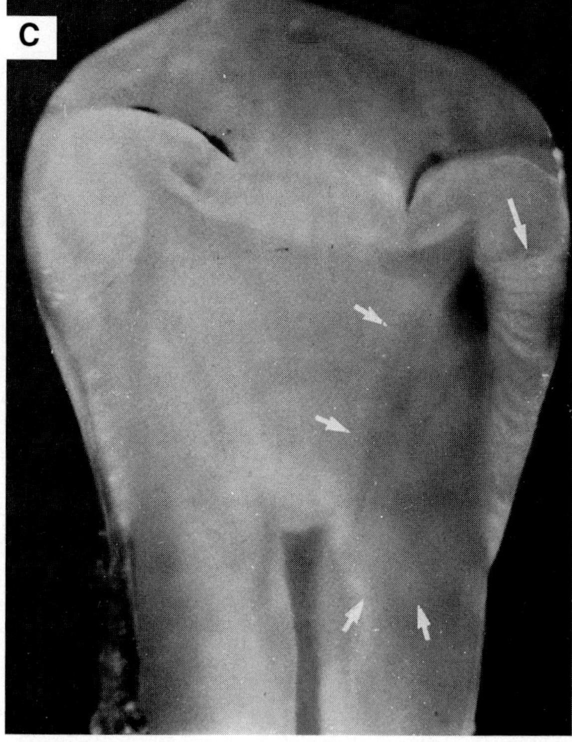

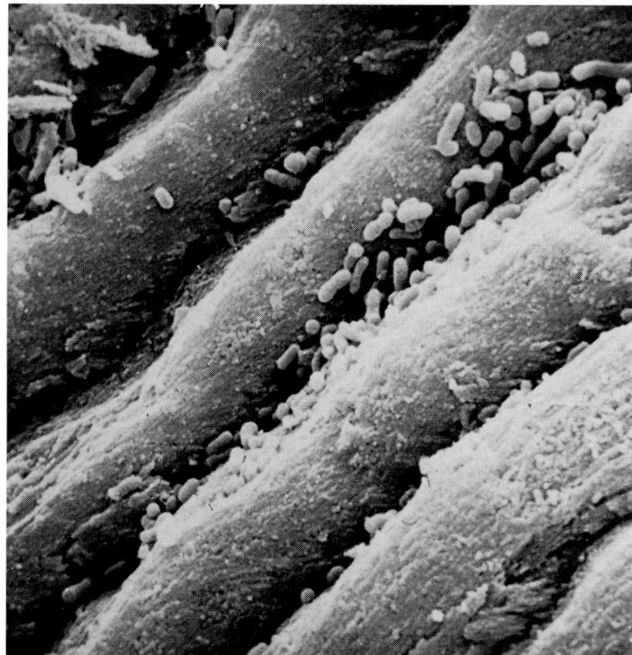

Figure 4-4 Round and rod-shaped microorganisms found between enamel prisms on the surface of a dull "white-spot" lesion. Bacteria extend to the dentinoenamel junction. Reproduced with permission from Brännström M.[3]

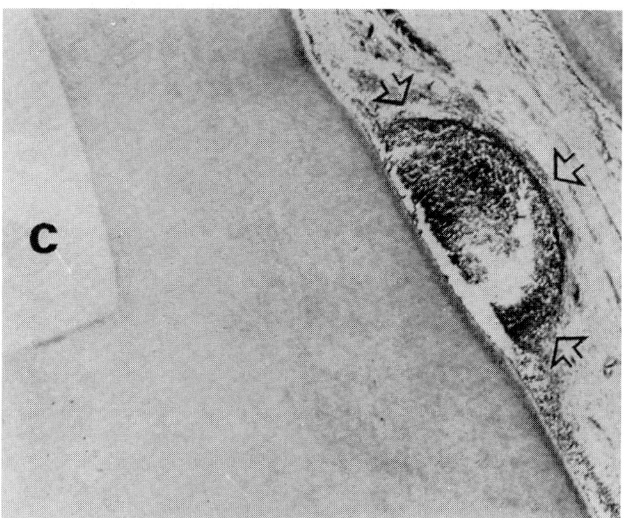

Figure 4-5 Localized abscess formation (**arrows**) subjacent to dentin cavity (C) after 32 hours of microbial provocation with lyophilized components from dental plaque bacteria. Reproduced with permission from Bergenholtz G.[345]

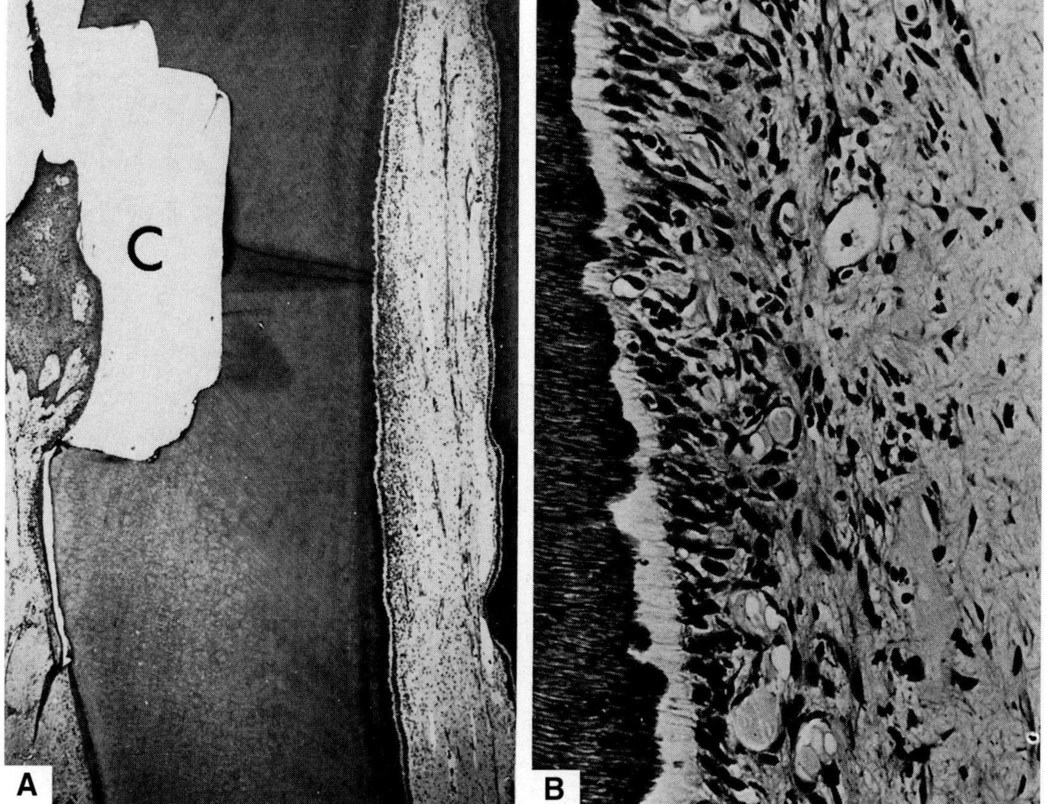

Figure 4-6 A, Histologic pulp changes defined as **slight**. Cavity (C) restored with gutta-percha for 8 days. B, Higher magnification of area subjacent to the cavity. A slight increase in cellularity results in obscuring of cell-free zone. Slight increase in capillaries. Reproduced with permission from Mjör IA and Tronstad L.[9]

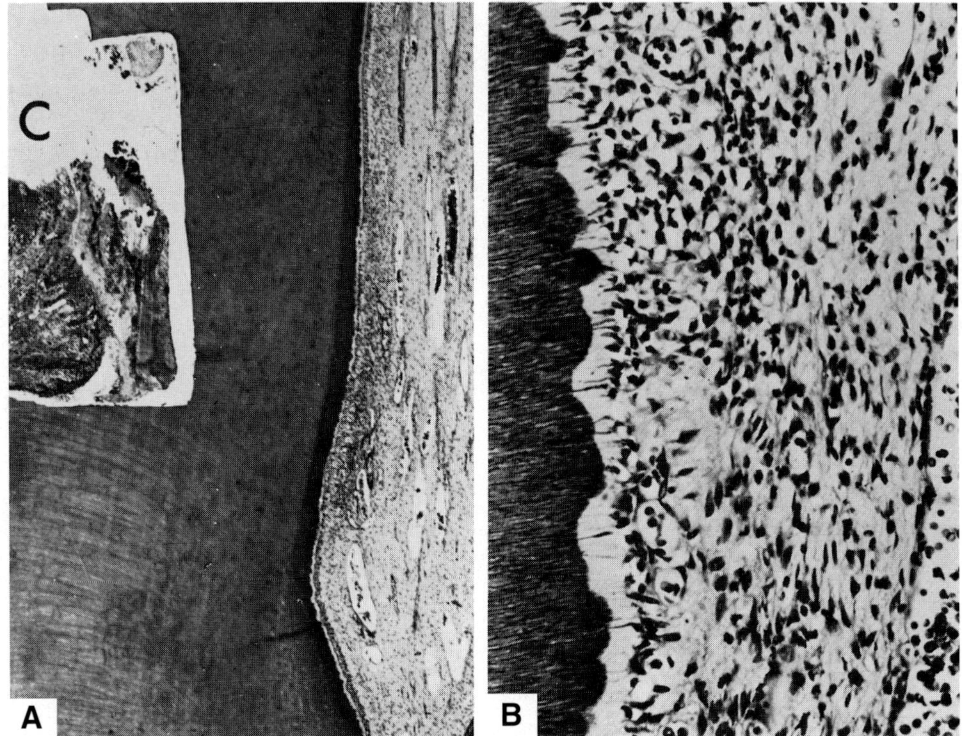

Figure 4-7 A, Histologic pulp changes defined as **moderate**. Cavity (C) left open for 8 days. **B**, Higher magnification of area subjacent to the cavity. Increased cellularity and disruption of odontoblastic layer with some odontoblast nuclei displaced into dentin tubules. Increase in vascularity. Reproduced with permission from Mjör IA and Tronstad L.[9]

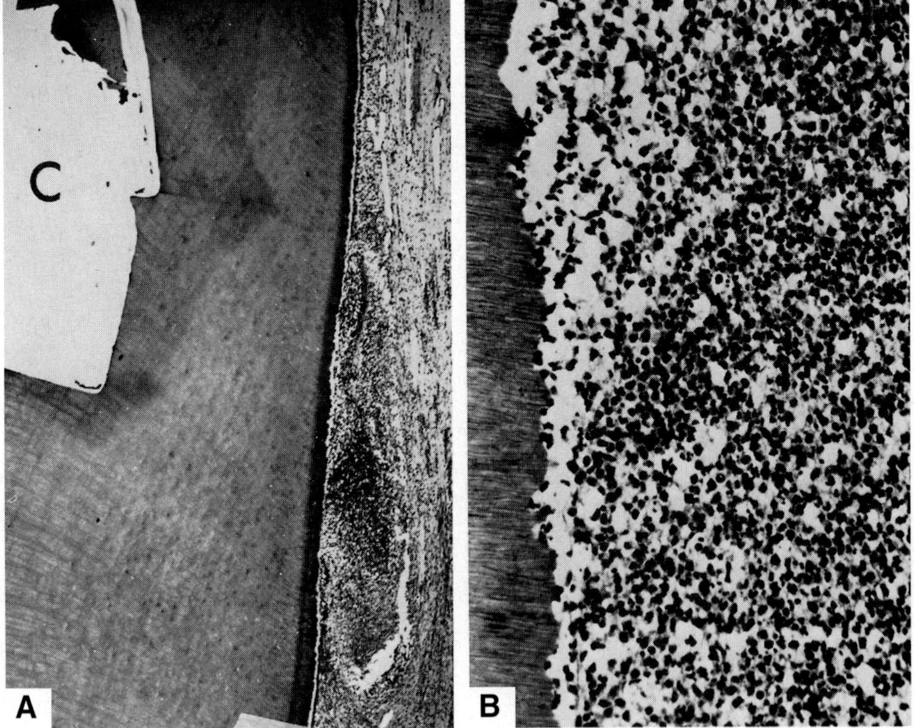

Figure 4-8 A, Histologic pulp changes defined as **severe**. Cavity (C) filled with soft, carious human dentin for 8 days. **B**, Higher magnification of area subjacent to cavity. Marked cellular infiltration and necrosis, odontoblast layer also destroyed, and predentin missing. Reproduced with permission from Mjör IA and Tronstad L.[9]

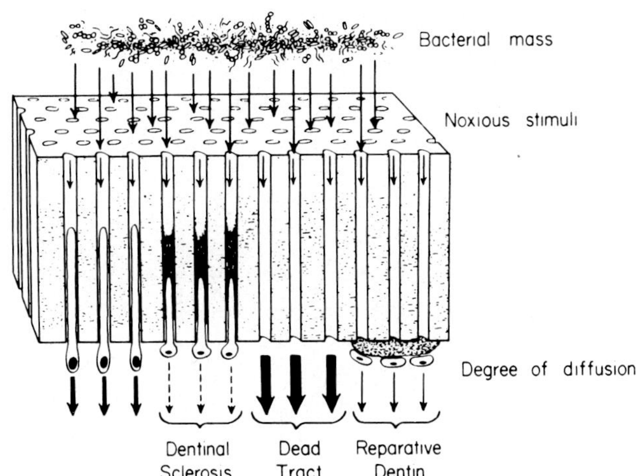

Figure 4-9 Dentin permeability, ranging from left to right: primary tubular, sclerotic, dead tract and reparative (irritation) dentin. The degree of noxious diffusion is denoted by the size of the arrows; dead tract noxious diffusion is the greatest and sclerotic noxious diffusion is the least. Reproduced with permission from Trowbridge HO.[11]

surprisingly rapid through enamel? As we shall see, demineralization appears to be the answer.

Mjör found that **bacteria** in soft carious dentin, sealed into class V preparations in intact teeth, had not penetrated to the pulp in 82 days.[12] In spite of this, severe pulpitis was present.

Massler and Pawlak described "affected" and "infected" dentin, based on the difference between the two conditions.[13] They quoted MacGregor, who said that the active carious lesion is composed of an outer **infected** layer and "a deeper (underlying) **affected** layer which has been demineralized by acids produced by the bacteria in the infected surface layer."[14] The entire protocol for indirect pulp capping therapy is based on the premise that the pulp is "affected" but not "infected" by bacteria; therefore, early pulpitis should be reversible.

Langeland, on the other hand, questioned the rationale of this supposition.[15] Using anaerobic culturing and electron microscopy, he demonstrated dead and live bacteria in all leathery dentin. Going farther into the dentin, he found bacteria "in the tubules of hard dentin below the meticulously cleaned cavity surface." In the pulps subjacent to this infected dentin, pathologic changes were occurring. In fact, bacteria were seen to penetrate "through the calciotraumatic line, the irritation dentin, and predentin to the pulp"—hardly the proper soil for reversibility of pulpitis.[15]

In view of these findings, Paterson and Pountney[16] and Watts and Paterson[17] have made some remarkable observations. Monoinfecting the mouths of gnotobiot-

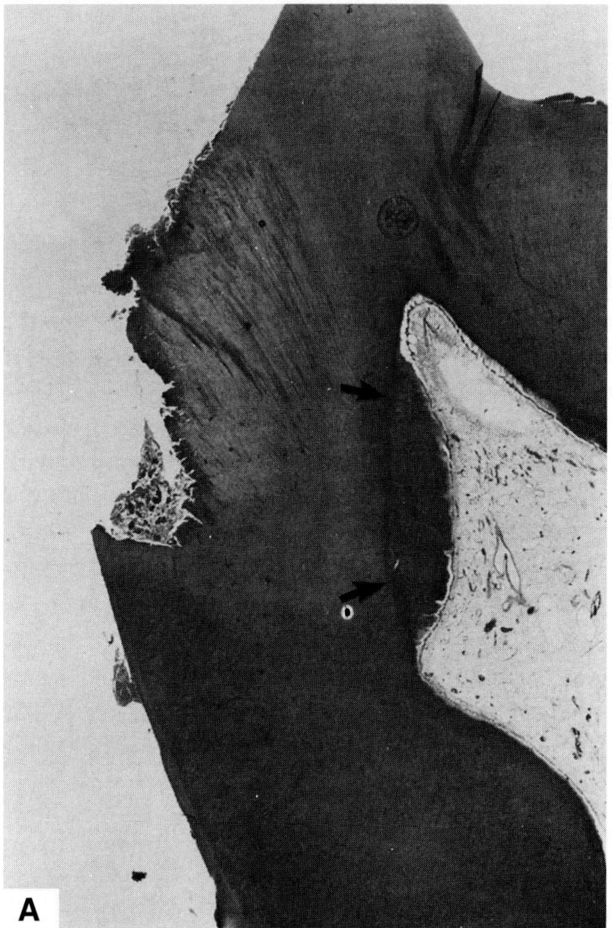

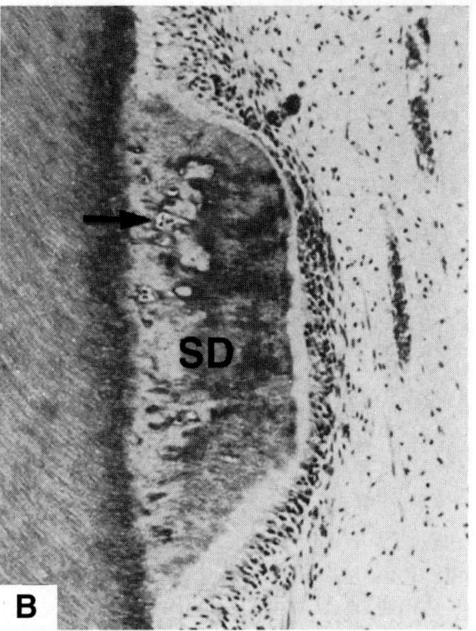

Figure 4-10 A, Irritation dentin formation (**arrows**) subjacent to carious lesion. Reproduced with permission from Trowbridge HO.[11] **B,** Higher magnification of irritation dentin subjacent to cavity first filled with human carious dentin (7 days) and then with zinc phosphate cement for 32 days. There is no evidence of inflammation. Cellular inclusion in irritation dentin (SD). Reproduced with permission from Lervik T.[142]

ic rats with either *Streptococcus mutans,* the known cause of dentin caries, or *Lactobacillus casei,* thought to contribute to enamel caries, the authors were surprised to detect **no** pulp inflammation: "Direct invasion of vital pulp tissue by bacteria did not occur, even when pulps were left exposed directly to saliva."[16,17] Necrosis in pulp horns did occur, however, in some very advanced lesions, which were "always associated with extensive irregular calcification."[16,17] Yet neither inflammation nor *S. mutans* was present; apparently, the pulp cells had phagocytized the microorganisms. It is Paterson's further contention "that the organisms commonly isolated from caries in dentine are not very harmful to the pulp: Secondary contamination with the mixed flora from saliva is the major source of pulp damage" (personal communication, August 11, 1982). For a more in-depth discussion of the role bacteria play in inflammation and necrosis of the pulp, the reader is referred to chapter 3.

Later studies by the Paterson group at Glasgow University carried these initial findings one step further.[18] After infecting pulp **exposures** in germ-free rats with *S. mutans*, Paterson and Watts further concluded that this caries-causing bacteria is relatively innocuous to the pulp tissue. Necrosis, **without inflammation,** seen in the pulps, was caused primarily by the crushing effect of food impaction on the pulp. Furthermore, after 28 days, in 79% of the infected pulps, "well-formed dentin bridges were present," which is hardly a sign of pulps overwhelmed by bacteria.[19]

Paterson and colleagues made the point that it seems "prudent to avoid the contamination of deep cavity floors with saliva." The rubber dam, they stated, is important, limiting the bacterial flora in deep cavities to the caries-causative germs, which are a "weak pathogen to the pulp."[18–20]

Seltzer stated that "there is a tremendous resistance against the penetration of microorganisms into the pulp."[21] Quite possibly, the pulp succumbs to mixed or anaerobic infections but not to single bacterial strains.

A major breakthrough in understanding the enigma of the movement of bacteria through the dentin and into the pulp was supplied by Olgart et al.[22] in Sweden and by Michelich et al.[23] in the United States. These latter investigators stated that "as long as the dentin is **not** acid-etched, bacteria seldom penetrate into the tubules, presumably because they are physically restricted from the tubule orifice by a thin layer of microcrystalline debris." Conversely, they found that "bacteria can penetrate **acid etched** dentinal tubules by growth or hydrostatic pressure," such as the pressure during mastication[23] (Figure 4-11). Meryon and her group in England later proved that three strains of bacteria were unable to penetrate through dentin because of the smear layer. When the smear layer was removed by citric acid etching, however, the bacteria readily penetrated through 500 microns (0.5 mm) of human dentin.[24]

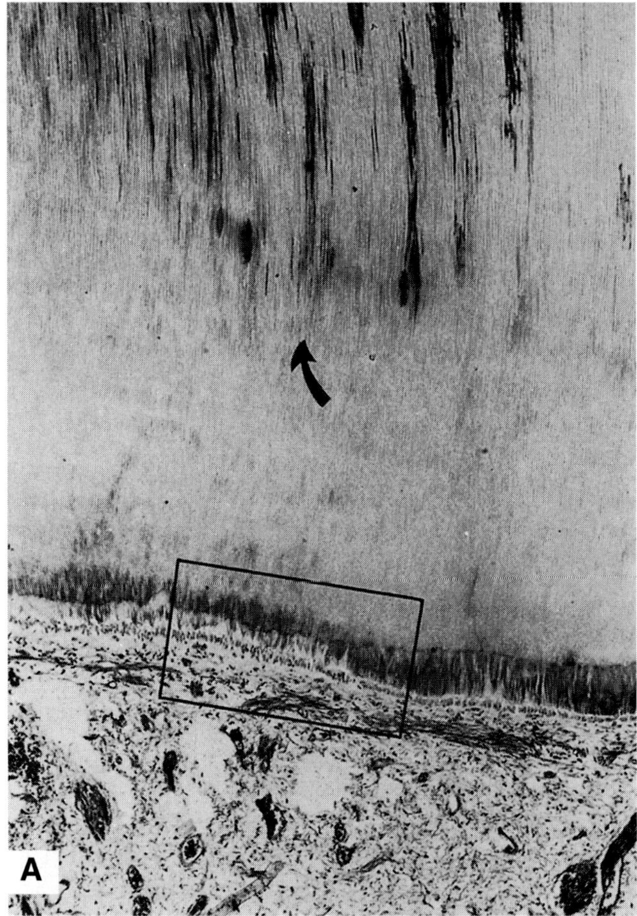

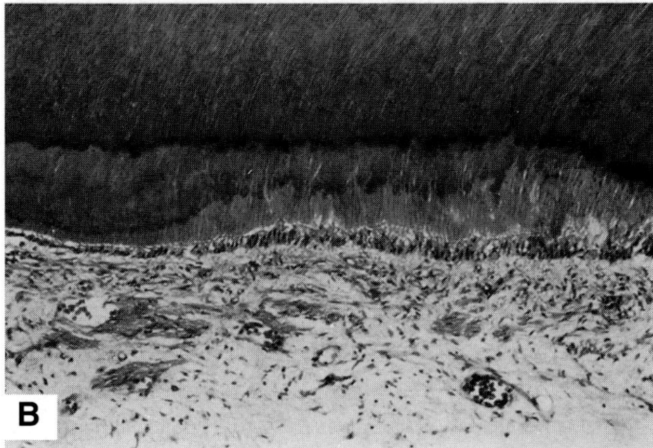

Figure 4-11 A, Bacterial penetration of dentin from carious lesion. Deepest point of penetration (**arrow**) 0.8 mm from pulp. B, Higher magnification of rectangle in A. Predentin activity, diffuse infiltration of chronic inflammatory cells, and deposition of collagen fibers. Reproduced with permission from Trowbridge HO.[11]

One could summarize, therefore, that "unetched dentin, while permitting fluid filtration, restricts bacterial penetration."[23] Hence the noxious **filtrates** from the carious lesion or dental plaque can penetrate into the tubules (where the odontoblast cell body is affected) and into the pulp, where inflammation rapidly develops. The **bacteria,** on the other hand, being grossly larger than the filtrate, cannot pass the calcific structures or the microcrystalline tubular debris unless preceded by an acid (which they produce) that decalcifies the dentin while clearing and widening the tubules.

The slowness with which dentin demineralization and subsequent bacterial transport occur is related to the higher **organic** content of dentin. Enamel, on the other hand, being highly **inorganic,** is demineralized readily (witness the total loss of enamel in histologic sections) by the bacteria, thus allowing an easier pathway for bacterial movement through enamel as noted by Brännström et al.[3]

In the end, Massler's and MacGregor's[13,14] "affected," **decalcified** leathery dentin might well provide the bacterial pathway for pulp invasion and infection. Whether the ensuing pulpitis is reversible or irreversible is still open to question. It is quite possibly **reversible** if the bacteria have not yet reached the pulp and quite possibly **irreversible** if the pulp has become infected by bacteria.[1]

Pulpal Healing. Bacteria are an obvious formidable enemy of the pulp, but possibly not so formidable as once supposed. In a review of the clinical management of the deep carious lesion, Canby and Burnett discussed the wisdom of **not** exposing the pulp under deep caries: "Removing all carious dentin and jeopardizing a **vital pulp with no significant untoward history or reaction** [emphasis added] would seem to be a questionable method and a needless contribution to the complexity of treatment..."[25]

This approach is also borne out by Muntz et al.[26] and by Seltzer et al.,[27] who predicted the possibility of pulp recovery if its ability to produce irritation dentin keeps ahead of the carious process. This could well happen. Irritation dentin is formed in monkey teeth at a rate of 2.9 μm per day, over three times the rate of secondary dentin, of which 0.8 μm is laid down daily.[28]

The healing capacity of the pulp, inflamed by bacterial toxins or bacteria *per se*, is still in dispute. As stated above, the pulp may well be able to keep ahead of **chronic** caries by constantly laying down irritation or sclerotic dentin while receding from the irritant to "lick its wounds," so to speak. But **acute** caries is another matter. If pulp inflammation begins within hours of irritation by **bacterial toxins,** can the pulp recover from this plight, or, in other words, is the pulpitis reversible?

Bergenholtz and Lindhe seemed to think so: "A moderate to severe inflammatory pulpal reaction may heal **if the irritating agents are removed from the dentin** [emphasis added]. Healing of a localized pulp reaction (abscess formation) may occur not only when the irritating agents are removed from the dentin, but also more important, healing may occur even with constant bacterial irritation of dentin."[7]

Bergenholtz and Lindhe had this histologic insight after removing dental plaque constituents from sealed class V preparations after 32 hours (see Figure 4-5) at 4, 10, or 30 days and substituting zinc oxide–eugenol (ZOE) cement.[7] They further surmised that **irritation dentin,** accompanying sudden (within 32 hours) bacterial irritation, "should be regarded as a scar tissue that develops after or along with the healing process of the pulp."[7] However, there was also evidence contrary to the healing process. In other cases, Bergenholtz and Lindhe found that "an acute inflammatory reaction of the dental pulp can result in total necrosis of pulp tissue..."[7]

Lervik and Mjör also noted healing in inflamed pulps after 7 to 8 days.[29] In a series of experiments in which they induced pulp inflammation within 2 to 3 days by sealing soft carious dentin into cavity preparations of intact teeth, they found that healing had begun 7 to 8 days later in the form of increased predentin formation. They were struck by the quality of the irritation dentin effort to establish a barrier against further noxious stimuli. Very **irregular** irritation dentin formed in one of their experimental teeth, which became necrotic after 82 days. Successful healing, on the other hand, was marked by quite **regular** dentin formation.[29]

Langeland et al., in marked contrast, have long felt atubular dentin to be less permeable and that pulp inflammation is readily found subjacent to atubular and tubular dentin.[30]

It has been pointed out that irregular, or basically atubular, dentin "results from destruction of the involved odontoblastic processes and the entire odontoblasts" and that "the cells immediately subjacent to the 'reparative' dentin more closely resemble fibroblasts than the original odontoblasts." Regular (tubular) dentin, on the other hand, derives from uninjured or newly formed odontoblasts. It is further stated that repair of dentin "is in no way indicative of the repair of the pulpal connective tissue" and that pulp repair can never be complete as long as chronic inflammation is present: "In fact, it may be this chronic subclinical pulpitis that results in acute endodontic emergencies..."[31]

Healing Attempts. Whether pulp inflammation can be reversed by treating the pulp, through the dentin, with various medicaments also has long been in dispute. Langeland was quite pessimistic about these attempts.[15] In a series of experiments testing the efficacy of penicillin combined with camphorated monochlorophenol, corticosteroids such as Mosteller's solution or Ledermix (Lederle, Germany), silver nitrate, and microcrystalline sulfathiazole, Langeland found them all ineffective antiphlogistics. It is true that these drugs initially reduced pulpal pain, but in the long run, inflammation persisted or worsened. Pulps exposed to camphorated phenol, formocresol, formaldehyde, glutaraldehyde, and procion dyes all suffered "coagulation necrosis, which was later followed by liquefaction necrosis and inflammation in the adjacent pulp tissue."[15]

If the production of irritation dentin is any measure of pulp health or recovery, researchers in Scotland reported significant development of tertiary (irritation) dentin following the application of various cavity lining materials.[32] "Tertiary dentin formation was greatest beneath cavities lined with calcium hydroxide and least beneath cavities lined with materials (Ledermix), [Lederle–Germany] containing corticosteroids."[32]

This phenomenon proves once again the value of a **mild irritant,** such as calcium hydroxide, in stimulating pulp recovery. On the other hand, severe irritants such as ZOE were not nearly as effective, and anti-inflammatory components such as corticosteroids actually slowed repair to about one-third that achieved by calcium hydroxide.[32]

SUMMARY: One might summarize by repeating that bacteria cause reparable as well as irreparable damage to the pulp. Taintor et al. best stated this particular point while commenting on the pitfalls of assuming repair:

> "Using the crude parameters of pulpal diagnosis (that is, cold, warm, electric pulp test, percussion, palpation, and radiographic evidence), an initial diagnosis must be made as to the status of the pulp. If it can be determined that the pulp is reversibly inflamed...['Ay, there's the rub'] the course of treatment should be to remove the cause. The diagnosis must be made on the basis of the above objective tests, the objective and subjective clinical signs and symptoms, and confirmation of the carious extent of the lesion by excavation (in one or more sittings). If bacterial invasion of the pulp has occurred, the excavation will and should result in opening to the pulp and endodontic therapy should be performed."[31]

Fractured Crown. *Complete Fracture.* Accidental coronal fracture into the pulp seldom devitalizes the pulp at that instant. However, the inevitable pulp death of the **untreated** coronal fracture results from infection by oral bacteria gaining ready access to the pulp. It does not matter how extensive the fracture is, only that the pulp has been exposed to a mixed bacterial insult.

Most coronal fractures involve the maxillary anterior teeth, although posterior teeth are sometimes fractured in severe automobile accidents or sheared in half in boxing accidents or fights. Classification of fractures and their treatment and restoration are covered in detail in chapter 15.

Incomplete Fracture. Incomplete fracture of the crown (infraction), often from unknown causes, frequently allows **bacterial entrance** into the pulp. Ritchey et al. reported 22 cases of toothache and pulp death associated with incomplete fracture in molars.[33] Pulp infection and associated inflammation depend on the extent of fracture, that is, whether the fracture is complete, extending into the pulp chamber, or only through the enamel. In the former, pulpitis is certain to develop (Figure 4-12); in the latter, the pulp is merely hypersensitive to cold and mastication.

Nonfracture Trauma. Grossman reported pulp canal infection from trauma without fracture of teeth. After carefully swabbing *Serratia marcescens* into the **gingival sulcus** of incisors of dogs and monkeys, Grossman dropped a weight onto individual teeth, which was heavy enough to traumatize but not to fracture the tooth. About one-third of the time, *S. marcescens* could be recovered from the affected root canals from 7 to 54 days later.[34]

Anomalous Tract. Anomalous tooth development, of both the crown and the root, accounts for a substantial number of pulp deaths, usually by bacterial invasion. In each case—dens invaginatus, dens evaginatus, and/or radicular lingual grooves—bacterial infection is the cause of pulp inflammation or tooth loss.

In the case of the internal (dens) anomalies, bacterial infection of the pulp through a development fault in the enamel cap or through caries in a deep pit is the route of invasion. In most of the external (developmental groove) defects, the bacterial invasion is down the defect in the root surface where the periodontal ligament cannot properly attach.

Dens Invaginatus. Most dens invaginatus defects are found in maxillary lateral incisors and range from a slight lingual pit in the cingulum area to a frank and obvious anomalous tract apparent visually or radiographically (Figure 4-13).

Oehlers classified these defects according to their severity[35] (Figure 4-14). Bhaskar described a coronal and radicular dens.[36] The coronal type may involve all of the layers of the enamel organ into the dental

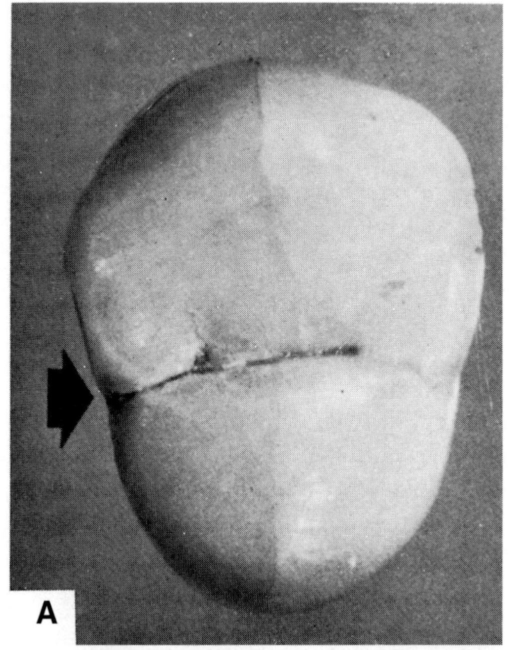

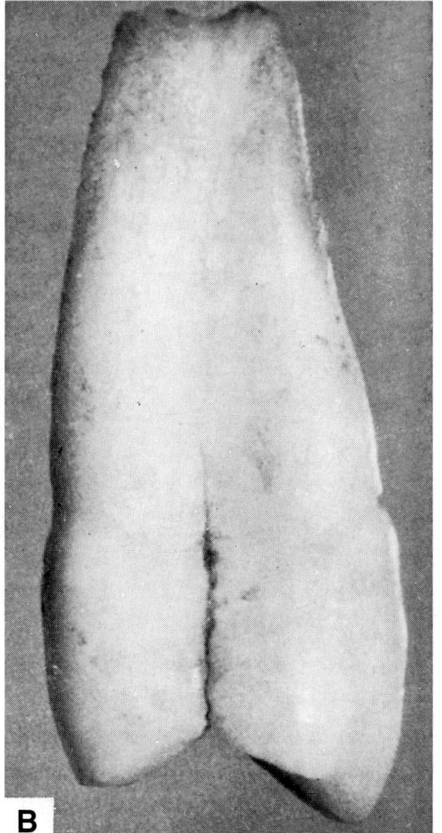

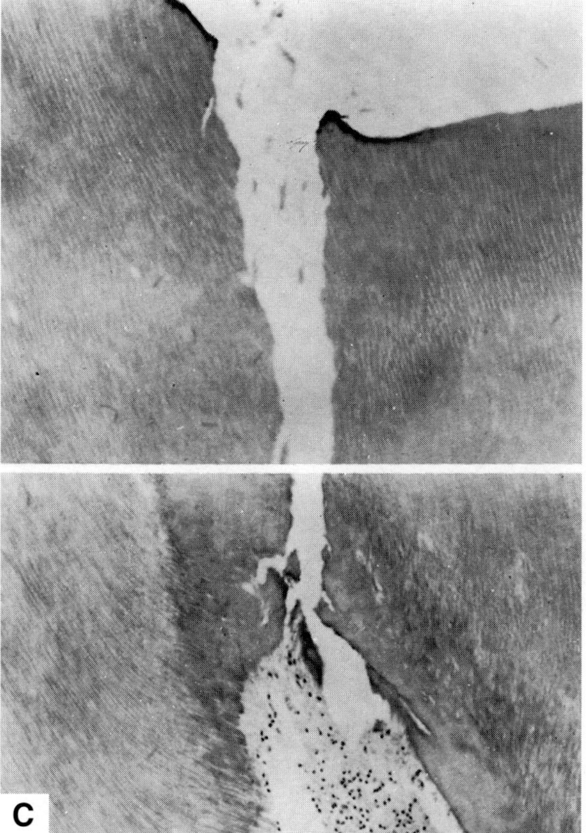

Figure 4-12 Undetected fracture in otherwise sound premolar. **A**, Precipitated iodine shows fracture (**arrow**). Buccolingual fracture was caused by forceps. **B**, Mesial view. Fracture extends into pulp that has become infected from invading bacteria. **C**, Photomicrograph of undisclosed fracture from floor of cavity to pulp. Inflammatory degeneration of pulp is apparent. (**A** and **B** courtesy of Dr. Dudley H. Glick; **C** courtesy of Dr. Harold Stanley.)

papilla. In these cases, the pulp may be exposed and thus open to bacterial invasion, inflammation, and necrosis. Periradicular lesions develop early. In the radicular dens, there is a fold in Hertwig's epithelial root sheath into the developing tooth, and enamel and dentin are produced there. This dens is Oehler's type 3 defect, which opens through from the crown to the apex (foramen caecum), ensuring bacterial invasion and infection (Figure 4-15).

Although most "dens in dentes" are unilateral, they may be bilateral as well.[37–39] Although they are most often found in the maxillary lateral incisors, where so

Figure 4-13 Developmental anomalies of maxillary incisors. A, Dens invaginatus of the cingulum (**arrow**) allows coronal bacterial ingress. B, Clinical appearance of palatogingival groove. Palatal periodontal pocket extends to the apex. C, Three examples of lingual anomalies leading to tooth loss: **left,** invagination and accessory root (**arrow**); **middle,** palatogingival groove to the apex; **right,** palatogingival groove to the midroot of the central incisor. D, Bifid root formation. Bacteria have invaded through the developmental tract not readily seen (**left**). Six months later (**right**), the coronal defect has been filled, but a huge infected cyst has developed following pulp necrosis. B and C reproduced with permission from Simon JHS et al.[61]

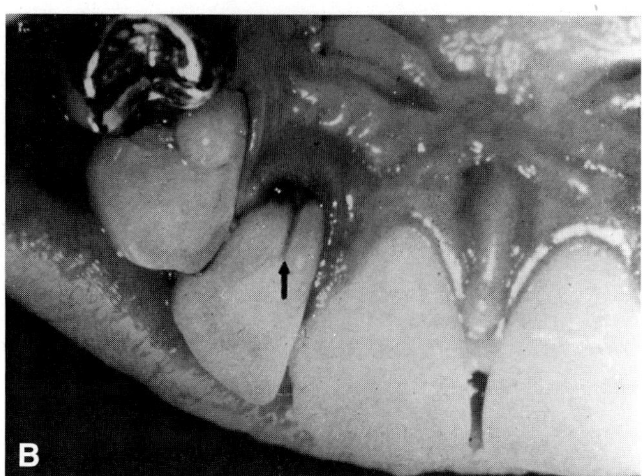

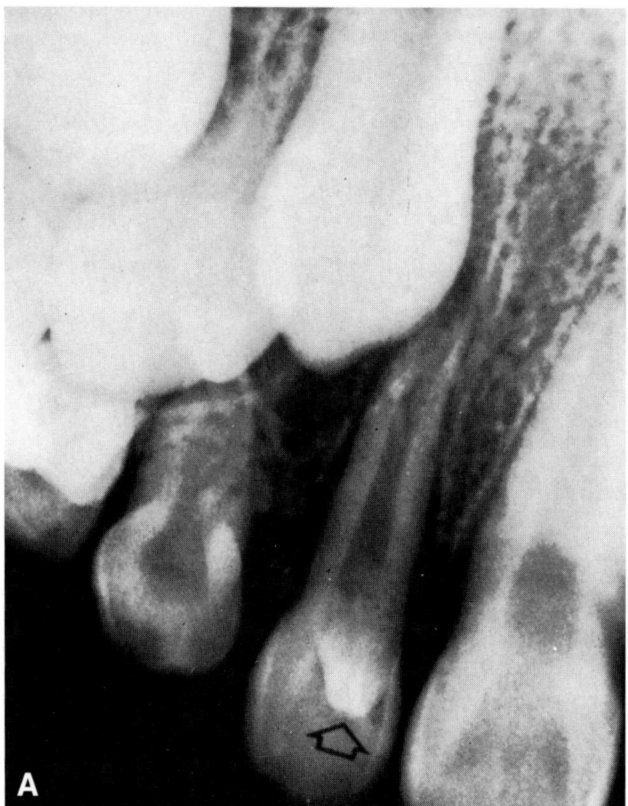

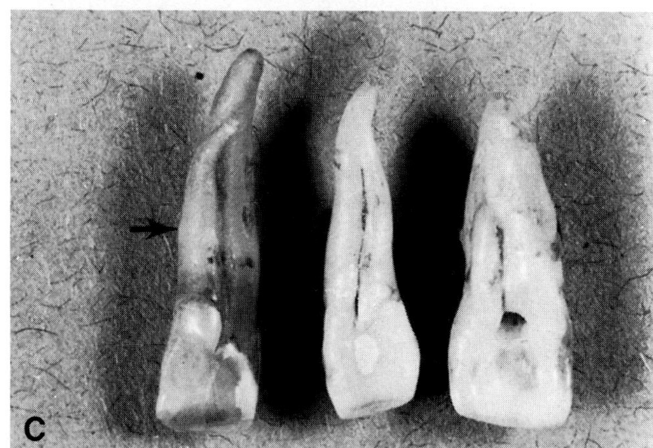

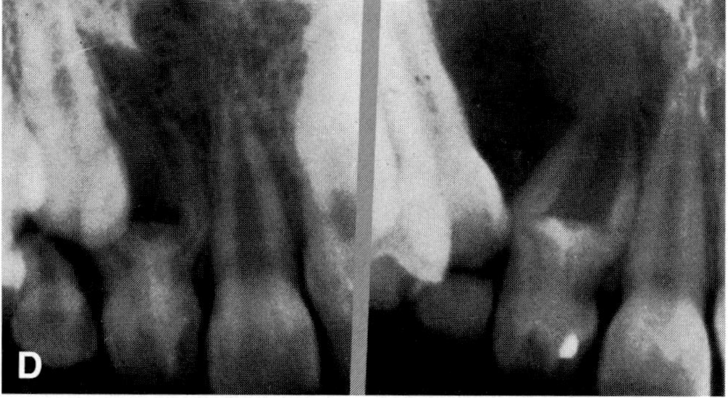

many other anomalies develop, they may also be found in the maxillary central incisors, the mandibular incisors,[37] and other teeth as well. Although not well documented, the clinical observation has been made of a higher than normal incidence of periradicular cysts associated with these cases.[38,40]

The prevalence of dens invaginatus may be higher than generally credited. Frequencies as low as 0.25%[41] but up to 6.9%[42] have been cited. Japanese researchers surveyed the dental radiographs from 766 dental students and reported an incidence of 9.66% overall, with 46.8% of the affected teeth "peg-shaped."[43]

Many dentists panic when faced with dens invaginatus, particularly if a huge periradicular lesion or radicular cyst is present. Extraction often follows panic. Most of these cases can be treated endodontically, including retrofillings.

Dens Evaginatus. Dens evaginatus has a tract to the pulp at its point of attachment. It is a fairly common occurrence in Asians.[44,45] It is usually found on mandibular premolars. Merrill also reported a high incidence (4.5%) of this anomaly in Alaskan Eskimos, an observation serving to illustrate their ethnic ties to Asian peoples.[46,47]

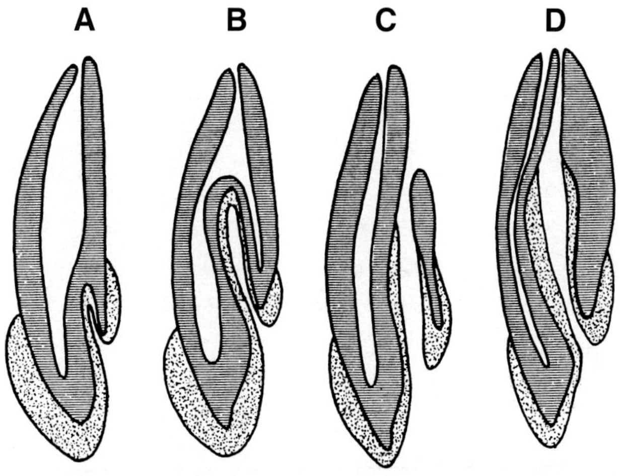

Figure 4-14 Classification of invaginated teeth according to Oehlers. A, Type 1, confined within the crown. B, Type 2, blind sac extending beyond the cementoenamel junction but not reaching the periodontal ligament (PDL) (subject to caries). C, Type 3, extends beyond the cementoenamel junction with the second foramen extending into the periradicular tissues. D, Type 3 with second foramen in the apical area. Reproduced with permission from DeSmit A and Demant L. JOE 1982;8:506.

Yip reported that 2.2% of 2,373 Singapore schoolchildren were afflicted with the condition, all of them of Asian stock and none East Indian in origin.[48] Senia and Regezi reported the condition in a Filipino woman,[49] and Sykaras reported a case in the maxillary premolars of a Greek girl.[50] Carlsen reported a case from the Royal Dental College in Denmark (personal communication, June 1972), and Palmer reported five evaginated odontomas in Caucasian children from England[51] (Figure 4-16). Lin et al. reported **bilateral** dens evaginatus in an 11-year-old Chinese girl,[52] as did Gotoh et al. in patients in Japan.[53] Gotoh et al. also reported a markedly lower incidence of dens evaginatus in the Japanese—only 0.12%. They found only 109 teeth in 53 patients of 42,177 examined.[53]

From the University of California at Los Angeles (UCLA), a report documented "dens evaginatus in several members of a family of Guatemalan Indian descent."[54] The authors believe that "autosomal dominant inheritance is probable." But the all time high for dens evaginatus must be the report from the US Army by Augsburger and Wong: seven of eight premolars in a 12-year-old girl from Guam were affected by dens evaginatus. Through early diagnosis, pulpotomy, root canal treatment, and composite reinforcement around the evaginations, all seven of the teeth were saved and still intact after 4 years.[55]

It seems obvious that although **in**vagination is found universally and primarily in maxillary lateral incisors, the **ev**aginated tubercle of the mandibular premolars is primarily an Asian condition. Dens evaginatus is the antithesis of dens invaginatus; it is "caused by the folding of a part of the inner enamel epithelium into the stellate reticulum...The evaginated enamel epithelium and the underlying cells of the dental papilla form an enamel tubercle with a dentin core which has a central canal connected with the pulp."[50] The tubercle gives the tooth its volcanic appearance (see Figure 4-16).

Radicular Lingual Groove. This anomaly, also found primarily in maxillary lateral incisors, is also known as the palatogingival or distolingual groove. The defect "usually starts in the region of the cingulum and proceeds apically and frequently toward the distal portion of the tooth for various distances along the surface of the root."[56] The "fold" extends as a twisting defect into the surface of the root for a depth of 2 or 3 mm[56] (Figure 4-17). In an electron microscopic study of 14 lateral incisors with radicular lingual grooves, Chinese researchers discovered accessory canals connecting to the pulp in the depths of the grooves. They suspected bacterial ingress through these canals.[57]

Radicular lingual groove is a fairly common and frequently overlooked developmental defect. Incidence ranges from 3[58] to 8.5%.[59] It may be found on maxillary central incisors as well, sometimes on the labial.

If the pulp is not directly connected to the depth of this groove, how does it become infected? Because of the nature of the groove, one suspects that cementum formation is disturbed or even absent—no cementum,

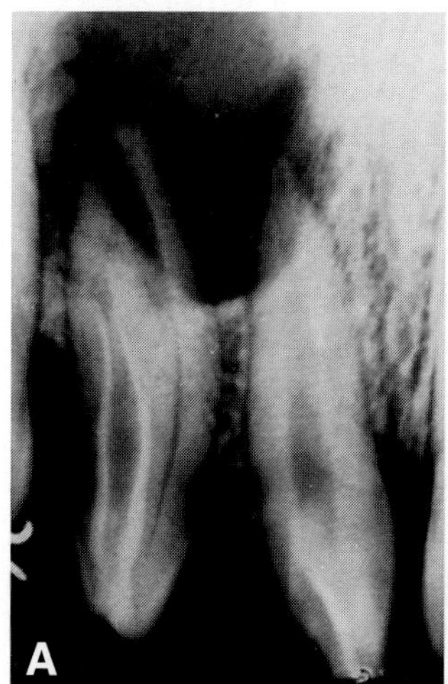

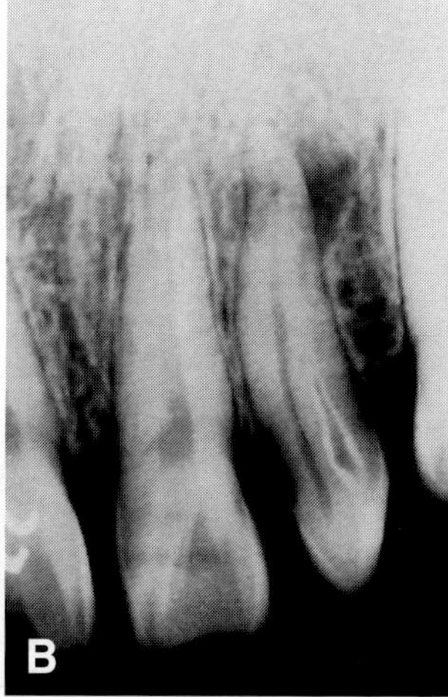

Figure 4-15 Twenty-year-old woman with bilateral dens invaginatus. A, Lateral incisor with Oehler's Type 3 dens. A huge cyst has developed. B, Oehler's Type 2 dens defect that apparently communicates with pulp, leading to necrosis and radicular lesion. Reproduced with permission from Gotoh T et al.[43]

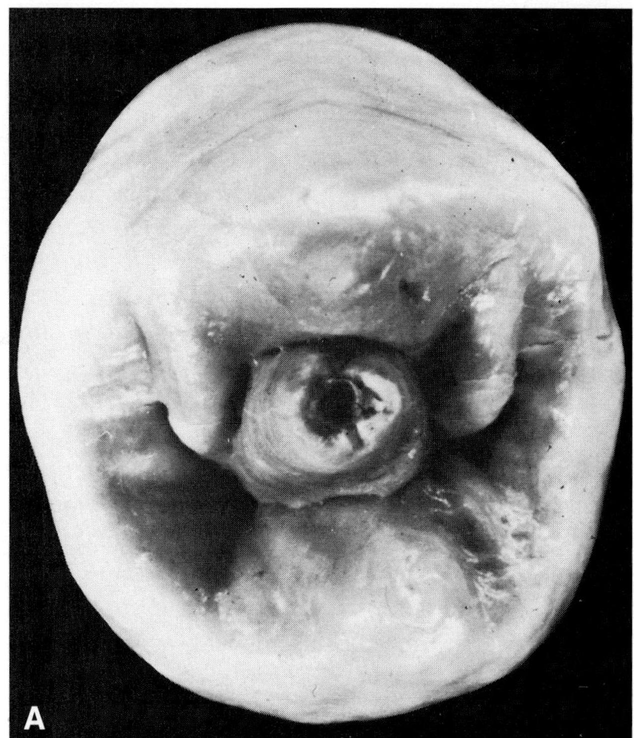

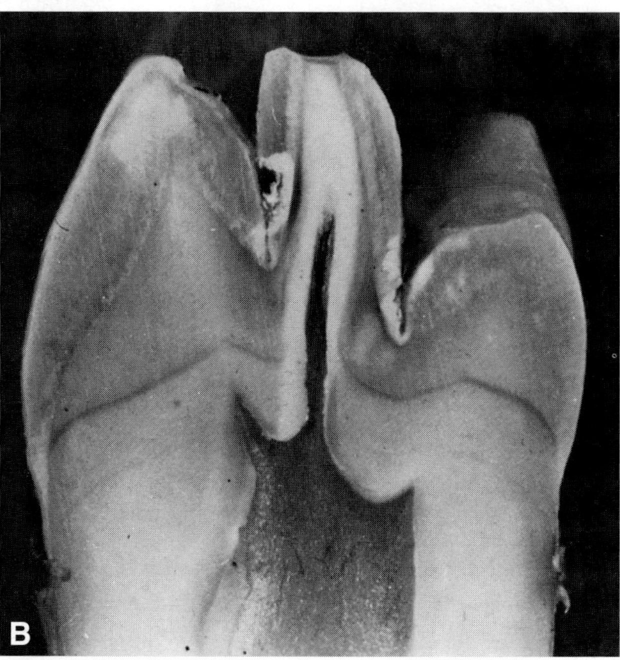

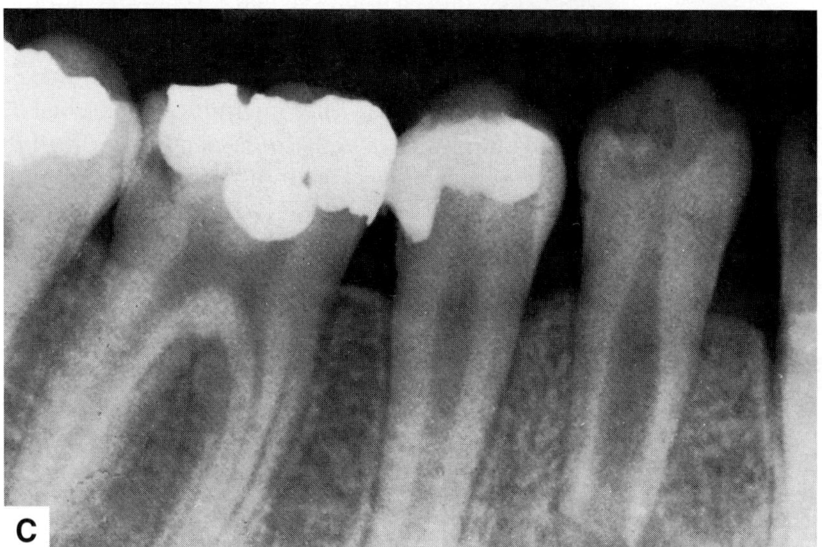

Figure 4-16 *Dens evaginatus.* **A**, Volcanic appearance of extra cusp. Direct ingress of bacteria to pulp is possible. **B**, Extension of pulp into evaginated defect. **C**, Mandibular first premolar with necrotic pulp. Patient is Asian with "extra cusp" and developmental tract through which bacteria invaded. (**A** courtesy of Dr. Ole Carlson, Copenhagen, Denmark; **B** reproduced with permission from Palmer ME. Oral Surg 1973;35:772.)

no attachment. The defect then becomes "a sluice, a funnel" for bacteria—a narrow winding periodontal pocket on the lingual.[60] If the groove is long enough, the infection and usually the palatal abscess that forms extend to the apex. Retrogenic pulp infection is then a common sequela (Figure 4-18).

If diagnosed early enough and the groove is not too long, too tortuous, or too deep, treatment may save the pulp and the tooth (see chapter 12). All too frequently, however, diagnosis is too little and too late, and treatment is of no avail. The tooth must be extracted.[61]

Radicular Ingress

Caries. Root caries is, of course, a less frequent occurrence than coronal caries, but it remains, nonetheless, a **bacterial source** of pulp irritation. Cervical root caries, particularly at the buccogingival, is a common sequela to gingival recession. Massler spoke of the increased incidence of cervical caries in the elderly.[62] Interproximal radicular caries often follows periodontal procedures if meticulous oral hygiene is not maintained. Caries in the furca also may follow periodontal involvement of this region (Figure 4-19).

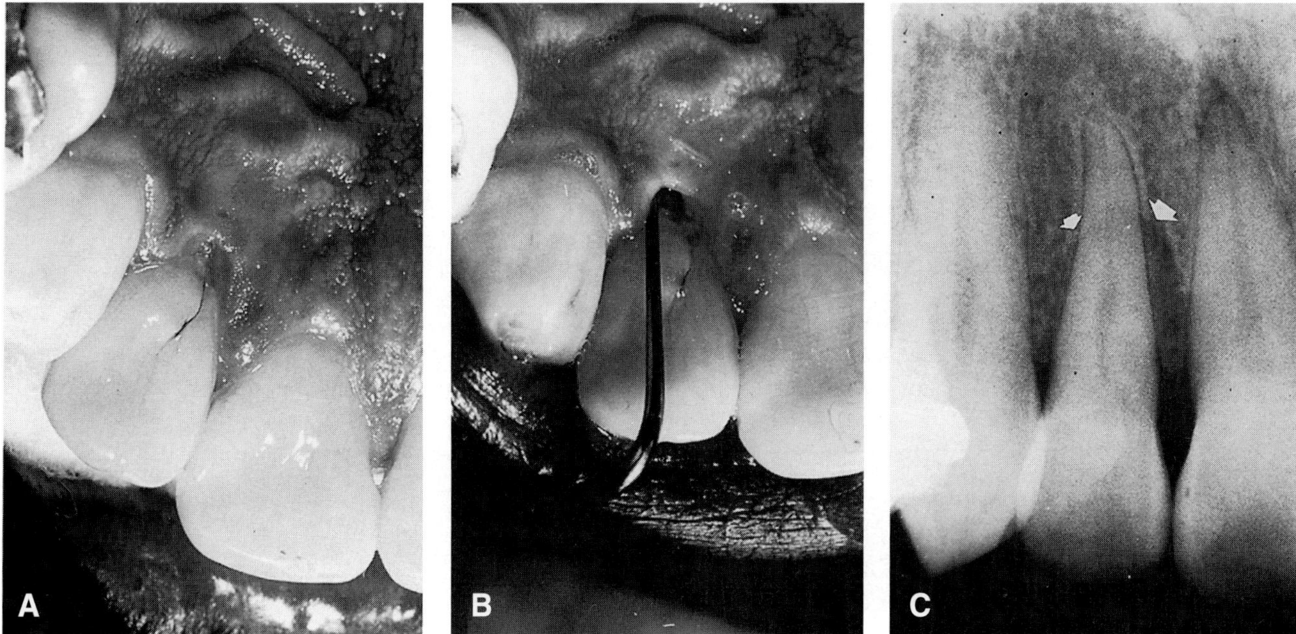

Figure 4-17 A, Radicular lingual groove seen extending from the cingulum to the inflamed gingival margin. B, Periodontal probing reveals the depth of pocket formation associated with the groove. C, Broad bone loss indicates chronic lesions. Narrow pockets, not easily discernible by radiograph, are associated with acute lesions. Reproduced with permission from Robison SF and Cooley RL.[60]

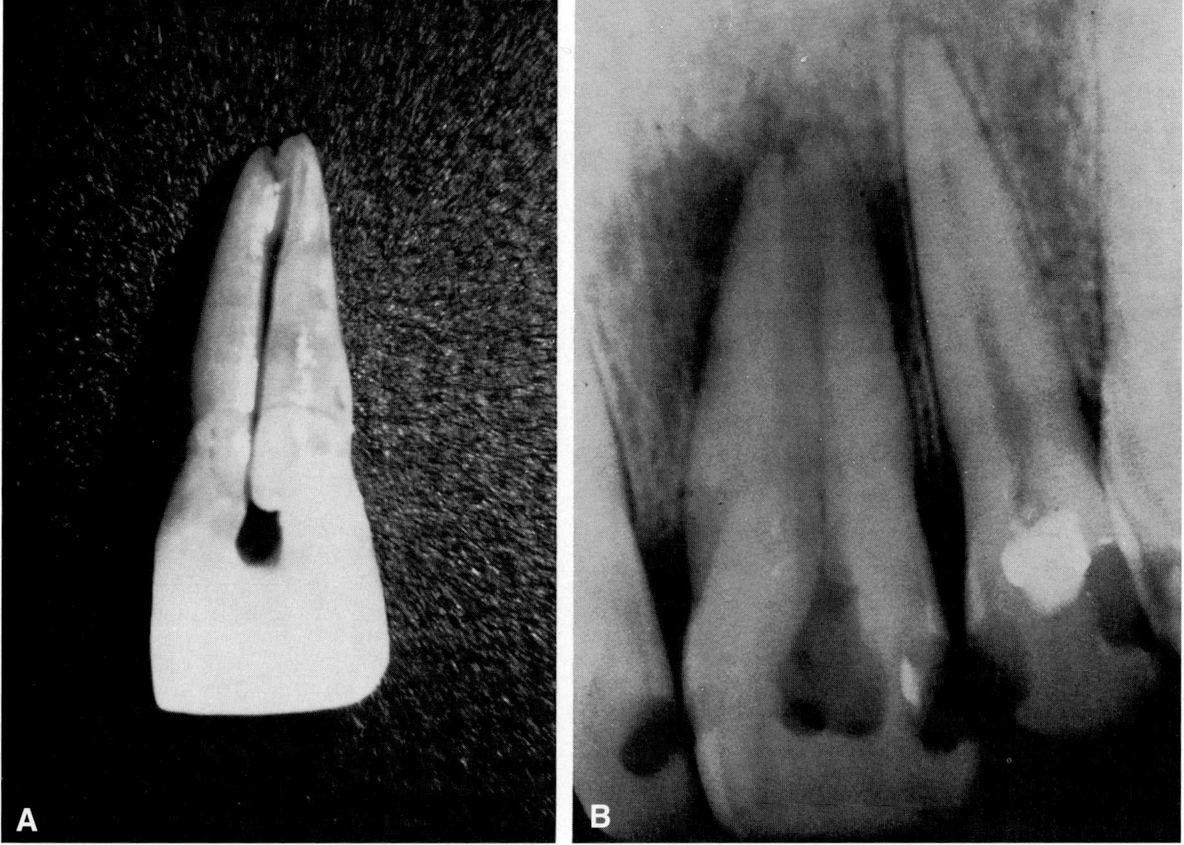

Figure 4-18 Radicular lingual groove extending to apex leading to irreversible pulpitis, palatal periodontal destruction, and tooth loss. A, Depth and severity of groove. B, Hopeless outcome of combined endodontal-periodontal lesion. (Courtesy of David S. August.)

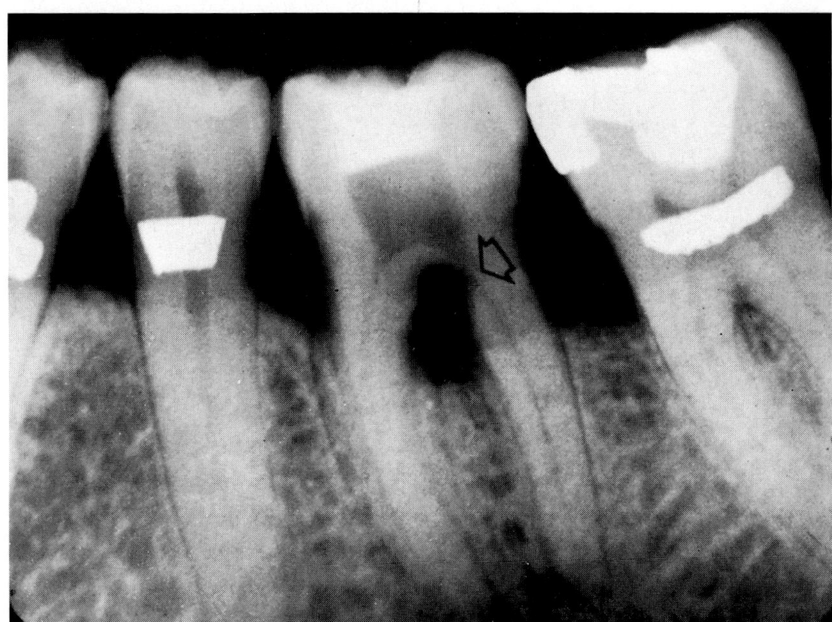

Figure 4-19 Carious invasion of pulp (**arrow**) at the furca of a periodontally involved tooth.

Retrogenic Infection. *Periodontal Pocket.* The fact that the pulp does not frequently become infected through the apical foramen or lateral accessory canals associated with a chronic periodontal pocket attests to its inherent ability to survive. Seltzer et al. have shown increased atrophy and dystrophic calcifications in the pulps of periodontally involved teeth but not necessarily infection.[63] Mazur and Massler, on the other hand, could not demonstrate these changes.[64]

Periodontists often encounter periodontal pockets that extend to and surround the apex (Figure 4-20), as well as lateral accessory canals, or accessory canals in the furca area of molars (Figure 4-21), which also extend into septic and infected pockets.[65] In view of the frequency of deep pocket occurrence, one is hard-pressed to explain why retrogenic pulp infection is not more common. Nonetheless, it does occur and, in combination with the dystrophic changes observed,[63] might well serve to explain why these pulps become necrotic. Langeland and colleagues observed that "pathologic changes occurred in the pulp tissue when periodontal disease was present, but the pulp did not succumb as long as the main canal—the major pathway of the circulation—was not involved."[66] They found that involved lateral canals or root caries damage the pulp, "but total disintegration apparently occurs only when all main apical foramina are involved in the bacterial plaque" (Figure 4-22). One should also be aware that accessory or lateral canals may not be truly functional, having been blocked internally by sclerosis or advancing irritation dentin.

Although it has long been held that bacteria retrogenically infecting dental pulps must be blood- or lymphborne and most likely arise from periodontal pockets, there has been no direct proof that this is so. Saglie and his associates at UCLA provided exquisite proof that such a transport is possible, with the bacteria passing through the pocket lining to reach the circulation.[67] Their scanning electron microscopic studies of human periodontal pockets clearly showed bacteria penetrating the ulcerated lining epithelium, squirming through "holes and tunnels" left by leukocytes migrating from the circulation and connective tissue below, as well as from desquamated cells (Figure 4-23). This bacterial movement toward the bloodstream could also explain the source of pulp infection when teeth are traumatized but not fractured.[34]

Periodontal Abscess. **Retrogenic pulp infection,** either accompanying or immediately following an acute periodontal abscess, is also an infrequent cause of otherwise unexplained pulp necrosis.

Hematogenic Infection. **Bacteria gaining access** to the pulp through vascular channels is entirely within reason. The anachoretic attraction of bacteria to a lesion readily applies to injured pulp tissue.[68] Anachoresis of bacteria from the vessels of the gingival sulcus, as explained above by Saglie et al.,[67] or from a **systemic transient bacteremia** also serves to explain the unusual number of infected pulp canals, following impact injury without fracture, to 46 intact teeth, observed by MacDonald et al.[69] and experimentally by Grossman.[34] The so-called "stressed pulp"

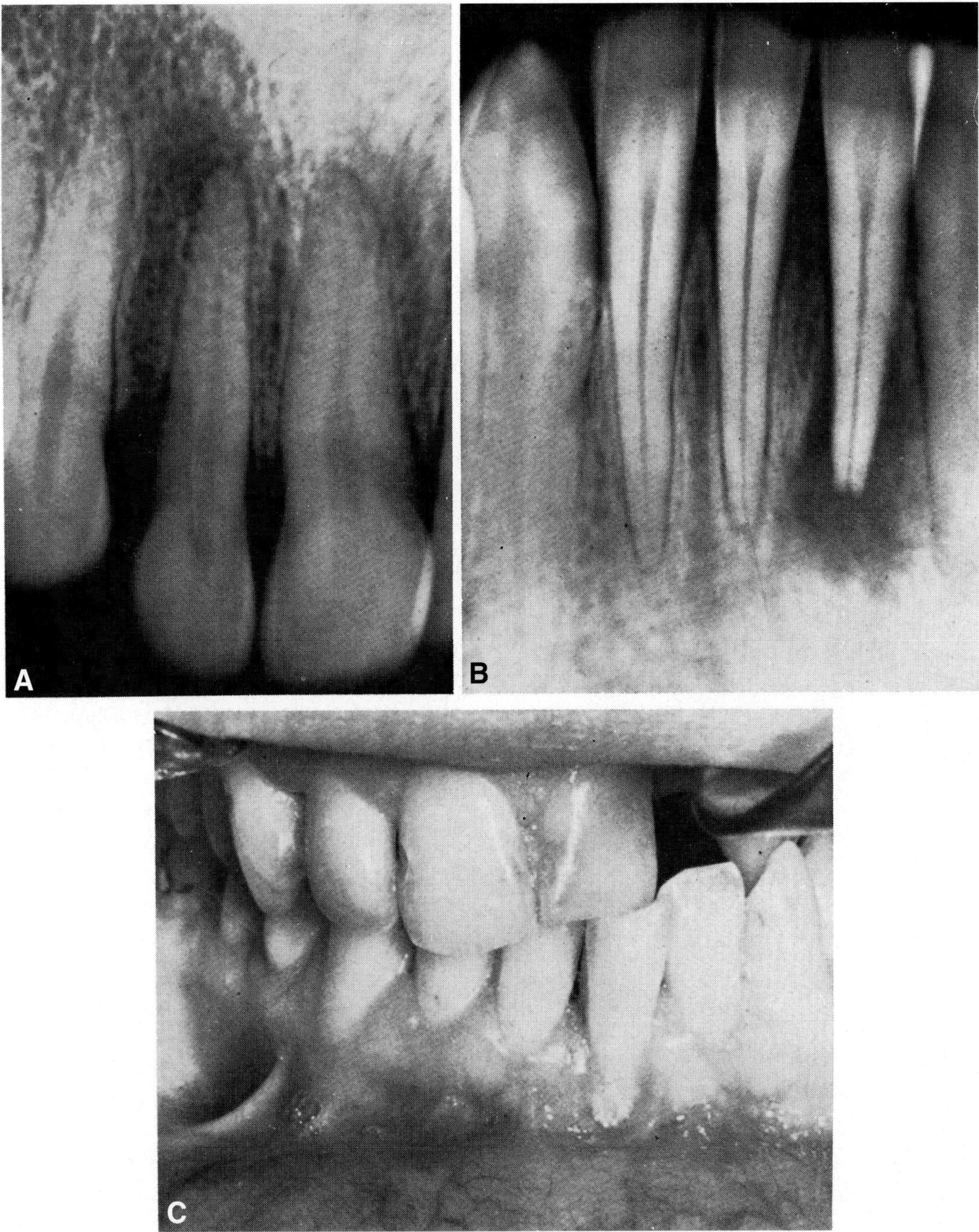

Figure 4-20 Differential diagnosis of retrogenic pulp infection from periodontal pocket. **A**, The pulp of the lateral incisor is infected and necrotic and apparently related to the distolingual pocket that extends to the apex. Occlusal traumatism may be a factor, although there was no history of impact trauma. **B**, Radiographic appearance mistakenly diagnosed as chronic apical periodontitis. Notice extreme incisal wear. Pulp is vital in the involved central incisor. **C**, Same case as **B**. The orifice to the labial periodontal lesion is apparent, as well as the traumatic relationship between the maxillary and mandibular incisors. The pulp is not involved in spite of the extensive pocket.

could well be a haven for blood- or lymphborne bacteria. Injured or scarred tissues appear to have an affinity for attracting bacteria, as shown by the bacterial plaques that form on heart valves scarred by rheumatic fever. In Greece, Tziafas produced a streptococcal bacteremia in dogs after having pulp-capped 36 teeth with Dycal (L.D. Caulk, Milford, Dela.), calcium hydroxide, or Teflon. Bacteria were not observed in the control teeth or in three of four of the Teflon cappings. But in all of the mildly inflamed calcium hydroxide cappings, however, "colonies of gram-positive cocci were found."[70]

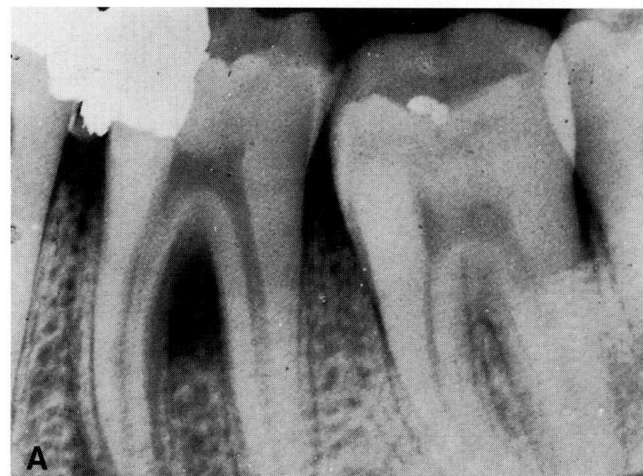

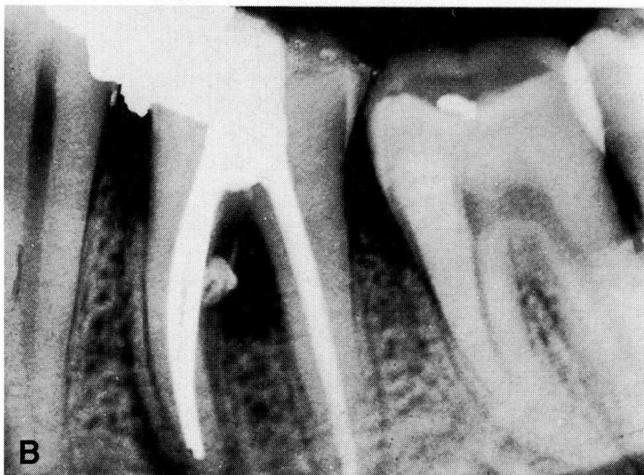

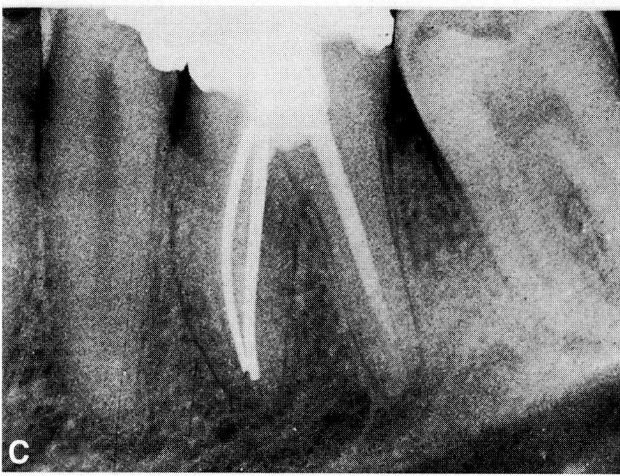

Figure 4-21 A, Bony lesion in furcation draining through buccal gingival sulcus. The molar pulp is necrotic. B, Obturation reveals the lateral accessory canal. C, Three-year recall radiograph. Total healing is apparent. No surgery was used. (Courtesy of Dr. Rafael Miñana, Madrid, Spain.)

TRAUMATIC CAUSES

Acute Trauma

Coronal Fracture. Most pulp death following coronal fractures is incidental to the bacterial invasion that follows the accident. There is no question, however, that severe impact injury to the coronal pulp initiates an inflammatory attempt toward repair. Untreated bacterial invasion negates any possibility of sustained vitality.

Radicular Fracture. Accidental fracture of the root disrupts the pulp vascular supply; thus the injured coronal pulp can lose its vitality. The apical radicular pulp tissue, however, usually remains vital.

One should not assume pulp death too soon after an accident. Complete repair of the fracture by callus formation of cementum has been known to occur (see chapter 15). Moreover, the blood supply may remain viable, either through the apical vessels or through the ingrowth of new vessels through the fracture site.

As with any other condition affecting the pulp, the younger the patient, the better the prognosis for pulp vitality. The extensive vascular supply through the incompletely formed root end provides a much greater opportunity for repair than the fractured root and disrupted blood supply of a fully formed tooth.

Vascular Stasis. The tooth that receives a severe impact injury, yet is not dislocated or fractured, is more apt to lose pulp vitality immediately than the tooth that fractures. Evidently, the pulp vessels are either severed or smashed at the apical foramen, resulting in ischemic infarction.

Pulp canal calcification by irritation dentin is another pulp response to trauma. Thus the pulp may either die from trauma or furiously eliminate itself by irritation dentin formation. Conversely, impact trauma may lead to internal resorption in which the pulp "attacks" the dentin rather than builds it. For a more complete discussion of pulp necrosis subsequent to pulp canal obliteration owing to trauma, see chapter 15.

Again, after trauma, the possibility exists for pulp repair and revascularization depending on the age of the patient. The developing tooth with an open flaring apex is quite apt to remain vital or regain vitality. In the older patient, the prognosis for repair is limited.

Luxation. Extrusive and lateral luxation and intrusion nearly always result in pulp death. Pulpal recovery is possible in young, immature teeth with wide, open apexes, however.

Avulsion. It goes without saying that pulp necrosis is the obvious consequence of total avulsion of a tooth. In spite of pulp death, however, the tooth should still be replanted (see chapter 15).

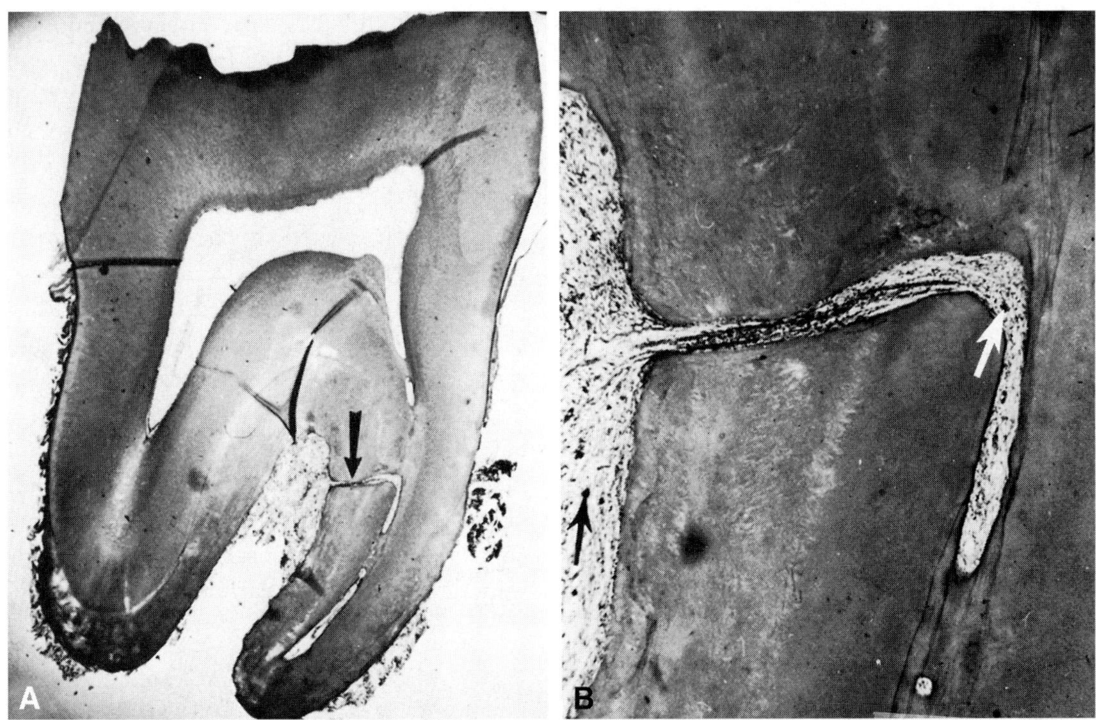

Figure 4-22 A, Accessory canal (**arrow**) from vital pulp into the inflamed tissue of molar bifurcation. **B,** Inflammation in the accessory canal with only slight inflammation in the canal pulp. Epithelial rests (**arrows**) are present in both bifurcation and pulp canal. Reproduced with permission from Rubach WC, Mitchell DF. J Periodontol 1965;36:34.

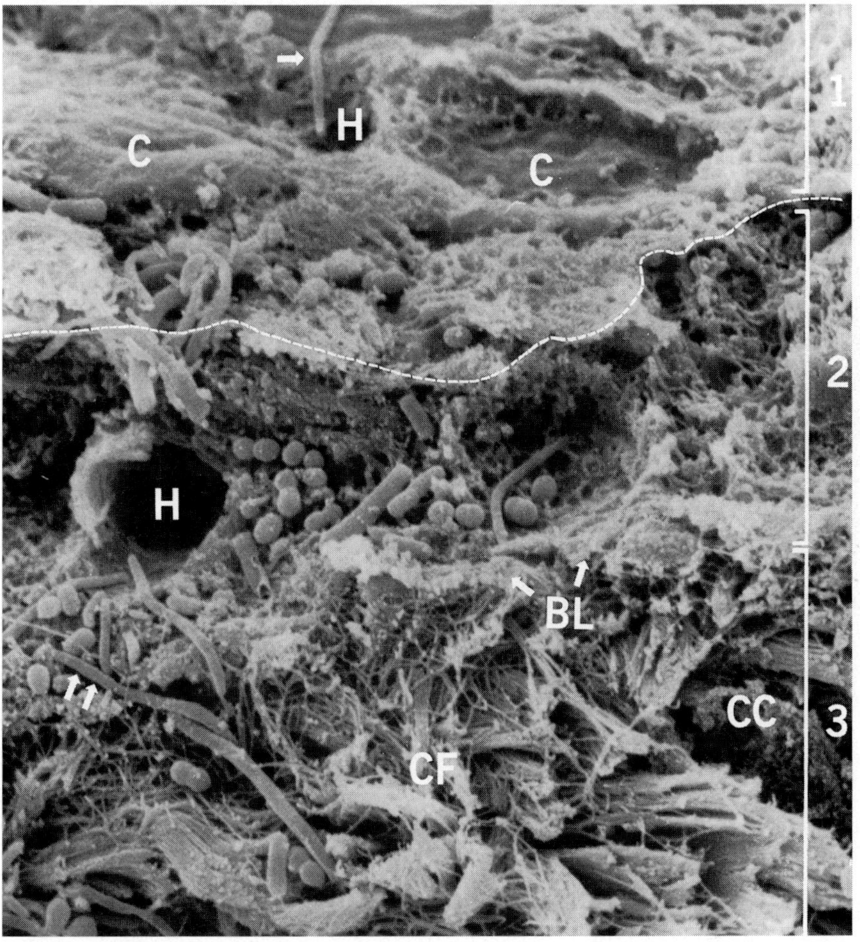

Figure 4-23 How bacteria move from a periodontal pocket into underlying connective tissue, the vascular system, and eventually the pulp. Scanning electron microscopic depiction of the inside of an ulcerated and infected pocket. **Area 1 (right border)** is the surface view of lining epithelium. C, epithelial cell. **Dotted line** demarcates the cut surface of the epithelium (**Area 2**). The basement lamina (BL) separates the epithelium from connective tissue (**Area 3**), which contains collagen fibers (CF) and connective tissue cells (CC). Bacteria (**top arrow**) enter a hole (H) in the epithelium (left by a desquamated cell) and travel through a "tunnel" to emerge into connective tissue through the hole. Abundant cocci, rods, and filaments are seen alongside the hole on the basement lamina. Filaments and cocci are then seen perforating the basement membrane (**double arrow**) to penetrate connective tissue and reach blood and/or lymph vessels. Reproduced with permission from Saglie R et al.[67]

Chronic Trauma

Adolescent Female Bruxism. Ingle and Natkin reported an unusual syndrome of osteoporosis and pulp death of mandibular incisors in adolescent females who compulsively grind their teeth in protrusive excursion.[71,72] Evidently, the trauma is so severe and sustained that pulp necrosis eventually develops (Figure 4-24). Cooke also reported the syndrome in an 18-year-old girl. Pulpitis with moderate pulpalgia was reversed within a year by the patient's wearing a night guard.[73]

Traumatism. The effect on the pulp from chronic occlusal trauma has been expressed by Landay and Seltzer.[74] Excessive occlusal force was placed on the molars of Wistar rats. Seven to 10 months passed before pulp changes appeared: "There was a significant concentration of macrophages and lymphocytes in the central area of the pulps." Irritational dentin and disrupted odontoblasts also appeared along the pulp chamber floor above the furcation. At 1 year, the pulp response to occlusal trauma had increased in spite of the fact that the periodontal damage had been repaired.[74] Cottone reported pulp necrosis in the lower incisors of skin divers, initiated by grasping the mouthpiece of their oxygen supply between their front teeth for long periods of time.[75]

Attrition or Abrasion and Erosion. Pulp death or inflammation related to incisal wear or gingival erosion is a rarity. The reparative power of the pulp to lay down dentin as it recedes ahead of this stimulus is phenomenal. Occasionally, however, a severely worn mandibular incisor is encountered, with a necrotic pulp and an observable incisal opening into the pulp chamber (Figure 4-25). Quite possibly, the pulps of this patient were devitalized at an earlier time, and attrition finally

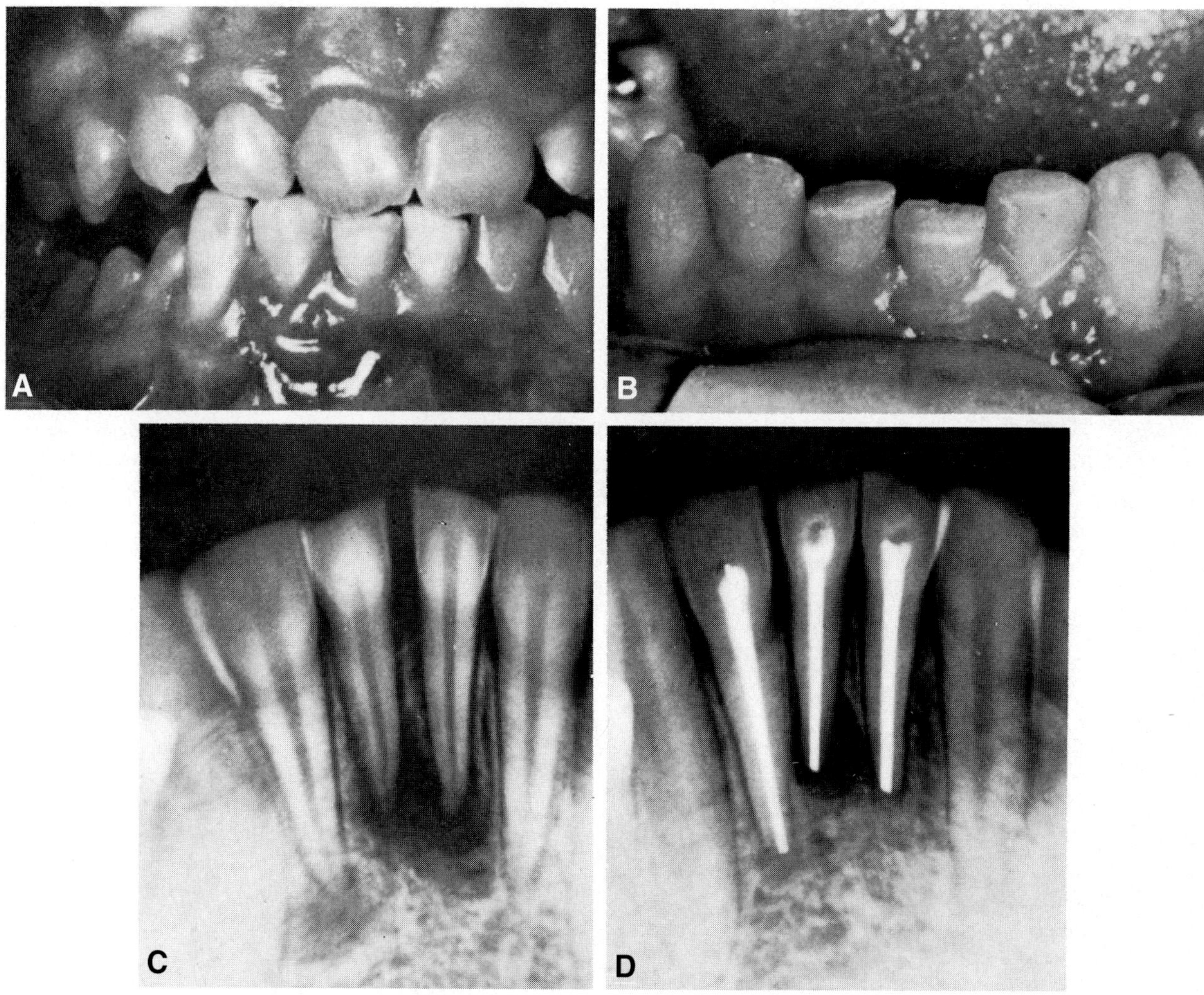

Figure 4-24 Osteoporosis and pulp death of mandibular incisors in a 14-year-old girl who compulsively ground her teeth in protrusive excursion. A, Position assumed during bruxism. B, Extensive wear of mandibular incisors caused by compulsive grinding. C, Pulps of three incisors have been devitalized by the force of traumatic habit. Acute abscess has separated central incisors. D, One year following root canal therapy, some repair has occurred; however, persistent habit prevents complete healing. Reproduced with permission from Natkin E and Ingle JI.[72]

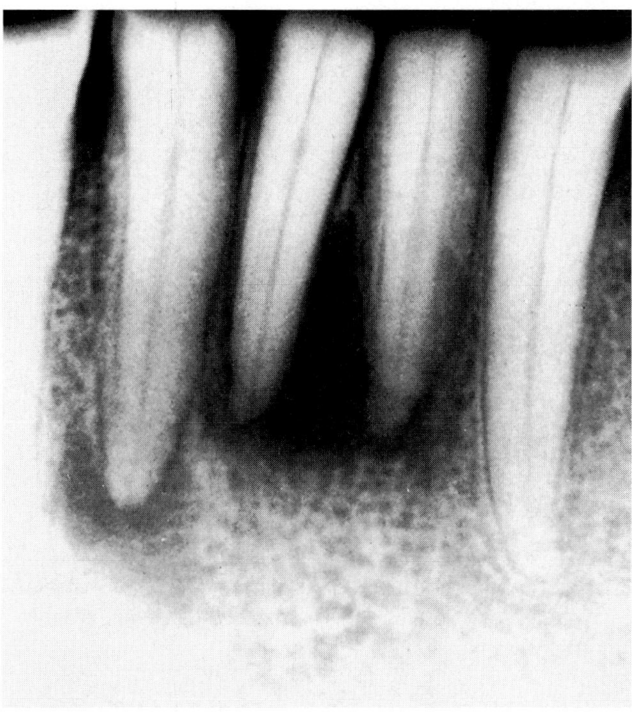

Figure 4-25 Incisal abrasion into pulp, leading to pulp necrosis of three mandibular incisors.

reached the chamber. Incisal attrition is more apt to develop opposite porcelain teeth. Seltzer et al. noted retrogressive and atrophic pulp changes, but not total necrosis, in relation to the constant irritation or attrition or abrasion.[63] Sognnaes and colleagues reported cervical erosion so severe that the pulps of maxillary incisors were invaded[76] (Figure 4-26).

Grippo reported a positive relationship between the occlusion and erosion. He termed it **abfraction erosion.** He noted that teeth with erosion are also teeth that show a good deal of attritional wear, or bruxism. Evidently, the constant minute flexure and material fatigue of the tooth cause abfraction or microscopic "flaking" away of the tooth structure.[77]

"Dentrifice abrasion" may also be so severe so as to invade the pulp space. Meister et al. reported a case in which the patient brushed vigorously once a day with liberal amounts of toothpaste and a hard toothbrush.[78] The plastic handle of the brush was seen to bend from the force used. Not only were the pulps of two teeth invaded by bacteria, but the teeth were nearly severed (Figure 4-27).

IATRAL CAUSES

Cavity Preparation

Heat of Preparation. The heat generated by grinding procedures of tooth structure has often been cited

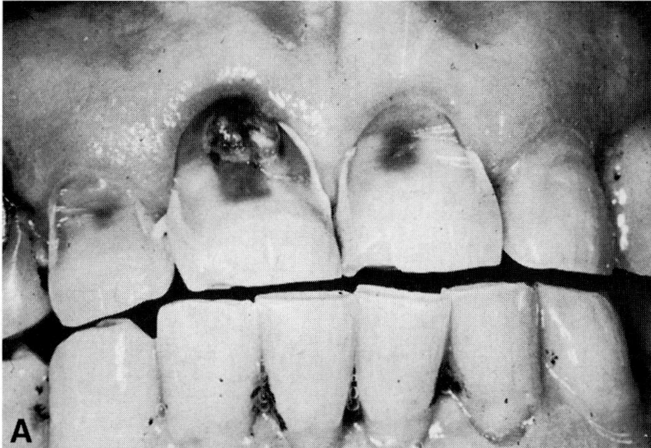

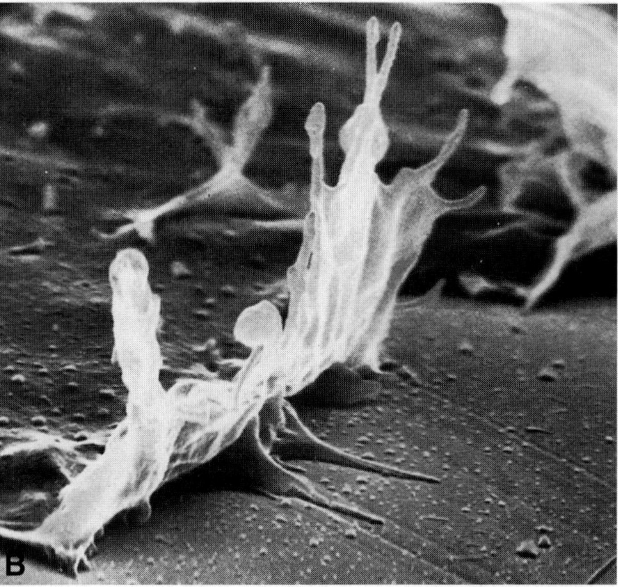

Figure 4-26 **A,** Dental erosion has exposed the pulps of the maxillary central incisors. Reproduced with permission from Sognnaes RF et al.[76] **B,** Possible cause of erosion. Fibroblastic cell perambulation by a process of "ruffling" may cause ablation of tooth or plastic surfaces. Reproduced with permission from Revell J-P. Engineering and Science, Pasdena, California Institute of Technology, Nov.-Dec., 1973.

as the greatest single cause of pulp damage during cavity preparation. As Kramer stated, "If the use of these instruments today is not to provide a harvest for the endodontist tomorrow, it is essential that the development of these high-speed handpieces should be accompanied by the development of adequate cooling mechanisms"[79] (Figure 4-28). The inevitable inflammation following cavity preparation, ranging from reversible to irreparable changes, has been well documented by many (Figure 4-29).[1,79–81] Zach and Cohen found that "...an intrapulpal temperature rise of 5.5°C (10°F) in rhesus Macaca monkeys caused 15% of the pulps to lose vitality."[82]

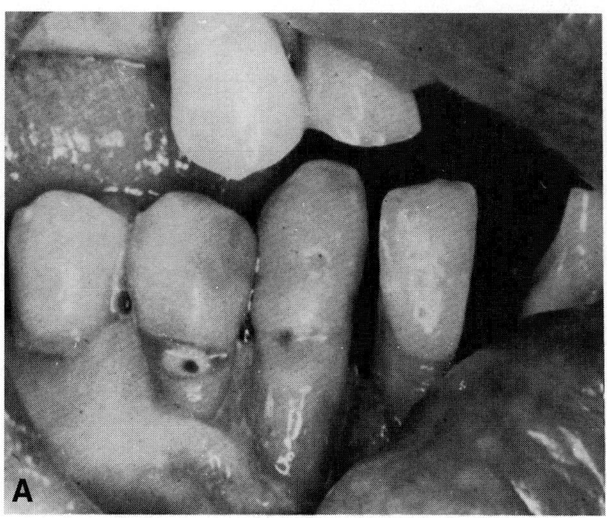

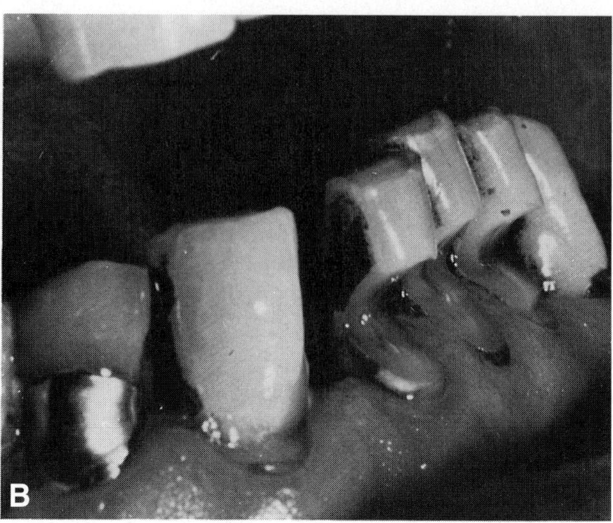

Figure 4-27 "Toothbrush" abrasion into the pulp cavity. **A**, The pulp canal is evident on the first premolar. A hard-bristle brush was used since childhood. Reproduced with permission from Gillette WB, Van House RL. JADA 1980;101:476. **B**, Attrition from "dentifrice" abrasion extends almost completely through the incisors. Reproduced with permission from Meister F, Braun RJ, Gerstein H. JADA 1981;101:651.

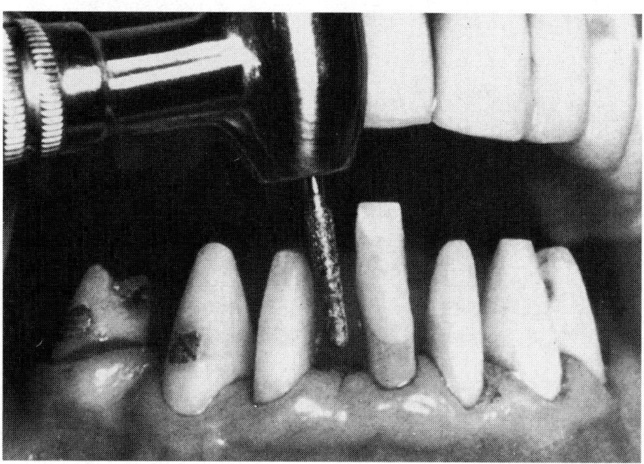

Figure 4-28 Iatral pulp death frequently occurs when teeth must be reduced to this extent. It is imperative that copious water coolant be used to protect pulp from heat damage and desiccation during preparation.

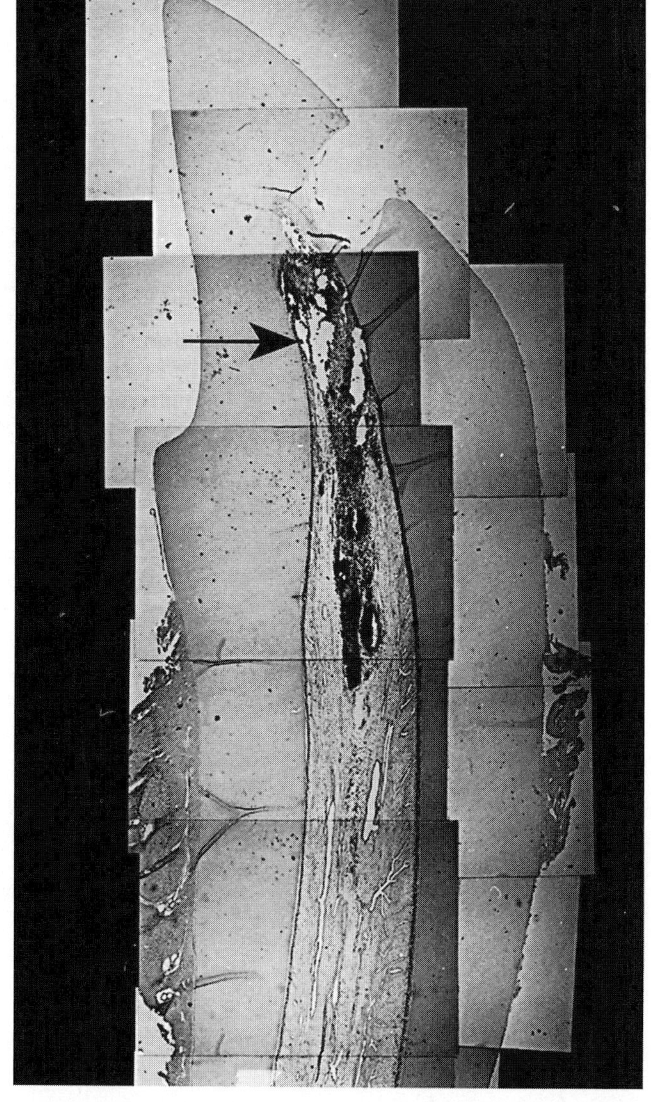

Figure 4-29 Severe pulpal inflammation and necrocytic area (**arrow**) induced by cavity preparation 4 hours previously with high-speed carbide bur at 400,000 rpm and no water coolant spray. The remaining dentin thickness is 0.5 mm. Reproduced with permission from Kogushi M et al. JOE 1988;14:475.

Swerdlow and Stanley pointed out the basic factors in rotary instrumentation that cause temperature rise in the pulp. In order of their importance, they are as follows:

1. Force applied by the operator
2. Size, shape, and condition of cutting tool
3. Revolutions per minute
4. Duration of actual cutting time[83]

One would surmise that the ultraspeed (300,000 rpm) instruments of today are more traumatic to the pulp than the low-speed (6,000 rpm) instruments of the past. Such is not the case if adequate air-water coolant is used. Stanley and Swerdlow concluded that speeds of 50,000 rpm and over were found to be less traumatic to the human pulp than techniques using 6,000 and 20,000 rpm.[80] They pointed out, however, that the value of coolants becomes more significant at higher speeds. It is possible to "burn" the pulp in 11 seconds of preparation time if air alone is used as a coolant at 200,000 rpm. This concurs with the findings of Vaughn and Peyton, who showed that the highest intrapulpal temperatures were reached within the first 10 seconds of grinding.[84] Peyton and Henry also demonstrated that the temperature rose up to 110°F at 15,000 rpm if no coolant was used while cutting with a No. 37 inverted cone diamond point at a 0.5 pound load.[85]

Stanley emphasized the destructive intervention of cavity preparation. In his experience, he found that "a pure **acute** inflammatory lesion seldom exists except following severe traumatic episodes or **cutting a cavity preparation** [emphasis added]" in an intact tooth. It is his contention that the demise of the pulp begins with a chronic lesion turned acute by the insult of cavity preparation (stressed pulp), so to speak. At that time, leukocytes are found in the pulp lesion.[86]

As Zach noted, "There is good histologic validation that an increase in intrapulpal temperature of 20°F may result in irreversible damage to a substantial number of pulps so assaulted."[87] Using four different techniques to prepare cavities, Zach found low-speed drilling with no coolant to be the least acceptable method, followed by ultraspeed with no coolant. He also found desiccation from **air cooling quite damaging**. Langeland and Langeland also noted that desiccation may accentuate the effects of cavity preparation in the pulp.[88]

Stanley and Swerdlow stated that the degree of cellular displacement of odontoblastic nuclei into the cut dentinal tubules is the best indication of the severity of pulp inflammation initially.[89] They felt that this displacement of the cells was caused by a buildup of intrapulpal pressure by an inflammatory response and that the edema, hyperemia, and exudation occurring in proximity to the pulp wall literally forced the odontoblast nuclei and blood cells into the dentinal tubules.

Confirming this thesis and using cellular displacement into the tubules as a criterion for pulp inflammation, Ostrom, in an ingenious experiment, was able to show that the heat of preparation causes pulp inflammation during preparation and that the cellular displacement into the tubules is the result of the pressure generated from intrapulpal inflammation following the temperature rise.[90]

After reviewing the research in this area, Goodacre concluded that "low speed produces less thermal elevation than high speed which produces less elevation than ultrahigh speed."[91] He also quoted Ottl and Lauer, who noted that "carbide burs generate less thermal change than diamond instruments" and that "coarse diamonds produce a more pronounced temperature increase than fine diamonds."[92]

Depth of Preparation. It can be stated categorically that the deeper the preparation, the more extensive the pulp inflammation. This has been shown by Seelig and Lefkowitz, who observed the degree of pulp response as **inversely** proportional to the remaining thickness of dentin.[93]

The effect on the pulp of merely cutting on the dentin was well demonstrated by Searls.[94] Carefully preparing cavities with a 33½ bur on rat incisors at 150,000 rpm under a jet stream of water, Searls noted that the uptake of labeled proline was substantially reduced in those odontoblasts the processes of which had been cut. A surprising finding was the reduced protein synthesis in the pulp adjacent to the cut tubules as well, as revealed by the tritiated proline.[94]

Pulp Horn Extensions. The close proximity of the pulp to the external surface of the tooth, particularly at the furcal plane area, where tooth preparation for full coverage of periodontally involved teeth is so critical, has been emphasized by Sproles[95] and by Stambaugh and Wittrock.[96] At some points, the pulp is only 1.5 to 2.0 mm away **before** preparation is even begun. Stanley and Swerdlow pointed out the increased importance of air-water coolant as the dentin is thinned and the pulp approached.[89]

In a remarkable investigation of the coronal pulp chambers of maxillary and mandibular molar teeth, Sproles discovered never-before-reported **cervical** pulp horns (Figure 4-30). Found 66.8 to 96.3% of the time in the first and second molar teeth (Table 4-1), this extra pulp horn presents a real danger in cavity preparation.[95]

Sproles pointed out that the exact location of this pulp extension is most frequently found at the

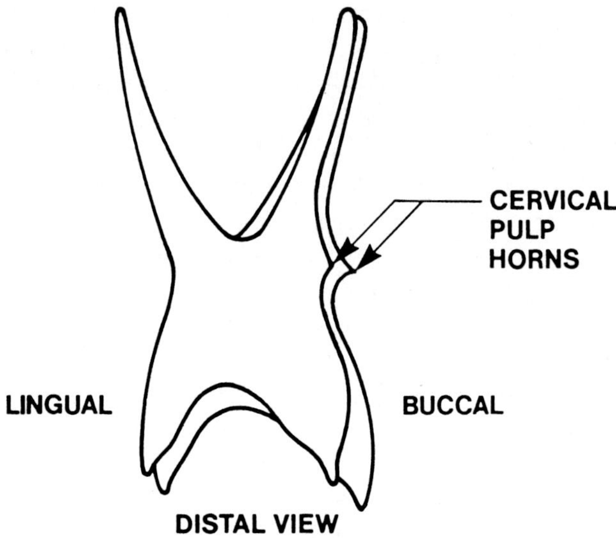

Figure 4-30 Sproles's cervical pulp horns, found in multiple locations in up to 96.3% of molar teeth, extend perilously close to the tooth surface near the cementoenamel junction. Reproduced with permission from Sproles RA.[95]

mesiobuccal: 65.1% in the maxillary molars and 61.3% in the mandibular molars (see Table 4-1). But he also noted that there may be multiple locations, that is, a number of cervical pulp horns on any one tooth, at each axial line angle or centered buccally or lingually.[95]

Sproles further stated that the high incidence of **pulp sensitivity** in these teeth, following gingival recession or Class V or full-crown restoration, could well be related to the very close proximity of these "extra" pulp horns: "Due to the high incidence of this horn on the mesiobuccal aspects, Class V and full crown preparations should perhaps be redesigned to be placed at a minimum depth in the mesial one-half of the preparation or perhaps entirely in the enamel."[95]

Seltzer et al. noted "huge amounts" of irritation dentin under **restorations,** much more than under caries.[63] They noted as well that irritation dentin under restorations was more amorphous and irregular and that the associated odontoblastic nuclei were grossly altered in structure.

Dehydration. Brännström documented the damaging effects on the pulp by dehydration of the exposed dentin.[97,98] **Constant** drying and chip blowing with warm air during cavity preparation under the rubber dam might well contribute to pulp inflammation and the possible necrosis that sometimes follows restorative dentistry, particularly in an already "stressed pulp." Basing his research on the simple biologic law that no cell can function in the absence of water, Langeland found the first stage of inflammation "when the dentin of the floor of the cavity is blown dry, even if the preparation has been carried out under a water spray."[99] He stated, "Any procedure that causes desiccation, under whatever conditions, hot or cold, will cause cellular damage" (personal communication, September 30, 1981).

Pulp Hemorrhage. Occasionally, during cavity preparation, particularly full-crown preparation of anterior teeth, the dentin is seen to suddenly "blush." Pulp hemorrhage has just taken place, quite possibly from an increase in intrapulpal pressure so great as to rupture a pulp vessel and force erythrocytes past the odontoblasts out into the dentinal tubules. This phenomenon, which has also been seen during class V cavity preparation, must be similar to the hemorrhage into the dentin following a severe, traumatic blow to the tooth. In the latter case, however, it is surmised that the blood is driven into the dentin by the hydraulic pressure developed from the blow.

Pulps suffering a total hemorrhage into the dentin can hardly be considered candidates for longevity,

Table 4-1 Percent of Occurrence*

Tooth	% of Total Examined	% Mesiobuccal	% Distobuccal	% Mesiolingual	% Distolingual
Maxilla					
1st molar	96.3	70.3	22.2	53.7	11.1
2nd molar	73.6	59.5	8.0	20.2	8.7
Mean	84.9	65.1	15.1	36.9	9.9
Mandible					
1st molar	71.8	61.5	24.4	14.1	19.3
2nd molar	66.8	61.1	31.6	12.2	8.1
Mean	69.3	61.3	28.0	13.1	13.7

*Occurrence of "extra" **cervical** pulp horns as first described by Sproles. Percentages do not add to 100 because multiple horns may appear on any single tooth. Moreover, the midbuccal or midlingual locations are not reported above.[97]

although the "blushing" has been seen to disappear in time. At a later time, most pulps that appear to have clinically recovered have actually succumbed to the violence of their initial response.

Microhemorrhages are probably a common occurrence during cavity reparation, a finding demonstrated by Orban as early as 1940.[100] Fortunately, recovery from these minor hemorrhages is the rule rather than the exception.

Pulp Exposure. The increased incidence of pulp death following pulp exposure has been experienced by all dentists. If at all possible, a layer of solid (not leathery) dentin should be allowed to remain as pulp cover.[25,31] The numerous methods devised and drugs used to "cap" pulp exposures, and the discouraging results reported for pulp capping, verify the importance of maintaining pulp integrity.

Occasionally, a pulp exposure is made unknown to the dentist because there is no bleeding. The first indication of a problem is the patient's complaint of pulpalgia when the anesthesia "wears off." A radiograph reveals the exposure and cement forced into the pulp (Figure 4-31).

Pin Insertion. Since the advent of pin placement into the dentin to support amalgam restorations, or as a framework for building up badly broken down teeth for full-crown construction, an increase in pulp inflammation and death has been noted. Undoubtedly, in some cases, the trauma of preparing and inserting the pins is insult enough to finish off an already stressed pulp. In other cases, however, the pins may have been inadvertently inserted directly into the pulp or so close to it that they acted as a severe irritant. It was revealed in 1989 that half of America's dentists used retentive pins in restoring compromised teeth. In 1988, they placed 11 million pins.[101] Research from North Carolina suggested that those 11 million pins may have caused somewhere between 4.4 million and 8.5 million pulp exposures. Chapel Hill researchers placed a range of pin sizes properly positioned in 60 extracted molar teeth. When **only one regular pin** was placed, they were appalled to find that cracks extended into the pulp **73% of the time.** Even the smallest pins caused pulp exposures 40% of the time.[102] If one extrapolates this 73% finding by using chance analysis, **two pins** would cause pulp exposures **93%** of the time and **three pins 98%** of the time.

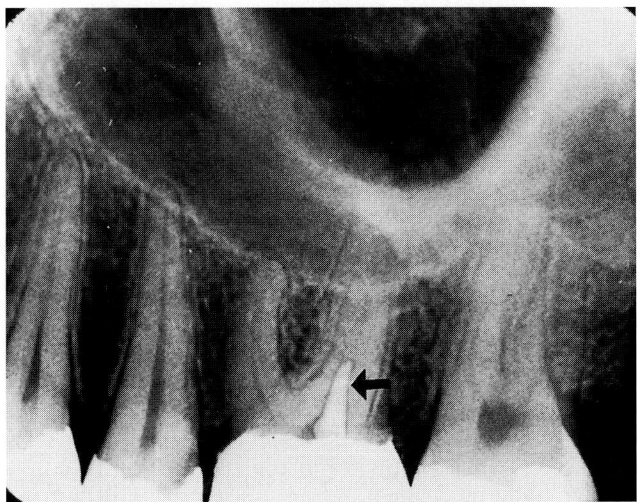

Figure 4-31 Cement forced into pulp during cementation. Pulpitis and severe pulpalgia resulted.

Suzuki and colleagues found pulp necrosis in their experimental specimens in which pulp exposure had occurred and in which the pins had been placed without the presence of calcium hydroxide[103] (Figure 4-32, A). In some cases, in which preparation and placement were too close to the pulp, dentinal fractures occurred with resultant pulp inflammation just beneath (Figure 4-32, B). When preparation and placement were near the pulp, and in the presence of calcium hydroxide, however, irritation dentin formed to protect the underlying pulp, which remained normal[103] (Figure 4-32, C).

Pulp damage from pins may become a moot point. Pins are gradually being replaced by dentin adhesives that bond buildup materials to tooth structure.

Impression Taking. Seltzer et al. showed that damaging pulp changes may develop when impressions are taken under pressure.[5] In one instance, bacteria placed into a freshly prepared cavity were forced into the pulp. One might well extrapolate these experimental findings to apply them to impressions taken with force, in deep cavities or full-crown preparations. Moreover, the negative pressure created in removing an impression may also cause odontoblastic aspiration.

Restoration

Insertion. Severe hypersensitivity and pulpalgia, symptomatic of underlying pulp inflammation and subsequent necrosis, have been noted following the insertion of gold foil and silver amalgam restorations. Foil insertion is evidently far more traumatic to the pulp than amalgam insertion using foil over amalgam in a ratio of 9 to 1 (University of Washington, unpublished data, 1964). James and Schour found gold foil to be the most irritating of eight filling materials.[104]

Patients sometimes report protracted pulpalgia or hypersensitivity following the insertion of **silver amalgam** restorations. Again, this could be related to the force of insertion or possibly to the expansion of the

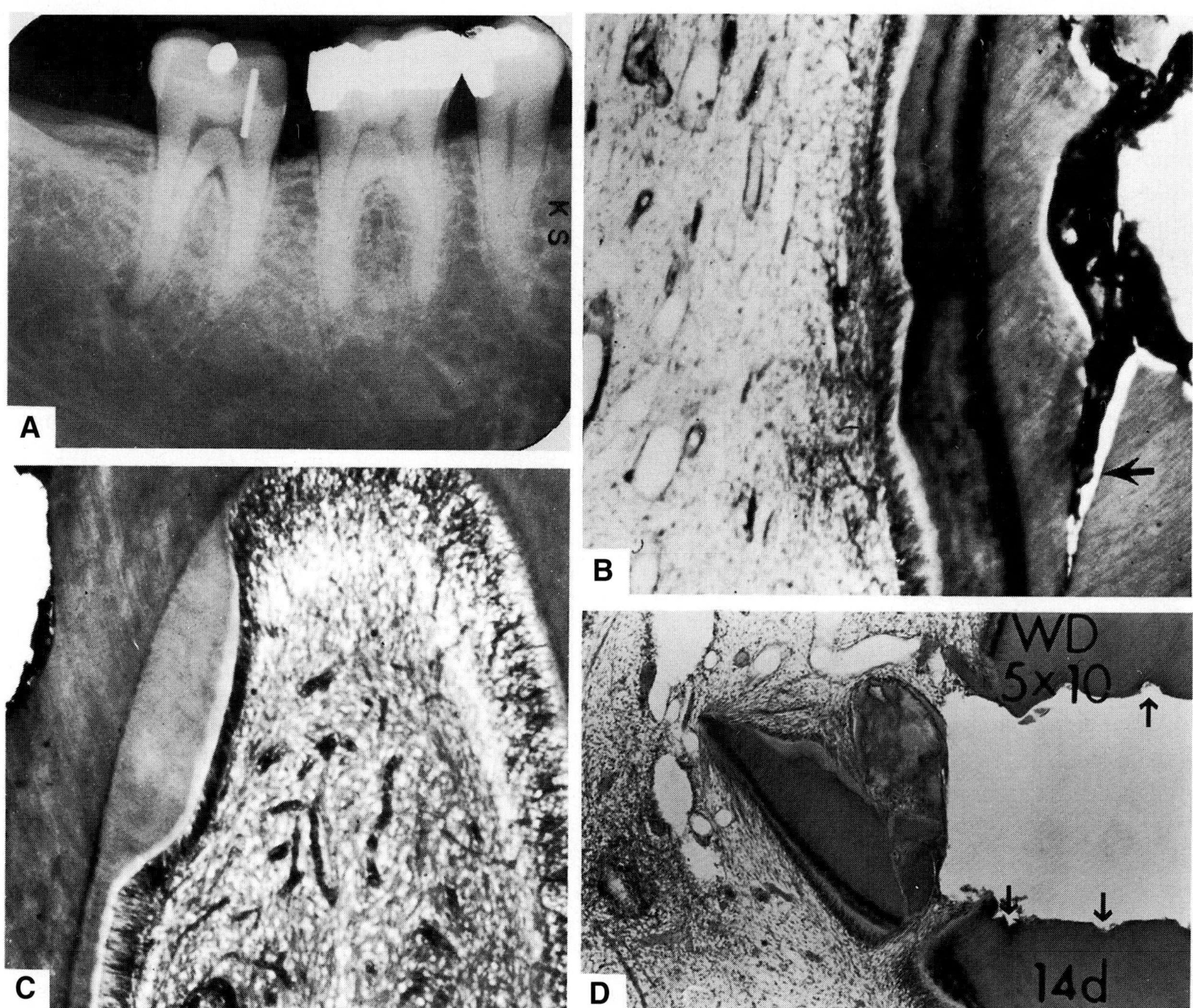

Figure 4-32 A, Pin placement directly into coronal pulp with subsequent pulpalgia, necrosis, and periradicular lesion. Reproduced with permission from Cooley RL, Lubow RM, Wayman BE. Gen Dent 1982;30:148. **B,** Pin placement with calcium hydroxide. Note dentinal cracks from the force of insertion (**arrow**). Cracks filled with calcium hydroxide. Moderate pulp inflammation under affected tubules. **C,** Pin placement with calcium hydroxide and no dentinal fracture. Irritation dentin response is apparent at 28 days. The remaining dentin thickness is 0.5 mm. **D,** Pin placement into pulp. Note the fractured roof of the pulp chamber, severe inflammation, and necrosis. **Arrows** indicate grooves cut in the dentin by a screw-type pin. **B, C,** and **D** reproduced with permission from Suzuki M, Goto G, Jordan RE. J Am Dent Assoc 1973;87:636.

amalgam after insertion. In any case, it seems reasonable to assume that pulp pain is an outgrowth of pulp inflammation. Swerdlow and Stanley reported pulp changes when amalgam was condensed into fresh cavities prepared with high-speed equipment.[105] No significant differences in pulp response were noted, however, between hand and mechanical condensation.

Pain following the insertion of glass ionomer cements and/or composite resins has also been reported. This phenomenon is dealt with in some depth later in the chapter.

Fracture. *Incomplete* fracture may be a sequela to restoration with either gold or silver. Patients sometimes complain of hypersensitivity or pulpalgia for months following the placement of a foil, inlay, or amalgam only to gain relief when a cusp finally fractures away or the crown fractures horizontally. Ritchey et al. listed 22 cases of pulpalgia related to incomplete fracture of posterior teeth restored with "soft gold" inlays.[33] Incomplete fracture is further complicated by bacterial invasion through the microscopic fracture line (see Figure 4-12, C).

There is no question about pulp insult when a complete fracture into the pulp develops as a result of inlay or three-quarter crown placement or removal. In addition to the typical vertical fracture, a number of **hori-**

zontal fractures have also been seen, developing at the gingival and following a cleavage line that was set up during the placing of a Class V foil.

Force of Cementing. Unanesthetized patients often complain of pulp pain when an inlay or crown is finally cemented. Occasionally, the pain does not "wear off," and the dentist realizes that the final cementation was the *coup de grâce* to a sick pulp. Undoubtedly, the chemical irritation of the cement liquid is a factor, but, on the other hand, the tremendous hydraulic force exerted during cementation could not help but drive the liquid toward the pulp. The pressure exerted would be similar to the force exerted in taking a full-crown impression.

The saving grace in most cases is the protection provided to the pulp by the "smear layer" produced during cavity preparation. Microcrystalline obstruction of the tubuli orifices can be negated, however, by scrubbing the dentin cavity surface or applying acid or ethylenediaminetetraacetic acid (EDTA) "cavity cleansers." Cavity liners, dentin bonding agents, or thin cement bases have much to recommend their use.

Heat of Polishing. Finally, but by no means last in order of iatral importance, the pulp damage caused by polishing restorations must be considered. This damage may be compounded by polishing with dry powders while the tooth is anesthetized. The subsequent temperature increase gives rise to the same pulp damage previously discussed under cavity preparation. Interproximal finishing of gold foils, silicates, or composites with 18-inch finishing strips without a constant air coolant must be condemned as well.

Summary. Having said all of this, there is little wonder that Felton and his colleagues at North Carolina found such a high incidence of pulpal morbidity and necrosis under restorations. They compared "1084 teeth restored with onlays, crowns, or bridges in service for 3-30 years with a similar number of unrestored control teeth." Statistical analysis ($p < .01$) "revealed a higher incidence of pulpal necrosis associated with full coverage restorations (13.3%) compared to partial veneer restorations (5.1%)."[106] If an amalgam or composite buildup was placed, the incidence of necrosis rose to 17.7 and 8.1%. They also found a positive relationship between the length of time the tooth was temporized and the number of pulps that became necrotic.[106] This latter finding could well be owing to **bacterial microleakage** and/or damage from the heat generated when plastic, temporary crowns are fabricated directly on the freshly cut preparation.[107]

Goodacre noted that several studies have pointed to the need for endodontic treatment following the placement of **fixed partial abutments** that range from 3% after 5 to 10 years, up to 21% after 6 years, to as high as 23% after only 2 years.[91] He further noted that the span—the length of the prosthesis—also affected the need for endodontic treatment; again, needs ranged from 7% following a 7-unit prosthesis to a 38% endodontic need in a 12-unit fixed bridge.[91] Also, following the concept of the "stressed pulp," he pointed out that 3% of the teeth with little or no caries required no endodontic treatment after 5 years, whereas 10% of the teeth with **deep carious lesions** required treatment.[91]

The number of pulps surviving the rigors of restoration is surprising when one considers the trauma to the pulp from cavity preparation, the desiccating effect of chip blowing, the chemical irritation of a cement base or luting cement, the trauma and prolonged operating time of insertion, and the heat generated in finishing. Those pulps that do not survive might well have been "stressed" to their limit by previous carious, traumatic, and treatment insult. The new round of "therapy" could be the proverbial "straw that broke the camel's back."

Intentional Extirpation and Root Canal Filling

A number of situations arise in restorative dentistry, particularly periodontal prosthesis, for which intentional extirpation of the pulp is indicated. Total root amputation or hemisection of periodontally involved roots also requires intentional extirpation of the remaining pulps. A number of situations have been documented by Bohannan and Abrams,[108] who listed the following indications for intentional extirpation: reorientation of the occlusal plane of tipped, drifted, or elongated teeth; (see Figure 4-28); reduction of the crown-root ratio in the face of advanced loss of bony support; and the establishment of parallelism of clinical crowns when a fixed prosthesis is being used. Add to these indications the necessity to use the root canal for dowel retention of a crown, plus intentional extirpation of the pulp of a tooth, badly drifted to the labial, that is now being restored with a jacket crown to a more esthetic relationship. The pulp must be entered to cut the preparation far enough back into the arch.

Abou-Raas also recommended intentional extirpation and root canal filling as a prelude to internal bleaching of teeth badly stained from prolonged tetracycline ingestion.[109]

Orthodontic Movement

Although orthodontists may deny the possibility, dental pulps can be devitalized during orthodontic movement. Not only devitalization but also hemorrhage can occur, for when the patient presents for endodontic therapy, the tooth may be discolored. Paradoxically, the maxillary canine, which is seldom devitalized by other trauma, appears to be the tooth most susceptible to pulp hemorrhage and necrosis under the forces of orthodontic movement; ischemic infarction is probably the best explanation.

As proof that orthodontic tooth movement does affect pulp viability, Hamersky and colleagues found a 27% depression in pulp tissue respiration as a result of orthodontic force application.[110]

Studies of the effects on the pulp from intrusive forces have also demonstrated compromised blood flow to the pulp in rats[111] and marked changes in the dentin and pulps in the teeth of 60 children undergoing intrusive forces.[112]

Periodontal Curettage

Although root planing and root curettage have been shown to stimulate the deposition of irritation dentin,[113] **extended** curettage can result in pulp devitalization. During curettage of a periodontal lesion that extends entirely around the apex of a root, the pulp vessels may be severed and the pulp devitalized. Pulp vitality is a small price to pay if the tooth can be retained by periodontal curettage followed by root canal therapy.

Electrosurgery

The possible damaging effects of electrosurgery on the pulp were explored by Robertson and his associates.[114] In their experiment with monkeys with and without Class V amalgam fillings, "electrosurgical current was delivered for **one second** with a fully rectified unit at an output intensity consistent with normal clinical usage. Electrosurgery, involving cervical restorations, consistently resulted in **coagulation necrosis** of the pulp and extensive resorption of cementum, dentin and interradicular bone in the furcation area of multirooted teeth."[114] Krejci and his associates produced similar results in beagles. No damage occurred at 0.4 seconds, but at 0.8 to 1.1 seconds, hemorrhagic necrosis of the pulp was found when Class V amalgams were contacted with the electrode.[115] These results certainly suggest that inadvertent contact with metallic restorations during electrosurgery may severely endanger the pulp and periodontal structures alike.

Laser Burn

Laser beams are sometimes used to weld dental materials intraorally, particularly gold and nickel-chromium alloys. Ruby laser radiation has been shown by Adrian and his colleagues to be most damaging to the pulp.[116] They found severe hemorrhage in the pulp chamber and focal necrosis of the odontoblasts when monkey teeth were subjected to 2,370 joules/cm. At 2,800 joules/cm, coagulation necrosis of the pulp occurred.

More recently, however, the neodymium laser has been considered a more effective welding agent than the ruby laser. Adrian again tested the effects on the pulp of the neodymium laser and found that although the damage was considerably less than that caused by the ruby laser, it was still enough for concern.[117] Even at two to three times the intensity of the ruby laser (6,772 joules/cm), "in no case did coagulation necrosis of the pulpal contents occur with the Nd (neodymium) laser although Grade 2 pulp inflammation did develop below enamel-dentin burns."[117]

In Paris, Melcer et al. tested the carbonic gas laser that emits energy densities between 10 and 25 joules/cm^2.[118] In the United States, Powell et al. conducted CO_2 laser tests on the enamel of dogs' teeth but used laser power densities as high as 102 joules per cm^2.[119] Miserendino et al. tested a CO_2 laser with 30 to 250 joules. They observed intrapulpal temperature increases ranging from 5.5 to 32°C. Laser exposures below 10 joules, however, produced rises below 5.5°C, an acceptable level.[120]

Low-density laser has been suggested for caries removal. In Class V cavities, French researchers subjected the pulpal floor to eight impacts of short duration, 0.2 second up to 2.0 seconds: "With an energy of 15 joules emitted in eight pulses of 3W, 0.6s, a new mineralized dentin formation was observed. In the pulp tissue, consisting of 70 percent to 80 percent water, the CO_2 laser beam was almost completely absorbed."[118] Powell et al. irradiated the enamel of dogs' teeth with up to 10 times the power used in dentin and reported no damage.[119] This was confirmed by another group of French researchers, who irradiated dogs' teeth at two levels: 285 joules per cm^2 and 570 joules per cm^2. In Class V cavities, they "obtained dentinal sealing without affecting the underlying pulp."[121]

It appears, therefore, "that the emission of the CO_2 laser beam, characterized by a low power and short periods of emission...produces a fast and constant reactional dentinogenesis without necrotic alteration..."[118]

Periradicular Curettage

A not infrequent result of periradicular surgery is the devitalization of the pulps of **adjacent vital teeth** during curettage of an extensive bony lesion (Figure 4-33). This iatral devitalization of normally vital pulps most frequently occurs in the mandibular incisor region. Two cases reporting the surgical removal of cementomas in the mental region are of note.[122,123] Keyes and

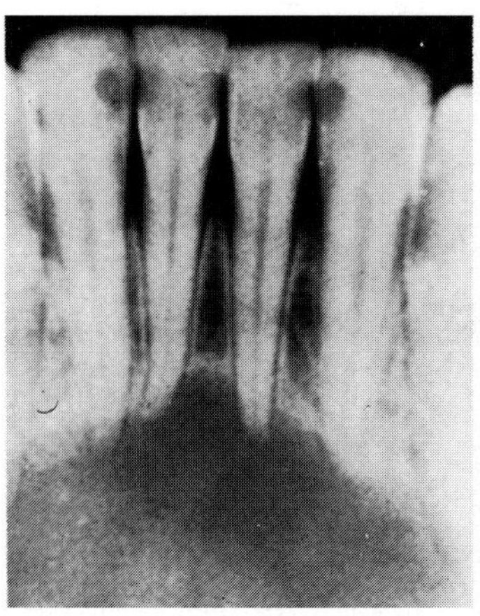
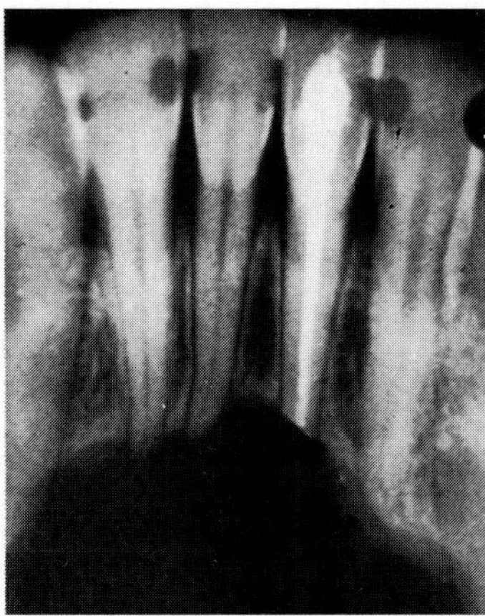
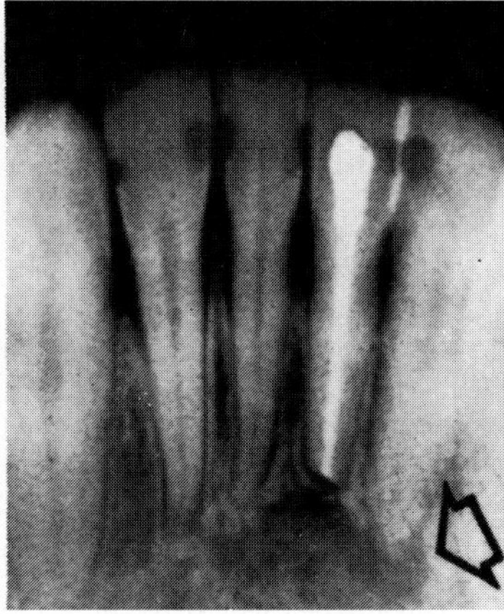

Figure 4-33 Pulp death caused by periradicular curettage during cyst enucleation. The huge apical cyst seen initially (**left**) is related to only one pulpless tooth that has been treated (**center**) and the cyst thoroughly enucleated. Examination of a 1-year postoperative radiograph (**right**) reveals radiolucency (**arrow**) apical to the lateral incisor devitalized during curettage.

Hildebrand reported a case of a 12-year-old girl with a huge third-stage cementoma associated with a nonvital mandibular central incisor. Root canal therapy failed to relieve the painful symptoms, so the cementoma was removed.[122] In the second case, reported from Jerusalem, all of the lower incisors involved in a relatively asymptomatic, second-stage, benign cementoma were vital. Following surgery, however, both lateral incisors were devitalized and required endodontic treatment.[123]

The possibility of this accident is good cause for the limitation of promiscuous periradicular surgery in this region. If endodontic surgery is absolutely indicated, accidental devitalization is less likely to occur if great care is exercised to avoid the tissue around adjacent teeth. A marsupial surgical technique has also been used.

Rhinoplasty

Nasal plastic surgery may be the cause of pulp death. Glick reported three cases of pulp death in maxillary anterior teeth following plastic reconstruction of the nose (personal communication, 1978). Root tips of maxillary central incisors have been fractured during this operation.

Osteotomy

Osteotomy of the maxilla or mandible, to reposition grossly malpositioned segments of the face, has grown to epidemic proportions. Early studies on the circulation of pulps in teeth involved in moved segments of the maxilla were quite encouraging.[124,125] However, research using histologic evaluation of pulpal health revealed that the majority of the pulps in the experimental animals showed cellular and circulatory pathologic changes, even in the presence of collateral circulation.[126,127] On the other hand, human studies by Bell and his surgical group in Dallas were most encouraging. After following 10 patients who had had Le Fort I osteotomies, as well as other maxillofacial surgery, Di et al. reported intact pulp circulation in teeth within the surgical sites and "no significant differences in tooth development between the surgical and control groups."[128] Surgery done with great care and precision appears to spell the difference.

Intubation for General Anesthesia

A relatively common operating room accident, the luxation of the mandibular incisors, may be caused by the heavy retraction against these teeth with an inflexible endotracheal tube. Cases have been seen following tonsillectomy with all four mandibular incisors luxated. A survey of 133 anesthesiology training programs revealed that the average incidence of dental injuries in 1,135,212 tracheal intubations was 1 in 1,000. Broken teeth accounted for the same number of complications as did cardiac arrest, 37.5%. As a matter of fact, "damaged teeth" was the most frequent anesthesia-related insurance claim from 1976 to 1983.[129]

CHEMICAL CAUSES

Filling Materials

Are we ready to rewrite the book on pulp inflammation induced by dental materials? For generations, the profession has labored under the misconception that most filling materials are highly toxic to the dental pulp.

In recent years, however, thanks in great part to British, American, and Scandinavian researchers, dentists have come to realize that it is primarily bacteria that cause continuing pulp inflammation, the so-called toxic effects long blamed on various liners, bases, and filling materials. These disclosures pose the question: How do the bacteria get into a position to irritate the pulp after a filling has been placed? Microleakage is one answer—microleakage around fillings once thought to fill the coronal cavities entirely. In addition, bacteria left behind in the smear layer may also contribute toxins if allowed to remain viable by being "fed" substrate through microleakage.

Some toxicity from materials does exist, however, mostly contributing to inflammation immediately after placement. With time, and in the absence of bacteria, this toxic effect fades unless, of course, the pulp was so stressed that it was already struggling for survival before this new insult was added. In any event, the various filling materials must still be considered, both from their toxicity standpoint and for their marginal sealing capabilities as well.

Cements. To the severe insult to the pulp from bacteria of dental caries, plus the iatral trauma from cavity preparations, must be added the chemical insult from the various filling materials. The commonly used cements today are zinc phosphate, ZOE, polycarboxylate, glass ionomer, and the immediate temporary cements. At one time, silicate cements were used a great deal but have been largely supplanted by composite resins.

Silicate cements have long been condemned both clinically and histologically as a pulp irritant. Because of this and their relative impermanence, silicates gradually slid into disfavor and disuse. Initially, Zander summarized his investigation of the pulp effects of silicate by stating that silicate cement is highly irritating to the pulp and that a nonirritating base, such as ZOE cement, should be used under silicates, especially in younger patients.[130] What Zander did not realize is that ZOE has been found to be even more irritating than silicate.[131] On the other hand, ZOE does have the capability of sealing the dentin against microleakage, sealing at least long enough to pass an extended experimental time span. Unfortunately, it will ultimately wash out. Over the years, Zander's work on silicates was confirmed by James and Schour,[132] Langeland,[99] and El-Kafrawy and Mitchell.[133]

The vulnerability of pulp under intact dentin is one thing; the protection of an irritation dentin barrier is another. The true value of calcification became apparent when Skogedal and Mjör placed silicate cement in unlined cavities below which **irritation dentin** had been induced.[134] After 1 month, 16 of 17 pulps showed "no or only slight reactions" subjacent to the extensive **irritation dentin** formation (Figure 4-34). The one remaining pulp was only "moderately inflamed."

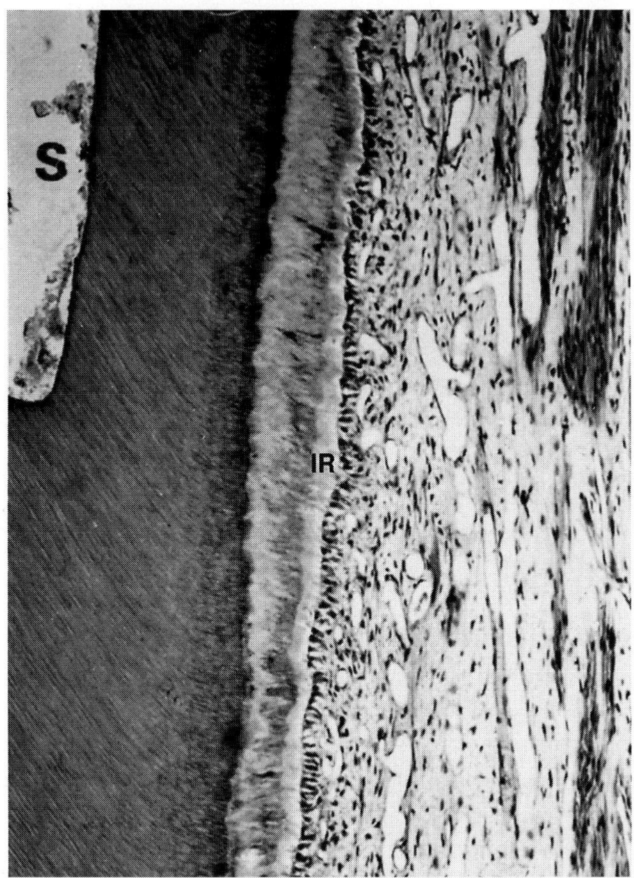

Figure 4-34 Silicate placed 1 month after irritation dentin (IR) has been allowed to form. Pulp reaction is slight, subjacent to silicate in cavity labeled S. Reproduced with permission from Skogedal O and Mjör IA.[134]

Microleakage. Similar findings were reported by Tobias et al., who used ZOE to seal over experimental silicates.[135,136] Their results suggest "that the majority of pulpal inflammation observed beneath...silicate cements is **associated with microbial leakage** at the material/cavity wall interface. The silicate cements themselves appear to have little toxic effect."[135]

Brännström and Olivera also stated that "the main cause of pulpal injury under silicate cement was the growth of bacteria that remained before insertion."[137] In fact, for "8 cavities without bacterial growth and with silicate cement placed directly on an exposed pulp," there were no serious injury and no inflammatory reactions" caused by the silicate (Figure 4-35).[137]

In a classic study, Cox and Bergenholtz achieved similar results when they inserted silicate directly into the pulp and prevented bacterial microleakage with a ZOE overlay.[138] In fact, at 21 days, they were amazed to find "new hard tissue directly adjacent to the interface ...a response that has been believed to be exclusive for calcium hydroxide..."[138]

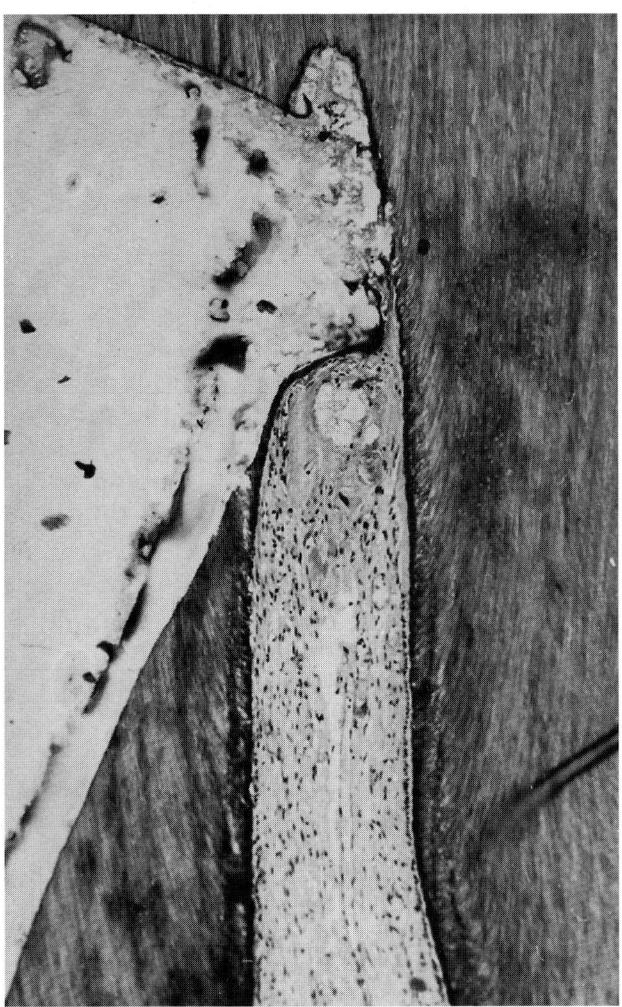

Figure 4-35 Tissue response to silicate cement forced through pulp exposure 1 month previously. Superficial necrosis in response to trauma but no inflammation and no bacteria under silicate. Reproduced with permission from Brännström M and Olivera V.[137]

Zinc phosphate cement has been both condemned[139,140] and praised as a cementing medium and an insulating and protective base. Langeland,[99] as well as Dubner and Stanley, were not too concerned over pulp reactions under zinc phosphate cement.[141] Cox and Bergenholtz drew the same conclusion when they inserted zinc phosphate cement **directly into the pulp.** At 21 days, and **when bacterial microleakage was prevented** by a ZOE surface seal, they found "complete tissue healing and hard tissue repair" right up against the cement.[138]

Investigation of the effect of zinc phosphate cement on the pulp has generally been done on teeth with healthy pulps. Will the "stressed" pulps of carious teeth react in a like manner? Lervik experimentally induced **pulpitis** in 56 teeth in monkeys and placed cements (zinc phosphate and carboxylates) in the Class V cavities.[142] After 32 days and 90 days (Figure 4-36), "healing, with the formation of secondary dentin and slight to no pulpal inflammation, was the usual end result."[142] Time heals **almost** everything!

Brännström and Nyborg, also testing zinc phosphate and polycarboxylate cements, found that "zinc phosphate cement used as a cementing medium does not cause inflammation of the pulp after one to six weeks." The same was true of polycarboxylate cement.[143] These authors are convinced that the **bacteria** left in the prepared cavity are responsible for any inflammation seen under zinc phosphate cement. Their "findings emphasize the importance of cleaning the prepared surfaces from grinding debris and bacteria before cementation,"[143] and, one might add, **preventing microleakage thereafter.**

One must also stress the difference between zinc phosphate cement, mixed to a putty-like consistency and used as a cement base, compared to thin-mix zinc phosphate used as a luting agent. In the latter case, because of the high percentage of unincorporated phosphoric acid, patients may suffer severe pain with cementation, the so-called "phosphoric acid sting." This is owing to the low pH of the mix and the hydraulic pressure of forcing the casting to place, which forces the acid into the dentinal tubules. A severely stressed pulp may not recover from this initial chemical shock.

"**Zinc oxide-eugenol** still remains the most effective temporary filling material when prevention of pulpal

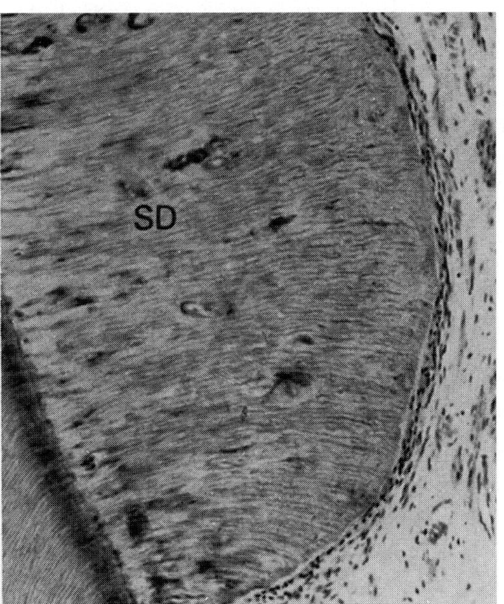

Figure 4-36 Irritation dentin subjacent to zinc-phosphate cement placed in a cavity 90 days previously. Pulpitis was previously induced by sealing soft carious dentin in the cavity. The cell-free zone cannot be differentiated subjacent to irritation dentin. Reproduced with permission from Lervik T.[142]

injury is of prime concern." This statement by Dubner and Stanley is echoed by virtually all of the early investigators in the field.[141] James and Schour suggested that ZOE "may even have exerted a palliative effect on the pulp."[132] Quite possibly, this so-called "palliative effect" is related to the **obtundent effect** eugenol exerts on sensory nerves, rendering them less capable of carrying the "pain message" to the brain.

In view of the strong lobby for ZOE's supposedly bland effect on the pulp, it is surprising to learn that Brännström and Nyborg believe ZOE to be more noxious than either zinc phosphate or polycarboxylate cements.[143] Mjör pointed out that ZOE cement "appears to have marked bacteriostatic and bacteriocidal effects" but cannot be counted on to sterilize infected carious dentin.[144] Das found ZOE cement toxic to human dental pulp cells in tissue culture. Moreover, he found that zinc oxide powder alone was toxic, as were gutta-percha points, which are heavily "filled" with zinc oxide.[145] This is not surprising in view of the findings of Meryon and Jakeman that the zinc released at 14 days from ZOE was a strong toxin *in vitro* against human fibroblasts. Absorption of the released zinc by the remaining dentin on the cavity floor is the pulp's saving grace.[146]

Meryon further tested ZOE to determine the toxic effect of eugenol. She found that eugenol could pass the dentin barrier. The thicker the remaining dentin thickness, however, the less toxic the effect of eugenol. Meryon stated that "eugenol release occurs as a result of hydrolysis of zinc eugenolate." Removal of the smear layer increased the passage of eugenol to the pulp.[147]

Brännström and Nyborg believe that ZOE also exerts a dehydrating effect. That effect, plus 5 seconds of air-drying the experimental cavities, could have caused the damage from desiccation apparent in their slides. In any event, they recommended that a calcium hydroxide liner be placed before ZOE cement is used as a base.[148]

In another study, Brännström and his associates found that IRM cement (Caulk-deTrey, USA and Switzerland) (ZOE strengthened with polymethylmethacrylate) produced "slight to moderate" pulp inflammation if the dentin thickness was less than 0.5 mm. Again they recommended calcium hydroxide as a cavity liner.[149]

In a fastidious study reported by Cook and Taylor, a number of ZOE cements were tested for toxicity.[150] Injected in their unset state into the belly walls of rats, the reaction areas were then examined histologically at 2, 16, and 30 days. After reviewing the numerous favorable reports on ZOE, Cook and Taylor seemed somewhat surprised to find the degree of toxicity caused by the ZOE cements in their study[150] (Figure 4-37). Valcke and his South African associates were also surprised to find ZOE cement to be more toxic than silicate.[131]

Cox and Bergenholtz had the same experience as Valcke using ZOE as a **control** against silicate, zinc phosphate, calcium hydroxide, amalgam, and two composites, **all inserted into the pulp**. However, ZOE came off the worst, with mononuclear cell infiltrates and no hard tissue repair at 21 days.[138]

In view of the more recent evidence that ZOE cement is not as soothing as long thought (periodontists gave up ZOE perio-pack years ago, and pedodontists and endodontists are fully aware of the damaging effects of ZOE cement against a pulp exposure), one must carefully consider the advice to use calcium hydroxide cavity liner when ZOE is used as a cement base or as a luting medium. Remember, in the same study showing ZOE cement and zinc oxide powder to be toxic, Das found calcium hydroxide nontoxic to human pulp tissue cells.[145]

Cavit (Premier Dental; Norristown, Pa.), the resin-reinforced, ZOE temporary cement used extensively in pulpless teeth, enjoys less favor in temporizing **vital** teeth because of the pulpal discomfort that ensues. When Cavit is placed against dentin covering a vital pulp, it causes desiccation. Although Cavit, like ZOE, is hydroscopic, it has a sixfold greater water absorption value than ZOE. The pain on insertion undoubtedly arises from fluid displacement in the dentin tubuli. Therefore, Cavit should always be placed in a moist cavity. Provant and Adrian found no statistical difference between Cavit and ZOE as far as pulp reaction was concerned.[151]

Red and black copper cements have been found to be quite irritating to the pulp and have practically passed from use.

Polycarboxylate cements, a mixture of resin and zinc phosphate cements, have been heavily advertised as adhesives. Evidently, they do adhere to enamel and also initially adhere to dentin, although this latter bond is soon broken. Langeland and colleagues tested two polycarboxylates against pulp reaction in monkey teeth,[152] as did Lervik[142] and Brännström and Nyborg.[148] All reported favorably on the carboxylates.

The results indicate that polycarboxylate cements *per se* are relatively inert. If used as a base or cavity liner, care should be taken to secure full coverage of all exposed dentin to prevent reactions from microleakage reaching the dentin.

Plastics. The commonly used plastic filling materials are amalgam (which is not usually thought of as a plastic, although it is so physically if not chemically),

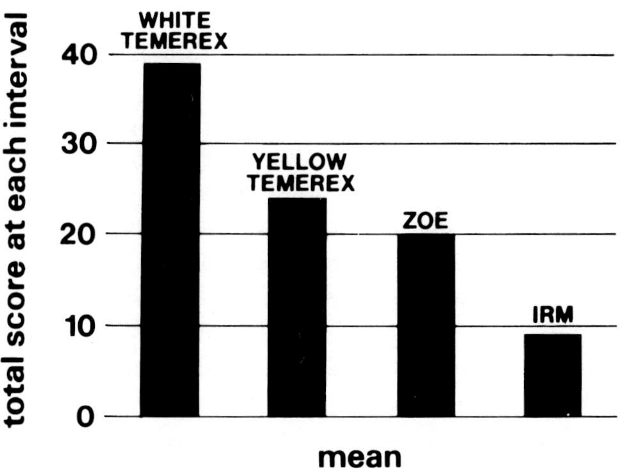

Figure 4-37 Levels of toxicity of four zinc oxide–eugenol–type cements injected into the belly wall of rats. Mean of responses from 2 to 30 days. White Temerex appears to be the most toxic and IRM the least. Reproduced with permission from Cook DJ, Taylor PPJ.[150]

the self-curing and light-cured resins, the composites, and gutta-percha or temporary stopping.

Amalgam. Silver alloy amalgam has been found to be a relatively nontoxic filling material, although Swerdlow and Stanley found twice as much inflammatory change under amalgam fillings than under ZOE controls.[105] Although they attributed this difference in inflammation to the "physical insertion of the amalgam," it might actually have been caused by bacteria from microleakage. Amalgam is notorious for its poor marginal seal, whereas ZOE has a deserved reputation for sealing dentin, if only for a limited time.

In recent years, amalgam has been undergoing both physical and chemical changes as materials science advances. Spherical alloys and the new higher copper alloys are only two of the changes: "The search for amalgams with low creep has led to the development of products with high Cu control."[153]

How does the pulp fare under such new products? According to Skogedal and Mjör, one of the alloys, Sybraloy (Kerr Co.; Orange, Calif.), did poorly.[154] Testing the pulpal inflammation potential of three higher copper alloys against a conventional alloy, these researchers found that Sybraloy, with a 30% copper content, caused unacceptable pulp damage in half of the test teeth, both at 1 week and at 2 to 3 months (Table 4-2). Disperalloy (Johnson & Johnson, New Brunswick, N.J.) (12% copper) and Indiloy (Shofu Dental, Japan) (13% copper), on the other hand, compared favorably with a conventional alloy with 5% copper content[152] (see Table 4-2).

Testing toxicity of amalgam alloys by soft tissue implantation studies was also carried out by Mjör and his group. Silver/tin/zinc alloys and silver/tin/copper alloys all caused a slight tissue reaction.[156]

Suspecting that copper and mercury are the culprits in pulpal irritation by amalgams, Leirskar and Helgeland placed samples of two mixed amalgams in Petri dishes seeded with human epithelial cells, as they did with silicate.[155] Both silver alloy and high copper alloy showed pronounced cytotoxic effects. They were surprised to find that **zinc** was released in substantial amounts from the so-called "silver" alloy (composed of silver, tin, copper, zinc).

Meryon and Jakeman also found that zinc was released from traditional amalgam. Compared with the zinc released from zinc phosphate cement, zinc from amalgam was "moderately" toxic.[146] This phenomenon was also noted by Omnell in periradicular tissue associated with amalgam retrofillings.[156]

Copper was rapidly released from the copper-containing amalgam in amounts far exceeding toxic levels. Mercury and cadmium were also released. Leirskar and Helgeland believe that the "leaching out of the metal ions from the amalgams can possibly help explain the reactions observed."[155]

Table 4-2 Pulp Reactions*

Amalgam	% Copper Control of Alloys	At 1 Week		At 2 to 3 Months		Formation of Irritation Dentin
		Acceptable	Unacceptable	Acceptable	Unacceptable	
Sybraloy	30	3	4	7	6	13
Disperalloy	12	5	1	14	0	7
Indiloy	13†	3	3	10	0	10
Royal Dental Alloy (control)	5	5	2	11	2	10

*Pulp reaction to various amalgams at 1 week and at 2 to 3 months observation period. Note that half of the reactions were unacceptable in teeth tested with **Sybraloy**, a 30% copper content alloy. **Disperaloy** (12% copper) and **Indiloy** (13% copper) fared as well as the conventional alloy, Royal Dental (5% copper).

†Contains 5% indium.

Scandinavian researchers strongly emphasized **the necessity of placing a base under each amalgam** filling, particularly under the high–copper content alloys.[144,153–158] Not only do the cements, which are less toxic, cover the dentinal tubules, they also protect against the incursion of bacteria from marginal leakage.

Herein may lie the clue to all of these studies—marginal leakage. In their classic study, Cox and Bergenholtz placed a dispersed-phase amalgam (Contour, Kerr Co.; Orange, Calif.) directly into pulp exposures. At 7 days, neither the surface-sealed (with ZOE) nor the unsealed amalgam pulp cappings had developed moderate pulpal inflammation (Figure 4-38). At 21 days, however, only the amalgam fillings sealed off from the saliva by a ZOE surface seal exhibited no pulpal inflammation. At the same time, "**three** out of the four 21 days, **unsealed**, amalgam-capped pulps presented moderate to severe inflammation." **Stained bacteria were found under all three of these amalgams.**[138]

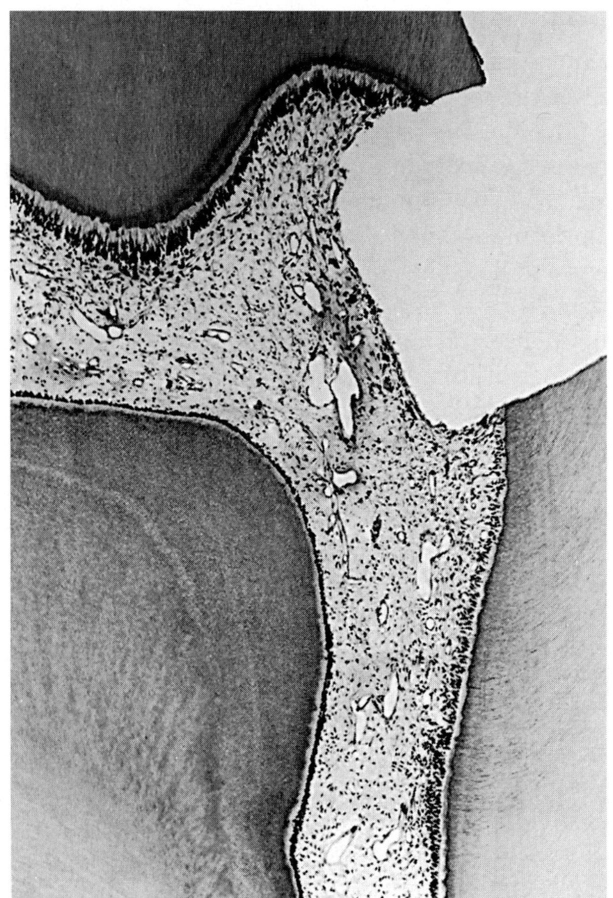

Figure 4-38 One of four unsealed amalgam pulp cappings at 7 days. Pulp reorganized with no inflammation. In marked contrast, the other three unsealed amalgam cappings exhibited marked inflammation. Reproduced with permission from Cox CF et al.[138]

Researchers at Birmingham (University of Alabama) also reported the pulpal impact **from microleakage** when they compared a conventional amalgam versus a high copper amalgam.[159] Both amalgams came off poorly when **unsealed** by a ZOE overseal. They pointed out that "freshly packed conventional amalgams leak initially, but with time a marginal seal is usually effected presumably due to the **corrosion** products at the interface of material and cavity wall."[159] They also noted that "high copper amalgams exhibit greater microleakage than conventional amalgams at 6 and 12 months."[159]

In any event, the problem of microleakage under amalgam may become a moot point if one considers two important factors impacting on the use of silver amalgam. On the one hand is the introduction of the 4-META (Parkell Co., Farmingdale, N.Y.) dental adhesives, which substantially bond amalgams to tooth structure. One would hope that this might eliminate microleakage entirely and thus enhance the use of this age-old and dependable filling material. On the other hand, a significant segment of the lay public and the profession has declared amalgam a toxic threat to health, if not life, because of the alleged release of mercury vapors into the mouth and eventually the bloodstream. There has even been a call to prohibit the further use of silver amalgam.

Resins. When the self-curing resins were introduced following World War II, great hopes were expressed for these materials. Unfortunately, a flurry of early reports appeared indicating the irritating effects of the resins on the pulp.

As straight filling materials, the self-curing **resins** have virtually disappeared. For constructing **temporary crowns**, however, these products are extensively used. Because many temporaries are made in the mouth, not in the laboratory, they have the potential to damage a dental pulp already traumatized by crown preparation. Early on, Seelig suggested that pulp injury under plastics might be caused by cavity preparation **or salivary leakage around the plastic.**[160] So, over 50 years ago, Seelig was forecasting the role that microleakage plays in pulp inflammation.

In spite of initial glowing reports on self-curing plastics,[161] Grossman recommended protective bases under self-curing plastics.[162] Following Grossman, Nygaard-Østby tested the effects on the pulp of five different plastics.[163] Severe inflammation was found under all five plastics. Langeland observed similar irreversible pulp changes under three plastics.[164] Some of the products were withdrawn from the market.[165]

It might well be that the initial toxic shock is so severe that the extensive use of mouth-curing plastics as temporary crowns accounts, in part, for the great number of latent pulp deaths under extensive restorative cases. One must also consider the damaging effect of the **heat generated** as the plastic material **self-cures** on the freshly cut preparation. Tjan and colleagues at Loma Linda University found as much as a 19°C temperature rise under some directly placed provisional crowns. They also found that the temperature increase could be significantly reduced if silicone putty impressions were used as a matrix.[107] A 5.5°C rise in temperature has been shown to be damaging to the pulp.[82]

To prove the point that there is a difference between *in vitro* and *in vivo* research results, a group in London tested two different methacrylate temporary crown materials on monkeys.[166] At 4 weeks, they found normal pulp tissue under both acrylics as well as "a small quantity of reparative dentin." The crowns, however, were well **sealed against microleakage.**

As far back as 1959, Zander voiced the fact that it was bacteria from microleakage that was the culprit causing pulp reactions, not the acrylics per se.[167,168]

Microleakage can best be controlled by marginal fit. Because temporary crowns are just that—temporary—not enough attention is paid to this important feature. The UCLA materials laboratory tested the marginal accuracy of nine popular brands of temporary restorative materials. They found SNAP (Parkell Co., USA) to give the best fit and Neopar (Kerr Co., USA) to be the worst. The other seven materials were scattered between.[169]

Composite Resins. In their *in vitro* study, Spangberg and colleagues determined that "Although when freshly prepared the composite materials cause less cell damage than the silicates or cold-curing plastics, the composites resemble the silicates in that they give off irritant components over a longer time than the cold-curing plastics."[170] The composites contain acrylic monomers in their catalyst system, and it can be assumed that the monomer would cause damage, as in the case of the cold-curing resins.

In addition to their principal and diluent monomers, composite resins contain other organic chemicals such as silane coupling agents, polymerization inhibitors, initiator-activator components (benzoyl peroxide), and ultraviolet stabilizers. Various inorganic fillers (glass beads and fibers, quartz, silicon dioxide, etc) are also added to modify the physical characteristics.

To determine their individual effect on the pulp, Stanley et al. separately tested each of the eight categories of chemical compounds that collectively form contemporary composite restorations.[171] They were surprised to find at 21 days that "none of the individual components could be considered significantly irritating." However, they knew, collectively, that the chemicals caused pulp inflammation. Pulp protection was therefore recommended.

In early *in vitro* testing of the composites, Dickey and colleagues found Adaptic as toxic as silicate.[172] It has since been removed from the market. Langeland also found no significant difference in pulp irritation between the silicates, cold-cure plastics, and composite resin materials.[173] Langeland et al. added, however, that "used with an adequate protective base, these materials are biologically acceptable, and because of their good physical properties, superior to other anterior tooth-filling material."[174] Quite possibly, Langeland's "adequate protective base" was in reality serving as a dentin sealant **preventing microleakage** and subsequent pulp inflammation.[174]

In spite of the laudatory reports regarding the physical and esthetic properties of the composites, problems have developed around the alleged irritation from their chemical constituents and attempts to improve their adhesive qualities. Stanley and his associates noted that, early on, investigators thought methacrylic acid was the primary pulp irritant.[175] Therefore, efforts were made to remove it from the newer composite formulations and to establish a neutral pH as well. It was shown, however, that removing methacrylic acid and adjusting the pH in composite liquid provided no improvement in pulp reaction. Stanley further stated that the composite manufacturers, apparently concerned with the toxicity of their products, have diverted their research efforts to improving color stability and physical properties or developing a better cavity liner or dentin bonding agent. He is adamant (as are most of the manufacturers) that any composite filling should be preceded by a protective base or, better yet, one of the new nontoxic cavity liners or bonding agents.[176] Stanley later noted that "only when the recently developed dual-cure resin cements are not adequately cured with visible light do significant pulpal lesions appear."[176]

In the previously quoted research effort, Cox and Bergenholtz placed composite resins directly into pulp exposures in deep cavities prepared in monkey teeth.[138] Under resin-capped exposures, **sealed against microleakage** by ZOE overfillings, they found "normal pulp tissue architecture against the composite interface, in all four teeth, at 21 days. **Hard tissue repair** was also present in the ZOE-sealed restorations" (Figure 4-39, A). All of the composite-capped (unsealed) exposures that **exhibited microleakage** "showed some degree of stained bacteria" as well as pulp tissue breakdown, severe inflammation, and necrosis (Figure 4-39, B).[138]

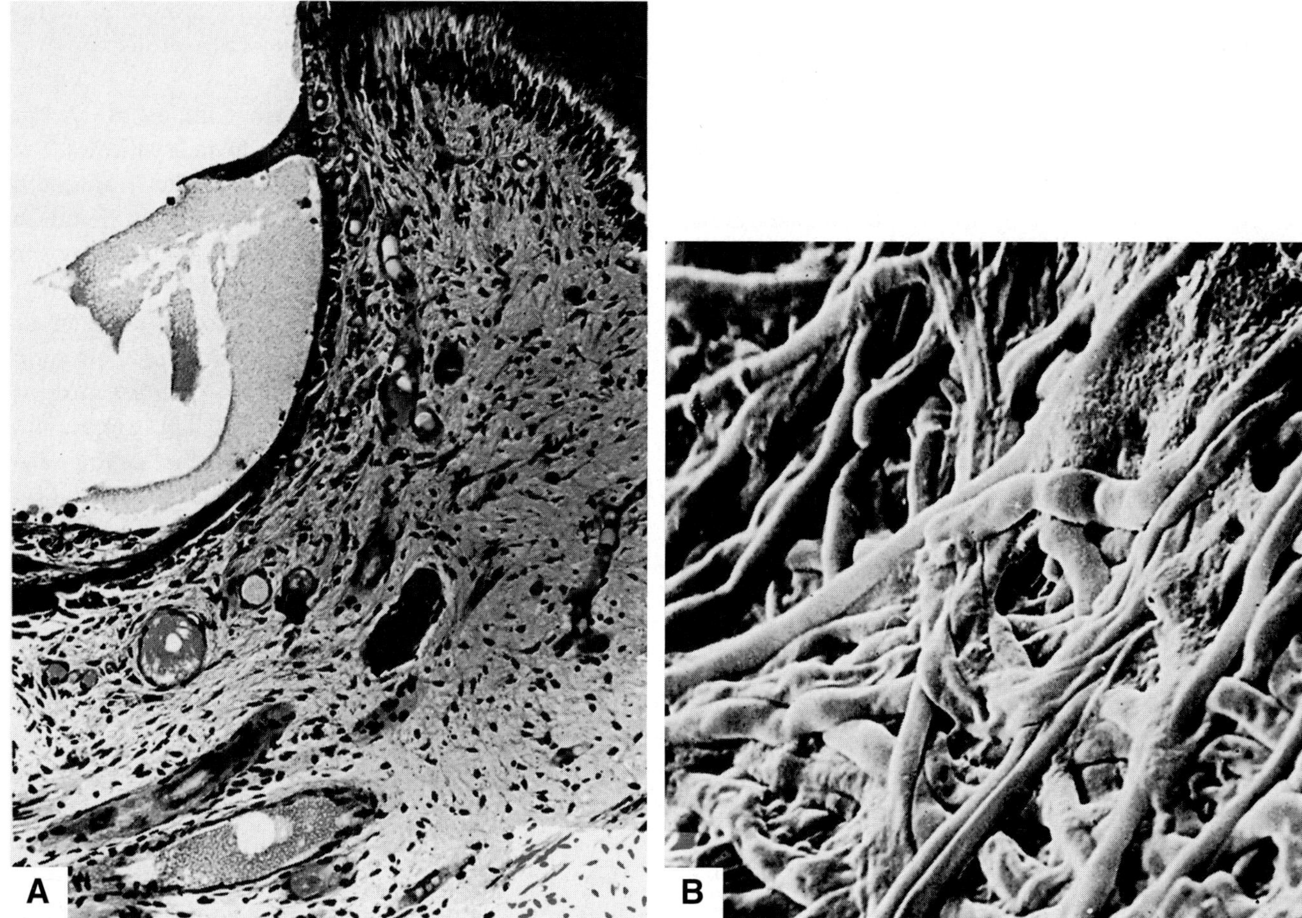

Figure 4-39 Prevention of microleakage prevents pulp irritation. **A**, Composite resin-capped pulp after 21 days sealed from oral bacteria by zinc oxide–eugenol overfilling. Note odontoblasts and new hard tissue adjacent to composite. There is no inflammation. Reproduced with permission from Cox CF et al.[138] **B**, If restoration is not sealed from saliva, microleakage allows a "tangle" of bacterial colonies to proliferate under composite resin, leading to pulpal inflammation. Reproduced with permission from Brännström M.[211]

Hörsted and his Danish colleagues conducted a similar study, preparing cavities in monkey teeth with a remaining dentin thickness of only 0.3 mm.[177] They then placed both a chemically cured composite and a light-cured composite in these deep cavities. Half of the cavities were lined with calcium hydroxide and half were not. Pulp inflammation was generally related to microleakage ("bacteria were found in all **unlined** cavities…"). The most pronounced inflammatory changes were seen beneath the pulpo-gingival corner of the cavity"—a common site for bacteria to accumulate and penetrate the tubuli."[177]

Speculating on this finding, Hörsted et al. emphasized the importance of carefully extending the protective dentin liner to proximal and gingival walls as well as the pulpal floor. They also urged care in acid-etching the enamel to prevent gaps at the enamel surface, which open to microleakage.[177]

Heys et al. of Michigan placed two microfilled composites and a conventional composite in monkey teeth as well.[178] No cavity liner, acid etchant, or bonding agent was used in cavities averaging 0.59 mm remaining dentin thickness. At 8 weeks, 6 of 27 teeth were acutely inflamed.

Again, **bacteria were indicted.** They were found along the cavity walls of all teeth. There was no penetration of bacteria into the tubuli, however. Pulp protection was undoubtedly afforded by an intact smear layer obstructing the tubuli in some cases. In spite of this evidence, Heys et al. made a pitch for a calcium hydroxide liner.[178]

In spite of the suggestions that calcium hydroxide be used as a cavity liner, a number of dental scientists have questioned its use under composite resins.[179] Lacy pointed out that "calcium hydroxide should be used only in instances when extra pulp protection or stimulation is needed."[179] Even then, a thin layer of one of the newer hard setting preparations is indicated. This allows for more depth and strength in the resin. Calcium hydroxide, however, should be protected by a layer of glass ionomer cement.[179]

The late Ron Jordan, one of North America's foremost authorities on the clinical use of composite resins, recommended glass ionomer cements, rather than calcium hydroxide, under composite fillings.[180] If calcium hydroxide must be used (in near exposures or actual exposures), hard, light-activated calcium hydroxide should be used and then covered by a glass ionomer base. In very deep cavities, calcium hydroxide should also be used under glass ionomers.[180] Eventually, the dentin bonding agents may completely replace glass ionomer cements in such situations.

Calcium Hydroxide Resin, Light Cured. Because it comes in a form of light-cured composite resin, calcium hydroxide will be discussed here as well. Stanley and Pameijer studied just such a material, Prisma VCL Dycal (L.D. Caulk Co., Milford, Dela.) which "consists of calcium hydroxide and fillers of barium sulfate dispersed in a specially formulated urethane dimethylacrylate resin" containing initiators (camphoroquinone) and activators. The resin is activated by light in the wavelength range of 400 to 500 mm.[181] Prisma VCL Dycal is similar to Cavalite (Kerr Co.; Orange, Calif.), which also contains a glass ionomer powder filler and 14% calcium hydroxyapatite.

Composite resin calcium hydroxide has a number of advantages over regular water or methylcellulose-based calcium hydroxide: "dramatically improved strength, essentially no solubility in acid, and minimal solubility in water."[181] To this can be added the control the clinician has over working time with any light-activated resin that "sets on command" and reaches its maximum physical properties almost immediately.[181]

Calcium hydroxide causes the deposition of minerals essential to the repair of pulp exposures by the stimulation that comes from its being a mild tissue irritant. It is necessary, therefore, that the calcium hydroxide not be so tightly bound in the resin that it cannot be released to act as an irritant. This is essentially what Stanley and Pameijer tested for, comparing Prisma VLC Dycal against water-soluble Advanced Formula II Dycal (L.D. Caulk Co.; Milford, Dela.). They found the resin-based Prism VLC Dycal to be over three times stronger than the water-based Dycal and its solubility in water to be less by half.[181]

Concerning pulp response to light-cured Dycal, "inflammation was of no consequence."[181] This is in contrast to regular Dycal, which "caused a thickness of pulp mummification (chemical cautery) of 0.3-0.7 mm at the exposure sites."[182]

The lower pH of Prisma VLC Dycal evidently precludes pulp necrosis but still provides sufficient irritation to stimulate the **formation of irritation dentin.** Stanley observed dentin bridging in all but one specimen in the study.[182] Cavalite, with an almost neutral pH, has been shown in capping studies to produce a dentin bridging and pulp reorganization. McComb placed Cavalite first, as the "best combination of strength, clinical handling and aesthetics."[183]

Stanley and Pameijer warned that care must be taken not to "bayonet" dentin chips into the pulp or force the capping agent therein. Either or both will form a "double bridge" of dentin deeper in the pulp, and the trapped tissue will become nonvital. One must also make sure that the covering restoration is not lifted from the exposure site by intrapulpal edema or the bridge will not form against the pulp tissue.[181]

Glass ionomer cements, a formulation of resin and silicates, were developed in 1972, in England, by Wilson and Kent and termed "ASPA" (an abbreviation for aluminosilicate-polyacrylic acid).[184] Since its original formulation, other acids have been added: itaconic acid to increase the reactivity of the polyacrylic acid, tartaric acid to extend the working time, and polymaleic and mesaconic acid to improve the cement's physical properties.

"Combining the strength, rigidity and fluoride release properties of a silicate glass powder with the biocompatibility and adhesive characteristics of a polyacrylic acid liquid..., glass ionomer cements may be characterized as strong, stiff, hard, materials that are adhesive to calcified tissue, have low toxicity, and are potentially anticariogenic."[185] Various manufacturers throughout the world were licensed to produce and market the glass ionomers as both a filling/basing cement and a luting cement.[186]

Initially, all of the testing of ASPA was for its physical and chemical properties. By 1975, Klotzer had tested its biologic effect on pulps in monkey teeth and concluded that ASPA II was an irritant, but less so than silicate.[187] The following year, Dahl and Tronstad found much the same.[188] They also noted that toxicity diminished with setting time and that at 24 hours it was completely set and nontoxic.[188]

In 1978, Tobias and Browne tested ASPA and concluded that pulpal reaction to ASPA was "similar to that of polycarboxylate cements."[189]

In 1980, Cooper tested ASPA IV and ASPA IVA in Class V cavities in premolars in humans, without a rubber dam, and filled them with either ASPA IV, ASPA IVA, silicate, or ZOE. He found irritation dentin protecting the pulp and proved these materials to be mild irritants, not toxic ones.[186]

Nordenval and colleagues also tested ASPA in etched and unetched cavities, and after 70 to 90 days found "no inflammation under any of the cavities including the two with pulp exposures."[190] **They also found no bacteria in the cavities.**

Kawahara et al. found that "[G]lass ionomer cement has no irritant effect upon the living pulp, but polycarboxylate and zinc oxide–eugenol cement kept their irritating effect after setting."[191] Meanwhile, in the United States, Pameijer et al. were testing glass ionomers in primates and concluded that they were biocompatible to the pulp and that a "protective base (Dycal) was not deemed necessary."[192] They also observed no bacteria on cavity walls or within the tubules. When a similar study was done without pressure and using Ketac-Cem (Premier Dental; Norristown, Pa.) luting cement, Pameijer and Stanley found minimal pulpal response.[193–195] By 1984, Meryon and Smith were reporting fluoride release from three glass ionomers, which they felt should serve as a "protection against secondary caries but may initiate some pulpal inflammation."[196]

In 1987, Fitzgerald et al. evaluated three luting cements, zinc phosphate, polycarboxylate, and G.C. Fuji glass ionomer (G.C. International, Japan/USA), **for bacterial leakage.**[197] Cultivable bacteria were found under all three cements but significantly less than would be suspected from the stained bacterial layer found later when all of the test crowns were eventually removed. At 10 days and 56 days, there was a **significant decrease** in the number of bacteria **under glass ionomer** cement but a **significant increase** in bacteria **under zinc phosphate.** Bacterial counts under polycarboxylate remained about the same.[197]

Fitzgerald et al. **blamed microleakage** for this increase in cultivable bacteria. They postulated, moreover, that the observed microleakage "might provide enough fluid movement across the cut dentin to elicit a painful response." They cited "the hydrodynamic theory of pulpal pain, small movements of fluid within dentinal tubules causing pulpal pain"[197] (see chapter 7). They concluded that "it is possible that glass ionomer cement had antibacterial actions (fluoride) that reduced the number of viable bacteria but not the amount of fluid penetration."[197]

It would appear that the presence of bacteria alone is not the prime cause of hypersensitivity, for if it were, zinc "phosphate should be the most sensitive."[197] Pameijer and Stanley concurred in this observation, pointing out that bacteria could not be responsible for early inflammation, which is more likely caused by cement acidity.[193]

To raise the abrasion resistance for glass ionomer cements, McLean and Gasser in England combined the glass with silver to produce a sintered metal–glass composite called **cermet.**[198] It is sold as Ketac-Silver (Premier-Espe; Norristown, Pa.), and McLean recommended its use for very conservative cavity preparations wherein the cermet, bonding to both enamel and dentin, reformed a monolithic structure with the tooth, returning it to its former strength.[199,200] McLean had no comment about pulp irritability from cermet, and, for the time being, one would cautiously assume it to be the same as regular glass ionomer cement.

The findings on glass ionomer cements presented here may be summarized by saying that they are no more toxic, and to some extent less so, than other filling or luting cements. They are recommended as a base or liner under composite resin fillings and amalgams. If handled properly and allowed to set without moisture, they are strong, do not shrink, and resist dissolution by either water, saliva, or acid. At this juncture, they have a decided advantage: they are the only **cements** that bond to dentin. To this a caveat must be added: If they are used as a base under composite resin fillings, this bond may be illusory. According to Garcia-Godoy, "Although glass ionomer adheres to dentin, the polymerization contraction of the composite bonded to it can break the original bond between the glass ionomer and the dentin," **allowing microleakage.**[201]

If placed in deep cavities or over extensive crown preparations, light-cured calcium hydroxide should first be used as a base under glass ionomers wherever a thin remaining dentin thickness is suspected. This is especially true in crown preparations if immediate and lasting hypersensitivity is to be avoided. Before placing **glass ionomers**, the dentinal tubuli must be **well occluded** to prevent either the **pulpal** flow of free polyacrylic acid or the flow of dentinal fluid in the tubuli, a movement that brings on pain by hydrodynamic stretching or crushing of the odontoblasts. This is particularly true if anhydrous ionomers are used for they draw the dentinal fluid away from the pulp, incurring immediate and lasting hypersensitivity.[193]

All in all, glass ionomer cements are a valuable addition to dentistry. They not only bond chemically to dentin (for how long is not known), they also do not shrink or leave a contraction gap between the cement and dentin. Furthermore, they have a compressive strength of 28,000 psi. On the other hand, they are technique sensitive. When using them as **luting agents,** however, the areas close to the pulp should be covered with visible light cure (VLC) calcium hydroxide. This protects the pulp in critical areas without losing the benefit of the bonding advantages. Stanley pointed out that glass ionomer cements "appear to be pulp irritants mainly when used as luting agents."[176]

Preparation of the Cavity to Receive Composite Filling Materials. Before any glass ionomer cement or composite material is placed, elaborate preparations must be made of the margins and surfaces of the enamel and dentin. Enamel rods are "opened" by acid etching. In spite of the many caveats about not using strong acid on freshly cut dentin, some dentists remove the dentinal smear layer with 37 to 50% citric or phosphoric acid.

Etching Agents. **Acid etching the enamel** to improve bonding is a necessary part of the composite technique. Based on the success of enamel bonding, it is also believed that etching the dentin will improve bonding while "cleansing and removing grinding debris, dentin chips, blood and denatured collagen from the cavity preparation."[173] To this one might add, **bacteria in the smear layer** as well.

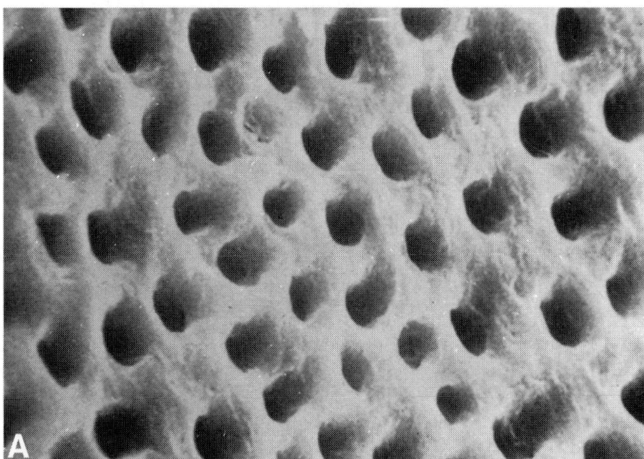

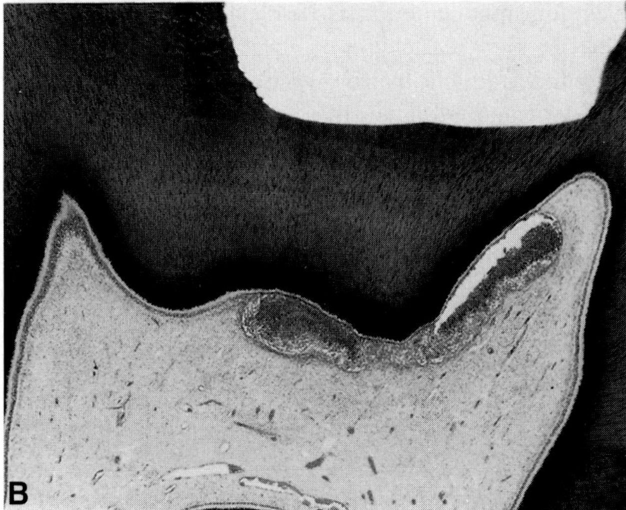

Figure 4-40 A, Cross-section of dentin tubules in the floor of a cavity treated with 50% citric acid cleaner for 2 minutes. Openings are unobstructed and enlarged. Note absence of tubular contents—microcrystalline debris or odontoblast processes. Reproduced with permission from Cotton WR and Sigel RL.[203] B, Severe inflammatory response and necrosis in pulp 7 days following acid etch of dentin for 1 minute and filled with composite. Dentin depth at horn 1.1 mm. (Courtesy of Dr. Y. Hirai and Prof. T. Ishikawa, Tokyo, Japan.)

Initially, citric and phosphoric acids were recommended on both enamel and dentin, apparently with no thought given to pulp reactions* (Figure 4-40). This was followed by a flurry of research efforts purporting to show the deleterious effects of acid treatment of the dentin.[174,175,202–208] In these experiments, a number of factors may have contributed to the pulpal inflammatory response to acid on dentin, including strength of acid (50%),[175] length of application time (up to 5 minutes[203,205]), remaining dentin thinness,[206] toxicity of the ZOE test filling materials,[131,138,207,208] and the irritating effects of **bacteria** bathing the dentin through **microleakage** under resin test restorations.[138]

But, gradually, the conventional wisdom regarding dentin acid treatment appeared to turn to favor the use of acids. Brännström recommended acid etching dentin and noted no lasting pulpal inflammation.[209] Pashley stated that "...this seemingly extreme procedure does not injure the pulp, especially if diluted acids are used for short periods of time."[210] White and Cox reported that "acid etching of vital dentin does not cause pulp inflammation."[211]

Fusayama in Japan[212] and Kanca[213–217] and Bertolotti[218] in the United States popularized dentin acid treatment, claiming no deleterious pulpal effects. An important *caveat*, however, is the subsequent application of a **dentin bonding agent, thus eliminating microleakage.** In histologic pulp studies in monkeys, testing the true effects of acid conditioning but eliminating other toxic irritants (ie, ZOE, microleakage, etc), White et al. found "that acid etching of vital dentin does not impair pulpal healing when placed in deep Class V cavities."[219]

To remove the smear layer and its incorporated bacteria, Kanca used 37% phosphoric acid gel applied for only 15 seconds.[217] Others used 10% polyacrylic acid (Smear clean/10, H.O. Denta, USA) for 10 seconds,[205] 10% citric acid (10-3 conditioner, Parkell Co., Farmingdale, N.Y.) for 10 seconds, 2.5% nitric acid, or EDTA. These diluted acids, left in place for a short period of time, fall within Pashley's "window of safety."[210] As a matter of fact, Nakabayashi showed that overetching the dentin weakens the bond between adhesives and the dentin.[220]

One must know that commercial etchants are seldom marketed as such but are euphemistically called "conditioners" or "primers." Whatever they are called, it

*One thinks of these etching acids as being highly acidic. Actually, they are virtually the same pH as fresh lemon juice, pH 1.4. They range from pH 1.3 to pH 2.6.

goes without saying that the dentin surface, cleaned of the smear layer and its bacteria, and the dentinal tubules opened, must then be protected by a cavity liner or base or, better yet, by a **dentin bonding agent** that adheres the final filling to the tooth structure, eliminating microleakage.

Cavity Liners, Bases, and Dentin Bonding Agents. When one usually thinks of cavity liners, the varnishes and resin monomers come to mind, including chemicals such as copal, polyvinyl, cyanoacrylate, the acrylics, and procion dye liners.[174] But the list is longer. It should also include cements: zinc phosphate, ZOE, glass ionomers, and polycarboxylate, as well as calcium hydroxide, particularly the new light-activated resin-type calcium hydroxide. Some of the new liners contain ingredients such as glutaraldehyde, hydroxyethylmethacrylate (HEMA), oxalate salts, and oleic acid. The dentin bonding agents may also be thought of as cavity liners, even though their initial responsibility is to bind final restorations, metal, porcelain, or resin to dentin.

What are the indications for using a base or a cavity liner? One might first suggest that a liner or base protects the pulp by acting as a barrier against thermal sensitivity and **against microleakage.** Liners should also reduce or eliminate dentin permeability. Some, like calcium hydroxide, act as mild stimulants to produce protective dentin. Others, such as ZOE, lull the pulp to "sleep."

Since "these materials are applied directly onto dentin, they should be nontoxic, nonirritating and cause no irreversible changes to the pulp."[221] At the same time, the liner or base must have sufficient compressive strength so that it will not collapse or crush down under biting pressure. If it does, it will allow the flexion of the major filling material above it, leading to distortion, marginal opening with eventual breakage of the marginal seal, or possibly fracture of the filling material itself, a cusp, or both. Flexion also causes pulpal pain. In addition to being biocompatible with the pulp, the base or liner must be chemically compatible with the final filling material as well.

For all of the above reasons, **ZOE is not a good base.** In the long run, it is not a biocompatible material. It is also soft, easily compressible, and chemically antagonistic to resins, and if microleakage occurs, ZOE washes out.

Calcium hydroxide, on the other hand, is an ideal pulp protectant but should be used only where indicated, **in a very thin layer,** over near or true pulp exposures (under dam) and should be the light-activated resin calcium hydroxide that features a high compressive strength.

Regular aqueous or methylcellulose calcium hydroxide also fails as a base. It is biocompatible with the pulp but, unfortunately, has a very low compressive strength, allowing the filling to be crushed into it.

There are other variations of pulp-stimulating cements that enjoy wide use, particularly in Europe: calcium hydroxide cements containing corticosteroids (Ledermix, Lederle, Germany) or sodium and potassium salts (Calxyl, Otto Co., Germany).

Baratieri and his colleagues found that Ledermix (calcium hydroxide cement containing triamcinolone, a corticosteroid) depresses the activity of the odontoblasts and thus slows and deters irritation dentin apposition.[222] The findings were comparable to those with dexamethasone (Decatron, Merck-Sharpe & Dohme; Hoddeson, Hertfordshire, U.K.), another corticosteroid,[222] Langeland et al. noted earlier,[223,224] as had Mjör and Nygaard Østby.[225] Calxyl, a calcium hydroxide mixture, in contrast to Ledermix, "allows the maintenance of normal dentinogenesis by protecting the pulp against the irritation from operative procedures."[222]

Finally, time-honored zinc oxyphosphate cement is an excellent base under inlays and amalgams, as is polycarboxylate cement. For strength of the final covering restoration, however, these bases should not exceed 1.0 mm in thickness.[226] In the long run, both cements have limited pulpal irritation qualities.

Liners. Time-honored (but not very) copal varnishes (Copalite, H. J. Bosworth Co.; Skokie, Ill.) may be used under zinc oxyphosphate cement bases or directly under amalgams but **never** under composite resins or glass ionomer cements. As Pashley and Depew pointed out, "Copalite reduces permeability to some degree. But Copalite residue is hydrophobic and tends to lie on top of cavity surfaces much like a gasket."[227] Although initially reducing microleakage, Copalite "tended to permit increased leakage after three months."[227] It has been shown that "pinholes" develop over each open tubule as fluid pushes through (Figure 4-41).

Around 1980, the methylcellulose-based liners were introduced and found to be efficacious as pulp protectants and also highly compatible under composite resins.[228] Stanley recommended that a thin coating of calcium hydroxide should be used under most resins (personal communication, September 1, 1981).

A dentin sealant, Barrier, also became available. A 50/50 polymer compound of dimerized oleic acid with ethylenediamine, it has an extremely high molecular weight and will completely block dentin tubuli. (Composite resin monomer has a very low molecular weight.) Tested for biocompatibility, Barrier was found to be completely nontoxic to the pulp at the end of 1 week.[229]

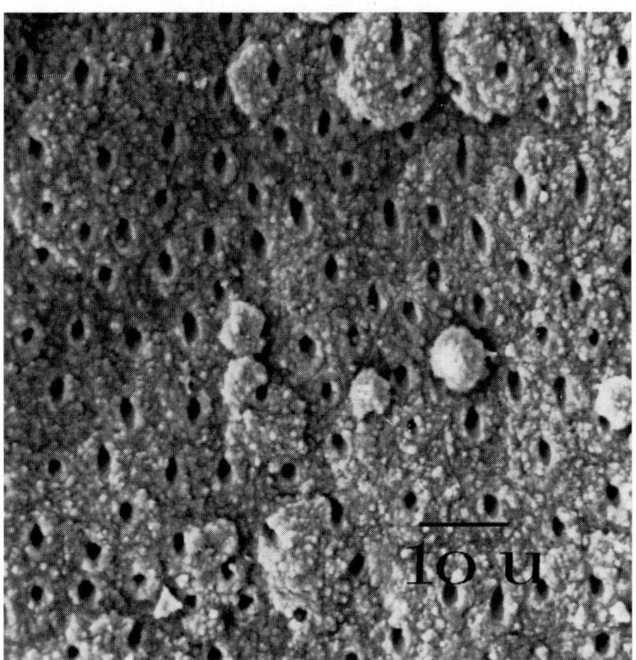

Figure 4-41 Dentin wall magnified ×1,000. Moisture-filled dentinal tubules cannot be sealed by varnish cavity liners, and pinholes develop through which toxic filling materials penetrate to irritate pulp. Reproduced with permission from Koenigs JF, Brilliant JD, Foreman DW. Oral Surg 1974;38:573.

Researchers at Loma Linda University compared all three of the "varnishes," Barrier, Universal, and CaviLine.[230] All three brands "demonstrated a statistically significant reduction in dentin permeability to free monomer." **Time Line** (L.D. Caulk Co.; Milford, Dela.), a visible light-cure liner to be used over the smear layer, was well received by Barkmeier, who stated that the "pulp response to this new resin base was excellent"(personal communication, April 24, 2002). Time Line also claims fluoride release.

These new cavity liners have been well received, practically replacing copal varnish. Outside of calcium hydroxide bases, however, they all stand a good chance of being replaced in turn by the newer adhesive bonding agents that adhere to the tooth and restoration as well.

Dentin Bonding Agents. The turning point in pulp protection may well come from **dentin bonding agents.** A host of these products have been rushed to the market, a number without adequate biologic evaluation or long-range intraoral testing. If any of them live up to promise, they will solve the problems of microleakage and/or filling retention.

Dentin bonding agents should serve a multiple purpose: they should chemically and/or physically bond to the enamel, cementum, dentin, and the intertubular dentin, as well as into the tubules; they should seal off the tubules to prevent invasion by chemical or bacterial toxins as well as the bacteria themselves; they should not wash out, allowing for later microleakage; and, if at all possible, they should also adhere to the filling material placed against them, either resins, ceramics, amalgam, gold, or semiprecious metals. In short, they should be the "glue" that dentistry has long sought, attaching everything to everything.

As far as endodontics is concerned, there should be three considerations in evaluating these products: (1) Do they themselves chemically damage the pulp? (2) Will they seal the dentin to prevent other toxins (bacterial or chemical) from irritating the pulp? (3) Will they permanently seal the dentin, cementum, and enamel surfaces to prevent future microleakage?

Rather than discuss all of the various products, most of which have one or more shortcomings when measured against the criteria listed above, one example will be used, 4-META/MMA-TBB polymer. 4-META is 4-methacryloxyethyl trimellitate anhydride, MMA is methyl methacrylate, and TBB is tri-N-butyl borane. This product, developed in Japan by Nakabayashi,[231] is sold in Japan as Superbond (Sun Medical Co., Japan) and in North America as C & B Metabond (Parkell Co.; Farmingdale, N.Y.). It has the desirable characteristic of bonding to dentin, enamel, and cementum on the one face and metals, ceramic, and resins on the other.

Its analogue, modified by adding HEMA and a fourth proprietary ingredient to the basic 4-META/MMA-TBB formula, presents a thinner film thickness and is used to bond fresh amalgams, as well as resins, to the tooth. Sold in Japan as **D-Liner** (Sun Medical Co.; Salem, Va.) and in North America as **Amalgambond** and **Amalgambond Plus** (Parkell Co.; Farmingdale, N.Y.), these products have the unique capability of uniting tooth and silver amalgam (as well as composites) into a monolithic structure rather than a filling inserted into the tooth. This is an added advantage over dentin bonding agents **that attach only** to resins.

An added advantage of 4-META is its hydrophilic and hydrophobic nature. As it sets, it will not shrink away from the pulpal fluid that gathers on the surface of etched dentin, as many dentin adhesive agents do. As a matter of fact, the catalyst (TBB) requires moisture to trigger polymerization. This is particularly important in deep cavities.[232] Pashley pointed out that the fluid content of dentin varies from 1% at the dentinoenamel junction to 22% near the pulp.[233] In addition, 4-META/MMA is self-curing and therefore does not suffer from the problems of shrinking toward the light source (and away from the tooth surface) as do light-cured dentin bonding agents.

Longitudinal studies of these new products are, of course, limited. Recently, however, Summitt and his associates presented the results of a 4-year study comparing 60 complex amalgam restorations in vital molar teeth, 30 teeth in each cohort. In half of the cases, pins were used for retention. In the other half, **Amalgambond Plus** was used for retention. At the end of 4 years, "the bonded restorations were performing as well as the pin-retained restorations," except three of the pin-retained restorations "suffered significant tooth fracture adjacent to the restoration."[234]

To achieve true dentin adherence with a dentin bonding agent, the smear layer must be removed. For this procedure, "10-3" is used: 10% citric acid and 3% ferric chloride applied for 10 seconds. When the base/catalyst, 4-META/MMA-TBB, is applied to the cleaned dentin surface, a "hybrid" layer of dentin and resin forms that is very adherent to the tooth. This bonding is a physical entanglement between the resin and the collagen fibers of the dentin matrix—collagen that has been frayed by the smear removal. The dentin bonding agent also flows into the tubules and mechanically locks there (Figure 4-42).

If the dentin is completely covered, and if this new acid-resistant, hybrid layer will last forever, the problem of microleakage would be solved and the pulp would be everlastingly protected from external attack. Time (and longitudinal, intraoral, clinical studies) will tell.

Placement. As far as immediate irritation from the placement procedures of 4-META/MMA is concerned, there is evidence that pulpal irritation is minor and brief. As previously stated, there does not appear to be any lasting pulpal damage from the use of 10% citric acid for 10 seconds.[233] As far as 4-META/MMA-TBB itself is concerned, Japanese researchers compared the new material (in dog dental pulp studies) with another dentin bonding agent and against controls of glass ionomer and polycarboxylate cements.[235] They found that the effects of the dentin bonding agents on the dental pulp were "less harmful" than the classic cements. Four other Japanese research groups found essentially the same, that "the system was found to be safe and pulp compatible."[236–238] Toshiaki et al. stated that the C & B Metabond was found to cause significantly less inflammation than either polycarboxylate or zinc phosphate cements.[239]

Pashley pointed out that if bonding agents do not completely polymerize, free monomer may irritate the pulp, especially in deeper cavities.[233] Prinsloo and Vander Vyver in South Africa found that "C&B Metabond shows a much higher degree of polymerization than dual-cure [self-cure and light-cure] cements—70% vs. 30% at 24 hours."[240]

Testing for any "leakage cytotoxic components" of five adhesives, Tell and his associates found that 4-META/MMA-TBB "demonstrated the least cytotoxic leachable components by producing no cell death after day 5."[241] Four other products tested leaked toxic components for 2 years.[243] Cox et al. and Yamami, Miyakoshi, and Matsura and their colleagues, in Japan,[243–245] also reported 4-META as less toxic.

On the basis of this evidence, one might conclude that this new dentin bonding agent (serving as an example of what is sure to evolve) is no more toxic on application than any other dentin bonding agent or composite resin. Furthermore, its acid-resistant nature

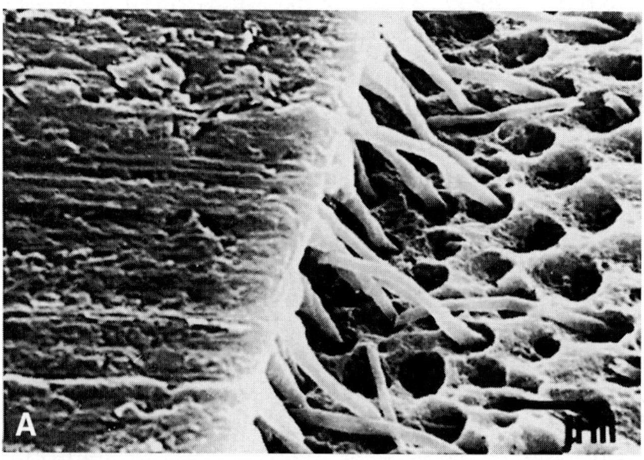

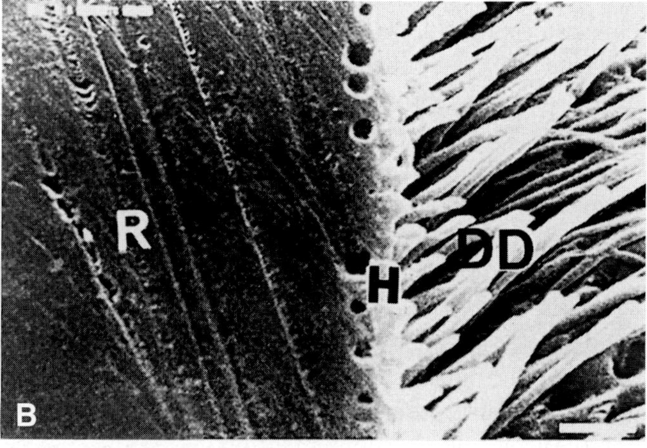

Figure 4-42 **A**, Dentin bonding agent 4-META penetrates tubules and bonds to collagen. The dentin is partially decalcified to show deep tubular penetration. Adhesive and collagen merge at the surface to form a "hybrid" layer. **B**, After composite resin (R) was bonded to dentin, the section was decalcified in acid, demonstrating acid-resistant hybrid layer (H). Decalcified dentin (DD) shows characteristic resin tags. Reproduced with permission from Nakabayashi N. Adhesive dental materials. Trans. Internat. Cong. on Dent. Mater., Acad., Dent. Mater., November 1989, p. 70.

and its dentin (as well as enamel, cementum, metal, ceramic, and resin) bonding capabilities might well be the preventive panacea to future pulp survival.

Tubule Blockage Agents. In Australia, Al-Fawaz and his researchers showed the transport of two components of a composite resin, HEMA and Bis-GMA, through the tubules of acid-etched dentin into the pulp during the crown cementation.[246] If toxic enough to "sting" a stressed pulp, either of these chemicals could start an inflammatory reaction that might not resolve. One way to ensure pulp protection from potentially toxic products is to block the dentinal tubules. This can be neatly accomplished by using oxalates on the dentin surface. Remember the "gritty" feeling in your mouth when you eat spinach or rhubarb? This is the same process—the oxalates precipitate calcium from the saliva in the one case or from the dentinal fluid in the other.

Pashley tested 3% half-neutralized oxalic acid plus 30% dipotassium oxalate for efficacy in plugging the tubules and blocking dentin permeability.[227] The insoluble calcium oxalate crystals that formed in the tubules led to a 98.25% reduction in dentin permeability, "lower than any other liner previously tested (Figure 4-43)."[227] Later, Stanley et al. tested in monkeys the pulpal effects of applying ferric oxalate hexahydrate (6.8% aqueous solution, pH 0.84) in Class V cavities for 60 seconds, rinsed and air-dried.[247] This technique was previously developed by Bowen (the "father" of composite resins) and Cobb.[248] Stanley and Bowen[247] found that "so little pulpal pathology is in accord with the concept that the ferric oxalate and other solutions bring about an obturation of the dentinal tubules without releasing noxious components." After testing in humans, Bowen et al. concluded that "the experimental material is safe and effective."[249]

One problem emerged with ferric oxalates, however: in some teeth, a marginal stain developed. This led to a search for other oxalic compounds, and aluminum oxalate emerged as acceptable. Once again, the Bowen/Stanley group reported no displacement of the odontoblasts and only "slight" to "no" inflammatory response. They concluded that the aluminum oxalate material appeared "safe for human clinical trials."[250]

At the US National Bureau of Standards, both ferric oxalate and aluminum oxalate were tested for **microleakage** against two commercial bonding agents. After being thermocycled for 7 days, all four materials exhibited gingival microleakage, although the oxalates "had lower microleakage scores than the two commercial systems tested."[251]

If the dentin can be rendered totally impermeable, then the toxicity to the pulp of any product placed on the fresh dentin surface does not matter. The tubule blocking agent, of course, cannot interfere with dentin adhesion or be so toxic itself that it causes pulp inflammation. Leinfelder pointed out that sealing the dentin surface with an adhesive bonding agent that produces a

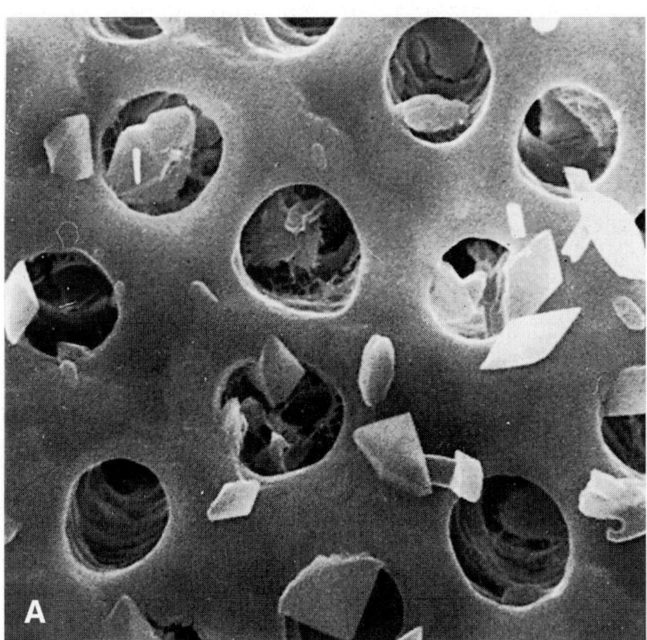

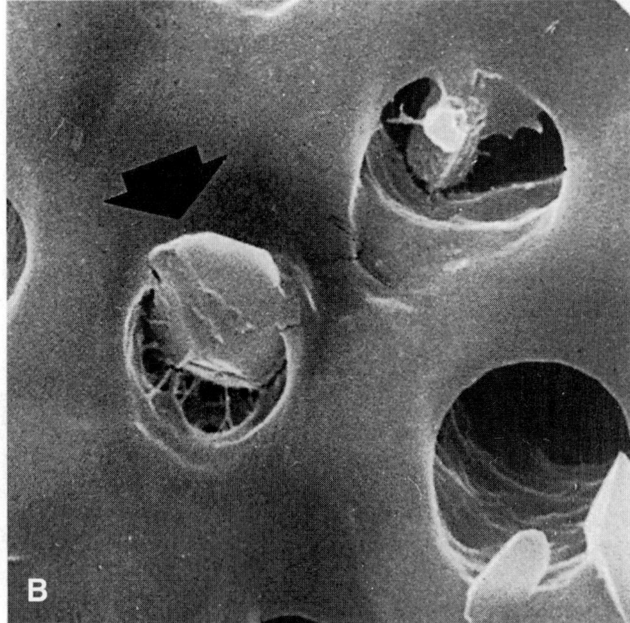

Figure 4-43 A, Dentin treated with 30% potassium oxalate reveals calcium oxalate crystals that closely match the size of tubule orifices. Note penetration of crystals into tubules. B, Higher magnification of A reveals strands of material connecting crystals to walls of tubules. Dentin permeability is reduced by 98.25%. Reproduced with permission from Greenhill JD, Pashley DH. J Dent Res 1981;60:686.

hybrid layer "effectively stops the fluid flow" and basically eliminates postoperative sensitivity.[252]

Disinfectants

The empiric habit of dentists attempting to sterilize prepared cavities before inserting a restoration is time honored. In spite of this, Black did not recommend that an antibacterial cavity agent be used, although his contemporaries were using caustic drugs.[253] Dorfman et al. and Stephan also questioned the value of the so-called "sterilization" of the cavity.[254,255] Many of the drugs were a poor choice.

Silver Nitrate and Phenol. Seltzer et al. found **silver nitrate** to be devastating to the pulps of monkey teeth when applied to shallow cavities.[5] They also described pulps in a "severely disturbed condition" months following the application of phenol to a deep cavity. As late as 6 months following the application of these drugs, recovery was questionable. Obviously, these older drugs were far too toxic to be used for so-called "cavity sterilization."

In more modern times, Brännström et al. strongly emphasized the importance of cleansing the prepared cavity. They pointed out that "bacteria can survive in grinding debris which forms a smear layer 2 to 5 microns thick that adheres to the prepared surfaces and cannot be removed by a water spray." They claimed that this **layer of bacteria** "appears to be the main cause of injury to the pulp observed under restorative materials..."[149]

Brännström and Nyborg recommended that a microbicidal, surface-active cavity cleanser, **Tubulicid** (red label; Tublicid Red [chlorhexidine digluconate dodecyldiaminoethyl-glycerine and sodium fluoride], Dental Therapeutics AB, Sweden) be scrubbed in the cavity with a cotton pellet and then left for 1 minute before removing it and air-drying the cavity for 5 seconds.[148] Surfaces treated in this manner have most of the **smear layer removed** without opening the outer orifices of the dentin tubuli plugged with microcrystalline smear. Removing the bacteria-laden smear layer with 10% polyacrylic acid (for 10 seconds) or 10% citric acid (for 10 seconds) is another very acceptable method.

Sodium Fluoride. The irritating effects on the dental pulp of sodium fluoride were noted early on by Lefkowitz and Bodecker[256] and by Rovelstad and St. John[257] but denied by Maurice and Schour.[258] Later, Furseth and Mjör applied 2% sodium fluoride for 2 minutes in freshly prepared dentin cavities in young human teeth and found virtually no adverse pulp reaction.[259]

The use of the fluorides as a desensitizing agent on the **external** tooth surface is probably well within reason, even when precipitated by electrolytic action. Walton and his associates applied sodium fluoride by iontophoresis to exposed dentin on **root surfaces** of young, permanent dog teeth.[260] Two levels of current were used: therapeutic levels and five times therapeutic levels. They found that "There were no demonstrable histologic or ultrastructure alterations of the underlying pulp..."

In spite of this "surface" evidence, it is questionable whether sodium fluoride should be precipitated by electrolysis on freshly cut dentin. By measuring beta-ray emissions from preparations from teeth subjected to electrolytic action of radioactive sodium chloride, Briscoe et al. demonstrated that the halogen was driven completely to the pulp.[261]

Desiccants

Alcohol, Ether, and Others. Time-honored desiccants, such as acetone, ethyl alcohol, ether, and chloroform, are probably not damaging to the pulp by their chemical action but rather by upsetting the physiologic equilibrium of the dental interstitial **fluid.** Use of the desiccants is also invariably followed by a blast of air. The irritation from dehydration must be indicted as well.

Products such as Cavidry (Parkell Co.; Farmingdale, N.Y.) or Cavilax (Premier Dental; King of Prussia, Pa.) may be used for "the rapid drying, cleaning or degreasing of intracoronal or extracoronal tooth preparations."[262] The active ingredients are methylethylketone and ethyl acetate. These products are especially useful in removing the light film of oil and moisture left by the air rotor handpiece. Cavidry evaporates in seconds without a blast of air. It should not be used in close proximity to the pulp, however.

IDIOPATHIC CAUSES

Aging

Inevitable retrogressive aging changes take place in the pulp as in all other body tissues. The decreased numbers and size of cells and increase in collagen fiber content have long been noted as an age change.[263] The constant recession of the normal pulp and its production of secondary and irritational dentin are as certain as death and taxes.

Seltzer et al. pointed out that atrophy of the pulp normally occurs with advancing age.[63] They described these dystrophic changes as the "burned out" appearance of an "exhaustion atrophy." This aged pulp seems less likely to resist insult than the young, "virile" pulp, although there is a paucity of published evidence to prove this.

Internal Resorption

Although internal resorption may occur in chronic pulpal inflammation, it also occurs as an idiopathic dystrophic change. Trauma in the form of an accidental blow, or **traumatic cavity preparation**, has often been indicted as a triggering mechanism for internal resorption. In this event, the metaplastic area of the pulp might develop from a localized hemorrhage. Dentin destruction follows (Figure 4-44).

An outstanding report from the Karolinska Institute in Sweden dealt with 13 teeth extracted because of internal resorption.[264] The researchers found that internal resorption progresses more rapidly in deciduous teeth. In addition, they were surprised to learn that 11 of the 13 teeth exhibited **caries** as the resorption triggering mechanism, and that only 2 of the teeth had been traumatized.

"Active internal resorption was found in all teeth. It was characterized by large multinucleated dentinoclasts in resorption lacunae on the pulpal dentin sur-

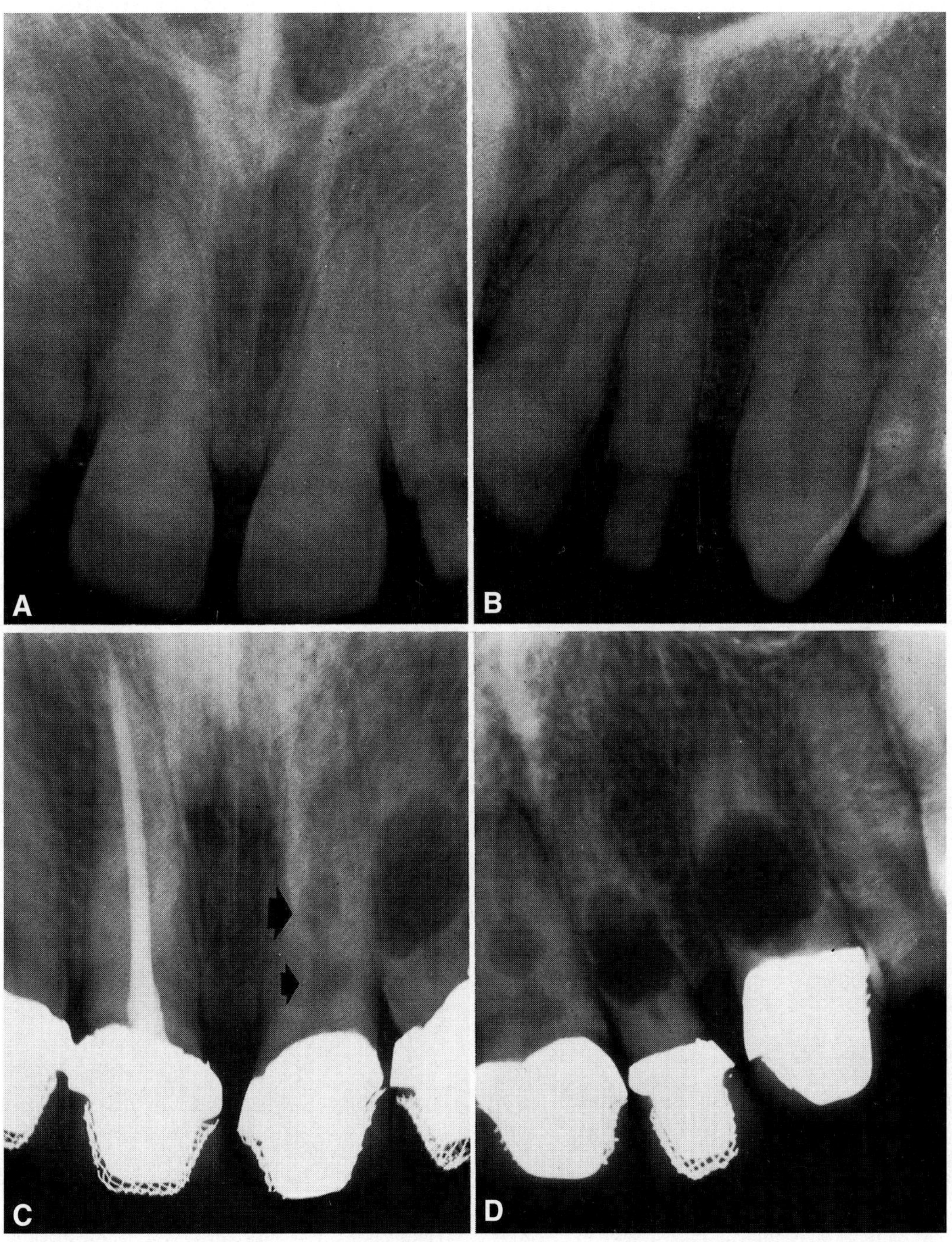

Figure 4-44 Extensive internal resorption apparently triggered by iatral causes. Normal condition of teeth prior to crown preparation is seen in "before" radiographs (**A** and **B**). Development of internal resorption from high-speed preparation without water coolant is seen 1 year later (**C** and **D**). (Courtesy of Dr. Dudley H. Glick.)

face" (Figure 4-45). The "nuclear domains" of these peculiar dentinoclasts were covered with numerous microvilli. Microscopically, these cells were similar to the cementoclasts observed in external root resorption (Figure 4-46).

In all teeth, there were varying degrees of inflammation, and in all but two teeth, bacteria could be detected where the coronal pulp tissue was necrotic. "Odontoblasts could not be observed in any of the teeth and predentin was rarely seen...The tissue that had replaced the normal pulp resembled periodontal membrane connective tissue...Mineralized tissue resembling bone or cellular cementum partly outlined the pulp cavity in all teeth."[264]

Based on the histochemical similarity, the Swedish researchers surmised that "internal resorption is engineered by clastic cells similar or identical to osteoclasts." They also concluded that the "tissue in the pulp cavities differed markedly from normal pulp tissue and appeared to have been replaced by ingrowing periodontal connective tissue or had undergone metaplasia of such tissue. The process appeared to alternate between resorption of dentin and apposition of mineralized tissue."[264]

Brooks reported an unusual case of internal resorption in the crown of an **unerupted** lower second premolar in an 11-year-old boy.[265]

External Resorption

One cannot say that external root resorption is a pulp dystrophy for its origin lies within the tissue of the periodontal membrane space. Common to all forms of tooth resorption is the removal of the mineralized and organic components of dental tissues by clastic cells. In the case of external root resorption, this may be a **transitory** response as in **surface resorption**[266] that may occur following trauma or orthodontic tooth movement.

All other forms of external root resorption are **progressive** and may have important implications from a pulpal viewpoint. **Inflammatory (infective) root resorption**[266] usually results from luxation or exarticulation injury and is caused by the transmission of bacterial toxins from a devitalized and infected pulp via dentinal tubules to an external root surface that has previously been partly denuded of the normally protective cementum-cementoid layer by surface resorption. Clastic cells are stimulated to the region by inflammatory mediators such as prostaglandins and cytokines, which are libertated as part of the inflammatory process.

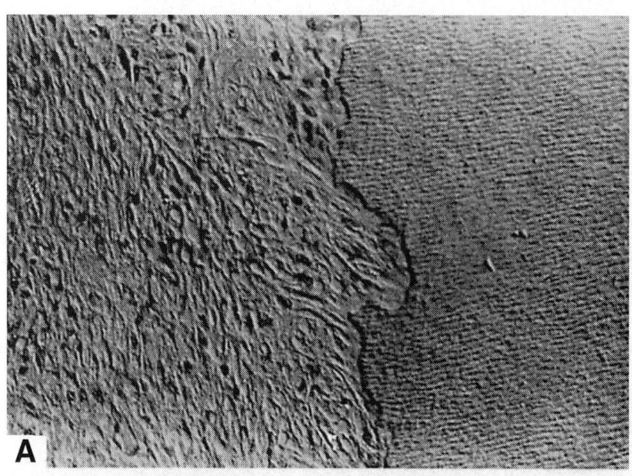

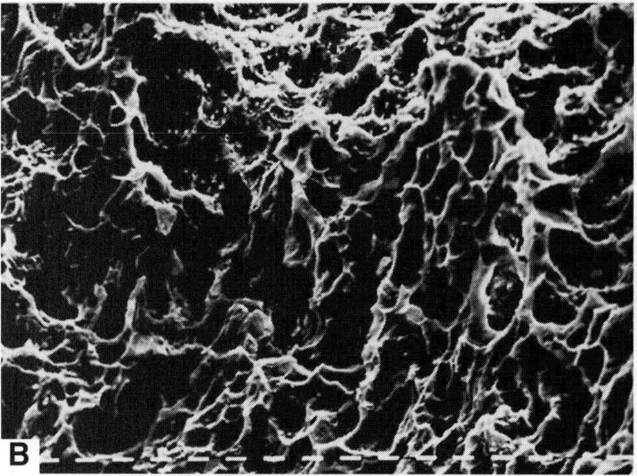

Figure 4-45 A, Internal resorption lacunae caused by dentinoclasts. B, Scanning electron micrograph of rough and uneven dentin surface with numerous resorption lacunae. Reproduced with permission from Wedenberg C. JOE 1987;13:255.

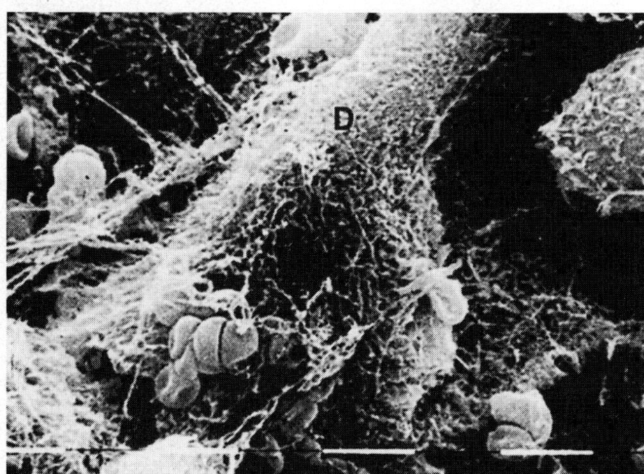

Figure 4-46 Dentinoclast (D) on dentin surface. The cell surface is covered with numerous microvilli. Cells also present: macrophage and erythrocytes. Reproduced with permission from Wedenberg C and Zettesqvist L.[264]

A diagnosis of **inflammatory root resorption**, which is characterized radiographically by bowl-like radiolucencies in both the tooth and the adjacent bone, is also diagnostic of an infected and probably totally necrotic pulp. Early root-canal débridement and medication with calcium hydroxide paste is recommended. Prophylactic pulpectomy is also recommended in cases of trauma for which there is a high expectation of pulp death, such as a replanted or intrusively luxated tooth with a mature apex. Intracanal medication with calcium hydroxide paste will generally control potential resorption.

Replacement resorption[266] occurs when there has been death of the periodontal ligament cells. Clastic cells, derived from the adjacent bone, cause a progressive replacement of dentin by bone. Inflammatory (infective) resorption may be superimposed on replacement resorption. Ultimately, the tooth is replaced by bone as it is progressively resorbed.

In the case of extracanal invasive resorption,[267] also termed **invasive cervical resorption** by Heithersay,[268] the pulp remains unaffected until late in the process owing to an apparently thin and resorption-resistant layer of dentin and predentin. This separates the pulp from the ingrowing tissue that is initially fibrovascular in character but becomes a fibro-osseous type of tissue. If exposed to the oral cavity, the pulp will be invaded by microorganisms. Although pulp vitality can be maintained if there is early diagnosis and treatment of this type of resorption, more extensive lesions require nonsurgical root canal therapy and resorption treatment if the tooth is to be retained.

When external resorption destroys enough dentin to reach the pulp, pulp inflammatory changes begin. The same infection problem also develops when internal resorption destroys enough tooth structure to reach the sulcus. Continued resorption takes place until the pulp either is removed or becomes necrotic.

Researchers at Kings College in London reported a case of multiple idiopathic external resorption involving 14 teeth.[269] Although electric pulp testing gave a vital response in all affected teeth, radiographs showed extensive apical root resorption in both arches (Figure 4-47). The teeth were symptomless and nonmobile. Although the patient was a morphine and heroin addict and had had hepatitis A, he did not have hypoparathyroidism or pseudohypoparathyroidism, diseases that lead to root resorption.

Hereditary Hypophosphatemia

An unusual and rare cause of pulpal dystrophy occurs in individuals afflicted with hereditary hypophosphatemia. This disease, which results in dwarfism and "tackle" deformity, was formerly called refractory rickets or vitamin D–resistant rickets. It is characterized dentally by the huge pulps (Figure 4-48) and incomplete calcification of the dentin. The pulps in the teeth of these dwarfs appear to be fragile and succumb to

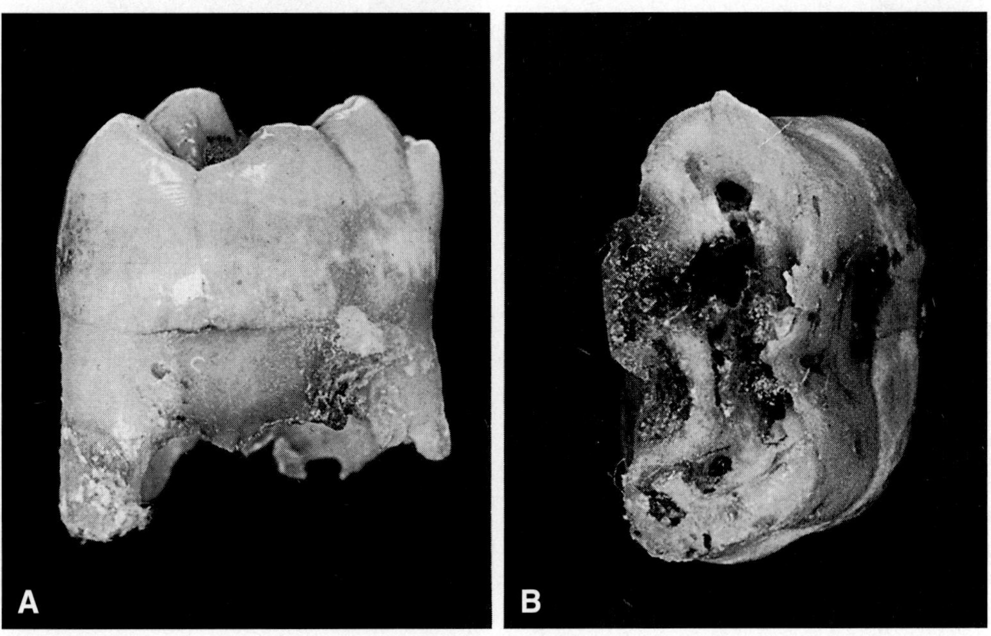

Figure 4-47 Idiopathic external root resorption leading to pulpal involvement in maxillary second molar, 1 of 14 teeth so affected. Reproduced with permission from Pankhurst CL et al.[269]

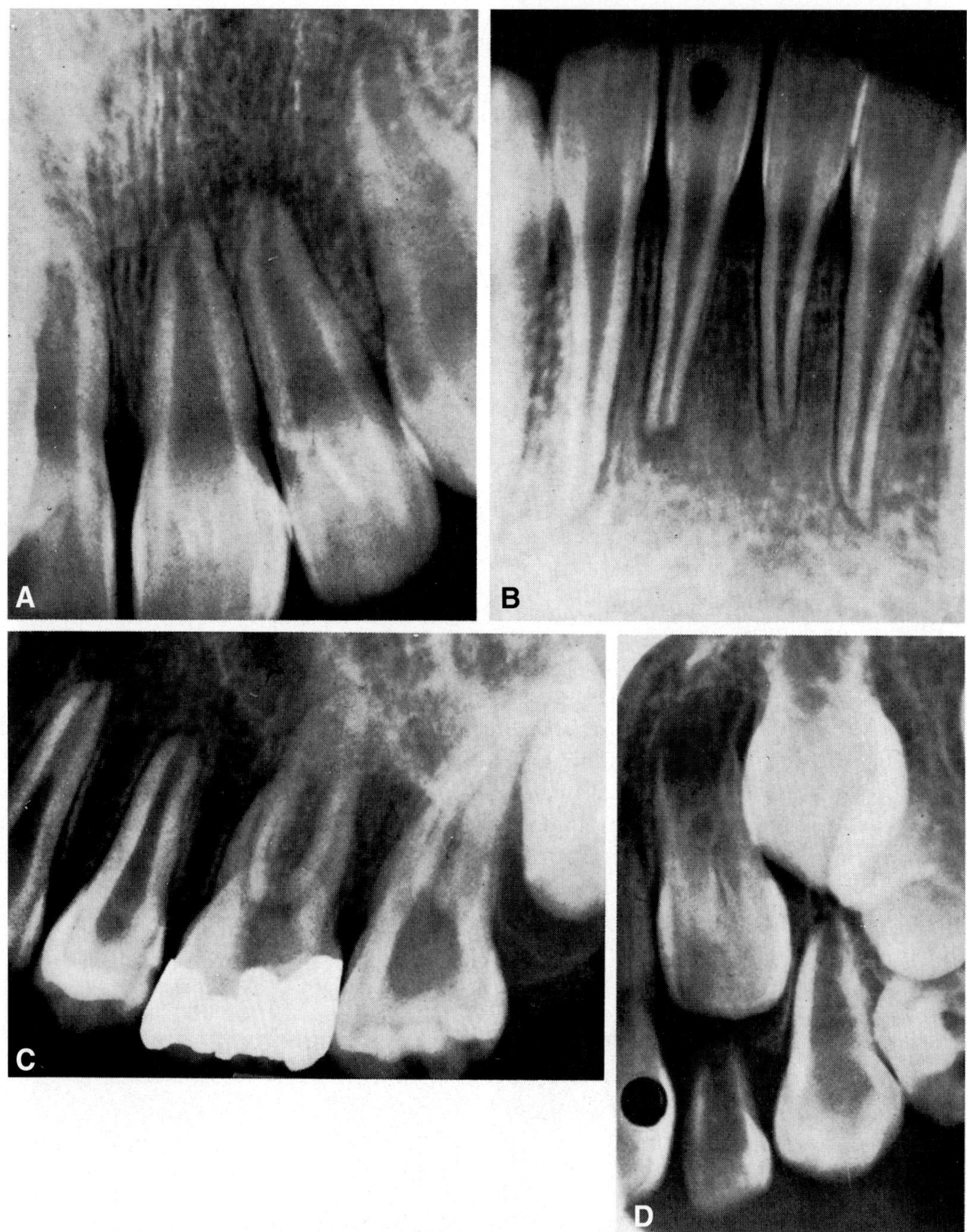

Figure 4-48 Unusual pulp dystrophy seen with hereditary hypophosphatemia. Incomplete calcification of dentin and huge pulps leave these teeth vulnerable to pulp infection and necrosis. **A**, Adult maxillary incisors at age 13. Note huge pulp. **B**, Mandibular incisors have been traumatized and pulp necrosis has developed. **C**, Huge pulps seen in premolar and molar teeth. Pulp of the first molar later became necrotic. **D**, Same pulp size and shape are apparent in deciduous dentition. Diagnosis of condition could have been made at this stage from dental radiographs. Early vitamin D therapy might have prevented dwarfing.

what would normally be minor irritating stimuli. In one case, the patient had 11 pulpless teeth that required endodontic treatment.

A report from Montreal pointed out that two different diseases are operative in producing this syndrome, namely autosomal dominant hypophosphatemic bone disease (HBD) and X-linked hypophosphatemia (XLH).[270] Although victims of HBD and XLH share similar dental abnormalities (large pulp spaces and pulp necrosis), patients with XLH have severe malocclusions as well. Unfortunately, the dental abnormalities are not prevented by early systemic treatment.[270]

From Holland, a study of 22 family members, blood related to a young woman exhibiting the characteristic signs and symptoms of hypophosphatemia, revealed several others who also had dental abnormalities. Of these, however, only one sister fulfilled the biochemical criteria for the disease.[271] Biochemical examination of an extracted tooth from this sister showed phosphate and alkaline phosphatase values that were **7 to 10 times lower** than normal.[271]

Sickle Cell Anemia

Sickle cell anemia, "a genetic disorder characterized by an abnormal hemoglobin molecule which distorts the erythrocyte into sickle-shaped cells," has been indicted as a cause of pulp death.[272] Three cases exhibiting periradicular radiolucent areas have been reported. One patient had five noncarious, nontraumatized teeth involved. The sickle cells are suspected of compromising the microcirculation of the pulp.

Herpes Zoster Infection

Goon and Jacobsen have reported a case of multiple pulp deaths caused by herpes zoster infection of the trigeminal nerve.[273] Immediately after suffering fifth nerve "shingles," the patient developed a "postzoster infection complex, that is, prodromal odontalgia, pulpless teeth, neuralgic and facial scarring." The causative agent is varicella-zoster virus residing in the ganglion cells sometime after a primary varicella (chickenpox) infection. Because the pulp contains terminal nerve endings, it is speculated that the reactivated virus travels the length of the nerve and infects the pulp vasculature, leading to infarction and pulp death. Gregory et al. also reported such a case,[274] as did Lopes and his associates in San Paulo, Brazil[275] (Figure 4-49).

Human Immunodeficiency Virus and Acquired Immune Deficiency Syndrome

"Dental pulp tissue from a patient with acquired immune deficiency syndrome (AIDS) was examined to determine the presence of human immunodeficiency virus (HIV). The results found a high concentration of proviral HIV DNA."[276] "Fibroblasts have been implicated as a major reservoir for HIV in the body."[277] Glick et al. suggested that other viruses, such as hepatitis B, may also reside in the pulp.[276]

THE FUTURE

Pulp death seems to be on the increase, or perhaps only an apparent increase owing to an awareness of the value of the treated pulpless tooth. With routine examination and early treatment, with a cautious, temperate approach to all restorative procedures, and with a sensible use of filling materials, the dentist can **prevent** a great deal of pulp death.

Prevention of Pulp Injury

In 1969, the American Dental Association (ADA) reported that American dentists extracted 56 million teeth, placed 213 million fillings, made 4 million bridges and 10 million complete and partial dentures, and completed 9 million root canal fillings. All of these 292 million cases of dental therapy (only a fraction of the dentistry being done today) had a direct relation to the dental pulp and testify either to its insult and injury or its disease or loss.[278]

That some of this injury might have been prevented seems apparent. Caries alone probably accounted for most of this dental treatment. Impact trauma undoubtedly accounted for a large proportion as well. That virtually unspoken third cause, "dentistogenic" (iatro-

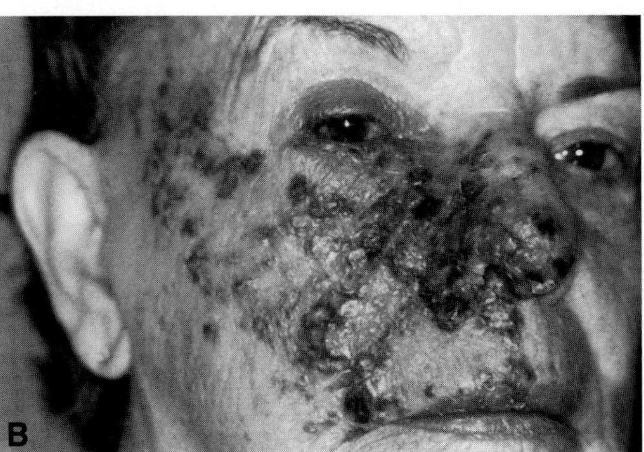

Figure 4-49 Herpes zoster (shingles) of the maxillary branch of the trigeminal nerve. **A**, Multiple vesicles on the face and involving the right eye 4 days after initial visit. **B**, Ten days after diagnosis. Lesions follow distribution of the fifth nerve. The patient recovered in 1 month. Reproduced with permission from Lopes MA, et al.[275]

genic), accounted for an embarrassingly high percentage of the pulp injury and death reflected in the ADA report. The University of Connecticut reported, for example, that "previous restorative treatment was the major etiologic factor leading to root canal therapy."[279]

There are many day-to-day insults levied against the pulp that can be **prevented:** (1) depth of cavity and crown preparation, (2) width and extension of cavity and crown preparation, (3) heat damage and desiccation during cavity preparation, (4) chemical injury through medicaments, (5) toxic cavity liners and bases, (6) toxic filling materials, and (7) **prevention of microleakage.**

Depth and Width of Cavity Preparation. Extreme pulp trauma results when the pulp is closely approached or the dentin is extensively removed. Overcutting cavity preparations, whether or not the pulp is exposed, are undoubtedly one of the greatest insults to the pulp. It should be quite obvious that full-crown preparations damage every single coronal odontoblast. Before one cavalierly decides on full coverage for a tooth, if a less extensive restoration will do, the latter should be a standard preventive consideration. When elective, shallow preparations are always the wiser choice over deep preparations. The integrity of the pulp is affected as rotary instruments approach the predentin, not just because of the immediate pulp damage but also because of the proximity of toxic filling materials. Udolph et al., for example, found that composite filling materials would not irritate the pulp if 2 mm of dentin remained between the pulp and the filling.[280] Although it is generally true that the risk of pulp damage diminishes with increasing distance,[281] there is no sacred distance beyond which no damage occurs. The surface width of the cavity may be as important as the depth. In fact, a cut into the dentin exposes the pulp to a variety of exogenous irritants.

Heat Damage and Desiccation during Cavity Preparation. The damage that results when high-speed rotary instruments are used, without an adequate water coolant, has been well documented by Takahashi, who induced acute pulpal inflammation by cavity preparation **without water spray**, using a high-speed carbide bur at 400,000 rpm.[282]

Goodacre summarized it best when he stated that "[T]o minimize the thermal effects, tooth preparations should be performed using an ultra highspeed handpiece (250,000–400,000 rpm) with an air-water spray from multidirectional water ports. Water flow rate should be at 50 ml/minute and the water should be regulated to be below body temperature (ideally 30–34°C). Deeper parts of the tooth preparation should be excavated using a slower speed handpiece (160,000 rpm or less) and new carbide burs. **Aggressive** tooth preparation should be accompanied by **supplemental water spray** from a syringe with a constant focus on the rotary instrument.[91] Coarse diamonds may be used with air-water spray for gross reduction. Fine diamond instruments or carbide burs are recommended for final smoothing of the tooth preparation.[92] To aid visibility, smoothing of finish lines and fine detail may be done with **only air** as a coolant. All tooth preparation should be accomplished using **intermittent 10 to 15-second contact** with the tooth."[91]

Also damaging is the custom of preparing cavities under a constant blast of air directed by an assistant. Here again, the desiccation of the dentin (and eventually the pulp) is most damaging. Odontoblastic nuclei and even erythrocytes can be seen microscopically, virtually "sucked up" into the desiccated tubules. Add to this damage the toxic effects of medicaments, liners or bases, and filling material to give the pulp the *coup de grâce.*

Chemical Injury through Medicaments Applied to the Dentin. One could say that pulp injury from chemical irritants can best be prevented by **not** applying chemicals to the dentin. This prohibition refers to silver nitrate, phenol, alcohol, ether, acetone, thymol, fluoride, and cyanoacrylate, to name a few irritants. Corticosteroids may be the exception to the rule. Van Hassel and McHugh reported that the "ability of prednisolone to suppress inflammatory vascular changes can prevent pressure-induced venous collapse beneath deep cavity preparations."[283] On the other hand, one should not place false hope on cortisone to suppress all inflammation. It has been shown that inflammation will continue in the pulp despite the application of corticosteroids, alone or in combination with other medicaments,[30] if pulp inflammation has "passed that point of no return." Cortisone reduces pain, but this may lull the dentist and patient into a false sense of security.

Cavity Liners and Bases. The very products made to protect the pulp might well be the toxins that bring about its demise. Spångberg and colleagues have shown that the commonly used cavity liners may be more cytotoxic in vitro against HeLa cells than the composite filling materials they are to protect against.[284] "It is reasonable to believe," they said, "that the early irritation is caused by the solvent of the liner," which might soon dissipate by evaporation.

Cavity liners have another disadvantage as well. As they cure against the dentin surface, "pinholes" develop that lead directly to the open tubules. Attempts at building up layers of the liner by multiple applications will not solve the pinhole problem. The toxic chemical in the restorative material leaks directly through to the tubules to irritate the pulp (see Figure 4-41). Spångberg summarized it simply: "For pulp protection, a base is necessary."[284]

In view of the fact that some cavity liners have been shown to be ineffective as well as toxic, it follows that their use cannot be recommended routinely as a preventive measure. Cement bases, on the other hand, can serve to prevent the toxic and/or thermal damage that may be generated by filling materials. The most common bases are oxyphosphate of zinc cement, polycarboxylate cement, and ZOE. All three have been shown to be irritants to the pulp, especially ZOE, but the two other cements may prevent greater damage from other more toxic fillings.

Placing a cement base may lull one into a false sense of security. The usual thought is protecting the pulp **floor** of a cavity, but it is easy to forget that if the smear layer is removed, all open dentinal tubules, even those on the walls, are connected to the pulp and may serve as toxic conduits. Pulp floor cement bases were developed for thermal protection but serve today as only partial protection against noxious chemical fillings. If in doubt, cover all of the dentin. Baume and Fiore-Donno suggested that in very deep preparations, a base containing calcium hydroxide best protects beneath composite resin restorations.[285] Aqueous or methylcellulose calcium hydroxide bases, however, do not adapt well after curing, even if applied sufficiently thick to be immediately impenetrable. Through microleakage, irritants may then work around the calcium hydroxide bases to reach the open tubules.[286] Light-cured, resin-based calcium hydroxide cement/liners are preferable and highly recommended.

Cement bases have one other bonus: they block open tubules from bacteria and their noxious by-products. Dickey and colleagues found severe pulp **necrosis** under a composite restorative material only when a bacterial plaque had formed on the cavity floors.[172] Bacterial entree was gained from marginal microleakage or cavity contamination prior to filling. The noxious role of bacterial plaque under restorations was confirmed by Brännström and Nyborg.[287] Spångberg and colleagues recommended a base for pulp protection from microleakage.[170] Unfortunately, bases of polycarboxylate cement, which is touted as being adhesive, actually allow bacterial plaque to form on the cavity floor under composite materials. More recently, dentin bonding agents have been found to reduce or eliminate this problem.

Filling Materials. What more can be said about the noxious role toxic filling materials might play in pulp inflammation? One cannot avoid them as a preventive measure for they have no substitutes for esthetic anterior restorations. One can only say, "Use a proper protective base or liner, one that covers all of the exposed dentin surface in the cavity." Care must also be taken in drying the dentin even before placement of the base. If desiccation precedes the introduction of any cement base, the irritant components of the base will replace the tissue fluid in the tubules, and the pulp reactions will be more severe than if care is taken during surface drying.

Biocompatibility and Postoperative Sensitivity. Under this title, the Council on Dental Materials, Instruments, and Equipment of the ADA issued an important report in 1988.[288] It deals with the perplexing problem that has been detailed in the preceding sections of this chapter. "Although there are data to indicate that these materials are biocompatible, there are also reported cases of postoperative sensitivity when restorations involve the use of composite resins, dentin bonding agents and glass ionomer cements." This report enlarged on and updated the Council report of 1984.[289]

As before, the report blamed **microleakage, bacterial invasion**, and hydraulic pressure for pulp discomfort. Added in 1988 was "pain caused by shrinkage stresses" during curing of resins. Dentin permeability might also be included as a culprit.

Microleakage and Bacterial Invasion. New studies on these associated problems are emerging. As previously stated, initial leakage under amalgams is extensive, but with time, a marginal seal is effected, "presumably due to the formation of corrosion products" under the amalgam.[155]

The effect on microleakage under amalgams by removing the smear layer has also been treated.[287] Researchers in South Africa found that "cavities without smear layers displayed significantly improved sealing properties." They contend that the "smear layer is unstable and leaches out."[290]

An English group studied microleakage under a range of filling materials—silicate, zinc phosphate, methylmethacrylate, glass ionomer, and ZOE—and found no bacteria under 77% of the cavities filled in humans.[291] In the remaining 23%, "the correlation between the amount of inflammation and bacterial microleakage for all materials was statistically significant." While blaming microleakage and bacteria for pulpal inflammation, they further contended "that chemical toxicity from the materials themselves is only of minor importance."[291]

Marginal Fit. Finally, one would be safe in saying that the integrity of marginal fit of the restoration, be it a crown, temporary crown,[169] inlay, or amalgam, is most essential in preventing leakage. This applies to composite resins as well, bonding to the cavity margin. The Achilles' heel of composite is its failure to bond to cementum.

A well-done study at the Medical College of Georgia compared for leakage Class V restorations placed entirely within root surfaces. The specimens were thermocycled in dye, thousands of times, between 5°C and 55°C.[292] Although leakage into the cementum margins was noted in all specimens, microleakage through to the dentin was worse around amalgams and glass ionomer cements. Surprisingly, the least leakage occurred around a light-cured composite resin (Aurafill, Johnson & Johnson; New Brunswick, N.J.) placed without a dentin-bonding agent.[292]

Smear Layer. Inside the cavity, the smear layer is "good news and bad news" or "damned if you do or damned if you don't." If the smear layer remains, it protects the pulp by plugging the tubules, preventing ingress of bacteria and their toxins as well as chemical toxins (Figure 4-50). On the other hand, if it is removed, it allows absolute adaptation of the restoration to the true dentin surface, essential in the case of resins and important in the case of amalgams. **Microleakage is increased if the smear layer remains, whereas dentin permeability is increased if the smear layer is removed.** Jodaikin and Austin recommended the removal of the smear layer under amalgams as early as 1981.[290]

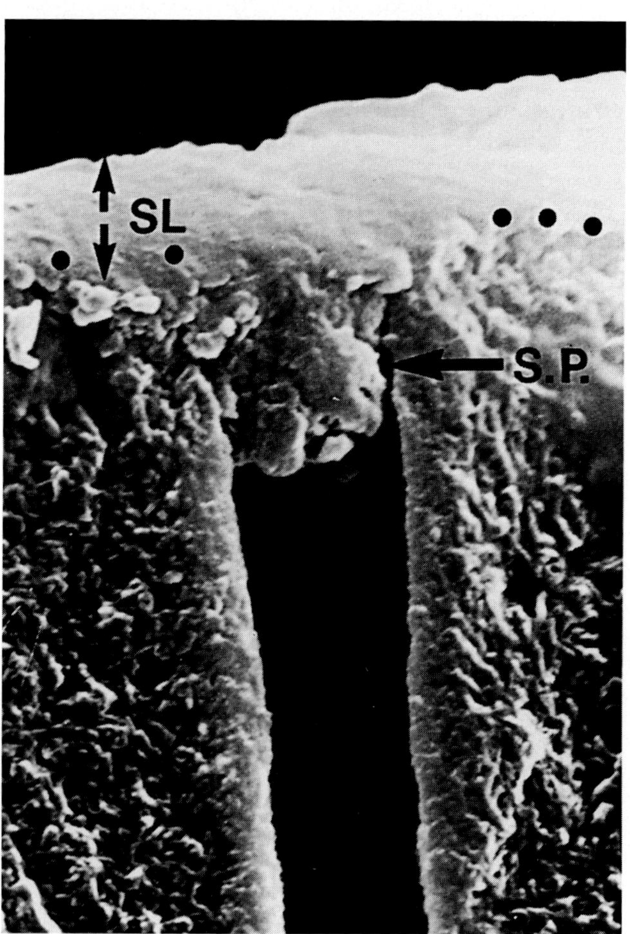

Figure 4-50 Longitudinal section of dentinal tubule containing a smear plug (S.P.) emerging from the smear layer (SL). Reproduced with permission from Pashley DH.[233]

How can one have it both ways: improved filling adaptation yet guaranteed pulp health? The answer seems to lie in agents that clean the dentin surface yet leave the tubules still plugged or, better yet, completely clean the dentin and the tubuli orifices and then "replug" the tubules with a precipitate or a bonding agent.

Duke and colleagues at Indiana stated that polyacrylic acid gave the best result in removing the smear layer.[293]

The Laboratory of the Government Chemist, Department of Industry in England (where glass ionomer cements were developed) recommended the use of surface conditioners of "high molecular weight."[294] They achieved their highest bond strengths with either polyacrylic acid, tannic acid (tanning agent for collagen), or a surface active microbicidal solution from Sweden, Tublicid (AB Bofors Nobelknut, Sweden), which contains EDTA, chlorhexidine gluconate, and a wetting agent. All are biocompatible. Citric acid, EDTA, and ferric chloride, were found to be much less effective.

Pashley and the English researchers[227,291] agree that if the tubules are opened, they must be reoccluded. This is accomplished by the new oxalates or, in the case of amalgam placement, castings, or jacket cementation, by one of the new liners such as Barrier or one of the new dentin adhesives such as 4-META.

Washout. If type 1 (luting agent) glass ionomer cements or type 2 (restorative material) ionomers are used, it is imperative that these cements do not wash out, particularly "when the gingival wall of the restoration is placed below the cementoenamel junction."[295] The Product Evaluation Laboratory of the University of California, San Francisco, thermocycled a number of these restorations with either polymer-type bonding agents or glass ionomer cements beneath composite fillings.[295] They were particularly careful to avoid hydration or dehydration of the glass ionomers. Dye penetration studies after severe thermocycling proved Gingivaseal (Parkell Co.; Farmingdale, N.Y.) to be the **most effective** glass ionomer as far as insolubility was concerned. The **least soluble** polymer liner was Urename (Cadeo, USA).

The Bullard group at Alabama found that an exact correlation exists between microleakage and the coefficient of thermal expansion of a filling material.[296] Arranged in order from the **least leakage** and the **lowest coefficient** of thermal expansion to the highest for each, they are (1) glass ionomer cement, (2) amalgam, (3) ZOE cement, (4) posterior composite resin, (5) microfilled composite resin, and (6) unfilled acrylic resin. The teeth were alternately cycled 125 times between baths of fuschin dye, one bath at 5°C and the other at 55°C. No acid-etching or bonding agent was used under any of the materials.

The Dental Advisor also tested glass ionomer cements for bond strength to dentin.[297] That group found Cement/Liner (Parkell Co.; Farmingdale, N.Y.) to be the highest, with a bond strength of 50.3 kg/cm^2.

All of the cement manufacturers emphasize the importance of protecting the glass ionomer cements from moisture, humidity, or even dry air while they are setting. Immediately after placement, they should be coated with a cavity liner material, particularly at the gingiva margin, where crevicular fluid may contaminate. Within the cavity, the liner is peeled off after the cement sets but before etching.

Hydraulic Pressure. The immediate sensitivity after cementation with glass ionomer luting agents may be attributed to its anhydrous nature. If the tubules are sealed, however, this should not happen unless unusual hydraulic pressure is exerted during cementation that breaks through the tubuli "plugs." Die spacing and/or internal relief of crowns before cementation could prevent this undue pressure. This can even be improved by placing an "internal escape channel," which also improves the gingival fit.[298]

The importance of hydrostatic pressure during crown cementation was dramatically demonstrated at Ohio State University,[299] when crowns were cemented by direct static pressure (biting down on an orangewood stick) and the crowns failed to seat fully by 203 microns. When **dynamic** pressure was applied, however, by **rocking the orangewood stick both vertically and horizontally**, the gingival space between tooth and crown was narrowed to an unbelievable **minus 14 microns.** By this simple procedure of dynamic seating, an unacceptable marginal discrepancy was dramatically reduced to a wholly acceptable one, 14 microns **beyond** the try-in position of the crown (Figure 4-51). This alone would significantly reduce gingival microleakage.[300]

Remaining Dentin Thickness. Finally, it goes without saying that proximity to the pulp and the remaining dentin thickness are probably the most crucial factors in this confusing equation. Microleakage, bacterial irritation or invasion, chemical toxicity, and even hydraulic pressure are all moot if an adequate thickness of dentin is left to protect the pulp. If the remaining dentin is thin, the pulp must be protected. If not protected, hypersensitivity or even inflammation leading to necrosis will develop.

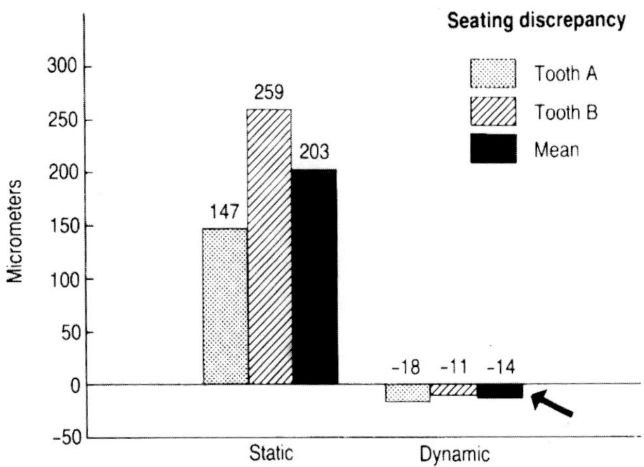

Figure 4-51 Comparison of static and dynamic cementation seating of complete cast crowns. The enormous mean discrepancy between +203 microns (static) and −14 microns (**arrow**) (dynamic) is highly significant statistically. Reproduced with permission from Rosenstiel SF and Gegauff AG.[299]

Shrinkage Stresses. The problem with composite resins is that they shrink. As they polymerize, they contract. This means that they pull away from margins, **leaving** marginal gaps, or their contraction may cause cusp flexure, leading to hypersensitivity or even fracture.[300] Using replacement of an MOD amalgam with esthetic composite resin in a maxillary premolar as an example, if the entire cavity is filled with composite resin and the material extends over onto the etched and chamfered enamel surfaces, as it should, the resin will shrink as it polymerizes under light activation. This contraction pulls the buccal and lingual walls toward each other (cuspal flexion), causing pain.[301] The dentinal fluid in the tubules will be disturbed, particularly when biting stresses tend to force the cusps outward. This pumping action is suspected as another source of pain.

To prevent the problem of polymerization shrinkage, the composite must be placed and cured in small increments. Each application of a new layer fills in the shrinkage gap from the previous layer. If the dentin has been covered with glass ionomer cement or a dental adhesive that bonds to the dentin, the layers of composite will then bond to the adhesive or the etched ionomer and then to each other (the "sandwich" technique). The result will be a monolithic restoration, the filling materials becoming a part of the tooth, not merely "sitting" in the tooth as an amalgam or an inlay will do.

If all of these protective measures are taken—in lining, basing, and incremental filling—there should be no cause for pulpal sensitivity or death.

Bertolotti also addressed the sensitivity problems that develop following crown or inlay cementation.[301] He pointed out that nearly all cases are in molars and that it seemingly makes no difference what the luting agent might be—resin cements, zinc phosphate, glass ionomer—the results are the same. Sensitivity dissipates in about 6 months.

Caries Control. By not exposing the pulp, the dentist can avoid inflicting iatral injury. Even in the face of deep caries, the dentin cover should be maintained if bacteria have not penetrated through to the pulp. Fauchard, in 1746, probably said it best: "...exposing the nerve and making the cure worse than the disease."[302] Sir John Tomes, in 1859, voiced a similar concern: "[it is] better to allow some carious dentin to remain over the pulp rather than run the risk of sacrificing the tooth."

The modern version of these warnings by Fauchard and Tomes has developed a technique of caries control, often **mistermed** "indirect pulp capping," which means leaving carious dentin **permanently** under the filling. In the modern version, however, **carious dentin is not purposely left under a permanent restoration** but is left there only temporarily as the pulp is allowed to recover and protect itself with a layer of irritation dentin. To a great extent, the success of this procedure will depend on the genus of bacteria in the remaining dentin. If they are facultative anaerobes, continued breakdown may be the end result. On the other hand, if healing progresses, irritation dentin may be produced in amounts that may fill an entire pulp horn; remember, however, that irritation dentin is still penetrable by microorganisms and medicaments.[303]

The technique is carried out in the following manner: (1) the rubber dam is applied, and (2) the soft carious dentin is removed along the walls of the cavity and as far pulpally as possible without exerting pressure on the pulp roof. (For this, Caridex might be used.) (3) The cavity is washed with lukewarm water and is then carefully dried without desiccation. (4) A layer of **calcium hydroxide** is applied over the **entire dentin surface.** (5) A thick mix of ZOE cement (chemically pure) is then applied without pressure over the pulp floor. (The ZOE should be prepared by incorporating as much zinc oxide into the mix as possible and then removing excess eugenol with a squeeze cloth.) (6) A good protective provisional filling is then placed. (7) Three to six months later, if there has been no discomfort, pulp vitality should be determined, and, if vital, the provisional filling and the ZOE base are removed and the softened dentin carefully excavated. Fusayama pointed out that carious softened dentin has two layers: a top part of dead tissue and a softened bottom layer that is still alive and capable of remineralization. By repeated applications of a red stain (**Caries Detector**, Kuraray, Japan), the "dead tissue" dentin is stained and carefully removed, leaving the "living dentin" to be capped.[304] (8) If acceptable, dentin is found covering the pulp, and a new base of calcium hydroxide is inserted in the cavity's deepest points. This base and the dentin walls should then be coated with a **dentin bonding agent** to prevent future microleakage. The bonding agent should then be covered by a thick cement base and a permanent restoration is placed. (9) On the other hand, if the pulp tests nonvital, if chronic pulpitis is suspected, or if an exposure is encountered, either from instruments or caries persisting under the base, appropriate endodontic treatment is performed based on the state of development of the pulp and the closure of the apical foramen.

It would seem that the success of "indirect pulp capping" is dependent on the health of the pulp (ie, has it already become infected and hence inflamed?). How thick is the remaining dentin, and is it infected or is it capable of remineralization? How effective is the calcium hydroxide dressing? Calcium hydroxide is the only factor that can be immediately controlled.

In this case, calcium hydroxide is not being used as a liner to protect the pulp but rather as an antibacterial agent and mild pulp stimulant to produce irritation dentin.

To accomplish these two objectives, **nonsetting** calcium hydroxide paste in water, saline, or methylcellulose best serves the purpose. In this form, the pH is at least 11, which is an antibacterial alkalinity. If a minute pulp exposure has been overlooked, it will serve as a pulp capping and "stimulate an increase in mineralization within the dentin."[305]

In this nonpermanent situation, British researchers found calcium hydroxide paste in saline to be much more effective than a commercial hard-setting calcium hydroxide cement (LIFE, Kerr Dental; Orange, Calif.). This group "had significantly larger volumes of inflamed pulp tissue than the...CH paste group." Not unexpectedly, there were also significantly more cases (16 versus 7) with bacteria under the hard-setting versus the soft calcium hydroxide.[305]

In an extensive review of calcium hydroxide, another British group pointed out that as a pulp dressing, calcium hydroxide stimulates healing "due to the antibacterial activity" rather than its mineralization effect.[306] They made the important point, however, that "the material has no beneficial effect on the healing of an inflamed pulp, and its use would appear to be indicated for the treatment of healthy or superficially contaminated pulps where bacteria have not penetrated into the deeper part."[306]

High success rates for "indirect pulp capping" are frequently reported but are based on clinical experimentation. The success criteria used are a lack of radiographically observable periradicular lesions and lack of pain. Periradicular radiolucency, however, takes longer to develop than the usual length of these studies, and lack of pain in the presence of inflammation is the rule rather than the exception. Thus, histopathologic and microbiologic studies that show continued, although often slow, breakdown of the pulp under remaining caries should be accepted as a reflection of the actual clinical condition. Many of these teeth eventually need endodontic treatment.

Summary

From this discussion, one can readily see that a number of measures and programs may be undertaken by the dentist and staff to prevent discomfort and sensitivity as well as insult and injury to the dental pulp. Most of all, one must follow the Hippocratic Oath and not inflict through one's ministrations additional trauma or irritation on the patient (the pulp).

PULPAL PATHOLOGY

Many clinicians believe that the pulpal response to injury, treatment, and trauma is unpredictable. As a result, dentists have been unable to correlate clinical signs and symptoms with a corresponding specific histologic picture.[307–311]

The pulp is basically connective tissue, as found elsewhere in the body. However, several factors make it unique and thus alter its ability to respond to irritation:

1. The pulp is almost totally surrounded by a hard tissue (dentin), which limits the area for expansion and restricts the pulp's ability to tolerate edema.
2. The pulp has almost a total lack of collateral circulation, which severely limits its ability to cope with bacteria, necrotic tissue, and inflammation.
3. The pulp possesses a unique cell, the odontoblast, as well as cells that can differentiate into hard tissue–secreting cells that form more dentin and/or irritation dentin in an attempt to protect the pulp from injury.

In spite of these circumstances, studies have indicated that an injured pulp has some capacity to recover, but the degree is uncertain. However, what is important to the clinician is whether the tooth requires endodontic treatment or is amenable to pulp maintenance or preventive therapy.

Pulpal pathosis is basically a reaction to bacteria and bacterial products. This can be a direct response to caries, microleakage of bacteria around fillings and crowns, or bacterial contamination after trauma, either physical or iatrogenic. The pulp responds to these challenges by the inflammatory process. Histologic changes associated with inflammation may occur even with a relatively mild stimulus to the tooth. The vibration of a bur across enamel or the early penetration of caries through the dentinoenamel junction may induce visible, but slight, inflammation in the underlying pulp.[312] The pulp reaction to caries is basically progressive. As the depth of caries increases, the degree of injury increases. Significantly, the inflammation and accompanying hard tissue reaction tend to localize at the base of the involved dentinal tubules that provide the primary passageway (Figures 4-52, 4-53, and 4-54). However, the pulp may withstand a very deep but nonpenetrating carious lesion (Figure 4-55).

HARD TISSUE RESPONSE TO IRRITATION

Irritation Dentin

The undisturbed odontoblast synthesizes and secretes dentin matrix and then induces it to mineralize. The formed dentin demonstrates predictable morphology and function with only slight variations. Before eruption and contact with the opposing tooth, the dentin formed is termed "primary." After occlusal contact, the dentin is termed "secondary." Although there are conflicting terminologies, some authors contend that there is a visible alteration in the dentin that differentiates secondary from primary dentin.[313] However, primary and secondary dentin are usually indistinguishable and possess similar properties. The term "secondary" is used for the continuous, slow formation of primary dentin after eruption.[314]

An odontoblast that is mildly stimulated may form dentin that closely resembles normal physiologic dentin. However, since **odontoblasts are incapable of mitosis,**[315] they must be replaced by underlying cells that mature from dividing undifferentiated precursors or by redifferentiation of fibroblasts[316] (Figure 4-56). These new cells are atypical, frequently without a process, and thus form an atypical irregular structure called irritation or reparative dentin[317] (Figure 4-57).

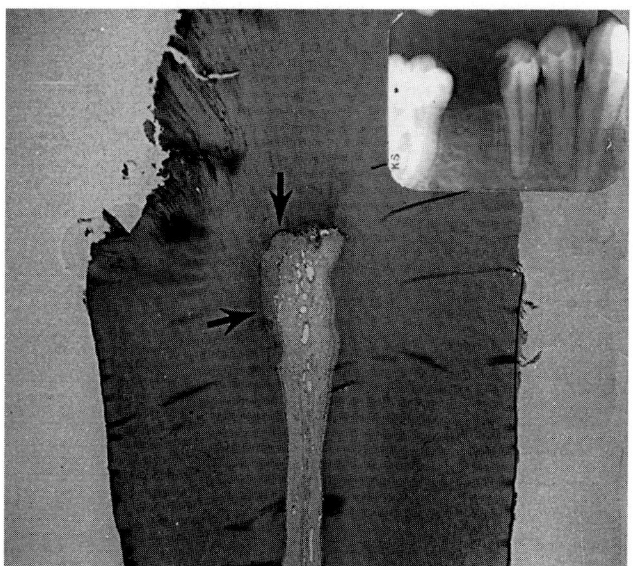

Figure 4-52 Adult human mandibular second premolar with a deep carious lesion on the distal surface. Note irritation dentin formation (**arrows**) under the affected tubules. **Inset** shows the radiographic appearance of tooth. The area indicated by the arrows is seen at higher magnification in Figure 4-53.

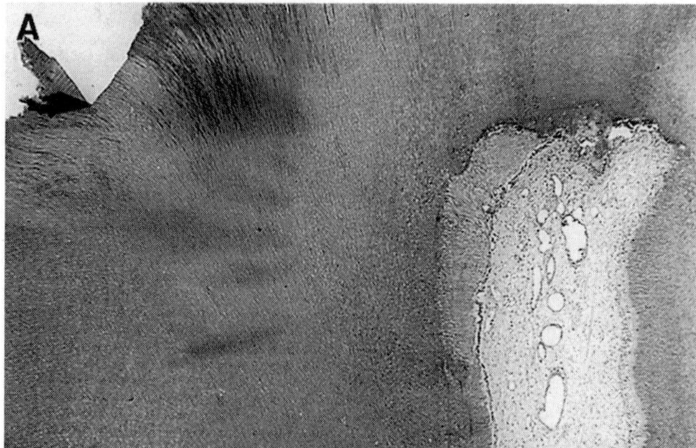

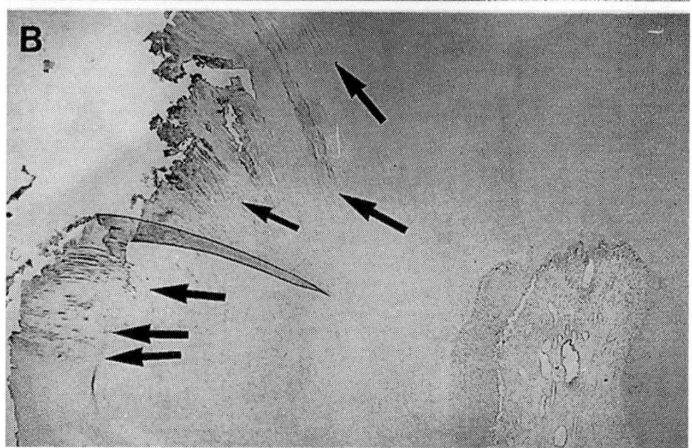

Figure 4-53 A, Intermediate magnification of the coronal area of the tooth from Figure 4-52. Note the amount of irritation dentin on the left (affected) side of the pulp relative to the right (unaffected) side. The pulp vessels are very dilated. Hematoxylin and eosin stain. B, Same specimen as shown in A, stained for bacteria. Note the invasion of microorganisms deep into some (**arrows**) but not all tubules. Bacteria have not penetrated as deeply as the hematoxylin and eosin stain (in A) suggests.

The term "irritation" dentin more appropriately describes the dentin's genesis than "reparative."[318] The term **irritation** is based on clinical, anatomic, and histologic findings. To designate this as **reparative** dentin is misleading; its formation may falsely indicate that the pulp is healing or repairing.[319] In fact, its formation occurs independently of the presence of inflammation and may form on the walls of an irreversibly damaged pulp.[320] Continued irritation dentin formation may depend on persistent injurious stimuli; such a condition is **neither** desirable nor reparative.[321]

An example of irritation dentin formation is the reaction following impact trauma and subluxation in which the blood supply is temporarily disrupted. It can be speculated that the marked changes following such an injury result from odontoblast replacement. As a result of the vascular impairment, the odontoblasts degenerate in large numbers. New cells arise, align themselves along exposed predentin, and rapidly form a very irregular hard tissue. The delineation between the old and new altered hard tissue is called the "calciotraumatic line"[322] (Figure 4-58). Frequently, there are inclusions of tissue or bacteria in this region that become entrapped in or under the forming irritation dentin. Newly differentiated cells apparently do not possess the inhibitory regulation of normal odontoblasts. Thus, these new cells are uncontrolled and continue to form irritation dentin until there is almost

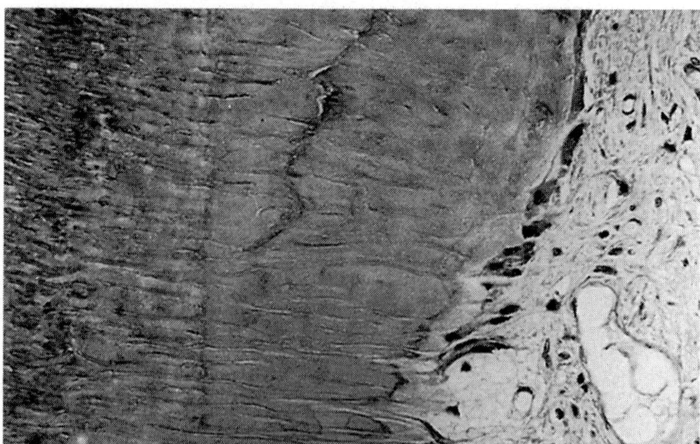

Figure 4-54 High magnification of irritation dentin formed under the carious lesion seen in Figure 4-52 and 4-53. Irritation dentin (**center**) is clearly less tubular than the original dentin seen on the left side of the micrograph. Note the lack of a well-defined odontoblastic layer and the irregular shape of cells at the pulp margin of the dentin.

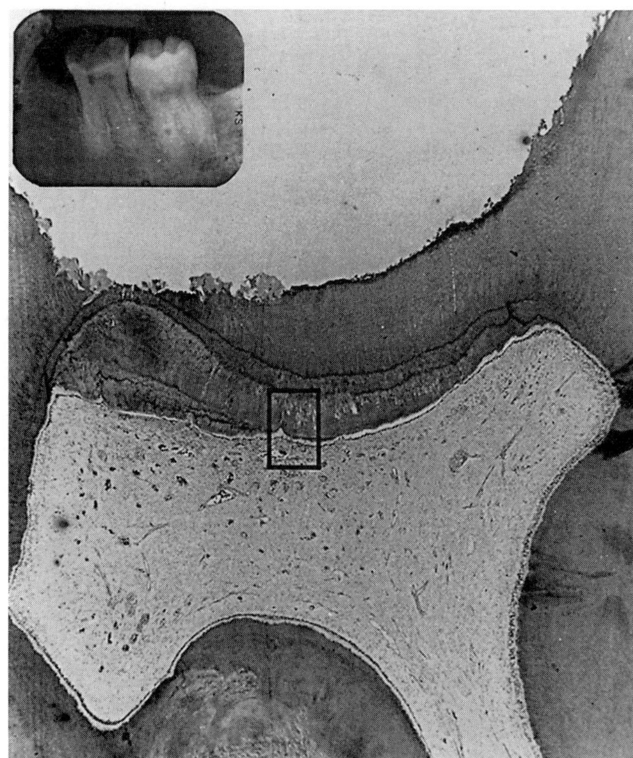

Figure 4-55 Adult human mandibular second molar with a very deep carious lesion. Carious material was excavated with a round bur prior to extraction without pulp exposure. Note the thickness (0.2 mm) and appositional appearance of the irritation dentin. The underlying blood vessels are dilated. **Inset** indicates the radiographic appearance of the tooth. Even a **very** thin layer of intact dentin often protects the underlying pulp from severe injury and irreversible inflammation.

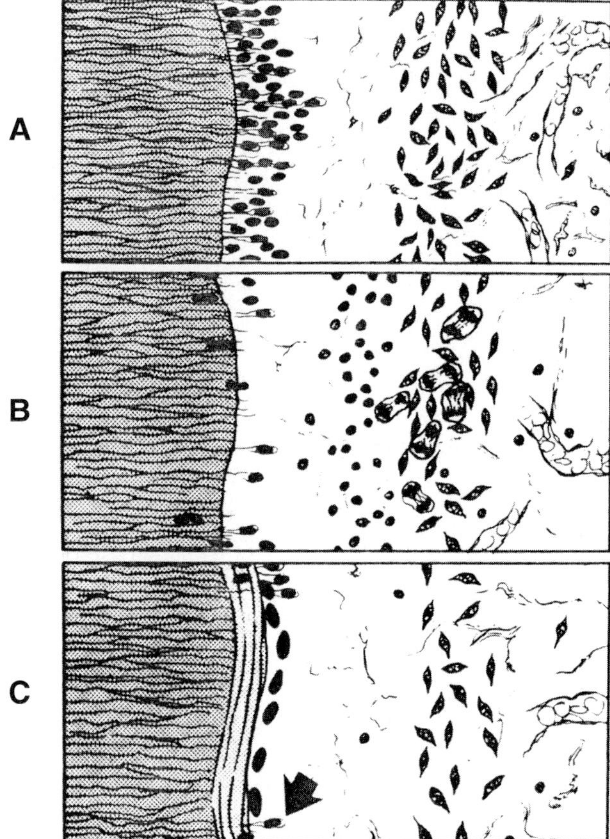

Figure 4-56 Schematic showing cellular response to injury to the odontoblast layer. **A**, Normal odontoblasts adjacent to the cell-free and cell-rich zones. **B**, Odontoblasts are largely destroyed with resultant inflammation in the cell-free zone and mitosis of undifferentiated mesenchymal cells in the cell-rich zone. **C**, Undifferentiated cells have matured and migrated to dentin surface to occupy space vacated by odontoblasts. These new cells, which are not true odontoblasts, form unique atubular hard tissue (irritation dentin). Few odontoblasts survive (**arrow**) and continue to form tubules. (Courtesy of Dr. Henry Trowbridge.)

total obliteration of the pulp called "calcific metamorphosis."[323–326]

A similar response may occur following pulpotomy in teeth with irreversible pulpitis. Odontoblasts are absent and replaced by these unique cells even at sites distant to the cut surface. The ensuing partial, but not complete, obliteration of the remaining canal space often makes endodontic treatment difficult since the canals are very small (Figure 4-59).

Anything that exposes or contacts dentin has the **potential** to stimulate formation of underlying irritation dentin. For example, caries and attrition usually cause inflammation and the formation of irritation dentin at the pulpal end of the involved tubules.[327–329] Cavity preparation without adequate coolant may also cause an injury that results in irritation dentin formation.

The morphology of irritation dentin has been studied, but little is known of its functions. Some attribute protective properties to this tissue and therefore recommend methods or materials to stimulate its formation.[330,331] Others doubt its ability to protect the

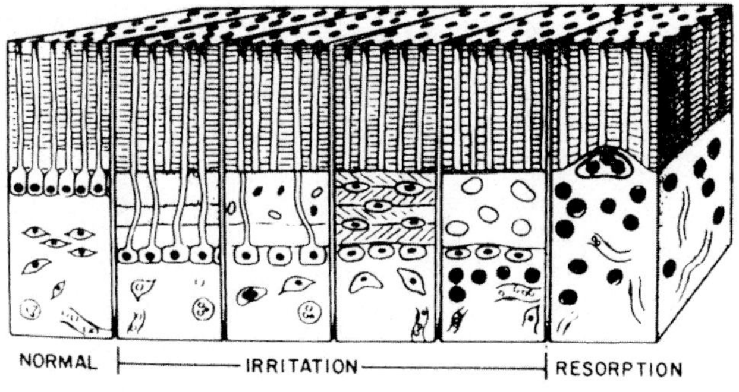

Figure 4-57 Hard tissue response to injury varies. Irritation dentin may have different structures according to relative numbers of odontoblasts surviving and numbers of new cells arising to form altered hard tissue. Resorption is also a common phenomenon. Factors stimulating resorption are yet unknown. (Courtesy of Dr. Henry Trowbridge.)

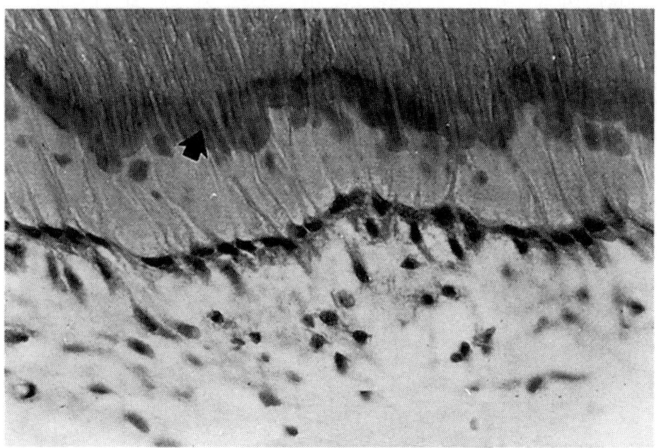

Figure 4-58 Calciotraumatic line (**arrow**) forming in response to recent injury from deep caries penetration. As a result of the injury to odontoblasts, mineralization has been delayed, indicated by widened predentin matrix. Irritation dentin is forming, demonstrated by a decrease in numbers of tubules. Cells aligned along predentin have been termed "replacement odontoblasts." Reproduced with permission from Trowbridge H.[11]

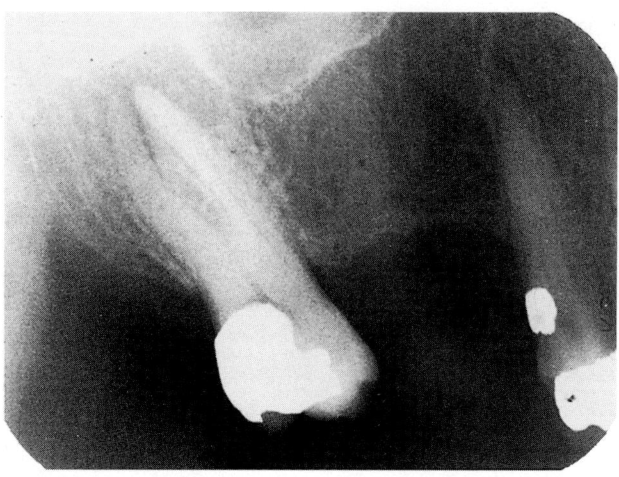

Figure 4-59 Obliteration of pulp canals that frequently follows pulpotomy or partial pulpectomy. Calcification may greatly reduce the canal size, making it invisible on radiographs and difficult to locate during root canal treatment. However, a pulp space containing necrotic material remains, as evidenced by the large periradicular inflammatory lesion. (The radiolucent lines over the roots are superimposed periodontal ligament spaces, **not** canals.)

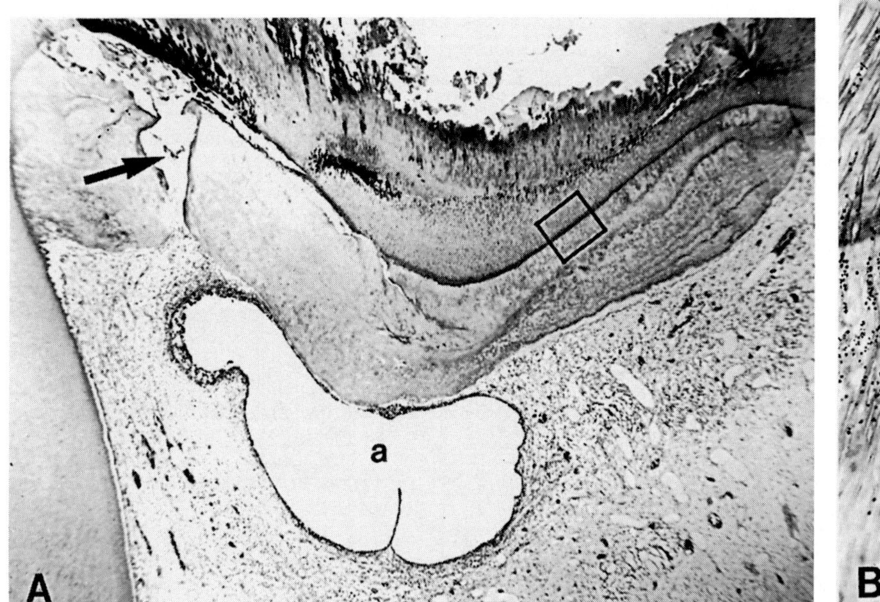

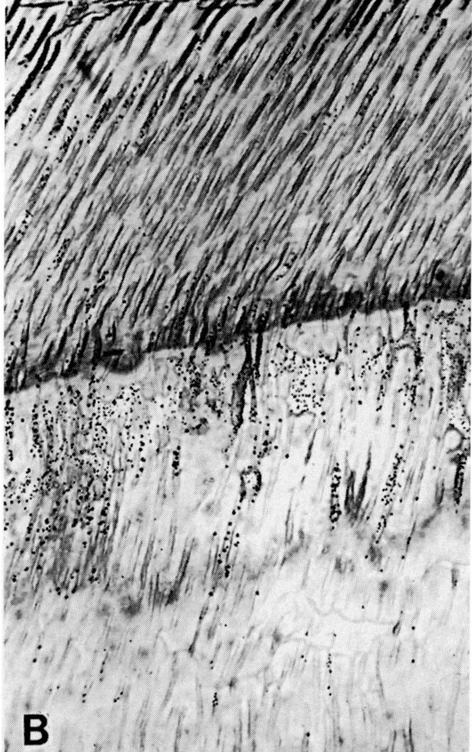

Figure 4-60 **A**, "Indirect pulp cap." Although extensive irritation dentin has formed under carious lesion, it has not protected the pulp from effects of irritants, as shown by microabscess (**a**). Frequently, the barrier is incomplete, as evidenced by the opening (**arrow**), forming communication between carious dentin and the underlying pulp. **B**, Area of box in **A**. Silver nitrate was placed on the surface of caries and can be seen passing through tubules in a pulpward direction. It readily crosses the calciotraumatic line, into underlying irritation dentin and eventually into pulp. Reproduced with permission from Langeland K. JOE 1982;7:148.

underlying pulp and believe its formation is dependent on the presence of irritation. They have demonstrated its permeability, permitting passage of chemicals and bacteria and other substances[332] (Figure 4-60). The exact degree of permeability remains to be demonstrated experimentally. Certainly, the presence of irritation dentin delays, but does not prevent, the eventual penetration of caries into the pulp. Unfortunately for the pulp, formation of irritation dentin and its morphology under caries do not occur predictably. Fingers of soft tissue may extend from the underlying pulp to penetrate deep into the hard tissue (see Figure 4-60). The barrier may therefore be incomplete and relatively nonprotective.[321,333] Its importance relative to maintenance of pulpal health is largely unknown and remains the subject of much speculation and considerable misinformation.

PULPITIS

The nature of the inflammatory response is related to both direct and immune mechanisms. Direct injury of the pulp from caries occurs via the dentinal tubules (Figure 4-61). Irritants (bacterial by-products, disintegrating elements of carious dentin, or chemicals from foods) either permeate through tubules (Figure 4-62) to contact and destroy odontoblasts and underlying cells or have an osmotic effect that also destroys cells by rapid, forceful fluid movement.[334]

The immune process and accompanying injury comprise another mechanism responsible for the develop-

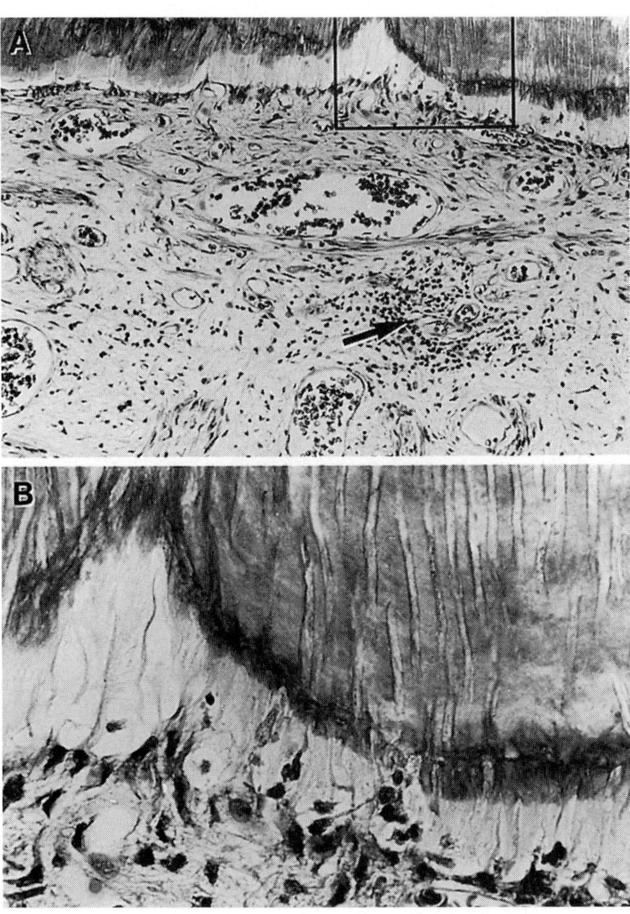

Figure 4-61 A, Magnification of region indicated by the box in Figure 7–4 under a deep carious lesion. Dentin seen in the micrograph is irritation dentin, and cells lining its surface are not typical odontoblasts but flattened, irregular, less differentiated cells. Note the dilated state of underlying blood vessels and accumulation of round cells (**arrow**). B, High-power micrograph of the area outlined by the box in A. Irritation dentin is almost as tubular as regular dentin and permits bacterial products to diffuse from carious lesion to pulp, where they can produce both inflammation and injury to odontoblasts.

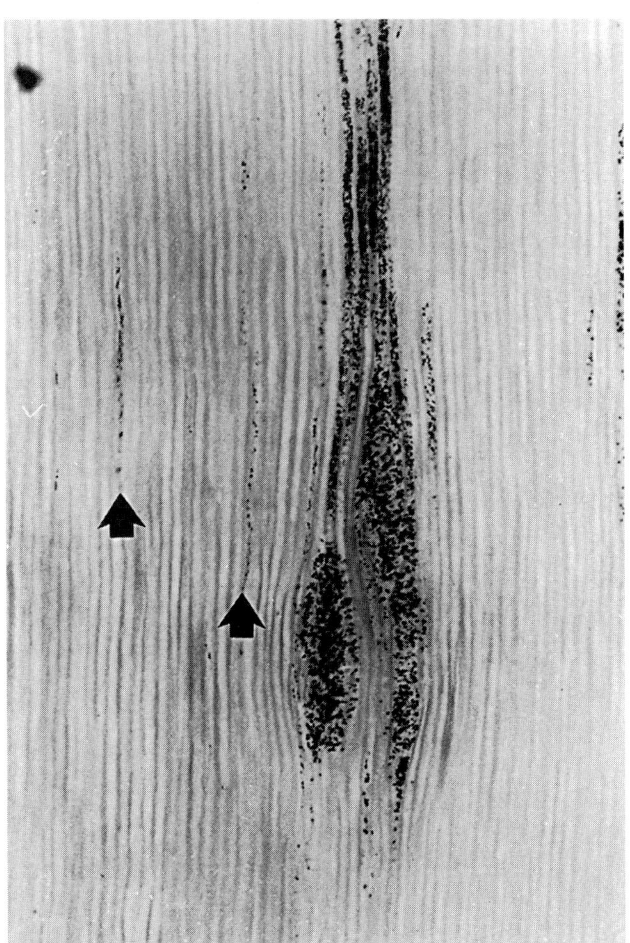

Figure 4-62 Section of human carious dentin showing colonization of individual tubules (**arrows**) and enlargement and fusion of adjacent tubules owing to bacterial action. Reproduced with permission from Trowbridge HT.[11]

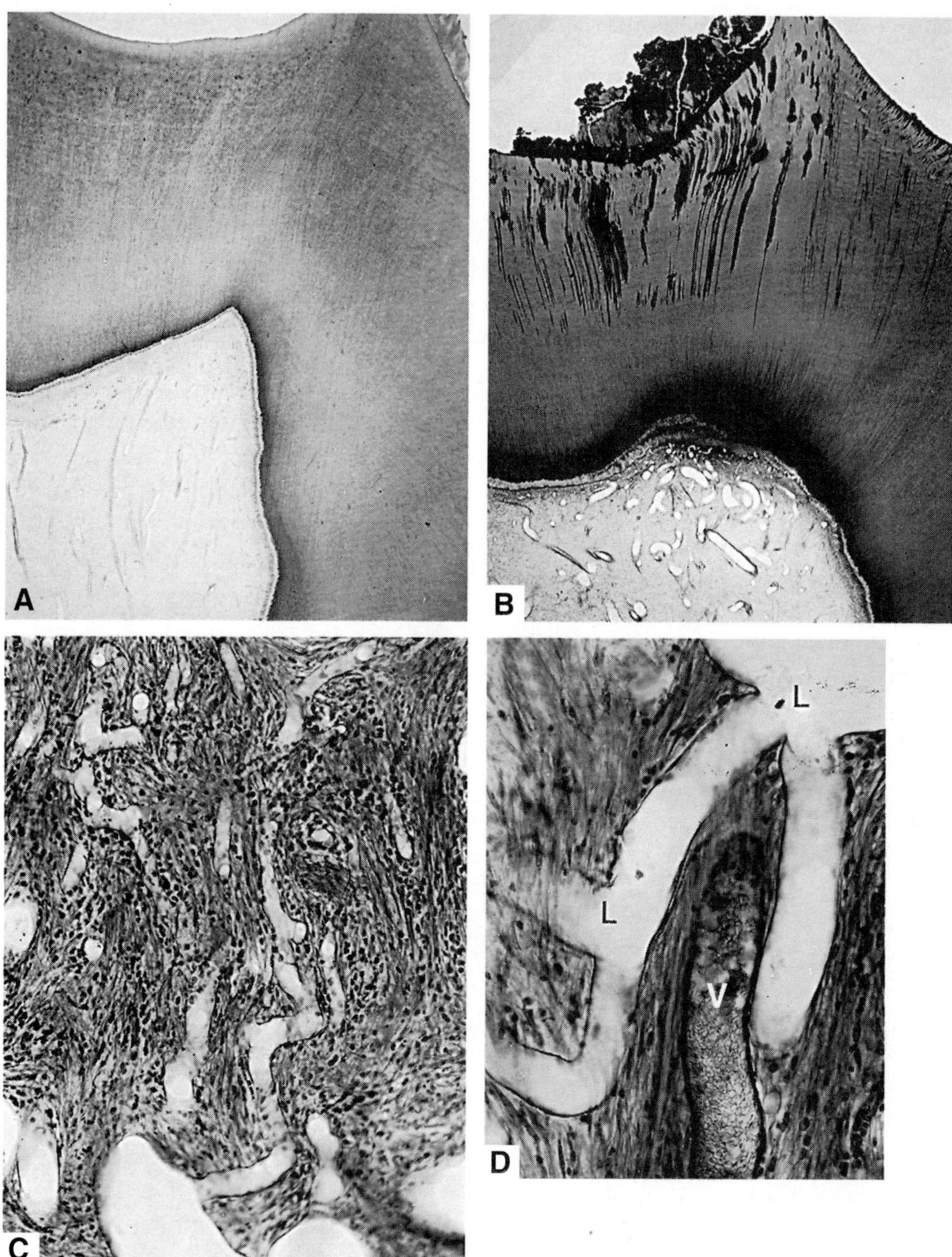

Figure 4-63 A, Section of **noncarious adult** molar. Note absence of any pulp changes under normal dentin. B, Section of **carious adult** molar. Carious process has invaded dentin. Note dilated vessels concentrated in a region of pulp under affected tubule. C, High magnification of inflammatory lesion in coronal pulp seen in B. D, Higher magnification of a portion of an inflammatory lesion. L = lymphatic vessel; V = venule filled with red blood cells. Reproduced with permission from Bernick S. JDR 1977;56:841.

ment of pulpitis.[335] Immunocompetent cells, immunoglobulins (antibodies), and complement factors have been identified in inflamed pulpal tissues. Both the humoral and cellular responses occur in the pulp.[336]

The end result, whether induced by direct irritation or from the immune system, is the release of chemical mediators that initiate inflammation. This is a vascular response. The increase in the permeability of vessels nearest the site of injury and extravasation of fluid into the connective tissue spaces (edema) cause an elevation in local pressure. This edema alters or destroys the odontoblast layer. Chemical modification of the ground substance also occurs, as evidenced by an increased eosinophilia.[337] Marked dilation of vessels (Figure 4-63) leads to slowing of erythrocytes and the margination of leukocytes along the walls (Figures 4-64

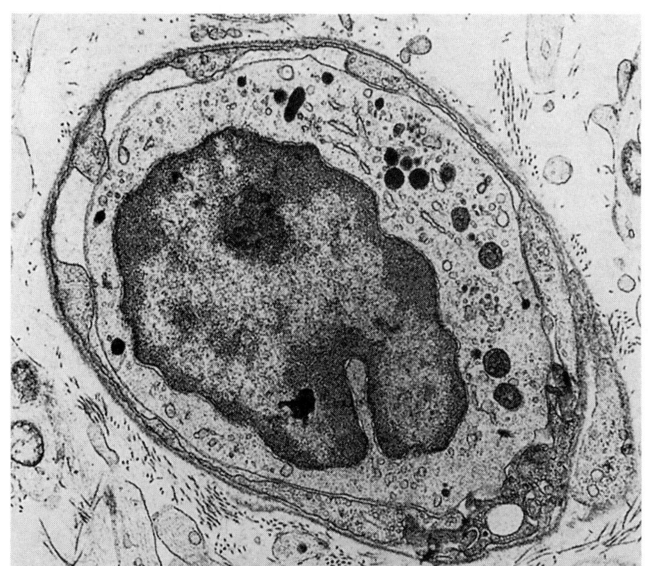

Figure 4-64 Electron micrograph of a pulpal capillary containing a lymphocyte. This chance observation is not typically found in capillaries within an inflammatory area. (Courtesy of Dr. Robert Rapp.)

and 4-65). The leukocytes then squeeze through the intracellular spaces of the vessel endothelia in response to chemotactic signals originating in the damaged tissue. This is called diapedesis.

The result of the inflammatory process is an infiltrate of leukocytes around the dilated vessels. The acute cells of the infiltrate dominate the scene at the expense of the original connective tissue cell population. In turn, these acute cells are supplanted by chronic mononuclear cells.[338]

The proportional representation of acute cells is variable. Leukocytes of all forms are present, but the "chronic" cells (small lymphocytes, macrophages, and plasma cells) quickly dominate. Neutrophils are commonplace when the inflammation is a localized process or the tissue destruction is marked,[339] but seldom is there a predominance of polymorphonuclear neutrophil leukocytes. It is for this reason that the true microscopic definition of "acute" inflammation is said to be absent or transient in pulp sections.

An interesting phenomenon, unique to the pulp, relates to the presence of mast cells, ordinarily a common inhabitant of loose fibrous connective tissue. This important cell type is rich in histamine and bradykinin; both are mediators of vascular changes associated with inflammation. For unexplained reasons, the **mast cell is rarely seen** in healthy pulps but appears in large numbers with inflammation.[340,341]

The sum total of the inflammatory response may cause more damage than the irritants alone. Immune and inflammatory reactions may destroy adjacent normal cellular and extracellular components. Trowbridge and Daniels reported a patient with an immunologic deficiency that permitted overwhelming bacterial colonization of a pulp, accompanied by only **minor** destruction and inflammation.[342] In a normal individual, the bacteria would be quickly eliminated but at destructive cost to the nearby tissues.

In general, the density of inflammatory cells and the size of the pulp lesion increase as the caries progresses in depth and width. The ability of the pulp to withstand injury is related to the severity of inflammation. Initially, the inflammation is reversible, but beyond a critical point it becomes irreversible.

Reversible Pulpitis

The condition of reversible pulpitis is characterized by the description of inflammation in the preceding paragraphs. The lesion is predominantly chronic, and the inflammation is localized at the base of the involved tubules (Figure 4-66).

By definition, this reactive inflammatory process resolves or diminishes with removal of the irritant. Experiments have shown that chronically inflamed and damaged pulps may heal when caries is removed from the overlying dentin.[343–349] It must be emphasized that these experimental injuries were not carious exposures (gross, direct bacterial invasion) and therefore represented sterile inflammation. Frank penetration of bacteria into the pulp is frequently the crossover point to irreversible pulpitis. This is not to say that irreversible pulpitis cannot occur **before** exposure.

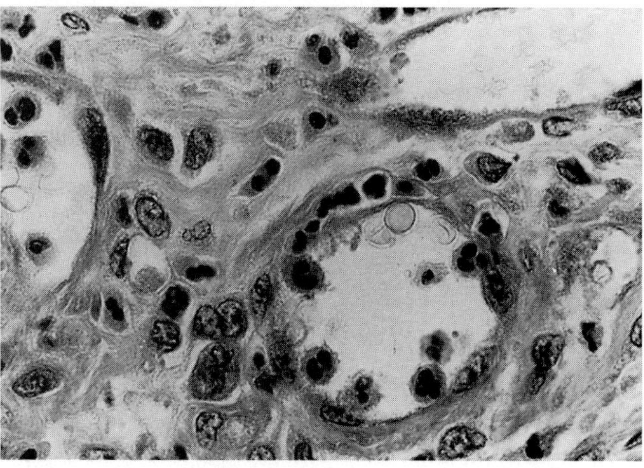

Figure 4-65 High magnification of dilated pulpal venules in area of inflammation. Note pavementing of leukocytes along the walls of vessels.

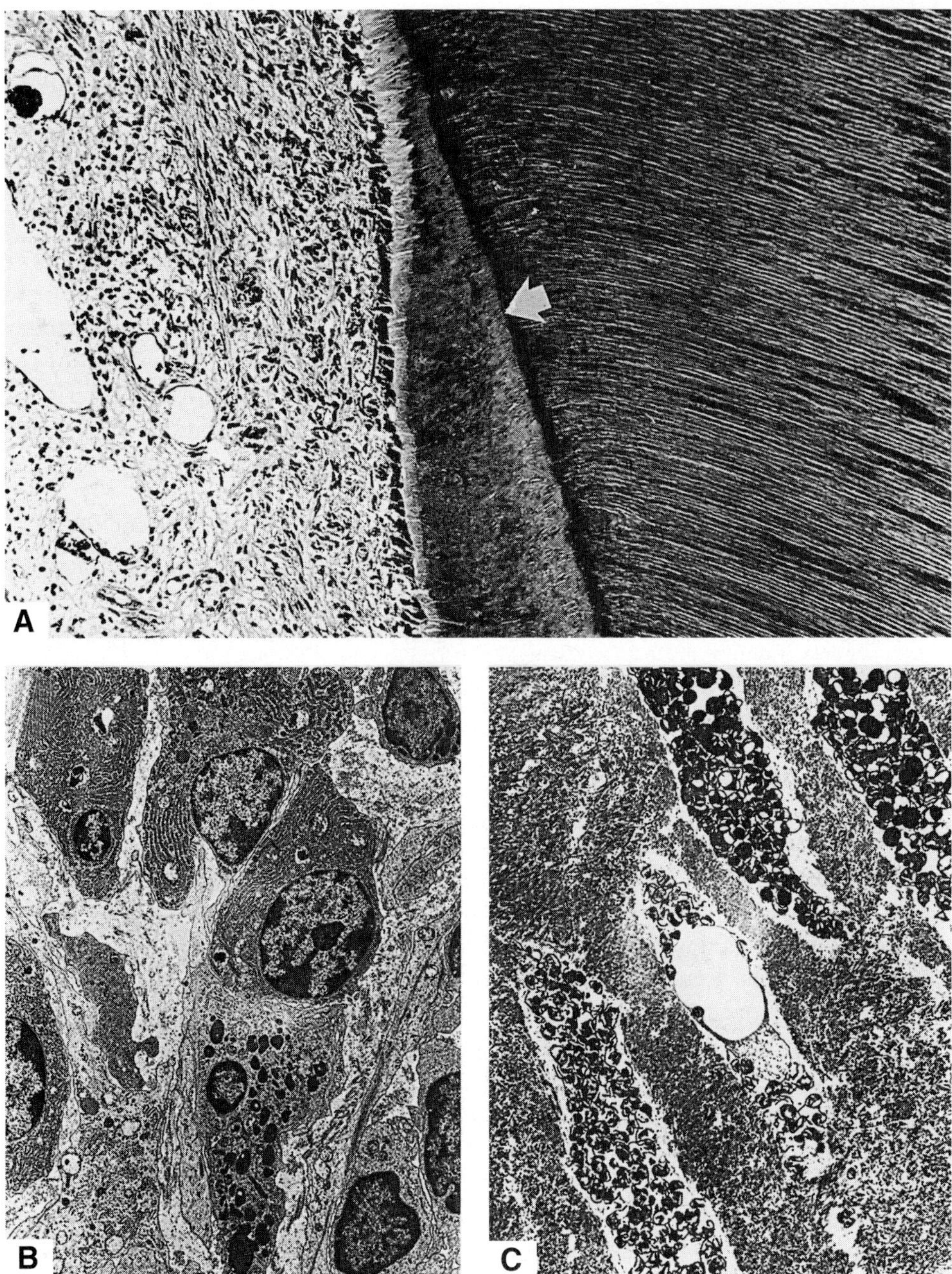

Figure 4-66 A, Micrograph of pulp and carious dentin in an adult molar. Dark areas in the right portion of dentin are microorganisms in dentinal tubules. The calciotraumatic line (**arrow**) divides dentin into original primary dentin and subsequent irritation dentin. The tubular pattern of irritation dentin is irregular, and the underlying pulp is infiltrated with chronic inflammatory cells. B, Transmission electron micrograph of pulp affected by dentinal caries showing chronic inflammatory cells. C, Transmission electron micrograph of carious dentin. Invasion of dentinal tubules with cocci-like microorganisms. Reproduced with permission from Torneck C. In: Roth G, Calmes R, editors. Oral biology. Toronto: CV Mosby; 1981. p. 138.

Irreversible Pulpitis

By definition, the pulp has been damaged beyond repair, and even with removal of the irritant it will not heal. The pulp will progressively degenerate, causing necrosis and reactive destruction.

The clinician sometimes assumes that pulp death will occur rapidly and tries to correlate severe pulp disease with significant symptoms. The process may be agonizing to the patient, but more frequently it is asymptomatic. Necrosis may occur quickly, or the process may require years. In the latter case, neither the patient nor the dentist is aware of the degree of devastation of the pulp because severe disease is often unaccompanied by pain. The dentist must be aware of and inform the patient that **pulp death often occurs slowly and without dramatic symptoms.**

Although carious exposure is not necessary for the pulp to become irreversibly inflamed, this stage is irreversible. A carious exposure is that point at which **infected,** altered dentin comes into contact with pulpal soft tissues (Figure 4-67). This penetration of caries allows large numbers of bacteria, carious dentin debris and breakdown products, salivary by-products, and chemicals from ingested foods direct access to the pulp. This infection leads to the development of a microabscess. Progression of the inflammatory process to the stage of acute abscess[328,347] signifies an irreversible pulpal condition.

Microabscesses of the pulp begin as tiny zones of necrosis within dense inflammatory cell infiltrates comprised principally of acute inflammatory cells. These lesions are frequently found immediately adjacent to carious exposures.

Commonly, an abscess contains concentrations of necrotic and degenerating cells, cellular elements, and microorganisms (Figure 4-68).[347,348] The cells and cellular debris appear to be primarily from disintegrating fibroblasts and inflammatory cells. The important inflammatory cell in the abscess is the neutrophil, which is drawn to the area but dies very quickly. Immediately surrounding the abscess may be a dense infiltration of lymphocytes, plasma cells, and macrophages. Bacteria usually do not penetrate owing to their ingestion by phagocytic cells (see Figure 4-68, B) and therefore are not seen beyond the region of necrosis.[345] Histologically **intact myelinated and unmyelinated nerves** may be observed in areas with dense inflammation and cellular degeneration.[349]

In histopathologic terms, the nature of the pulpal response to caries is variable. The duration of involvement and the resistance of the pulp are significant. One pulp may have a carious exposure and contain a single abscess, whereas another with a similar carious lesion may contain numerous abscesses (Figures 4-69 and 4-70). Other pulps may give evidence of having undergone a rapid transition from localized abscess to widespread necrosis. This latter response is often accompanied by bacterial growth within the pulp chamber.

Some pulps, on the other hand, respond to carious exposure by surface "ulceration" that exposes the pulp to the oral cavity. Because it is open and no longer in a confined space, it can be theorized that a "safety valve" exists that delays the spread of injury. Excess fluid (transudates and exudates) produced as part of the inflammatory response does not accumulate but rather drains into the oral cavity. Therefore, the intrapulpal

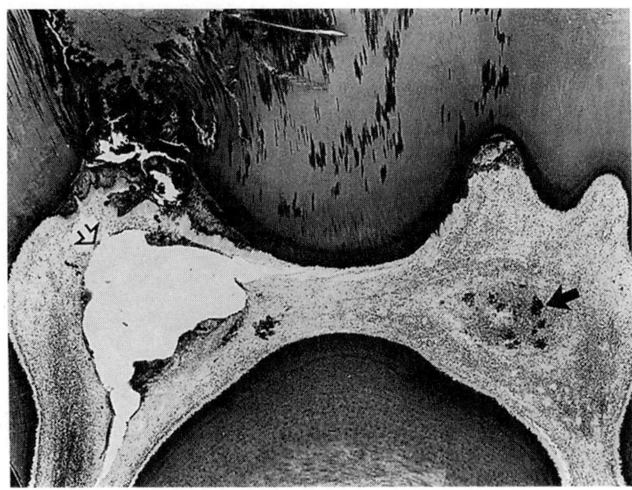

Figure 4-67 Massive, rapidly advancing pulp necrosis in an adult molar. Bacterial penetration resulted in development of microabscess (**open arrow**). Much pulp became necrotic without undergoing typical liquefaction. Small dots (**solid arrow**) are bacterial masses. Reproduced with permission from Matsumiya S et al.[350]

pressure does not rise. In addition, the fluid transudation from the open lesion is probably maximal. This high turnover of interstitial fluid must literally flush toxins, inflammatory mediators, hydrolytic enzymes, etc from the pulp, keeping their concentration too low to cause further tissue damage. Thus, the open pulp apparently responds similarly to inflamed gingiva. Under this condition, the pulp is able to offer long-term resistance and to delay extensive breakdown of the soft tissue mass.

Although the entire occlusal surface of the coronal pulp is open and ulcerated, the deeper connective tissue may be normal (Figure 4-71). Beneath the necrotic surface of the ulcer lies a zone of dense leukocytic infiltration. Beyond this, a zone of proliferating fibroblasts and collagenous fibers serves to delineate the process. At some point, the injurious agents breach the fibrous zone, and inflammatory changes spread to increasingly deeper layers of the pulp. **The end result is necrosis.**

Hyperplastic Pulpitis

Hyperplastic pulpitis (pulp polyp) is the most visually dramatic of all pulp responses. Rising out of the carious shell of the crown is a "mushroom" of living pulp tissue that is often firm and insensitive to the touch (Figure 4-72 and 4-73).

The chronically inflamed young pulp, widely exposed by caries on its occlusal aspect, is the forerunner of this unique growth. Proliferative growth of inflamed connective tissue resembles a pyogenic granuloma of the gingiva. This is an unusual response for adult pulps.

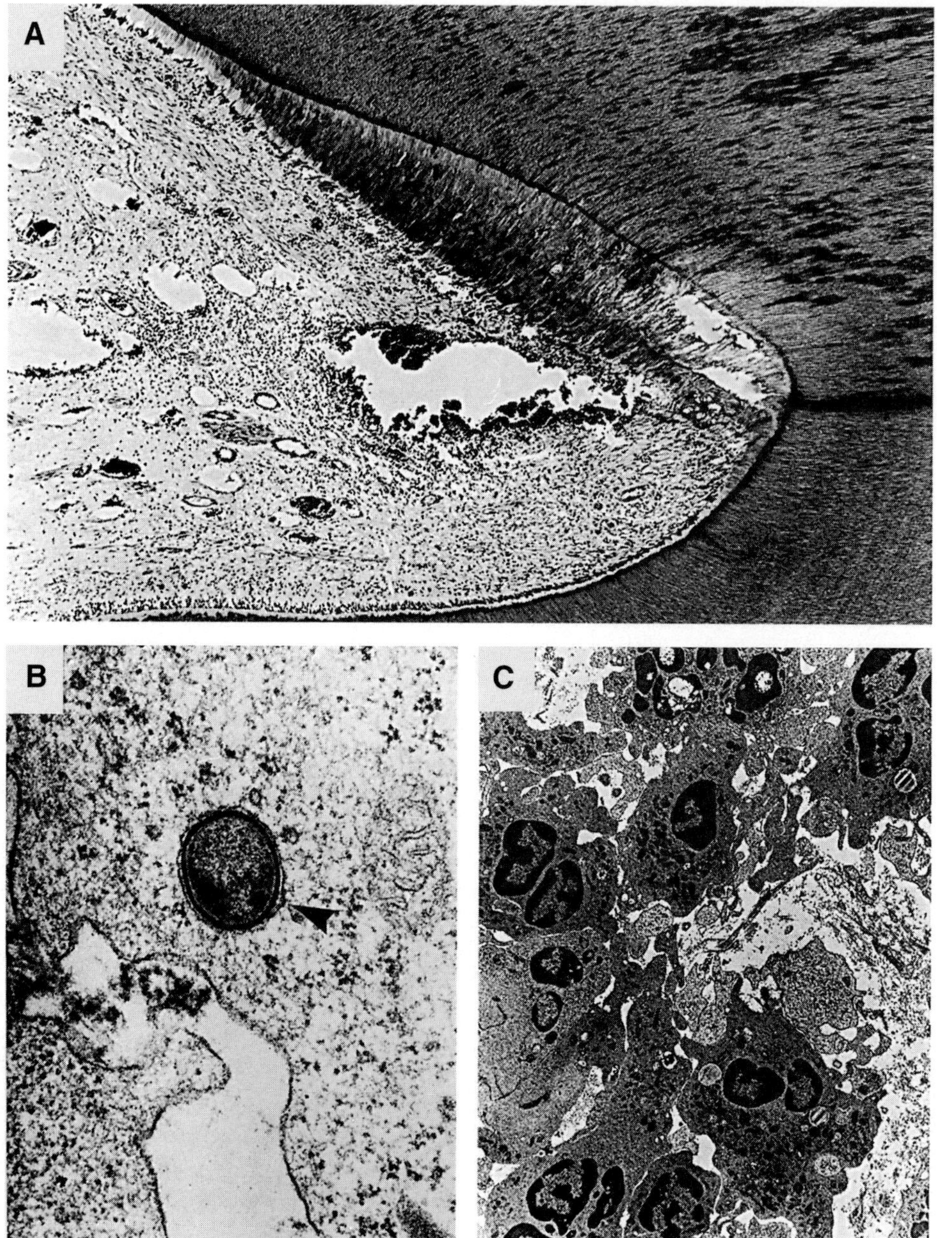

Figure 4-68 A, Micrograph of carious exposure in an adult molar. Microorganisms have penetrated the full thickness of primary and irritation dentin. Small focal microabscess is present in pulp tissue subjacent to exposure. Peripheral portion of the microabscess displays numerous polymorphonuclear leukocytes, and the surrounding pulp displays infiltration with polymorphonuclear leukocytes and mononuclear cells. **B**, Transmission electron micrograph of gram-positive coccus (**arrow**) within phagosome of macrophage in human pulp exposed to dental caries. **C**, Transmission electron micrograph of polymorphonuclear response in pulp subjacent to carious exposure. Reproduced with permission from Torneck C. J Oral Pathol 1977;6:82.

Microscopically, the pulp polyp is a complex of new capillaries, proliferating fibroblasts, and inflammatory cells. Support for the protruding mass is supplied by collagenous fibers rooted in the deeper pulp tissue of the chamber. Sensory nerve elements are almost totally absent near the surface, in contrast to the rich innervation and exquisite sensitivity of an exposed pulp that is not hyperplastic.

Before the lesion has grown to any extent, its surface layer consists of massed necrotic cells and leukocytes with chronic inflammatory cells beneath forming a zone of variable width. As the tissue expands, it may acquire a stratified squamous epithelial cover that may form by a true cell graft. Cells of the oral mucosa floating free in the saliva may grow over the surface of the highly vascularized young connective tissue, or a direct migration of

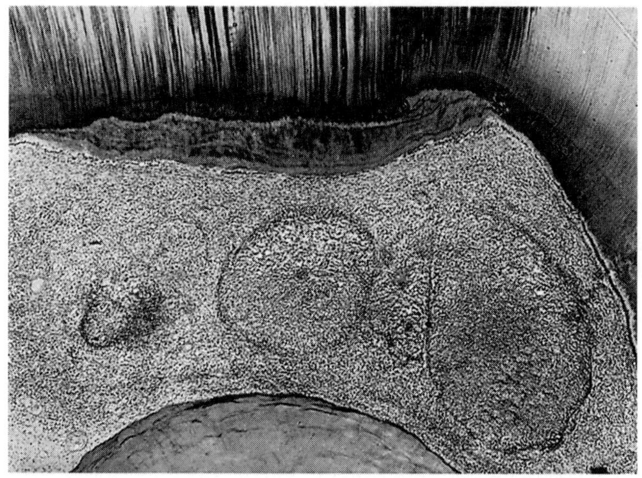

Figure 4-69 Adult molar with deep caries. The entire coronal pulp demonstrates chronic inflammation with several "encapsulated" microabscesses. Irritation dentin was probably produced **before** pulp developed microabscesses. Reproduced with permission from Matsumiya S et al.[350]

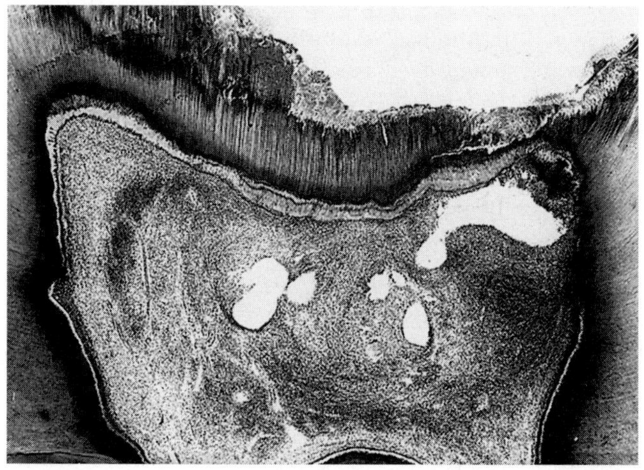

Figure 4-70 Multiple microabscesses in molar pulp. Caries penetration has been extensive, and inflammatory change in pulp connective tissue is far advanced. Inflammatory cells are everywhere. Space in the center of each abscess represents lysed and necrotic material lost in the preparation of the section. Reproduced with permission from Matsumiya S et al.[350]

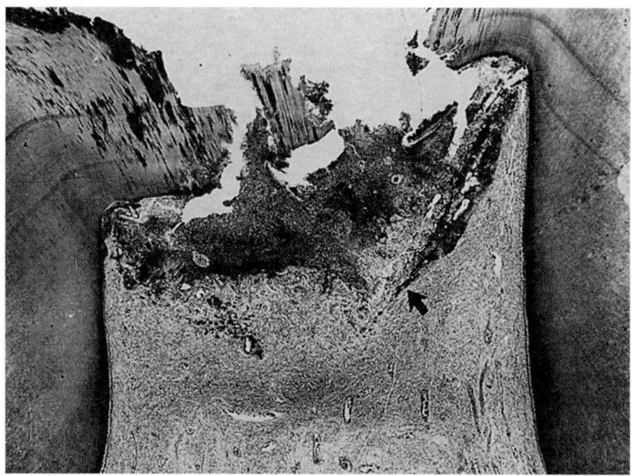

Figure 4-71 Ulceration of entire surface of human pulp in response to carious exposure. Beneath the necrotic surface of ulcer is a zone of dense leukocytic infiltration. Below this is a zone of proliferating fibroblast cells and collagenous fibers, that is, a "collagenous" or fibrous zone. Irregular calcifying masses (**arrow**) are sometimes found in this area. Toward the floor of the pulp chamber, the connective tissue is relatively normal. Reproduced with permission from Matsumiya S et al.[350]

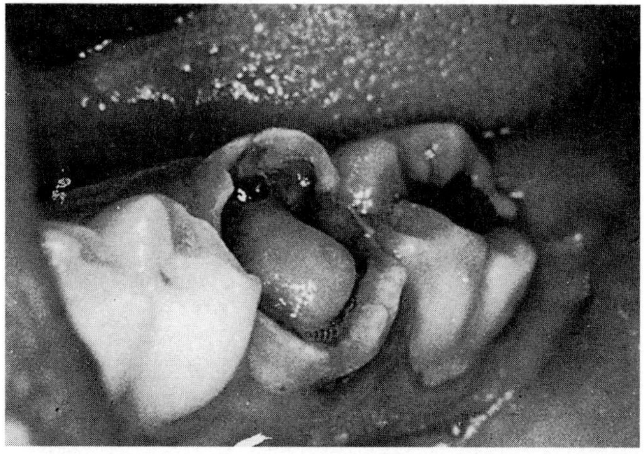

Figure 4-72 Pulp polyp in a mandibular first molar. Although, histologically, pulp is classified as having hyperplastic pulpitis, clinically, tissue rising out of the crown is firm and insensitive. (Courtesy of Dr. G. Norman Smith.)

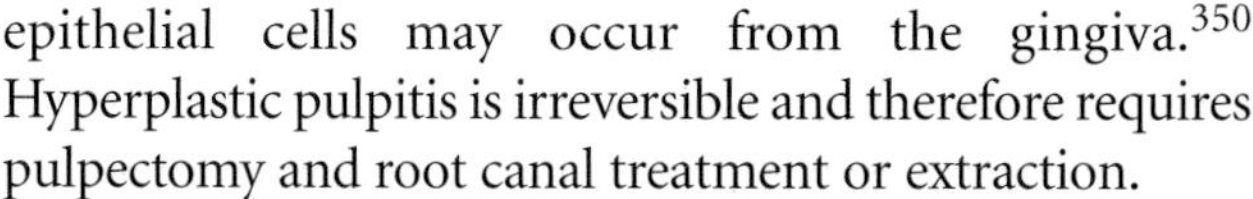

epithelial cells may occur from the gingiva.[350] Hyperplastic pulpitis is irreversible and therefore requires pulpectomy and root canal treatment or extraction.

Necrosis

As inflammation progresses, tissue continues to disintegrate in the center to form an increasing region of liquefaction necrosis (Figure 4-74). Because of the lack of collateral circulation and the unyielding walls of the dentin, there is insufficient drainage of inflammatory fluids. This results in localized increases in tissue pressures, causing the destruction to progress unchecked until the entire pulp is necrotic (Figure 4-75). The rate of progress of liquefaction necrosis varies. The speed may correlate with the ability of the tissue to drain or absorb fluids, thus minimizing increases in intrapulpal pressure. To demonstrate the importance of a "closed" lesion, experiments were performed in which pulps in

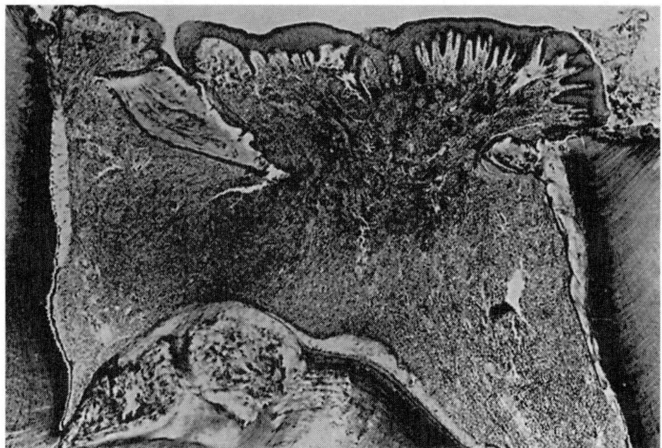

Figure 4-73 Completely epithelialized pulp polyp. Stratified squamous epithelium covers the entire surface. Mass beneath the epithelium in the upper left is a large fragment of dentin. Reproduced with permission from Matsumiya S et al.[350]

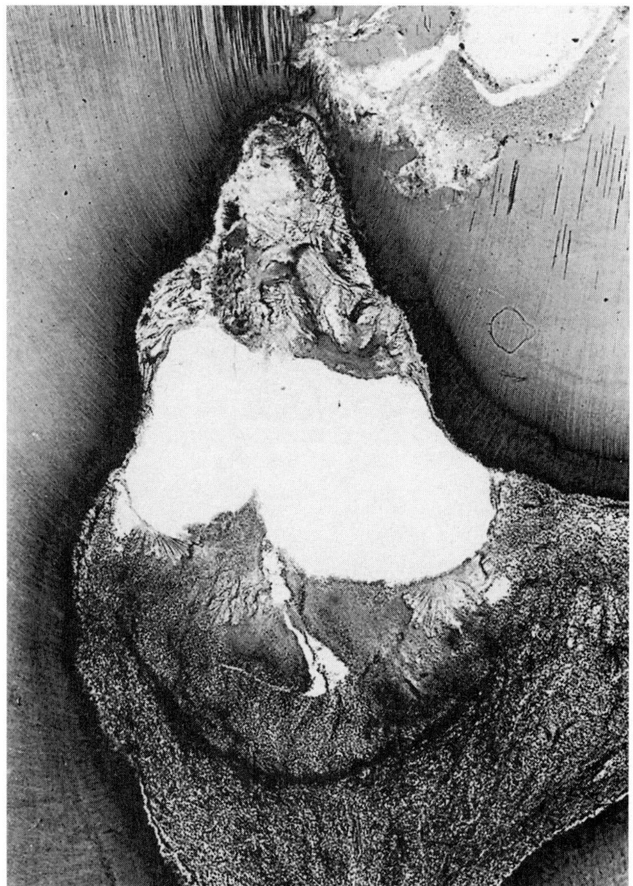

Figure 4-74 Liquefaction necrosis (microabscess) in pulp horn in response to carious exposure. This is the **usual** occurrence; therefore, pulps cariously exposed are irreversibly inflamed. Necrosis will expand to eventually involve the entire pulp. The space is an artifact—liquefied contents washed out during histologic preparation. Reproduced with permission from Matsumiya S et al.[350]

monkey teeth were opened to the oral cavity and then closed after a few days. This procedure consistently induced very rapid and total pulp necrosis. Periradicular pathosis quickly followed,[351] demonstrating the impact of the combination of tissue damage from the bur and irritants (bacteria) from the oral cavity combined with a lack of pressure release.

The region of necrosis contains irritants from tissue destruction and microbes, both anaerobic and aerobic. These irritants contact peripheral vital tissue and continue to exert damage.[352] Bacteria penetrate to the boundaries of necrosis but are not observed in adjacent inflamed tissue.[348] However, their toxins and enzymes are continually permeating surrounding tissues and inciting inflammation.[353] Where liquefaction necrosis contacts dentin, the predentin is lost, probably by the action of collagenase.[354] Since this permits bacteria to penetrate into dentinal tubules[348] (Figure 4-76), it is necessary to remove these dentin layers on all walls during canal instrumentation.

Adjacent to the liquefaction necrosis is a zone of chronic inflammation. Although the width of this zone may vary, generally it is rather narrow (Figure 4-77). Periradicular inflammation would not be expected to develop until the pulp is nearly totally necrotic. However, sometimes there is vital, inflamed pulp and histologically normal radicular pulp with radiographic evidence of periradicular inflammation. Although it has not been demonstrated experimentally, irritating factors must diffuse from the coronal tissues, pass through the radicular pulp, and elicit a periradicular inflammatory response with reactive bone resorption. This clinical entity is usually seen in children, teenagers, or young adults (Figure 4-78) and can present a diagnostic puzzle.[355]

Inflammatory Resorption

The opposite response to formation of dentin (resorption of dentin) may occur. The term internal or intracanal resorption is applied to the destruction of predentin and dentin. It is insidious, usually asymptomatic, and unidentifiable on radiographs until the lesion has progressed considerably (Figure 4-79 and 4-80). It may begin in the pulp chamber or the root canal. If allowed to continue untreated, it can perforate either above bone or into the periodontal ligament within bone. Sometimes it is impossible to say with accuracy that the resorption was not originally external. Regardless of the site of initial resorption, such communication of the pulp and periodontium creates severe, irreversible pathosis (Figure 4-81).

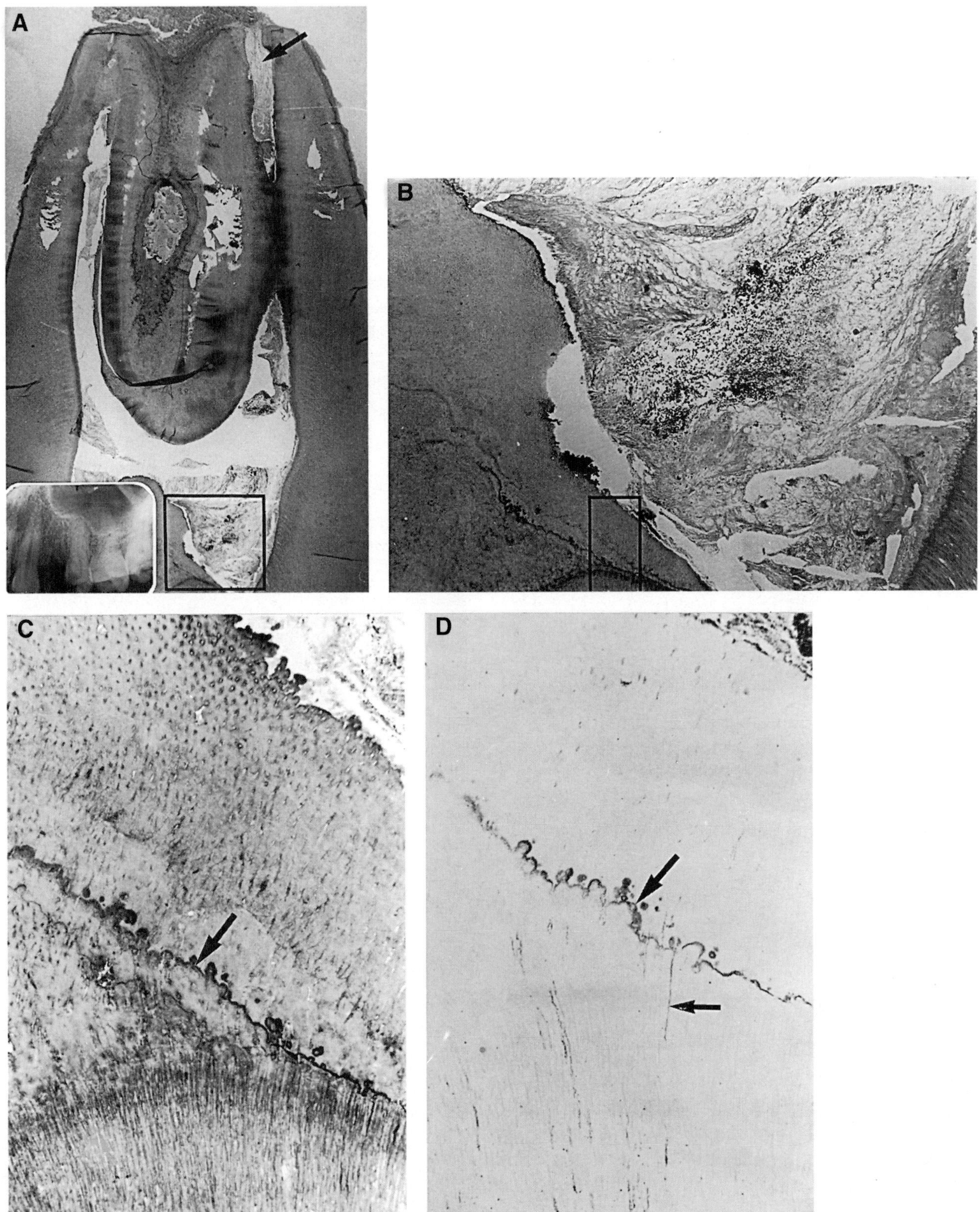

Figure 4-75 A, Pulp necrosis. The pulp of a maxillary premolar has undergone necrosis, although an area of vitality persists near the apex in one canal (**arrow**). Note the periradicular abscess, although the radiograph of this tooth (**lower left**) demonstrates no periradicular bony changes. B, Region indicated by box in A. Pulp horn contains amorphous debris and concentration of bacteria. C, Region indicated by box in B. **Arrow** indicates the so-called calciotraumatic line separating regular tubular dentin from irregular, less tubular, irritation dentin. D, Histologic section adjacent to C, stained for bacteria. Bacteria, streaming down tubules (**small arrow**), are concentrated in the calciotraumatic line (**large arrow**). Bacteria are less numerous in underlying irritation dentin.

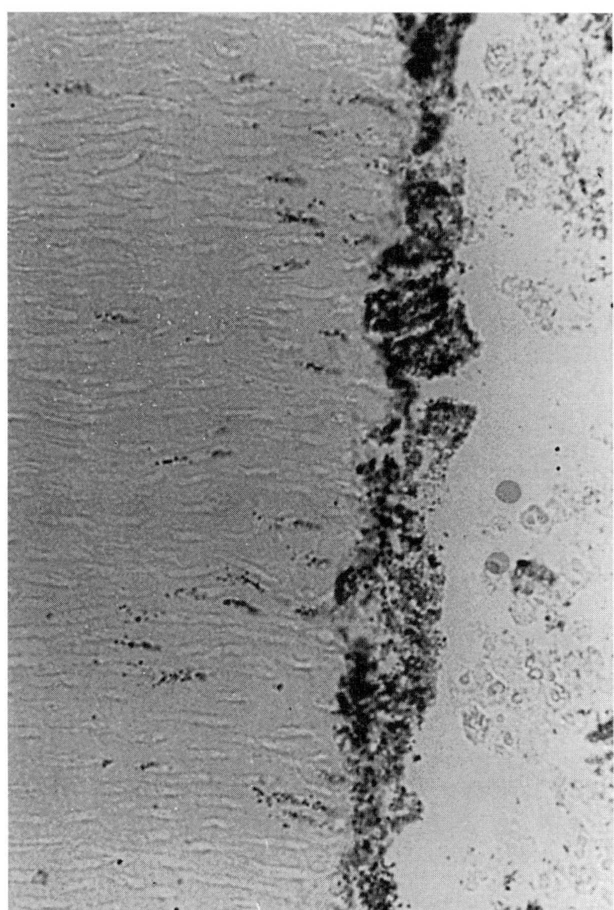

Figure 4-76 Bacterial penetration into tubules (**left**). Their source is masses of bacteria in the canal space (**right**).

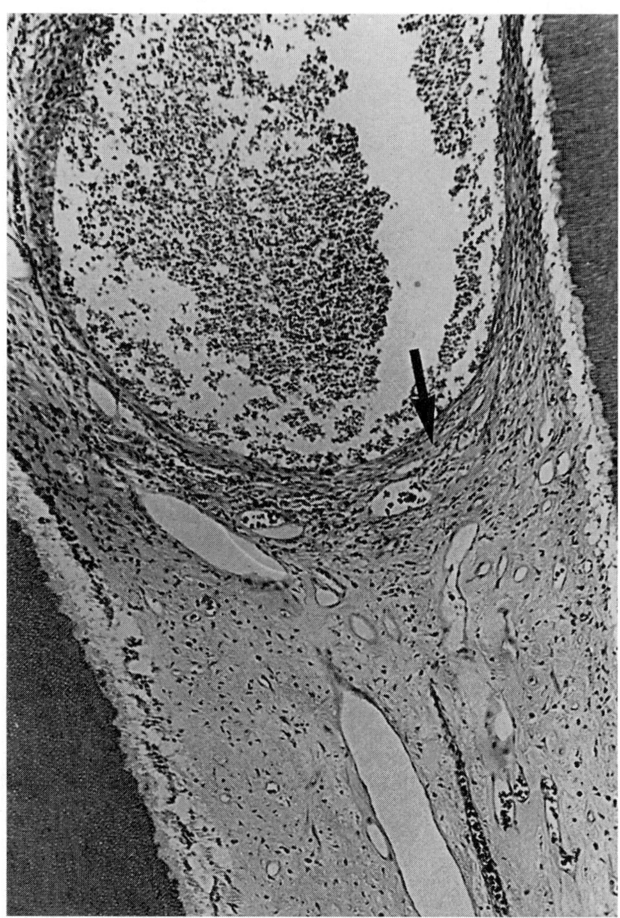

Figure 4-77 Narrow zone of response adjacent to region of liquefaction necrosis. Collagen is arranged peripherally (**arrow**) around the abscess, separating this irritant from underlying vital pulp tissue. Inflammatory response in this tissue is surprisingly mild, with few scattered cells.

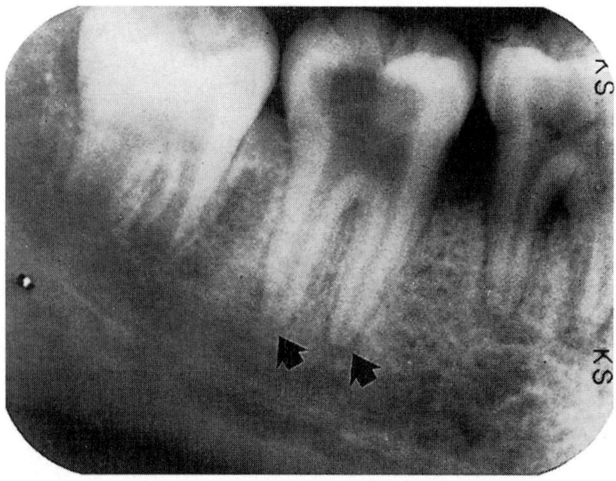

Figure 4-78 A **vital** coronal pulp and associated periradicular resorptive lesions (**arrows**), most likely to occur in young persons, as demonstrated by a newly erupted, but cariously involved, second molar in a 15-year-old patient. Usually, a periradicular lesion is associated with necrotic pulp, as is the case on the **first** molar.

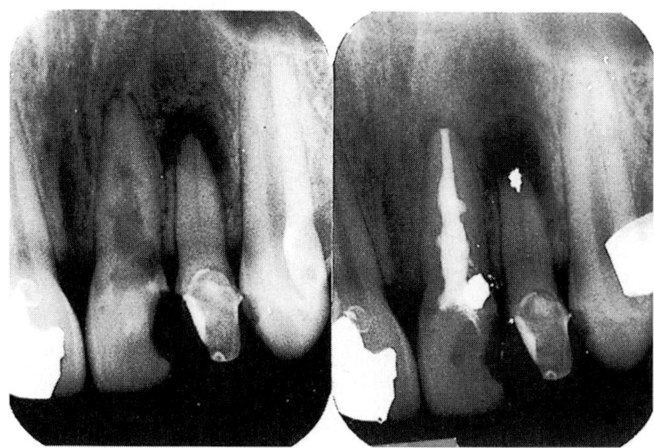

Figure 4-79 Differing pulp responses to trauma. Both incisors suffered impact as well as caries and restorative trauma. It is not clear why one pulp may react with extensive internal resorption and why another pulp may form calcifications. Treatment was successful in the central incisor but unsuccessful in the lateral incisor; the "cork-in-a-sewer" retrofilling failed.

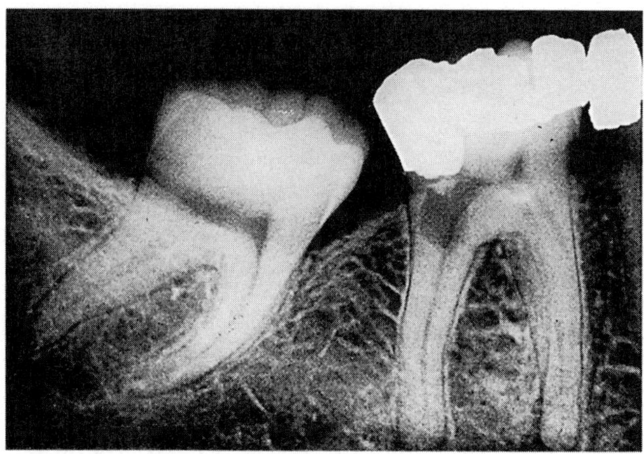

Figure 4-80 Advanced internal resorption of a first molar. The process spread distally from the pulp to undermine restoration and perforate externally. The pulp is now necrotic, as evidenced by inflammatory lesion at apex. The cause of internal resorption may be from deep caries, pulp cap, or trauma from extraction of the second molar.

Serial sectioning of many teeth in the early stages of pulp disease has shown that internal resorption frequently occurs in inflamed pulps. Also, resorption and apposition of dentin on the pulp wall are usually related to existent pulpitis[356, 357] and the presence of bacteria.[358] A history of trauma from either a blow or restorative procedures can sometimes be implicated, but the precise etiology is unknown. Resorption often moves swiftly but sometimes appears to arrest after a time and be quiescent. Also, the resorptive process stops when the pulp becomes necrotic.

Internal (inflammatory) resorption is partially the work of specialized multinucleated giant cells.[359,360] These cells are identical to osteoclasts,[361] but because they are resorbing dentin, they are sometimes termed "dentinoclasts."[362–364] They are found in close apposition to the dentin surface and often within "bays" of their own creation. The lost predentin and dentin are replaced by chronic inflammatory tissue or occasionally by apposition of a hard tissue that looks like bone. Because the process of internal resorption is frequently intermittent, repair may follow resorption. During the lull in resorption, cells differentiate from the mesenchymal cells of the pulp and produce tissue resembling both dentin and bone. Clinicians should be aware that, once internal resorption is visible on radiographs or can be seen as a pink area through the intact enamel, it is considered a form of **irreversible pulpitis**. Radiographic evidence of internal resorption requires root canal therapy to stop the process. For additional information on internal resorption, see chapter 6.

PULPAL SEQUELAE TO IMPACT TRAUMA

Pulpal responses to trauma can be categorized as repair, calcification, resorption, or necrosis. The response depends on type, duration, severity, and susceptibility of the pulp to injury. The result may be adaptation, reversible injury, or death.[365] It is not understood at present how a particular traumatic injury may produce pulpal calcification in one tooth, whereas the adjacent tooth may respond with internal inflammatory resorption. Each process can be produced by trauma (Figure 4-82 and 4-83).

Trauma to teeth from a sudden impact (eg, a blow or a missile) can produce any one, or a combination, of the injuries classified by the World Health Organization (see chapter 15). Those associated with pulp hypoxia are the luxation injuries, avulsions, and alveolar fractures involving tooth sockets. Several investigators[366-369] have shown the association of pulp necrosis to these injuries.

Pulp hypoxia is produced by damage to the vessels entering the apical root canal system. With minimal collateral circulation, the pulp will soon show the effects of impaired blood flow.[370]

Damage can range from compressing and crushing to complete severing of vessels entering the apical foramina. Reduced or inadequate blood flow causes ischemia, leading to an infarct of the pulp. An infarct is defined as tissue death owing to hypoxia. Pulp tissue apparently has the ability to survive for a relatively long period of time without oxygen,[370] which is probably related to the availability of adenosine triphosphate (ATP). When cellular depletion of ATP occurs, the cell presumably ceases to function, and cell death occurs.[365] There is no detectable sharp line between reversible

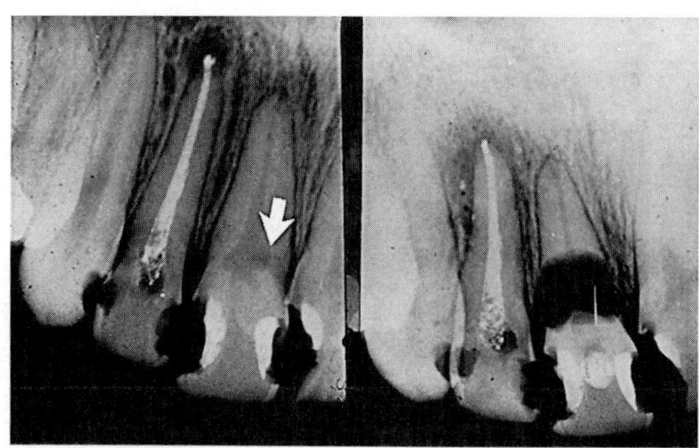

Figure 4-81 Early internal resorption (**arrow**) of a maxillary central incisor. Presumably, pulpitis preceded resorption. Extensive destruction was seen in 6 months. The initial limited area of resorption changed to a massive lesion, virtually severing the crown from roots.

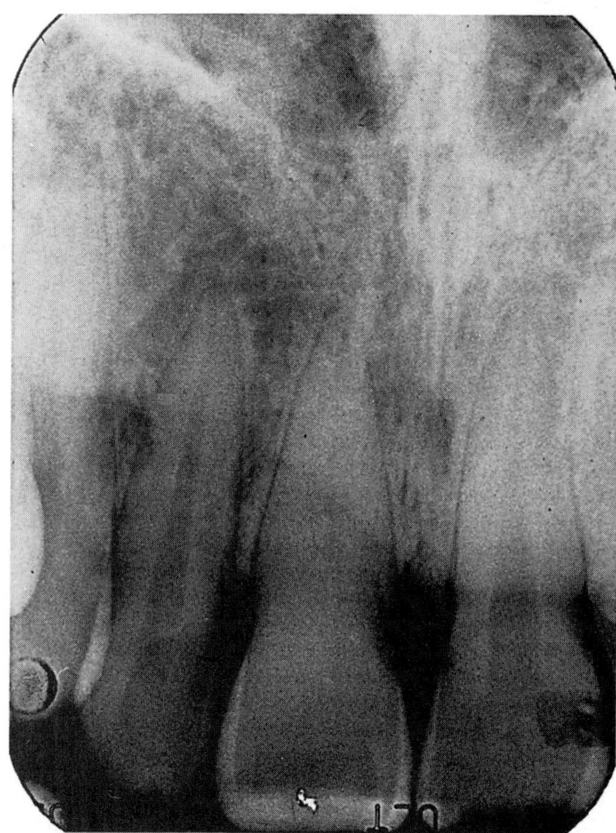

Figure 4-82 Radiograph of a maxillary right central incisor. The pulp chamber and canal have been obliterated with irritation dentin (calcific metamorphosis). (Courtesy of Dr. James Simon.)

and irreversible injury of a cell. However, three events are recognized as being associated with cell death: depletion of ATP, damage to the cell membrane, and an influx of calcium into the cell, causing disruption of function. Any one or all three—and probably additional—factors may be involved.

Cell death (and pulp tissue death) can be recognized histologically only after necrotic changes have taken place. This can be understood in the light of how one examines cells and tissues histologically. From biopsy and before necrosis occurs, tissues are fixed chemically, and what is seen under the microscope is presumably the way cells appear when alive. Thus, tissue sections are "dead" but not "necrotic" unless the sample is from already necrotic tissue.

Necrosis of the infarcted pulp begins soon after tissue death occurs (Figure 4-84).[370] First, lactic acid accumulates, lowering the pH, which, in turn, activates intracellular lysosomes to digest the cell. However, enzymatic digestion is not a major occurrence in necrosis owing to hypoxia. This is in contrast to tissue death, in which bacteria and inflammatory cells are present. In such cases, heterolytic enzymatic digestion predominates, resulting in liquefaction necrosis and pus. In hypoxic tissue death, coagulation necrosis occurs as a result of protein denaturation. The basic outline of the coagulated cell will be preserved for some time. This occurs because the acidosis in the cell causes denaturation of the structural proteins and the enzymatic proteins, thereby blocking proteolysis. When coagulation necrosis occurs elsewhere in the body, the infarct will eventually be removed by scavenger cells, but not in the pulp. Thus, an infarcted pulp may remain unchanged for a long time until bacteria enter the pulp space.[371]

When pulp tissue that has undergone coagulation necrosis is removed, it has the shape and form of a pulp but does not bleed. This has been called a "fibrotic pulp" or a "collagen skeleton." The collagen remains fibrotic, but there are no cells, nerves, or blood vessels (Figure 4-85 and 4-86).

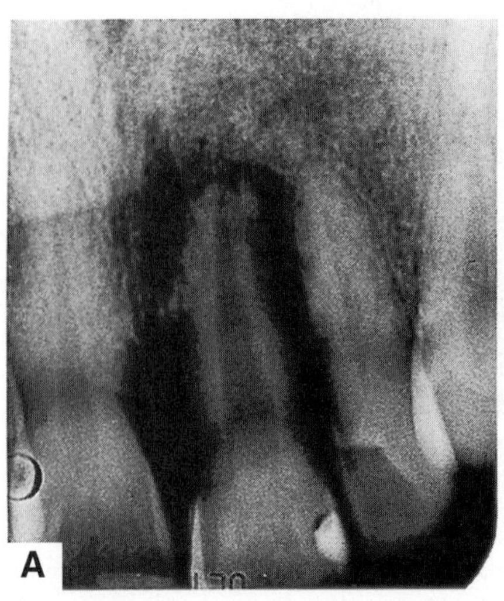

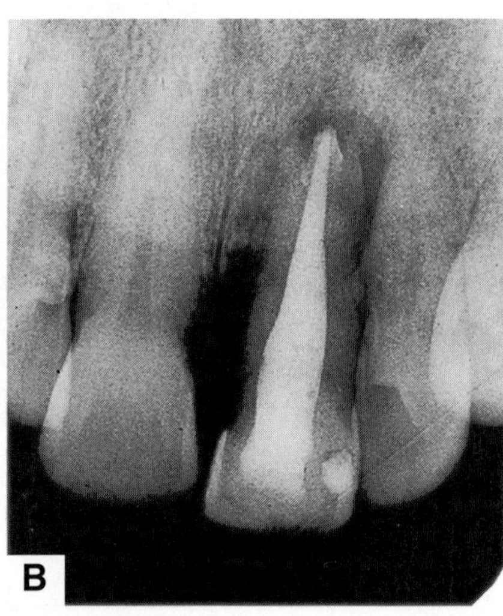

Figure 4-83 A, Radiograph of a maxillary left central incisor. The canal is large because the trauma stopped root development when the pulp became necrotic. Note inflammatory resorption of the apex. B, After endodontic therapy. (Courtesy of Dr. James Simon.)

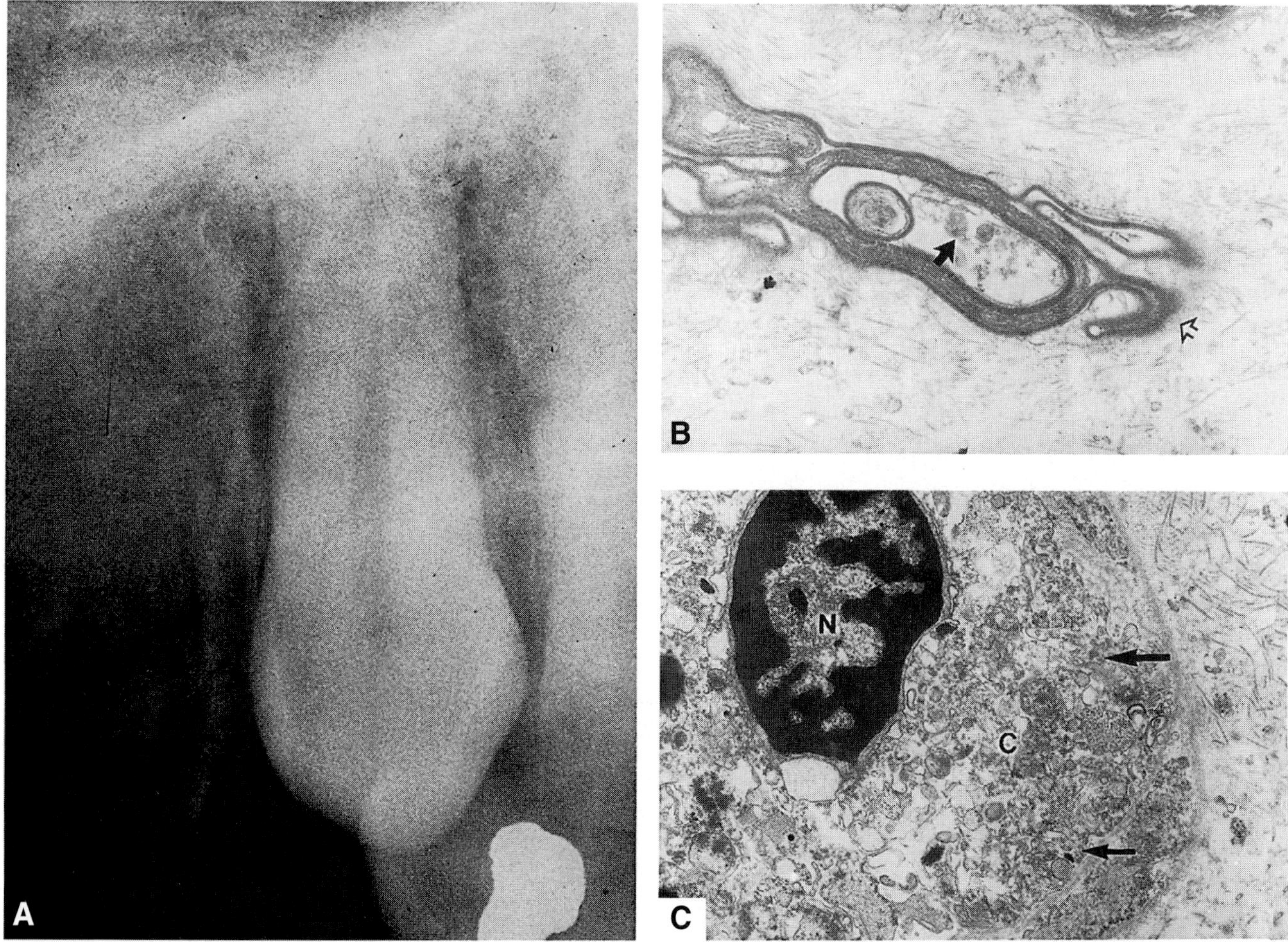

Figure 4-84 **A,** Radiograph of canine intruded by trauma. **B,** Effect of hypoxia on pulp owing to intrusion. Myelinated nerve showing vacuolization of axon (**closed arrow**), disruption and smudging of myelin sheath (**open arrow**), and loss of cellular detail. C, Loss of cellular detail in the nucleus (N) and cytoplasm (C). Note cell clumping in nucleus and loss of organelles with rupture of lysosome (**arrow**) in cytoplasm. (Courtesy of Dr. James Simon.)

As cell necrosis (both coagulation and liquefaction necrosis) progresses, histologic changes occur in the nucleus and the cytoplasm.[372–374] The nucleus undergoes karyolysis, pyknosis, and karyorrhexis. Karyolysis is progressive fading of the nucleus. Pyknosis describes gradual shrinkage, and karyorrhexis is nuclear fragmentation, the end result being disappearance of the nucleus. The process is much slower in coagulation than in liquefaction necrosis.

The cytoplasm of the cell undergoing necrosis shows signs of clumping owing to denaturation of cytoplasmic proteins. The histologic appearance is one of an acidophilic, granular, opaque mass. As the necrotic process continues, the pulp tissue gradually loses its recognized morphology and ends up as a diffuse tissue mass containing the outline of cells and remnants of fibers, vessel walls, and nerves.[371]

Since the blood supply to the pulp is compromised and possibly absent, the removal of the necrotic pulp by phagocytic cells is difficult if not impossible. That leaves two possible sequelae: dystrophic calcification at the apical openings entombing the necrotic pulp indefinitely or invasion by bacteria, resulting in a gangrenous necrosis. This term is an old one, but it describes the result of bacterial invasion of tissue that died secondary to hypoxia— a similar situation to that seen in gangrene of an extremity such as a leg from coagulation necrosis owing to impaired circulation followed by bacterial ingrowth into the dead tissue.

Dystrophic calcification may occur at the apical canal openings, where coagulation necrosis attracts calcium salts from the surrounding environment. This is similar to calcification subjacent to layers of coagulation necrosis produced by caustic pulp-capping agents.

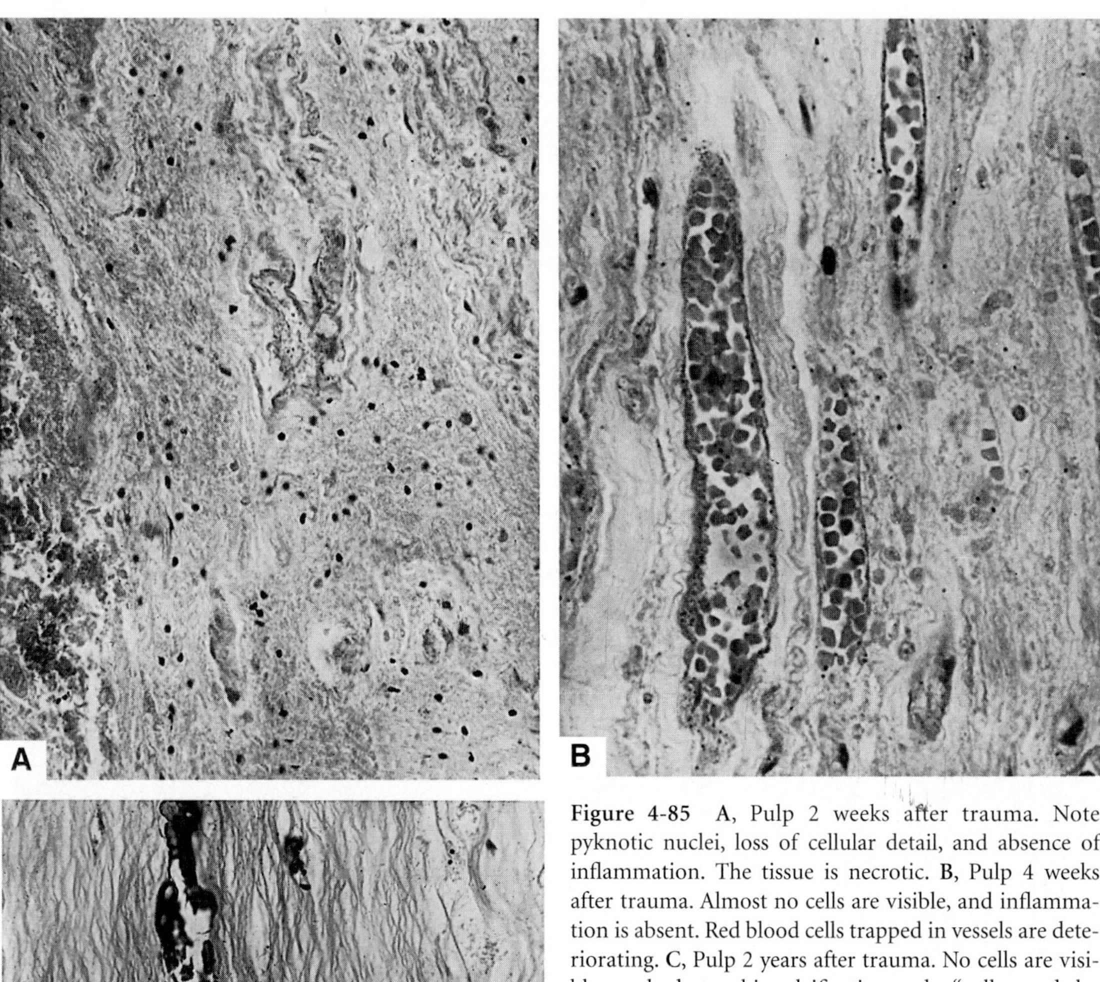

Figure 4-85 **A**, Pulp 2 weeks after trauma. Note pyknotic nuclei, loss of cellular detail, and absence of inflammation. The tissue is necrotic. **B**, Pulp 4 weeks after trauma. Almost no cells are visible, and inflammation is absent. Red blood cells trapped in vessels are deteriorating. **C**, Pulp 2 years after trauma. No cells are visible—only dystrophic calcification and a "collagen skeleton." (Courtesy of Dr. James Simon.)

Gangrenous necrosis of the pulp results from bacteria entering the pulp space containing coagulation necrotic tissue. Bacterial invasion cannot occur by anachoresis because the blood circulation to the pulp is now nonexistent; it must occur through the open apex or through pathways in the hard tissues of the tooth. Also, tooth infractions, where cracks extend from the enamel or cementum through dentin, would be another possible pathway. Another may be lateral canals, either already exposed to the oral environment by periodontal disease or subsequently opened by scaling procedures. It is also possible that bacteria may enter through exposed dentinal tubules. With the tubules either empty or containing necrotic odontoblastic processes, bacteria can grow in a pulpal direction and toward a ready food source.

Once bacteria have invaded the necrotic pulp, they release enzymes to break down the necrotic tissue for assimilation of the available nutrients; by the process of heterolysis, liquefaction (also called "wet gangrene") occurs. This activity produces an abundance of by-products, which eventually leak into periradicular tissues, causing inflammatory and immunologic reactions. These are commonly referred to as acute exacerbations with pain and swelling: a periradicular abscess. If the egress is slow, the reaction may be more gradual and chronic, resulting in an abscess that drains through a fistulous tract.

The events involved in pulpal infarcts owing to hypoxia have been described. The clinical implication is that coagulation necrosis may go undetected for various lengths of time, but when bacteria gain access to

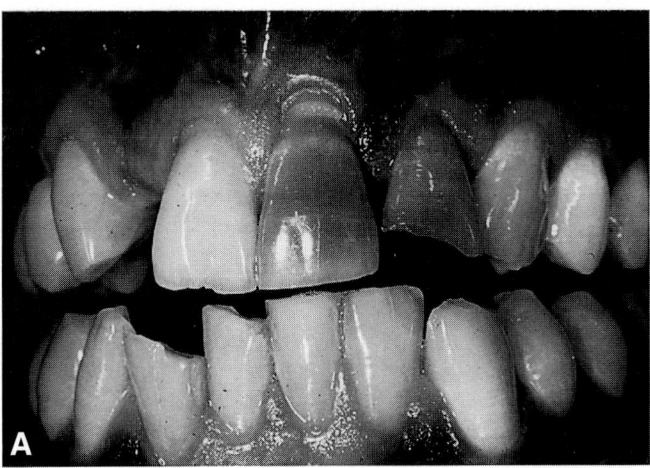

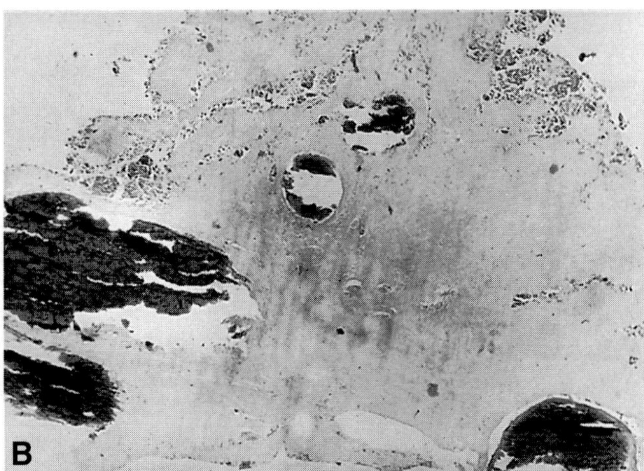

Figure 4-86 **A**, Discolored left central and lateral incisors. The patient reported accidental trauma 20 years earlier. **B**, Pulp tissue from the lateral incisor appeared fibrotic. Histologic picture shows uniformly amorphous tissue with dystrophic calcification. (Courtesy of Dr. James Simon.)

this necrotic pulp, the potential for a flare-up is strong. Since it is not predictable when and if such an event will occur, the necrotic pulp should be removed even in the absence of symptoms.

The end result of inflammatory disease is necrosis of the pulpal tissue. The end result of noninflammatory oxygen deprivation is necrosis or a noncellular collagen skeleton replacing the vital cellular pulp tissue. Extirpation of the necrotic tissue is necessary in either pathologic process.

REFERENCES

1. Langeland K. Histologic evaluation of pulp reactions to operative procedures. Oral Surg 1959;12:1235.
2. Brännström M, Lind PO. Pulpal response to early caries. J Dent Res 1965;44:1045.
3. Brännström M, et al. Invasion of microorganisms and some structural changes in incipient enamel caries. Caries Res 1980;14:276.
4. Douglass CW, et al. Clinical efficacy of dental radiographs in the detection of dental caries and periodontal diseases. Oral Surg 1986;63:330.
5. Seltzer S, Bender IB, Kaufman IJ. Histologic changes in dental pulps of dogs and monkeys following application of pressure, drugs and microorganisms on prepared cavities. Part II. Changes observable more than one month after application of traumatic agents. Oral Surg 1961;14:856.
6. Skogedal O, Tronstad L. An attempt to correlate dentin, and pulp changes in human carious teeth. Oral Surg 1977;43:135.
7. Bergenholtz G, Lindhe J. Effect of soluble plaque factors on inflammatory reactions in the dental pulp. Scand J Dent Res 1975;83:153.
8. Langeland K. Tissue changes in the dental pulp. Odont Tidskr 1957;65:239.
9. Mjör IA, Tronstad L. Experimentally produced pulpitis. Oral Surg 1972;34:102.
10. Reeves R, Stanley HR. The relationship of bacterial penetration and pulpal pathosis in carious teeth. Oral Surg 1966;22:59.
11. Trowbridge HO. Pathogenesis of pulpitis resulting from dental caries. JOE 1981;7:52.
12. Mjör IA. Bacteria in experimentally infected cavity preparations. Scand J Dent Res 1977;85:599.
13. Massler M, Pawlak J. The affected and infected pulp. Oral Surg 1977;43:929.
14. MacGregor AB. The position and extent of acid in the caries process. Arch Oral Biol 1961;4:86.
15. Langeland K. Management of the inflamed pulp associated with deep carious lesions. JOE 1981;7:169.
16. Paterson RC, Pountney SK. Pulp response to dental caries induced by *Streptococcus mutans.* Oral Surg 1982;53:88.
17. Watts A, Paterson RC. Migration of materials and microorganisms in the dental pulp of dogs and rats. JOE 1982;8:53.
18. Paterson RC, Watts A. Further studies on the exposed germ-free dental pulp. Int Endondont J 1987;20:112.
19. Paterson RC, Pountney SK. The response of the dental pulp to mechanical exposure in gnotobiotic rats monoinfected with a strain of *Streptococcus mutans.* Int Endodont J 1987;20:159.
20. Paterson RC, Pountney SK. Pulp response to *Streptococcus mutans.* Oral Surg 1987;64:339.
21. Seltzer S. Discussion of vascular permeability and other factors in the modulation of the inflammatory response. JOE 1977;3:214.
22. Olgart L, Brännström M, Johnson G. Invasion of bacteria into dentinal tubules. Acta Odontol Scand 1974;32:61.
23. Michelich VJ, Schuster GS, Pashley DH. Bacterial penetration of human dentin in vitro. J Dent Res 1980;59:2398.
24. Meryon SD, Jakreman KJ, Browne RM. Penetration in vitro of human and ferret dentine by three bacterial species in relation to their potential role in pulpal inflammation. Int Endodont J 1986;19:213.
25. Canby CP, Burnett GW. Clinical management of deep carious lesions. Oral Surg 1963;16:999.
26. Muntz JA, Dorfman A, Stephan RM. In vitro studies of sterilization of carious dentin. I. Evaluation of germicides. J Am Dent Assoc 1943;30:1893.
27. Seltzer S, Bender IB, Ziontz M. The dynamics of pulp inflammation: correlations between diagnostic data and actual histologic findings in the pulp. Oral Surg 1963;16:969.

28. Wennberg A, Mjör IA, Heide S. Rate of formation of regular and irregular secondary dentin formation in monkey teeth. Oral Surg 1982;54:232.
29. Lervik T, Mjör IA. Evaluation of techniques for the induction of pulpitis. J Biol Buccale 1977;5:137.
30. Langeland K, Tobon G, Langeland LK. The effect of corticosteroids on the dental pulp. In: Grossman LI, editor. Fourth International Conference on Endodontics. Philadelphia: University of Pennsylvania Press; 1968. p. 15.
31. Taintor JF, Biesterfeld RC, Langeland K. Irritational or reparative dentin. Oral Surg 1981;51:442.
32. Ivanovic V, Santini A. Rate of formation of tertiary dentin in dogs' teeth in response to lining materials. Oral Surg 1989;67:684.
33. Ritchey B, Mendenhall R, Orban B. Pulpitis resulting from incomplete tooth fracture. Oral Surg 1957;10:665.
34. Grossman LI. Origin of microorganisms in traumatized, pulpless, sound teeth. J Dent Res 1967;46:552.
35. Oehlers FA. *Dens invaginatus.* Variations of the invagination process and associated crown forms. Oral Surg 1957; 10:1204.
36. Bhaskar SN. Synopsis of oral pathology. St. Louis: CV Mosby; 1977.
37. Conklin WW. Bilateral *dens invaginatus* in the mandibular incisor region. Oral Surg 1978;45:905.
38. Angsburger RA, Brandebura J. Bilateral *dens invaginatus* with associated radicular cysts. Oral Surg 1978;46:260.
39. Burton DJ, et al.: Multiple bilateral *dens in dente* as a factor in the etiology of multiple periradicular lesions. Oral Surg 1980;49:496.
40. Conklin WW. *Dens in dente* as a factor in the etiology of a radicular cyst. Oral Surg 1962;15:588.
41. Poyton GH, Morgan GA. *Dens in dente.* Dent Radiogr Photogr 1966;39:27.
42. Amos EE. Incidence of the small *dens in dente.* J Am Dent Assoc 1955;51:31.
43. Gotoh T, et al. Clinical and radiographic study of *dens invaginatus.* Oral Surg 1979;48:88.
44. Kato K. Contributions to the knowledge concerning the cone-shaped supernumerary cusp in the center of the occlusal surface on the premolars of Japanese. Nippon Skika Gaku Eassi 1937;30:23.
45. Lau TC. Odontogenesis of the axial cone type. Br Dent J 1955;99:219.
46. Merrill RG. Occlusal anomalous tubercles on biscuspids of Alaskan Eskimos and Indians [thesis]. Univ. of Washington; 1959.
47. Merrill RG. Occlusal anomalous tubercles on bicuspids of Alaskan Eskimos and Indians. Oral Surg 1964;17:484.
48. Yip WK. The prevalence of *dens evaginatus.* Oral Surg 1974;38:90.
49. Senia ES, Regezi JA. *Dens evaginatus* in the etiology of bilateral pathologic involvement of caries-free premolars. Oral Surg 1974;38:465.
50. Sykaras SN. Occlusal anomalous tubercle on premolars of a Greek girl. Oral Surg 1974;38:88.
51. Palmer ME. Case reports of evaginated odontomes in Caucasians. Oral Surg 1973;35:772.
52. Lin LM, Chance K, Skribner J, Langeland K. *Dens evaginatus*: a case report. Oral Surg 1987;63:86.
53. Gotoh T, et al. Clinical and radiographic study of *dens evaginatus.* Dentomaxillofac Radiol 1979;8:78.
54. Stewart RE, et al. *Dens evaginatus* (tuberculated cusps): genetic and treatment considerations. Oral Surg 1978;46:831.
55. Augsburger RA, Wong MT. Pulp management in *dens evaginatus.* JOE 1996;22:323.
56. August DS. The radicular lingual groove: an overlooked differential diagnosis. J Am Dent Assoc 1978;96:1037.
57. Zhirong G, et al. Scanning electron microscopic investigation of maxillary lateral incisors with a radicular lingual groove. Oral Surg 1989;68:462.
58. Everett F, Kramer G. The disto-lingual groove in the maxillary lateral incisor: a periodontal hazard. J Periodontol 1972;43:352.
59. Withers J, et al. The relationship of palatogingival grooves in localized periodontal disease. J Periodontol 1981;52:41.
60. Robison SF, Cooley RL. Palatogingival groove lesions: recognition and treatment. Gen Dent 1988;36:340.
61. Simon J, Glick DH, Frank AL. Predictable endodontic and periodontic failures as a result of radicular anomalies. Oral Surg 1971;37:823.
62. Massler M. Cervical caries in the very elderly. Presented at the Alpha Omega Convention, Boston, December, 1985.
63. Seltzer S, Bender IB, Ziontz M. The dynamics of pulp inflammation: correlation between diagnostic data and actual histologic findings in the pulp. Oral Surg 1963;16:846.
64. Mazur B, Massler M. Influence of periodontal disease on the dental pulp. Oral Surg 1964;17:592.
65. Johnston HB, Orban B. Interradicular pathology as related to accessory root canals. JOE 1948;3:21.
66. Langeland K, Rodrigues H, Dowden W. Peridontal disease, bacteria, and pulpal histopathology. Oral Surg 1974;37:257.
67. Saglie R, Newman MG, Carranza FA Jr, Pattison GL. Bacterial invasion of gingiva in advanced periodontitis in humans. J Periodontol 1982;53:217.
68. Robinson HBG, Boling L. The anchoretic effect in pulpitis. I. Bacteriologic studies. J Am Dent Assoc 1941;28:265.
69. MacDonald JB, Hare GC, Wood AWS. The bacteriologic status of the pulp chambers in the intact teeth found to be nonvital following trauma. Oral Surg 1957;10:318.
70. Tziafas D. Experimental bacterial anachoresis in dog dental pulps capped with calcium hydroxide. JOE 1989;15:591.
71. Ingle JI. Alveolar osteoporosis and pulpal death associated with compulsive bruxism. Oral Surg 1960;13:1371.
72. Natkin E, Ingle JI. A further report on alveolar osteoporosis and pulpal death associated with compulsive bruxism. J Am Soc Periodont 1963;1:360.
73. Cooke HG. Reversible pulpitis with etiology of bruxism. JOE 1982;8:280.
74. Landay MA, Seltzer S. The effects of excessive occlusal force on the pulp. Oral Surg 1971;32:623.
75. Cottone JA. Palm Springs Seminar, January 1990.
76. Sognnaes RF, Wolcott RB, Xhonga FA. Dental erosion. J Am Dent Assoc 1972;84:571.
77. Grippo JO. Abfractions: a new classification of hard tissue lesions of teeth. J Esthet Dent 1991;3:14.
78. Meister F, Braun RJ, Gerstein H. Endodontic involvement resulting from dental abrasion or erosion. J Am Dent Assoc 1980;101:651.
79. Kramer IRH. Pulp changes of non-bacterial origin. Int Dent J 1959;9:435.
80. Stanley HR, Swerdlow H. Reaction of the human pulp to cavity preparation: results produced by eight different operative technics. J Am Dent Assoc 1959;58:49.

81. Brännström M. Cavity preparation and the pulp. Dent Prog 1961;2:4.
82. Zach L, Cohen G. Thermogenesis in operative techniques. Comparisons of four methods. J Prosthet Dent 1962;12:977.
83. Swerdlow H, Stanley HR. Higher speeds in dentistry. J District Columbia Dent 1959;34:4.
84. Vaughn RC, Peyton FA. The influence of rotational speed on temperature rise during cavity preparation. J Dent Res 1951;30:737.
85. Peyton FA, Henry EE. The effect of high speed burs, diamond instruments and air abrasives in cutting tooth tissue. J Am Dent Assoc 1954;49:426.
86. Stanley HR. Importance of the leukocyte to dental health. JOE 1977;3:334.
87. Zach L. Pulp lability and repair: effect of restorative procedures. Oral Surg 1972;33:111.
88. Langeland K, Langeland L. Pulp reactions to crown preparation, impression, temporary crown fixation, and permanent cementation. J Prosthet Dent 1965;15:129.
89. Stanley HR, Swerdlow H. Aspiration of cells into dentinal tubules? Oral Surg 1958;11:1007.
90. Ostrom CA. Pulp damage by induced inflammation. Dent Prog 1963;3:207.
91. Goodacre C. Principles of tooth preparation. Presented at the American Academy of Fixed Prosthodontics, Chicago, IL, February 19, 1999.
92. Ottl P, Lauer HC. Temperature response in the pulpal chamber during ultrahigh speed tooth preparation with diamond burs of different grit. J Prosthet Dent 1998;80:12.
93. Seelig A, Lefkowitz W. Pulp response to filling materials. N Y State Dent J 1950;16:540.
94. Searls JC. Radioautographic evaluation of changes induced in the rat incisor by high-speed cavity preparation. J Dent Res 1975;54:174.
95. Sproles RA. Coronal pulp anatomy [thesis]. Los Angeles: Univ. of Southern California; 1975.
96. Stambaugh RV, Wittrock JW. The relationship of the pulp chamber to the external surface of the tooth. J Prosthet Dent 1977;37:537.
97. Brännström M. Dentinal and pulpal response. II. Application of an air stream to exposed dentin. Short observation period. Acta Odontol Scand 1960;18:17.
98. Brännström M. Dentinal and pulpal response. III. Application of an air stream to exposed dentin. Long observation period. In: Anderson DJ, editor. Sensory mechanisms in dentine. New York: Macmillan; 1963. p. 235–52.
99. Langeland K. Histologic evaluation of pulp reactions to operative procedures. Oral Surg 1959;12:1357.
100. Orban B. Migration of leukocytes into the dentinal tubules. J Am Dent Assoc 1940;27:239.
101. Informetrics, National Research Center, Consumable Products Tracking Study. January 1989.
102. Webb EL, et al. Tooth crazing associated with threaded pins: a 3-dimensionable model. J Prosthet Dent 1989;61:624.
103. Suzuki M, Goto G, Jordan RE. Pulpal response to pin placement. J Am Dent Assoc 1973;87:636.
104. James VE, Schour I. Early dentinal and pulpal changes following cavity preparations and filling materials in dogs. Oral Surg 1955;8:1305.
105. Swerdlow H, Stanley HR. Response of the human dental pulp to amalgam restorations. Oral Surg 1962;15:499.
106. Felton D, et al. Long term effects of crown preparation on pulp vitality [abstract]. JDR 1989;68:1009.
107. Tjan AHL, et al. Temperature rise in the pulp chamber during fabrication of provisional crowns. J Prosthet Dent 1989;62:622.
108. Bohannan HM, Abrams L. Intentional vital pulp extirpation in periodontal prosthesis. J Prosthet Dent 1961;11:781.
109. Abou-Raas M. The elimination of tetracycline discoloration by intentional endodontics and internal bleaching. JOE 1982;8:101.
110. Hamersky PA, et al. The effect of orthodontic force application on the pulpal tissue respiration rate in the human premolar. Am J Orthodont 1980;77:368.
111. Stenvik A, McClugage SG. The effect of experimental tooth intrusion on pulp and dentin. Oral Surg 1971;32:639.
112. Guevara JJ, McClugage SG. Effects of intrusive forces upon the microvasculature of the dental pulp. Angle Orthodont 1980;50:129.
113. Hattler AB, Listgarten MA. Pulpal response to root planing in a rat model. JOE 1984;10:471.
114. Robertson PB, Luscher B, Spångberg LS, Levy BM. Pulpal and periodontal effects of electrosurgery involving cervical metallic restorations. Oral Surg 1978;46:702.
115. Krejci RF, et al. The effects of electrosurgery on dog pulps under cervical metallic restorations. Oral Surg 1982;54:575.
116. Adrian JC, Bernier JL, Sprague WG. Laser and the dental pulp. J Am Dent Assoc 1971;83:113.
117. Adrian JC. Pulp effects of neodymium laser. Oral Surg 1977;44:301.
118. Melcer J, Chaumette MT, Melcer F, et al. Preliminary report on the effect of the CO_2 laser beam on the dental pulp of the *Macaca mulatta* primate and the beagle dog. JOE 1985;11:1.
119. Powell GL, et al. Pulpal response to irradiation of enamel with continuous wave CO_2 laser. JOE 1989;15:581.
120. Miserendino LJ, et al. Thermal effects of continuous wave CO_2 laser exposure on human teeth: an in vivo study. JOE 1989;15:302.
121. Bonin P, et al. Dentinal permeability of the dog canine after exposure of a cervical cavity to the beam of a CO_2 laser. JOE 1991;17:116.
122. Keyes G, Hildebrand K. Successful surgical endodontics for benign cementoblastoma. JOE 1987;13:566.
123. Stabholz A, Friedman S, et al. Maintenance of pulp vitality following surgical removal of a symptomatic cementoma. JOE 1988;14:43.
124. Bell WH, et al. Bone healing and revascularization after total maxillary osteotomy. J Oral Surg 1975;33:253.
125. Pepersach WJ. Tooth vitality after alveolar segmental osteotomy. J Maxillofac Surg 1973;1:85.
126. Nanda R, Legan HL, Langeland K. Pulpal and radicular response to maxillary osteotomy in monkeys. Oral Surg 1982;53:624.
127. Ohzei H, Takahazshi S. Histological pulp changes in the dental osseous segment following anterior maxillary osteotomy. Bull Tokyo Dent Coll 1980;21:21.
128. Di S, Bell WH, et al. Long-term evaluation of human teeth after LeFort I osteotomy: a histologic and developmental study. Oral Surg 1988;65:379.
129. Lockhart PB, et al. Dental complications during and after tracheal intubation. J Am Dent Assoc 1986;112:480.

130. Zander HA. The reaction of dental pulps to silicate cements. J Am Dent Assoc 1946;33:1233.
131. Valcke CF, Cleaton-Jones PE, et al. The pulpal response to a direct filling resin without an inorganic filler: Isopast. J Oral Rehabil 1980;7:1.
132. James VE, Schour I. Early dentinal and pulpal changes following cavity preparation and filling materials in dogs. Oral Surg 1955;8:1305.
133. El-Kafrawy AH, Mitchell DF. Pulp reactions to open cavities later restored with silicate cement. J Dent Res 1977;85:575.
134. Skogedal O, Mjör IA. Pulp reactions to silicate cement in teeth with healing pulpitis. Scand J Dent Res 1977;85:575.
135. Tobias RS, Plant CG, Browne RM. Reduction in pulpal inflammation beneath surface-sealed silicates. Int Endodont J 1982;15:173.
136. Tobias RS, Plant CG, Browne RM. A comparative pulpal study of the irritant effects of silicate cements. Br Dent J 1981;150:119.
137. Brännström M, Olivera V. Bacteria and pulpal reactions under silicate cement restorations. J Prosthet Dent 1979;41:290.
138. Cox CF, et al. Biocompatibility of surface sealed dental materials against exposed pulps. J Prosthet Dent 1987;57:1.
139. Gurley WB, Van Huysen G. Histologic changes in teeth due to plastic filling materials. J Am Dent Assoc 1937;24:1806.
140. Massler M. Effects of filling materials on the pulp. N J Dent 1956;26:183.
141. Dubner R, Stanley HR. Reaction to the human pulp to temporary filling materials. Oral Surg 1962;15:1009.
142. Lervik T. The effect of zinc phosphate and carboxylate cements on the healing of experimentally induced pulpitis. Oral Surg 1978;45:123.
143. Brännström M, Nyborg H. Pulpal reactions to polycarboxylate and zinc phosphate cements used with inlays in deep cavity preparations. J Am Dent Assoc 1977;94:308.
144. Mjör IA. Histologic demonstration of bacterial subjacent to dental restorations. Scand J Dent Res 1977;85:169.
145. Das S. Effect of certain dental materials on human pulp in tissue culture. Oral Surg 1981;52:76.
146. Meryon SD, Jakeman KJ. The effects *in vitro* of zinc release from dental restorative materials. Int Endodont J 1985;18:191.
147. Meryon SD. An *in vitro* study of factors contributing to the blandness of zinc oxide-eugenol preparation *in vivo*. Int Endodont J 1988;21:200.
148. Brännström M, Nyborg H. Pulp reaction to a temporary zinc oxide/eugenol cement. J Prosthet Dent 1976;35:185.
149. Brännström M, Nordenvall KJ, Torstenson B. Pulpal reaction to IRM cement: an intermediate restorative material containing eugenol. J Dent Child 1981; July-Aug p. 259.
150. Cook DJ, Taylor PP. Tissue reactions to improved zinc oxide-eugenol cements. J Dent Child 1973;40:199.
151. Provant DR, Adrian JC. Dental pulp reaction to Cavit temporary filling materials. Oral Surg 1978;45:305.
152. Langeland LK, Walton RE, Rodrigues HH et al. Pulp response to polycarboxylate and composite resin [abstract]. J Dent Res 1972; [abstract 383].
153. Mjör IA, Eriksen HM, Haugen E, Skogedal O. Biologic assessment of copper-containing amalgams. Int Dent J 1977;27:333.
154. Skogedal O, Mjör IA. Pulpal response to dental amalgams. Scand J Dent Res 1979;87:346.
155. Leirskar J, Helgeland K. Mechanism of toxicity of dental materials. Int Endodont J 1981;14:42.
156. Omnell KA. Electrolytic precipitation of zinc carbonate in the jaw. Oral Surg 1959;12:846.
157. Mjör IA, Lervik T. Pulp healing subjacent to corticosteroid covered and amalgam covered dentin. Oral Surg 1975;40:789.
158. Möller B. Reaction of the human dental pulp to silver amalgam restorations. Acta Odontol Scand 1975;33:233.
159. Tobias RS, Plant CG, Browne RM. A comparative study of two dental amalgam alloys. Int Endodont J 1987;20:8.
160. Seelig A. The effect of direct filling resins of the tooth pulp. J Am Dent Assoc 1952;44:261.
161. Lefowitz W, Seelig A, Zachinsky L. Pulp response to a self-curing acrylic filling material. N Y State Dent J 1949;15:376.
162. Grossman LI. Pulp reaction to the insertion of self-curing resin filling materials. J Am Dent Assoc 1953;46:265.
163. Nygaard-Østby B. Pulp reaction to direct filling resins. J Am Dent Assoc 1955;50:7.
164. Langeland, K.: Pulp reactions to resin cements. Acta Odontol Scand 1956;13:239.
165. Suarez CL, Stanley HR, Gilmore HW. Histopathologic response of the human dental pulp to restorative materials. J Am Dent Assoc 1970;80:792.
166. Pearson GJ, Picton DCA, et al. The effect of two temporary crown materials on the dental pulp of monkeys. Int Endodont J 1986;19:121.
167. Zander HA. The effect of self-curing acrylics on the dental pulp. Oral Surg 1951;4:1563.
168. Zander HA. Pulp response to restorative materials. J Am Dent Assoc 1959;59:911.
169. Crispin BJ, Watson JF, Caputo AA. The marginal accuracy of treatment restorations: a comparative analysis. J Prosthet Dent 1980;44:283.
170. Spångberg L, Rodrigues H, Langeland LK, Langeland K. Toxicity of anterior tooth restorative materials on HeLa cells in vitro. Oral Surg 1973;36:713.
171. Stanley HR, Bowen RL, Folio J. Compatibility of various materials with oral tissues. II. Pulp responses to composite ingredients. J Dent Res 1979;58:1507.
172. Dickey DM, El-Kafrawy AH, Mitchell DF. Clinical and microscopic pulp response to a composite restorative material. J Am Dent Assoc 1974;88:108.
173. Langeland K. Prevention of pulpal damage. Dent Clin North Am 1972;16:709.
174. Langeland K, Dowden WE, Tronstad L, Langeland K. Human pulp changes of iatrogenic origin. Oral Surg 1971;32:943.
175. Stanley HR, Going RE, Chaunch HH. Human pulp response to acid pre-treatment of dentin and to composite restorations. J Am Dent Assoc 1975;91:817.
176. Stanley HR. Effects of dental restorative materials. J Am Dent Assoc 1993;124:76.
177. Hörsted PB, Simonsen AM, Mogens JL. Monkey pulp reactions to restorative materials. Scand J Dent Res 1986;94:154.
178. Heys RJ, Heys DR, Fitzgerald M. Histological evaluation of microfilled and conventional composite resins on monkey dental pulps. Int Endodont J 1985;18:260.
179. Lacy AM. A critical look at posterior composite restorations. J Am Dent Assoc 1987;114:357.
180. Jordan RL. Glass ionomer cements. Palm Springs Seminar, Palm Springs, CA, March 1988.

181. Stanley HR, Pameijer CH. Pulp capping with a new visible light curing calcium hydroxide composition (Prisma VLC Dycal). Oper Dent 1985;10:156.
182. Stanley HR, Lundy T. Dycal therapy for pulp exposures. Oral Surg 1972;34:818.
183. McComb D. Liners and bases—current concepts and materials. Alpha Omegan 1988;81:42.
184. Wilson AD, Kent BE. A new translucent cement for dentistry: the glass ionomer cement. Br Dent J 1972;132:133.
185. Smith DC. Composition and characteristics of glass ionomer cements. J Am Dent Assoc 1990;120:20.
186. Cooper IR. The response of the human dental pulp to glass ionomer cements. Int Endodont J 1980;13:76.
187. Klötzer WT. Pulp reactions to a glass ionomer cement. J Dent Res 1975;54:678.
188. Dahl BL, Tronstad L. Biological tests on an experimental glass ionomer cement. J Oral Rehabil 1976;3:19.
189. Tobias RS, Browne RM, et al. Pulpal response to a glass ionomer cement. Br Dent J 1978;144:345.
190. Nordenval K, Brännström M, Torstensson B. Pulp reactions and microorganisms under ASPA and Concise composite fillings. J Dent Child 1979;46:449.
191. Kawahara H, Imanishi Y, Oshima H. Biological evaluation of glass ionomer cement. J Dent Res 1979;58:1080.
192. Pameijer CH, Segal E, Richardson J. Pulpal response to a glass-ionomer cement in primates. J Prosthet Dent 1981;46:36.
193. Pameijer CH, Stanley HR. Primate pulp response to anhydrous chembond. J Dent Res 1984;63:171.
194. Stanley HR. Pulpal responses to ionomer cements—biological characteristics. J Am Dent Assoc 1990;120:25.
195. Pameijer CH, Stanley HR. Biocompatibility of a glass ionomer luting agent in primates—part I. Am J Dent 1988;1:71.
196. Meryon SD, Smith AJ. A comparison of fluoride release from three glass ionomer cements and a polycarboxylate cement. Int Endodont J 1984;17:16.
197. Fitzgerald M, Heys RJ, et al. An evaluation of a glass ionomer luting agent: bacterial leakage. J Am Dent Assoc 1987;114:783.
198. McLean JW, Gasser O. Glass-cermet cements. Quintessence Int 1985;16:333.
199. McLean JW. New concepts in cosmetic dentistry using glass-ionomer cements and composites. Calif Dent Assoc J 1986;14:20.
200. McLean JW. Cermet cements. J Am Dent Assoc 1990;120:43.
201. Garcia-Godoy F. Microleakage of a posterior composite resin lined with glass ionomer. Gen Dent 1988;36:514.
202. Eriksen HM, Leidal TI. Monkey pulpal response to composite restorations in cavities treated with various cleansing agents. Scand J Dent Res 1979;87:309.
203. Cotton WR, Seigel RL. Human pulpal response to citric acid cavity cleanser. J Am Dent Assoc 1978;96:639.
204. Eriksen HM. Protection against harmful effects of a restorative procedure using an acidic cavity cleanser. J Dent Res 1976;55:281.
205. Jordan RL. Posterior composites. Palm Springs Seminar, Palm Springs, CA, March 1988.
206. Lee H, Orlowski J, et al. Effects of acid etchants on dentin. JDR 1973;52:1228.
207. Retief D, et al. Pulpal response to phosphoric acid. J Oral Pathol 1974;3:114.
208. Macko D, Rutberg M, Langeland K. Pulpal response to the application of phosphoric acid to dentin. Oral Surg 1978;45:930.
209. Brännström M. Dentin and the pulp in restorative dentistry. London: Wolfe Medical Publications; 1982.
210. Pashley DH. Smear layer: physiological considerations. Oper Dent Suppl 1984;3:18.
211. White KC, et al. Histologic pulpal response of acid-etching vital dentin [abstract]. JDR 1992;71:188.
212. Fusayama T. Factors and prevention of pulp irritation by adhesive composite resin restorations. Quintessence Int 1987;8:633.
213. Kanca J III. Bonding to tooth structure: a rational rationale for clinical protocol. J Esthet Dent 1989;1:135.
214. Kanca J III. An alternative hypothesis to the cause of pulpal inflammation in teeth treated with phosphoric acid on the dentin. Quintessence Int 1990;21:83.
215. Kanca J III. One-year evaluation of a dentin-enamel bonding system. J Esthet Dent 1990;2:100.
216. Kanca J III. Pulpal studies: biocompatibility or effectiveness of marginal seal? Quintessence Int 1990;21:775.
217. Kanca J III. A method of bonding to tooth structure. JDR 1990;69:231.
218. Bertolotti RL. Total etch—the rational dentin bonding protocol. J Esthet Dent 1991;3:1.
219. White KC, Cox CF, et al. Pulp response to adhesive resin systems applied to acid-etched vital dentin. Quintessence Int 1994;25:259.
220. Nakabayashi N. Dentin Adhesives Palm Springs Seminar, Los Angeles, January 11, 1991.
221. Tagger M, Tagger E. Pulpal reactions to a dentin bonding agent: Dentin Adhesit. JOE 1987;13:113.
222. Baratieri A, Minani C, Deli R. A study on the pulpodentinal response to lining material using tetracycline labelling technique. Int Endodont J 1981;14:4.
223. Langeland K, Langeland L. Indirect capping and the treatment of deep carious lesions. Int Dent J 1968;18:326.
224. Langeland K, Langeland L, Anderson DM. Corticosteroids in dentistry. Int Dent J 1977;27:217.
225. Mjör IA, Nygaard Østby B. Experimental investigations on the effect of Ledermix on normal pulps. J Oral Therapeut Pharmacol 1966;2:367.
226. Eames WB, Scrabeck JG. Bases, liners and varnishes: interviews [illegible]ith contemporary authorities. Gen Dent 1985;33[illegible].01.
227. Pashley DH, Depew DD. Effects of the smear layer, Copalite, and oxalate on microleakage. Oper Dent 1986;11:95.
228. Jendresen MD, Stanley HR. A composite resin compatible cavity varnish. J Dent Res 1981;60A:477.
229. Kaufman C, Pelznes RB, et al. An evaluation of the protective properties of a new varnish. Quintessence Int 1982;6:1.
230. Tjan AHL, Grant BE, Nemetz H. The efficacy of resin compatible cavity varnishes in reducing dentin permeability to free monomer. J Prosthet Dent 1987;57:179.
231. Nakabayashi N, et al. Studies on dental self-curing resins: Adhesion to dentin by mechanical interlocking. J Jpn Soc Dent Mater Dev 1982;1:74.
232. Tao L, Tagami J, Pashley DH. The effect of simulated pulpal pressure on shear bond strength of C and B Metabond to dentin [abstract]. J Dent Res 1989;68:321.
233. Pashley DH. Clinical considerations of microleakage. JOE 1990;16:70.

234. Summitt J, Burgess J, et al. Four year evaluation of Amalgambond Plus and pin-retained amalgam restorations. Presented at the IADR annual meeting, March 2000.
235. Yamani T, et al. Histopathological evaluation of the effects of a new dental adhesive on dog dental pulp. J Jpn Prosthet Soc 1986;30:671.
236. Watanabe M, et al. The pulp response to the new composite resin system, "Metafil." Jpn J Conserv Dent 1988;31:428.
237. Itoh K, et al. Pulp response of adhesive dental resins. J Jpn Soc Dent Mater Devices 1986;5:287.
238. Matsura T. Histopathological study of pulpal irritation of dental adhesive resin: part 2, Super Bond C and B. J Jpn Prosthet Soc 1987;31:418.
239. Toshiaki Y, et al. Histopathological evaluation on dog dental pulp. J Jpn Prosthet Soc 1986;30:671.
240. Prinsloo LC, Vander Vyver PJ. Degree of polymerization of modern adhesive resin cements [abstract]. JDR 1996;75:1312.
241. Tell RT, et al. Long-term cytotoxicty of orthodontic direct bonding adhesives. Am J Orthod Dentofacial Orthop 1988;93:419.
242. Cox CF, et al. Pulp response following in vivo etching and 4-META bonding [abstract]. JDR 1993;72:213.
243. Yamami T, et al. Histopathological evaluation of the effects of a new dental adhesive resin on the dog dental pulp. J Jpn Prosthet Soc 1986;30:671.
244. Miyakoshi S, et al. Interfacial interactions of 4-META-MMA/TBB resin and the pulp [abstract]. JDR 1993;72:220.
245. Matsura T, et al. Histopathological study of pulpal irritation of dental adhesive resin. J Jpn Prosthet Soc 1987;31:418.
246. Al-Fawaz A, Gerzina TM, Hume WR. Movement of resin cement components through acid-treated dentin during crown cementation in vitro. JOE 1993;19:219.
247. Stanley HR, Bowen RL, Cobb EN. Pulp responses to a dentin and enamel adhesive bonding procedure. Oper Dent 1988;13:107.
248. Bowen RL, Cobb EN. A method for bonding to dentin and enamel. J Am Dent Assoc 1983;107:734.
249. Bowen RL, et al. Clinical trials of a material adhesive to dentin and enamel [abstract]. J Dent Res 1988;67:284.
250. Blosser RL, et al. Pulpal response to two new dentin and enamel bonding systems [abstract]. J Dent Res 1988;67:134.
251. Chohayeb A, Rubb NW. Marginal leakage of bonded composite resins [abstract]. JOE 1988;14:197.
252. Leinfelder KF. Current developments in dentin bonding systems. J Am Dent Assoc 1993;124:40.
253. Black GV, Black's operative dentistry. 9th ed. Vol II. South Milwaukee (WI): Medico-Dental Publishing Co; p. 113.
254. Dorfman H, Stephan RM, Muntz JA. In vitro studies on sterilization of carious dentin. II. Extent of infection in carious lesions. J Am Dent Assoc 1943;30:1901.
255. Stephan RM. Consultant symposium: our empiric cavity sterilization. Part III. N Y State Dent J 1960;26:183.
256. Lefkowitz W, Bodecker CF. Sodium fluoride: its effect on the dental pulp. Preliminary report. Ann Dent 1945;3:141.
257. Rovelstad GH, St. John WE. The condition of the young dental pulp after application of sodium fluoride to the freshly cut dentin. J Am Dent Assoc 1949;39:670.
258. Maurice CG, Schour I. Effects of sodium fluoride upon the pulp of the rat molar. J Dent Res 1956;35:69.
259. Furseth R, Mjör IA. Pulp studies after 2 per cent sodium fluoride treatment of experimentally prepared cavities. Oral Surg 1973;36:109.
260. Walton RE, Leonard LA, Sharwy M, Gangerosa LP. Effects on pulp and dentin of iontophoresis of sodium fluoride on exposed roots in dogs. Oral Surg 1979;48:545.
261. Briscoe WT, Monson DL, Ingle JI. Electrolysis in tooth structure [thesis]. Seattle: Univ. of Washington; 1956.
262. Parkell product information: Cavidry package insert. Farmingdale (NY): Parkell; 2002.
263. Sicher H. Orban's oral histology and embryology. 5th ed. St. Louis: CV Mosby; 1962.
264 Wedenberg C, Zettesqvist L. Internal resorption in human teeth—a histological scanning electron microscopic and enzyme histochemical study. JOE 1988;13:255.
265. Brooks JK. An unusual case of idiopathic internal root resorption beginning in an unerupted permanent tooth. JOE 1986;12:309.
266. Andreasen JO, Andreasen FM. Textbook and color atlas of traumatic injuries to the teeth. 3rd ed. Copenhagen: Munskgaard; 1994.
267. Frank AL, Bakland LK. Supra osseous extracanal invasive resorption. JOE 1987;13:348.
268. Heithersay GS. Clinical, radiologic, and histopathologic features of invasive cervical resorption. Quintessence Int 1999;30:27.
269. Pankhurst CL, Eley BM, Monzi C. Multiple idiopathic external root resorption. Oral Surg 1988;65:754.
270. Schwartz S, et al. Oral findings in patients with autosomal dominant hypophosphatemic bone disease and X-linked hypophosphatemia: further evidence that they are different diseases. Oral Surg 1988;66:310.
271. Macfarlane JD, Swart JGN. Dental aspects of hypophosphatasia: a case report, family study and literature review. Oral Surg 1989;67:521.
272. Andrews CH, England MC Jr, Kemp WB. Sickle cell anemia: an etiological factor in pulpal necrosis. JOE 1983;9:249.
273. Goon WWY, Jacobsen PL. Prodromal odontolgia and multiple devitalized teeth caused by a herpes zoster infection of the trigeminal nerve: report of a case. J Am Dent Assoc 1988;116:500.
274. Gregory WB, Brooks LE, Penick EC. Herpes zoster associated with pulpless teeth. JOE 1975;1:32.
275. Lopes MA, de Souza FJ, Filho JJ Jr, de Almeida OP. Herpes zoster infection as a differential diagnosis of acute pulpitis. JOE 1998;24:143.
276. Glick M, et al. Detection of HIV in the dental pulp of a patient with AIDS. J Am Dent Assoc 1989;119:649.
277. Levy JA. Human immunodeficiency virus and the pathogenesis of AIDS. JAMA 1989;261:2997.
278. American Dental Association. Facts about the dental market [pamphlet]. Chicago: Journal of the American Dental Association Press; 1975.
279. Cyr G, et al. Major etiologic factors leading to root canal procedure [abstract]. JOE 1985;11:145.
280. Udolph CH, Kopel HM, Melrose RJ, Grenoble DE. Pulp response to composite resins with or without calcium hydroxide bases. J Calif Dent Assoc 1975;3:56.
281. Langeland LK, Guttuso J, Jerome DR, Langeland K. Histologic and clinical comparison of Addent with silicate cement and cold-curing materials. J Am Dent Assoc 1966;72:373.
282. Takahashi K. Changes in pulpal vasculature during inflammation. JOE 1990;16:92.
283. Van Hassel HJ, McHugh JW. Effect of prednisolone on intrapulpal pressure [abstract 499]. J Dent Res 1972.

284. Spångberg L, Rodrigues H, Langeland K. Effect of cavity liners on HeLa cells in vitro. Oral Surg 1974;37:284.
285. Baume LJ, Fiore-Donno G. Response of the human pulp to a new restorative material. J Am Dent Assoc 1968;76:1016.
286. Langeland K. Criteria for biologic evaluation of anterior tooth filling materials. Int Dent J 1967;17:405.
287. Brännström M, Nyborg H. Pulpal reaction to composite resin restorations. J Prosthet Dent 1972;27:181.
288. Council on Dental Materials, Instruments, and Equipment. Biocompatibility and postoperative sensitivity. J Am Dent Assoc 1988;116:767.
289. Council on Dental Materials, Instruments, and Equipment. J Am Dent Assoc 1984;109:476.
290. Jodaikin A, Austin JC. The effects of cavity smear layer removal on experimental marginal leakage around amalgam restorations. J Dent Res 1981;60:1861.
291. Browne RM, Tobias RS, et al. Bacterial microleakage and pulpal inflammation in experimental cavities. Int Endodont J 1983;16:147.
292. Wenner A, Austin JC. Microleakage of root restorations. J Am Dent Assoc 1988;17:825.
293. Duke ES, Phillips RW, Blumenshine R. Effects of various agents in cleaning out dentin. J Oral Rehabil 1985;12:295.
294. Powis DR, Folleras T, Merson SA, Wilson AD. Improved adhesion of a glass ionomer cement to dentin and enamel. J Dent Res 1982;61:1416.
295. Kemples D, et al. Reports from the Product Evaluation Laboratory, University of California, San Francisco. Dentin bonding systems: an update. Dent-E-Val 1986;3:25.
296. Bullard RH, Leinfelder KF, Russell CM. Effect of coefficient of thermal expansion on microleakage. J Am Dent Assoc 1988;16:871.
297. Product review, glass ionomer bases. Dental Advisor 1987;4: #2, 8.
298. Tjan AHL, Miller GD, et al. Internal escape channels to improve the seating of full crowns and various marginal configurations: a follow up study. J Prosthet Dent 1985; 53:759.
299. Rosenstiel SF, Gegauff AG. Improving the cementation of complete cast crowns: a comparison of static and dynamic seating methods. J Am Dent Assoc 1988;117:845.
300. Eick JD, Welch FH. Polymerization shrinkage of posterior composite resins and its possible influence on postoperative sensitivity. Quintessence Int 1986;17:103.
301. Bertolotti RL. Luting and sensitivity. Adhesion Dentistry 1990.
302. Fauchard P. The surgeon dentist or treatise on the teeth. Lindsay L, translator. Pound Ridge (NY): Milford House; 1969.
303. Langeland K, Dowden WE, Tronstad L, Langeland LK. Human dental pulp. Siskin M, editor. St. Louis: CV Mosby; 1973. p. 122–59.
304. Fusayama T. G.V. Black's principles get a fresh look. Lecture, ADA Annual Session, November 6, 1990.
305. Warfving J, et al. Effect of calcium hydroxide treated dentine on pulpal responses. Int Endodont J 1987;20:183.
306. Foreman PC, Barnes IE. A review of calcium hydroxide. Int Endodont J 1990;23:283.
307. Seltzer S, Bender IB, Ziontz M. The dynamics of pulp inflammation: correlations between diagnostic data and actual histologic findings in the pulp: I and II. Oral Surg 1963;16:846, 969.
308. Mumford JM. Relationship between pain-perception threshold of human teeth and their histologic condition of the pulp. JDR 1965;44:1167.
309. Seltzer S, Bender IB. The Dental Pulp. Ed: Hargreaves, KM, Goodis, HE. Chicago, Quintessence Publish Co. 2002.
310. Garfunkel A, Sela J, Ulmansky M. Dental pulp pathosis: clinicopathologic correlations based on 109 cases. Oral Surg 1973;35:110.
311. Seltzer S, Bender IB. The Dental Pulp. Edited by Hargreaves KM and Goodis HG. Chicago, Quintessence Publishing Co., 20002.
312. Brännström M, Lind P. Pulpal response to early caries. JDR 1965;44:1045.
313. Scott J, Symons N. Introduction of dental anatomy. 8th ed. Edinburgh: Livingstone; 1977.
314. Baume L. The biology of pulp and dentine. Vol 8: monographs in oral science. Basel: Karger; 1980.
315. Cotton W. Pulp response to cavity preparation as studied by thymidine-3H autoradiography. In: Finn SB, editor. Biology of the dental pulp organ. Birmingham: Univ. of Alabama Press; 1968. p. 219.
316. Feit J, Metelora M, Sindelka Z. Incorporation of 3H thymidine into damaged pulp of rat incisors. JDR 1970;49:783.
317. Mjör IA, Karlsen K. The interface between dentine and irregular and secondary dentine. Acta Odontol Scand 1970;28:363.
318. Taintor JF, Biesterfeld RC, Langeland K. Irritational or reparative dentin. Oral Surg 1981;51:442.
319. Seltzer S, Bender I. Inflammation in the odontoblastic layer of the dental pulp. J Am Dent Assoc 1959;59:720.
320. Tronstad L, Mjör I. Capping of the inflamed pulp. Oral Surg 1972;34:477.
321. Langeland K. Tissue changes in the dental pulp. An experimental histologic study. Odontol T 1956;65:375.
322. Scott NJ, Webber DF. Microscopy of the junctional region between human coronal primary and secondary dentin. J Morphol 1977;154:133.
323. Holcomb J, Gregory W. Calcific metamorphosis of the pulp: its incidence and treatment. Oral Surg 1967;24:825.
324. Andreasen J, Hjörting-Hansen E. Intra-alveolar root fractures: radiographic and histological study of 50 cases. J Oral Surg 1967;25:414.
325. Lundberg M, Cvek M. A light microscopy study of pulps from traumatized permanent incisors with reduced pulp lumen. Acta Odontol Scand 1980;38:89.
326. Jacobsen I, Kerekes K. Long-term prognosis of traumatized permanent anterior teeth showing calcifying processes in the pulp cavity. Scand J Dent Res 1977;85:588.
327. Reeves R, Stanley HR. The relationship of bacterial penetration and pulpal pathosis in carious teeth. Oral Surg 1966;22:59.
328. Corbett M. The incidence of secondary dentine in carious teeth. Br Dent J 1963;114:142.
329. Shovelton D. A study of deep carious dentin. Int Dent J 1968;18:392.
330. Miller WA, Massler M. Permeability of active and arrested carious lesions in dentine. Br Dent J 1962;112:187.
331. Thomas J, Stanley HR, Gilmore H. Effects of gold foil condensation of human dental pulp. J Am Dent Assoc 1969;78:788.
332. Langeland K. Responses of the adult tooth to injury. In: Finn SB, editor. Biology of the dental pulp. Birmingham: Univ. of Alabama Press; 1968. p. 169.

333. Berk H. Preservation of the dental pulp in deep seated cavities. J Am Dent Assoc 1957;54:226.
334. Trowbridge HT. Pathogenesis of pulpitis resulting from dental caries. JOE 1981;7:52.
335. Naidorf I. Correlation of the inflammatory response with immunological and clinical events. JOE 1977;3:223.
336. Morse DR. Immunologic aspects of pulpal periradicular disease. Oral Surg 1977;43:437.
337. Stanley HR, Weaver K. A technique for the preparation of human pulpal tissue. In: Finn SB, editor. Biology of the dental pulp organ. Birmingham: Univ. of Alabama Press; 1968.
338. Seltzer S. Discussion of vascular permeability and other factors in the modulation of the inflammatory response. JOE 1977;3:214.
339. Furseth R, Mjör IA, Skogedal O. The fine structure of induced pulpitis in a monkey. Arch Oral Biol 1979;24:883.
340. Zacharisson B, Skogedal O. Mast cells in inflamed human dental pulp. Scand J Dent Res 1971;79:488.
341. Miller GS, et al. Histologic identification of mast cells in human pulp. Oral Surg 1978;46:559.
342. Trowbridge H, Daniels T. Abnormal immune response to infection of the dental pulp. Oral Surg 1977;43:902.
343. Mjör IA, Tronstad L. The healing of experimentally induced pulpitis. Oral Surg 1974;38:115.
344. Spångberg LS, et al. Pulpal and periodontal effects of electrosurgery involving based and unbased cervical restorations [abstract]. JDR 1980;59:375.
345. Bergenholtz G. Inflammatory response of the dental pulp to bacterial irritation. JOE 1981;7:100.
346. Bergenholtz G. Effect of bacterial products on inflammatory reactions in the dental pulp. Scand J Dent Res 1977;85:122.
347. Torneck, C. A report of studies into changes in the fine structure of the dental pulp in human caries pulpitis. JOE 1981;7:8.
348. Lin L, Langeland K. Light and electron microscopic study of teeth with carious pulp exposures. Oral Surg 1981;51:292.
349. Torneck C. Changes in the fine structure of the dental pulp in human caries pulpitis. Part 1. Nerves and blood vessels. J Oral Pathol 1974;3:71.
350. Matsumiya S, Kondo S, Takuma S, et al. Atlas of oral pathology. Tokyo: Tokyo Dental College Press; 1955.
351. Walton R, Garnick J. Induction of pulpal necrosis and periradicular pathosis in monkeys [abstract]. JDR 1984;63:332.
352. Dahlén G, Bergenholtz G. Endotoxic activity in teeth with necrotic pulps. JDR 1980;59:1033.
353. Sunquish G, Johansson E. Neutrophil chemotaxis induced by anaerobic bacteria isolated from necrotic dental pulps. Scand J Dent Res 1980;88:113.
354. Morand M, Schilder H, et al. Collagenolytic and elastinolytic activities from diseased human dental pulps. JOE 1981;7:156.
355. Jordan R, Suzuki M. Indirect pulp capping of carious teeth with periradicular lesions. J Am Dent Assoc 1978;97:37.
356. Schroff FR. Pathology of the dental pulp. Aust Dent J 1955;59:95.
357. Simpson HE. Internal resorption. J Can Dent Assoc 1964;30:355.
358. Wedenberg C. Development and morphology of internal resorption in teeth—a study in humans, monkeys and rats. Stockholm: Kongl Carolinska Medico Chirurgiska Institutet; 1987.
359. Warner GR, Orban B, Hine MK, Ritchey BT. Internal resorption of teeth: interpretation of histologic findings. J Am Dent Assoc 1947;34:468.
360. Sullivan HR, Jolly M. Idiopathic resorption. Aust Dent J 1957;61:193.
361. Fish E. Calcified tissue of repair. Proc R Soc Med 1932;32:609.
362. James VS, Englander HR, Massler M. Histologic response of amputated pulps to calcium compounds and antibiotics. Oral Surg 1957;10:975.
363. Nyborg H. Healing processes in the pulp on capping. Acta Odontol Scand 1955;13 Suppl 16:9–130.
364. Kalnins V, Frisbie HE. The effect of dentin fragments on the healing of exposed pulp. Arch Oral Biol 1960;2:96.
365. Curriculum Guidelines in endodontics. J Dent Educ 1993;57:251.
366. Nanda R, Legan HL, Langeland K. Pulpal and radicular response to maxillary osteotomy in monkeys. Oral Surg 1982;53:624.
367. Andreasen FM. Histological and bacteriological study of pulps extirpated after luxation injuries. Endodont Dent Traumatol 1988;4:170.
368. Andreasen FM, Vestergaard Pedersen B. Prognosis of luxated permanent teeth—the development of pulp necrosis. Endodont Dent Traumatol 1985;1:207.
369. Andreasen FM, Zhijie Y, Thomsen BL. Relationship between pulp dimensions and development of pulp necrosis after luxation injuries in the permanent dentition. Endodont Dent Traumatol 1986;2:90.
370. Bender IB. Pulp biology conference: a discussion. JOE 1978;4:37.
371. Stanley HR, et al. Ischemic infarction of the pulp: sequential degenerative changes of the pulp after traumatic injury. JOE 1978;4:325.
372. Rubin E, Farber JL. Cell injury. In: Rubin E, Farber JL, editors. Pathology. Philadelphia: JB Lippincott; 1988. p. 2–33.
373. Robbins SL, Angell M, Kumar V. Basic pathology. 3rd ed. Philadelphia: WB Saunders; 1981.
374. Lundberg M, Cvek M. A light microscopy study of pulps from traumatized permanent incisors with reduced pulpal lumen. Acta Odontol Scand 1980;38:89.

Chapter 5

PERIRADICULAR LESIONS

Mahmoud Torabinejad and Richard E. Walton

As a consequence of pathologic changes in the dental pulp, the root canal system can harbor numerous irritants. Egress of these irritants from infected root canals into the periradicular tissues can initiate formation and perpetuation of periradicular lesions. Depending on the nature and quantity of these irritants, as well as the duration of exposure of the periradicular tissues, a variety of tissue changes can occur. When the irritants are transient in nature, the inflammatory process is short-lived and self-limiting. However, with an excessive amount of irritants or persistent exposure, the nonspecific and specific immunologic reactions can cause destruction of periradicular tissues.[1] Radiographically, these lesions appear as radiolucent areas around the portal(s) of exit of the main canal or lateral and/or accessory canals. Histologically, depending on their stage of development, the lesions contain numerous inflammatory cells such as polymorphonuclear neutrophil leukocytes (PMNs), macrophages, lymphocytes, plasma cells, mast cells, basophils, and eosinophils. The interaction between the irritants and the host defensive mechanisms results in release of numerous mediators that curtail progression of infection and development of severe local infection (**osteomyelitis**) and systemic complication such as septicemia. Numerous studies, conducted within the past 30 years, elucidate the reactions and mediators of pathogenesis of human periradicular lesions. This chapter contains information about the etiologic factors involved in the development of periradicular lesions, mediators that participate in the pathogenesis of the changes, a classification of periradicular pathosis with emphasis on their clinical and histologic features, and repair of periradicular lesions following root canal therapy. In addition, some nonendodontic lesions with clinical and/or radiographic signs and appearances similar to endodontic lesions of pulpal origin will be discussed.

PERIRADICULAR LESIONS OF PULPAL ORIGIN

Irritants

Irritation of pulpal or periradicular tissues results in inflammation. The major irritants of these tissues can be divided into living and nonliving irritants. The living irritants are various microorganisms and viruses. The nonliving irritants include mechanical, thermal, and chemical irritants. Mild to moderate injuries of short duration cause **reversible** tissue damage and **recovery** of these tissues. Persistent and/or severe injuries usually cause **irreversible** changes in the pulp and development of periradicular lesions.

Microbial Irritants

Microbial irritants of pulp and periradicular tissues include bacteria, bacterial toxins, bacterial fragments, and viruses. These irritants egress apically from the root canal system into the periradicular tissues and initiate inflammation and tissue alterations. A number of studies have shown that pulpal and/or periradicular pathosis do not develop without the presence of bacterial contamination. Kakehashi and associates created pulpal exposures in conventional and germ-free rats.[1] Pulpal necrosis and abscess formation occurred by the eighth day in the conventional rats. In contrast, the germ-free rats showed only minimal inflammation throughout the 72-day investigation. Möller and coworkers made pulpal exposures in monkeys and lacerated the pulp tissue with endodontic instruments.[2] In one group, all procedures were carried out in a sterile environment and the access cavities were sealed. In the other group, after pulp exposure the teeth were left open to intraoral contamination. Six months later, only mild inflammation was apparent in the periradicular tissues in the first group. In contrast, the periradicular tissues in the second group were severely inflamed.

Other investigators examined the flora of previously traumatized teeth with necrotic pulps with and without periradicular pathosis.[3,4] Teeth without apical lesions were aseptic, whereas those with periradicular lesions had positive bacterial cultures. Korzen et al. demonstrated the importance of the amount of microbial inoculum in the pathogenesis of pulpal and periradicular lesions.[5] They showed that higher levels of contamination lead to greater inflammatory responses.

In addition to bacterial irritation, the periradicular tissues can be mechanically irritated and inflamed. Physical irritation of periradicular tissues can also occur during root canal therapy if the canals are instrumented or filled beyond their anatomic boundaries. Periradicular tissues can be irritated by impact trauma, hyperocclusion, endodontic procedures and accidents, pulp extirpation, overinstrumentation, root perforation, and overextension of filling materials.

Chemicals are used as adjuncts for better débridement and disinfection of the root canal system. An in vitro study, however, has shown that many of these chemicals are highly concentrated and not biocompatible.[6] Irrigating solutions such as sodium hypochlorite and hydrogen peroxide, intracanal medications, and chelating agents such as ethylenediaminetetraacetic acid (EDTA) can also cause tissue injury and inflammation if inadvertently extruded into the periradicular tissues. Some components in obturation materials can irritate the periradicular tissues when extruded beyond the root canal system.

Periradicular Reaction to Irritation

The periradicular tissues consist of apical root cementum, periodontal ligament, and alveolar bone. The apical periodontium is also richly endowed with cellular and extracellular components containing blood and lymphatics, as well as sensory and motor nerve fibers supplying both pulp and periodontium. Other structural elements of the periodontal ligament include ground substance, various fibers, fibroblasts, cementoblasts, osteoblasts, osteoclasts, histiocytes, undifferentiated mesenchymal cells, and the epithelial cell rests of Malassez.

Irritation of periradicular tissues results in inflammatory changes taking place. The vascular response to an injury includes vasodilation, vascular stasis, and increased vascular permeability. The latter leads to extravasation of fluid and soluble components into the surrounding tissues. These vascular changes cause redness, heat, swelling, and pain, which are the cardinal signs of inflammation. The inflammatory cells involved in various stages of tissue injury and repair include platelets, PMNs, mast cells, basophils, eosinophils, macrophages, and lymphocytes,[7] all of which have specific roles in inflammatory responses.

Mediators of Periradicular Lesions

The inflammatory process is not completely understood, but a number of substances have been implicated as mediators of inflammation. They include neuropeptides, fibrinolytic peptides, kinins, complement fragments, arachidonic acid metabolites, vasoactive amines, lysosomal enzymes, cytokines, and mediators of immune reactions.

Neuropeptides. These are proteins generated from somatosensory and autonomic nerve fibers following tissue injury. They include substance P (SP), calcitonin gene–related peptide (CGRP), dopamine hydrolase, neuropeptide Y originating from sympathetic nerve fibers, and vasoactive intestinal polypeptides generated from parasympathetic nerve fibers.[8]

Substance P is a neuropeptide present in both the peripheral and central nervous systems. The release of SP can cause vasodilation, increased vascular permeability, and increased blood flow during inflammation. In addition, it can cause the release of **histamine from mast cells** and potentiate inflammatory responses.

Calcitonin gene–related peptide has been localized in small to medium sensory nerve fibers. Like SP, it is a potent vasodilator and may play a role in the regulation of blood flow in bone, periosteum, and other sites. Substance P and CGRP have been found in pulp and periradicular tissues.[9]

Fibrinolytic Peptides. The fibrinolytic cascade is triggered by the Hageman factor, which causes activation of circulating plasminogen, previously known as fibrinolysin and digestion of blood clots. This results in release of fibrinopeptides and fibrin degradation products that cause increased vascular permeability and leukocyte chemotaxis.[10]

Kinins. Release of kinins causes many signs of inflammation.[11] They include chemotaxis of inflammatory cells, contraction of smooth muscles, dilation of peripheral arterioles, increased vascular permeability, and pain. The kinins are produced by proteolytic cleavage of kininogen by trypsin-like serine proteases, the kallikreins. The kinins are subsequently inactivated by removal of the last one or two C-terminal amino acids by the action of peptidase.[12] The kallikreins are also able to react with other systems, such as the complement and coagulation systems, to generate other trypsin-like serine proteases.[13] Elevated levels of **kinins** have been detected in **human periapical lesions.**[14]

Complement System. The complement system consists of a number of distinct plasma proteins capable of interacting with each other and with other systems to produce a variety of effects.[15] Complement is able to cause cell lysis if activated on the cell membrane and also to enhance phagocytosis through interaction with complement receptors on the surface of phagocytic cells. Complement can also increase vascular permeability and act as a chemotactic factor for granulocytes and macrophages. The complement system is a complex cascade that has two separate activation pathways that converge to a single protein (C3) and complete the cascade in a final, common sequence. Complement can be activated through the classic pathway by antigen-antibody complexes or through the alternative pathway by directly interacting with complex carbohydrates on bacterial and fungal cell walls or with substances such as plasmin.

Several investigators have found **C3 complement** components in human **periradicular lesions.**[10] Activators of the classic and alternative pathways of the complement system include immunoglobulin (Ig) M, IgG, bacteria and their by-products, lysosomal enzymes from PMNs, and clotting factors. Most of these activators are present in periradicular lesions. Activation of the complement system in these lesions can contribute to bone resorption either by destruction of already existing bone or by inhibition of new bone formation via the production of prostaglandins (PGs).

Arachidonic Acid Metabolites. Arachidonic acid is formed from membrane phospholipid as a result of cell membrane injury and phospholipase A_2 activity and is further metabolized.

Prostaglandins are produced as a result of the activation of the cyclooxygenase pathway of the arachidonic acid metabolism. Their pathologic functions include increased vascular permeability and pain. Torabinejad and associates demonstrated in an animal model that periradicular bone resorption could be inhibited by administration of **indomethacin (Indocin), an antagonist of PGs.**[16] **High levels of PGE_2 were found in periradicular lesions** of patients with **symptomatic apical periodontitis** (SAP).[17] Takayama et al.[18] and Shimauchi and coworkers[19] confirmed these findings by demonstrating lower levels of PGE_2 associated with asymptomatic large lesions or cessation of symptoms subsequent to emergency cleaning and shaping of root canals. Miyauchi et al. used immunohistochemical staining and found PGE_2, $PGF_{2\alpha}$, and 6-keto-$PGF_{1\alpha}$ in the experimentally induced periapical lesions in rats.[20]

Leukotrienes (LTs) are produced as a result of the activation of the lipoxygenase pathway of the arachidonic acid metabolism. Polymorphonuclear neutrophil leukocytes and mast cells are the major sources for production of LTs.[21] Leukotriene B_4 is a powerful chemotactic agent from PMNs. Increased levels of **LTB_4** have been found in **symptomatic** human **periapical lesions.**[22] Other leukotrienes such as LTC_4, LTD_4, and LTE_4 are chemotactic for eosinophil and macrophage, cause increased vascular permeability, and stimulate lysozyme release from PMNs and macrophages.[15]

Vasoactive Amines. Vasoactive amines are present in mast cells, basophils, and platelets. **Histamine,** the major one of these substances, is found in all three cell types, whereas **serotonin** is present only in platelets.[21] Release of these materials causes increased vascular permeability, as well as muscle contraction of airways and gastrointestinal tracts. Numerous **mast cells** have been detected in human **periradicular lesions.**[23,24] Physical or chemical irritation of periradicular tissues during root canal therapy can cause mast cell degranulation. The discharged vasoactive amines can initiate an inflammatory response or aggravate an existing inflammatory process in the periradicular tissues.

Lysosomal Enzymes. Lysosomal enzymes are stored preformed in membrane-bound bodies within inflammatory cell cytoplasm. Lysosomal bodies are found in PMNs, macrophages, and platelets and contain acid as well as alkaline phosphatases, lysozyme, peroxidase, cathepsins, and collagenase. They can be released via exocytotic type events during cell lysis or secreted during phagocytosis. Release of these enzymes into the tissues causes increased vascular permeability, leukocyte chemotaxis, generation of C5a from C5, and **bradykinin** formation.[15] Aqrabawi and associates examined human periradicular lesions for the presence of lysosomal hydrolytic arylsulfatase A and B and found higher levels of these substances in lesions of endodontic origin compared to the control tissues.[25]

Cytokines. The major cytokines that have been implicated in bone resorption are various **interleukins (ILs)** and **tumor necrosis factors (TNFs).**[15]

Interleukin-1 is produced primarily by monocytes and macrophages.[26,27] Human monocytes produce at least two IL-1 species, IL-1α and IL-1β.[28] Interleukin-1β is the major form secreted by human **monocytes.** The chief component of osteoclast activating factor was purified and found to be identical to IL-1β.[29] Interleukin-1β is the most active of the cytokines in **stimulating bone resorption** in vitro, 15-fold more potent than IL-1α and 1,000-fold more potent than TNFs.[30] Interleukin-1 has been associated with increased bone resorption in vivo in several diseases. *Interleukin-1* has been implicated in the **bone resorp-**

tion for periodontal disease and **periradicular lesions.**[31–39]

Interleukin-6 is produced by a number of cells with a wide range of cell targets.[40] It is produced by osteoblasts, but in response to other bone resorptive agents such as parathyroid hormone, IL-1, and 1,25-hydroxyvitamin D_3.[41] **Interleukin-6** is produced during immune responses and may play a role in human resorptive diseases such as **adult periodontitis**[42] and **rheumatoid arthritis.**[43] Recent studies have shown that **IL-6** may play a significant role in the **pathogenesis of human periradicular lesion.**[44,45]

Tumor necrosis factor-α and TNF-β have bone resorption activities similar to that of IL-1. Their effects on osteoclasts are indirect and are mediated through osteoblasts.[46] The effect of TNF-α on bone resorption is dependent on PG synthesis.[47] **Tumor necrosis factors** have been detected in **periradicular lesions** of experimental animals and humans.[38,39,48,49]

Immunologic Reactions. In addition to the nonspecific mediators of inflammatory reactions, immunologic reactions also participate in the formation and perpetuation of periradicular pathosis.[10,15,35] These reactions can be divided into antibody- and cell-mediated responses. The major antibody-mediated reactions include IgE mediated reactions and antigen-antibody (immune complex)–mediated reactions.

Immunoglobulin E–mediated reactions occur as a result of an interaction between antigens (allergens) and basophils in the blood or mast cells in the tissues. Vasoactive amines such as **histamine or serotonin** are present in preformed granules **in basophils and mast cells** and are released by a number of stimuli including physical and chemical injuries, complement activation products, activated T lymphocytes, and bridging of membrane-bound IgE by allergens. Numerous mast cells have been detected in human periradicular lesions.[23,24] IgE molecules have also been found in human periapical lesions.[10] Presence of potential antigens in the root canals, IgE immunoglobulin, and mast cells in pathologically involved pulp and periradicular lesions indicate that IgE-mediated reactions can occur in periradicular tissues. Irritation of periradicular tissues during cleaning, shaping, or obturation of the root canal system with antigenic substances can cause mast cell degranulation. The discharged vasoactive amines can initiate an inflammatory response or aggravate an existing inflammatory process in the periradicular tissues.[15]

Antigen-Antibody or Immune Complex Reactions. Antigen-antibody or immune complex reactions in periradicular tissues can be formed when extrinsic antigens such as bacteria or their by-products interact with either IgG or IgM antibodies. The complexes can bind to the platelets and cause release of vasoactive amines, increased vascular permeability, and chemotaxis of PMNs. The pathologic effects of immune complexes in periradicular tissues have been demonstrated in experimental animals. Torabinejad and associates placed simulated immune complexes in feline root canals and showed a rapid formation of periradicular lesions and accumulation of numerous PMNs and osteoclasts.[16] These findings were confirmed when Torabinejad and Kiger immunized cats with subcutaneous injections of keyhole-limpet hemocyanin and challenged the animals with the same antigen via the root canals.[50] Radiographic and histologic observations showed the development of periradicular lesions consistent with characteristics of an **Arthus-type reaction.**

Immune complexes in human periradicular lesions have been found using the anticomplement immunofluorescence technique, localized immune complexes in human periradicular specimens.[51] Torabinejad and associates measured the serum concentrations of circulating immune complexes in patients with asymptomatic and symptomatic periradicular lesions. The results indicated that immune complexes formed in chronic periradicular lesions are confined within the lesions and do not enter into the systemic circulation. However, when the serum concentrations of circulating immune complexes in patients with **acute abscesses** were compared with those of people without these lesions, they found that these complexes **entered the circulation** in patients with **symptomatic periradicular abscesses.** The concentrations of these complexes came back to normal levels after either root canal therapy or extraction of involved teeth.[52,53]

Cell-Mediated Immune Reactions. Numerous B and T lymphocytes have been found in human periradicular lesions by the indirect immunoperoxidase method,[54] with the T cells outnumbering the B cells significantly. A number of investigators have found approximately equal numbers of T-cell subsets in chronic lesions (T helper/T suppressor ratio < 1.0).[55–58] Stashenko and Yu demonstrated in developing lesions in rats that T helper cells outnumber T suppressor cells during the acute phase of lesion expansion. In contrast, T suppressor cells predominate at later time periods when lesions are stabilized.[58] Based on these results, it appears that T helper cells may participate in the initiation of periradicular lesions, whereas T suppressor cells prevent rapid expansion of these lesions.

The specific role of T lymphocytes in the pathogenesis of periradicular lesions has been studied by several investigators.[39,59,60] Wallstrom and Torabinejad exposed the pulps of mandibular molars of athymic and conventional rats and left them open to the oral flora for 2, 4, or 8 weeks.[59] Statistical analysis of the tissue reactions to this procedure showed no significant difference between periradicular tissue responses of the two species of animals. Waterman and associates compared periradicular lesion formation in immunosuppressed rats with that in normal rats and found no significant histologic differences between the two groups.[60] Fouad studied the progression of pulp necrosis and the histomorphometric features of periapical lesions in mice with severe combined immunodeficiencies.[39] He found no significant differences between the reaction and progression of pulp and periapical tissues between these animals and those in normal mice. These findings suggest that the pathogenesis of periradicular lesions is a multifactorial phenomenon and is not totally dependent on the presence of a specific group of cells or mediators.

CLINICAL CLASSIFICATION OF PERIRADICULAR LESIONS

Periradicular diseases of pulpal origin have been named and classified in many different ways. These lesions do not occur as individual entities; there are clinical and histologic crossovers in the terminology regarding periradicular lesions as the terminology is based on clinical signs and symptoms as well as radiographic findings. In this chapter, periradicular lesions are divided into three main clinical groups: **symptomatic (acute) apical periodontitis, asymptomatic (chronic) apical periodontitis, and apical abscess.** Since there is no correlation between histologic findings and clinical signs, symptoms, and duration of the lesion,[10,21] the terms ***acute*** and ***chronic***, which are histologic terms, will not be used in this chapter. Instead, the terms ***symptomatic*** and ***asymptomatic***, which describe clinical conditions, will be used.

APICAL PERIODONTITIS

Depending on clinical and radiographic manifestations, these lesions are classified as ***symptomatic*** or ***asymptomatic*** periodontitis.

Symptomatic Apical Periodontitis

Symptomatic apical periodontitis (SAP) is a localized inflammation of the periodontal ligament in the apical region. The principal causes are irritants diffusing from an inflamed or necrotic pulp. Egress of irritants such as bacteria, bacterial toxins, disinfecting medications, debris pushed into the periradicular tissues, or physical irritation of the periapical tissues can cause SAP. Impact trauma can also cause SAP (see chapter 15).

Sensitivity to percussion is the principal clinical feature of SAP. Pain is pathognomonic and varies from slight tenderness to excruciating pain on contact of opposing teeth. Depending on the cause (pulpitis or necrosis), the involved tooth may or may not respond to vitality tests. Regardless of the causative agents, SAP is associated with the exudation of plasma and emigration of inflammatory cells from the blood vessels into the periradicular tissues. The release of mediators of inflammation causes breakdown of the periodontal ligament and resorption of the alveolar bone. A minor physical injury, such as penetrating the periradicular tissues with an endodontic file, may cause a transient inflammatory response. However, a major injury, causing extensive tissue destruction and cell death, can result in massive inflammatory infiltration of the periradicular tissues. Although the dynamics of these inflammatory lesions are poorly understood, the consequences depend on the type of irritant (bacterial or nonbacterial), degree of irritation, and host defensive mechanisms. The release of chemical mediators of inflammation and their action on the nerve fibers in the periradicular tissues partially explain the presence of pain during SAP. Also, since there is little room for expansion of the periodontal ligament, increased interstitial tissue pressure can also cause physical pressure on the nerve endings, causing an **intense, throbbing,** periradicular pain. Increased pressure may be more important than the release of the inflammatory mediators in causing periradicular pain. The effect of fluid pressure on pain is dramatically demonstrated on opening into an unanesthetized tooth with this condition. The release of even a small amount of fluid provides the patient with immediate and welcome relief. Radiographs show little variation, ranging from normal to a "thickening" of the periodontal ligament space (Figure 5-1) in teeth associated with SAP.

Asymptomatic Apical Periodontitis

Asymptomatic apical periodontitis (AAP) may be preceded by SAP or by an apical abscess. However, the lesion frequently develops and enlarges **without any subjective signs and symptoms.** Inadequate root canal treatment may also cause the development of these lesions. Generally, a necrotic pulp gradually releases noxious agents with **low-grade pathogenicity** or in low concentration that results in the development of AAP. This pathosis is a long-standing, "smoldering" lesion and is usually accompanied by radiographically visible periradicular **bone resorption.**

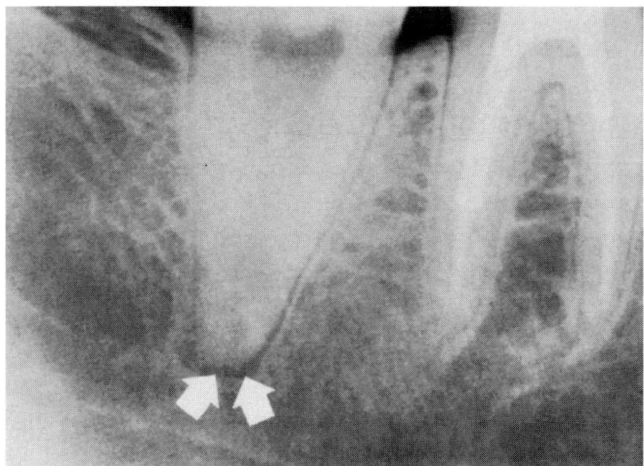

Figure 5-1 Radiographic features of symptomatic apical periodontitis. "High" amalgam restoration was placed on the occlusal surface of a second mandibular molar. The periodontal ligament space is widened at the apex (**arrows**). Clinically, the tooth is extremely sensitive to percussion.

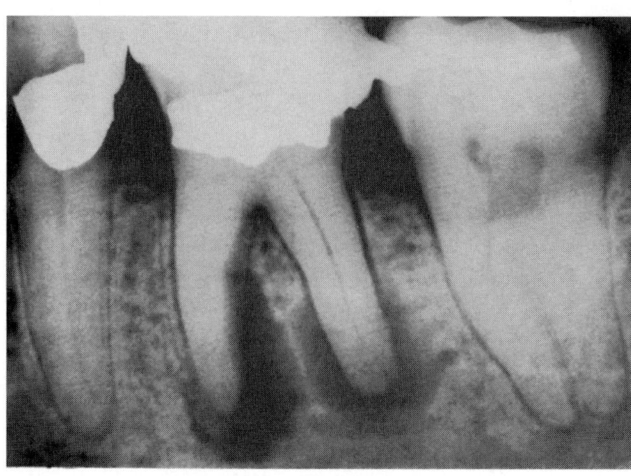

Figure 5-2 Radiographic appearance of asymptomatic apical periodontitis. Two distinct lesions are present at the periradicular regions of a mandibular first molar with necrotic pulp.

This condition is almost invariably a sequela to pulp necrosis.

The clinical features of **AAP** are unremarkable. The patient usually reports no significant pain, and tests reveal little or no pain on percussion. If **AAP** perforates the cortical plate of the bone, however, palpation of superimposed tissues may cause discomfort. The associated tooth has a **necrotic pulp** and therefore should not respond to electrical or thermal stimuli.

Radiographic findings are the diagnostic key. **Asymptomatic apical periodontitis** is usually associated with periradicular radiolucent changes. These changes range from thickening of the periodontal ligament and resorption of the lamina dura to destruction of apical bone resulting in a well-demarcated radiolucency (Figure 5-2).

Asymptomatic apical periodontitis has **traditionally** been classified histologically as either a periradicular **granuloma** or a periradicular **cyst.** Various clinical methods have been used to attempt to differentiate these two clinically similar lesions.[61–66] The only accurate way to distinguish these two entitles is by histologic examination.

Periradicular Granuloma. Nobuhara and del Rio showed that 59.3% of the periradicular lesions were granulomas, 22% cysts, 12% apical scars, and 6.7% other pathoses.[67] Histologically, the periradicular granuloma consists predominantly of granulation inflammatory tissue[68] with many small capillaries, fibroblasts, numerous connective tissue fibers, inflammatory infiltrate, and usually a connective tissue capsule (Figure 5-3). This tissue, replacing the periodontal ligament, apical bone, and sometimes the root cementum and dentin, is infiltrated by plasma cells, lymphocytes, mononuclear phagocytes, and occasional neutrophils. Occasionally, needle-like spaces (the remnants of cholesterol crystals), foam cells, and multinucleated foreign body giant cells are seen in these lesions (Figure 5-4).[69] Animal studies have shown that cholesterol crystals can cause failure of some lesions to resolve following nonsurgical root canal therapy.[70] Nerve fibers

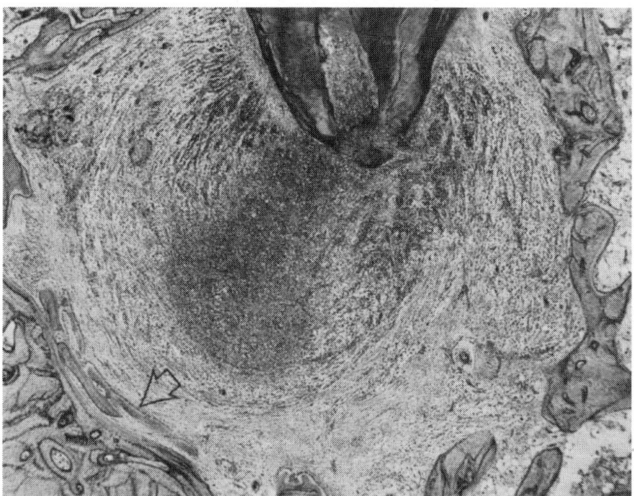

Figure 5-3 Apical periodontitis (granuloma) in its more classic form. The central zone is dense with round cells (plasma cells and small lymphocytes). Beyond is a circular layer of fibrous capsule. Limited bone regeneration (**arrow**) can be clearly seen at outer margin of capsule. Human tooth. Reproduced with permission from Matsumiya S. Atlas of oral pathology. Tokyo: Tokyo Dental College Press; 1955.

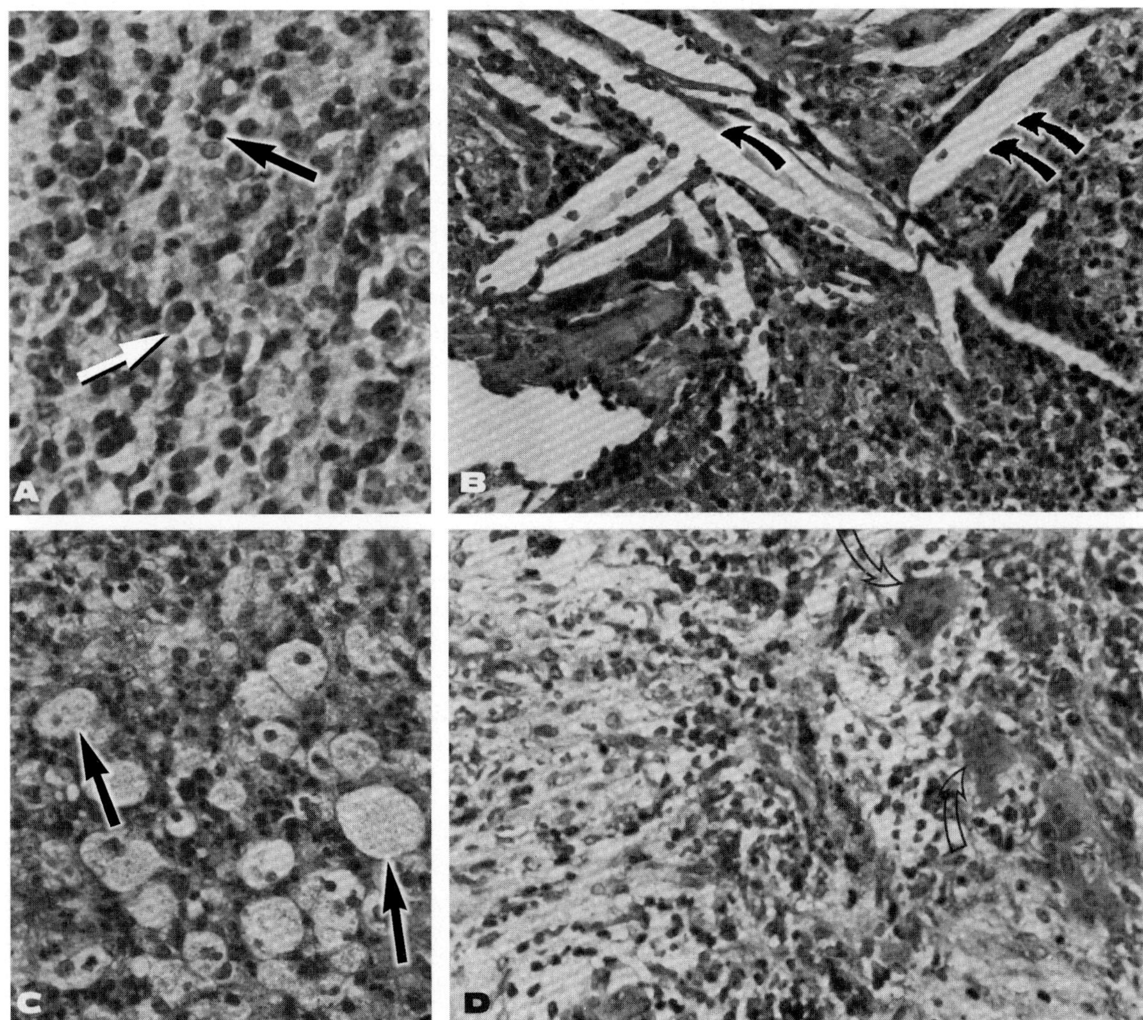

Figure 5-4 Histopathologic examination of apical periodontitis (granuloma) reveals A, the presence of many plasma cells (**white arrow**) and lymphocytes (**black arrow**); B, cholesterol slits (**black arrows**); C, foam cells (**black arrows**); D, multinucleated giant cells (**open arrows**). All of these features may not be seen in one specimen of a chronic periradicular lesion.

have also been demonstrated in these lesions.[71,72] Epithelium in varying degrees of proliferation can be found in a high percentage of periradicular granulomas (Figure 5-5).[69]

Periradicular Cyst. Histologic examination of a periradicular cyst shows a central cavity lined by stratified squamous epithelium (Figure 5-6). This lining is usually incomplete and ulcerated. The lumen of the periradicular cyst contains a pale eosinophilic fluid and occasionally some cellular debris (Figure 5-7). The connective tissue surrounding the epithelium contains the cellular and extracellular elements of the periradicular granuloma. Inflammatory cells are also present within the epithelial lining of this lesion. Histologic features of periradicular cysts are very similar to those of periradicular granulomas except for the presence of a central epithelium-lined cavity filled with fluid or semisolid material.

Local Effects of Asymptomatic Apical Periodontitis. Bone and periodontal ligament can be replaced by inflammatory tissue. This process is associated with formation of new vessels, fibroblasts, and sparse, immature connective tissue fibers. As long as egress of irritants from the root canal system to the periradicular tissues continues or macrophages fail to eliminate the materials they have phagocytosed,[73] destructive as well as healing processes will occur simultaneously in asymptomatic apical lesions. The extent of the lesion depends on the potency of the irritants within the root canal system and the activity level of defensive factors in this region. If a balance between these forces is maintained, the lesion continues in an asymptomatic manner indefinitely. On the other hand, if the causative factors overcome the defensive elements, a **symptomatic** periradicular lesion may be **superimposed** on the

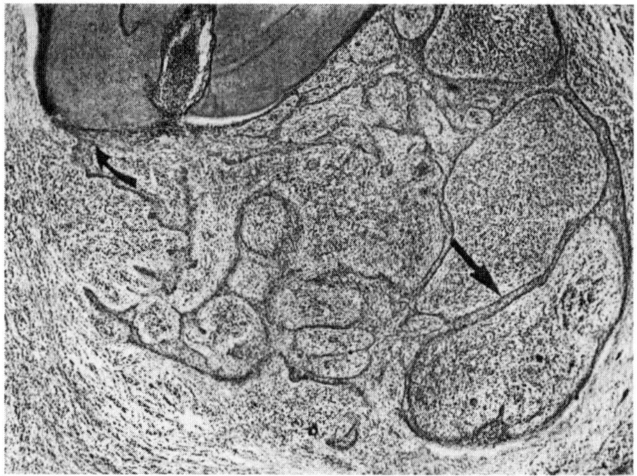

Figure 5-5 Apical periodontitis (granuloma) with contained epithelium. Epithelial cells of periodontal ligament have proliferated within new inflammatory tissue. The epithelium tends to ramify in a reticular pattern (**straight arrow**) toward receding bone. It also may, as in this case, apply itself widely to the root surface (**curved arrow**). Infiltration of epithelium by round cells is everywhere apparent. Human tooth. Reproduced with permission from Matsumiya S. Atlas of oral pathology. Tokyo: Tokyo Dental College Press; 1955.

asymptomatic one. This is one example of the so-called **phoenix abscess.**

Systemic Effects of Asymptomatic Apical Periodontitis. When the serum concentrations of circulating immune complexes (immunoglobulins G, M, and E) and the C3 complement component of patients with large periradicular lesions were measured and compared with those of patients with no lesions, investigators found no statistical difference between the two groups and concluded that **asymptomatic periradicular lesions cannot act as a focus to cause systemic diseases** via immune complexes.[51] However, when the same components were measured in patients with **symptomatic apical abscesses (SAAs)**, they found a statistically **significant difference** between the levels of immune complexes, IgG and IgM, and the C3 complement component between the two groups.[52] In addition, significant differences were also noted in the mean levels of concentration of immune complexes, IgG, IgM, and IgE, and the C3 complement component of these patients before and after root canal therapy or extraction of involved teeth. On the

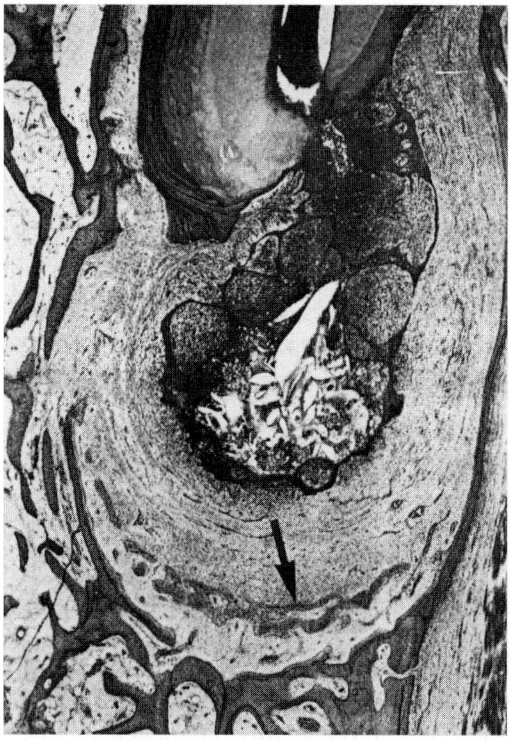

Figure 5-6 Apical cyst with marked inflammatory overlay. Round cells permeate both the epithelium and the connective tissue immediately deep to it. Spaces indicate where crystalline cholesterol has formed within the cyst. Bone formation is evident (**arrow**). This may reflect narrowing of the width of the connective tissue zone, as occurs in some apical cysts. Human tooth. Reproduced with permission from Matsumiya S. Atlas of oral pathology. Tokyo: Tokyo Dental College Press; 1955.

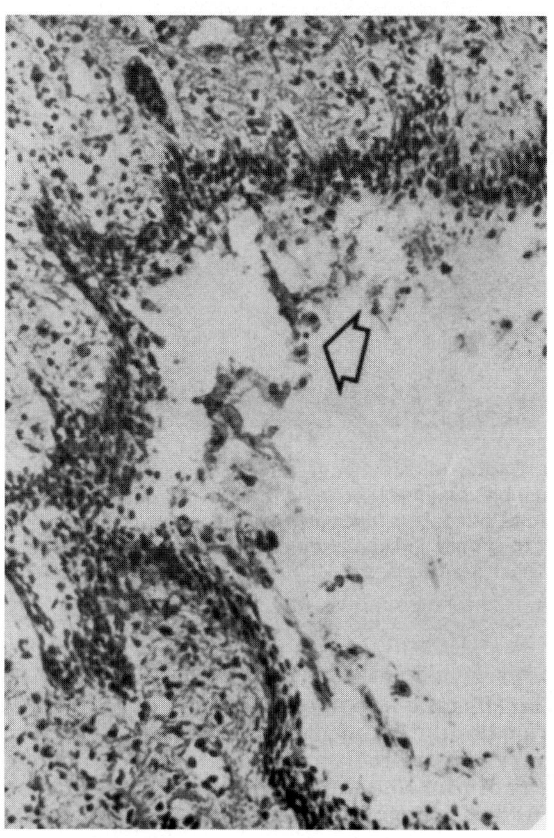

Figure 5-7 Central cavity, epithelial lining, and some of the connective tissue wall of human apical cysts. Both epithelial cells and leukocytes are floating free within the cyst cavity (**open arrow**). The epithelial lining is thin and penetrated by many round cells. Connective tissue shows moderate chronic inflammation.

basis of this study, it appears that symptomatic periradicular lesions may lead to measurable systemic immunologic reactions, but the clinical significance of these changes remains unclear.

Theories of Apical Cyst Formation. Histologic examination of normal human periodontal ligament shows remnants of Hertwig's epithelial root sheath along its length (the so-called epithelial cell rests of Malassez). Inflammation in the periradicular tissues, on the other hand, is associated with proliferation of these normally quiescent cells.[74] This explains why proliferating epithelium has been found in a significant percentage of periradicular granulomas.[75,76] The main difference between periradicular granulomas and cysts is the presence of a cavity lined by stratified squamous epithelium. The cyst lining probably arises from offspring of the proliferating epithelium present in apical granulomas.

The pathogenesis of apical cysts is not fully understood. The two prevailing theories for cavity formation in proliferating epithelium are the "breakdown" theory[69,77,78] and the "abscess cavity" theory.[79,80] The **breakdown theory** postulates that a continuous growth of epithelium removes central cells from their nutrition; consequently, the innermost cells die, and a cyst cavity forms. Because there is no evidence for lack of blood supply and the proliferating epithelium is usually invaginated by connective tissue, this theory is somewhat unsatisfactory. The **abscess cavity theory** states that a cyst results when an abscess cavity is formed in connective tissue and epithelial cells cover the exposed connective tissue, as in an ordinary wound. Because of inherent differences between the epithelial cell rests of Malassez and the epithelial cells of skin, and because of the numerous discontinuities in the linings of apical cysts, this theory does not fully explain cyst formation either.

Available evidence indicates that the development of these cavities in proliferating epithelium may be mediated by immunologic reaction. These reactions include the presence of immunocompetent cells in the proliferating epithelium of periradicular lesion,[81–83] the presence of Igs in cyst fluid,[84] and the discontinuity in the epithelial linings of most apical cysts.[85,86] Activated epithelial cell rests of Malassez can obtain antigenicity or become recognized as antigens and consequently elicit immunologic reactions.[87]

Regardless of its pathogenesis, the apical cyst evidently carries its own seeds of destruction. It survives by virtue of the irritants supplied to inflamed periradicular tissues and usually disintegrates spontaneously following elimination of those irritants.[88] Its destruction may be owing to the presence of antigenic epithelium.[87]

Condensing Osteitis

Inflammation of periradicular tissues of teeth usually stimulates concurrent osteoclastic and osteoblastic activities. Osteoclastic (resorptive) activities are usually more prominent than osteoblastic (formative) activities, and **periradicular inflammation** therefore is usually associated with **radiolucent changes.** In contrast, condensing osteitis is associated with predominant osteoblastic activity; the reason for this is unknown. Condensing osteitis is possibly attributable to a special balance between host tissues and the root canal irritants.

Condensing osteitis, or chronic focal sclerosing osteomyelitis, is a radiographic variation of AAP and is characterized as a localized overproduction of apical bone. A **low-grade inflammation** of the periradicular tissues is usually related to condensing osteitis. Radiographically, this lesion is usually observed around the apices of mandibular posterior teeth with pulp necrosis or chronic pulpitis.

Condensing osteitis may manifest with varied signs and symptoms because it is associated with a variety of pulpal and periradicular lesions. The tooth associated with condensing osteitis may be asymptomatic or sensitive to stimuli. Depending on the pulpal status, the tooth may or may not respond to electrical and thermal stimuli. The radiographic appearance of condensing osteitis, a well-circumscribed radiopaque area around one or all of the roots, is often **indicative of chronic pulpitis** (Figure 5-8). The radiopaque periradicular changes return to normal after successful root canal therapy (Figure 5-9).[89]

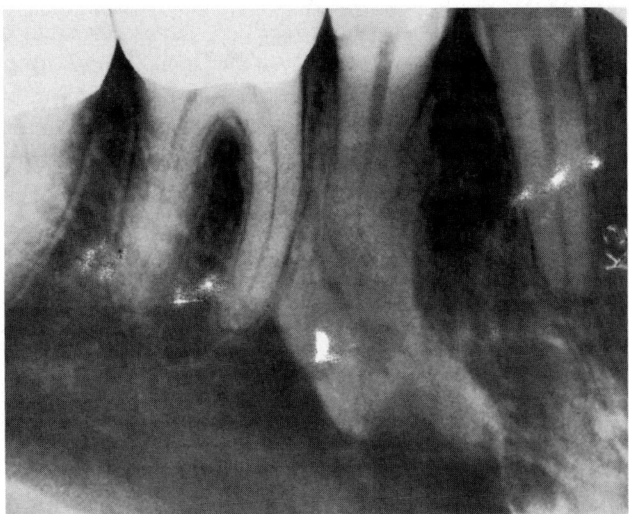

Figure 5-8 Apical condensing osteitis that developed in response to chronic pulpitis. Additional bony trabeculae have been formed and marrow spaces have been reduced to a minimum. The periodontal ligament space is visible, despite increased radiopacity of nearby bone.

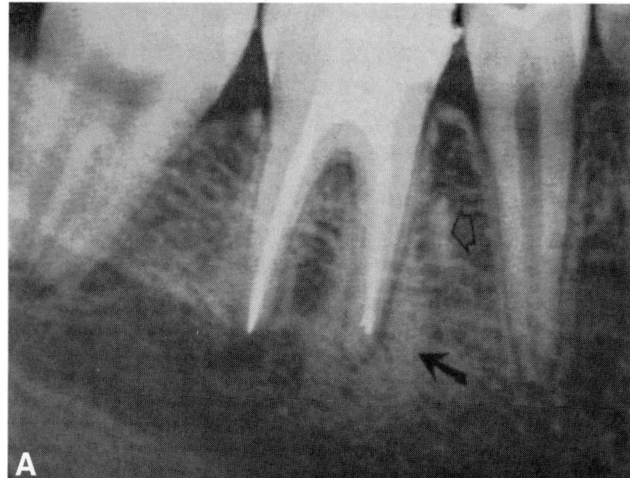

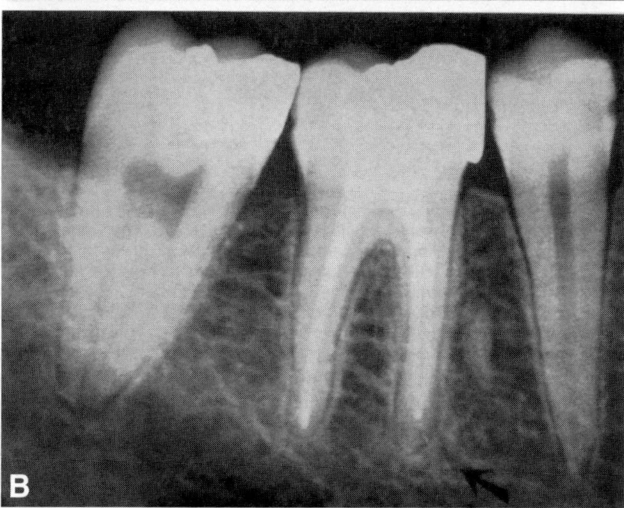

Figure 5-9 A, Apical condensing osteitis associated with chronic pulpitis. Endodontic treatment has just been completed. Obvious condensation of alveolar bone (**black arrow**) is noticeable around the mesial root of the first molar. Radiolucent area is evident at the apex of the distal root of the same tooth. The retained primary molar root tip (**open arrow**) lies within the alveolar septum mesial to the molar. B, Resolution (**arrow**) of apical condensing osteitis shown in A, 1 year after endodontic treatment. From a radiographic standpoint, complete repair of both periradicular lesions has been obtained. Reversal of apical condensing osteitis and disappearance of radiopaque area are possible.

APICAL ABSCESSES

An abscess is a localized collection of pus in a cavity formed by the disintegration of tissues.[90] Based on the degree of exudate formation and its discharge, the severity of pain, and the presence or absence of systemic signs and symptoms, apical abscesses can be divided into symptomatic or asymptomatic conditions.

Symptomatic Apical Abscess

A sudden egress of bacterial irritants into the periradicular tissues can precipitate an SAA and its more severe sequelae, acute osteitis and cellulitis. The clinical and histopathologic features of these conditions appear to be related to either the concentration and toxicity of the irritant or the local proliferation of invading organisms with their destructive activities. Chemical or bacterial irritation of the periradicular tissues through immunologic or nonimmunologic reactions can cause release of biologic substances similar to those involved in SAP and produce the same microvascular changes.

An SAA is an inflammatory process in the periradicular tissues of teeth, accompanied by exudate formation within the lesion. A frequent cause of **SAA** is a rapid influx of microorganisms, or their products, from the root canal system.

An SAA may occur without any obvious radiographic signs of pathosis. The lesions can also result from infection and rapid tissue destruction arising from within AAP, another example of the so-called phoenix abscess.

The patient may or may not have swelling. When present, the swelling may be localized or diffuse. Clinical examination of a tooth with SAA shows varying degrees of sensitivity to percussion and palpation. There is no pulp reaction to cold, heat, or electrical stimuli as the involved tooth has a necrotic pulp. Radiographic features of the SAA vary from a thickening of the periodontal ligament space to the presence of a frank periradicular lesion (Figure 5-10).

Spread of inflammatory response into the cancellous bone results in apical bone resorption. Since inflammation is not confined to the periodontal ligament but has spread to the bone, the patient now has an acute osteitis. These **patients are in pain** and may have systemic symptoms such as fever and increased white blood cell count. Because of the pressure from the accumulation of exudate within the confining tissues, the pain can be severe. Spread of the lesion toward a surface, erosion of cortical bone, and extension of the abscess through the periosteum and into the soft tissues is ordinarily accompanied by **swelling** and some relief. Commonly, the swelling remains localized, but it also may become diffuse and spread widely (**cellulitis**) (Figure 5-11). The extent of swelling reflects the amount and nature of the irritant egressing from the root canal system, the virulence and incubation period of the involved bacteria, and the host's resistance. The location of the swelling is determined by the relation of the apex of the involved tooth to adjacent muscle attachments.[91]

Immunologic or nonimmunologic inflammatory responses contribute to the breakdown of the alveolar bone and cause disruption of the blood supply, which,

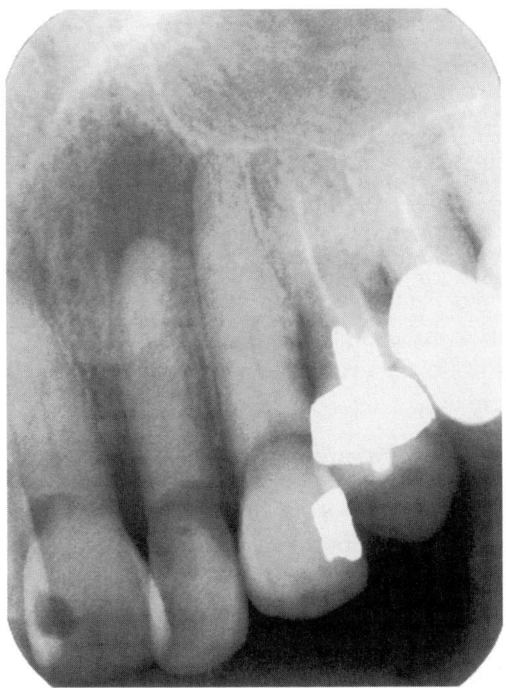

Figure 5-10 Radiographic features of symptomatic apical abscess. The patient developed sudden symptoms of pain and facial swelling. Radiographically, a lesion is apparent apically to the maxillary left lateral incisor, that did not respond to vitality tests, confirming pulpal diagnosis of necrosis.

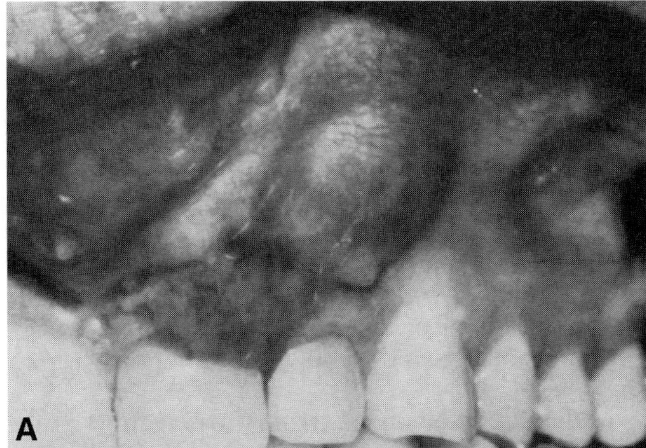

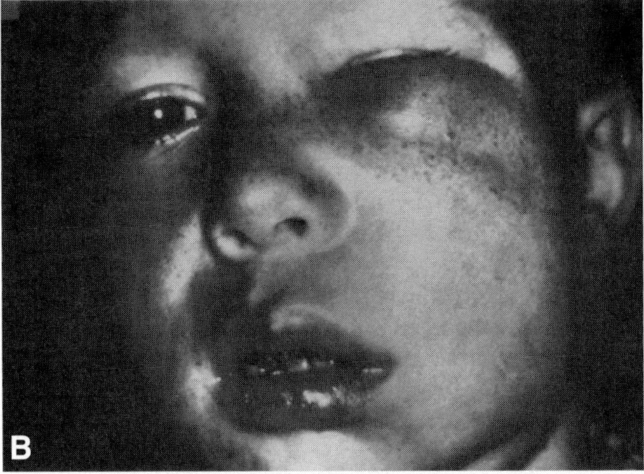

Figure 5-11 A, Localized abscess resulting from an incomplete root canal treatment on a maxillary lateral incisor. B, Cellulitis caused by a maxillary first molar with necrotic pulp. (Courtesy of Dr. Mohammad Baghai.)

in turn, produces more soft and hard tissue necrosis. The **suppuration** process finds lines of least resistance and eventually **perforates the cortical plate.** When it reaches the soft tissue, the pressure on the periosteum is relieved, usually with an abatement of symptoms. Once this drainage through bone and mucosa is obtained, **suppurative apical periodontitis** or an asymptomatic periradicular abscess is established.

Asymptomatic Apical Abscess

Asymptomatic apical abscess (AAA), also referred to as **suppurative apical periodontitis,** is associated with a gradual egress of irritants from the root canal system into the periradicular tissues and formation of an exudate. The quantity of irritants, their potency, and their host resistance are all important factors in determining the quantity of exudate formation and the clinical signs and symptoms of the lesion. **Asymptomatic apical abscess** is associated with either a continuously or intermittently **draining sinus tract.** This is visually evident as a **stoma** on the oral mucosa (Figure 5-12) or occasionally as a fistula on the skin of the face (Figure 5-13). The exudate can also drain through the gingival sulcus of the involved tooth, mimicking a periodontal lesion with a "pocket." This is not a true periodontal

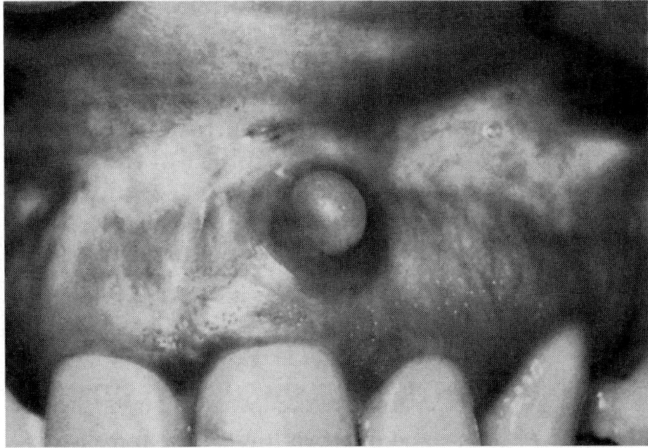

Figure 5-12 Apical abscess and its stoma. Initially, the abscess was asymptomatic, but when the opening of the sinus tract from the maxillary left central incisor became blocked, the accumulation of drainage caused pain.

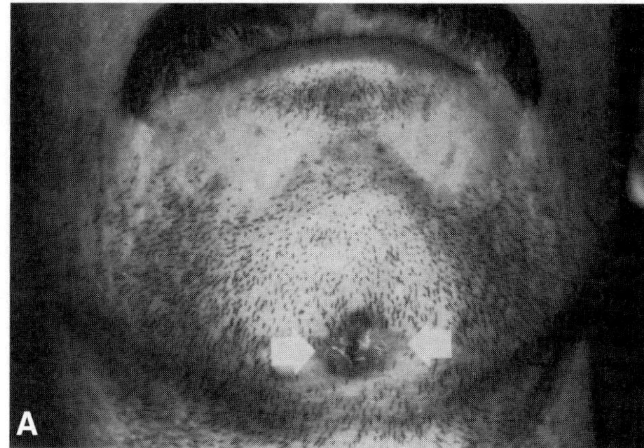

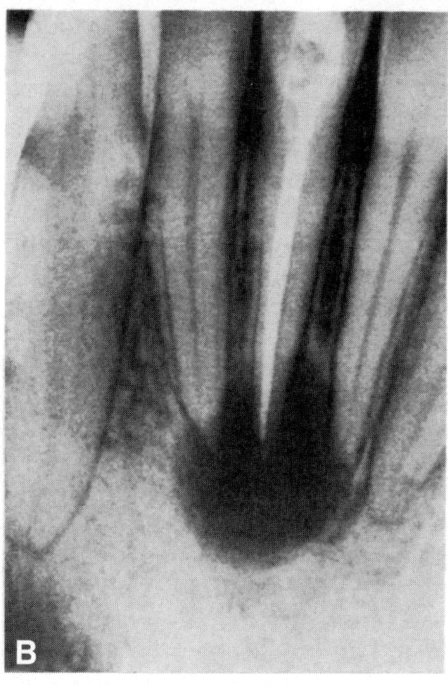

Figure 5-13 A, Apical abscesses occasionally drain extraorally (**white arrows**). After several years of treatment for "skin infection" with no results from topical application of numerous antibiotics, the problem was traced to the central incisor with previous root canal treatment. B, The tooth was retreated nonsurgically and the chin lesion healed within a few weeks with some scarring. (Courtesy of Dr. Leif K. Bakland.)

pocket as there is not a complete detachment of connective tissue from the root surface.[92] If left untreated, however, it can be covered with an epithelial lining and becomes a true periodontal pocket.

An AAA is usually associated with little discomfort. If the sinus tract drainage becomes blocked, however, varying levels of pain and swelling will be experienced. Correspondingly, clinical examination of a tooth with this type of lesion reveals a range of sensitivity to percussion and palpation, depending on whether the tract is open, draining, or closed.

Vitality tests are negative on teeth with AAA because of the presence of necrotic pulps. Radiographic examination of these lesions shows the presence of bone loss at the apexes of the involved teeth (Figure 5-13, B).

The sinus tract that leads away from this suppurative core to the surface may be partially lined with epithelium or the inner surface composed of inflamed connective tissue.[93] The sinus tract, like the periradicular cyst, arises and persists because of irritants from the pulp. Similarly, these sinus tracts, whether lined or not, resolve following root canal treatment removing the etiology.

REPAIR OF PERIRADICULAR LESIONS

Removal of irritants from the root canal system and its total obturation result in repair of inflamed periradicular tissue.[94] Depending on the extent of tissue damage, repair varies from a simple reduction and resolution of inflammation to a more complex regeneration, involving remodeling of bone, periodontal ligament, and cementum. Repair of the lesion, therefore, may take days to years. Periradicular inflammatory lesions usually arise from irritants of a necrotic pulp. Endodontic treatment may initiate or amplify the inflammation by extruded debris, overextended instruments, or filling materials extended into the periradicular tissues. As a result, the periodontal ligament and its surrounding tissues are replaced by chronic inflammatory tissue. As long as irritation continues, simultaneous destruction and repair of these periradicular tissues continue.

This pattern of breakdown/repair was demonstrated by Fish,[95] who produced infected lesions in guinea pigs by drilling holes in the bone and packing wool fibers saturated with microorganisms. He described four reactive zones to the bacteria: **infection, contamination, irritation,** and **stimulation**. The central **infection** zone had microorganisms and neutrophils. **Contamination** was a zone of round-cell infiltrate. The zone of **irritation** was characterized by the presence of macrophages and osteoclasts. The outermost area was the zone of **stimulation,** containing fibroblasts and forming collagen and bone.

Extrapolations of Fish's findings to the tooth with a necrotic pulp have been made. Egress of microorganisms and the other irritants from the root canal system into the periradicular tissues causes the central zones of tissue destruction near the zone of infection. As the toxicity of irritants is reduced in the central zones, the number of reparative cells increases peripherally.[96] **Removal of the irritants and their source by root canal débridement and proper obturation permits the reparative zone to move inward.**

The healing of periradicular tissues after root canal treatment is often associated with formation and organization of a fibrin clot, granulation tissue formation and maturation, subsidence of inflammation, and, finally, restoration of normal architecture of the periodontal ligament. Since the inflammatory reactions are usually accompanied by microscopic and macroscopic resorption of the hard tissues, bone and cementum repair occurs as well.

Periradicular lesions repair from the periphery to the center. If the cortical plate is perforated by resorption, the healing process is partially **periosteal** in nature. Boyne and Harvey, after creating cortical plate perforations in the jaws of humans, showed that labial defects measuring 5 to 8 mm in diameter healed completely within 5 months.[97] When they studied apical defects measuring 9 to 12 mm, they found that these lesions had limited labial cortex formation and instead were filled with avascular fibrous connective tissue up to 8 months following surgery.

If lesions have not involved the periosteum, the healing response will be **endosteal**, with formation of bony trabeculae extending inward from the walls of the lesion toward the root surface. On the periphery, osteoblasts appear and elaborate bone matrix (osteoid), which gradually mineralizes as it matures. If cementum or dentin has been resorbed by the inflammation, remodeling and repair are by secondary cementum.

The last to form is likely the fibrous component interposed between newly formed bone and the cemental root surface. These fibers have basically two orientations. One is a true periodontal ligament arrangement, whereas the other is an alignment of collagen parallel to the root surface. Both orientations represent complete healing.

The sequence of events post–endodontic treatment leading to complete repair of periradicular tissues, after inflammatory destruction of the periodontal ligament, bone, or cementum, has not been validated. Most information is based on repair of extraction sites or healing of bone cavities following periradicular curettage. These may or may not be accurate as to patterns of nonsurgical apical repair. A blood clot forms following extraction or apicoectomy, which becomes organized into recognizable granulation tissue. This tissue contains endothelium-lined vascular spaces, vast numbers of fibroblasts, and associated collagen fibers. The granulation tissue is infiltrated by neutrophils, lymphocytes, and plasma cells. On the periphery of the granulation tissue, osteoblasts and osteoclasts abound. With maturation, the number of cells decreases, whereas collagen increases. Ultimately, mature bone forms from the periphery toward the center.[98]

Do different types of endodontic periradicular lesions have different patterns of healing? Possibly there are variations, but this has not been conclusively demonstrated. Of the three general lesion types—granuloma, cyst, and abscess—it is likely that the granuloma follows the pattern described above.[99] The abscess may be slower; the exudates and bacteria must be cleared from the tissues before regeneration occurs. A variation of the abscess, the sinus tract (intraoral and extraoral) will heal following root canal treatment.[100] It has been suggested that the periradicular cyst with a cavity that does not communicate with the root canal is less likely to resolve following root canal treatment[101]; this has yet to be proven.

There is some evidence that at least some lesions may heal with formation of scar tissue.[102] Although the frequency of healing by scar tissue is unknown, it is likely that it seldom occurs following root canal treatment, being much more common after periradicular surgery on maxillary anterior teeth.[103]

NONENDODONTIC PERIRADICULAR LESIONS

Bhaskar, in his textbook on radiographic interpretation, listed 38 radiolucent lesions and other abnormalities of the jaws.[104] Three of these lesions, dental granuloma, radicular cyst, and abscess, are categorized as being related to necrotic pulps. In addition, Bhaskar identifies 16 radiopaque lesions of the jaws, 3 of which, condensing osteitis, sclerosing osteomyelitis, and Garré's osteomyelitis, are also related to pulpal pathosis. The dentist must therefore differentiate between the endodontic and the nonendodontic lesions, ruling out those that trace their origin from non–pulp-related sources. Additional confusion in radiographic diagnosis relates to normal radiolucent and radiopaque structures that lie within or over apical regions.

Differential diagnosis of periradicular pathosis is essential and, at times, confusing. There is a tendency for the clinician to assume that a radiolucency is an endodontically related lesion and that root canal treatment is necessary without performing additional confirmatory tests. **Avoid this pitfall!**

The dentist must therefore be astute as well as knowledgeable when diagnosing bony lesions. It is important that teeth with sound pulps not be violated needlessly because of the mistaken notion that radiolucencies in the apical region always represent endodontic pathema. The reverse is also true; endodontic lesions may mimic nonendodontic pathosis.

Significantly, **most** radiolucent lesions do indeed trace their origin to pulpal disease. Therefore, the dentist is likely to encounter many more endodontic lesions, because of their sheer numbers, than other types of pathosis. However, many of the nonendodontic lesions mimic endodontic pathema, with similar symptoms and radiographic appearance.[105] On the other hand, many of the nonendodontic lesions are symptomless (as endodontic lesions frequently are) and are detected only on radiographs. To avoid errors, the dentist must approach all lesions with caution, whether symptomatic or not.

This section will deal with lesions of the jaws categorized as **odontogenic** or **nonodontogenic** in origin. Odontogenic lesions arise from remnants of odontogenesis (or the tooth-forming organ), either mesenchymal or ectodermal in origin. Nonodontogenic lesions trace their origins to a variety of precursors and therefore are not as easily classified.

Not all bony lesions that occur in the jaws will be discussed as many are extremely rare or do not ordinarily mimic endodontic pathosis. An oral pathology text should be consulted for clinical features and histopathology of missing entities. Furthermore, the lesions that are included are not discussed in detail. Of primary concern are the clinical findings causing them to resemble endodontic pathema, as well as those factors leading to accurate differential diagnosis.

Differentiating between lesions of endodontic and nonendodontic origin is usually not difficult. **Pulp vitality testing**, when done with accuracy, is the primary method of determination; nearly all nonendodontic lesions are in the region of vital teeth, whereas endodontic lesions are usually associated with pulp necrosis, giving negative vitality responses. Except by coincidence, nonendodontic lesions are **rarely** associated with pulpless teeth. Other significant radiographic and clinical signs and symptoms, however, aid in differential diagnosis.

Odontogenic Cysts

Dentigerous Cyst. Also called follicular cysts, dentigerous cysts are derived histogenetically from the reduced enamel epithelium of an impacted or embedded tooth. Therefore, they are most often associated with the crowns either of **impacted third molars,** maxillary canines, or mandibular second premolars. The majority are found in the mandible.[106,107] Although most remain small and asymptomatic, dentigerous cysts have the potential to become aggressive lesions. Continued enlargement may involve large areas of the jaws, particularly the mandible, with displacement of teeth and expansion of cortices.[108]

Dentigerous cysts may be confused with endodontic lesions by either radiographic or other clinical findings. Routine periradicular or panographic films might reveal its presence at the apex of adjacent teeth, sometimes causing root resorption. An unusual variant is the **circumferential dentigerous cyst** (Figure 5-14). The tooth may erupt through the dentigerous cyst, with the resulting radiolucency occurring periradicularly, thus closely mimicking periradicular pathosis of pulp origin.[109] The dentigerous cyst occasionally may become secondarily infected and inflamed, often via a pericoronal communication. The swelling and pain clinically resemble disease of pulpal origin.

This cyst is readily differentiated from chronic apical periodontitis or acute apical abscess in that the adjacent erupted tooth invariably demonstrates pulp vitality.

Lateral Periodontal Cyst. This uncommon cyst arises at the lateral surface of a tooth, usually in the mandibular premolar-canine area (Figure 5-15). This lesion is currently thought to arise from remnants of the dental lamina and probably represents the intraosseous analog of the gingival cyst of the adult.[110] Clinically, the lesion is asymptomatic, and again the

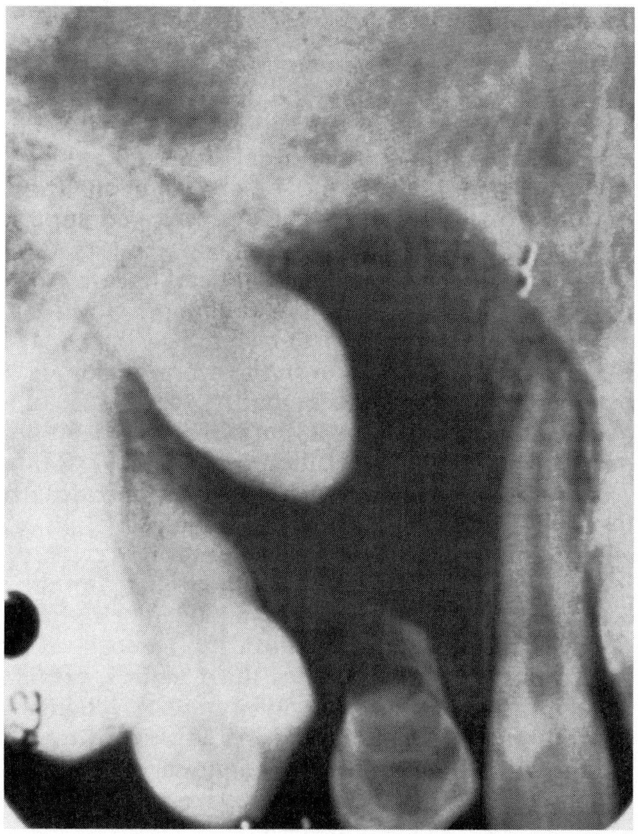

Figure 5-14 Circumferential dentigerous cyst developed around the crown of an unerupted canine. The cyst may be enucleated (care must be taken to avoid the incisor) and the canine brought into position with an orthodontic appliance. (Courtesy of Dr. Russell Christensen.)

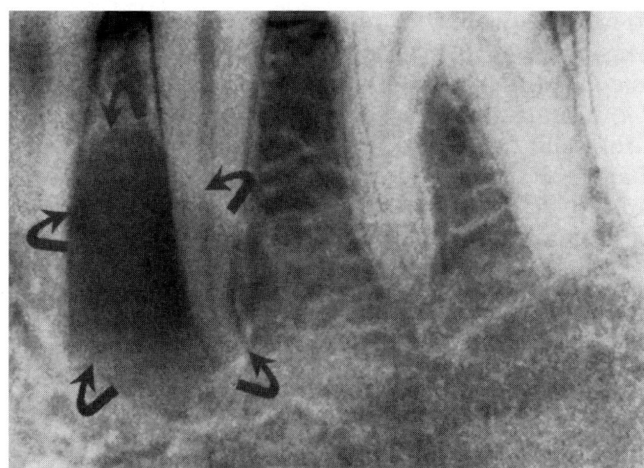

Figure 5-15 Lateral periodontal cyst. Well-circumscribed radiolucent area in apposition to the lateral surfaces of the lower premolars (**black arrows** demarcate the extent of lesions). No clinical signs or symptoms were noted. Pulps tested vital.

pulp of the involved tooth is vital. Radiographically, the lesion is usually less than 1 cm in diameter and may or may not have a surrounding rim of dense bone. It resembles the **lateral radicular cyst,** which is an endodontic inflammatory lesion related to a necrotic pulp.[111] Differentiation is made on the basis of pulp vitality testing.

Odontogenic Keratocyst. The odontogenic keratocyst is a relatively common lesion, probably arising from remnants of the dental lamina.[112] Clinically and radiographically, this lesion may resemble a periradicular lesion.[113] The keratocyst may confuse the clinician by manifesting pain, soft tissue swelling, or expansion of bone. Radiographically, the lesion may appear as a unilocular or multilocular radiolucency in the lateral or apical region of teeth, usually in the mandible[114] (Figure 5-16). However, other keratocysts mimic (and may have their origins in) dentigerous and lateral periodontal cysts in their radiographic appearance.

Differentially, the adjacent teeth respond to vitality testing. The keratocyst is easily differentiated from lesions of pulp origin on the basis of its pathognomonic histologic features. The lesion has a **marked tendency to recur** following surgical removal,[115] indicating that the keratinized epithelium has a greater growth potential than does ordinary cyst epithelium.[116]

Residual Apical Cyst. The residual apical cyst or residual dentigerous cyst reportedly represents a persistent apical cyst that was associated with an extracted pulpless tooth. It has been theorized that an apical cyst has the potential to develop from epithelial remnants after extraction and to be a self-perpetuating lesion.[108] Contradicting this theory is the evidence that apical cysts usually resolve spontaneously following nonsurgical root canal treatment.[117] The cyst wall may, in fact, carry the seeds of its own destruction. Toller[118] and Torabinejad[87] have presented evidence that the epithelium may be antigenic and speculate that it would therefore be eliminated by the immune mechanism.

Consequently, only a few specimens of residual cyst have been carefully described. Kronfeld noted the basic epithelium, cavity, and capsule.[119] He stressed the absence of inflammatory cells in both the epithelial lining and the connective tissue zone, which further casts doubt that this would truly be a "residual" apical cyst. Very uncommon (if it exists at all) and uncomplicated, the lesion offers few problems.

Bone Pathology: Fibro-osseous Lesions

In a comprehensive publication, Waldron and Giansanti classified and reviewed fibro-osseous lesions of the jaws.[120] These represent a phenomenon in which normal bone is replaced by a tissue compound of fibroblasts and collagen, containing varying amounts of a bony or cementum-like calcification. The radiographic appearance varies according to size and relative amounts and mixtures of fibrous tissue/hard tissue. Because of these radiographic appearances and their location over and around apices, some types of fibro-osseous lesions are often confused with endodontic lesions. These will be discussed further.

Periradicular Cemental Dysplasia. Also termed periradicular osteofibrosis or, more commonly, periapical cementoma, periradicular cemental dysplasia

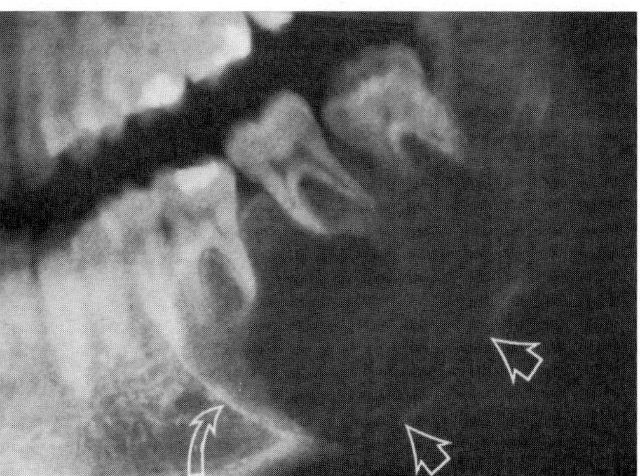

Figure 5-16 Odontogenic keratocyst. A multilocular radiolucency with sclerotic border (**arrows**) in the mandible. All of the molars in this case responded to a vitality test. (Courtesy of the Department of Oral Pathology, Loma Linda University.)

demonstrates lesions that are often multiple, usually involve the mandibular incisors, and occur most often in middle-aged African American women. However, they can and do occur elsewhere in the jaws and in any race and at other ages. Their etiology is unknown.

Periradicular cemental dysplasia has an interesting evolution.[121] The progression is from normal alveolar bone to **bone resorption and fibrosis** and finally to **dense, atypical reossification.** The initial stage (osteolytic stage) is characterized histologically by a proliferation of fibroblasts and collagen fibers in the apical region of the periodontal ligament. The resultant mass induces resorption of the medullary bone surrounding the apex, resulting in a radiolucent lesion closely mimicking a lesion of pulpal origin (Figure 5-17). During this stage of radiolucency, errors are frequently made,[122] emphasizing the necessity of pulp testing.

Unlike apical periodontitis or an apical cyst, this new growth is free of inflammation. Furthermore, nerves and vessels are unimpeded as they make their passage to and from the root canal.

In time, cementoblasts differentiate within the soft tissue, and a central focus of calcification appears (**intermediate stage**) (Figure 5-18). This deposition of

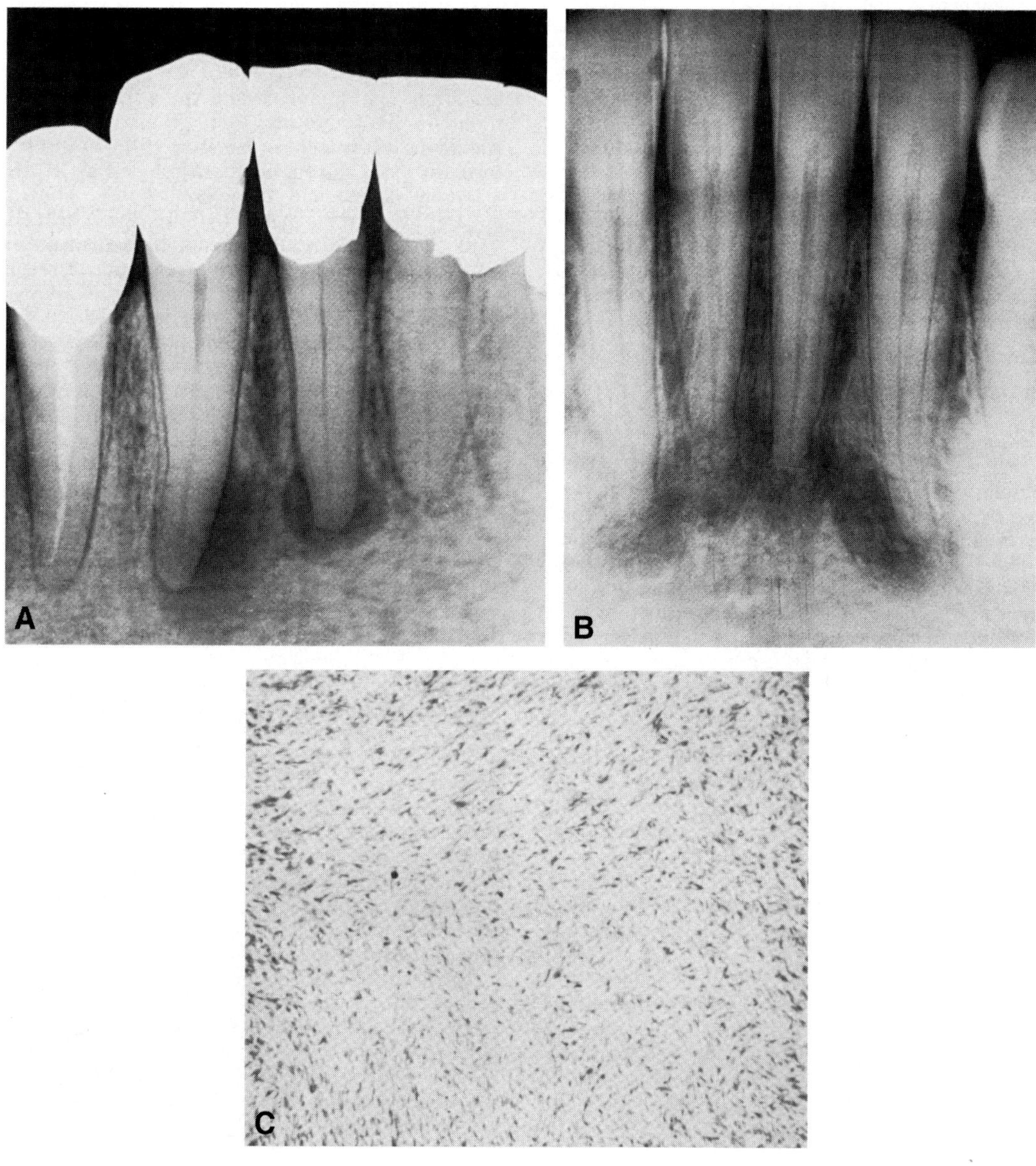

Figure 5-17 A, Periradicular cemental dysplasia (osteofibrosis), **initial stage**. Pulps in both teeth are vital. **B**, Transition to the **second stage** is developing. **C**, Biopsy of periradicular osteofibrosis, initial stage. Fibrous connective tissue lesion has replaced cancellous bone. (Photomicrograph courtesy of Dr. S. N. Bhaskar and the Walter Reed Army Institute of Research. US Army photograph.)

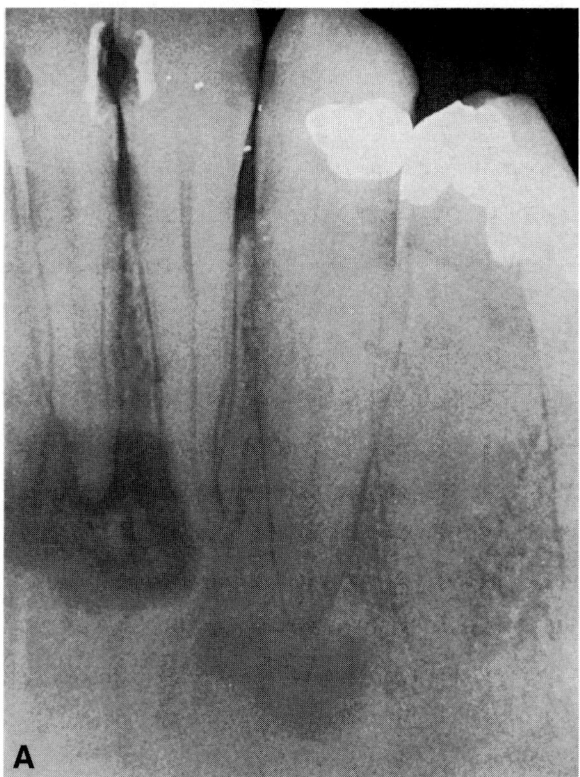

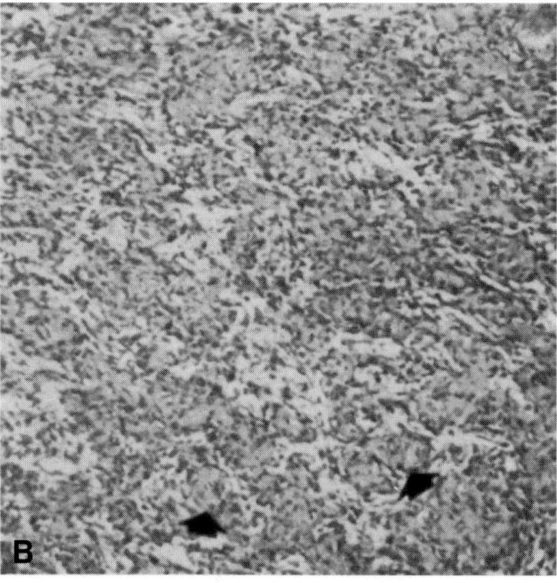

Figure 5-18 A, Periradicular cemental dysplasia, **intermediate stage,** central incisor and canine. Slight calcification of the fibrotic lesion is now developing. The pulps are vital. **B,** Biopsy of the intermediate stage with foci (**arrows**) of calcification appearing throughout the lesion. (Photomicrograph courtesy of Dr. S. N. Bhaskar and the Walter Reed Army Institute of Research, US Army photograph.)

hard tissue may be continued over the years until nearly all of the fibrous tissue is reossified. When this occurs, the evolution has reached its third and final stage (**mature stage**) (Figure 5-19). The reossification is characterized radiographically by increasing radiopacity.

Problems of **differential diagnosis** arise in conjunction with the **initial radiolucent stage** of periradicular cemental dysplasia (see Figure 5-17). Clinically, the lesions are **always asymptomatic**, and the adjacent teeth respond to vitality testing. Radiographically, **an intact lamina dura** is usually (but not always) visible around the apices if carefully looking "through" the radiolucency.

Osteoblastoma and Cementoblastoma. These are apparent **benign neoplasms** and are closely related lesions. Some believe that a cementoblastoma is, in reality, an osteoblastoma with an intimate relationship with the root (Figure 5-20). The benign cementoblastoma (or true cementoma) is an uncommon neoplasm thought to represent a neoplasm of cementoblasts.[123] Radiographically, the lesion is characteristically associated and continuous with the roots of the teeth, usually a mandibular first molar.[124] The tumor mass is often surrounded by a thin, radiolucent zone that is continuous with the periodontal ligament space. Histologically, the tumor shows fusion with the root cementum.

Differentiation between cementoblastoma and condensing osteitis is based on differences in radiographic appearance; **condensing osteitis is diffuse,** shows no well-defined borders, and is associated with **chronic pulpal disease.** Furthermore, the lamina dura and normal periodontal ligament space may remain intact in condensing osteitis.

Cementifying and Ossifying Fibroma. The central ossifying fibroma is a benign, neoplastic, fibro-osseous lesion. Circumstantial evidence indicates that central ossifying fibromas originate from elements of the periodontal ligament.[120] Most of these lesions arise in the periradicular region and therefore **can be easily confused** radiographically with endodontic periradicular lesions (Figure 5-21). They tend to occur in **younger patients** and in the **premolar-molar region of the mandible.** Because they are **asymptomatic,** the lesions are frequently undetected. They attain a large size, often with visible expansion of the overlying cortex.

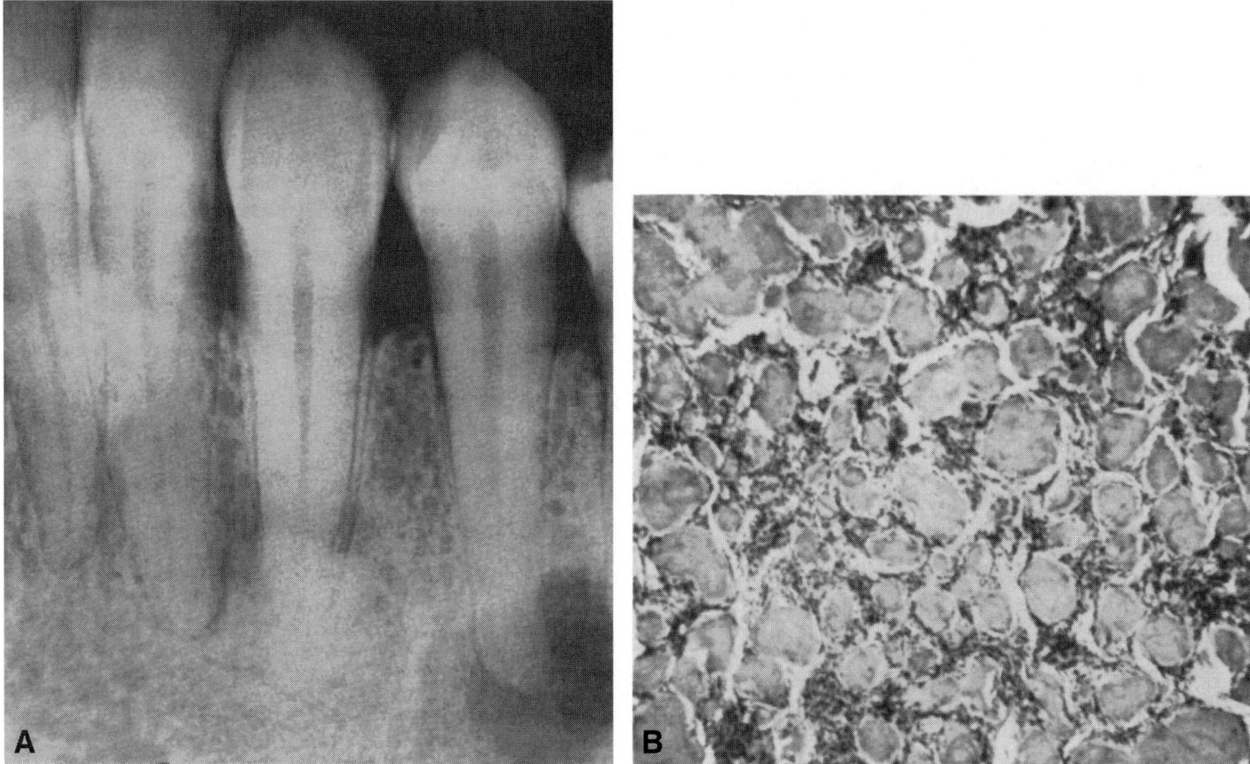

Figure 5-19 A, Periradicular cemental dysplasia, **mature stage**, canine. Osseous calcification associated with vital pulp. Fibrotic stage is seen at the periapex of the first premolar. **B**, Biopsy of the final stage with advanced, dense calcification. (Photomicrograph courtesy of Dr. S. N. Bhaskar and the Walter Reed Army Institute of Research. US Army photograph.)

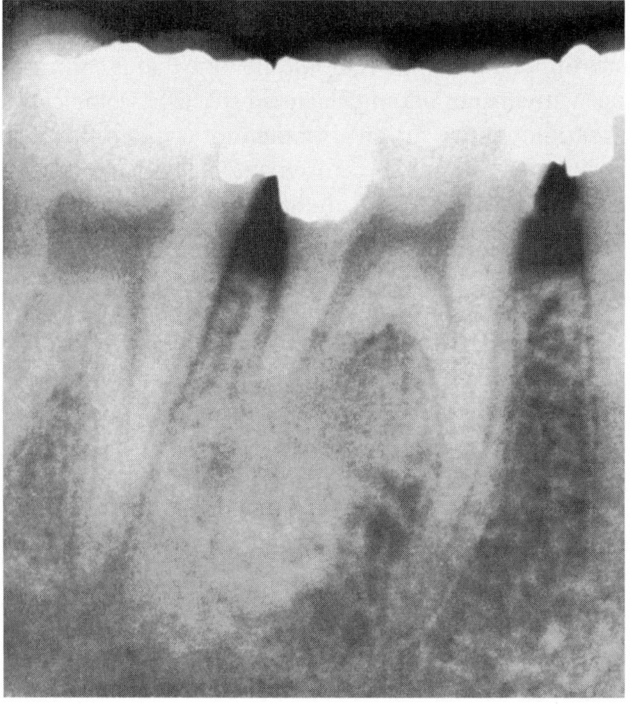

Figure 5-20 Cementoblastoma. The lesion is a fairly well-defined radiopaque mass surrounded by a thin radiolucent line. It has also replaced the apical portions of the distal root of the first molar.

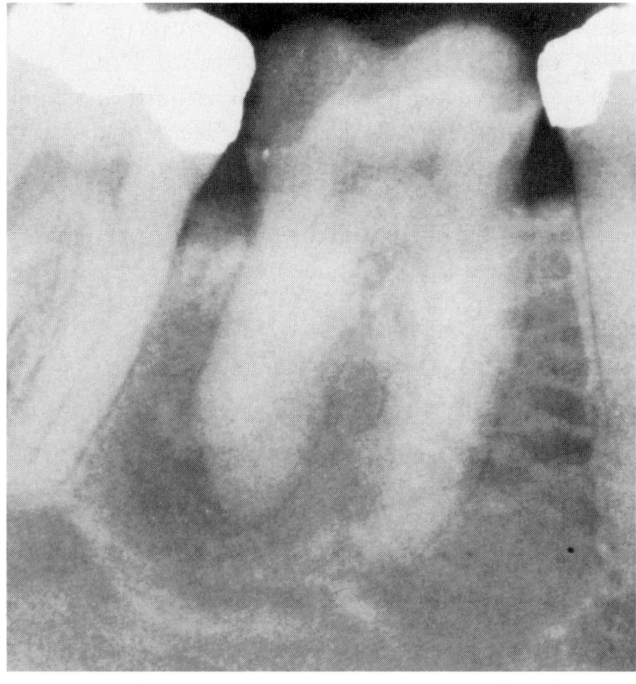

Figure 5-21 Ossifying fibroma. The patient presented with pain. The pulp was vital, indicating that this was not an endodontic pathosis. Root canal treatment was followed by root end removal and excision of the lesion. Biopsy confirmed the diagnosis.

The central ossifying fibroma has a characteristic progression of radiologic findings. During the **early stage**, which is **osteolytic**, bone is resorbed and replaced by fibrous tissue. Ossifying fibromas usually appear as solitary radiolucencies that may or may not be in contact with the apices of adjacent teeth (Figure 5-22). Because the lesion is ossifying (or cementifying), the lesion, with time, demonstrates calcified components in its center. These components enlarge and coalesce, until eventually most of the lesion appears radiopaque (see Figure 5-22).

Differentiating the ossifying fibroma from periradicular lesions is not difficult unless the dentist depends on radiographic findings alone. Characteristically, **the pulps** in the teeth in the region of the lesion are vital. Final diagnosis is by excision and biopsy, which show elements of calcified structures within the stroma.[125]

Odontogenic Tumors

Ameloblastoma. The ameloblastoma is a rare but **destructive lesion**. It is a locally invasive and sometimes dangerous lesion classified as an odontogenic tumor. It is **usually painless** and grows slowly. Clinically, it may resemble a periradicular lesion, demonstrating similar signs. As the lesion expands, it can cause displacement and increased mobility of teeth (Figure 5-23). Radiographically, it is usually multilocular but may appear as a solitary lesion, frequently associated with the apices of teeth, particularly in the mandibular posterior region. Often there is **associated root resorption.**[126]

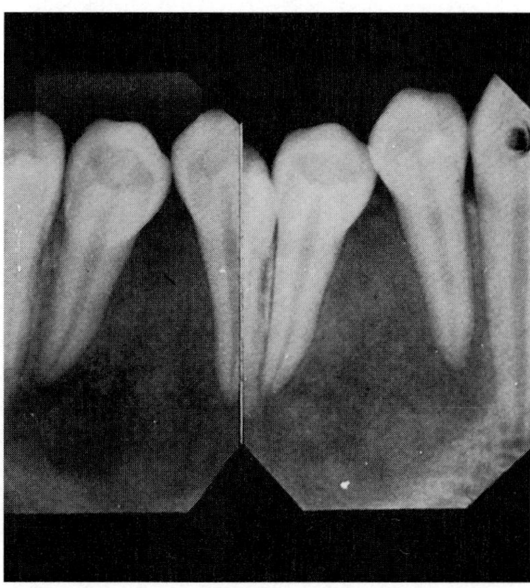

Figure 5-22 Central ossifying fibroma gradually calcifying with time. The asymptomatic lesion discovered in a radiographic survey initially resembled endodontic pathosis. (Courtesy of Dr. Raymond J. Melrose.)

The lesion may manifest endodontic-like clinical symptoms. An ameloblastoma may cause expansion of the jaws or erode the cortical bone and invade adjacent soft tissue. It is then visible and detectable on palpation. Some lesions are solid, whereas others are soft and fluctuant. If the lesion has undergone cystic degenera-

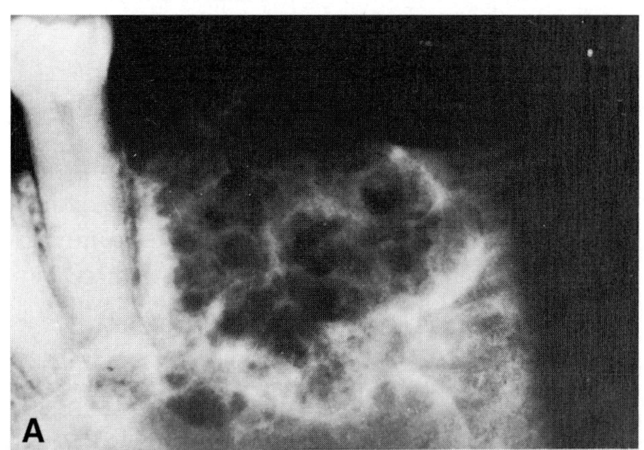

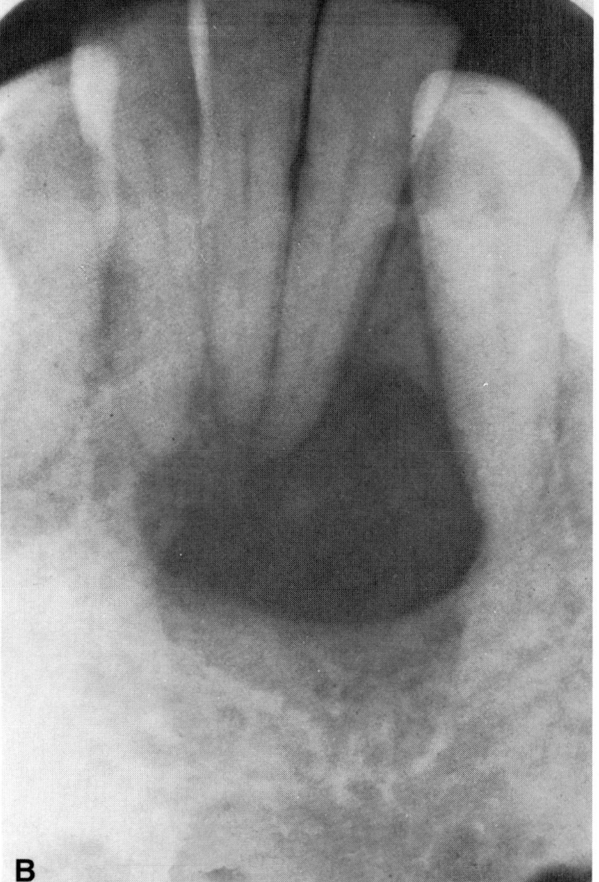

Figure 5-23 Two examples of ameloblastoma. **A**, Surgical specimen of infiltrating ameloblastoma of mandible. **B**, "Unicystic" ameloblastoma. This solitary lesion has displaced teeth much as an apical cyst would do. The teeth are vital. (Courtesy of Dr. Raymond J. Melrose.)

tion, **straw-colored fluid may be aspirated**, which gives the appearance of an apical cyst.

Again, the **differential diagnosis** depends on a more careful examination than radiographs alone. Radiographically and clinically, the **ameloblastoma** may resemble many other types of bony lesions, including periradicular lesions. **The critical test is the vitality of pulps** of adjacent teeth. Unless the ameloblastoma has caused significant damage by invading and disrupting sensory nerves (which is seldom), the teeth will respond to pulp testing.

Nonodontogenic Lesions

Central Giant Cell Granuloma. Of unknown etiology, the central giant cell granuloma is an expansile destructive lesion of the bone.[127] It most commonly **occurs in children and young adult females** and appears radiographically as a unilocular or multilocular radiolucency in the anterior-premolar region of the mandible. Clinically, the lesion is **usually asymptomatic**, but the involved region **may be painful** and show **bony expansion.**[123] Radiographically, it often **surrounds apices** and occasionally may produce **root resorption** or tooth displacement (Figure 5-24). Histologically, the stroma is characterized by fibroblastic tissue with foci of hemorrhage, many vascular spaces, and concentrations of multinucleated giant cells (Figure 5-25). Significantly and diagnostically, the pulps are usually vital, although the teeth are occasionally nonresponsive, apparently because of sensory nerve damage.

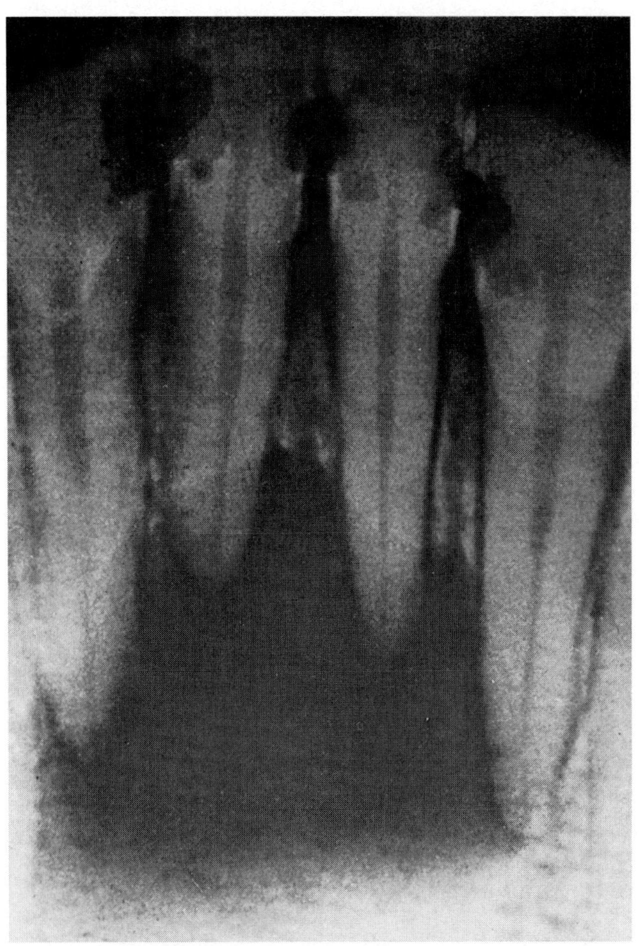

Figure 5-24 Central giant cell granuloma. A relatively smooth radiolucent lesion in the anterior region of the mandible. No resorption or displacement of teeth is noted. The teeth responded to vitality tests. (Courtesy of the Department of Oral Pathology, Loma Linda University.)

Because the pulps of adjacent teeth often have their blood supply interrupted during curettage of the lesion, root canal treatment is often necessary before or after surgical removal.

Nasopalatine Duct Cyst. Also known as the incisive canal cyst and median anterior maxillary cyst, the nasopalatine duct cyst is one of the more common pathologic entities arising in the anterior region of the maxilla. Because of its location, radiographic appearance, and symptoms, it is **easily confused with a periradicular lesion** (Figure 5-26). It arises from remnants of the embryologic nasopalatine duct and so is considered a developmental cyst.

Clinically, the lesion is usually asymptomatic but may show swelling or, if secondarily infected, discharge of pus in the incisive papilla region.[128] Radiographically, a well-defined radiolucent area is seen interradicularly or apically to the maxillary central incisors. It is often **heart shaped** owing to superimposition of the anterior nasal

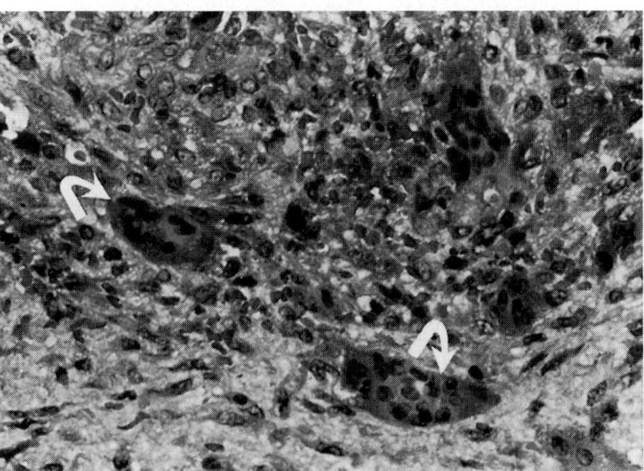

Figure 5-25 Central giant cell granuloma—relatively loose connective tissue with numerous fibroblasts and a few giant cells (**white arrows**).

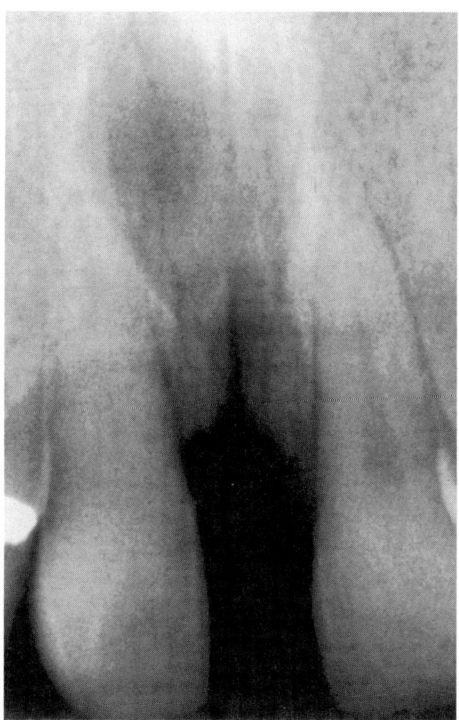

Figure 5-26 Nasopalatine duct cyst. This could be confused with endodontic pathosis. There was a history of trauma, with calcific metamorphisis of the right central incisor. Note the heart-shaped appearance of the lesion. (Courtesy of Dr. Richard Walton).

spine (see Figure 5-26). Growth of the cyst may cause **divergence of roots.**

As with other periradicular radiolucencies, **pulp testing** is the critical diagnostic determinant. A radiolucency associated with vital teeth indicates a nasopalatine duct cyst. A radiolucency associated with a nonvital pulp, although it resembles a nasopalatine duct cyst, is likely to be an endodontic lesion. In addition to pulp testing, **exposing radiographs from different** horizontal angles can help in differentiation. If the radiolucency is caused by a necrotic pulp, it will not be separated from the apex by the change in angles. However, if the radiolucency is caused by a large normal or a cystic nasopalatine duct, it will be moved from the apices with different horizontal angles of the cone (Figure 5-27).

Simple Bone Cyst. Also referred to as the solitary, traumatic, or hemorrhagic bone cyst or idiopathic bone cavity,[106] the simple bone cyst is most frequently found in the posterior mandible of young people, with fewer in older age groups. There is no sex predilection.[129] The etiology is unknown.

Simple bone cysts usually present a well-defined radiolucency but may also manifest radiopacities.[130] They may have **characteristically scalloped superficial**

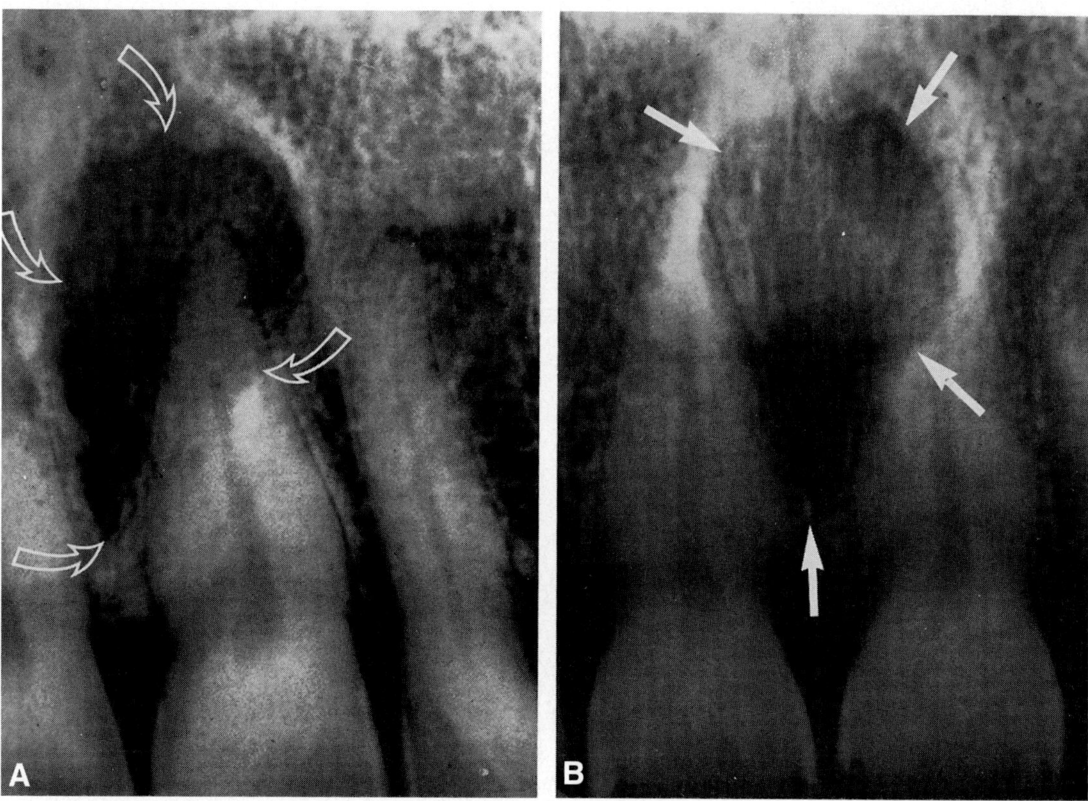

Figure 5-27 Nasopalatine duct cyst. **A**, A radiolucent lesion was noted near the apex of the vital maxillary central incisor (**open arrows**). **B**, By change of angulation, the radiolucent area "moves" between the two central incisors (**white arrows**). The lesion was asymptomatic.

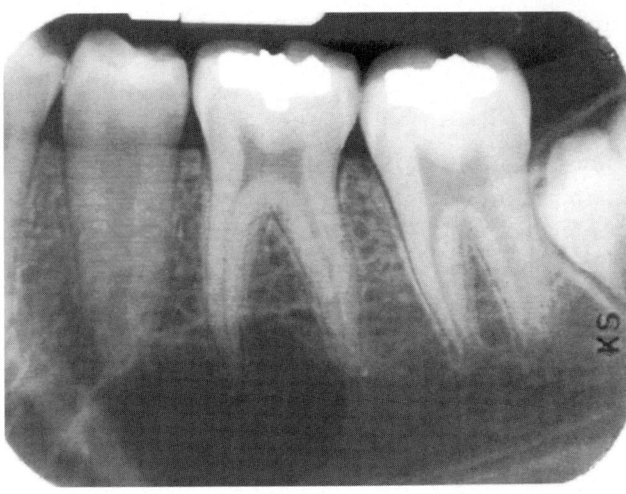

Figure 5-28 Simple bone cyst. Radiolucency superimposed over the mesial root apex of the first molar demonstrates the typical scalloped appearance. The teeth respond to pulp testing. Characteristically, the bony cavity is empty on surgical exposure.

borders as the lesions extend between the roots of the teeth. Superimposed over the root apices, they closely resemble **periradicular lesions** (Figure 5-28). The differentiation is not easily made on radiographs alone. In the case of the traumatic bone cyst, the lamina dura often remains intact, and the associated teeth respond to pulp testing.

An empty or fluid-filled cavity with a scanty granulation tissue lining is encountered at surgery. Treatment consists of **establishing hemorrhage** into the defect. **These lesions should not be curetted in their entirety** because this may sever the blood supply to the pulps in the overlying teeth and result in pulp necrosis.

Globulomaxillary Cyst. Although the globulomaxillary cyst has been classically regarded as a fissural cyst,[131] histologic and clinical evidence seemed to indicate that this lesion does not, in fact, exist as a separate entity.[132,133] Recently, D'Silva and Anderson questioned this assumption, stating that "the globulomaxillary cyst should again be considered an identifiable clinicopathologic entity."[134] The radiograph in Figure 5-29, A, may well represent an example of the so-called "true" lesion.

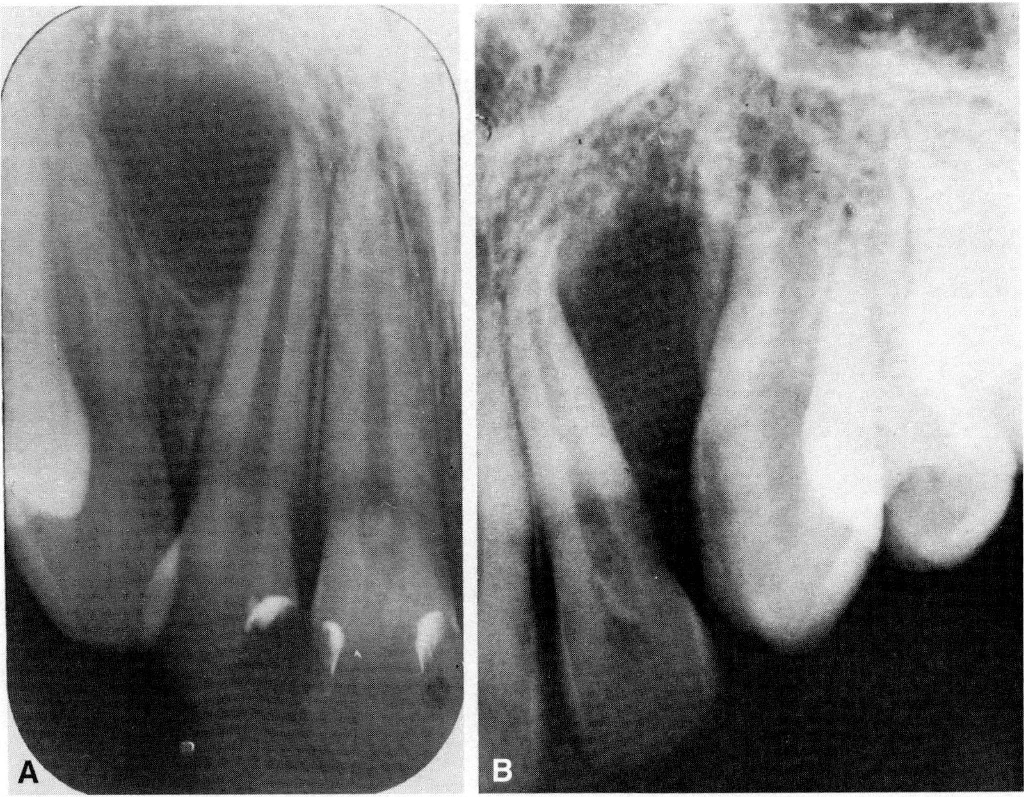

Figure 5-29 Two examples of a so-called "globulomaxillary" cyst. **A,** Although having every appearance of a true apical cyst, this lesion is associated with **vital** anterior teeth. This may be a true globulomaxillary cyst. (Courtesy of Dr. Richard E. Walton.) **B,** Necrotic pulp in the lateral incisor with dens en dente. The resultant lesion simulates a globulomaxillary cyst and is a frequent occurrence with anomalous incisors. (Courtesy of Dr. Raymond J. Melrose.)

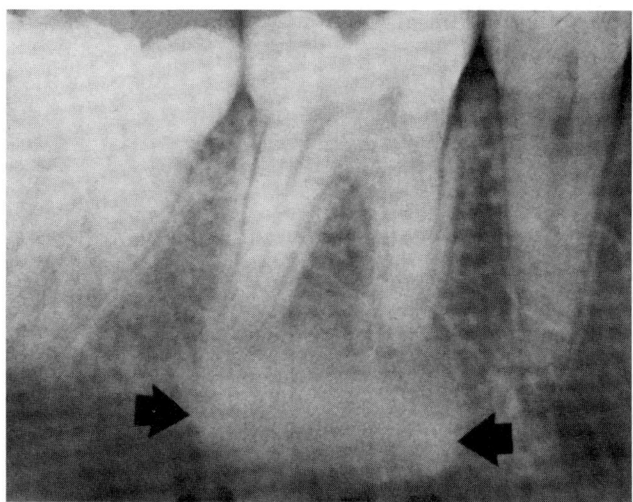

Figure 5-30 Enostosis. Also known as sclerotic bone. The radiopaque mass (**arrows**) probably represents an outgrowth of cortical bone on the endosteal surface. It is associated with neither pulpal nor periradicular pathosis and can be differentiated radiographically from condensing osteitis (see Figure 5-9) by its well-defined borders and homogeneous opacity.

Contrary to this classic assumption, Wysocki and Goldblatt have countercharged that D'Silva and Anderson are wrong, that the "so-called globulomaxillary cyst is extinct" and is, in all reality, related to **necrotic pulps in maxillary lateral incisors**[135] (Figure 5-29, B).

Careful diagnosis, in particular **pulp vitality testing**, should **always** be performed on teeth in the region of the globulomaxillary cyst.

Enostosis. The general group of radiopacities seen under the classification of enostosis must be **differentiated from** the common **condensing osteitis** frequently found in association with necrotic or inflamed pulps. There is confusion in the literature concerning the nature and classification of these lesions. Some authors consider them to be an osteoma or osteosclerosis,[136] whereas others refer to them as enostosis.[137] The term "enostosis" is preferable as these radiopacities probably represent developmental entities analogous to exostosis. They are **not** malignant neoplasms, as would be implied by the term "teoma."

Clinically and radiographically, enostoses usually can be readily differentiated from condensing osteitis. **Enostoses are not pathosis**; therefore, they are **asymptomatic** and cause no outward manifestations of jaw enlargement or soft tissue swelling. The growth is central and therefore on the endosteal surface and resides within the trabecular space. Radiographically, these are usually better defined (Figure 5-30) and less diffuse than condensing osteitis, which tends to have a concentric radiopaque appearance around the apices of involved teeth. Because **condensing osteitis is an inflammatory endodontic lesion**, it may be associated with the signs and symptoms that accompany pulpal or periradicular pathosis and may repair following root canal treatment (see Figure 5-9).

Malignancies

Carcinomas or sarcomas of various types are found in the jaws, rarely as primary but usually as metastatic lesions (Figures 5-31 and 5-32). Since they may manifest a variety of clinical and radiographic findings, this

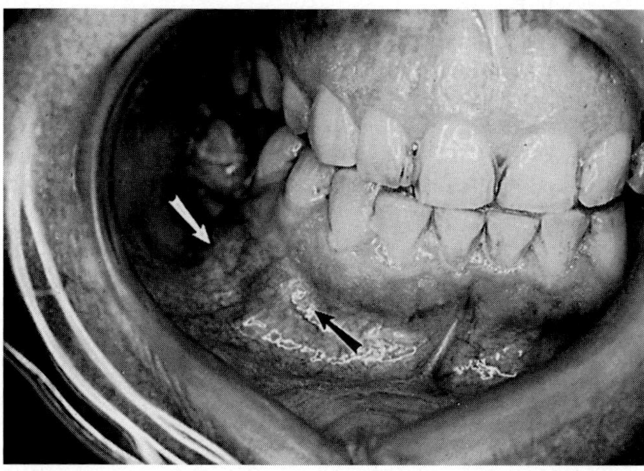

Figure 5-31 Vestibular-buccal swelling from metastatic breast cancer. Appearance and symptoms can be confused with apical abscess. (Courtesy of Drs. Raymond J. Melrose and Albert Abrams.)

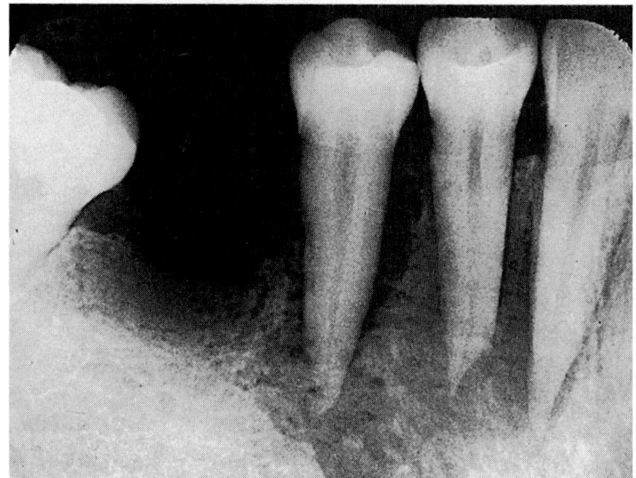

Figure 5-32 Metastatic breast cancer. All three teeth are nonresponsive to pulp testing. Unusual chisel edge and moth-eaten resorption are not typical of inflammatory osseous lesion. A biopsy proved lesion malignant. (Courtesy of Drs. Raymond J. Melrose and Albert Abrams.)

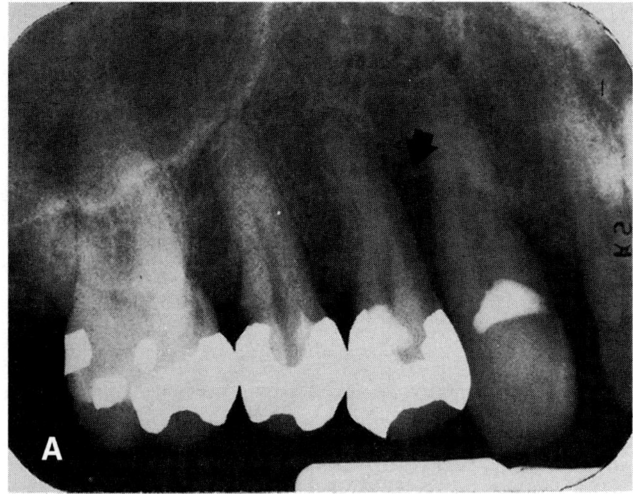

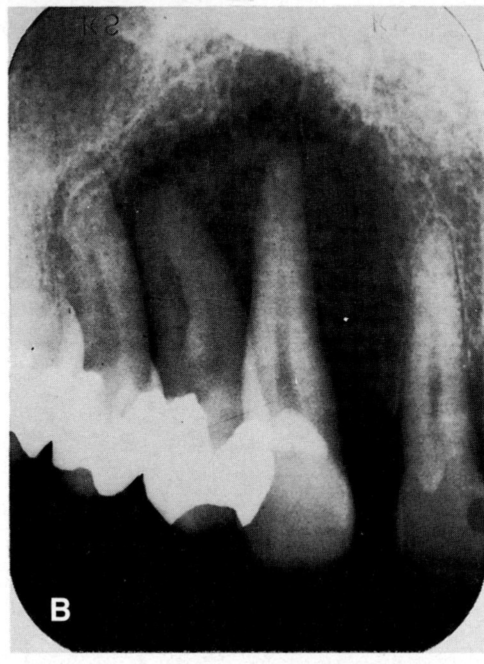

Figure 5-33 Squamous cell carcinoma of the gingiva. **A**, Vertical bone loss closely resembling a periodontal lesion (**arrow**). The lesion did not respond to periodontal therapy. **B**, After 2 months, radiolucency was considerably more extensive and thought to be of pulpal origin; however, adjacent teeth responded to pulp tests. Biopsy proved the lesion to be squamous cell carcinoma of the gingiva. (Courtesy of Dr. Mahmoud Torabinejad.)

discussion will be limited to a few of the more important aspects.[123]

Sarcoma. When seen in the jaws, these usually represent metastasis from other sites, although occasionally a primary lesion will arise in the mandible or maxilla. The osteosarcoma may have an appearance that **resembles a periradicular lesion.** It is frequently accompanied by pain and swelling and may cause extensive **bone loss and mobility of teeth** in areas of its growth. A common early manifestation is the symmetric **widening of the periodontal ligament space,** which closely resembles acute apical periodontitis.[138] The rapidly growing lesion may cause extensive root resorption and loss of pulp vitality in the associated teeth.

Carcinoma. Generally found in older patients, involvement of the jaws (usually the mandible) is **by metastasis** from a primary lesion elsewhere. Occasionally, the diagnosis of a jaw metastasis is the initial indication of a primary lesion at another site.[139] Therefore, the dentist must be alert to this possibility. These jaw lesions are usually radiolucent but may be mixed with radiopacities. **The prognosis for these patients is poor**; most do not survive more than a year.

Carcinoma lesions of the jaw may also manifest pain and swelling, loosening of teeth, or paresthesia, similar to endodontic pathosis.[140] Overall, however, metastatic carcinoma of the jaws usually has enough dissimilarities to endodontic periradicular pathosis to make the dentist suspicious. But because of similarities, differential diagnosis of the malignant lesions from periradicular pathosis is not always simple (Figure 5-33). Radiolucent jaw malignancies have been mistaken for periradicular lesions.[141]

REFERENCES

1. Kakehashi S, Stanley HR, Fitzgerald R. The effects of surgical exposures of dental pulps in germ-free and conventional laboratory rats. Oral Surg Oral Med Oral Pathol Oral Radiol Endod 1965;20:340.
2. Möller AJR, Fabricius L, Dahlen G, et al. Influence on periapical tissues of indigenous oral bacteria necrotic pulp tissue in monkeys. Scand J Res 1981;89:475.
3. Bergenholtz G. Micro-organisms from necrotic pulps of traumatized teeth. Odont Revy 1974; 25:347.
4. Sundqvist G. Bacteriological studies of necrotic dental pulps [PhD thesis]. Umea (Sweden): University Odontol Dissertation, 1976;7:1.
5. Korzen BH, Krakow AA, Green DB. Pulpal and periradicular tissue responses in conventional and monoinfected gnotobiotic rats. Oral Surg 1974;37:783.
6. Masillamoni CRM, Kettering JD, Torabinejad M. The biocompatibility of some root canal medicaments and irrigants. Int Endodont J 1981;14:115.
7. Torabinejad M, Finkelman RD. Inflammation and mediators of hard tissue resorption. In: Anderson J, Anderson F, editors. Textbook and color atlas of traumatic injuries to the teeth. 3rd ed. St. Louis: CV Mosby; 1994. p. 113.
8. Wakisaka S. Neuropeptides in the dental pulps: distribution, origin, and correlation. JOE 1990;16:67.
9. Byers MR, Taylor PE, Khayat BG, Kimberly CL. Effects of injury and inflammation on pulpal and periapical nerves. JOE 1990;6:78.
10. Torabinejad M, Eby WC, Naidorf IJ. Inflammatory and immunological aspects of the pathogenesis of human periapical lesions. JOE 1985;11:479.

11. Marceau F, Lussier A, Regoli D, Giroud JP. Pharmacology of kinins: their relevance to tissue injury and inflammation. Gen Pharmacol 1983;14:209.
12. Plummer TH, Erodos EG. Human plasma carboxypeptidase. Methods Enzymol 1981;80 P C:442.
13. Kaplan AP, Silverberg M, Dunn JT, Ghebrehiwet B. Interaction of the clotting, kinin-forming, complement and fibrinolytic pathways in inflammation. C-reactive protein and the plasma protein response to tissue injury. Ann N Y Acad Sci 1982;389:23.
14. Torabinejad M, Midrou T, Bakland L. Detection of kinins in human periapical lesions. J Dent Res 1986;68:201.
15. Torabinejad M. Mediators of acute and chronic periradicular lesions. Oral Surg 1994;78:511.
16. Torabinejad M, Clagett J, Engel D. A cat model for evaluation of mechanism of bone resorption: induction of bone loss by simulated immune complexes and inhibition by indomethacin. Calcif Tissue Int 1979;29:207.
17. McNicholas S, Torabinejad M, Blankenship J, Bakland L. The concentration of prostaglandin E2 in human periradicular lesions. JOE 1991;17:97.
18. Takayama S, Miki Y, Shimauchi H, Okada H. Relationship between prostaglandin E2 concentrations in periapical exudates from root canals and clinical findings of periapical periodontitis. JOE 1996;12:677.
19. Shimauchi H, Takayama S, Miki Y, Okada H. The change of periapical exudate prostaglandin E2 levels during root canal treatment. JOE 1997;23:755.
20. Miyauchi M, Takata T, Ito H, et al. Immunohistochemical detection of prostaglandins E_2, $F_{2\alpha}$, and 6-keto-prostaglandin $F_{1\alpha}$ in experimentally induced periapical inflammatory lesions in rats. JOE 1996;22:635.
21. Trowbridge HO, Emling RC. Inflammation: a review of the process. 4th ed. Chicago: Quintessence Publishing; 1993.
22. Torabinejad M, Cotti E, Jung T. Concentration of leukotriene B_4 in symptomatic and asymptomatic periapical lesions. JOE 1992;18:205.
23. Mathiesen A. Preservation and demonstration of mast cells in human apical granulomas and radicular cysts. Scand J Dent Res 1973;81:218.
24. Perrini N, Fonzi L. Mast cells in human periapical lesions: ultrastructural aspects and their possible physiopathological implications. JOE 1985;11:197.
25. Aqrabawi J, Schilder H, Toselli P, Franzblau C. Biochemical and histochemical analysis of the enzyme arylsulfatase in human lesions of endodontic origin. JOE 1993;19:335.
26. Mizel SB. Interleukin 1 and T cell activation. Immunol Rev 1982;63:51.
27. Gery I, Lupe-Zuniga JL. Interleukin 1: uniqueness of its production and spectrum of activities. Lymphokines 1984; 9:109.
28. March CJ, Mosley B, Larsen A, et al. Cloning, sequence and expression of two distinct human interleukin-1 complementary DNAs. Nature 1985;315:641.
29. Tatakis DN, Schneeberger G, Dziak R. Recombinant interleukin-1 stimulates prostaglandin E2 production by osteoblastic cells: synergy with parathyroid hormone. Calcif Tissue Int 1988;42:358.
30. Bertolini DR, Nedwin GE, Bringman TS, et al. Stimulation of bone resorption and inhibition of bone formation *in vitro* by human tumor necrosis factors. Nature 1986; 319:516.
31. Masada MP, Persson R, Kenney JS, et al. Measurement of interleukin-1α and -1β in gingival crevicular fluid: implications for the pathogenesis of periodontal disease. J Periodontal Res 1990;25:156.
32. Wang Cy, Stashenko P. The role of interleukin-1α in pathogenesis of periapical bone destruction in a rat model system. Oral Microbiol Immunol 1993;8:50.
33. Barkhordar RA, Hussain MZ, Hayashi C. Detection of IL-1β in human periapical lesions. Oral Surg 1992;73:334.
34. Lim GC, Torabinejad M, Kettering J, et al. Interleukin 1β in symptomatic and asymptomatic human periradicular lesions. JOE 1994;20:225.
35. Stashenko P, Teles R, D'Souza R. Periapical inflammatory responses and their modulation. Crit Rev Oral Biol Med 1998;9:498.
36. Matsumoto A, Anan H, Maeda K. An immunohistochemical study of the behavior of cells expressing interleukin-1 alpha and interleukin-1 beta within experimentally induced periapical lesions in rats. JOE 1998;24:811.
37. Kuo ML, Lamster IB, Hasselgren G. Host mediators in endodontic exudates. I. Indicators of inflammation and humoral immunity. JOE 1998;24:498.
38. Wang CY, Tani-Ishii N, Stashenko P. Bone-resorptive cykotine gene expression in periapical lesions in the rat. Oral Microbiol Immunol 1997;12:65.
39. Fouad AF. IL-1 alpha and TNF-alpha expression in early periapical lesions of normal and immunodeficient mice. J Dent Res 1997;76:1548.
40. Billiau A, Van Damme J, Ceuppens J, Baroja M. Interleukin 6, a ubiquitous cytokine with paracrine as well as endocrine functions. In: Fradelizi D, Bertoglio J, editors. Lymphokine receptor interactions. London: John Libby Eurotext; 1989. p. 133–42.
41. Feyen JHM, Elford P, Di Padova FE, Trechsel U. Interleukin-6 is produced by bone and modulated by parathyroid hormone. J Bone Miner Res 1989;4:633.
42. Kono Y, Beagley KW, Fujihashi K, et al. Cytokine regulation of localized inflammation. Induction of activated B cells and IL-6-mediated polyclonal IgG and IgA synthesis in inflamed human gingiva. J Immunol 1991;146:1812.
43. Al-Balaghi S, Strom H, Möller E. B cell differentiation factor in synovial fluid of patients with rheumatoid arthritis. Immunol Rev 1984;78:7.
44. Swolin-Eide D, Ohlsson C. Effects of cortisol on the expression of interleukin-6 and interleukin-1 beta in human osteoblast-like cells. J Endocrinol 1998;156:107.
45. Barkhordar RA, Hayashi C, Hussain MZ. Detection of interleukin-6 in human dental pulp and periapical lesions. Endod Dent Traumatol 1999;15:25.
46. Thomson BM, Mundy GR, Chambers TJ. Tumor necrosis factors α and β induce osteoblastic cells to stimulate osteoclastic bone resorption. J Immunol 1987;138:775.
47. Tashjian AH Jr, Voelkel EF, Lazzaro M, et al. Tumor necrosis factor-α (Cachectin) stimulates bone resorption in mouse calvaria via a prostaglandin-mediated mechanism. Endocrinology 1987;120:2029.
48. Safavi KE, Rossomando EF. Tumor necrosis factor identified in periapical tissue exudates of teeth with apical periodontitis. JOE 1991;17:12.
49. Kawashima N, Stashenko P. Expression of bone-resorptive and regulatory cytokines in murine periapical inflammation. Arch Oral Biol 1999;44:55.

50. Torabinejad M, Kiger RD. Experimentally induced alterations in periapical tissues of the cat. J Dent Res 1980;59:87.
51. Torabinejad M, Kettering JD. Detection of immune complexes in human periapical lesions by anticomplement immunofluorescence technique. Oral Surg 1979;48:256.
52. Torabinejad M, Theofilopoulos AN, Kettering JD, Bakland LK. Quantitation of circulating immune complexes, immunoglobulins G and M, and C3 complement in patients with large periapical lesions. Oral Surg 1983;55:186.
53. Kettering JD, Torabinejad M. Concentration of immune complexes, IgG, IgM, IgE, and C3 in patients with acute apical abscesses. JOE 1984;10:417.
54. Torabinejad M, Kettering JD. Identification and relative concentration of B and T lymphocytes in human chronic periapical lesions. JOE 1985;11:122.
55. Cymerman JJ, Cymerman DH, Walters J, Nevins AJ. Human T lymphocyte subpopulations in chronic periapical lesions. JOE 1984;10:9.
56. Babal P, Soler P, Brozman M, et al. In situ characterization of cells in periapical granulomas by monoclonal antibodies. Oral Surg 1987;64:548.
57. Barkhordar RA, Resouza YG. Human T lymphocyte subpopulations in periapical lesions. Oral Surg 1988;65:763.
58. Stashenko P, Yu SM. T helper and T suppressor cells reversal during the development of induced rat periapical lesions. J Dent Res 1989;68:830.
59. Wallstrom JB, Torabinejad M. The role of T cells in the pathogenesis of periapical lesions. Oral Surg 1993;76:2;213.
60. Waterman PA, Torabinejad M, McMillan PJ, Kettering JD. Development of periradicular lesions in immunosuppressed rats. Oral Surg 1998;85:720.
61. Priebe WA, Laxansky JP, Wuehrmann AH. The value of the roentgenographic film in the differential diagnosis of periradicular lesions. Oral Surg 1954;7:979.
62. Wais FT. Significance of findings following biopsy and histologic study of 100 periradicular lesions. Oral Surg 1958;11:650.
63. Forsberg A, Hagglund G. Differential diagnosis of radicular cyst and granuloma: use of x-ray contrast medium. Dent Radiogr Photogr 1960;33:84.
64. Cunningham CJ, Penick EG. Use of a roentgenographic contrast medium in the differential diagnosis of periradicular lesions. Oral Surg 1968;26:96.
65. Howell FV, de La Rosa VM, Abrams AM. Cytologic evaluation of cystic lesions of the jaws: a new diagnostic technique. J South Calif Dent Assoc 1968;36:161.
66. Morse DR, et al. A rapid chairside differentiation of radicular cysts and granulomas. JOE 1976;2:17.
67. Nobuhara WK, del Rio CE. Incidence of periradicular pathoses in endodontic treatment failures. JOE 1993;19:315.
68. Weiner S, McKinney R, Walton R. Characterization of the periradicular surgical specimen. Oral Surg 1982;53:293.
69. Shafer W, Hine M, Levy B. A textbook of oral pathology. 3rd ed. Philadelphia: WB Saunders; 1974.
70. Nair PN, Sjogren U, Sundqvist G. Cholesterol crystals as an etiological factor in nonresolving chronic inflammation: an experimental study in guinea pigs. Eur J Oral Sci 1998;106(2 Pt 1):644.
71. Bynum JW, Fiedler DE. Demonstration of nerve tissue in periradicular inflammation lesions [abstract]. J Dent Res 1960; 39:737.
72. Martinelli C, Rulli MA. The innervation of chronic inflammatory human periradicular lesions. Arch Oral Biol 1967;112:593.
73. Spector WG. Chronic inflammation. JOE 1977;3:218.
74. Ten Cate AR. The histochemical demonstration of specific oxidative enzymes and glycogen in the epithelial cell rests of Malassez. Arch Oral Biol 1965;10:207.
75. Linenberg WB, et al. A clinical, roentgenographic, and histopathologic evaluation of periradicular lesions. Oral Surg 1964;17:467.
76. Simon JH. Incidence of periradicular cysts in relation to the root canal. JOE 1980;6:845.
77. Hill TJL. The epithelium in dental granuloma. J Dent Res 1930;10:323.
78. Ten Cate AR. The epithelial cell rests of Malassez and the genesis of the dental cyst. Oral Surg 1972;34:956.
79. McConnell G. The histopathology of the dental granuloma. J Am Dent Assoc 1921;8:390.
80. Summers L. The incidence of epithelium in periradicular granulomas and mechanisms of cavitation in apical dental cysts in man. Arch Oral Biol 1974;19:1177.
81. Shear M. The histogenesis of the dental cyst. Dent Pract 1963;13:238.
82. Shear M. Inflammation in dental cysts. Oral Surg 1964;17:756.
83. Toller PA, Holborrow EJ. Immunoglobulins and immunoglobulin-containing cells in cysts of the jaws. Lancet 1969;2:178.
84. Toller PA. Protein substances in odontogenic cyst fluids. Br Dent J 1970;128:317.
85. Toller PA. Epithelial discontinuities in cysts of the jaws. Br Dent J 1966;120:74.
86. Valderhaug J. A histologic study of experimentally produced intraoral odontogenic fistulae in monkeys. Int J Oral Surg 1973;2:54.
87. Torabinejad M. The role of immunological reactions in apical cyst formation and the fate of epithelium after root canal treatment: a theory. Int J Oral Surg 1983;12:14.
88. Bhaskar SN. Nonsurgical resolution of radicular cysts. Oral Surg 1972;34:458.
89. Hedin M, Polhagen L. Follow-up study of periradicular bone condensation. Scand J Dent Res 1971;79:436.
90. Dorland's illustrated medical dictionary. 26th ed. Philadelphia: WB Saunders; 1981. Abscess; p. 4.
91. Goldberg MH, Topazian RG. Odontogenic infections. In: Topazian RG, Goldberg MH, editors. Oral and maxillofacial infections. 3rd ed. Philadelphia: WB Saunders; 1994. p. 212.
92. Valderhaug J. Epithelial cells in the periodontal membrane of teeth with and without periradicular inflammation. Int J Oral Surg 1974;3:7.
93. Harrison J, Larson W. The epithelialized oral sinus tract. Oral Surg 1976;42:511.
94. Green TL, et al. Radiographic and histologic periapical findings of root canal treated teeth in cadaver. Oral Surg 1997;83:707.
95. Fish EW. Bone infection. J Am Dent Assoc 1939;26:691.
96. Bergenholtz G, et al. Morphometric analysis of inflammatory periradicular lesions in root filled teeth [abstract]. J Dent Res 1982;61:96.
97. Boyne PH, Harvey WL. The effects of osseous implant materials on regeneration of alveolar cortex. Oral Surg 1961; 14:369.

98. Amler MH. The time sequence of tissue regeneration in human extraction wounds. Oral Surg 1969;27:309.
99. Fouad AF, Walton RE, Rittman BR. Healing of induced periapical lesions in ferret canines. JOE 1993;19:123.
100. Johnson BR, Remeikis N, VanCura J. Diagnosis and treatment of cutaneous facial sinus tracts of dental origin. J Am Dent Assoc 1999;130:832.
101. Nair PNR. Review: new perspectives on radicular cysts: do they heal? Int Endod J 1998;31:155.
102. Nair PNR, et al. Persistent periapical radiolucencies of root-filled human teeth, failed endodontic treatments, and periapical scars. Oral Surg 1999;87:617.
103. Molven O, Halse A, Grung B. Incomplete healing (scar tissue) after periapical surgery: radiographic findings 8 to 12 years after treatment. JOE 1996;22:264.
104. Bhaskar SN. Radiographic interpretation for the dentist. 2nd ed. St. Louis: CV Mosby; 1975.
105. Ardekian L, Peled M, Rosen D, et al. Clinical and radiographic features of eosinophilic granuloma in the jaws. Oral Surg 1999;87:238.
106. Pindborg JJ, Hjorting-Hansen E. Atlas of diseases of the jaws. Philadelphia: WB Saunders; 1974.
107. Dachi S, Howell F. A survey of 3,874 routine full-mouth radiographs. II. A study of impacted teeth. Oral Surg 1961; 14:1165.
108. Shafer W, Hine M, Levy B. A textbook of oral pathology. 4th edition. Philadelphia: WB Saunders; 1983.
109. Thoma KH. The circumferential dentigerous cyst. Oral Surg 1964;18:368.
110. Wysocki G, et al. Histogenesis of the lateral periodontal cyst and the gingival cyst of the adult. Oral Surg 1980;50:327.
111. Kerezoudis N, Donta-Bakoyianni C, Siskos G. The lateral periodontal cyst: aetiology, clinical significance and diagnosis. Endod Dent Traumatol 2000;16:144.
112. Brannon RB. The odontogenic keratocyst. Oral Surg 1977;43:233.
113. Wright BA, et al. Odontogenic keratocysts presenting as periradicular disease. Oral Surg 1983;56:425.
114. Pindborg J, Hansen J. Studies on odontogenic cyst epithelium. 2. Clinical and roentgenographic aspects of odontogenic keratocysts. Acta Pathol Microbiol Scand 1963;568(A):283.
115. Tau CH. Odontogenic keratocyst. Oral Surg 1998;86:573.
116. Pindborg JJ, Hjorting-Hansen E. Atlas of diseases of the jaws. Philadelphia: WB Saunders; 1974. p. 134.
117. Morse D, et al. Nonsurgical repair of electrophoretically diagnosed radicular cysts. JOE 1975;1:158.
118. Toller P. Newer concepts of odontogenic cysts. Int J Oral Surg 1972;1:3.
119. Kronfeld R. The epithelium in chronic apical periodontitis. In: Proceedings of the Ninth Australian Dental Congress; 1937. p. 578.
120. Waldron C, Giansanti J. Benign fibro-osseous lesions of the jaws: a clinical-radiologic-histologic review of sixty-five cases. II. Benign fibro-osseous lesions of periodontal ligament origin. Oral Surg 1973;35:340.
121. Zegarelli E, et al. The cementoma: a study of 230 patients with 435 cementomas. Oral Surg 1964;17:219.
122. Wilcox LR, Walton R. A case of mistaken identity: periapical cemental dysplasia in an endodontically treated tooth. Endod Dent Traumatol 1989;5:298.
123. Neville B, Damm D, Allen C, Bouquot J. Oral and maxillofacial pathology. Philadelphia: WB Saunders; 1995: p. 476.
124. Cherrick H, et al. Benign cementoblastoma: a clinicopathologic evaluation. Oral Surg 1974;37:54.
125. Wood N, Goaz, P. Differential diagnosis of oral lesions. 2nd ed. St. Louis: CV Mosby; 1980.
126. Struthers P, Shear M. Root resorption by ameloblastoma and cysts of the jaws. Int J Oral Surg 1976;5:128.
127. Whitaker SB, Waldron C. Central giant cell lesions of the jaws. Oral Surg 1993;75:199.
128. Abrams A, Howell F, Bullock W. Nasopalatine cysts. Oral Surg 1963;16:306.
129. Kaugars G, Cale A. Traumatic bone cyst. Oral Surg 1987;63:318.
130. Matsumura S, Murakami S, Kakimoto N, et al. Histopathologic and radiographic findings of the simple bone cyst. Oral Surg 1998;85:619.
131. Gorlin R, Goldman H. Thoma's oral pathology. 6th ed. St. Louis: CV Mosby; 1970.
132. Christ T. The globulomaxillary cyst: an embryologic misconception. Oral Surg 1970;30:515.
133. Hollingshead MB, Schnieder L. A histologic and embryologic analysis of the so-called globulomaxillary cyst. Int J Oral Surg 1980;9:281.
134. D'Silva NJ, Anderson L. Globulomaxillary cyst revisited. Oral Surg 1993;76:182.
135. Wysocki GP, Goldblatt LI. The so-called "globulomaxillary cyst"' is extinct. Oral Surg 1993;76:185.
136. Stafne E, Gibilisco F. Oral roentgenographic diagnosis. 4th ed. Philadelphia: WB Saunders; 1975.
137. Worth HM. Principles and practice of oral radiologic interpretation. Chicago: Year Book Medical Publisher; 1963.
138. Garrington C, et al. Osteosarcoma of the jaws: analysis of 56 cases. Cancer 1967;20:377.
139. Svirsky JA, Epstein R, Dent D, Avillion G. Small cell carcinoma of the lung metastatic to the wall of a radicular cyst. JOE 1994;20:512.
140. Selden HS, Manhoff DT, Hatges NA, Michel RC. Metastatic carcinoma to the mandible that mimicked pulpal/periodontal disease. JOE 1998;24:267.
141. Torabinejad M, Rick G. Squamous cell carcinoma of the gingiva. J Am Dent Assoc 1980;10:870.

Chapter 6

ENDODONTIC DIAGNOSTIC PROCEDURES

John I. Ingle, Geoffrey S. Heithersay, Gary R. Hartwell, Albert C. Goerig, F. James Marshall, Robert M. Krasny, Alfred L. Frank, and Cyril Gaum

"For I seek the truth by which no man has ever been harmed."
–Marcus Aurelius, Meditations VI. 21, 173 AD

Before initiating treatment, one must first assemble collective information regarding signs, symptoms, and history. That information is then combined with results from the clinical examination and tests. This process is **diagnosis.** Stated another way, diagnosis is the procedure of accepting a patient, recognizing that he has a problem, determining the cause of the problem, and developing a treatment plan that will solve or alleviate the problem.

The diagnostician must have a thorough knowledge of examination procedures—percussion, palpation, probing, and pulp testing; a knowledge of pathosis and its radiographic and clinical manifestations; an awareness of the various modalities of treatment; and, above all, a questioning mind. To be added to these critical skills is the most basic skill of all, **listening** to the patient.

Of all of the important diagnostic tools, the **art of listening** is the most underrated. Yet careful and attentive listening establishes patient-dentist rapport, understanding, and trust. Such a relationship also enhances the patient's reliability as a historian.[1]

REQUIREMENTS OF A DIAGNOSTICIAN

Diagnosis is a personal and cognitive experience; therefore, many of the qualities of a good diagnostician are of an interpersonal nature and are based on knowledge, experience, and diagnostic tools. Diagnosing orofacial disease is similar to other medical diagnosis. Pulp tests, radiographs, percussion, palpation, and other tests and procedures can facilitate the diagnosing of dental/facial disease, just as the electrocardiograph, electroencephalograph, echocardiograph, computed axial tomographic and magnetic resonance imaging scan, and a host of other radiographs can facilitate medical diagnosis.

A dentist can develop a number of assets to become a successful diagnostician. The most important of these are **knowledge, interest, intuition, curiosity**, and **patience.** The successful diagnostician must also have acute senses and the necessary equipment for diagnosis.

Knowledge

Primarily, a dentist must depend on himself, not the laboratory. Therefore, knowledge is the most important asset the dentist must possess. This includes familiarity with all local orofacial causes of pain, as well as numerous systemic, neurogenic, and psychological causes. In addition, the dentist must be aware of the many physical, perceptual, emotional, and behavioral changes brought about by chronic pain. He must know that constant overwhelming pain can affect the function of every organ of the body. Chronic pain patients can develop increased blood pressure, heart rate, kidney function, decreased bowel activity, and hormone levels. They can have many symptoms, such as nausea, vomiting, photophobia, tinnitus, and vertigo. The astute clinician gathers knowledge about the patient and his problem through a thorough history and an examination. The history and examination include evaluating the physical, emotional, behavioral, and perceptual aspects of the patient's pain experience.

Under **knowledge** must also be listed the important asset of **knowing when and where to refer the patient** for additional consultation. This comes with experience and the help of physicians, psychologists, and fellow dentists who may be depended on to assist in diagnosis. Often the patient is referred because examination reveals a problem clearly in the province of the neurologist or otolaryngologist. Sometimes the patient is referred because the examiner has exhausted his knowledge and needs help in diagnosis. The recognition of fallibility and limitation—knowing when to yell for help—is also a major asset to the dentist.

Interest

The second important asset possessed by a good diagnostician is **interest.** The dentist must have a keen interest in the patient and his or her problem and must evidence this interest by handling the patient with understanding. If this attitude is not natural to the dentist, he will render the patient and the profession a service by referring all diagnostic problems to an interested and competent fellow practitioner.

Intuition

In addition to **interest** and **knowledge,** the good diagnostician is blessed with **intuition** or "sixth sense," so to speak. Good diagnosticians intuitively sense the presence of something unusual. This ability, which sometimes allows for "instant" diagnosis, is developed through broad experience with pain problems having unusual and multiple diagnoses.

Intuition tells the dentist when the patient is holding back information or is not telling the complete truth. Moreover, intuition immediately makes the examiner subtly aware of the patient who "knows too much," that is, all of the words and symptoms related to a certain condition. Intuition allows the dentist to suspect the unusual, but it also goes hand in hand with still another prime asset of a good diagnostician, **curiosity.**

Curiosity

The dentist must pursue or develop a natural curiosity about the patient and his condition if perseverance is to be maintained in arriving at a diagnosis. Dr. Harry Sicher often likened dental diagnosis to the actions of a good detective, and curiosity is a detective's greatest asset (personal communication, 1954). Medawar described diagnosis as the "use of the hypothetico-deductive system."[2] Again, **curiosity** goes with **interest,** and the dentist who is bored by the painstaking methods of diagnosis will never have the **curiosity** to delve a little deeper, probe a little further, or ask the unusual. All of this takes time and thus requires **patience.**

Patience

Often a definitive diagnosis of unusual pain may take hours, days, or even months to develop. Some patients complaining of unusual pain may have suffered this pain for years, so the dentist cannot expect to make a quick diagnosis in a matter of minutes. This is the reason, as stated earlier, why a difficult diagnosis may be unrewarding financially but very rewarding emotionally. Again, if the dentist is not willing to sacrifice the time to attempt to help these individuals, he is urged to **refer the patient** for diagnosis rather than make an incorrect, quick diagnosis that may result in improper treatment, such as reaching for the forceps or removing a healthy pulp.

The dentist obviously cannot abandon other patients to see one person repeatedly. Too frequently, the problem patient is asked to return at the end of the day, when both dentist and patient are tired and irritable. A better solution is to see the patient in the morning, before office hours. The dentists who are not willing to assume this imposition, and they are many, are urged to refer the patient to their more altruistic colleagues.

Senses

The good diagnostician must have the astuteness to grasp what his **senses** reveal. First, he has a voice to ask questions and ears to hear the answer; he has eyes to see and hands to probe and palpate. In short, the dentist has senses with which to communicate with the sick patient. But, as Friedman pointed out, "One must learn to listen with the third ear and see with the third eye" (personal communication, 1972).

Controlling these senses, however, is the **mind,** and if the mind does not inquire and then reason, or has not accumulated the knowledge necessary to inquire and finally to analyze, then the senses are useless. The mind must list all of the possible causes of the pain and then, more often than not, eliminate them one by one until the correct diagnosis is made.

HISTORY

Anamnesis, "recollection" or "calling to memory," is the first step in developing a diagnosis. The importance of obtaining and recording this "history" goes beyond medicolegal protection. A complete history (Table 6-1) will not determine treatment but may influence modifications in endodontic treatment modalities. It will seldom deny treatment. A complete medical history should contain, as a baseline, the vital signs; give early warning of unsuspected general disease; and define risks to the health of the staff as well as identify the risks of treatment to the patient. The medical history must be updated regularly, especially if there have been any changes in the patient's health status.

The procedure developed by the American Society of Anesthesiologists is a good system for organizing and assigning risk (Table 6-2). Once the status of the patient's general health has been established, a dental diagnosis is best developed by following the time-honored formula of determining the **chief complaint,** enlarging on this complaint with questions about the **present dental illness,** relating the history of past dental illness to the chief complaint, and combining this

Table 6-1 Medical History Form*

MEDICAL HISTORY

Name ______ Sex ______ Date of Birth ______
Address ______
Telephone ______ Height ______ Weight ______
Date ______ Occupation ______ Marital Status ______

MEDICAL HISTORY	CIRCLE	
1. Are you having pain or discomfort at this time?	YES	NO
2. Do you feel very nervous about having dentistry treatment?	YES	NO
3. Have you ever had a bad experience in the dentistry office?	YES	NO
4. Have you been a patient in the hospital during the past 2 years?	YES	NO
5. Have you been under the care of a medical doctor during the past 2 years?	YES	NO
6. Have you taken any medicine or drugs during the past 2 years?	YES	NO
7. Are you allergic to (ie, itching, rash, swelling of hands, feet, or eyes) or made sick by penicillin, aspirin, codeine, or any drugs or medications?	YES	NO
8. Have you ever had any excessive bleeding requiring special treatment?	YES	NO

9. Circle any of the following which you have had or have at present:

Heart Failure	Emphysema	AIDS or HIV
Heart Disease or Attack	Cough	Hepatitis A (infectious)
Angina Pectoris	Tuberculosis (TB)	Hepatitis B (serum)
High Blood Pressure	Asthma	Liver Disease
Heart Murmur	Hay Fever	Yellow Jaundice
Rheumatic Fever	Sinus Trouble	Blood Transfusion
Congenital Heart Lesions	Allergies or Hives	Drug Addiction
Scarlet Fever	Diabetes	Hemophilia
Artificial Heart Valve	Thyroid Disease	Venereal Disease (Syphilis, Gonorrhea)
Heart Pacemaker	X-ray or Cobalt Treatment	Cold Sores
Heart Surgery	Chemotherapy (Cancer, Leukemia)	Genital Herpes
Artificial Joint	Arthritis	Epilepsy or Seizures
Anemia	Rheumatism	Fainting or Dizzy Spells
Stroke	Cortisone Medicine	Nervousness
Kidney Trouble	Glaucoma	Psychiatric Treatment
Ulcers	Pain in Jaw Joints	Sickle Cell Disease
		Bruise Easily

10. When you walk up stairs or take a walk, do you ever have to stop because of pain in your chest, or shortness of breath, or because you are very tired?	YES	NO
11. Do your ankles swell during the day?	YES	NO
12. Do you use more than two pillows to sleep?	YES	NO
13. Have you lost or gained more than 10 pounds in the past year?	YES	NO
14. Do you ever wake up from sleep short of breath?	YES	NO
15. Are you on a special diet?	YES	NO
16. Has your medical doctor ever said you have a cancer or tumor?	YES	NO
17. Do you have any disease, condition, or problem not listed?	YES	NO
18. WOMEN: Are you pregnant now?	YES	NO
Are you practicing birth control?	YES	NO
Do you anticipate becoming pregnant?	YES	NO

To the best of my knowledge, all of the preceding answers are true and correct. If I ever have any change in my health, or if my medicines change, I will inform the doctor of dentistry at the next appointment without fail.

______ ______ ______
Date *Dentist Signature* *Signature of Patient, Parent, or Guardian*

MEDICAL HISTORY/PHYSICAL EVALUATION **UPDATE**

Date	Addition	Signatures	
______	______	______	______
______	______	______	______
______	______	______	______

This comprehensive medical history responds to contemporary advances in physical evaluation and to increasing malpractice claims.

*Reproduced with permission from McCarthy FM. A new patient administered history developed for dentistry. J Am Dent Assoc 1985;111:595.

Table 6-2 American Society of Anesthesiologists (ASA) Physical Status Classification*

ASA Class	Patient Description	Clinical Examples	Clinical Management
1	A normally healthy patient	No organic, physiologic, biochemical, or psychiatric disturbance; treatment is for localized disorder	Routine care
2	A patient with mild systemic disease	Controlled essential hypertension, pronounced obesity, psychiatric disturbance	Routine care but limit procedural stress and length of appointment
3	A patient with severe systemic disease that is not incapacitating	Severe diabetes mellitus, congestive heart failure, chronic obstructive pulmonary disease	Strict limitation of complex procedures; careful anxiety control
4	A patient with an incapacitating systemic disease that is a constant threat to life	Acute myocardial infarction; advanced pulmonary, cardiac, hepatic, or renal insufficiency	Emergency or palliative care, usually in a hospital
5	A moribund patient who is not expected to live 24 hours with or without operation	Uncontrolled massive internal bleeding, rapidly progressing cardiac insufficiency with renal failure	Emergency life support only

*Used to categorize patients following history and examination. Classification should be entered prominently in chart. Assigning risk from treatment and level of clinical management follows classification. American Society of Anesthesiologists. New classification of physical status. Anesthesiology 1963;24:111.

with information about the patient's general health (**medical history**) and the examination results.

Chief Complaint

The chief complaint, usually in the patient's own words, is a description of the dental problem for which the patient seeks care. The verbal complaint may be accompanied by the patient pointing to the general area of the problem.

After establishment and recording of the **chief complaint**, the examination process is continued by obtaining a history of the **present illness.**

A patient in acute distress should undergo diagnosis and examination as quickly as possible so the chief complaint may be treated as expeditiously as possible. At a later time, when the patient is pain free and more rational, a complete treatment plan may be established. No treatment should be rendered unless the examiner is certain of the diagnosis. Patients with severe pain from pulpitis have difficulty in cooperating with the diagnostic procedures, but until the diagnosis has been made and the correct tooth identified, treatment must not be started (see chapter 7).

Present Dental Illness

A history of the present illness should indicate the severity and the urgency of the problem. If the problem is long-standing, proceed with detailed questions about past episodes of pain or swelling and any previous treatment performed to remedy the condition.

Pain is frequently the main component of the patient's complaint. A history of pain that persists without exacerbation may indicate a problem not of dental origin. If the chief complaint is "toothache" but the symptoms are too vague to establish a diagnosis, analgesics can be prescribed to help the patient tolerate the pain until the toothache localizes. If the patient arrives self-medicated with analgesics or sedatives, a diagnosis may be difficult to establish.[3]

The initial questions should help establish two basic components of pain: time (chronicity) and severity (or intensity). Start by asking such questions as "**How** long have you had this problem?" "**How** painful is it?" and "**How** often does it hurt?" Continue the questioning with "**When** does it hurt?" "**When** does it go away?" "**What** makes it hurt?" "**What** makes it hurt worse?" and "**What** makes it hurt less or go away?"

A history of painful responses to thermal changes suggests a problem of pulpal origin and will need to be followed up with clinical tests, using the thermal test that would most closely duplicate the patient's complaint: use ice if the complaint is pain with cold, and use a hot stimulus if the complaint is pain with such things as hot drinks.[4] It could also be important to learn that a tooth has been sensitive to thermal changes but no longer responds to such stimuli; this would indicate that the tooth may have a pulp that is now necrotic.[5]

A history of painful response to eating and biting or pain on pressing the gingiva is also helpful. Minor sensitivities or swellings, [illegible]y noticeable to the patient, can initially be overlooked by the examiner. These may prove to be very important diagnostic clues and should be noted. A collection of data such as that shown in Figure 6-1 is helpful in directing the examination procedures and sometimes in pinpointing the problem. The type and number of past dental treatments should reveal the degree of sophistication of previous therapy and help in evaluating the expectations of the patient as well. The presence of obvious dental neglect or the unwillingness of the patient to have a pulpless tooth restored may rule out endodontic therapy.

The question, **"What kind of treatment have you had?"** might elicit a history of pulp capping, deep fillings with sedative bases, or indirect pulp caps. These teeth, as well as those that have received impact trauma, may exhibit calcific metamorphosis or dystrophic calcifications and may be a difficult endodontic treatment

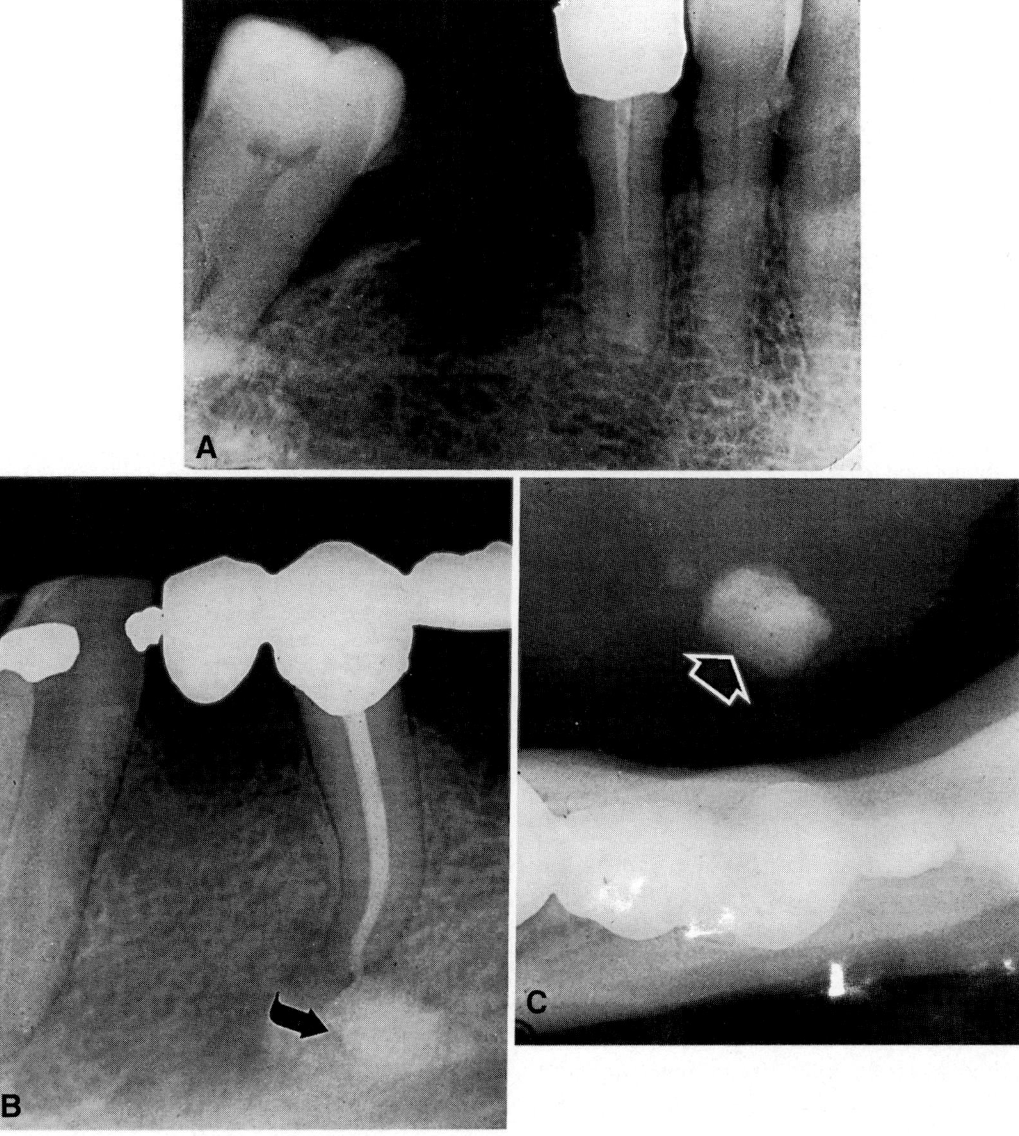

Figure 6-1 A, Chief complaint of vague discomfort directed attention to an incomplete root canal filling. However, the examination was redirected to calculus and periodontal disease, when it was revealed that the treatment was 50 years old. **B**, Radiograph taken immediately after filling suggests gross overfill (**arrow**). **C**, An occlusal radiograph, however, shows a sialolith, that was not initially suspected (**arrow**). Repeated surgery for this condition had not been elicited in the past dental history. Reproduced from Marshall FJ. Dent Clin North Am 1979;23:495.

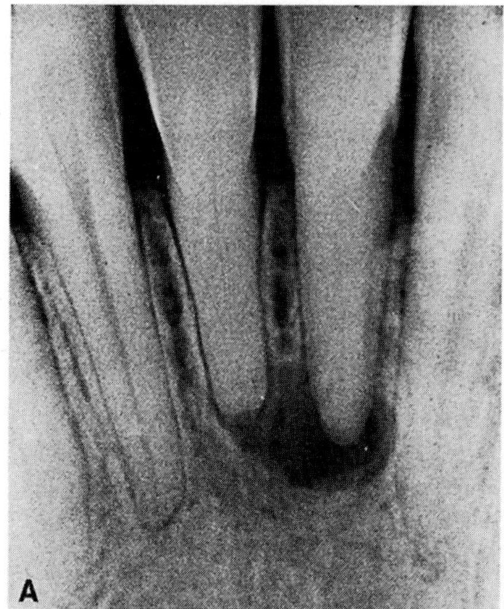

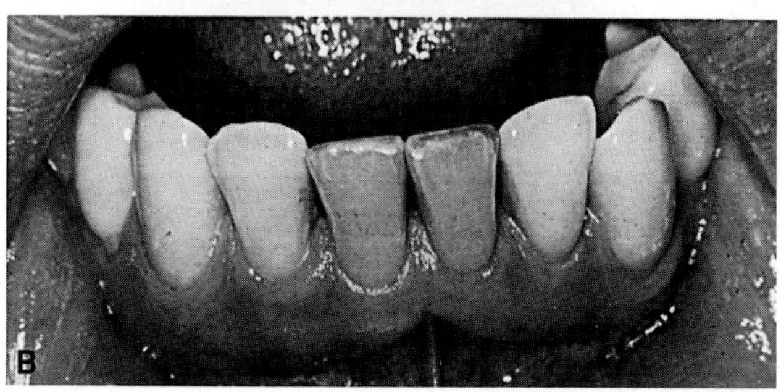

Figure 6-2 A, Mandibular incisors with sclerosed canals and chronic apical periodontitis. Surgical treatment was required. B, Same case. "Dark teeth" caused the patient to seek treatment. If immediate post-trauma and follow-up radiographs had been made regularly, nonsurgical therapy could have been attempted when change was first noted. Reproduced from Marshall FJ. Dent Clin North Am 1979;23:495.

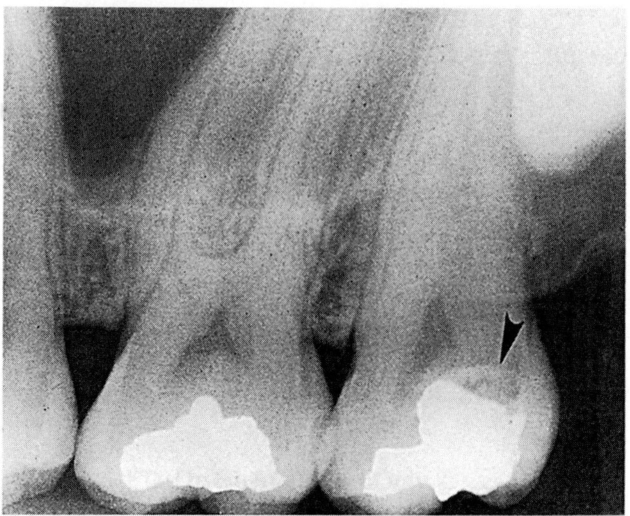

Figure 6-3 Radiolucent material (possibly a pulp cap) shows under occlusal amalgam of a second molar. Patient had complained of pain for 4 months, referring over the entire maxilla and mandible. Pain was not relieved completely by infiltration anesthesia over the second molar and persisted in the mandible. However, a posterior superior alveolar block relieved pain in both areas, demonstrating the fallibility of anesthesia in diagnosing referred pain. Reproduced with permission from Marshall FJ. Dent Clin North Am 1979;23:495.

problem (Figure 6-2). Although a positive and accurate answer may not result, the question will prompt a closer look at radiographs for the presence or absence of cement bases or for recurrent caries or caries remaining under restorations (Figure 6-3).

Full-crown restorations should also raise questions to the patient regarding "wet" or "dry" drilling. "Dry drilling" may result in an increased incidence of inflammation and even internal resorption (see Figure 4-44). Patients who have undergone orthodontic treatment may have areas of resorption or pulpal changes. In the past decade, there has been an increased interest in adult orthodontics, and recent studies indicate that the adult pulp may be more susceptible than younger pulps to such iatral trauma[6] (Figure 6-4).

The question, **"How many times has this tooth or have these teeth been treated?"** is also pertinent. A tooth with a history of repeated restorations and multiple occurrences of caries ("stressed pulp") should be evaluated carefully with respect to pulpal status before procedures such as full crowns or bridge abutment restorations are initiated. Root canal therapy prior to restorations in such teeth is often indicated. The question, **"How recently has this tooth or area been treated?"** may provide information that the problem of thermal sensitivity is merely a reaction to a recently placed restoration. If the pain is of low intensity, a patient may tolerate it in the hope that it will subside. Pain existing for several months may have become part of the patient's lifestyle.[7]

A history of long-standing, severe pain should raise suspicion that the condition may be other than pulpal in origin. Additional examinations for myofascial or neurologic pain, as well as cardiac referred pain or possibly psychogenic pain, should be considered. A more detailed discussion of this subject is found in chapter 8.

Finally, the patient must be asked about past reactions to dental procedures; to pain, both dental and general; and to expectations for treatment. A patient with a history of low pain threshold and strong analgesic dependency, as well as many previous attempts to solve the problem, may require special treatment or referral.

It should be noted that history taking is a process of questions and answers and that many questions are

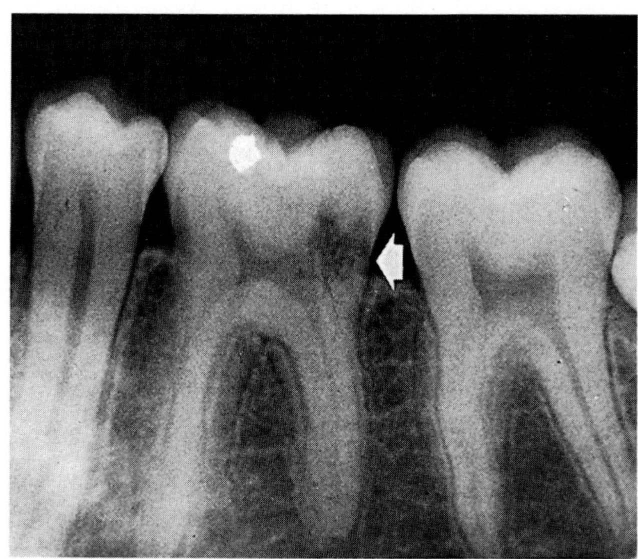

Figure 6-4 Invasive resorption (**arrow**) triggered by orthodontic movement of molar tooth. (Courtesy of Robert M. Krasny.)

repeated. These repeated questions are not redundant but are deliberate attempts to confirm data and validate the diagnosis.

Medical History

Patients need to share their medical problems with their dentists so the data can be used in planning treatment.[8] This begins when the patient completes some standard form (see Table 6-1 or 6-2), usually at the same time as the receptionist records other basic data. The confidence needed to share these data builds slowly in some people. Thus, there is a need to review carefully and sincerely the answers the patient has recorded on the health history form. This review may be more comfortable for the patient after asking about the chief complaint.

In reviewing the medical history, particular emphasis must be placed on **illnesses, history of bleeding, and medications. Illness** often means hospitalization to patients; consequently, they may not list weight changes, accidents, or problems related to stress and tension. Patients who are African American should be questioned about sickle cell anemia; there is a report of pulp necrosis occurring in patients with this distressing condition.[9]

The term **bleeding** is usually interpreted by the patient to mean frank blood and seldom elicits answers related to bruising or healing time, chronic use of aspirin[10] (not considered a drug by many people), or a history of liver disease. These should all be specifically mentioned in the medical history form.

Medication means to many people only those items obtained by written prescription. Dentists must also ask about "pills" and "drugs." With the availability of home remedy "medical" texts, many people are self-medicating with diet pills, sleep inducers, and vitamins, as well as "recreational drugs," to mention only a few. Even if these self-administered medications do not influence treatment directly, the knowledge that patients have a tendency to "do their own thing" may be helpful in planning treatment.

Women should be asked if they are pregnant or if they have menstrual or menopausal problems. Positive answers to these questions must be weighed and evaluated along with the other responses to determine the risk of treatment against the risk of nontreatment.

When the history uncovers a serious problem, and a review of the systems involved (cardiac, respiratory, etc) does not explain the problem, the patient's physician must be consulted.

During these interviews, the dentist-patient relationship tends to crystallize. A rapport is established that is relevant and meaningful to all future relationships. This is the time when anxious, frightened patients may be calmed and reassured even though they may not be completely at ease until the first treatment is completed and they learn that dental procedures can be uneventful and nontraumatic.

Kindness and attention to their concerns or problems (chief complaint) during the history-taking will greatly reduce most patients' emotional trauma and stress, particularly when this phase is followed by a thorough, painless examination.

CLINICAL EXAMINATION

In general, the clinical examination should follow a logical sequence from the general to the specific, from the more obvious to the less obvious, from the external to the internal. The results of the examination, along with the information from the patient's history, will be combined to establish the diagnosis, formulate a treatment plan, and determine the prognosis.

Vital Signs

The first step in examination is to record the patient's vital signs, thus establishing a baseline or a **"norm"** for each patient during treatment, whether routine or emergency. Patients with test values outside the range of acceptable norms are at risk, as is the dentist who treats them.[8] Common sense suggests that this risk should be shared with the patient's physician by a telephone conversation at least. Information received should be recorded in the chart and dated.

The vital signs may be recorded by any trained member of the office team. However, abnormal values must be evaluated by the doctor. The person of first contact should also record, for later evaluation, any additional observations of abnormalities such as breathlessness, color change, altered gait, or unusual body movements observed during the initial meeting.

Blood Pressure (normal: 120/80 mm Hg for persons under age 60; 140/90 mm /Hg for persons over age 60). Routine use of the sphygmomanometer not only establishes a baseline blood pressure but occasionally brings to light unsuspected cases of hypertension in patients who are not regularly seeing a physician or are not maintaining prescribed regimens of therapy. Halpern reported that only 18% of the dental clinic patients attending Temple University Dental School "were seeing their physicians."[8] At times, however, elevated blood pressure is caused only by the stress and anxiety of the moment and can be dealt with by reassurance or, if necessary, pretreatment sedation. Even more important, however, is the emphasis that this face-to-face procedure places on an examination. Both the patient and the doctor are inclined to be more serious in their questions and answers when the examination begins with blood pressure records. It must be stressed that no patient, with or without a dental emergency, should be treated when his **diastolic** blood pressure is over 100 mm.[11]

Pulse Rate and Respiration (normal: pulse, 60 to 100 beats/minute; respiration, 16 to 18 breaths per minute). When these examinations are added to the recording of blood pressure, the dentist increases the opportunity to know the patient better. These examinations also show the patient, by physical contact, how further examination will proceed—deliberately, gently, and completely. Pulse and respiration rates may also be elevated owing to stress and anxiety; in fact, these signs may be even better indicators of stress than is blood pressure. Tests with markedly positive findings should be repeated later in the appointment or at a subsequent appointment.

Temperature (normal: body temperature, 98.6°F [37°C]). The taking and recording of body temperature is a simple, significant procedure. An elevated temperature (fever) is one indication of a total body reaction to inflammatory disease. If the body temperature is not elevated, one can assume that the body is "managing" its defenses well, that whatever the local signs are (pain, swelling, abscess formation, etc), systemic treatment, with its attendant risks, will likely not be required. A temperature above 98.6° but less than 100°F indicates localized disease.[12] Localized disease can usually be treated by removing the cause (eg, cleaning the root canal) and/or incision and drainage.

Cancer Screen (soft tissue examination: lumps, bumps, white spots). Every new patient must be routinely screened for cancer and other soft tissue nonodontogenic conditions as part of the examination. And they must be informed of the results! This examination should include a survey of the face, lips, neck, and intraoral soft tissues. When such examinations are made routinely, without secrecy, they will usually dispel the unstated fears of the cancerphobe and add to the confidence and rapport of all patients with their dentists. The sooner this examination is completed the better.

It is sometimes argued that dentists are liable if they inform patients that they are performing an examination and then miss finding disease when it is present. In fact, dentists are even more liable if they miss reporting the disease because they have not made an examination.

Extraorally, a cancer survey includes palpation for masses and examination for asymmetry and color changes. Intraorally, this examination is repeated with the additional care of directed lighting and of moving the tongue in such a manner so that all areas can be clearly seen (Table 6-3). Detailed procedures are presented elsewhere.[13]

Extraoral Examination

Inflammatory changes originating intraorally and observable extraorally may indicate a serious, spreading problem.[14] The patient must be examined for asymmetries, localized swelling, changes in color or bruises, abrasions, cuts or scars, and similar signs of disease, trauma, or previous treatment. Positive findings combined with the chief complaint and information about past injuries or previous treatments to teeth or jaws will begin to clarify the extent of the patient's problem.

The extraoral examination includes the face, lips, and neck, which may need to be palpated if the patient reports soreness or if there are apparent areas of inflammation. Painful and/or enlarged lymph nodes are of particular importance. They denote the spread of

Table 6-3 Oral Cancer Warning Signals*

Swelling, lump, or growth anywhere in or about the mouth
White, scaly patches inside the mouth
Any sore that does not heal
Numbness or pain anywhere in the mouth area
Repeated bleeding in the mouth without cause

*"Open Wide." Reproduced with permission from the American Cancer Society, New York.

inflammation as well as possible malignant disease. The extent and manner of jaw opening can provide information about possible myofascial pain and dysfunction.[15] The temporomandibular joint should be examined during function for sensitivity to palpation, joint noise, and irregular movement.[16]

Intraoral Examination

The intraoral examination is begun with a general evaluation of the oral structures. The lips and cheeks are retracted while the teeth are in occlusal contact and the oral vestibules and buccal mucosa are examined for localized swelling and sinus tract or color changes. With the patient's jaws apart, the dentist should evaluate in a similar manner the lingual and palatal soft tissues. Also, the presence of tori should be noted. Finally, as part of the general inspection, carious lesions, discolorations, and other obvious abnormalities associated with the teeth, including loss of teeth and presence of supernumerary or retained deciduous teeth, should be noted.

Often the particular tooth causing the complaint is readily noted during this visual examination if it has not already been pointed out by the patient. Complaints associated with discolored or fractured teeth, teeth with gross caries or large restorations, and teeth restored by full coverage are for the most part readily located. True "puzzlement" begins when the complaint centers on teeth fully crowned and part of extensive bridges or splints, or when only a few teeth are restored, and then only with minimal restorations.

Transillumination with a fiber-optic light, directed through the crowns of teeth, can add further information.[17] By this method, a pulpless tooth that is not noticeably discolored may show a gross difference in translucency when the shadow produced on a mirror is compared to that of adjacent teeth. Transillumination may also locate teeth with vertical cracks or fractures.

If the involved tooth is not readily identified, it may be necessary to thoroughly examine all of the teeth in the half arch or opposing arch, depending on how specifically the patient can localize the area of pain. Although the size of a carious lesion or the presence of a crown or large restoration may point to the involved tooth, the symptoms may be referred pain or pain from an adjoining tooth with problems. Adjacent teeth with large restorations or crowns can be assumed to be equally at risk. Regardless of the presence or absence of findings, the patient's premonitions and descriptions should not be ignored in favor of what appears to be obvious. For the record and for the possibility of additional later treatment, the condition of all teeth in the immediate vicinity should also be recorded. This is especially true following an accident. In fact, the general state and care of the entire mouth must be noted along with the particular tooth's restorability and strategic importance.

If the patient's **chief complaint** includes symptoms that occur following specific events (eg, chewing, drinking cold liquids), the specific intraoral examination should include tests that duplicate or reproduce these symptoms. For example, if the chief complaint is pain with hot liquids, the clinical tests may include testing the suspected tooth with a hot stimulus. A positive response (development of the chief complaint) will be important evidence in establishing the diagnosis.

In the following sections, various tests will be described, detailing how to perform them and how to evaluate the results. The correct diagnosis can be established more readily the more information that is developed from all sources: history, clinical examination, radiographic evaluation, and clinical tests.

Coronal Evaluation. For psychological reasons and to expedite treatment, the most obviously affected tooth is examined first, particularly when the patient, the history, or the general examination calls attention to a certain tooth.

Using a mouth mirror and an explorer, and possibly a fiber-optic light source, the dentist carefully and thoroughly examines the suspected tooth or teeth for caries, defective restorations, discoloration, enamel loss, or defects that allow direct passage of stimuli to the pulp. Sometimes sealing off such leakage with temporary cements or periodontal dressings can be diagnostic (Figure 6-5). Vertical and horizontal fractures located by transillumination should be further investigated by hav-

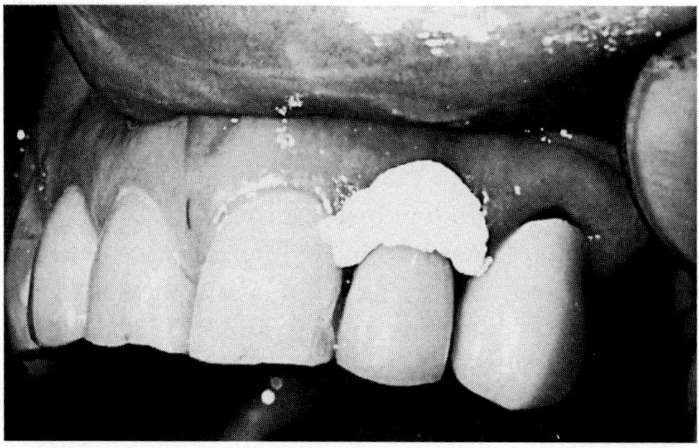

Figure 6-5 Zinc oxide–eugenol temporary cement packed buccally and lingually to seal margins of a porcelain-fused-to-metal crown against external stimulus (leakage). If the patient's complaint stops, then the margins can be permanently sealed or the crown remade. This technique is particularly helpful when several teeth are crowned. (Courtesy of Dr. F. James Marshall.)

ing the patient bite on some firm object such as the Tooth Slooth (Laguna Niguel, Calif.), or a wet cotton roll.[18] Occlusal wear facets and parafunctional patterns are also sought out, as is tooth mobility.

Pulpal Evaluation

The clinical condition of the pulp can be evaluated by thermal stimuli, percussion, palpation, and vitality tests. Generally, pain of endodontic origin results from pulp inflammation that spreads from the coronal pulp apically to the periodontal ligament, which then spreads to the periosteum overlying the apical bone and beyond. Pulpal and periradicular symptoms, therefore, sometimes combine, making pulpal assessment difficult.

The purpose of evaluating the pulpal condition is to arrive at a diagnosis—namely, the nature of the disease involving the pulp. After determining the diagnosis, there are specific treatment options for each pulpal condition. Irreversible pulpitis and pulp necrosis require removal of the pulp (pulp extirpation and root canal treatment, or extraction of the tooth), whereas a tooth with a normal pulp or with reversible pulpitis may be treated by preserving the pulp (vital pulp therapy). The various methods of pulpal evaluation, then, do not dictate treatment but provide information that can be used with other information (history and radiographs) to establish a diagnosis. Pulp tests alone are usually not adequate for establishing a diagnosis but can provide very useful information.[19,20]

Clinical Endodontic Tests

There are several ways to obtain information about the condition of a tooth's pulp and supporting structures. Probably no one test is sufficient in itself; the results of several tests often have to be obtained to have enough information to support a likely diagnosis or perhaps a list of differential diagnoses.

Thermal Tests. Two types of thermal tests are available, cold and hot stimuli. Neither is totally reliable in all cases, but both can provide very useful information in many cases of pulpal involvement.

The cold test may be used in differentiating between reversible and irreversible pulpitis and in identifying teeth with necrotic pulps. It can also alleviate pain brought on by hot or warm stimuli, a finding that patients sometimes discover can provide them with much relief.

When cold is used to differentiate between reversible and irreversible pulpitis, one must try to determine if the effect of stimulus application produces a lingering effect or if the pain subsides immediately on removal of the stimulus from the tooth. The "lingering" quality of pain to a cold stimulus might be considered in cases in which the patient clearly feels that the pain is still present several seconds after stimulus removal. In testing, if the pain lingers, that is taken as evidence for irreversible pulpitis; if pain subsides immediately after stimulus removal, hypersensitivity or reversible pulpitis is the more likely diagnosis.

Cold as a test for pulp vitality (pulp necrosis versus vital pulp) is probably not entirely reliable since teeth with calcified pulp spaces may have vital pulps, but cold stimuli may not be able to excite the nerve endings owing to the insulating effect of tertiary/irritation dentin.

Cold testing can be made with an air blast, a cold drink, an ice stick, ethyl chloride or Fluori-Methane (Gebauer Chemical Co., Cleveland, Ohio) sprayed on a cotton swab, or a carbon dioxide (CO_2) dry "ice" stick.[21] Fuss et al. found CO_2 "snow" or Fluori-Methane more reliable than ethyl chloride or an ice stick.[22] Rickoff et al. reported that CO_2 snow applied to a tooth for as long as 5 minutes did not jeopardize the health of the pulp,[23] nor does it damage the surface of the enamel.[24] On the other hand, CO_2 does cause "pitting" of the surface when applied to porcelain on porcelain-fused-to-metal restorations for as little as 5.4 seconds.[25]

The CO_2 dry ice stick is preferred for testing because it does not affect adjacent teeth, whereas the air blast and the ice stick do, and because it gives an intense, reproducible response[26] (Figure 6-6). This has been confirmed by Peters et al. in their studies on the effects of CO_2 used as a pulpal test.[24,27–29] Small icicles can be made in the office by freezing water in anesthetic needle covers.

When testing with a cold stimulus, one must begin with the most posterior tooth and advance toward the anterior teeth. Such a sequence will prevent melting ice water from dripping in a posterior direction and possibly excite a tooth not yet tested, giving a false response.

Hot testing can be made with a stick of heated gutta-percha or hot water. Both have advantages, but hot water may be preferable because it allows simulation of the clinical situation and also may be more effective in penetrating porcelain-fused-to-metal crowns.[30]

The use of a hot stimulus in the form of hot water can help locate a symptomatic tooth with a necrotic (or dying) pulp. The effect tends to be lingering, and the main reason for using the test is to localize which tooth is symptomatic. Often other evidence (patient's own opinion, radiographs, history, clinical appearance) will indicate which tooth is suspected. This tooth is then **isolated with a rubber dam** so the hot water will flow only around the tooth. A positive response of pain, similar to the chief complaint, provides the information needed to identify the problem tooth.

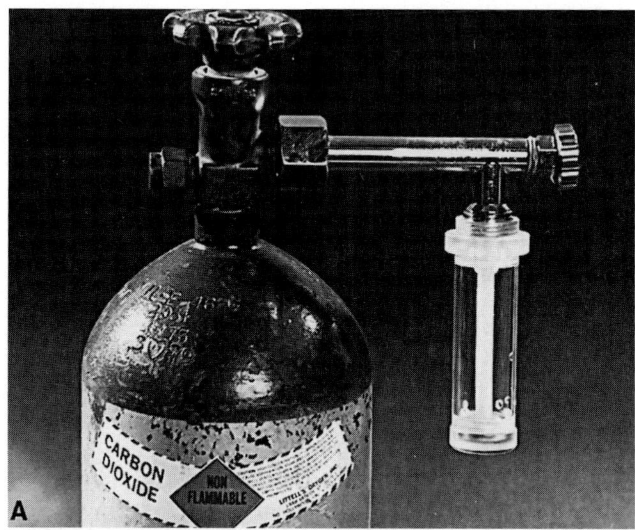

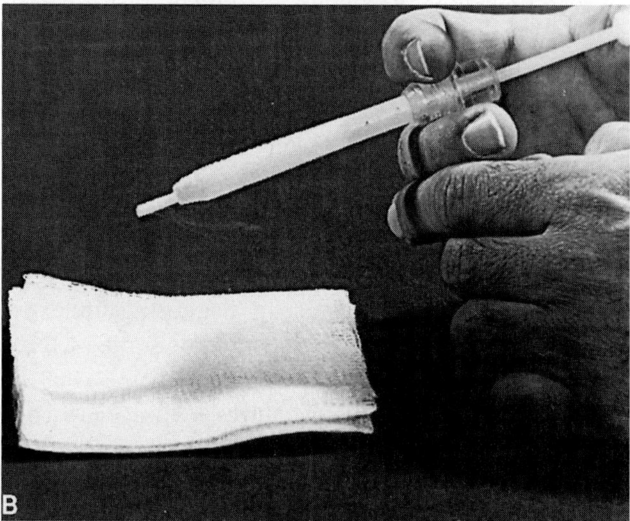

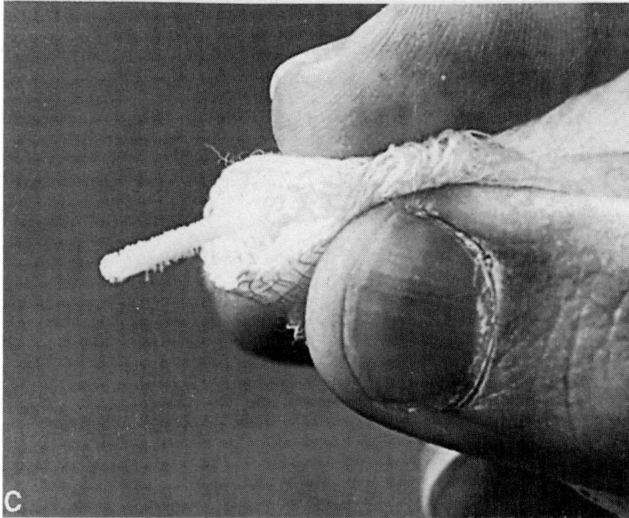

Figure 6-6 Carbon dioxide dry ice "pencil" for thermal testing developed by H. Obwegeser. **A**, Metal arm and plastic ice former attached to tank of siphoned CO_2 (siphoned type of CO_2 should be used). **B**, Loaded ice former is removed and plunger inserted to extrude the CO_2 ice pencil. **C**, Ice pencil held in gauze to prevent CO_2 "burns." (Courtesy of Union Broach Co.)

For routine heat testing, gutta-percha, preferably baseplate gutta-percha, is warmed, formed into a cone, applied to a warmed instrument, reheated, and applied to the moistened tooth (so it will not adhere.) It is reheated for each tooth. If the patient is complaining of a severe toothache, one must be ready to apply cold immediately following a dramatic response to heat. The diagnosis is made!

Thermal testing, hot or cold, can be used for testing teeth with full coverage, to differentiate between vital and necrotic pulps, and requires only a "yes" or "no" response: is the stimulus perceived or not?[21,30]

Percussion. Apical periodontitis is usually an extension of pulpal inflammation, but it may also result from impact trauma, traumatic occlusion, or sinusitis affecting maxillary teeth.[31] However, since apical periodontitis is so frequently associated with pulpal inflammation, percussion tests are included when evaluating pulpal conditions even though the percussion produces a response in the periodontium rather than the pulp.

The procedure for testing is simple: use a mirror handle and **very gently** tap the occlusal/incisal surfaces of several teeth in the area in question. Sometimes a tooth is so painful that merely touching it with a fingertip produces pain, so careful evaluation, prior to testing, is important.

The difficulty in evaluating percussive responses is one of quantity and quality. Does the pain signal inflammation with abscess formation, or is it just mild inflammation from an inflamed pulp? It has been stated that the percussive sound offers clues: a dull note signifies abscess formation, a sharp note merely inflammation.[32] It is probably doubtful that such differentiation can be made consistently. Perhaps the most useful information from percussion is to identify which tooth may be the problem tooth, whereas the final diagnosis requires additional information.

Palpation. Sensitivity to finger pressure (palpation) on the mucosa over the apex of a tooth, buccal or lingual, signals the further spread of inflammation from the periodontal ligament to the periosteum overlying the bone. This examination is most effective when it can be made bilaterally at the same time (Figure 6-7). Besides the pain response to this test, information can also be obtained about asymmetry and fluctuation in the areas examined. Sometimes because of excessive swelling and associated severe pain, it is difficult to diagnose fluctuation (subperiosteal abscess).

Electric Pulp Test. Although any stimulus can initiate a neural response, be it thermal change or physical contact with the dentin and pulp, the most frequent

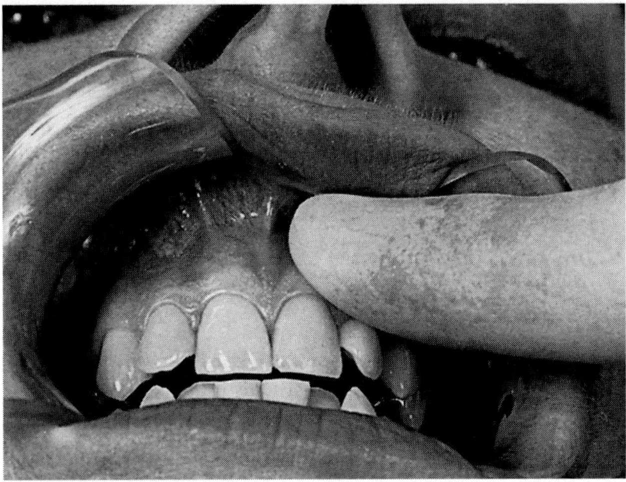

Figure 6-7 During palpation with the index finger, the dentist should watch for the patient's eyelid blink or forehead wrinkling as the first sign of pain.

testing device has been some form of electric pulp tester.[33] Presently, there are a number of very efficient, battery-powered, and easily controlled devices on the market. All have sophisticated circuitry and digital display. Price is the major difference between the various brands, foreign or domestic. Examples are the Digitest and Gentle Pulse (Parkell Products; Farmingdale, N.Y.) Vitality Scanner and Endoanalyzer (Sybron Analytic Technology; Orange, Calif.), Trilite (Evident/Pulpdent, UK and USA), Pulppen (Hygenic Corp., USA), Sirotest (Siemens AG, Germany), Digipex II (Mada Equip. Co., Japan and USA), Neotest (Amadent; Cherry Hill, N.J.), and the Dentometer (Dahlin, Denmark, UK, and USA).

In contrast to the older types of electric pulp testers, these devices produce little discomfort, even when operated by inexperienced examiners[34–39] (Figure 6-8). It is important to follow the manufacturer's instructions to establish positive contact.

The testing procedure must be explained to the patient. An apprehensive or confused patient or a malingering patient may give erratic responses and invalidate the testing. It may be necessary to practice testing on teeth other than the ones being examined to help the patient get used to the procedure. As with most tests, electric pulp testing (EPT) should not be used as the only method for diagnosis.

Electric pulp testing provides limited, though often very useful, information, whether or not the pulpal nerve fibers are responsive to electric stimulation. Many factors affect the level of response: enamel thickness, probe placement on the tooth[40,41] (see Figure 6-8, A and B), dentin calcification, interfering restorative materials, the cross-sectional area of the probe tip,[36] and the patient's level of anxiety. Comparison of EPT results among various teeth is done primarily for the purpose of identifying teeth with no response (or doubtful response, ie, responses at the high end of the scale). Moreover, one needs to keep in mind that both false-positive and false-negative results happen fairly frequently, so EPT results must be evaluated carefully. A consistently negative (or doubtful) response indicates a necrotic pulp. There are exceptions, of course.

A recently erupted tooth frequently gives a negative response, yet never in its lifetime will the pulp be more vital. In recent studies, it has been found that the newly erupted teeth have more large unmyelinated axons than do mature teeth, the speculation being that some of these large fibers may ultimately become myelinated.[42–45] Since it is principally the pulpal "A" fibers that respond to EPT, variability in the number of A fibers entering the tooth offers a possible explanation as to why EPTs tend to be unreliable in young teeth.[42,43]

A young tooth traumatized by impact may not respond to testing, yet when the pulp is opened, the rush of blood illustrates the error of the test. Multirooted teeth often give bizarre pulp test readings when one canal may have vital pulp tissue and other canals necrotic tissue. Practice in diagnosing and experience with the EPT will help overcome some of these difficulties.

Electric Pulp Testing Procedures. To achieve consistent results with an electric pulp tester, one must follow a standard procedure. Dry the teeth to be tested and isolate them with cotton rolls. Cover the tip of the electrode with toothpaste or a similar electrical conductor.

To stimulate the pulp nerve fibers, the electric current must complete a circuit from the electrode through the tooth, through the patient, and back to the electrode. When gloves were not routinely used by dentists, the ungloved fingers of the dentists completed the current by contacting both the electrode and some part of the patient's face, usually the cheek. With gloved hands, that connection is interrupted.

To establish a complete circuit using rubber gloves, one of two methods must now be followed. A ground attachment may be clipped on the patient's lip (see Figure 6-8, D), or the patient may complete the circuit by placing a finger on the metal electrode handle. The latter method has the advantage of giving the patient more control: simply lifting the finger off the electrode handle when a sensation is felt will immediately interrupt the current and terminate the stimulation[46,47] (see Figure 6-8, C).

A record must be made of the results of each tooth tested. If repeat tests are indicated, it is probably better

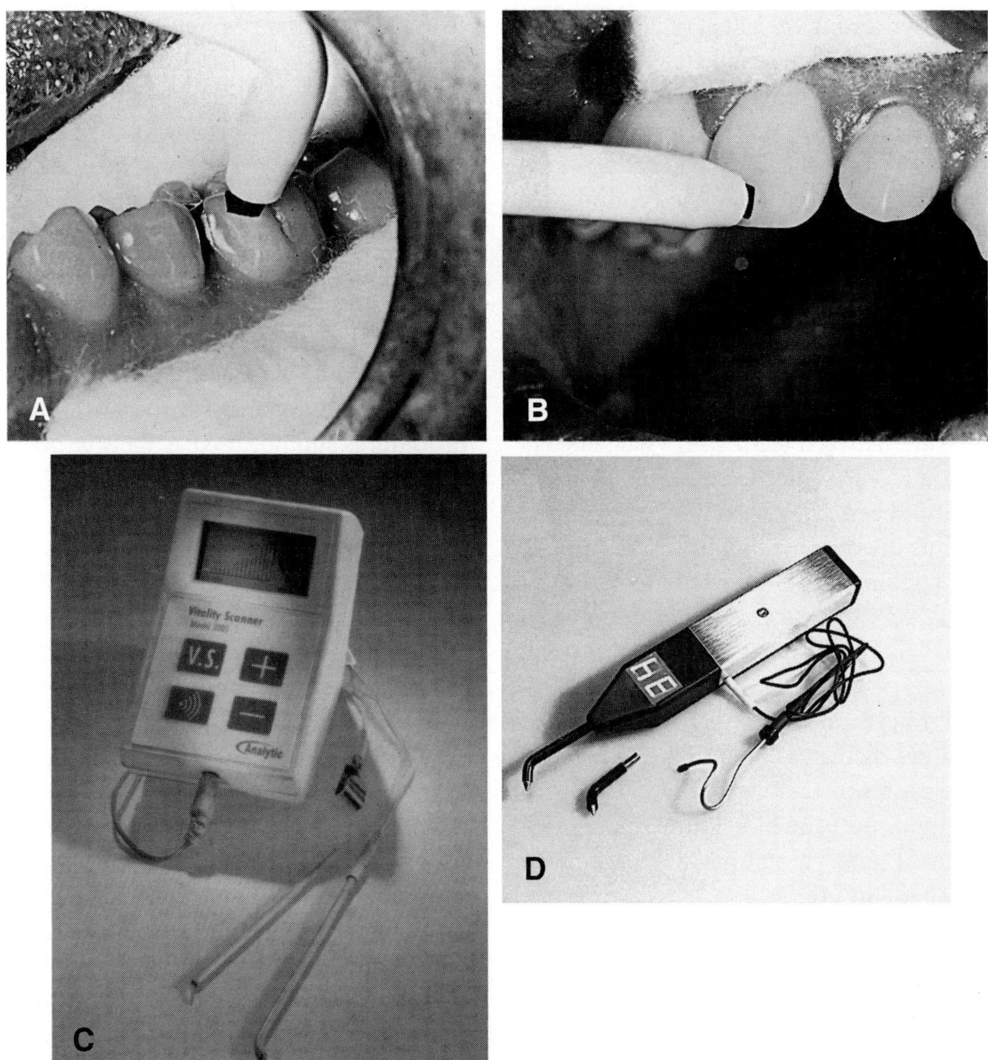

Figure 6-8 Use of an electric pulp tester. **A**, Posterior teeth should be isolated and dried. Mylar strips can be used to separate connecting metallic fillings. Using toothpaste as a conductor, contact should be made on the occlusal third. **B**, Isolated and dried anterior teeth are contacted on the incisal third to avoid false stimulation of gingival tissue. **C**, Vitality Scanner pulp tester. To complete the circuit, the patient may touch the metal handle. **D**, Digitest pulp tester with lip contact to complete circuit. Both pulp testers have a digital readout. The difference lies in size and price. **A** and **B** reproduced with permission from Marshall FJ. Dent Clin North Am 1979;23:495. **C** courtesy of Analytic Technology. **D** courtesy of Parkell Products.

to use the same pulp tester each time for more accurate comparison. Being able to quantify results numerically is a decided advantage of EPT over thermal testing.

Multirooted teeth may need to be tested by placing the electrode on more than one crown location. It may happen that two areas on a molar will give a negative response, but a positive test within the normal range may be gained in another area. This may indicate that the pulp in two canals is necrotic, whereas the pulp in the third canal is still vital.

If CO_2 dry ice testing is not possible and if it is imperative that a tooth fully covered by gold or porcelain be electrically pulp tested, a cavity is prepared without anesthesia, through the restorative material, **until the dentin is reached.** During preparation, penetration to the dentin may be sufficient enough to elicit a response. If not, the probe is placed directly on dentin and the response noted. To avoid contacting the metal of the crown, a tiny piece of "spaghetti" tubing can be used to insulate the tester probe. Analytic Technology also makes a Mini-Tip for this purpose, or a small instrument such as an endodontic file may be used as a "bridging" device.[48]

Precautions in Use of an Electric Pulp Tester. It has been suggested that using an electric pulp tester on patients who have an indwelling cardiac pacemaker is contraindicated. After testing the effect of electric pulp testers on dogs with artificial pacemakers, Woolley and associates concluded that currents of the magnitude of 5 to 20 milliamps are sufficient to modify normal pacemaker function.[49] After testing one battery-powered device and three using line current, they found that only one caused interference with pacemaker action. They also warned against devices such as desensitizers and electrosurgical units that could produce unknown current leaks, as one of the pulp testers did.

Liquid Crystal Testing. Cholesteric liquid crystals have been used by investigators[50] to show the difference in tooth temperature between teeth with vital (hotter) pulps and necrotic (cooler) pulps. The **laser Doppler flowmeter** has also been shown to measure pulpal blood flow and thus the degree of vitality.[51–53] Already used in medicine (retina, renal cortex), this experimental device might well spell the difference between reversible and irreversible pulpitis—the stressed pulp, if you will.

The **Hughes Probeye camera,** which is capable of detecting temperature changes as small as 0.1°C, has also been used to measure pulp vitality experimentally.[54] All three of these methods measure blood flow in the pulp, the true measurement of pulpal status. One may emerge as the pulp tester of the future.

Occlusal Pressure Test. A frequent patient complaint is pain on biting or chewing. The causes for such symptoms include apical periodontitis, apical abscess, and incomplete tooth fractures (infractions). A clinical test that simulates the chief complaint is the occlusal pressure test (or biting test). Several methods exist, such as biting on an orangewood stick, a Burlew rubber disk, or a wet cotton roll. All have the ability to simulate a bolus of food and allow pressure on the occlusal surfaces.

The orangewood stick, the **Tooth Slooth,** and Burlew disks allow pinpoint testing of individual cusp areas, whereas the wet cotton roll has the advantage of adapting to the occlusal surface, allowing for pressure over the entire occlusal table. This test is useful in identifying teeth with symptoms of apical periodontitis, abscess, or cracks. An interesting clinical observation in patients with tooth infractions (cracked tooth syndrome) is pain often experienced when biting force is released rather than during the downward chewing motion.

Anesthetic Test. Pain in the oral cavity is frequently referred from one tooth to an adjacent one or even from one quadrant to the opposing one. The anesthetic test can help identify the quadrant from whence the focus of pain originates. The suspected tooth should be anesthetized, and, if the diagnosis is correct, the referred pain should disappear, even when it is referred to the opposite arch.

Test Cavity. This test is often a last resort in testing for pulp vitality. It is important to explain the procedure to the patient because it must be done without anesthesia. Make a preparation through the enamel or the existing restoration until the dentin is reached. If the pulp is vital, the heat from the bur will probably generate a response from the patient; however, it may not necessarily be an accurate indication of the degree of pulpal inflammation. As with other tests, the cavity test must be used in conjunction with the history and other testing procedures and not used as the sole determinant.

The Stressed Pulp

Abou-Rass has directed the attention of the profession to what he calls "the stressed pulp."[5] This is the pulp that over the years has been stressed by both disease and treatment (caries and periodontis; trauma—impact, occlusal, and iatral; chemicals—cements, resins, and amalgams). This is the tooth that has decayed and been restored then re-restored, cut down, heated up—all of the insults a pulp is subjected to over a long span of time.

In addition, when the tooth is now ready to be used as an abutment for an important partial denture, fixed or removable, still more iatral insult follows. Careful as one might be, the tooth must still be reduced some more, heated up, cooled off, and injured by impressions, try-ins, and temporaries. The final insult is permanent cementation followed by **microleakage**.

Is it any wonder that a number of these stressed pulps finally give up by either aching and dying or just quietly dying? But the tragedy is that the tooth is now covered by a beautiful new restoration that will have to be weakened or destroyed to reach the ailing pulp. Would it not have been better, asked Abou-Rass, to have determined the quality of life of the pulp before treatment and have taken action before, not after, the final commitment has been made?[5]

How does one determine which pulps are stressed? By taking a careful history and examination, of course. The dentist must consider the patient's lengthy report on this particular tooth, the radiographic outline of the pulp cavity, and the examination findings. The examination includes transilluminating; probing; percussing; examining for cracks, crazing, and abrasion; and the response to pulp testing, thermal and electrical.

Any negative results should be viewed with suspicion, including past trauma, orthodontic movement, multiple or deep restorations, poor systemic health, irradiation in the area, tooth coloration, structural cracks, defective restorations, condensing osteitis (see Figure 6-49), pulp stones, irritation dentin, narrow canals, nearby pins, pulp capping, delayed response to heat and cold, or even a negative response to the electric pulp tester. All of these data must then be considered and acted on before committing **this** tooth with **this** pulp to the forthcoming stressful events.

If one determines that a pulp has been severely stressed, would it not be better to intentionally remove the pulp and perform root canal therapy before proceeding with treatment, rather than having to cut back through a fine restoration to perform the inevitable?

Clinical judgment comes with clinical experience. But when dealing with "pulps that have received repeated previous injury and survived with diminished responses and lessened repair potential,"[5] it might be wiser to act sooner rather than later.

Periodontal Evaluation

No dental examination is complete without careful evaluation of the teeth's periodontal support. Periodontal probing and recording pocket depths provide information with respect to possible etiology and prognosis (see following sections).

There is little question that pulpal necrosis can lead to loss of periodontal support. Whether periodontal disease can cause pulpal degeneration is a question not clearly answered. There is agreement, however, that a potential interaction exists between the pulp and periodontium. For the purposes of endodontic treatment of a single tooth, probing may be limited to the tooth involved and at least the adjacent teeth. As part of a total oral examination, all teeth should be included in the probing evaluation. The number of probing locations may vary depending on the tooth's location. Four to six areas surrounding the tooth should provide a good picture of periodontal support. Gingival and sulcular bleeding and drainage, along with the presence of plaque and calculus, should also be noted.

FACTORS INFLUENCING PROGNOSIS

Endodontic diagnosis should not be the sole determinant of treatment planning. Other factors contribute to determine whether a suspicious tooth should be restored or a pulpally involved tooth should be treated. Periodontal health, restorative considerations, and radiographic evidence of anatomic complexities associated with the tooth will have a major impact on any treatment decision.

Periodontal Disease

Periodontal stability is a basic requirement for any tooth being considered for endodontic therapy. This stability is determined by the amount of bony support, the health of that support, and the health of the overlying soft tissue. Examination alone cannot guarantee the future health of these tissues, but usually it can determine existing disease. Isolated bone loss or tooth mobility may or may not signify periodontal disease. It may be owing to periradicular disease of pulpal origin, or it may be combined periodontal-endodontal disease.[55] Generalized bone loss of periodontal disease will definitely affect prognosis and therefore the treatment plan.

As part of the examination, probe the sulcus of the tooth or teeth in question and record the pocket measurements. Also test for mobility and record the data using a system of 0 through 3. Grade 0 means normal mobility, grade 1 slight mobility, grade 2 marked mobility, and grade 3 mobility and depressable. Also record if bleeding occurs on probing. Particular note should be made of palatal grooves in single rooted teeth (Figure 6-9), furcas in multirooted teeth, and other anomalies (enamel projections, etc), as these may aggravate gingival conditions and make for unstable future periodontal health. These examinations will establish approximate bone levels and the crown-root ratio. The presence of 3 to 5 mm pockets of a first-degree mobility indicates "moderate periodontitis" (Figure 6-10). When this is found, the entire mouth should be screened for periodontal disease and treated accordingly.[56]

Pockets deeper than 5 mm, or mobility graded 2 or 3, indicate "severe periodontitis," and periodontal treatment is imperative. Referral to a periodontist should be considered. Regardless of the extent of the periodontal disease or who renders the treatment, the patient must be advised of the effect that periodontal disease can have on the prognosis for endodontic therapy. Hiatt reported 20-year follow-up on two cases involving a number of teeth treated with combined periodontal/endodontal therapy. Only one tooth was lost, because of root resorption.[57]

Restorability

The restorability of a tooth requiring endodontic treatment depends on the amount of sound tooth structure remaining and the effect that the restoration will have on the periodontal tissues—not invading the "biologic width" between restoration and the periodontal ligament (PDL), for example. Prior to any endodontic treatment, and after all present coronal restorations and caries are removed, the remaining tooth structure should be re-examined with a fiber-optic light for **fractures** and **perforations**. At this time, teeth with vertical fractures or severe perforations are generally untreatable.

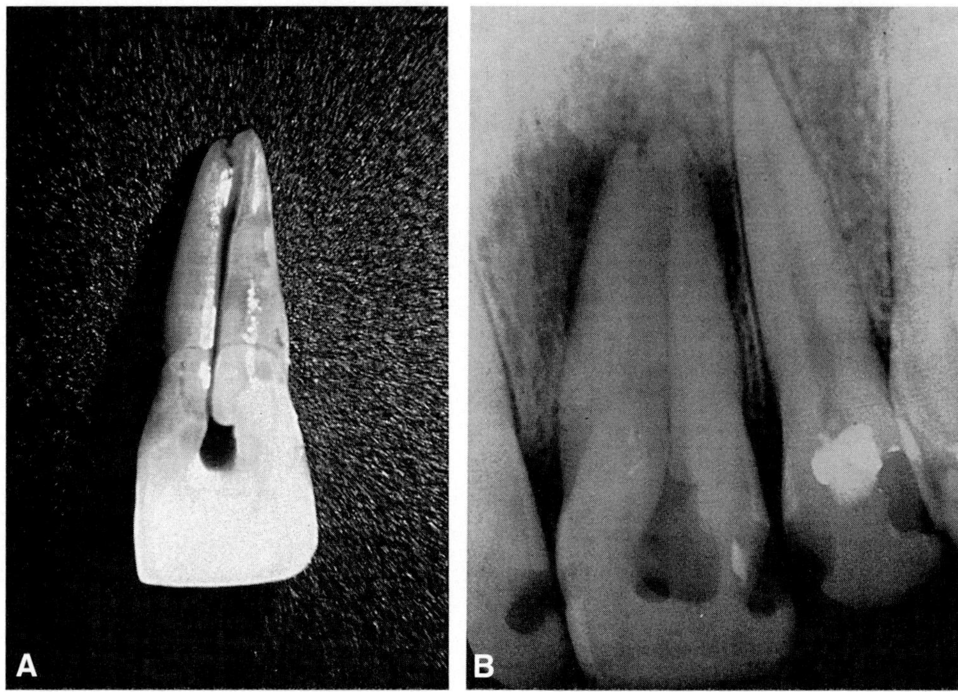

Figure 6-9 Deep palatal groove anomaly leading to irreversible pulpitis and periodontal disease and tooth loss. A, Depth and severity of the groove. B, Combined endodontal-periodontal lesion. (Courtesy of Dr. David S. August.)

It should also be noted that pulpless teeth are not strengthened by the use of posts.[58] Posts are for the retention of crown build-up. Retention of the crown and strength of the restoration depend on the design of the restoration, placing margins well onto solid tooth structure.

RADIOGRAPHIC EXAMINATION

In the sequence of examination, radiographic evaluations should come last. In practical terms, one usually takes a look at the radiographs first and then proceeds with the other evaluation. Following the examination, in

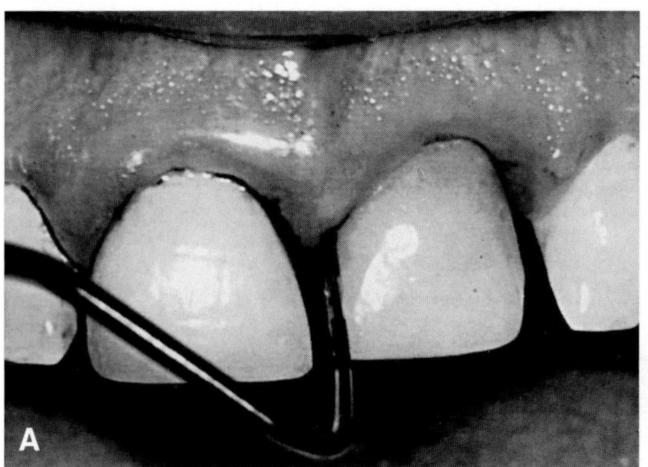

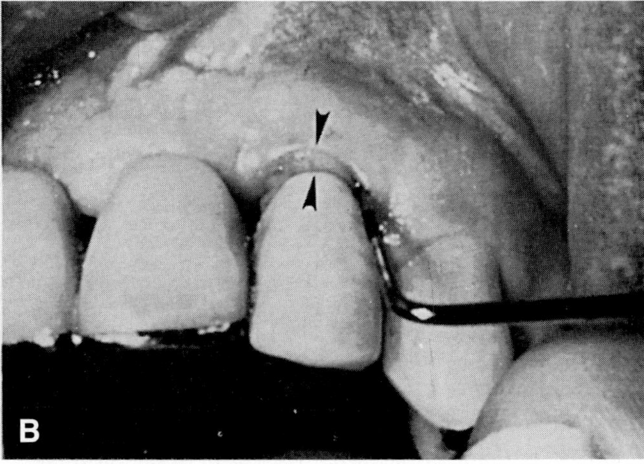

Figure 6-10 A, Five mm pocket, first-degree mobility, and bleeding indicate moderate periodontitis associated with pulpless tooth. Successful periodontal treatment may well be necessary to retain the endodontically treated tooth. A complete periodontal examination is indicated. B, A pulpless tooth is periodontally involved as well. Recession (**arrows**) is undoubtedly related to crown preparation invading the biologic width of the periodontal ligament attachment. (Courtesy of Dr. F. James Marshall.)

hindsight, radiographs can be better interpreted when the results of the previous examination are available.

First, a few words about endodontic radiographs. The radiographic image is a shadow and has the elusive qualities of all shadows. First and foremost, it is **a two-dimensional representation of a three-dimensional object** (Figure 6-11). Also, like any shadow, it may be too light or too dark, too short or too long. The central beam must be carefully oriented to give detail where detail is required (Figure 6-12). This usually requires the central beam to be aimed directly through the periapex rather than a compromise position at the crest of the alveolar process.

In addition to central beam positioning, two or more exposures are frequently necessary to check out detail from more than one horizontal angle (Figure 6-13). This is especially true in the case of the normal bony foramens. The mental foramen may be directly superimposed over the apex of the mandibular premolars, for example (Figure 6-14). The nasopalatine foramen also may be superimposed on the apex of the maxillary central incisors. Because these foramina are actually some distance from the apices of these teeth, their shadows may be shifted far to the mesial or the distal merely by shifting the **horizontal angle** of the cone of the x-ray machine to the mesial or distal during separate exposures (Figure 6-15). On the other hand, if the radiolucent area in the radiograph is actually a lesion truly associated with the periapex of the involved tooth, its shadow will remain "attached" to the root end and will remain so in spite of a mesial or distal shift in separate films. For details regarding the "horizontal shift," the reader is referred to chapter 9.

Interpretation

The finest radiologist will be severely handicapped in securing valuable information from a film that has not been properly placed, exposed, and processed. Conversely, the finest film is of limited value if the interpreter is inadequately trained.

Neaverth and Goerig have emphasized the necessity of knowing the normal structures before interpreting the abnormal (personal communication, 1995). Using radiographs of unusual clarity, they have delineated the anatomic structures of the posterior mandible and

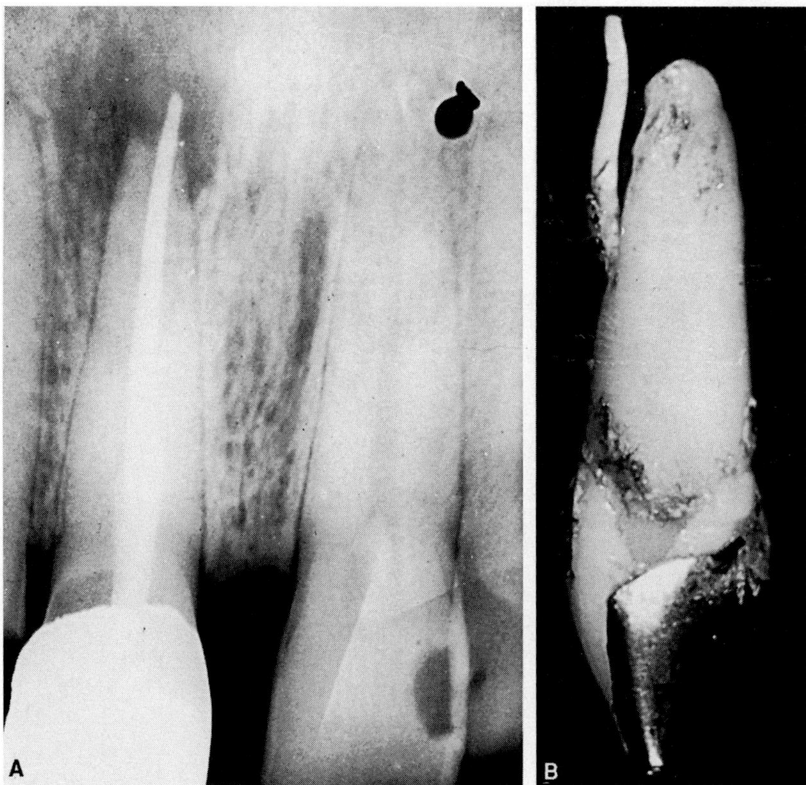

Figure 6-11 Misleading radiograph related to lack of a third dimension. **A**, Failing root canal therapy in the maxillary central incisor appears to be grossly overfilled. **B**, The extracted tooth seen in the radiograph proves that the case is not overfilled. Perforation was by huge enlarging instruments used through restricted access cavity. (Courtesy of Dr. Eugene Meyer.) Reproduced with permission from Luebke RG, Glick DH, Ingle JI. Oral Surg 1964;18:97.

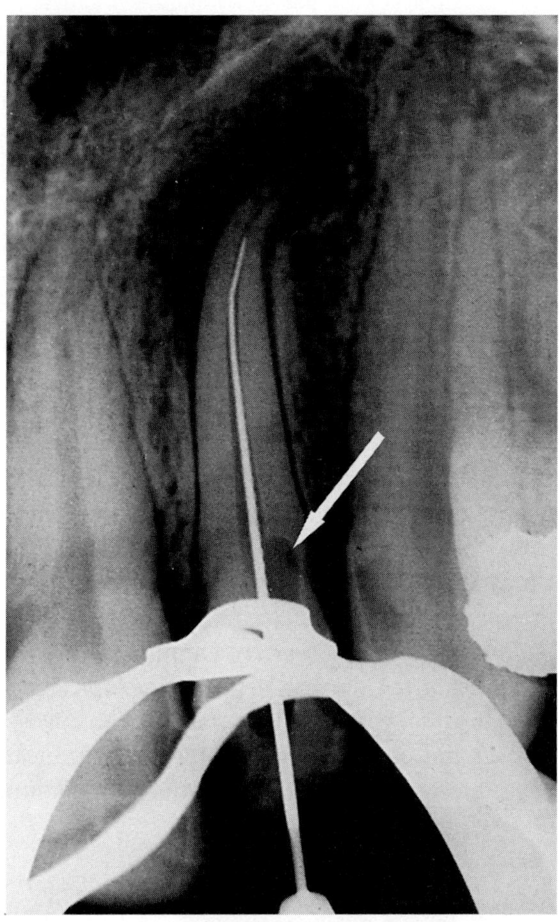

Figure 6-12 The importance of an adequate radiograph. A number of important details may be learned from this film: (1) size and character of periradicular lesion, (2) curvature of root end, (3) relationship of root to adjacent roots, (4) mesial or distal inclination of root, (5) approximate length of tooth, (6) relationship of exploring instrument to root curve, (7) size of canal, and (8) divergence of coronal cavity (**arrow**). Periodontal lesions and root fractures could also be apparent. A central beam, directed through the periradicular region, gives clarity to this important area.

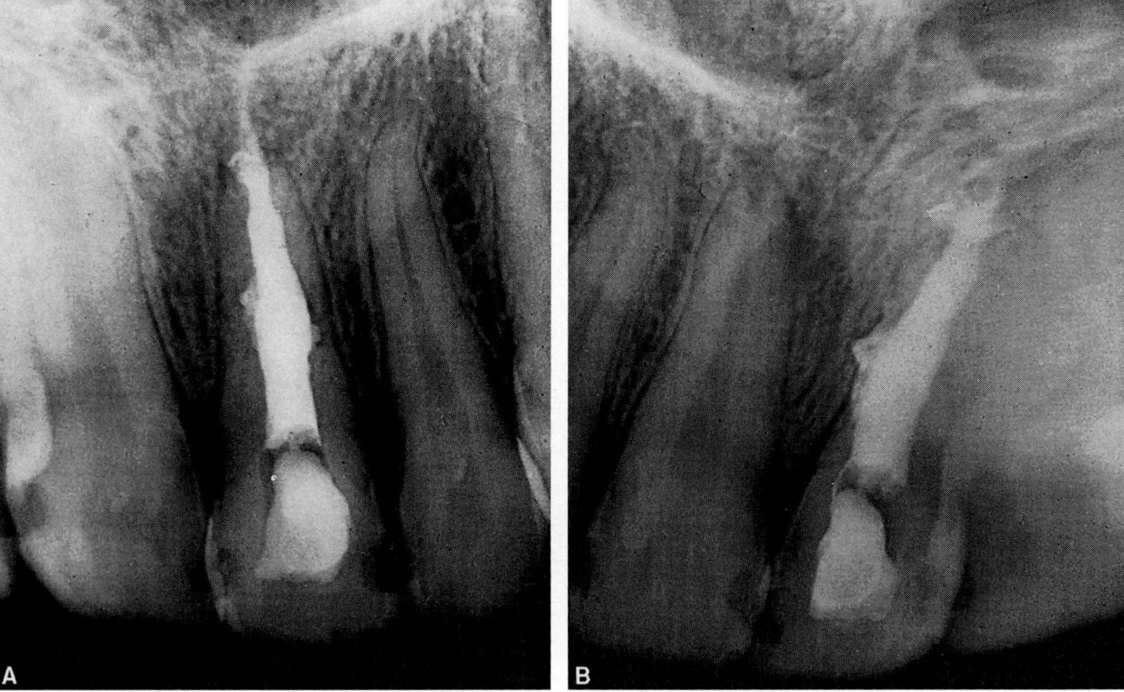

Figure 6-13 Variations in horizontal angle improve radiographic interpretation. **A,** In this straight-on, labial-lingual projection, an internal resorption defect is seen. **B,** In a mesially directed projection, the extension of the resorptive defect to the mesial-lingual is apparent.

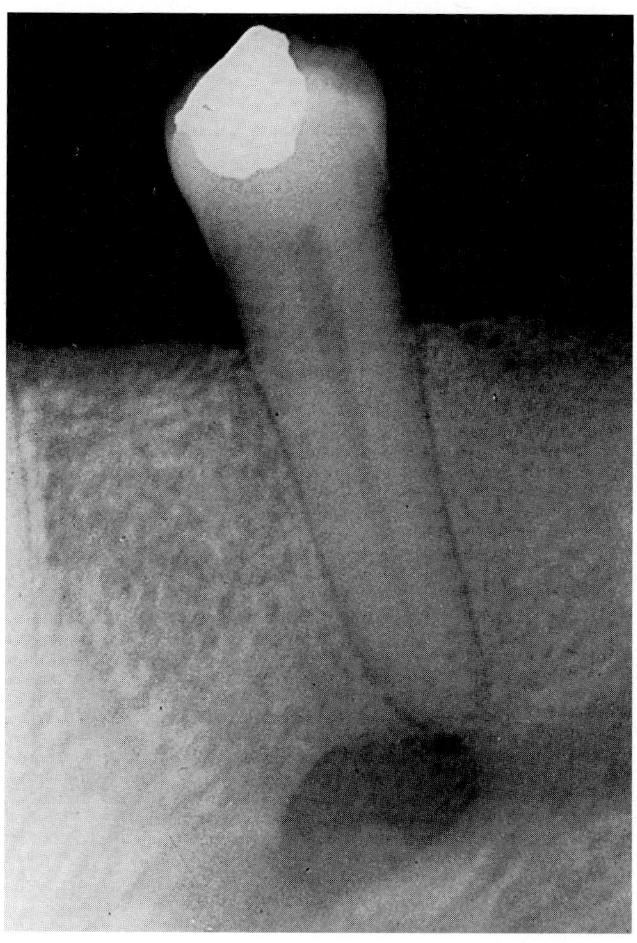

Figure 6-14 Mental foramen is superimposed exactly at the apex of a vital mandibular premolar and may easily be mistaken for a periradicular lesion.

maxilla (Figure 6-16). Many times, these structures can imitate or hide lesions of endodontic or nonendodontic origin. It is also important to identify structures such as the mandibular canal and maxillary sinus and approach them with caution during endodontic treatment and surgery. Encroachment into these areas has led to numerous lawsuits.[59]

An organized method of evaluating and interpreting radiographs, from a single film to a full-mouth set or a panographic plate, has been suggested by Wuehrmann.[60] This technique recommends **reviewing one structure at a time,** such as the lamina dura. Follow this structure all the way around the first tooth on the left and then around the next tooth and the next until the full-film or full-mouth survey is scanned. The findings are recorded as normal or changed.

Brynolf has paid special attention to the continuum of the lamina dura and the periodontal ligament space.[61] She has pointed out the normal appearance of the lamina dura at the apex, which, under magnification, can be seen dipping down into the apical orifice. If there is slight inflammation at the apex, the lamina dura is lost as the PDL space widens[62] (Figure 6-17). Kaffe and Gratt at Tel Aviv University found much the same as Brynolf, that the best radiographic features for accuracy in diagnosis were lamina dura continuity and PDL width and shape.[63]

Following Wuehrmann's suggestion, one proceeds to the next structure, for instance, the crowns of the teeth.[60] Each crown is evaluated independently. The

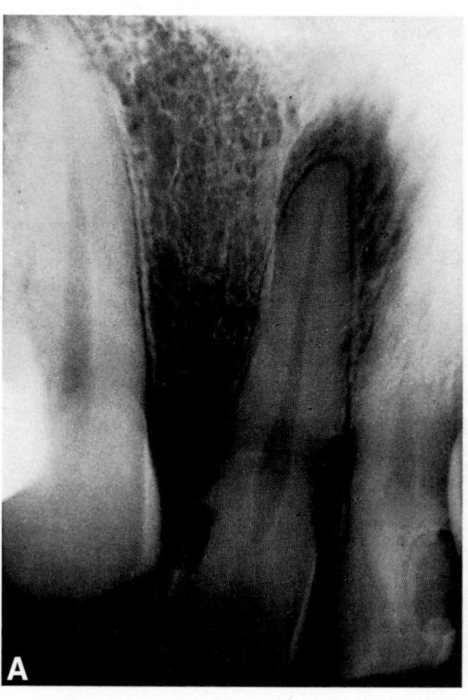

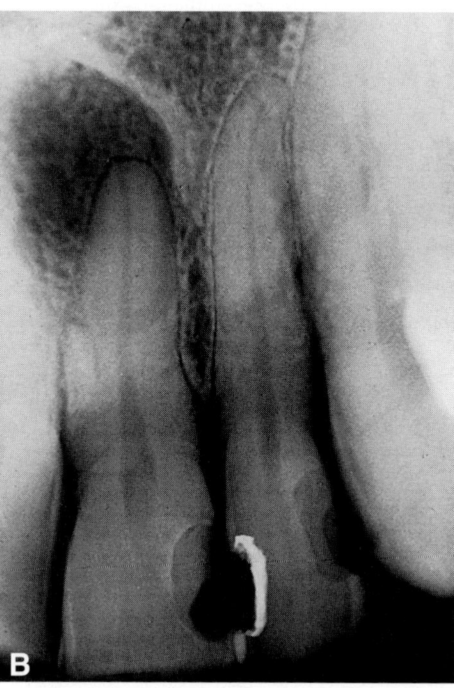

Figure 6-15 Example of a method used to determine the relationship of radiolucency to the periapex of a tooth. A, The nasopalatine foramen is superimposed over the periapex of a **right** central incisor. The right lateral incisor is missing. B, By changing the horizontal projection, the shadow of the nasopalatine foramen may also be superimposed over the periapex of the **left** central incisor, proving that the radiolucent area is some distance lingual to the apex of both teeth.

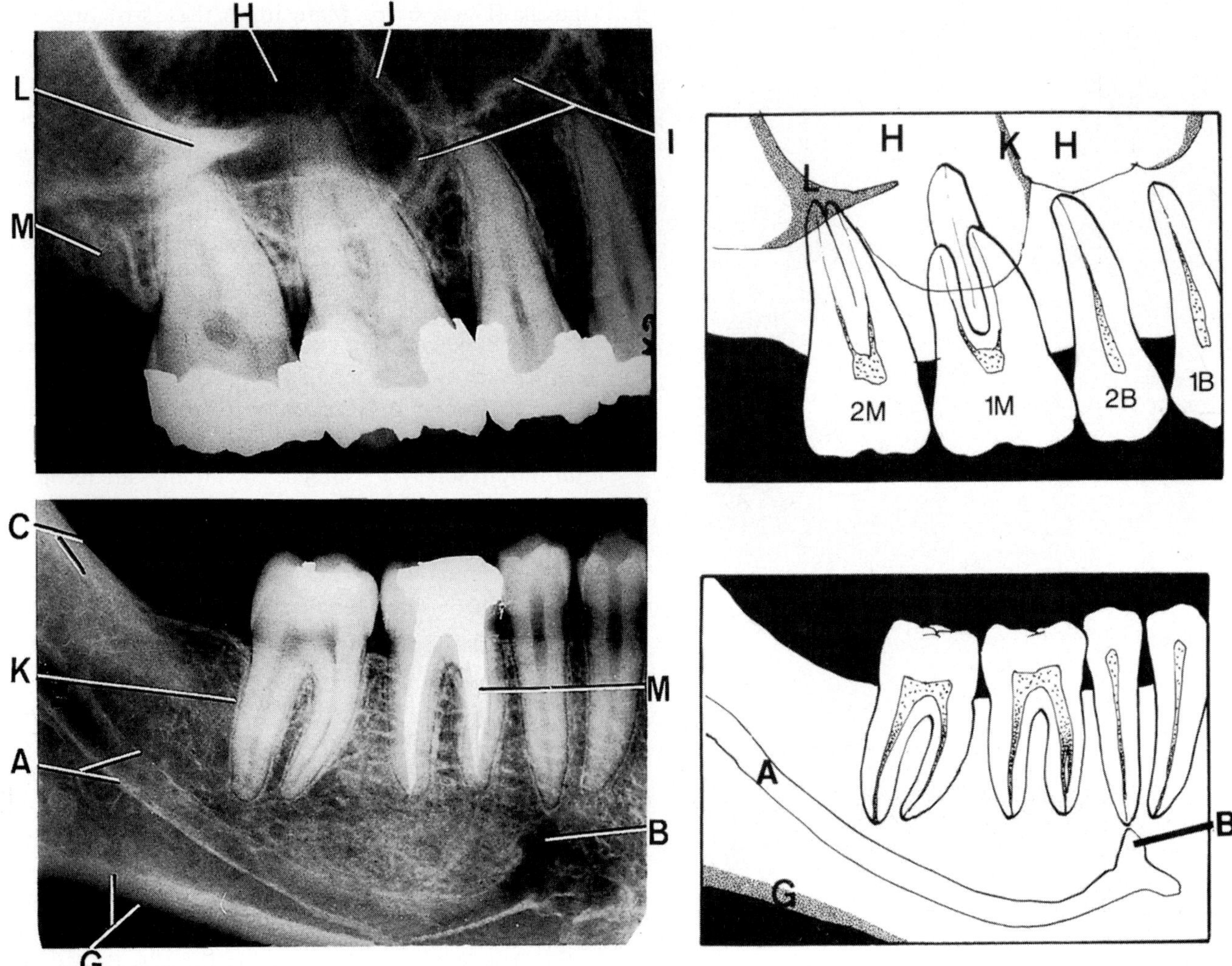

Figure 6-16 **Above,** Anatomic landmarks in a **maxillary** arch. H = maxillary sinus; I = floor of the maxillary sinus; J and K = bony septum in the maxillary sinus; L = zygomatic process; M = maxillary tuberosity. **Below,** Anatomic landmarks in the **mandibular** arch. A = mandibular canal; B = mental foramen; C and G = cortical bone, border of the mandible; K = lamina dura; M = root canal filling. (Courtesy of Drs. Albert C. Goerig and Elmer J. Neaverth.)

crest of the alveolar process should then be followed from left to right, upper to lower, and all of the structures outside the alveolar process should be evaluated as well—the sinuses, floor of the nose, foramina, and so on. In short, radiographic interpretation should be done in **an organized habitual way** so that nothing is overlooked.

Tracing the dark periodontal membrane space will reveal the number, size, and shape of the roots and their juxtaposition. While observing the roots, one must look for periradicular lesions and root defects such as anomalies, fractures, and external resorption. The number, curvature, size, and shape of all of the canals and chambers should be noted along with internal resorption, pulp stones, linear calcification, and open apices.

For example, if a large pulp chamber is seen in a single adult tooth while other chambers are narrowing, one should suspect a necrotic pulp, even though a periradicular lesion might not be apparent. In marked contrast, Swedish dentists have reported dramatic narrowing of pulp chambers in patients with serious renal disease, particularly those with transplanted kidneys who are on high doses of corticosteroids.[64]

Radiographic coronal evaluation includes depth of caries and restorations with respect to the pulp, as well as evidence of pulp cappings or pulpotomy, dens *invaginatus* or *dens evaginatus,* and the size of the preparations under porcelain or resin jacket crowns.

Evaluation, however, comes down to a matter of personal interpretation, as demonstrated by Goldman and

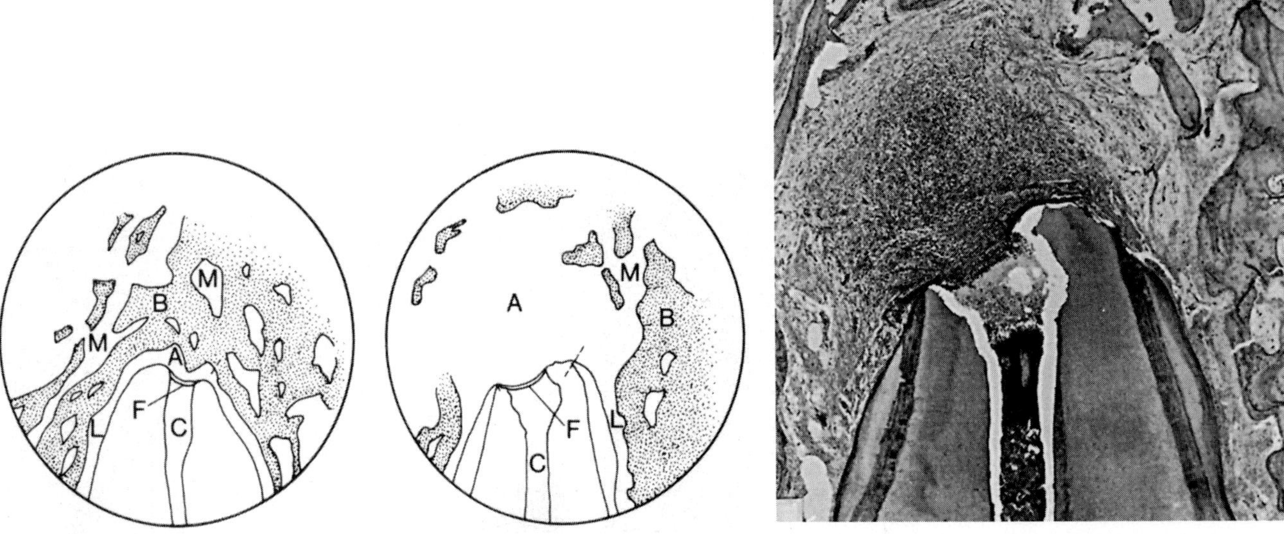

Figure 6-17 Brynolf's interpretation of the normal and resorbed **lamina dura**. **Left**, Radiographic appearance of a normal **lamina dura** under magnification. Note the "tit" of bone (opposite A) thrusting toward the foramen (F). **Center**, Loss of **lamina dura** at the apex along with apical inflammatory resorption from the necrotic canal (C). A = apical soft tissue; B = bone trabeculae; C = root canal; F = foramen; L = PDL space; M = medullary space. **Right**, necropsy of specimen detailed in **Center**. Reproduced with permission from Brynolf I[61] and Brynolf I. Odontologisk Revy 1967;18 Suppl 11:27.

his colleagues.[65,66] The radiographs of 253 cases, originally examined by three faculty members at Tufts University, were re-examined by them 6 to 8 months later. These endodontists agreed with **themselves** from 72 to 88% of the time. Ten years later, however, the same group repeated essentially the same experiment with 79 other dentists and found that they not only disagreed with each other over half the time but, worse yet, **disagreed with themselves** 22% of the time.[67] Much the same was found by researchers in Israel[63] and Greece.[68]

Antrim found that holding the radiograph up to a view box produced more consistent agreement among examiners than either projecting the radiograph or using a magnifying glass.[69] However, Weine has claimed that projecting the image produces the best interpretative result.[70]

One of the reasons for these discrepancies, of course, deals with how one interprets bony lesions. Shoha et al. were able to demonstrate the variables in this interpretation.[71] They found that lesions were always larger than their radiographic image, especially in the mandibular molar region. Lesions in the premolar area were only slightly larger than their radiographic image. Lesions found by hindsight were often difficult to detect initially because of their vague outline. In Holland, it was found that **cortical** bone had to be damaged by an osseous lesion before radiolucency could be detected and that loss of cancellous bone alone was not enough to be visible radiographically.[72]

Bender has illustrated this dramatically with a radiograph of a molar tooth showing increased density of the bone at the periapex[73] (Figure 6-18, A). Yet when the tooth was extracted, a huge granuloma was attached, which was not at all apparent in the film (Figure 6-18, B).

Root Anatomy

The radiographic examination provides essential information relative to normal and abnormal root formation. Since mandibular incisors frequently have two canals and, at times, two roots, adding an additional radiographic view from the mesial or distal can aid in detecting such anatomic variances.

One can expect anatomic variations in all tooth locations. Mandibular premolars and molars are no exception (Figure 6-19). By both radiographic and mechanical means (Figure 6-20), the number of canals and foramina should be determined before canal enlargement is completed. Because of frequent variations, it is a good habit to examine radiographs with a magnifying glass so as not to miss an extra canal or other variations.

Maxillary first premolars with three roots or canals are seen more clearly if the projected horizontal direction of the central beam is slightly from the mesial

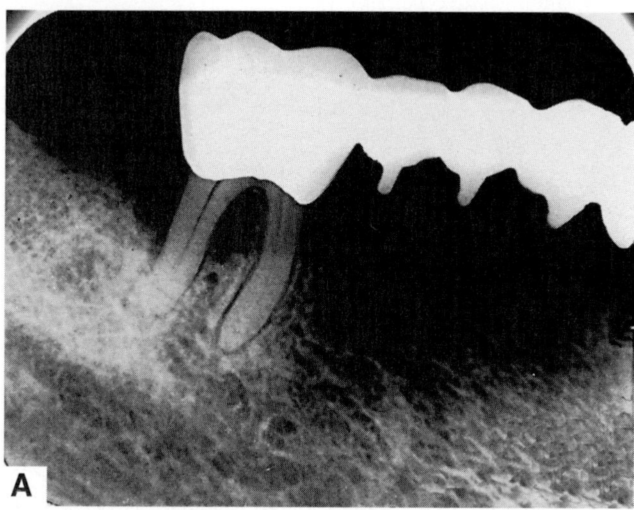

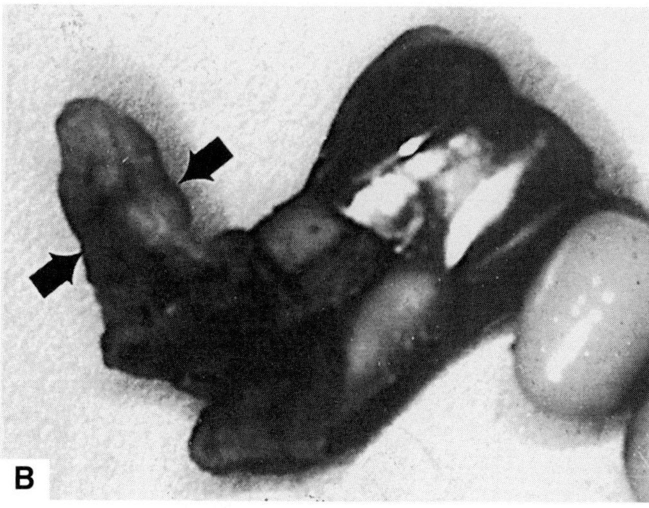

Figure 6-18 Radiographic deception owing to the thickness of the cortical bony plates. **A**, Osteosclerosis distal to the second molar completely masks a huge bony lesion within spongy bone. **B**, Same tooth extracted with an enormous space-occupying granuloma (**arrows**), not in the least suspected radiographically. Reproduced with permission from Bender IB.[73]

(Figure 6-21). The normal two roots or two canals of the maxillary first premolar also are easier to find **if the beam is directed from the mesial.** A recent *in vivo* study showed that two canals are present in maxillary **second** premolars 59% of the time, more than had been reported previously.[74–77] The mesial angulation technique is therefore beneficial in detecting the second canal in maxillary second premolars. In this case, the lingual root **always** appears to the mesial on the film (the SLOB rule—Same Lingual-Opposite Buccal).[78]

Slowey has demonstrated how difficult it is to detect extra roots, let alone extra canals.[79] One particularly baffling case involved a maxillary lateral incisor with an unusual second root. In the post-treatment radiograph, a bony lesion could be seen to the distal (Figure 6-22, A), but it was assumed that the lesion was related to invagination from the cingulum. Because the lesion did not heal, the tooth was extracted, and only then was the extra root revealed (Figure 6-22, B and C). A radiograph of the contralateral incisor revealed what appeared to be a bilateral anomaly (Figure 6-22, D). As Slowey pointed out, "whenever the outline of the root is unclear, has an unusual contour, or strays in any way from the expected radiographic appearance, one

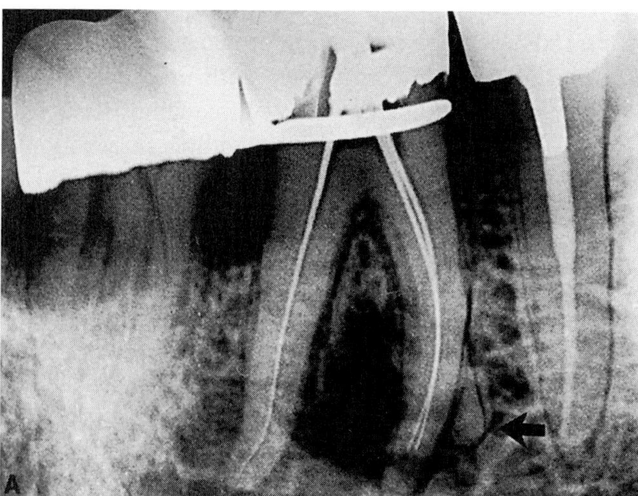

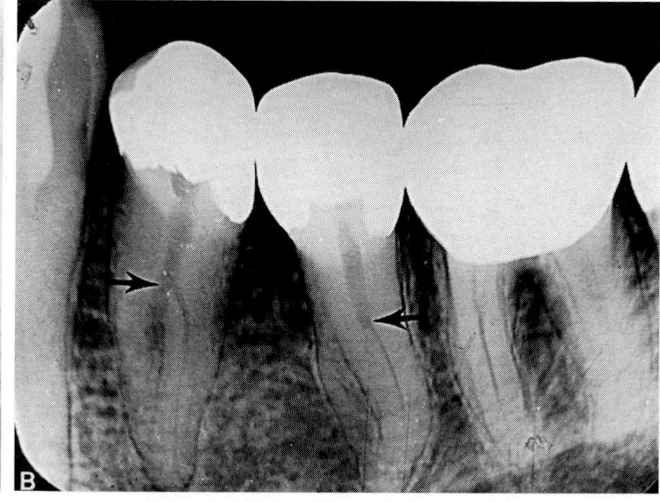

Figure 6-19 **A**, Mesial root of first molar has not only two separate canals but an additional root as well (**arrow**). **B**, Two premolars with an unusual root and canal formation. "Fast break" in canal radiodensity (**arrows**) indicates canal bifurcation. Both teeth have three and possibly four canals, but the number of apical foramens can be determined only by instrument placement (see Figure 6-21). Reproduced with permission from Slowey RR.[79]

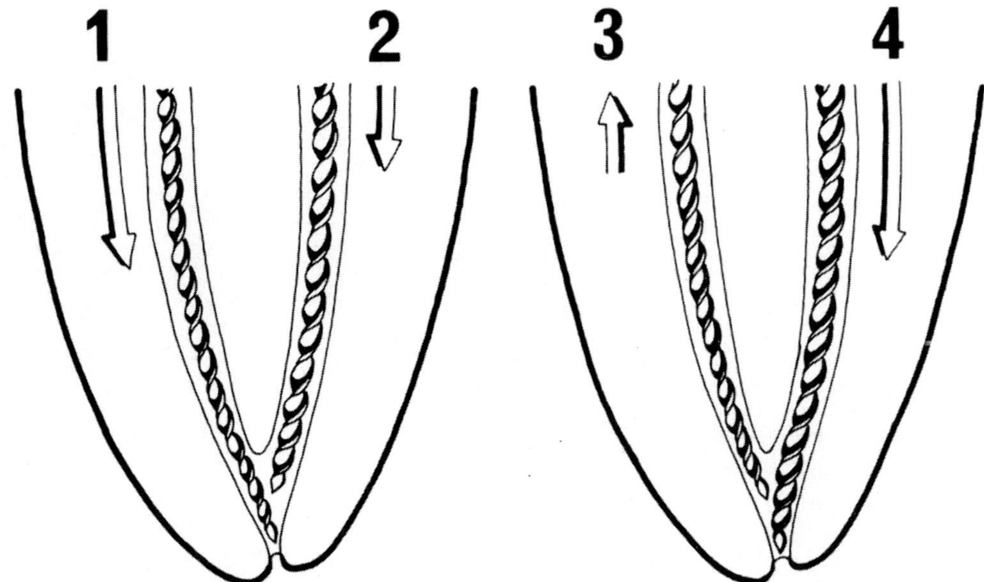

Figure 6-20 Mechanical means of determining separate or common foramina for two canals. The instrument is placed to full depth in either canal (1) and the instrument in the second canal (2) is prevented from going fully to place. Single foramina can then be confirmed by raising the first instrument (3), allowing the second instrument to go fully to place (4). If turned, the instruments can be felt to grate against each other. Reproduced with permission from Serene TP, Krasny RM, Ziegler PE, et al. Principles of preclinical endodontics. Dubuque (IA): Kendall/Hunt Publishing Co.; 1974.

should suspect an additional root canal…"[79] He quoted Worth, who said, "Look at the corners of the radiograph and the center will take care of itself."[79]

The mystery of extra canals within the normal number of roots is more perplexing than the extra root problem itself. Slowey has also given us some tips on how to detect the undetected.[79] One method is to follow the image of the test file in the length-of-the tooth film, particularly in the coronal part of the root. If an **extra dark line** is apparent in the coronal third of the root, running parallel to the instrument (Figure 6-23), one should suspect a second canal. This is especially true in the mesiobuccal root of maxillary first molars, where a fourth canal is found 51.5 to 69% of the time in vitro[75,76,80–83] but only 18.6 to 33.3% in vivo.[82–84] Fourth canals frequently occur in the distal roots of mandibular first molars as well[84] (Figure 6-24).

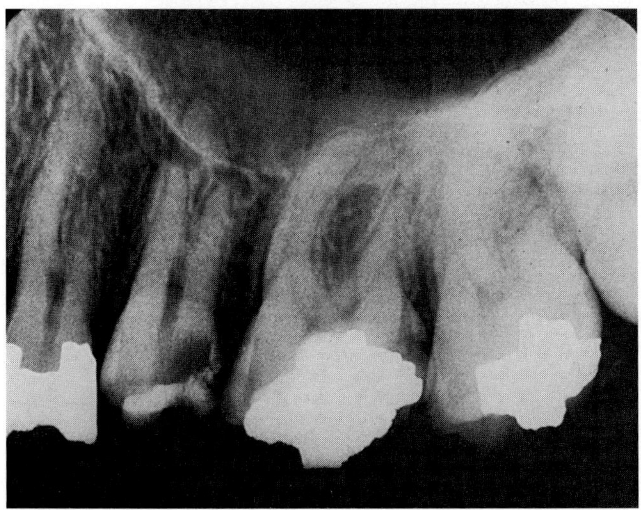

Figure 6-21 Three-rooted maxillary first premolar (**arrow**) and second premolar are readily discerned in this radiograph. Clarity of root structure can be improved by "aiming" a central beam directly through the **apical** region.

Another diagnostic clue was pointed out by Slowey.[79] It could be called "the fast break." When viewing a radiograph, if there is a **sudden change** in the radiolucency within a canal, this change in density probably signals the beginning of an additional canal (Figure 6-25), a frequent occurrence in maxillary first premolars. In mandibular canines (Figure 6-26, A), such observations should be followed up by taking additional radiographs from a different horizontal angle (Figure 6-26, B) and possibly searching out the extra canals with the length-of-tooth instrument films (Figure 6-26, C).

Frequently, root formation results in severe curvature. When the curvature is to the mesial or distal, so frequently seen in the maxillary lateral incisors or occasionally in premolars (Figure 6-27), there is little problem

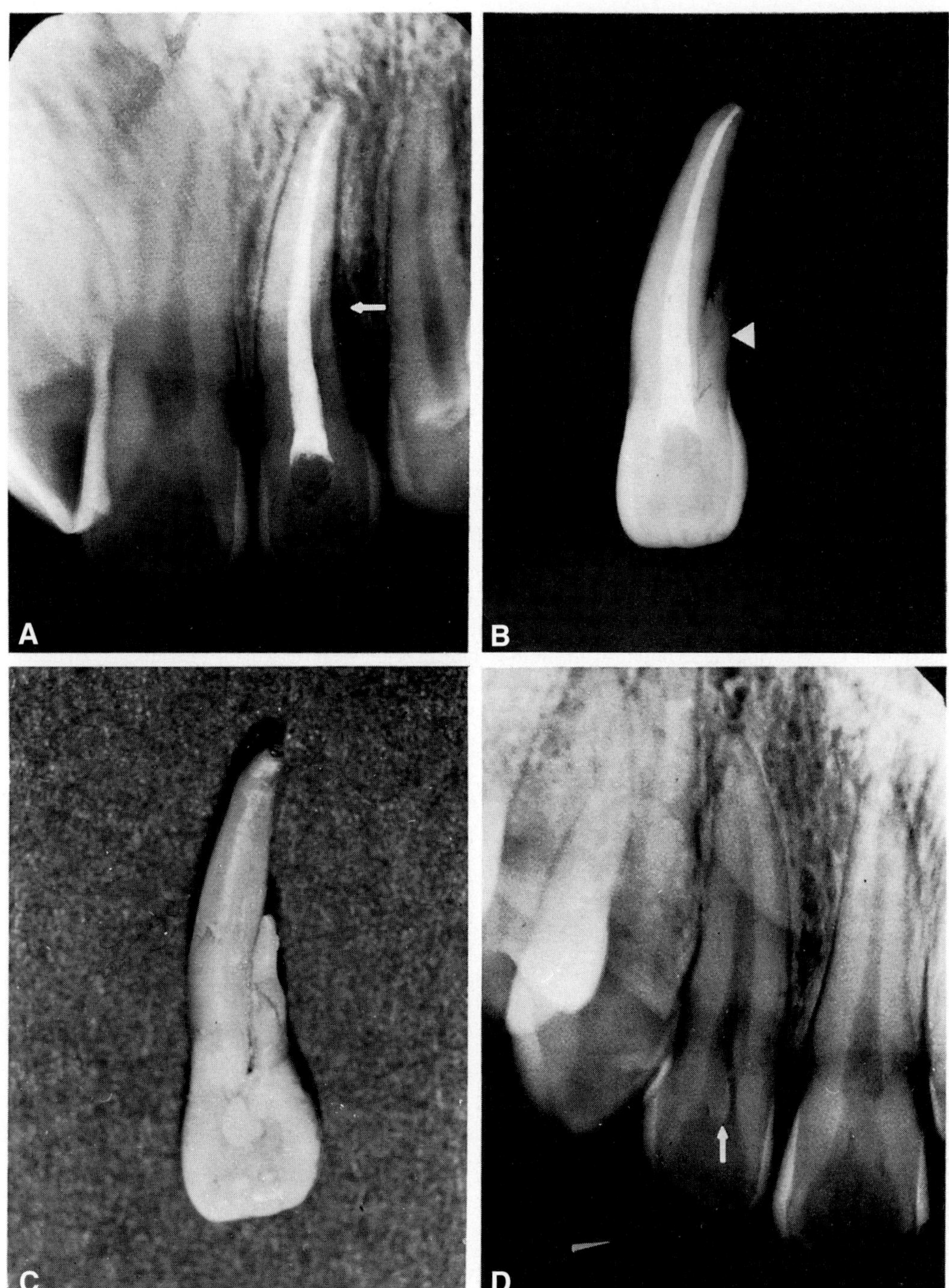

Figure 6-22 A, Continuing lateral lesion (mesial) and acute abscess (**arrow**). The tooth is finally extracted. B, Benchtop radiographic view reveals a second root and an unfilled canal (**arrow**), not seen in the original films. C, Lingual view of second root and invagination from the cingulum. **D**, On the contralateral side, a similar anomaly exists. Reproduced with permission from Slowey RR.[79]

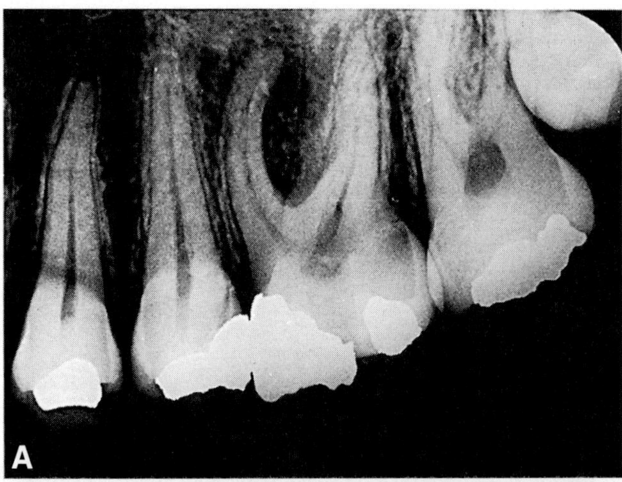

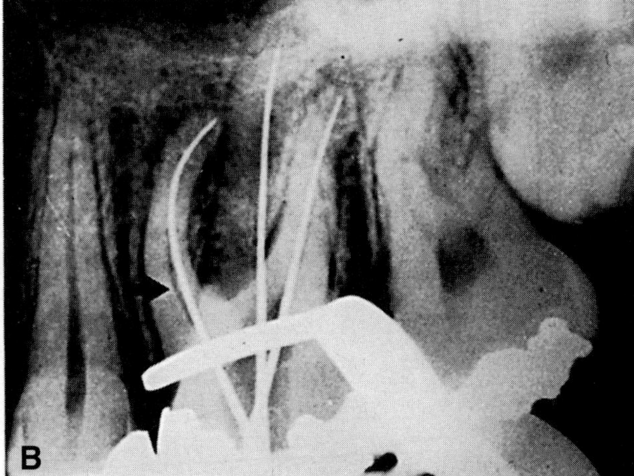

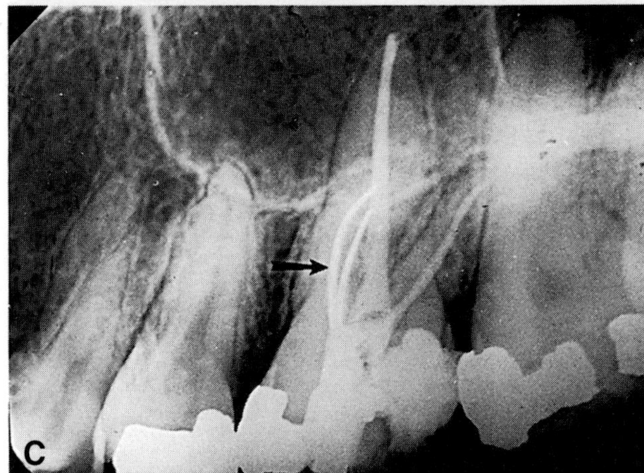

Figure 6-23 A, From viewing the initial film, one would not suspect that there are two canals in the mesiobuccal root of the first molar. **B**, An extra dark line alongside the exploring instrument (**arrow**) signals the possibility of a second canal. **C**, Final film showing two separate mesiobuccal canals (**arrow**) apparently arising from a common orifice. Reproduced with permission from Slowey RR.[79]

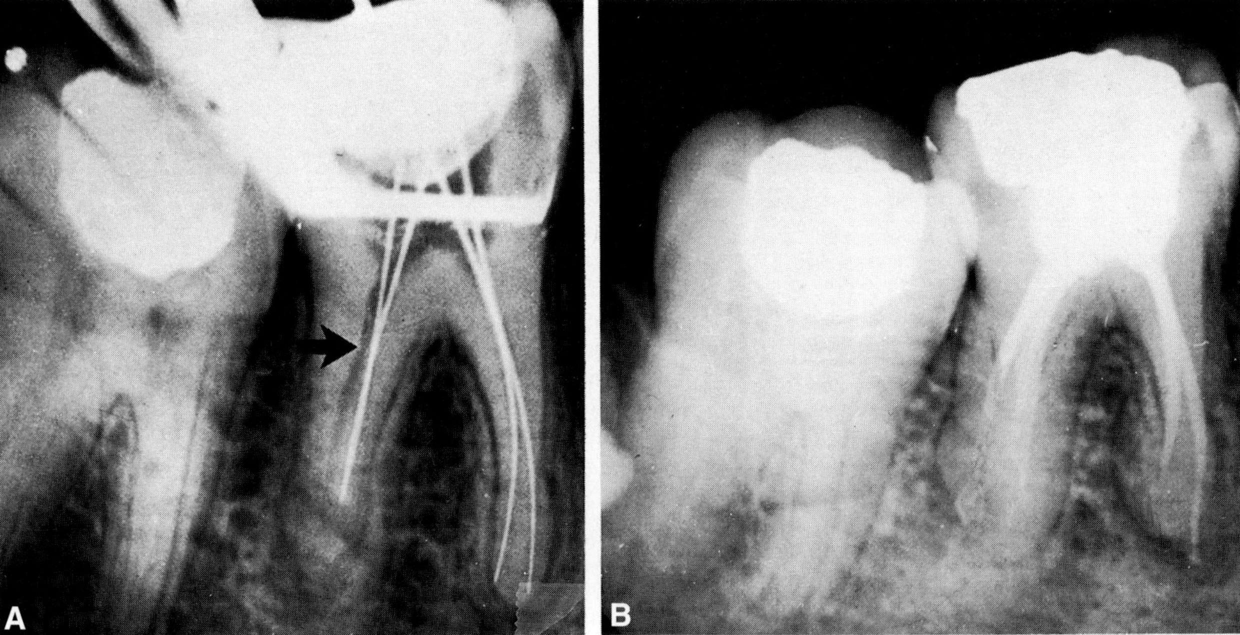

Figure 6-24 **A**, Two instruments in a single canal, but a wide, extra dark line (**arrow**) indicates an additional canal. **B**, Final filling proves four canals. Reproduced with permission from Slowey RR.[79]

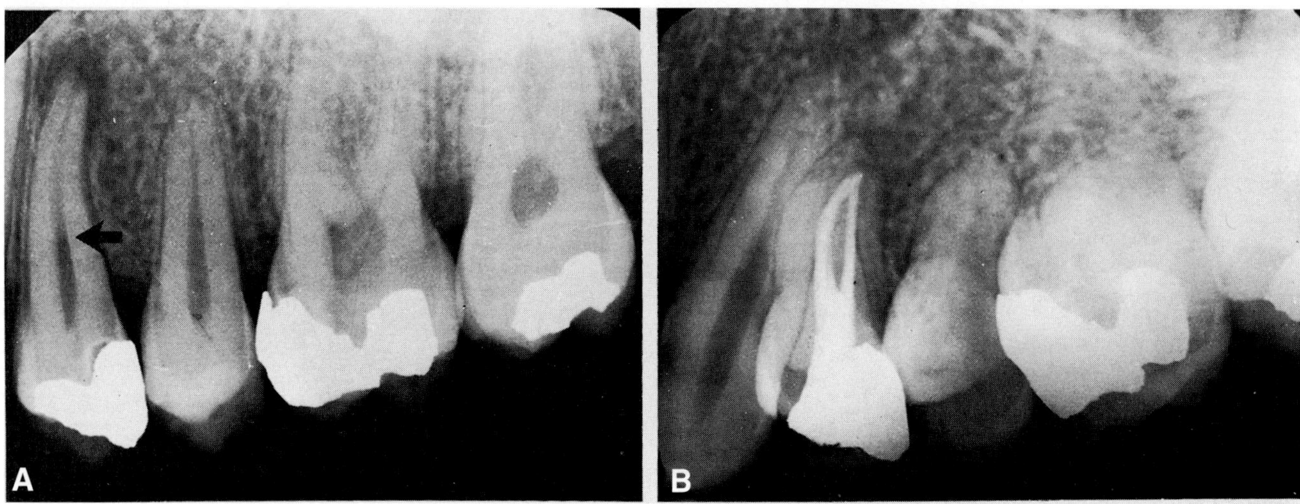

Figure 6-25 A, Sudden change in radiographic density (**arrow**) signals probable canal bifurcation at that point. **B**, Change from right-angle horizontal projection (A) to 20-degree projection from the distal clearly reveals two canals but a single foramen. Reproduced with permission from Slowey RR.[79]

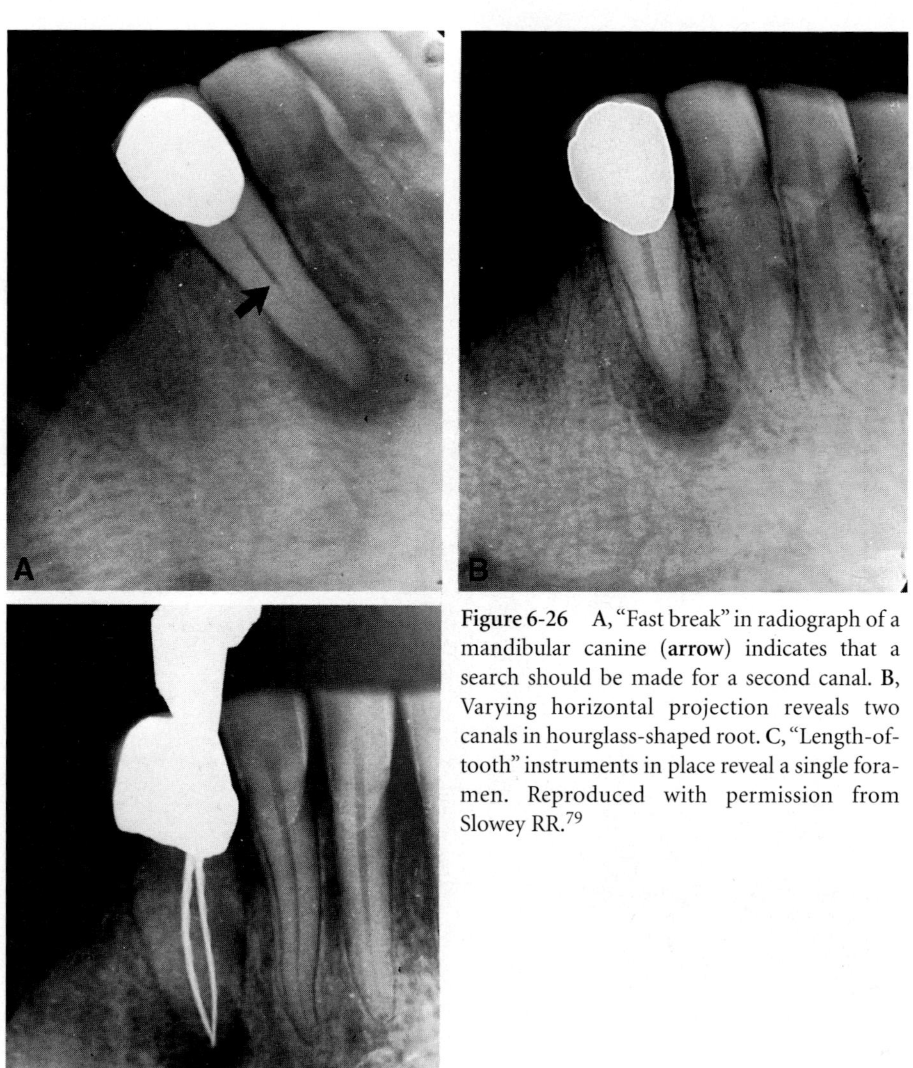

Figure 6-26 A, "Fast break" in radiograph of a mandibular canine (**arrow**) indicates that a search should be made for a second canal. **B**, Varying horizontal projection reveals two canals in hourglass-shaped root. **C**, "Length-of-tooth" instruments in place reveal a single foramen. Reproduced with permission from Slowey RR.[79]

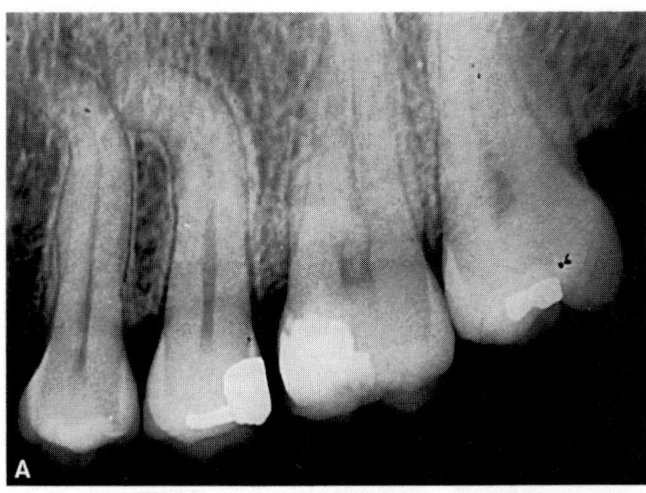

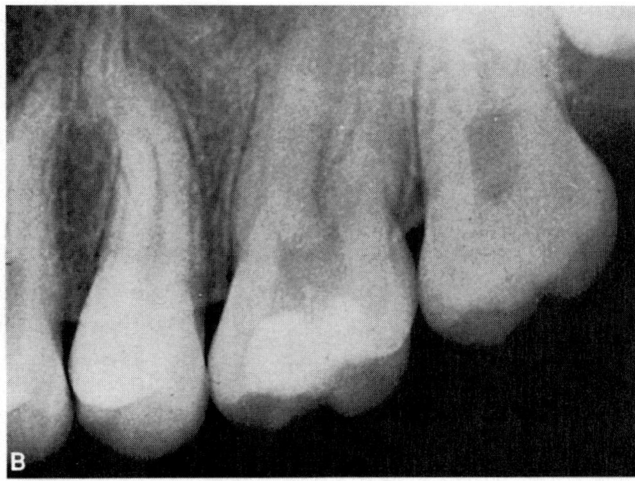

Figure 6-27 Unusual **mesial** and bayonet curvature seen in three maxillary premolars and easy to detect.

in detecting the curvature. However, when the curvature is to the **buccal** or **lingual**—in the same plane as the central x-ray beam—the curvature is more difficult to detect (Figure 6-28). Careful examination may reveal increased radiopacity at the root end as the root doubles back on itself and is literally "x-rayed" twice. In its extreme, a peculiar "target" or "bull's-eye" appearance will show in the film (Figure 6-29).

In addition to "normal" variances in tooth form, such as curvatures and extra roots, anomalies that may

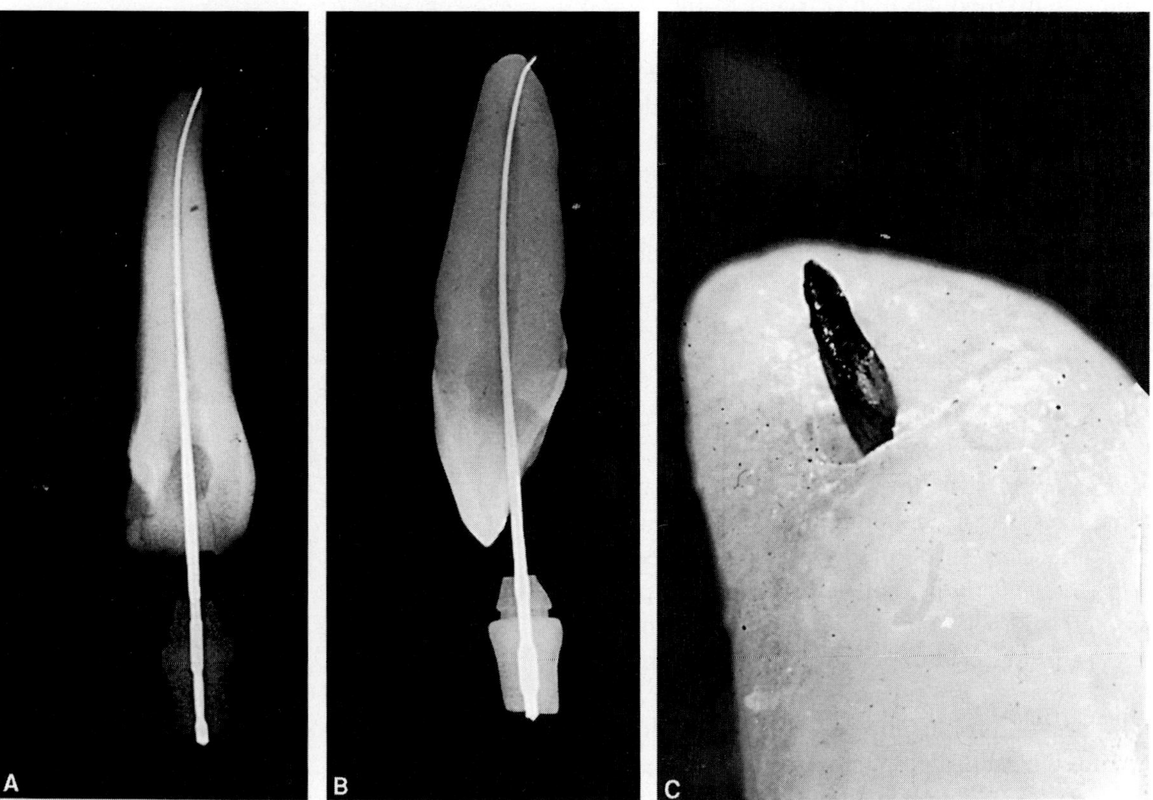

Figure 6-28 Double root canal curvature in a maxillary lateral incisor. **A**, Radiograph with instrument proves that the canal exits to distal. **B**, Mesiodistal view of the same tooth shows that the canal also exits to the lingual. **C**, Apical photograph of the same tooth demonstrates an instrument perforating the lingual far short of the apex. (Courtesy of Drs. Howard Clausen and John R. Grady.)

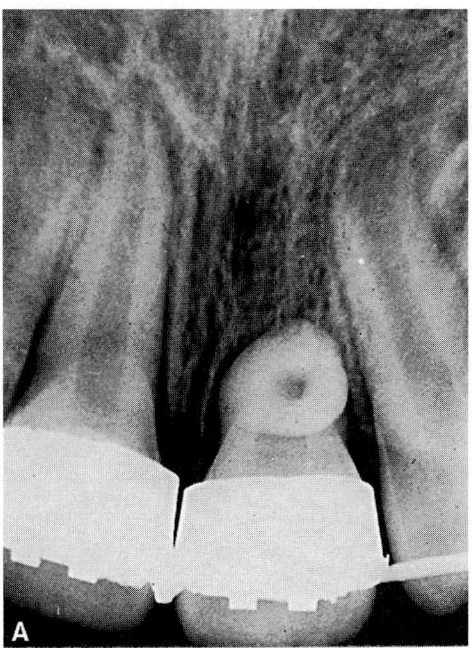

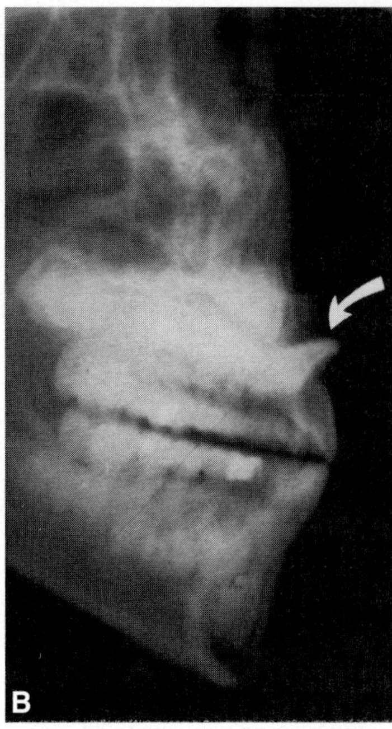

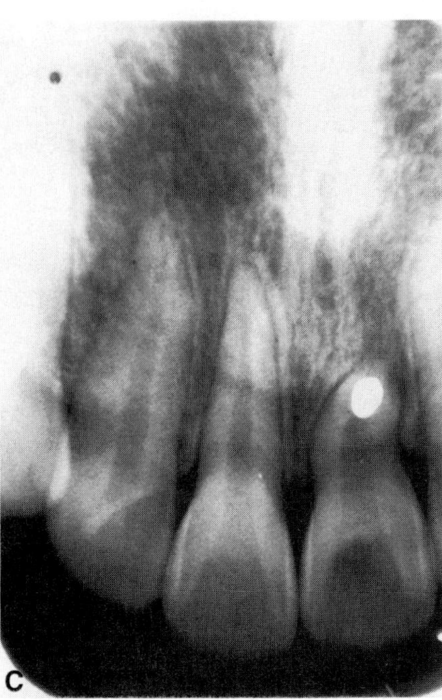

Figure 6-29 "Target" or "bull's-eye" phenomena seen in roots that severely curve to the buccal or lingual, that is, in the direction of the central beam. **A**, Central incisor with a dilacerated root under orthodontic realignment. **B**, Lateral head film in which the labially dilacerated root (in A) is apparent (**arrow**). C, Resection and retrofilling of the dilacerated root seen in **A** and **B**. (**A** and **B** courtesy of Dr. Alfred T. Baum; C courtesy of Dr. Dudley H. Glick.)

affect pulp vitality may also be detected in the radiographs. **Invagination** and palatal radicular groove (see Figure 6-9) are conditions that frequently have anomalous tracts leading from the enamel surface directly to the pulp (Figure 6-30). Such defects may involve the root, either partially or all the way to the apex. These grooves permit bacterial invasion of the pulp, which leads to periradicular lesions and pulp necrosis. Other anomalies such as odontome and microdont may also lead to pulp necrosis (Figure 6-31).

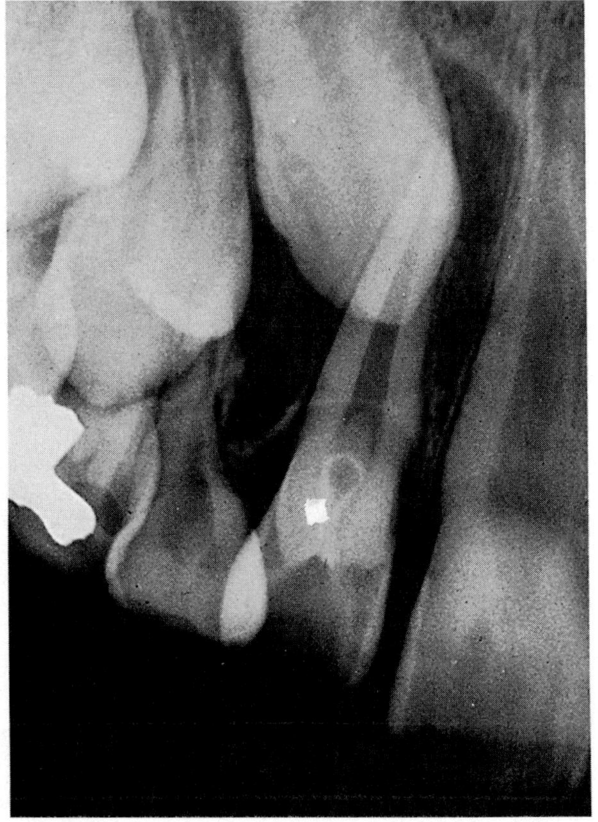

Figure 6-30 *Dens invaginatus* in the cingulum area of a maxillary lateral incisor. Anomalous tract seen in this radiograph has led to pulp infection and periradicular pathosis.

Conditions Inside the Tooth

Pulpal changes such as inflammation and necrosis cannot be detected radiographically within the canal. Only changes in calcific structures can be demonstrated. However, the results of pulp tissue changes are observable, that is, internal resorption as a result of irreversible pulpitis, periradicular bony changes resulting from pulp necrosis, and lack of continued root formation in immature teeth subjected to pulp destructive traumatic injuries.

Pulp Stones. Chronic pulpal disease may facilitate the formation of pulpal calcifications such as pulp stones (Figure 6-32). However, the mechanism of pulp stone formation and the various factors necessary in the calcific process are not well known at this time, a fact illustrated by the observations that pulp stones are

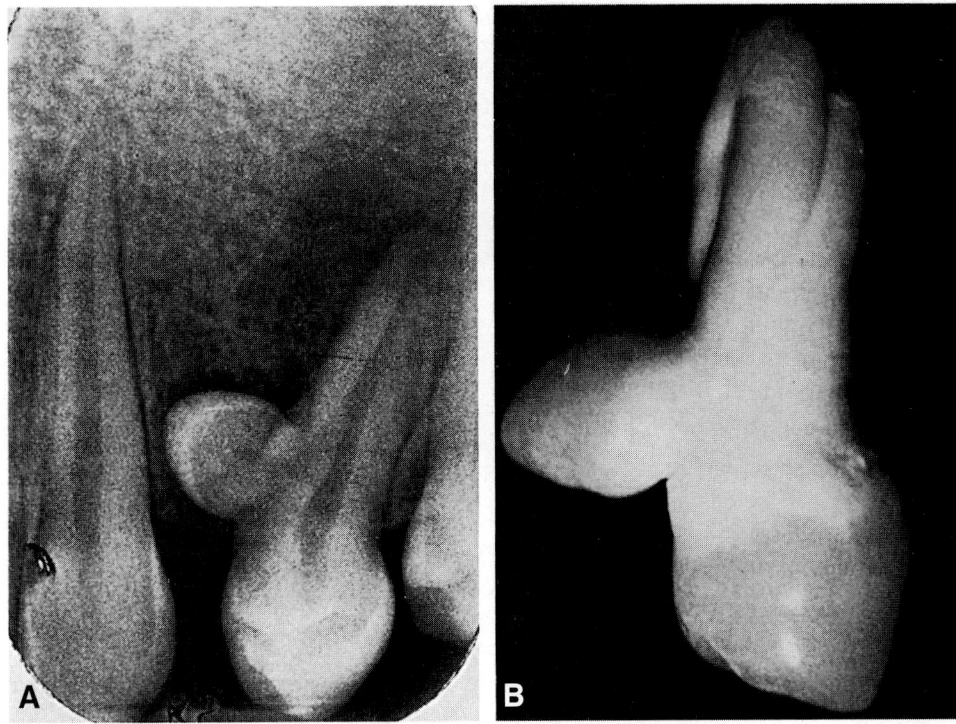

Figure 6-31 A, Radiograph reveals 7 mm irregular radiolucency with a sclerotic border associated with an acute abscess. **B,** An extracted fused supernumerary microdont that had a cyst attached. Reproduced with permission from Samuels DS. Oral Surg 1992;73:131.

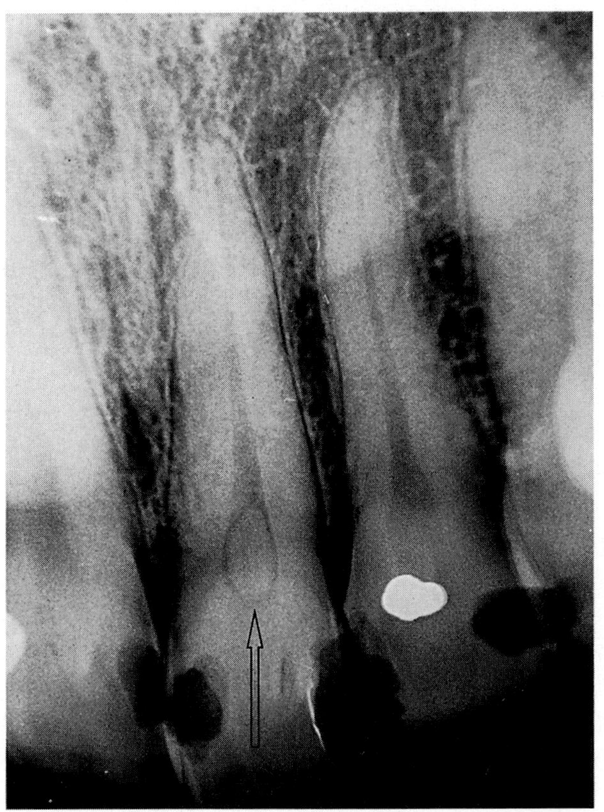

Figure 6-32 Huge pulp stone (**arrow**) that has developed in association with chronic pulpitis. This "ball and socket" type of stone must be fragmented to be removed.

found in apparently normal teeth with healthy pulps (Figure 6-33). Careful examination of radiographs may reveal other problems beside pulp stones—root fractures, calcification, early pulp death (Figure 6-34), and internal and external resorption.

Internal Resorption. Following traumatic injuries and/or caries, internal resorption may be detected on radiographs (Figure 6-35). Differentiation between internal and external resorption may be made radiographically.[85] First, the lesion of internal resorption usually has sharp smooth margins that can be clearly defined (see Figure 6-35, A). However, it need not be symmetric. Another diagnostic sign is the manner in which the pulp "disappears" into the lesion, not extending **through** the lesion in its regular shape (Figure 6-35, B).

At times, an area of resorption may be confused with dental caries radiographically. However, dental caries is less sharply defined than is internal resorption. Neither caries nor internal resorption should be ignored; internal resorption can progress to the point of extensive tooth destruction and perforation.[86]

Wedenberg and Lindskog, after experimentally producing internal resorption in monkey incisors, concluded that there are two types of internal resorption: transient, which may repair itself, and progressive, "the latter requiring continuous stimulation by infection."[87]

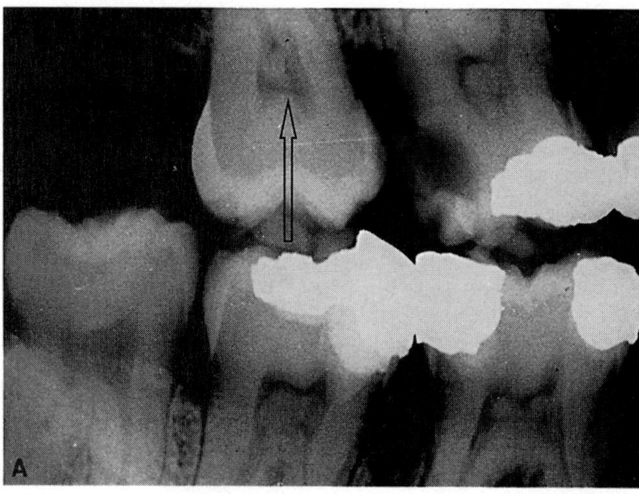

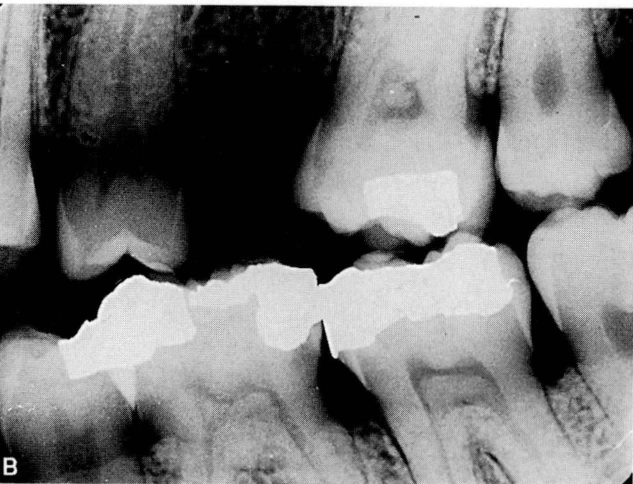

Figure 6-33 Left (A) and right (B) bitewing radiographs reveal multiple pulp stones that have developed in the molar teeth of one patient. Many stones are related to advanced carious lesions and large restorations. **A,** One stone (**arrow**) has also developed in an intact tooth.

From London, Lynch and Ahlberg reported bilateral idiopathic internal resorption. The radiolucent areas were cleanly defined, punched-out lesions. The pulp was seen to disappear into the lesion.[88]

Herpes zoster was linked to resorption in other cases. The varicella-zoster virus lies dormant for years in a nerve ganglion, from an earlier "chickenpox" attack, and can suddenly reactivate to infect the pulp.[89]

Conditions Outside the Tooth

One of the most common occurrences seen radiographically on the outside of the root of the tooth is **external resorption.**

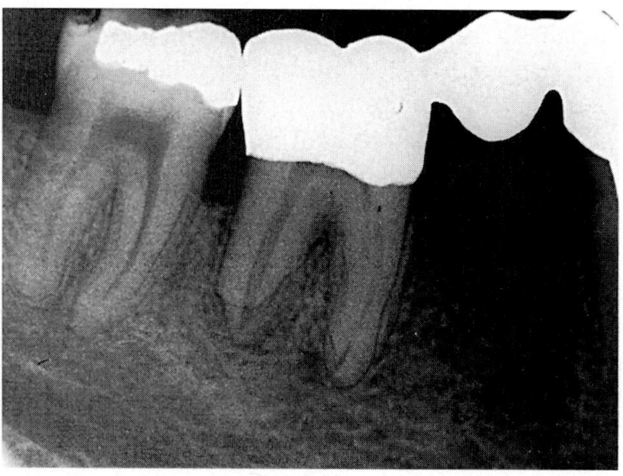

Figure 6-34 Diagnostic radiograph of a first molar reveals early pulp death in the distal canal and calcification followed by necrosis in the mesial canals leading to a periradicular lesion. Chisel-shaped resorption of the distal root typical of long-standing chronic inflammation. (Courtesy of Dr. Craig Malin.)

External Resorption. Andreasen has stated that following traumatic injuries there are three main types of external root resorption: **surface, inflammatory, and replacement resorption. Surface resorption** is caused by acute injury to the periodontal ligament and root surface. Cell proliferation mediation removes the traumatized structures. If injury is not repeated, healing takes place with new cementum and PDL. **Inflammatory resorption** may occur from combined injury to the PDL and cementum complicated by bacteria from the infected root canal, which, in turn, stimulate the osteoclasts. Resorption usually ceases if the root canal is thoroughly débrided and obturated unless stimulation has provoked the third type of resorption, **replacement resorption.** In this type, ankylosis between bone and tooth occurs without the intervening PDL, and the constantly remodeling bone slowly removes the tooth and replaces it with bone. This is often seen in unsuccessful replant cases.[90]

Frank has delineated another type of external root resorption that he terms **extra-canal invasive resorption,** totally different from regular external or internal resorption.[91] This phenomenon has interested clinicians and researchers over the last century and has been variously called *odontoclastoma,*[92] *idiopathic external resorption,*[93] *peripheral cervical resorption,*[94] *cervical external resorption,*[95] *peripheral inflammatory root resorption,*[96,97] *cervical resorption,*[98] and, more recently, *invasive cervical resorption.*[99]

Frank et al. made the point that **extra-canal invasive** is the more descriptive term[100] (rather than "external-internal," which Frank originally used) because of the external origin of this resorptive defect, before it invades the dentin (Figure 6-36), but, more

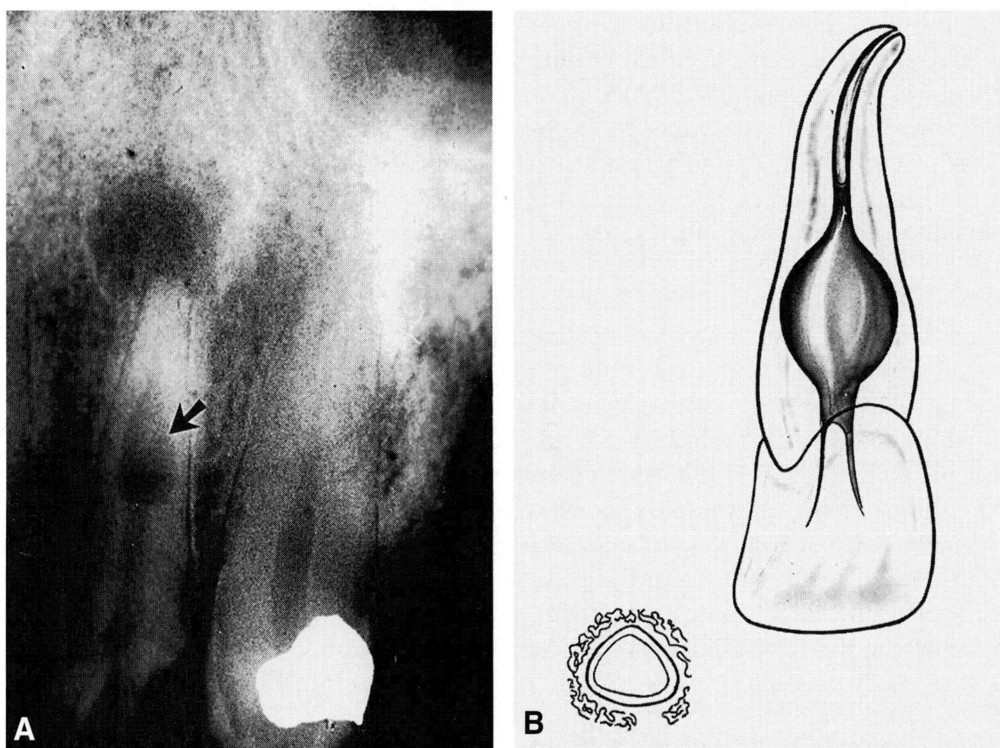

Figure 6-35 A, Radiograph of lesion of **internal** resorption (**arrow**). Note sharp smooth margins. (Courtesy of Drs. A. H. Gartner, T. Mack, R. Somerlott, and L. Walsh.) **B**, Drawing of internal resorption shows how the shadow of the pulp "disappears" into the huge lesion. Reproduced with permission from a drawing modified from Lepp FH. Oral Surg 1969;27:185.

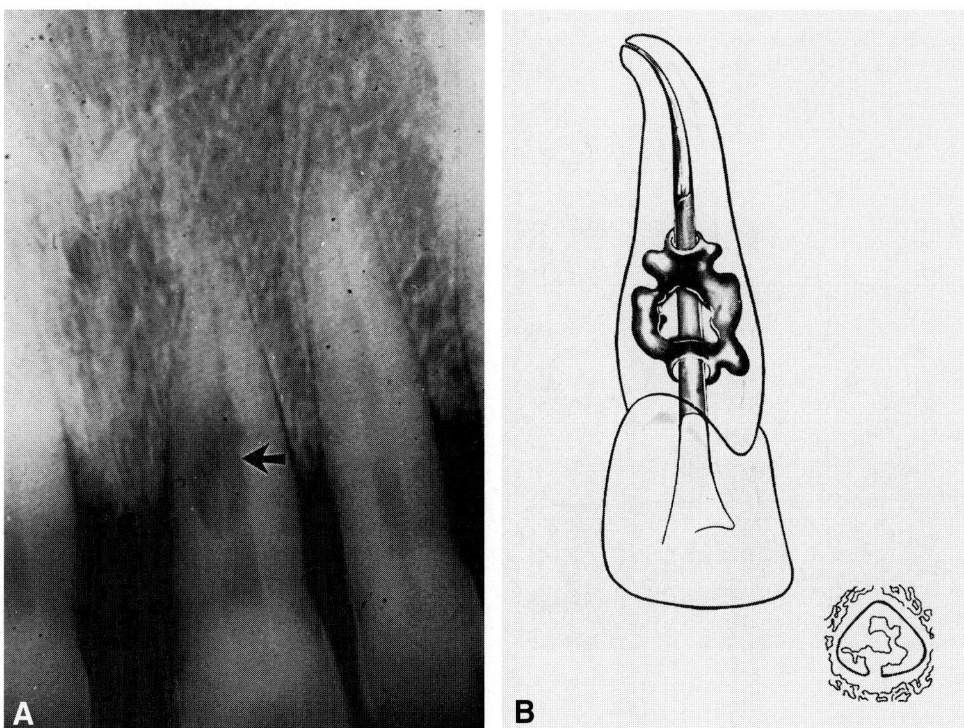

Figure 6-36 A, Radiograph of lesion of **extra-canal invasive** resorption (**arrow**). Note the ragged margins of the lesion. (Courtesy of Drs. A. H. Gartner, T. Mack, R. Somerlott, and L. Walsh.) **B**, Drawing of resorption shows how the shadow of pulp "passes through" the lesion unaltered. Inset depicts external lesion perforating into and resorbing dentin. Reproduced with permission from a drawing modified from Lepp LH. Oral Surg 1969;27:185.

important, that the destruction surrounds the root canal **without necessarily involving the pulp** (Figure 6-37). This, of course, gives an entirely different radiographic appearance than internal resorption. In extra-canal invasive resorption, the pulp appears to pass through the lesion (Figure 6-38), whereas the pulp "disappears" in the internal resorptive lesion (see Figure 6-35).

The histopathologic characteristics of this insidious and often aggressive form of invasive tooth resorption are of interest and significance to clinicians. Although the invading tissue is derived from **ectomesenchymal** precursor cells within the periodontal ligament, it differs both in structure and behavior from the periodontal ligament. In early lesions, the invading tissue is fibrovascular (Figure 6-39), which accounts for the pinkish appearance that may be evident near the gingival margin of the affected teeth.[99] Later, as resorption extends more deeply into radicular tooth structure, the histopathologic appearance may be described as fibro-osseous—bone-like depositions being evident—both within the fibrovascular tissue and laid directly onto resorbed dentin surfaces (Figure 6-40). Of clinical significance is the deeply infiltrating channels that often interconnect with the periodontal ligament. **Effective treatment can be achieved only if all ramifications are inactivated or removed** (see chapter 12).

Jaacob examined 18 of these cases and determined that the pulp spaces were separated from the resorptive areas by a "resistant dentin shell."[101] Quite possibly, this phenomenon of not invading the pulp relates to the character of the dentin surrounding the pulp. Clastic cells generally attack **well-calcified structures** such as bone, dentin, and cementum. The pulp, however, is surrounded by **uncalcified predentin**—uncalcified material not readily amenable to cellular clastic action. In addition, there is evidence for an anti-invasive factor in tooth dentin.[102]

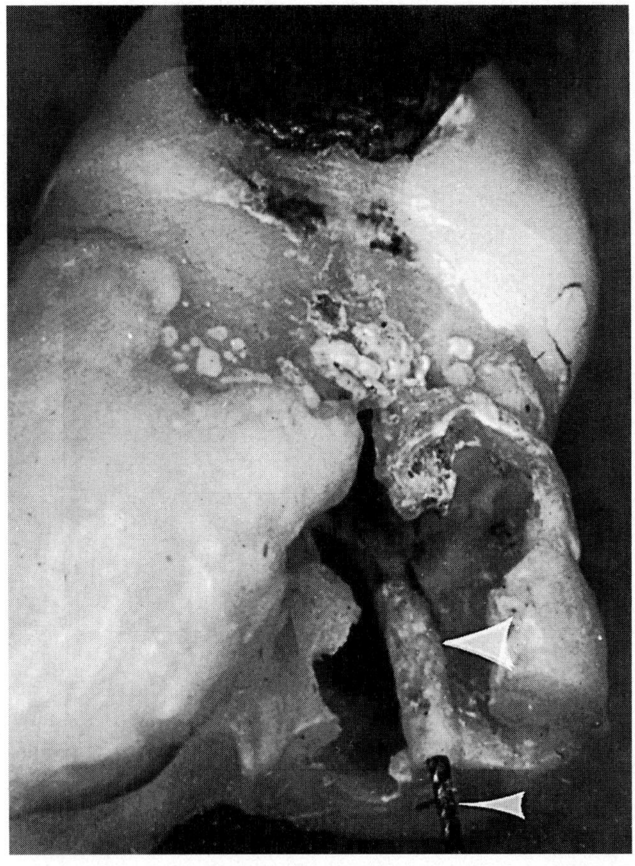

Figure 6-37 Extra-canal invasive resorption. The integrity of the root canal is evident in the extracted molar (**larger arrow**). Note the file (**smaller arrow**) extending into the canal. (Courtesy of Dr. Harold Gerstein.)

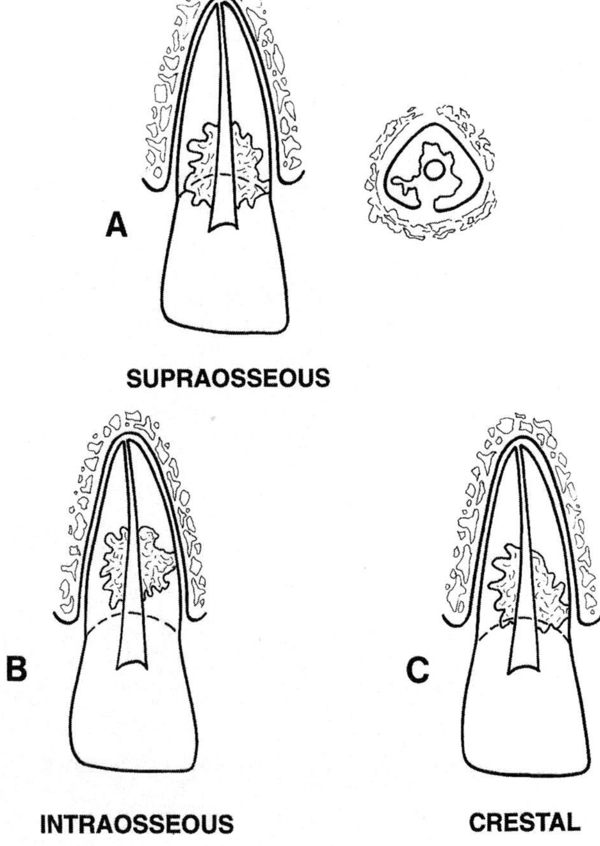

Figure 6-38 Frank's classification of extra-canal invasive resorption. **A**, Supraosseous, the most frequent form. Inset depicts external invasion and dentin destruction, yet intact pulp. Note that the cross-section does not invade the pulp. **B**, Intraosseous: it is difficult to determine the point of origin radiographically. **C**, Crestal, which may be related to orthodontic movement. (Courtesy of Dr. Alfred L. Frank.)

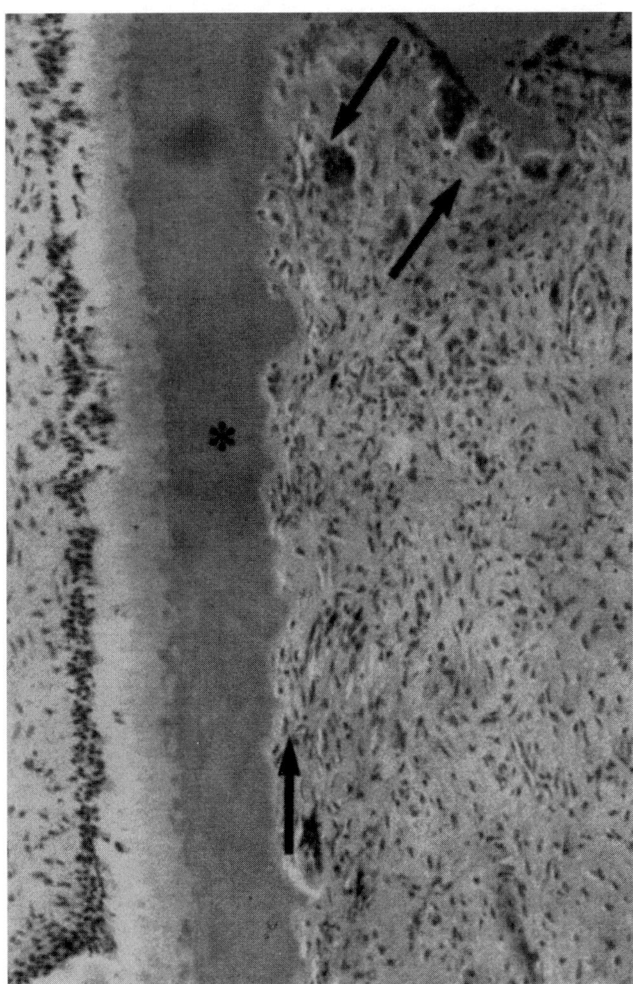

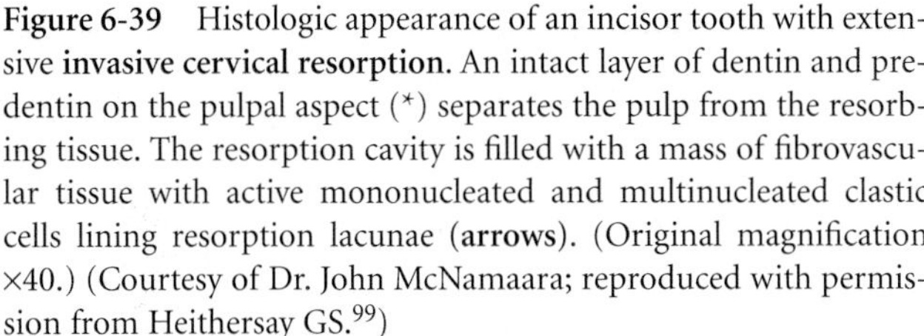

Figure 6-39 Histologic appearance of an incisor tooth with extensive **invasive cervical resorption.** An intact layer of dentin and predentin on the pulpal aspect (*) separates the pulp from the resorbing tissue. The resorption cavity is filled with a mass of fibrovascular tissue with active mononucleated and multinucleated clastic cells lining resorption lacunae (**arrows**). (Original magnification ×40.) (Courtesy of Dr. John McNamaara; reproduced with permission from Heithersay GS.[99])

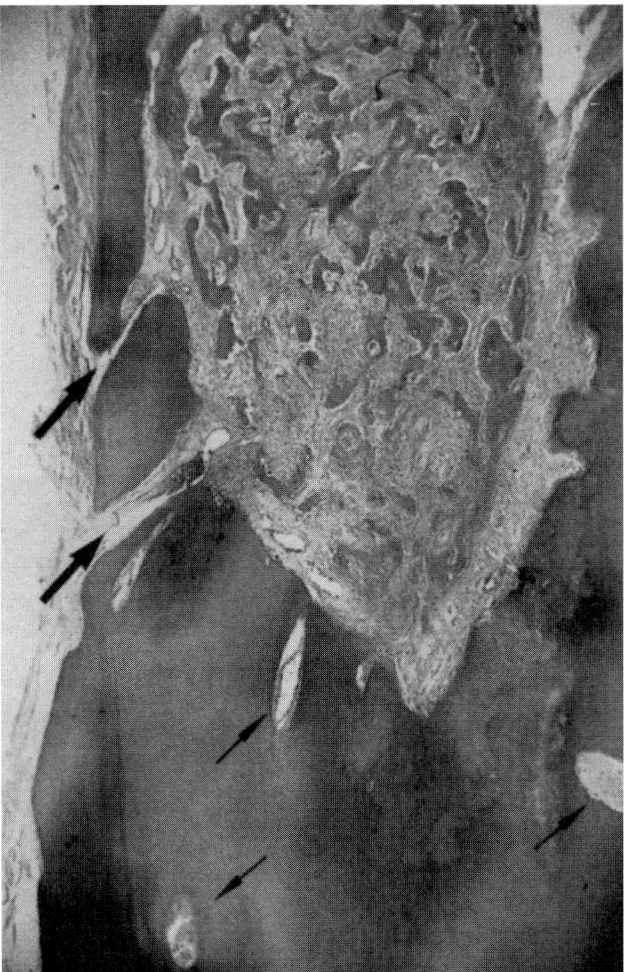

Figure 6-40 Histologic appearance of an extensive **invasive cervical resorption** with radicular extensions. Masses of ectopic calcific tissue are evident both within the fibrovascular tissue occupying the resorption cavity and on resorbed dentin surfaces. In addition, communicating channels can be seen connecting with the periodontal ligament (**large arrows**). Other channels can be seen within the inferior aspect of the radicular dentin (**small arrows**). (Original magnification × 30.) Reproduced with permission from Heithersay GS.[99]

Although most extra-canal invasive root resorption occurs at the immediate subgingival level — **supraosseous,** if you will (see Figure 6-38, A)—Frank et al. described an additional intraosseous variation that is difficult to locate radiographically since it is **not** accompanied by periodontal breakdown.[100] There may, however, be an open lesion just at or beneath the gingival sulcus (Figure 6-41, A). In addition, the resorption may extend into the coronal tooth structure, and a "pink tooth" may result (Figure 6-42), much the same as with coronal internal resorption. This may be more apt to happen with what Frank described as a **crestal** variety of invasive resorption (see Figure 6-38, C).[91] If the lesion is visible radiographically, but not apparent visually, it may be probed for with a curved explorer.

The **intraosseous** variety of extra-canal invasive resorption (see Figure 6-38, B) is characterized radiographically as having an irregular moth-eaten appearance within the tooth—the more advanced, the more radiolucent (see Figure 6-41, B). Again, close examination will show the outline and integrity of the canal that appears to "pass through" the lesion unaltered (Figure 6-43). The pulp usually tests vital and has been asymptomatic. The radiographic appearance of these lesions varies. In early lesions, a small radiolucency may

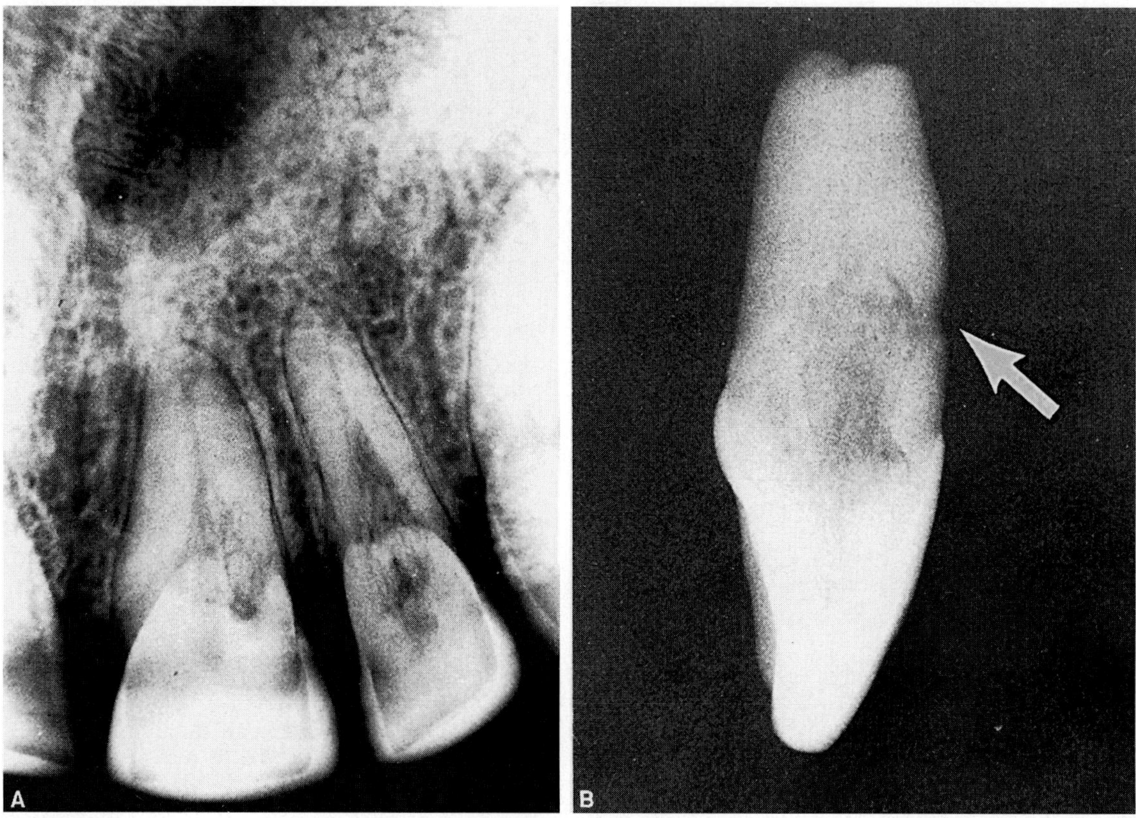

Figure 6-41 **A,** Extra-canal invasive resorption, supraosseous, of the central and lateral incisors. The integrity of the root canals remains intact. **B,** Extra-canal invasive resorption, intraosseous, of the maxillary lateral incisor. **Arrow** marks the labial site of origin. (Courtesy of Dr. Alfred L. Frank.)

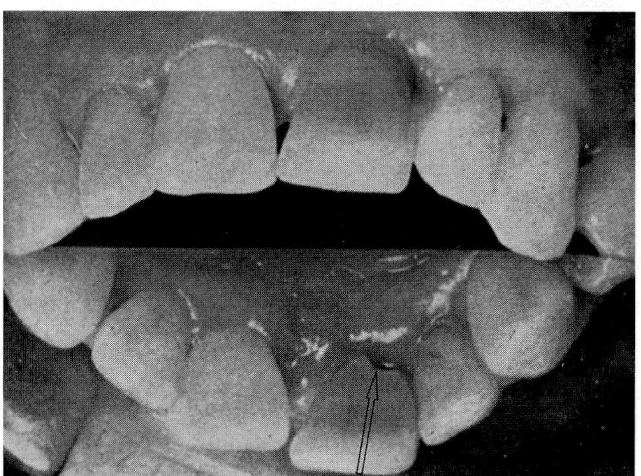

Figure 6-42 Frontal and mirror views of a "pink tooth," supraosseous extra-canal invasive resorption of a crown (**arrow**) following impact trauma.

emerge—somewhat irregular in appearance—that may, on occasion, resemble dental caries.

Extra-canal invasive resorption may also radiographically resemble internal resorption (see Figure 6-43, A). To differentiate, off-angle mesial and distal radiographs will "move" the extra-canal type of resorption, whereas the **internal resorptive defect will not move** on the film (see Figure 6-43, B).

Although the etiology of extra-canal invasive resorption is unknown, several potential causative factors have been identified and recently analyzed. Heithersay studied 222 patients, with a total of 257 teeth, exhibiting varying degrees of invasive cervical resportion[103] (Figure 6-44). Orthodontics alone was the most significant causative factor[104–106] (21.2% of patients, 24.1% of teeth), whereas trauma was the next most identifiable potential cause accounting for 14.0% of patients and 15.1% of teeth. Often this type of resorption was associated with a combination of factors, for example, trauma and bleaching. Bleaching as a sole factor was found in 4.5% of patients and 3.9% of teeth.

Other factors identified as potential predisposing factors, but at a low level, were surgery, periodontics,

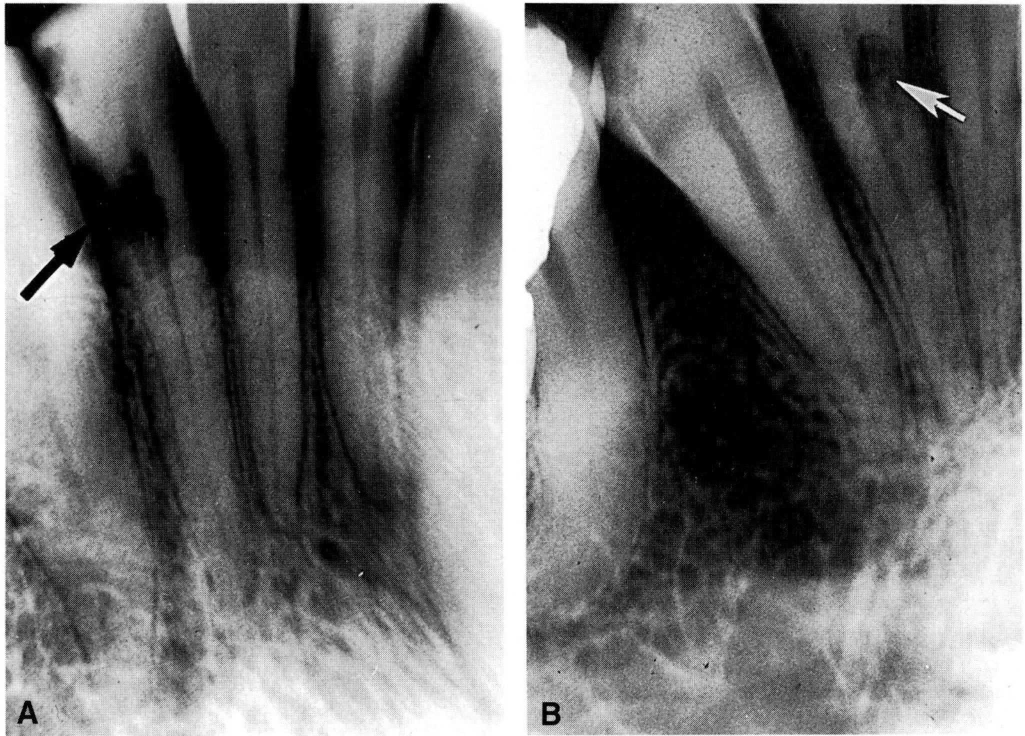

Figure 6-43 Extra-canal invasive resorption, supraosseous. **A**, Lesion (**arrow**) superimposed over the canal. **B**, Same tooth, radiographed from the mesial; the lesion "shifts" (**arrow**) within the tooth. Pulp tests are vital. (Courtesy of Dr. Alfred L. Frank.)

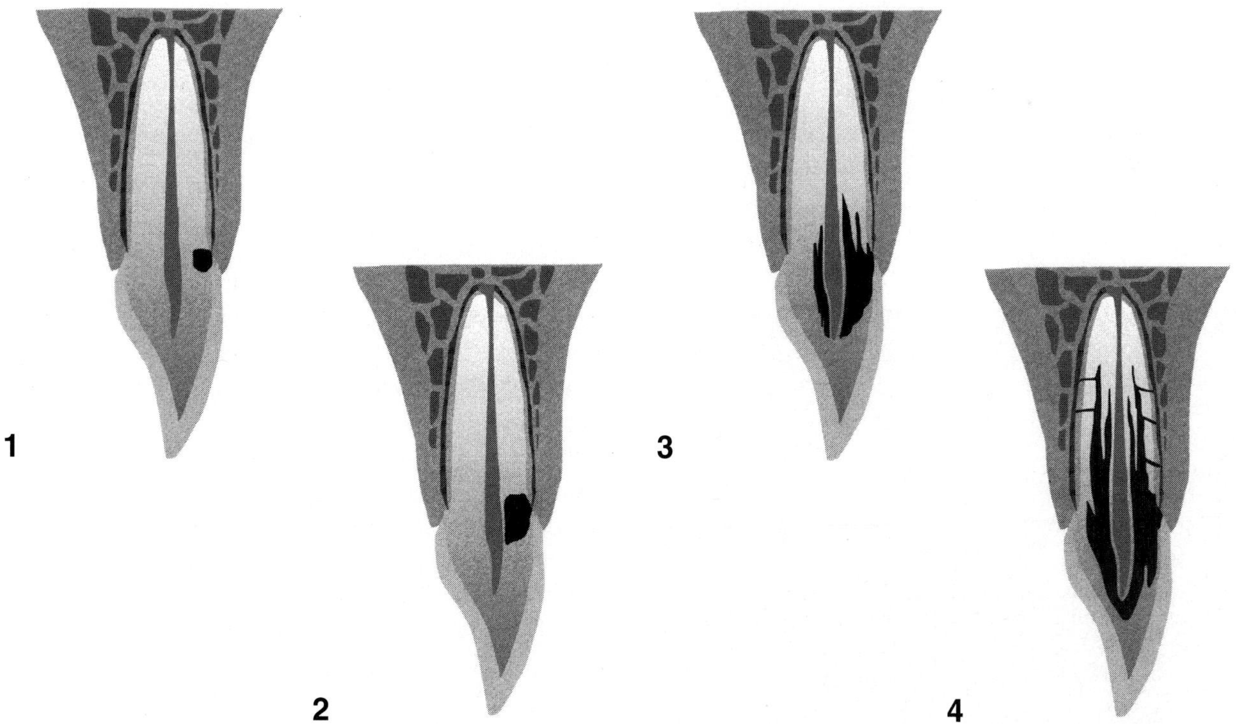

Figure 6-44 Heithersay's clinical classification of **invasive cervical resorption: Class l:** A small invasive resorptive lesion near the cervical area with shallow penetration into the dentin. **Class 2:** A well-defined invasive resorptive lesion that has penetrated close to the coronal pulp chamber but shows little or no extension into the radicular dentin. **Class 3:** A deeper invasion of dentin by resorbing tissue, not only involving the coronal dentin but also extending at least to the coronal third of the root. **Class 4:** A large invasive resorptive process that has extended beyond the coronal third of the root canal. Reproduced with permission from Heithersay GS.[99]

bruxism, delayed eruption, developmental defects, and interproximal stripping. The potential for invasion via a crack in extensively restored teeth was identified. The clinical classification in Figure 6-44 is also of importance when assessing teeth suitable for treatment, as discussed in chapter 12. Suffice it to say, Class 1 to 3 lesions must be completely débrided and inactivated and, if not pulp invasive, filled with a suitable restorative material such as dentin adhesive and composite resin (Figure 6-45), glass ionomer cement, or, in some situations, mineral trioxide aggregate. The extensive Class 4 lesions are not suitable for current therapy, and no treatment or extraction is recommended.[107]

Radiographic Diagnosis: Periradicular Lesions

Pulpal inflammation and necrosis eventually produce periradicular changes. The earliest is a widening of the periodontal ligament space, usually at the apex.

Periradicular Lesions. Most often a widened PDL space and inflammatory apical root resorption are associated with pulp necrosis and infection. Occasionally, however, these signs may be associated with occlusal traumatism (Figure 6-46). This emphasizes the need for additional tests beyond radiographs. A widened PDL space may also be expected with other conditions: acute apical periodontitis, a beginning acute apical abscess, or, occasionally, acute pulpitis.

Apical External Resorption. With this condition, the apex may range in appearance from slightly blunted (Figure 6-47, A) to grossly resorbed (Figure 6-47, B), caused by the pressure from orthodontic movement.[104–106] It also may be obliquely resorbed (Figure 6-48, A) or have a cupped-out appearance (Figure 6-48, B), or it may resemble the chewed appearance of a tree felled by a beaver (Figure 6-48, C). In any event, if apical resorption has taken place, the apical foramen will be in the center of the root. If the root resorption has a "moth-eaten" appearance, it is possible that the tooth, by accident, was ripped loose from its ligaments and/or was replanted. Sometimes an unexplained lesion in the region strongly suggests a malignancy (see Figure 5-32).

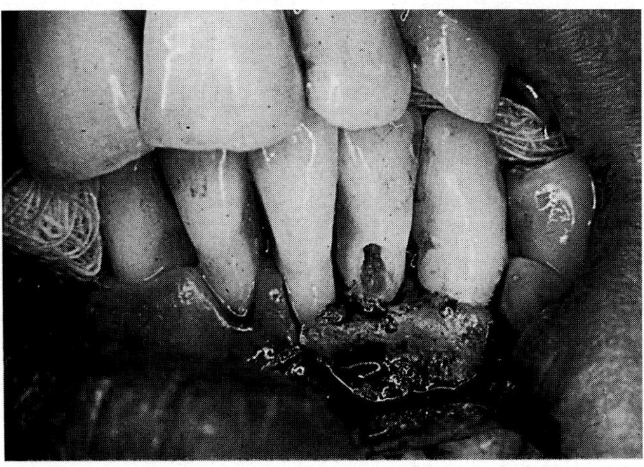

Figure 6-45 Supraosseous extra-canal invasive resorptive lesion (seen radiographically in Figure 6-43). The defect does not invade the pulp and may be restored with the dentin bonding agent and composite resin. (Courtesy of Dr. Alfred L. Frank.)

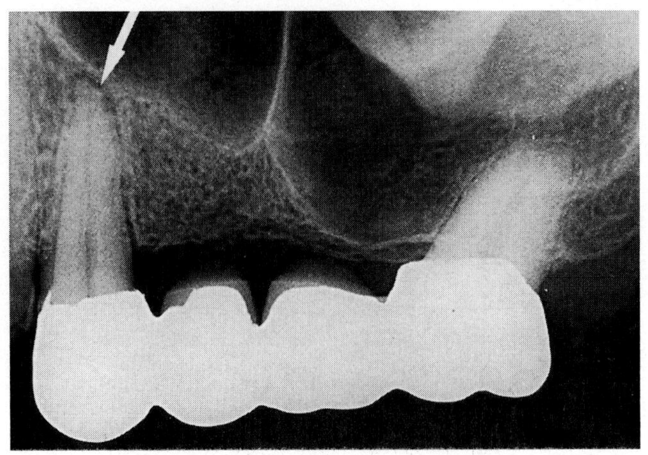

Figure 6-46 Periradicular changes associated with traumatism (**arrow**) are often mistaken for lesions of pulp origin. The first premolar is vital but highly mobile.

Condensing Osteitis. The exact opposite of root resorption is condensing osteitis. Teeth with **chronic pulpal inflammation** sometimes exhibit increased apical bone calcifications, which have a radiopaque appearance on x-ray films (Figure 6-49). Initially, the root may have been blunted by inflammatory resorption, and then this space is filled by osteosclerotic bone. Following successful root canal therapy, the regional radiopacity slowly changes back to a normal appearance[108] (see Figure 5-9). Both idiopathic and sclerosing osteomyelitis result in bone hypercalcification as well.[109,110]

Radiographic Changes as Sequelae to Pulp Necrosis. The severe periradicular osseous lesions that develop as sequelae of pulp necrosis are by far the most frequently observed changes.

Associated with **asymptomatic apical periodontitis** (AAP) is a well-circumscribed osseous lesion. Radiographically, it appears as a radiolucent area, varying in size from a few millimeters to a centimeter or larger in size. The bony perimeter of the lesion may appear radiopaque (Figure 6-50). These lesions do not always appear at the periapex. Occasionally, they are seen on the lateral surface of the root associated with an accessory canal (Figure 6-51).

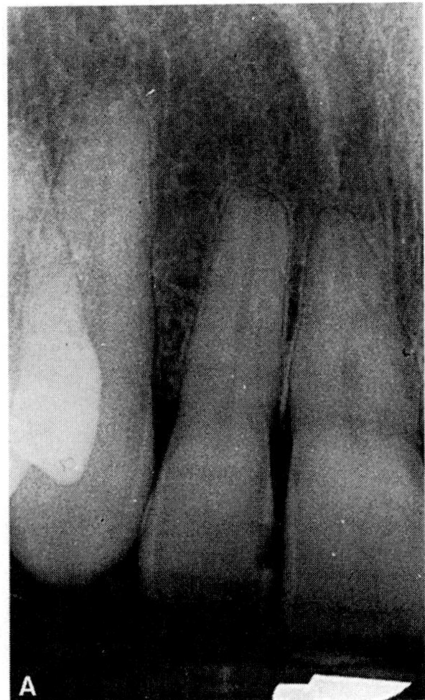

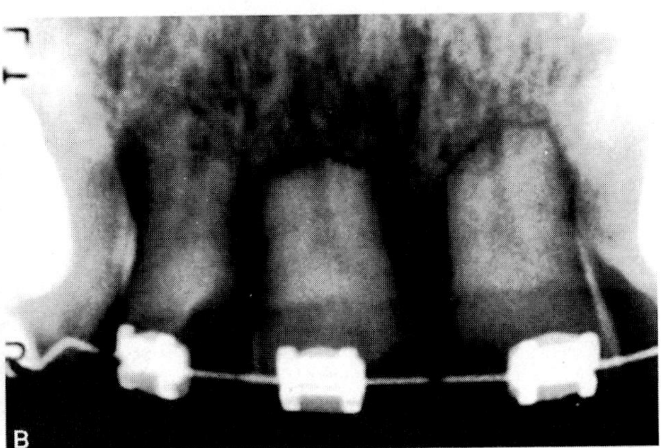

Figure 6-47 A, Blunted apices of teeth moved orthodontically more than 60 years ago. B, Massive root resorption associated with orthodontic tooth movement. Note the development of periodontitis as well. (B courtesy of Dr. Bradley H. Gettleman.)

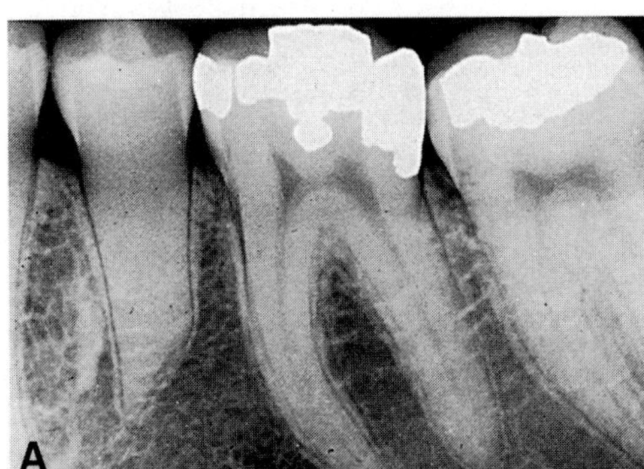

Figure 6-48 A, Total pulp calcification and external root end resorption following injury of a mandibular second premolar. B and C, Two forms of apical external resorption. B, A resorptive defect leaves a flaring apical foramen that could not be adequately obturated by conventional methods. C, Advanced external resorption of the apex makes conventional instrumentation hazardous. B and C reproduced with permission from Luebke RG, Glick DH, Ingle JI. Oral Surg 1964;18:97.

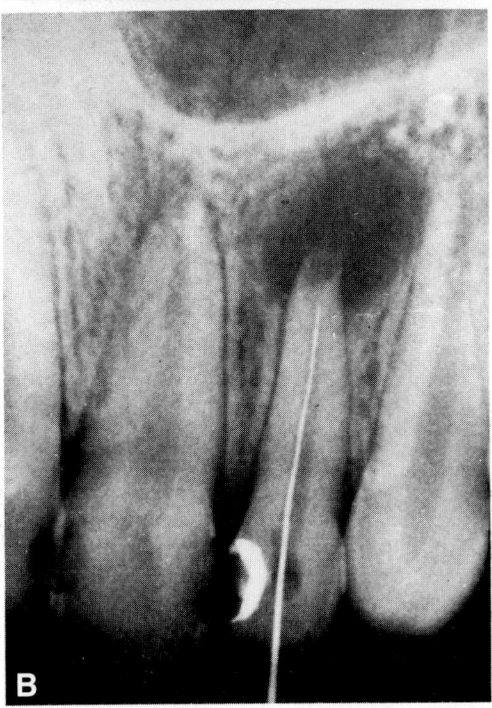

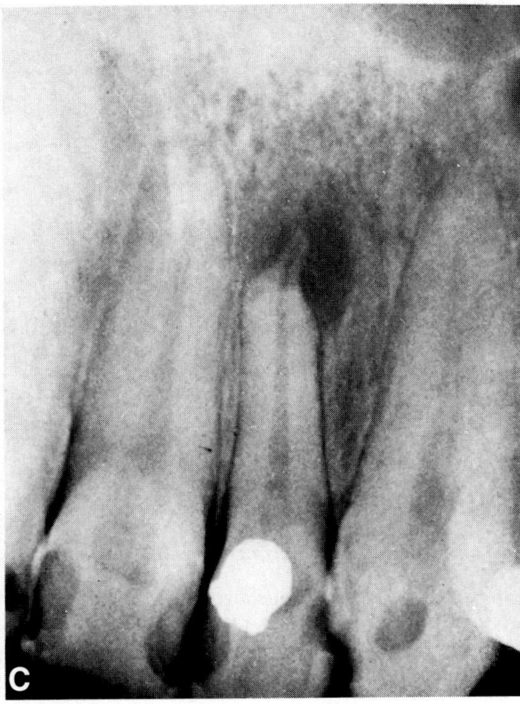

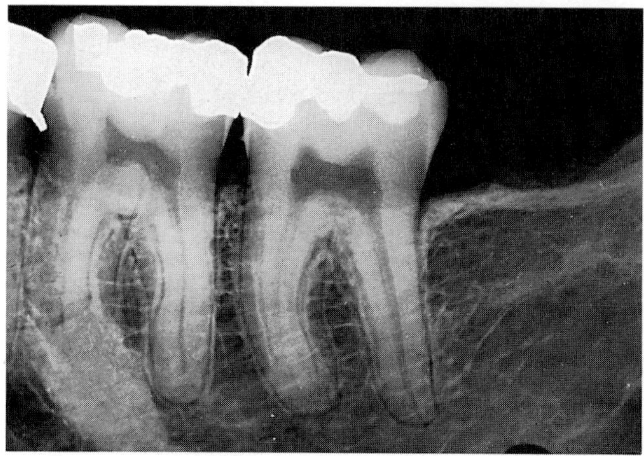

Figure 6-49 Condensing osteitis, external resorption, and pulp stones associated with chronic pulpitis of the first molar. Condensing osteitis will disappear following successful endodontic therapy.

The radiographic appearance of a **asymptomatic apical abscess** (AAA) is generally that of a larger, more diffuse, and irregular radiolucent lesion (Figure 6-52). This lesion may also drain into the mouth through a sinus tract or extraorally onto the neck or chin (Figure 6-53). An **apical cyst** may also develop out of a chronic abscess. In this case, the lesion appears more circumscribed, more like a "granuloma" in appearance (Figure 6-54, A). It is also pathognomonic of cysts to move the roots of teeth laterally (Figure 6-54, B). Natkin et al.

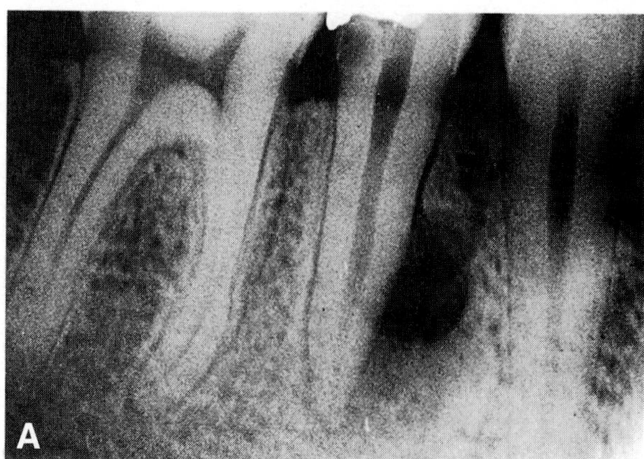

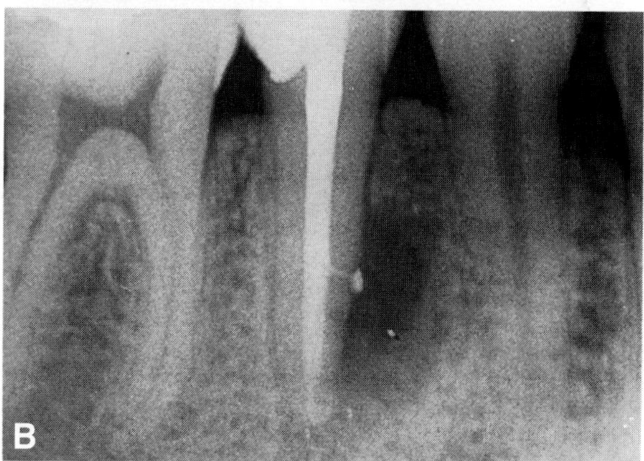

Figure 6-51 **A,** Lateral lesion denotes pulp necrosis and drainage through the lateral accessory canal. **B,** Filling material extrudes, denoting the accessory canal. (Courtesy of Drs. Albert C. Goerig and Elmer J. Neaverth.)

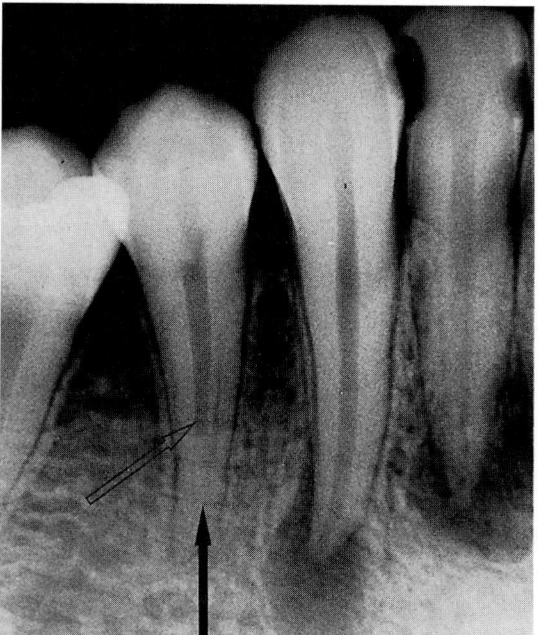

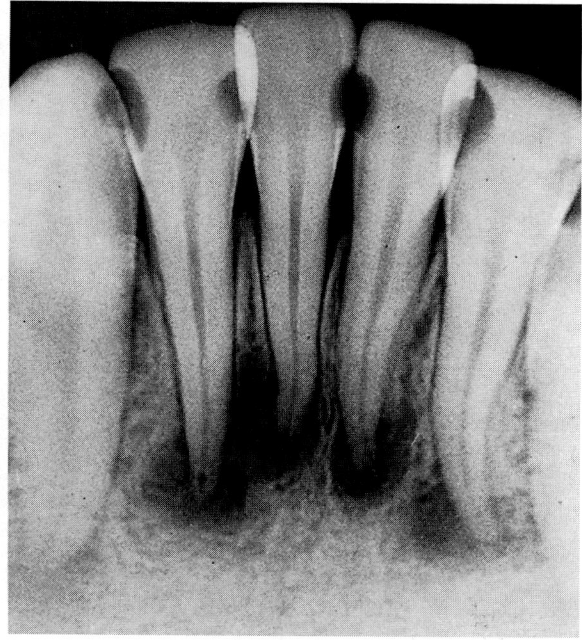

Figure 6-50 **Chronic** apical periodontitis involving five mandibular anterior teeth. Pulp death from impact trauma. Well-circumscribed lesions and pear-shaped configuration periradicular to the canine are typical of chronic apical periodontitis. These may be confused with an apical cyst. A bifurcated canal (**black arrow, left**) is also apparent. A sudden change in radiolucency in the canal (**open arrow**) denotes point of separation of canals.

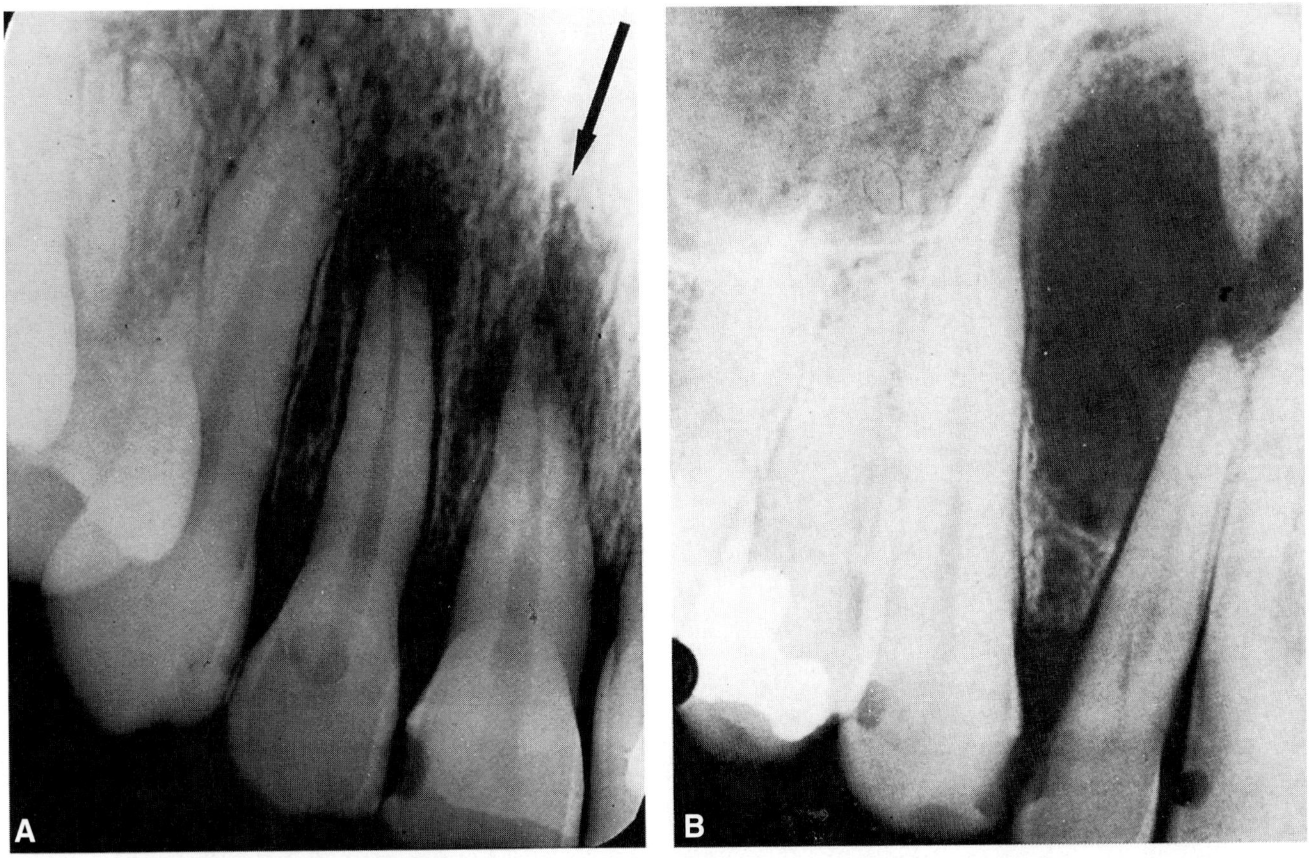

Figure 6-52 A, Diffuse radiolucent appearance (**arrow**) of an asymptomatic apical abscess (AAA) (with stoma) is here contrasted with an asymptomatic apical periodontitis (AAP) associated with a lateral incisor (no stoma). **B**, Asymptomatic apical abscess with drainage through buccal stoma following chronic infection of an apical cyst. Huge diffuse radiolucency is typical of AAA. The root of the tooth is displaced laterally by pressure from the cyst.

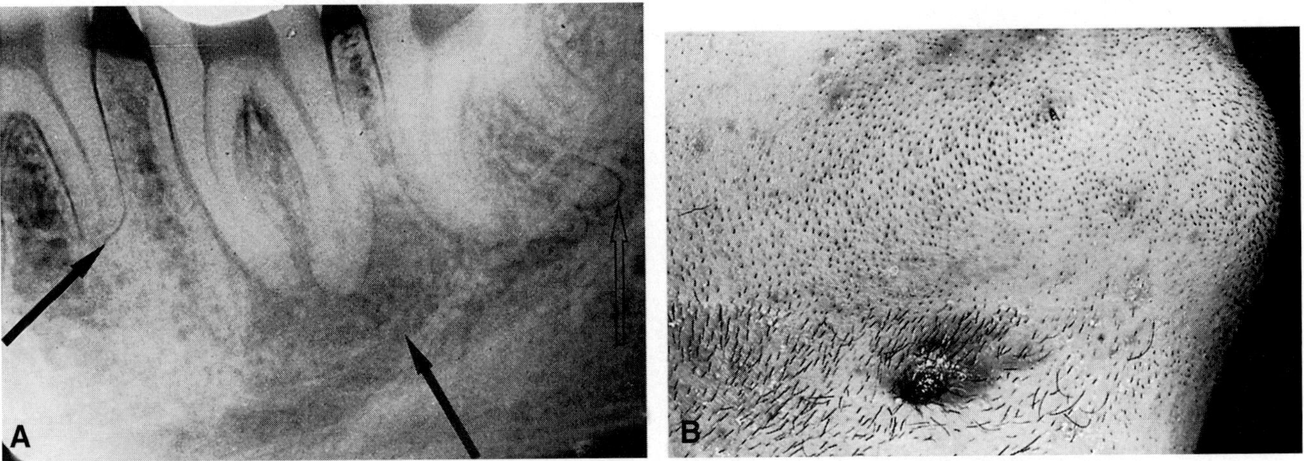

Figure 6-53 A, Diffuse radiographic appearance (**right arrow**) of an asymptomatic apical abscess may be overlooked owing to radiopacity of the heavy cortical bone. Also noted are condensing osteitis and external root resorption from chronic pulpitis (**left arrow**), as well as an anomalous third root of the third molar. **B**, Extraoral stoma (**neck**) of 8 years duration, draining from the chronic apical abscess seen in A. Immediately following root canal therapy, the discharge ceased, and the stoma healed to a "navel" of scar tissue.

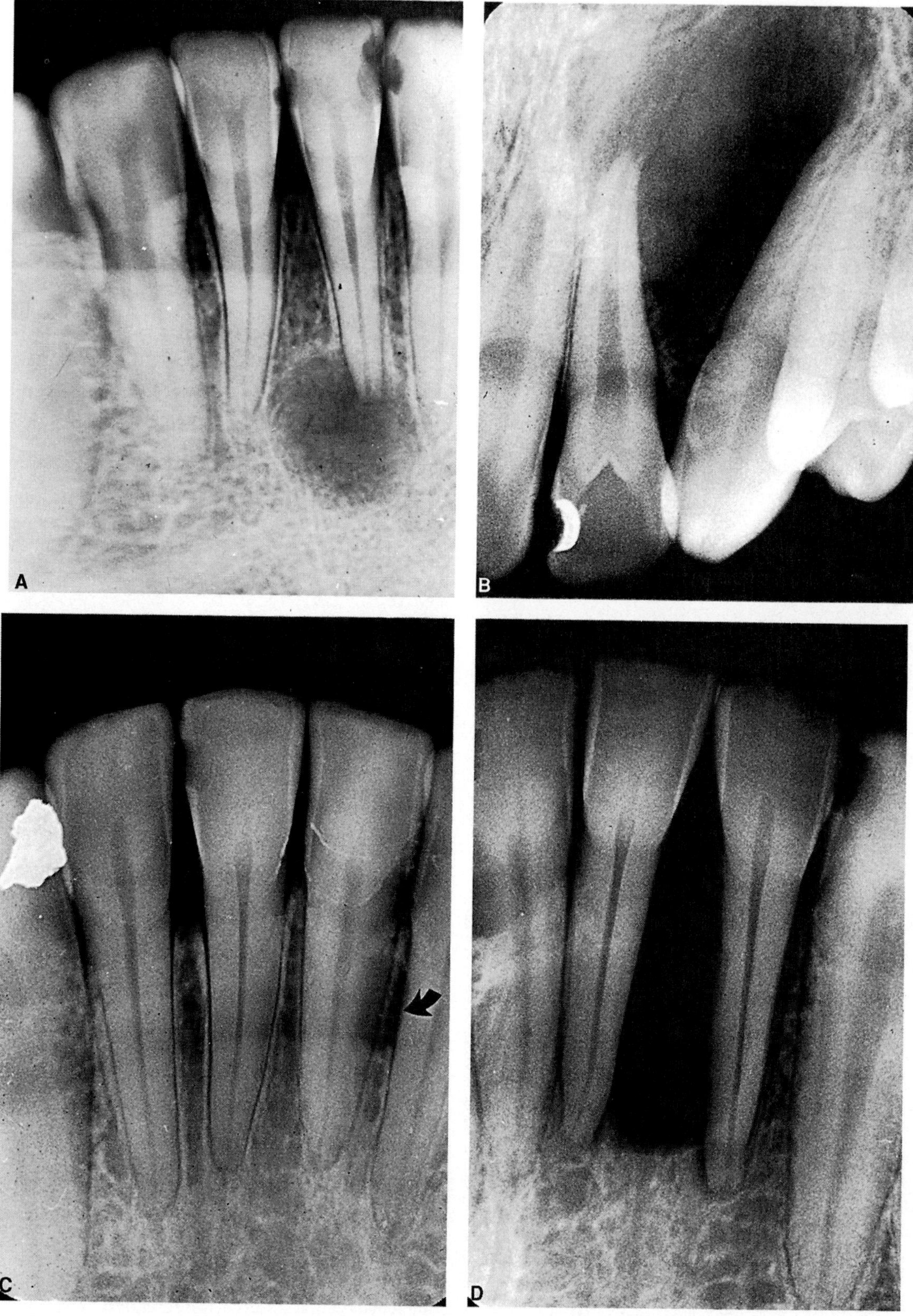

Figure 6-54 Movement of teeth is pathognomonic of a cyst. **A**, Root separation beginning from modest cyst development. Typical circumscribed radiopaque perimeter may be confused with asymptomatic apical periodontitis. **B**, Pulpless lateral incisor with infected apical cyst. The canine has been particularly displaced. **C**, Lateral cyst (**arrow**) not involved with a pulpless tooth. **D**, Same case, 14 months later. Teeth remain vital. Biopsy, lateral periodontal cysts. **C** and **D** reproduced with permission from Degering CI. Oral Surg 1971;32:498.

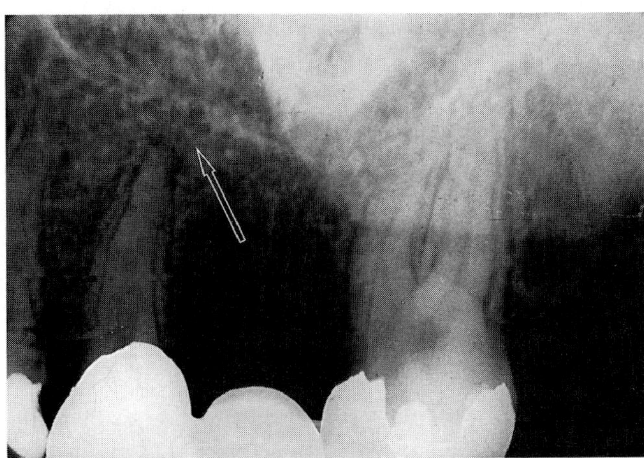

Figure 6-55 A chronic apical abscess (**arrow**) has perforated the floor of the antrum, causing chronic unilateral maxillary sinusitis, which healed following endodontic therapy.

postulated that the larger the lesion, the more apt it is to be a cyst.[111]

In the event that one of these inflammatory lesions is in contact with the floor of the maxillary sinus, chronic sinusitis may result (Figure 6-55).

Lesions of Nonendodontic Origin. A number of pathologic changes in and near the alveolar process may be mistaken for periradicular lesions of pulpal origin. First to consider would be the nonodontogenic cysts: the so-called "globulomaxillary" cyst, the midline palatal cyst, and the cyst of the nasopalatine canal or foramen. Because these cysts are not associated with the exact root end, they may be "moved" radiographically around and away from the root ends if the horizontal direction of the central x-ray beam is varied from side to side (Figure 6-56). Residual cysts, as well as globulomaxillary cysts, may be found along the lateral surface of the root (see Figure 5-29).

To be further considered in the differential diagnosis of cysts is the vitality of the pulps of associated teeth. The pulp of a tooth with an **apical** cyst should test nonvital. This may not be true of the teeth near nonodontogenic cysts, unless traumatic injuries caused pulp death and also triggered sutural cyst formation. Weine and Silverlade pointed out that residual cysts may masquerade as periradicular lesions as well.[112] It should be noted that there is controversy as to whether globulomaxillary cysts exist as a clear entity.

Periodontal lesions may be mistaken for periradicular lesions of endodontic origin (Figure 6-57). The periodontal probe and pulp tester are invaluable in determining the origin of the lesion. An additional method is to place a silver or gutta-percha point in the periodontal pocket and take a radiograph. If the lesion is traceable to the apex of a tooth but the pulp responds to pulp testing, the evidence for primary periodontal involvement is strong.

Common errors in diagnosis center around the lesions of **periradicular osteofibrosis** or **cementoblastoma,** particularly during stage 1, when radiolucency is so apparent (Figure 6-58, A and B). By the time the lesion begins to calcify into a sclerotic lesion (Figure 6-58, C to E), little doubt should exist about the nature of the lesion. Errors will still be made, however, in spite of all evidence to the contrary. The pulp tester will invariably help determine the diagnosis. A group in Great Britain has noted that osteofibrosis can be associated with hyperparathyroidism, which, in turn, may be familial.[113]

In marked contrast, Marks and Dunkelberger have pointed out that Paget's disease of bone (osteitis defor-

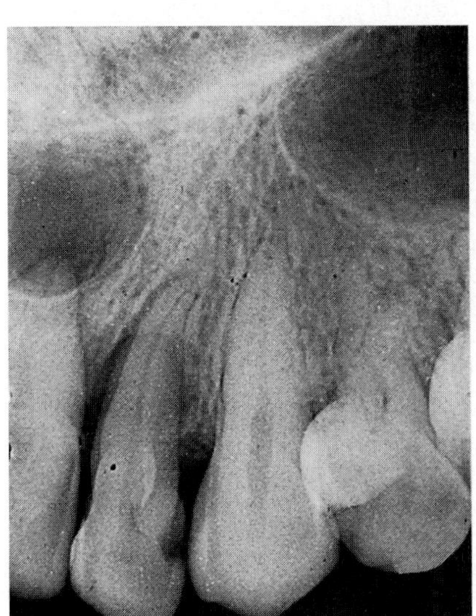

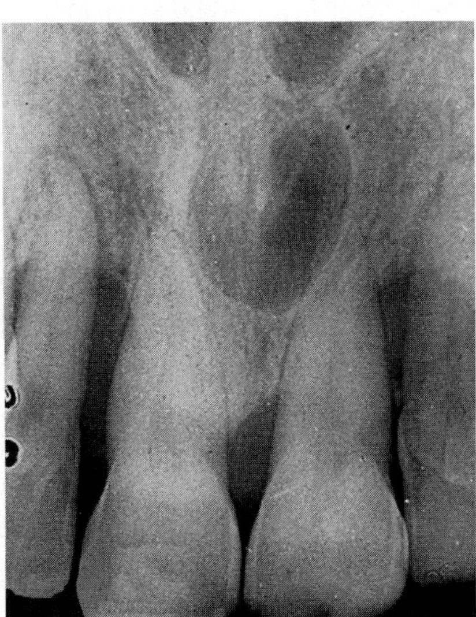

Figure 6-56 A cyst of the nasopalatine canal that may be "moved" from side to side by varying the horizontal angle of x-ray exposure. The lesion appears to be directly over the apex of the central incisor (**left**) but has "moved" to the middle-line position in direct labiolingual projection (**right**). Periodontal disease complicates the case.

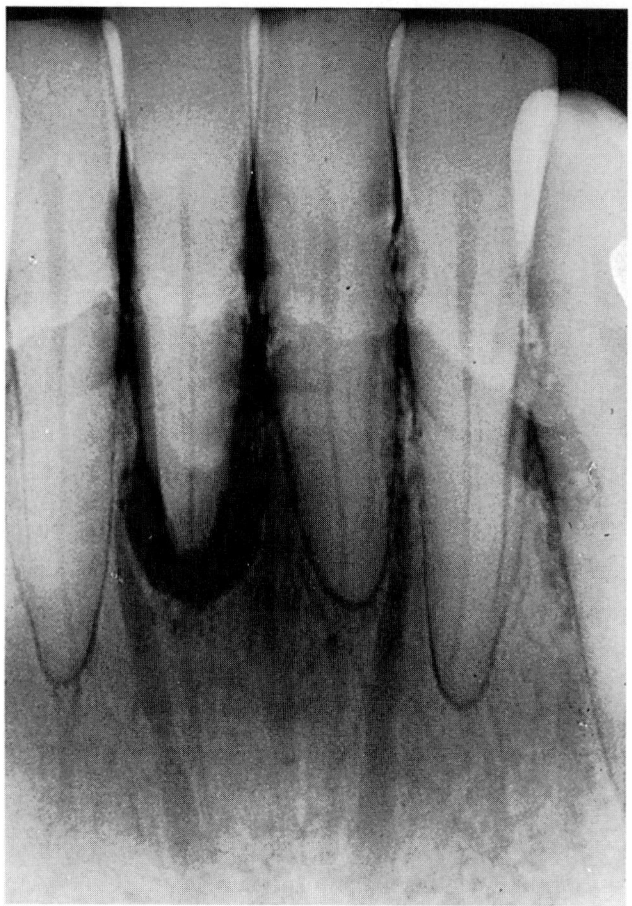

Figure 6-57 A periodontal lesion appears as a periradicular lesion. The involved central incisor is vital. A peculiar radiolucent, horizontal band lies between heavy supragingival calculus and the crest of the alveolar process. (Courtesy of Dr. Jerome Zech.)

mans) often presents oral findings—atypical facial neuralgia and/or paralysis, **hypercementosis,** generalized pulp calcification, loss of lamina dura, root blunting by resorption, and loss of normal bony trabeculation[114] (Figure 6-59, A and B). Any one sign or symptom can easily be confused with a host of localized diseases.

Importance of Endodontic Radiography

Radiography is of paramount importance to the practice of endodontics. It would be virtually impossible to obtain good results from treatment without the use of radiographs. One needs excellent diagnostic films before treatment begins, during treatment (in spite of the availability of electronic apex locators), and to evaluate treatment results after completion of endodontic therapy. On the other hand, one must not become totally dependent on the radiograph. It is mandatory that other tests be used in conjunction with radiographs. Figure 6-60 is a good case in point—a serious error in diagnosis avoided by additional films and vitality testing. In marked contrast, Figure 6-61 illustrates a tragic misdiagnosis owing to a singular dependence on radiographs. A simple vitality test would have alerted the dentist to an error in diagnosis.

Furthermore, it should **not** be assumed that a fistula is necessarily associated with the tooth to which it lies opposite. The draining sinus tract may arise some distance from its orifice. Radiographing a gutta-percha or annealed silver point along the length of the tract may totally change an initial snap diagnosis (Figure 6-62).

Initial Radiograph. Initial diagnostic radiographs must be studied carefully, not only as an aid in diagnosis but also as a "blueprint" for what to expect during treatment (Figure 6-63, A).

First, one must note the size and shape of the pulp chamber and the direction and angulation of the canals as they leave the chamber, as well as obstructions such as pulp stones. One realizes how valuable the initial radiograph is each time a tooth with a full crown is treated when the radiopaque metal crown eliminates a preview of coronal pulp anatomy.

Curvature of the roots and the approximate length of the tooth are next noted. Curvatures in the buccal or lingual directions are difficult to detect, but additional radiographic angulations may help. Distal or mesial inclination of the roots is usually apparent on the radiograph; that information can be used to prevent gouging and perforation of the root canals.

Confirmatory Radiographs. The radiograph is not only a valuable diagnostic tool, it is also an indispensable working tool. It provides pertinent information about treatment progress.

If, after the initial entry into the crown, the access opening appears to be headed away from the canal orifices, a **confirmatory film** should be taken to evaluate alignment (see Figure 6-11). Such progress films also provide assistance in searching for calcified canals.

The **confirmatory length-of-tooth film** is undoubtedly the second most valuable film to be taken after the initial diagnostic radiograph (Figure 6-63, B). In addition to information about the position of the file tip in relation to the root apex, it can also show whether the file is in the canal as intended or has entered a root perforation.

The **confirmatory trial point radiograph** serves two important purposes. First, it confirms the visual and "tugback" judgment of the fit of the initial filling point. Second, it provides the final opportunity to judge the advance of instrumentation. If an error in the length of the tooth has been made, and the canal has been instrumented short or long, here is an opportunity to correct the error.

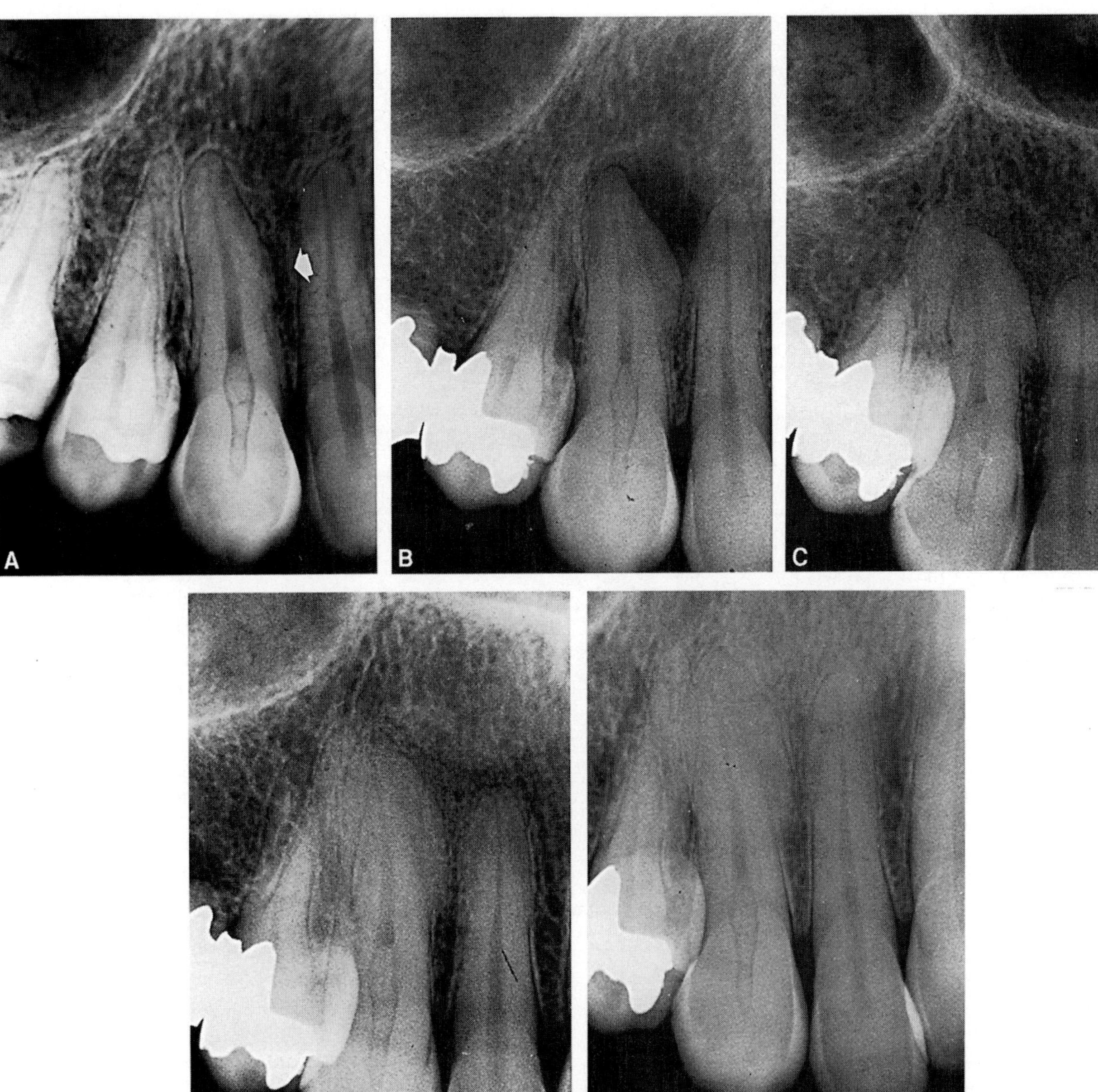

Figure 6-58 Chronologic development of a suspected cementoblastoma over a 25-year period. A, **Initial** radiograph with a lesion apparent as a radiolucent area (**arrow**), as well as excess cemental formation. Note the huge pulp stone. The pulp is vital. B, **Ten years later**, a huge radiolucent lesion is present as well as a gross increase in cementoma. C, **Fifteen years later**, a decrease in radiolucency and an increase in cementoma. D, **Twenty years later**, virtual disappearance of radiolucency along with a gross increase in hypercementosis. E, **Twenty-five years later**, total cementoblastoma. The pulp remains vital. (Courtesy of Dr. Maurice J. Friedman.)

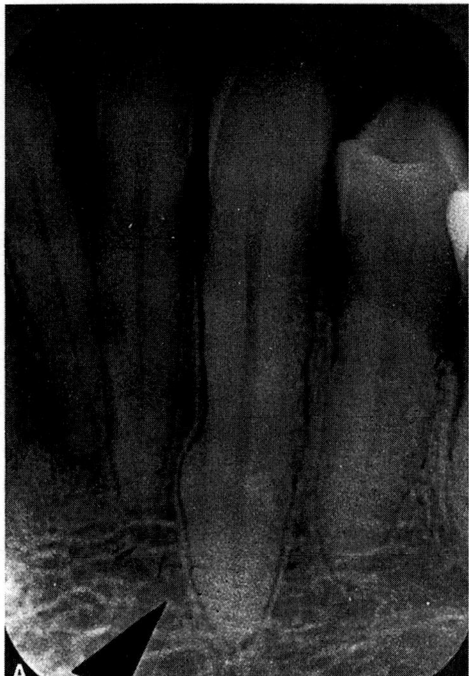

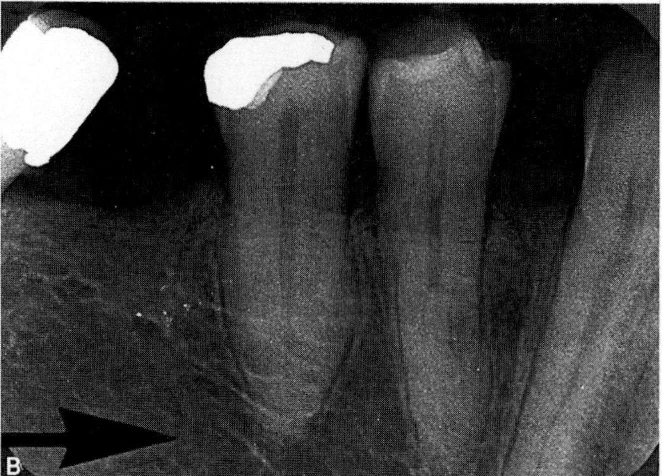

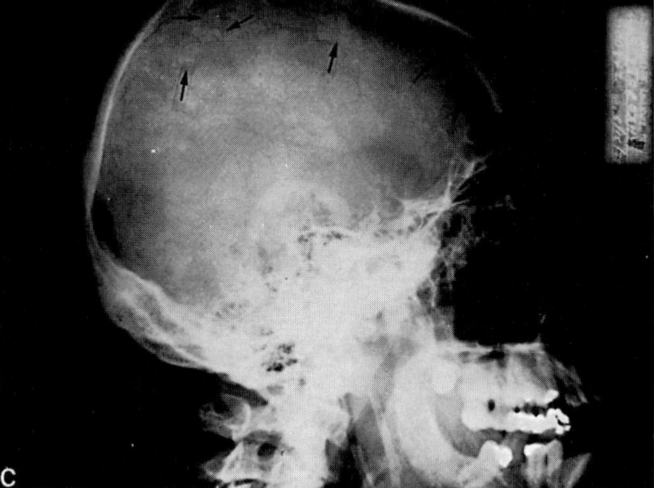

Figure 6-59 Confusion surrounding the oral radiologic appearance of Paget's disease. **A**, Hypercementosis and pulp calcification in the right mandibular canine (**arrow**). **B**, Same condition in the left premolar. Note loss of trabeculation and formation of pulp stones (**arrow**). **C**, "Cottonwool" appearance (**arrows**) in the skull view confirms Paget's disease. Reproduced with permission from Marks JM and Dunkelberger FB.[114]

The **confirmatory post-treatment film** follows completion of the root canal filling. It should be made before a coronal restoration is placed because some correction in the canal filling may have to be made. Ideally, the final film for the record, and the duplicate film to be returned if a referring dentist is involved, should be taken without the rubber dam clamp (Figure 6-63, C).

Confirmatory progress films are also important during surgery. Searching for root tips, lost filling material, location of root apexes during trephination or apicoectomy—these are only a few of the uses made of confirmatory radiographs.

Post-Treatment Evaluation Radiograph. Historically, post-treatment evaluations have been a part of clinical endodontic practice. This radiograph allows an opportunity to evaluate changes taking place periradicularly as a result of root canal therapy (Figure 6-63, D). A 1-year interval is a realistic time frame for most endodontic cases such as those with initial apical lesions or those with potential post-treatment problems. If any abnormal or unusual findings are noted, it may be necessary to re-treat, either surgically or nonsurgically, or if changes are uncertain, further re-evaluation may be indicated. Patients, however, may not consider post-treatment evaluation to be important, particularly if they are asymptomatic. Riley surveyed 159 diplomates of the American Board of Endodontics, who reported that fewer than half of their patients returned on recall.[115]

Re-treatment Radiography. Before initiating re-treatment, particularly a referred patient, the dentist must always have a "fresh film." Films sent with the patient by the referring dentist may be outdated and may also have been taken prior to a procedure such as access preparation. A new film may supply surprising information about the tooth, perforations, broken instruments, failure to obturate, ineffective surgery, and a number of conditions well below the standard of care (Figure 6-64).

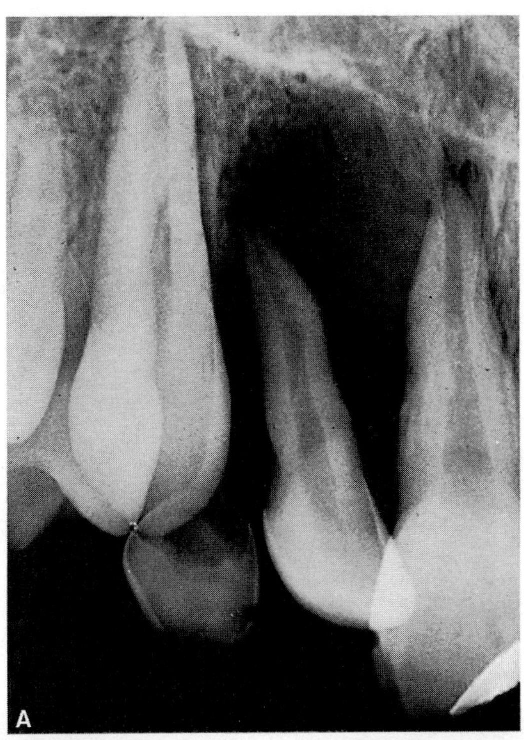

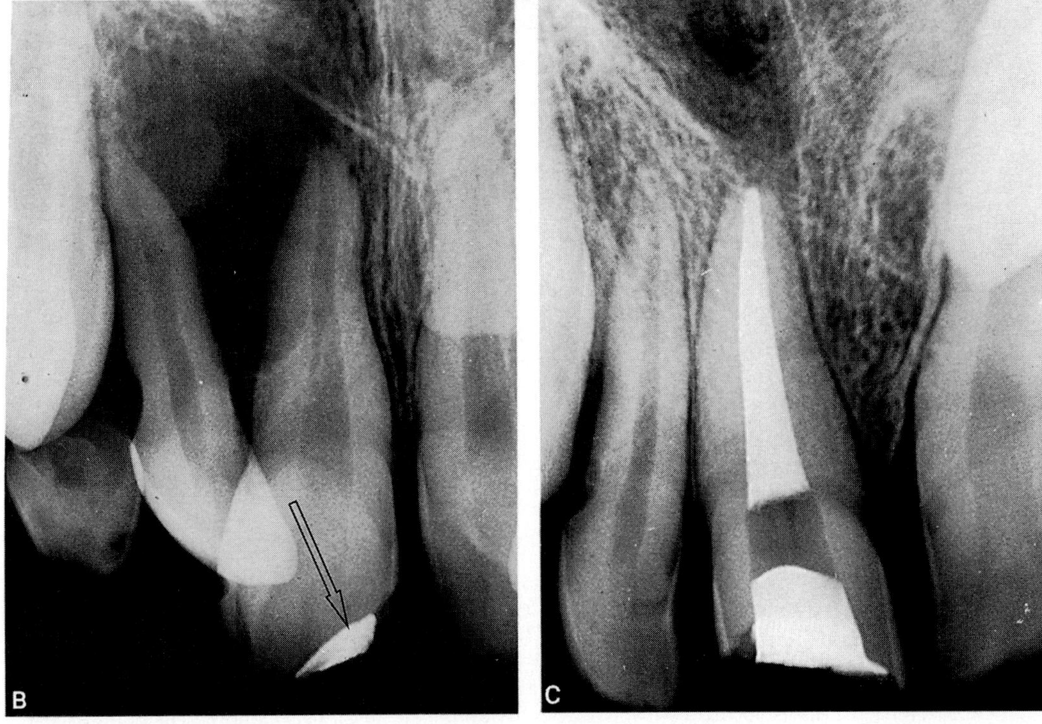

Figure 6-60 Importance of multiple roentgenographic exposures. **A**, Lateral incisor appears to be the principally involved tooth in this direct buccolingual projection. **B**, Projection through the central incisor shows that it is involved in the lesion as well. The lateral incisor is vital and the central incisor is nonvital, pulp death having developed from trauma (**arrow**). **C**, Following therapy, new bone develops throughout the area, and both teeth reattach. (Courtesy of Dr. Pierre R. Dow.)

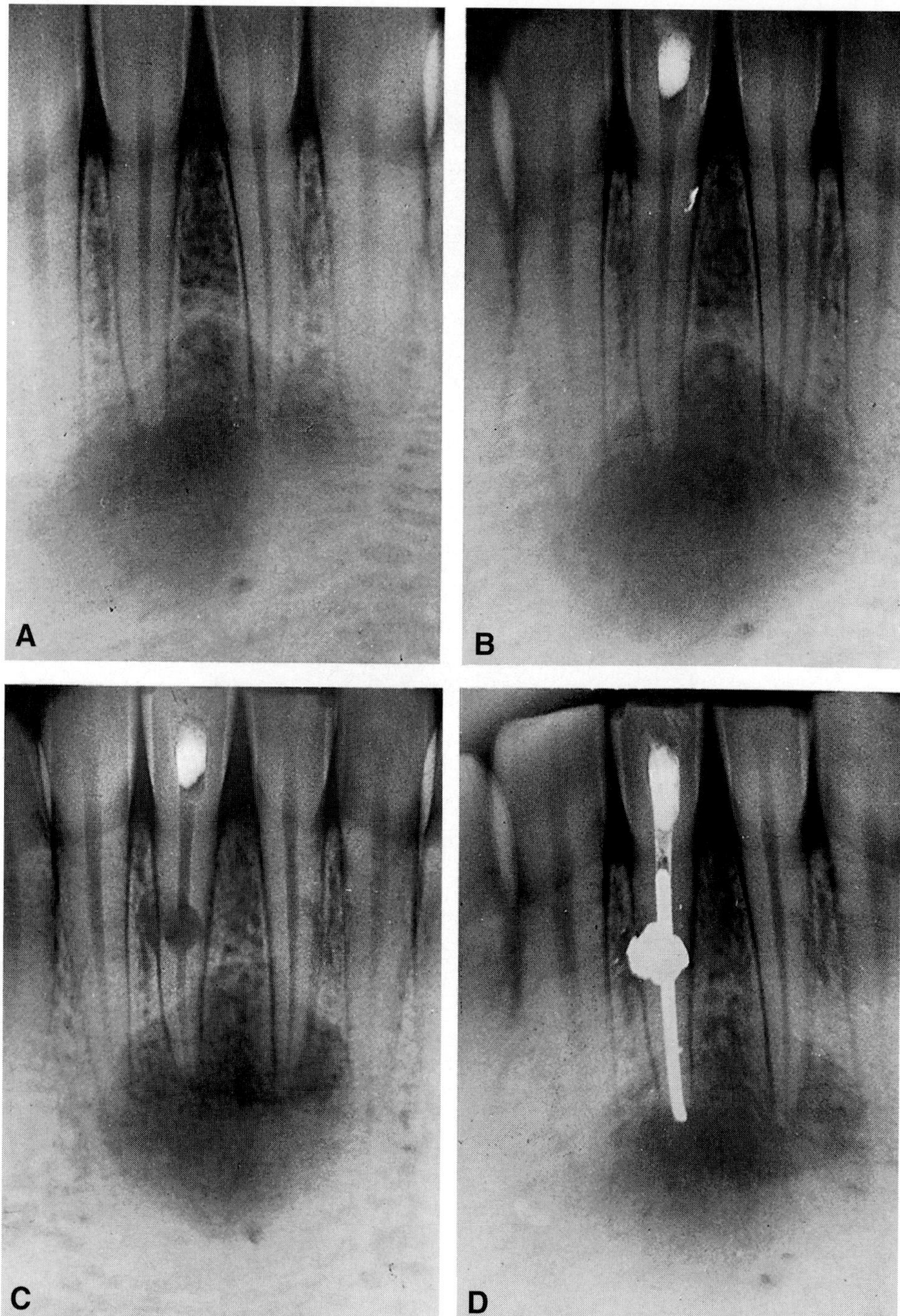

Figure 6-61 Chronologic development of an internal resorptive defect that has become external as well. The patient is an adolescent female with bruxism (see chapter 4 and Figure 4–24). **A**, Mandibular incisors apparently involved with asymptomatic apical periodontitis. The pulps of both teeth are vital. **B**, The referring dentist mistakenly opened into vital pulp of the right central incisor. Detecting his error, he placed a temporary filling and dismissed the patient. **C**, Six months later, internal resorption from the stimulated pulp has perforated the root, and external resorption has also begun. **D**, Total pulpectomy, root canal therapy, and amalgam repair of the resorptive lesion save the incisor. The left central incisor remains vital. Alleviation of trauma from bruxism will allow healing.

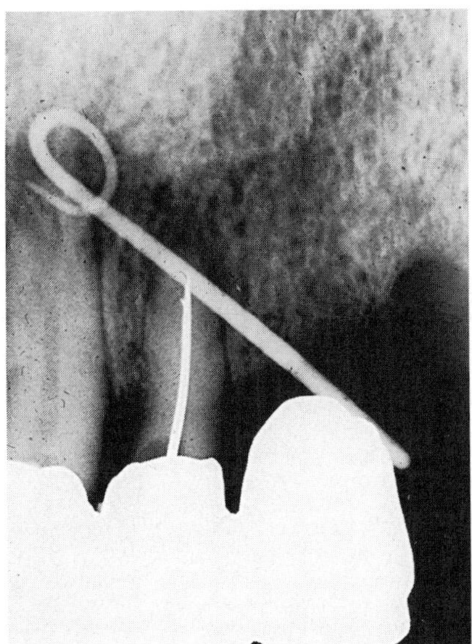

Figure 6-62 Although the stoma of the draining sinus tract was over the canine pontic and the treated lateral incisor was suspected as the origin, it was actually the more distant central incisor causing the problem. (Courtesy of Dr. Cyril Gaum.)

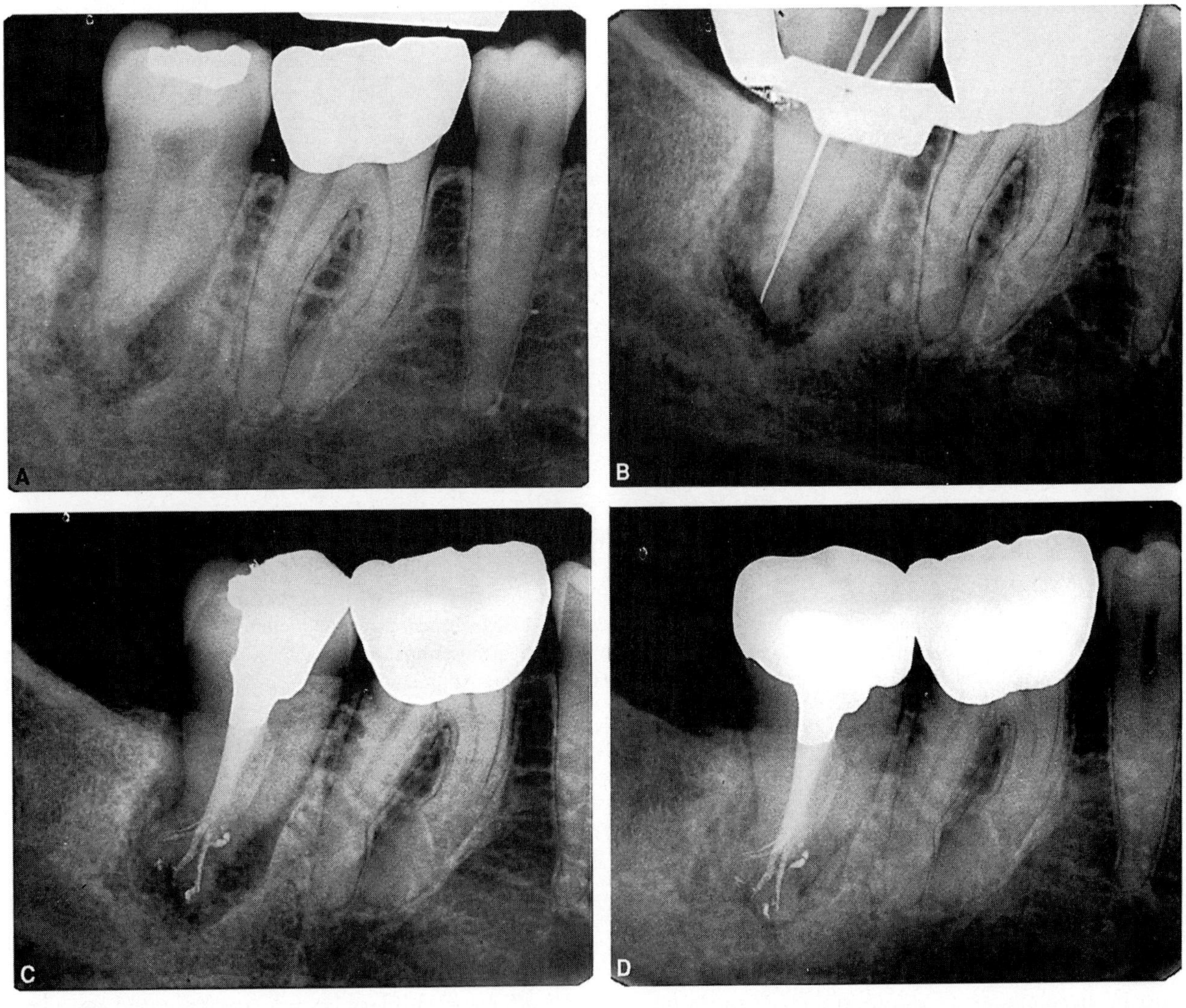

Figure 6-63 Importance of initial and confirmatory radiographs. **A**, The initial film alerts the dentist to confusing canal anatomy and a significant periradicular and lateral root lesion. **B**, Confirmatory length of the tooth radiograph reveals the presence of a C-shaped canal. **C**, Immediate postoperative confirmatory film shows a complicated root canal system obturated by vertical compaction of warm gutta-percha. Obtura II was used for back-filling. **D**, Confirmatory 1-year follow-up film shows the degree of healing. (Courtesy of Dr. Michael J. Scianamblo.)

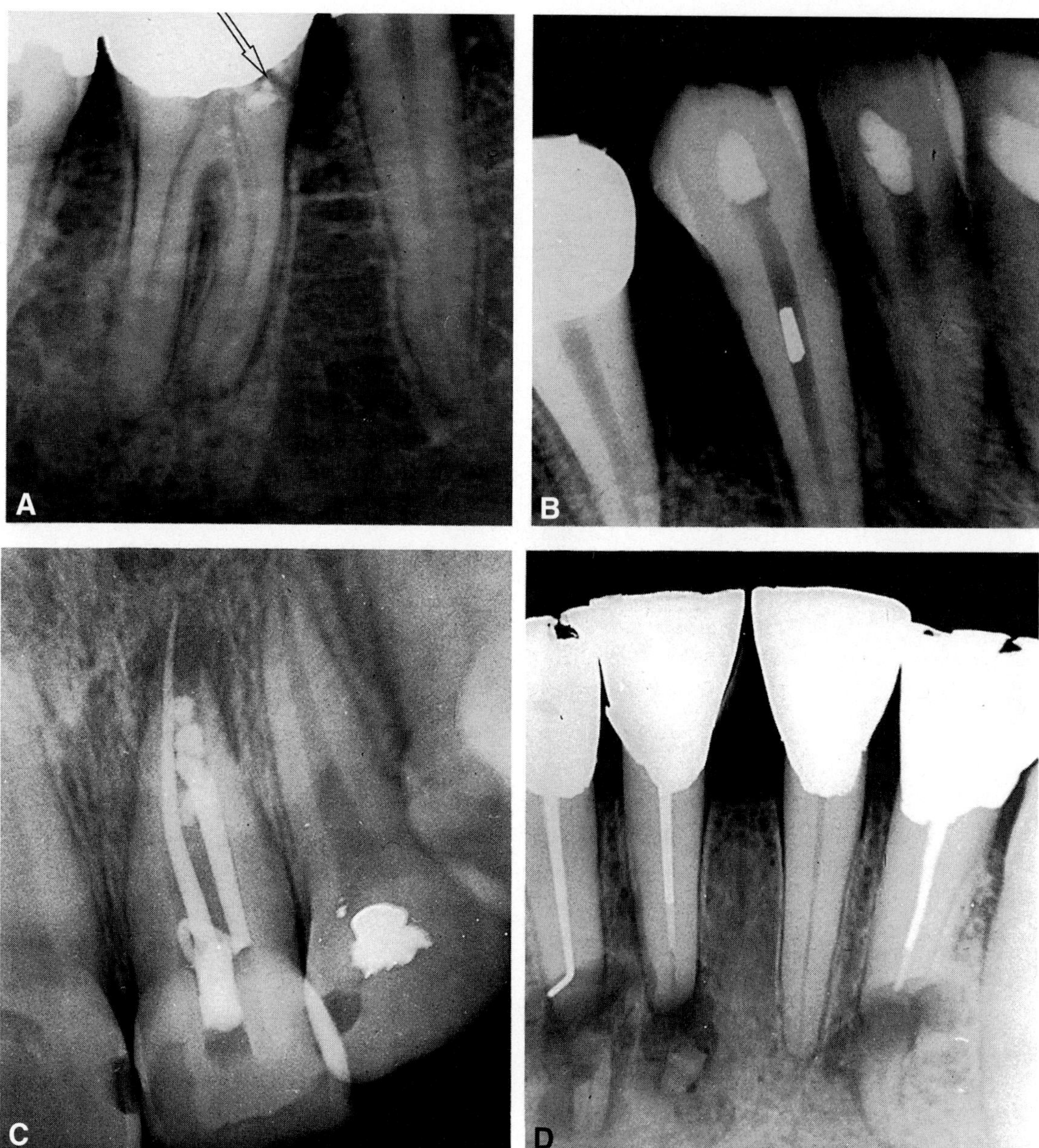

Figure 6-64 A, Root perforation (**arrow**) and associated periodontal lesion are revealed by radiography. Condensing osteitis and external root resorption are related to chronic pulpitis, the initial complaint. **B**, **C**, and **D**, Treatment errors and failures revealed by radiographs. **B**, Fissure bur broken in the canal; **C**, totally ineffective canal obliteration. An inadequate coronal access cavity is smaller than the canal and the apex to be débrided and obliterated; **D**, complete "butchery" and total failure in attempted multiple apicoectomies. The canals are inadequately filled, and amputated root tips have been left in place.

DIAGNOSTIC PERPLEXITIES

Even after a careful history and examination, some dental problems still defy immediate diagnosis. The most frequent among these have been cataloged as diagnostic perplexities: (1) sinus tract, (2) numbness, (3) persistent discomfort, (4) cracked tooth syndrome, (5) bizarre radiographic appearance, (6) idiopathic root resorption, and (7) treatment failures.

Sinus Tract

The stoma of a sinus tract may not always exist opposite the lesion. An example is the case of drainage in the area of an extracted canine (see Figure 6-62). Initially, the adjacent pulpless lateral incisor would be suspect. However, when a tracer gutta-percha point was inserted through the stoma to the depth of the sinus tract, it pointed to the pulpless central incisor. Harris revealed

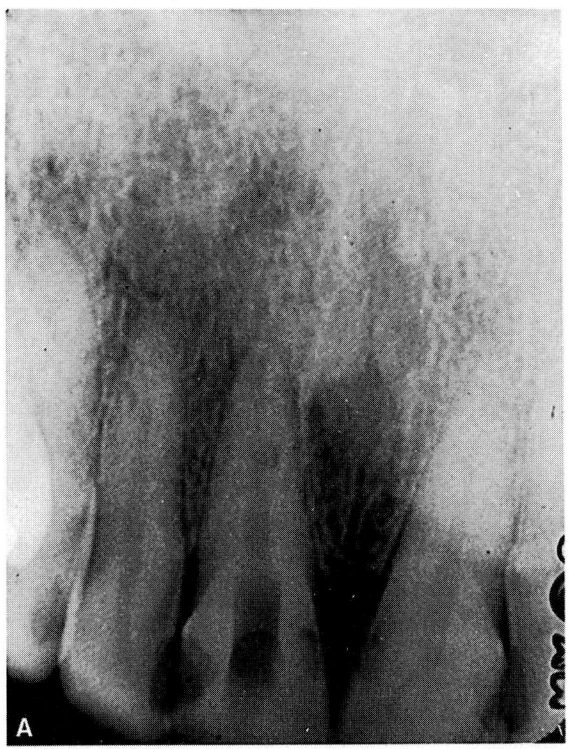

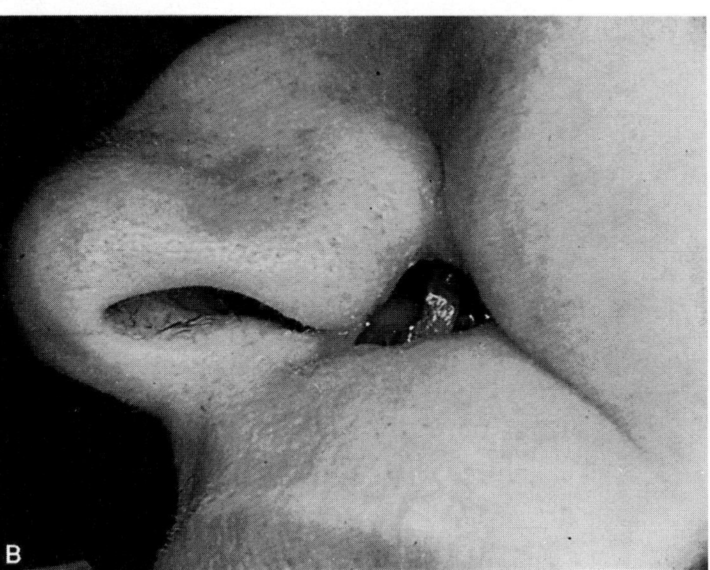

Figure 6-65 A, Pulpless central incisor with vague periradicular osseous changes. B, Draining fistula associated with the infected pulpless incisor in A. Reproduced with permission from Harris WE.[116]

a pulpless maxillary central incisor that was draining extraorally through a stoma as far as the angle of the *ala nasi*[116] (Figure 6-65). A similar situation, draining directly into the nostril from a periradicular lesion of a central incisor, was reported from Israel.[117]

Sinus tracts related to cracked teeth are most perplexing and often can be diagnosed only by the laying of a surgical flap. In one particular case, the fracture was not discernible in the initial radiograph, but following obturation of the root canal, the horizontal fracture became readily apparent (Figure 6-66).

Numbness

A symptom occasionally associated with endodontic cases is numbness in either the area containing the tooth or paresthesia of a distant part, such as the lip. When numbness occurs, one should also be concerned with trigeminal neuropathies—tumors or cysts that involve the innervation.

Numbness can also be related to large periradicular lesions encroaching on the mandibular canal (Figure 6-67, A). In this case, after root canal therapy, the numbness subsided, and within 14 months the lesion had healed and normal sensation had returned (Figure 6-67, B). Numbness associated with an acute alveolar abscess is often noted, but in such cases, the diagnosis should be quite obvious. Paresthesia may follow gross overfilling in the mandible, which invades the inferior alveolar canal. Paresthesia may also follow surgery in the region of the lower premolars.

Sixty-one cases of facial numbness were reviewed by researchers at the Mayo Clinic,[118] who found that 83% of the cases had a definite cause, including 48% in which the numbness was of dental origin. Thrush and Small reported seven cases of facial numbness, only one case of which was dental—typical mandibular numbness following a most profound local anesthesia and molar extraction.[119] The remaining cases of numbness were caused by carcinoma of the nasopharynx, tumor invasion of the gasserian ganglion, adenocarcinoma of the brainstem, and cerebrovascular accident. All of these patients exhibited numbness of the jaws, lips, tongue, or palate. They summarized their report by saying, "The most important task is to exclude neoplasia." They recommended basal views of the skull and examination of the nasopharynx.[119]

Persistent Discomfort

After completion of treatment, either nonsurgical or surgical, some patients continue to have symptoms. Others develop discomfort some time later. A patient in the latter category was examined radiographically months after root canal therapy and placement of a bridge abutment. The discomfort was "midtooth," and the radiograph revealed a bony lesion in that area along with external root resorption and a poorly obturated

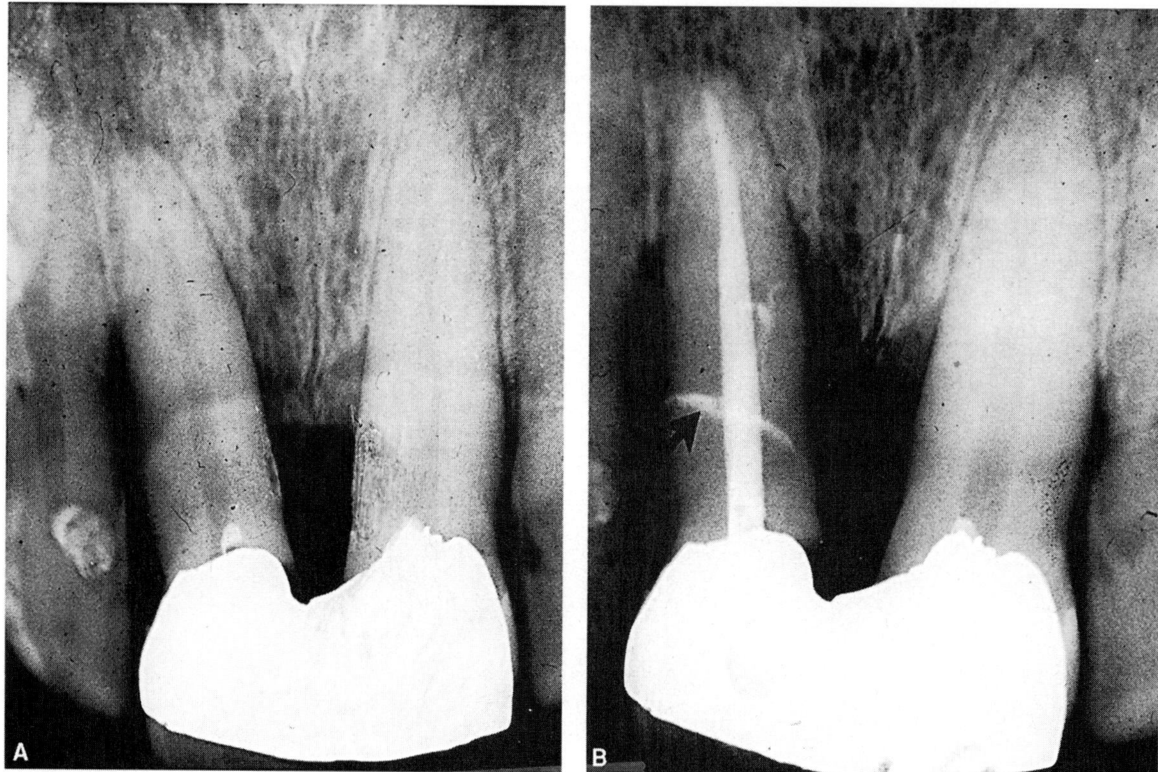

Figure 6-66 A, Preoperative film reveals no fracture line associated with chronic fistula. B, Cement is extruded (**arrow**) into the fracture line. (Courtesy of Dr. Cyril Gaum.)

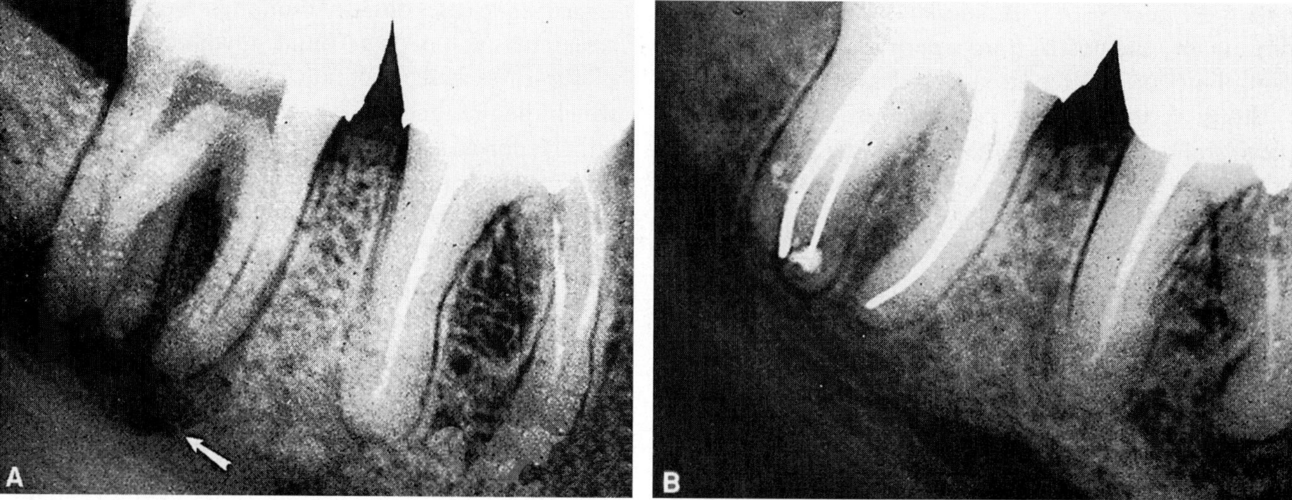

Figure 6-67 A, Extensive periradicular lesion encroaching on the mandibular canal (**arrow**). Numbness results. B, Successful endodontic result, 14 months later. Numbness disappeared as healing advanced. Note the two distal canals and lateral canal as well. (Courtesy of Dr. Cyril Gaum.)

midcanal (Figure 6-68, A). After re-treatment through the crown, the discomfort subsided (Figure 6-68, B). Failing root canal therapy appears to be one of the causes of post-treatment discomfort.

Glick reported a number of cases of persistent discomfort following root canal filling along with the bizarre symptom of continued sensitivity to cold.[120] After careful examination ruled out the possibility of pulpitis in an adjacent tooth, Glick concluded that an additional canal must be present in the treated tooth, one that was missed during treatment. Reopening the pulp chamber and searching for the extra canal was not

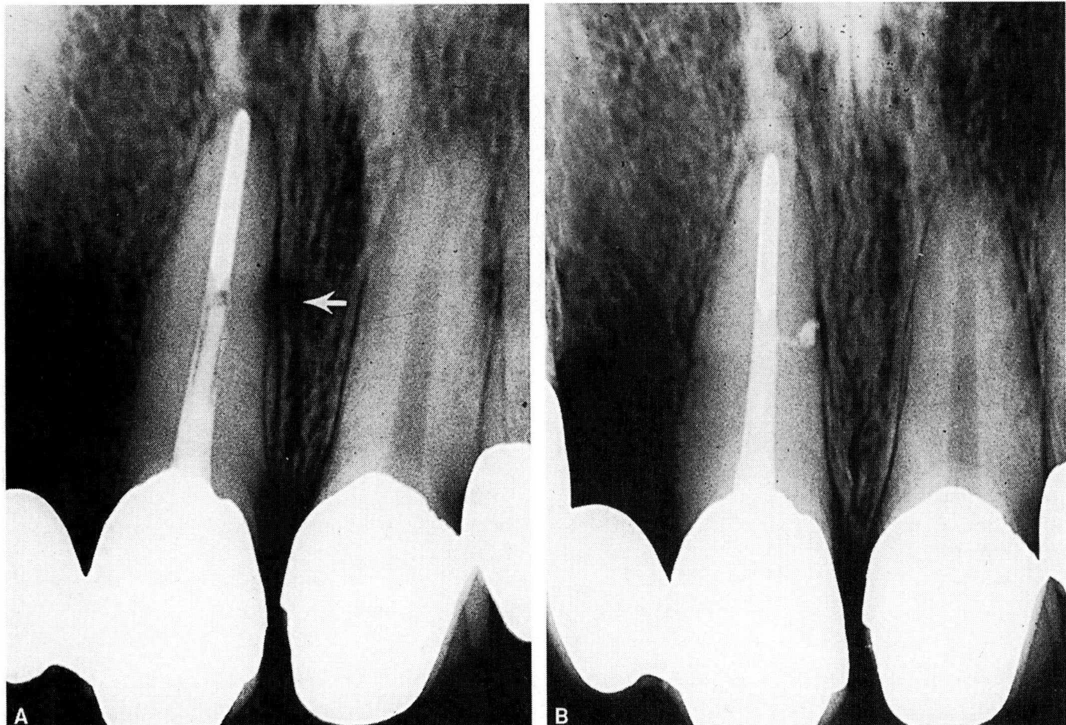

Figure 6-68 A, Persistent discomfort after endodontic treatment and bridge placement. The lesion (**arrow**), midroot with some resorption, indicates a patent accessory canal. **B**, Re-treatment obturates the accessory lateral canal, healing occurs, and discomfort is alleviated. (Courtesy of Dr. Joel L. Dunsky.)

productive. In desperation, Glick sealed formocresol in the chamber, which immediately and permanently eliminated the pain. Although not advocating this as a routine procedure, Glick has found it effective on a number of occasions.

In another report (Figure 6-69), cotton and Cavit (3M/Espe; St. Paul, Minn.) were sealed in a post-space preparation of a distal canal of a mandibular molar, resulting in continuous pain. When the post space was not used for the intended post and core, the space was refilled with gutta-percha and sealer. The cause of discomfort immediately became apparent when sealer was forced out of a minute fracture line.

In a most perplexing and life-threatening situation reported by Verunac,[121] a young submariner consistently developed massive facial emphysema each time the submarine dived. The swelling would become pronounced after the submarine was deeply submerged for 15 hours (Figure 6-70). Within 4 or 5 days after surfacing, the swelling would disappear. Navy physicians had given him antibiotics to no avail and had recommended his discharge from the service. Examination by a dentist revealed a lingual cusp fractured away from a maxillary first premolar, exposing the lingual canal that was patent through the foramen. The air under submerged pressure was being forced through this tiny hole into the entire side of the face and neck (see Figure 6-70).

In a recent study, the phenomenon of **barodontalgia** (aka aerodontologia) was also reported during simulated high-altitude flights and in actual flights. Endodontically treated teeth or teeth with necrotic

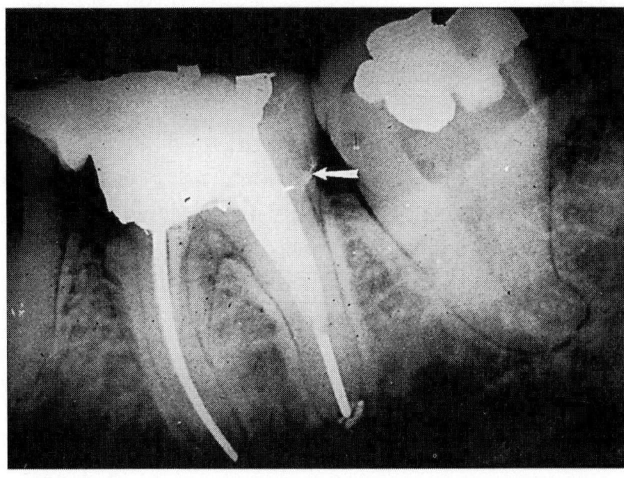

Figure 6-69 Cement extruded through an undisclosed hairline fracture (**arrow**) reveals the source of persistent discomfort. (Courtesy of Dr. Cyril Gaum.)

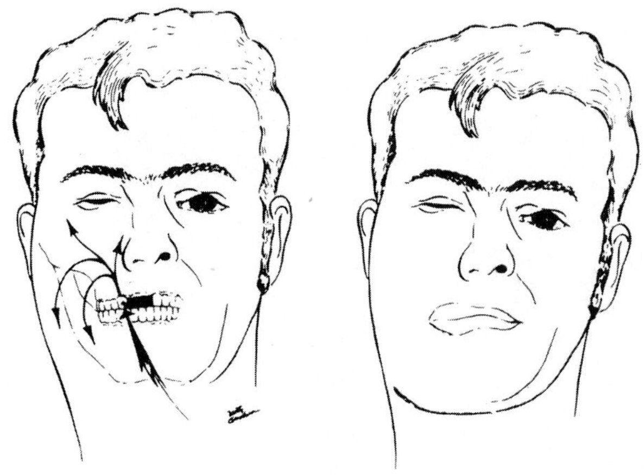

Figure 6-70 During transient periods of increased pressure in a deeply submerged submarine, extracorporeal air entered facial interstitial spaces through an empty root canal. Reproduced with permission from Verunac JJ.[121]

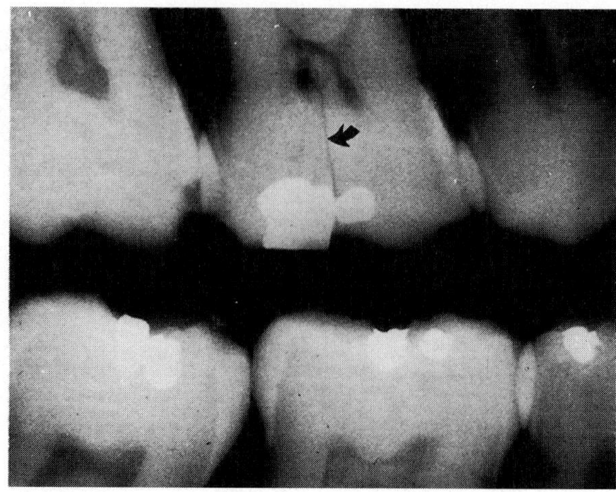

Figure 6-71 Vertical fracture of the crown (**arrow**) revealed in the bitewing film was not apparent in the periradicular film. (Courtesy of Dr. Cyril Gaum.)

pulps did not respond painfully in pressure chamber simulation. Only teeth with inflamed vital pulps reacted to pressure change.[122]

Another cause of persistent discomfort reported earlier in this text relates to root-filled teeth wherein the apex perforates a **fenestration** of the buccal bone. A similar report from Paris noted that the discomfort was relieved when the root end was exposed surgically and the portion of the root extending through the fenestration was "trimmed back" to within the bony housing.[123]

Cracked Tooth Syndrome

Infraction of tooth structure (cracked tooth syndrome) accounts for many perplexing diagnostic problems. A typical situation is that of a patient who experienced intermittent episodes of acute pain radiating over the entire side of the face. The periradicular radiograph revealed a periradicular lesion, and vitality testing proved the pulp to be nonvital. Before endodontic therapy was started, a bitewing radiograph was taken, revealing a vertical fracture into the pulp (Figure 6-71). It is interesting that the crack could not be seen in the periradicular film but did show in the bitewing. Crown fractures, **if in a buccolingual direction**, may be more easily detected by bitewing radiographs.

Bizarre Radiographic Appearances

Radiographs have many limitations, one of which is that many conditions can produce similar appearances on x-ray films. Just such a case is illustrated in a film of a maxillary incisor. The tooth was exquisitely tender to percussion and was mobile. In the radiograph, a horizontal radiolucency appeared above the margin of the porcelain jacket crown (Figure 6-72, A), diagnosed as a fracture with pulp involvement. The crown was removed, and what appeared to be a fracture turned out to be a high chamfer crown preparation. This was verified with a second radiograph (Figure 6-72, B). The pulp was necrotic.

Idiopathic Tooth Resorption

It is difficult at times to determine the cause (or causes) for cases of root resorption. One such case involved the roots of a mandibular molar bridge abutment, where resorption began shortly after root canal therapy (Figure 6-73, A). Within 2½ years, the roots had completely resorbed away (Figure 6-73, B to D). One might speculate that this resorption could have been related to the patient's breast cancer. It has been postulated that a parathyroid-like hormone is secreted by tumor cells, and there is a high incidence of hypercalcemia in patients with breast cancer.

Breast cancer could not have been an etiologic factor in a similar case reported by Poliak (personal communication, 1975). His patient was a middle-aged male motion picture producer who developed an unexplained resorption 5 years following therapy of an endodontically treated mandibular second molar. Within 2 years, the entire root structure had essentially resorbed away. From England, Pankhurst et al. reported a number of teeth in the same patient with idiopathic resorption.[124]

Treatment Failures

The examination of the treatment failures is important because if the cause of failure can be determined and corrected, the failure may be reversed.

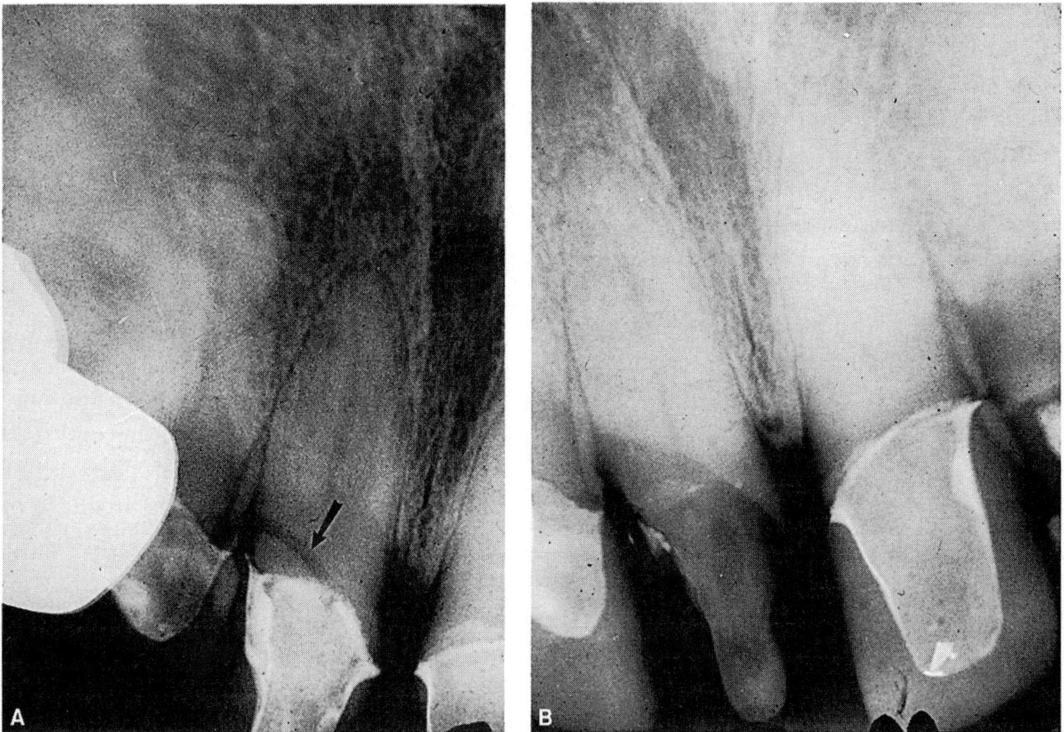

Figure 6-72 A, Radiolucent line (**arrow**) is suspected of being a fracture under the jacket crown. **B**, The jacket crown is removed, and the "fracture" becomes a high chamfer preparation. (Courtesy of Dr. Cyril Gaum.)

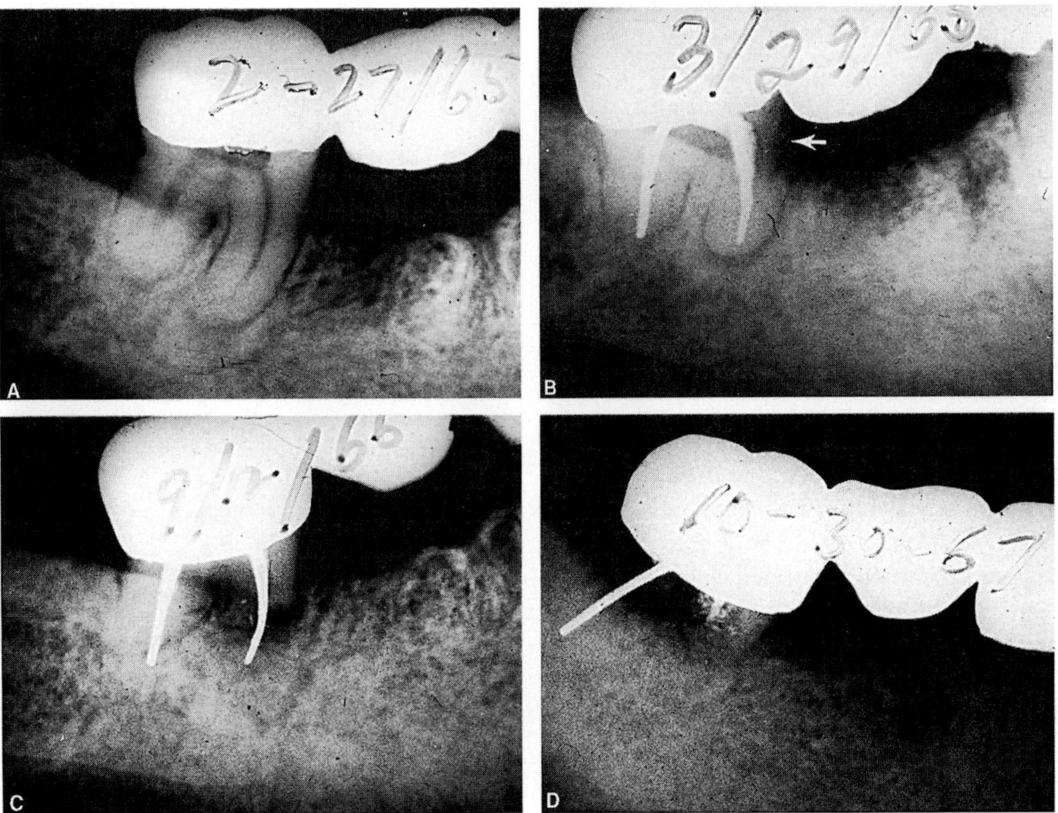

Figure 6-73 Unexplained root resorption of bridge abutment in a patient with breast cancer. **A**, Initial film. **B**, One month later. **C**, Seven months later. **D**, Two and a half years later. (Courtesy of Dr. Cyril Gaum.)

Before proceeding with a detailed examination, the most obvious causes of failure should be eliminated: is the canal incompletely cleaned and filled, or, on the other hand, is there an obvious perforation of the root, obvious overfilling, or a crown or root fracture? If all of the obvious factors can be eliminated, then some other obscure cause of failure must be present. Remember, hoof beats usually means horses, not zebras!

The examiner should then begin a detailed examination following a four-stage procedure. One of these four steps in the examination should reveal the cause of failure:

1. Complete a thorough radiographic study of the involved tooth with exposure from three different horizontal projections, the standard buccal-to-lingual projection, 20 degrees from the mesial, and 20 degrees from the distal. **The central beam must pass directly through the apex.** If this does not reveal incomplete obturation of the apical one-third of the canal, a canal obviously not filled, a perforated canal, or an **extra canal** or root, then proceed to
2. Examine the involved tooth for signs of occlusal traumatism. Test the mobility of the tooth and, using the forefinger, test for movement under the forces of centric closure and both lateral excursions. Be certain to check the tooth for trauma in the **non-functional,** lateral position or "balance." Look for telltale wear facets on occluding surfaces. If the tooth is not being traumatized by bruxism or an extraoral habit, then proceed to
3. Check the vitality of adjacent teeth to be sure that the periradicular lesion is not being maintained by an adjacent necrotic pulp. If all of these points of examination check out as normal, then
4. Check the involved tooth and adjacent teeth for a coexistent periodontal lesion. This step should be left until last because the area may have to be anesthetized to complete the periodontal probing to depth.

If all of these causes are checked and eliminated by examination, one may assume that failure is owing to an unusual factor such as a vertical root fracture or an incomplete root canal preparation and filling that does not show radiographically. If the unusual can be eliminated by careful questioning, observation, and examination, the examiner should finally suspect incomplete canal treatment, and steps should be taken to eliminate the cause.

Crump has summarized this very well, using the mnemonic device of **POOR PAST**, an acronym in which each letter stands for the failure to search for the following[125]:

P = Perforation	P = Periodontal disease
O = Obturation incomplete	A = Another tooth
O = Overfill	S = Split tooth
R = Root canal overlooked	T = Trauma

By using the recall of POOR PAST as a check list, the clinician can go through all of the etiologic possibilities until finally arriving at the culprit. Unless the situation is hopeless, as with advanced periodontal disease or a vertical fracture, re-treatment will often reverse a failure into a success (see chapter 13). Occasionally, to get additional information, occlusal films or lateral head films are necessary to "reach" beyond the limits of the standard periradicular film. Teeth that "disappear" from traumatic intrusion may be shown on these films but off the scope of a periradicular film.

REFERENCES

1. Krasny RM. Seven steps to better doctor-patient communications. Dent Econ 1982;60:26.
2. Medawar PD. The art of the soluble. London: Metheun;
3. Bolden TE, et al. Effect of prolonged use of analgesics on pulpal responses: a preliminary investigation. J Dent Res 1975;54:198.
4. Cecic PA, Hartwell GR, Bellizzi R. Cold as a diagnostic aid in cases of irreversible pulpitis. Oral Surg 1983;56:647.
5. Abou-Raas M. The stressed pulp condition: an endodontic restorative diagnostic concept. J Prosthet Dent 1982;48:264.
6. Hamersky PA, et al. The effect of orthodontic force application on the pulpal tissue respiration rate in the human premolar. Am J Orthodont 1980;77:368.
7. Sternbach RA. Pain patients: traits and treatments. New York: Academic Press; 1974.
8. Halpern IL. Patient's medical status—a factor in dental treatment. Oral Surg 1975;39:216.
9. Andrews CH, et al. Sickle cell anemia: an etiological factor in pulpal necrosis. JOE 1983;9:249.
10. Biesterfeld RC, et al. Aspirin: an update. JOE 1978;4:198.
11. Abbey LM, Hargrove B. Guidelines for a dental office high blood pressure screening program. Virg Dent J 1974;51:52.
12. Summers G.W. The diagnosis and management of dental infections. Otolaryngol Clin North Am 1976;8:717.
13. American Cancer Society. Oral cancer examination procedure. New York: The American Cancer Society.
14. Tarsitano JJ. The use of antibiotics in dental practice. Dent Clin North Am 1970;14:697.
15. Cohen SR. Follow-up evaluation of 15 patients with myofascial pain-dysfunction syndrome. J Am Dent Assoc 1978;97:825.
16. Guralnick W, Kaban LB, Merrill RB. Temporomandibular joint affliction. N Engl J Med 1978;299:123.
17. Hill CM. The efficacy of transillumination in vitality tests. Int Endod J 1986;19:198.
18. Cameron CE. The cracked tooth syndrome. J Am Dent Assoc 1976;93:971.
19. Fulling HJ, Andreasen JO. Influence of splints and temporary crowns upon electric and thermal pulp-testing procedures. Scand J Dent Res 1976;84:291.

20. Dachi SF, et al. Standardization of a test for dental sensitivity to cold. Oral Surg 1976;29:687.
21. Ehrman EH. Pulp testers and pulp testing with particular reference to the use of dry ice. Aust Dent J 1977;22:272.
22. Fuss Z, et al. Assessment of reliability of electric and thermal pulp testing agents. JOE 1986;12:301.
23. Rickoff B, et al. Effects of thermal vitality tests on human dental pulp. JOE 1988;14:482.
24. Peters DD, et al. Evaluation of the effects of carbon dioxide used as a pulp test. Part III. *In vivo* effect on human enamel. JOE 1986;12:13.
25. Krell KV, et al. The effects of CO_2 ice on PFM restorations [abstract]. JOE 1985;11:
26. Erdelsky I, Dedik J. An apparatus to determine pulp vitality by cold. Pract Zub Lek 1976;24:555.
27. Augsburger RA, Peters DD. In vitro effects of ice, skin refrigerant, and CO_2 show on intrapulpal temperature. JOE 1981;7:110.
28. Peters DD, et al. Evaluation of the effects of utilizing carbon dioxide as a pulpal test. Part I. In vitro effect on human enamel surface. JOE 1983;9:219.
29. Ingram TA, Peters DD. Evaluation of the effect of carbon dioxide used as a pulpal test. Part II. In vivo effect on canine enamel and pulpal tissue. JOE 1983;9:296.
30. White JH, Cooley RL. A quantitative evaluation of thermal pulp testing. JOE 1977;3:453.
31. Bellizzi R, et al. Sinusitis secondary to pregnancy rhinitis mimicking pain of endodontic origin. A case report. JOE 1983;9:60.
32. Weisman MI. Reverberation—an aid in endodontic diagnosis. JOE 1981;7:459.
33. Matthews B, Searle BN. Some observations on pulp testers. Br Dent J 1974;137:307.
34. Kidder RS, Michelich RJ, Walton RE. Clinical study of patient reaction to pulp testing instruments. Presented at the meeting of the American Association of Endodontists in Los Angeles, California, April 18, 1980.
35. Kitamura T, Takahashi T, Horiuchi H. Electrical characteristics and clinical application of a new automatic pulp tester. Jpn J Conserv Dent 1979;22:202.
36. Dummer PMH, et al. A laboratory study of four electric pulp testers. Int Endodont J 1986;19:161.
37. Dummer PMH, Tanner M. The response of caries-free, unfilled teeth to electrical excitation: a comparison of two new pulp testers. Int Endodont J 1986;19:172.
38. Cooley RL, et al. Evaluation of a digital pulp tester. Oral Surg 1984;58:437.
39. Davies AL, Rawlinson A. A comparison between two electric vitality testers and ethyl chloride with special reference to a newly available device. Int Endodont J 1988;21:320.
40. Jacobson JJ. Probe placement during electric pulp testing procedures. Oral Surg 1984;58:242.
41. Bender IB, et al. The optimum placement—site of the electrode in electric pulp testing of the 12 anterior teeth. J Am Dent Assoc 1989;118:305.
42. Johnson DC, et al. Quantitative assessment of neural development in human premolars. Anat Rec 1983;205:421.
43. Fulling HJ, Andreasen JO. Influence of maturation status and tooth type of permanent teeth upon electrometric and thermal pulp testing. Scand J Dent Res 1976;84:286.
44. Fuss A, et al. Assessment of reliability of electrical and thermal pulp testing agents. JOE 1986;12:301.
45. Trowbridge HO. Review of dental pain—history and physiology. JOE 1986;12:445.
46. Cailleteau JG, Ludington JR. Using the electric pulp tester with gloves: a simplified approach. JOE 1989;15:80.
47. Anderson RW, Pantera EA. Influence of a barrier technique on electric pulp testing. JOE 1988;14:179.
48. Pantera EA, Anderson RW. Use of dental instruments for bridging electric pulp testing. JOE 1992;18:37.
49. Woolley L, et al. A preliminary evaluation of the effect of electric pulp testers on dogs with artificial pacemakers. J Am Dent Assoc 1974;89:1099.
50. Howell RM, Duell RC, Mullancy TD. The determination of pulp vitality by thermographic means using cholesteric liquid crystals. Oral Surg 1970;29:763.
51. Gazelius B, et al. Non-invasive recordings of blood flow in human dental pulp. Endodont Dent Traumatol 1986;2:219.
52. Wilder-Smith PEEB. A new method for the noninvasive measurement of pulpal blood flow. Int Endodont J 1988;21:307.
53. Rowe AHR, Pitt-Ford TR. The assessment of pulpal vitality. Int Endodont J 1990;23:77.
54. Pogrel MA, et al. Studies in tooth crown temperature gradients with the use of infrared thermography. Oral Surg 1989;67:583.
55. Biesterfield RC, et al. The endodontal-periodontal relationship. Gen Dent 1981;29:118.
56. Morgulis JR, Oliver RC. Developing a periodontal screening examination. J Calif Dent Assoc 1979;7:59.
57. Hiatt WH. Histologic and clinical assessment of long-term pulpal-periodontal therapy. Oral Surg 1982;54:436.
58. Trabert KC, et al. Tooth fracture—a comparison of endodontic and restorative treatments. JOE 1978;4:341.
59. Cohen S, Schwartz S. Endodontic complications and the law. JOE 1987;13:191.
60. Wuehrmann AH. Radiation hygiene and its practice in dentistry are related to film viewing procedures and radiographic interpretation. J Am Dent Assoc 1970;80:346.
61. Brynolf I. Radiography of the periradicular region as a diagnostic aid. I. Diagnosis of marginal changes. Dent Radiogr Photogr 1978;51:21.
62. Brynolf I. Seminar on radiology, Loma Linda University, Loma Linda, California, November 14, 1985.
63. Kaffe I, Gratt BM. Variations in the radiographic interpretation of the periapical dental region. JOE 1988;14:330.
64. Nasstrom K, et al. Narrowing the dental pulp chamber in patients with renal disease. Oral Surg 1985;59:242.
65. Goldman M, et al. Reliability of radiographic interpretations. Oral Surg 1974;38:287.
66. Goldman M, et al. Endodontic success—who's reading the radiograph? Oral Surg 1972;33:432.
67. Gelfand M, Sunderman EJ, Goldman M. Reliability of radiological interpretations. JOE 1983;9:71.
68. Lambrianidis T. Observe variations in radiographic evaluation of endodontic therapy. Endodont Dent Traumatol 1985;1:235.
69. Antrim DD. Reading the radiograph: a comparison of viewing techniques. JOE 1983;9:502.
70. Weine FS. Lecture on endodontics, Palm Springs Seminar, Palm Springs, California, February 5, 1990.
71. Shoha RR, Dowson J, Richards AG. Radiographic interpretations of experimentally produced bony lesions. Oral Surg 1974;38:294.
72. van der Stelt PF. Experimentally produced bone lesions. Oral Surg 1985;59:306.

73. Bender IB. Factors influencing the radiographic appearance of bony lesions [published erratum appears in JOE 1982;8:332].
74. Bellizzi R, Hartwell G. Radiographic evaluation of root canal anatomy of *in vivo* endodontically treated maxillary premolars. JOE 1985;11:37.
75. Pineda F, Kuttler Y. Mesiodistal and buccolingual roentgenographic investigation of 7,275 root canals. Oral Surg 1972;33:101.
76. Green D. Double canals in single roots. Oral Surg 1973;35:689.
77. Vertucci FJ, et al. Root canal morphology of the human maxillary second premolars. Oral Surg 1972;38:456.
78. Goerig AC, Neaverth EJ. A simplified look at the buccal object rule in endodontics. JOE 1987;13:570.
79. Slowey RR. Radiographic aids in the detection of extra root canals. Oral Surg 1974;37:762.
80. Weine FS, Healy HJ, Gerstein H, Evanson L. Canal configuration in the mesiobuccal root of the maxillary first molar and its endodontic significance. Oral Surg 1969;28:419.
81. Pineda F. Roentgenographic investigation of the mesiobuccal root of the maxillary first molar. Oral Surg 1973;36:253.
82. Seidberg BH, et al. Frequency of two mesiobuccal root canals in maxillary permanent first molars. J Am Dent Assoc 1973; 87:852.
83. Pomeranz HH, Fishelberg G. The secondary mesiobuccal canal of maxillary molars. J Am Dent Assoc 1974;88:119.
84. Hartwell G, Bellizzi R. Clinical investigation of *in vivo* endodontically treated mandibular and maxillary molars. JOE 1982;8:555.
85. Gartner AH, Sommerlott R, Walsh L. Differential diagnosis of internal and external resorption. Paper presented at the meeting of the American Association of Endodontists, New Orleans, LA. April 25, 1975.
86. Wedeberg C, Zettesqvist L. Internal resorption in human teeth—a histological scanning electron microscopic and enzyme histochemical study. JOE 1988;13:255.
87. Wedenberg C, Lindskog S. Experimental internal resorption in monkey teeth. Endodont Dent Traumatol 1985;1:221.
88. Lynch EJ, Ahlberg KF. Bilateral idiopathic root resorption of upper first premolars. Int Endodont J 1984;17:218.
89. Solomon CS, et al. Herpes zoster revisited: implicated in root resorption. JOE 1986;12:210.
90. Andreasen JO. External root resorption: its implication in dental traumatology, paedodontics, periodontics, orthodontics, and endodontics. Int Endodont J 1985;18:109.
91. Frank AL. External-internal progressive resorption and its nonsurgical correction. JOE 1981;7:473.
92. Fish EW. Benign neopolasias of tooth and bone. Proc R Soc Med 1941;34:427.
93. Wade AB. Basic periodontology. Bristol (UK): Wright & Sons; 1980.
94. Southan JC. Clinical and histopathological aspects of peripheral cervical resorptions. J Periodontol 1987;38:534.
95. Makkes PC. Thoden van Velzen SK. Cervical external root resorption. J Dent 1975;3:217.
96. Gold SI, Hasselgren G. Peripheral inflammatory root resorption: a review of the literature with case reports. J Clin Periodontol 1992;19:523.
97. Tronstad L. Root resorption: etiology and terminology and clinical manifestrations. Endod Dent Traumatol 1988;4:241.
98. Trope M, Chivian N. Root resorption. In: Cohen S, Burns R, editors. Pathways of the pulp. 6th ed. St. Louis: CV Mosby; 1994. p. 493–503.
99. Heithersay GS. Clinical, radiologic, and histopathologic features of invasive cervical resorption. Quintessence Int 1999;30:27.
100. Frank AL, Simon JHS, Glick DH, Abou-Raas M. Clinical and surgical endodontics: concepts in practice. Philadelphia: JB Lippincott; 1983.
101. Jaacob HB. The resistant shell of teeth suffering from idiopathic external resorption. Aust Dent J 1980;25:73.
102. Wedenberg C, Lindskog S. Evidence for a resorption inhibitor in dentin. Scand J Dent Res 1987;95:270.
103. Heithersay GS. Invasive cervical resorption: analysis of potential predisposing factors. Quintessence Int 1999;30:83.
104. Gaudet EL Jr. Tissue changes in the monkey following root torque with the BEGG technique. Am J Orthodont 1970;58:164.
105. Remington DN, et al. Long-term evaluation of root resorption occurring during orthodontic treatment. Am J Orthodont Dentofac Orthoped 1989;96:43.
106. Cwyk F, et al. Endodontic implications of orthodontic tooth movement [abstract]. JOE 1984;10:
107. Heithersay GS. Treatment of invasive cervical resorption: an analysis of results using topical application of trichloracetic acid, curettage, and restoration. Quintessence Int 1999;30:96.
108. Eliasson S, et al. Periapical condensing osteitis and endodontic treatment. Oral Surg 1984;57:195.
109 Geist JR, Katz JO. The frequency and distribution of idiopathic osteosclerosis. Oral Surg 1990;69:388.
110. Eversole LR, et al. Focal sclerosing osteomyelitis/focal periapical osteopetrosis; radiographic patterns. Oral Surg 1984;58:456.
111. Natkin E, et al. The relationship of lesion size to diagnosis, incidence, and treatment of periapical cysts and granulomas. Oral Surg 1984;57:82.
112. Weine FS, Silverlade LB. Residual cysts masquerading as periapical lesions. J Am Dent Assoc 1983;106:833.
113. Warnakulasuriya S, et al. Familial hyperparathyroidism associated with cementifying fibroma of the jaws in two siblings. Oral Surg 1985;59:269.
114. Marks JM, Dunkelberger FB. Paget's disease. J Am Dent Assoc 1980;101:49.
115. Riley RR. Endodontic recall procedures. Oral Surg 1974;37:118.
116. Harris WE. Unusual endodontic complication: report of a case. J Am Dent Assoc 1971;83:358.
117. Heling I, Rotstein I. A persistent oronasal sinus tract of endodontic origin. JOE 1989;15:132.
118. Goldstein N, Gibilisco J, Rushton J. Trigeminal neuropathy and neuritis. JAMA 1963;184:458.
119. Thrush DC, Small M. How benign a symptom is facial numbness? Lancet 1970;11:851.
120. Glick DH. Presentation before the American Association of Endodontists, Hollywood, FL, April 1983.
121. Verunac JJ. Recurrent severe facial emphysema in a submariner. J Am Dent Assoc 1973;87:1192.
122. Senia S, Cunningham KW, Marxe RE. The diagnostic dilemma of barodontalgia. Oral Surg 1985;60:212.
123. Boucher Y, Sobel M, Sauveur G. Persistent pain related to root canal filling and apical fenestration. JOE 2000;26:242.
124. Pankhurst CL, et al. Multiple idiopathic external root resorption. Oral Surg 1988;65:754.
125. Crump MC. Differential diagnosis in endodontic failure. Dent Clin North Am 1979;23:617.

Chapter 7

DIFFERENTIAL DIAGNOSIS AND TREATMENT OF DENTAL PAIN

John I. Ingle and Dudley H. Glick

"For there was never yet a philosopher who could endure the toothache patiently."

–William Shakespeare,
Much Ado About Nothing, Act V, Scene 1

Orofacial pain is a major public health problem. This fact was recently emphasized by a report from the US National Center for Health Statistics (NCHS). Although their figures and estimates apply only to the United States, they may generally be extrapolated worldwide.

The NCHS interviewed "45,711 households in the US civilian population." This was the 1989 National Health Interview Survey (NHIS). Using the statistics developed from this survey, the National Institute of Dental Research reported in 1993 that "about 39 million people or about 22% of the U.S. population 18 years of age or older are estimated to have experienced at least one of five types of orofacial pain more than once during the past six months."[1]

This alarming cohort of 39 million can be further broken down into 22 million toothaches (12.2%), 15 million oral sores (8.4%), 9.5 million "jaw joint" pains (1.4%), and 1.3 million burning mouth pains (0.7%). The total adds up to more than 39 million because some respondents suffered from more than one type of orofacial pain.[1] Of the 45,711 households interviewed, 9,072 people reported orofacial pain. These figures, extrapolated nationwide, may actually be too low because the Armed Forces, institutions (prisons, etc), and children under age 18 were not included in the statistics.

The shocking revelation that 22 million people in the United States suffer from a toothache within a 6-month period is an overall prevalence rate of 12,261 persons per 100,000 population. The prevalence for African Americans (14,584) and Hispanics (14,226) was even higher.[1]

By all odds, the most frequently seen "pain" patient will be experiencing acute, true intraoral pain, toothache and its sequelae being the most common. Pain accompanying intraoral lesions and infections is the next most commonly seen. After that, the field thins somewhat, with top priority going to the **acute** pains of everyday general, endodontic, and oral surgery practice.

Less commonly seen, but a good deal more baffling, are the chronic pains found in and around the mouth, a number of them referred there from faraway sites. These are the craniofacial pains to be discussed in detail in Chapter 8. Because these two types of oral and perioral pain are so different in diagnosis and management, they will be dealt with separately, even though there is often a confusing overlap.

The first premise in diagnosis is to "play the percentages," thinking first of the most commonly occurring. As the old saying goes, "If you hear hoofbeats, think of horses, not zebras." If an obvious diagnosis is not immediately apparent, a good diagnostician begins with the most frequent cause of this type of pain, not some obscure, seldom seen syndrome. Systematically working down through the pain roster, from most common to least common, a logical diagnosis is finally arrived at.

A well-trained dentist may render many services that gain him a deep personal satisfaction. Foremost among these are the diagnosis and relief of excruciating or long-lasting pain. These are the occasions patients remember most vividly: "the night you came back at midnight and relieved my terrible toothache," or "…you diagnosed the constant pain I had for 3 years, Doctor, and after everyone else had given up."

Solving these problems is rarely rewarding financially, but they are the few moments we as a profession enjoy that set us apart from the lay public. These problems also try one's patience and ingenuity; only the skilled are successful in diagnosing and managing the really difficult cases.

Diagnosis is a personal and cognitive experience; therefore, many of the qualities of a good diagnostician are of an interpersonal nature and based on knowledge, experience, and diagnostic tools. Diagnosing orofacial disease is similar to medical diagnosis. The pulp test, radiographs, percussion, palpation, and other tests and procedures can facilitate the diagnosing of facial disease, just as the electrocardiograph, electroencephalograph, liver and kidney function tests, echocardiograph, computed axial tomographic scanners, and a host of other radiographs can facilitate medical diagnosis.

REQUIREMENTS OF A DIAGNOSTICIAN

A dentist can develop a number of assets to become a successful diagnostician. Again, the most important of these are **knowledge**, **interest**, **intuition**, **curiosity**, and **patience**. The successful diagnostician must also have acute senses and the necessary tools for diagnosis. For a detailed discussion of these assets, see Chapter 6.

HISTORY, EXAMINATION, DIAGNOSTIC TESTS, AND CONSULTATIONS

The important steps leading to a diagnosis and establishing a plan of treatment have been dealt with in depth in the previous chapter. Additional information, necessary to establish a diagnosis in chronic extracranial and intracranial pain complexes, will be detailed in the next chapter dealing with craniofacial pain.

PULP PAIN

Pulp pain, or **pulpalgia,** is by far the most commonly experienced pain in and near the oral cavity and may be classified according to the degree of severity and the pathologic process present:

1. Hyperreactive pulpalgia
   a. Dentinal hypersensitivity
   b. Hyperemia
2. Acute pulpalgia
   a. Incipient
   b. Moderate
   c. Advanced
3. Chronic pulpalgia
   a. Barodontalgia
4. Hyperplastic pulpitis
5. Necrotic pulp
6. Internal resorption
7. Traumatic occlusion
8. Incomplete fracture

The mildest pulp discomfort, experienced when no inflammation is present, is **hyperreactive pulpalgia.**

Hyperreactive Pulpalgia

Hyperreactive pulpalgia is characterized by a **short, sharp, shock**—that is, "pain" best described as a sensation of sudden **shock.** The sensation is as sharp as it is sudden and **must be elicited** by some exciting factor. **It is never spontaneous.** The pain is of short duration, lasting only slightly longer than the time during which the irritating element is in contact with the tooth. In some manner, the odontoblastic cellular body within the dentin must be excited by a noxious stimulus, either hot or cold, sweet or sour, or touch. Excitation of the odontoblast conducts the excitation to the pulp nerves. These "dentinal receptors have the characteristics of slow adaptation."[3]

It is difficult to explain to a patient that the severe pain experienced when eating ice cream—a blinding pain that extends upward through the eye and into the forehead—is really normal and not pathologic. In "lay terms," one can only tell the patient that the cold "excites" the nerve in the tooth, and the pain is so severe it is referred upward through the eye.

The dentist, however, requires a more sophisticated explanation. Although this is hard to come by, the best explanation revolves around thinking of the fluid in the dentinal tubules, along with the odontoblast cells, as a "pump"—a hydrodynamic theory, if you will, that proposes that the fluid moves back and forth to stretch, compress, and excite the pulp nerves.[4]

Brännström pointed out that "the displacement of tubule contents, if the movement occurs rapidly enough, may produce deformation of nerve fibers in the pulp or predentin or damage to the cells; both of these effects may be capable of producing pain."[4] Such a mechanical transmission of the stimulus would account for the hitherto inexplicably great sensitivity of the dentin to pain, in spite of the apparent absence of nerve fibers in this tissue.[4]

Brännström further confirmed the damage and pain generated by blowing air over exposed dentin.[5] A short air blast evaporates from 0.1 to 0.3 mm of fluid from the dentinal tubule. This results in immediate capillary fluid replacement from the pulp's blood supply, sucking the odontoblasts and nerve fibers up into the tubule. The nerves are stretched or even torn off, eliciting pain (Figure 7-1).

On continued exposure to an air blast, however, a plug of fluid protein builds up in the tubule, preventing fluid outflow. This plug "closes the pump" and leads to dentin **in**sensitivity. When water is applied to the dentin surface, however, the plug "melts" and sensitivity returns (see Figure 7-1).

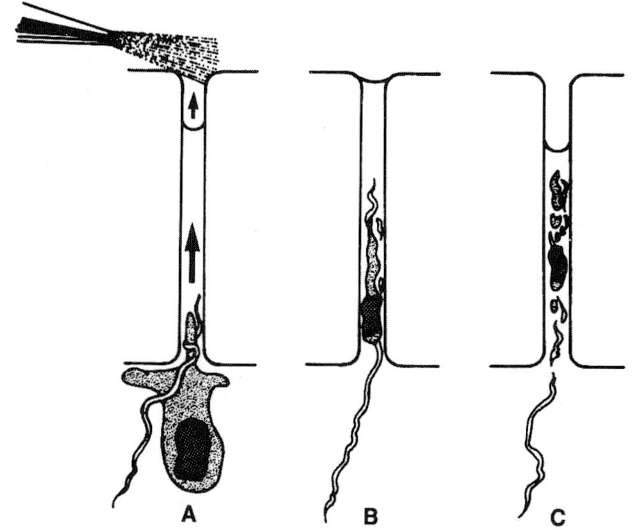

Figure 7-1 Pain produced by air blast. A, Air evaporates dentinal fluid, causing rapid outflow (arrows) owing to capillary pressure from the pulp's vessels. B, Odontoblast and accompanying nerve fiber aspirated into tubule, stretching nerve and causing pain. C, Prolonged air blast caused a protein plug to form in the tubule, preventing outward flow. Redrawn with permission from Brännström M. Dentin and pulp in restorative dentistry. Nacka (Sweden): Dental Therapeutics AB; 1981. p. 15.

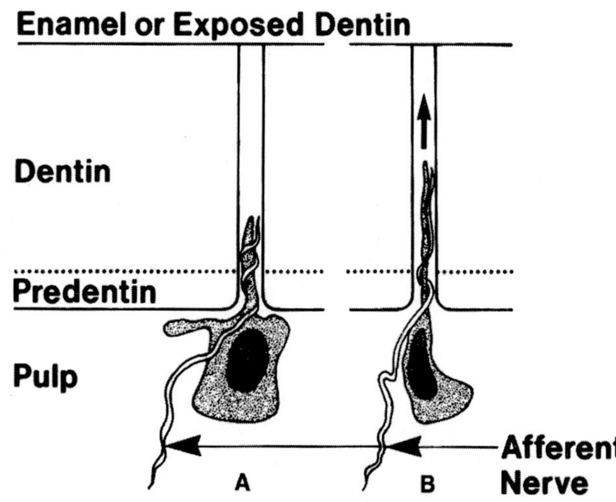

Figure 7-2 The effect of cold stimulus on the pulp. A, Cold is applied to the tooth, causing a contraction of fluid in tubule. B, Pulp capillary pressure forces replacement fluid into the tubule along with the odontoblast and afferent nerve. Stretching of nerve (arrow) produces intense pain. Redrawn with permission from Brännström M. Dentin and pulp in restorative dentistry. Nacka (Sweden): Dental Therapeutics AB; 1981. p. 17.

The same phenomenon is produced by the dental drill, the frictional heat and surface pressure displacing the tubule fluid and causing pain. Scraping or chiseling the dentin produces similar pressure and pain.

Pulp pain produced by cold is a similar phenomenon. When cold is applied, the fluid in the tubules contracts, thus redirecting the fluid volume. Fluid contraction within the tubules again produces fluid outflow owing to the normal pulp pressure, and the nerves are once again stretched into the tubules along with the odontoblasts (Figure 7-2).[5] Beveridge measured a fall in intrapulp pressure when cold was applied to a tooth[6] (Figure 7-3). Researchers in Israel found this to be an "interstitial" pressure fall, whereas the "arterial transmural" pressure rose.[7]

Hyperreactive pulpalgia owing to the application of heat is more easily explained. Again, Beveridge easily demonstrated a true increase in intrapulp pressure when heat was applied to the tooth (Figure 7-4). An increase of pressure within the pulp serves to excite the sensory pulp nerves.[6]

Three different types of response to heat have also been recorded from pulp nerve fibers: (1) a transient type of response when pulp nerve fiber was excited by heat over 43°C (the response ceased as soon as the temperature fell below the firing points), (2) a long-lasting type of response that started at over 45°C and continued even after the temperature had returned to the initial level for a few minutes, and (3) a pulsating type of response in which the discharge of the fiber was synchronized with the heartbeat.[8]

Brännström added to the understanding of the "pumping" excitation by dentinal fluid when he pointed out, "Fluids have a considerably greater coefficient of expansion than solids—a sudden rise in temperature of 20°C at the outer one-third of the closed tubule

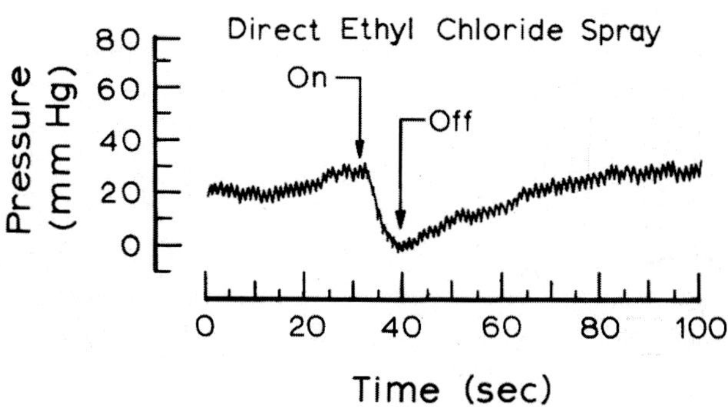

Figure 7-3 Effect of intrapulp pressure by application of cold ethyl chloride spray to anesthetized mandibular premolar in a 13-year-old boy. Within 8 seconds, intrapulp pressure had dropped from 30 mm Hg to nearly zero. After the irritant was removed, pressure returned to initial baseline within 1 minute. Reproduced with permission from Beveridge EE, and Brown AC.[14]

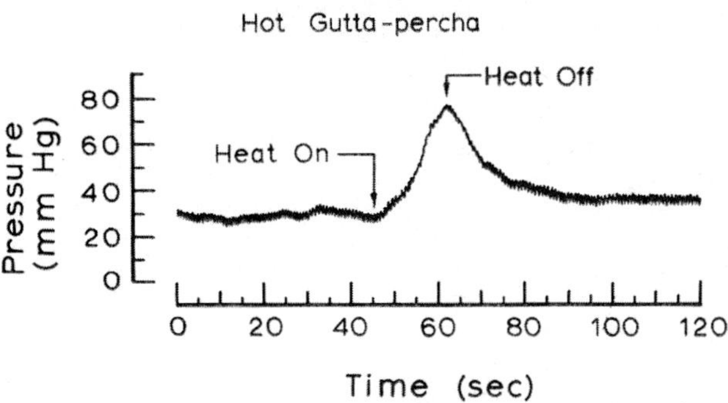

Figure 7-4 Effect on intrapulp pressure by application of hot gutta-percha to an anesthetized maxillary premolar in a 12-year-old girl. Within 15 seconds, the intrapulp pressure had more than doubled. After heat was removed, the intrapulp pressure dropped precipitously but not to the original baseline. Reproduced with permission from Beveridge EE, and Brown AC.[14]

might result in an immediate pulpward movement of about 5 micra of the content of the tubules,"[9] once again stretching the afferent nerves.

Hyperreactive pulpalgia is common following the placement of a new restoration. Patients also complain after root planing and curettage or following periodontal surgery, which exposes the root surface. Hyperreactive pulpalgia also may be present in the tooth with a carious lesion. Teeth traumatized by bruxism or incompletely fractured teeth are generally more hyperreactive, as are the maxillary teeth involved in maxillary sinusitis.

It is possible, with our present level of knowledge, to divide the sensations of hyperreactive pulpalgia into hypersensitivity and hyperemia.

Dentinal Hypersensitivity

The exciting factors of a hypersensitive pulp are usually cold food or drink or cold air, contact of two dissimilar metals that will yield a galvanic shock, or stimulation of the exposed dentin on the root surface by cold, sweet or sour substances, vegetable or fruit acid, salt, or glycerine, or often just touching the surface with a fingernail, a toothbrush, an interdental stimulator, or an explorer. One should not be surprised at this latter reaction when the microanatomy of the dentin and pulp is reviewed. The cementum covering the gingival root dentin frequently is missing or has been removed by curettage or brushing, exposing the dentinal tubules. It has also been reported that the use of the new "calculus-removing" toothpastes leads to an increased dentinal hypersensitivity. Evidently, these agents remove the surface smear layer and open the dentinal tubuli orifices (Palm Springs Seminars, Palm Springs, California, 1990, Lecture, Ingle JI.).

When one considers that "one square millimeter of dentin contains approximately 30,000 tubules*[10] and that "approximately 25% of the volume of the dentin is occupied by fluid, most of which is in the dentinal tubules,"[11] one must be struck by the capacity for fluid dynamic hypersensitivity emanating from exposed dentin.

This is a frequent complaint following periodontal surgery when whole areas of root are exposed by the apically repositioned gingiva. Add to this the careful root preparation that removes most of the cementum covering the dentin. The problem is then compounded by two other avenues leading to irritation: the use of citric acid on the root surface to remove the smear layer that may "plug" the tubuli and the formation of dental plaque on the root surfaces.[12] The acid-releasing bacteria in the plaque set up a steady barrage of irritation into the dentinal tubules.

This is a "catch-22" equation: the hypersensitive dentin is "painful" to brush and floss and therefore is avoided by the patient. The bacterial plaque that then forms causes greater sensitivity, so the area is avoided all the more during home care, which, in turn, leads to more plaque and greater sensitivity. Relieving the sensitivity is the only solution to the problem.

One is led to conjecture about the pulp sensation stimulated by sour substances, fruit juices, sugar, salt, and dissimilar metals, which may be described as an electric current flowing between the oral cavity and the pulp. Sicher postulated that the oral cavity is positively charged and the pulp is negatively charged (personal communication, 1958). Any electrolyte, such as salt or fruit acid, upsets this ionic balance, and the resultant current stimulates the nerve endings to the odontoblasts. The sensation disappears as soon as the electrolyte is diluted away or metal (such as aluminum foil) is removed. In addition to the current flow theory, Anderson believes that "pain can be evoked from dentin by applying to it solutions which exert high osmotic pressure."[13] Brännström pursued this idea further, although he believes it is not simply a question of osmosis but relates again to the hydrodynamic "pump"—concentrated solutions of sugar, salt, etc dehydrate the tubule contents, causing their rapid outflow and deformation of the nerves within the tubule.[4,5] Brännström also pointed out that a similar mechanism is operant when cracks develop in the dentin—that is, as a cusp flexes with biting pressure, the fluid in the tubules is pumped back and forth (especially on release), which stimulates the pain response.[5]

*This figure varies between 10,000 and 30,000 depending on the location in the tooth—crown or root.

Hyperemia

All minor pulp sensations were once thought to be associated with **hyperemia**, an increased blood flow in the pulp. The investigations of Beveridge and Brown demonstrated, however, that an increase in intrapulp tissue pressure is produced only when heat is applied to the tooth, not when cold is applied.[6,14] The increased pressure against the sensory nerve endings in the pulp might well produce the sensation associated with hyperemia. Quite possibly, this will explain why the pain appears to be of a different intensity and character with applications of cold or heat, the cold producing a sharp hypersensitivity response and the heat producing true transient hyperemia and a dull pain.

This difference in the character of the painful response between cold and hot might well be explained by the difference in the nerve fibers supplying the pulp:

> The pulp contains both myelinated A nerve fibers and unmyelinated C nerve fibers. The former [A] are fast-conducting and have a low response threshold, whereas the latter [C] are slow-conducting with a higher activation threshold. Activation of the A fibers...will cause a sharp localized response, whereas activation of C fibers will cause a dull, poorly localized response.[10]

Cold stimulates the fast-conducting A fibers, producing the sharp, localized pain. Continued heat application, on the other hand, will more likely stimulate the slower-conducting C fibers, deeper in the pulp, with a resulting dull pain of longer duration, the pain also experienced with early pulpitis.[10] Trowbridge concurred in reviewing the action of the A and C fibers and pointed out that approximately 25% of the dentinal tubules contain nerve fibers.[11]

The converse of "pain from pressure" also appears to be true. Beveridge and Brown have shown the **effect of pain** on intrapulp pressure.[14] Paradoxically, pulp pain causes first a fall and then, when removed, a rise in intrapulp tissue pressure (Figure 7-5): "This again raises the question of the role of neural control in the regulation of intrapulp pressure."[14] It was also discovered that intrapulp pressure decreased when the patient fell asleep and increased when she awakened.

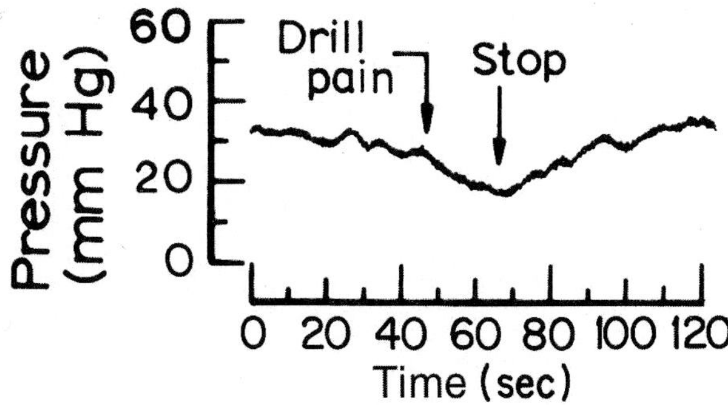

Figure 7-5 Effect on a partially anesthetized pulp from pain elicited by cavity preparation on the maxillary premolar of an 11-year-old girl. Intrapulp pressure dropped about 10 mm Hg within 25 seconds, during which the patient experienced pain. When drilling ceased, intrapulp pressure climbed slowly to a level slightly higher than the original baseline. Reproduced with permission from Beveridge EE, and Brown AC.[14]

Examination

Determining which tooth is hyperreactive by examination is not always as simple a step as it might seem. A patient may complain of the symptoms of hypersensitivity on taking cold water into the mouth. On the other hand, ice on the suspected tooth during examination may not elicit an unusual reaction. In this case, the entire tooth must be surrounded by cold for the pulp to react. This particular condition is best checked by isolating the teeth adjacent to the suspected tooth behind a heavy rubber dam and then playing a stream of ice water onto the tooth being examined.

If the tooth has had a recent restoration, it usually responds to applications of ice, carbon dioxide "ice," or Fluori-Methane (Gebauer Chemical Co., Cleveland, Ohio) or ethyl chloride sprayed on a large cotton pellet. Cervical dentin exposed by scratching with an explorer may also elicit a pain response.

Hyperreactive teeth are also said to be more sensitive to the pulp tester; that is, "they require lower levels of electrical stimulation to produce a response."[10] "Electrical stimulation is different from other types of stimuli in that it does not cause movement of the fluid within the dentinal tubules."[10] The sensation derived from electrical stimulation has been described as a "prepain" sensation—"tingling, hot, sharp or warm; rarely is it described as painful."[10]

Some of the fast-conducting A fibers are initially stimulated by electricity and are described by Nahri as A beta fibers with conduction velocities well beyond the A delta fibers stimulated by tubule fluid movement. At higher levels of electrical stimulation, the slower C fibers "kick in" so that the summation of A and C fibers produces the painful response "associated with higher electrical stimulation."[15]

Treatment

Grossman has stated, "The best treatment for hyperemia lies in its prevention."[16] This is sound advice. Application of the new resin adhesives or placement of an insulating base under metallic restorations will materially reduce most hypersensitivity. Moreover, this sensation usually diminishes gradually as irritation dentin builds to protect the dental pulp.

There is, however, another source of continuing irritation often overlooked—microleakage.[17] Virtually every restoration placed—amalgam, resin, cemented restorations—will share some degree of microleakage around and under the filling. The bacteria collected here will again produce acidic irritants that could affect the pulp through the dentinal fluid. The resulting degree of sensitivity will, in great measure, depend on the presence or absence of a smear layer that obstructs the tubuli.[17] Removal of the smear layer (which is very fragile to acids such as those found in soda drinks and fruit juices) and its replacement with one of the new resin bonding agents will materially overcome the problem of microleakage. These adhesives have been shown to be a substitute for an insulating cement base.

Since a true hyperreactive pulp is not a pathologic condition, it may continue to be sensitive for years, acting as a distress signal, warning against insult to a particular tooth. The patient learns to avoid the involved tooth and often becomes a unilateral masticator in the process. The pulp seems well able to accept constant insult, and the statement that long-standing "hyperemia" eventually terminates in pulp inflammation and death is patently false. Apparently, something more than hypersensitivity or hyperemia must be present to lead to necrosis. One would suspect inflammation and/or infection.

Recent interest in eliminating dentinal hypersensitivity has stimulated the revival or development of a number of modalities—physiologic, chemical, or mechanical in nature. **Physiologic** methods are remineralization of the dentinal tubulii from the "calcium phosphate-carbohydrate-protein complex" in the saliva and/or from the formation of irritation dentin from the pulp. Both of these techniques can take place naturally over long periods of time, but artificially stimulating salivary flow and/or pulp activity are too time consuming and painful to be practical.[18]

For **chemical/mechanical obstruction,** "the ideal desensitizing agent should be non-irritating to the pulp; be relatively painless on application; be easily applied; be rapid in action; have long-term or permanent effectiveness; and produce no staining."[19] Krauser pointed out the obverse, "that an agent may be effective (1) in one individual but not in another, (2) on one tooth but not on others, and (3) against one stimuli but not others."[20]

"Various agents have been used in attempts to seal the peripheral ends of tubules in sensitive dentin."[18] Agents that have been tried and found wanting are calcium hydroxide, formalin, and silver nitrate. Tubule-sealing agents that have proved successful are potassium oxalate, strontium chloride, sodium and stannous fluoride, and the resins, including the new adhesives. Another approach, using potassium nitrate, blocks sensory nerve activity at the pulpal end of the tubules by altering the excitability of the nerves.

Potassium oxalate as a desensitizing agent was developed by Greenhill and Pashley.[21] It is sold commercially as PROTECT (John O. Butler Co., Chicago, Ill.). Applying potassium oxalate to the dentin surface, which, in turn, produces "calcium oxalate crystals of different particle sizes within the dentinal tubules, is a means of obstructing the tubules' apertures (Figure 7-6)." "Calcium oxalate is poorly soluble and is formed when the potassium oxalate contacts the calcium ions in the dentinal fluid."[18] A single-dose applicator permits pinpoint delivery, to the sensitive area, of monopotassium-monohydrogen oxalate. Although the degree and duration of relief will vary from patient to patient, the effectiveness of a single application by the dentist can last up to 6 months.

One rather crude study was less than enthusiastic about oxalate dentin desensitization after 3 months using a monopotassium-monohydrogen oxalate agent,[22] whereas a more sophisticated American and two Japanese reports conveyed a good impression of the oxalate solution for densensitization.[23–25]

Strontium chloride is contained in two toothpastes on the market, Sensodyne (Block Drug Co., Jersey City, N.J.) and Thermadent (Mentholatum Co., Buffalo, N.Y.). Strontium combines "with phosphate in the dentinal fluid and exchanging for calcium in the hydroxyapatite of the dentinal tubule walls may produce strontium phosphate crystals and dentinal tubules closure."[18] Goodman believes that the strontium ion alters neural transmission, which may account for the immediate improvement in relieving sensitivity.[26] Strontium may also stimulate the formation of irritation dentin, and it has been reported "as well to bind to the matrix of the tubule, thus reducing its radius."[27]

The **fluorides, sodium** and **stannous,** have been used as desensitizing agents longer than any of the other mineral salts. Initially, sodium fluoride was used in paste form (33%) and burnished into the sensitive areas. Repeated applications were necessary. Neither stannous nor sodium fluoride anticaries rinses or toothpastes, however, are particularly effective desensitizers.

Goodman has stated that, "Fluoride is thought to work by reaction between the fluoride ion and ionized calcium in the tubular fluid to form an insoluble calci-

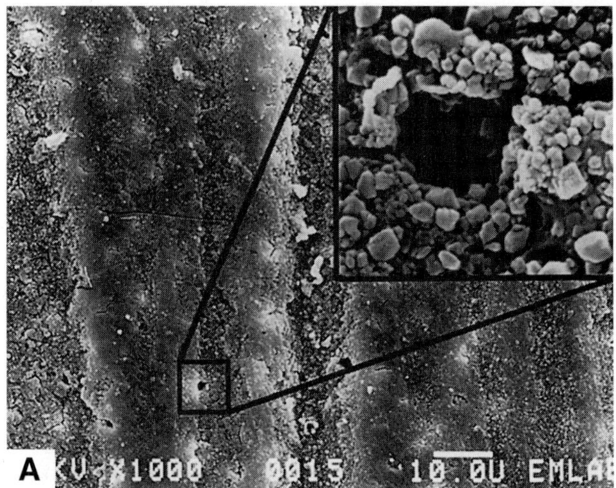

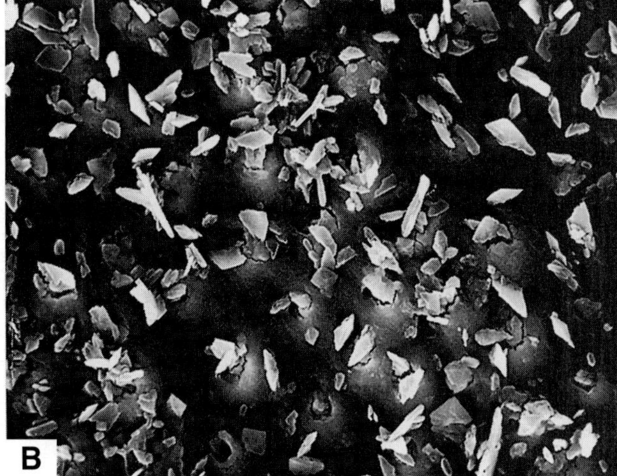

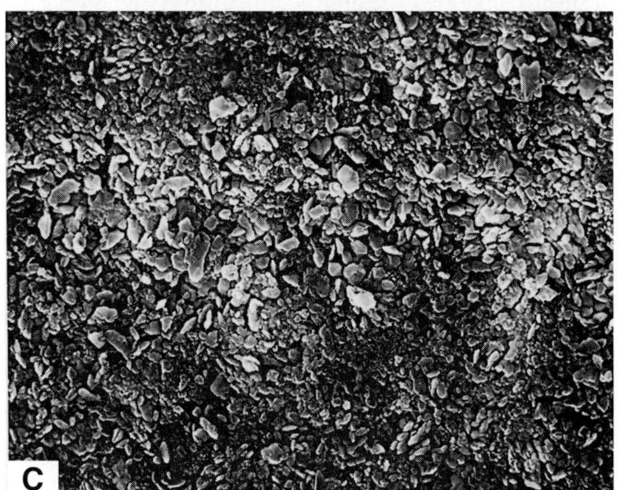

Figure 7--6 **A**, Smear layer–covered dentin treated with 3% monopotassium-monohydrogen oxalate for 30 seconds (original ×1,000 magnification). Enlarged inset (×10,000 original magnification) reveals a crack over the tubule. Much of the surface is angular crystals of calcium oxalate. (Courtesty of David H. Pashley.) **B**, Smear layer treated with neutral 30% dipotassium oxalate. Note large crystals growing out of the smear layer. **C**, Surface of **B** treated with 3% monopotassium-monohydrogen oxalate, pH 2.0, acid etches the smear layer away but reacts with calcium from tubular fluid to release a host of finer crystals effectively plugging the tubules. **B** and **C** reproduced with permission from Pashley DH, Galloway SE. Arch Oral Biol 1985;30:731.

um fluoride precipitate."[26] It may also stimulate the formation of irritation dentin.

Stannous fluoride with carboxylmethylcelluose in a glycerine gel was found to be significantly more effective than a placebo gel in reducing hypersensitivity,[18] and an acidulated sodium fluoride solution decreased conduction in the tubuli by 24.5%. If sodium fluoride was applied by iontophoresis, hydraulic conduction in the dentinal tubules was decreased by 33%.[21]

Fluoride iontophoresis has been recognized for years as a consistently successful treatment for dentinal hypersensitivity. Gangerosa is credited with popularizing this treatment when he introduced the Electro Applicator. The Desensitron (Parkell Products, Farmingdale, N.Y.) has also proved effective.

To use these battery-powered devices, the patient holds the positive electrode in his hand and the dentist, using the negative electrode, applies a 2% solution of sodium fluoride to the sensitive areas of the teeth. Using this technique, Simmons reported 94 to 99% reduction in hypersensitivity.[28] According to a report from India,[29] a comparative evaluation of the desensitizing effects of the topical application of 33.3% sodium fluoride paste, of iontophoresis with a 1% solution of sodium fluoride, and of iontophoresis with the patient's own saliva was made. Iontophoresis with sodium fluoride produced immediate relief after one application, whereas topical application required two to three applications. The authors concluded that "iontophoresis with 1% sodium fluoride is the method of choice for the treatment of hypersensitive dentin, as it meets all the requirements of an ideal desensitizing agent except permanency of effect, which requires further investigation" (Table 7-1).[29]

Gangerosa reported very similar results as well as recommending the iontophoretic application of the fluoride in a tray to desensitize a number of teeth.[30–33] Carlo and colleagues reported 100% desensitization after two iontophoretic fluoride treatments 73.9% of the time.[34] Brough et al., on the other hand, found **one**

Table 7-1 Comparison of Desensitizing Method[29]

	Group		
Degree of Relief	I* (%)	II† (%)	II‡ (%)
Good	33.33	55.55	—
Moderate	52.94	44.45	35.13
None	13.73	—	64.87

*Treatment by topical application using a 33.3% solution of sodium fluoride.
†Treatment by ionophoresis using a 1% solution of sodium fluoride.
‡Treatment by ionophoresis with patient's own saliva.

application of 2% sodium fluoride by iontophoresis to be no more effective to cold response than a similar application with distilled water or 2% sodium fluoride without iontophoresis.[35]

Potassium nitrate as a desensitizing agent was developed by Hodash, who reported the use of saturated solutions and pastes to be used for home care that contain up to 5% potassium nitrate.[36] These pastes are sold over the counter as Promise and Sensodyne Fresh Mint (Block Drug Co., Jersey City, N.J.) and Denquel (Vicks Oral Health Group, Wilton, Conn.).

Hodash reported that "Relief of hypersensitivity was notable and rapid in most instances," and that "Potassium nitrate is also an extremely safe chemical."[36] Goodman has shown some impressive clinical results using dentifrices containing potassium nitrate.[26] He suggested that desensitization may occur either by the oxidizing nature of potassium nitrate or by crystallization, which blocks the tubules, or both.[26] Pashley, on the other hand, believes that potassium nitrate does not block the tubules but instead reduces the sensitivity of the mechanoreceptor nerves to the movement of dentinal fluid in the tubuli, which normally would produce painful stimuli. Although the fluid still shifts, according to Pashley, "the nerves would not fire because they would be rendered unexcitable."[37] Goodman also believes that the "potassium ion depolarizes the nerve fiber membrane...in which few or no action potentials can be evoked."[26] Patients should be encouraged to use the desensitizing dentifrices frequently.

Composite resins and bonding adhesives have also been used very successfully to reduce or eliminate dentinal hypersensitivity. Early on, isobutyl cyanoacrylate was found to be effective by blocking the dentinal tubules. Bahram stated that "Cyanoacrylate should be repeated after 6 weeks."[38]

In another study, a light-curing dentin bonding agent, Scotchbond (3-M Co., St. Paul, Minn.), was painted onto sensitive areas of exposed dentin and light-cured for 20 seconds.[27] After one treatment, all sensitivity was eliminated in 89% of the extremely sensitive surfaces and in 97% of the moderately sensitive surfaces. "After 6 months, 85 percent of these teeth were [still] without sensitivity and only 15 percent exhibited any sensitivity at all."[27] In contrast, a "control" group treated with a sodium fluoride/strontium chloride solution received virtually no relief.[27] More recently, Amalgambond (Parkell Products, Farmingdale, N.Y.), a 4-META bonding agent, was tested: "Initially all teeth treated had an immediate response of no sensitivity." At 6 months, 18 of 19 treated teeth showed decreased sensitivity, 15 of those showing no sensitivity. All control teeth remained sensitive.[39] A similar study, in which "several coats of a dentin primer (NPG-GMA, BPDM) were applied to root sensitive teeth, achieved similar six months results—all patients symptomless except one who was slightly sensitive to ice."[40]

The authors of this study are very positive that the success of resin adhesive therapy depends on careful preparation of the root surface and application of the resin before curing. If or when the resin wears away and sensitivity returns, additional application should eliminate the discomfort once again. Many of the manufacturers of dental adhesives are making extended claims for the effectiveness of their product to reduce hypersensitivity, and this appears justified.

In conclusion, there are a number of alternative modalities that will desensitize hypersensitive dentin. It "boils down" to what works best in the dentist's and/or the patient's hands. One must remember that the placebo effect is always present and that at least 30% of the time, **anything** that is done will achieve a result, for example, the relief achieved over 3 months using only water.[35]

It should also be remembered that "molars are usually less sensitive than cuspids or premolars, which are, in turn, usually less sensitive than incisors...older teeth are less sensitive than younger teeth."[18] Also, dental plaque elimination should be the first priority before any treatment is undertaken.

Acute Pulpalgia

True pulpalgia begins with the development of pulp inflammation or pulpitis. Beveridge and Brown have shown that an increased intrapulp tissue pressure is possible.[14] It may be postulated that this pressure might well be the stimulus that is applied to the sensory nerves of the pulp and leads to severe toothache.

Incipient Acute Pulpalgia. The mild discomfort experienced as the anesthetic wears off following cavity preparation is a good example of **incipient pulpalgia.** The patient may be vaguely aware that the tooth feels different, "as though it has been worked on," but the sensation disappears by the next morning.

Stanley and Swerdlow have shown extravascular migration of inflammatory cells following even modest irritation by a controlled and cooled cavity preparation.[41] It is most fortunate that, from the incipient stage, pulpitis is **reversible**, and the discomfort vanishes. One would suspect that incipient pulpalgia is so mild that the pulpitis it predicts is often ignored by the patient until it is too late. This could well be true of the initial sensation developing with a new carious lesion, the slight ache in response to cold or sweets (see Figures 6–2 and 6–3).

Excitation. Incipient acute pulpalgia must be stimulated by an irritant such as cavity preparation, cold, sugar, or traumatic occlusion.

Examination. If the pulpalgia follows cavity preparation, the involved tooth is obvious. If dental caries is the noxious stimulus, the cavity is found by an explorer and radiographs. The lesion may be quite small, just into the dentin. The patient can usually tell which quadrant is involved and may even point out the involved tooth. Cold is the best stimulus to initiate incipient acute pulpalgia. The pulp tester is of questionable value in these cases.

When traumatic occlusion is causing the pain, the diagnosis becomes more difficult (see "Traumatic Occlusion," below).

Treatment. Removal of the carious lesion followed by calcium hydroxide application and a sedative cement for a few days may be all that is required to arrest **incipient acute pulpalgia.** Watchful waiting following cavity preparation should not extend to procrastination, leading to moderate or advanced acute pulpalgia. Corticosteroids placed in the cavity following preparation or used on the dentin surface prior to cementation of extensive restorations have proved effective for reducing postoperative pain (HR Stanley, personal communication, 1984).

Moderate Acute Pulpalgia. The pain of **moderate acute pulpalgia** is a true toothache, but one the patient can usually tolerate. Many patients report for dental attention after hours, or sometimes days, of discomfort from the developing pulpitis. The pain is frequently described as a "nagging" or a "boring" pain, which may at first be localized but finally becomes diffuse or referred to another area. The pain differs from that of a hyperreactive pulp in that it is not just a short, uncomfortable sensation but an extended pain. Moreover, the pain does not necessarily resolve when the irritant is removed, but the tooth may go on aching for minutes or hours, or days for that matter.

Excitation. **Moderate pulpalgia** may start spontaneously from such a simple act as lying down. This alone accounts for the seeming prevalence of toothache at night. Some patients report that the pulp aches each evening, when they are tired. Others say that leaning over to tie a shoe or going up or down stairs—any act that raises the cephalic blood pressure—will start the pain. The list of inciting irritants would not be complete without mentioning hot food or drink, sucking on the cavity, and biting food into the cavity. Most pain of **moderate pulpalgia,** however, is started by eating, usually something cold.

Hahn and his associates have reported a correlation between thermal sensitivity in irreversible pulpitis cases and the microorganisms present in deep carious lesions. Using anaerobic testing methods, they found that *Fusobacterium nucleatum* and *Actinomyces viscosus* were associated with sensitivity and prolonged pain induced by cold. Other bacteria produced heat-sensitive responses.[42]

A warm water rinse does not usually relieve the pain, and cold water makes it worse. The patient may find, however, that two or three aspirin or acetaminophen tablets bring relief. He may continue to take analgesics for days, while wishfully thinking that the pulp will recover. Too many dentists also practice this same game of self-deception.

Examination. Attempting to determine which tooth is involved with **moderate acute pulpalgia** is often a difficult experience. The patient may report after days of discomfort, and by this time the pain, though still present, may be widespread and vague. The patient believes he can pinpoint the exact tooth, but then he becomes confused. The typical statement, "the tooth stopped aching as soon as I entered the office," is commonly heard. No amount of irritation will start it again. If the patient is on heavy analgesics or mild narcotics, it is best to postpone examination until responses will not be clouded by drugs.

If the pain has been constant for some time, all of the pulps on the affected side seem to ache, and, frequently, two or three give approximately the same response to the pulp tester or thermal testing. This is where intuition comes into play. The examiner gets a "feeling" about a particular tooth. It might respond a bit sooner to the pulp tester, or it may ache just a bit longer after cold is applied. The restoration seen in the radiograph may be just a little deeper. All too frequently, in this day of "full coverage," a number of teeth may be restored with full crowns, a situation that manifestly compounds the problem.

If the pain is only vague when the patient is first seen, the dentist should attempt, by careful questioning, to obtain a general idea of the area of the pain. Usually, the patient can tell which side is involved and frequently whether pain is in the maxilla or the mandible. This may not be absolute, however, for the pain may be referred from one arch to the other. The patient may remember where the pain started initially, hours or days before. Examination of the suspected area may immediately reveal the involved tooth, made obvious by a large carious lesion or huge restoration. Then again, nothing unusual may be present.

Radiographs may give an immediate clue in the form of a huge interproximal cavity or a restoration impinging on the pulp chamber. If nothing is learned from radiographic examination, the electric pulp tester is then employed, but generally without great success.

A tooth involved in **moderate acute pulpalgia** is hypersensitive and will respond sooner, or lower, on the scale of the pulp tester. Then again, all of the teeth in the area may be hypersensitive and respond in the same way to pulp testing so that no definite conclusions may be drawn from this test. This leaves the thermal test as the final arbiter since percussion and palpation rarely reveal any response, although the tooth may be slightly sensitive to percussion.

The first thermal evaluation to use is the cold test because the pulp is more likely to respond to this stimulus. The tooth under the greatest suspicion should be tested first. The examiner should block the adjacent teeth with his fingers, being careful that melting ice does not run onto these teeth. The immediate response to cold may be quite sudden, violent, and lasting. On the other hand, the initial pain may go away immediately when the cold is removed. **This is the time to stop!** Do not test any more teeth for about 5 minutes. The reason for this is quite obvious: The pain in the tested tooth that stops aching may **rebound** within a few minutes, and if the dentist has proceeded to test other teeth, neither he nor the patient will be able to differentiate the aching tooth. If the pulp starts to ache, however, reapplying the cold should increase and prolong the pain.

Infrequently, heat is the stimulus that starts the symptoms. Sometimes, however, nothing will start the ache, and the patient must be dismissed and asked to return when the tooth is again painful.

Occasionally, the search is narrowed down to a maxillary **and** a mandibular tooth, both prime suspects because both are aching. One molar is the problem tooth and the other the "referred" tooth. If an anesthetic is injected into the **suspected** arch, and the hunch was correct, the pain should stop in both teeth. If the pain does not stop, the offending tooth is in the opposite arch. Again, by means of the anesthetic test, aching mandibular **premolars** may be differentiated from molars by the use of a mental injection that will anesthetize from the second premolar toward the midline. A zygomatic injection in the maxillary arch for the maxillary molars, or a careful slow infiltration for the maxillary premolars injected well forward toward the canine, may differentiate between these confusingly similar pains. Nor should one forget the **interligamentary injection** (see chapter 9). Injecting down through the periodontal ligament allows each individual tooth, even each individual root, to be anesthetized. Although this analgesia may not be profound enough for pulpectomy, it may prove adequate to stop pulpalgia from referring. The anesthetic test is a last resort and should be used after all other means have been exhausted.

In diagnosing **moderate acute pulpalgia,** above all, the examiner must **think,** must be shrewd, and must not panic. If in doubt, hesitate! Often one more day may make a difference. The patient should be warned to return to the office without having taken any analgesics.

Treatment. The treatment for **moderate pulpalgia** is quite simple: pulpectomy and endodontic therapy if the tooth can and should be saved or extraction if the tooth should be sacrificed. If endodontic therapy is indicated, it may be completed in one appointment.

Hodosh and colleagues, who reported favorably on the use of potassium nitrate as a desensitizing agent,[36,43] also used the chemical mixed with carboxylate cement as a pulp-capping medium in teeth with pulpitis. In a preliminary report, they noted that all of the teeth became asymptomatic immediately but that 2 of 86 failed.[43]

Glick used Formocresol to treat pulps that continue to ache after root canal therapy has been completed. His supposition is that vital, inflamed tissue still exists in a canal that is impossible to locate. The tooth may even respond to thermal and electric testing. The Formocresol "embalms" the microscopic remainder of the pulp, and the pain is alleviated.[44] In the same vein, a US Army dentist reported two endodontically treated teeth that still ached when heat was applied. After re-entry, a careful search revealed additional untreated canals. Total pulpectomy and root canal filling completely eliminated the postoperative pain.[45]

In the Orient, toothache has long been alleviated with acupuncture. A favorite site to place the acupuncture needle is the Hoku point—midway in the web of tissue between the thumb and index finger on either hand. Temporary relief of pain is achieved after a few minutes of "needling" this point. The respected pain center group at McGill University has reported similar results by massaging the Hoku point for about 5 minutes with an ice cube wrapped in a handkerchief. "Ice, an analgesic, helps overload the circuits, quickly 'closing the pain gate,' according to the researchers."[46] This simple method of pain control might well be recommended to a patient unable to appear immediately at the dental office.

Advanced Acute Pulpalgia. There is never any question about the patient suffering the pain of advanced acute pulpalgia. He is experiencing one of the most excruciating acute pains known to humanity, comparable to otic abscess, renal colic, and childbirth. If every dentist personally experienced the pain of **advanced acute pulpalgia,** he would be a more sympathetic practitioner for the experience.

This patient is in exquisite agony and sometimes becomes hysterical from the pain. The patient often is crying and virtually unmanageable. One patient, who had to drive 40 miles to a dentist, reported that he could stand the pain no longer, so he stopped the car, took out a pair of pliers, and pulled his own tooth. Patients have confessed contemplating suicide to escape the pain.

The relief for this pain is embarrassingly simple: **cold water,** preferably iced. Cold water rinsed over the tooth is all that is usually needed to arrest the pain temporarily. The patient might discover this fact while taking an analgesic and, in so doing, receive immediate relief. He then reports to the dentist with a thermos or jar of ice water in hand, only stopping to sip as the pain gradually returns. Frequently, he times the periods of relief much as the expectant mother times her labor pains. The relief often lasts 30 to 45 seconds.

When a patient telephones reporting a toothache, especially late at night, the dentist should always inquire, "Have you tried **rinsing** cold water on the tooth?" If the answer is negative, request that the patient do so and return to the telephone to report results. If the cold gives relief, the compassionate professional meets the patient as soon as possible to provide permanent relief. If cold aggravates the pain, the patient has moderate pulpalgia, which might well become **advanced pulpalgia** by morning. The patient with **advanced pulpalgia** would have to continue rinsing with cold water throughout the night, and, even then, the cold may no longer give relief. Thus, a tired and "frazzled" patient becomes a hysterical one.

Examination. The examination for advanced acute pulpalgia, in comparison to that for moderate pulpalgia, is relatively simple, even if the tooth is not aching when the patient presents himself. The involved tooth always has a closed pulp chamber, as revealed by the radiograph. Otherwise, the tremendous intrapulp pressure could not develop. In addition, the radiograph may reveal a thickened periodontal membrane space at the apex as the inflammation spreads out of the pulp.

The history is self-incriminating. The symptoms are violent! The involved tooth usually can be pointed out by the patient and is sometimes tender to percussion as well. These teeth are said to be less sensitive to the pulp tester (requiring a higher reading), but the performance of this test is merely "gilding the lily." Heat is the merciless offender. Hahn reported that cavities filled with "black pigmented *Bacteroides*, *Streptococcus mutans*, and total anaerobic colony counts were positively related to the heat sensitivity" in irreversible pulpitis cases.[42]

Because the inflamed pulp reacts so violently to heat, the most decisive test is the heat test, although one must have a cold water syringe in the other hand, ready to give immediate relief. As soon as the hot gutta-percha touches the involved tooth, the patient develops what Sicher has called the **subgluteal vacuum;** he suddenly rises up in the chair as if stabbed. Cold water is instantly applied, and the pain subsides.

The thermal test is conclusive! When the patient is again comfortable, however, the adjacent teeth should also be tested to ascertain that no more than one tooth is involved or that the suspected tooth gives the most violent reaction. The patient should be assured that the involved tooth will not again be warmed.

Local anesthesia gives blessed relief, and the dentist has, from that moment, made a friend for life. The friendship will be more lasting if the tooth is saved by endodontic therapy rather than extracted.

Treatment. The treatment for **advanced pulpalgia** is the same as for moderate pulpalgia: pulpectomy and endodontic therapy for the salvageable tooth and extraction for the hopeless one.

Complete anesthesia of an inflamed pulp may be difficult even though all outward signs would indicate the conduction or infiltration injection to be successful. In this case, an intrapulp injection of lidocaine or pressure anesthesia with lidocaine or an interligamentary injection may be necessary.

Following pulpectomy, the pulpless tooth should be relieved of occlusal contact by grinding. Endodontic therapy should be completed at a later appointment.

Chronic Pulpalgia

The discomfort from **chronic pulpalgia** is best described as a "grumble," a term commonly used by patients who withstand the mild pain for weeks, months, or years. Often the pain can easily be kept under control with one or two analgesic tablets, two or three times daily. Frequently, the patient seeks relief only when the pulp begins to ache every night.

The pain from **chronic pulpalgia** is quite diffuse, and the patient may have difficulty locating the source of annoyance. Patients frequently say that they have a "vague pain in my lower jaw." **Chronic pulpalgia** is likely to cause referred pain, which is also mild. Other patients may appear with beginning acute apical abscess and confess to knowing that something was "wrong" with the tooth for months. Other patients comment on the bad taste or odor constantly noted.

Excitation. The pulp involved in **chronic pulpalgia** is not affected by cold but may ache slightly on contact with hot liquids. The most common report is that the tooth is sore to bite on." If meat or a bread crust, for example, is crushed into the cavity, the pain lasts until the irritant is dislodged. The patient may report that the tooth begins to hurt late in the day, "when I'm tired," or, more frequently, "when I lie down."

Barodontalgia. One patient confessed to discomfort each Monday morning and Friday evening. These were the times each week when he crossed a 4,000-foot mountain pass in his travel across Washington state. Here the slight difference in barometric pressure was enough to excite the pain response. The same may be true during an airplane flight. (Planes are actually pressurized at 5,000 feet, not sea level.)

Kollman tested 11,617 personnel of the German Luftwaffe who participated in simulated high-altitude flights up to 43,000 feet: "Only 30 (0.26%) complained of toothache (barodontalgia)." Chronic pulpitis was the principal culprit, followed by maxillary sinusitis.[47]

Rauch classified **barodontalgia** (formerly called aerodontalgia) according to the chief complaint.[48] If the patient has pulpitis, he will have pain on **ascent**—sharp momentary pain (Class I) in the case of acute pulpitis, and dull throbbing pain (Class II) in the case of chronic pulpitis. These pains are caused by the extraoral decompression of the ambient pressure in the plane, which, in turn, allows for a compensating increase of pressure within the pulp chamber and root canal. Descent (compression of the ambient pressure) brings relief in the pulpitic tooth. If the pulp is necrotic, the reverse is true, a dull throbbing pain (Class III) on **descent** (compression) and asymptomatic on **ascent** (decompression). In a case of periradicular abscess or cyst, severe persistent pain (Class IV) occurs with **both** ascent and descent.

Rauch pointed out that "even though the highest incidence factor is less than 2 percent, because of the vast number of people" who fly, barodontalgia must be considered in the differential diagnosis of oral pain.[48]

Examination. Determining which tooth is involved with **chronic pulpalgia** is often ridiculously simple and, on other occasions, most difficult. Frequently, a large carious lesion is present, or an amalgam restoration is fractured at the isthmus. Another common offender is recurrent caries under a restoration, usually an inlay. These are the lesions that are painful when compressed by food packed into the cavity.

The leathery dentin covering these lesions may be removed with a spoon excavator, often without anesthesia and with no great discomfort. The pulp lies revealed, covered with a gray scum of surface necrosis. Biopsy would show degeneration of the remainder of the pulp, accounting for the lack of severe pain.

The **chronic pulpalgia** that is the most difficult to diagnose lies under a full crown because it is impossible to pulp test electrically, or under a three-quarter crown, where recurrent caries is not revealed by radiographs. In these cases, carbon dioxide "ice" should be used as the stimulant.

The pulp tester and the radiograph are the best tools for locating the tooth involved with **chronic pulpalgia,** which will sometimes respond as "necrotic" to electric testing—that is to say, it will take the maximum discharge from the tester. In any case, a high reading on the rheostat should be expected. England and colleagues demonstrated intact nerve fibers, with some variations from normal, in pulp specimens with "irreversible pulpitis."[49] In the necrotic pulp, dissolution of the fibers was apparent.

The radiograph often reveals interproximal or root caries, or recurrent caries under a restoration. In **chronic pulpalgia,** the so-called "thickened" periodontal membrane also may be present, indicating that the inflammatory process is not confined completely to the pulp. These cases may also demonstrate **condensing osteitis** of the cancellous bone at the apices. Interestingly, this osteosclerosis disappears after successful endodontic therapy (see Figure 5-9).

The apices of the involved roots also show external resorption, although this condition is more prevalent following pulp necrosis and complete periradicular involvement (see Figure 6–49).

Thermal tests are of little value in a positive sense in diagnosing **chronic pulpalgia,** although, in some cases, slight pain may be experienced in response to extreme heat. This is in accord with the patient's history of no response to iced drinks but an occasional response to hot coffee.

Percussion has a good deal to offer in many of these cases. Often the patient is vaguely aware that something feels "different" about the involved tooth when it is percussed. Palpation is virtually useless. However, having the patient bite on an applicator stick sometimes reveals soreness of a particular tooth.

Chronic pulpalgia has the aggravating habit of referring its vague pains throughout the region. The patient may insist that a mandibular molar is aching, whereas examination reveals that a maxillary molar is the offender. Often anesthetizing the involved tooth is the only convincing proof to the patient that he is wrong. Patients have reported with aching of a maxillary molar when the maxillary lateral incisor has been found to be the offender. If the tooth suspected by the patient appears normal to all examination and testing, the examiner should be suspicious of **chronic pulpalgia** in another tooth on the same side. The mandibular molar involved in **chronic pulpalgia** is not as apt to refer pain to the ear as it is in acute pulpalgia.

Treatment. The treatment for **chronic pulpalgia** is quite basic: pulp extirpation and endodontic therapy if the tooth is to be saved and extraction otherwise. Anesthesia is no problem.

Hyperplastic Pulpitis. The exposed tissue of a **hyperplastic pulp** is practically free of symptoms unless stimulated directly.

Excitation. The discomfort of a **hyperplastic pulp** is quite simple. It "erupts" out of its open bed of caries for all to see. Differential diagnosis is concerned with only one problem, namely that of discerning whether the polyp is pulp or gingival in origin because both are covered by epithelium (see Figures 4-72 and 4-73).

The pulp polyp may be lifted away from the walls with a spoon excavator and the pedicle of its origin thus revealed. It is remarkably painless to handle and may even be excised with a sharp spoon excavator with no great discomfort.

Treatment. Frequently, the teeth involved in **hyperplastic pulpitis** are so badly decayed that restoration is virtually impossible. Hence, extraction is usually indicated. On the other hand, if the tooth can be restored, pulpectomy and endodontic therapy are recommended prior to restoration. Glick reported limited success with pulpotomy in these cases, done originally as an experiment on three cases with good bleeding (personal communication, 1964). He was surprised to see periradicular repair take place.

Necrotic Pulp. There are no true symptoms of complete **pulp necrosis** for the simple reason that the pulp, with its sensory nerves, is totally destroyed. Often, however, only partial necrosis has occurred, and the patient has the same vague, comparatively mild discomfort described for chronic pulpalgia.

The examiner also must bear in mind that the pulp in one or two canals in multirooted teeth may be necrotic, and the pulp in a second or third canal may be vital and quite probably involved in acute or chronic pulpitis. The results of examination in these cases are most bizarre because each level of pulp vitality is represented by a confused response.

Examination. A routine radiographic survey or coronal discoloration may present the first indication that something is amiss in the case of the tooth with a necrotic pulp. On questioning, the patient may recall an accident of years ago or a bout of pulpalgia long since forgotten.

Many cases of **pulp necrosis** are discovered because of the discoloration of the crown. This applies primarily to the anterior teeth and ranges from a vague discoloration, visible only to the trained eye, to frank discoloration of the darkened tooth. A discernible difference may sometimes be demonstrated by transillumination with a fiber optic.

The radiograph may be helpful if a periradicular lesion exists because its presence usually indicates associated pulp death. Radiographically, the tooth with the **necrotic pulp** may exhibit only slight periradicular change; in other words, a radiolucency is usually found by hindsight rather than foresight. Then again, a sizable periradicular bony lesion may accompany the **necrotic pulp.** No changes in the canal are noted radiographically to indicate necrosis.

One of the first lessons to be learned, however, is **never** to trust a radiograph alone in diagnosing pulp necrosis. A snap judgment of the periradicular radiolucency that exists with periradicular osteofibrosis associated with perfectly normal, vital pulps will lead to error if the examiner depends on radiograph evidence alone. It is imperative **always to pulp-test the tooth.**

The electric pulp tester, therefore, is the instrument of choice for determining pulp necrosis. With complete necrosis, no response will be given at any level on the tester. With partial necrosis, a vague response that can easily be tolerated may be elicited at the top of the scale. The tooth with a necrotic pulp may also be slightly painful to percussion.

Treatment. There is no treatment for pulp necrosis per se because the necrotic pulp has long since been destroyed. If the tooth can be saved, endodontic therapy is indicated.

Internal Resorption. Internal resorption is an insidious process when the afflicted pulp is completely free of symptoms. On the other hand, this condition has been known to mimic moderate acute pulpalgia in pain intensity. The usual case, however, closely resembles the chronic pulpalgia syndrome, that is, mild pain at the tolerable level. When confined to the crown, enough tooth structure may be destroyed for the pulp to show through the enamel—hence the synonym for **internal resorption,** "pink tooth."

Excitation. Symptoms of **internal resorption** depend primarily on whether the process has broken through the external tooth surface. If the pulp destroys enough tooth structure to finally erupt into the oral cavity, it responds much as the hyperplastic pulp, painful only to pressures of mastication.

Because the pulp is undergoing dystrophy localized to a single area, it is not as likely to be excited by the drinking of hot or cold fluids. The pulp that erodes through the root surface may give vague symptoms, primarily with mastication, but the patient usually remembers these symptoms in retrospect after the condition is pointed out on the radiograph.

Examination. Two methods of examination reveal the case of **internal resorption:** visual examination if the crown is involved and radiographic examination for the crown and root. Thermal tests and the electric pulp tester may provide confirming, yet only partially reliable, evidence.

The case of **internal resorption** that is truly difficult to diagnose is the one of coronal involvement often hiding behind the full or three-quarter crown and thus not revealed in the radiograph. The patient complains of vague symptoms and referred pain, but the response of the involved pulp to the testing procedures may be similar to that of the other teeth. Percussion may be of slight value. In these cases, an intuitive hunch is needed. If one is fortunate, the correct tooth, when tested, may exhibit slight variances from the other teeth in the area. On the basis of these minor variances, the suspected tooth is chosen; however, the presence of **internal resorption** is not confirmed until the coronal pulp is entered.

Treatment. Pulpectomy is the only treatment for **internal resorption.** As long as the pulp remains, it is most likely to continue its destructive process. If the tooth can be saved by endodontic restoration, the defect can best be obturated by thermoplasticized and compacted gutta-percha.

Traumatic Occlusion. A tooth **traumatized** by bruxism or **traumatized** because a restoration is in hyperocclusion often responds much like the tooth with mild pulpalgia. First, the pulp is usually hypersensitive, reacting primarily to cold. In addition, the pain may be vague, reminiscent of chronic pulpalgia.

The patient may complain of being bothered by pulp discomfort on awakening in the morning or possibly of being awakened by the discomfort. The story of pain at the end of a rather trying day is also characteristic. Pathognomonically, the patient reports relief after only one aspirin. Moreover, he usually says that the tooth is not painful on mastication; at least this is not his chief complaint.

Paradoxically, even a **well-treated** pulpless tooth being traumatized by bruxism presents the vague symptoms of pseudopulpalgia. It, of course, does not respond to thermal stimuli but still feels like a mild toothache.

Examination. From the patient's history usually comes the clue to diagnosing the pain from trauma. History of "toothache" on awakening is an unusual symptom and should direct one's thinking toward bruxism at night. The discussion of a tense daily situation is another clue. The vagueness of the pain is most important because one expects to be dealing with chronic pulpalgia, and yet the thermal and pulp tester response is often like that of a normal or hyperreactive pulp. The fact that a low dosage of a mild analgesic can control the pain is pathognomonic.

If one suspects pain from trauma, one should look for facets of wear on the tooth. Articulating paper may be helpful; however, the point of contact may not be readily apparent. One young patient shifted her mandible forward during sleep and ground the distal of the mandibular second molar against the mesial of the maxillary first molar, a protrusive shift of a full centimeter. It was difficult to believe that the two well-worn facets would match, and yet, when the youngster was teased into protruding her mandible to this extent, causing contact between the two surfaces, her eyes lighted in delight, and she began compulsive bruxism.[†]

It should be remembered that the mandible also may be retruded in sleep, causing facets distal to masticatory facets to be involved. Examination for these annoying contacts should be carried out with the patient supine in the dental chair.

Too many dentists examine the median occlusion position (centric) and the lateral excursion of **function** (working bite) and completely neglect to examine for **nonfunctional** (balancing bite) **traumatic contacts.** So

---

[†]Contraction or stretch of muscles (as in yawning) is often pleasurable!

often the nonfunctional contact is the patient's compulsive position. Some patients even bring diagrams to the office to describe the point of interference, demonstrating an abnormal and exaggerated oral awareness.

Peculiarly enough, the involved tooth or teeth are frequently not sensitive to percussion but are sensitive to mastication. Biting or chewing on a narrow cotton roll or Burlew disk will sometimes elicit discomfort.

The radiograph may show no periradicular changes or may exhibit a widened periodontal space and apical external root resorption (see Figure 6–46).

Treatment. Treatment for these cases obviously involves relieving the point of occlusal trauma by judicious grinding to reshape the involved tooth and its opponent. Actually, the tooth should be completely disoccluded to give the inflamed tissue a chance to recover.

Many times, the dentist is unsure of his diagnosis, especially in cases that closely resemble or actually are pulpitis. The pulp should be given the benefit of the doubt, particularly if a fully restored crown is involved and complete testing is difficult. If symptoms and signs are vague, the case should first be handled as a problem of traumatic occlusion, especially if there is some evidence that this might be true. If, after careful adjustments, the pulp does not respond with almost immediate relief, the possibility of pulpitis should be reconsidered, but only after all of the excursions of the mandible and the patient's history are rechecked.

Sometimes the patient reports relief as soon as the occlusion corrections are completed, even before leaving the chair.

Incomplete Fracture or Split Tooth. The tooth that is **split** or **cracked** but not yet fractured presents some of the most bizarre symptoms encountered in practice. These symptoms range from those of a constant, unexplained hypersensitive pulp to constant, unexplained toothache.

The tooth may be uncomfortable only occasionally during mastication, and at that time the pain may be one quick, unbearable stab. This is when the crack in the dentin suddenly spreads as the cusp separates from the remainder of the tooth. The pulp may only be hypersensitive, possibly for years. In one case, follow-up continued for 8 years, and the pulp hypersensitivity immediately ceased when the buccal cusp fractured away.

Many of the cases involve noncarious, unrestored teeth; hence it is hard to believe that anything could be wrong with the tooth. If the **split** has extended through the pulp, bacterial invasion occurs, and true pulpitis results. These cases are comparatively easy to diagnose because of the obvious symptoms.

The most frequent complaint is that of a tooth painful to bite on, with an occasional mild ache. One case was diagnosed over the telephone on the basis of a report of these classic symptoms by the harassed referring dentist. The patient confirmed the diagnosis by reporting the same day with the buccal cusp of a maxillary premolar in hand.

Excitation. The discomfort of the **split** tooth is elicited by biting on the tooth or contacting cold fluids. If the pulp is involved in fracture, any exciting agent for pulpalgia will bring on discomfort.

Examination. First, one thinks of carefully examining the tooth, dried and under good light, to find the crack in the enamel. Usually, the search goes unrewarded because the examiner sees no cracks at all or finds similar enamel crazing in every tooth.

The pulp tester customarily gives a normal reading unless the pulp is involved. Thermal tests may be valuable if a cold or hot stream is played on the tooth or hot or cold fluids are rinsed against the possible culprit. Hot gutta-percha or a stick of ice, on the other hand, is usually valueless.

Percussion alone, surprisingly enough, is usually not helpful, yet biting on an applicator stick or cotton roll may give the spreading action needed to elicit pain.

The crown may also be painted with tincture of iodine, which is washed off after 2 minutes. The crack often appears as a dark line (see Figure 4–12).

A piece of Burlew rubber disk can be used to stress a possibly fractured tooth. Held in a locking pliers, it can be shifted around to different positions on the occlusal surface while the patient is asked to bite on it. An even more definitive device is the Tooth Slooth (Laguna Niguel, California, USA), a triangular plastic tip on a handle (Figure 7-7). With this device, it can be determined quite accurately which cusp is splitting away.

The radiograph records an obvious split only if it is in correct alignment to the central rays (Figure 7-8). It will completely fail to reveal the almost microscopic split, which elicits the really bizarre syndrome.

Treatment. If an **incomplete fracture** is suspected but the pulp is not involved, the crown should be pre-

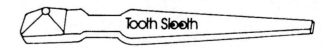

Figure 7-7 The Tooth Slooth, a fracture detector. The concave area at the peak of the pyramid is placed on the tip of the suspected cusp. The patient bites down on the plastic device, and the dentist watches for changes in facial expression or verbal reaction. Several cusps should be tested.

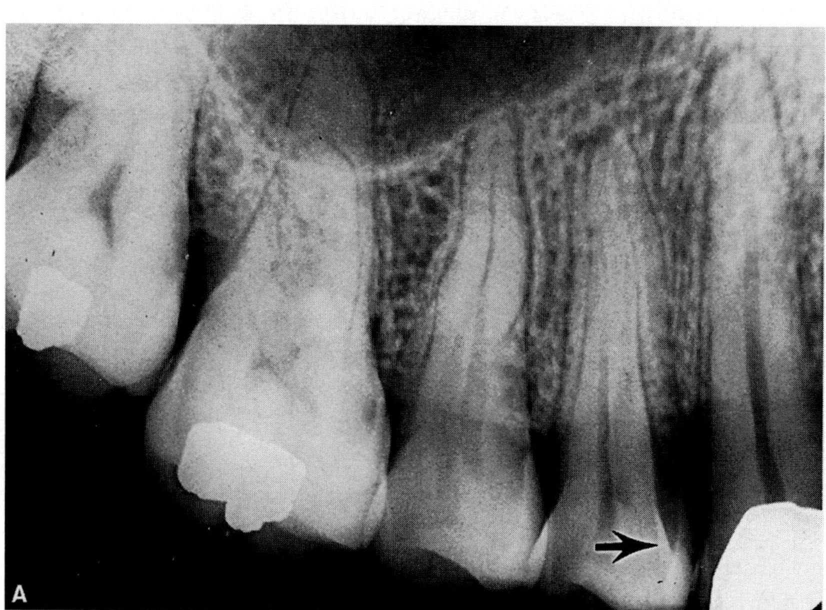
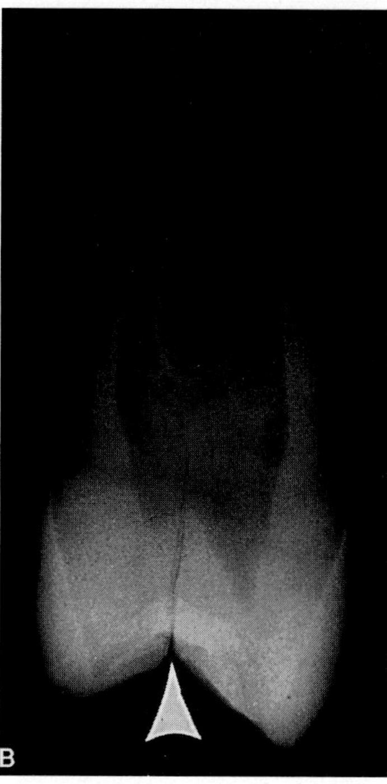

Figure 7-8 Radiographs are usually useless in diagnosing undetected fracture. **A**, The point of fracture (**arrow**) cannot be seen in a clinical radiograph. **B**, After the tooth is extracted and radiographed in a mesial-distal direction, fracture into the pulp (**arrow**) becomes apparent. Also note lateral canals. (Courtesy of Dr. Dudley H. Glick.)

pared for a full crown, which should then be cemented temporarily with zinc oxide–eugenol cement. The full crown binds the remaining tooth structure much as the hoops contain the staves of a barrel.

If the **incomplete fracture** has entered the pulp and a true pulpalgia indicates that pulpitis is present, then root canal therapy should be completed first, followed by full coverage to prevent a total fracture. If the fracture has extended completely through, into the periodontal ligament and pulp, the chances of saving the entire tooth are remote indeed. The possibility of saving a portion of the tooth is discussed in chapter 12.

POSTOPERATIVE PAIN: INCIDENCE, PREVENTION, AND TREATMENT

There is no question that a good deal of postoperative pain is associated with endodontic therapy. This is one of the factors that continues to affect the public adversely concerning root canal therapy. Some of these problems are unavoidable, but many are iatral. Apical overextension of necrotic debris (infected or otherwise), instruments, paper points, medicaments, and filling materials lead to postoperative pain. Apical perforation is a common occurrence that can mainly be avoided by careful attention to establishing and maintaining correct working length.

In surveying 1,204 teeth treated endodontically, Dutch investigators reported an incidence of 30% postoperative pain: 7% with severe symptoms and 23% with moderate symptoms.[50] By far the greatest number of cases of postoperative pain (65%) were related to patients who reported at the first appointment **with preoperative pain.** In contrast, only 23% of those who developed postoperative pain were free of pain initially. Most postoperative pain occurred on the first day after initiating endodontic treatment. Emergency treatment was necessary in 57% of the patients to relieve the pain. Analgesics satisfied the rest.[50]

In a subsequent study, the Dutch team further analyzed a subsection of the cohort of 803 patients with 1,204 teeth, mostly completed in one appointment—1 hour for single canal cases and 2 hours for molars.[51] A positive correlation was found "in the case of a nonvital pulp in conjunction with preoperative pain on the day of treatment [and] when a radiolucency larger than 5 mm in diameter is present." The chance of postoperative pain also increases with the number of root canals in the tooth. The probability of postoperative pain was reduced in any case with a vital pulp.[51]

A US Navy group has also reported that patients who were asymptomatic at the start of treatment experienced a low incidence of postoperative pain.[52] As one would expect, they also found that pulpectomy significantly reduced **post**operative pain in patients who had reported initially with **pre**operative pain. More recently, it was reported that complete pulpectomy was the most effective method of preventing postoperative pain in those patients presenting with preoperative toothache in teeth with vital pulpitis. The next most effective method was pulpotomy and the least effective was partial pulpectomy, which was twice as likely to allow pain to continue.[53]

Chronic postoperative pain following endodontic surgery is quite unusual, even though immediate postsurgical acute pain is expected. One survey, however, classified 5% (6 cases) of a cohort of 118 cases as endodontic failures because of continuing pain for an average of 21 months.[54] It was determined that three of the six patients may have suffered from post-traumatic dysesthesia, "pain associated with the manipulation of the root or apical bone…If nerve injury occurs, an abnormal repair process is possible." The remaining three "failures" were thought to be phantom tooth pain. The duration of pain in this group **prior** to treatment was 1, 4, and 36 months, respectively.[54]

PREOPERATIVE THERAPY

A number of studies have been done evaluating the efficacy of preoperative medication of cases suspected as potential "troublemakers."[52,54–58] The Navy group (above) found that the preoperative administration of flurbiprofen (a nonsteroidal anti-inflammatory drug [NSAID]) significantly reduced postoperative pain compared to placebos.[52] A group in Pittsburgh also recommended the use of an NSAID, the shorter-acting ibuprofen, as a preoperative prophylactic against the possibility of postoperative pain.[59]

Morse and his group at Temple University achieved similar results with the prophylactic administration of diflunisal (a long-acting NSAID).[55] They also found that the intracanal use of a corticosteroid solution following pulpectomy was efficacious.[56] These results were similar to those of their previous studies with antibiotics.[57]

The value of oral dexamethasone (corticosteroid) following initial endodontic treatment has also been reported.[58]

Questioning the time-honored procedure of prophylactically relieving the occlusion of posterior teeth being treated endodontically, a group at Iowa University found that there was no statistically significant difference between routine occlusal relief and placebo relief.[60] Although they could state that their results "cast doubt on the practice of routinely relieving the occlusion of posterior teeth receiving endodontic treatment," they did not imply that occlusal relief should be abandoned in cases of acute apical abscess (AAA) or acute apical periodontitis (AAP).[60]

PERIRADICULAR PAIN

Periradicular pain may be almost as excruciating as pulp pain and may often continue for a longer period of time. Periradicular lesions that may produce discomfort are (1) SAP, (2) SAA, (3) asymptomatic apical abscess (AAA), and (4) apical cyst. The adjective "acute," as used here, refers to the severity and the rapidity of the course of the lesion. **Acute apical periodontitis** is by far the most distressing periradicular lesion.

Symptomatic Apical Periodontitis

Symptoms. This acute form of periradicular pain can be most excruciating and sometimes lasts for days. The tooth is exquisitely painful to touch, and even contacting the tooth in closure may bring a flood of tears. The pain is most persistent, lasting 24 hours a day.

The pain has been described as constant, gnawing, throbbing, and pounding. Eventually, the patient may gain blessed relief, only to bite on the tooth while eating or during sleep, which starts the pain cycle once more. Many patients beg to have the tooth extracted. Yielding to their wishes, this has been done only to have the pain continue for another 48 hours owing to osteitis.

There is no overt swelling involved, just a grossly painful tooth elevated slightly in its socket. One week of discomfort is to be expected if nothing is done!

Etiology. The degree of discomfort described in the preceding paragraphs may be iatral. That is, the clinician perforates the root apex during endodontic therapy, forces caustic medicaments or irritating solutions through the apical foramen, or forcibly deposits necrotic, infected, and toxic canal contents into the periradicular tissue. These irritants produce a violent inflammatory reaction. If bacteria are present in the canal and are extruded apically, an acute abscess also develops to complicate the picture.

Typically, **SAP** follows initial endodontic treatment. The mandibular premolars and molars are the teeth most frequently and violently involved, the premolars especially. This fact could be attributed to their invitingly straight, tapered canals, which encourage abuse of the periapex with a reamer or file. Furthermore, the thick bony cortex and the small amount of cancellous bone found in this area limit the space allowable for swelling. This limitation greatly increases the pressure in the area and hence the pain.

Examination. Diagnosis of SAP is relatively easy; the patient is in severe pain, and the involved tooth is exquisitely painful to touch. The tooth is in supraocclusion, and the mandible cannot be closed without initial impact on the involved tooth.

Treatment. The soundest treatment of AAP is its prevention. Care in **instrumentation** is the most significant preventive measure. Care in **medication** is another precautionary measure. Overmedication and irritating medicaments cause a high percentage of these exasperating cases. Virtually all of the intracanal medicaments used today are toxic to periradicular tissue. It is essential, therefore, that medicaments be confined to the pulp chamber, that canals **not** be "flooded" with medicaments, and that paper points saturated with a drug **not** be sealed in canals.

In spite of precautionary measures, SAP may still develop. When it does, the greatest problem involves maintaining the patient in comfort for the entire period of healing and repair. To allow a patient to remain in violent, uncontrolled pain borders on criminal neglect.

When the patient reports with these acute symptoms, the tooth need only be touched to determine the location. To relieve the pain, an immediate injection of a **long-lasting** local anesthetic, such as bupivacaine (Marcaine) with epinephrine 1:200,000, should be given.

As soon as the tooth is comfortable under anesthesia, the occlusion should be adjusted to free the tooth completely from contact in closure or in any excursion. If possible, occlusal **corrections should be made in the opposite arch** to prevent more insult to the affected tooth.

A rubber dam should then be placed and the temporary filling removed very carefully. The tooth must be supported with the fingers to prevent further trauma. Using paper points with great care, the **chamber and canal should be cleared of any liquid contents.** An instrument is placed in the canal, **short** of the registered tooth length, and a radiograph is taken to check the original tooth length. The present determination of **accurate tooth length** is most important. Earlier instrumentation at an elongated, inaccurate tooth length may be the basis for the present serious trouble. When the length of the tooth is re-established, a reamer with an instrument stop should be set for this exact length and then employed to **just barely** perforate (trephine) through the apical foramen. Sometimes this brings forth a flow of blood and fluid, which materially reduces the periradicular pressure. This must be done in a dry, clean canal and with the greatest caution not to further traumatize the periradicular tissue.

The advent of the corticosteroids as **anti-inflammatory** agents has improved the treatment of SAP. Hydrocortisone, combined with neomycin (Neo-Cortef 1.5% eye/ear drops, sterile suspension, Upjohn Co., Peapack, N.J.), is recommended as an anti-inflammatory/antibacterial medicament. The canal is flooded with this liquid suspension and then, very gently, the fluid is "teased" out of the trephined apex with a fresh sterile instrument. A loose cotton pellet is then placed in the chamber and a **thin** temporary filling placed without undue pressure. The canal should **not** be filled to overflowing with the corticoid solution to allow space for inflammatory swelling. There will be some "lag time" before the antiphlogistic effect of the hydrocortisone takes place.

If the tooth continues to be painful after the analgesia wears off, the patient is instructed to return to the office to have the procedure repeated. Removing the temporary (with a dam in place) once again allows for drainage, and the canal is again medicated with neomycin 1.5%. The temporary is replaced to prevent secondary contamination. Each time the rubber dam is removed, the occlusion should again be checked. Frequently, further adjustment is necessary because the tooth has again been elevated in the alveolus. The patient is warned not to eat on this side; however, the warning is usually superfluous.

When the patient is leaving the office, he should be instructed that if the pain becomes unbearable at night, he can remove the temporary at home. He should be shown in a mirror how to pick out the thin temporary filling by using a safety pin that has been straightened into a right angle. Exposed to the saliva, the canal, of course, becomes contaminated. This is a modest problem, however, compared to a sleepless night of pain that might be suffered by the patient.

In a further attempt to reduce or eliminate post-treatment pain, Liesinger and colleagues reported the successful use of dexamethasone (corticosteroid), injected intraorally or intramuscularly, to suppress pain.[61,62] In a more objective laboratory study, a group at San Antonio, Texas, quantitated the effect of dexamethasone as an anti-inflammatory drug.[63] After producing acute periradicular lesions in rat molars by overinstrumentation, they injected either dexamethasone or a saline control in the buccal vestibule opposite the no-insulted teeth. They found that the "dexamethasone produced a significant anti-inflammatory effect" as measured by the number of polymorphonuclear neutrophil leukocytes that were counted in the area.[63]

The patient should also be carried on systemic antibiotics and an anti-inflammatory drug, such as ibuprofen (Motrin), naproxen (Naprosyn), diflunisol (Dolobid), or piroxicam (Feldene), for 4 days. By that time, the problem should have been resolved. For greater detail, see chapter 18.

The patient should also be given a narcotic for analgesia: 30 to 60 mg (0.5 to 1 grain) of codeine is the initial prescription, taken every 3 hours with 10 g aspirin. If the patient does not obtain relief from codeine or cannot tolerate the drug, 50 to 100 mg meperidine (Demerol) is prescribed every 4 hours, depending on the patient's age and weight. A few patients have had such intense, prolonged pain that they required morphine. Other patients have found it necessary to return every 5 or 6 hours for injections of local anesthetic into the affected area.

Alveolar trephination is another means of relieving the severe pain of **SAP.** Trephination, or surgical fistulation, is thoroughly discussed in Chapter 12.

In any event, the patient should be seen daily until the symptoms have resolved. Endodontic therapy should not be undertaken until the tooth is comfortable.

Acute Apical Abscess. The pain of **AAA** is similar to that described for AAS but somewhat lower in intensity. After all, necrosis is an extension of the inflammatory cycle, which begins with acute apical periodontitis and continues to the abscess state if not checked.

Necrosis of the **acute abscess** usually destroys enough tissue to permit fluid dispersement. The extravasated fluid breaks out into the soft tissue and marrow spaces where swelling is not as confined as it was at the periapex. This is not to say that the **AAA** is not painful. On the contrary, it is quite painful, but in comparison with SAP, the unbearable pain has gone and in its place is a full systolic throbbing pain, particularly on palpation. The involved tooth is also painful to movement or mastication.

Etiology. The discomfort of **AAA** develops gradually as the abscess grows in size. The condition is invariably related to bacterial invasion of the periradicular region from a necrotic, infected pulp canal. The **abscess** may develop spontaneously from an infected pulpless tooth or may follow initial endodontic treatment if bacteria are forced into the periradicular tissue.

In any event, the initial discomfort may be mild but gradually builds in intensity as the abscess becomes indurated or hardened. When the alveolar plate is "eroded" by the process and the abscess gathers into frank pus, the entire area softens and feels fluctuant to palpation, and the pain is greatly reduced.

Examination. Diagnosis of AAA is a relatively simple matter. The patient has pain and, invariably, swelling. Although the swelling may not always be observable to the examiner, the patient feels the tenseness of the swollen area. The degree of swelling varies from the initial, undetected swelling to gross cellulitis and massive asymmetry (see Figure 5–11). The involved tooth also is extremely painful to percussion or palpation. Radiographically, the picture may vary from a widened periodontal space to a large alveolar radiolucency. Actually, the radiograph is not the best means of diagnosis because it frequently reveals nothing of true diagnostic value.

Outside of percussion, electric pulp testing is the best method of diagnosis because the pulp of the tooth involved in AAA is invariably necrotic. The vitality test, moreover, is the best criterion to differentiate an **AAA** from an **acute periodontal abscess.** In the case of the periodontal abscess, the pulp of the involved tooth is not likely to be necrotic, although, by chance, it could be. Percussion proves that the **periodontal abscess** is not as painful as the apical abscess. The reason is quite clear. The periodontal abscess is a "lateral" abscess, found on the side of the root, so that percussion causes little increase in pressure. On the other hand, percussion against the inflamed **periapex** of the tooth with **AAA** induces a great increase in pressure owing to the wedging effect of the tapering root.

The adjacent teeth involved in the swollen area may also be painful to percussion, and they register an increased reading on the pulp tester owing to the collateral edema. The adjacent teeth, however, are not nearly as painful to percussion as the involved tooth and usually register within normal limits in pulp testing. Multiple loss of vitality may follow an accident so that a number of adjacent teeth could test nonvital, but usually only one is abscessed.

In contrast to percussion, thermal tests have little value. Extremes of heat may increase gas expansion in the area and thereby increase the pain momentarily. Cold may give slight relief but usually does nothing at all. Palpation of the area reveals the swelling, and the pressure increases the discomfort.

Treatment. Under a special section devoted to these problems in Chapter 12, treatment of the AAA is discussed in detail. Suffice it to say here that drainage is established through the root canal if the abscess is in its initial stage, or by incision if the abscess is fluctuant. Trephination may also be performed to establish drainage and relieve pressure. The occlusion is relieved and a regimen of systemic antibiotics and either hot rinses or cold applications is prescribed for the patient depending on the stage of development of the abscess.

The pain often can be controlled with mild analgesics such as acetaminophen. However, hydrocodone or meperidine (Demerol) must be prescribed for severe cases.

Endodontic therapy or extraction, whichever is indicated, is completed after the acute symptoms have subsided and while the patient is still receiving antibiotics. Periradicular surgery is rarely necessary in treating these cases.

Chronic Apical Periodontitis. **Chronic apical periodontitis** is seldom painful and is thoroughly discussed in chapter 5 under "Periradicular Pathology."

Treatment. Endodontic therapy is usually indicated for the tooth involved with **CAP.** This is sometimes followed by periradicular surgery, but only where indicated.

Chronic Apical Abscess. Also called **suppurative apical periodontitis,** CAA is generally free of symptoms. There may be stages in the long history of such a lesion when a draining fistula closes, and mild swelling and discomfort ensue. The patient reports that the abscess drains daily or that opening the abscess with a needle relieves the discomfort.

Many cases of **suppurative apical periodontitis** are so painless that they go undetected for years until revealed by radiography.

Etiology. **Chronic apical abscess** is the inflammatory response to an infection by bacteria of low virulence from the root canal. As stated previously, the only discomfort associated with a CAA is that related to the occasional closing of the draining fistula with attendant pressure. This chronic lesion, however, may develop an acute exacerbation, the **phoenix abscess,** and when this happens, the patient has all of the problems of an AAA. In this event, the pain and swelling are magnified owing to the large preexisting lesion.

Examination. On questioning, the patient with a previously undetected **CAA** may remember a particularly stormy session in the involved area or perhaps a traumatic incident in which the pulp was devitalized by a blow. There has been no discomfort since, however.

Chronic apical abscess is frequently associated with long-standing dental restorations such as full gold or jacket crowns, large composites or amalgams, and extensive bridgework. Occasionally, a routine radiograph reveals a CAA, associated with a discolored anterior tooth. This may appear as an area of **diffuse radiolucency** around the apex of the tooth in question and may vary from a minor lesion to a massive loss of bone. External resorption of the root end is also a common finding.

The lesion of CAA, easiest to detect, has an associated draining fistula, usually intraoral, seldom cutaneous. This sinus tract, lined with inflammatory tissue, drains the abscess through a stoma into the oral cavity. It is the closing of this tract that causes the patient discomfort.

Treatment. If the tooth involved with **CAA** can be saved, it may be retained by endodontic therapy. Periradicular surgery is sometimes indicated for these pathologic lesions. The chronic lesion that becomes acutely infected must be treated as an AAA until the symptoms have subsided. The tooth may then be handled as an endodontic case or extracted, as conditions indicate.

Apical Cyst. The **apical cyst,** per se, is painless unless it becomes infected. In that event, the case should be handled as an AAA. The apical cyst is discussed in chapter 5 under "Periradicular Pathology."

Treatment. When treated endodontically, the apical cyst may be enucleated during periradicular surgery.

PERIODONTAL LESION PAIN

Few periodontal lesions are severely painful. The causes of these lesions are divided into diseases that attack just the gingiva and those that involve the deeper periodontal complex. Two uncomfortable lesions that involve the gingiva and mucosa are **acute necrotizing ulcerative gingivitis** and **herpes simplex.** These diseases offer no severe problems in the differential diagnosis of pain because both lesions are diagnosed from their appearance and/or odor.

Two painful conditions that involve the pericemental structures and must be differentiated are the **acute gingival or periodontal abscess** and **pericoronitis.**

Acute Gingival or Periodontal Abscess

The patient with an **acute periodontal abscess** seeks treatment for a tooth that is painful to move or to bite on. The pain, however, is not as deep-seated or throbbing as that of an AAA. Although some localized swelling is present, it is not as extensive as with the AAA.

Etiology. The **acute periodontal or gingival abscess** develops from a virulent infection of an existing periodontal pocket or as an apical extension of infection from a gingival pocket. Most **gingival abscesses** are associated with traumatic injury to the gingiva or periodontium by a mechanical force. Both types of abscess are frequently seen in patients who have compulsive clenching or bruxism.

Examination. Although the involved tooth may be painful to movement, it is not as painful as the tooth involved in an AAA. Furthermore, the location of the abscess is usually different; the **periodontal abscess "points" opposite** the **coronal third** of the root, whereas the **apical abscess** generally **"points" opposite** the **apex.**

The electric pulp tester is the surest method of differentiation. The necrotic, infected pulp causing an apical abscess always gives an essentially negative response to testing, whereas the tooth involved with the

periodontal abscess is generally vital. Use of the periodontal probe often reveals a tract from the gingival sulcus to the abscess.

Treatment. The reader is referred to a periodontics text for information on treatment.

Pericoronitis

The common complaint of the patient with **pericoronitis** is severe radiating pain in the posterior mouth and the inability to comfortably open or close the mandible. Not only is it painful to close against the inflamed operculum distal to the erupting mandibular molar, but the pain of muscle trismus limits translation of the mandible as well. The tissue distal to the erupting molar is most painful to touch, especially during eating. The pain radiates through the region, down into the neck, and up into the ear and can easily be confused with pulp pain. Occasionally, an erupting third molar elicits the same deep, spreading pain well before the tooth breaks through the oral epithelium.

Etiology. Pericoronitis is caused by injury and infection of the pericoronal tissue associated with erupting molars, usually mandibular third molars. The tissue may be injured during eating by trauma from food such as peanuts or bread crust. The infection begins under the operculum and extends with attendant swelling around the entire unerupted crown. This area is frequently a source of primary infection with *Borrelia vincentii* and *Fusiformis dentium.*

Examination. The history of trismus and discomfort on opening or closing the mandible is indicative of **pericoronitis.** When the operculum is palpated or probed, it is found to be swollen and exquisitely painful. The patient usually assumes that it is the tooth that is painful.

Pericoronitis must sometimes be differentiated from a periodontal abscess commonly occurring along the distal aspect of the second molars. Again, the periodontal abscess is not nearly as painful as **pericoronitis.**

Treatment. The reader is referred to an oral surgery text for information on treatment of **pericoronitis.**

REFERRED PAIN

Referred Pulp Pain

One of the most frequently encountered and most baffling phenomena with which the dental diagnostician must deal is the problem of referred pulp pain. Texts and articles discussing this subject frequently give "pat rules" of pain reference with the implication that if pain is to be referred from a tooth, it is always referred in a particular pattern. This is not so, as anyone active in diagnosis soon discovers. Quite bizarre reference pathways are frequently encountered, and the clinician soon comes to realize that almost any reference, except across the midline, is possible.

Symptoms. Glick has well illustrated referred pain from pulpalgia—from tooth to tooth and from tooth to nearby cutaneous and deep structures.[64] Figures 7-9 and 7-10 illustrate this information to facilitate diagnosis by visual association.[64]

The leading published scientific study on pulp pain and referred pain is that of Robertson et al.[65] These authors produced toothache by placing stimulating electrodes into defects in the enamel of their own teeth. They found that by delivering up to 10.0 volts to the teeth, severe pain could be induced. Moreover, they discovered that when they maintained the shock for 10 minutes, the pain would be referred out of the teeth and over the entire distribution of the involved division of the nerve. Systematically and cleverly, these researchers mapped and described the reference pain from a number of teeth, mandibular and maxillary alike (Figures 7-11 and 7-12).

What Roberston et al. described from experimentation has been seen countless times by dentists—the patient with advanced acute pulpalgia who is suffering localized and referred pain with all of the attendant systemic signs and symptoms. They further experimented with the reduction of referred pain first by injecting anesthetics into the **area of referred pain** on the face and scalp and, second, into the area of the original "noxious stimulation," that is, the tooth.[65] As Figure 7-13 demonstrates, only **partial** relief from pain developed following procaine injection into the **referred** area; however, **complete** relief from pain was experienced when the region of the **original** source of pain was anesthetized.

Robertson et al. also found that protracted pain, as found in osteomyelitis of the mandible, led to sustained contraction and pain of the muscles of the face, head, and neck. In this case (Figure 7-14), when the source area of pain in the mandible was anesthetized, the referred pain area involved with the third division of the fifth nerve was abolished. On the other hand, the pain areas owing to spasm of the muscles of the neck continued. The phenomenon of myofascial trigger point pain and dysfunction developing as a result of pulpalgia is exactly the reverse of referred tooth or jaw pain from spasm of the trapezius muscle or the muscles of mastication as described by Travell (see Figures 8-28, 8-29, and 8-30).[66]

The interesting research of Ray and Wolff would seem to confirm the reference of deep pulp pain into more superficial and cutaneous associated regions but could hardly be construed to explain the pain referred

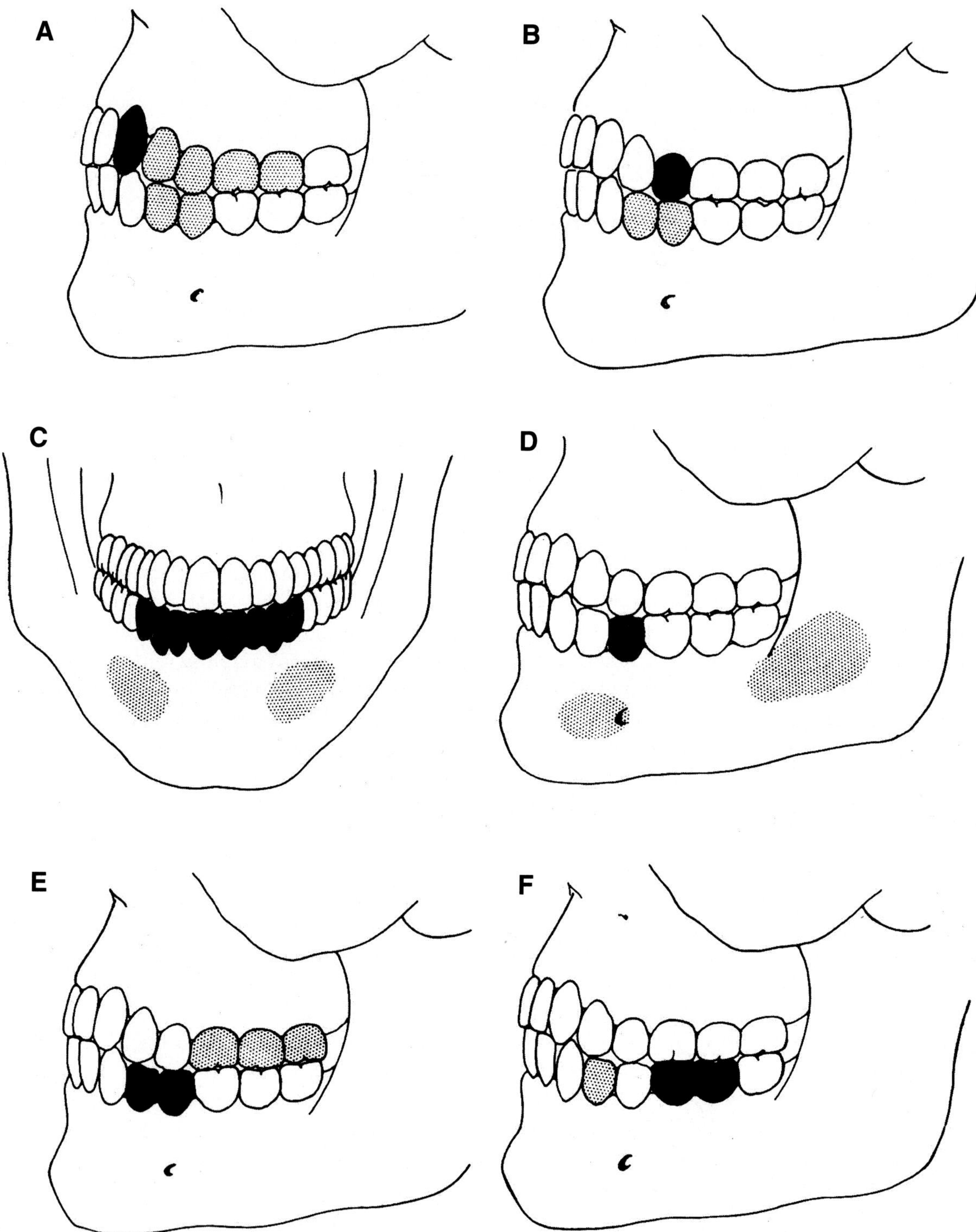

Figure 7-9 Referred pain pathways from teeth involved with pulpalgia to other teeth as well as to the immediate area. **Black** signifies tooth with pulpalgia; **stippled** areas, the site of referred pain. **A**, The maxillary canine may refer to the maxillary first or second premolars and/or the first or second molars, as well as to the mandibular first or second premolars. **B**, Maxillary premolars may refer pain to the mandibular premolars. The reverse is also true. **C**, Mandibular incisors, canine, and first premolar may refer pain into the mental area. **D**, The mandibular second premolar may refer pain into the mental and midramus area. **E**, Mandibular first or second premolars may also refer pain into maxillary molars. **F**, Mandibular molars may refer pain forward to the mandibular premolars. Adapted with permission from Glick DH.[64]

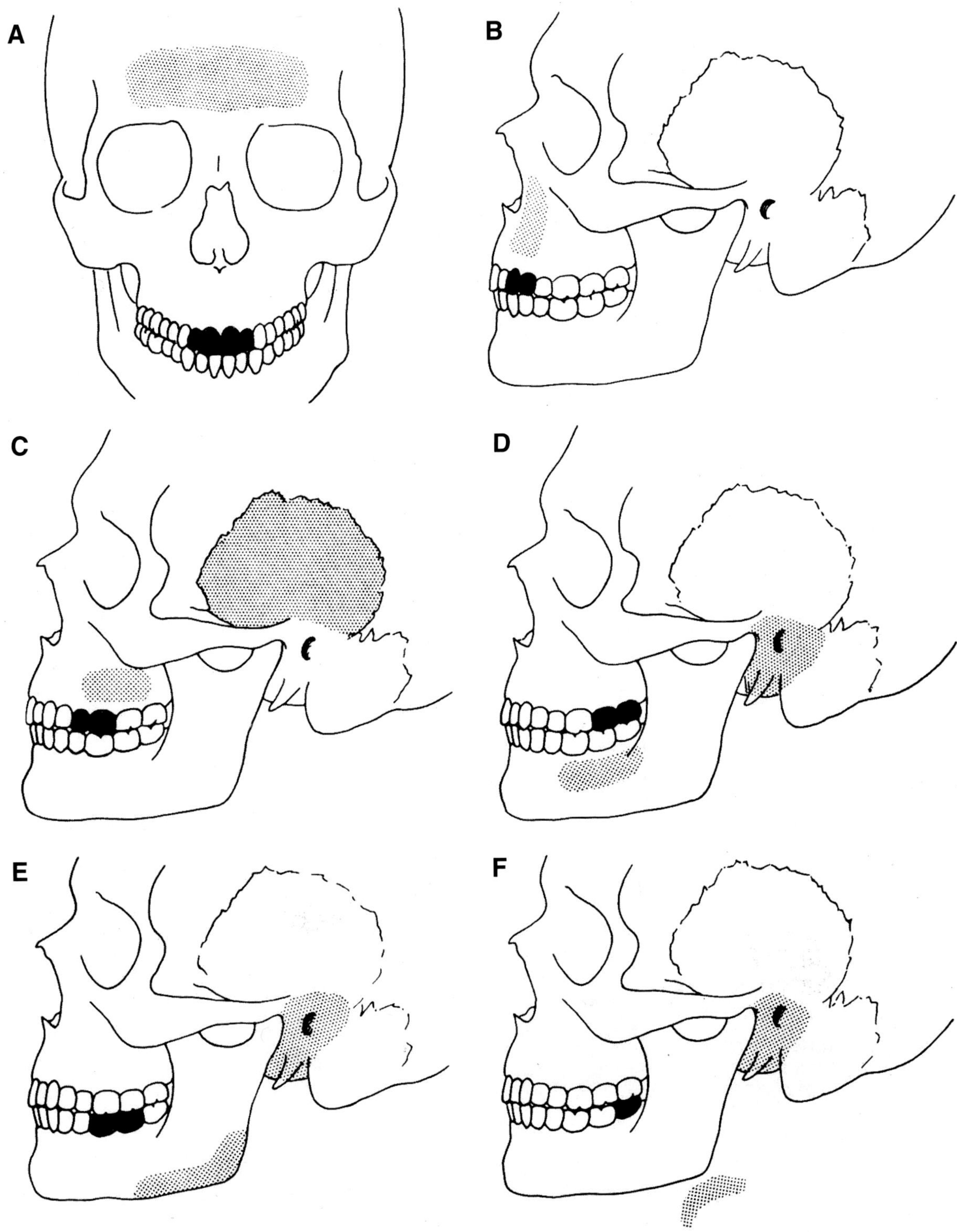

Figure 7-10 Pain referred from pulpalgia to structures remote from the involved tooth. **Black** indicates teeth involved in pulpalgia; **stippled** areas, remote areas of referred pain. **A**, Maxillary incisors may refer pain to frontal area. **B**, Maxillary canine and first premolar may refer pain into the nasolabial area and orbit. **C**, The maxillary second premolar and first molar may refer pain to the maxilla and back to the temporal region. **D**, Maxillary second and third molars may refer pain to mandibular molar area and occasionally into the ear. **E**, Mandibular first and second molars may commonly refer pain to the ear and to the angle of the mandible. **F**, The mandibular third molar may refer pain to the ear and occasionally to the superior laryngeal area. Adapted with permission from Glick DH.[64]

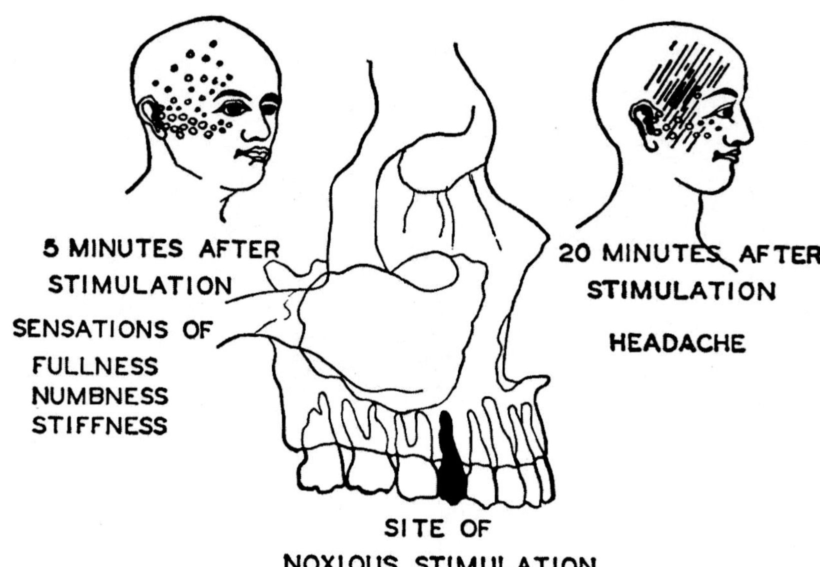

Figure 7-11 Pain referred from a maxillary second premolar. Pain was initially experienced locally in the tooth following noxious stimulation by 10 volts of electricity. Within 5 minutes, numbness, fullness in the ear, and muscle stiffness had developed, in addition to steady pain along the homolateral temporal, zygomatic, and supraorbital areas. The headache reached its maximum distribution and intensity within 20 minutes after cessation of toothache. Reproduced with permission from Wolff HG. Headache and other head pain. New York: Oxford University Press; 1950.

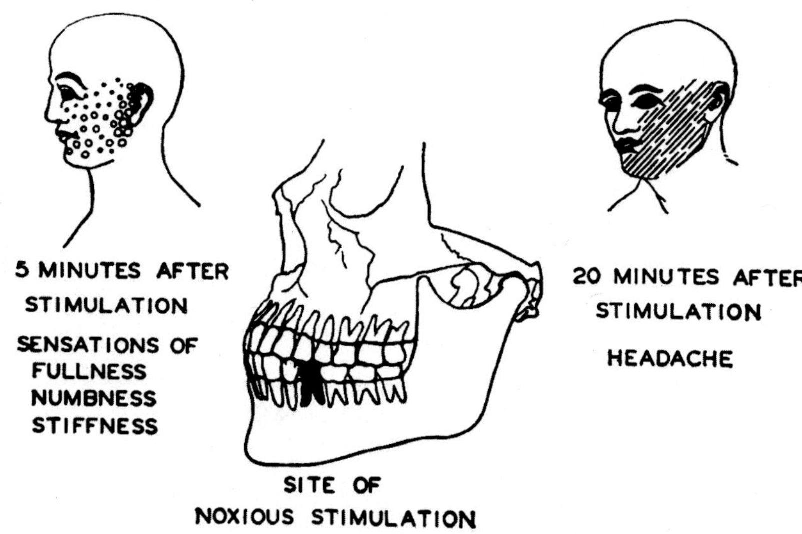

Figure 7-12 Electrical stimulation of a lower first molar maintained severe toothache for 10 minutes. Pain was referred into the ear canal and throughout the upper and lower jaws, over the zygoma and temple, to the top of the ear; a sensation of fullness and ache persisted in the ear. Numbness and stiffness of the masseter muscle developed. Twenty minutes after stimulation, severe "lower-half" headache developed throughout the region. Reproduced with permission from Wolff HG. Headache and other head pain. New York: Oxford University Press; 1950.

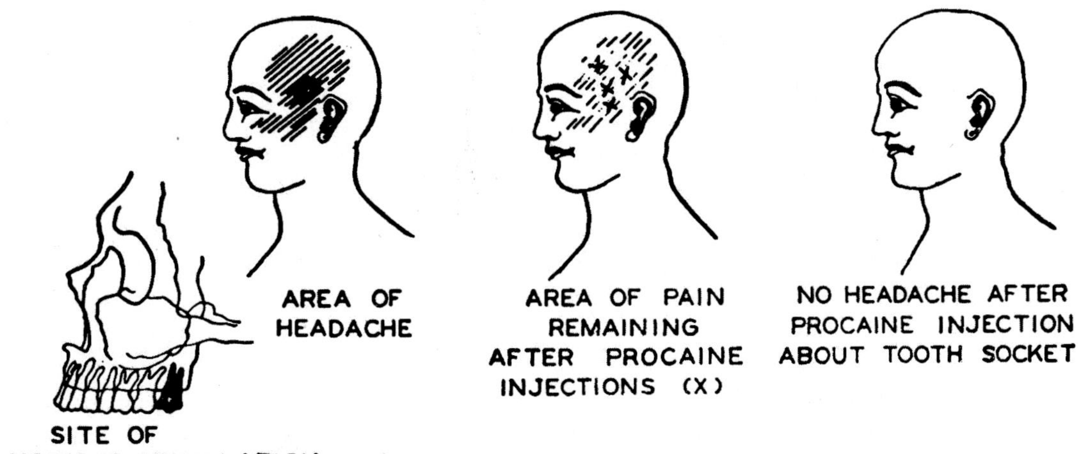

Figure 7-13 Broad area of referred pain developed from maxillary third molar pulpalgia. Injecting procaine into the **referred area** alleviated pain only at the site of injections. All primary and referred pain was totally eliminated by injecting at the site of primary noxious stimuli (third molar). Reproduced with permission from Wolff HG. Headache and other head pain. New York: Oxford University Press; 1950.

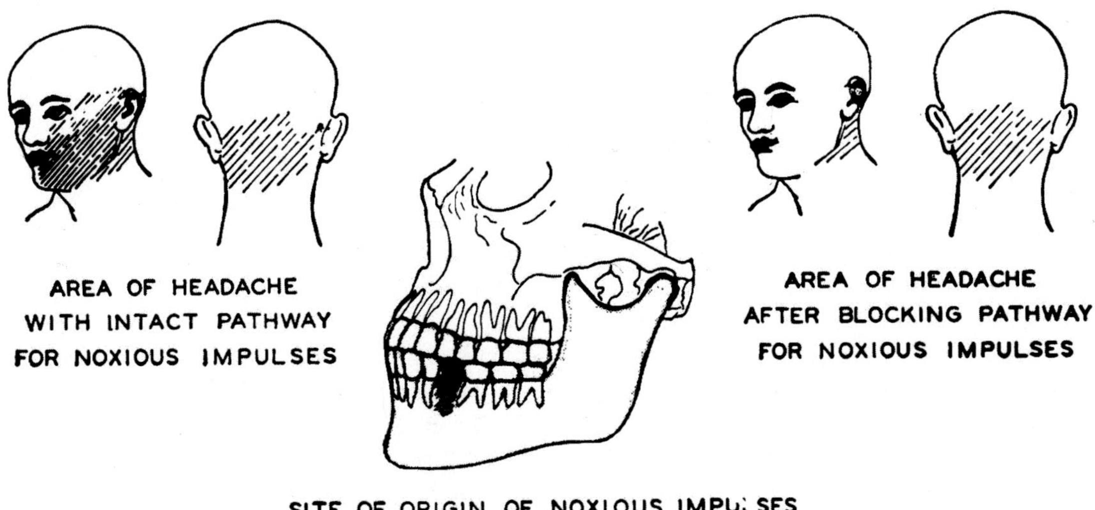

Figure 7-14 Protracted pain from a lower premolar caused not only widespread referred pain (see Figure 7-10) but also pain from spasm of muscles of the face, head, and neck. Anesthetizing the primary source of pain alleviated pain referred along two divisions of the fifth nerve but did not relieve spasm and pain of muscles of the neck. The reverse is also true. Myofascial pain from these muscles will refer into the oral cavity. Reproduced with permission from Wolff HG. Headache and other head pain. New York: Oxford University Press; 1950.

from one tooth to another or from the paranasal tissue into the teeth.[67] This type of referred pain has been discussed by Ruch and Fulton as **habit reference.**[68] "Evidence that reference of sensation is a learned phenomenon," they stated, "can be found in the clinical observation that a pain may be referred not to its usual point of reference but to the site of a previous surgical operation, trauma, or localized pathological process."[68]

"Habit reference" was verified by Hutchins and Reynolds, who demonstrated that teeth filled **without** benefit of local anesthesia could be made to ache when the homolateral nasal wall was stimulated by a needle prick in the vicinity of the maxillary sinus ostium.[69] Ruch and Fulton, in reviewing the research of Hutchins and Reynolds, looked on the traumatized sensory nerves of involved dental pulps as a "learned response."[68] They stated further, "The pain impulses from the sinus, conducted in an overlapping pathway, were simply given the previously learned reference for impulses in that path."[68]

This same thought may be projected to explain how pain in one tooth (possibly even in the opposing homolateral arch) could be referred there from pulpitis in another tooth some distance away. The pulp of the referred tooth might well have been previously traumatized by caries, a blow, or a dental procedure without anesthesia. This injured pulp then becomes the fertile ground on which the seeds of referred response could be sown in the future. This might also explain why pain is referred to teeth when the patient has mumps or inflammation of the temporomandibular joint.

Continuing further with their studies, Reynolds and Hutchins found that they could virtually eliminate referred pulp pain by procaine block anesthesia.[70] This was done by repeating their previous experiment in which they performed traumatic dental work **without anesthesia** on both sides of the **maxillary arch** and later demonstrated that **pain** was referred to these teeth from a pinprick of the maxillary ostium in the nose. After this fact was well established, the teeth on the **right** side were all **anesthetized.** Two weeks following these injections, the **right** side was again tested with stimulation of the ostium. Amazingly, no referred pain could be elicited on any tooth that had been previously anesthetized. On the **left** side, however, which had **not been anesthetized,** the teeth still responded with referred pain when the left maxillary ostium was stimulated. Therefore, the importance of rendering dental treatment under local anesthesia is emphasized by Reynolds and Hutchins since pain was not referred to teeth treated under local anesthesia.[70]

EXTRAORAL PAIN

As explained above, pain from sources outside the oral cavity may refer into the oral cavity. The reverse is also true.

These diagnostic and treatment problems will be dealt with in some depth in chapter 8. To complete the record, however, these sites will merely be mentioned at this point.

Atypical Toothache

Rees and Harris described a disorder that they called **atypical odontalgia.**[71] Patients present themselves with all of the typical features of an acute toothache—severe, throbbing, continuous pain starting in one quadrant but spreading even across the midline. Also referred to as "dental migraine" or "phantom tooth pain," this condition is often associated with patients suffering from unipolar, or common, depression. A recent review of 28 cases, followed since 1979 from a cohort of 120 cases, revealed that 81% of the patients were female and ranged from 13 to 80 years of age (mean 42.6 years). The pain was located in the teeth, jaws, or gingiva 93% of the time. However, 14% said that the pain affected areas of the face—the cheek and around the eyes and ears. Only 4% reported tongue pain. The onset of the pain was precipitated by dental procedures 31% of the time. Tricyclic and monoamine oxidase inhibitor antidepressant therapy relieved pain in many of the cases.[72] Because it falls within the descriptive area of "**atypical facial neuralgia,**" this type of pain will be discussed further in that section of chapter 8.

Salivary Gland Disorders

The salivary glands can be affected by many diseases, including obstruction, infection, degeneration, and tumor growth. Pain and tenderness, however, are usually found in association with inflammation of the gland itself. In Sjögren's syndrome, parotitis is also accompanied by diminished salivation and lacrimation and some other connective tissue disorder, such as lupus erythematosus or rheumatoid arthritis.[73] Pain from any of these conditions will refer to the teeth. For further details, see chapter 8.

Ear Pain

Pain within the ear can be caused by a disease within the ear and related structures as with otitis media or mastoiditis. Pain may also be referred to the ear from many other head and neck structures including the teeth, temporomandibular joint, tonsils, tongue, throat, trachea, and thyroid.[74] This is because the ear is innervated by cranial nerves V, VII, VIII, IX, X, XI, and C1, C2, and C3.

Sinus and Paranasal Pain

Sinusitis is a common cause of dull, constant pain.[75] The location of this pain can vary from the maxilla and maxillary teeth in maxillary sinusitis to the upper orbit and frontal process in frontal sinusitis, between and behind the eyes in ethmoid sinusitis, and at the junction of the hard and soft palate, occiput, and mastoid process in sphenoid sinusitis. Pain from the sinuses may be referred into the oral cavity, the teeth in particular. The reverse is also true; that is, pain from the teeth or from periradicular lesions may be discerned as sinus pain or may be the source of maxillary sinus disease.[75] Selden has pointed out, in discussing the oral-antral syndrome, that about 25% of chronic maxillary sinusitis is secondary to dental infections.[76] Because of the extraoral nature of sinus and paranasal pain and disease, it will be considered in greater depth in chapter 8.

Myocardial Infarction, Coronary Thrombosis, Angina Pectoris, and Thyroid Disease.

It is hard to imagine that a site as distant from the oral cavity as the heart may refer pain into the teeth and jaws. But refer it does, in a most confusing manner. The diagnostician must be quite astute to recognize that the "toothache" described by the patient is actually reflecting serious cardiac disease.

Other sources of referred pain to the jaws are cardiospasm (spasm of the esophageal cardiac sphincter associated with hiatal hernia of the diaphragm) and thyroid disease. In addition to these pain references, women have reported oral discomfort associated with the menopause—43% of peri- and postmenopausal women reporting oral pain compared with only 6% of premenopausal women.[77] Two-thirds of the menopausal women reporting discomfort were relieved of their symptoms after hormone replacement therapy.[77]

Also reported is pain from non-Hodgkin's lymphoma disguised as odontogenic pain. There is a higher incidence of this disease in patients with acquired immune deficiency syndrome (AIDS).[78]

Because of the extraoral nature of these sources of referred oral pain, they will be discussed further in chapter 8.

CONCLUSION

In conclusion, one could state that the vast majority of patients who present themselves in pain are suffering acute pain. It would also be fair to state that most of these patients are suffering from a toothache (dental pulpalgia).

The dentist who is experienced in pain diagnosis will systematically examine and test to narrow down the suspected source of the pain. The inexperienced often push ahead and blunder into a serious error in misdiagnosis and treatment. One must deal with certainty, and if one is uncertain of the tooth or condition involved, the perplexing case should be referred to an expert diagnostician.

Chronic pain is an entirely different matter. Diagnosis and treatment of these cases might involve a team of experts at a tertiary care pain center. For this reason, an entire chapter, chapter 11, is devoted to these baffling cases.

REFERENCES

1. Lipton JA, Ship JA, Larach-Robinson D. Estimated prevalence and distribution of reported orofacial pain in the United States. J Am Dent Assoc 1993;124:115.
2. Medawar PB. The art of the soluble. London: Methuen; 1967.
3. Yamana M. In: Anderson DJ, editor. Sensory mechanism in dentine. New York: Macmillan; 1963. p. 78.
4. Brännström M. In: Anderson DJ, editor. Sensory mechanism in dentine. New York: Macmillan; 1963. p. 78.
5. Brännström M. The hydrodynamic theory of dentinal pain: sensation in preparations, caries, and the dentinal crack syndrome. JOE 1985;12:453.
6. Beveridge EE. Measurement of human dental intrapulpal pressure and its response to clinical variables [master's thesis]. Seattle (WA): Univ. of Washington; 1964.
7. Shoher I, Mahler Y, Samueloff S. Dental pulp photoplethysmography in human beings. Oral Surg 1973;36:915.
8. Funakoshi M, Zotterman Y. In: Anderson DJ, editor. Sensory mechanism in dentine. New York: Macmillan; 1963. p. 69.
9. Brännström M. In: Anderson DJ, editor. Sensory mechanism in dentine. New York: Macmillan; 1963. p. 72.
10. Kleinberg I. Dentinal hypersensitivity, part I: the biologic basis of the condition. Compend Contin Educ 1986;7:182.
11. Trowbridge HO. Review of dental pain—histology and physiology. JOE 1986;12:445.
12. Wallace JA, Bissada NF. Pulpal and root sensitivity related to periodontal therapy. Oral Surg 1990;69:743.
13. Anderson DJ. Sensory mechanisms in dentine. New York: Macmillan; 1963. p. 89.
14. Beveridge EE, Brown AC. The measurement of human dental intrapulpal pressure and its response to clinical variables. Oral Surg 1965;19:655.
15. Nahri MVO. The characteristics of intradental sensory units and their responses to stimulation. JDR 1985;64:564.
16. Grossman LI. Endodontic practice. 8th ed. Philadelphia: Lea & Febiger; 1974. p. 45.
17. Brännström M. The cause of postrestorative sensitivity and its prevention. JOE 1986;12:475.
18. Kleinberg K. Dentinal hypersensitivity, part II: treatment of sensitive dentin. Compend Contin Educ 1986;7:281.
19. Reis-Schmidt T. Dentinal hypersensitivity: a question of comfort. Dent Prod Rep 1988; p. 21.
20. Krauser JT. Hypersensitive teeth, part II: treatment. J Prosthet Dent 1986;56:307.
21. Greenhill JD, Pashley DH. The effect of desensitizing agents on the hydraulic conductance of human dentin *in vitro*. JDR 1981;60:686.
22. Cooley RL, Sandoval VA. Effectiveness of potassium oxalate treatment on dentin hyper-sensitivity. Gen Dent 1989;37:330.
23. Muzzin KB, Johnson R. Effects of potassium oxalate on dentin hypersensitivity *in vivo*. J Periodontol 1989;60:151.
24. Ikeda H, et al. Effects of potassium oxalate solution on the dentin hypersensitivity. Jpn J Conserv Dent 1988;31:1202.
25. Suda H, et al. Dentin sensitivity reduced by the application of chemical solutions. Jpn J Conserv Dent 1988;31:1210.
26. Goodman CH. Therapeutic modalities in the treatment of dentinal hypersensitivity. In: Proceedings on dentinal hyper-sensitivity. Jersey City (NJ): Block Drug Co.; 1987. p. 18.
27. Jensen ME, Doering JV. A comparative study of two clinical techniques for treatment of root surface hypersensitivity. Gen Dent 1987;35:128.
28. Simmons JJ. Ionic desensitization of teeth. Tex Dent J 1961;79:11.
29. Murthy KS, Talim ST, Singh I. A comparative evaluation of topical application and iontophoresis of sodium fluoride for desensitization of hypersensitive dentin. Oral Surg 1973;36:448.

30. Gangerosa LP, Park NH. Practical considerations in iontophoresis of fluoride for desensitizing dentin. J Prosthet Dent 1978;39:173.
31. Gangerosa LP, Heuer GA. A practical technique for treating tooth hypersensitivity. Dent Surg 1978;55:37.
32. Gangerosa LP. Iontophoretic application of fluoride by tray technique for desensitization of multiple teeth. J Am Dent Assoc 1981;102:50.
33. Gangerosa LP, et al. Double-blind evaluation of duration of dentin sensitivity reduction by fluoride iontophoresis. Gen Dent 1989;37:361.
34. Carlo GT, et al. An evaluation of iontophoretic application of fluoride for tooth desensitization. J Am Dent Assoc 1982;105:452.
35. Brough KM. The effectiveness of iontophoresis in reducing dentin hypersensitivity. J Am Dent Assoc 1985;111:761.
36. Hodosh M. A superior desensitizer—potassium nitrate. J Am Dent Assoc 1974;88:831.
37. Pashley DH. Dentin permeability, dentin sensitivity, and treatment through tubule occlusion. JOE 1986;12:465.
38. Bahram J, et al. Cyanoacrylate—a new treatment for hypersensitive dentin and cementum. J Am Dent Assoc 1987;114:486.
39. Calamia J, et al. Effect of Amalgambond (a 4-meta bonding agent) on cervical sensitivity [abstract]. JDR 1992;71:132.
40. Ianzano JA, Gwinnett J. Polymeric sealing of dentinal tubules to control sensitivity. JDR 1992;71:205.
41. Stanley HR, Swerdlow H. Reactions of the human pulp to cavity preparation: results produced by eight different operative grinding techniques. J Am Dent Assoc 1959;58:49.
42. Hahn C-L, et al. Correlation between thermal sensitivity and microorganisms isolated from deep carious lesions. JOE 1993;19:26.
43. Hodosh M, et al. Potassium nitrate: an effective treatment for pulpitis. Oral Surg 1983;55:419.
44. Glick DH. Lecture before the American Association of Endodontists, April 1983.
45. Kier DM, et al. Thermally induced pulpalgia in endodontically treated teeth. JOE 1991;17:38.
46. Newsviews. Ice the pain. Calif Dent Assoc J 1988;16:51.
47. Kollman W. Incidence and possible causes of dental pain during simulated high altitude flights. JOE 1993;19:154.
48. Rauch JW. Barodontologia—dental pain related to ambient pressure change. Gen Dent 1985;33:313.
49. England MC, et al. Histopathologic study of the effect of pulpal disease upon the nerve fibers of the human dental pulp. Oral Surg 1974;38:783.
50. Genet JM, et al. The incidence of postoperative pain in endodontic therapy. Int Endodont J 1986;19:221.
51. Genet JM, et al. Preoperative and operative factors associated with pain after the first endodontic visit. Int Endodont J 1987;20:53.
52. Flath RK, et al. Pain suppression after pulpectomy with preoperative flurbiprofen. JOE 1987;13:339.
53. Oguntebi BR, et al. Postoperative pain incidence related to the type of emergency treatment of symptomatic pulpitis. Oral Surg 1992;73:479.
54. Campbell RL, et al. Chronic facial pain associated with endodontic therapy. Oral Surg 1990;69:287.
55. Morse DR, et al. Comparison of prophylactic and on-demand diflunisal for pain management of patients having one-visit endodontic therapy. Oral Surg 1990;69:729.
56. Moskow A, et al. Intracanal use of a corticosteroid solution as an endodontic anodyne. Oral Surg 1984;58:600.
57. Morse DR, et al. Prophylactic penicillin versus penicillin taken at the first sign of swelling in cases of asymptomatic pulpal-periradicular lesions: a comparative analysis. Oral Surg 1988;65:228.
58. Krasner P, Jackson E. Management of post-treatment endodontic pain with oral dexamethasone: a double-blind study. Oral Surg 1986;62:187.
59. Jackson EL, et al. Preoperative anti-inflammatory medication for the prevention of postoperative dental pain. J Am Dent Assoc 1989;119:641.
60. Creech JL III, et al. Effect of occlusal relief on endodontic pain. J Am Dent Assoc 1984;109:64.
61. Liesinger LW, Marshall FJ, Marshall JG. Effect of variable doses of dexamethasone on post-treatment pain. JOE 1993;19:35.
62. Marshall JG, Liesinger AW. Factors associated with endodontic posttreatment pain. JOE 1993;19:573.
63. Nobuhara WK, et al. Anti-inflammatory effects of dexamethasone on periradicular tissues following endodontic overinstrumentation. JOE 1993;19:501.
64. Glick DH. Locating referred pulpal pains. Oral Surg 1962;15:613.
65. Robertson S, Wolff, Goodell. The teeth as a source of headache and other pain. Arch Neurol Psychiatry 1947;57:277.
66. Travell, J. Temporomandibular joint dysfunction: temporomandibular joint pain referred from muscles of the head and neck. J Prosthet Dent 1960;10:745.
67. Ray BS, Wolff HG. Experimental studies on headache. Pain sensitive structures of the head and their significance in headache. Arch Surg 1940;41:813.
68. Ruch TC, Fulton JF. Medical physiology and biophysics. 18th ed. Philadelphia: WB Saunders; 1960.
69. Hutchins HC, Reynolds OE. Experimental investigation of the referred pain of aerodontalgia. J Dent Res 1947;26:3.
70. Reynolds OE, Hutchins HC. Reduction of central hyper-irritability following block anesthesia of peripheral nerve. Am J Physiol 1948;152:658.
71. Rees RT, Harris M. Atypical odontalgia. Br J Oral Surg 1978–79;16:212.
72. Schnurr RF, Brooke RI. Atypical odontolgia. Oral Surg 1992;73:445.
73. Arthritis Foundation: primer on the rheumatic diseases. JAMA 1973;224:663.
74. Birt D. Headaches and head pains associated with diseases of the ear, nose and throat. Med Clin North Am 1978;62:523.
75. Boles R. Paranasal sinuses and facial pain. In: Alling CC, Mahan PE, editors. Facial pain. 2nd ed. Philadelphia: Lea & Febiger; 1977. p. 115–34.
76. Selden HS. Annual meeting, American Association of Endodontists, April 1990.
77. Wardrop RW, et al. Oral discomfort at menopause. Oral Surg 1989;67:535.
78. Bavitz JB, et al. Non-Hodgkin's lymphoma disguised as odontogenic pain. J Am Dent Assoc 1992;123:99.

Chapter 8

NONODONTOGENIC TOOTHACHE AND CHRONIC HEAD AND NECK PAINS

Bernadette Jaeger

Pain is perfect misery, the worst of evils; and excessive, overturns all patience.

–John Milton, Paradise Lost

Patients with chronic oral or facial pain, or headache, present a true diagnostic and therapeutic challenge to the practitioner. For many in the dental profession, the only solution to problems of pain lies with a scalpel, forceps, or ever-increasing doses of analgesics, narcotics, or sedatives. Many patients with chronic pain have suffered this mistreatment and stand as an indictment of a poorly trained, insecure, and disinterested segment of dentistry. Attending to patients who have been unable to obtain resolution of their pain complaint, despite extensive evaluation and treatment, requires a compassionate reappraisal and fresh approach. Fortunately, accurate diagnosis and successful management of these patients can be among the most rewarding experiences in dental or medical practice.

WHAT IS PAIN?

Pain is not a simple sensation but rather a complex neurobehavioral event involving at least two components. First is an individual's discernment or perception of the stimulation of specialized nerve endings designed to transmit information concerning potential or actual tissue damage (nociception). Second is the individual's reaction to this perceived sensation (pain behavior). This is any behavior, physical or emotional, that follows pain perception. Culture or environment often influences these behaviors. Beyond this is the suffering or emotional toll the pain has on any given individual. Suffering is so personal that it is difficult to quantify, evaluate, and treat.

The fact that pain is difficult to define, quantify, and understand is reflected in the numerous ways in which it has been described. *Dorland's Medical Dictionary* defines pain as "a more or less localized sensation of discomfort, distress, or agony resulting from the stimulation of specialized nerve endings."[1] In this definition, the behavioral reaction to nociception is already assumed to be distress or agony, which is not always the case. Take, for example, the observations made by Beecher in 1956 that only 25% of soldiers wounded in battle requested narcotic medications for pain relief, compared to more than 80% of civilian patients with surgical wounds of a similar magnitude.[2] Clearly, the behavioral reaction to similar nociceptive stimuli varies from person to person and depends on a number of factors, including the significance of the injury to that individual. The wounded soldier may be relieved to be out of a life-threatening situation; the surgical patient may be concerned about recurrence of a tumor just removed. *Dorland's* definition also implies that stimulation of nociceptors is required for perception of pain, yet the dental patient who has been anxious for weeks in anticipation of the "needle" at the dentist's office may jump in agony at the slightest touch of his cheek.

Fields defined pain as "an unpleasant sensation that is perceived as arising from a specific region of the body and is commonly produced by processes that damage or are capable of damaging bodily tissue."[3] He emphasized the need to be able to localize the painful source in order to distinguish it from psychological pain and suffering, for example, the "pain" of a broken heart.

A more complete definition is cast by the **International Association for the Study of Pain (IASP)** in its taxonomy of painful disorders.[4] That definition of pain is as follows: "An unpleasant sensory and emotional experience associated with actual or potential tissue damage, or described in terms of such damage." Added to this definition, however, is the following, emphasizing the subjective nature of pain that distinguishes and separates it from the simple stimulation of nociceptors:

Pain is always subjective. Each individual learns the application of the word through experiences related to injury in early life. It is unquestionably a sensation in a part of the body, but it is also always unpleasant and therefore also an emotional experience. Many people report pain in the absence of tissue damage or any likely pathophysiological cause, usually this happens for psychological reasons. There is no way to distinguish their experience from that due to tissue damage, if we take the subjective report. If they regard their experience as pain and if they report it in the same ways as pain caused by tissue damage, it should be accepted as pain. This definition avoids tying pain to the stimulus. Activity induced in the nociceptor and nociceptive pathways by a noxious stimulus is not pain, which is always a psychological state, even though we may well appreciate that pain most often has a proximate physical cause.[4]

The IASP definition of pain makes the point that **pain is pain even if a nociceptive source is not readily identified.** Pain owing to psychological causes is as real as any pain associated with actual nociception and should be treated as such.

To understand pain better, this chapter first looks at what is currently known about the anatomy and physiology of the nociceptive pathways and some of the modulating influences that modify the nociceptive input into the central nervous system. Following this, various psychological and behavioral factors that influence the perception of and reaction to pain are reviewed.

NEUROPHYSIOLOGY OF PAIN

The following summarizes what is known about the basic anatomy and physiology of pain under normal physiologic conditions[5]:

Acute Pain Pathways

The body has specialized neurons that respond only to noxious or potentially noxious stimulation. These **neurons** are called **primary afferent nociceptors** and are made up of small-diameter thinly myelinated A delta and unmyelinated C fibers (Figure 8-1). They **synapse in the substantia gelatinosa** of the dorsal horn of the spinal cord with neurons known as second-order pain transmission neurons. From here the signals are transmitted along specialized pathways (spinothalamic and reticulothalamic tracts) to the medial and lateral

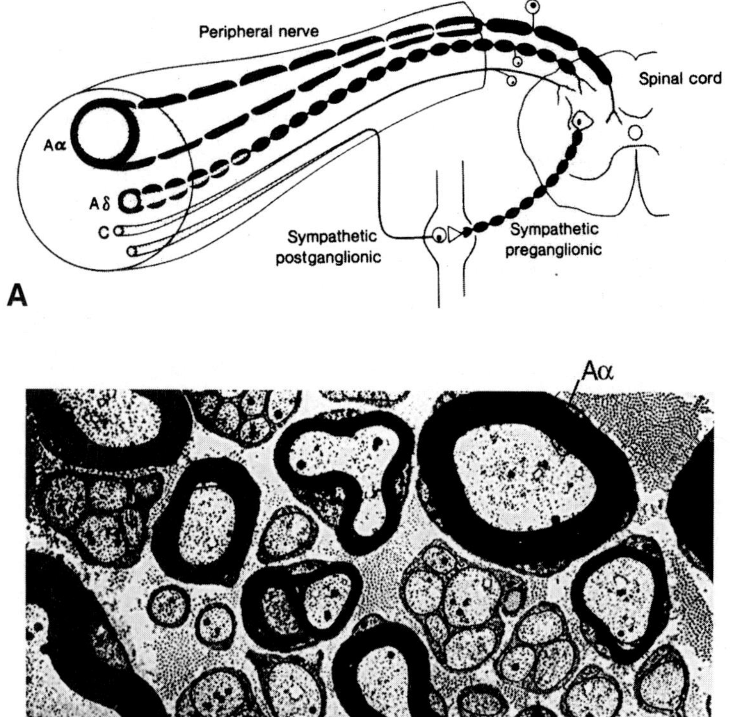

Figure 8-1 Components of a typical cutaneous nerve. **A** illustrates that there are two distinct functional categories of axon: primary afferents with cell bodies in the dorsal root ganglion and sympathetic postganglionic fibers with cell bodies in the sympathetic ganglion. Primary afferents include those with large-diameter myelinated (Aα), small-diameter myelinated (Ad), and unmyelinated (C) axons. All sympathetic postganglionic fibers are unmyelinated. **B**, Electron micrograph of cross-section of a cutaneous nerve illustrating the relative size and degree of myelination of its complement of axons. The myelin appears as black rings of varying thickness. The unmyelinated axons (C) occur singly or in clusters. Reproduced with permission from Ochoa JL. Microscopic anatomy of unmyelinated nerve fibers. In: Dyck PJ, et al, editors. Peripheral neuropathy. 1st ed. WB Saunders; Philadelphia (PA): 1975.

regions of the thalamus (Figure 8-2). Perception of nociception may occur in the thalamus and cortex, but the exact location is unknown, and the contribution of the cortex to pain perception is controversial.[3]

Fields divided the processing of pain from the stimulation of primary afferent nociceptors to the subjective experience of pain into four steps: transduction, transmission, modulation, and perception.[3] **Transduction** is the activation of the primary **afferent** nociceptor. Primary afferent nociceptors can be activated by intense thermal and mechanical stimuli, noxious chemicals, and noxious cold. They are also activated by stimulation from endogenous algesic chemical substances (inflammatory mediators) produced by the body in response to tissue injury. Damaged tissue or blood cells release the polypeptide **bradykinin** (**BK**), potassium, histamine, serotonin, and arachidonic acid. Arachidonic acid is processed by two different enzyme systems to produce **prostaglandins** and **leukotrienes,** which, along with BK, act as inflammatory mediators (Figure 8-3). Bradykinin acts synergistically with these other chemicals to increase plasma extravasation and **produce edema**. Plasma extravasation, in turn, replenishes the supply of inflammatory chemical mediators. Whereas prostaglandins stimulate the primary afferent nociceptor directly, the leukotrienes contribute indirectly by causing **polymorphonuclear neutrophil leukocytes** to release another chemical, which, in turn, stimulates the nociceptor. Bradykinin further contributes by causing the **sympathetic** nerve terminal to release a prostaglandin that also stimulates the nociceptor.[6] Additionally, in an area of injury or inflammation, the **sympathetic nerve terminal** will release yet another prostaglandin in response to its own neurotransmitter, **norepinephrine**. The presence of such an ongoing inflammatory state causes physiologic **sensitization** of the primary afferent nociceptors.[6] Sensitized nociceptors display ongoing discharge, a lowered activation threshold to **normally nonpainful stimuli** (**allodynia**), and an **exaggerated response** to noxious stimuli (**primary hyperalgesia**).[7]

In addition to sending nociceptive impulses to synapse in the dorsal horn of the spinal cord, activation of cutaneous C fibers causes their cell bodies to synthesize the neuropeptides, **substance P** and **calcitonin gene–related peptide** (CGRP). These neuropeptides are then antidromically transported along axon branches to the periphery by an axon transport system where they induce further plasma extravasation and increase inflammation. The release of these algogenic substances at the peripheral axon injury site produces the flare commonly seen around an injury site and is referred to as **neurogenic inflammation** or the **axon reflex**[7–9] (Figure 8-4).

Transmission refers to the process by which peripheral nociceptive information is relayed to the central

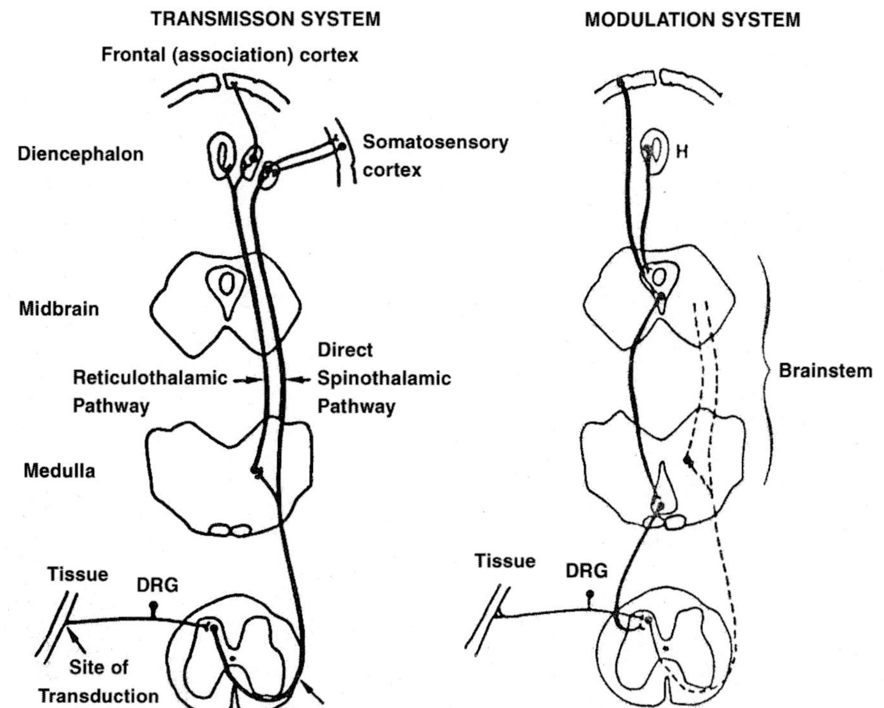

Figure 8-2 Diagrammatic outline of major neural structures relevant to pain. Sequence of events leading to pain perception begins in the transmission system with transduction (lower left), in which a noxious stimulus produces nerve impulses in the primary afferent nociceptor. These impulses are conducted to the spinal cord, where primary afferent nociceptors contact central pain transmission cells, which relay the message to the thalamus either directly via the spinothalamic tract or indirectly via the reticular formation and the reticulothalamic pathway. From the thalamus, the message is relayed to the cerebral cortex and the hypothalamus (H). The outflow is through the midbrain and medulla to the dorsal horn of the spinal cord, where it inhibits pain transmission cells, thereby reducing the intensity of perceived pain. Reproduced with permission from Pain and disability, copyright 1987 by the National Academy of Sciences. Published by National Academy Press, Washington, DC.

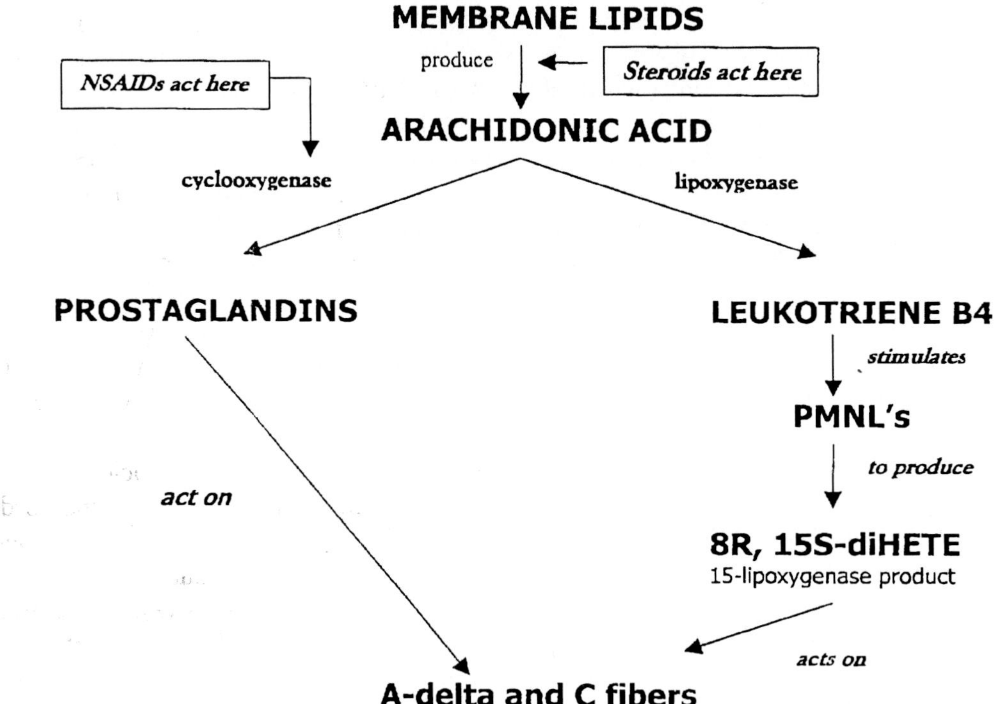

Figure 8-3 Membrane lipids produce arachidonic acid, which is converted to prostaglandins by the cyclooxygenase enzyme and to leukotriene B_4 by the lipoxygenase enzyme. Prostaglandins act directly on the primary afferent nociceptor to lower the firing threshold and therefore cause "sensitization." Leukotriene B_4 cause polymorphonuclear neutrophil leukocytes (PMNLs) to produce another leukotriene that, in turn, acts on the primary afferent nociceptor to cause sensitization. Steroids prevent the synthesis of arachidonic acid altogether, thus inhibiting both pathways of prostaglandin production. Nonsteroidal anti-inflammatory drugs (NSAIDs), on the other hand, inhibit only the cyclooxygenase pathway.

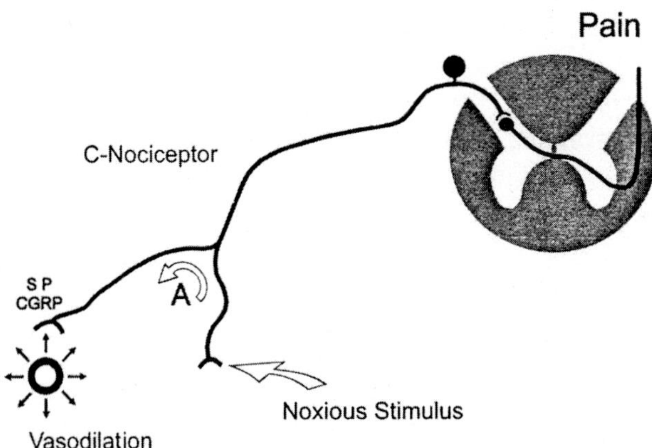

Figure 8-4 The axon reflex. Activation of cutaneous nociceptive C fibers elicits impulses that are conveyed centrally to induce pain and antidromically via axon branches (A). The antidromically excited peripheral C-fiber terminals release vasoactive substances, for example, calcitonin gene–related peptide (CGRP) and substance P (SP), causing cutaneous vasodilation, which produces the flare that develops around the site of noxious stimulation. Reproduced with permission from Fields HL, Rowbotham M, Baron R. Neuralgia: irritable nociceptors and deafferentation. Neurobiol Dis 1998;5:209.

nervous system. The primary afferent nociceptor synapses with a second-order pain transmission neuron in the dorsal horn of the spinal cord where a new action potential heads toward higher brain structures (see Figure 8-2). It is at this point that repeated or intense C fiber activation causes specific changes involving substance P and excitatory amino acids acting on N-methyl-D-aspartate (NMDA) receptors that results in **central sensitization.**[7] Long-term changes in the response of second-order pain transmission neurons to nonpainful and painful input are induced with intense or prolonged nociceptive stimuli.[7] The response of these spinal cord dorsal horn neurons increases progressively and is enhanced with repeated identical noxious cutaneous input from the periphery, a process called "wind-up."[10–12] In addition, the size of the receptive field of the second-order pain transmission neuron increases.[13] The subjective correlate of wind-up is "**temporal summation,**" for which a slowly repeated noxious stimulus is associated with a progressive increase in the intensity of perceived pain.[7,14] In addition, with central sensitization, stimulation of A beta fibers (large-diameter low-threshold mechanoreceptors that normally respond only to painless tactile stimuli) will also activate second-order nociceptive dorsal horn neurons, producing what is called a "**secondary mechanical hyperalgesia**" in the area surrounding the initial tissue injury[7,15] (Figure 8-5).

Modulation refers to mechanisms by which the transmission of noxious information to the brain is reduced. Numerous **descending inhibitory** systems that originate supraspinally and strongly influence spinal nociceptive transmission exist.[16] In the past, only midline structures such as the periaqueductal gray and nucleus raphe magnus were known to be involved in descending nociceptive modulation (Figure 8-2). Now many sites previously thought to be primarily involved in cardiovascular function and autonomic regulation (eg, nucleus tractus solitarius; locus ceruleus/subceruleus, among others) have also been shown to play a role in pain modulation.[16] The ascending nociceptive signal that synapses in the midbrain area activates the release of **norepinephrine (NE)** and **serotonin,** two of the main neurotransmitters involved in the descending inhibitory pathways.[16] Activity in the pain modulation system means that there is less activity in the pain transmission pathway in response to noxious stimulation.

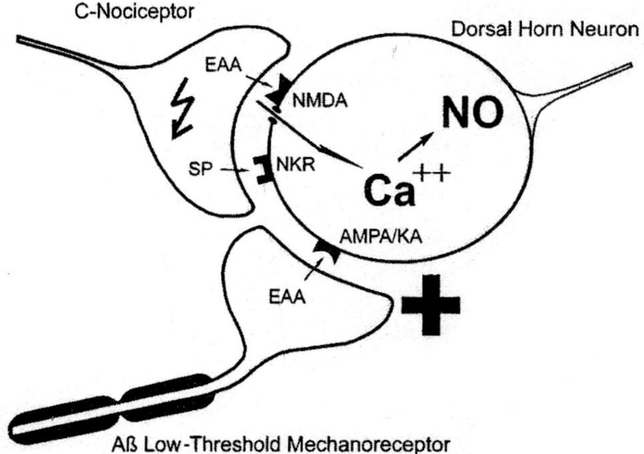

Figure 8-5 Central sensitization and allodynia. Input from C-nociceptors enhances the response of dorsal horn pain-signaling neurons to subsequent afferent inputs (central sensitization). This involves neuropeptides such as substance P (SP) acting at neurokinin receptors (NKR) and excitatory amino acids (EAA) acting at both the AMPA/KA and N-methyl-D-aspartate (NMDA) receptors, triggering secondary NO (nitric oxide) mechanisms. Large-diameter low-threshold mechanoreceptive primary afferents (A beta fibers) respond maximally to innocuous tactile stimuli and normally produce tactile sensation. When central sensitization is present, A beta fibers become capable of activating central nervous system pain-signaling neurons (+), leading to touch-evoked pain (allodynia). Reproduced with permission from Fields HL, Rowbotham M, Baron R. Neuralgia: irritable nociceptors and deafferentation. Neurobiol Dis 1998;5:209.

An endogenous opioid system for pain modulation also exists.[17] **Endogenous opioid peptides** are naturally occurring pain-dampening neurotransmitters and neuromodulators that are **implicated in pain suppression** and modulation because they are present in large quantities in the areas of the brain associated with these activities (subnucleus caudalis and the substantia gelatinosa of the spinal cord).[17,18] They reduce nociceptive transmission by preventing the release of the excitatory neurotransmitter substance P from the primary afferent nerve terminal. The presence of these natural opioid receptors for endogenous opiates permits morphine-like drugs to exert their analgesic effect.

The final step in the subjective experience of pain is **perception.** How and where the brain perceives pain is still under investigation. Part of the difficulty lies in the fact that the pain experience has at least two components: the sensory-discriminatory dimension and the affective (emotional) dimension. The affective dimension of pain is made up of feelings of unpleasantness and emotions associated with future implications related to the pain.[19] Although functional magnetic resonance imaging (MRI) studies have demonstrated the involvement of the thalamus and multiple cortical areas in the perception of pain, it is clear from the intersubject variability in the activation of any one of these areas that affective reactions and possibly motor responses are also involved.[20]

Of significance is the fact that, with high levels of modulation, or with damage in the pain transmission system, it is possible to have nociception without pain perception. Conversely, with certain types of damage to the nervous system, there may be an overreaction to pain stimuli or pain perception without nociception.[3]

Referred Pain

Pain arising from deep tissues, muscles, ligaments, joints, and viscera is often perceived at a site distant from the actual nociceptive source. Thus, the pain of **angina pectoris** is often felt in the left arm or the **jaw**, and diaphragmatic pain is often perceived in the shoulder or neck. Whereas cutaneous pain is sharp, burning, and clearly localized, referred pain from musculoskeletal and visceral sources is usually deep, dull, aching, and more diffuse.

Referred pain presents a diagnostic dilemma. If left unrecognized, it may result in a clinician telling a patient that his pain is psychogenic in origin. Treatments directed at the site of the pain are ineffective and, if invasive, subject the patient to unnecessary risks, expense, and complications. However, referred pain is dependent on a primary pain source and will cease if this source is eliminated.

The mechanism of referred pain is still somewhat enigmatic. The two most popular theories are convergence-projection and convergence-facilitation:

1. **Convergence-projection theory**: This is the most popular theory. Primary afferent nociceptors from both visceral and cutaneous neurons often converge onto the same second-order pain transmission neuron in the spinal cord,[21] and convergence has been well documented in the trigeminal brainstem nuclear complex.[22–25] The trigeminal spinal tract nucleus also receives converging input from cranial nerves VII, IX, and X, as well as the upper cervical nerves.[26,27] The brain, having more awareness of cutaneous than of visceral structures through past experience, interprets the pain as coming from the regions subserved by the cutaneous afferent fibers (Figure 8-6).
2. **Convergence-facilitation theory**: This theory is similar to the convergence-projection theory, except that the nociceptive input from the deeper structures causes the resting activity of the second-order pain transmission neuron in the spinal cord to increase or be "facilitated." The resting activity is normally created by impulses from the cutaneous afferents. "Facilitation" from the deeper nociceptive impulses causes the pain to be perceived in the area that creates the normal, resting background activity. This theory tries to incorporate the clinical observation that blocking sensory input from the reference area, with either local anesthetic or cold, can sometimes reduce the perceived pain. This is particularly true with referred pain from **myofascial trigger points** (**TrPs**), for which application of a vapocoolant spray is actually a popular and effective modality used for pain control.

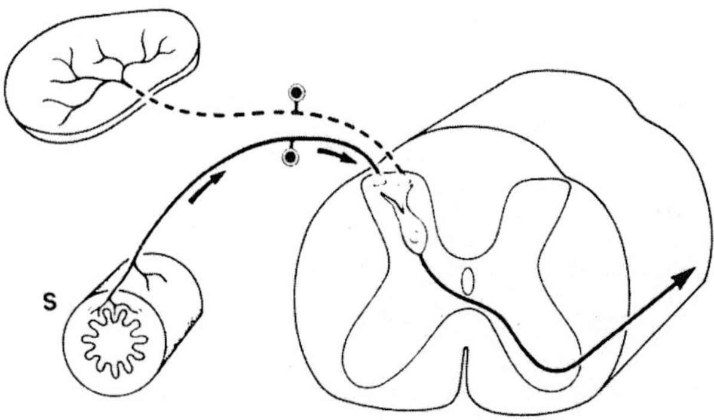

Figure 8-6 The convergence-projection hypothesis of referred pain. According to this hypothesis, visceral afferent nociceptors (S) converge on the same pain-projection neurons as the afferents from the somatic structures in which the pain is perceived. The brain has no way of knowing the actual source and mistakenly "projects" the sensation to the somatic structure. Reproduced with permission from Fields HL.[3]

The mechanism of referred pain from myofascial TrPs is also under speculation. According to Mense, the convergence-projection and convergence-facilitation models of referred pain do not directly apply to muscle pain because there is little convergence of neurons from **deep** tissues in the dorsal horn.[28] Based on experimentally induced changes in the receptive field properties of dorsal horn neurons in the cat in response to a deep noxious stimulus[29] (Figure 8-7), Mense proposed that convergent connections **from other spinal cord segments** are "unmasked" or opened by nociceptive input from skeletal muscle and that referral to other myotomes is owing to the release and spread of substance P and CGRP to adjacent spinal segments[28] (Figure 8-8). Simons has expanded on this theory to specifically explain the referred pain from TrPs[30] (Figure 8-9). Myofascial pain (MFP) is discussed in more detail later in the chapter.

Trigeminal System

An appreciation of the arrangement of the trigeminal nociceptive system provides some insight into the interesting pain and referral patterns that are encountered in the head and neck region. The primary afferent nociceptors of the fifth cranial nerve synapse in the nucleus caudalis of the brainstem. The nucleus caudalis is the caudal portion of the trigeminal spinal tract nucleus and corresponds to the substantia gelatinosa of the rest of the spinal dorsal horn (Figure 8-10). From here the nociceptive input is transmitted to the higher centers via the trigeminal lemniscus. Of significance is the arrangement of the trigeminal nerve fibers within this nucleus and the fact that the nucleus descends as low as the third and fourth cervical vertebrae (C3–4) in the spinal cord. Fibers from all three trigeminal branches are found at all levels of the nucleus, arranged with the mandibular division highest and the ophthalmic division lowest.[31] In addition, they are arranged in such a manner that fibers closest to the midline of the face synapse in the most cephalad portion of the tract. The more lateral the origin of the fibers on the face, the more caudal the synapse in the nucleus (Figure 8-11). Understanding this "laminated" arrangement helps to explain why a maxillary molar toothache may be perceived as pain in a mandibular molar on the same side (referred pain) but not in an incisor. Similarly, pain perceived in the ear may actually be owing to (or referred from) an infected third molar.

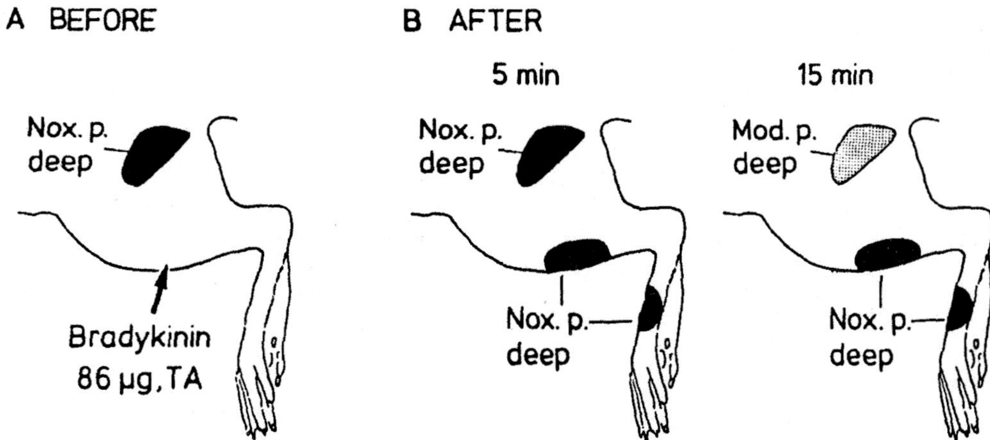

Figure 8-7 Changes in receptive field (RF) properties of a dorsal horn neuron following intramuscular injection of a painful dose of bradykinin (BKN). A, Location and size of the original RF (**black**) before BKN injection. The neuron required noxious deep pressure stimulation (Nox. p. deep) of the proximal biceps femoris muscle for activation. The **arrow** points to the injection site in the anterior tibial muscle (TA). **B, left**, 5 minutes after the BKN injection, two new RFs were present (**black**), both of which were located in deep tissues and had a high mechanical threshold. **B, right**, 15 minutes after the BKN injection, the original RF displayed a lowering in mechanical threshold and now responded to moderate (innocuous) deep pressure (Mod. p. deep). Reproduced with permission from Mense S.[28]

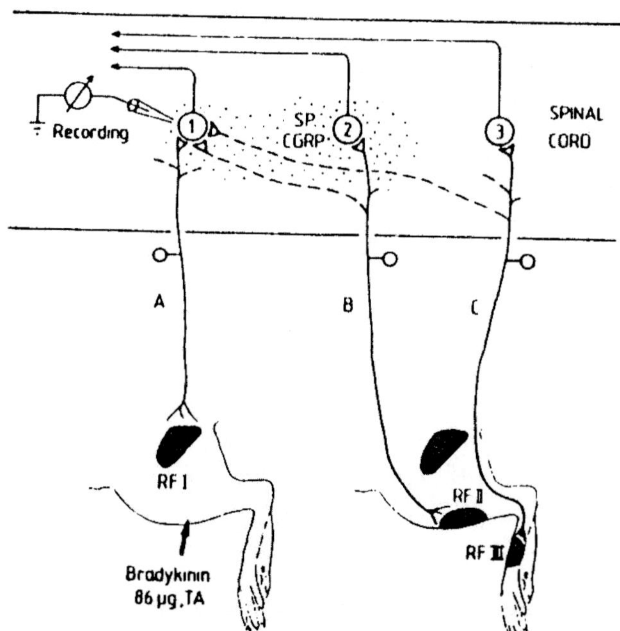

Figure 8-8 Neuroanatomic model explaining the appearance of new receptive fields (RFs) (see Figure 8-7) by unmasking latent connections in the dorsal horn. The activity of neuron 1 was recorded with a microelectrode introduced into the spinal cord. The neuron is connected by pathway A to its original RF in the biceps femoris muscle (RF I). Synaptically effective connections are drawn as **solid lines**, ineffective (latent) connections as **dashed lines**. The injection of bradykinin was made outside RF I into the tibialis anterior (TA) muscle, which contains the RF of neuron 2 (RF II). The bradykinin-induced excitation of nociceptive fibers of pathway B is assumed to release substance P (SP) and calcitonin gene–related peptide (CGRP) in the dorsal horn, which diffuse (stippling) to neuron 1 and increase the efficacy of latent connections from pathways B and C to this cell. Now neuron 1 can be activated also from RF II and RF III. (Menses, unpublished data). Reproduced with permission from Mense S.[28]

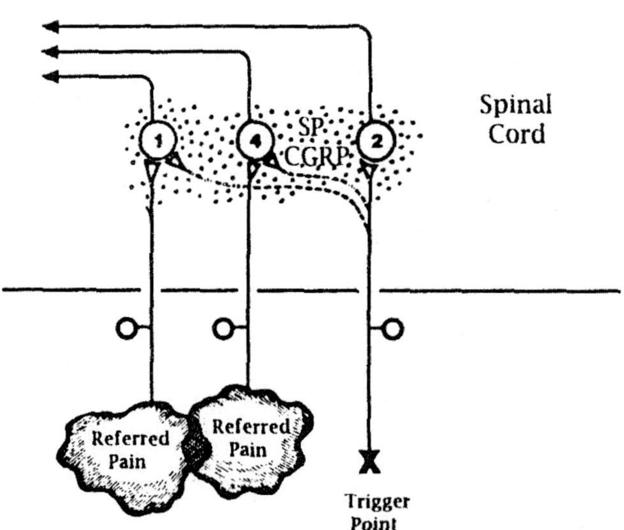

Figure 8-9 Extension of the neuroanatomic model presented in Figure 8-7 of Mense's model of deep referred pain. Although no direct experimental evidence substantiates this modification, it is compatible with the mechanisms described by Mense and helps to explain some trigger point characteristics not accounted for by his model. Neurons 1 and 2 correspond to neurons 1 and 2 in the Mense model. Neurons 1 and 4 are connected by solid lines to their respective receptive fields. These fields are the areas that would be identified as the source of nociception when neurons 1 and 4 are activated. Nociceptive input from the trigger point would activate neuron 2 and could account for the initial localized pain in response to pressure applied to the trigger point. This activity is assumed to release substance P (SP) and calcitonin gene–related peptide (CGRP) in the dorsal horn that diffuses (**stippling**) to neurons 1 and 4. This increases the efficacy of latent connections (**dashed lines**) to these cells. Now neurons 1 and 4 can be activated by nociceptive activity originating in the trigger point and would be perceived as referred pain. Reproduced with permission from Simons DG.[30]

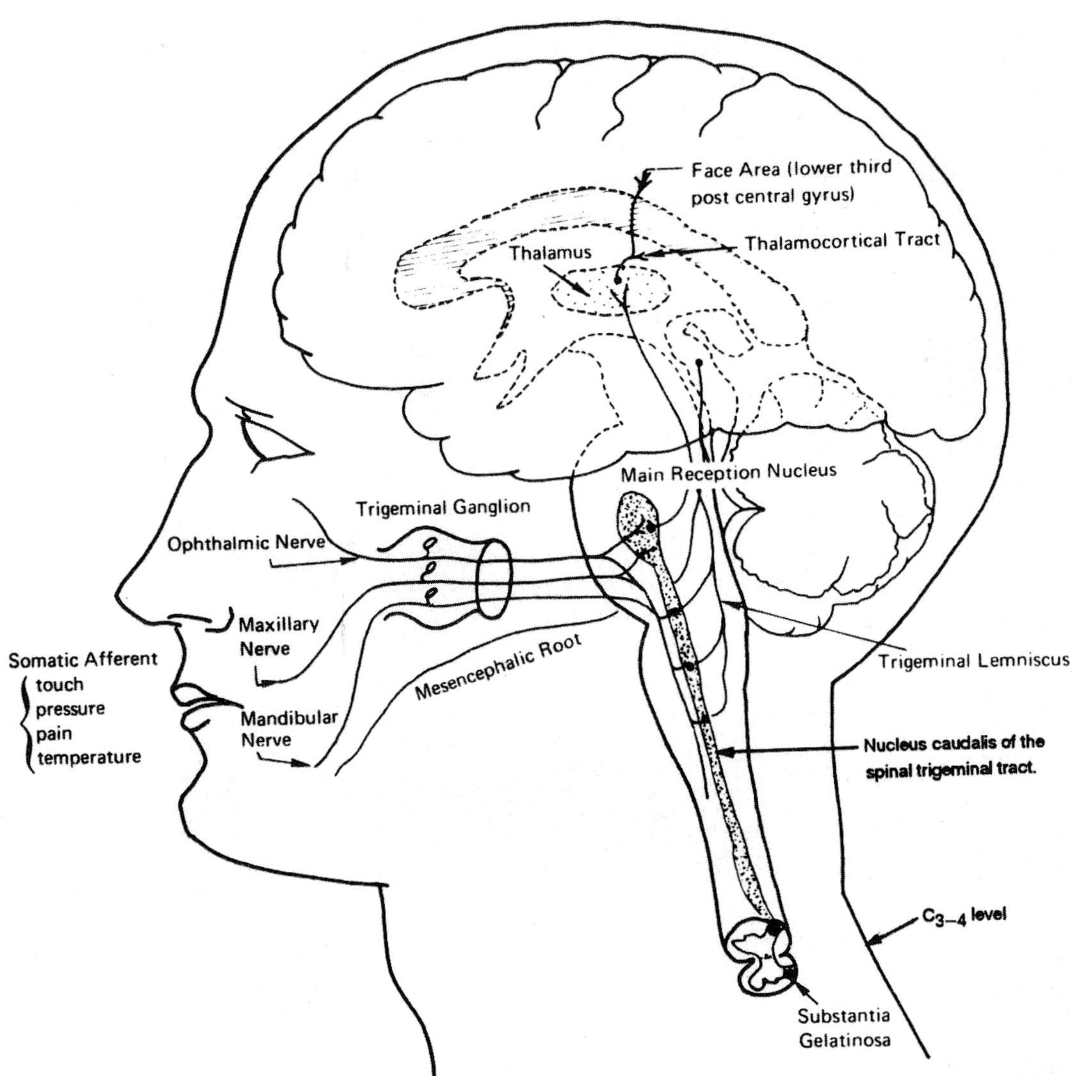

Figure 8-10 Primary afferent nociceptive fibers of the trigeminal nerve (cranial nerve V) synapse in the nucleus caudalis of the spinal trigeminal tract. The nucleus caudalis descends as low as C3–4 in the spinal cord. Many nociceptors from deep cervical structures synapse on the same second-order pain transmission neurons as the trigeminal nerve. This may explain why cervical pain disorders are often perceived as facial pain or headache.

Because the trigeminal nucleus descends to the C3–4 level in the spinal cord, primary afferent nociceptors from deep cervical structures synapse on the same second-order pain transmission neurons that subserve the fifth cranial nerve.[32] This convergence of primary afferent nociceptors from the trigeminal region and the cervical region provides a basis for understanding why **cervical pain** disorders may be perceived as pain in the head and face, particularly in the forehead and temple—the lateral ophthalmic trigeminal fibers synapse the lowest (see Figure 8-11).

Chronic Pain

Pain becomes complicated and difficult to manage when it is prolonged. Often the clinician is frustrated by the apparent discrepancy between the identifiable nociceptive source, which may seem very small, and the amount of suffering and disability seen. It becomes easy to label these patients as "crazy" or "malingering" (deliberately, fraudulently feigning an illness for the purpose of a consciously desired outcome).[1] Yet there are both physiologic and psychological mechanisms that may increase pain perception—mechanisms that help to explain why there may be a discrepancy between actual nociception, perceived pain, and the apparent resultant suffering and disability.

Physiologic Mechanisms Modifying Pain. *Sensitization.* As previously discussed, primary afferent nociceptors become sensitized through the release of endogenous substances caused by tissue injury. As a

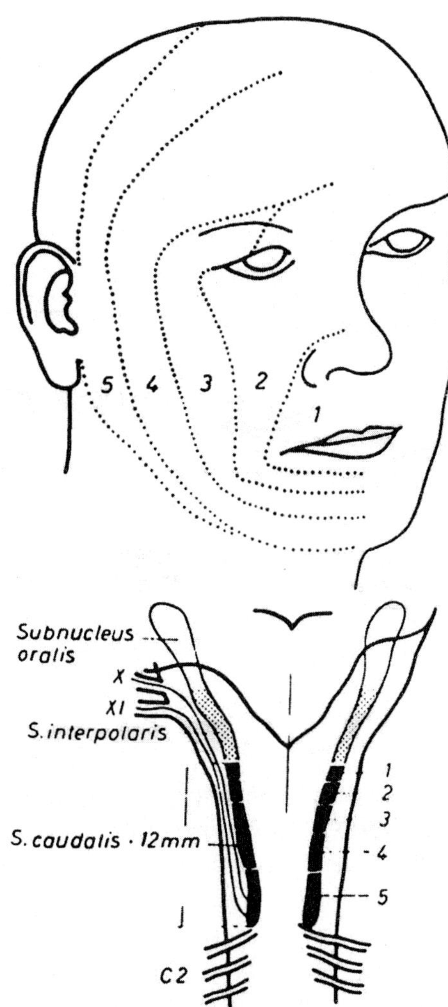

Figure 8-11 The arrangement of the trigeminal nociceptive fibers of the spinal trigeminal tract is significant. Fibers from all three trigeminal branches are found at all levels of the nucleus, arranged with the mandibular division highest and the ophthalmic division lowest. Fibers closest to the midline of the face synapse in the most cephalad portion of the tract. The more lateral the origin of the fibers on the face, the more caudal the synapse in the nucleus. Reproduced with permission from Kunc Z.[31]

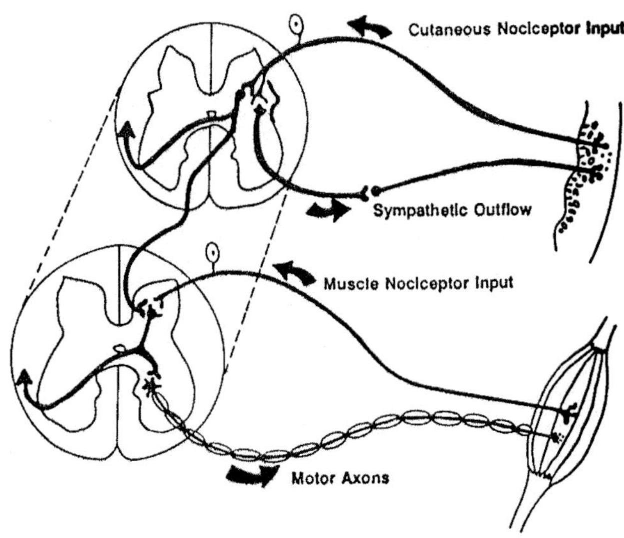

Figure 8-12 Reflex activation of nociceptors in self-sustaining pain. There are two important reflex pathways for pain. The **top loop** illustrates the sympathetic component. Nociceptor input activates sympathetic reflexes, which activate or sensitize nociceptor terminals. The **bottom loop** illustrates the muscle contraction loop. Nociceptors induce muscle contraction, which, in some patients, activates muscle nociceptors that feed back into the same reflex to sustain muscle contraction and pain. Reproduced with permission from Pain and disability, copyright 1987 by National Academy of Sciences. Published by National Academy Press, Washington, DC.

result, **normally innocuous stimuli become painful.**[6] For example, acute arthritis of the temporomandibular joint (TMJ) results in pain on joint movement or with increased pressure from chewing, normally innocuous events. Similarly, a minor burn on the tongue from hot tea makes it almost impossible to eat anything even mildly spicy.

Spreading Muscle Spasm. Sustained muscle contraction (spasm) may arise as the result of a primary noxious stimulus. This is a spinal reflex and a protective response to tissue injury (Figure 8-12). An example of this would be masticatory elevator muscle spasm (trismus) secondary to an infected third molar. The spasm may actually be the chief complaint, and yet, initially, it is dependent on the primary pain source. However, if the muscle spasm results in ischemia and accumulation of potassium ions, muscle nociceptors may be activated, resulting in the development of an independent, self-perpetuating primary pain source in the muscle (see Figure 8-12). Successful treatment of the infection or removal of the painful third molar will no longer correct the muscle pain problem since use of the muscle produces pain, causing more spasm, causing more pain. In addition, studies have shown that this type of deep musculoskeletal pain causes spasm and pain in other muscles innervated by the same spinal segment.[33,34] Long-standing conditions of this sort may result in recruitment of more muscles and more pain, with the ultimate establishment of a vicious spreading pain cycle. This may partly explain the development and some of the characteristics of myofascial TrPs, to be discussed in detail later in the chapter.

Autonomic Factors. Just as primary afferent nociceptive input may activate motoneurons, so may it also activate the sympathetic nervous system (see Figure 8-12). Efferent discharge from the sympathetic nervous system has been shown, in animals at least, to activate primary afferent nociceptors, especially when injured.[35] Thus, a peripheral injury may set up a positive feedback loop through **activation of the sympathetic nervous system** that will perpetuate the activation of the primary afferent nociceptors. The extreme result of this type of sympathetic hyperactivity is a condition known as **"reflex sympathetic dystrophy"** (discussed in more detail later in this chapter). In this syndrome, the pain, even from a minor injury, does not subside and, in fact, develops into a progressive, excruciating burning pain with cutaneous hypersensitivity. The pain may occur in a site larger than and different from that of the original injury; autonomic signs such as vasoconstriction or sweating of the painful area are usually present. The sympathetic nervous system is strongly implicated because sympathetic blockade abolishes the pain. Mild forms of this self-perpetuating loop of sympathetic activity and primary nociceptive response may explain why pain sometimes worsens, even when the injury has healed.

Psychological Factors Modifying Pain. Three thresholds for sensation and pain help in understanding the **subjective experience** of pain. "**Sensory threshold**," "**pain threshold**," and "**pain tolerance**" (or "**response threshold**") refer to the specific levels in the sensory continuum where intensity of stimulation meets a change in conscious experience. Joy and Barber used an example of a human subject, stimulated with an increasing-intensity electrical current to the finger, to help distinguish each of the thresholds.[36]

The first time the subject reports perception of any sensation is termed the "**sensory threshold**." This is defined as the **lowest level** of stimuli that will cause any sensation—the summation of large sensory fibers from receptors for touch, temperature, and vibration. As the current is increased, the sensation becomes stronger until the subject states that it is **"painful."** This is the "**pain threshold**" and has been shown to be fairly constant among individuals.[15,37] Neurologically, when the summation of firing of primary afferent nociceptive fibers reaches a certain point, pain is perceived. If the intensity of the electrical current is increased above pain threshold, a level of pain will be reached that the subject **can no longer endure.** This is "**pain tolerance**" or the "**response threshold.**" At this point, the individual makes an attempt to withdraw from the stimulus.

The range between the pain threshold and response threshold is termed a person's **tolerance to pain,** that is, the amount of pain that can be tolerated after pain is first perceived. Although the pain threshold is relatively constant among different people, pain tolerance varies greatly. This is because perception of sensations and tolerance to pain vary in relation to many cognitive, affective (emotional) factors.

Cognitive and Affective Factors. Sensory factors include the detection, localization, quantification, and identification of the quality of a particular stimulus. Reaction to the stimulus, the intensity of desire to terminate the stimulus, is determined by cognitive and affective variables. **Cognitive variables** include such things as an individual's **past experience** with similar stimuli, their **psychological makeup**, and **societal** and **cultural** factors. **Affective variables** relate to emotions and feelings and determine how unpleasant the stimulus is to the individual. Affective descriptors of a sensory experience might include words such as "nagging," "uncomfortable," "intense," or "killing," in contrast to sensory features such as "mild burning," "localized to the palate," or "aching over the TMJ."

Affective variables may be accompanied by **anxiety or depression** and are influenced by expectation and suggestion. For example, most people are not particularly distressed about having a headache since the vast majority of headaches are not pathologic. Yet someone whose sibling recently died of a brain tumor might be much more worried and anxious about this same symptom, even if it is very mild. Similarly, recurrence of pain owing to cancer carries with it the knowledge that the disease may be progressing and may remind the individual of his mortality. This type of pain will have many more emotional components and may be perceived as much more severe.

Another good example is the anxious dental patient who jumps in agony at the first touch of the cheek. Even though the sensation of touch is well below his experimental pain threshold, the patient perceives it and reacts to it as painful. Conversely, a person experiencing analgesia through hypnosis may perceive no sensations or only nonpainful sensations while undergoing normally painful procedures such as tooth extraction or pulp extirpation.[38,39]

Frontal lobotomy reduces or abolishes the affective component to pain, without disturbing pain threshold or pain intensity,[23] supporting the idea that affective components of pain are processed in different areas of the brain from sensation.

Behavioral Factors. Suffering and pain are communicated through actions such as moaning, limping, grimacing, guarding, pill taking, or visiting the doctor. These actions are termed **pain behaviors.** Pain behaviors follow basic learning principles and tend to increase unconsciously if they are **rewarded by positive consequences**. Positive consequences may include attention from loved ones and/or the medical/dental system and avoidance of various aversive tasks and responsibilities. Since chronic pain conditions, by definition, last a long time, they provide an opportunity for unconscious learning to occur. The pain behaviors observed in a patient with chronic pain may be the cumulative result of intermittent **positive reinforcement** over months or years. In addition, **well behaviors** are often totally ignored and nonreinforced, causing them to decrease.

Just as positive reinforcement causes an increase in particular behaviors, so will nonreinforcement cause a decrease. Thus, even when the nociceptive source has diminished or healed, pain perception and attendant disability may be maintained through **learned pain behaviors** along with physical, cognitive, and affective factors.[40] A more complete description of learned behavior in pain is given in the section on psychogenic pain.

PAIN ASSESSMENT TOOLS

Pain is a subjective experience that is communicated to us only through words and behaviors. Unlike measuring blood pressure, temperature, or erythrocyte sedimentation rate, measuring pain intensity is extremely difficult. As discussed above, there are several physiologic and psychological factors that will influence the intensity of pain perceived. Other cognitive, affective, behavioral, and learning factors affect how this pain is communicated.

Nonetheless, **measuring pain** is important, not just for studying pain mechanisms in a laboratory but also to **assess treatment outcome**. To this end, a number of instruments have been developed and tested for their reliability and validity in measuring different aspects of the pain experience.

Quantifying the Pain Experience

Visual Analog Scales. A visual analog scale is a line that represents a continuum of a particular experience, such as pain. The most common form used for pain is a **10 cm line,** whether horizontal or vertical, with perpendicular stops at the ends. The ends are anchored by "No pain" and "Worst pain imaginable" (Figure 8-13). **Numbers should not be used** along the line to ensure a better, less biased distribution of pain ratings. Otherwise, a disproportionately high frequency of 5s and 10s will be chosen.[41] Patients are asked to place a slash mark somewhere along the line to indicate the intensity of their current pain complaint. For scoring purposes, a millimeter ruler is used to measure along the line and obtain a numeric score for the pain ratings. Most people understand this scale quickly and can easily rate their pain. Children as young as 5 years are able to use this scale.[42] Its reliability and validity for measuring pain relief have been demonstrated.[43,44]

The use of the scale should be clearly explained to the patient. For measuring treatment outcome, relief scales (a line anchored with "no pain relief" and "complete pain relief") may be superior to asking absolute pain intensities.[45] Similarly, if a pain intensity visual analog scale was used, patients may be more accurate if they are allowed to see their previous scores.[46] Caution is advised with photocopying because this process usually lengthens the line and introduces error.

McGill Pain Questionnaire. The McGill Pain Questionnaire (Table 8-1) is a verbal pain scale that uses a vast array of words commonly used to describe a pain experience. Different types of pain and different diseases and disorders have different qualities of pain. These qualitative sensory descriptors are invaluable in providing key clues to possible diagnoses. Similarly, patients use different words to describe the affective component of their pain.

To facilitate the use of these words in a systematic way, Melzack and Torgerson set about categorizing many of these verbal descriptors into classes and subclasses designed to describe these different aspects of the pain experience. In addition to words describing the sensory qualities of pain, affective descriptors including such things as fear and anxiety and evaluative words describing the overall intensity of the pain experience were included.[47]

The words are listed in 20 different categories (see Table 8-1). They are arranged in order of magnitude **from least intense to most intense** and are grouped according to distinctly different qualities of pain. The patients are asked to circle only one word in each category that applies to them. Patients are usually happy to select from this list of pain-describing adjectives, often

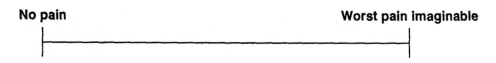

Figure 8-13 Visual analog pain scale used to indicate patient's level of daily pain. The patient places a mark at the perceived level of discomfort. The scale is 10 cm, so direct measurement can subsequently be made.

Table 8-1 Sample of Classic McGill Pain Questionnaire

Terms Describing Pain				
Sensory				
1	2	3	4	5
Flickering	Jumping	Pricking	Sharp	Pinching
Quivering	Flashing	Boring	Cutting	Pressing
Pulsing	Shooting	Drilling	Lacerating	Gnawing
Throbbing		Stabbing		Cramping
Beating		Lancinating		Crushing
Pounding				
6	7	8	9	10
Tugging	Hot	Tingling	Dull	Tender
Pulling	Burning	Itchy	Sore	Taut
Wrenching	Scalding	Smarting	Hurting	Rasping
	Searing	Stinging	Aching	Splitting
			Heavy	
Affective				
11	12	13	14	15
Tiring	Sickening	Fearful	Punishing	Wretched
Exhausting	Suffocating	Frightful	Gruelling	Blinding
		Terrifying	Cruel	
			Vicious	
			Killing	
Evaluative	**Miscellaneous**			
16	17	18	19	20
Annoying	Spreading	Tight	Cool	Nagging
Troublesome	Radiating	Numb	Cold	Nauseating
Miserable	Penetrating	Drawing	Freezing	Agonizing
Intense	Piercing	Squeezing		Dreadful
Unbearable		Tearing		Torturing

saying, "Now I can tell exactly how it feels. Before I couldn't think of just the right words."

The first 10 categories represent different sensory descriptors that cover various temporal, spatial, pressure, and thermal qualities of pain. The next five categories are affective or emotional descriptors, category 16 is evaluative (ie, how intense is the pain experience), and the last four categories are grouped as miscellaneous.

To score the questionnaire, the words in each category are given a numeric value. The first word in each category ranks as 1, the second as 2, etc. The scores for each category are added up separately for the sensory, affective, evaluative, and miscellaneous groupings. Then the total number of words chosen is also noted. Using this questionnaire, it is possible to obtain a sense of the quality of a patient's pain complaint (categories 1 through 10), its intensity (category 16), and the amount of emotional or psychological overlay accompanying the pain (categories 11 through 15). Changes in a patient's pain experience can be monitored by administering the questionnaire at various time points during treatment and follow-up.

Melzack used this master list of words to derive quantitative measures of clinical pain that can be treated statistically; if used correctly, it can also detect changes in pain with different treatment modalities.[48]

Psychological Assessment

Chronic pain is the most complicated pain experience and the most perplexing and frustrating problem in medicine and dentistry today. Because chronic pain syndromes have such a complex network of psychological and somatic interrelationships, it is critical to view the patient as an integrated whole and not as a sum of individual parts. Determining the emotional, behavioral, and environmental factors that perpetuate chronic pain is as essential as establishing the correct physical diagnosis or, in many chronic cases, multiple diagnoses.

Almost all patients with chronic head and neck pain have physical findings contributing to their complaint. Similarly, almost all patients with chronic head and neck pain have psychological components to their pain as well. Contributing to the complex neurobehavioral aspects of pain is the fact that chronic pain is not self-limiting, seems as though it will never resolve, and has little apparent cause or purpose. As such, multiple psychological problems arise that confuse the patient and perpetuate the pain. Patients feel helpless, hopeless, and desperate in their inability to receive relief. They may become hypochondriacal and obsessed about any symptom or sensation they perceive. Vegetative symptoms and overt depression may set in, with sleep and appetite disturbances. Irritability and great mood fluctuations are common. Loss of self-esteem, libido, and interest in life activities adds to the patient's misery. All of this may erode personal relationships with family, friends, and health professionals. Patients focus all of their energy on analyzing their pain and believe it to be the cause of all of their problems. They shop from doctor to doctor, desperately searching for an organic cure. They can become belligerent, hostile, and manipulative in seeking care. Many clinicians make gallant attempts with multiple drug regimens or multiple surgeries, but failure frustrates the clinician and adds to the patient's ongoing depression.

Near the end of this progression, in addition to their continuing pain, many of these patients have multiple drug dependencies and addictions or high stress levels; they may have lost their jobs, be on permanent disability, or be involved in litigation.

Herein lies the importance of proper **psychological diagnosis** as well as accurate physical diagnosis. An appropriate evaluation should include consideration of all factors that reinforce and perpetuate the pain complaints. Examining factors contributing to pain aggravation can include a look at stress (current and cumulative), interpersonal relationships, any secondary gain the patient may be receiving for having the pain, perceptual distortion of the pain, and poor lifestyle habits such as inadequate diet, poor posture, and lack of exercise. This information may well point to the reasons why patients have been unsuccessfully treated in the past. Obtaining baseline measures of pain levels, drug intake, functional impairment, and emotional state is important and will help monitor a patient's progress through rehabilitation.

Systematic assessment of psychosocial difficulties that interfere with work and interpersonal activities is important but often neglected. The dentist should include questions to elicit information about oral habits, depression, anxiety, stressful life events, lifestyle changes, and secondary gain (operant pain) in the clinical interview. To decide which patient should be referred for a full psychological assessment, the clinician evaluating a patient with chronic pain may choose to use simple questionnaires that are easy to administer, do not take long to fill out, and are reliable and adequate psychological screening tools. The Multidimensional Pain Inventory (**MPI**),[49] Beck Depression Inventory (**BDI/BDI-II**),[*50,51] and Chronic Illness Problem Inventory (**CIPI**)[†52] fulfill this purpose, although many other reliable instruments also exist. Patients who score high on any of these inventories should be sent to a psychologist or psychiatrist familiar with chronic pain for a more complete workup. Psychologists or psychiatrists may use the Minnesota Multiphasic Personality Inventory (**MMPI/MMPI-II**),[53] in addition to the BDI-II and other psychological instruments, as part of their comprehensive assessment.

MAKING A DIAGNOSIS

Diagnosing orofacial disease and headaches follows the same principles as any medical diagnosis. Of primary importance is a careful and exhaustive **history**. This alone will often point directly to a specific diagnosis or at least reveal a diagnostic category. The history is followed by a **physical examination**, which should help to confirm or rule out the initial diagnostic impression. If necessary, further **diagnostic studies** such as pulp testing, nerve blocks, radiographs, or blood tests may be carried out or ordered at this time. These may help rule out serious disorders and provide information complementing the history and physical examination. Finally, if doubt concerning the diagnosis persists, or pathosis out of one's area of expertise exists, other medical specialists and health care providers may provide valuable consultation.

---

*The BDI and BDI-II can be obtained by contacting the Psychological Corporation, 555 Academic Court, San Antonio, TX 78204.

†Copies of the CIPI can be obtained by contacting Dr. Bruce Naliboff, PhD, Clinical Professor, Department of Psychiatry and Biobehavioral Sciences, Co-Director, CURE Neuroenteric Disease Program, UCLA Division of Digestive Disease, VA Greater Los Angeles Healthcare System, Building 115, Room 223, 11301 Wilshire Boulevard, Los Angeles, CA 90073; Tel: 310-268-3242; Fax 310-794-2864.

Begin by pondering the scenario of the following case.

Case History

A 33-year-old woman presents herself for evaluation of intense left-sided facial pain. The pain is described as a constant burning sensation that radiates from the left preauricular area to the orbit, zygoma, mandible, and, occasionally, shoulder. Her pain is exacerbated by cold air, cold liquids, chewing, smiling, and light touch over certain areas of her face. She also reports a constant "pinching" sensation over her left eyebrow and mandible and photophobia in the left eye. She is currently taking high doses of narcotics with little relief.

The pain began 1 year previously, after the extraction of a left maxillary molar. The extraction site apparently developed a "dry socket" (localized osteomyelitis of the alveolar crypt). This was treated appropriately but without relief of the patient's symptoms. Subsequently, two mandibular molars on the same side were extracted in an attempt to relieve the pain. These extraction sites likewise developed "dry sockets" and were treated, again without pain relief. Local anesthetic injections twice daily for many months and a 4-week course of cephalosporin, given empirically for possible periodontal infection or osteomyelitis of the mandible, were also unsuccessful.

To properly evaluate these rather confusing signs and symptoms, additional information is necessary.

Classification

In evaluating orofacial pains and headaches, an easy-to-use, practical, and clinical classification of these pains will facilitate diagnosis (Table 8-2). In developing such a classification, it is important to remember that local pathosis of the extracranial or intracranial structures and referred pain from pathema of more distant organs such as the heart must be ruled out first. This covers a wide variety of infectious, inflammatory, degenerative, neoplastic, or obstructive processes that can affect any organ in the head, neck, and thorax, including the brain (see Tables 8-7 through 8-9). Most dentists and physicians are well trained to evaluate a patient for such pathosis.

There are other disorders, however, that cause pain in the head and neck region that cannot be attributed to any obvious diseases of the craniofacial, craniocervical, thoracic, or intracranial organs. These disorders are less well appreciated and, for ease of clinical use, are best classified according to the apparent tissue origin of the pain (see Table 8-2). For an exhaustive classification of headaches and facial pain that includes very specific diagnostic criteria, the reader is referred to the International Headache Society's publication.[54]

The primary distinguishing feature of these diagnostic categories is the **quality** of the pain. For example, **vascular** pain, such as with migraine, generally has a throbbing, pulsing, or pounding quality; **neuropathic** pain, for example, trigeminal neuralgia, is usually described as sharp, shooting, or burning and is restricted to the peripheral distribution of the affected nerve branch; **muscle** pain is usually deep, steady, and aching or produces a sensation of tightness or pressure.

In contrast, **extracranial** or **intracranial** pathema may present with any quality of pain. An inflamed tooth pulp may throb with each heartbeat. A tumor pressing on a nerve may cause sharp, lancinating, neuralgic-like pain. A sinus infection may be dull and aching. **Referred pain** tends to be deep and poorly localized and have an aching or pressing quality.

Once organic pathosis has been ruled out, a preliminary diagnostic category can be chosen based on the

Table 8-2 Practical Clinical Classification of Craniofacial Pain

General Classification	Origin of Pain	Basic Quality of Pain
Local pathosis of extracranial structures	Craniofacial organs	Any
Referred pain from remote pathologic sites	Distant organs and structures	Aching, pressing
Intracranial pathosis	Brain and related structures	Any
Neurovascular	Blood vessels	Throbbing
Neuropathic	Sensory nervous system	Shooting, sharp, burning
Causalgic	Sympathetic nervous system	Burning
Muscular	Muscles	Deep aching, tight
Unclassifiable	Etiology as yet unknown	Any

location and the quality of the pain. Therefore, when taking a pain history, the first questions to ask are "**Where,** exactly, do you feel your pain?" "**How,** exactly, does your pain feel to you?" "Please mark on this line how severe you consider your pain to be at its worst, usual, and lowest." This will help guide further questioning to confirm or rule out a specific diagnosis within that group. For example, a patient may complain of a constant dull ache in front of the ear and a paroxysmal lancinating pain that shoots from the ear to the chin and tongue. In this situation, two patterns of pain are described. One points to a possibly myofascial or rheumatic diagnosis for the ear pain and the other to a paroxysmal neuralgia for the shooting pain. Further history, examination, and diagnostic tests will help establish more definitive physical diagnoses. This systematic approach is particularly helpful in chronic pain, in which there are often multiple diagnoses, and psychological distress and pain behavior may confuse the diagnostic process.

If the patient in the case outlined above does not have any ongoing pathologic lesions of the extracranial or intracranial structures, which categories of pain would fit her description best? Based on the limited information given, namely, a constant burning quality, the most likely preliminary diagnostic categories are neuropathic or sympathetic. To make a specific diagnosis within a category, more specific information regarding the pain, its temporal pattern (timing of occurrence), associated symptoms, and aggravating and alleviating factors is needed.

History

The key elements of taking a history for a pain complaint are delineated in Table 8-3.

Establishing the patient's chief complaint requires listening carefully as the patient describes each type of pain or complaint present, including the **location, quality, and severity** of each symptom. Chronic pain patients often have multiple pain complaints with different descriptions, which may indicate that multiple diagnoses are involved. When this is the case, obtaining complete information on each pain complaint separately simplifies the diagnostic process.

The patient in the case scenario complains of only one pain. The location is over the left side of the face, radiating from the preauricular area. The quality of the pain is described primarily as burning. Her usual pain intensity on a 0 to 10 scale is 8, 5 being the lowest and 9 being the highest.

Table 8-3 History of Pain

- Chief complaint
- Characteristics of pain
  - Location
  - Quality
  - Temporal patterns
    - Constant or intermittent
    - Duration of each attack if intermittent
    - Diurnal variation in intensity if constant
    - Seasonal variation of symptoms if any
  - Associated symptoms
  - Precipitating factors if intermittent
  - Aggravating factors
  - Alleviating factors
  - Symptoms severity range (lowest, usual, and highest pain intensities)
  - Onset and history
  - Past and present medications or other treatments for pain
- Past medical and dental history
- Family history
- Social history
- Review of systems

Different pains also have different **temporal patterns** or patterns of occurrence. For example, a patient may complain of an intermittent, unilateral throbbing head pain. This would be the hallmark of a diagnosis in the vascular category. The exact pattern of the pain will help determine which vascular headache the patient is suffering. For example, **migraines** last from 4 to 48 hours and occur once or twice a year up to several times per month. **Cluster headaches** last less than 90 minutes each but occur several times a day, for several months, before going into remission. Similar distinctions can be made with neuropathic pains. The pain of trigeminal neuralgia is seconds in duration and may be triggered frequently throughout the day. The pain of a post-traumatic neuropathy or postherpetic neuralgia is constant.

The temporal pattern for this patient's burning pain is constant, with little daily variation.

Often there are associated symptoms such as nausea, vomiting, ptosis, nasal congestion, tingling, numbness, blurred vision, or visual changes that may precede or accompany the pain. These symptoms may point to a specific diagnosis. For example, visual changes may precede a migraine with aura. Nausea and vomiting often accompany severe headaches, especially migraine.

Generalized malaise may accompany a temporal arteritis. Autonomic changes, such as ptosis, nasal congestion, or conjunctival injection, almost always accompany cluster headaches or chronic paroxysmal hemicrania. Tingling and numbness may occur with deafferentation (nerve damage) pains such as postherpetic or post-traumatic neuralgias.

Unexplained neurologic symptoms, however, such as cognitive or memory changes, transient sensory or motor loss of the face or extremities, tinnitus, vertigo, loss of consciousness, or any of the above symptoms not fitting an appropriate pain picture, must alert the health professional to the possibility of an intracranial lesion, requiring further workup. Some of these symptoms may be normal bodily sensations enhanced through distorted perceptions. Similarly, others, such as tinnitus, vertigo, or sensory tingling, may be associated with the referred symptoms of **myofascial TrP pain.**[55] Further diagnostic tests or consultations may be needed to rule out more serious pathosis.

Associated symptoms for this patient include a constant "pinching" sensation over her left eyebrow and mandible and photophobia of the left eye. She also describes occasional "electric" attacks that radiate out from the left TMJ. The "electric" attacks she describes last anywhere from 30 minutes to 24 hours.

Precipitating, aggravating, and alleviating factors also add clues to the origin of pain. Foods rich in tyramine may trigger a migraine attack.[56] Light touch, shaving, or brushing teeth may precipitate an attack of trigeminal neuralgia. Cold weather, maintaining any one body position for a prolonged period of time, or overexercise will aggravate MFP. A dark room and rest will alleviate migraine but aggravate cluster headache. Heat and massage will alleviate muscular pain and MFP but may aggravate an inflamed joint.

The burning pain is constant, without precipitating factors. Aggravating factors include cold air, cold liquids, chewing, smiling, and light touch. The "electric" attacks are precipitated by light touch over the preauricular area. At this stage, nothing alleviates the pain. High doses of narcotics barely serve to "take the edge off."

Gathering information about the **onset** and **history** of the problem will provide further clues as to the etiology of the complaint. Of interest are the events surrounding the initiation of the pain, how the pain has changed since onset, and what evaluations and treatment have been tried in the past. For example, a history of skin lesions and malaise (herpes zoster) typically precedes postherpetic neuralgia. Acute trauma may precede a myofascial TrP pain complaint. In contrast, psychological stress can trigger almost any type of pain complaint.

Knowing which specialists the patient has seen, which tests and radiographs have already been completed, what the previous diagnostic impressions have been, and which treatments have been tried helps the practitioner in several ways. First, which workups are still needed? Did the past workups adequately rule out organic or life-threatening pathema? How long ago were these workups completed? Have the symptoms changed since then? Do any of these workups need to be repeated? Second, what diagnoses were considered in the past? Were appropriate medications or treatments tried, in adequate doses and for long enough periods of time? With acute pain, the history is usually quite short, but **with chronic pain, the history may take hours to obtain,** the patient having seen many different health care providers in the past. With chronic pain, the effect of past medications, surgeries, and other treatments may provide insight not only into the etiology of the pain but also the psychological or behavioral status of the patient.

The pain began 1 year previously, after the extraction of a left maxillary molar. The extraction site apparently developed a "dry socket." This was treated appropriately but without relief of the patient's symptoms. Subsequently, two left mandibular molars were extracted in an attempt to relieve the pain. These extraction sites likewise developed "dry sockets" and were treated, again without pain relief. Local anesthetic injections twice daily for many months and a 4-week course of cephalosporin given empirically for possible periodontal infection or osteomyelitis of the mandible were also unsuccessful.

This history tells us that, initially, local tooth pathosis was suspected as the etiology of the pain. However, extraction of teeth provided no relief. Osteomyelitis and possibly periodontal disease had also been suspected, but high-dose antibiotic treatment for osteomyelitis also failed to provide pain relief. Are there other extracranial or intracranial pathemas that may need to be ruled out?

A **family history** should include information regarding the patient's parents and siblings. Are they alive and well? If not, why not? Does anyone in the immediate family suffer from a similar pain problem? For example, 70% of migraine patients have a relative who also has or had migraine. Does anyone in the family have a chronic illness? This person may provide a model for pain behavior and coping.

The patient's parents and siblings are alive and well. There is no history of similar illness or chronic illness in her family.

A **social history** not only should cover demographic information, marital status, household situation, and occupation but should also seek to uncover any potential perpetuating factors to the pain. Look for potential stressors at work and at home and ask about postural habits, body mechanics, dietary habits, environmental factors, and drug and alcohol use.

This patient lives in a rural farm area, has been married to the same man for 15 years, and has three children. She used to work on the farm but has been unable to do so for the last 6 months because of the pain. The patient has smoked one pack a day for 18 years. She does not drink alcohol. Currently she spends most of her day in bed because of the pain.

Since the patient lives in a rural area, the possibility of a coccal infection must be considered and ruled out.

The **past medical history** may reveal some underlying illness such as lupus erythematosus or hypothyroidism that may predispose the patient to developing pain. Past surgeries and medications for other purposes, any psychiatric history, allergies, hospitalizations, and other illnesses must be included and may reveal health care abuse.

The patient states that she is otherwise in good health. She had the usual childhood diseases, has no known allergies, and has been hospitalized only for the birth of her children. There is no history of trauma other than the tooth extractions previously mentioned.

A **review of systems** screens the person's present state of health. It includes asking about any recent symptoms related to the head and neck; the skin; and the cardiovascular, respiratory, gastrointestinal, genitourinary, endocrine, neurologic, obstetric-gynecologic, and musculoskeletal systems.

The patient complains of decreased energy and sleep disturbance secondary to the pain. She has no other complaints.

In acute pain problems, a firm diagnosis may be established almost immediately from the history. In contrast, **diagnosis** of a chronic pain complaint **may take months** of tests or trials despite an exhaustive history.

The next step in diagnosis is a thorough **physical examination.**

Physical Examination

The physical examination for craniofacial pain may vary slightly, depending on its location and the apparent cause. Pathosis of extracranial structures, particularly the oral cavity, must be sought and ruled out first. This usually involves inspection, palpation, percussion, transillumination, and auscultation of the tissues and structures suspected of causing pain. Intraoral examination, which must include inspection of all intraoral tissues, teeth, and periodontium, is discussed in detail in chapters 6 and 7. Once acute pathema has been ruled out, the physical examination must be augmented to include evaluation of the cranial nerves, temporomandibular joint, cervical spine, and head and neck muscles. In specific cases, a more comprehensive neurologic examination may be indicated. The basic components of a physical examination are listed in Table 8-4.

General inspection can reveal a great deal about a patient to the alert clinician. A slouching posture can point to **depression.** Rigidity in posture or clenching is an indication of excess **muscle tension** in the neck, shoulders, or jaws. **Asymmetry, swelling, redness,** and other signs may indicate a neoplastic or infectious process. Closer **inspection of the head and neck** may reveal scars of past surgeries, trophic skin changes associated with reflex sympathetic dystrophy, or color changes from local **infection,** systemic **anemia,** or **jaundice.**

The examination of the **TMJs** involves testing the range and quality of motion of the mandible, palpating and listening for joint noises, and palpating the lateral

Table 8-4 Physical Examination

General inspection
Head and neck inspection
Stomatognathic examination
Cervical spine examination
Myofascial examination
Cranial nerve examination
Neurologic screening examination

and dorsal joint capsules for tenderness. The normal range of jaw opening is 40 to 60 mm. Laterotrusive and protrusive movements should be 8 to 10 mm. The path of opening and laterotrusive and protrusive movements should be straight, without deflections or deviations. Joint capsule palpation anterior to the tragus of the ear for the lateral capsule and from the external auditory meatus for the dorsal capsule may be "uncomfortable" but should not be painful.

As discussed later in the chapter, the cervical spine is often the source of persistent referred pain to the orofacial and TMJ regions. Similarly, poor posture is one of the most important contributing factors to TMJ dysfunction and **myofascial TrP** pain. For these reasons, the cervical spine and posture must be evaluated in any chronic head and neck or facial pain problem. Examination of the cervical spine includes testing its range and quality of motion as a whole, as well as testing the range and quality of motion of the first two cervical joints individually.[57–59] Posture, especially anterior head positioning, must also be systematically evaluated. For details on how and why this is important, the reader is referred to Travell and Simons' *Trigger Point Manual.*[55]

Myofascial TrP examination requires a thorough, systematic palpation of all of the masticatory and cervical muscles, looking for tight muscle bands and the focal tenderness associated with myofascial TrPs. **Myofascial TrP is the most prevalent cause of chronic pain,** both in the head and neck region and in general.[60–64] Also, it is frequently an accompanying diagnosis to other chronic pain conditions.

A **cranial nerve examination** (Table 8-5) is indicated when the history points to a neuropathic type of pain; if disturbances in touch, taste, smell, sight, hearing, motor function, balance, or coordination are suspected; or if there are any subjective complaints or objective signs of cranial nerve involvement. Lesions of the cranial nerve nuclei or their efferent or afferent pathways will result in an abnormal examination. For example, meningitis may cause double vision; an acoustic neuroma may cause hearing loss. Symptoms of numbness or tingling may accompany nasopharyngeal carcinoma or other intracranial pathema. Sensory deficits can be verified using accurate two-point discrimination testing, pinprick tests, and light touch tests. Complaints of transient or persistent paralysis, weakness, or spasticity of any of the head and neck muscles dictate the need for evaluation of the nerves that control their motor function.

The motor function of the head and neck is mediated through several cranial nerves. The **trigeminal nerve, cranial nerve V**, controls the masticatory mus-

Table 8-5 Cranial Nerve Examination

I.	Olfactory Test sense of smell of each nostril separately by using soap, tobacco, or coffee with patient's eyes closed
II.	Optic Test visual acuity Examing fundi ophthalmoscopically Test visual fields
III, IV, VI.	Oculomotor, Trochlear, Abducens Test pupillary reactions to light and accommodation Test extraocular movements Check for ptosis or nystagmus
V.	Trigeminal Motor—Palpate masseter and temporalis during contraction Sensory—Test discrimination of pinprick, V1, V2, V3 temperature, V1, V2, V3 and light touch, V1, V2, V3 Test corneal reflex
VII.	Facial Observe patient's face during rest and conversation Check for symmetry, tics Examine for symmetric smile, ability to wrinkle forehead, hold air in cheeks, and tense the platysma muscle
VIII.	Acoustic Whisper, rub fingers or hold watch next to ear, use tuning fork for Rinne & Weber tests
IX, X.	Glossopharyngeal, Vagus Check for symmetric movement of soft palate and uvula when patient says "Ah" Check gag reflex by touching back of throat Note any horseness
XI.	Spinal accessory Have patient shrug shoulders against resistance (trapezius) (partially inervated by C4) Have patient turn head against resistance (SCM)
XII.	Hypoglossal Observe tongue in mouth: check for atrophy or asymmetry Check for deviation by having patient stick tongue out

cles. The **facial nerve, cranial nerve VII**, controls the muscles of facial expression. The **hypoglossal nerve, cranial nerve XII**, controls the tongue. The **spinal accessory nerve, cranial nerve XI**, controls the trapezius and sternocleidomastoid muscles. Detailed information on how to perform a cranial nerve examination is available in Bates's textbook on physical examination and history taking.[65] If intracranial pathosis is suspected, a complete **neurologic examination**, including mental status; cerebellar, motor, and sensory function; and reflexes, is indicated. This requires referral to a competent neurologist.

General inspection *of the patient reveals an obese female in moderate distress.* **Closer inspection of the head and neck** *reveals slight swelling of the left cheek with a distinct increase in skin temperature over this site.*

On intraoral examination, *the intraoral tissues are firm, pink, and stippled without lesions. The patient is missing teeth #15, 16, 17, 18, and 19.* **Temporomandibular joint examination** *reveals an active oral opening of only 33 mm with little translation of the left condyle (the jaw deflects to the left with opening). Definitive intraoral or extraoral palpation is impossible because the patient complains of pain at the slightest touch.*

The patient has full range of motion of the cervical spine. *The first two cervical joints similarly show good range and quality of motion. Her posture is slightly abnormal, with elevation of the left shoulder and a forward head position.*

Myofascial TrP examination *is restricted to the cervical muscles and unaffected side owing to the extreme sensitivity of the left side of the face. Even so, active myofascial TrPs are found in the left upper trapezius that intensify the patient's pain over the left temple and angle of the jaw.*

Cranial nerve examination *is normal except for the extreme cutaneous sensitivity on the left side of the face.* **Neurologic examination** *is similarly unremarkable.*

At this stage, one must still rule out acute pathologic change. Pathosis of the various organs and structures of the head and neck should always be suspected first in any orofacial pain. The teeth, pulp and periodontium, TMJs, eyes, ears, nose, throat, sinuses, and salivary glands should be thoroughly evaluated (see Table 8-7). As mentioned previously, the quality of pain from this group varies depending on the etiology. Equally important are many **referred pain** problems (see Table 8-8). These are very often difficult to diagnose and include pathologic conditions such as the tight, pressing pain of coronary artery disease that may be felt in the sternum and the jaws.

This patient demonstrates swelling and temperature change as well as cutaneous hyperesthesia over the painful area. She could still have a chronic osteomyelitis despite the previous course of antibiotics. She could have a retropharyngeal abscess or neoplastic disease affecting or surrounding the fifth cranial nerve, either intracranially or extracranially. She could also have a localized coccal infection since she lives in a rural area. The limited range of motion of the left temporomandibular joint and the fact that much of her pain seems to emanate from there bring up the possibility of severe degenerative joint disease or neoplastic disease involving the joint. The myofascial TrPs in the left trapezius have probably developed in response to the chronic pain problem. It is unlikely that myofascial TrP pain is the primary cause of this patient's pain.

The next step involves choosing appropriate diagnostic studies to help rule out the pathema suspected.

Diagnostic Studies

Table 8-6 is a list of some of the more common diagnostic studies available to help facilitate diagnosis.

Panoramic and periradicular radiographs reveal an area of bony sclerosis in the mandibular extraction sites, consistent with the history of curettage of dry sockets and not at all typical of osteomyelitis. Temporomandibular joint tomograms reveal flattening of the left condyle consistent with mild to moderate degenerative joint disease. Computed tomographic (CT) scans of the brain, mandible, and retropharyngeal area are normal. A gallium scan, which is used to identify soft tissue inflammation, is normal also. Skin tests for coccal infection are negative. Complete blood count and erythrocyte sedimentation rate also fail to show any signs of infection or inflammation. No pathosis of the extracranial and intracranial structures can be identified.

What, then, could be causing this patient's pain? At this point in the workup of a pain patient, practitioners are often tempted to ascribe the pain to some "psychogenic" problem. Clearly, if there is no obvious pathologic process, and the patient is in severe distress or does

Table 8-6 Common Diagnostic Studies

Pulp testing
Radiography
Tomography
Laboratory studies (blood, urine)
CT or MRI scan
Bone scan
Gallium scan
Arthrography
Thermography
Nerve conduction studies
EEG
Lumbar puncture
Differential diagnostic analgesic blocking

not respond well to treatments, then she must be suffering from a "psychogenic" pain. Don't be too sure!

"Psychogenic" Pain

Many clinicians use the term "psychogenic" to refer to patients with a chronic pain problem that has a strong emotional component or to patients who do not respond well to somatic treatment. It must be reemphasized, however, that psychological factors are intimately involved in the expression of all pain, regardless of etiology or time course.

By definition, chronic pain has been present for a protracted period (at least 6 months), and the patient has usually received multiple treatments with little or no results. This creates an emotional strain for the patient and frustration for the clinician, sometimes resulting in the inappropriate label of "psychogenic pain." Patients with chronic pain invariably have a somatic diagnosis. What frustrates the clinician is often the discrepancy between the identifiable somatic cause and the disproportionate amount of perceived pain and disability that accompanies this cause.

True "psychogenic pain" is a **rare** diagnosis that must be restricted to those patients in whom thorough, sophisticated medical evaluations and tests fail to uncover any somatic basis for their pain **and** in whom psychological evaluation reveals psychopathology that may actually account for their presentation. Myofascial TrP pain is frequently overlooked as an organic finding and is thus often mislabeled as psychogenic pain.[66] Occasionally, there are patients in whom no etiology for their pain can be identified and who have no psychological findings consistent with a psychological disorder. This situation simply speaks to the limitations of our current medical knowledge and the complexity of the human nervous system and is not an indication of the mental state of the patient.

Conversion Reaction. A true conversion reaction is **very rare**. It is thought to represent the successful substitution of a more valid somatic symptom for emotional turmoil in a patient's life. This symptom is most frequently blindness or deafness, and the condition is more common in young women.[67] However, patients can be of any age or sex, and, occasionally, the symptom substitution may involve pain. When this occurs, the quality of the pain can be related in very descriptive, affective terms such as "lightning-like explosions," "heavy weight pressing on my head," "spike into my head," "rope choking my throat," "ugly pain," and others.

The pain is usually described as continuous or unrelenting. It is rarely affected by external events; however, it can be changed by emotions. Despite the elaborate terms used to describe the pain, these patients often appear indifferent about it.

Clinically, there are usually no physical findings, including no myofascial TrPs. A careful history may reveal that patients either grew up with a parent or relative who was ill or they themselves had a history of a prolonged childhood illness. Mental status may be normal; however, these patients generally have been and are under intense emotional stress, have poor social relationships, and may be occupationally incapacitated.

The reasons for a conversion reaction vary. Causes may include handling nonspecific stress, anticipating a major life change, dealing with a catastrophic life situation, and the manifestation of a severe body image problem. The patient subconsciously converts an apparently **socially unacceptable** psychological illness to the **socially acceptable** physical complaint of pain.

Somatic Delusions. Somatic delusions may occur in patients with psychiatric diagnoses such as psychosis or schizophrenia. These patients lose rational thought and attachment to reality and display uncontrolled obsessions of pain or problems with their health. Psychiatric care or hospitalization is strongly indicated since the possibility of suicide may be great.

Operant Pain (Pain Behavior). Although pain behaviors (the behavioral manifestations of pain, distress, and suffering) likely result from a complex interaction of various psychological and physical factors,[40] understanding the basic concepts of learning and "operant" conditioning is essential to understanding the chronic pain patient.

In combination with cognitive and affective factors, learned behavior and **"operant conditioning"** are powerful psychological or "psychogenic" factors that play an important role in any patient with a chronic or persistent pain problem. Fordyce and Steger described operant pain and conditioning as follows:

> ...in chronic pain, the normal responses to a noxious stimulus, such as moaning, complaining, grimacing, limping, asking for medication, or staying in bed, are present for a long enough period of time to allow learning to occur. By using the above set of actions, termed operants, the patient either purposely or unintentionally communicates to those around him that he has pain. The significance of these operants is that they can be influenced by certain consequences. For example, if a certain behavior or action is consistently followed by a favorable consequence (a positive reinforcer), then the probability that the behavior or action will be repeated again in response to a similar stimulus is increased (as in Pavlov's dog). If, however, a certain behavior or action is not consistently followed by a favorable consequence, the behavior will diminish in frequency and disappear. This is known as "extinction."[68,69]

It is generally accepted that all chronic pain begins at some point with a true pathologic or nociceptive stimulus. This stimulus elicits a pain response or "pain behavior." Most people live in an environment that systematically and positively reinforces pain behaviors while ignoring or punishing healthy behaviors.[69] In acute pain, these behaviors and their rewards subside quickly, but in chronic or persistent pain, pain behaviors become more prominent and may persist even after the noxious stimulus is gone: "The degree of pain behavior has little or no direct relationship to pathogenic [or nociceptive] factors."[69]

It is easy to label the behavioral manifestations of pain, distress, and suffering as pain of psychogenic origin. Unfortunately, this term usually implies some kind of personality disorder such as **hypochondriasis** (excessive concern with one's health and bodily functions) or **hysteria** (also known as conversion reaction), and often this is not present, or, if it is, it generally has little or nothing to do with the pain. As Fordyce said, "It is not necessary to have personality problems to learn a pain habit, because learning occurs automatically if the conditions are favorable."[69] Therefore, other psychological labels, such as **somatization** (conversion of mental states into bodily symptoms similar to hysteria but with more elaborate complaints), **malingering** (conscious exhibition of pain or illness for secondary gain), and **Munchausen syndrome** (a type of malingering characterized by habitual presentation for hospital treatment of an apparent acute illness with a plausible and dramatic but fictitious history),[1] are also usually inappropriate. The astute clinician will try to ascertain which environmental factors are acting to maintain and reinforce a particular behavior instead of assuming that the patient has a character disorder.

It is important to realize that, whether or not the pain has an ongoing organic basis, **it is still very real to the patient** and can be as intense as any somatic pain. Management typically requires a multidisciplinary approach that includes identification and elimination of any positive reinforcers to the pain behaviors. All treatment and follow-up visits, medications, exercises, rest, etc must be scheduled on a time-contingent and **NOT** a pain-contingent basis, regardless of the somatic diagnosis. The family must also be educated to reinforce well behaviors and ignore sick behaviors. Then activity levels must be increased and medications gradually decreased and eliminated. The help of a behaviorally oriented psychologist or psychiatrist familiar with chronic pain patients is highly recommended.

Occasionally, situational insight, supportive therapy, guidance, or counseling is sufficient to resolve the problem. Other cases may require more long-term outpatient psychotherapy. Sometimes medications such as antidepressants, antipsychotics, hypnotics, or tranquilizers will help alleviate the pain. Inpatient psychiatric care is indicated for anyone at risk of committing suicide or inflicting bodily injury on themselves or others.

An interview with a psychologist and the MMPI did not reveal a psychopathologic state in this particular patient. So, clearly, there must be other factors that have not been considered that are causing this patient's pain.

Instead of falling into the trap of calling unidentified pain "psychogenic," one should go back to the classification of pain (see Table 8-2) to answer this question. Based on the burning quality of pain, it is clear that neuropathic or sympathetic pains would be the categories most likely to carry a diagnosis that accounts for this patient's pain. These pains and specific diagnoses within each category are described in more detail later in the chapter.

SPECIFICS FOR EACH BROAD CATEGORY OF PAIN ORIGIN

The remainder of the chapter will be devoted to discussing many of the specific diagnoses that fall into each broad diagnostic category. This classification is by no means exhaustive. The disorders discussed are those with which **dentists should be familiar.** An exhaustive treatise of orofacial pains has been published by Bell[70] and an official classification with diagnostic criteria by the International Headache Society.[54]

Extracranial Pathosis

Local pathosis of extracranial structures and referred pain from remote pathologic *sites* are listed in Tables 8-7 and 8-8.

Acute pain arising from pathosis of the extracranial structures is commonly seen in dental practice. Some extracranial acute pain is well localized, easily identifiable, and straightforward to treat. However, some pains from local pathema are more elusive because they are referred to other head and neck structures. Similarly, pathosis of some distant structures such as the heart and thyroid may refer pain into the head, neck, or jaws. These more unusual pains will be discussed.

Tooth Pulp, Periodontium, Periradicular Structures, Gingiva, Mucosa. Diseases of the intraoral structures, including referred pain from pulpalgia, are fully discussed in chapter 7 and will not be covered here.

Salivary Gland Disorders. The salivary glands can be affected by many diseases, including ductal obstruction, infection, inflammation, cystic degeneration, and tumor growth. Pain and tenderness are typically found in association with ductal obstruction, inflammation, or infection.

Etiology. The most common causes are mumps and acute parotitis in children and blockage of salivary flow by a mucus plug or a sialolith in adults. The latter results in pressure from salivary retention and may cause ascending infection. Sjögren's syndrome, a disease of unknown etiology typically seen in older women, is characterized by dry eyes, dry oropharyngeal mucosa, and enlargement of the parotid glands.[71] This disorder also may cause salivary gland pain if the glands become inflamed.

Table 8-7 Local Pathosis of Extracranial Structures

Structures	Diseases
Tooth pulp, periradicular structures	Inflammation
Periodontium, gingival, mucosa	Infection
Salivary glands	Degeneration
Tongue	Neoplasm
Ears, nose, throat, sinuses	Obstruction
Eyes	
Temporomandibular joints	

Table 8-8 Referred Pain from Remote Pathologic Sites

Structures	Diseases
Heart	Angina pectoris, myocardial infarction
Thyroid	Inflammation
Carotid artery	Inflammation, other obscure causation
Cervical spine	Inflammation, trauma, dysfunction
Muscles	Myofascial trigger points

Symptoms. Salivary gland pain is typically localized to the gland itself, and the gland is tender to palpation. Precipitating and aggravating factors to the pain are salivary production prior to meals, eating, and swallowing. Mouth opening may aggravate the pain because of pressure on the gland from the posterior border of the mandible during this movement. This, and increased pain with chewing, may lead the clinician to mistake the pain as being from the masticatory system. Associated symptoms include salivary gland swelling and, occasionally, fever and malaise. Salivary flow from the affected gland may be minimal or nonexistent.

Examination. The pain can be localized fairly well by palpation. Other signs of inflammation may be present. With parotid gland disorders, to determine diminished or absent flow, the gland can be manually milked while observing salivary flow from the parotid duct.

Diagnostic Tests. Radiographs of the gland and ducts may reveal a calcific mass in the region of the gland. Sialography (radiographic examination of a gland using a radiopaque dye injected into the ductal system) may also show obstruction or abnormal ductal patterns.

Treatment. The mucus plug or sialolith should be removed in the case of obstruction. Antibiotics may be needed if infection accompanies the pain.

Ear Pain. Most patients who have a primary complaint of ear pain will seek the help of their primary care physician or an ear, nose, and throat (ENT) specialist. Ear pain is typically seen with disorders such as otitis media, otitis externa, and mastoiditis and may be associated with headache. When a medical workup is negative, patients may be referred to the dentist for evaluation of ear pain. Astute physicians will want to know whether the TMJ or the pulpalgia is referring the symptoms. Patients may also present themselves to the dentist with another primary pain complaint such as toothache or headache, whereupon when taking a careful history, ear pain is found to be an associated symptom. The dentist needs to rule out dental disease or temporomandibular disorders as a cause of ear pain. Additionally, the dentist must decide when a referral for a medical workup of ear pain is indicated.

Etiology. The ear is innervated by cranial nerves V, VII, VIII, IX, X, and XI and also branches of the upper cervical roots that supply the immediate adjacent scalp and muscles. Therefore, pain can be referred to the ear from inflammatory or neoplastic disease of the **teeth**, tonsils, larynx, nasopharynx, thyroid, TMJ, and cervical spine, as well as from inflammation or tumors in the posterior fossa of the brain.[72] Ear pains are also associated with neuralgias such as herpes zoster of cranial nerve V or VII, glossopharyngeal neuralgia, and nervus intermedius neuralgia. These will be discussed later.

Symptoms. Primary ear pains are usually described as a constant aching pressure. Their onset is usually recent. Inflammatory or infectious disorders may be associated with fever and malaise. These complaints should be diagnosed and managed by an ENT specialist.

Patients with otitis externa (inflammation of the external auditory canal) may present themselves to the dentist first because this pain is aggravated by swallowing. Otitis externa may be misdiagnosed as arthralgia of the TMJ if the condyle is palpated through the external auditory canal without first evaluating the ear. Glossopharyngeal neuralgia, also aggravated by swallowing, may need to be considered if ear and dental pathosis are absent.

Examination. The dentist must carefully examine the dentition for pulpal disease and the oropharyngeal mucosa for inflammation to rule out referred ear pain from oral or dental sources. Myofascial TrPs in the lateral and medial pterygoid muscles frequently refer pain to the ear as well.

If primary ear pain is suspected, referral to a competent ENT specialist should be made. However, screening examination should include visual inspection of the ear and ear canal. Use of an otoscope facilitates this examination. Wiggling the auricle itself or tugging on the earlobe will aggravate otitis externa and will help distinguish an ear lesion from a TMJ problem. Pumping on the ear with the palm of the hand will exacerbate pain from otitis media. Hearing can be grossly evaluated by rubbing the fingers together in front of each ear or using a watch tick or coin click. The practitioner can use his own hearing as a control.

Treatment. Primary ear pain should be diagnosed and managed by an ENT specialist. Dental sources of ear pain are treated by treating the oral pathema. Of importance is the fact that primary ear pain may also induce **secondary myospasm** and development of **myofascial TrPs**, which may persist beyond the course of primary ear disease. These TrPs and resulting masticatory dysfunction are self-perpetuating, even after the acute ear problem resolves. Appropriate treatment of this secondary masticatory dysfunction will be required for resolution of the complaint.

Case History

A good example of this phenomenon is a 27-year-old woman who presented with an 18-month history of right-sided facial pain that started after a middle ear infection. During the initial illness, she experienced dizziness, and a spinal tap was performed to rule out viral meningitis. This was negative, and a diagnosis of a viral syndrome was made. Several months later, persistent pain led the patient to seek a further ENT consultation. A cyst discovered in the right maxillary sinus was removed through a Caldwell-Luc procedure, with only transient relief of symptoms, however.

On evaluation, the patient complained of intermittent, deep, dull, aching pain in the right side of her face, including her eye, ear, and neck. The pain was associated with blurred vision, ptosis, and redness of both eyes. She also complained of unilateral hearing loss and nasal congestion on the symptomatic side. The pain occurred one or two times per week and lasted 24 to 48 hours.

Examination revealed multiple active myofascial TrPs in the right masseter, temporalis, medial pterygoid, sternocleidomastoid, and suboccipital muscles that reproduced all of her symptoms, including blurred vision. In contrast, there were essentially no TrPs in any of the muscles on the asymptomatic side. Treatment directed at rehabilitation of the involved muscles provided significant reduction in the intensity and frequency of her pain.

Sinus and Paranasal Pain. The most common extraoral source of dental pain arises from the maxillary sinus and associated pain-sensitive nasal mucosa. Many teeth have been mistakenly extracted because of an incorrect diagnosis of this syndrome.

Symptoms. Contrary to popular belief, infection and inflammation of the sinuses rarely cause facial pain or headache. Chronic sinusitis may cause symptoms of fullness or pressure but rarely pain. The location of these symptoms may vary from the maxilla and maxillary teeth in maxillary sinusitis to the upper orbit and frontal process in frontal sinusitis, between and behind the eyes in ethmoid sinusitis, and at the junction of the hard and soft palate, occiput, and mastoid process in sphenoid sinusitis.

The sinusitis patient who reports to the dentist does so with a chief complaint of "toothache." In this case, constant but rather mild pain in a number of posterior maxillary teeth on one side is almost pathognomonic. All of the teeth on this side, the roots of which are related to the floor of the sinus, may be aching mildly.

The teeth feel elongated, as if they "touch first" when the patient closes. The teeth are also tender, and the patient clenches against them, saying it "hurts good" to do so. These same maxillary teeth are hypersensitive to cold fluids. Occasionally, all of the maxillary teeth on the involved side, to the midline, feel uncomfortable and elongated. The pain, mild but deep and nonpulsating, radiates out of this area onto the face, upward toward the temple, and forward toward the nose. A referred frontal headache and cutaneous hyperalgesia along the side of the face and scalp may also be present. The patient frequently reports that the pain begins in the early afternoon or may give a history of increased pain at altitude when crossing a high mountain pass or when making a plane flight. Patients may also complain of a "stuffy nose," blood- or pus-tinged mucus, postnasal drip, fever, and malaise.

Etiology. The sinuses themselves are relatively pain-insensitive structures. Studies done by both Wolff and Reynolds et al. demonstrate that most so-called "sinus" pain actually arises from the nasal mucosa or from stimulation of the nasal ostia.[73,74] Nasal spurs have also been implicated as a cause of facial pain or headache.[75] The nasal mucosa and the pain-sensitive ostia become irritated and inflamed when inflammatory exudate from the antrum spills out onto these structures.[76] Direct stimulation of the ostia has also been shown to refer pain to the teeth.[76,77]

Allergies may also cause boggy, edematous nasal mucosa. This may cause swelling of the turbinates, which may, in turn, block off the ostia of the maxillary sinuses. This has been implicated in causing referred symptoms to the teeth (Figure 8-14).

Sicher also pointed out that the superior alveolar nerves, supplying the maxillary molar and premolar teeth, pass along the thin wall of the sinuses.[78] The canaliculi of the teeth often open toward the sinus, and pulpal nerves may be in direct contact with the inflamed mucoperiosteum of the sinus lining. Their direct irritation may cause dental symptoms. The reverse is also true. Inflammation or infection from the root of a tooth in contact with the sinus floor may cause sinusitis. This, in turn, will not resolve until the dental problem is corrected.

Examination. The dentist's contribution will be to rule out dental disease as the cause of the pain and correctly refer the patient for complete diagnosis and treatment.

The extraoral examination should include palpation of the maxillary sinuses under the zygomatic process bilaterally. If maxillary sinusitis is present and unilateral, the cheek on the involved side, from the canine fossa back to the base of the zygomatic process, will be tender to heavy palpation. The patient may say it feels as if he has been hit in the area, or "frostbitten" is another term used in northern climes. It may also hurt to smile.

If the patient complains of frontal headache, the dentist should check the frontal sinuses for tenderness by pressing up against the inferior surface of the supraorbital ridge on each side of the nose. All of the anterior sinuses, maxillary, frontal, and anterior ethmoidal, may be involved at one time. Such pansinusitis may follow an upper respiratory infection.

The intraoral examination should include mobility, percussion, thermal and electric pulp tests, and radiographs. The teeth adjacent to the affected maxillary sinus often are mobile when moved between the two

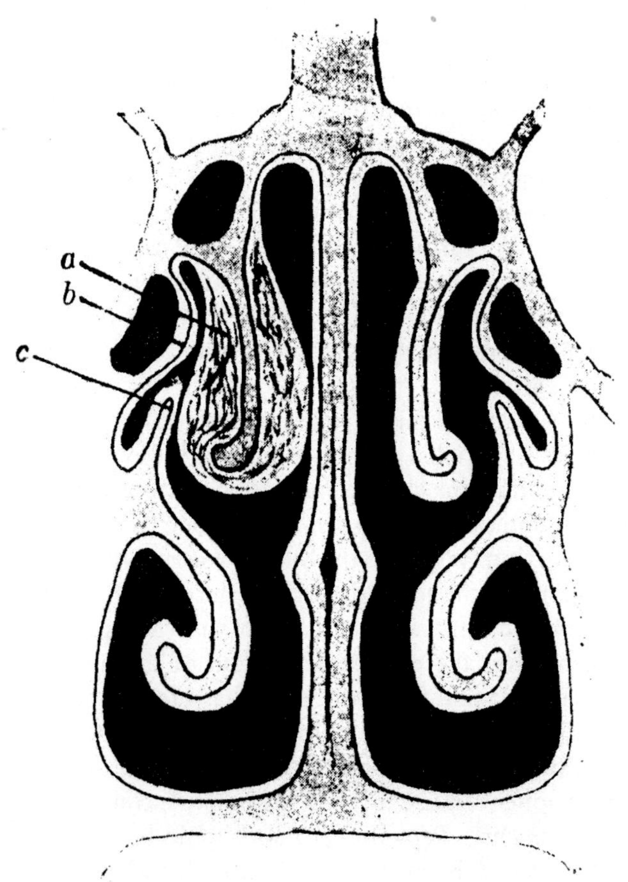

Figure 8-14 Inflammation of nasal mucosa causes swelling of the turbinate and blocks off the ostium of the maxillary sinus. Pain referred to maxillary teeth may then develop. Reproduced with permission from Ballenger JJ.[77]

index fingers. Furthermore, the teeth are painful and sound "mushy" when percussed and may be hypersensitive to cold or when pulp tested electrically compared to the uninvolved side. Illuminating the sinuses with a fiber optic in a darkened room may reveal changes in the affected sinus. Direct inspection of the nasal passages with a speculum will reveal engorged nasal mucosa and turbinates.

Radiographically, the involved teeth are likely to be normal, reconfirming that nothing is wrong orally. The roots of the teeth, however, may be found extending well up into or against the sinus floor, which would account for their involvement. On the other hand, the radiograph and pulp test may show a pulpless tooth with a periradicular lesion. As stated previously, this could be the cause of a unilateral sinus inflammation. Nenzen and Walander found "local hyperplasia of the maxillary sinus mucosa" in 58% (14 of 24) of the patients who had pulpless teeth with periradicular lesions associated with the floor of the sinus.[79]

Persistent pain in this area may be caused by a cyst or neoplasm of the maxillary sinus. In these cases, the pain syndrome is the same as for sinusitis but more long-standing. A radiographic study of the area may reveal the lesion.

The diagnosis of maxillary sinusitis may be confirmed by spraying 4% lidocaine anesthetic from a spray bottle into the nostril on the affected side. This will anesthetize the sensitive area around the ostium. The pain from the congested nasal mucosa and accompanying maxillary sinusitis should be substantially reduced within a minute or two.

Treatment. Complete diagnosis and treatment of maxillary sinusitis are left to the ENT specialist. Treatment usually consists of the use of decongestants and analgesics. If there is persistent purulent discharge, cultures should be taken and appropriate antibiotics prescribed.

Temporomandibular Joint Articular Disorders. Before discussing TMJ disorders, a distinction must be made between pain and dysfunction arising from the TMJ itself, temporomandibular disorder (TMD), and MFP owing to trigger points. Temporomandibular disorder is an umbrella term that refers to various painful and nonpainful conditions involving the TMJ and the associated masticatory musculature. Myofascial pain is a distinct muscle pain disorder that produces various local and referred symptoms from TrPs in taut bands of skeletal muscle and may or may not be associated with a TMJ disorder. Myofascial pain is reviewed in detail later in this chapter.

Historically, there has been much confusion around TMD and the differential contribution of pain from the joint versus the muscles and MFP. In a study conducted at the University of Minnesota TMJ and Facial Pain Clinic, doctors evaluated 296 consecutive patients with chronic head and neck pain complaints.[66] Only 21% of these patients had a TMJ disorder as the primary cause of pain. In all 21%, the joint disorder included an inflammation of the TMJ capsule or the retrodiscal tissues. Myofascial pain owing to TrPs was the primary diagnosis in 55.4% of the patients in the Minnesota study, almost three times the incidence of primary joint pain. Nonpainful internal derangements of the TMJs were felt to be a perpetuating factor to the myofascial TrPs in 30.4%.[60]

Considering these data, it is important to make a distinction between true TMJ pain, MFP owing to TrPs alone, and MFP owing to TrPs that is being perpetuated by a noninflammatory or intermittently inflammatory joint condition. Treatment priorities will be affected accordingly.

Table 8-9 provides a simple breakdown of TMJ disorders, the **vast majority** of which are **nonpainful.** Included in this category are inflammatory disorders, disk derangement disorders, and osteoarthritis. It is possible to have several of these diagnoses affecting one joint. It is also very common to find myofascial TrP pain associated with TMJ pathosis.

Table 8-9 Temporomandibular Joint Articular Disorders

Inflammatory disorders
Capsulitis/synovitis
Polyarthritides
Disk derangement disorders
Disk displacement with reduction
Disk displacement without reduction
Osteoarthritis (noninflammatory disorders)
Primary
Secondary
Congenital or developmental disorders
Aplasia
Hypoplasia
Hyperplasia
Neoplasia
Temporomandibular joint dislocation
Ankylosis
Fracture (condylar process)

Adapted from Okeson.[61]

The term **internal derangement** applies to all joints and encompasses those disorders causing mechanical interference to normal joint function. In the TMJs, this primarily involves displacement and distortion of the articular disk, as well as remodeling of the articular surfaces, and joint hypermobility.[80] Many of the articular disorders affecting the TMJs involve an abnormal or restricted range of motion and noise but are relatively painless. These include the **congenital or developmental disorders, disk derangement disorders, osteoarthritis, and ankylosis** listed in Table 8-9. Any pain associated with these disorders is usually momentary and associated with pulling or stretching of ligaments. In the case of **ankylosis**, pain ensues if the mandible is forcibly opened beyond adhesive restrictions. Forcible opening can cause acute inflammation. Primary or secondary **osteoarthritis**, unless accompanied by synovitis, is also associated with minimal pain or dysfunction,[61] although crepitus and limited range of motion may be present.

As far as the incidence of TMJ pain in the general population is concerned, the National Institute of Dental Research, reporting on the National Center for Health Statistics' 1989 survey of 45,711 US households over 6 months, has estimated that 9,945,000 Americans were suffering from what they termed "jaw joint pain." They further estimated that 5.3% of the US population were experiencing this condition at any one time. Twice as many women as men complained of jaw pain.[81]

Inflammatory Disorders of the Joint. It is the inflammatory joint disorders that cause pain. Included in this group are **capsulitis and synovitis** and **polyarthritides** (Table 8-9).[82,83]

Symptoms. **Capsulitis and synovitis** present with similar signs and symptoms and are difficult to differentiate. The chief symptom is continuous pain over the joint, aggravated by function. Swelling may be evident, and the patient may complain of an acute malocclusion ("back teeth on the same side don't touch"), restricted jaw opening, and ear pain. There is usually a history of trauma, infection, polyarthralgia, or chronic, nonpainful degenerative arthritis that is now in an acute stage.[61,83] Because the pain is fairly constant, the clinical picture is often complicated by referred pain, masticatory muscle spasm, or myofascial TrP pain.[83] The pain tends to wax and wane with the course of the inflammation. Inflammatory disorders of the joint may occur alone or in combination with an internal derangement.

Polyarthritides are relatively uncommon and occur with other rheumatologic diseases, such as rheumatoid arthritis. Symptoms may include pain at rest and with mandibular function, crepitus, and a limited range of motion.

Etiology. **Inflammation of the capsule or synovium** may occur secondary to localized trauma or infection, through overuse of the joint, or secondary to other joint disorders. **Synovitis** may also occur secondary to primary osteoarthritis. The inflammatory conditions occur most commonly in young people with a history of trauma, clenching, bruxism, or internal derangement.[84]

Inflammation and degenerative changes in the TMJ caused by systemic rheumatologic illnesses that affect multiple joints are called **polyarthritides.** They include most commonly rheumatoid arthritis, juvenile rheumatoid arthritis, psoriatic arthritis, and gout. The autoimmune disorders and mixed connective tissue diseases such as scleroderma, Sjögren's syndrome, and lupus erythematosus may also affect the TMJ.[61]

Examination. For **capsulitis and synovitis,** palpation over the joint itself is painful. Posterior or superior joint loading and any movement that stretches the capsule may also increase the pain. Range of motion is not usually restricted except owing to pain. Initiation of mandibular movement after a period of rest may be slow and "sticky." Inflammatory effusion in the joint may cause acute malocclusion with slight disclusion of the homolateral posterior teeth. Although clenching may be painful, biting on a tongue depressor may reduce the pain by preventing intercuspation and full closure.

In the **polyarthritides,** palpation of the joint is also painful. Range of motion is not affected except owing to pain and may be accompanied by crepitus; malocclusion is related to inflammatory effusion or lateral pterygoid muscle spasm secondary to the primary pain.[83] In severe cases of rheumatoid arthritis, rapid resorption of the condyles causes an acute anterior open bite.[61] Ankylosis may also occur.

Diagnostic Tests. Plain films and tomography will show few, if any, bony changes in the joint with **capsulitis or synovitis** unless these are secondary to osteoarthritis. Magnetic resonance imaging, on the other hand, will show a bright T_2-weighted signal secondary to the presence of fluid.

The **polyarthritides** will show extensive TMJ changes on radiographic examination. Radiographic changes include more gross deformities than are seen in osteoarthritis, including erosions, marginal proliferations, and flattening. Of particular diagnostic value in the polyarthritides are various serologic tests screening for evidence of rheumatoid disease such as antinuclear antibodies, elevated erythrocyte sedimentation rate, rheumatoid factor, or anemia, although not all rheumatologic diseases are seropositive. Definitive diagnosis and management of the polyarthritides are left to the rheumatologist. The dentist's role is to manage concomitant TMJ symptoms should they occur.

Treatment. In treating inflammatory TMJ disorders, palliative care is an appropriate first step. This includes jaw rest, a soft diet, and **nonsteroidal anti-inflammatory drugs (NSAIDs)**. Intermittent application of ice or moist heat may also be helpful. Office physical therapy, including ultrasonography, may be indicated in some patients. Single supracapsular or intra-articular injections of steroids may be effective in reducing inflammation and pain if simpler methods prove ineffective. Pain relief from steroid injection can be expected to last 1½ to 2 years provided that the patient limits joint use appropriately. It is generally accepted that steroid injections into the TMJ should be limited: no more than two in 12 months, and two or three in a lifetime. This is because of concern about inducing joint deterioration owing to the steroid.[85] More recent data suggest that these injections may be better tolerated than previously thought.[86]

Definitive therapy is aimed at reducing the causative or contributing factors. This must involve the patient, who alone controls the functional demands placed on the joint. The dentist must enlist his help and compliance. This is best achieved through reassurance and education. The patient must be motivated to reduce joint use and eliminate abusive habits. Home exercises, application of heat and ice, and massage are also important. In addition to the self-help program, construction of a **stabilization splint may help reduce bruxism** and decrease intra-articular pressure on the joint. If necessary, a psychological approach to decrease **bruxism or clenching** may also be instituted. Surgery is seldom, if ever, indicated.

If the condition is owing to **polyarthritis**, management is similar to treating the systemic disease itself. It includes analgesics and anti-inflammatory agents such as aspirin, indomethacin, ibuprofen, corticosteroids such as prednisone, gold salts, and penicillamine. Physical therapy, home exercises, appropriate jaw use, reduction of abusive habits, occlusal stabilization, and periodic intra-articular steroid injections are other supportive measures. Surgical intervention is limited to severe cases with marked dysfunction.

Disk Derangement Disorders. The disk derangement disorders include disk displacement with and without reduction.

Symptoms. Both of these disorders are typically **painless**. With **disk displacement with reduction**, pain, when present, is intermittent and related to interference or "jamming" of the disk and function of the condyle against ligaments. Patients may complain of difficulty in opening the jaws, particularly in the morning. Sometimes they have to manipulate their jaws, with a resultant loud crack, before they can function normally for the rest of the day.

Patients who present with ***disk displacement without reduction*** usually relate a history of TMJ clicking that stopped when the joint "locked." In addition to the limited range of motion, they may also complain of mild hyperocclusion on the affected side. Acutely, there may be pain that is usually secondary to attempts to open the mouth. Over time, the mandibular range of motion gradually improves and the pain subsides, often being replaced with a feeling of stiffness.

Etiology. The development of a disk displacement disorder is often attributed to external trauma, such as a blow, or to chronic microtrauma, such as **habitual parafunction (especially bruxism)** in a TMJ in which structural or functional incompatibilities exist. Occlusal disharmony, such as loss of posterior teeth or occlusal interferences in retruded and lateral movements, may contribute to the problem but is rarely causative.

Discrete clicks and pops are the result of the rapid reduction of an anteriorly displaced disk on opening (Figure 8-15). Locking results when the disk is so severely displaced or deformed that it can no longer relocate itself on top of the condyle during normal opening movements (Figure 8-16).

Examination. With **disk displacement with reduction**, there is a normal mandibular range of movement. Palpation of the joint on opening and closing will reveal a fairly distinct click or pop that is often accompanied by a slight deviation of mandibular movement. These clicks and pops are usually found at approximately 25 to 30 mm of opening, the point at which the condyle shifts from rotation to translation in the opening cycle. Often these joint noises are reciprocal. That is, there is another, very soft click just at the end of the closing path. It is at this time that the disk once again slips off the condyle and into its anterior position.

With **disk displacement without reduction**, there is clear restriction of jaw range of motion to approximately 25 to 30 mm. If only one joint is locking, the midline will deviate toward the affected joint. **Forced opening results in pain.** Laterotrusive movement is restricted to the unaffected side; bilateral restriction exists if the disorder affects both joints.

Diagnostic Tests. For **both disk displacement with and without reduction**, tomograms of the joints may

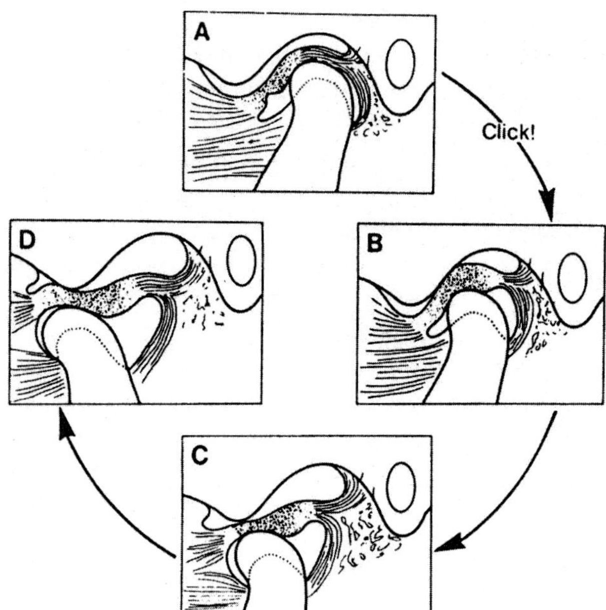

Figure 8-15 Internal temporomandibular joint derangement—the early click. Notice in the closed position (**A**) that the disk (**stippled**) is situated completely anterior to the articulating surface of the condyle. As the condyle begins to translate anteriorly, it passes beneath the thickened rim of the disk at the same time the patient notices a "click" within the joint. At one fingerbreadth opening (**B**), and throughout the remaining opening sequence (**C** and **D**), the relationship between the disk and bony structure is normal and not painful. Reproduced with permission from Wilkes CH. Arthrography of the temporomandibular joint. Minn Med 1978;61:645.

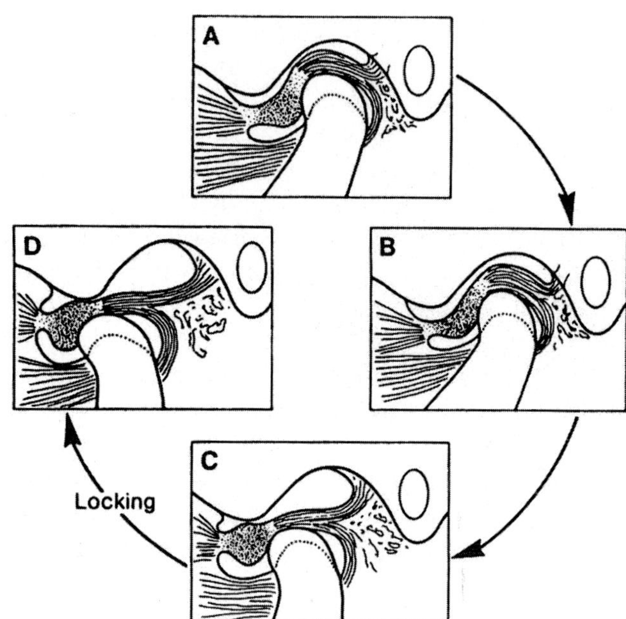

Figure 8-16 Severe disk derangement—the closed lock situation. In the closed projection (**A**), notice that the stippled disk has been deformed from a normal biconcave wafer to an amorphous mass. The disk is situated entirely anterior to the condylar articulating surface. During jaw opening (**B** and **C**), the condyle progressively forces the disk mass anteriorly, causing greater deformation. At no point in the sequence does the condyle negotiate its way past the thickened posterior aspect of the disk to acquire a normal relationship. Locking (**D**) and discomfort ensue. Reproduced with permission from Wilkes CH. Arthrography of the temporomandibular joint. Minn Med 1978;61:645.

reveal a mild posterior displacement of the condyle in the glenoid fossa, although this is not a consistent finding and should not be used alone to make a diagnosis. Bony contour of the condyle will usually show only mild degenerative changes. Arthrography or MRI reveals anterior displacement of the articular disk in both conditions. In **disk displacement with reduction,** the anterior displacement typically normalizes during jaw function.

Treatment. Because most disk displacement disorders are **non**painful, many patients only require an explanation for their symptoms and reassurance. There is no clear evidence that all disk displacement disorders are progressive[87] or that intervention prevents progression. In fact, **most TMDs are self-limiting.**[88–90]

Specific treatment, when indicated, will depend on the specific nature of the derangement. Conservative, reversible treatments such as patient education and self-care, physical therapy, behavior modification, orthopedic appliances, and medications are appropriate. Since most TMDs are self-limiting and resolve without serious long-term effects,[81–90] extensive occlusal rehabilitation or surgery should be avoided except in carefully selected cases.[91]

Osteoarthritis (noninflammatory) is found in many of the joints of the body and is classified according to perceived etiology. **Primary osteoarthritis** is so called because its etiology is unrelated to any other currently identifiable local or systemic disorder.[92] It may affect the TMJ alone or may include other joints of the body.[90,93,94] When other joints are involved, any of the weight-bearing joints in the body may be affected. Heberden's nodes of the terminal phalangeal joints are a clinical feature.

Secondary osteoarthritis, on the other hand, is considered to be the result of a specific precipitating event (such as trauma or infection) or other disease or disorder (such as rheumatoid arthritis, endocrine disturbance or gout, or a TMJ disk derangement disorder).

Symptoms. Despite their classification as noninflammatory disorders, **primary and secondary osteoarthritis** may be associated with a secondary synovitis. As a result, **the patient may complain of pain** with function and tenderness over the joint. In the absence of synovitis, crepitus and limited range of motion are the most likely complaints.

Etiology. **Osteoarthritis** is a degenerative joint condition characterized by joint breakdown involving erosion and attrition of articular tissue along with remodeling of the underlying subchondral bone[95] (Figure 8-17). Degenerative change is thought to be induced when the joint's natural physiologic remodeling capabilities are exceeded owing to factors that overload and stress the joint.[95,96]

Examination. The distinguishing clinical feature of **osteoarthritis** is crepitus: grating or multiple cracking noises within the joint during opening and closing. There may also be limitation of movement of the condyle and deviation to the affected side with opening. **When accompanied by synovitis, there is pain with function** and point tenderness over the joint on palpation.

Diagnostic Tests. Radiographic examination of the condyle may reveal decreased joint space, subchondral sclerosis, cystic formation, surface erosions, osteophytes, or marginal lipping. The articular eminence may be flattened or eroded or may contain osteophytes (see Figure 8-15). All clinical laboratory findings are usually within normal limits.

Treatment. Since most osteoarthritis is nonpainful and dysfunction is minimal, patients often do well with appropriate explanation of their symptoms and reassurance without specific treatment. When accompanied by synovitis and pain, treatment strategies for the acute inflammatory disorders are appropriate. Identification in **secondary osteoarthritis** of a precipitating disease or event may simplify treatment since correction of the underlying cause may facilitate resolution of any symptoms associated with the osteoarthritis.

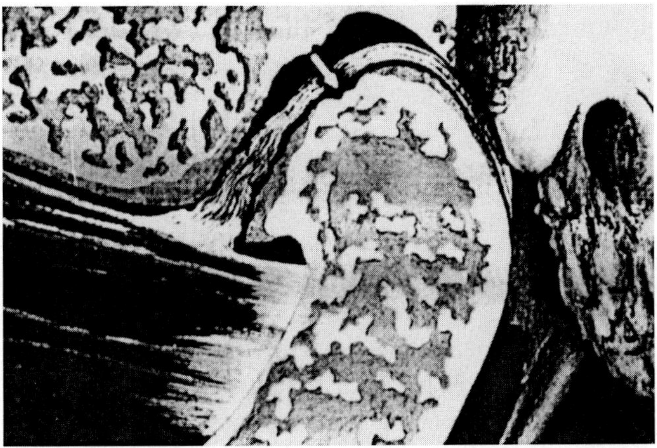

Figure 8-17 Degenerative joint changes that occur to the disk and condylar surfaces. Disk perforation (**arrow**), allowing bone-to-bone contact, may cause crepitus and pain on opening and closing. (Courtesy of Dr. Samuel Higdon.)

Congenital or developmental disorders such as **aplasia**, **hypoplasia**, and **hyperplasia** tend to cause esthetic and functional problems and are rarely accompanied by pain.

Temporomandibular joint dislocation refers to that situation when a patient is unable to close his mouth because the condyle is trapped either anterior to the articular eminence or anterior to a posteriorly dislocated disk.[97] Elevator muscle spasm usually aggravates the situation by forcing the condyle superiorly and opposing attempts to relocate the condyle in the glenoid fossa or on the articular disk. There is usually a history of nonpainful hypermobility and sometimes of previous dislocations that the patient was able to reduce himself.

Symptoms. The patient is distressed because of the inability to close the mouth and sometimes **associated pain. There is acute malocclusion.**

Examination. This reveals an anterior open bite with only the posterior teeth in contact. Visual inspection or palpation of the articular fossa may reveal a depression where the condyle would normally be.[98]

Diagnostic Tests. Radiographic examination shows the condyles anterior to the articular eminence or anteriorly displaced within the fossa.

Treatment. Reduction of the mandibular displacement is the goal and usually requires some kind of manual manipulation of the mandible. Initial steps include reassurance followed by gentle jaw opening against resistance to relax the elevator muscles. Manipulation procedures to reduce the mandible range from simple downward and posterior pressure on the chin during voluntary yawning, to downward and backward pressure on the mandibular molar teeth during yawning, to the administration of muscle relaxants or local anesthetic or even intravenous sedation followed by manual manipulation. Patients can expect some mild residual pain for one to several days following reduction.

Ankylosis in the TMJ refers to a fibrous or bony union between the condyle, disk, and fossa causing restricted mandibular range of motion with **deflection of the mandible to the affected side but no pain.** Ankylosis may follow joint inflammation caused by direct trauma, mandibular fracture, surgery, or a systemic disease such as arthritis. Treatment depends on the degree of dysfunction: arthroscopy and physical therapy may improve function for fibrous ankylosis (most common); open joint surgery is needed to create a new articulating surface in bony ankylosis (relatively rare). Elevator muscle shortening must be addressed as part of the management protocol for both conditions.

Referred Pain from Remote Pathologic Sites

Angina Pectoris and Myocardial Infarction. Severe pain referred into the mandible and maxilla from a region outside the head and neck is most commonly from the heart. The opposite pain reference has also been reported—pain from pulpalgia referring down the homolateral neck, shoulder, and arms.[99] That cardiac pain can be referred as far away as the jaws is fascinating. Yet remembering that dorsal root ganglion cells have been shown to branch in the periphery[100,101] and that, in the rat at least, the dorsal root ganglion cell supplying the heart also supplies the arm[100] helps to provide a possible explanation to this referred pain phenomenon (Figure 8-18). Potential convergence of nerve fibers from different sensory dermatomes in the dorsal horn of the spinal cord provides a basis for a "convergence-projection" phenomenon for the pain referral (see Figure 8-6). Ruch and Fulton defined a dermatome or sensory root field as "...the area of skin supplied with afferent fibers by a single posterior root."[102] They went on to say, "Dermatomes of adjacent roots overlap greatly so that always two and sometimes three roots supply a single point on the skin." Figure 8-19 shows how the thoracic dermatomes, innervating the chest and arms, overlap with the cervical dermatomes, some of which innervate the arm and shoulder, as well as part of the lower face.[102] The second cervical dermatome, in turn, slightly overlaps with the fifth cranial nerve, which innervates the entire oral complex.

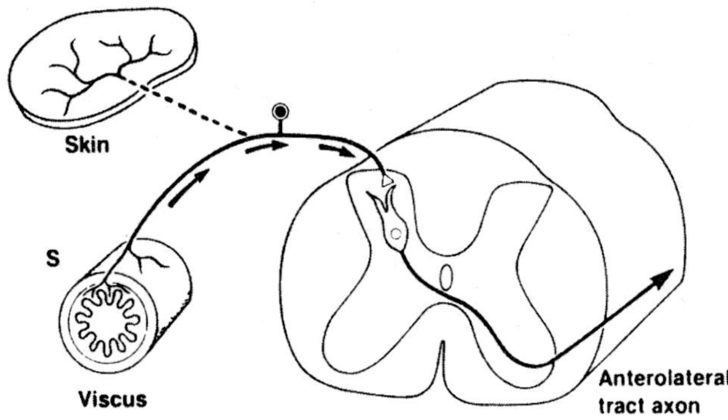

Figure 8-18 Branched primary afferent hypothesis of referred pain. According to this theory, a single primary afferent branches to supply both the deep structure stimulated and the structure(s) in which the pain is perceived. Reproduced with permission from Fields HL.[3]

Repetition of a previous paragraph may help to explain this phenomenon more clearly:

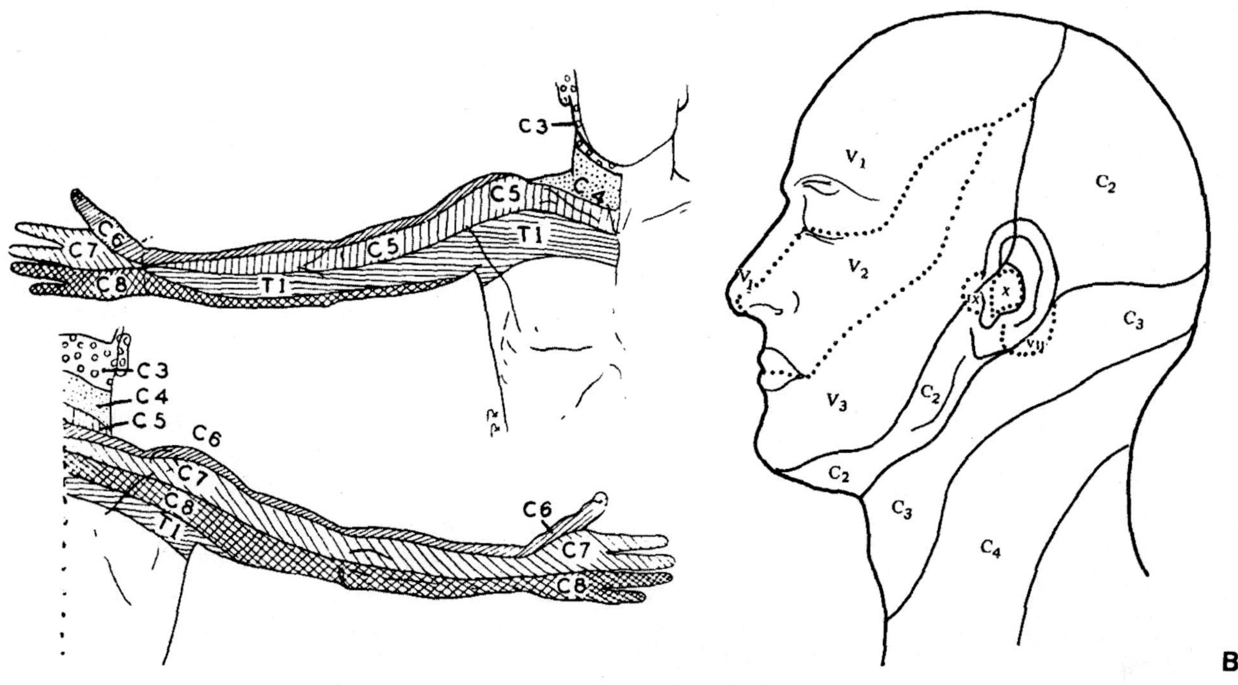

Figure 8-19 A, Dermatome chart of upper extremity of man. Pain referred out of the chest from the first thoracic dermatome advances by overlapping dermatomes to the third cervical dermatome, which, in turn, overlaps the third division of the fifth cranial nerve. This has been offered as a possible explanation for reference of deep visceral pain from the myocardium into the jaws and teeth and down the left arm. **B**, Detailed map of sensory nerve responsibility. Note how C2 overlaps with V3 (trigeminal-mandibular). **A** reproduced with permission from Keegan J, Garrett FD. The segmental distribution of the cutaneous nerves in the limbs of man. Anat Rec 1948;102:409. **B** reproduced with permission from Clemente CD. Anatomy: a regional atlas of the human body. Philadelphia: Lea & Febiger; 1975.

Primary afferent nociceptors from both visceral and cutaneous neurons often converge onto the same second-order pain transmission neuron in the spinal cord. The brain, having more awareness of cutaneous than of visceral structures through past experience, interprets the pain as coming from the regions subserved by the cutaneous afferent fibers (see Figure 8-6).

Hence, branching and/or convergence of thoracic, cervical, and fifth cranial nerve fibers might well explain the bizarre pain referral patterns from the heart.

Symptoms. **Angina pectoris** is typically characterized by heaviness, tightness, or aching pain in the mid or upper sternum. These symptoms may radiate upward from the epigastrium to the mandible—the left more frequently than the right. In addition, the inner aspects of the arms may ache, again the left more frequently and extensively than the right. This pattern is similar to that seen with myocardial infarction (Figure 8-20, A). Precipitating factors include exertion and emotional excitement or ingestion of food.[103] Angina attacks are usually short-lasting, rarely longer than 15 minutes. A number of patients with recurrent angina pectoris, who know they have the disease and who use nitroglycerine to control the attacks, have reported left mandibular pain with each spasm. Anginal pain referred to the left posterior teeth was well documented by Natkin et al.: "In certain instances pain was experience with concomitant chest pain, and in other instances, pain was confined to the teeth."[104]

Myocardial infarction is characterized by a symptom complex that includes a sudden, gradually increasing precordial pain, with an overwhelming feeling of suffocation. The squeezing pain radiates in a pattern similar to that described for angina pectoris (see Figure 8-20, A). Accompanying these symptoms may be a sense of impending doom, nausea, and the attendant signs of shock: sweating, cold clammy skin, and a gray complexion. In advanced stages, the patient becomes unconscious and cyanotic. If conscious, the patient generally complains of the severe pain and rubs the chest, jaw, and arm. These are the advanced signs and symptoms of a heart attack.

Severe pain in the left maxilla and mandible related to angina pectoris or myocardial infarction may occur without any other symptoms. Bonica reported **an incidence as high as 18% for the presentation of cardiac pain as jaw or tooth pain alone.**[105] The distribution of this cardiac pain may vary. One patient had the unusual symptoms of referred pain in the left maxilla and right arm but no chest pain. Matson reported a case of coronary thrombosis during which the patient experienced "pain in both sides of the mandible and neck, which radiated to the lateral aspects of the zygoma and temporal areas. She specifically denied having chest, shoulder or arm pains..."[106] Norman discussed four unusual cases of myocardial infarction with pain referred to the right and left jaws.[107] The left maxilla is also a common site. Batchelder and her colleagues[103] also reported a case in which mandibular pain was the sole clinical manifestation of coronary insufficiency. Krant reported referred pain in the left mandibular molars that proved to be a manifestation of a malignant mediastinal lymphoma.[108] It is these patients with jaw pain in the absence of other symptoms of heart disease who report to the dental office for diagnosis.

Etiology. **Angina pectoris** refers to pain in the thoracic region and surrounding areas owing to transient and reversible anoxia of the myocardium secondary to exertion or excitement.[109] Coronary atherosclerosis is the most common cause of this anoxia.

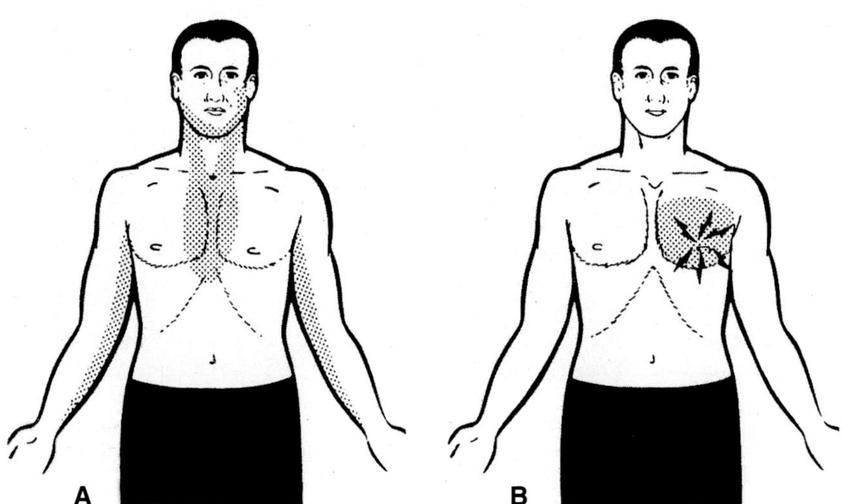

Figure 8-20 **A,** Pattern of pain and referred pain emanating from myocardial infarction. Central necktie pattern and greater left jaw and arm pain than on the right side are typical. **B,** Harmless noncardiac pain in the left chest. Reproduced with permission from Turner GO. Medical World News, April 6, 1973.

Aortic stenosis and coronary arterial spasm are other, less frequent causes.

Myocardial infarction refers to necrosis of the cardiac muscle secondary to a severe reduction in coronary blood supply.[109] Coronary artery occlusion may develop from gradual closure of the vessel by atherosclerotic deposits on the vessel wall or may be caused by hemorrhage under an atherosclerotic plaque, raising the plaque to obstruct the vessel lumen. Predisposing factors include heredity, obesity, tobacco use, lack of physical exercise, diet, emotional stress, and hostility and anger.[110]

Examination. A careful history is important in diagnosing the referred oral pain of myocardial infarction. Usually, the patient has a rather unusual story to tell, with fairly severe pain that began rather suddenly in the left jaw and grew in intensity. The symptoms may sound very much like a pulpitis. The pain might even have moved from mandible to maxilla. The dentist must rule out dental pathosis quickly and efficiently.

Diagnostic Tests. Radiographs and pulp testing of all of the teeth in the site of pain or rinsing with ice water will be equivocal. Analgesic block of the involved tooth or teeth will fail to relieve the pain.

After localized dental or TMJ origins have been ruled out, referred pain from the chest must be considered.

Treatment. If cardiac pain is suspected, the patient must be referred to an emergency room immediately. It is wise to call the hospital and have them ready to receive the patient. If pain is severe, 5 to 10 mg of morphine sulfate should be administered intramuscularly or intravenously. Further exertion by the patient should be avoided to minimize oxygen demands placed on the heart.

If the patient loses consciousness, the "ABCs" of cardiopulmonary resuscitation should be applied until help arrives.

Thyroid. The thyroid is a butterfly-shaped gland situated in the neck superficial to the trachea at or below the cricoid cartilage. Thyroid hormone regulates the metabolic state of the body. Disorders of the thyroid gland are prevalent in medical practice, second only to diabetes as an endocrine disorder.[109] **Subacute thyroiditis** (viral inflammation of the thyroid gland) is of interest to the dentist because it may refer **pain to the jaws and ears.**

Symptoms. The typical symptom picture includes pain over at least one lobe of the thyroid gland or pain radiating up the sides of the neck and **into the lower jaws, ears, or occiput. Swallowing may aggravate the symptoms.** This is usually associated with a feeling of pressure or fullness in the throat. There may be mild fever, asthenia, and malaise.[109] Symptoms may wax and wane over a period of months and then finally resolve with return of normal thyroid function.

Etiology. Subacute thyroiditis is reported to occur 2 to 3 weeks after an upper respiratory infection and is viral in origin.[111]

Examination. The thyroid gland may be visibly enlarged and will be tender to palpation with nodularity (Figure 8-21). If thyroiditis or other thyroid disease is suspected, referral to the patient's physician should be made for a complete medical workup.

Diagnostic Tests. A complete blood count may show an elevated leukocyte count. The erythrocyte sedimentation rate will be substantially elevated. Further workup and treatment are in the realm of the physician and will likely include various thyroid function tests.

Treatment. Subacute thyroiditis may resolve spontaneously. Aspirin and occasionally steroids are used to control the pain and inflammation. Thyroid supplements are sometimes indicated.[112]

Carotid Artery. Stimulation of various parts of the carotid artery in the region of the bifurcation has been shown to cause pain in the **ipsilateral jaw, maxilla, teeth, gums**, scalp, eyes, or nose.[113] In the absence of other demonstrable pathema, unilateral dull, aching, sometimes throbbing pain **in the jaws**, temple, and neck may be attributable to a carotid system arteritis, also known as **carotidynia** (carotid pain). This pain syndrome may be more prevalent than previously reported in the literature because the constellation of symptoms and findings may be confused with TMJ pain, MFP, salivary gland obstruction, and other extracranial sources of pain.

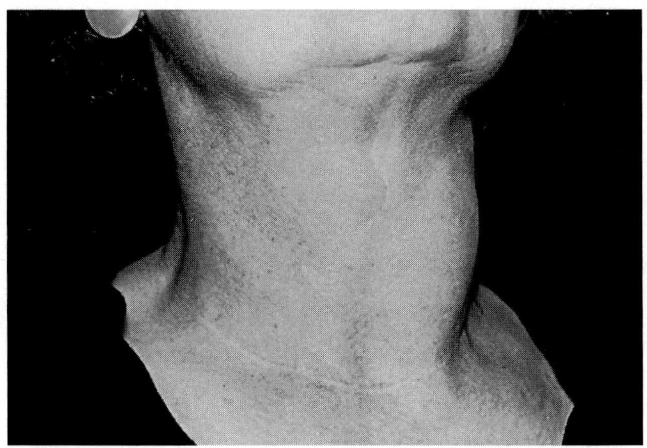

Figure 8-21 Benign thyroid tumor that recurred following thyroidectomy is referring pain into the mandibular first molar on the homolateral side.

Symptoms. The patient with **carotidynia** will most likely complain of constant or intermittent dull, aching, rarely pulsing **jaw and neck pain,** with intermittent sore throat or swollen glands. The pain may also involve the **temple and TMJ region** and radiate forward into the **masseter muscle** with occasional concomitant tenderness and fullness. Aggravating factors may include **chewing, swallowing**, bending over, or straining. Females outnumber males approximately 4 to 1.[114–117] The syndrome may develop at any age but is most common over age 40. There may be a family history of migraine.

Etiology. The nerves innervating the adventitial and intimal walls of the carotid artery are considered part of the visceral nervous system.[118] The convergence-projection theory of referred visceral pain discussed earlier in this chapter may explain why pain is referred from the carotid artery to the skin and muscles of the head and neck region.

Some authors feel that the artery and its peripheral branches are inflamed and that biopsy may reveal the presence of inflammatory and giant cells.[118] Precipitating factors may include an inflammatory response secondary to physical trauma or bacterial or viral infection, drugs, or alcohol.[118]

Others have found no evidence of inflammation and feel that the pain syndrome is owing to a pathophysiologic mechanism similar to migraine.[114] Elongation of the stylohyoid process is **not** thought to be a cause of this pain.[116]

Examination. Examination may reveal tenderness and swelling over the ipsilateral carotid artery along with pronounced throbbing of the carotid pulse.[115] Palpation may aggravate the pain. Similarly, the external branches of the carotid system and surrounding areas may also be tender. This may include the masticatory and cervical muscles, which may contain myofascial TrPs and lead to an **erroneous diagnosis** of musculoskeletal pain. Palpation over the sternocleidomastoid may aggravate the pain because of incidental irritation of the carotid vessel. The thyroid is nontender. All other tests and examinations are normal.

Treatment. Medications used in the treatment and prevention of migraine headaches have been shown to be effective in controlling the symptoms of carotidynia.[114] Some authors advocate the use of steroids and NSAIDs.[117] Concomitant treatment of any myofascial TrPs will ameliorate the symptoms to some extent.[116]

Cervical Spine. Disorders of the cervical spine and neck area may refer pain into the **facial region** owing to convergence of cervical and trigeminal primary afferent nociceptors in the nucleus caudalis of the spinal trigeminal tract. The normal cervical spine has 37 individual joints, making it the most complicated articular system in the body.[119] Most of the structures in the neck have been shown to produce pain when stimulated.[120] Pain may be elicited through several different pathologic processes including trauma; inflammation or misalignment of the vertebral bodies; inflammation or herniation of the intervertebral disks; trauma or strains to the spinal ligaments; and strains, spasms, or tears of the cervical muscles.

Nonmusculoskeletal pain-producing structures of the neck include the cervical nerve roots and nerves and the vertebral arteries.[120] Trauma, inflammation, and compression are implicated in the etiology of pain from these structures as well.

Acute trauma and primary pathologic processes of the neck are obviously not in the realm of the dentist to diagnose and treat; therefore, these will not be discussed. However, the cervical spine must be recognized as a potential source of dermatomal and referred pain into the head and **orofacial** region. Chronic subclinical dysfunction of the cervical spine may produce complaints that first appear in the dental office. This dysfunction may serve as a powerful perpetuating factor in temporomandibular and facial pain disorders and must be screened for and appropriately managed for successful treatment outcome.

Cervical Joint Dysfunction. Cervical joint dysfunction refers to a lack of normal anatomic relationship and/or restricted functional movement of individual cervical vertebral joint segments.

Etiology. In the craniocervical region, cervical joint dysfunction may occur as the result of trauma (eg, a **whiplash injury**), degenerative osteoarthritis, or chronic poor postural habits that result in sustained muscular contraction and immobility. As the cervical spine loses mobility and adapts to abnormal positions, nerve compression, nerve root irritation, neurovascular compression, posterior vertebral joint irritation, and peripheral entrapment neuropathies may result.[59,121] Entrapment or chronic irritation of the nerve roots in the C4 to C7 area generally produces pain in the respective dermatomes in the shoulder and arm regions (see Figure 8-19). Although C1, C2, and C3 nerve roots are not thought to be involved in compression or peripheral entrapment-type problems,[122] they do become inflamed through mechanical irritation by other neighboring structures such as the vertebral processes, muscles, or connective tissue capsules. When this occurs, pain may be experienced in the craniofacial, **orofacial, mandibular**, and **temporomandibular** regions (the C2–C3 dermatomes) (see Figure 8-19 and

Figure 8-22). Pain impulses from the first four upper cervical roots are thought to be referred to the trigeminal region (mainly V1 and V2) as a result of the proximity of the nucleus caudalis in the spinal trigeminal tract.[32] The nucleus caudalis descends into the spinal cord as far as C3–C4 (see Figure 8-8). These dermatomal and referred pain syndromes are particularly important to the dentist.

Symptoms. Local symptoms of cervical dysfunction may include stiffness, pain, and a limited range of motion of the head and neck.[120] The patient may also complain of throat tightness and difficulty swallowing.[121] **Dermatomal pains** may have an aching or neuritic quality and typically follow the distribution of the cervical nerve root involved. **Referred pains** are usually deep and aching and may present as a unilateral headache, as in a headache syndrome known as "cervicogenic headache."[32,123] This headache has a clinical picture similar to migraine except that the pain is strictly or predominantly unilateral and always on the same side. The patient may note that cervical movement or pressure on certain spots in the neck will precipitate a headache.

Examination. Postural evaluation is essential for all facial pain patients. Of particular importance is anterior head position. Examination of the cervical spine should include range of motion in flexion, extension, lateral flexion, and rotation. Additionally, the movement of the individual upper cervical segments (occiput—C1 and C1–C2) should be evaluated.[57,59] Range of motion is often restricted with cervical dysfunction. Upper cervical dysfunction may be unilateral or bilateral.

Radiographic evaluation may reveal osteoarthritis or show a decreased cervical lordosis, evidence of soft tissue spasm, or muscular shortening. Most commonly, however, no pathologic radiographic findings are present. More sophisticated radiographic techniques can pick up decreased cervical mobility.[124]

Treatment. Physical therapy, including cervical joint mobilization along with a comprehensive home exercise program and postural retraining, is required to treat pain of cervical origin.

Local treatment of referred symptoms does not provide long-lasting, if any, relief. If the patient has a true dental or TM disorder *and* dysfunction of the cervical spine, both problems must be addressed. Very often craniofacial pain will resolve once the cervical problem is corrected. If pain exists in both regions, it is likely that the cervical problem is perpetuating the facial pain. It is extremely rare for pain to be referred in a caudal direction.[70] Thus, **facial pain only rarely causes neck pain.**

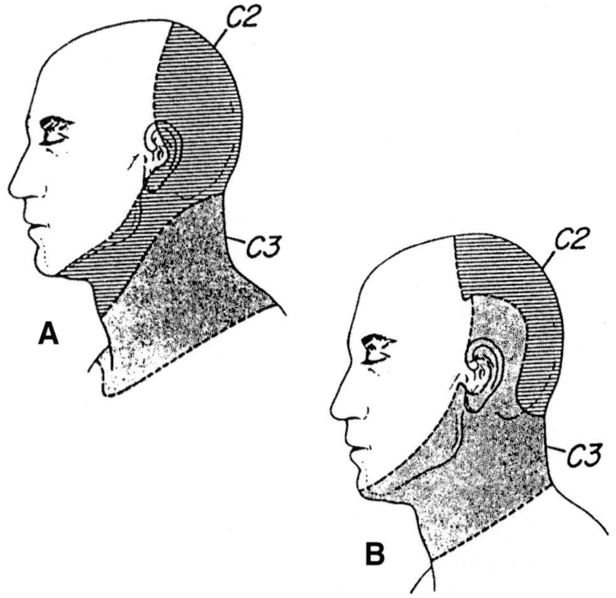

Figure 8-22 A study by Poletti revealed a slightly different distribution of C2–C3 dermatomes for pain than those previously defined by using tactile criteria. The upper figure (A) depicts the C2 and C3 tactile dermatomes previously defined by Foerster. The lower figure (B) depicts C2 and C3 pain dermatomes as defined by Poletti. Reproduced with permission from Poletti CE. C-2 and C-3 pain dermatomes in man. Cephalalgia 1991;11:158.

Case History

The following is a classic example of misdiagnosis of a referred cervical pain problem. A 38-year-old woman presented herself to the Pain Management Center at the University of California at Los Angeles (UCLA) with a 14-year history of severe left hemicranial headaches that had forced her to give up working. Because of the unilateral distribution, they had previously been misdiagnosed and unsuccessfully treated as migraine. However, the pain was strictly unilateral and was present on a continuous daily basis (unlike migraine), with intermittent exacerbations. The quality of the pain was described as dull and aching, progressing to throbbing only when severe. The patient also had an endodontic history involving the upper left second premolar, reportedly still sensitive. The dental examination revealed slight hyperocclusion of the involved premolar, which was corrected. Thorough musculoskeletal examination of the TMJ and cervical spine revealed a very prominent dysfunction of atlas on axis on the left. There was no evidence of any internal derangement of the TMJ. Myofascial examination revealed several active TrPs that reproduced her pain complaint.

Physical therapy, including cervical joint mobilization along with a comprehensive home exercise program and postural retraining, was instituted. As treatment progressed, the painful area began to decrease in size until all that remained was the left TMJ and left lower-border mandible pain— the precise distribution of the C2 tactile dermatome (see Figure 8-19, B and Figure 8-22, A) and C3 pain dermatome (see Figure 8-22, B).

Myofascial TrP injections into the left splenius capitis muscle in conjunction with further physical therapy and a continued home program completely resolved the C1–C2 dysfunction and the associated dermatomal pain. The patient has now been pain free for 18 years.

The case of this patient illustrates how easy it would be to search in the TMJ and dental area for a cause for the pain when the true culprit is actually the neck. The role of cervical dysfunction and myofascial trigger points in this type of pain presentation has been thoroughly discussed.[125]

A TMJ disorder is unlikely to be causing all of our patient's pain. However, on examination, a restricted mandibular range of motion was found, as well as radiographic evidence of degenerative joint disease. Perhaps these are incidental findings. Alternatively, if the internal derangement is painful or the joint is inflamed, it may also be a contributing factor.

Muscles. Myofascial TrP pain is discussed under "Muscular Pains" in this chapter.

INTRACRANIAL PATHOSIS

Although rare, intracranial lesions can cause pain referral to all areas of the head, face, and neck, including the oral cavity. Neurologic or neurosurgical evaluation is critical to rule out space-occupying lesions, intracranial infections, or neurologic syndromes.

Intracranial causes of head and neck pain can be classified into two groups: those caused by **traction on pain-sensitive structures** (which include the venous sinuses, dural and cerebral arteries, pia and dura mater, and cranial nerves) and those caused by **specific central nervous system syndromes**, such as neurofibromatosis, meningitis, or thalamic pain[126,127] (Table 8-10). Different types of cerebrovascular accidents and venous thrombosis may also cause painful central nervous system lesions. Most of these problems will, however, not be seen in the dental office and therefore will not be discussed in detail.

Table 8-10 Intracranial Causes of Pain

Neoplasm	Neurofibromatosis
Aneurysm	Meningitis
Hematoma/hemorrhage	Thalamic pain
Edema	
Abscess	Cerebrovascular accidents
Angioma	Venous thrombosis

Intracranial lesions are rarely painful, but when they are, the pain is severe and difficult to treat.[128] The quality of pain may vary from a generalized throbbing or aching to a more specific paroxysmal sharp pain. **Neurofibromatosis**, a condition in which there are numerous pedunculated tumors of neurolemmal tissue all over the body, is not painful unless the tumors press on nerves. Intracranial lesions are usually associated with different focal neurologic signs or deficits such as weakness, dizziness, difficulty in speaking or swallowing, ptosis, areas of numbness, memory loss, or mental confusion. If such neurologic signs or deficits appear with a pain complaint, pain from intracranial sources must be ruled out. This will require referral to a competent neurologist or neurosurgeon. Treatment will depend on the diagnosis and may range from antibiotic or antiviral therapy for infective processes to surgical intervention for aneurysms and tumors to palliative pain management for inoperable cases.

In our patient, presented earlier, extensive examinations and sophisticated imaging techniques have already ruled out extracranial and intracranial pathosis as causes for her pain, although she does have active myofascial TrPs in the trapezius muscle referring pain into the angle of the jaw. This, however, does not account for her entire pain presentation. The other sources of pain must still be sought.

NEUROVASCULAR PAINS

This category of pain encompasses several of the primary headache disorders (headaches not of pathologic origin) such as migraines, cluster headache syndromes, and simple intracranial vasodilation, as well as some headaches associated with pathologic vascular disorders, such as temporal arteritis (Table 8-11). The list includes only those headaches that have a higher likelihood of presenting in the dental office.

Table 8-11 Neurovascular Pains

Migraines
Migraine with aura (classic)
Migraine without aura (common)
Migraine with prolonged aura (complicated)
Cluster headaches and chronic paroxysmal hemicrania
Cluster headache
Episodic
Chronic
Chronic paroxysmal hemicrania
Miscellaneous headaches unassociated with structural lesion
External compression headache
Cold stimulus headache
Benign cough headache
Benign exertional headache
Headache associated with sexual activity
Headaches associated with vascular disorders
Arteritis
Carotid or vertebral artery pain
Hypertension
Headaches associated with substances or their withdrawal
Acute substance use/exposure (nitrates, monosodium glutamate, carbon monoxide, alcohol)
Chronic substance use/exposure (ergotamine, analgesics)
Acute use withdrawal (alcohol)
Chronic use withdrawal (ergotamine, caffine, narcotics)
Headaches associated with metabolic disorder
Hypoxia
Hypoglycemia
Dialysis

Adapted from Headache Classification Committee of the International Headache Society.[54]

In general, these headache types share the following features. They all have primarily a deep, throbbing, pulsing, or pounding quality, occasionally sharp, and occasionally with an aching or burning background. The pain is exclusively or **predominantly unilateral** with pain-free or almost pain-free periods between attacks. The main difference between the different headache types lies in their temporal patterns (Figure 8-23) and their associated symptoms.

Migraine

Symptoms. Migraine with aura, commonly known as "classic" migraine, is distinguished by the occurrence of transient focal neurologic symptoms (the aura), 10 to 30 minutes prior to the onset of headache pain. Visual auras are most common and may present as flashing lights, halos, or loss of part of the visual field. Somatosensory auras are also common and consist of dysesthesias that start in one hand and spread up to involve the ipsilateral side of the face, nose, and mouth.[129] The headache itself is predominantly unilateral in the frontal, temporal, or retrobulbar areas, although it may occur **in the face or in a single tooth.** The pain may begin as an ache but usually develops into pain of a throbbing, pulsating, or beating nature. Associated symptoms may include nausea, vomiting, photo- and phonophobia, cold extremities, water retention, and sweating. The headaches are episodic and can last anywhere from several hours to 3 days, with variable pain-free periods (days to years).

Migraine without aura or "common" migraine is similar to migraine with aura except that the headache occurs without a preceding aura.

Migraine headaches are more common in females and may begin in early childhood. The usual onset is

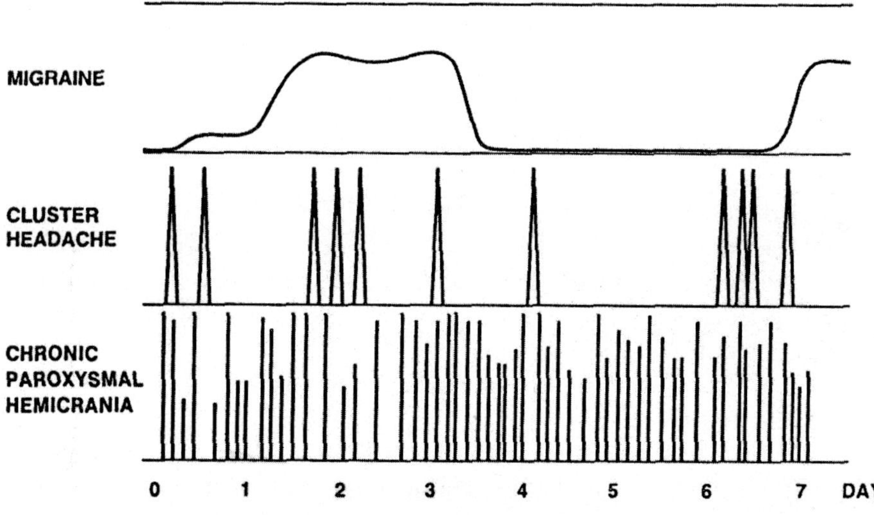

Figure 8-23 Comparison of temporal pattern of three main "vascular" headache types.

between the ages of 20 and 40 years, with 70% of these patients reporting **a family history** of migraine. Some factors that may precipitate the headache include stress and fatigue, foods rich in tyramine (ripe cheese) or nitrates, red wines and alcohol, histamines, and vasodilators. Often patients with migraine, especially migraine without aura, have **overlying MFP**, causing additional dull, aching headache pain.

Case History

The following is an example of an unusual presentation of a migraine headache of particular interest to the dentist. The patient was a 52-year-old woman who had a 7-year history of pain in the upper right quadrant, second premolar area, radiating to the right temple. The quality of pain was described as pulsing, sharp, and penetrating. The temporal pattern was intermittent, with 2 to 3 days of pain followed by 1 to 2 weeks without pain. The symptoms occurred without any identifiable precipitating factor, although loud noise seemed to make the pain worse. Associated autonomic symptoms were absent. Previous unsuccessful treatments included endodontic treatment of the right maxillary second premolar and an exploratory open flap in the same area, looking for fractures or external resorption. Topical anesthetics over the gingiva surrounding tooth #4 were similarly ineffective in relieving the symptoms. A diagnosis of migraine without aura was made based on the quality and temporal pattern of the pain and the absence of dental pathema to explain the symptoms. Treatment with abortive migraine medications proved quite successful.

Etiology. The exact etiology and pathogenesis of ***migraine with aura*** headaches remain controversial. The prevailing view is that migraine pain originates from the vascular and nervous tissues in and around the brain. The pain is thought to be *referred* to the more superficial cranial structures through convergence of vascular and somatic nerve fibers on single second-order pain transmission neurons in the trigeminal nucleus caudalis.[130] A sterile neurogenic inflammation caused by the release of vasoactive neuropeptides from nerves surrounding the affected intracranial vasculature is thought to be the nociceptive source. It is postulated that documented cerebral blood flow changes seen in various studies[131,132] may be a trigger for the events leading to the inflammation. The efficacy of the **ergot** alkaloids and a newer family of drugs called **"triptans"** appears to be attributable to the ability of these drugs to block neurogenic plasma extravasation and sterile inflammation.[133] It is currently not clear whether the ability of these drugs to cause vasoconstriction has anything to do with pain relief.[134]

Many headache researchers and clinicians feel that ***migraine without aura*** is the same as migraine with aura, except that the aura is absent or not dramatic enough to be noted. Thus, the mechanism is thought to be similar. There is, however, fairly good evidence that the ***pain*** of migraine without aura may actually be owing to muscle tenderness and referred pain from myofascial TrPs rather than cerebral vascular changes.[135,136] In fact, the same blood flow studies that showed intracranial vascular blood flow changes in migraine with aura failed to show any significant changes in migraine without aura.[137]

Examination. The diagnosis of migraine can usually be made by history. Nonetheless, examination of the patient complaining of undiagnosed intermittent toothache or facial pain should include a thorough dental, TMJ, and muscle evaluation. Once obvious dental and joint pathology has been ruled out, and the qualitative and temporal pattern of the pain raises the possibility of dental or facial migraine, referral to an orofacial pain dentist should be made. **Dental heroics should be avoided.**

Diagnostic Tests. There are no diagnostic tests that will confirm a diagnosis of migraine headache. If the headache is of recent onset, a neurologic evaluation including a CT scan or an MRI may be indicated. Thermography during an acute attack of migraine does show areas of increased blood flow on the side of the headache.[138,139]

Treatment. Long-term management of migraine headache typically requires identification and control of any obvious precipitating factors. Restriction of alcohol intake and elimination of tyramine-containing foods[140] are simple yet sometimes effective means of decreasing the frequency of migraine attacks. Regular meals and good sleep hygiene also help prevent the onset of migraine. If myofascial TrPs or musculoskeletal dysfunction are present, competent treatment of these will significantly reduce the frequency of the vascular headache symptoms and reduce the need for migraine medications. For those patients in whom stress, depression, or anxiety play a role, psychological interventions such as stress management and relaxation training, biofeedback, or cognitive behavioral therapy may be indicated.

Medications used in the treatment of migraine include abortive and prophylactic drugs, the choice of which depends on the frequency of migraine attacks.

Individuals who suffer less than three or four migraines per month may do well with abortive drugs that are taken during the onset of the headache or migrainous facial pain. Abortive drugs are particularly useful in migraine with aura for which the aura warns the patient that a headache is pending. The newest abortive drugs are the **"triptans,"** of which **Imitrex (sumatriptan)** was the first. Various ergotamine preparations, long the drugs of first choice for migraines, are also available. The latter are effectual and somewhat less expensive, but nausea and vomiting are frequent, undesirable side effects. Prophylactic medications are used when headache frequency exceeds three or four per month since the **triptans may cause coronary vasospasm or ischemia** and **ergot preparations, potent peripheral vasoconstrictors, may cause peripheral vascular problems.** Prophylactic medications include β-blockers, tricyclic antidepressants, calcium channel blockers, and others.

Cluster Headache and Chronic Paroxysmal Hemicrania

These headaches are classified together because they share several clinical characteristics and may have similar etiologic mechanisms. Nonetheless, they are easily distinguishable clinically and clearly differ from migraine.

Symptoms. **Cluster headaches** derive their name from their temporal pattern. They tend to occur in "clusters," a series of one to eight 20- to 180-minute attacks per day lasting for several weeks or months, followed by remissions of months or years[54,141,142] (see Figure 8-23). These headaches are found five to eight times more frequently in men than in women, particularly in **men** aged 20 to 50 years **who smoke.** The pain is a severe, unilateral, continuous, intense ache or burning that often occurs at night. Movements that increase blood flow to the head may result in throbbing. The most common sites are either around and behind the eye radiating to the forehead and temple or around and behind the eye radiating infraorbitally **into the maxilla and occasionally into the teeth,** rarely to the lower jaw and neck. Because of the oral symptoms, serious diagnostic errors are committed by dentists. Researchers from UCLA reported that 42% of 33 patients suffering cluster headache had been seen by dentists and that 50% of these patients **received inappropriate dental treatment.**[143]

Prodromal auras are absent with cluster headaches, but nasal stuffiness, lacrimation, rhinorrhea, conjunctival injection, perspiration of the forehead and face, and Horner's syndrome (ptosis of upper lid and miosis) are characteristic. Precipitating factors may include alcohol or other vasodilating substances, such as nitroglycerine. Cluster headache patients typically pace the floor during their headaches owing to the intensity of pain. This is in contrast to the migraine patient, who retreats to a dark room to sleep.

Cluster headaches may progress from the more classic episodic form, occurring in periods lasting 1 week to 1 year, with at least 2-week pain-free periods between, to a chronic form in which remissions are absent or last less than 2 weeks.[54] Rarely is the chronic form present from the onset.

Case History

The following history was obtained from a 42-year-old man who had suffered from cluster headaches for 27 years. The pain, located retro-orbitally on the right side, was described as intermittent, sharp, excruciating, and knife-like. Associated symptoms included tearing of the right eye, stuffiness of the right nostril, numbness on the right side of the face, and right conjunctival injection. The pain occurred one or two times per year in "cluster periods" of 1 to 5 weeks duration. The headaches typically lasted 60 to 75 minutes and could occur multiple times per day. During an attack, the patient would pace the floor and hit his head against doors and walls. He noted that red wine could precipitate an attack and avoided alcohol during headache periods. Past trials of various migraine medications were all without benefit. Oxygen inhalation at the onset of a headache attack, however, immediately relieved the pain. Of importance was a past medical history of myocardial infarction at age 35 and poorly controlled hypertension. These factors impacted treatment and will be discussed.

Chronic paroxysmal hemicrania (**CPH**), as the name implies, is typically an unremitting, unilateral headache disorder, although episodic versions have been identified.[144] Chronic paroxysmal hemicrania is characterized by short-lasting (2 to 45 minutes), frequently occurring attacks of pain (five per day for more than half of the time).[54,145] The quality of pain is throbbing or pounding, with an intensity that parallels that of cluster headaches, the patient often choosing to pace the floor during an attack. Pain location is predominantly oculotemporal and frontal, always on the same side, and can spread to involve the entire side of the head and the neck, shoulder, and arm.[145] Cases involving CPH presenting as **intermittent toothache** have been reported.[146] Turning or bending the head forward may precipitate an attack in some cases.[147] Associated symptoms include unilateral lacrimation, nasal stuffiness, and conjunctival injection. Nausea and vomiting are usually absent, as are visual or somatosensory auras. In contrast to cluster headache, CPH is seen **predominantly in women.**[148] Age at onset appears to be 20 years, although a variable pre-CPH period may exist.[148]

Case History

A 21-year-old woman presented with a 3-year history of right-sided supraorbital headaches. These headaches had a full, tight, aching quality with shooting, stabbing exacerbations brought on by rapid head movement, sneezing, or running. Associated symptoms included ptosis and tearing of the right eye. The pain lasted approximately 1 hour and occurred three to four times per day. The longest the patient had ever been without pain since the onset of the headaches was less than 5 days. The headache was completely responsive to indomethacin (NSAID), which is typical of CPH. Of interest was a family history of cluster headaches in her father and a cousin of her mother.

Etiology. *Cluster Headaches.* The exact etiology or mechanism of ***cluster headaches***, and CPH for that matter, is as yet unknown. Over the years, many theories have been advanced to try to explain the pronounced sympathetic and parasympathetic symptomatology, the trigeminal distribution of the pain, and the periodicity. To date, no consensus has been reached. Vasodilation, once considered an important element in the pathogenesis of cluster, is now thought to be secondary to trigeminal activation.[142] This is because the pain of cluster headache typically precedes any extracranial blood flow changes, and intracranial blood flow studies have shown inconsistent results.[142] The unusual temporal pattern of cluster headaches implicates the hypothalamus, which regulates autonomic functions and also largely controls circadian rhythms, as possibly triggering the primary neuronal discharge resulting in cluster headache pain.[142,149] Studies of circadian changes in various hormone levels in cluster patients versus controls do support activation of the hypothalamic gray matter region during cluster headache.[142,150,151] Others propose a complex neuroimmunologic mechanism.[152]

Chronic Paroxysmal Hemicrania. The pathophysiology of CPH is also unknown. Because of the autonomic and temporal similarities of CPH with cluster headache, similar mechanisms are implicated, yet studies of the cardiovascular and sweat responses as well as cognitive processing in the two headaches suggest that they are different.[153,154]

Examination. *Cluster Headaches.* Diagnosis is based on signs and symptoms. There are no diagnostic tests to confirm a diagnosis of cluster headache. Either the patient presents with a typical history and no abnormalities on physical and neurologic examination or the examination may cause suspicion of organic lesions with an ultimately normal neuroimaging scan.[54] Mild ptosis and miosis with or without periorbital swelling and conjunctival congestion may be present on the side of the headache if the patient is seen during or shortly after an attack.[142]

Chronic Paroxysmal Hemicrania. As with cluster headache, a careful history is the primary basis for diagnosis. Organic lesions should always be ruled out with any new headache disorder.

Treatment. Definitive treatment of cluster headaches and CPH is best left to the orofacial pain dentist or other health care provider with a specific interest in headache management.

Cluster Headaches. Many of the treatments used for migraine therapy are also useful in cluster headaches, including symptomatic use of subcutaneous sumatriptan.[155,156] In general, however, prophylactic medications are more appropriate in cluster headache because of the frequency of attacks and because prodromal warning symptoms are rare. Cluster headache patients are often wakened from sleep, and the pain reaches its high intensity very quickly. Once the cluster period subsides, patients are weaned from medications until the headaches recur.

Oxygen inhalation (100% 7 to 8 L per minute with a nonrebreathing mask), given at the very beginning of an attack for 15 minutes, may be successful in aborting an attack. Oxygen and subcutaneous sumatriptan are also useful as abortive options for the patient taking prophylactic medications who is experiencing breakthrough headaches. In rare cases of resistant chronic cluster headache, trigeminal ganglion lysis or gamma knife treatment may be considered.[157–160]

Chronic Paroxysmal Hemicrania. Indomethacin is the medication of choice for CPH. If the pain does not resolve with this medication, it is unlikely to be CPH. Aspirin and naproxen have a partial effect, but the relief is not as dramatic as with indomethacin.[145]

Miscellaneous Headaches Unassociated with Structural Lesion

Symptoms. These headaches, which include external compression headache, cold stimulus headache, benign cough headache, benign exertional headache, and headache associated with sexual activity,[54] are usually bilateral, short-lasting, and clearly related to a well-defined precipitating factor. For example, cold stimulus headache may result from exposure of the head to cold or from ingestion of cold substances.

The latter headache, also known as **"ice cream headache,"** typically occurs in the middle of the forehead after cold food or drink passes over the palate and lasts less than 5 minutes. **Benign cough headache** is a bilateral headache of extremely short duration (1 minute) that is precipitated by coughing. Physical exertion may also result in bilateral throbbing headaches that may last anywhere from 5 minutes to 24 hours. In some individuals, **sexual excitement** precipitates bilateral headache. This headache intensifies with increasing sexual arousal and may become "explosive" at orgasm.

Etiology. **External compression headache** is precipitated by prolonged stimulation of the cutaneous nerves through pressure from a tight band, hat, swim goggles, or sunglasses. **Cold stimulus headaches** are caused by exposure of the head to cold or from sudden stimulation of the nasopalatine or posterior palatine nerves with cold foods such as ice cream.[54] **Benign cough** and **exertional headaches**, as well as headaches associated with sexual activity, seem to occur more commonly in people with a history of migraine. The exact mechanism underlying these headaches is unknown but may be related to increased venous pressure in the head, transient hypertension, muscle contraction, increased sympathetic tone, or possibly the release of vasoactive substances.[161]

Treatment. Most of these headaches can be prevented by avoiding the precipitating cause (eg, pressure from swim goggles, exposure of the head to cold, rapid ingestion of cold substances, exertion). If necessary, frequent exertional headaches can be treated with prophylactic medications such as propranolol or NSAIDs.[161]

Headaches Associated with Vascular Disorders

This category includes headaches that are attributable to demonstrable pathosis, such as giant cell arteritis or acute hypertension. Other pathologic vascular causes of headache include vertebral or carotid artery dissection and intracranial ischemia owing to intracranial hematoma, subarachnoid hemorrhage, arteriovenous malformations, or venous thrombosis (see Table 8-11). Headaches owing to such intracranial pathosis are unlikely to appear in the dental office and are therefore not further described. **Giant cell arteritis**, however, which does, on occasion, present with **dental symptoms**, may produce serious, irreversible consequences if left unrecognized and untreated.

Giant Cell Arteritis (Temporal Arteritis)

Headache or facial pain from giant cell arteritis is relatively rare, but the dentist must know about this disorder and be able to recognize it because blindness is a serious potential complication.

Symptoms. The patient with giant cell arteritis is usually over 50 years old and may have other rheumatic symptoms, such as polymyalgia rheumatica. Involvement of the temporal artery may bring the patient in to see the dentist first because **pain with mastication ("jaw claudication") may be the first or only symptom.** Friedlander and Runyon reported patients with **a burning tongue and claudication of the muscles of mastication.**[162] Guttenberg et al. reported a case mimicking dental pain that led to **inappropriate, ineffective endodontic surgery.**[163]

The pain is usually unilateral and in the anatomic area of the artery but may also radiate down to the ear, **teeth**, and occiput with generalized scalp tenderness. Temporal arteritis may resemble a migraine attack because it, too, has a persistent throbbing quality that may last hours to days and the location is unilateral, over the temple area.[114] **Temporal arteritis,** however, has an **additional burning, ache-like quality.** The pain increases with lowering of the head, **mastication**, and movements that create increased blood flow to that artery. The patient may present with complaints of malaise, fatigue, anorexia, and weight loss if the arteritis occurs as a febrile illness. In advanced cases, patients may complain of transient visual loss on the side of the headache. This is particularly severe and requires immediate, aggressive treatment since thrombosis of the ophthalmic artery may result in partial or complete blindness.

Etiology. Arterial inflammation, which may often be associated with immunologic disorders, is the causative factor in this headache. Arterial biopsy often reveals frayed elastic tissues and giant cells in the vessel walls on histologic examination.[164]

Examination. Dental examination is negative. The temporal artery may be tender to palpation, thickened, and enlarged and may lack a normal pulse. Digital pressure with occlusion of the common carotid artery on the same side will frequently alleviate the symptoms. Ophthalmologic examination or evaluation of optic ischemia is mandatory.

Diagnostic Tests. Erythrocyte sedimentation rate, although a nonspecific test, will be significantly elevated above 60 mm/hour Westergren in giant cell arteritis. Definitive diagnosis is based on arterial biopsy. The entire temporal artery is typically removed to ensure sampling of diseased sections; skip lesions are common. Biopsy of the artery is essential because treatment involves high doses of steroids, but treatment is never delayed if visual disturbance is present.

Treatment. The dentist who suspects temporal arteritis should immediately refer the patient to a rheumatologist or internist for complete workup. If optic symptoms are present, emergency ophthalmologic examination is essential without delay.

Treatment of the condition consists of emergency dosages of steroids. When the elevated sedimentation rate has been reduced, maintenance doses of **prednisone** are administered as clinically determined.

Carotid or Vertebral Artery Pain. Dissection of the carotid or vertebral arteries causes headache and cervical pain on the same side as the dissection. This serious, life-threatening condition is typically acute and accompanied by symptoms of transient ischemic attack or stroke. Since patients with this problem are unlikely to appear in the dental office, there need be no further discussion of this type of syndrome.

Idiopathic carotidynia was discussed under the category of referred pain from remote pathosis.

Hypertension

Symptoms. Generalized throbbing headache may be a symptom of acute hypertension, especially if the diastolic pressure rises 25%.[54]

Etiology. Usually, abrupt increases in blood pressure are associated with ingestion of a substance that causes vasoconstriction or a systemic disorder such as pheochromocytoma, preeclampsia or eclampsia in pregnancy, or malignant hypertension. Chronic arterial hypertension is not reported to cause headache.[165]

Examination. A routine blood pressure check is useful to rule out hypertension as a medical problem requiring treatment.

Treatment. Patients with acute or chronic hypertension should be referred to their family practitioner for management. Associated headaches resolve within 24 hours to 7 days after resolution of the hypertension.

Headache Associated with Substances or Their Withdrawal and Headache Associated with Metabolic Disorders

These headache types are unlikely to present as a primary complaint in the dental office and thus will not be discussed further here.

Our patient's pain had none of the characteristics described in this category of pain. Therefore, vascular headaches can be excluded in the differential diagnosis.

NEUROPATHIC PAINS

Neuropathic pains are caused by some form of structural abnormality or pathosis affecting the peripheral nerves themselves. This is in contrast to the normal transmission of noxious stimulation along these nerves from organic disease or trauma. The structural abnormality or pathosis affecting the nerve(s) may have many different etiologies, including genetic disorders such as porphyria; mechanical damage from compression, trauma, entrapment, traction, or scarring; metabolic disorders such as diabetes, alcoholism, nutritional deficiencies, or multiple myeloma; toxic reactions to drugs, metals, or certain organic substances; or infectious or inflammatory processes such as herpes, hepatitis, leprosy, or multiple sclerosis.

Not all neuropathies are painful. When they are, they may be dramatically so. The distinguishing feature of peripheral neuropathic pains in the head and neck region is the quality of pain, which is burning, sharp, shooting, lancinating, or electric-like. The distribution of the pain is limited to the anatomic pathways of the nerve involved and is almost always unilateral. Sensory abnormalities may include diminished pain sensation in the presence of hypersensitivity to typically nonpainful stimuli.

In general, neuropathic pains in the head and neck can be divided into two main groups, paroxysmal or continuous, based on their temporal pattern (Table 8-12).

Paroxysmal Neuralgias

Symptoms. Paroxysmal, lancinating, sharp, unilateral pain that follows a distinct dermatomal pattern is common to all paroxysmal neuralgias. The pain is often

Table 8-12 Neuropathic Pains

Paroxysmal
Trigeminal neuralgia
Glossopharyngeal neuralgia
Nervus intermedius neuralgia
Occipital neuralgia
Neuroma
Continuous
Postherpetic neuralgia
Post-traumatic neuralgia
Anesthesia dolorosa

described as electric-like, shooting, cutting, or stabbing. The attacks may last only a few seconds to minutes, with virtually no discomfort between attacks. Sometimes patients notice vague prodromata of tingling and occasionally ache or burn after an attack. The attacks may occur intermittently, with days to months between a series of attacks. Usually, patients complain of "trigger areas" that, when stimulated, precipitate an attack. These are frequently located within the distribution of the nerve affected, usually on the skin or oral mucosa. Neural blockade of the trigger area almost always relieves the pain for the duration of action of the local anesthetic. Should neural blockade fail to relieve the symptoms, either the diagnosis or the nerve block technique must be questioned.

Each type of paroxysmal neuralgia has its own distinct characteristics.

Trigeminal neuralgia, or tic douloureux, usually affects one or at most two divisions of the fifth cranial nerve.[54] The **mandibular and maxillary** divisions are most commonly **involved together**, causing pain to shoot down the mandible and across the cheek into the teeth or tongue. The maxillary or mandibular divisions alone are the next most frequently affected, with ophthalmic division neuralgias being the least common. The pain is unilateral 96% of the time. Touching and washing the face, tooth brushing, shaving, chewing, talking, or even cold wind against the face may set off the trigger and result in pain. Deep pressure or painful stimuli are usually tolerated without a painful episode. Patients go to extraordinary lengths, such as not shaving, washing, or brushing their teeth, to avoid stimulating the trigger area. Between attacks, patients are completely pain free. Long remissions for months or years are not uncommon but tend to decrease with increasing age.

Trigeminal neuralgia is **almost twice as common in women** as in men and usually starts after the age of 50.[166] Anyone under the age of 40 with this disorder should be referred to a neurologist to be worked up for a structural lesion or multiple sclerosis.

A syndrome of pain preceding the onset of true paroxysmal trigeminal neuralgia, known as **pretrigeminal neuralgia** (PTN), has been described.[167,168] Patients may present themselves up to 2 years before developing trigeminal neuralgia, with pain usually **localized to one alveolar quadrant** and sometimes a sinus. They may describe this pain as dull, aching and/or burning, or as **a sharp (burning) toothache, not unlike pain arising from the dental pulp**. Some patients may also report a "pins and needles" sensation. Duration of PTN pain may be 2 hours to several months, with variable periods of remission. Movement, usually opening of the mouth, may trigger the pain.

Dental pathosis may be minimal or absent. Retained root tips are the most common finding, and their removal has been associated with remission of pain. Obvious dental pathosis should be treated, but **dental heroics in the absence of clinical or radiographic findings should be avoided.** A UCLA group reported that 61% of the cases with PTN or trigeminal neuralgia were incorrectly diagnosed and treated for dental conditions.[168] Onset of classic trigeminal neuralgia may be quite sudden and occurs in the same division affected by the PTN symptoms. Onset may follow remission produced by previous dental treatment.

Case History

A 67-year-old man underwent extensive dental treatment, including endodontic therapy and hemisection of tooth #30, followed by the placement of two different intraoral stabilization appliances, for a pain complaint that turned out to be trigeminal neuralgia. He had also seen a general medical practitioner and a neurologist, who were unable to identify a cause for his pain. A diagnosis of psychogenic pain was made. The reason the true diagnosis was not obvious was because the patient described the pain as constant and related to tooth #30, worsened by eating and talking. Careful questioning, however, revealed that the pain was not constant. Indeed, if he sat very still without talking or moving his mouth, he was pain free. Movement of the tongue, touching the lower lip, and biting anywhere in the mouth seemed to be precipitating factors. Observation of an attack during the history and physical examination confirmed the diagnosis: the patient became very quiet, his lips began to tremble, and tears came to his eyes because the pain was so intense. The whole episode lasted less than a minute, after which the patient resumed normal conversation.

Glossopharyngeal neuralgia is 70 to 100 times less common than trigeminal neuralgia.[169] The symptoms include unilateral and rarely nonconcurrent bilateral stabbing pain in the lateral posterior pharyngeal and tonsillar areas, **the base of the tongue**, down into the throat, the eustachian tube or ear, and down the neck.[170] Sometimes pain radiates into the vagal region and **may be associated with salivation**, flushing, sweating, tinnitus, cardiac arrhythmias, hypertension, vertigo, or syncope. **Throat movements**, pressure on the tragus of the ear, **yawning, or swallowing** may trigger the pain. Again, local anesthesia of the trigger area temporarily prevents precipitation of attacks. This can be accomplished by spraying the posterior pharynx with a topical anesthetic.

Eagle's syndrome may be the cause of symptoms similar to those of glossopharyngeal neuralgia,[171–173] although some believe that this syndrome is not sufficiently validated.[54] The symptoms, which include a "sore throat" and **posterior tongue and pharyngeal pain,** are thought to be related to compression of the area of the glossopharyngeal nerve by a calcified elongation of the **stylohyoid process** of the temporal bone. Precipitating factors include fast rotation of the head, **swallowing, and pharyngeal motion from talking and chewing.** Blurring of vision and vertigo are rarely seen.

Nervus intermedius neuralgia is extremely rare.[174] The pain is described as a lancinating "hot poker" in the ear.[170] It can occur anterior to, posterior to, or on the pinna; in the auditory canal; or, occasionally, in the soft palate. A duller background pain may persist between attacks. Attacks may be accompanied by **salivation, tinnitus,** vertigo, or **dysgeusia.**[175] The trigger area is usually in the external auditory canal. This neuralgia has also been termed **Ramsay Hunt syndrome,** geniculate neuralgia, or Wrisberg's neuralgia and is often associated with **herpes zoster** (or shingles).

Superior laryngeal neuralgia is also a rare neuralgia with paroxysmal neuralgic pains of varying duration, minutes to hours, located in the throat, in the submandibular region, or under the ear. Triggering factors include swallowing, turning the head, loud vocalizations, or stimulating the site overlying the hypothyroid membrane where the nerve enters the laryngeal structures.

Occipital neuralgia occurs in the distribution of the greater or lesser occipital nerves to the back of the head and mastoid process. The **ear and the underside of the mandible** may be involved because of the dermatomal patterns of C2 and C3 (see Figures 8-19, B, and 8-22). The pain often radiates into the **frontal and temporal regions,** occasionally with the same sharp, electric-like character of the other neuralgias, but may last hours instead of seconds. Sometimes the pain takes on a more continuous burning, aching nature. A case of maxillary right posterior quadrant **dental pain** owing to occipital neuralgia has been reported.[176] Trauma, especially rotational injuries to the neck, may precede the onset. Trigger zones, such as those seen with trigeminal neuralgia, are rare. The pain may be associated with neck and back pain, and emotional stress is a common aggravating factor.

Etiology. The paroxysmal neuralgias are considered **symptomatic** if a specific pathologic process affecting the involved nerve can be identified and **idiopathic** if not. Paroxysmal neuralgias rarely occur in young people unless there is a distinct compression of the nerve by a tumor or other structural lesion. Compression of the nerve either peripherally or centrally by bone, scar tissue, tumors, aberrant arteries, or arteriovenous malformations causes **focal demyelination,** which is postulated to result in ectopic firing and reduced segmental inhibition of the low-threshold mechanoreceptors and wide-dynamic-range relay neurons.[177] The net effect is a **lowered threshold** of neuronal firing for which ordinary orofacial maneuvers such as chewing, swallowing, talking, or smiling may precipitate a neuralgic attack.

Trigeminal neuralgia, along with other paroxysmal cranial neuralgias, is typically considered idiopathic, although nerve compression by intracranial arteries that have become slack and tortuous with age is thought to be the likely culprit.[178] The **demyelinating** lesions associated with **multiple sclerosis** may also precipitate trigeminal neuralgia in younger individuals. The symptoms of trigeminal neuralgia associated with diabetic polyradiculopathy have also been reported.[179]

Despite the apparent idiopathy of trigeminal neuralgia, there are numerous published observations that suggest that some cases may have an intraoral etiology. From Ratner et al.'s jaw bone cavities, also known as **"residual infection in bone"** or "chronic, smoldering, nonsuppurative osteomyelitis," to Bouquot et al.'s "neuralgia-inducing cavitational osteonecrosis" (**NICO lesions**), there are several anecdotal reports in the literature of successful relief of trigeminal neuralgia–like pain with surgical exposure and curettage of jaw bone cavities.[180–187] Microbiologic sampling of these cavities using aseptic precautions revealed, in many cases, the presence of a wide variety of both nonpathologic and pathologic oral microorganisms.[180] Microscopic examination of tissue removed from these bone cavities has revealed neuromas in 50% of cases and frequent **myelin degeneration.**[188,189] Bouquot et al. examined 224 tissue samples removed from alveolar bone cavities in 135 patients with trigeminal neuralgia or atypical facial neuralgia. They reported evidence of chronic intraosseous inflammation in all of the samples.[184] Retrospective identification and follow-up by questionnaire of 190 patients who had had jaw bone curettage of histologically confirmed inflammatory jaw bone lesions for neuralgic pain showed 74% with significant improvement over 4 years. Approximately one-third of these had required additional curettage.[190]

Although these findings are provocative, they are surrounded by controversy. Loeser, a neurologist, noted that many normal subjects also have bone cavities and that not all patients with trigeminal neuralgia or unexplained facial pains have these cavities.[191] A surprising number of dentists, and particularly oral surgeons, concur with Loeser.

In marked contrast, Raskin, also a neurologist, has addressed this problem and has stated,

> [I am speaking] of the people who have nondescript pain when I can't make any further diagnosis. If they have a tooth extraction site on the side of their pain, I have the oral surgeon do a local anesthetic block. If that stops their pain, they then get that mandibular or maxillary bone explored and curetted. If I can cure trigeminal neuralgia with a 45 minute dental procedure rather than [the patient] taking Tegretol, I'm all for it. I would rather have some negative explorations, if that's what it takes, to save someone either a posterior fossa operation or taking some drug for the next 20 years. I go hard on this. It is still contentious I know. I am quite impressed, and I don't think we can afford to ignore this data.[192]

Glossopharyngeal neuralgia is much more frequently a frankly symptomatic neuralgia. Tumors are found in 25% of cases. Local infection, neck trauma, elongation of the styloid process (Eagle's syndrome), and compression of the nerve root by a tortuous vertebral or posterior inferior cerebellar artery[193] are other symptomatic causes of this ninth-nerve neuralgia. Unlike trigeminal neuralgia, glossopharyngeal neuralgia is almost never associated with multiple sclerosis.[169]

Occipital neuralgia may be secondary to hypertrophic fibrosis of subcutaneous tissue around the occipital nerve following trauma, irritation of the nerve by the atlantoaxial ligament, spondylosis of the upper cervical spine, spinal cord tumors, or tubercular granulomas.[194] Myofascial TrPs in the semispinalis capitis and splenius cervicus muscles may mimic this type of pain or may cause neuralgia-like symptoms owing to entrapment of the greater occipital nerve as it passes through the tense semispinalis muscle fibers.[55] Since treatment of myofascial TrPs is noninvasive, with very low morbidity and no mortality, they must be carefully ruled out before neurectomy or other neuroablative techniques are considered.[195]

Examination. A patient presenting with symptoms of ***trigeminal neuralgia*** must be worked up for dental disorders, sinus disease, and head and neck infections or neoplasms.[61,196,197] Since nerve compression from intracranial tumors, aneurysms or vascular malformations, or central lesions from multiple sclerosis may also cause symptomatic trigeminal neuralgia,[198,199] all patients with trigeminal neuralgia–like symptoms should be worked up with an **imaging study** of the head, either contrast-**enhanced CT or MRI,** in addition to routine films.

Diagnosis of ***pretrigeminal neuralgia*** is based on the clinical presentation of constant dull toothache pain in the absence of dental or neurologic findings and normal radiographic, CT, or MRI examinations.

Since ***glossopharyngeal neuralgia*** is more often associated with nasopharyngeal, tonsillar, or posterior fossa tumors or other pathosis than is trigeminal neuralgia, imaging studies including skull films, panoramic films, and MRI are essential.

In ***Eagle's syndrome***, the diagnosis is usually established on the basis of radiographs, as well as intraoral finger palpation of the posterior pharyngeal area. Panoramic films should reveal a **stylohyoid process that is so long** that its image projects beyond the ramus of the mandible. Anything shorter is not significant, and other causes for the patient's pain should be sought. Pain is alleviated temporarily by neural block of the suspected compressive area. Treatment is primarily surgical shortening of the styloid process either through an intraoral or an extraoral approach.[171]

Occipital neuralgia requires a thorough musculoskeletal evaluation in addition to a cervical spine radiographic series to rule out neoplasms or other local destructive lesions. Digital palpation of the greater occipital nerve along the nuchal line may be painful. Caudal pressure to the vertex of the head while it is flexed and rotated toward the side of the pain may reproduce cervical compression symptoms.[200] Sensory loss is rare. Because myofascial TrPs may mimic or accompany this disorder, careful palpation of the posterior cervical muscles for the tight bands and focal tenderness with referred pain, characteristic of myofascial TrPs, is essential.[196]

Treatment. Obviously, if a neuralgia is "symptomatic" or the result of identifiable pathema or structural lesion, treatment is directed at correction of the cause. For example, stylohyoid resection may be indicated if this is the cause of glossopharyngeal neuralgia. However, for idiopathic paroxysmal neuralgias, the first treatment of choice is the drug **carbamazepine (Tegretol)**. Carbamazepine is most efficacious in trigeminal neuralgia but has some success in glossopharyngeal or nervus intermedius neuralgias as well. **Baclofen (Lioresal), gabapentin (Neurontin),** and

diphenylhydantoin (Dilantin) are also used, alone or in combination. All of these medications may cause varying degrees of dizziness, drowsiness, and mental confusion. In addition, carbamazepine may cause hematopoietic changes and baclofen may affect liver enzymes. Although such side effects are not as common as once thought and are less common with gabapentin and diphenylhydantoin, patients taking any of these medications must be monitored very closely initially.

In those infrequent instances for which these medications or combinations thereof are ineffective, or the patient becomes refractory to the medications or cannot tolerate them, either owing to severe drowsiness or frank allergy, neurosurgical intervention remains an option. In **trigeminal neuralgia**, gamma knife radiosurgery is the newest alternative for treatment. **Gamma knife radiosurgery** is a neurosurgical technique using a single-fraction high-dose ionizing radiation focused on a small (4 mm), stereotactically defined intracranial target.[201] The targeted cells necrotize without apparent harm to adjacent tissues. In **trigeminal neuralgia**, the beam is focused on the trigeminal sensory root adjacent to the pons. The results have been so good[202,203] that some authors advocate **gamma knife radiosurgery as the "safest and most effective form of treatment currently available for trigeminal neuralgia."**[202] The procedure carries with it low morbidity (infrequent reports of delayed onset of facial tactile hypesthesia or paresthesias) and no mortality.[201] Nonetheless, the long-term effects of this form of treatment have yet to be evaluated, and more traditional approaches to the surgical treatment of trigeminal neuralgia are still used, especially in younger patients.

Younger, healthier patients may choose to undergo **suboccipital craniotomy with microvascular decompression.**[204] In this major neurosurgical procedure, which in some centers is now performed endoscopically, an attempt is made to relieve any pressure on the trigeminal sensory root from blood vessels or other proximal structures. The superior cerebellar artery is the most common offender because it tends to kink under the ganglion itself. Muscle or sponge may be used to hold the vessel away from the nerve root. In this way, pain relief may be obtained with no or minimal loss of sensation or damage to the fifth cranial nerve.[204–206]

For older or medically infirm patients, alternatives to gamma knife radiosurgery include injection of glycerol into the arachnoid cistern of the gasserian ganglion or radiofrequency neuroablation of the trigeminal sensory root to destroy A delta and C pain fibers.[207] Both of these procedures involve the percutaneous insertion of a needle through the cheek into Meckel's cave. They are usually carried out by a neurosurgeon under local anesthesia with fluoroscopic control and take less than 45 minutes. The patient is conscious for both of these percutaneous procedures. Because they are relatively simple procedures, with low morbidity and mortality, they can easily be repeated should the symptoms return. Rare complications include corneal anesthesia, anesthesia dolorosa, injury to the carotid artery, and sixth cranial nerve palsy.[208,209]

Therapies, especially medications, used to treat true trigeminal neuralgia have been reported to work for **pretrigeminal neuralgia** as well.[210]

Idiopathic **glossopharyngeal neuralgia** may be managed with the same medications used for trigeminal neuralgia. If these fail, microvascular decompression has been reported effective.[211] Nerve section in the posterior fossa[212] and percutaneous thermocoagulation have also been described, with mixed results.[213,214]

Because of its predominantly musculoskeletal etiology, **occipital neuralgia** lends itself best to nonpharmacologic and nonsurgical treatments. Consequently, physical therapy, postural re-education, corrected ergonomics, home neck-stretching exercises, TrP injections, and even C2 nerve blocks, with or without corticosteroids, are the first line of approach.[195] Surgical interventions, such as neurectomy,[215] rarely provide long-term relief.[216]

Surgical section of the nervus intermedius or the chorda tympani has been reported to relieve the pain of **nervus intermedius neuralgia**, as has neurectomy in the case of recalcitrant **superior laryngeal neuralgia.**[217,218]

Neuromas are non-neoplastic, nonencapsulated, tangled masses of axons, Schwann cells, endoneurial cells, and perineurial cells in a dense collagenous matrix (Figure 8-24).

Etiology. Neuromas tend to develop when a nerve axon is transected, as might occur with a dental extraction, surgery, or trauma. The proximal stump of a transected nerve is still connected to its cell body and, in a few days postinjury, will start to sprout axons, in an attempt to re-establish continuity with its distal segment. Usually, this process is unsuccessful, especially in soft tissue; therefore, a tangled mass of tissue results.[219] In the orofacial region, neuromas most commonly develop in the area of the mental foramen, followed by the lower lip, tongue, and buccal mucosa, all easily traumatized sites. Neuromas are least likely to occur in the inferior alveolar canal because the bone guides the tissue growth.

In a seminal research effort, Hansen found neuromas forming quite routinely in the extraction sockets of the rat alveolus. Four months after extraction, he noted

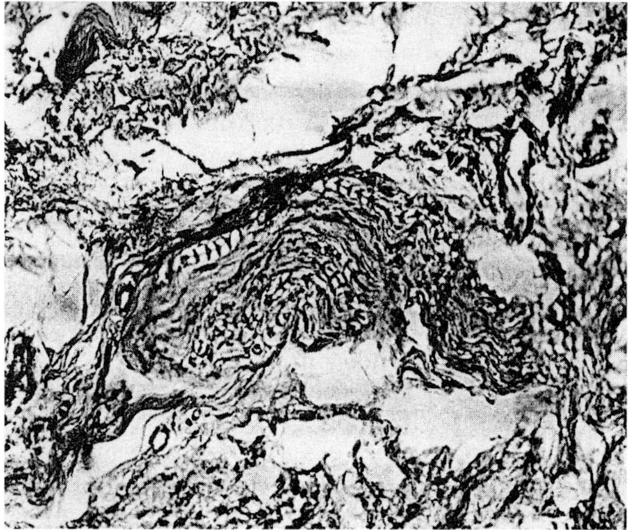

Figure 8-24 Amputation neuroma revealed by biopsy. Strikingly clear-cut, tangled, and well-myelinated fibers, cut at various angles, are massed with irregular sheath and perineural connective tissue into an abnormal aggregate of varying size and surrounded by well-vascularized fibrous tissue. Biopsy was occasioned by sharp, intermittent pricking "nerve pain," 6 months in duration, becoming more diffuse and steady. (Courtesy of Dr. Gordon Agnew.)

axon and myelin sheath degeneration at the bottom of the alveolus. At 10 months, the appearance was that of a small traumatic neuroma.[220] If this same phenomenon occurs as frequently in humans as in experimental animals, it might well account for persistent postextraction pain, for which the patient is finally classified as neurotic and the pain as psychogenic. Of 45 oral traumatic neuromas reviewed for clinicopathologic features, 15 were painful, and 53% of these demonstrated inflammatory infiltrate under light microscopy.[221] This was in contrast to only 17% of asymptomatic neuromas. Only 4 (9%) in this series were associated with extractions. Anoxia and local scar formation are thought to contribute to the production of pain.[222]

Symptoms. A neuroma may be completely asymptomatic, and, in fact, approximately 25% of them are. However, neuromas are capable of generating very prolonged electrical impulses in response to a variety of stimuli.[219] They may even discharge spontaneously.

The diagnostic features of a neuroma include a history of prior surgery or a lacerating injury at the site of the pain, along with precipitation of the pain with local pressure or traction. The pain is short-lasting, with a burning, tingling, radiating quality. A drop of local anesthetic will abolish the response. If the neuroma has developed on the inferior alveolar nerve, it may be visible radiographically as a widening of the mandibular canal.

Neuromas may also occur in the **TMJ postsurgically** or post–lacerating trauma.[70] Symptoms include restricted joint movement owing to adhesions and pain with neuropathic qualities (sharp, shooting, itching, burning) on stretching of the adhesions. The deep aching pain of musculoskeletal disorders is lacking.

Examination. In the oral cavity, neuromas may appear as nodules of normal surface color but usually are not visible or palpable. Of greater interest is the presence of a scar, indicating previous injury or surgery. In the TMJ, movement against adhesive restrictions, as with jaw opening, should elicit short-lasting neuropathic pain.

Treatment. A one-time excision of a sensitive neuroma located in accessible scar tissue is worth trying provided that the pain is localized and can be relieved by infiltration with a local anesthetic.[70] Unfortunately, neuroma excision and other peripheral neuroablative procedures provide significant relief in very few patients.[223] **Neuromas often re-form**, and the pain may return. Medications such as carbamazepine (Tegretol) or amitriptyline (Elavil) may be helpful but should be used only if the patient feels that the pain is severe enough to warrant tolerating the side effects that may accompany these medications.

Continuous Neuralgias

Continuous neuralgias typically occur after some kind of peripheral nerve damage or "deafferentation." This category includes **postherpetic, post-traumatic,** and **postsurgical neuralgias**, as well as **anesthesia dolorosa.** As with paroxysmal neuralgias, the continuous neuralgias follow the distribution of the damaged nerve but differ in that the pain is more or less continuous, with some fluctuation over time. Patients report altered sensations, dysesthesias, or pain in the distribution of the nerve that varies from tingling, numbness, and twitching to prickling or burning. They may also report **"formication,"** which is a sensation of worms under the skin or ants crawling over the skin. The dysesthesias are generally discomforting to the patient because they are continuous and exacerbated by movement or touching of the area. As with paroxysmal neuralgias, local anesthetic blocks of the nerve eliminate all paresthesias except numbness.

Postherpetic Neuralgia (PHN). *Etiology.* Postherpetic neuralgia follows an acute attack of **herpes zoster** ("shingles"). Herpes zoster is an acute viral infection produced by the deoxyribonucleic acid (DNA) virus varicella zoster. Varicella zoster causes chickenpox in the young and afterward remains in the ganglia of sensory nerve endings in a dormant "provirus" form. Periodically, the virus reverts to its infectious state and is held in check by circulating antibodies. If an individual is immunocompromised or is older and has a low antibody titer, the infectious virus is able to retrace its path down the sensory nerve and escape into the skin, where it causes the typical skin eruptions and vesicles of zoster. Acute hemorrhagic inflammation with demyelination and axonal degeneration of dorsal root ganglion cells has been demonstrated in early and more recent pathologic studies.[224–228]

Acute herpes zoster affects individuals over 70 years of age 12 times more frequently than persons under 10 presumably because their antibody titer decreases as their exposure to children with chickenpox diminishes. One or two of every 100 elderly people suffer an attack of shingles in a single year. They may have repeated attacks, often in the same distribution; 3.4 per 1,000 individuals develop PHN annually.[229]

Symptoms. Continuous pain in the distribution of the affected nerve and malaise commonly precede the eruption of **acute herpes zoster**, sometimes along with paresthesia and shooting pains. Vesicles form, become infected, scab over, and heal. Small and sometimes severe scars are left behind. The scars are usually anesthetic, the skin between being hyperesthetic.

Ten to 15% of patients with herpes zoster develop lesions in the head and neck region, and 80% of these are in the ophthalmic division of the trigeminal nerve[54,70] (Figure 8-25). C1–3 are also sometimes affected. When cranial nerve V1 is affected, vesicles may appear on the cornea, and the risk of impaired vision is high. If the infection affects the maxillary division of the trigeminal nerve, intraoral eruptions may develop concomitantly with those on the skin. Involvement of the oral mucosa without cutaneous involvement may occur and must be differentiated from aphthous stomatitis.[70] Multiple devitalized teeth, isolated in a single quadrant, have been reported as a rare complication of herpes zoster infection.[230] If the **facial nerve (cranial nerve VII)** is involved, facial palsy may occur owing to pressure on the nerve from inflammatory swelling in the bony canal. The pupil may become permanently paralyzed, and the upper eyelid may droop. Involvement of the geniculate ganglion causes lesions to erupt in the external auditory canal, may cause acoustic symptoms, and is known as Ramsey Hunt syndrome.[70]

Postherpetic neuralgia results when the pain of acute zoster does not subside as the acute eruption clears. The pain of PHN often has several distinct components.[7] Patients complain of a steady, deep, aching pain along with superimposed sharp, stabbing pains similar to trigeminal neuralgia. In addition, many complain of **allodynia**, which is pain in response to light brushing of the skin, an innocuous event under normal

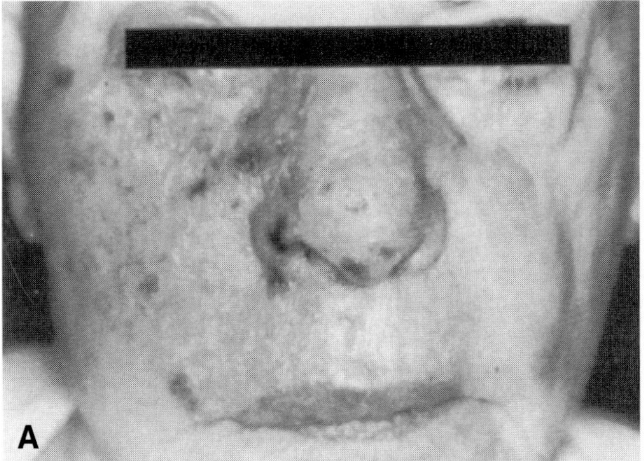

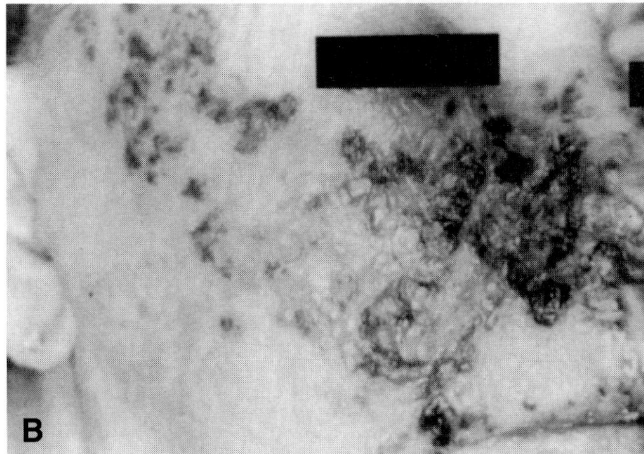

Figure 8-25 Herpes zoster infection (shingles). **A**, Multiple vesicles on the face and involvement of the right eye 4 days after initial visit. **B**, Ten days afer diagnosis, lesions follow distribution of the trigeminal nerve. Reproduced with permission from Lopes MA, Filho FJ de S, Junior JJ, de Almeida OP. Herpes Zoster infection as a differential diagnosis of acute pulpitis. J Endodon 1998;24:144.

circumstances. The pain is limited to the distribution of the affected nerve, and there is usually also cutaneous scarring and sensory loss.[231,232] Complaints of **formication** are not infrequent. Since this pain is severe and unrelenting, it places a large emotional burden on the elderly patients who suffer from it. Interruption of sleep, drug reliance, depression, and even contemplation of suicide are common.

Examination. The history of acute zoster infection and the obvious scars it leaves behind make diagnosis relatively simple in most cases. Postherpetic neuralgia, on the other hand, may occur up to a month or two after the vesicular stage of herpes zoster has healed. If the patient knows he has had severe herpes zoster infection, the diagnosis may well be self-evident. The dentist, however, should carefully check the mouth to ascertain that a concomitant severe pulpitis is not superimposed on the condition.

Difficulty in diagnosis arises when the severe vesicular herpetic attack is not manifested but rather one or two small aphthous ulcers appear in the oral cavity or on the lips or face. This mild attack is often forgotten by the patient, and a careful history is essential.[233]

Treatment. In the future, new vaccines may reduce the overall incidence of chickenpox in the population or boost immunity to varicella-zoster virus in middle-aged persons, thus preventing the emergence of the virus from its latent phase.[234] Although age is the most important risk factor for development of this painful chronic disorder, early treatment during the ***acute phase of herpes zoster*** with antiviral agents or certain tricyclics (antidepressants), combined with psychosocial support, may be effective in preventing the development of PHN.[235] Although sympathetic nerve blocks do tend to reduce acute herpetic pain, they have not been proven to be effective in preventing PHN.[231,236,237]

Treatment of **PHN** is often difficult and unrewarding. The longer the infection continues and the longer the patient has PHN, the more difficult pain management becomes. **Tricyclic antidepressants, gabapentin,** and **opioids** are the only medications that have shown efficacy in randomized clinical trials.[235] Topical agents also work[238] but are rarely effective alone.[235] **Amelioration of the depression** that invariably accompanies this condition is as significant in therapy as reduction of the primary pain.

Post-traumatic Neuralgias. Traumatic injury to the peripheral nerves often results in persistent discomfort that is qualitatively different from PHN.

Symptoms. The pain is described as a continuous tingling, numb, twitching, or prickly sensation but without the intense, burning hyperesthesia usually seen with PHN or painful neuromas. Onset is following damage to the nerve by trauma or surgery. The discomfort can be self-limited, but total nerve regeneration is a slow, inaccurate process and can result in permanent dysesthesias or the formation of a neuroma.

Etiology. Peripheral degeneration or scarring of the nerve may be found on histopathologic examination. Substance P has been implicated as a mediator of the pain, and depletion of this neurotransmitter has been shown to reduce the pain.

Treatment. Treatment of traumatic trigeminal dysesthesias may be met with varying success and can include any of the pharmacologic therapies used for the other neuralgias as well as acupuncture, transcutaneous electrical nerve stimulation, and hypnosis. Capsaicin, a substance P depleter with significant long-term effects, has been used topically in the treatment of post-traumatic neuralgia with some success.[239] All of the available therapies may be used individually or in combination with other interventions. In some cases of trigeminal neuropathy, in which peripheral nerve damage has resulted in continuous severe pain, electrical stimulation of the gasserian ganglion via an implanted electrode has been shown to provide good pain relief.[240]

Anesthesia Dolorosa. This literally means "painful anesthesia" or pain in a numb area.

Etiology. Anesthesia dolorosa is considered a complication of deafferentation procedures such as trigeminal rhizotomy or thermocoagulation used to treat trigeminal neuralgia. It may also follow trauma or damage to the trigeminal nuclear complex or after vascular lesions of the central trigeminal pathways.[54]

Symptoms. Patients complain of pain in an area that is otherwise numb or has decreased ability to detect tactile or thermal stimuli. Onset follows deafferentation of part or all of the trigeminal nerve, and the pain typically follows the distribution of the deafferented branches.

Examination. The painful area is numb or has diminished sensation to pinprick.

Treatment. Anesthesia dolorosa is a chronic intractable pain syndrome[70] that is very difficult to treat. Centrally acting medications such as tricyclics or anticonvulsants may provide some relief.

Our patient, described initially, has complaints that have characteristics of both the continuous and paroxysmal neuralgias. The constant burning pain could be a continuous neuralgia. Since there is no history of viral infection or herpes zoster outbreak, it is unlikely to be PHN. Since there is no history of deafferentation procedures, anesthesia dolorosa is also unlikely. However, multiple extractions and repeated dry sockets may have resulted in the development of deafferentation pain in V2 and V3; it does not explain the pain in V1.

What about the sharp, shooting, electric-like pains the patient complained about? These are reminiscent of trigeminal neuralgia. However, the temporal pattern is inconsistent. Trigeminal neuralgia attacks are over in seconds to minutes; this patient complains of pains lasting 30 minutes to 24 hours. Also, the patient is too young for an idiopathic trigeminal neuralgia, and CT scans have failed to show any structural lesion that could account for such a pain. Thus, at this point, there is one possible diagnosis on our differential list, namely, post-traumatic deafferentation pain.

CAUSALGIC PAINS

Causalgia is a word derived from the Greek words *kausos*, meaning "heat," and *algia*, meaning "pain." Causalgia was first described by Mitchell in 1864 as a pain that appears following damage to a major peripheral nerve by a high-velocity missile injury.[241] Consequently, it is typically seen in the extremities. In 1947, Evans[240] used the term "reflex sympathetic dystrophy" (**RSD**) to describe the same burning pain.[242] He noted that the pain had many features of sympathetic stimulation such as redness, swelling, sweating, and atrophic changes in the skin, muscles, and bones. He also found that minor injuries, such as fractures or sprains, could precipitate this pain, not just major nerve trauma. That same year, Bingham published the first report of RSD of the face.[243]

Today RSD and, in particular, causalgia are considered the most dramatic forms of a class of pains called **sympathetically maintained pains (SMPs)**, RSD occurring without and causalgia with a definable nerve lesion. Because the exact contribution of the sympathetic nervous system to RSD and causalgia is still under investigation, an effort was made in the mid-1990s to rename these types of pain disorders as **"complex regional pain syndromes," type I and type II**, respectively.[244] These terms eliminate the implied causal association of the sympathetic nervous system to these pain disorders. This terminology, along with clinical criteria, was included in the second edition of the IASP Classification of Chronic Pain Syndromes but has shown marginal reliability when tested clinically,[245,246] and the terms SMP, RSD, and causalgia continue to be used.

Symptoms

The characteristic **pain is a constant, hot, burning sensation** with painful cutaneous hypersensitivity (hyperalgesia) and muscle tenderness.[3] The pain is worse with light touch, heat, cold, or emotional stress.

Typically, **RSD** begins a few days to several weeks after an injury to or an inflammation of sensory afferent pathways.[247] In the head and neck region, RSD has been reported to develop after maxillofacial surgery for cancer, head injury, ***molar extraction***, and sinus surgery.[248] If allowed to progress undiagnosed or untreated, RSD passes through an initial or "traumatic" stage characterized by a burning ache, edema, and hyperthermia to a second or "dystrophic" stage, with cool, cyanotic skin, spreading pain, and edema. The third or "atrophic" stage is evidenced by muscle atrophy; osteoporosis; smooth, glossy, mottled-appearing skin; and intractable pain. However, because of the abundant collateral blood circulation in the head and neck region, the bony, vascular, and trophic changes so typical in the extremities are less common in the face.[248]

Etiology

The exact pathophysiologic mechanisms of RSD are unknown. What is known is that after experimental nerve injury, surviving primary afferent nociceptors develop noradrenergic receptors and become sensitive to noradrenalin,[233,248,250] as do primary afferents that are experimentally cut and surgically repaired.[251] Other experimental studies suggest that some regenerating primary afferents may anastomose with the regenerating postganglionic sympathetic axons that run with them.[252,253] Post-traumatic sympathetic-afferent coupling also appears to occur in the dorsal root ganglion where sympathetic fibers that innervate the vasculature subserving the dorsal root ganglion begin to sprout around the primary afferent fibers[254,255] (Figure 8-26).

Clinically, the sympathetic nervous system is implicated in these pains because sympathetic blockade provides profound relief, and electrical stimulation of sympathetic outflow makes the pain worse.[256] Neither of these conditions exists in a normal individual. Changes in central pain pathways are also implicated in the RSD picture.[3]

Examination

The patient with **causalgia/RSD** complains of pain at the slightest touch and is difficult to examine. The skin may be flushed and dry or cold and sweaty, and a temperature difference may be discernible.

Diagnostic Tests

Definitive diagnosis of the condition in the head and neck can be accomplished through **immediate reduction of pain** and hyperesthesia with a successful **local anesthetic block of the stellate ganglion.** This procedure requires a trained anesthesiologist since the stellate ganglion is located in close proximity to several vital structures, including the vertebral artery and the apex of the lung.

Treatment

Repeated sympathetic blocks are the treatment of choice for sympathetically maintained pains. Early intervention is best. For the upper extremities and the head and neck region, this involves **repeated blocks of the stellate ganglion.**[248] Oral medications such as calcium channel blockers or low-dose tricyclic antidepressants with or without an anticonvulsant or systemic local anesthetic may be a useful adjunct.[257] Biofeedback

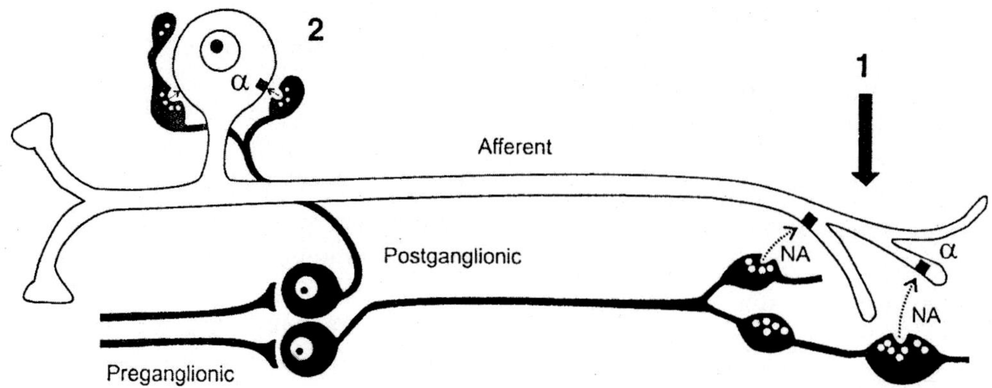

Figure 8-26 Influence of sympathetic activity and catecholamines on sensitized and damaged primary afferents. Normally primary afferent neurons do not have catecholamine sensitivity, and their activity is unaffected by sympathetic outflow. After nerve lesion (1) or in the presence of inflammation, afferent terminals in the periphery or afferent somata in the dorsal root ganglion acquire sensitivity to noradrenaline (NA) by expressing α-receptors at their membrane. Activity in postganglionic sympathetic neurons is now capable of activating afferent neurons by the release of NA. In addition, sympathetic postganglionic neurons sprout around dorsal root ganglion cells (2). Reproduced with permission from Fields HL, Rowbotham M, Baron R. Neuralgia: irritable nociceptors and deafferentation. Neurobiol Dis 1998;5:209.[7]

and relaxation techniques may help reduce generalized sympathetic activity. Transcutaneous electrical nerve stimulation or acupuncture in combination with physical therapy may be helpful in providing relief and increasing function. Surgical removal of the upper sympathetic chain is the last resort procedure when all else has failed. If an inadequate sympathectomy is performed, the pain may return.

Our patient complains of pain with many of the characteristics described for RSD and causalgic pain. The pain has a burning quality. The skin is hypersensitive. The affected side of the face is warmer to touch and slightly swollen. The pain is made worse with any type of stimulation. She has a history of tooth extraction with alveolar osteitis (dry socket). Reflex sympathetic dystrophy of the face is definitely worth listing as a possible diagnosis.

When dealing with any neuropathic or sympathetically maintained pain, referral to a neurologist should be considered if there are any subjective complaints or objective findings of cranial nerve deficits such as areas of facial hypesthesia, persistent motor weakness or paralysis, or a depressed corneal reflex.

MUSCULAR PAINS

Pain of muscular origin is generally described as a continuous, deep, dull ache or as tightness or pressure. It is undoubtedly the **most prevalent cause of pain in the head and neck region.**[62,63,258] According to Bell, "a good rule to follow in diagnosing pains about the face and mouth is initially to assume that the pain is dental until proved otherwise, then muscular until proved otherwise."[70] **Myospasm, myositis, and myofascial TrP pain** will be discussed as part of this group (Table 8-13). **"Local myalgia— unclassified"** includes **muscle splinting,** which is grouped with other muscle disorders such as delayed-onset muscle soreness or pain owing to ischemia, bruxism, or fatigue. This is because there are few clinical characteristics that differentiate these muscle disorders from each other.[61]

Myospasm

Etiology. Myospasm, **involuntary** continuous contraction of a muscle or group of muscles, may occur owing to acute overuse, strain, or overstretching of muscle previously weakened through protective reflex contraction (see Figure 8-11). Commonly termed a "charley horse," muscle spasm may occur, for example, **after sustained opening of the patient's mouth for dental treatment.** Deep pain input from other sources such as joint inflammation, dental infection, or myofascial TrPs may also result in reflex spasm of associated mus-

Table 8-13 Muscular Pains

Myospasm pain
Myositis pain
Local myalgia—unclassified
Myofascial pain
Tension-type headaches
Coexisting migraine and tension-type headaches

Adapted from Okeson.[61]

cles. In the absence of an obvious etiology, patients should be questioned regarding medication use. Medications such as **Compazine** (prochlorperazine) and **Stelazine** (trifluoperazine) or other major tranquilizers **may cause muscle spasm.** Prolonged use of this type of medication may also result in **tardive dyskinesia**, an irreversible condition consisting of involuntary movement of the tongue and/or lips.

Symptoms. An acutely shortened muscle with gross limitation of movement and constant pain is characteristic. The pain has a dull, aching quality with occasional sharp, lancinating pains in the ear, temple, or face. Depending on which muscles are involved, acute malocclusion may result. Patients may complain of increased pain on chewing or functioning of the spastic muscle. Headache may also result.

Examination. A normal jaw opening of 40 to 60 mm may be reduced to 10 to 20 mm with spasm. Malocclusion and abnormal jaw opening may be evident.

Diagnostic Tests. Electromyography (EMG), surface, needle, or fine wire, will show substantially increased muscle activity even at rest.[61,259] Injection of suspected muscles with plain 0.5% or 1% procaine or lidocaine should provide relief and confirm the diagnosis.

Treatment. If left untreated, the pain will subside. However, as a result of decreased function, there is a risk of developing contracture. Many episodes of "lock jaw" and torticollis (wry neck) are attributable to contracture. Therefore, patients should continue to use the jaw within pain-free limits. Heat may provide symptomatic relief. As the pain decreases, gradual active stretching of the muscle over a period of 3 to 7 days, with simultaneous application of counterstimulation or injection of the muscle with a weak solution of plain procaine or lidocaine, may facilitate restoration of normal function.

Myositis

Myositis is ***inflammation*** of muscles that, in the head and neck region, most frequently involves the masseter and medial pterygoid muscles. According to Bell, "the familiar **trismus** [our emphasis added] associated with dental sepsis, injury, surgery, or needle abscess typifies this condition."[70]

Etiology. Myositis is usually the result of external trauma (eg, contact sports), excessive muscle overuse, or spreading infection (eg, dental abscess).[70,260] In fact, many of the same things that cause myospasm may cause myositis if prolonged or severe enough. The associated mandibular dysfunction is related to pain and to the presence of inflammatory exudate in the muscles. Myositis may progress to fibrous scarring or contracture.[70,260]

Symptoms. Characteristically, the patient complains of continuous pain over the muscle aggravated by jaw opening, limited jaw opening, and swelling over the involved muscle. **There is usually a history of trauma or infection.** If the cause is attributable to infection, the patient may also complain of malaise and fever.

Examination. Myositis can be distinguished from myospasm owing to the presence of swelling. The muscle is diffusely tender. Mandibular range of motion is severely restricted. **Regional lymphadenitis** is present if there is infection.

Treatment. Treatment of both myositis and contracture is similar to that used for myospasm, except that **NSAIDs** are also recommended. Exercises, massage, and injections are contraindicated until acute symptoms have subsided.

Local Myalgia—Unclassified

Myospasm and myositis present with specific characteristics that allow a definite clinical distinction to be made. Other kinds of myalgias owing to ischemia, muscle overuse (fatigue and postexercise muscle soreness), or protective "splinting" or co-contraction also exist. However, currently, there is little scientific information to allow clear distinction between these disorders, and for this reason they are grouped together as unclassified myalgias.[61]

Myofascial Pain

Myofascial pain, a regional referred pain syndrome associated with focally tender **TrPs** in muscle, is a prevalent cause of pain in all parts of the body and has been reported as a common source of pain in numerous medical specialties.[62,64] For example, almost 30% of patients presenting themselves with a complaint of pain in an internal medicine practice[62] and over 80% of patients in a chronic pain center[64] had MFP as a primary diagnosis. It is also the most prevalent cause of painful symptoms in TMDs.[63,258]

In a study conducted at the University of Minnesota TMJ and Facial Pain Clinic, doctors evaluated 296 consecutive patients with chronic head and neck pain complaints.[258] Myofascial pain was the primary diagnosis in 55.4% of these patients. Nonpainful internal derangements of the TMJs were felt to be a perpetuating factor to the MFP in 30.4%. In contrast, only 21% of these patients had a TMD disorder as the primary cause of pain. In this 21%, the joint disorder included inflammation of the TMJ joint capsule or the retrodiscal tissues.

Despite its prevalence and the recent surge in scientific documentation, **MFP** remains poorly understood and frequently unrecognized by most health care providers. Many physicians and dentists alike insist on calling it myo*facial* pain and think of it as a myalgia of the facial muscles and masticatory muscles. Others feel that it is a syndrome that involves some internal derangement of the TMJ plus associated local muscle soreness.

Symptoms. In **MFP**, the presenting pain complaint is usually a ***referred symptom*** with a **deep, dull aching quality** located in or about normal muscular or, importantly, nonmuscular structures. In the head and neck region, the patient may complain of such things as **toothache**, sinus pain, TMJ pain, or headache, yet evaluation of these areas does not yield any pathologic change. In fact, ***any undiagnosed deep, dull, aching pain may be myofascial in origin.*** The intensity of MFP should not be underestimated: the pain intensity has been documented to be equal or slightly greater than that of pain from other causes.[62]

Associated symptoms, thought to be owing to the physiologic sensory, motor, and autonomic effects seen with prolonged pain, are common and may confuse the clinical picture.[261–263] These effects were discussed earlier in the section under "Neurophysiology of Pain." Associated sensory complaints may include tenderness in the referred pain site, such as scalp pain on brushing the hair, or abnormal sensitivity of the teeth.[264] Motor effects include increased EMG activity in the pain reference zone,[262,263,265,266] although patients rarely complain about this specifically. Autonomic changes such as localized vasoconstriction (pallor),[262] sweating, lacrimation, coryza, increased salivation, and nausea and vomiting have also been reported.[55]

Patients note worsening of symptoms with increased psychological stress, cold weather, immobility, and overuse of involved muscles. Hot baths, rest, warm weather, and massage are typical alleviating factors.

Etiology. Myofascial TrPs can be primary or secondary. When primary, injury to the muscle owing to **macrotrauma** or **cumulative microtrauma** is typically involved. Macrotrauma is easily identified and includes injuries such as those caused by falls, blows, sports injuries, motor vehicle accidents, or even **prolonged jaw opening** at the dental office. Microtrauma is more insidious and includes muscle overuse owing to poor posture and body mechanics, abnormal strain, and repetitive motion–type injuries.

Secondary myofascial TrPs develop in response to prolonged underlying disease, especially if painful, for which any process that activates nociceptors may induce secondary muscle contraction and TrP development (**described under "Physiologic Mechanisms Modifying Pain" at the beginning of this chapter**). Secondary MFP may prolong and complicate pain owing to other causes.[261] Examples include migraine, inflammatory disorders of the TMJ, chronic ear infections, **persistent pulpalgia**, PHN, cancer, or any other chronic painful condition including **bursitis of the tensor villi palatini muscle** as it passes over the hamulus.[261,267] Myofascial pain needs to be identified and treated to reduce pain and improve response to other therapies. Patients with what appears to be primary MFP, in whom TrPs and pain recur despite appropriate initial response to TrP therapies and compliance to home exercise, must be re-evaluated for occult underlying disease or other perpetuating factors.

In MFP, the presenting pain complaint is always associated with a TrP located in a taut band of skeletal muscle that is often distant from the site of pain. Trigger points are focally tender, firm, nodular areas in muscle, that, with the application of 2 to 4 kg of pressure for 6 to 10 seconds, produce spontaneous referred pain or intensify existing pain in local or distant locations.[268] Patients are typically unaware of the existence of these TrPs. Trigger points are considered active when the referred pain pattern and associated symptoms are clinically present and latent when they are not. Trigger points will vacillate between active and latent states depending on the amount of psychological stress the individual is under and the amount of muscle overload placed on the affected muscle.

The location of TrPs and their associated referred pain patterns are predictable and reproducible from patient to patient[55,269–271] (Figures 8-27 to 8-30). A meticulous discussion of MFP, as well as a complete compendium of the pain referral patterns for most muscles of the body, has been brilliantly detailed by Travell and Simons.[55,271]

Pathophysiology. With some training, myofascial TrPs are relatively easy to palpate. Despite the comparative ease of clinical identification of TrPs, controversy still exists about their structure and exact pathophysiology. Muscle biopsy studies using light and electron microscopy, as well as histochemical analyses, have not shown consistent abnormalities, and there is no evidence for inflammation.[272,273] However, careful monopolar needle EMG evaluation has revealed some interesting information.

Although EMG findings in the muscle surrounding the TrP are normal, higher EMG microvoltages, called "spontaneous electrical activity" or "SEA," are found in the TrPs themselves.[274] Spontaneous electrical activity is significantly higher in subjects with clinical pain owing to active TrPs than in subjects without clinical pain who have latent or no TrPs. Spontaneous

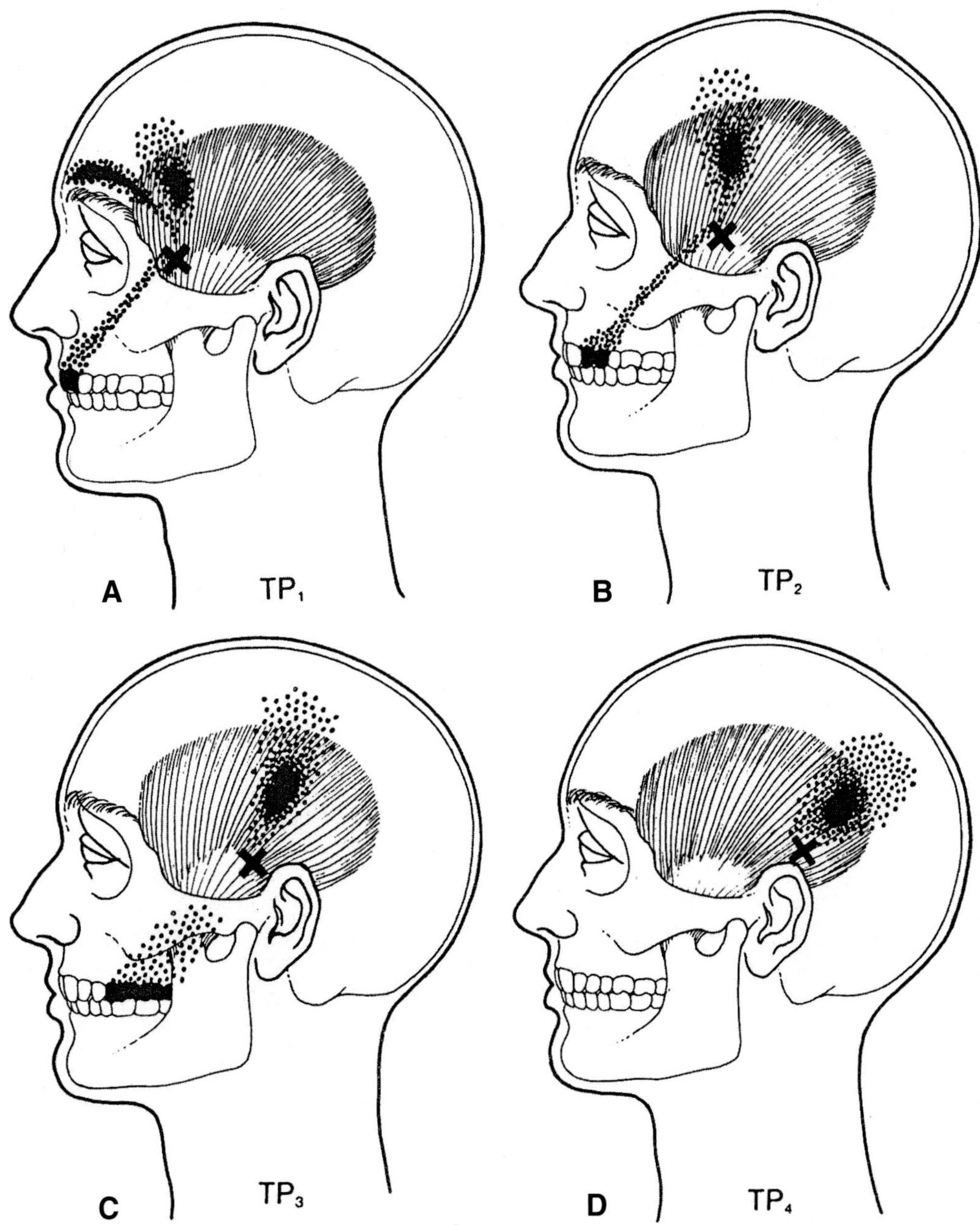

Figure 8-27 Referred pain patterns from trigger points (**crosses**) in the temporalis muscle (essential zone, **black**; spillover zone, **stippled**). **A,** Anterior "spokes" of pain arising from anterior fibers (trigger point, TP_1). Note reference to anterior teeth. **B** and **C,** middle "spokes of TP_2 and TP_3 referring to maxillary posterior teeth, sinus, and zygomatic area. **D,** Posterior, TP_4, supra-auricular "spoke" referral. Reproduced with permission from Simons DG et al.[55]

electrical activity can be recorded only if the needle is precisely placed in the nidus of the TrP; movement of the needle tip as little as 1 mm is enough to lose the signal. Spontaneous electrical activity has been interpreted by Hubbard and others as arising from muscle spindles[274,275]; Simons et al. and Hong and Simons believe that dysfunctional muscle motor end plates are to blame.[55,276]

Muscle spindles are 1.5 mm × 5 mm mechanoreceptors that signal muscle length. They are found between and parallel to skeletal muscle fibers and are more numerous in the cervical and axial muscles, where TrPs more commonly occur.[52,277] They contain intrafusal fibers that are innervated by the sympathetic nervous system and are pain and pressure sensitive. Psychological stress, which causes increased sympa-

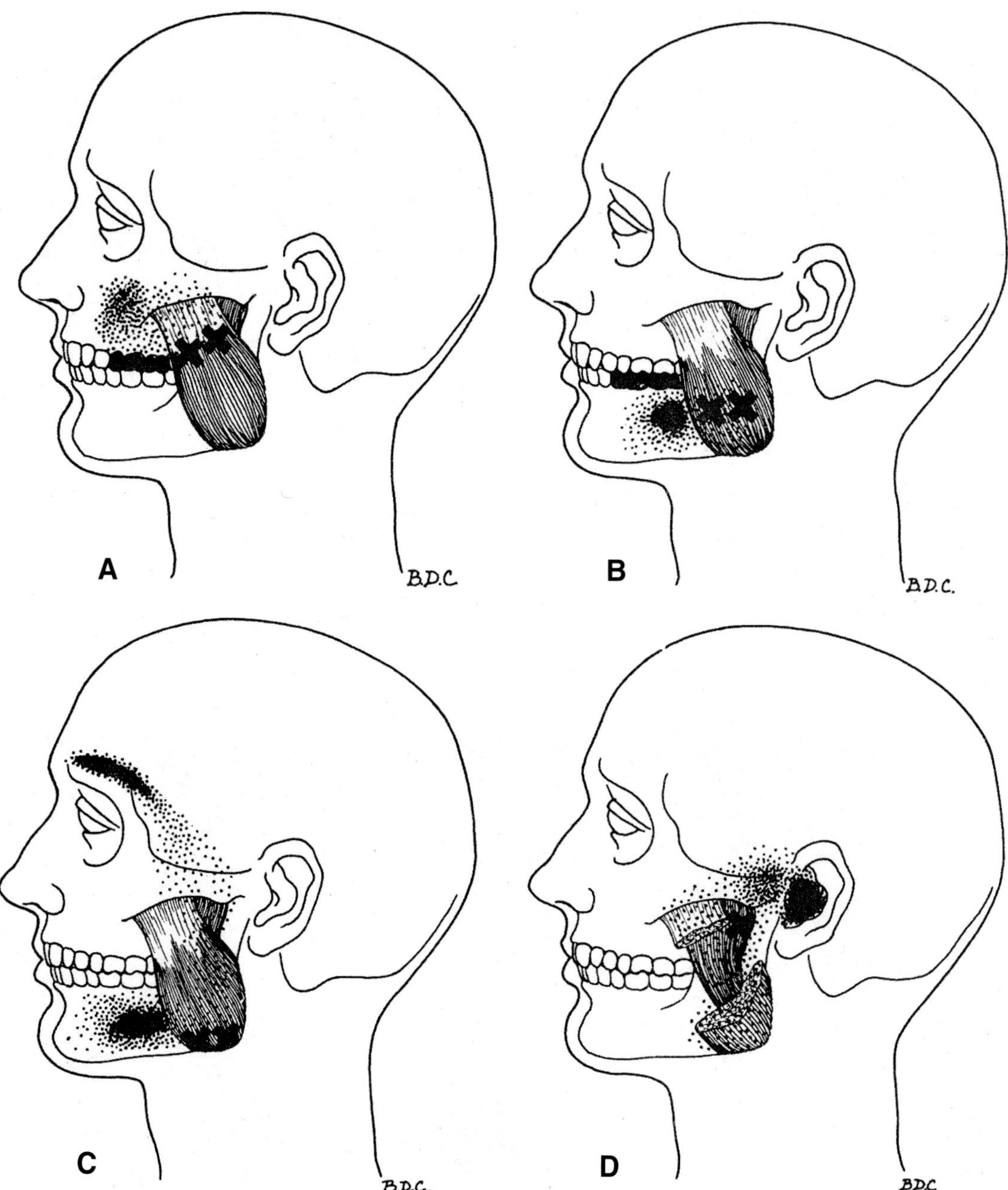

Figure 8-28 Central and referred pain from the masseter muscle. The **crosses** locate trigger points in various parts of the masseter; the **black areas** show essential referred pain zones and **stippled areas** are spillover pain zones. **A**, Superficial layer, upper portion. Note reference to maxillary posterior teeth. **B**, Superficial layer, midbelly. Note spillover reference to mandible and posterior teeth. **C**, Superficial layer; lower portion refers to the mandible and frontal "headache." **D**, Deep layer; upper part refers to the temporomandibular joint area and ear. Reproduced with permission from Simons DG et al.[55]

thetic output, has been shown to increase the SEA recorded from TrPs, whereas the EMG activity of adjacent non-TrP sites remains unchanged.[275] These data parallel the clinical observation that emotional stress activates or aggravates pain from TrPs and supports the spindle hypothesis of TrPs. Similarly, intramuscular or intravenous administration of sympathetic blocking agents effectively abolishes the SEA,[274,277,278] whereas curare and botulinum toxin, postsynaptic and presynaptic cholinergic blockers, respectively, have no effect on SEA in randomized, controlled studies.[274,279] A solitary human EMG-guided biopsy specimen contained a single muscle spindle (Figure 8-31).

The existence of afferent pain receptors in muscle spindles does provide an explanation for TrP palpation tenderness. Hubbard and Shannon argued that based

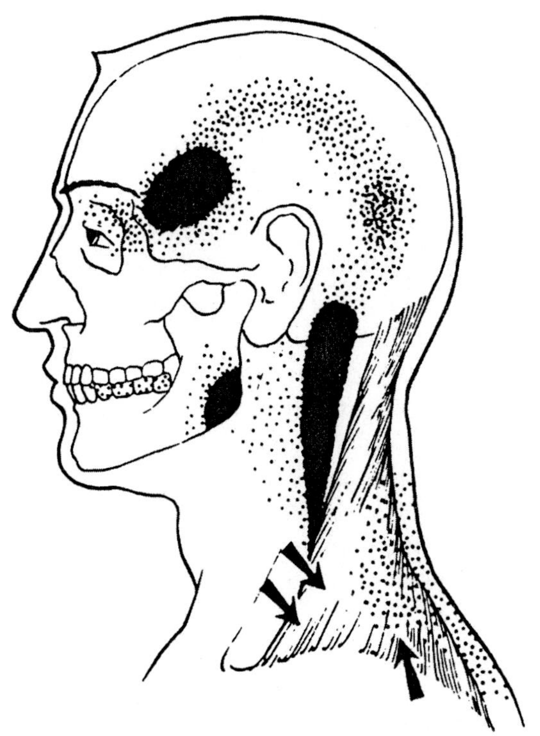

Figure 8-29 Composite pain reference pattern of trapezius muscle, suprascapular region. Trigger points are indicated by **arrows**, essential pain reference zones by **black** on posterior teeth. Spillover pain zones are **stippled**. Note temporal "tension headache" and reference to the angle of the mandible with spillover to posterior teeth. Reproduced with permission from Travell JG.[264]

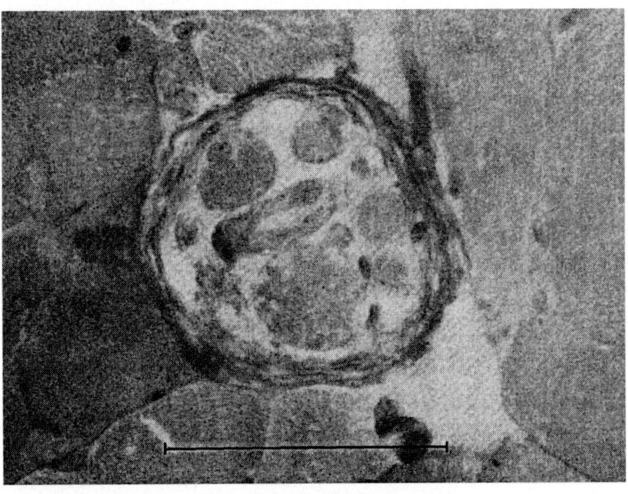

Figure 8-31 Photomicrograph of a cross-section of the muscle spindle found in the electromyographically guided trapezius biopsy specimen. van Gieson's stain. Bar represents 50 micrometers. Reproduced with permission from Hubbard DR.[277]

on its size and structure, a muscle spindle would feel like a grain of rice in the muscle and could be the TrP nodule that is palpable clinically (personal communication, 1999). Similarly, contracted muscle spindles could also produce taut bands (D Hubbard and S Shannon, personal communication, 1999).

Motor end plates are where the efferent motor nerve fibers attach to muscle fibers. The motor end-plate theory proposes that SEA is owing to excess acetylcholine release into the synaptic cleft by dysfunctional end plates at the neuromuscular junction.[55,280]

Based on the psychophysical evidence available to date and the observation that myofascial TrPs are frequently located in and around the motor end-plate area of muscles,[281] Simons and Reeves et al. hypothesized that the myofascial TrP represents an area of isolated sustained muscle contraction, uncontrolled metabolism, and localized ischemia that is initiated by acute muscle injury or strain.[266,282] This theory does provide a credible explanation for the palpable nodules and taut muscle bands associated with TrPs. The TrP

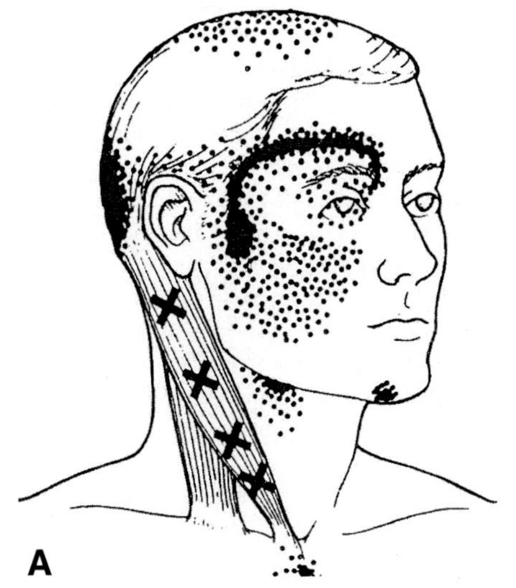

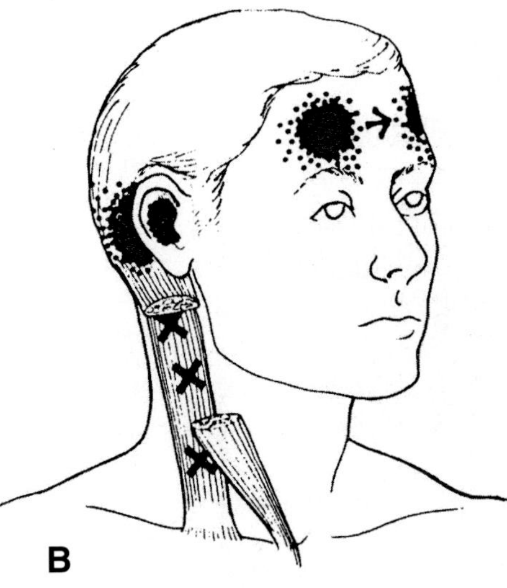

Figure 8-30 Pain reference from sternocleidomastoid muscle. Trigger points (**crosses**), essential reference zones (**black**), and spillover areas (**stippled**). **A**, The sternal division. **B**, The clavicular (deep) division refers most common frontal "tension headaches." Reproduced with permission from Simons DG et al.[55]

nodule is described as a group of "contraction knots" in which a number of individual muscle fibers are maximally contracted at the end-plate zone, making them shorter and wider at that point than the noncontracted neighboring fibers. If enough fibers are so activated, a **palpable nodule** could result. As for the taut band, both ends of these affected muscle fibers would be maximally stretched out and "taut," producing the palpable taut band (Figure 8-32).

Clinically, data exist documenting that TrPs are truly focally tender areas in muscle; pain with palpation is not owing to generalized muscle tenderness.[282,283] Indeed, tenderness to palpation over **non**-TrP sites in subjects with MFP does not differ significantly from normals.[282] Also, muscle bands containing TrPs will display a local **twitch response,** a transient contraction of the muscle band with deep "snapping" digital palpation. This response, best appreciated in more superficial muscle fibers, has also been substantiated experimentally.[284] A rabbit model of the twitch response has documented that, at least in rabbits, the twitch response is a spinally mediated reflex.[285,286]

The mechanism of referred pain from myofascial TrPs is also under speculation. According to Mense[28] and Vecchiet et al.,[287] the convergence-projection and convergence-facilitation models of referred pain (described earlier under "Referred Pain") do not directly apply to muscle pain because there is little convergence of neurons from deep tissues in the dorsal horn.[28] These authors propose that convergent connections from other spinal cord segments are "unmasked" or opened by nociceptive input from skeletal muscle and that referral to other myotomes is owing to the release and spread of substance P to adjacent spinal segments[28,288] (see Figures 8-6 and 8-7). Simons has expanded on this theory to specifically explain the referred pain from TrPs[30] (see Figure 8-9).

The following is an excellent example of myofascial TrP pain developing in response to an acutely inflamed TMJ.

Case History

A 47-year-old man with a long-standing history of painless osteoarthrosis of both TMJs presented

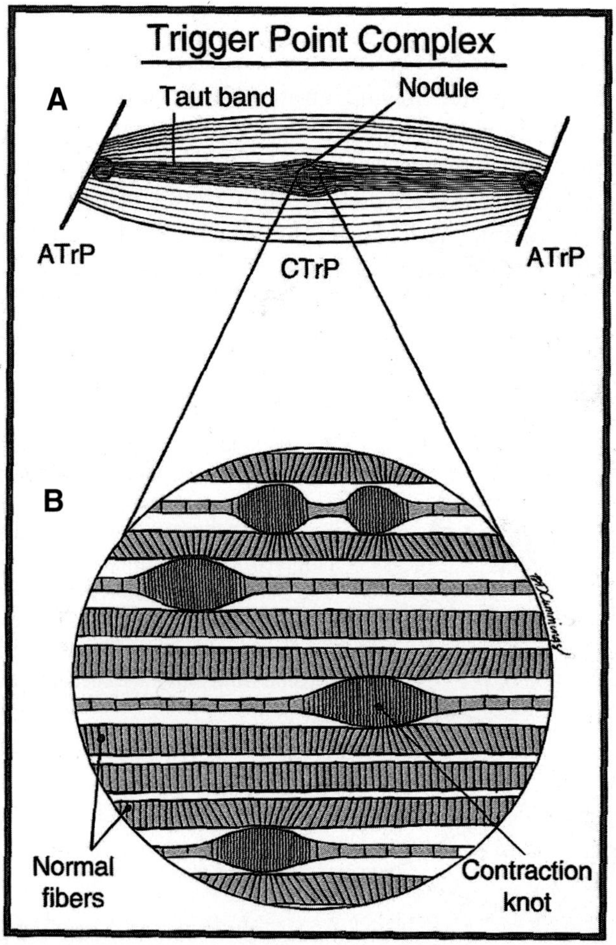

Figure 8-32 Schematic of a trigger point (TrP) complex of a muscle in longitudinal section. **A**, The central TrP, which is drawn in the muscle end-plate zone, contains numerous "contraction knots," maximally contracted individual muscle fibers that are shorter and wider at the end plate than the noncontracted neighboring fibers. **B** is an enlarged view of part of the central TrP showing the distribution of five contraction knots. The vertical lines in each muscle fiber identify the relative spacing of its striations. The space between two striations corresponds to the length of one sarcomere. Each contraction knot identifies a segment to muscle fiber experiencing maximal contracture of its sarcomeres. The sarcomeres within these contraction knots are markedly shorter and wider than the sarcomeres of the neighboring normal muscle fibers. In fibers with these contraction knots (note the lower three individual knots), the sarcomeres on the part of the muscle fiber that extends beyond both ends of the contraction knot are elongated and narrow compared with normal sarcomeres. At the top of this enlarged view is a pair of contraction knots separated by an interval of empty sarcolemma between them that is devoid of contractile elements. This configuration suggests that the sustained maximal tension of the contractile elements in an individual contraction knot could have caused mechanical failure of the contractile elements in the middle of the knot. If that happened, the two halves would retract, leaving an interval of empty sarcolemma between them. In patients, the central TrP would feel nodular as compared to the adjacent muscle tissue because it contains numerous "swollen" contraction knots that take up additional space and are much more firm and tense than uninvolved muscle fibers. If enough fibers are so activated, a palpable nodule could result. As for the taut band, both ends of these affected muscle fibers would be maximally stretched out and "taut," producing the palpable taut band. Reproduced with permission from Simons DG et al.[55]

himself with an acute left TMJ inflammation. This was conservatively treated with rest, soft diet, and anti-inflammatory medications. Severe symptoms subsided, but the patient continued to complain of persistent "aching of the left jaw." Clenching the teeth together produced a high-pitched ringing in his left ear. Careful history revealed that the pain was no longer specifically over the joint but was actually inferior and anterior to the left TMJ over the masseter muscle. Active range of motion of the mandible had increased from 41 to 47 mm, and the joint was nontender to palpation. Despite the negative joint examination, the less astute clinician may still direct his or her energies toward treating the TMJs, especially since there is documented osteoarthrosis bilaterally, worse on the left. However, the source of the pain is now from myofascial TrPs and not the joint. Palpation of the masseter muscle, particularly the deep fibers, reproduced the patient's current symptoms, including the ringing in his left ear (Figure 8-33). Trigger points in this part of the masseter muscle have also been reported to cause unilateral tinnitus[55] and accounted for the high-pitched sound the patient complained of with clenching. Treatment must be directed at rehabilitating the masseter muscle and not at the asymptomatic joint.

Examination. Because the patient's pain complaint is typically a referred symptom, it is usually distant from the muscle containing the guilty TrP,[55,288] although some TrPs also cause more localized pain symptoms. Multiple TrPs can produce overlapping areas of referred pain (Figure 8-34). The pattern of pain can be used in reverse to identify possible etiologic TrPs. *Systematic fingertip examination* of suspected muscles and their contralateral counterparts, looking for taut bands and focal tenderness, is ***essential.*** **Effective TrP palpation is a skill that must be learned and practiced.** Depending on the muscle, the tip of the index finger should be used for flat palpation or the index finger and thumb for pincer-type palpation (Figure 8-35). Once a TrP is found, 2 to 4 kg/cm^2 of pressure should be applied for 6 to 10 seconds to elicit the referred pain pattern, if any. The examination may replicate the patient's pain so precisely that there is no doubt about the diagnosis. If uncertainty exists, specific TrP therapies, such as "spray and stretch" or TrP injections, described below, may be used diagnostically. ***All head and neck muscles should be routinely examined*** in patients with a persistent pain complaint. This will help identify both primary and secondary MFP in addition to helping identify TrPs in key muscles (eg, upper trapezius or sternocleidomastoid) that may be inducing or perpetuating satellite TrPs in muscles located in the pain referral sites (eg, temporalis).[55,263]

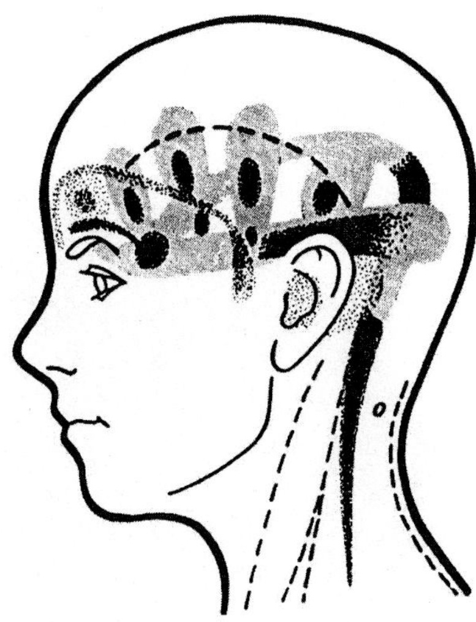

Figure 8-34 Overlapping pain referral patterns from the temporalis, sternocleidomastoid, upper trapezius, and suboccipital muscles produce a clinical picture of "tension-type headache." Unilateral symptoms may mimic migraine without aura.

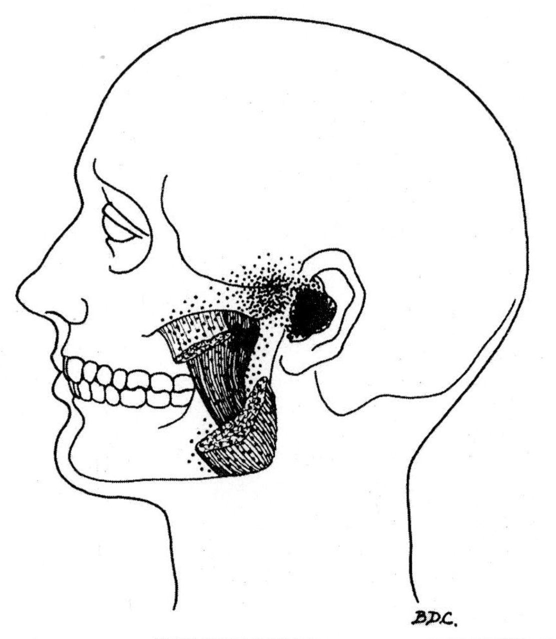

Figure 8-33 Deep layer, upper part of the masseter muscle refers pain to the temporomandibular joint area and ear. Reproduced with permission from Simons DG et al.[55]

Treatment. Recommended treatment of MFP involves most importantly identification and control of causal and perpetuating factors, patient education, and specific home stretching exercises. Therapeutic techniques such as "spray and stretch," voluntary contract-

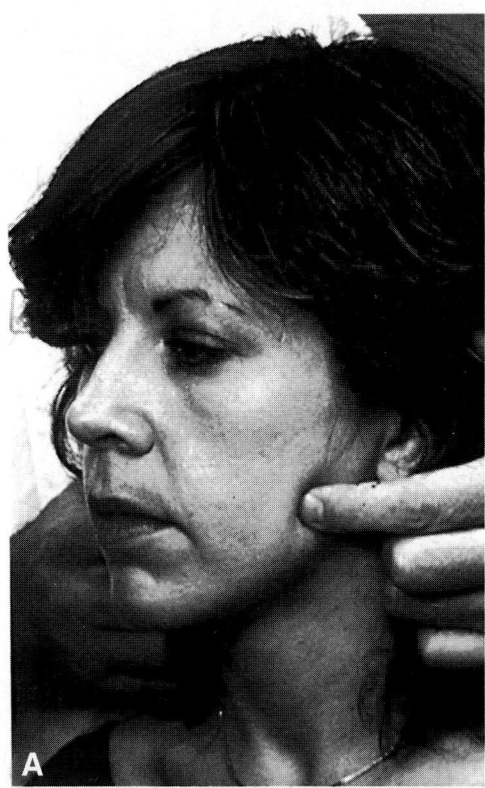

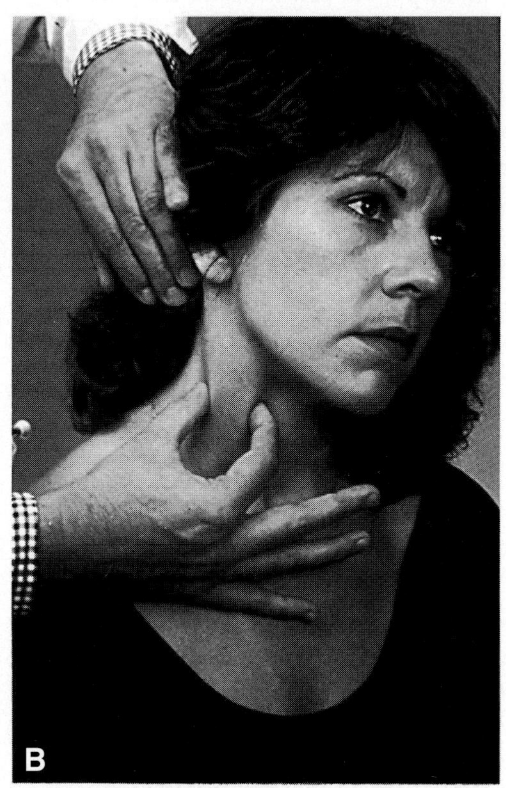

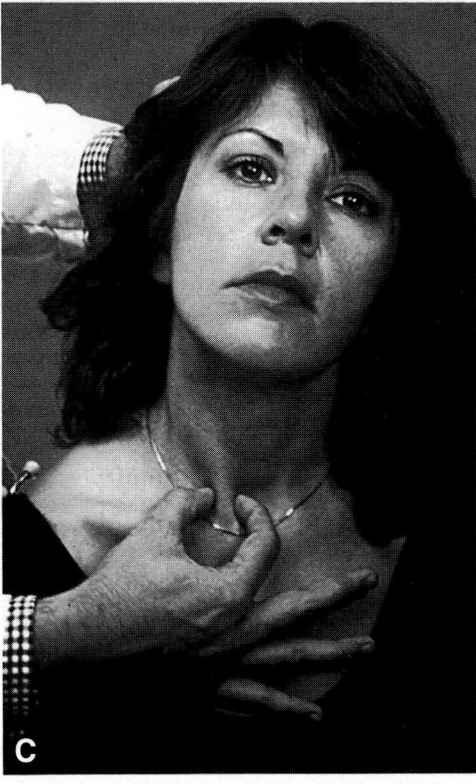

Figure 8-35 Muscle palpation for myofascial trigger points. A, "Flat" fingertip palpation of masseter muscle looking for taut bands and focal tenderness characteristic of myofascial trigger points. The flat palpation technique is also useful for temporalis, suboccipital, medial pterygoid, and upper back muscles. B, "Pincer" palpation of the deep clavicular head of the sternocleidomastoid muscle. C, "Pincer" palpation of the superficial sternal head. Heads should be palpated separately. The upper border of the trapezius also lends itself to pincer palpation.

release, TrP pressure release, and TrP injections[289,290] are useful adjunctive techniques that usually facilitate the patient's recovery. **Myofascial TrP therapists** are especially adept at TrP examination, spray and stretch, and TrP pressure release techniques.

Perpetuating factors most commonly include mechanical factors that place an increased load on the muscles. Teaching patients good posture and body mechanics will go a long way in reducing referred pain from myofascial TrPs, especially in the head and neck region.[291] An **intraoral stabilization splint** may be indicated to decrease the frequency of clenching or bruxing as a perpetuating factor.

Psychological factors, such as **stress** that has been shown to cause TrP activation or **depression** that lowers pain thresholds, will contribute to MFP. Sleep disturbance and inactivity are also common perpetuating factors. Simple stress management and relaxation skills are invaluable in controlling involuntary muscle tension if this is a problem. Mild depression and sleep disturbance can be treated with low doses of **tricyclic antidepressant drugs** and a structured exercise/activation program.

Other perpetuating factors include metabolic, endocrine, or nutritional inadequacies that affect muscle metabolism.[55] Patients should be screened for general good health and referred to their physician for management of any systemic abnormalities. In secondary MFP, the primary concomitant painful disorder, such as TMJ capsulitis, pulpitis, or PHN, must also be treated or managed.

Spray and stretch is a highly successful technique for the treatment of myofascial TrPs that uses a vapocoolant spray (Gebbauer, Co.; Cleveland, OH) to facilitate muscle stretching. Muscle stretching has been shown to reduce the intensity of referred pain and TrP sensitivity in patients with myofascial pain.[292] Vapocoolant is applied slowly in a systematic pattern over the muscle being stretched and into the pain reference zone (Figure 8-36). This technique and alternatives not using vapocoolant are described in detail in Simons et al.'s text.[55]

Needling of TrPs with or without injection of solution has also been shown to be helpful in reducing TrP activity to allow stretching.[290,292–296] Although dry needling is effective, use of a local anesthetic reduces postinjection soreness.[292] If a local anesthetic is to be injected, 0.5% procaine or 0.5% lidocaine is recommended. Longer-acting amide local anesthetics or local anesthetics containing epinephrine cause permanent muscle damage.[297] Injection must always be followed by stretch.[55] Trigger point injection in the absence of a home program that addresses relevant perpetuating factors will provide only temporary relief.

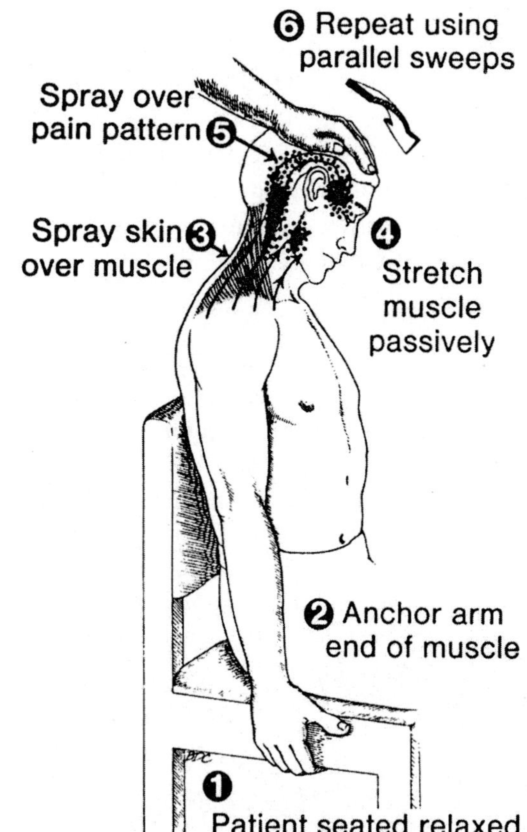

Figure 8-36 Sequence of steps when stretching and spraying any muscle for myofascial trigger points, here applied to the upper trapezius. **1**, Patient supported in a comfortable relaxed position. **2**, One end of the muscle is anchored. **3**, Skin sprayed with three to four parallel sweeps of vapocoolant over the length of the muscle in the direction of the pain pattern (**arrows**). **4**, Immediately after the first sweep of spray, pressure is applied to stretch the muscle and continues as the spray is applied. **5**, Sweeps of spray cover the referred pain pattern of the muscle. **6**, Steps 3, 4, and 5 repeated only two or three times or less. Hot packs and several cycles of full active range of motion follow. Reproduced with permission from Simons DG et al.[55]

Tension-type headaches are usually bilateral, with a pressing, nonpulsating quality. They last 20 minutes to 7 days when episodic and may be daily without remission when chronic.[54] Overlapping referred pain patterns from myofascial TrPs can produce a typical tension-type headache (see Figure 8-33). Studies have documented the presence of focally tender points and referred pain in this type of headache.[136,298] Thus, the same treatment strategies used for MFP also work well for the reduction of tension-type headache.[289,298]

Coexisting migraine and tension-type headache, previously termed mixed headache, tension-vascular headache, or combination headache and now often described under the term transformed migraine, combine features of both tension-type and neurovascular headaches. These patients have varying degrees of each of these two headache types. Typically, they complain of dull, aching, pressing head pain that progresses into a throbbing headache. This type of headache has an even higher incidence of pericranial muscle tenderness and referred pain than tension-type headache.[136] Treatment requires management of the MFP as well as judicious use of abortive or prophylactic migraine medications.

Although our patient did not complain specifically of deep, aching pains, secondary MFP does occur with most types of chronic pain input into the central nervous system. Therefore, it is likely that secondary myofascial TrPs have developed. In fact, when the patient was initially examined, TrPs were found in the upper trapezius muscle that referred pain to the side of the temple and face (see Figure 8-36). Even if this is not the primary cause of the pain, it is likely to be a contributing factor.

UNCLASSIFIABLE PAINS/ ATYPICAL FACIAL PAINS

Mock et al. have stated, "The diagnoses atypical facial pain and atypical facial neuralgia are often applied interchangeably to the patient with poorly localized, vaguely described facial pain, nonanatomic in distribution with no evidence of a defined organic cause."[299] Technically, these are not "atypical" pains but idiopathic pains, pains for which we do not yet have a diagnosis or sufficient understanding. Yet if we look at retrospective analysis of data collected on 493 consecutive patients who presented to a university orofacial pain clinic, a different picture emerges.[300] A diagnosis of atypical facial pain was made if patients had persistent orofacial pain for more than 6 months for which previous treatments had been unsuccessful and the diagnosis was unknown on referral to the clinic. Of the 493 patient charts reviewed, 35 (7%) met these criteria. Using the American Academy of Orofacial Pain diagnostic criteria,[61] all but 1 (97%) had diagnosable physical problems and sometimes multiple overlapping physical diagnoses causing the pain. Over half (19 of 35 or 54%) were found to have **MFP owing to TrPs** as a primary cause or significant contributing factor to the pain. Eleven (31%) had periodontal ligament sensitivity, 8 had referred pain from dental pulpitis, 3 had neuropathic pain, and 1 each had burning mouth from oral candidiasis, sinus pathology, burning tongue from an oral habit, pericoronitis, or an incomplete tooth fracture.

There is currently significant controversy in the field about the diagnosis and classification of atypical facial pain. Myofascial TrP pain is clearly under-recognized,[301,302] and trigeminal neuropathies or "dysesthesias," which many believe to be at fault for various "atypical" facial pains, are still inadequately understood.[301] Although proposals for nomenclature and classification changes abound,[301–303] this "atypical" nomenclature is likely to haunt the dental/orofacial pain profession for several years to come.

Two types of atypical pain that commonly appear in the dental office are **atypical odontalgia** (idiopathic toothache, phantom odontalgia,[303] or trigeminal dysesthesia) and **burning mouth syndrome** (Table 8-14). Although deafferentation (neuropathic pain) is believed to play a role in both of these pain syndromes, the mechanism and etiology are still largely speculative. Therefore, it is as yet difficult to reliably classify them under any of the diagnostic categories already discussed.

Atypical Odontalgia

In 1979, Rees and Harris described a disorder they called atypical odontalgia.[304] Synonymous or almost synonymous terms include phantom tooth pain,[303] idiopathic orofacial pain,[305] vascular toothache,[70] and, more recently, trigeminal dysesthesia. Patients present with chronic toothache or tooth site pain with no obvious cause. **It is extremely important for dentists to be aware of the existence of this syndrome** to avoid performing unnecessary dental procedures and extractions. It has been postulated that as many as **3 to 6% of endodontic patients** may suffer from this type of tooth pain, especially if they had pain prior to pulp extirpation.[303]

Symptoms. The chief complaint is a deep, dull, aching pain in a tooth or tooth site that is unchanging over weeks or months. The pain is fairly constant, with some diurnal fluctuation, and usually worsens as the day progresses. The molars are most commonly involved, followed by premolars. Anterior teeth and canines are less frequently affected.[306] The vast majority of patients present themselves with unilateral pain, although other quadrants may become involved and other oral and facial sites may hurt.

Most patients are **female** and **over 40 years** of age. Table 8-15 lists the clinical characteristics of patients with atypical odontalgia as reported by several different authors. Onset of the pain may coincide with or devel-

Table 8-14 Unclassifiable Pains

Atypical odontalgia
Burning mouth syndrome

Table 8-15 Clinical Characteristics of Patients with Atypical Odontagia*

N = 30
Age 58.4 y
Duration 4.4 y
90% female

*Seen at the University of Florida College of Dentistry.[309]

op within a month or so after dental treatment (especially endodontic therapy or extraction) or trauma or medical procedures related to the face.[303] Patients may have a history of repeated dental therapies that have failed to resolve the problem. Chewing or clenching on painful teeth, heat, cold, and stress are typical but inconsistent aggravating factors.

Etiology. The true etiology of atypical odontalgia remains elusive. Bell classified it as a vascular disorder,[70] as did Rees and Harris, who postulated a "painful migraine-like disturbance" in the teeth and periodontal tissues, possibly triggered by depression.[304] There are no data to support this idea, although a study using subcutaneous sumatriptan in 19 atypical facial pain patients did show some small temporary positive effects, possibly supporting a vascular contribution to the pain.[307,308] Others have suggested depression or some other psychological disorder as the cause[309,310] since many patients with atypical odontalgia report depressive symptoms on clinical interview.[303,311,312] However, these results must be questioned owing to poor, uncontrolled study methodology and because there is a generally higher incidence of depression in patients with chronic pain. Of interest is the fact that standard **MMPI scores** for patients with **atypical odontalgia** compared with standard scores for a chronic headache group (matched for age, sex, and chronicity) were similar, and scales for both groups were within normal ranges,[306,313] making a psychological cause unlikely.

A more probable cause of atypical odontalgia is **deafferentation** (partial or total **loss of the afferent nerve supply** or sensory input) with or without sympathetic involvement. **Atypical odontalgia usually follows a dental procedure**, and most dental procedures, including cavity preparation, cause varying degrees of deafferentation. Studies supporting this theory are also lacking, yet the symptoms and clinical presentation are consistent with post-traumatic neuropathic pain. Many cases respond to sympathetic blocks[306] or phentolamine infusion,[314] implying that at least some may be sympathetically mediated or maintained. This theory would also explain why the pain remains even after the painful tooth is extracted. In addition, the preponderance of females suffering from this disorder raises the question of the role of estrogen and other female hormones as a risk factor in atypical odontalgia and related idiopathic orofacial pains.[315]

Examination. Intraoral and radiographic examination are typically unrevealing. If the pain is in a tooth as opposed to an extraction site, responses to percussion, thermal testing, and electric pulp stimulation are variable. Clinically, there is no observable cause, yet **thermographic evaluation is always abnormal.**[316] The majority of patients report little or no relief with diagnostic local anesthetic blocks,[306,317] although sympathetic blocks seem to be helpful.[306]

Treatment. Invasive, irreversible treatments, such as endodontic therapy, exploratory surgery, extraction, or even occlusal adjustments, **are contraindicated.**[303,317] This is because, despite possible transient relief, the pain is likely to recur with equal or greater intensity.

The current treatment of choice is the use of **tricyclic antidepressant agents** such as **amitriptyline or imipramine.**[303,306,317] If the pain has a **burning quality**, the addition of a **phenothiazine**, such as **trifluoperazine**, may be helpful.[303,317] Tricyclic antidepressants have analgesic properties independent of their antidepressant effects and often provide good pain relief at a fraction of the dose typically used to treat depression.[312,318] Pain relief normally occurs at doses from 50 to 100 mg. Dry mouth is an expected and usually unavoidable side effect. A history of significant cardiac arrhythmias or recent myocardial infarction, urinary retention, and glaucoma are contraindications for the use of tricyclic medications because of their atropine-like action. Patients may need reassurance that the pain is **real and not psychogenic** but that invasive procedures will not help.

If a patient complains of associated gingival hyperesthesia, use of topical agents such as local anesthetic or capsaicin have been shown to be beneficial.[314] Unwanted stimulation of the area can be reduced by construction of an acrylic stent that can also be used to help apply any topical medication.

Burning Mouth Syndrome

Burning mouth syndrome is an intraoral pain disorder that most commonly **affects postmenopausal women.** The National Institutes of Dental and Craniofacial Research (NIDCR) report on the national Centers for Disease Control household health survey stated that 1,270,000 Americans (0.7% of the US population) suffered from this disorder.[81] When it primarily affects the tongue, it is referred to as **burning tongue** or **glossody-**

nia. Grushka and her colleagues have conducted several studies to systematically characterize the features of this syndrome.[319–322]

Symptoms. Patients complain of intraoral burning, the tip and sides of the tongue being the most common sites, followed by the palate. Dry mouth, thirst, taste and sleep disturbances, headaches, and other pain complaints are frequently associated symptoms. **Onset is often related to a dental procedure**. The intensity of pain is quantitatively similar to that of toothache, although the quality is burning rather than pulsing, aching, or throbbing. The pain increases as the day progresses and tends to peak in early evening. Patients with burning mouth syndrome may complain of spontaneous tastes or **"taste phantoms" (dysgeusia)**.[323]

Etiology. There are many obvious oral and systemic conditions that are associated with mucogingival and glossal pains. These include candidiasis, geographic tongue, allergies to dental materials, denture dysfunction, xerostomia, various anemias and vitamin deficiencies (iron, vitamin B_{12}, or folic acid), diabetes mellitus, several dermatologic disorders (lupus, lichen planus, erythema multiforme), human immunodeficiency virus, or systemic medications (either directly or indirectly through resultant xerostomia).[81,324] However, in **burning mouth syndrome,** controlled studies have documented that the oral mucosa appears normal, and no obvious organic cause can be identified.[322] There is evidence for a higher incidence of immunologic abnormalities in burning mouth syndrome patients than would be expected in a normal population, and several burning mouth syndrome patients have been shown to have Sjögren's syndrome.[319]

Recent research supports the following theory on the etiology of pain and phantom tastes in burning mouth syndrome patients. The special sense of taste from the tongue is mediated by cranial nerves VII (anterior two-thirds) and IX (posterior one-third). Cranial nerve VII innervates the fungiform papillae of the tongue, which, in turn, are surrounded by pain fibers from cranial nerve V. Cranial nerve VII normally inhibits both cranial nerve V (pain fibers) and cranial nerve IX (taste). Damage or partial deafferentation of cranial nerve VII appears to release inhibition of both cranial nerves V and IX, producing both pain and taste phantoms, respectively.[324,325]

Burning mouth syndrome is not to be confused with postmenopausal oral discomfort, which has a burning component. In the latter condition, estrogen replacement therapy is effective about half of the time.[326]

Psychological factors, although present in some of this population, do not appear to be etiologic.[327,328]

Examination. The patient with burning mouth syndrome generally has a negative intraoral examination. Obvious tissue-irritating causes such as denture soreness, rough crowns or teeth, and other causes of tissue irritation such as candidiasis or true vitamin deficiencies must, of course, be ruled out.

Tests. Candidiasis should be tested for even if the mucosa looks normal. **Local anesthetic rinse** will decrease the pain of other conditions such as geographic tongue or candidiasis but **increase the pain of burning mouth.** This increase in pain is thought to be owing to further loss of A beta fiber inhibition. Sedimentation rate may be mildly elevated, and, in view of the higher incidence of immunologic abnormalities, rheumatologic evaluation should be considered.

Treatment. Studies assessing therapeutic outcome are lacking. Low-dose tricyclic antidepressants, such as amitriptyline, have had some success,[324] but newer open label studies suggest that clonazepam, both orally and topically, may be more useful.[329,330] Topical application of 0.5 or 1 mg clonazepam two or three times daily provided complete to significant relief in 19 of 25 patients.[330] Orally, low (0.25 to 0.75 mg) daily doses of **clonazepam** provided relief for 70% of 30 patients.[329] Addition of low doses of **valproic acid or imipramine** may be useful if more pain relief is required.[329]

The pain our patient complains of has none of the characteristics of either atypical odontalgia or burning mouth syndrome except for the burning quality. It is therefore unlikely that these diagnoses are causing her pain.

Thus, we have the following differential:

1. *Rule out reflex sympathetic dystrophy (sympathetically maintained pain) of the left side of the face.*
2. *Rule out post-traumatic neuralgia of cranial nerve V1–V3 on the left.*
3. *Myofascial TrP pain is likely to be contributing to the pain complaint.*
4. *There is internal derangement of the left TMJ with questionable contribution to the total pain complaint.*

How can one differentiate between 1 and 2? Sensory blocks of the trigeminal nerve in the past have provided temporary but not long-lasting relief. In fact, the pain returned with the return of sensation. To differentiate between a purely sensory neuralgia and RSD (sympathetically maintained pain), the definitive test is a stellate gan-

glion block. This will provide dramatic relief if the pain is sympathetically mediated and no relief if it is owing to a neuralgia.

Left sympathetic stellate ganglion block does indeed relieve this patient's pain, and the pain relief outlasts the duration of the local anesthetic. Although the patient is pain free, it is possible to complete a thorough musculoskeletal examination. Range of motion is restricted in the left TMJ, with deviation of the jaw to that side on opening. At 30 mm of mandibular depression, a loud crack is audible, and the patient is able to open wider. Active myofascial TrPs that refer pain into the forehead and along the side of the face are found in the upper trapezius, masseter, and lateral pterygoid muscles.

Management of this patient's pain will require repeated sympathetic blockade to control the sympathetically maintained pain. In addition, postural and stretching exercises, along with an intraoral stabilization splint, are indicated to reduce the MFP and stabilize the left TMJ. Spray and stretch, TrP pressure release, and/or TrP injections may facilitate the resolution of the MFP even further. Ultimately, dental treatment to restore left posterior dental support is indicated. Stress management and relaxation training may further help this patient control her pain. This is true because somatic and psychological factors are never separate in maintaining pain. Stress and anxiety will increase sympathetic activity, which will activate both the RSD and myofascial TrPs, both of which are intimately involved in this patient's pain.

This case illustrates the complexity of dealing with patients with persistent orofacial head and neck pain complaints. Multiple diagnoses and contributing factors are common. Multidisciplinary treatments are often required for rehabilitation. Rehabilitation includes treatment of the pathema causing the pain, as well as altering lifestyle habits and psychological concomitants that perpetuate the problem. A good liaison with a competent psychologist and physical therapist is invaluable when evaluating and treating these patients.

CONCLUSION

In conclusion, it is a time-consuming and difficult task to understand and manage people **suffering chronic pain.** Many interdisciplinary pain clinics employ orofacial pain dentists; physicians; psychologists; nurses; physical, occupational, and myotherapists; and other health professionals to coordinate patient care and to provide a comprehensive healthy environment for rehabilitation. Chronic pain management, including orofacial pain, has become a growing specialty in health care. It takes years of training and experience to gain adequate insight into these complex cases. Several dental schools across the United States now offer 2-year postgraduate orofacial pain programs to train interested dentists in the field of orofacial pain. Dentists with competence in this field can be identified by contacting the American Board of Orofacial Pain. This organization awards diplomate status to qualified dentists who pass their certification examination. Orofacial pain dentists, armed with knowledge, interest, curiosity, and patience, and, finally, the instruments of diagnosis, enjoy a most rewarding experience—identifying the source of pain and relieving the suffering of a fellow human being. **The orofacial pain dentist**, oriented toward looking at the patient as a whole person, can gain much satisfaction from arriving at a correct diagnosis and saving teeth or preventing unnecessary surgery.

The complex and personal nature of good diagnosis cannot be overemphasized. This is the area in which the dentist is most likely, on a professional basis, to earn the respect and friendship of his colleagues, both dental and medical, as well as that of his patients.

REFERENCES

1. Dorland's illustrated medical dictionary. Philadelphia: WB Saunders; 1974. Pain; p. 1119.
2. Beecher HK. Relationship of significance of wound to the pain experienced. JAMA 1956;161:1609.
3. Fields H. Pain. New York: McGraw-Hill Information Services Company, Health Professions Division; 1987.
4. Classification of chronic pain. Descriptions of chronic pain syndromes and definitions of pain terms. Pain 1986;3 Suppl 1.
5. The anatomy and physiology of pain. In: Osterweis M, Kleinman A, Mechanic D, editors. Pain and disability. Clinical, behavioral, and public policy perspectives, Institute of Medicine, Committee on Pain Disability, and Chronic Illness Behavior. Washington (DC): National Academy Press; 1987.
6. Basbaum AI, Levine JD. The contribution of the nervous system to inflammation and inflammatory disease. Can J Physiol Pharmacol 1991;69:647.
7. Fields HL, Rowbotham M, Baron R. Neuralgia: irritable nociceptors and deafferentation. Neurobiol Dis 1998;5:209.
8. Chapman LF. Mechanisms of the flare reaction in human skin. J Invest Dermatol 1977;69:88.
9. Pernow B. Substance P. Pharmacol Rev 1983;35:85.
10. Mendell LM, Wall PD. Responses of single dorsal cord cells to peripheral cutaneous unmyelinated fibers. Nature 1965;206:97.
11. Price DD, et al. Spatial and temporal transformations of input to spinothalamic tract neurons and their relation to somatic sensations. J Neurophysiol 1978;41:933.

12. Dickenson AH. Central acute pain mechanisms. Ann Med 1995;27:223.
13. Cervero F, Laird JM, Pozo MA. Selective changes of receptive field properties of spinal nociceptive neurones induced by noxious visceral stimulation in the cat. Pain 1992;51:513.
14. Price DD, Hu JW, Dubner R, Gracely RH. Peripheral suppression of first pain and central summation of second pain evoked by noxious heat pulses. Pain 1977;3:57.
15. Simone DA, Sorkin LS, et al. Neurogenic hyperalgesia: central neural correlates in responses of spinothalamic tract neurons. J Neurophysiol 1991;66:226.
16. Jones SL. Descending noradrenergic influences on pain. Prog Brain Res 1991;88:381.
17. Basbaum AI, Fields HL. Endogenous pain control systems: brainstem spinal pathways and endorphin circuitry. Annu Rev Neurosci 1984;7:309.
18. Kanjhan R. Opioids and pain. Clin Exp Pharmacol Physiol 1995;22:397.
19. Price DD. Psychological and neural mechanisms of the affective dimension of pain. Science 2000;288:1769.
20. Davis KD. The neural circuitry of pain as explored with functional MRI. Neurol Res 2000;22:313.
21. Milne RJ, et al. Convergence of cutaneous and pelvic visceral nociceptive inputs onto primate spinothalamic neurons. Pain 1981;11:163.
22. Sessle BJ, Greenwood LF. Inputs to trigeminal brain stem neurons from facial, oral, tooth pulp and pharyngolaryngeal tissues: I. Responses to innocuous and noxious stimuli. Brain Res 1976;117:211.
23. Hyashi H, Sumino R, Sessle BJ. Functional organization of trigeminal subnucleus interpolaris: nociceptive and innocuous afferent inputs. Projections to thalamus, cerebellum, and spinal cord, and descending modulation from periaqueductal gray. J Neurophysiol 1984;51:890.
24. Broton JG, Hu JW, Sessle BJ. Effects of temporomandibular joint stimulation on nociceptive and nonnociceptive neurons of the cat's trigeminal subnucleus caudalis (medullary dorsal horn). J Neurophysiol 1988;59:1575.
25. Kojima Y. Convergence patterns of afferent information from the temporomandibular joint and masseter muscle in the trigeminal subnucleus caudalis. Brain Res Bull 1990;24:609.
26. Sessle BJ. The neurobiology of facial and dental pain: present knowledge, future directions. J Dent Res 1987;66:962.
27. Kerr FWL. Facial, vagal and glossopharyngeal nerves in the cat: afferent connections. Arch Neurol 1962;6:624.
28. Mense S. Referral of muscle pain. New aspects. Am Pain Soc J 1994;3:1.
29. Hoheisel U, Mense S, Simons DG, Yu X-M. Appearance of new receptive fields in rat dorsal horn neurons following noxious stimulation of skeletal muscle: a model for referral of muscle pain? Neurosci Lett 1993;153:9–12.
30. Simons DG. Neurophysiological basis of pain caused by trigger points. APS J 1994;3:17–19.
31. Kunc Z. Significant factors pertaining to the results of trigeminal tractotomy. In: Hassler R, Walker AE, editors. Trigeminal neuralgia: pathogenesis and pathophysiology. Stuttgart: Georg Thieme Verlag; 1970. p. 90–100.
32. Pfaffenrath V, et al. Cervicogenic headache—the clinical picture, radiological findings and hypotheses on its pathophysiology. Headache 1987;27:495.
33. Head H. On disturbance of sensation with special reference to the pain of visceral disease. Brain 1893;16:1.
34. Kellgren JH. Observations on referred pain arising from muscle. Clin Sci 1938;3:175.
35. Devor M. The pathophysiology and anatomy of damaged nerve. In: Wall PD, Melzack R, editors. Textbook of pain. Edinburgh: Churchill Livingstone; 1984.
36. Joy ED, Barber J. Psychological, physiological, and pharmacological management of pain. Dent Clin North Am 1977;21:577.
37. Willis WD. The pain system. Basel: S. Karger; 1985.
38. Barber J. Rapid induction analgesia: a clinical report. Am J Clin Hypn 1977;19:138.
39. Barber TS. Toward a theory of pain: relief of chronic pain by prefrontal leukotomy, opiates, placebos, and hypnosis. Psychol Bull 1959;56:430.
40. Turk DC, Okifuji A. Evaluating the role of physical, operant, cognitive, and affective factors in the pain behaviors of chronic pain patients. Behav Modif 1997;21:259.
41. Scott J, Huskisson EC. Graphic representation of pain. Pain 1976;2:175.
42. Scott J, et al. The measurement of pain in juvenile chronic polyarthritis. Ann Rheum Dis 1977;36:186.
43. Huskisson EC. Visual analog scales. In: Melzack R, editor. Pain measurement and assessment. New York: Raven Press; 1973. p. 33–7.
44. Price DD, et al. The validation of visual analogue scale measures for chronic and experimental pain. Pain 1983;17:45.
45. Huskisson EC. Measurement of pain. Lancet 1974;ii:127.
46. Scott J, Huskisson EC. Accuracy of subjective measurements made with or without previous scores: an important source of error in serial measurements of subjective states. Ann Rheum Dis 1979;38:558.
47. Melzack R, Torgeson WS. On the language of pain. Anesthesiology 1971;34:50.
48. Melzack R. The McGill Pain Questionnaire: major properties and scoring methods. Pain 1975;1.
49. Rudy TE. Multiaxial assessment of pain. Multidimensional Pain Inventory: user's manual. University of Pittsburgh (PA): Departments of Anesthesiology and Psychiatry, Pain Evaluation and Treatment Institute; 1989.
50. Steer RA, Rissmiller DJ, Beck AT. Use of the Beck Depression Inventory-II with depressed geriatric patients. Behav Res Ther 2000;38:311.
51. Beck AT, Steer RA, Shaw BF, Emery G Psychometric properties of the Beck Depression Inventory: twenty-five years of evaluation. Clin Psychol Rev 1988;8:77.
52. Kames LD, et al. The Chronic Illness Problem Inventory: problem-oriented psychosocial assessment of patients with chronic illness. Int J Psychiatry Med 1984;14:65.
53. Hathaway SR, McKinley JC. The Minnesota Multiphasic Personality Inventory manual. New York: Psychological Corporation; 1967.
54. Headache Classification Committee of the International Headache Society. Classification and diagnostic criteria for headache disorders, cranial neuralgias and facial pain. Cephalalgia 1988;8 Suppl 7.
55. Simons DG, Travell JG, Simons LS. Travell and Simons' myofascial pain and dysfunction. The trigger point manual. Vol 1. Upper half of body. 2nd ed. Baltimore: Williams and Wilkins; 1999.
56. Lance JW. Mechanism and management of headache. 3rd ed. Boston: Butterworths; 1978.

57. Clark GT. Examining temporomandibular disorder patients for cranio-cervical dysfunction. J Craniomandib Pract 1984;2:55.
58. Hoppenfield S. Physical examination of the spine and extremities. New York: Appleton-Century Crofts; 1976.
59. Janda V. Some aspects of extracranial causes of facial pain. J Prosthet Dent 1986;56:484.
60. Fricton JR, Kroening R, Haley D, Siegert R. Myofascial pain syndrome of the head and neck: a review of clinical characteristics of 164 patients. Oral Surg 1985;160:615.
61. Okeson JP, editor. Orofacial pain. Guidelines for assessment, diagnosis, and management. American Academy of Orofacial Pain. Chicago: Quintessence; 1996.
62. Skootsky SA, Jaeger B, Oye RK. Prevalence of myofascial pain in general internal medicine practice. West J Med 1989;151:157.
63. Solberg WK. Myofascial pain and dysfunction. In: Clar JW, editor. Clinical dentistry. Hagerstown (MD): Harper and Row; 1976.
64. Fishbain DA, et al. Male and female chronic pain patients categorized by DSM-III psychiatric diagnostic criteria. Pain 1986;26:181.
65. Bates B. A guide to physical examination and history taking. 4th ed. Philadelphia: JB Lippincott; 1987.
66. Jaeger B, Skootsky SA. Male and female chronic pain patients categorized by DSM-III psychiatric diagnostic criteria [letter]. Pain 1987;29:263.
67. Munford P, Liberman RP. Behavior theory of hysterical disorders. In: Roy A, editor. Hysteria. New York: John Wiley & Sons; 1982.
68. Fordyce WE, Steger JC. Chronic pain. In: Pomerleau OF, Brady JP. Behavioral medicine: theory and practice. Baltimore: Williams & Wilkins; 1978. p. 125–54.
69. Fordyce WE. An operant conditioning method for managing chronic pain. Postgrad Med 1973;53:123.
70. Bell WE. Orofacial pains: classification, diagnosis, management. 3rd ed. Chicago: Year Book Medical Publishers; 1985.
71. Arthritis Foundation. Primer on the rheumatic diseases. JAMA 1973;224:663.
72. Birt D. Headaches and head pains associated with diseases of the ear, nose and throat. Med Clin North Am 1978;62:523.
73. Wolff HG. Headache and other head pain. New York: Oxford University Press; 1950.
74. Reynolds OE, Hutchins HC, et al. Aerodontalgia occurring during oxygen indoctrination in low pressure chamber. US Naval Med Bull 1946;46:845.
75. Gerbe RW, et al. Headache of nasal spur origin: an easily diagnosed and surgically correctable cause of facial pain. Headache 1984;24:329.
76. Dalessio DJ. Wolff's headache and other head pain. 3rd ed. New York: Oxford University Press; 1972.
77. Ballenger JJ. Diseases of the nose, throat and ear. 11th ed. Philadelphia: Lea & Febiger; 1969.
78. Sicher H. Problems of pain in dentistry. Oral Surg 1954;7:149.
79. Nenzen B, Walander U. The effect of conservative root canal therapy on local mucosal hyperplasia of the maxillary sinus. Odontol Rev 1967;18:295.
80. Solberg WK. Temporomandibular disorders. Br Dent J 1986.
81. Lipton JH, Ship JA, Larach-Robinson D. Estimated prevalence and distribution of reported orofacial pain in the United States. J Am Dent Assoc 1993;124:115.
82. American Academy of Orofacial Pain. McNeill C, editor. Temporomandibular disorders: guidelines for classification, assessment, and management. Chicago: Quintessence; 1993.
83. Bell W. Clinical management of temporomandibular disorders. Chicago: Yearbook Medical Publishers; 1982.
84. Guralnick W, Raban LB, Merrill RG. Temporomandibular joint afflictions. N Engl J Med 1978;123:299.
85. Gangarosa LP, Mahan PE. Pharmacologic management of TMD-MPDS. Ear Nose Throat J 1982;61:670.
86. Wenneberg B, Kopp S, Grondahl HG. Long-term effect of intra-articular injections of a glucocorticosteroid into the TMJ: a clinical and radiographic 8-year follow-up. J Craniomandib Disord 1991;5(1)11.
87. Rasmussen OC. Description of population and progress of symptoms in longitudinal study of temporomandibular arthropathy. Scand J Dent Res 1981;89:196.
88. Fricton JR. Recent advances in temporomandibular disorders and orofacial pain. J Am Dent Assoc 1991;122:25.
89. Greene CS, Laskin DM. Long term evaluation of treatment of myofascial pain-dysfunction syndrome: a comparative analysis. J Am Dent Assoc 1983;107:235.
90. Magnusson T, Carlsson GE, Egermark I. Changes in subjective symptoms of craniomandibular disorders in children and adolescents during a 10 year period. J Orofac Pain 1993;7:76.
91. Greene CS, Laskin DM. Long-term status of TMJ clicking in patients with myofascial pain and dysfunction. J Am Dent Assoc 1988;117:461.
92. Brandt KD, Slemenda CW. Osteoarthritis: epidemiology, pathology, and pathogenesis. In: Schumacher HR, editor. Primer on the rheumatic diseases. 10th ed. Atlanta: Arthritis Foundation; 1993. p.184–8.
93. Kreutziger KL, Mahan PE. Temporomandibular degenerative joint disease. Part I. Anatomy, pathophysiology, and clinical description. Oral Surg 1975;40:165.
94. Christian CL. Diseases of the joints. Part VII. In: Wyngaarden JB, Smith LH Jr. Cecil textbook of medicine. 15th ed. Philadelphia: WB Saunders; 1979. p. 185–93.
95. De Bont LGM, Boering G, Liem RSB, et al. Osteoarthritis of the temporomandibular joint: a light microscopic and scanning electron microscopic study of the articular cartilage of the mandibular condyle. J Oral Maxillofac Surg 1985;43:481.
96. Stegenga B, de Bont LGM, Boering G, et al. Tissue responses to degenerative changes in the temporomandibular joint: a review. J Oral Maxillofac Surg 1991;49:1079.
97. Katzberg RW, Westesson PL. Diagnosis of the temporomandibular joint. Philadelphia: WB Saunders; 1993.
98. Bell WE. Temporomandibular disorders: classification, diagnosis and management. 3rd ed. Chicago: Year Book; 1990.
99. Senia ES, Clarich JD. Arm pain of dental origin. Oral Surg 1974;38:960.
100. Alles A, Dom RM. Peripheral sensory nerve fibers that dichotomize to supply the brachium and the pericardium in the rat: a possible morphological explanation for referred cardiac pain? Brain Res 1985;342:382.
101. Laurberg S, Sorensen KE. Cervical dorsal root ganglion cells with collaterals to both shoulder skin and the diaphragm. A fluorescent double labeling study in the rat. A model for referred pain? Brain Res 1985;331:160.
102. Ruch TC, Fulton JF. Medical physiology and biophysics. 18th ed. Philadelphia: WB Saunders; 1960.

103. Batchelder BJ, et al. Mandibular pain as the initial and sole clinical manifestation of coronary insufficiency: report of case. J Am Dent Assoc 1987;115:710.
104. Natkin E, Harrington GW, et al. Anginal pain referred to the teeth. Oral Surg 1975; 40:678.
105. Bonica JJ. The management of pain. Vol II. Philadelphia: Lea & Febiger; 1990.
106. Matson MS. Pain in orofacial region associated with coronary insufficiency. Oral Surg 1963;16:284.
107. Norman JE de B. Facial pain and vascular disease: some clinical observations. Br J Oral Surg 1970;8:138.
108. Krant KS. Pain referred to teeth as the sole discomfort in undiagnosed mediastinal lymphoma. J Am Dent Assoc 1989;118:587.
109. Andreoli TE, et al, editors. Cecil essentials of medicine. Philadelphia: WB Saunders; 1986.
110. Russel HI. Roles of heredity, diet and emotional stress in coronary heart disease. JAMA 1959;171:503.
111. Wartofsky L, Ingbar SH. Diseases of the thyroid. In: Harrison's principles of internal medicine. 12th ed. Boston: McGraw-Hill; 1991.
112. Greene JN. Subacute thyroiditis. Am J Med 1971;63:729.
113. Fay T. Atypical facial neuralgia, a syndrome of vascular pain. Ann Otol Rhinol Laryngol 1932;41:1030.
114. Lovshin LL. Carotidynia. Headache 1977;17:192.
115. Hill LM, Hastings G. Carotidynia: a pain syndrome. J Fam Pract 1994;39:71.
116. Sheon RP, et al. Soft tissue rheumatic pain. Philadelphia: Lea & Febiger; 1987.
117. Cannon CR. Carotidynia: an unusual pain in the neck. Otolaryngol Head Neck Surg 1994;110:387.
118. Troiano NF, Gerald WG. Carotid system arteries: an overlooked and misdiagnosed syndrome. J Am Dent Assoc 1975;91:589.
119. Bland JH. Disorders of the cervical spine. Philadelphia: WB Saunders; 1987.
120. Edmeads V. Headaches and head pains associated with diseases of the cervical spine. Med Clin North Am 1978;62:533.
121. Rocabado M. Diagnosis and treatment of abnormal craniocervical and craniomandibular mechanics. In: Head, neck and temporomandibular joint dysfunction manual. Tacoma (WA): Rocabado Institute; 1981. p. 1–21.
122. Bogduc N. The anatomy of occipital neuralgia. J Clin Exp Neuropsychol 1981;17:167.
123. Sjaastad O, Saunte C, et al. "Cervicogenic" headache. A hypothesis. Cephalalgia 1983;3:249.
124. Pfaffenrath V, Dandekar R, et al. Cervicogenic headache: results of computer-based measurements of cervical spine mobility in 15 patients. Cephalalgia 1988;8:45.
125. Jaeger B. Are "cervicogenic" headaches due to myofascial pain and cervical spine dysfunction? Cephalalgia 1989;9:157.
126. Jannetta PJ. Pain problems of significance in head and face, some of which often are misdiagnosed. Curr Probl Surg 1973;47:53.
127. Walker AE. Neurosurgical aspects of head pain. In: Appenseller O, editor. Pathogenesis and treatment of headache. Wallingford (CT): Spectrum; 1976. p. 148–9.
128. Nurmikko TJ. Mechanisms of central pain. Clin J Pain 2000;16(2 Suppl):S21.
129. Spierings ELH. Recent advances in the understanding of migraine. Headache 1988;28:655.
130. Moskowitz MA. Basic mechanisms in vascular headache. Neurol Clin 1990;8:801.
131. Olesen J, et al. Focal hyperemia followed by oligemia and impaired activation of rCBF in classic migraine. Ann Neurol 1981;9:344.
132. Lauritzen M, et al. Changes in regional cerebral blood flow during the course of classic migraine attacks. Ann Neurol 1983;13:633.
133. Saito K, et al. Ergot alkaloids block neurogenic extravasation in dura mater: proposed action in vascular headaches. Ann Neurol 1988;24:732.
134. Lance JW. Current concepts of migraine pathogenesis. Neurology 1993;43 Suppl 3 :S11.
135. Tfelt-Hansen P, et al. Prevalence and significance of muscle tenderness during common migraine attacks. Headache 1981;2:45.
136. Lous I, Olesen J. Evaluation of pericranial tenderness and oral function in patients with common migraine, muscle contraction headache and combination headache. Pain 1982;12:385.
137. Hachinski VC, et al. Cerebral hemodynamics in migraine. Can Sci Neurol 1977;4:245.
138. Rapoport AM, et al. Correlations of facial thermographic patterns and headache diagnosis. In: Abernathy M, Uematsu S, editors. Medical thermology. Washington (DC): American Academy of Thermology; 1986. p. 56.
139. Volta GD, Anzola GP. Are there objective criteria to follow up migrainous patients? A prospective study with thermography and evoked potentials. Headache 1988;28:423.
140. Diamond S, Dalessio DJ. Migraine headache. In: Diamond S, Dalessio DJ, editors. The practicing physician's approach to headache. 4th ed. Baltimore: Williams and Wilkins; 1986. p. 50–6.
141. Diamond S, Dalessio DJ. Cluster headache. In: Diamond S, Dalessio DJ, editors. The practicing physician's approach to headache. 4th ed. Baltimore: Williams and Wilkins; 1986. p. 66–75.
142. Goadsby PJ. Cluster headache: new perspectives. Cephalalgia 1999;19 Suppl 25:39–41.
143. Bittar G, Graff-Radford SB. A retrospective study of patients with cluster headache. Oral Surg 1992;73:519.
144. Benoliel R, Sharav Y. Paroxysmal hemicrania. Case studies and review of the literature. Oral Surg Oral Med Oral Pathol Oral Radiol Endod 1998;85:285–92.
145. Sjaastad O, Dale I. A new(?) clinical headache entity, "chronic paroxysmal hemicrania." Acta Neurol Scand 1976;54:140.
146. Delcanho RE, Graff-Radford SB. Chronic paroxysmal hemicrania presenting as toothache. J Orofac Pain 1993; 7:300–6.
147. Sjaastad O, et al. Chronic paroxysmal hemicrania: mechanical precipitation of attacks. Headache 1979;19:31.
148. Sjaastad O, et al. Chronic paroxysmal hemicrania (CPH). The clinical manifestations. A review. Ups J Med Sci 1980;31 Suppl:27.
149. Dodick DW, Rozen TD, Goadsby PJ, Silberstein SD. Cluster headache. Cephalalgia 2000;9:787–803.
150. Waldenlind E, et al. Decreased nocturnal serum melatonin levels during active cluster headache periods. Opus Med 1984;29:109.
151. May A, Bahra A, Buchel C, et al. Hypothalamic activation in cluster headache attacks. Lancet 1998;352:275–8.

152. Martelletti P, Giacovazzo M. Putative neuroimmunological mechanisms in cluster headache. An integrated hypothesis. Headache 1996;36:312.
153. Russel D. Clinical characterization of the cluster headache syndrome. In: Olesen J, Edvinnson L, editors. Basic mechanisms of headache. Amsterdam: Elsevier Science; 1988. p. 21.
154. Evers S, Bauer B, Suhr B, et al. Cognitive processing is involved in cluster headache but not in chronic paroxysmal hemicrania. Neurology 1999;53:357–63.
155. Ekbom K. Treatment of cluster headache: clinical trials, design and results. Cephalalgia 1995;15 Suppl 15:33–6.
156. Gobel H, Lindner V, Heinze A, et al. Acute therapy for cluster headache with sumatriptan: findings of a one-year long-term study. Neurology 1998;51:908–11.
157. O'Brien MD, et al. Trigeminal nerve section for unremitting migrainous neuralgia. In: Rose FC, Zilkha KJ, editors. Progress in migraine research I. London: Pittman Books; 1981. p. 185.
158. Delassio DJ. Surgical therapy of cluster headache. In: Mathew N, editor. Cluster headache. New York: Spectrum; 1984. p. 119.
159. Salvesen R. Cluster headache. Curr Treat Option Neurol 1999;1:441.
160. Ford RG, Ford KT, Swaid S, et al. Gamma knife treatment of refractory cluster headache. Headache 1998;38:3–9.
161. Kunkel RS. Complications and rare forms of migraine. In: Olesen J, Edvinnson L, editors. Basic mechanisms of headache. Amsterdam: Elsevier Science; 1988. p. 82.
162. Friedlander AH, Runyon C. Polymyalgia rheumatic and temporal arteritis. Oral Surg 1990;69:317.
163. Guttenberg SA, et al. Cranial arteritis odontogenic pain: report of a case. J Am Dent Assoc 1989;119:621.
164. Diamond S, Dalessio DJ. The practicing physician's approach to headache. 4th ed. Baltimore: Williams & Wilkins; 1986.
165. Waters WE. Headache and blood pressure in the community. BMJ 1971;1:142.
166. Penman J. Trigeminal neuralgia. In: Vinken PJ, Bruyn GW, editors. Handbook of clinical neurology. Vol 5. Amsterdam: Elsevier; 1968. p. 296–322.
167. Mitchell RG. Pre-trigeminal neuralgia. Br Dent J 1980;149:167.
168. Merrill RL, Graff-Radford SB. Trigeminal neuralgia: how to rule out the wrong treatment. J Am Dent Assoc 1992;123:63.
169. Rushton JG, et al. Glossopharyngeal (vagoglossopharyngeal) neuralgia. Arch Neurol 1981;38:201.
170. Walker AE. Neuralgias of the glossopharyngeal, vagus and nervus intermedius nerves. In: Knighton PR, Dumke PR, editors. Pain. Boston: Little, Brown; 1966. p. 421–9.
171. Balbuena L Jr, Hayes D, Ramirez SG, Johnson R. Eagle's syndrome. South Med J 1997;90:331.
172. Massey EW, Massey J. Elongated styloid process (Eagle's syndrome) causing hemicrania. Headache 1979;19:339.
173. Sivers JE, Johnson GK. Diagnosis of Eagle's syndrome. Oral Surg 1985;59:575.
174. Dubuisson D. Nerve root damage and arachnoiditis. In: Wall PD, Melzack R, editors. Textbook of pain. New York: Churchill Livingstone; 1984. p. 436.
175. White UC, Sweet WH. Pain and the neurosurgeon. Springfield (IL): Charles C. Thomas; 1969.
176. Sulfaro MA, Gobetti JP. Occipital neuralgia manifesting as orofacial pain. Oral Surg 1995;80:751.
177. Fromm GH, Terrence CF, Maroon JC. Trigeminal neuralgia. Current concepts regarding etiology and pathogenesis. Arch Neurol 1984;41:1204.
178. Janetta PJ. Surgical treatment: microvascular decompression. In: Fromm GH, Sessle BJ, editors. Trigeminal neuralgia: current concepts regarding pathogenesis and treatment. Boston: Butterworth-Heinemann; 1991. p. 145–57.
179. Casamassimo PS, et al. Diabetic polyradiculopathy with trigeminal nerve involvement. Oral Surg 1988;66:315.
180. Ratner EJ, Person P, Klieman DJ, et al. Jawbone cavities and trigeminal and atypical facial neuralgias. Oral Surg 1979;48:3.
181. Roberts AM, Person P. Etiology and treatment of idiopathic trigeminal and atypical facial neuralgias. Oral Surg 1979;48:298.
182. Roberts AJ, Person P, et al. Further observations on dental parameters of trigeminal and atypical facial neuralgias. Oral Surg 1984;58:121.
183. Ratner JR, et al. Alveolar cavitational osteopathosis: manifestations of an infectious process and its implication in the causation of pain. J Periodontol 1987;58:77.
184. Bouquot JE, Roberts AM, Person P, Christian J. Neuralgia-inducing cavitational osteonecrosis (NICO). Osteomyelitis in 224 jawbone samples from patients with facial neuralgia. Oral Surg 1992;73:307.
185. Spolnik KJ. Ratner bone cavity: something to consider in differential diagnosis. Presentation before the American Association of Endodontists, Chicago, IL, April 29, 1993.
186. Shaber EP, Krol AJ. Trigeminal neuralgia—a new treatment concept. Oral Surg 1980;49:286.
187. Mathis BJ, et al. Jawbone cavities associated with facial pain syndromes: case reports. Mil Med 1981;146:719.
188. Sist T. Lecture on orofacial pain, Eisenhower Hospital, Rancho Mirage, CA, September 1983.
189. Lin L, Langeland K. Innervation of the inflammatory periradicular lesions. Oral Surg 1981;51:535.
190. Bouquot JE, Christian J. Long-term effects of jawbone curettage on the pain of facial neuralgia. J Oral Maxillofac Surg 1995;53:387; discussion 397.
191. Loeser JD. Tic douloureux and atypical facial pain. RCDC symposium. J Can Dent Assoc 1985;51:917.
192. Raskin N. Residual infection in bone. Presentation before the American Association for the Study of Headache and Facial Pain, Quebec City, QC, June 19, 1987.
193. Laha RK, Jannetta PJ. Glossopharyngeal neuralgia. J Neurosurg 1977;47:316.
194. Andrychowski J, Nauman P, Czernicki Z. Occipital nerve neuralgia as postoperative complication. Views on etiology and treatment. Neurol Neurochir Pol 1998;32:871.
195. Graff-Radford SB, Jaeger B, Reeves JL. Myofascial pain may present clinically as occipital neuralgia. Neurosurgery 1986;19:610.
196. Pinsaesdi P, Seltzer S. The induction of trigeminal neuralgia-like pain and endodontically treated teeth. JOE 1988;14:360.
197. Francica F, et al. Trigeminal neuralgia and endodontically treated teeth. JOE 1988;14:360.
198. Fromm GH. Etiology and pathogenesis of trigeminal neuralgia. In: Fromm GH, editor. The medical and surgical management of trigeminal neuralgia. Mount Kisco (NY): Futura; 1987. p. 31–41.
199. Cheng TMW, Cascino TL, Onofrio BM. Comprehensive study of diagnosis and treatment of trigeminal neuralgia secondary to tumors. Neurology 1993;43:2298.

200. Druigan MC, et al. Occipital neuralgia in adolescents and young adults. N Engl J Med 1962;267:1166.
201. Varady P, Dheerendra P, Nyary I, et al. Neurosurgery using the gamma knife. Orv Hetil 1999;14;140:331.
202. Young RF, Vermulen S, Posewitz A. Gamma knife radiosurgery for the treatment of trigeminal neuralgia. Stereotact Funct Neurosurg 1998;70 Suppl 1:192.
203. Pollock BE, Gorman DA, Schomberg PJ, Kline RW. The Mayo Clinic gamma knife experience: indications and initial results. Mayo Clin Proc 1999;74:5.
204. Burchiel KJ, et al. Comparison of percutaneous radiofrequency gangliolysis and microvascular decompression for the surgical management of tic douloureux. Neurosurgery 1981;9:111.
205. Lee KH, Chang JW, Park YG Chung SS. Microvascular decompression and percutaneous rhizotomy in trigeminal neuralgia. Stereotact Funct Neurosurg 1997;68(1–4 Pt 1):196.
206. Broggi G, Ferroli P, Franzini A, et al. Microvascular decompression for trigeminal neuralgia: comments on a series of 250 cases, including 10 patients with multiple sclerosis. J Neurol Neurosurg Psychiatry 2000;68:59.
207. Cappabianca P, Spaziante R, Graziussi G, et al. Percutaneous retrogasserian glycerol rhizolysis for treatment of trigeminal neuralgia. Technique and results in 191 patients. J Neurosurg Sci 1995;39:37.
208. Lunsford LD. Treatment of tic douloureux by percutaneous retrogasserian glycerol injection. JAMA 1982;248:449.
209. Sweet WH, Wepsie JG. Controlled thermocoagulation of the trigeminal ganglion and rootlets for differential destruction of pain fibers. J Neurosurg 1974;40:143.
210. Fromm GH, et al. Pretrigeminal neuralgia. Neurology 1990;40:1493.
211. Kondo A. Follow-up results of using microvascular decompression for treatment of glossopharyngeal neuralgia. J Neurosurg 1998;88:221.
212. Meglio M, Cioni B. Percutaneous procedures for trigeminal neuralgia: microcompression versus radio-frequency thermocoagulation. Pain 1989;38:9.
213. Lazorthes Y, Verde JC. Radiofrequency coagulation of the petrous ganglion in glossopharyngeal neuralgia. Neurosurgery 1979;4:512.
214. Laha JM, Tew JM Jr. Long-term results of surgical treatment of idiopathic neuralgias of the glossopharyngeal and vagal nerves. Neurosurgery 1995;36:926.
215. Hunter CR, Mayfield SH. Role of the upper cervical roots in the production of pain in the head. Am J Surg 1949;78:743.
216. Campbell JK, Cassel RD. Headache and other craniofacial pain. In: Bradley WG, Daraf RL, Finical GM, Marston CD, editors. Neurology in clinical practice. Boston: Butterworth-Heinemann; 1989. p. 1543.
217. Lovely TJ, Jannetta PJ. Surgical management of geniculate neuralgia. Am J Otol 1997;18:512.
218. Bruyn GW. Nervus intermedius neuralgia (Hunt). Superior laryngeal neuralgia. In: Rose FC, editor. Headache. Handbook of clinical neurology. Vol 4. Amsterdam: Elsevier; 1986. p. 487–500.
219. Devor M. The pathophysiology and anatomy of damaged nerve. In: Wall PD, Melzack R, editors. Textbook of pain. New York: Churchill-Livingstone; 1984. p. 51.
220. Hansen HJ. Neuro-histological reactions following tooth extractions. Int J Oral Surg 1980;9:411.
221. Peszkowski MJ, Larsson A. Extraosseous and intraosseous oral traumatic neuromas and their association with tooth extraction. J Oral Maxillofac Surg 1990;48:963.
222. Robinson M, Slavkin H. Dental amputation neuromas. J Am Dent Assoc 1965;70:662.
223. Burchiel KJ, Johans TJ, Ochoa J. The surgical treatment of painful traumatic neuromas. J Neurosurg 1993;78:714.
224. Head H, Campbell AW. The pathology of herpes zoster and its bearing on sensory location. Brain 1900;23:353.
225. Lhermitte J, Nicholas M. Les lésions spinales du zona. La myelte zosterienne. Rev Neurol 1924;1:361.
226. Denny-Brown D, et al. Pathologic features of herpes zoster: a note on "geniculate herpes." Arch Neurol Psychiatry 1944;77:337.
227. Watson CP, Evans RJ, Watt VR. Post-herpetic neuralgia and topical capsaicin. Pain 1988;33:333.
228. Watson CP, Deck JH, Morshead C, et al. Post-herpetic neuralgia: further post-mortem studies of cases with and without pain. Pain 1991;44:105.
229. Tyring SK. Advances in the treatment of herpesvirus infection: the role of famciclovir. Clin Ther 1998;20:661.
230. Goon WWY, Jacobsen PL. Prodromal odontalgia and multiple devitalized teeth caused by a herpes zoster infection of the trigeminal nerve: report of case. J Am Dent Assoc 1988;116:500.
231. Baron R, Saguer M. Postherpetic neuralgia. Are C-nociceptors involved in signaling and maintenance of tactile allodynia? Brain 1993;116:1477.
232. Nurmikko T, Bowsher D. Somatosensory findings in postherpetic neuralgia. J Neurol Neurosurg Psychiatry 1990;53:135.
233. Barrett AP, et al. Zoster sine herpete of the trigeminal nerve. Oral Surg 1993;75:173.
234. Johnson RW. Herpes zoster and postherpetic neuralgia. Optimal treatment. Drugs Aging 1997;10:80.
235. Beydoun A. Postherpetic neuralgia: role of gabapentin and other treatment modalities. Epilepsia 1999;40 Suppl 6:S51–6.
236. Diamond S. Postherpetic neuralgia. Prevention and treatment. Postgrad Med 1987;81:321.
237. Boas RA. Sympathetic nerve blocks: in search of a role. Reg Anesth Pain Med 1998;23:292.
238. Juel-Jenson BE, et al. Treatment of zoster with idoxuridine in dimethyl sulphoxide. Results of two double blind controlled trials. BMJ 1970;IV:776.
239. Canavan D, Graff-Radford SB, Gratt B. Traumatic dysesthesia of the trigeminal nerve. J Orofac Pain 1994;4:391.
240. Meyerson BA, Hakanson S. Suppression of pain in trigeminal neuropathy by electrical stimulation of the gasserian ganglion. Neurosurgery 1986;18:59.
241. Mitchell SW, et al. Gunshot wounds and other injuries of nerves. Philadelphia: JB Lippincott; 1864.
242. Evans JA. Reflex sympathetic dystrophy: report on 57 cases. Ann Intern Med 1947;26:417.
243. Bingham JAE. Causalgia of the face. Two cases successfully treated by sympathectomy. BMJ 1947;1:804.
244. Stanton-Hicks M, Janig W, Hassenbusch S, et al. Reflex sympathetic dystrophy: changing concepts and taxonomy. Pain 1995;63:127.
245. Galer BS, Bruehl S, Harden RN. IASP diagnostic criteria for complex regional pain syndrome: a preliminary empirical validation study. International Association for the Study of Pain. Clin J Pain 1998;14(1):48.

246. Bruehl S, Harden RN, Galer BS, et al. External validation of IASP diagnostic criteria for complex regional pain syndrome and proposed research diagnostic criteria. International Association for the Study of Pain. Pain 1999;81:147.
247. Detakats G. Sympathetic reflex dystrophy. Med Clin North Am 1963;49:117.
248. Jaeger B, Singer E, Kroening R. Reflex sympathetic dystrophy of the face: report of two cases and a review of the literature. Arch Neurol 1986;43:693.
249. Janig W, Levine JD, Michaelis M. Interactions of sympathetic and primary afferent neurons following nerve injury and tissue trauma. Prog Brain Res 1996;113:161.
250. Sato J, Perl ER. Adrenergic excitation of cutaneous pain receptors induced by peripheral nerve injury. Science 1991;251:1608.
251. Habler HJ, Janig W, Koltzenburg M. Activation of unmyelinated afferents in chronically lesioned nerves by adrenaline and excitation of sympathetic efferents in the cat. Neurosci Lett 1987;82:35.
252. Aguayo AJ, Bray GM. Pathology and pathophysiology of unmyelinated nerve fibers. In: Dyck PJ, Thomas PK, Lambert EH, editors. Peripheral neuropathy. Philadelphia: WB Saunders; 1975. p. 363–78.
253. Belenky M, Devor M. Association of postganglionic sympathetic neurons with primary afferents in sympathetic-sensory co-cultures. J Neurocytol 1997;26:715.
254. Chung K, Yoon YW, Chung JM. Sprouting sympathetic fibers form synaptic varicosities in the dorsal root ganglion of the rat with neuropathic injury. Brain Res 1997;751:275.
255. McLachlan EM, Jang W, Devor M, Michaelis M. Peripheral nerve injury triggers noradrenergic sprouting within dorsal root ganglia. Nature 1993;363:543.
256. Walker AE, Nulson F. Electrical stimulation of the upper thoracic portion of the sympathetic chain in man. Arch Neurol Psychiatry 1948;59:559.
257. Lipman AG. Analgesic drugs for neuropathic and sympathetically maintained pain. Clin Geriatr Med 1996;12:501.
258. Friction J, et al. Myofascial pain and dysfunction of the head and neck: a review of the clinical characteristics of 164 patients. Oral Surg 1985;60:615.
259. Layzer RB. Diagnostic implications of clinical fasciculations and cramps. In: Rowland LP, editor. Human motor neuron diseases. New York: Raven; 1982. p. 23–7.
260. Roth G. The origin of fasciculations. Ann Neurol 1982;12:542.
261. Jaeger B. Myofascial referred pain patterns: the role of trigger points. Can Dent Assoc J 1985;13:27.
262. Travell J, et al. Effects of referred somatic pain on structures in the reference zone. Fed Proc 1944;3:49.
263. Carlson CR, Okeson JP, Falace DA, et al. Reduction of pain and EMG activity in the masseter region by trapezius trigger point injection. Pain 1993;55:397.
264. Travell J. Temporomandibular joint dysfunction: temporomandibular joint pain referred from muscles of the head and neck. J Prosthet Dent 1960;10:745.
265. Lewit K. Manipulative therapy in rehabilitation of the locomotor system. 2nd ed. Oxford: Butterworth Heinemann; 1991.
266. Simons DG. Referred phenomena of myofascial trigger points. In: Vecchiet L, Albe-Fessard D, Lindblom U, Giamberardino MA, editors. New trends in referred pain and hyperalgesia. Pain research and clinical management. No 27. Amsterdam: Elsevier Science; 1993. p. 341–57.
267. Salins PC, et al. Bursitis: a factor in the differential diagnosis of orofacial neuralgias and myofascial pain dysfunction syndrome. Oral Surg 1989;68:154.
268. Hong C-Z, Chen Y-N, Twehous D, Hong DH. Pressure threshold for referred pain by compression on the trigger point and adjacent areas. J Musculoskel Pain 1996;4:61.
269. Kleinegger CL, Lilly GE. Cranial arteritis: a medical emergency with orofacial manifestations. J Am Dent Assoc 1999; 130:1203.
270. Simons DG. Myofascial pain syndrome of head, neck, and low back. In: Dubner R, Gebhart GF, Bond MR, editors. Pain research and clinical management. Vol 3: proceedings of the Fifth World Congress on Pain. Amsterdam: Elsevier Science; 1988.
271. Travell JG, Simons DG. Myofascial pain and dysfunction. The trigger point manual. Vol 2. The lower extremities. Baltimore: Williams and Wilkins; 1992.
272. Miehlke K, et al. Clinical and experimental studies on the fibrositis syndrome. Z Rheumaforsch 1960;19:310.
273. Yunus M, Kalyan-Raman UP. Muscle biopsy findings in primary fibromyalgia and other forms of non-articular rheumatism. Rheum Dis Clin North Am 1989;15:115.
274. Hubbard DR, Berkoff GM. Myofascial trigger points show spontaneous needle EMG activity. Spine 1993;18:1803.
275. McNulty WH, Gevirtz RN, Hubbard DR, Berkoff GM. Needle electromyographic evaluation of trigger point response to a psychological stressor. Psychophysiology 1994;31:313.
276. Hong C-Z, Simons DG. Pathophysiologic and electrophysiologic mechanisms of myofascial trigger points. Arch Phys Med Rehabil 1998;79:863.
277. Hubbard DR. Chronic and recurrent muscle pain: pathophysiology and treatment, and review of pharmacologic studies. J Musculoskel Pain 1996;4:123–124..
278. Chen JT, Chen SM, Kuan TS, et al. Phentolamine effect on the spontaneous electrical activity of active loci in a myofascial trigger spot of rabbit skeletal muscle. Arch Phys Med Rehabil 1998;79:790.
279. Wheeler AH, Goolkasian P, Gretz SS. A randomized double-blind prospective pilot study of botulinum toxin. Injection for refractory unilateral cervical-thoracic paraspinal myofascial pain syndrome. Spine 1998;23:1662.
280. Simons D. Clinical and etiological update of myofascial pain from trigger points. J Musculoskel Pain 1996;4:93.
281. Simons DG, Hong C-Z, Simons LS. Nature of myofascial trigger points, active loci [abstract]. J Musculoskel Pain 1995;3 Suppl 1:62.
282. Reeves JL, Jaeger B, Graff-Radford SB. Reliability of the pressure algometer as a measure of trigger point sensitivity. Pain 1986;24:313.
283. Vecchiet L, Giamberardino MA, de Bigontina P, Dragani L. Comparative sensory evaluation of parietal tissues in painful and non-painful areas in fibromyalgia and myofascial pain syndrome. In: Gebhart GF, Hammond DL, Jensen TS, editors. Proceedings of the 7th World Congress on Pain. Progress in pain research and management. Vol 2. Seattle: IASP Press; 1994. p. 177–249.
284. Fricton JR, et al. Myofascial pain syndrome: electromyographic changes associated with local twitch response. Arch Phys Med Rehabil 1986;66:314.
285. Hong C-Z, Torigoe Y, Yu J. The localized twitch responses in responsive taut bands of rabbit skeletal muscle fibers are related to the reflexes at spinal cord level. J Musculoskel Pain 1995;3:15.

286. Hong C-Z, Torigoe Y. Electrophysiological characteristics of localized twitch responses in responsive taut bands of rabbit skeletal muscle. J Musculoskel Pain 1994;2:17.
287. Vecchiet L, Vecchiet J, Giamerardino MA. Referred muscle pain: clinical and pathophysiologic aspects. Curr Rev Pain 1999;3;489.
288. Travell JG, et al. The myofascial genesis of pain. Postgrad Med 1952;11:425.
289. Graff-Radford SB, Reeves JL, Jaeger B. Management of head and neck pain: the effectiveness of altering perpetuating factors in myofascial pain. Headache 1987;27:186.
290. Sola A. Trigger point therapy. In: Roberts JR, Hedges JR, editors. Clinical proceedings in emergency medicine. 2nd ed. Philadelphia: WB Saunders; 1991. p. 828.
291. Komiyama O, Kawara M, Arai M, et al. Posture correction as part of behavioural therapy in treatment of myofacial pain with limited opening. J Oral Rehabil 1999;26:428.
292. Jaeger B, Reeves JL. Quantification of changes in myofascial trigger point sensitivity with the pressure algometer. Pain 1986;27:203.
293. Hong C-Z. Lidocaine injection versus dry needling to myofascial trigger point. The importance of the local twitch response. Am J Phys Med Rehabil 1994;73:256.
294. Frost FA, et al. A control, double-blind comparison of mepivacaine injection versus saline injection for myofascial pain. Lancet 1980;1:499.
295. Hameroff SR, et al. Comparison of bupivacaine, etidocaine, and saline for trigger-point therapy. Anesth Analg 1981;60:752.
296. Lewit K. The needle effect in the relief of myofascial pain. Pain 1979;6:83.
297. Benoit PW. Microscarring in skeletal muscle after repeated exposures to lidocaine with epinephrine. J Oral Surg 1978;36:530.
298. Jaeger B. Tension-type headache and myofascial pain. In: Fricton JR, Dubner R, editors. Advances in pain research and therapy. Vol 21. New York: Raven Press; 1995.
299. Mock D, et al. Atypical facial pain: a retrospective study. Oral Surg 1985;59:472.
300. Fricton JR. Atypical orofacial pain disorders: a study of diagnostic subtypes. Curr Rev Pain 2000;4:142–7.
301. Graff-Radford SB. Facial pain. Curr Opin Neurol 2000;13:291–6.
302. Pfaffenrath V, Rath M, Pollmann W, Keeser W. Atypical facial pain—application of the IHS criteria in a clinical sample. Cephalalgia 1993;13 Suppl 12:84–8.
303. Marbach JJ, Raphael KG. Phantom tooth pain: a new look at an old dilemma. Pain Med 2000;1(1):68.
304. Rees RT, Harris M. Atypical odontalgia. Br J Oral Surg 1978–9;16:212.
305. Woda A, Pionchon P. A unified concept of idiopathic orofacial pain: clinical features. J Orofac Pain 1999;13:172.
306. Solberg WK, Graff-Radford SB. Orodental considerations in facial pain. Semin Neurol 1988;8:318.
307. al Balawi S, Tariq M, Feinmann C. A double-blind, placebo-controlled, crossover, study to evaluate the efficacy of subcutaneous sumatriptan in the treatment of atypical facial pain. Int J Neurosci 1996;86:301.
308. Harrison SD, Balawi SA, Feinmann C, Harris M. Atypical facial pain: a double-blind placebo-controlled crossover pilot study of subcutaneous sumatriptan. Euro Neuropsychopharmacol 1997;7:83.
309. Marbach JJ. Is phantom tooth pain a deafferentation (neuropathic syndrome)? Part I. Oral Surg 1993;75:95.
310. Marbach JJ. Is phantom tooth pain a deafferentation (neuropathic syndrome)? Part II. Oral Surg 1993;75:225.
311. Reik L. Atypical facial pain. Headache 1985;25:30.
312. Feinman C. Pain relief by antidepressants: possible modes of action. Pain 1985;23:1.
313. Graff-Radford SB, Solberg WK. Is atypical odontalgia a psychological problem? Oral Surg 1993;75:579.
314. Vickers ER, Cousins MJ, Walker S, Chisholm K. Analysis of 50 patients with atypical odontalgia. A preliminary report on pharmacological procedures for diagnosis and treatment. Oral Surg 1998;85:24.
315. Woda A, Pioncho P. A unified concept of idiopathic orofacial pain: pathophysiologic features. J Orofac Pain 2000;14:196.
316. Graff-Radford SB, Ketelaer MC, Gratt BM, Solberg WK. Thermographic assessment of neuropathic facial pain. J Orofac Pain 1995;9:138.
317. Bates RE Jr, Stewart CM. Atypical odontalgia: phantom tooth pain. Oral Surg 1991;72:479.
318. McQuay HJ, Tramer M, Nye BA, et al. A systematic review of antidepressants in neuropathic pain. Pain 1996;68:217.
319. Grushka M. Clinical features of burning mouth syndrome. Oral Med 1987;63:30.
320. Grushka M, et al. Psychophysical evidence of taste dysfunction in burning mouth syndrome. Chem Senses 1986;11:485.
321. Grushka M, et al. Pain and personality profiles in burning mouth syndrome. Pain 1987;28:155.
322. Grushka M, Sesse BJ. Demographic data and pain profile of burning mouth syndrome (BMS). J Dent Res 1985;64:1648.
323. Bartoshuk LM, Grushka M, Duffy VB, et al. Burning mouth syndrome: a pain phantom in supertasters who suffer taste damage? [abstract]. San Diego (CA): American Pain Society; 1998.
324. Mott AE, Grushka M, Sessle BJ. Diagnosis and management of taste disorders and burning mouth syndrome. Dent Clin North Am 1993;37:33.
325. Grushka M, Bartoshuk LM. Burning mouth syndrome and oral dysesthesia. Can J Diagn 2000;17:99.
326. Forabosco A, et al. Efficacy of hormone replacement therapy in postmenopausal women with oral discomfort. Oral Surg 1992;73:570.
327. Grushka M, Sessle BJ. Burning mouth syndrome. Dent Clin North Am 1991;35:171.
328. Bogetto F, Maina G, Ferro G, et al. Psychiatric comorbidity in patients with burning mouth syndrome. Psychosom Med 1998;60:378.
329. Grushka M, Epstein J, Mott A. An open-label, dose escalation pilot study of the effect of clonazepam in burning mouth syndrome. Oral Surg 1998;86:557.
330. Woda A, Navez ML, Picard P, et al. A possible therapeutic solution for stomatodynia (burning mouth syndrome). J Orofac Pain 1998;12:272.

Chapter 9

PREPARATION FOR ENDODONTIC TREATMENT

John I. Ingle, Richard E. Walton, Stanley F. Malamed, Jeffrey M. Coil, John A. Khademi, Frederick H. Kahn, Barnet B. Shulman, James K. Bahcall, and Joseph T. Barss

Before the actual operative aspects of root canal therapy are begun, a number of preparatory procedures must first be completed:

1. Radiography is needed, first as an aid to diagnosis, then periodically during treatment. Endoscopy, orascopy, and the surgical microscope are supplemental aids to visual enhancement.
2. Specialized endodontic instruments and equipment must be arranged for ready use.
3. Local anesthesia of the involved tooth or area may be necessary. Special problems of anesthesia also may arise, particularly with mandibular molars and in the case of an inflamed pulp.
4. Rubber dam placement sometimes requires special handling in endodontics.

ENDODONTIC RADIOGRAPHY*

No single scientific development has contributed as greatly to improved dental health as the discovery of the amazing properties of cathode rays by Professor Wilhelm Konrad Roentgen in November 1895. The significant possibilities of their application to dentistry were seized upon 14 days after Roentgen's announcement, when Dr. Otto Walkoff took the first dental radiograph in his own mouth.[1] In the United States, within 5 months, Dr. William James described Roentgen's apparatus and displayed several radiographs. Three months later, Dr. C. Edmund Kells gave the first clinic in this country on the use of the x-ray for dental purposes. Three years later (1899), Kells was using the x-ray to determine tooth length during root canal therapy.

"I was attempting to fill the root canal of an upper central incisor," Kells later said. "It occurred to me to place a lead wire in this root canal and then take a radiogram to see whether it extended to the end of the root or not. The lead wire was shown very plainly in the root canal."

One year later (1900), Dr. Weston A. Price "called attention to incomplete root canal fillings as evidenced in radiographs." By 1901, Price was suggesting that radiographs be used to check the adequacy of root canal fillings.[2] Price is also credited with developing the bisecting angle technique, whereas Kells described what today is called the paralleling technique, made popular some 40 years later by Dr. Gordon Fitzgerald.

Although these early attempts were rarely of diagnostic quality, they were the beginning of a new era for all of dentistry. For the first time, dentists could see the accumulation of past dental treatment—therapy done without knowledge of what lay beneath the gingiva. Needless to say, the calamitous findings must have disheartened the conscientious practitioner. Yet even today, with all of the modern engineering refinements, the sleekness of operation, and the reduction of hazards, a discouraging segment of our profession continues to deprive the public by failing to use radiography to its full potential.

The total application of roentgen rays and the disciplined interpretation of the product are beyond the scope of this textbook. Only the utilization of radiography in endodontics will be discussed here. Suffice it to say that **radiography is absolutely essential for root canal therapy.**

Application of Radiography to Endodontics

The roentgen ray is used in endodontic therapy to (1) aid in the diagnosis of hard tissue alterations of the

*Abstracted in part from Walton RE.[27]

teeth and periradicular structures; (2) determine the number, location, shape, size, and direction of roots and root canals; (3) estimate and confirm the length of root canals before instrumentation; (4) localize hard-to-find, or disclose unsuspected, pulp canals by examining the position of an instrument within the root (Figure 9-1); (5) aid in locating a pulp that is markedly calcified and/or receded (Figure 9-2); (6) determine the relative position of structures in the facial–lingual dimension; (7) confirm the position and adaptation of the primary filling point; (8) aid in the evaluation of the final root canal filling; (9) aid in the examination of lips, cheeks, and tongue for fractured tooth fragments and other foreign bodies (except plastic and wood) following traumatic injuries; (10) aid in localizing a hard-to-find apex during periradicular surgery; (11) confirm, following periradicular surgery and **before suturing**, that all tooth fragments and excess filling material have been removed from the apical region and the surgical flap; and (12) evaluate, in follow-up films, the outcome of endodontic treatment.

Limitations of Radiographs

Radiographs have their limitations! They are suggestive only and should not be considered the singular final evidence in judging any clinical problem. There must be correlation with other subjective and objective findings. The greatest fault with the radiograph relates to its physical state; it is a record of a shadow, and as such only two dimensions are shown on a single film. As with any shadow, these dimensions are easily distorted through improper technique, anatomic limitations, or processing. In addition, the buccal-to-lingual dimension is absent on a single film and is frequently forgotten, although techniques are available to define the third dimension. These techniques are described later in detail.

Radiographs are not infallible. Various states of pulpal pathosis are indistinguishable in the x-ray shadow. Neither healthy nor necrotic pulps cast an unusual image. Correspondingly, the sterile or infected status of hard or soft tissue is not detectable other than by inference. Only bacteriologic evidence can determine this. Furthermore, periradicular soft tissue lesions cannot be accurately diagnosed by radiographs; they require histologic verification. Chronic inflammatory tissue cannot, for example, be differentiated from healed, fibrous, "scar" tissue, nor can a differential diagnosis of periradicular radiolucencies usually be made on the basis of size, shape, and density of the adjacent bone.[3–7] A common misconception is that an inflammatory lesion is present only when there is at least a perceptible "thickening" of the periodontal ligament space. In fact, investigators have demonstrated that lesions of the **medullary bone** are likely to go undetected until the resorption has expanded into and eroded a portion of the **cortical plate.**[8–11]

The difficulties and inherent errors in radiographic interpretation were clearly demonstrated by Goldman et al.,[12] who submitted recall radiographs of endodontic treatments, for clinical evaluation, to a group of radiologists and endodontists. They assessed success and failure by observation of radiodensities. There was **more disagreement than agreement** among the examiners.

Radiographs are an essential aid to diagnosis but must be used with discretion. However, radiographs are the

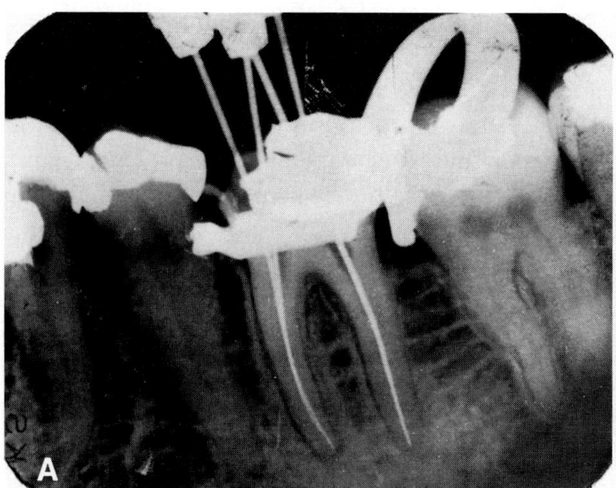

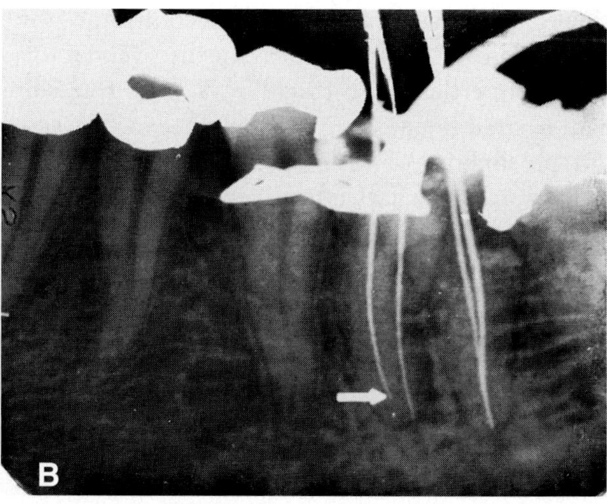

Figure 9-1 Disclosing canals by radiography. **A,** Right-angle horizontal projection reveals four files in separate canals superimposed. **B,** Horizontal angulation varied 30 degrees mesially reveals all four canals and file short of working length in mesiolingual canal (**arrow**). Reproduced with permission from Walton RE.[27]

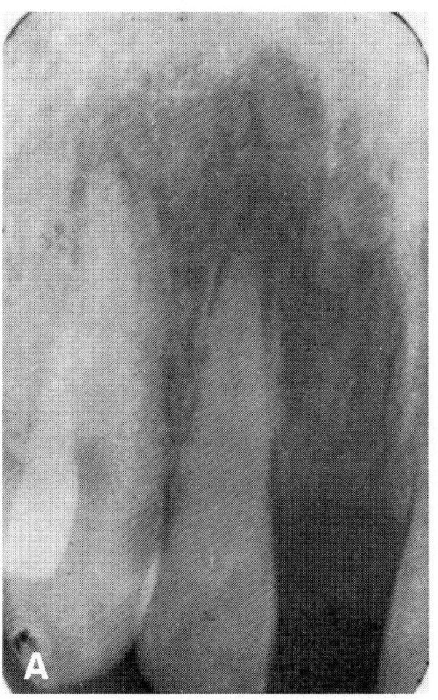

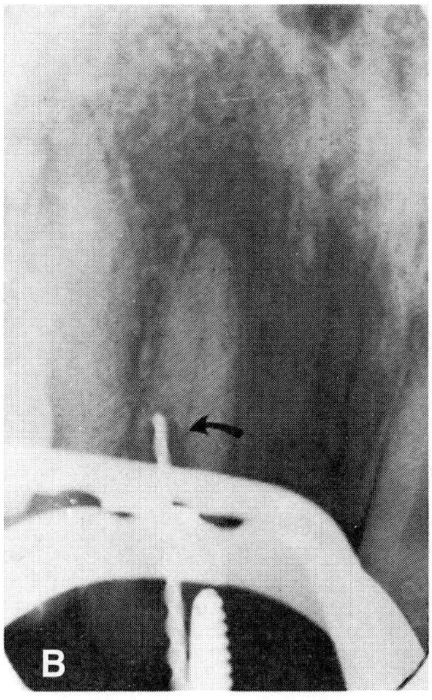

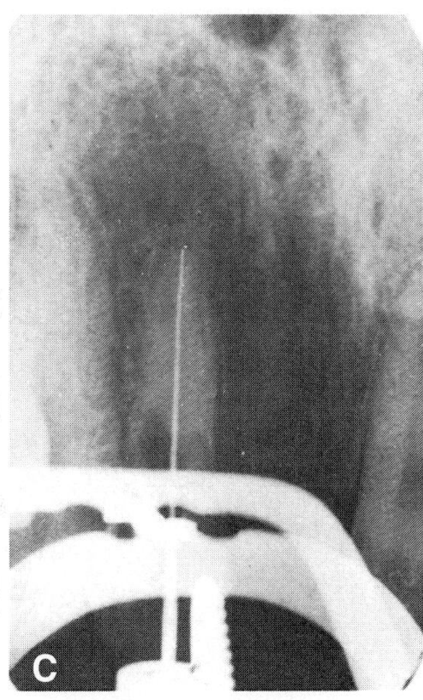

Figure 9-2 Locating canal of the receded pulp. **A,** Advanced calcification and receded pulp. **B,** Radiograph reveals angulation of preparation and canal (**arrow**) at mesial of cut. **C,** Canal, seen in radiograph, is discovered with a fine file. (Courtesy of Dr. Steven Koehler.)

only method whereby the dentist can "visualize" that which he cannot see or feel during the process of diagnosis and treatment. He will discover that, as his radiographic techniques and interpretation improve, so will the ease and success of his root canal treatment. The techniques outlined in the following sections have proved to be successful and predictable. If followed, they will greatly simplify difficulties in root canal treatment.

INSTRUMENTATION

Systems

There are two radiographic approaches. The traditional approach is the x-ray exposure of film, which is then **chemically processed** to produce an image. The newer digital radiography systems rely on an electronic detection of an x-ray-generated image that is then **electronically processed** to produce an image on a computer screen, an image that is similar in interpretative quality to the traditional radiograph.[13–16] Advantages of digital radiography include reduced radiation of the patient, speed of obtaining the image, enhancement of the image, computer storage, transmissibility, and a system that does not require chemical processing.[17] Disadvantages are cost and ease of use, although endodontists are not finding these to be a determent to their practice, in which speed and the preceding features are important. As costs decrease and technology improves, use of the digital system will undoubtedly increase by all practitioners. Digital radiography is discussed in full later in the chapter.

Traditional Machines

Two basic types of x-ray machines are commonly used in dental offices. One type has a range of kilovoltage and two milliamperage settings with which the long (16-inch) cone is frequently used. The other type offers only one kilovoltage and milliamperage setting and only the short (8-inch) cone. Either type provides adequate radiographs. However, each has advantages that, under different circumstances, will yield a more satisfactory result. The long-cone system is superior for diagnostic radiographs, whereas the flexible short-cone machine is more appropriate for treatment or "working" films. Any x-ray machine must be properly shielded and collimated by means of a lead diaphragm and filtered by aluminum disks to ensure proper radiation safeguards for the patient and professional personnel. An additional protective measure is the draping of the patient with a lead apron to block scatter radiation.

Long Cone. Because of the clarity of detail and minimum distortion inherent in the long-cone parallel technique,[18–21] the long-cone machine is preferred for exposing diagnostic, final, and follow-up radiographs.

Short Cone. Because of the number of working radiographs taken in the course of endodontic therapy, the practitioner treating more than the occasional tooth will find that a short-cone machine, with a small, easily manipulated head, saves much time, energy, and frustration (Figure 9-3).

Film. Industrial technological advances have allowed film exposure time to be reduced to fractions of

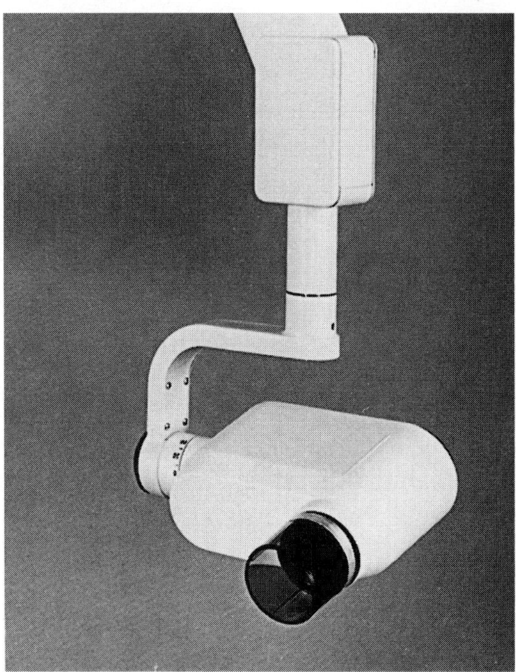

Figure 9-3 Working head of the flexible, compact, short-cone x-ray machine, the GX-770, ideal for exposing endodontic "working" films but of adequate quality for diagnostic, archival, or follow-up purposes. (Courtesy of Gendex Corp., USA.)

a second. Recent improvements in emulsion thickness allow rapid processing of the new films, which are used for diagnostic and "working films" alike. A study of Kodak Ektaspeed film ("E" film), which is coated with larger silver bromide crystals and has one half the exposure time of standard Kodak Ultraspeed film, concluded that the "Ektaspeed film had comparable accuracy with the Ultraspeed film in measuring root length," even though the new Ektaspeed is somewhat grainier.[22] A double-blind study found the slower Ultraspeed film superior "in terms of contrast, image, quality, and rater satisfaction."[23] However, a US Army study found both films "adequate for routine endodontic use."[24]

An even faster film (F speed) has very recently been introduced. This film requires 20% less radiation but appears grainier. There are no published studies to date on the suitability of this new film for endodontic use.

For dentists with a referral endodontic practice, duplicate film packets are recommended for the diagnostic, final treatment, and recall radiographs—one set for the permanent office record, the other for the referring dentist. One must know, however, that the front film in the double pack, the one closest to the x-ray machine, "had significantly superior image quality compared to back films."[25]

The standard periradicular size film is used for most situations. In addition, every office should have 2 × 3-inch **occlusal** film available for use when (1) periradicular lesions are so extensive that they cannot be demonstrated in their entirety on one periradicular film; (2) there is interest in or involvement of the nasal cavity, sinuses, or roof or floor of the mouth; (3) trauma or inflammation prohibits normal jaw opening required to place and hold a periradicular film; (4) a handicapped person is unable to hold a periradicular film by the usual means; (5) detection of fractures of the anterior portion of the maxilla or mandible is needed; and (6) very young children are being examined.

Film Placement. Film placed parallel to the long axis of the teeth and exposed by cathode rays at a right angle to the surface of the film yields accurate images, free of shortening or elongation[26] (Figure 9-4). If this principle is applied, it is unnecessary to memorize fixed cone angulations. In a modern, comfortable operating chair, moreover, with the patient in a semireclined position, she need not be returned to an upright position for each exposure.

Because of the complicating presence of the rubber dam, the methods for placement of **working** films dif-

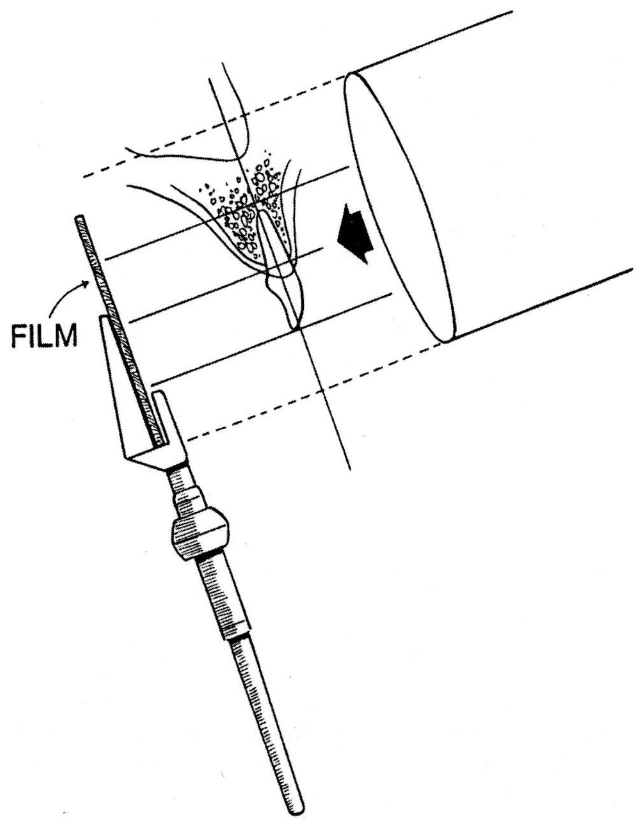

Figure 9-4 Radiographic parallelism. The long axis of the film, the long axis of the tooth, and the leading edge of the cone are parallel and perpendicular to the x-ray central beam. Reproduced with permission from Goerig AC. In: Besner E, et al., editors. Practical endodontics. St. Louis (MO): Mosby; 1993. p. 56.

fer somewhat from the methods for placement of diagnostic, final, and follow-up films.

Diagnostic Radiographs. These must be the **best radiographs possible.** To achieve this goal, there are advantages to parallelism, which permits more accurate visualization of structures as well as reproducibility. This facilitates comparison of follow-up radiographs.

There are a number of devices on the market that ensure film placement and parallelism. The **Rinn XCP** (Dentsply/Rinn Elgin, Ill.) virtually guarantees distortion-free films but cannot be used with the rubber dam in place. The **Rinn Endoray II endodontic film holder** is designed specifically to ensure parallelism yet avoid rubber dam clamps while allowing space for files protruding from the tooth (Figure 9-5). Film holders are preferred to finger retention of the film. A **straight hemostat** is an excellent film holder.

Working Radiographs. One great difficulty in root canal therapy is the clumsy, aggravating method of taking treatment radiographs with the rubber dam in place. Some dentists remove the rubber dam frame for access in film placement, and saliva enters to contaminate the operating field. It is therefore imperative that a film-placement technique be used so that the **rubber dam frame need not be removed.** Use of a radiolucent **N-Ø** (Nygaard–Østby) frame (Coltene/Whaledent/Hygenic; Mahwah, N.J.), **le Cadre Articulé**-type frame (Jored, Ormoy, France, or Trophy, USA) (see Figures 9-57 and 9-58), or the **Star VisiFrame** (Dentaleze/ Star, USA) will ensure that apices are not obscured.

With the rubber dam in place, a **hemostat-held** film has significant advantages over the finger-retained film: (1) the film placement is easier when the opening is restricted by the rubber dam and frame; (2) the patient may close with the film in place, a particular advantage in **mandibular posterior areas** where closing relaxes the mylohyoid muscle, permitting the film to be positioned farther apically; (3) the handle of the hemostat is a guide to align the cone in the proper vertical and horizontal angulation (Figure 9-6); (4) there is less risk of distortion of the radiograph caused by too much finger pressure bending the film; and (5) patients can hold a hemostat handle more securely with less possibility of film displacement. In addition, any movement can be detected by the shift of the handles and corrected before exposure.

In all instances of film placement, the **identifying dimple** should be placed at the incisal or occlusal edge to prevent its obscuring an important apical structure.

Cone Positioning. It is a mistake to rely on only one film. There is much to be learned from additional exposures taken from varied horizontal or vertical projections.

Vertical Angulation. Ordinarily, it is preferable to align the cone so the beam strikes the film at a right angle. This alignment ensures a fairly accurate vertical image. Elongation of an image, however, **may be corrected by increasing the vertical angle** of the central

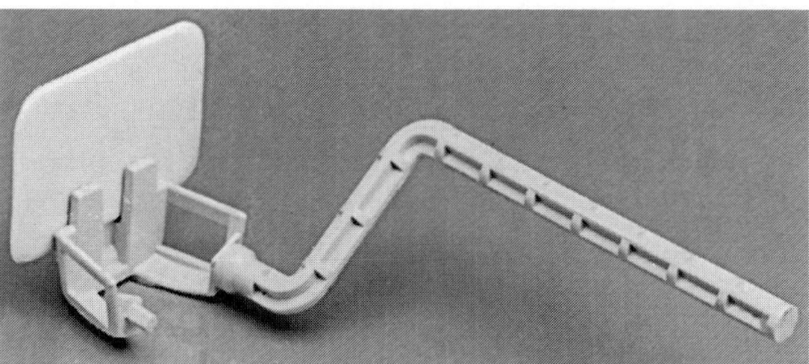

Figure 9-5 The universal Rinn EndoRay plastic film holder is designed for horizontal posterior films or anterior vertical films, maxilla or mandible, right or left. Here it is set for a maxillary posterior view. The "cupped-out" area accommodates the tooth, clamp, and extruding endodontic files. The parallel sighting rod/handle can be moved from right to left. (Courtesy of Rinn Corp., USA.)

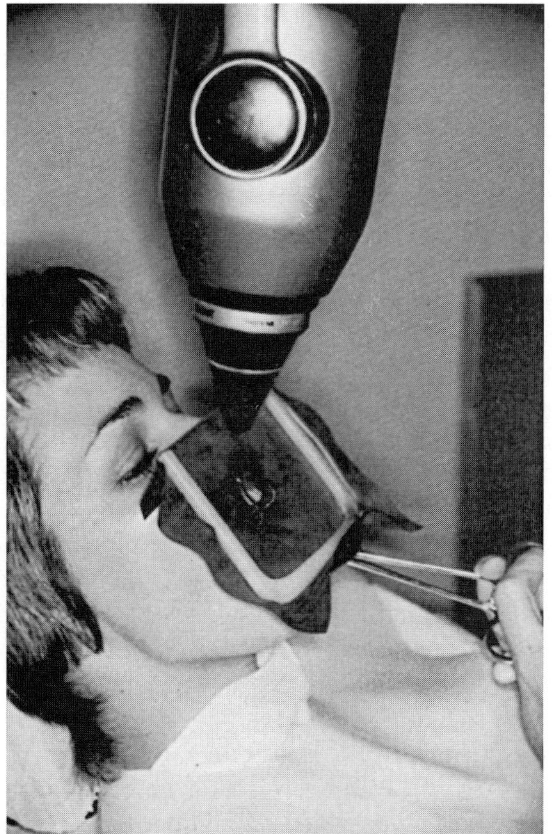

Figure 9-6 "Working" film properly placed and held under rubber dam with hemostat. Cone is aligned at right angle to handle. (Courtesy of Dr. Richard E. Walton.)

ray. Conversely, **foreshortening is corrected by decreasing** the vertical angle of the central ray. To remember this, one should think of the sun: it casts a shortened shadow at noon when it is at its zenith, or increased vertical angle.

Frequently, an impinging palatal vault prevents parallel alignment of the film and the teeth. However, if the film angle is no greater than 20 degrees in relation to the long axis of the teeth, and the beam is directed at a right angle to the film, no distortion occurs, although there is a less effective orientation of structures.[26] The resulting radiograph is still adequate.

Horizontal Angulation. Walton introduced an important refinement in dental radiography that has materially improved the endodontic interpretive film.[27] He demonstrated a simple technique whereby the **third dimension** may be readily visualized. Specifically, the anatomy of superimposed structures, the roots and pulp canals, may be better defined.

The basic technique is to vary the **horizontal angulation** of the central ray of the x-ray beam. By this method, overlying canals may be separated, and by applying Clark's rule,[28] the separate canals may then be identified. Clark's rule states that **"the most distant object from the cone (lingual) moves toward the direction of the cone."** Stated in another way, using a helpful mnemonic, Clark's rule has been referred to as the SLOB rule (Same Lingual, Opposite Buccal): the object that moves in the Same direction as the cone is located toward the Lingual. The object that moves in the Opposite direction from the cone is located toward the Buccal. The SLOB rule, simply stated, is "The lingual object will always follow the tube head." Goerig and Neaverth cleverly applied the SLOB rule to determine, from a single film, from which direction a radiograph was taken: mesial, straight on, or distal. Knowing the direction, one is then able to determine lingual from buccal[29] (Figure 9-7). Stated more simply, Ingle's rule is **MBD:** Always "shoot" from the Mesial and the Buccal root will be to the Distal.

Horizontal Angulation Variations. *Mandibular Molars.* As previously emphasized, the film must be positioned parallel to the lower arch. The **standard** horizontal x-ray projection then is at a right angle to the film (perpendicular), as shown in Figure 9-8. The two mesial canals are superimposed one upon the other and appear as a single line.

Through the **Walton projection,** however, the canals can be made to "open up." This is done by directing the central beam 20 to 30 degrees from the mesial (Figure 9-9, A). In Figure 9-9, B (**black arrows**), the two canals in each root can now be readily discerned.

The contrast gained by varying the horizontal projection can best be seen in a clinical case with four canals. Figure 9-10, A, taken at a right angle, clearly shows the four instruments superimposed on one another. Figure 9-10, B, on the other hand, taken from a 30-degree variance in horizontal projection, emphasizes the third dimension: the separation of the instruments in the canals. By applying Ingle's rule (MBD: shoot from the **mesial**), one also determines that the **buccal** canals are toward the **distal.**

Another point should be made at this time concerning a frequent mistake in "reading" periradicular radiographs. It can best be illustrated by a cross-sectional drawing of molar root structure. Roots containing two canals are often hourglass-shaped, as Figure 9-11, A, indicates. When an x-ray beam passes directly through this structure, the buccal and lingual portions of the root are in the same path (**arrows**). Because a double thickness of tooth structure is penetrated by the x-rays, it is seen in the film as a radiopaque root outline in close contact with the **lamina dura.** This is readily apparent on the radiograph (Figure 9-11, B).

By aiming the cone 20 degrees from the mesial, however, the central beam passes through the hourglass-shaped root at an angle (Figure 9-12, A). In this case, the two thicknesses of the root are projected separately onto the film. Since less tooth structure is penetrated by the x-ray, the image on the film is less dense. A radiolucent line is clearly seen in Figure 9-12, B (**open arrow**). This radiolucent line can be erroneously "read" as a root canal. One should take care to follow up the length of the line. Instead of entering the pulp chamber, it can be traced to emerge at the gingival surface of the root. This simple interpretive error can easily lead to gross mistakes in endodontic cavity preparation.

Mandibular Premolars. The importance of varying the horizontal angulation when radiographing mandibular premolars is demonstrated in Figure 9-13, A, wherein the central ray is directed at a right angle to the film. What appears to be a single straight canal is discernible in each premolar (Figure 9-13, B). There is an indication, however, in the image of the first premolar that the canal might bifurcate at the point of the abrupt change in density (**arrow**).

Directing the central ray 20 degrees from the mesial in the **first premolar** (Figure 9-14, A) causes the bifurcation to separate into two canals (Figure 9-14, B). The tapering outline of the tooth, seen in both projections, would indicate, on the other hand, that the two canals undoubtedly rejoin to form a common canal at the apex. In both the right-angle and 20-degree variance projections, the **second premolar** appears as a single canal.

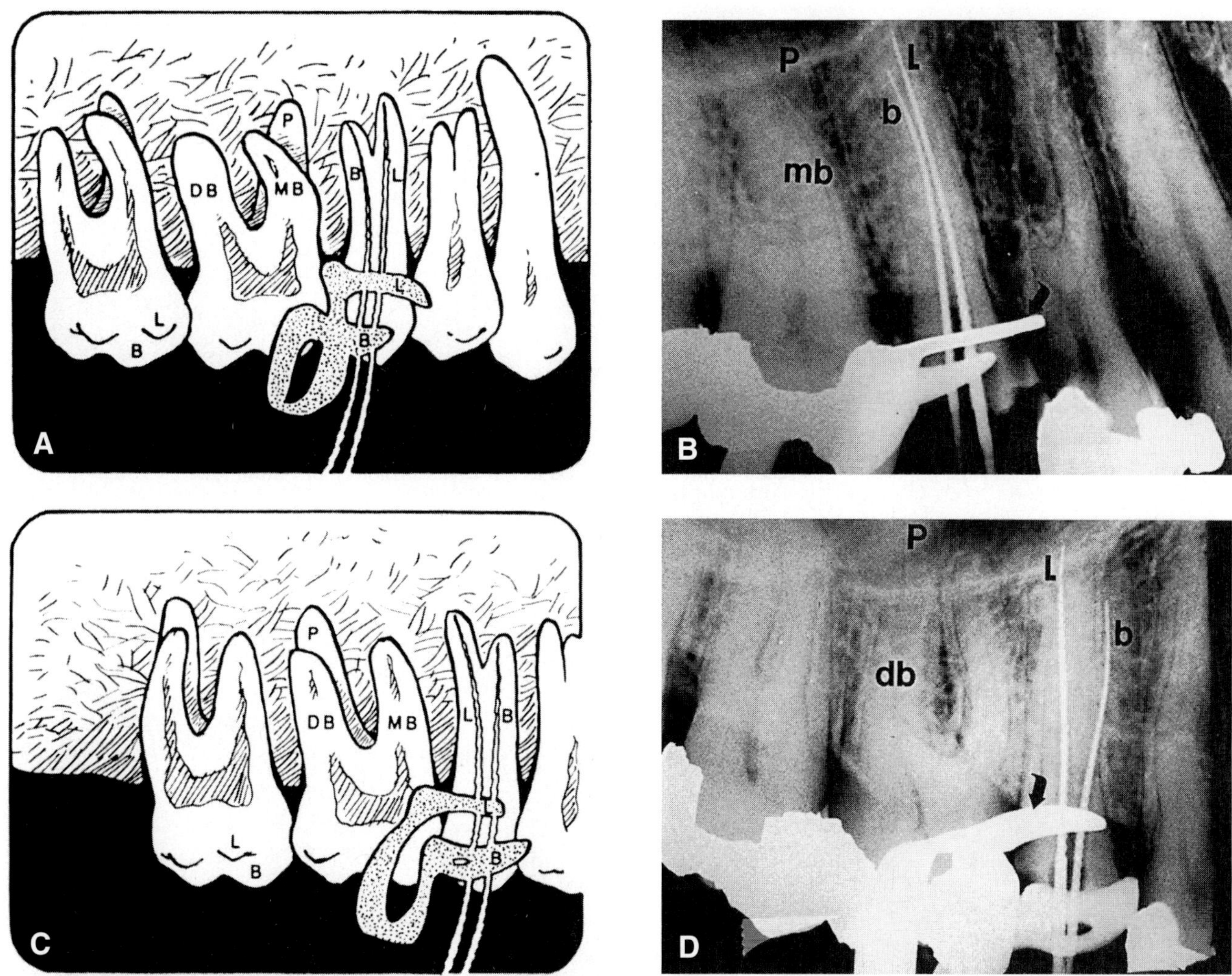

Figure 9-7 Applying the SLOB rule to determine the direction from which the film was taken. Anyone knowing the direction can tell lingual from buccal. Clues that the film is taken from the mesial: **A** and **B**, The mesial-buccal (MB) root lies over the palatal (P) root, that is, the lingual (palatal) root has moved mesially; the lingual arm of the rubber dam clamp (**arrow**) has moved mesially. The canine is visible. Once it has been determined that the radiograph was taken from the mesial, the lingual root (toward the mesial) of the premolar is defined. C and D, Radiograph of the same teeth taken from the distal. Clues are reversed. There is no canine visible in the film, and the lingual premolar canal is now toward the distal. Reproduced with permission from Goerig AC. In: Besner E, et al., editors. Practical endodontics. St. Louis (MO): Mosby; 1993. p. 54.

Maxillary Molars. Maxillary molars are consistently the most difficult to radiograph because of (1) their more complicated root and pulp anatomy, (2) the frequent superimposition of portions of the roots on each other, (3) the superimposition of bony structures (sinus floor, zygomatic process) on root structures, and (4) the shape and depth of the palate, which can be a major impediment.

As is true of the mandible, the complex root anatomy and superimpositions may be dealt with **by varying the horizontal** angulations. Film placement must again be parallel to the posterior maxillary arch, not to the palate.

The standard right-angle projection for a maxillary first molar that is illustrated in Figure 9-15, A, produces the image seen in Figure 9-15, B, wherein the zygomatic process is superimposed on the apex of the palatal root (**arrow**) and the distobuccal root appears to overlie the palatal root. The sinus floor is also superimposed on the apices of both the first and second molars.

When the horizontal angulation is varied by 20 degrees to the mesial (Figure 9-16, A), the zygomatic process is moved far to the distal of the first molar and the distobuccal root is cleared of the palatal root (Figure 9-16, B, **arrows**).

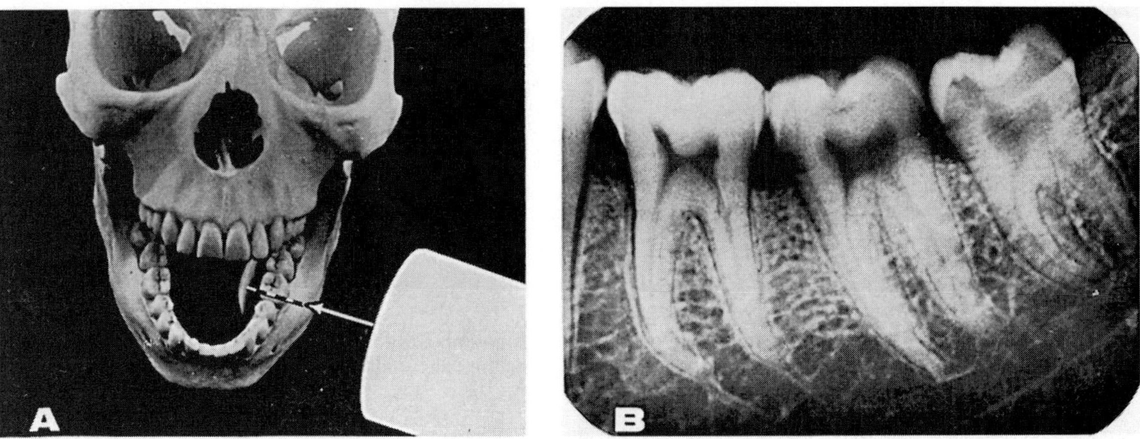

Figure 9-8 Mandibular molars. **A,** Central ray directed at right angle to film positioned parallel to arch. **B,** Limited information is gleaned from radiograph because of superimposition of structures and canals. Reproduced with permission from Walton RE. [27]

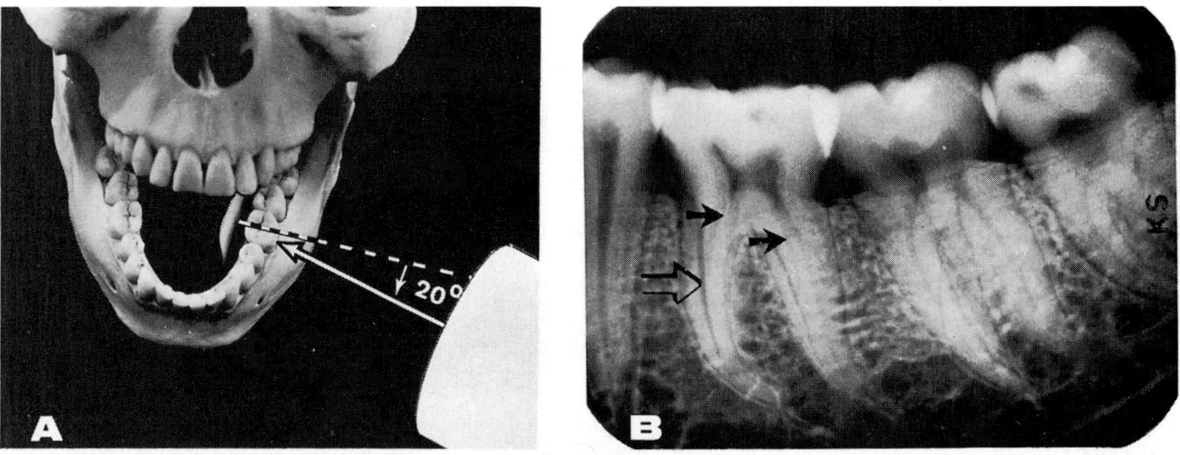

Figure 9-9 Mandibular molars. **A,** Central ray directed at 20 degrees mesially to film positioned parallel to arch. **B,** Two canals are now visible in both roots of the first molar (**black arrows**). **Open arrow** indicates confusing root outlines. Reproduced with permission from Walton RE.[27]

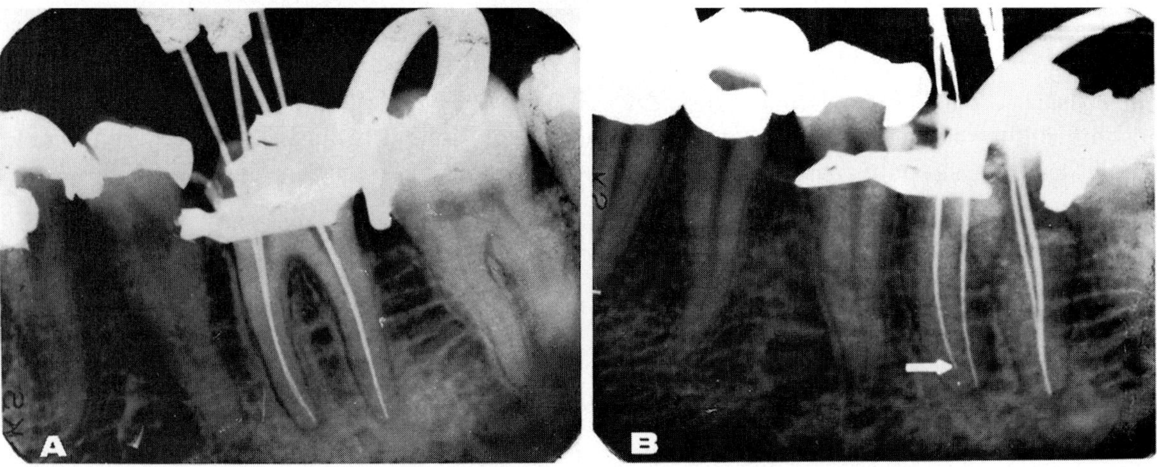

Figure 9-10 Mandibular molars. **A,** Right-angle horizontal projection superimposes four files, one on the other. **B,** Horizontal variance of 30 degrees separates four canals. SLOB rule proves lingual canals are to the mesial. Reproduced with permission from Walton RE. [27]

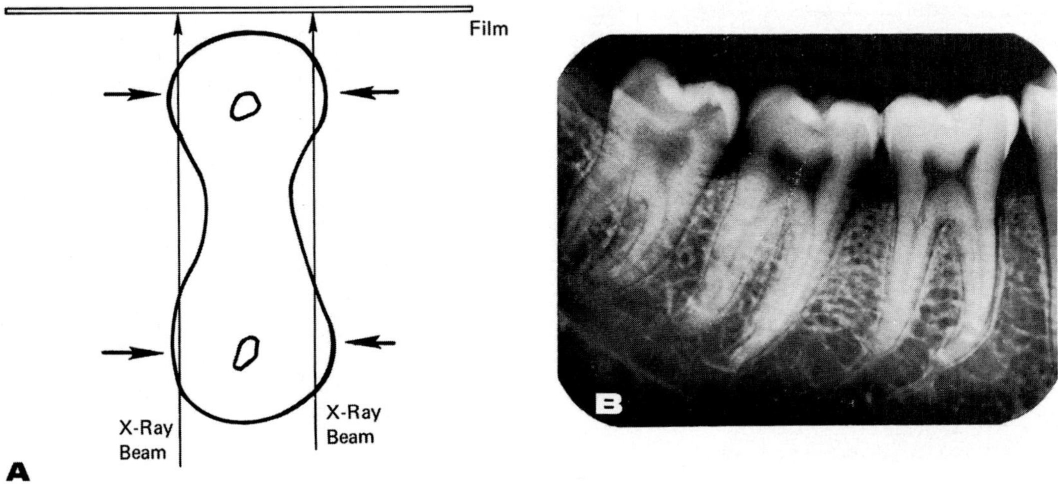

Figure 9-11 A, X-ray beam passing directly through two thicknesses of root structure presents intensified image on film. **B**, Note radiopaque root outline inside lamina dura. **B** reproduced with permission from Walton RE.[27]

The **opposite projection** also can be used to isolate the mesiobuccal root of the first molar, that is, the central ray may be projected from **20 degrees distal** to the right angle (Figure 9-17, A). Although this projection distorts the shape of the mesiobuccal root, it also isolates it (Figure 9-17, B), so that the canal is readily discernible (**arrow**). Also note that the zygomatic process is moved completely away from any root structure, including the second molar.

The same technique illustrated here for the maxillary first molar can be applied to the second or third molars by directing the central beam at a horizontal variance through those teeth.

Maxillary Premolars. Variance in the horizontal projection has great value in maxillary premolar radiography, particularly for the **first** premolar, which generally has two canals, but sometimes three. The clinical efficacy of the Walton technique is well illustrated in Figure 9-18. The right-angle horizontal projection produces the single canal image seen in Figure 9-18, A. By varying the angulation by 20 degrees, however, the two canals are separated (Figure 9-18, B), giving an unobstructed view of the quality of the fillings in both canals.

Mandibular Anterior Teeth. Aberrations in canal anatomy in the **mandibular** anterior teeth are infamous. Variance of the horizontal x-ray projections in this region will bring out the differences. Figure 9-19, A, illustrates the standard x-ray projection bisecting the film held parallel to the arch. The incisor teeth appear

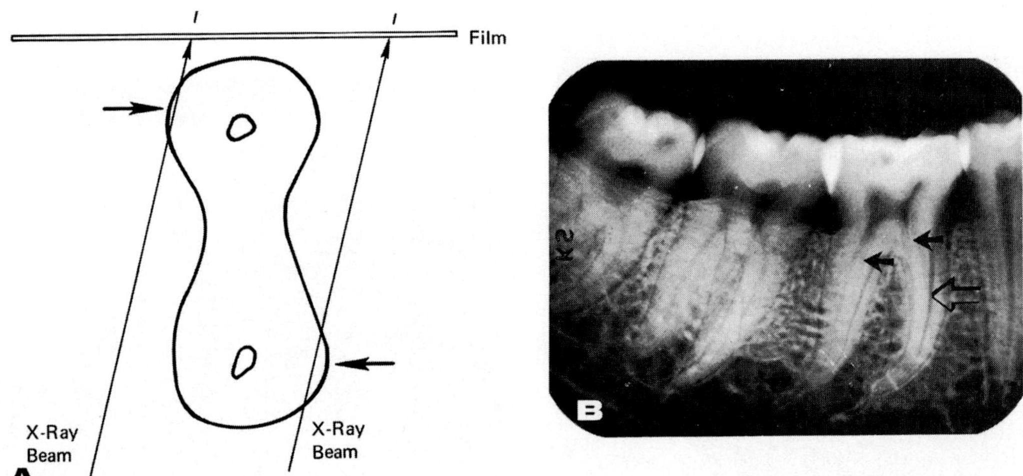

Figure 9-12 A, X-ray beam aimed 20 degrees mesially passes through single thicknesses of hourglass root, leaving less dense impression on film. **B**, Radiolucent line is apparent (**open arrow**) and may be confused with root canal. Note that it emerges at gingival, not into pulp chamber. **Black arrows** indicate regular canals. **B** reproduced with permission from Walton RE.[27]

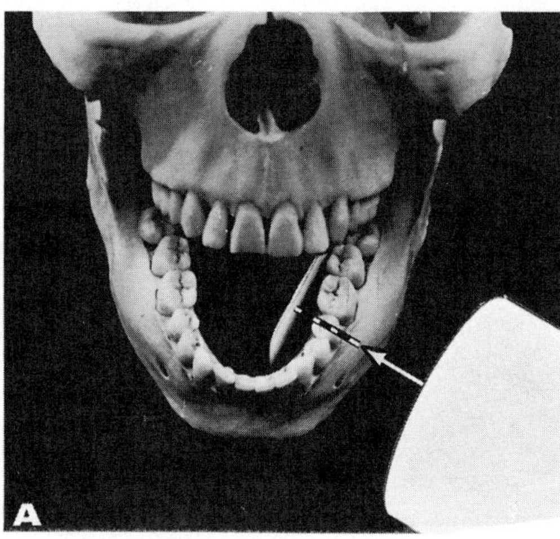

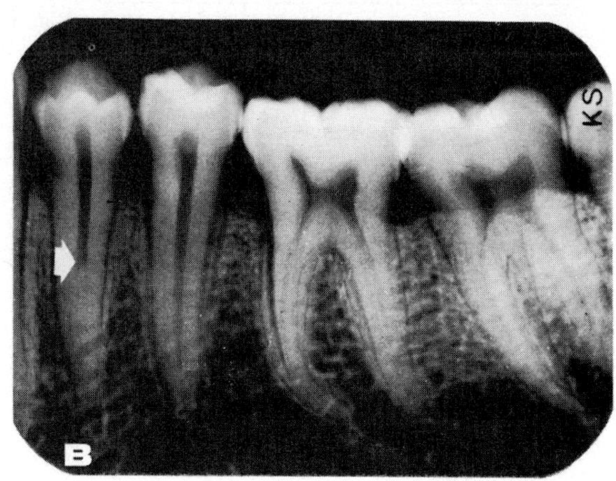

Figure 9-13 Mandibular premolars. **A,** Central ray directed at right angle to film positioned parallel to arch. **B,** Radiograph reveals one canal in each premolar, although abrupt change in density (**arrow**) may indicate bifurcation. Reproduced with permission from Walton RE. [27]

to have single canals. But a broad single canal is seen in the distorted canine image (Figure 9-19, B).

By varying the film placement and projecting directly through the canine, as seen in Figure 9-20, A (which is about 30 degrees variance for the incisors), separate canals appear in the incisors (Figure 9-20, B, **arrow**) and are then seen to coalesce at the apex. This would be expected, however, when one views the tapered incisor roots seen in both horizontal projections, roots far too narrow to support two separate canals and foramina. Once again, the abrupt change in canal radiodensity in the premolars (**arrow**) should make one suspicious of canal bifurcation, a fact that has already been confirmed in Figure 9-14, B.

Maxillary Anterior Teeth. Although canal or root aberrations appear less frequently in the maxillary anterior teeth, root curvature in the maxillary lateral incisors is a particularly vexing problem. Grady and Clausen have shown, for example, how difficult it is to determine when foramina exit to the labial or lingual.[30] Their radiographs of extracted teeth matched with photographs of instrument perforation short of the apex are a warning to all (Figure 9-21).

Processing. Another deterrent to full endodontic utilization of radiography has been the length of time required in most offices to process films. Old, weakened solutions greatly increase the time required for processing. Moreover, adherence to the manufacturer's recommended temperature and time (68°F for 5 to 7 minutes) for developing and clearing has retarded "on-the-spot" processing and viewing in most busy practices.

Ingle, Beveridge, and Olson demonstrated, in a well-controlled blind study, the effects of varied processing temperatures. A processing temperature of 92°F yielded, in less than 1 minute, the most acceptable

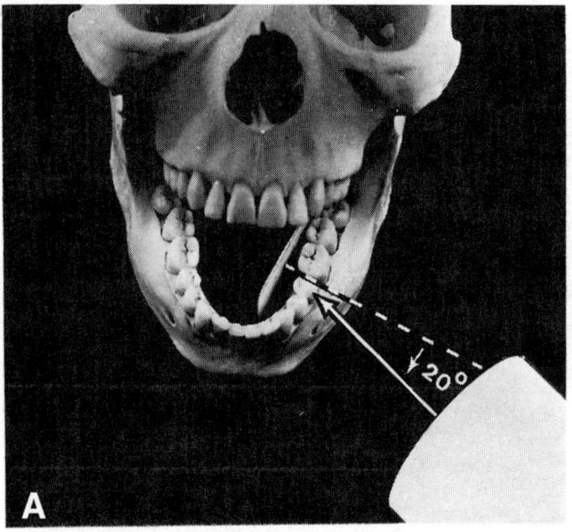

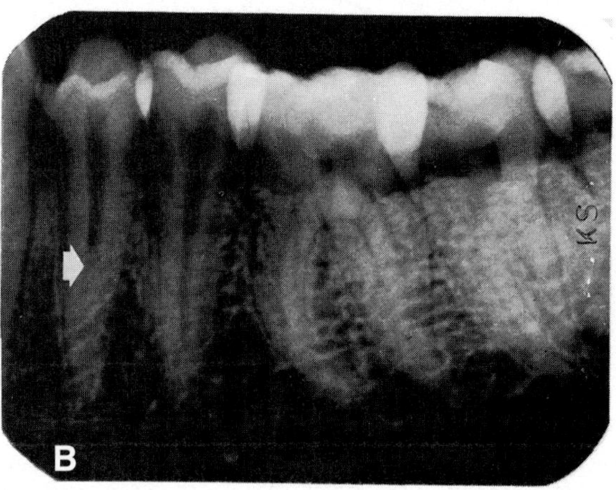

Figure 9-14 Mandibular premolars. **A,** Central ray directed at 20 degrees mesially to film, parallel to arch. **B,** In first premolar, two canals that are clearly visible (**arrow**) probably reunite, as indicated by sharply tapered root. Reproduced with permission from Walton RE. [27]

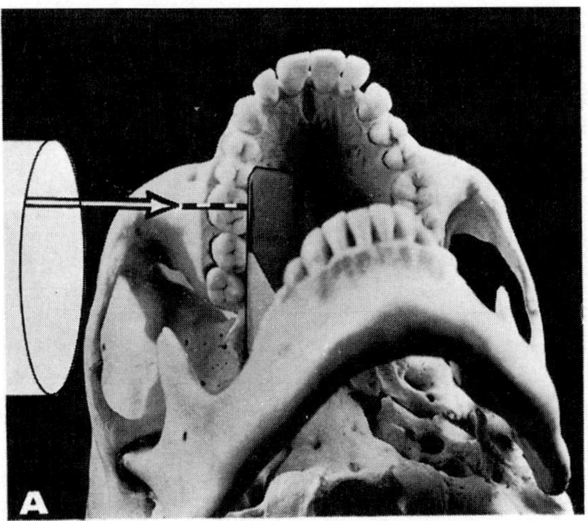

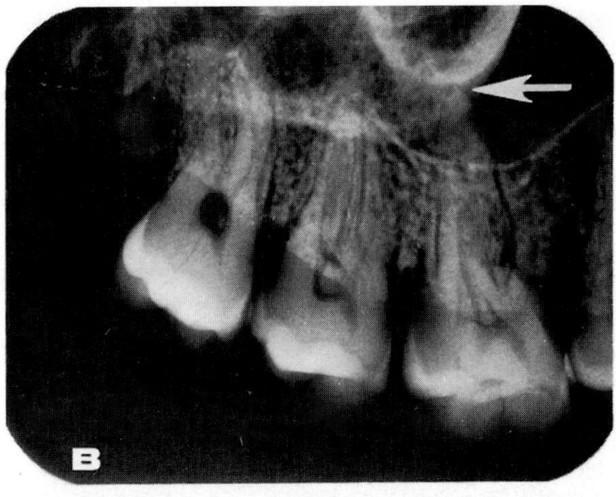

Figure 9-15 Maxillary molars. A, Central ray is directed through maxillary molar at right angle to inferior border of film. **Arrow** and **dotted line** passing through malar process indicate it will superimpose over first molar. B, Superimposition of first molar roots, sinus floor, and malar process (**white arrow**) confuse the diagnosis. Reproduced with permission from Walton RE.[27]

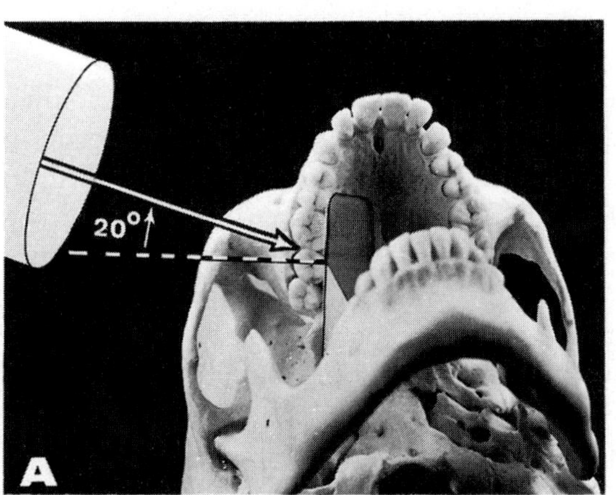

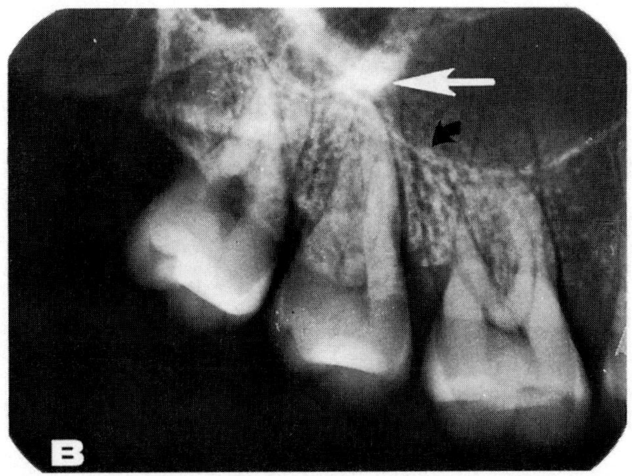

Figure 9-16 Maxillary molars. A, Central ray directed at 20 degrees **mesially** skirts malar process, projecting it distally. B, Distobuccal root is cleared of palatal root and malar process is projected far to distal (**white arrow**). Between right-angle and 20 degrees projection, all three roots are clearly seen. Reproduced with permission from Walton RE.[27]

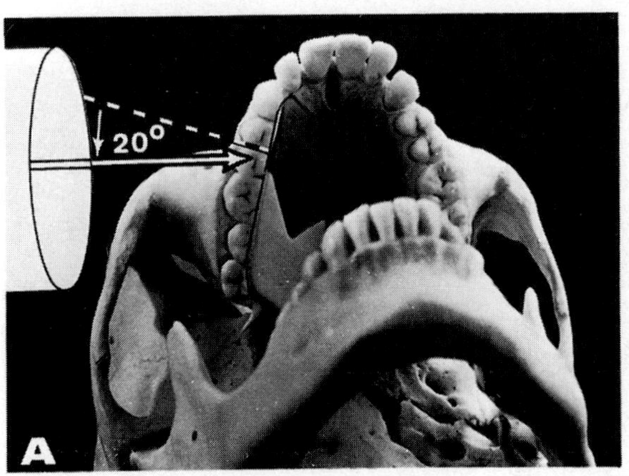

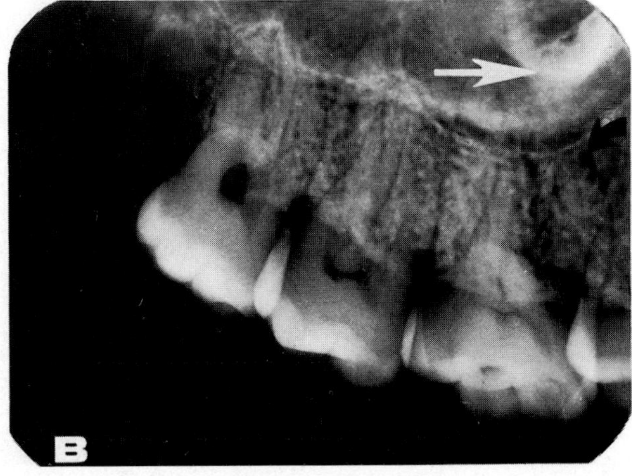

Figure 9-17 Maxillary molars. A, Central beam projected 20 degrees from the **distal.** B, Mesiobuccal root of the first molar is isolated (**black arrow**) and second and third molars are cleared of malar process, which is projected forward (**white arrow**). Sinus floor may be "lowered" or "raised" by changing vertical angulation. Reproduced with permission from Walton RE.[27]

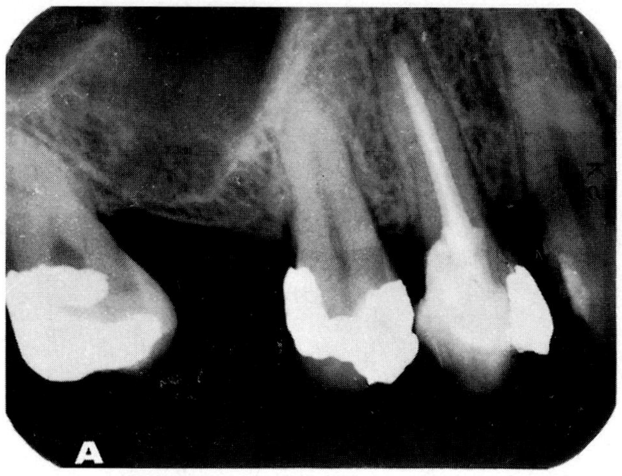

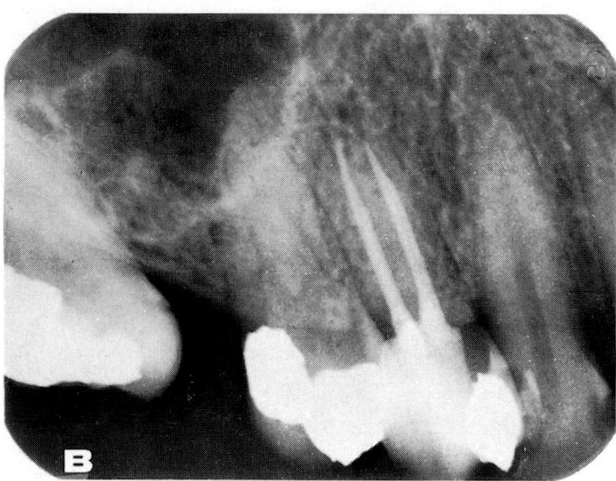

Figure 9-18 Maxillary premolars. **A,** Horizontal right-angle projection produces illusion that maxillary first premolar has only one canal. **B,** Varying horizontal projection by 20 degrees mesially separates two canals. Lingual canal is toward mesial. Reproduced with permission from Walton RE.[27]

radiographs.[31] A group of 37 physicians and dentists selected as "best" the films developed at 92°F from a coded selection of films processed at 4°F intervals in the range of 68 to 100°F. At 92°F, using Kodak developer and fixer mixed to company specifications, **development required only 30 seconds** and fixation required 25 to 35 seconds, with no loss of quality.

By comparison, the 70°F temperature, recommended at that time by the manufacturer, required 5 minutes developing time and 10 minutes fixing time for Ultraspeed film. Ektaspeed is slightly better: 72 to 80°F for 2½ to 4 minutes developing and 2 to 4 minutes fixing time. Finally, all films need to be **final washed** for at least 30 minutes.

In a practice limited to endodontics only, small quart-size tanks are adequate and economical. Frequent change of solutions is recommended.

Rapid Processing. Concentrated rapid-processing chemicals, such as **Kodak's Rapid Access** solution, have become very popular in endodontic practice. Although they are more expensive ounce for ounce, they save measurable time, requiring only 15 seconds developing and 15 seconds clearing time in the fixer at room temperature.

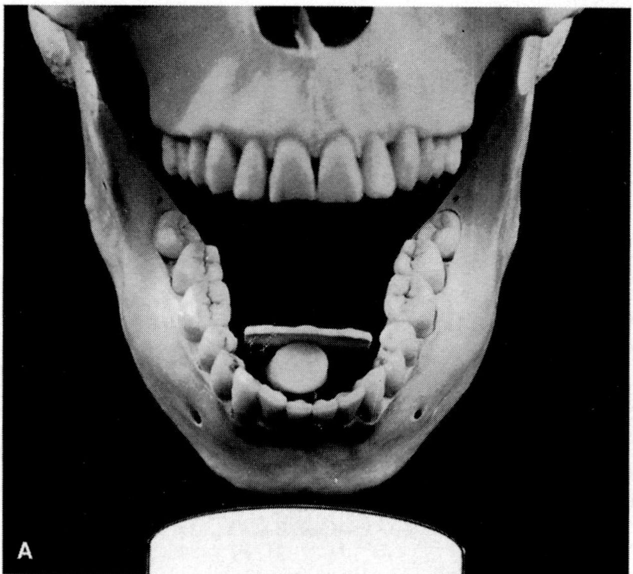

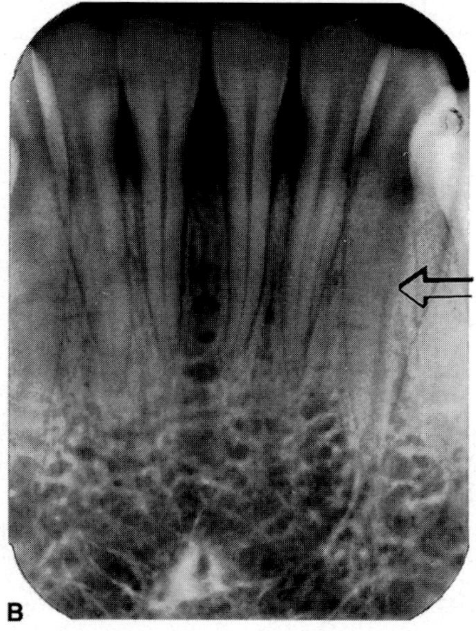

Figure 9-19 Mandibular anterior teeth. **A,** Film placement for bisecting-angle technique. Horizontal central beam projection at right angle to film. **B,** Single canals seen in central incisors with only suggestion of two canals in lateral incisor. In distorted image of canine, note broad labiolingual canal dimension (**arrow**). Reproduced with permission from Walton RE.[27]

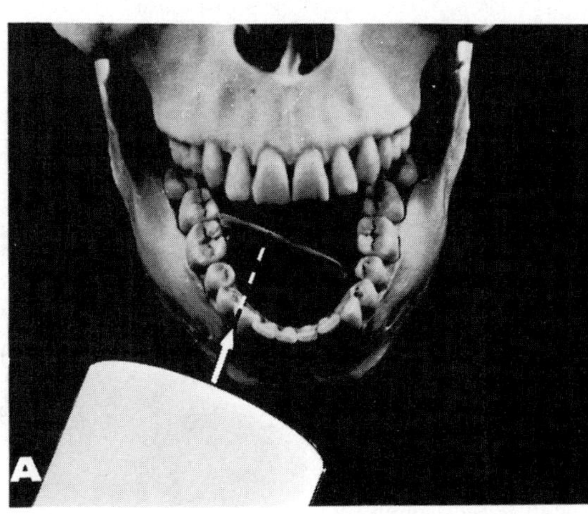

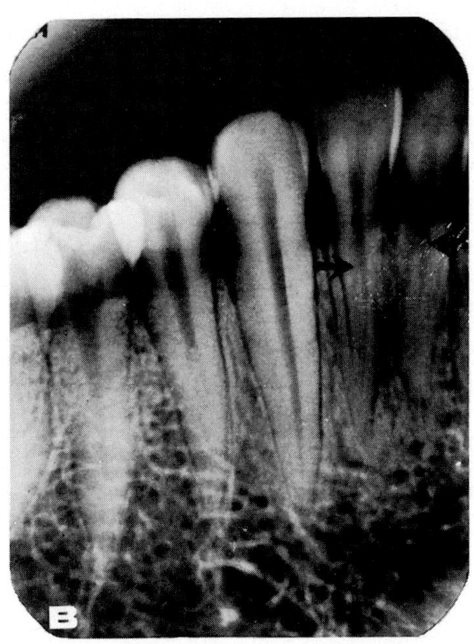

Figure 9-20 Mandibular anterior teeth. **A,** Film is positioned for canine radiograph using bisecting-angle technique. Horizontally, central beam is projected at right angle to film. **B,** Canine image is single straight canal, but incisor image reveals bifurcated canals that reunite in narrow tapered root (**arrows**). Note "bonus" image of bifurcated canals, first premolar. Reproduced with permission from Walton RE.[27]

A Tel Aviv/UCLA study tested four rapid-developing solutions, processing both Ultraspeed and Ektaspeed films. Film fog became a problem as the solutions deteriorated with time. Kodak Rapid Access had to be changed every day, whereas the other solutions, Colitts (Buffalo Dental; Syosset, N.Y.), IFP (M & D International), and Instaneg (Neo-Flo, Inc., USA), would deteriorate over 60 days. They also found that precise developing time and 3 to 5 seconds rinse time between developing and fixing are absolutely essential.[32]

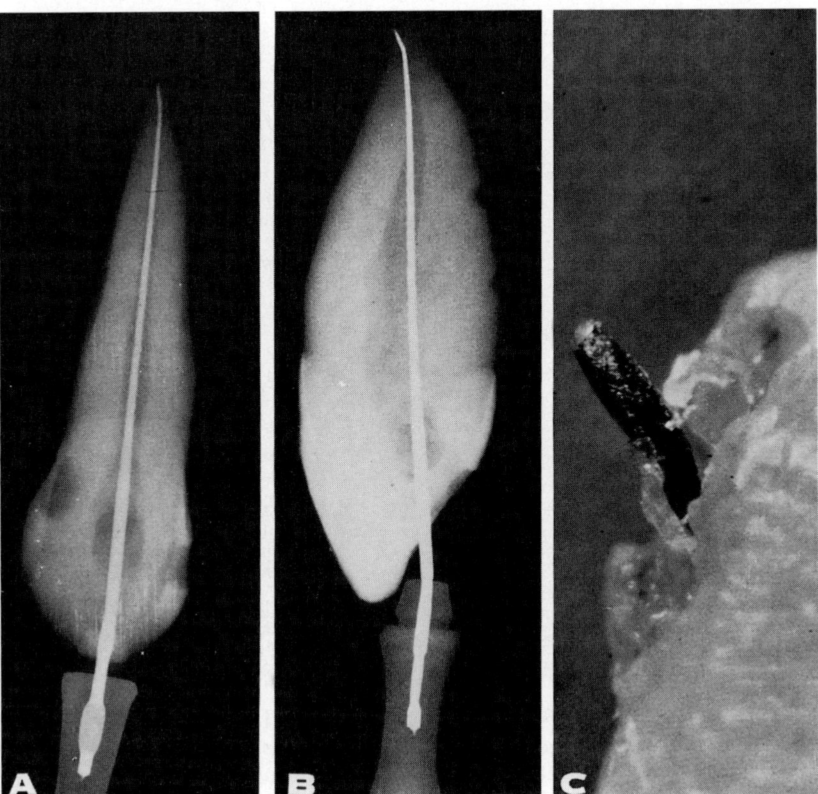

Figure 9-21 **A,** Labiolingual projection through canine shows instrument apparently at apex with slight distal curvature. **B,** Mesiodistal projection reveals instrument actually emerging from labial short of apex. **C,** Instrument perforating foramen to labial well short of radiographic root end. (Courtesy of Dr. John R. Grady and Dr. Howard Clausen.)

Warning: These rapidly processed films will fade or discolor with time.[33,34] This change can be prevented, after viewing, by returning the wet film for a few minutes of fixation, followed by washing for 30 minutes, and then drying. The films will then retain their quality indefinitely.

Table-Top Developing. For really rapid response and ease of processing, combining rapid-speed solutions with a **table-top processing hood** (Figure 9-22) greatly improves radiographic reporting, particularly working films. These hoods are often used right in the operatory. The operator places his hands through lightproof cuffs and observes hand movement inside the hood through the red Plexiglas cover. The rapid solutions and rinse water can be in small cups no deeper than a periradicular film (see Figure 9-22).

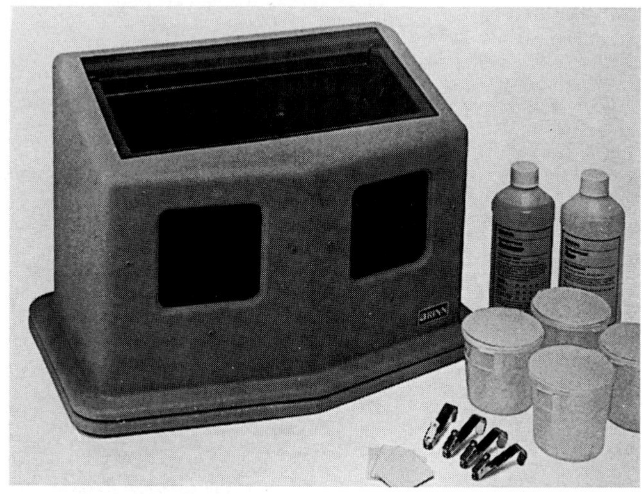

Figure 9-22 Counter-top x-ray developing hood along with rapid developer/fixer, solution cups, and single film holders. Light-tight handholes and lightproof lid for viewing. (Courtesy of Densply/ Rinn Corporation.)

Direct Digital Radiography

As dentistry parallels photography, in the move from silver halide film to digital photography and computer processing, the profession will undergo continued growth toward **digital radiographic systems.** Digital radiography used in dentistry is available in three variations: direct digital, storage phosphor, and indirect digital.

The **direct digital systems** use a solid-state sensor such as a charge coupled device (CCD) similar to the chips in home camcorders. These systems have a cable that connects the sensor to the computer and in turn to the screen monitor (Figure 9-23).

The **storage phosphor systems** use a photo-stimulable phosphor plate that stores the latent image in the phosphor for subsequent readout by an extraoral laser scanner (Figure 9-24).

Indirect digital systems use a scanning device connected to a computer for digitizing traditional silver halide dental films.

In clinical endodontics, the most applicable technology is the **direct digital** (wired) type of digital radiographic system. In a general practice, however, it can be advantageous to have the **film-scanning** capability.

Direct digital radiography (DDR) is the **direct replacement** of an x-ray film with an electronic image receptor or **sensor** and an image displayed on a **computer** (see Figure 9-23). In traditional dental radiography, as in photography, film is used to capture an image on a chemical emulsion. In the last 10 years, however, **photo film** is being replaced by the electronic digital camera. The **CCD** technology, used in digital cameras and camcorders, has been adapted for **intraoral** cameras and radiography. Both of these technologies share the same underlying operating principles.

DDR makes use of a rigid solid-state sensor, typically a **CCD,** a complementary metal oxide silicon, or a charge injection device, connected by a cable to a computer, a monitor, and a printer. The typical **DDR** sensor is packaged in a hard aluminum or plastic shell that encases several components (Figure 9-25). X-radiation (light), generated from any modern x-ray head, is converted by a screen to green light that is transmitted through an optical fiber to the **CCD** sensor. The **CCD**

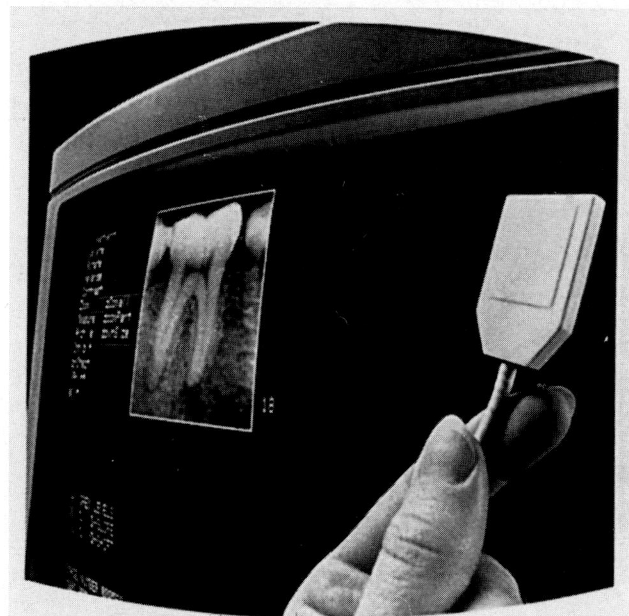

Figure 9-23 Digital radiography. VIXA intraoral sensor against the video screen showing last image in place. The sensor should be covered with a rubber finger-cot to preserve sterility.

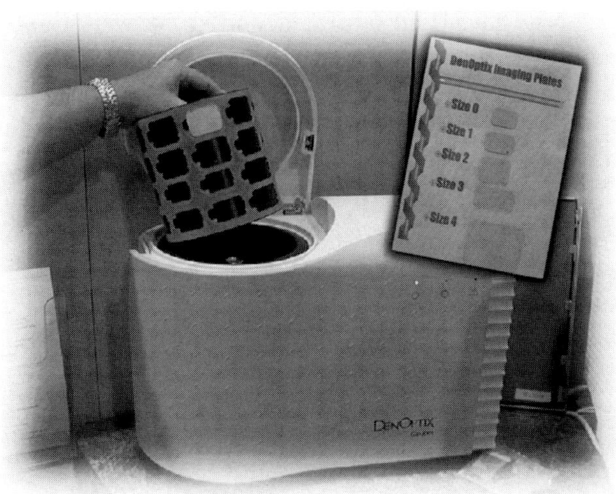

Figure 9-24 DenOptix Storage Phosphor system from Gendex with laser scanner. (Courtesy of Dentsply/Gendex.)

then converts the green light to electrons that are deposited in electron wells for subsequent readout, line by line by the electronics.[35–37]

The most significant advantage to the **DDR**-style devices is the near instantaneous (a few seconds) availability of the images after exposure **without removing** the sensor from the mouth.

This **allows multiple angles to be taken** to help in location of canals, identification of root curvatures, verification of working lengths, and verification of intermediate obturation results. Treatment delays caused by missed apices, cone cuts, and poor exposure are reduced from several minutes to seconds. This can be accomplished with one half to one-eighth of the radiation normally used in exposing a single silver halide dental film.

Tangible Benefits. There are several immediate benefits to using DDR for endodontic procedures. No darkroom or processing equipment is needed. Infection control procedures are reduced, and duplicates are instantly made with absolutely no loss in image quality. Additionally, the sensitivity of the receptors and the digital nature of the image permit **reduction** of the patient's x-ray exposure. **Computers can be used to store and enhance the image** or to transmit it over a telephone line to an insurance company or to a colleague for instant consultation. Most important is the trust and credibility gained by displaying a huge image that the patient can see and understand, using a familiar delivery medium—a "TV" picture (Figure 9-26). The radiographic picture on the computer screen helps the clinician explain needed treatment. This is particularly important for specialists as they may have only one or two visits to gain the patient's trust,

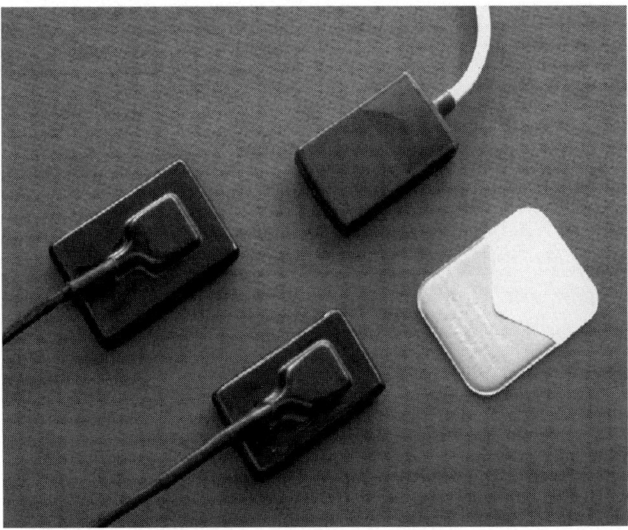

Figure 9-25 Trophy sensors. Clockwise from x-ray film (**right**), DMD size #1, DMD size #2, Trophy Universal. (Courtesy of John A. Khademi.)

explain the need for treatment, obtain informed consent, and complete their care.

Time Savings. Time saved by not waiting for film processing is certifiable with digital radiography. Automatic chemical processing takes 4 to 6 minutes, whereas the slowest digital system takes only 7 seconds. Yet this does not tell the whole story. The **real time** for a radiographic "event" is measured from the time the clinician first prescribes the radiograph until the time the image is ready for viewing. The assistant must drape the patient with the lead apron and position the sensor or film, which takes a few minutes. Then the film is removed from the mouth, chemically processed, rinsed, and dried. Thus the real time for film radiography is about 6 minutes, whereas digital radiography is closer to

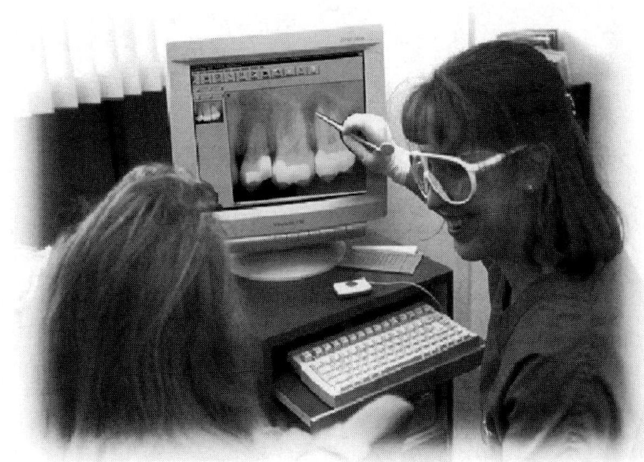

Figure 9-26 The patient can readily see her clinical situation on the computer screen. (Courtesy of John A. Kahdemi.)

3 minutes, including the draping. With **DDR**, however, there is no "dead time" during the radiographic event and no need to mentally "re-enter" the case.

Retakes. Ease of retakes is often overlooked when discussing time savings. Ease of retakes is the real time saver. With film, a retake requires another 6 minutes or more, whereas with digital, a retake takes an instant. An even greater benefit is that the x-ray head, patient, and sensor are all still in place. This simplifies interpretation and adjustment to different angles. There is no need to "remember" the case or wonder at what angle the last radiograph was taken.

Dose Reduction. Lower x-ray dosage is another quantifiable benefit of all digital radiography systems. Almost all of the digital systems are capable of reducing exposure to 50% of conventional E-speed film. Exposure can be further decreased to less than 20% if image quality is slightly compromised. This is accomplished by **underexposing the sensor** and then using the **computer-processing functions** to visually improve the image quality.

With the growing concern of patients regarding radiation exposure, digital systems help defuse their concerns about radiography.

Computer Processing. Although the software programs provided with the different digital radiography systems have a dazzling array of image-processing algorithms, only a few are of primary importance in endodontics. The most important image-processing tool is the **brightness/contrast tool**. Images that are washed out or underexposed can often be computer processed to increase their contrast and decrease the brightness (Figure 9-27). However, as useful as this tool is, it cannot correct a **badly overexposed** image because the pixels have been saturated, and no recovery can be made other than re-exposing the sensor.

From a patient education perspective, another computer enhancement that is quite useful is the **Pseudo-3D feature** shown in the **Trophy** software (Figure 9-28). The radiograph is converted to a contour map while maintaining the relative gray levels. The radiolucency at the periapex of the tooth is dark, relative to the surrounding structures, and thus appears as a "hole in the bone" in the Pseudo-3D view. This allows the clinician to communicate, in a more understandable manner, the loss of periapical bone.

Digital Radiographic Technique for Endodontics

The assistant enters the patient's demographics into the computer and selects the "exam type" from the menu that appears on the screen. The **sensor** is then sheathed in a latex "finger cot" (for sanitary reasons) (Figure 9-29) and correctly positioned intraorally. The x-ray head is then positioned, the computer software is activated, and x-ray exposure is made. The computer has captured and stored the image as it appears on the monitor screen (Figure 9-30). If adjustments are needed, the sensor and/or the x-ray beam (head) may be repositioned while the sensor is still in place. Again, the corrected image appears on the screen to guide the dentist and/or instruct the patient. All of the images will be "stored" and may later be recalled to complete the patient's record. The "before and after" images can then be transported by "hard copy" or electronic mail to the referring dentist.

Tooth Length Measurement. The ability to accurately measure preoperative working length is another useful tool. Since the pixel sizes making up the digital

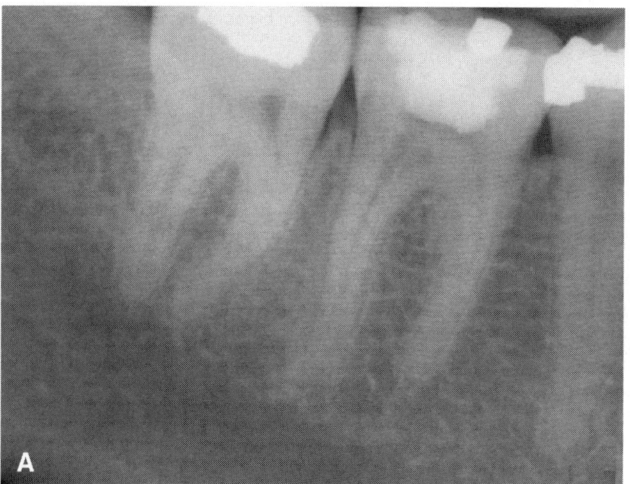

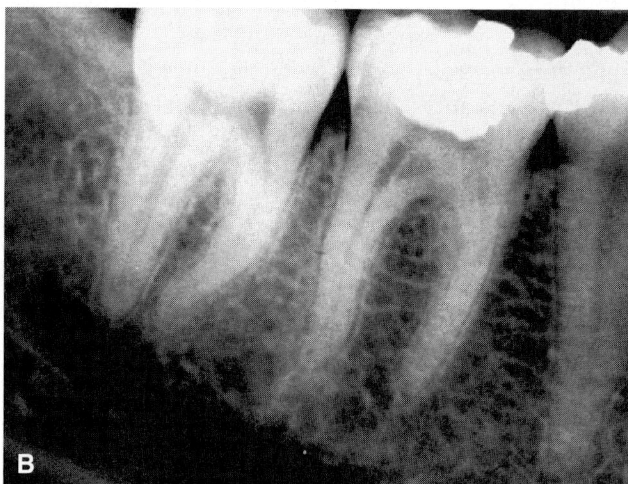

Figure 9-27 Computer processing to enhance image. **Left,** Slightly underexposed, unprocessed image. **Right,** Computer-processed image highlights resorptive defect over the distal root. (Courtesy of John A. Kahdemi.)

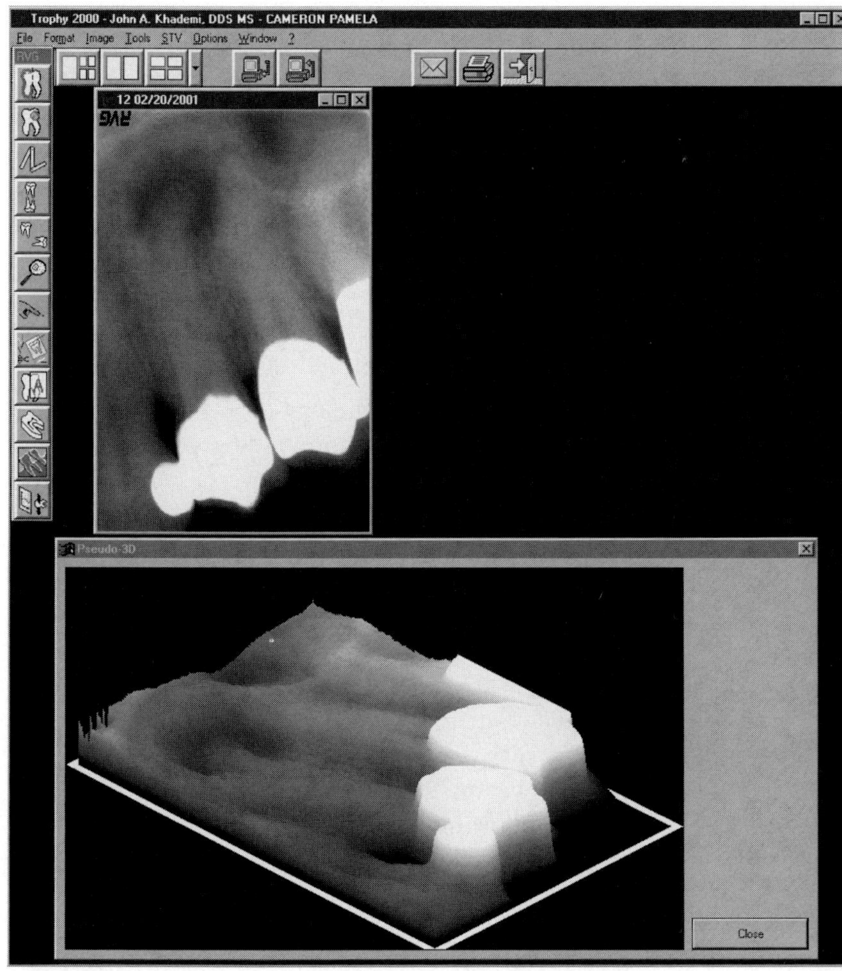

Figure 9-28 Computer enhancement using **Pseudo-3D feature of Trophy** software that converts a traditional two-dimensional radiograph into a "third-dimensional" contour map that is better understood by the patient. Note the periapical lesion as a "dark hole." (Courtesy of John A. Khademi.)

image are known, it is easy for the computer to calculate a preoperative length, even around curvatures. (Figure 9-31). Most digital radiography programs allow the clinician to start at either the coronal or apical reference point and enter (by clicking a mouse) several points along the anticipated canal path. These preoperative lengths are within 0.5 mm more than 95% of the time.

Sensor Sizes. Endodontic imaging needs can be met by a single sensor size. Generally, the smaller sensor size (size 1 equivalent) is the most useful in an endodontic setting (see Figure 9-25). The smaller size is more comfortable for the patient and easier for the assistant to place. The larger sensors can be more difficult to place because of their rigidity. An extra sensor should be available in the event of sensor failure.

Holders. Properly designed "paddle"-style holders greatly facilitate infection control procedures. Correct sensor positioning and angulation lead to better images. These holders can be easily bent to manage tipped and rotated upper and lower molars. **Snap-A-Ray** and **Rinn Endoray II**-style holders can also be

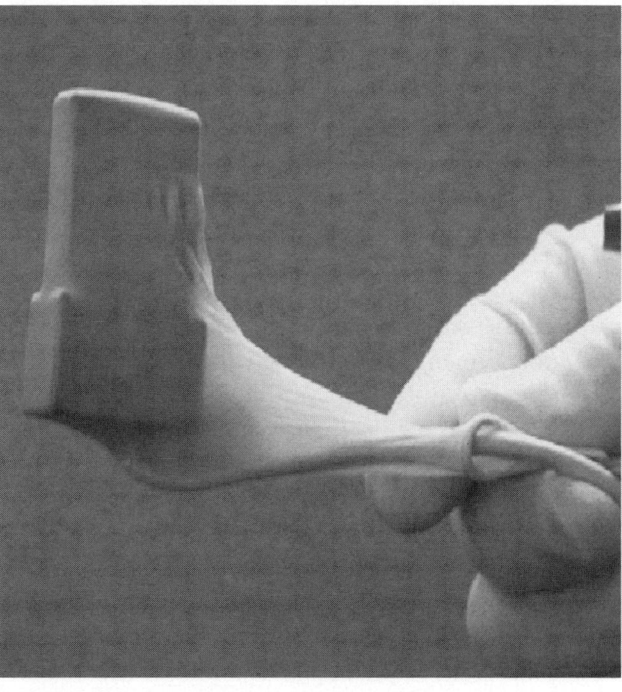

Figure 9-29 For sanitary reasons, the sensor is sheathed in a latex "finger-cot." (Courtesy of John A. Khademi.)

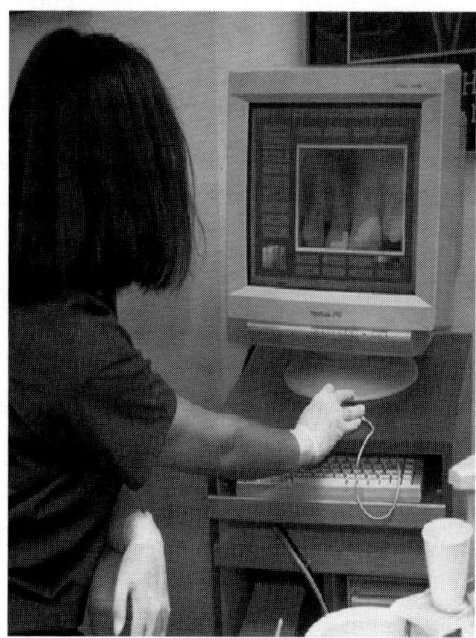

Figure 9-30 All of the radiographic images are stored in the computer and may be called up at any time for diagnosis, patient education, or printing. (Courtesy of John A. Khademi.)

used, but they are bulkier and harder to sheath. Occasionally, the aiming guides are in the way during angled radiography or interfere with the rubber dam.

Exposure. There is considerably less latitude with regard to correct exposure with digital systems than with film. Although this may seem counterintuitive, given that the digital images can be reprocessed, **overexposure** results in permanent loss, on the screen, of anatomic structures. With digital images, one should err on the side of **underexposure**—the opposite of film images. Additionally, some x-ray heads do not have a low enough setting; to further decrease exposure, the x-ray head is moved away from the patient by 6 to 12 inches.

Buyer's Guide

The prime technical factors to consider in the purchase of a digital radiography system for use in endodontics are the ease of use of the software and the availability of appropriately sized sensors, a sensor replacement warranty, and efficient holders. Multiple image processing and enhancement tools, although appealing, contribute little to the day-to-day use of the system and can often be in the way. The differences in **image quality** between the present systems are relatively narrow.

Computer Systems. This new technology to replace film requires a **Windows NT or Windows 2000 server** with Fault-Tolerant hard drives (RAID). Uninterruptible power supplies should be installed on the server and all clinical workstations. Images should be automatically **backed up** and stored off-site.

Monitors. Large, high-quality computer monitors allow maximum resolution of the image to be displayed as well as the ability to display multiple images. Larger monitors are often brighter, which allows for easier interpretation in the well-lit dental operatory. Flat panels or liquid crystal displays are becoming increasingly popular as the dental operatory becomes starved for space. One would be well advised, however, that some flat panels have very limited viewing angles, and the image is almost invisible when viewed off-angle.

FUTURE TRENDS

Digital Subtraction Radiology

Digital Subtraction Radiology (DSR) uses a computer to assess, in two or more radiographs, pathologic **changes** that have taken place over a period of time. With conventional radiography, detection of a change, such as an increase or decrease in lesion size, is done by viewing two films, side by side, on a view box. Unfortunately, this is a very insensitive technique for detecting small bony changes. With **conventional radiography**, a 30 to 50% radiodensity difference is needed for reliable detection of change, and cancellous bone changes may not be visible at all.[9] **DSR** can significantly improve one's diagnostic accuracy of periapical lesions, allowing for earlier intervention and more accurate detection of active disease.[38–42]

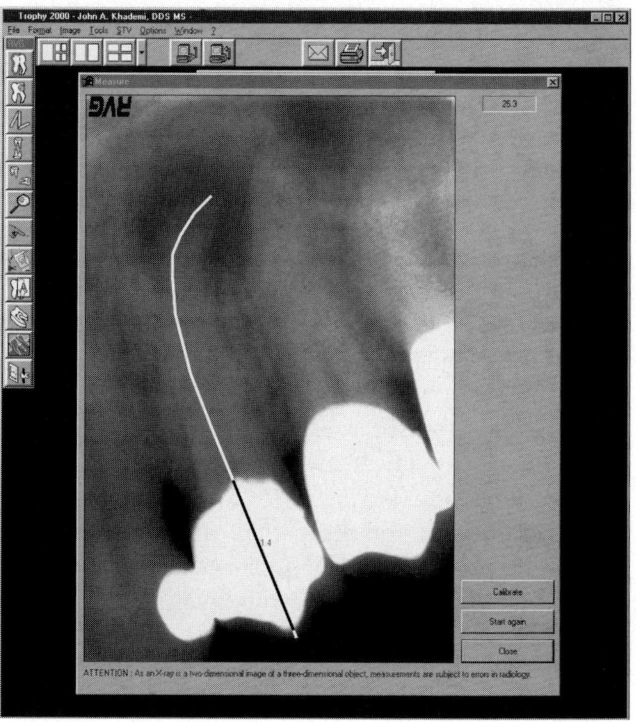

Figure 9-31 By beginning at the apex and advancing the cursor toward the crown with the "mouse," the computer will accurately calculate the working length of the tooth in millimeters, even around curvatures. (Courtesy of John A. Khademi.)

To use the DSR technique, the **two digital images** to be compared are brought into the computer software. Since they are digital images, they are stored in a numeric format in the computer memory and can be **compared mathematically**. Typically, the background images that have not changed—crowns, fillings, and so forth—are subtracted, which in turn highlights areas that have changed—lesion size and/or density, for instance.[43]

Tomography

Another exciting development is the generation of dental **tomographic images**[44] (E Hebranson and P Brown, personal communication, 1999). Tomography is a radiographic technique that essentially "slices" the teeth into thin sections. Computers then reassemble the sections to generate a three-dimensional image. When these techniques are refined, pulp spaces and roots will be visualized in the third dimension. Buccolingual curvatures will be evident, as well as the shape of the canal space and the location of the apical foramen (Figure 9-32). An additional advantage would be the elimination of specialized angled radiography; all angled views will be simultaneously captured in one exposure.

RADIOGRAPHIC INTERPRETATION

Since properly positioned, exposed, and processed radiographic or digital images (Figure 9-33) are of value only if they are properly interpreted, every advantage must be taken to obtain the most information from the image. For the student and seasoned practitioner alike, **a good magnifying glass** has often brought to light an extra root, root canal, or hard-to-find apex.

A superlative method for examining radiographs is the Brynolf magnifier-viewer.[45] This device enhances the viewing of individual films in two ways: the image is magnified several times, and all peripheral light is effectively blocked out. Masking the light source around a radiograph **greatly** increases the ability of the viewer to distinguish grades of density.[46] A film that has been slightly overexposed, if magnified and inspected over a strong light, yields a remarkable amount of unsuspected information. In a re-treated case, endodontic success had been denied for 9 years until inspection under magnification of the original radiograph disclosed a previously **overlooked third root** on a maxillary first premolar.

Many departures from classic radiographic procedures have been strongly advocated for endodontic

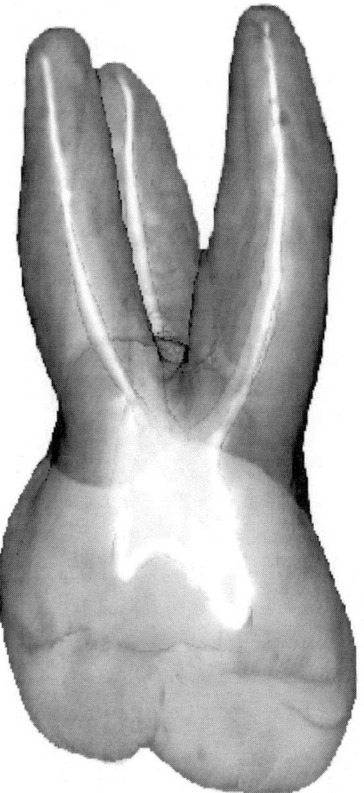

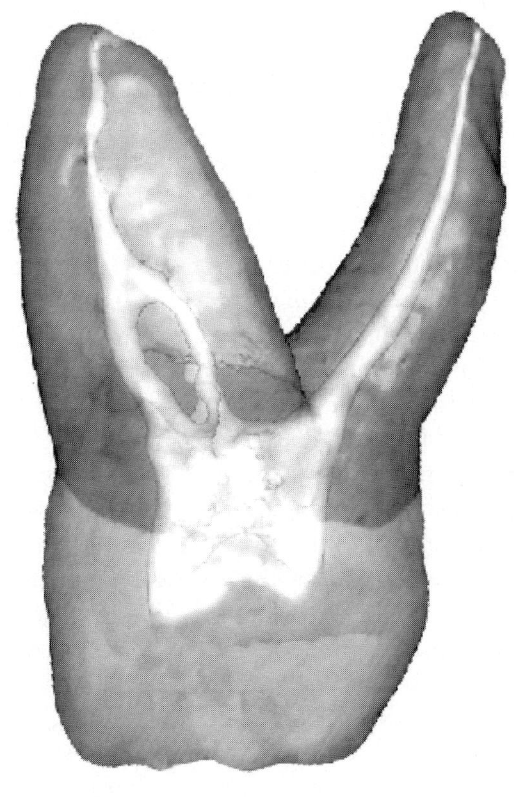

Figure 9-32 **Tomographic images** of a maxillary molar reconstructed by computer. Tomography essentially "slices" the image into thin sections and then "reassembles" them into a three-dimensional image. **A**, Buccal view. **B**, Mesial view. (Courtesy of John A. Khademi.)

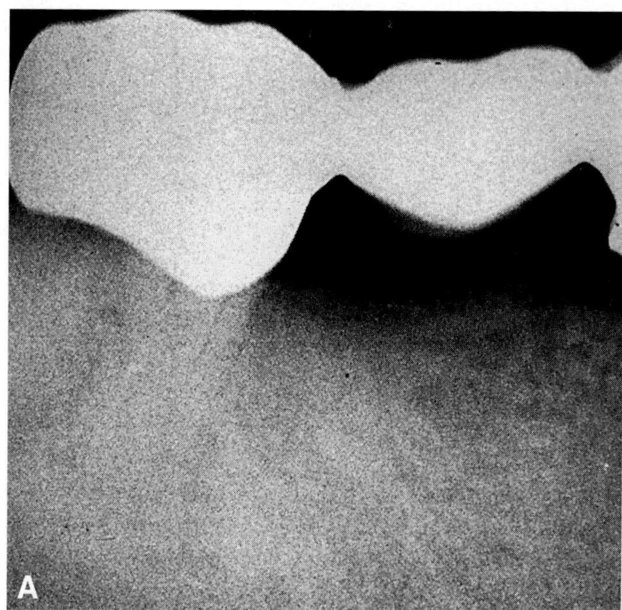

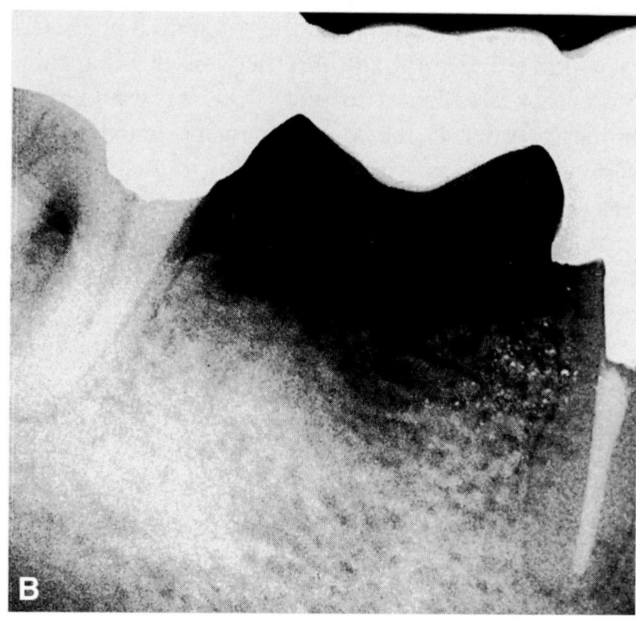

Figure 9-33 **A,** Poorly processed radiograph lacks definition for proper diagnosis. **B,** Properly processed radiograph of same case yields diagnostic details lacking in **A.** (Courtesy of A. C. Goerig and E. J. Neaverth.)

therapy. Any variation that makes the exposure and processing of radiographs easier, faster, and better, and the interpretation more thorough, increases the value of these "eyes beneath the surface." It is when we do not see what we are doing that failures increase.

VISUAL ENHANCEMENT

Endoscopy

Light and magnification are key factors in endodontics because what cannot be seen cannot be properly treated. The **Endoscope** (Karl Storz, Germany/USA) and the **Orascope** (Sitca, Inc., USA) provide both light and magnification for better access and location of canal orifices, fractures, failing silver points, separated instruments, and posts. They are also extremely useful in endodontic surgery, including apicoectomy, retrofillings of the root end, location and repair of perforations, and internal and external resorptive defects.

Endoscopy is the inspection of body cavities and organs using an endoscope. This device consists of a tube and an optical system with a high-intensity light. The image captured by the endoscopic camera is projected onto a video monitor for viewing (Figure 9-34). In endodontics, one can visualize access openings, canal orifices (Figure 9-35), the canal interior, fractures, resorptive defects, and surgical sites, all highly magnified.

Endoscopy dates back to the time of Hippocrates II (460–375 BC) when physicians of the time used tubes inserted into body openings to view interior structures. Abulkasim, in AD 1012, used a mirror to reflect light through the hollow tube. Aranzi, in 1585, used reflected solar rays to peer into nasal cavities. Bonzzani (1804) used a candle as a light source, and Segalas in 1826 added a cannula for ease of insertion. Desormeaux (1835) is considered the father of endoscopy, using kerosene lamplight reflected through a mirror system. He used this system as a cystoscope and a urethroscope. Panteleone (1869) refined the Desormaux scope for looking into the uterus. In 1877, Nitze added an optical lens system to the tube. Dittel (1887) added a small incandescent bulb at the end of a cystoscope as a light source. (Thomas Edison invented the incandescent lamp in 1880.) By the end of the nineteenth century, there existed cystoscopy, proctoscopy, laryngoscopy, and esophagoscopy. In 1901, Ott was the first to make a small incision into the abdomen and use a mirror head to reflect light. Also in 1901, Kelling injected air through a separate needle during a cystoscopic procedure in a dog as the first closed endoscopic procedure. Takagi (Tokyo 1918) was the first to examine the knee joint. In 1952, Hopkins used **quartz rods** in the tube of the scope to project light into the operating field, and in 1968 fiber optics were added, and the system that is used today came into being.[47]

The first use of the endoscope in endodontics was to observe fractures in teeth.[48] Held et al.[49] and Shulman and Leung[50] in 1996 reported the use of the endoscope for both conventional and surgical endodontics. Bahcall et al. recently described using the endoscope

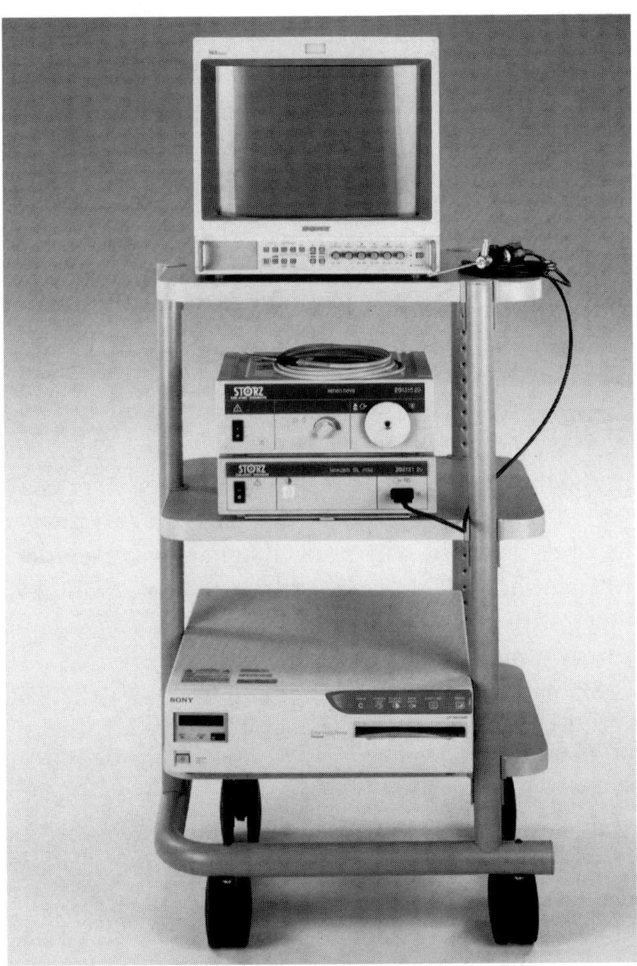

Figure 9-34 **Endoscope** set-up on mobile cart. **Top shelf,** Monitor, and to the **right, camera head** with **scope** attached. **Middle shelf, Xenon** light source on top of **Telecam**, the camera control unit, which is the heart of the system attached by cable to the camera scope **above. Bottom shelf,** Color **printer.** (Courtesy of Karl Storz & Co. Germany/USA.)

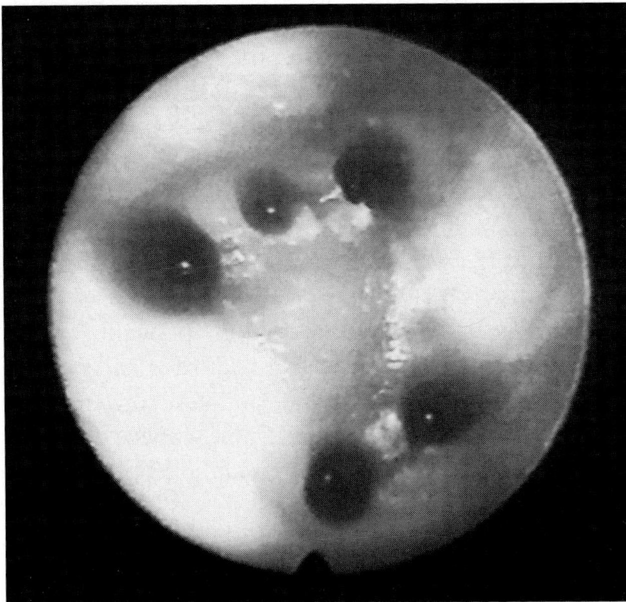

Figure 9-35 A 1.8 mm fiber-optic probe examination of the pulpal floor, revealing orifices of five canals of mandibular first molar. (Courtesy of J. K. Bahcall and J. T. Barss.)

for increased magnification and visualization during endodontic microsurgical procedures.[51]

There are many **advantages** to using the endoscope in endodontics: direct illumination of the field, brightness with no loss of resolution, and the ability to view inaccessible areas by seeing around corners and beneath and behind areas. The endoscope may be easily positioned 0.5 to 10 mm from the working field, where it will remain in focus. There is also a short learning curve of 2 weeks to 3 months, no eyestrain, freedom of body movement, and **no need** for the use of a mirror to reflect the image as is needed with the surgical microscope.

Magnification can be from 10 to 50 times the original, depending on the equipment. The endoscope is also cost effective compared with the microscope. It is easily transportable on a cart (see Figure 9-34) and can also be used as an **intraoral camera**. Both the dentist and assistant have full view of the operating field on the television monitor. Either the dentist or the assistant can hold the scope in place while the procedure is being performed.

There are **few disadvantages** to the endoscope. The operating field is not seen in three dimensions; however, this has not been shown to be an important limiting factor in either medical or dental endoscopy. Inadvertent damage to the quartz rods inside the scope can occur. A **nonbendable sheath** covering the scope is used to create rigidity and protect the rods from damage. The scope can be scratched by burs or various instruments if the tip of the scope is held in very close proximity to the operating field. However, these are unusual occurrences because the endoscope can be easily positioned so that it is not in direct proximity to the field of operation.

The equipment that makes up the endoscope system is the endoscope itself, a camera coupler/lens, a video camera, fiber-optic cables to carry light from a halogen or xenon light source, a camera control unit, a video recorder and/or a video color printer, and a video monitor to view the procedure (Figure 9-36). Although the video recorder and printer are not necessary for operation of the endoscope, they are useful for documentation and patient education. Furthermore, an endodontist may send a referring dentist a color print of a completed surgical procedure instead of, or along with, a radiograph.

Endoscopes for endodontics can be obtained in 4- and 8-inch lengths. The tube of the working end of the endoscope contains quartz rods, some of which bring light into the field of operation and some of which return the image to the camera that projects the image onto the video monitor. The working end of the scope can be obtained in a wide variety of angulations: 0, 30, 45, 90, and 135 degrees. The most useful endoscope for endodontics is the one having a 30-degree angle.

The endoscope comes in a variety of widths, from 0.7 to 10 mm. The most useful width for endodontic **surgical procedures is 4 mm,** and for **conventional** endodontic treatment, a **0.7 to 4 mm scope** is best.

The source of light is delivered to the scope by fiber-optic cables. Hundreds of glass fibers are bundled together to carry light to the quartz rods inside the scope. Light can come from either a halogen or a xenon source. **A halogen light** will provide from 150 to 300 watts of illumination with a slightly yellow hue. A **xenon light** source at 300 watts will provide light with a white hue that will have greater consistency and brightness. The xenon light is also more penetrating than is the halogen.

The camera coupler/lens attaches to the end of the scope. The coupler can be equipped with a **zoom control** that allows a closer view in the form of a **zoomed picture** that will usually **fill the entire monitor screen.**

Cameras are produced in one- and three-chip models. A one-chip camera will deliver 450 lines per second of image to a video monitor. A three-chip camera delivers 800 lines per second. For comparison, a standard television delivers 265 lines per second. For endodontic procedures, at this time, a **one-chip camera will provide sufficient definition and clarity.**

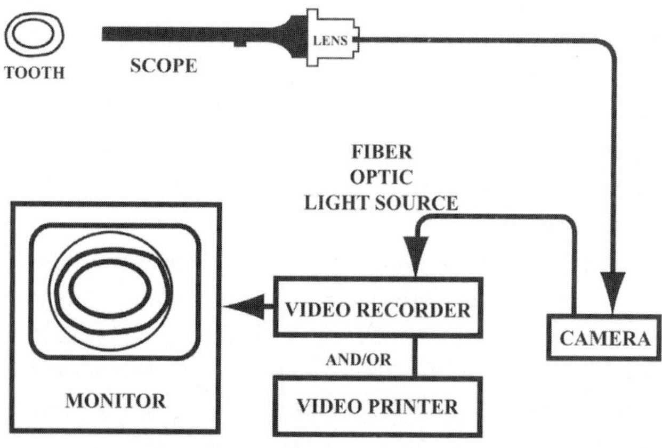

Figure 9-36 The Endoscope System. The **Scope**, surveying tooth, contains quartz rods that convey the image. They, in turn, are surrounded by a fiber-optic **light source.** The Scope is attached to the **camera** by a camera coupler, which in turn connects to the **computer** and **printer** as well as to the **monitor.** Images appear on the monitor and are stored in the computer for later printing if desired. (Courtesy of F. H. Kahn and B. B. Shulman.)

The camera control unit controls color density and shutter control. Automatic gain control ensures clarity of the picture. The **signal degenerates** with a longer cable and the devices (video recorder and printer) through which the signal has to travel before it reaches the monitor where it can be viewed. Any size monitor can be used; however, as the screen increases in size, the sharpness of the image decreases.

A **video recorder** can be used **to capture** an endodontic procedure. The best quality image for analog video is the Hi 8 system. The **highest quality image,** however, is recorded by using a **digital video recorder,** wherein the images can be edited and copied multiple times, with no loss of resolution, as will occur with an analog system.[50]

Stability of the scope itself is important. A variety of **sheaths** inserted over the tube of the scope are used to provide **rigidity**, support, and stability. They also protect the tip from potential damage from instruments. **Shulman** has described a stabilization technique for endodontic surgical procedures. He suggests placement of the end of the rigid sheath **on the surface of the bone,** adjacent to the surgical site, thus producing a **stable video image.**[50]

The sheaths come with a variety of working ends. Canal orifices, calcified canals, perforations, and resorptive defects can be viewed using a **forked-ended sheath** that can rest on access openings, a marginal ridge, or the buccal or lingual surface of the tooth being treated or an adjacent tooth (Figure 9-37, A). Sheaths with retractors that have **serrated ends** that are a similar shape to that of a handheld retractor can be anchored on bone to provide support and flap and cheek retraction during surgery (Figure 9-37 B). A sheath shaped like a tongue retractor is used to move the patient's tongue aside while viewing the lingual aspect of a tooth. The scope can be anchored in position by the sheath and the **lens/camera coupler can then be rotated 360 degrees** to completely view all aspects being treated.

During procedures involving rotary instruments, the tip of the endoscope can become covered with debris and the video picture can become blurred. Saline in a syringe or sterile water from a **triplex** or **Stropko syringe** (see chapter 12, "Endodontic Surgery") can be used to rinse away the debris and clear the viewing field on the monitor. A cotton swab saturated with saline solution can also be used to accomplish debris removal.

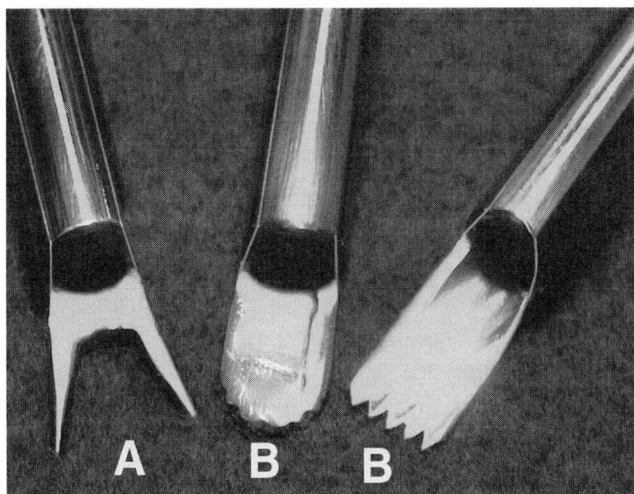

Figure 9-37 **Protective metal sheaths** that slip over the scope provide rigidity and allow the scope to be held in a stable position. **A,** Fork-ended sheath fashioned to rest on access openings and/or marginal ridges. **B,** Sheaths with serrated ends are used as retractors anchored in bone. Stability provides constant focus. (Courtesy of B. B. Shulman.)

After use, the sheaths should be placed in an ultrasonic cleaner to remove debris and sterilized in an autoclave with ethylene oxide or glutaraldehyde. **The scope cannot be placed in an ultrasonic cleaner** but can be easily cleaned by soaking in an enzymatic cleaner or washed gently with soap and distilled water and then sterilized in glutaraldehyde for 12 hours. Autoclavable scopes are also available. The lens head/camera coupler can be cleaned with a mild soap and distilled water and sterilized by soaking in glutaraldehyde. It is best protected with a disposable plastic tube—wrap during use to keep it sterile and free of debris.

The **Orascope** (Sitca, Inc., USA) is an evolutionary extension of dental endoscopy: **Orascopy**. Currently, there are two diameter sizes of flexible fiber-optic probes: the 1.8 mm and the 0.7 mm (Figure 9-38) The 1.8 mm probe has 30,000 fibers and the 0.7 has 10,000. A ring of light transmitting fibers surrounds the visual fibers (Figure 9-39). Both probes have a large depth of field and do not need to be refocused after the initial focus. The 1.8 mm probe is used to visualize conventional and surgical sites.[51] The **0.7 mm probe** is used for that and for **intracanal visualization** as well (Figure 9-40). Canal cleanliness, location of accessory canals, perforations, broken instruments, and resorptive defects are easily examined.[52,53] **The 0.7 mm probe must be used in a dry canal.** It will not penetrate blood, exudate, or irrigant. The **coronal two-thirds** of the canal should be flared to at least a size 70 instrument. **Jedmed** is planning to release an endoscopic system called **Endodontic Endoscopic Systems (E.E.S.).**

Future Possibilities

Many advances being made in medical endoscopy can easily be adapted to endodontic endoscopic procedures. Software can piece two-dimensional images together to create a virtual **three-dimensional** fly-through. **Virtual reality** technique training will enhance and speed the learning curve for difficult endodontic procedures. Video and audio conferencing using a **webcam,** which is **an endoscope** to project video images, digital radiographs, and patient files, can be sent over the Internet so that dentists anywhere in the world are able to confer and obtain the best diagnosis and treatment planning for their patients. **Future possibilities are unlimited.**

SPECIALIZED ENDODONTIC INSTRUMENTS AND EQUIPMENT

"The lack of proper equipment" is a reason often given by dentists who do not practice root canal therapy, and it well might be. Not only are special instruments imperative for endodontic treatment, but a special arrangement of these instruments is necessary.

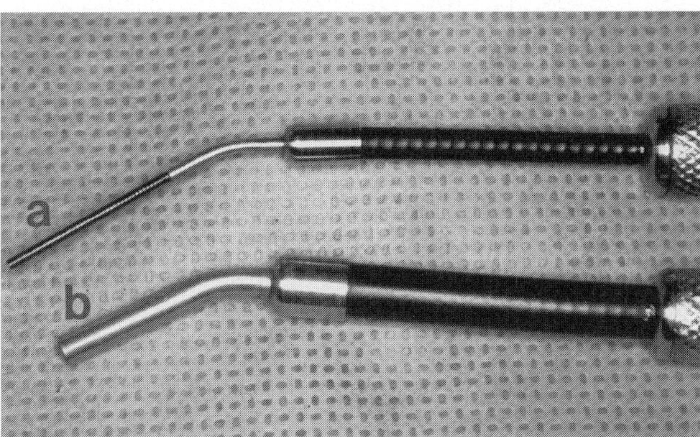

Figure 9-38 Unsheathed **Orascopic fiber-optic probes** in two sizes: ***a,*** 0.7 mm, and ***b,*** 1.8 mm. (Courtesy of Sitca, Inc., USA.)

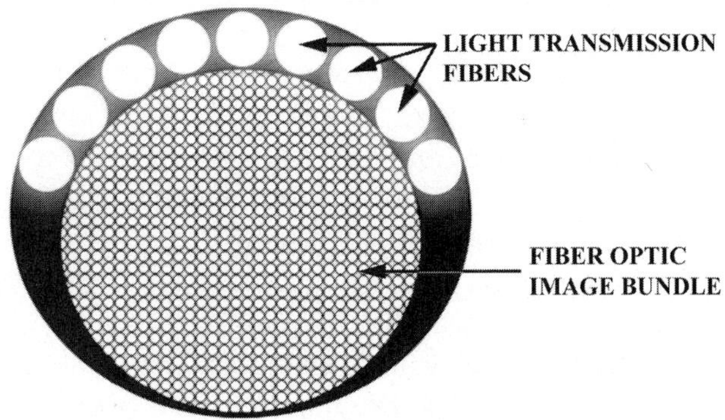

Figure 9-39 Cross-section of Orascopic probe showing the distribution of the fiber-optic image bundle and the light transmission fibers. (Courtesy of Sitca, Inc., USA.)

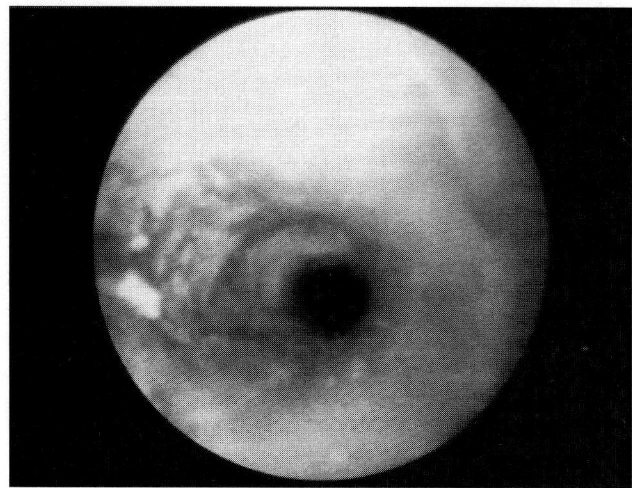

Figure 9-40 **Orascopic** view of the apical foramen and canal walls taken with a 0.7 mm **flexible probe** that contains 10,000 visual fibers plus light fibers (Courtesy of J. K. Bahcall and J. T. Barss.)

Impractical, inefficient scurrying around the office to gather together a collection of unsterile, ill-adapted equipment completely discourages the practitioner from endodontic therapy. These problems may be solved by **procuring** the correct equipment and supplies; by **packaging** the hand equipment into sterilized towel kits, into canisters, or on prearranged trays; and finally, by **storing** the small endodontic instruments in an **organized,** compartmentalized instrument case.

Sterilized Towel Kit

Standard dental instruments, along with a few special instruments necessary for root canal therapy, are wrapped into a pack in two layers of towel and fastened with a banker's pin or autoclave tape. This rolled kit can then be sterilized and stored, ready for use (Figure 9-41).

When treatment is to begin, the towel kit is unrolled on the working surface and the instruments arranged on the sterile surface according to their frequency of use. The following instruments are contained in the towel kit:

- Three dappen dishes
- One Luer syringe, 3 mL (disposable)
- One Luer type 27-gauge ProRinse needle
- One mouth mirror, "Front Surface"
- Two cotton pliers
- One DE spoon excavator, Starlite #31
- One plastic instrument, Glick #1, Star Dental
- One measuring gauge or millimeter ruler (metal)
- One pair of scissors, embroidery, 3¼-inch overall length
- One D-G explorer, Star Dental
- Three gauze sponges, 2 inch
- Three cotton rolls #3, 1-inch long

In any number of receptacles, ranging from a simple banker's sponge soaked in germicide to sophisticated stainless and plastic holders, the assistant may arrange the root canal instruments in numerical order and properly measured to length. It is impractical, if not impossible, to pass the short-handled instruments to the operator: hence the orderly arrangement for easy acquisition. For dentists working alone, the **Endoring** (Jordco/Almore International Inc., USA) is recommended (Figure 9-42).

Handpieces

The only regular dental equipment needed, other than anesthetic syringes and rubber dam equipment, are the two contra-angle handpieces: one high speed, the other conventional speed. All handpieces must be sterilized. The assistant should then place the correct burs in the contra angles, sized according to the tooth to be treated.

The burs, stored in the sterile instrument case, are removed from the case with the sterile cotton pliers and placed in the contra angle with the pliers (Figure 9-43). While the shaft of the bur is held with the pliers, the foot control of the conventional handpiece is just tapped. As the bur spins, it will drop down into place, and the latch may be closed.

For the high-speed handpiece, the burs can be dropped down into the chuck, which is then tightened. The handpiece must be absolutely concentric. Whipping of the end of the bur, experienced with a worn chuck, will fracture teeth and is particularly dan-

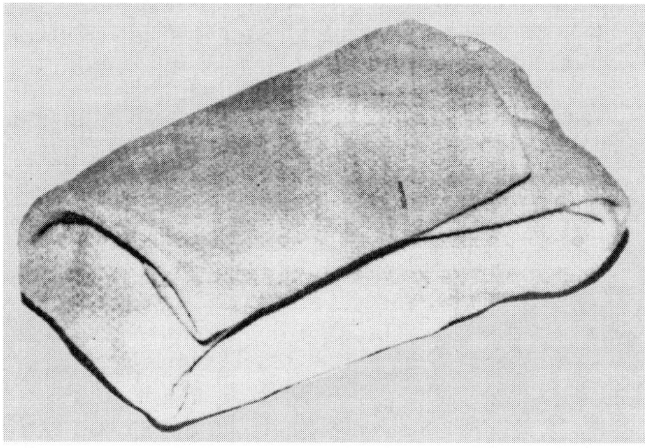

Figure 9-41 Sterilized towel kit or pack that contains standard dental instruments necessary for endodontic treatment. Colored towels are used to identify special endodontic instrument pack, which has been sterilized and conveniently stored for future use.

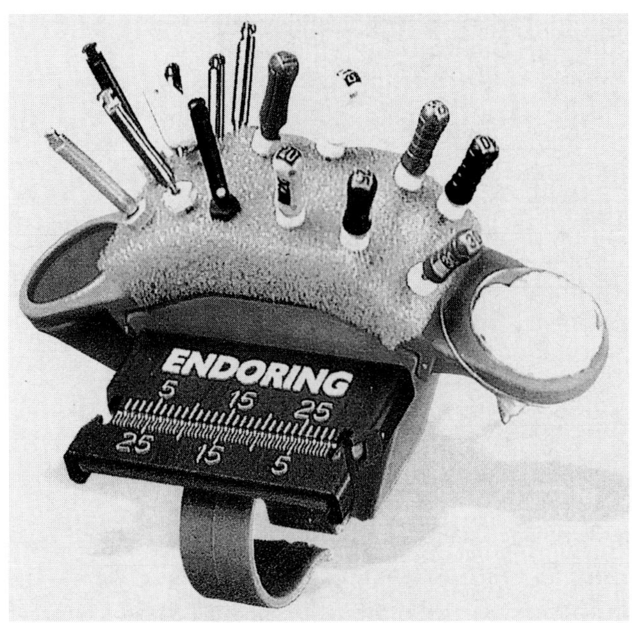

Figure 9-42 Handy Endoring worn by dentist working alone. Premeasured instruments are arranged in order in sterile, disposable plastic sponge. (Courtesy of Jordco, Inc.)

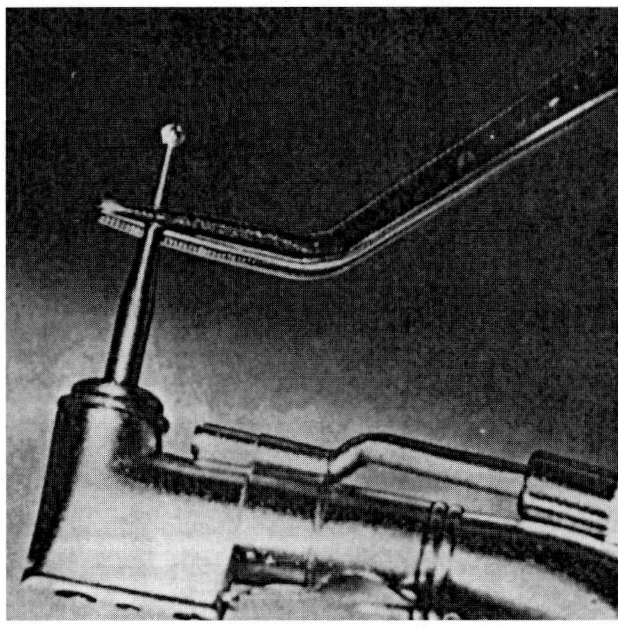

Figure 9-43 Sterile burs are placed in contra-angle handpiece with sterile pliers. Bur is "dropped" into place by holding shaft of bur with pliers and spinning foot control.

gerous when an extra long bur is being used to amputate an entire root.

Endodontic Instrument Case

The collection of tiny endodontic instruments must be kept in an organized arrangement yet lend itself readily to sterilization. The metal endodontic instrument case meets these requirements. Storage cases have long been available but never as refined as the modern cases (Figure 9-44). All of the reamers, files, broaches, burs, and filling equipment, as well as paper points and cotton pellets, are stored and sterilized in the case. The dentist or assistant removes these with **sterile pliers** only as needed.

The instrument case may be placed beside the dentist on a Mayo stand, or the assistant may obtain material from the case kept on the cabinet top. Supplies are transferred from the case to the open towel kit, which is the working surface. The case needs to be resterilized only when one of the instrument sizes is depleted. New instruments should replace sizes 10 through 25, which should be used only once. The larger instruments may be thoroughly cleaned and reused when the case is replenished before sterilization. A thorough discussion of endodontic instruments is found in chapter 10.

A selection of instruments is available from the various distributors of endodontic supplies. **These selections** have been developed for the clinician who treats all types of endodontic problems in a **general practice of dentistry**. The case and its contents are sterilized according to the directions given under "**Asepsis in Endodontic Practice**," chapter 3. The surgical armamentarium is dealt with in "Endodontic Surgery," chapter 12. Table 9-1 lists the contents of the endodontic instrument case.

PAIN CONTROL IN ENDODONTICS

In no other area of dentistry is the management of pain of greater importance than in endodontics. All too often the patient in need of endodontic therapy has endured a prolonged period of ever-increasing discomfort before seeking dental care. The reasons for this discomfort are manifold; however, there is one simple explanation in the overwhelming majority of these patients: They are scared! They are afraid of dentistry, which might be the reason for their dental problems in the first place; they are frightened of "root canal work" because of the common perception that "it hurts"; and they are often terrified at the thought of receiving local anesthetics, or "shots," in patient parlance.

It is possible to achieve clinically effective pulpal anesthesia on all teeth, infected or not, in any area of the oral cavity, with a very high degree of success and without inflicting any additional pain on the patient in the process.

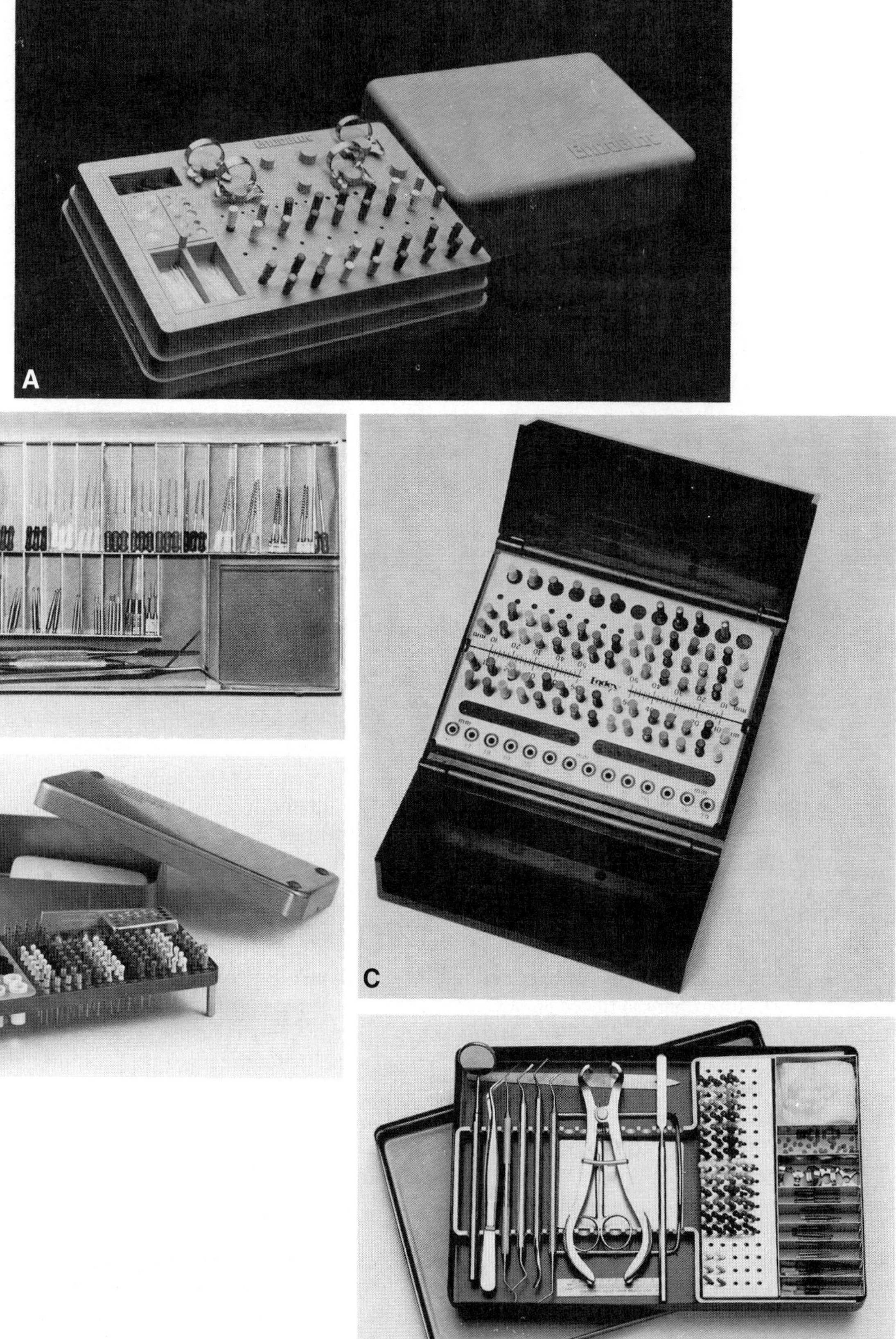

Figure 9-44 Five examples of instrument kits. **A,** ENDO-BLOC. **B,** University Case. **C,** ENDEX Endodontic System. **D,** Guldener SPLIT-KIT. **E,** TEXAS Case. (**A,** Courtesy of Endobloc, Inc., Cincinnati, OH; **B,** Courtesy of Union Broach, New York; **C,** Courtesy of Whaledent International, New York; **D,** Courtesy of Dentsply/Maillefer; **E,** Courtesy of University of Texas, San Antonio, TX.)

In the following section, common (and some uncommon) local anesthesia techniques that are used to provide effective pain control during dental treatment are presented.

Although it is possible (and probable) that the administration of local anesthesia will be both atraumatic to the patient and clinically effective, many endodontic patients (and, unfortunately, some professional colleagues) do not share that feeling. Given that a significant percentage of these patients are dental phobics, and that one of the greatest fears they harbor is the fear of pain, it is not unusual for these patients to experience "pain" at any and all times during treatment, warranted or not. There are the patients who jump when air is blown into the mouth; who exhibit an overactive gag reflex when anything is placed on the tongue or palate; who are "moving targets" during administration of the local anesthetic; who complain of "pain" constantly during treatment, even when the treatment being performed is truly **incapable** of provoking a true pain response (eg, cutting enamel or removal of an existing restoration).

The pain reaction threshold (**PRT**), defined as that point at which a person will interpret a stimulus as being painful, can be altered significantly in a given patient. These alterations can be to the patient's benefit (elevation of the PRT) or disadvantage (lowering of the PRT). Given that there is significant variation in individual response to stimulation (as described by the normal distribution curve), approximately 70% of a given population will respond appropriately to a given stimulus (eg, may say "ow" when receiving a mild painful stimulus). An additional 15% will under-react to the same stimulus. Their interpretation of this mildly painful stimulus will be that it did not hurt at all. This 15% of the population is called **"hypo-responders."** Thus, approximately 85% of a normal population will respond as expected to mildly painful stimuli. It is the remaining 15% of patients who are the **"hyper-responders."** Hyper-responding persons will interpret as painful what are usually nonpainful stimuli. And then there are the truly remarkable persons—the Indian fakir who is capable of walking across hot coals or lying on a bed of nails without experiencing any pain, or the stoic dental patient who withstands excruciating pain during every aspect of treatment.

With endodontic therapy, the number of patients who will hyper-respond to stimulation is significantly increased. Factors that lower the pain reaction include (1) the presence of pain at the start of treatment, (2) fatigue, and (3) fear and anxiety. To varying degrees, all may be present in endodontic patients.

Table 9-1 Contents of the Endodontic Instrument Case

Style "B" Hand Instruments	.02–.04 Tapers*
1 × 6 file, B, #08	1 × 6 file, B, #50
1 × 6 file, B, #10	1 × 6 file, B, #55
1 × 6 file, B, #15	1 × 6 file, B, #60
1 × 6 file, B, #20	1 × 6 file, B, #70
1 × 6 file, B, #25	1 × 6 file, B, #80
1 × 6 file, B, #30	1 × 6 file, B, #90
1 × 6 file, B, #35	1 × 6 file, B, #100
1 × 6 file, B, #40	1 × 6 file, B, #120
1 × 6 file, B, #45	1 × 6 file, B, #140
1 × 6 file, B, Golden Mediums, # 12–37	
1 × 12 files Hedstrom, assorted # 25–110	
Burs	
1 × 3 bur, carbide #701U, RA	
1 × 6 bur, #2 (3 surgical, 3 standard, RA)	
1 × 6 bur, #4 (3 surgical, 3 standard, RA)	
1 × 6 bur, #6 (3 surgical, 3 standard, RA)	
Broaches	
1 × 6 barbed broaches, fine	
1 × 6 barbed broaches, medium	
1 × 6 barbed broaches, coarse	
1 × 6 barbed broaches, extra coarse	
Obturation Instruments	
2 only cement spatula, #3	
2 only glass mixing slab, opal	
Paper points: fine, medium, and coarse	
Cotton pellets: large and small	
Special Towel Kits	
6 only: double-ended, hand style, M-spreader/pluggers	
8 only: Schilder pluggers,	
8–12 Cold sterilized or presterilized gutta-percha points and cones, assorted sizes (Dentsply/Tulsa, USA)	

*The same selection can be made for engine-driven nickel-titanium (NITI) instruments, sizes 15–80. Both stainless and NITI files have color-coded handles.

To increase the likelihood of pain-free endodontic treatment and to ensure the patient a "comfortable" experience, every dentist should make an effort to modify any of the factors acting to lower the PRT.

Chapter 18 covers a subject of great importance to the endodontist (analgesics), but also of importance to the endodontic patient is the matter of **sedation.** Fear and pain are a potent combination, capable of provoking some of the most catastrophic situations in the dental office, such as cardiac arrest. In surveying the incidence of medical emergencies in the dental environment, Malamed found that 54.9% occurred **during** the administration of the local anesthetic and an additional 22.0% occurring during dental treatment.[54] When the medical emergency arose during treatment, 65.8% of the occasions were either the **extirpation of the pulp (38.9%)** or extraction of a tooth (26.9%). The acute precipitating cause of the medical emergency was **inadequate pain control.** Although the patient had received the local anesthetic and had experienced subjective symptoms of anesthesia (eg, "numb" lip and tongue), as the extraction proceeded, or as the preparation came closer to the pulpal floor, sudden, unexpected pain occurred. The sudden elevation in blood catecholamine (epinephrine and norepinephrine) levels provoked significant elevations in both the blood pressure and heart rate and an exacerbation of the patient's underlying medical problems. This resulted in seizures, acute episodes of angina pectoris or asthma, cerebrovascular accident ("stroke"), syncope ("fainting"), hyperventilation, and psychiatric convergence reactions.

Management problems occurring during local anesthetic administration can be almost entirely prevented if consideration is given by the doctor to the patient's "feelings" about receiving "shots." Most persons do not relish the thought of receiving intraoral local anesthetic injections, demonstrated by the high incidence of adverse reactions occurring at this time. Interestingly, 53.9% of all emergencies reported by Malamed were "fainting," and over 54% of all emergencies occurred **during** the administration of the local anesthetic. Syncope during injection can be prevented virtually 100% of the time by following a few simple steps to make all local anesthetic injections as comfortable (atraumatic) as is possible (Table 9-2). Although all of the steps are important, three stand out: (1) placement of the patient who is to receive an intraoral local anesthetic into the **supine position** before the injection, (2) the **slow administration** of the local anesthetic solution, and (3) the use of **conscious sedation** before the administration of the local anesthetic.

The very simple concept behind the successful use of **conscious sedation** is that fearful patients are overly focused on everything that happens to them in the dental chair. Simply by administering a drug (central nervous system depressant) that takes the patient's awareness away from the dental milieu, the patient no longer over-responds to stimulation, does not care about the procedure, and in effect becomes a "normal" patient.

The administration of inhalation sedation with **nitrous oxide and oxygen (N_2O–O_2)**, carefully titrated, alleviates any fears of injections in the majority of needle-phobic dental patients. Continued administration of N_2O–O_2 during the endodontic procedure is entirely appropriate if the patient is at all apprehensive. In addition to relieving patients' anxieties, N_2O acts to elevate the PRT, providing a beneficial effect throughout the endodontic procedure. N_2O–O_2 is the safest of all conscious sedation techniques and, when properly used, is also one of the most effective.

When inhalation sedation is contraindicated (eg, patient is a mouth breather, patient has a "cold" or upper respiratory infection, or sedation has proved ineffective in the past in eliminating the patient's fears), other techniques of conscious sedation should be considered. These include the administration of central nervous system-depressant drugs (eg, benzodiazepines) orally, intramuscularly, intravenously, or intranasally. The safest and most effective, when used properly, is **intravenous conscious sedation.** With the availability of two benzodiazepines, **diazepam (Valium) and midazolam (Versed)**, administered via titration, it is possible to eliminate the dental fears of virtually all patients. Additionally, these drugs provide varying degrees of

Table 9-2 Atraumatic Local Anesthesia Technique

1.	Use a sterilized, sharp needle.
2.	Check the flow of local anesthetic solution before insertion of needle into tissues.
3.	Determine whether to warm the anesthetic cartridge and/or syringe.
4.	Position the patient (supine recommended).
5.	Dry the tissue.
6.	Apply topical antiseptic (optional).
7a.	Apply topical anesthetic (minimum 1–2 minutes).
7b.	Communicate with the patient.
8.	Establish a firm hand rest.
9.	Make the tissue taut.
10.	Keep syringe out of the patient's line of sight.
11a.	Insert needle into the mucosa.
11b.	Watch and communicate with the patient.
12.	Slowly advance the needle toward target.
13.	Deposit several drops of local anesthetic before touching periosteum.
14.	Aspirate.
15a.	Slowly deposit local anesthetic solution.
15b.	Communicate with the patient.
16.	Slowly withdraw syringe. Make needle safe and discard.
17.	Observe patient after injection.
18.	Record injection on the patient's chart.

Adapted from Malamed SF.[57]

amnesia, the patient having no recall of events occurring during their treatment ("it didn't happen").

Because of the prevalence of fear in endodontic patients, the use of conscious sedation should become increasingly more popular. Unfortunately, the use of conscious sedation by endodontists is extremely rare. The benefits to be gained from the proper use of conscious sedation greatly outweigh the very slight risks involved with their use.

Local Anesthetic Techniques

Problems arising in achieving profound pulpal anesthesia invariably develop in the mandible (Table 9-3). A survey by Walton and Abbott of 120 missed local anesthetic injections demonstrated that maxillary teeth were the problem 32% of the time.[55] On the other hand, on **two of three** occasions when anesthesia was ineffective, **mandibular teeth** were involved. **Mandibular molars** were the culprit **47%** of the time. Repeating the same survey, Malamed found significantly different results.[56] When inadequate local anesthesia developed, maxillary teeth were the problem only 9% of the time, whereas **91% of the offending teeth were in the mandible.** Of even greater significance is the fact that **mandibular teeth, other than molars, were never the problem (0%).**

Why the relative lack of anesthesia problems in the maxilla compared with the mandible? The very different composition of the cortical plate of bone on the buccal aspect of maxillary and mandibular teeth is one factor. In the adult mandible, the buccal cortical plate of bone is significantly thicker than that found overlying maxillary teeth. This added thickness makes the use of supraperiosteal anesthesia ineffective in the mandible, obviating the use of the easiest and most effective injection—infiltration.

Mandibular Anesthesia

To provide effective pulpal anesthesia in the **mandible,** one must administer the local anesthetic drug at a site where the nerve is still accessible (eg, before the nerve enters the mandibular foramen and into the mandibular canal). Thus, one is limited to two injection sites. One site is the lingual aspect of the mandibular ramus, where three techniques may be used: the **inferior alveolar (IA) nerve block** (the traditional "mandibular block"); the **Gow-Gates mandibular nerve block (GGMNB),** and the **Akinosi-Vazirani closed-mouth mandibular nerve block.** A second site of access to the mandibular nerve is available on the mandible, the **mental foramen,** located (usually) between the two premolars. Local anesthetic administered at this site will provide profound pulpal anesthesia of the premolar, canine and incisor teeth virtually 100% of the time, even when infection is present.

Table 9-3 Teeth Requiring Supplemental Injections

Teeth	Maxillary: Walton	Maxillary: Malamed	Mandible: Walton	Mandible: Malamed
Anteriors	2%	2%	9%	0%
Premolars	18%	2%	12%	0%
Molars	12%	5%	47%	91%

Adapted from Walton RE and Abbott BJ[55]; Malamed SF.[56]

On those occasions when these three mandibular nerve block injections fail to provide successful pulpal anesthesia, one of several supplemental techniques may be considered. These include the **periodontal ligament (PDL) injection, intraosseous (IO) anesthesia,** and **intrapulpal injection.** The IO technique has proved to be of tremendous benefit in endodontics, particularly as a means of providing anesthesia to the "hot" mandibular molar.

Maxillary Anesthesia

Although profound anesthesia of **maxillary teeth** is normally easier to obtain, problems, if they occur, usually do so following the administration of an infiltration injection to a central incisor, canine, or molar. The apex of the central incisor may lie under the cartilage of the nose, making infiltration less effective (as well as more uncomfortable). Canines that have longer than usual roots may not be anesthetized when the anesthetic is deposited below the apex (needle is not inserted far enough). Infiltration anesthesia of maxillary molars will fail in situations where the palatal root flares greatly toward the midline of the palate. Most local anesthetics infiltrated into the buccal fold will not diffuse far enough toward the midline to provide adequate pulpal anesthesia in this situation. Additionally, where periapical infection is present, the success rate of injected local anesthetics is diminished, sometimes considerably.

Fortunately, maxillary anesthesia can readily be achieved through the administration of nerve blocks. Three nerve blocks, the **posterior superior alveolar (PSA), middle superior alveolar (MSA),** and **anterior superior alveolar (ASA, "infraorbital"),** successfully provide pulpal anesthesia to maxillary teeth, even in the presence of infection.

Mandibular Techniques

The techniques are described briefly and their advantages and disadvantages highlighted. For a more in-

Table 9-4 Inferior Alveolar Nerve Block

Teeth Anesthetized	Recommended Needle	Volume of Anesthetic	+ Aspiration	VAS*
All mandibular teeth in quadrant	25 gauge: long	1.5 mL	10–15%	1–4

*VAS = visual analog scale, a rating of pain sensation. A score of "0": felt nothing; "1": minor, no problem; "3": some discomfort; "10": worst pain ever experienced.

depth description of these techniques, the reader is referred to local anesthesia textbooks by Malamed[57] and Jastak and Yagiela.[58]

Inferior Alveolar Nerve Block (IANB) (Table 9-4). This traditional mandibular nerve block provides, when successful, pulpal anesthesia of all mandibular teeth in the quadrant, along with buccal soft tissues and bone anterior to the mental foramen and the lingual soft tissues and anterior two-thirds of the tongue. Many approaches exist to this technique, all of which are acceptable, with two provisos: (1) the success rate for pulpal anesthesia should be at least 85% (with one injection depositing approximately 1.5 mL of anesthetic), and (2) the technique should not increase risk of harm to the patient.

The aim in the classic **Halstad** approach to the **IANB** is to deposit local anesthetic at the mandibular foramen, the site where the IA nerve enters the mandibular canal. Although still taught as the primary mandibular technique in most dental schools, the 85% success rate for pulpal anesthesia encountered with this technique is the lowest of any injection administered in dentistry. The most common reason the IANB is missed is caused by depositing the anesthetic solution **below** the mandibular foramen. As the IA nerve has already entered into the thick bony canal, pulpal anesthesia is not produced. The experienced doctor will **re-administer** additional local anesthetic at the site slightly (5 mm) higher than the initial site. The patient should be in a supine position during the IANB, but it is recommended that they be returned to a more upright (comfortable) position following drug administration and while awaiting the onset of anesthesia.

Gow-Gates Mandibular Nerve Block[59–61] (Table 9-5). The GGMNB is a true third division (V^3) nerve block, providing pulpal anesthesia to all mandibular teeth in the quadrant, as well as the same soft tissue distribution as the IANB. Additionally, the GGMNB provides sensory anesthesia of the buccal nerve as well as the mylohyoid nerve, eliminating one cause of partial anesthesia seen in mandibular first molars in approximately 1% of patients.

Local anesthetic is deposited on the lateral aspect of the neck of the mandibular condyle (Figure 9-45). V^3 has just exited the foramen ovale and, with the patient's mouth maintained in a wide-open position, the nerve lies near the condylar neck. First discussed in 1973, the GGMNB has slowly become more and more popular. Once learned, the GGMNB will provide a greater success rate for mandibular pulpal anesthesia.[61] Unfortunately, a learning curve does exist, and some doctors, frustrated by early failures, abandon this excellent technique. The major problem encountered in learning the GGMNB is the inability to contact bone at the neck of the mandibular condyle. The primary reason for this failure is closure (even slight closure) of the patient's mouth while the needle is being advanced (Figure 9-46).

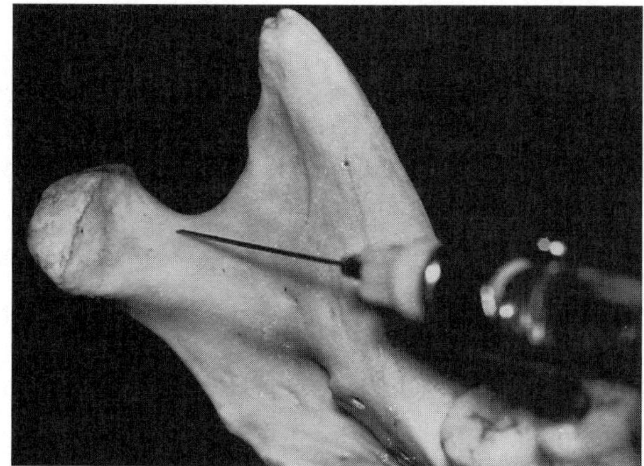

Figure 9-45 Gow-Gates mandibular block injection needle at the target area, the lateral aspect of the neck of the condyle. (Courtesy of Drs. Colin and Gwenet Lambert.)

Table 9-5 Gow-Gates Mandibular Nerve Block

Teeth Anesthetized	Recommended Needle	Volume of Anesthetic	+ Aspiration	VAS
All mandibular teeth in quadrant	25 gauge: long	1.8–3.0 mL	1–2%	1–3

VAS = visual analog scale.

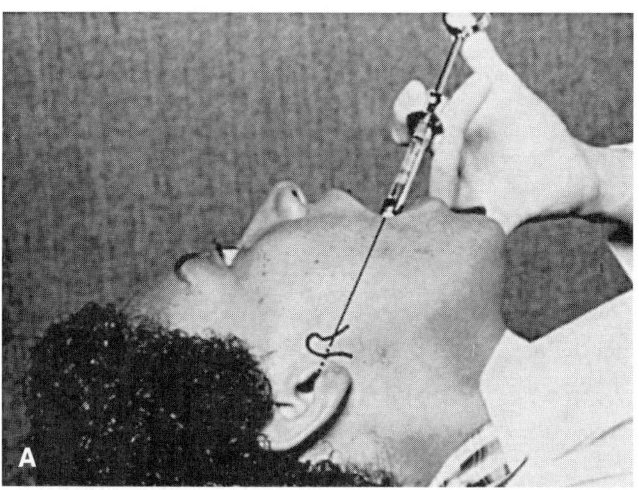

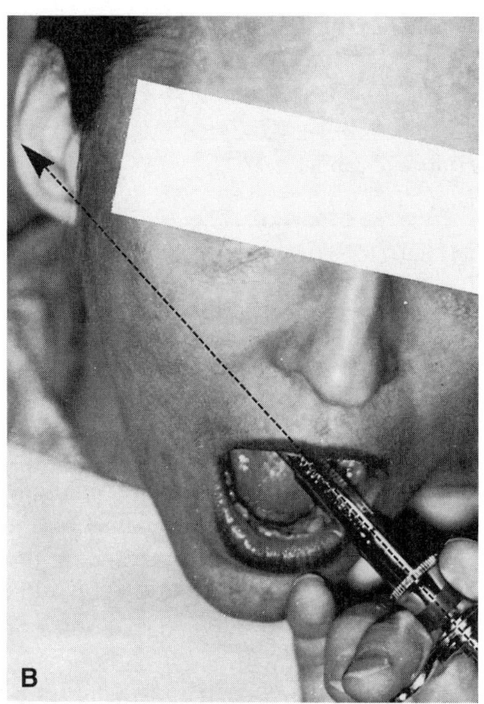

Figure 9-46 Gow-Gates injection technique. **A,** Patient is supine, mouth opened widely and head extended. Syringe is aligned with a plane from the intertragic notch on the ear and the opposite corner of the mouth. **B,** Laterally the syringe is aligned with flare of the tragus of the ear to the face and usually lies over the mandibular canine or premolars on opposite side. (Courtesy of Drs. Colin and Gwenet Lambert.)

As with the IANB, patients receiving the GGMNB should be supine during the injection, but returned to a more upright, comfortable position at the conclusion of the injection and while awaiting the onset of anesthesia. It is important that the mouth be maintained in a wide-open position throughout the injection and for 2 minutes following its completion.

Akinosi-Vazirani Mandibular Nerve Block (Closed-Mouth Technique)[62,63] **(Table 9-6).** Described in 1977, this mandibular block technique is of benefit in situations in which **unilateral trismus** is present, secondary to repeated mandibular injections at a previous dental visit. The patient is unable to open the mouth more than a few millimeters, preventing the administration of intraoral local anesthesia, as well as the performance of dental treatment. Since V^3 is both a sensory and motor nerve (to the muscles of mastication), blockade of V^3 provides relief of the muscle spasm, permitting the patient's mouth to open and the planned dental care to proceed.

The teeth are kept lightly in contact throughout the injection and the cheek is retracted. A long needle, either a 25- or a 27-gauge is placed, with its bevel facing the midline, into the **buccal fold** on the side of injection at the **height of the mucogingival junction of the last maxillary molar** (this injection is intermediate in height between the GGMNB and IANB). Soft tissue on the lingual aspect of the mandible is penetrated at a site immediately adjacent to the **maxillary tuberosity and the needle is advanced 25 mm,** where the local anesthetic is deposited. Motor paralysis usually develops before soft tissue and pulpal anesthesia. The patient, supine during the injection, should be repositioned more upright (comfortable) following injection and while awaiting onset of anesthesia.

Incisive Nerve Block (INB) (Mental NB) (Table 9-7). The **INB** is an underused technique, but one that provides pulpal anesthesia to the five mandibular anterior teeth on a very reliable basis, even in the presence of infection. Soft tissue anesthesia of the lower lip, skin of the chin, and buccal soft tissues anterior to the mental foramen is achieved 100% of the time. Local anesthesia is infiltrated **outside** the mental foramen and then, with the use of finger pressure, forced into the foramen and mandibular canal where the **incisive nerve** (a terminal

Table 9-6 Akinosi-Vazirani Mandibular Nerve Block ("Closed-Mouth" Technique)

Teeth Anesthetized	Recommended Needle	Volume of Anesthetic (Adult)	+ Aspiration	VAS
All mandibular teeth in quadrant	25 or 27 gauge: long	1.8 mL	< 10%	0–2

VAS = visual analog scale.

Table 9-7 **Incisive Nerve Block**

Teeth Anesthetized	Recommended Needle	Volume of Anesthetic (Adult)	+ Aspiration	VAS
Mandibular incisors and canine and premolars	27 gauge: long	0.6 mL	5.7%	0–2

VAS = visual analog scale.

branch of the IA nerve) is located. Pressure should be applied to the area for at least 1 minute, preferably 2 minutes, following deposition of the anesthetic. Lingual soft tissues, including the tongue, are not anesthetized in the incisive nerve block. Should lingual soft tissue anesthesia be required for placement of a rubber dam clamp, it can be achieved painlessly by advancing the needle through the already **anesthetized buccal papilla** toward the lingual while depositing small volumes of local anesthetic *en route.* With proper technique (eg, finger pressure for 2 minutes), the **INB** is virtually 100% successful, painless (there is no need for the needle to contact bone), and can be used successfully from the outset (there is **no learning curve** for this injection).

Maxillary Techniques

Posterior Superior Alveolar Nerve Block (PSANB) ("Zygomatic" NB) (Table 9-8). When successful pulpal anesthesia of maxillary teeth is not achieved through supraperiosteal injection, nerve block anesthesia usually succeeds. **PSANB** provides consistently reliable pulpal anesthesia to the three maxillary molars, even in the presence of infection or widely flared palatal roots. Buccal soft tissues and bone overlying this area are also anesthetized. As no bone is contacted in PSANB, the injection is extremely comfortable; however, the absence of bony contact increases the risk of developing a hematoma following the injection. This usually develops when the needle is advanced too far into the tissues. From the needle penetration site in the buccal fold by the **second maxillary molar,** the **short needle** is advanced to a depth of 16 mm in an inward, upward, and backward direction. This places the needle tip into the pterygomaxillary space, where the PSA nerves are located. In some patients, the mesiobuccal (MB) root of the first molar may not be anesthetized with the PSANB but may be anesthetized by an MSA nerve block, described in the following paragraph.[64]

Middle Superior Alveolar Nerve Block (MSANB) (Table 9-9). When present, the MSA nerve provides pulpal anesthesia to the two premolars and the **MB root of the first molar** (as well as the buccal soft tissues and bone overlying this area). Advancing the tip of the needle well above the **apex of the second premolar** and administering 0.9 mL of anesthetic will provide successful anesthesia almost 100% of the time.

Anterior Superior Alveolar Nerve Block (ASANB) ("Infraorbital" NB) (Table 9-10). In a technique technically similar to the incisive nerve block ("mental") in the mandible, the ASANB provides pulpal anesthesia to the incisors, canine, and both premolars on the side of injection, as well as their overlying soft tissues. The ASA is highly successful in the presence of infection (unless the infection is present in the region of the infraorbital foramen). The needle is inserted into the **buccal fold by the first premolar** and aimed for the infraorbital foramen, which is located by palpation. A volume of 0.9 mL of local anesthetic is deposited outside the infraorbital foramen and then forced into the foramen by the application of finger pressure for 2 minutes (1 minute minimally).

Supplemental Injection Techniques

Periodontal Ligament (PDL) Injection and Intraligamentary Injection (ILI)[65–67] (Table 9-11). When pulpal anesthesia of a single tooth is required, the **PDL** injection should be considered. This is of special importance in the mandible, where nerve block anesthesia is the

Table 9-8 **Posterior Superior Alveolar Nerve Block**

Teeth Anesthetized	Recommended Needle	Volume of Anesthetic (Adult)	+ Aspiration	VAS
Maxillary molars	25 or 27 gauge: short	0.9 mL	3.1%	0–2

VAS = visual analog scale.

Table 9-9 Middle Superior Alveolar Nerve Block

Teeth Anesthetized	Recommended Needle	Volume of Anesthetic (Adult)	+ Aspiration	VAS
Maxillary premolars + MB root first molar	27 gauge: short	0.9 mL	< 3%	0–2

MB = mesiobuccal; VAS = visual analog scale.

norm. In the maxilla, supraperiosteal injection infiltrated above the apex of any tooth will provide successful pulpal anesthesia with a success rate of > 95%. Because of the thickness of the **mandibular cortical plate** of bone (in adults), **infiltration** techniques are **doomed to failure.** Therefore, although the PDL may be successfully administered to any tooth, its use is most often reserved for mandibular teeth, specifically mandibular molars.

Although special syringes have been developed to assist in delivery of the local anesthetic in the PDL injection, a regular syringe may be used quite effectively. A volume of 0.2 mL of local anesthetic solution must be deposited interproximally on each root of the tooth to be treated. The **bevel of the needle should be placed against the root of the tooth** while it is advanced down into the PDL space until resistance prevents any further penetration (Figure 9-47 and Figure 9-48). As the anesthetic is slowly deposited, it should be noted that there is significant resistance to the administration of the solution and that the soft tissues in the area become ischemic. Presence of these two signs usually connotes successful anesthesia. Onset of clinical action is immediate; however, the duration of pulpal anesthesia is quite variable, although it is most often long enough to permit access to the pulp chamber of a previously sensitive tooth.

Two contraindications exist to administration of the PDL injection: **primary teeth** and the presence of **periodontal infection.** The presence of pocket infection in the site of needle insertion increases the risk of osteomyelitis developing subsequent to the injection (Figure 9-49).

Intraosseous (IO) Anesthesia[68–71] **(Table 9-12).** In true IO anesthesia, local anesthetic is injected directly into the bone surrounding the root of a tooth. Conceptually the **IO** injection is quite simple: the impediment to local anesthetic diffusion through bone in the adult mandible is the thickness of the cortical plate. Where a foramen is present, such as the mental foramen, the drug can gain access to the nerve and produce conduction blockade. Unfortunately, no such foramen is found on the **buccal aspect of the mandible** distal to the mental foramen, making it more difficult to obtain consistently reliable pulpal anesthesia on mandibular molars (see Table 9-3).

In the **IO** technique, **a small perforation** or foramen is made **through the cortical plate** of bone with a tiny dental bur, into which a needle is inserted and local

Table 9-10 Anterior Superior Alveolar Nerve Block

Teeth Anesthetized	Recommended Needle	Volume of Anesthetic (Adult)	+ Aspiration	VAS
Maxillary incisors, canine premolars + MB root first molar	25 gauge: long	0.9 mL	0.7%	0–2

MB = mesiobuccal; VAS = visual analog scale.

Table 9-11 Periodontal Ligament Injection and Intraligamentary Injection

Teeth Anesthetized	Recommended Needle	Volume of Anesthetic (Adult)	+ Aspiration	VAS
1 tooth	27 gauge: short	0.2 mL per root	0%	0–10

VAS = visual analog scale.

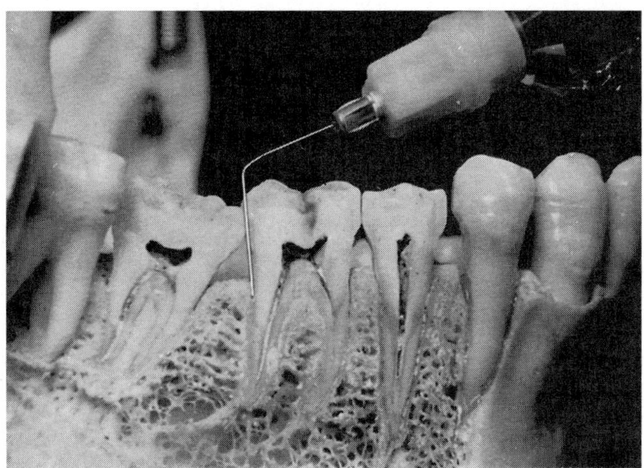

Figure 9-47 Needle penetrating distal periodontal ligament space of mandibular molar. (Courtesy of Drs. Colin and Gwenet Lambert.)

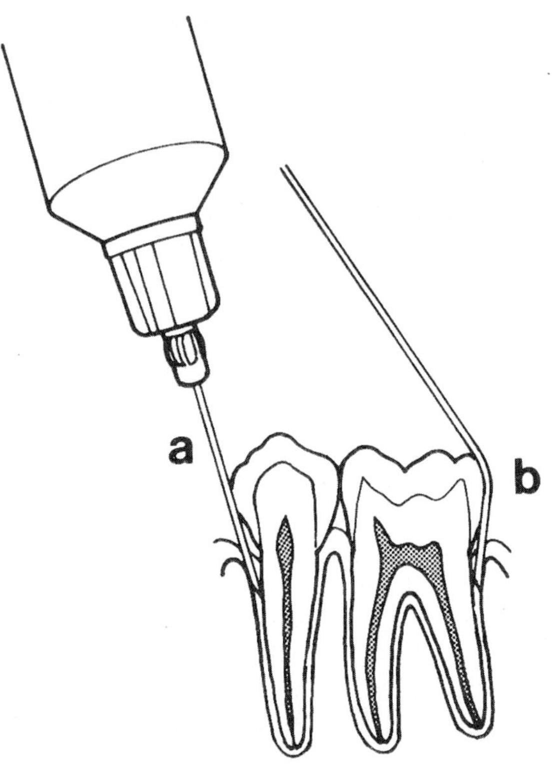

Figure 9-48 Insertion of needle for periodontal ligament injection. **a**, Correct insertion, bevel faces cribriform plate. **b**, Incorrect insertion directing stream toward tooth. (Courtesy of Drs. Colin and Gwenet Lambert.)

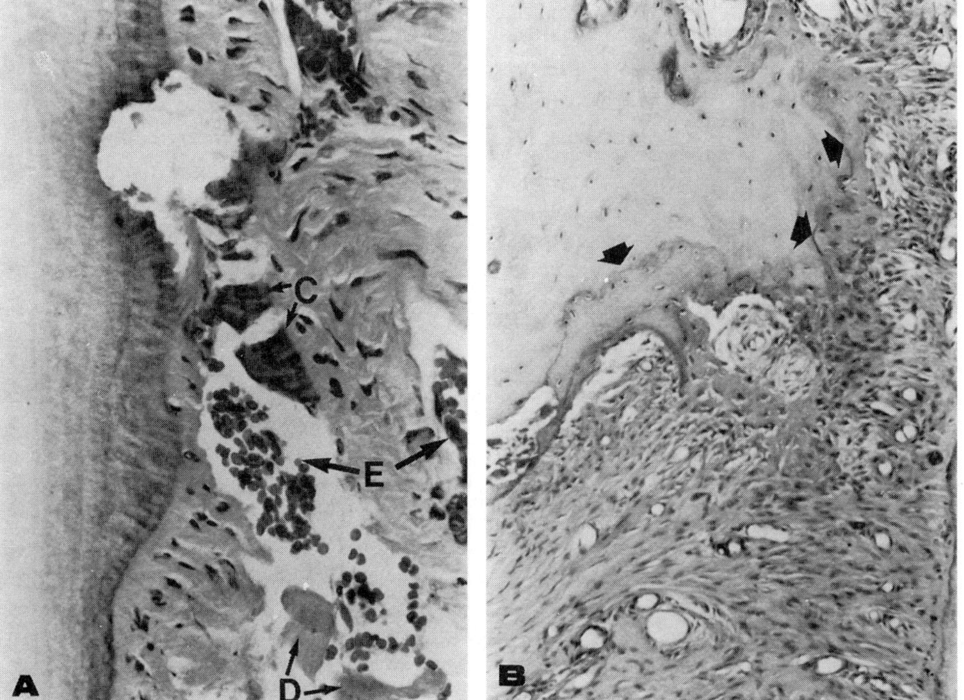

Figure 9-49 Damage and repair to periodontal structures from intraligamental injection. **A**, Needle tract from **lower right** into gouged cementum, **top left**. Chips of cementum (C), erythrocytes (E), and debris (D) carried in by needle indicate severity at time of injury. **B**, Tissue repair 25 days after intraligamental injection. New bone (**arrows**) has replaced bone resorbed following injection. Reproduced with permission from Walton RE, Garnick JJ. JOE 1982;8:22.

Table 9-12 Intraosseous Anesthesia

Teeth Anesthetized	Recommended Needle	Volume of Anesthetic (Adult)	+ Aspiration	VAS
1 or 2 teeth	27 gauge: short	0.45 to 0.6 mL	0%	0–2

VAS = visual analog scale.

anesthetic is administered. Intraosseous injections can provide anesthesia of but a single tooth or of multiple teeth in a quadrant, depending on the site of injection and the volume of anesthetic administered. When treating one or two teeth, 0.45 to 0.6 mL is usually used. IO anesthesia has proved to be of great benefit in endodontics when traditional injection techniques fail. Nusstein et al. found that 81% of mandibular and 12% of maxillary teeth in 51 patients diagnosed with **irreversible pulpitis required IO anesthesia** because of failure to gain pulpal anesthesia with infiltration or IA nerve block. IO anesthesia "was found to be **88% successful** in gaining total pulpal anesthesia for endodontic therapy."[70]

Parente et al. administered IO anesthesia to 37 patients with irreversible pulpitis.[71] Thirty-four were mandibular molars, 2 were maxillary molars, and 1 was a maxillary anterior tooth. Maxillary teeth received infiltration anesthesia, whereas mandibular teeth received the IA injection with a minimum of 3.6 mL of local anesthetic. **IO anesthesia** successfully provided pulpal anesthesia in **91% of mandibular molars** (31/34) and for two of three maxillary teeth.

There are **two concerns** regarding the **IO injection.** First, the local anesthetic is administered into a highly vascular site, where absorption into the cardiovascular system is quite rapid. Administration of an overly large volume of local anesthetic could lead to **elevated blood levels of the anesthetic** and signs and symptoms of **overdose.** The **second concern** regards the inclusion of **vasopressors** (eg, epinephrine) in the local anesthetic solution. This can lead to a rapid absorption into the cardiovascular system leading to an **"epinephrine reaction"** in which patients experience mild tremors of the extremities, palpitations, and diaphoresis after receiving the IO injection. Use of a **vasopressor-containing** local anesthetic in a patient with **significant cardiovascular disease** could provoke potentially life-threatening complications. It is recommended that a "plain" **non-epinephrine local anesthetic solution be used in the IO technique.**

Intrapulpal Anesthesia[72] **(Table 9-13).** When the pulp chamber has been exposed and, because of exquisite sensitivity, treatment cannot proceed, intrapulpal anesthesia should be considered. With the increased interest in the very successful IO technique, however, the need for intrapulpal anesthesia should diminish.

A small needle is inserted into the pulp chamber until resistance is encountered (Figure 9-50). The local anesthetic **must** be injected under pressure. **There will be a brief moment of intense discomfort** as the injection is started, but anesthesia usually supervenes almost immediately, and instrumentation can proceed painlessly. Because of the discomfort involved in intrapulpal anesthesia, the patient must be advised of this before the injection is begun. The concurrent administration of **inhalation sedation** (N_2O–O_2) or **intravenous Versed** will minimize patient response by **alleviating the PRT.**

Summary

Clinically effective pain control can be achieved in the vast majority of patients requiring endodontic therapy. When problems achieving pain control occur, it is usually at **the initial visit,** when a frightened patient, who has been hurting for some period of time, finally seeks relief from pain yet oftentimes is unable to manage the fears of dentistry. Through a combination of thoughtful caring for the patient, the use of **conscious sedation,** when indicated, and the effective administration of **local anesthesia,** endodontic treatment can proceed in

Table 9-13 Intrapulpal Injection

Teeth Anesthetized	Recommended Needle	Volume of Anesthetic (Adult)	+ Aspiration	VAS
1 tooth	27 gauge: short	0.2 to 0.3 mL	0%	5–10

VAS = visual analog scale.

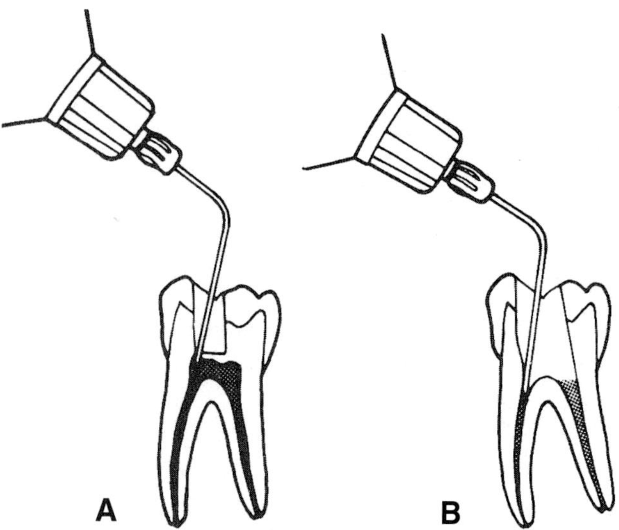

Figure 9-50 Intrapulpal pressure anesthesia with lidocaine. **A**, Coronal injection through pinhole opening in dentin. **B**, Pulp canal injection for each individual canal. Needle is inserted tightly and one drop of solution is deposited. (Courtesy of Drs. Colin and Gwenet Lambert.)

a more relaxed and pleasant environment for both the patient and dental staff.

ENDODONTIC PRETREATMENT

Root canal therapy does not necessarily begin with the placement of the rubber dam but with the **restorative or periodontic procedures necessary to simplify its placement.** These procedures determine the restorability of the tooth and establish a healthy periodontal relationship between tooth, gingiva, and bone. Pretreatment encompasses all procedures that ensure the ease of root canal treatment directed toward restoring and maintaining the involved tooth. The type of pretreatment varies with each case, but certain fundamental objectives must be considered:

1. Prevention of postoperative discomfort and the inopportune fracture of teeth. **Gross occlusal reduction** should be performed on any decayed or filled posterior tooth undergoing root canal therapy. All such teeth will be required to have capped cusp restorations or full crowns on completion of treatment. This reduction should be done **before** rubber dam placement to check occlusal clearance in all excursive movements. It should also be done **before** the first endodontic treatment, rather than after, in order **not to disturb** cuspal reference points used to establish proper **length of the tooth.** Exempt from this pretreatment are posterior teeth that have been adequately restored and anterior teeth.
2. Prevention of bacterial contamination from salivary leakage and prevention of percolation of intracanal medication. All **faulty restorations** and carious defects must be removed and replaced with temporary filling material (**TERM**) (L. D. Caulk; Milford, Dela.) or with alloy in the case of two or three surface fillings.

   To restore a minimal defect on the proximal, TERM can be placed after the endodontic appointment is completed and before the removal of the rubber dam.[73] On subsequent appointments, normal access can be made through the TERM temporary, but if such access weakens the filling, the entire temporary should be replaced at each visit.

   The use of **Cavit** (Premier-Espe; Norristown, Pa.) is limited by its slow-setting property, requiring 1 hour in a wet environment to reach a complete set.[74] It is also inadequate in large two- and three-surface temporary restorations and will never last beyond a week in any case.[75]

   Pretreatment often requires that a tooth be built up with temporary cement before the placement of the rubber dam. For example, a carious defect may extend subgingivally, permitting salivary leakage from beneath the rubber dam. In this situation, a fast, hard-setting filling, such as TERM or **Ketac-Fil** cement (Espe, USA), or alloy will permit the immediate placement of the rubber dam clamp and will withstand repeated application of the clamp.
3. **Provision of a sound margin of tooth structure for rubber dam placement.** The sound margin may be exposed by periodontal procedures or the crown may be restored with a temporary band.

Periodontal Therapy

Gingival hyperplasia or hypertrophy can be easily removed by gingivectomy or by the use of electrosurgery or laser. Both techniques are expedient but have the disadvantage in some cases of producing large surface wounds that may hemorrhage and must heal by secondary intention.

In such situations, and in cases in which the crown has been fractured or destroyed to the gingival level, a more refined mucogingival technique is indicated. The inflamed gingival margin is removed by means of an internally beveled horizontal incision. This measure eliminates an external wound and permits a rubber dam application immediately on completion of the procedure without the problem of hemorrhage control. Two vertical relaxing incisions, extended from the gingival margin **into the alveolar mucosa,** create a mucogingival flap and permit the free movement of this **flap to be repositioned apically** and sutured to place. This technique permits the exposure of additional root surface for the placement of the rubber dam clamp and final restoration. In some cases, corrective osseous recontouring may be necessary (Figure 9-51).

Copper Bands

The preceding periodontal procedures are expedient and can usually be limited to the endodontically involved tooth. However, there are some problems that cannot be easily corrected by periodontal therapy. Gross subgingival caries may be better treated by the cementation of a copper band custom fitted to the particular carious defect (Figure 9-52). The extraction of a partially erupted third molar may leave a bony defect and a deep carious lesion on the distal root of the second molar (Figure 9-53). A copper band may be readily adapted to extend subgingivally in this area, where anatomic considerations preclude definitive periodon-

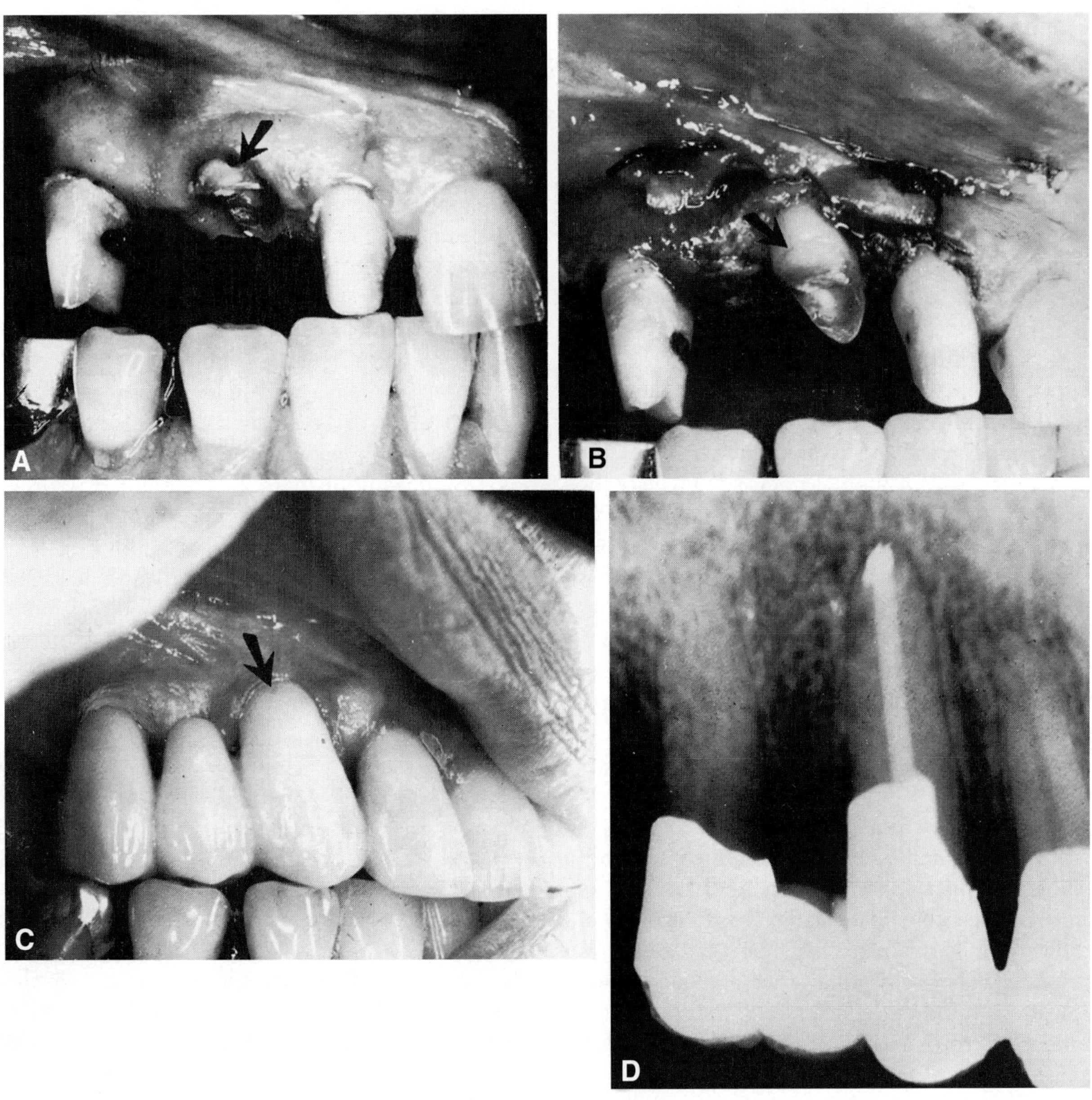

Figure 9-51 **A,** Preoperative view of maxillary canine whose crown is totally destroyed by caries under defective bridge abutment. Level of gingival tissue (**arrow**) in relation to remaining root is apparent. **B,** View following root canal therapy and apical repositioning of attached gingiva. Elongation of clinical crown is seen (**arrow**) in comparison with view in **A. C,** View of final restoration. Important canine abutment (**arrow**) is salvaged by combined endodontic–periodontic procedures. (Restoration by Dr. James Haberman.) **D,** Retrofilling of pulpless canine abutment was done during mucogingival surgery. Previous endodontic filling was incomplete. (Endodontic–periodontic therapy by Dr. Edward E. Beveridge.)

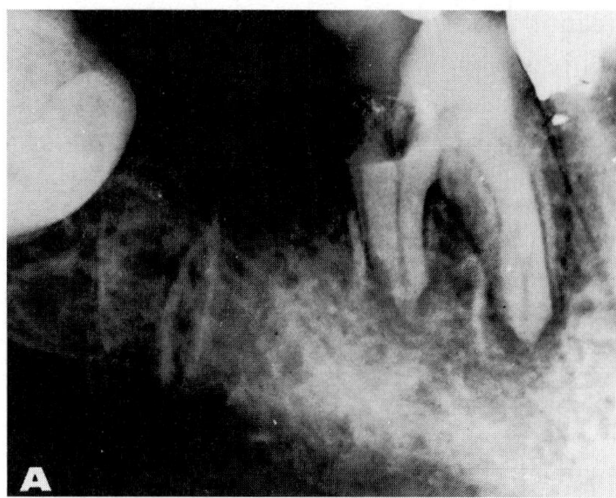

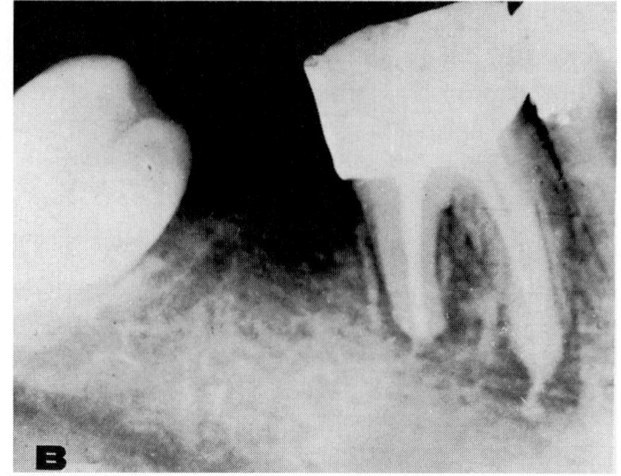

Figure 9-52 A, Badly broken-down pulpless molar with root resorption. Before endodontic treatment, cavity must be sealed off. B, Custom-fitted copper band allows for full treatment. (Courtesy of Dr. James D. Zidell.)

tal therapy. In severe cases, the periodontal or carious defect may be beyond repair, requiring **hemisection** of the distal root of the lower second molar. Banding may then be helpful to seal off the bisected pulp chamber.

Orthodontic Bands

Whereas the copper band is custom-fitted to adapt to a carious defect extending **well below** the gingival margin, the orthodontic band is prefabricated to fit the tooth supragingivally. Thus, it is not used to replace the copper band but to help retain a large temporary filling or support a tooth with undermined enamel walls. It is an essential step in the treatment of a tooth that is thought to be cracking or split (Figure 9-54). It serves as an excellent temporary restoration to prevent splitting during extended treatment, or after treatment, when final restoration has to be postponed. All bands are cemented with zinc oxyphosphate cement.

Temporary Crowns and Restorations

Aluminum shell crowns and plastic crowns or bridges cemented with zinc oxide–eugenol cement are not acceptable as proper pretreatment temporization. The placement of the rubber dam clamp and the tension of the rubber dam displace these temporary crowns, as does repeated rubber dam application and endodontic manipulation. In addition, access attempted through the temporary crown and cement may easily be misdirected against one of the axial walls of the preparation instead of directly into the pulp chamber.

RUBBER DAM APPLICATION

Rubber dam application is an essential prerequisite for providing nonsurgical endodontic treatment. For root canal treatment, rapid, simple, and effective methods of dam applications have been developed. In all but the most unusual circumstances, the rubber dam can be placed in less than 1 minute.

Although the modern endodontic approach to the use of the dam has changed, the importance and purposes of the dam remain the same:

1. It provides a dry, clean, and disinfected field.
2. It protects the patient from the possible aspiration or swallowing of tooth and filling debris, bacteria, necrotic pulp remnants, and instruments or operating materials[76–78] (Figure 9-55).
3. It protects the patient from rotary and hand instruments, drugs, irrigating solutions, and the trauma of repeated manual manipulation of the oral soft tissues.

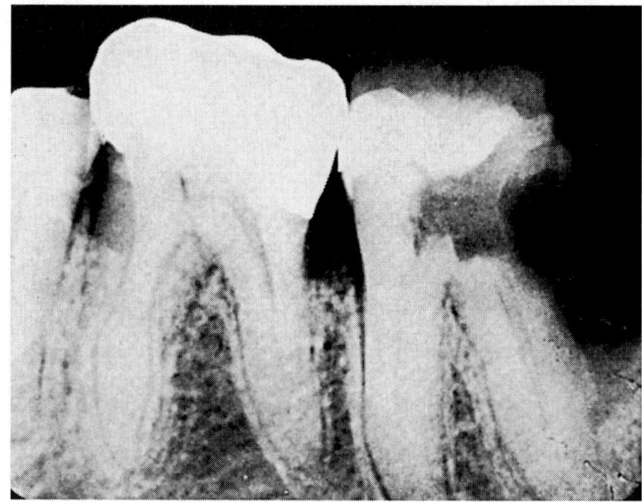

Figure 9-53 Destruction caused by partially erupted third molar and caries. Extended copper band will isolate crown for endodontic treatment. (Courtesy of Dr. James D. Zidell.)

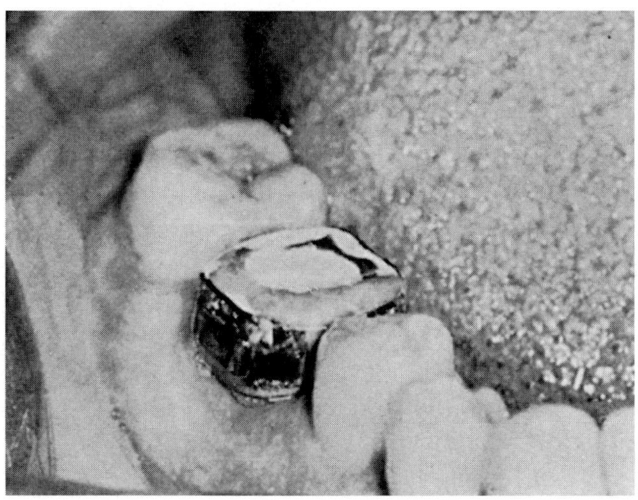

Figure 9-54 Prefabricated orthodontic band for supragingival containment of large temporary proximal filling or to support weakened enamel walls. (Courtesy of Dr. James D. Zidell.)

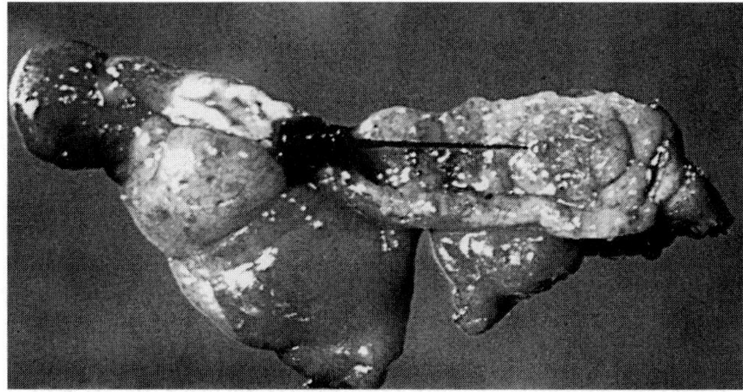

Figure 9-55 Swallowed endodontic file ended up in appendix and led to acute appendicitis and appendectomy. Rubber dam would have prevented this tragedy. Reproduced with permission from Thomsen LC, et al. Gen Dent 1989;37:50.

4. It is faster, more convenient, and less frustrating than the repeated changing of cotton rolls and/or saliva ejectors.

The rubber dam also provides a fluid seal from saliva from the working field. It has been recently shown *in vivo* that intraoral and extraoral microorganisms contaminating the root canal system will lead to eventual failure. [79]

Equipment

Time-and-motion studies have stressed the efficacy of kit or tray preparations that pool instruments and materials to be used in a given procedure. Applied to rubber dam application, this system encourages its more routine use.

Dam Material. Rubber dam is available in a variety of thicknesses, colors, sizes, methods of packaging, and material. The **medium-weight thickness** is recommended for general all-around use. It has the advantage of cupping around the cervical of teeth, providing a fluid seal without the use of floss ligature ties around each tooth. Also, it does not tear or rip easily and provides an unusual degree of protection from injury for the underlying soft tissues. It exerts a greater retracting force on the lips and cheeks than does the thinner material, thus affording greater access and improved vision.

There are advantages, however, in using the thin weight dam on mandibular anterior teeth and partially erupted posterior teeth. The problem of retaining a clamp on these tapered teeth, with little or no cervical undercut, is solved by applying the thinner dam, which exerts less dislodging force on the clamp. The disadvantage is that it is easily torn.

Dam materials may be purchased in 5- or 6-inch-wide rolls to be cut to size; precut sheets, either 5 inches × 5 inches, 5 inches × 6 inches, or 6 inches × 6 inches unsterilized and boxed; or precut and individually sterilized and packaged. A sheet 6 inches × 6 inches will fill all needs of various applications and is large enough to fit any size frame.

The choice of light or dark-colored material is largely up to the individual. However, dark material provides a contrasting color as a background for the light-colored tooth.

Rubber dam is available in latex and nonlatex material. The prevalence of allergies to latex has been increasing; it is important to recognize patients who may have an allergy to latex.[80] Latex-free dams, such as **silicone rubber** (Coltene/Whaledent/Hygenic Corporation, USA], are currently available. Additionally, the digits can be cut from a **vinyl glove**, and the remainder can be adapted to act as a rubber dam in patients who exhibit hypersensitivity to latex.

Punch. Any rubber dam punch that is convenient for the operator and creates a sharp clean hole in the dam material is satisfactory. All too often the punch has not been correctly centered over a hole, and a "nick" on the cutting margin results, producing an incomplete jagged cut in the dam material. This is easily corrected by "sharpening" the cutting edge of the hole with carborundum stone. Failure to correct this punching error will result in salivary leakage and contamination of the field at the site of the ragged hole in the dam.

Personnel at the Karolinska Institute were amazed to learn that "[M]icrobiologic leakage between the rubber dam and the tooth, in routine endodontic treatment, was found in 53% of the cases that, clinically, appeared to be free from saliva leakage."[81] They indicted the "time factor"—the longer the dam was in place, the greater the chance of contamination. Stretching the dam while taking radiographs and capillary forces also contributed. Leakage was significantly reduced by application of a wound dressing, Nobecutane (Astra Pharmaceutical, Sweden) and silicone medical adhesives (Dow Corning Medical Products, USA) to seal the dam and the tooth.[81]

Others have sealed this interface with cyanoacrylate,[82] rubber base adhesive,[83] Super Poli-Grip Denture Adhesive (Dentico, Inc., USA), and Oraseal (Ultradent Products, USA), made specifically to seal the rubber dam, including tears in the dam (Figure 9-56).

Frames. In addition to supporting the dam, frames should be **radiolucent** to prevent obliteration of an important area on the endodontic working radiograph. There are a variety of rubber dam frames that meet these requirements. The U-shaped **Young's frame** is made of either metal for use in restorative dentistry or of radiolucent plastic for endodontic applications. It is easily manipulated and is widely used. This frame holds the dam against the patient's face, and an absorbent napkin under the dam can be used for patient comfort.

The **Nygaard-Østby (N-Ø)** rubber dam frame (Coltene/Whaledent/Hygenic Corp.; Mahwah, N.J.) is shield shaped, made of radiolucent nylon, and may be in place while a tooth is subjected to x-ray without interfering with the radiographic image (Figure 9-57). It tends to hold the dam away from the patient's face and is thus cooler, drier, more comfortable, and requires no absorbent napkin. Because of its shape, it also directs the breath from the nostrils away from the operative field, thus minimizing possible root canal contamination by nasal staphylococci* (see Figure 9-57).

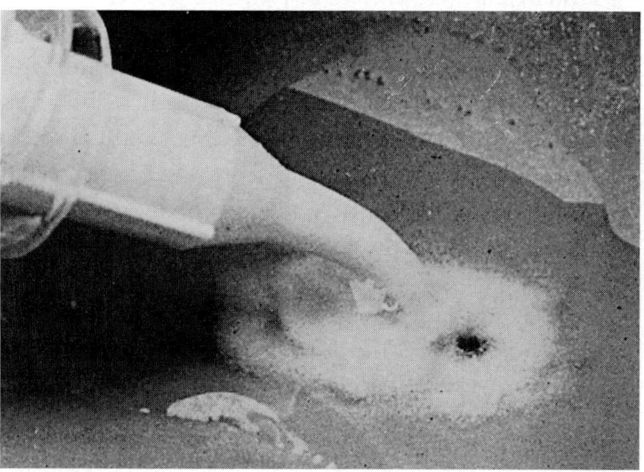

Figure 9-56 **Oraseal** ejected from tube seals tear in rubber dam, despite moisture from saliva. (Courtesy of Ultradent Prod., USA.)

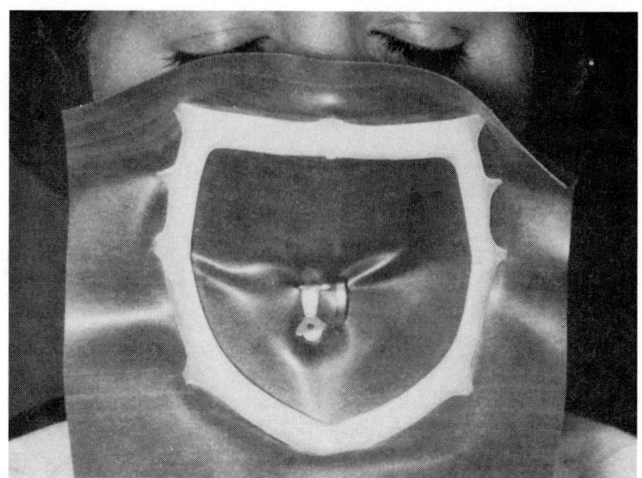

Figure 9-57 N-Ø rubber dam frame, developed in nylon by Nygaard-Østby, is radiolucent and will not impede x-rays. Frame is curved to fit patient's face and may be positioned so that patient breathes behind dam and not into operative field, as one would with a Wizard frame. (Courtesy of Coltene/Whaledent/Hygenic Corp.)

Another U-shaped frame, the **Starlite VisiFrame** (Interdent Inc.; Culver City, Calif.), is also made in radiolucent plastic. Because of its shape, it exerts less tension on the dam and is easier to use than the N–Ø frame when taking radiographs of molars. Like the N–Ø frame, it requires no absorbent napkin, and stands away from the face.

An innovative, articulated frame developed to facilitate endodontic radiography is **le Cadre Articulé** (the articulated frame) (Jored, Ormoy, France, and Trophy, USA). Developed in France by Dr. G. Sauveur, it is curved to fit the face (Figure 9-58, A) and is hinged in the middle to fold back, allowing easier access for radiographic film placement (Figure 9-58, B).

Clamps. Although a basic selection of five to seven clamps will permit most dentists to place a clamp and dam on a majority of teeth encountered, the more experienced operator builds up a larger collection over the years. Teeth that are rotated, partially erupted, malaligned, fractured, anomalous in crown form, or with severe carious involvement all present problems requiring special clamps or clamping techniques.

Table 9-14 lists a suggested assortment of metal clamps for the various teeth. Incisor and premolar clamps that are losing their tension should be retained as they often make excellent clamps for unusual molar applications.

---

*This most important point bears emphasis. All of the dental office personnel should have nose cultures, and if staphylococci are present, should apply Neosporin or Mycitracin to their nostrils each day.

Table 9-14 Rubber Dam Clamp Selection

Maxillary Teeth	
Central incisor	Ivory 00 or 2, 212 or 9A, Hu-Friedy 27, Ash A
Lateral incisor	Ivory 00, 212 or 9A, Ash C
Canine	Ivory 2 or 2A, 212 or 9A
Premolars	Ivory 2 or 2A, Hu-Friedy 27
Molars	Ivory 3 or 4, Ivory 8A, 12A or 13A, 14 or 14A, Ash A
Mandibular Teeth	
Incisors	Ivory 0 or 00, 212 or 9A, Ash C
Canine	Ivory 2 or 2A, 212 or 9A
Premolars	Ivory 2 or 2A, Hu-Friedy 27
Molars	Hu-Friedy 18, Ivory 8A, 12A or 13A, 14 or 14A, 26, Ash A, fatigued Ivory 2A

Plastic clamps (Moyco/Union Broach, USA) are also available in two sizes, large and small, and are used in selected cases. When metal clamp obstruction is a problem in radiography, **radiolucent plastic clamps** allow for an unobstructed view of the tooth. Plastic clamps can also be used to isolate teeth during vital tooth bleaching, using a heat lamp to avoid excessive heat buildup that occurs with conventional metal clamps.

Metal rubber dam clamps may damage tooth structure, restorations, and the **porcelain surface** of crowns or veneers. Conflicting reports have recently been published on the effect of rubber dam retainers on the surface of porcelain. One study reported that damage to the porcelain surface resulted when metal rubber dam retainers were in contact with porcelain-fused-to-metal (PFM) restorations.[84] Another study demonstrated that neither the broad contact of a plastic retainer beak nor the point contact under a metal retainer beak damaged the contact area of porcelain surface of a PFM cylinder.[85] However, repeated applications of rubber dam clamps, in multiple appointments necessary to complete endodontic procedures, is likely to increase the risk of damage.

For endodontic treatment particularly, the use of clamps with wings allows a more rapid, efficient means of applying the rubber dam. A well-trained assistant is able to perform much of the usual technical procedure of application described later in this section. The wings allow the dentist to place the clamp, dam, and frame in one operation (Figure 9-59). In addition, the wings cause a broader buccal-lingual deflection of the dam from the involved tooth, allowing increased access.

Rubber dam clamps undergo stress with repeated use and sterilization. Additionally, clamps that are used during endodontic procedures may be chemically stressed and subject to fracture if in contact with the irrigant sodium hypochlorite.[86] It is a good safety measure to place dental floss ligatures around both ends of the clamp bows so that if the clamp fractures, both portions can be retrieved.

Forceps. Either the Ash- or Ivory-style clamp forceps is satisfactory. One advantage of the **Ivory forceps,**

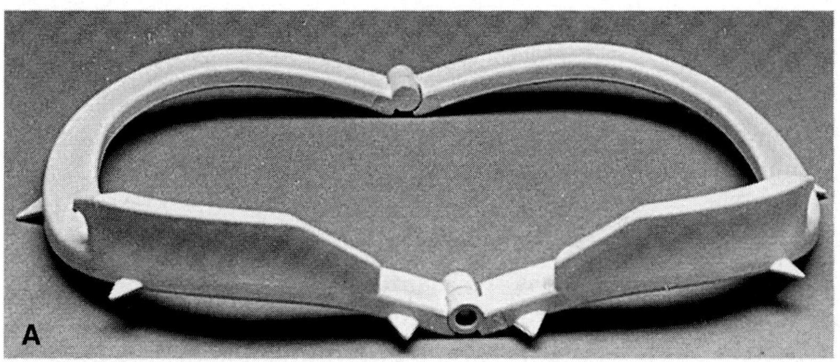

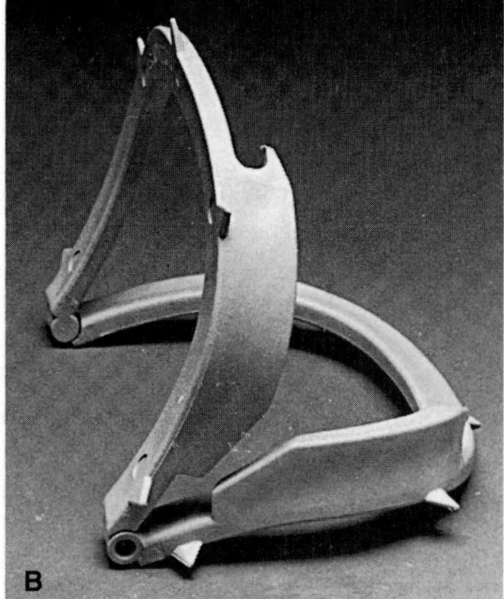

Figure 9-58 Le Cadre Articulé rubber dam frame. **A,** In closed position, frame is curved to fit face. **B,** Open position, from either side, allows passage of radiographic film holder. (Courtesy of Jored, Ormoy, France, and Trophy, USA.)

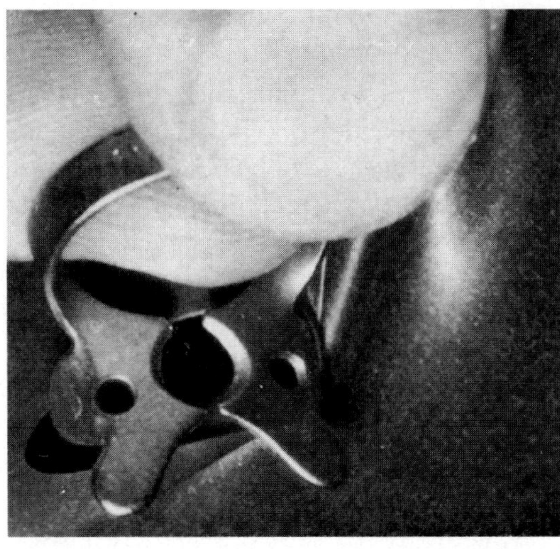

Figure 9-59 Placement of wings of clamp by assistant before positioning dam on frame. Bow of clamp is oriented to the distal.

however, is the **projections** from the **engaging beaks.** These allow the operator the opportunity to **exert a gingivally directed force**, which is often necessary to direct the clamp beyond the height of contour and into proximal undercuts.

The projections on the beaks also allow positive control, enabling the jaws of clamps to be tipped to depress either the "toe" or "heel" of the clamp. The **Ash-style forceps** beaks, on the other hand, afford a fulcrum point for posterior or anterior rotation of the clamp.

Tucking Instrument. A plastic or cement instrument is used to shed the rubber dam off the wings of the clamp once the clamp has been positioned. It is also used, along with a stream of air, to invert or "tuck" the edges of the dam into the gingival sulci, thus ensuring a moisture-proof seal. This is particularly necessary in multiple-tooth applications.

Dental Floss. At one time it was recommended that dental floss be routinely used as a ligature placed around the cervix of each tooth to invert or "tuck" the dam and provide a seal. Through the use of medium or heavy dam material, this is no longer necessary. **Floss** is still essential, however, for the **testing of contacts** before dam application and for **passing the dam** material through the contacts. In both instances, the operator should release his lingual grasp of the floss and **pull it out to the buccal**, rather than back through the contact point.

Saliva Ejector. Any disposable/**radiolucent** saliva ejector is acceptable. It should always be placed **underneath** the dam for endodontic use, in contrast to the procedure of cutting a hole through the dam. This will prevent possible salivary contamination of the field and be less of a hindrance while taking radiographs with the dam in place.

Technique of Application

Three methods of applying a rubber dam, two for a single-bowed clamp and one for a double-bowed clamp, are described in the following sections.

Preparation of Rubber Dam Application Using a Single-Bowed Clamp

Dentist.

1. Remove supra- and subgingival calculus and dental plaque. **Mark the tooth** to be treated with a **marker pen.**
2. Select the clamp to be used.
3. Test contacts with floss to ensure passability and to test for sharp edges that might tear the dam.

Assistant.

1. Punch one appropriate-sized hole just off center of a 6 inch × 6 inch piece of dam material. Rotate the dam to match the tooth to be treated: upper or lower, right or left. Traditionally, **only the teeth receiving therapy** should be included in the dam application.

2a. Stretch the dam over the frame and place the **wings** of the selected clamp in the punched hole with the bow of the clamp to the distal (Figure 9-60), **or**

2b. **Place only the bow** of the clamp through the punched hole of the rubber dam.

3. Place the forceps in the clamp holes with tension and hold in readiness for the dentist (see Figure 9-60).

Application by the Team Dentist.

4. Place an index finger in the vestibule to retract the lip and cheek. The patient is instructed to place the tongue on the opposite side.
5. Sight the tooth to be clamped between the jaws of the clamp (Figure 9-61, A). Direct vision is essential.
6. Place the clamp into the cervical proximal undercuts on the tooth as the index finger is removed from the vestibule (Figure 9-61, B). Finger pressure is sometimes used to ensure seating of the clamp

7a. For 2a above, shed the dam off the clamp wings with the tucking instrument (Figure 9-61, C). Care is taken not to rip the dam, **or**

7b. For 2b above, loosely apply the rubber dam frame to the corners of the rubber dam with the aid of the assistant. Then stretch the dam under the wings of the clamp with the tucking instrument and tighten the rubber dam over the entire frame.

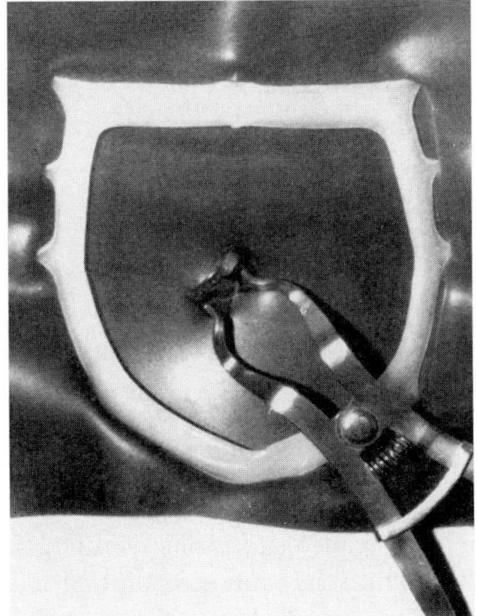

Figure 9-60 Assistant has mounted rubber dam on frame and has positioned wings of clamp in dam. She presents assembled unit with forceps to dentist, ready for placement. Notice that hole is punched just off center of 6 × 6-inch rubber dam. Position of hole is identical for each tooth and dam is rotated for either right or left side, upper or lower.

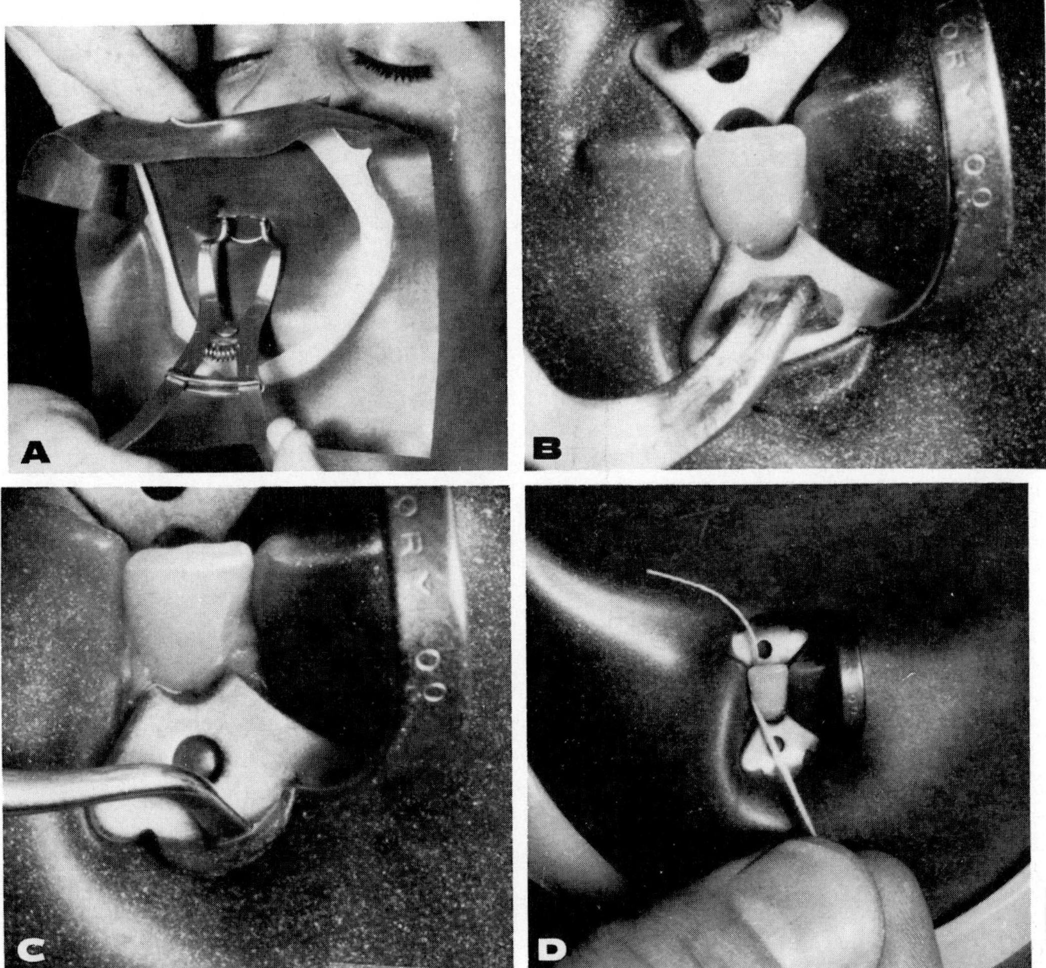

Figure 9-61 **A,** Dentist retracts lip and cheek with thumb and index finger of left hand and sites tooth to be clamped (here a maxillary premolar) between bows of the clamp. Care must be taken not to clamp wrong tooth. **B,** Clamp is carried into gingival undercuts. If undercuts are slight, clamp may be rotated on tooth to take advantage of undercuts along labial and lingual-proximal long axis. **C,** Dam is shed from clamp wings with tucking instrument, which is also used to carry lip of dam under gingival sulcus after tooth is air-dried. **D,** Dental floss is used to carry dam past interproximal contacts. Floss should then be pulled to buccal rather than removed back past contact.

8. Use floss to aid in passing the dam through contacts. Pull the floss through the labial or buccal rather than pulling back through the contacts (Figure 9-61, D).
9. In multiple-tooth applications, tuck the dam into the gingival sulci of the unclamped teeth, using the tucking instrument.

Assistant.

10. Use compressed air to dry the teeth; this aids in tucking.
11. Aid in tightening the rubber dam over the frame once the clamp is on the tooth and after the rubber dam is stretched under the wings of the clamp.
12. Place the saliva ejector under the dam. On a maxillary dam application, many patients do not need the saliva ejector.

Preparation of Rubber Dam Application Using a Double-Bowed Clamp

Dentist.

Same as for a single-bowed clamp.

Assistant.

1. Punch one large hole just off center of a 6 inch × 6-inch piece of dam material.
2. Stretch the dam over the frame

Application by the Team Dentist.

1. After the assistant has positioned the dam over the involved and **marked tooth** (Figure 9-62, A), place the clamp into the cervical proximal undercuts on the tooth.
2. Use floss to aid in passing the dam through the contacts (Figure 9-62, B).

Assistant.

1. Stretch the rubber dam over the **marked tooth** to be isolated (see Figure 9-62, A).
2. Ensure that the rubber dam is not blocking the patient's nose.
3. Place the saliva ejector under the dam.

Completed dam application should take less than 30 seconds of the dentist's time in all but the unusual cases. In applying the dam to a single tooth, however, the dentist must **take great care that the correct tooth is clamped.** After placement, the record is checked and the teeth are counted under the dam, first by the dentist and then independently by the assistant.

The team that is hesitant about clamping the wrong tooth must be cautioned about using the time-honored **system of first placing the clamp, then the dam, then the frame.** This sequence of rubber dam application may lead to accidental swallowing of a rubber dam clamp. There are several reports in the literature on the ingestion of rubber dam clamps.[87–89] This further emphasizes the importance of using floss ligatures around rubber dam clamps so that dislodged clamps and broken clamps can be retrieved quickly.[87-90]

Removal of Dam

1. For single-tooth applications, simply remove the clamp with the forceps and remove the dam.
2. In multiple-tooth applications, first remove the clamp, then place a finger under the dam in the vestibule, and stretch the dam to the facial, away from the teeth. Cut the stretched interproximal dam with scissors and then remove the dam. After removal, it is essential that the dam be inspected to

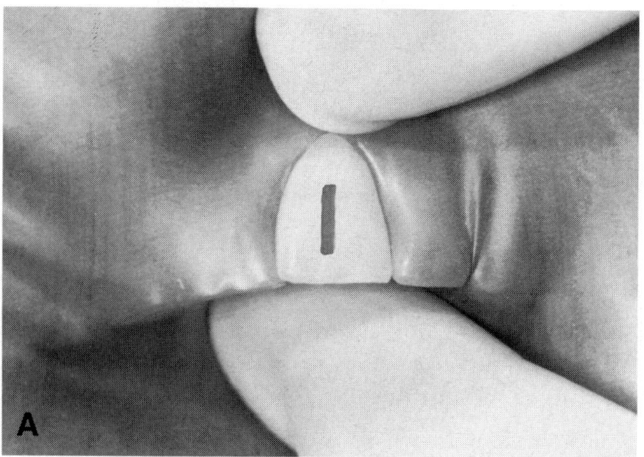

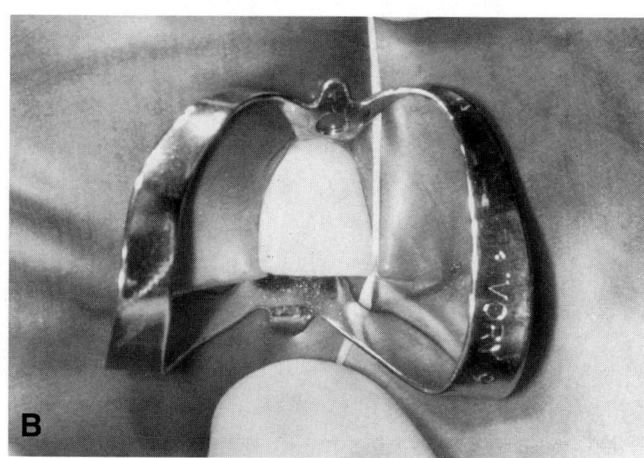

Figure 9-62 **A,** Rubber dam in place, exposing involved tooth previously marked with a marking pen. **B,** Clamp placement in gingival undercuts. Dental floss carries dam past interproximal contacts and is removed by pulling to buccal rather than back through contacts. (Courtesy of Jeffrey M Coil.)

ensure that no interproximal dam septum has been left between the teeth.

Circumstances Requiring Variations from the Usual Application

A number of circumstances require a variation from the standard dam application.

First Circumstance. A well-done gingival gold filling or PFM veneer crown on the involved tooth that could be damaged by clamps.

Variation. **Clamp one tooth posterior to**, and extend the rubber dam **one tooth anterior** to, the involved tooth.

Second Circumstance. Multiple adjacent teeth requiring treatment.

Variation. The posterior tooth is clamped normally while the clamp is reversed (with the bow pointing mesially) on the more anterior tooth. By another approach, the most posterior tooth is clamped normally, while the anterior portion of the dam is retained and retracted without a clamp. Neaverth has suggested that a ¼-inch-wide strip of dam can be stretched thin to simulate dental floss (personal communication, Feb. 2000). It is then passed through the contact and, when released, acts as a wedge holding the dam in place (Figure 9-63).

Third Circumstance. Bridge abutments, splints, and orthodontic bands with wires.

Variation. Punch a larger-than-usual hole in the dam. Smear **Oraseal** around the hole on the underside of the dam. This mucilaginous material prevents leakage. Clamp the tooth in the normal manner. In addition, place a round toothpick through the gingival embrasure next to the pontic. If leakage is still a problem, add more Oraseal around the abutment at the site of the leakage.

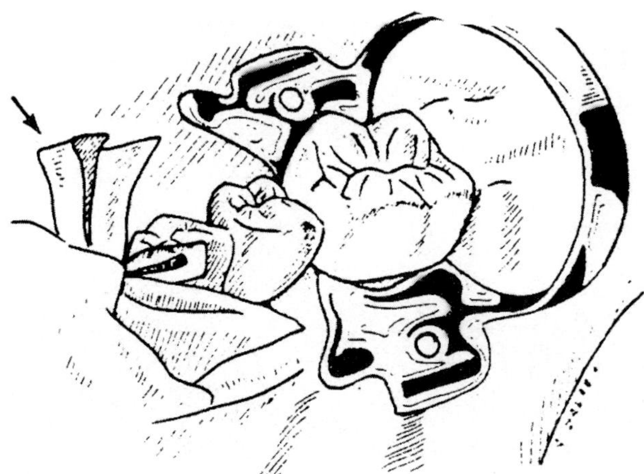

Figure 9-63 Narrow strip of rubber dam (**arrow**) passed through contact point acts as wedge to hold dam anteriorly without additional clamp. (Courtesy of Dr. E.J. Neaverth.)

Fourth Circumstance. Partially erupted tooth.

Variation. An **Ivory #14A** or **Ash #A** clamp forced subgingivally into the cervical undercut will often hold. On occasion, an Ash #C clamp, placed **on the oblique,** will suffice. For supragingival retention, **when no undercut** is present, Japanese researchers have recommended placing a small amount **of self-curing composite** resin on the labial and lingual **unetched enamel** surfaces. The clamp is set in this scaffold of the cured resin. After use, the resin can be lifted off with an excavator.[91]

Fifth Circumstance. Caries, resulting in a **subgingival restorative margin** of the involved tooth (Figure 9-64, A).

Variation. Clamp one tooth posterior to, and extend rubber dam one or two teeth **anterior to, the involved tooth.** The **furthest anterior tooth isolated** may receive a rubber dam clamp with its **bow pointing mesially.** If floss shreds through, or the rubber dam rips between the contacts, **Oraseal** may be necessary to develop a fluid seal (Figure 9-64, B). This multiple-tooth isolation facilitates easy placement of an **interproximal**

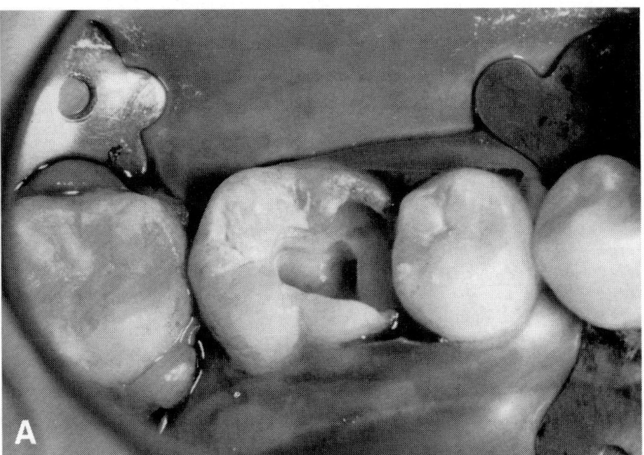

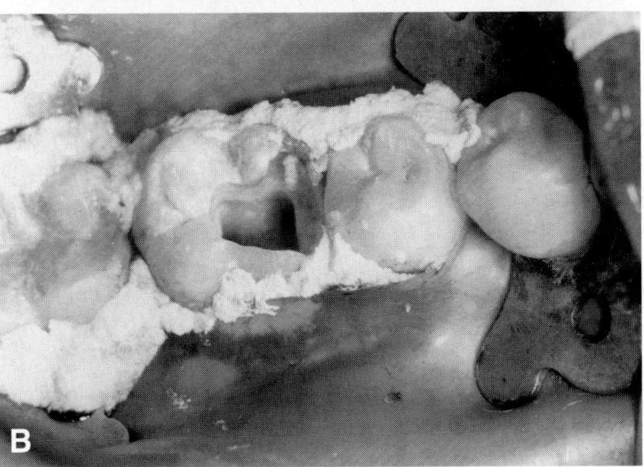

Figure 9-64 **A,** Four-tooth and two-clamp dam isolation in patient with Dilantin hyperplasia. **B,** Possible leakage toward the buccal and lingual is controlled by **Oraseal.** (Courtesy of Jeffrey M. Coil.)

matrix used during final restoration, without interference from a rubber dam clamp on the involved tooth.

Sixth Circumstance. Hemisected maxillary or mandibular molars.

Variation. Hemisected mandibular molars are treated as a premolar. Those that are wide buccolingually are best clamped with a fatigued **Hu-Friedy** or **Ivory #2 or #2A.**

A hemisected maxillary molar with the lingual root remaining is also best treated as a large premolar. A **Hu-Friedy #27** clamp frequently adapts well. When the two buccal roots of a maxillary molar remain, it is then best treated as a small molar, and an **Ash #A** frequently suffices. Often the hemisected maxillary molar can be clamped only by placing the clamp obliquely.

Seventh Circumstance. Full-crown preparation without a cervical undercut to retain the clamp.

Variations. A proper full-crown preparation will shed toward the occlusal, and the clamp may not provide adequate resistance to the tension of the rubber dam. It may be necessary to place **parallel horizontal grooves** on the buccal and lingual axial walls of the preparation near the gingival margin to permit the clamp to grasp onto the preparation. The **Ivory #2 or #2A** clamp will fit into these grooves for retention. It has also been suggested that applying composite resin on the buccal and lingual **unetched surfaces** might be superior to cutting grooves.[91]

Eighth Circumstance. Posterior teeth with minimal tooth structure for clamp retention.

Variation. The tension of the rubber dam as it is stretched taut over the frame exerts pressure, or a force of displacement, on the bow of the clamp. The **clamp may be reversed** on the working tooth; **a second clamp is placed over the rubber dam** on the next tooth posterior to absorb the pressure of the rubber dam.

Periodontal crown lengthening to "elongate" the crown of a fractured or badly decayed tooth was discussed in the section "**Endodontic Pretreatment.**"

Ninth Circumstance. Extensive caries resulting in subgingival buccal and/or lingual margin(s).

Variation. The involved tooth can undergo periodontal crown lengthening, addition of restorative material to allow for supragingival clamp placement, or gingival surgery to expose more tooth structure to allow for clamp placement (see Figure 9-51).

Tenth Circumstance. Fractured cusp with subgingival margin on buccal or lingual surface.

Variation. Use **three-tooth** rubber dam isolation **as in second circumstance.** By placing a **short cotton roll** under the wing of the rubber dam clamp, additional reflection of the rubber dam can be achieved (Figure 9-65). Note that the clamp would otherwise be unstable if placed on the involved tooth in the traditional single-tooth isolation.

Eleventh Circumstance. Tooth with calcified pulp chamber and canal(s).

Variation. Use **three-tooth** rubber dam isolation **as in second circumstance. Involved tooth is without a clamp,** allowing the operator to better visualize the CEJ region of the tooth. There are no clamp wings to obstruct one's view. A periodontal probe can be traced along the root surface to orientate oneself to the **crown–root angulations** during difficult-access cavity preparations. Additionally, the image in working films is unlikely to be obstructed by the clamp (Figure 9-66).

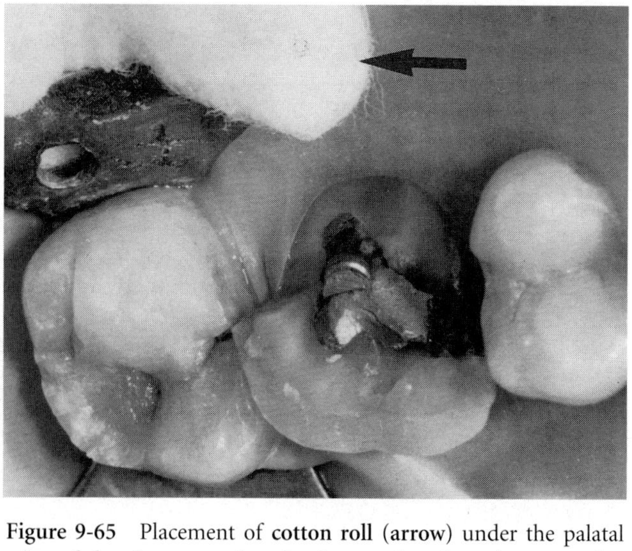

Figure 9-65 Placement of **cotton roll (arrow)** under the palatal wing of the clamp stretches the dam against the palate, exposing more of the fractured tooth surface. Seal can be augmented with **Oraseal.** (Courtesy of Jeffrey M. Coil.)

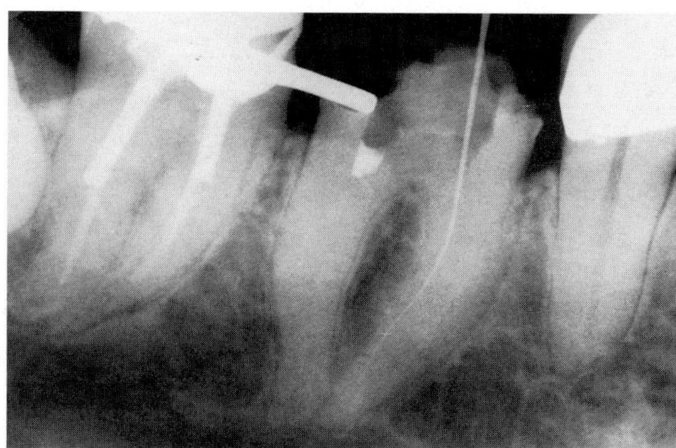

Figure 9-66 Fractured first molar isolated in three-tooth dam placement with clamp on second molar, allowing unobstructed view of canal orifices in first molar. Distal canal marked by gutta-percha to visualize correct drilling direction. (Courtesy of Jeffrey M. Coil.)

SUMMARY

Students, recent graduates, and veteran practitioners alike will find restorative and endodontic practice more rewarding and less frustrating as their mastery of rubber dam applications increases. The use of simplified techniques, improved materials, and organized procedures, as well as patience, practice, and perseverance, will hasten this mastery. **Remember, it is imperative that a rubber dam be used for all endodontic procedures!**

REFERENCES

1. Ennis LM, Berry HM. Dental roentgenology. 5th ed. Philadelphia: Lea & Febiger; 1959. p. 13.
2. Glenner RA. Eighty years of dental radiography. J Am Dent Assoc 1975;90:549.
3. Priebe WA, Lazansky JP, Wuehrmann AH. The value of the roentgenographic film in the differential diagnosis of periradicular lesions. Oral Surg 1954;7:979.
4. Baumann L, Rossman SR. Clinical roentgenologic and histopathologic findings in teeth with apical radiolucent areas. Oral Surg 1956;9:1330.
5. Wais FT. Significance of findings following biopsy and histologic study of 100 periradicular lesions. Oral Surg 1958;11:650.
6. Linenberg WP, et al. A clinical roentgenographic and histologic evaluation of periradicular areas. Oral Surg 1964;17:467.
7. LaLonde ER. A new rationale for the management of periradicular granulomas and cysts: an evaluation of histopathological and radiographic findings. J Am Dent Assoc 1970;80:1056.
8. Ardran GM. Bone destruction not demonstrable by roentgenography. Br J Radiol 1951;24:107.
9. Bender IB, Seltzer S. Roentgenographic and direct observation of experimental lesions of bone. J Am Dent Assoc 1961;62:153.
10. Ramadam AE, Mitchell DF. A roentgenographic study of experimental bone destruction. Oral Surg 1962;15:934.
11. Schwartz SF, Foster JK. Roentgenographic interpretation of experimentally produced bony lesions. Oral Surg 1971; 32(Pt I):606.
12. Goldman M, Pearson A, Darzenta N. Endodontic success—who's reading the radiograph? Oral Surg 1972;23:432.
13. Holtzman D, Johnson W, Southard T, et al. Storage-phosphor computed radiography versus film radiography in the detection of pathological periradicular bone loss in cadavers. Oral Surg 1998;86:90.
14. Sullivan J, Di Fiore P, Koerber A. RadioVisiography in the detection of periapical lesions. JOE 2000;26:32.
15. Burger C, Mork T, Hutter J, et al. Direct digital radiography versus conventional radiography for estimation of canal length in curved canals. JOE 1999;25:260.
16. Scarfe W, Czerniejewski W, Farman A, et al. *In vivo* accuracy and reliability in color-coded image enhancements for the assessment of periradicular lesion dimensions. Oral Surg 1999;88:603.
17. Baker W, Loushine R, West L. Interpretation of artificial and *in vivo* periapical bone lesions comparing conventional viewing versus a video conferencing system. JOE 2000;26:39.
18. Fitzgerald GM. Dental roentgenography I: an investigation in adumbration, or the factors that control geometric unsharpness. J Am Dent Assoc 1947;34:1.
19. Fitzgerald GM. Dental roentgenography II: vertical angulation, film placement and increased object-film distance. J Am Dent Assoc 1947;34:160.
20. Waggener DT. The right-angle technique using the extension cone. Dent Clin North Am 1968;783.
21. Forsberg J. A comparison of the paralleling and bisecting-angle radiographic techniques in endodontics. Int Endod J 1987;20:177.
22. Girsch WJ, Matteson SR, McKee MN. An evaluation of Kodak Ektaspeed periradicular film for use in endodontics. JOE 1983;9:282.
23. Kleier DJ, et al. Two dental x-ray films compared for rater preference using endodontic views. Oral Surg 1985;59:201.
24. Donnelly JC, et al. Clinical evaluation of Ektaspeed x-ray film for use in endodontics. JOE 1985;11:90.
25. Jarvis WD, et al. Evaluation of image quality in individual films of double film packs. Oral Surg 1990;69:764.
26. Barr JH, Gron P. Palate contour as a limiting factor in intraoral x-ray technique. Oral Surg 1959;12:459.
27. Walton RE. Endodontic radiographic techniques. Dent Radiogr Photogr 1973;46:51.
28. Clark CA. A method of ascertaining the relative position of unerupted teeth by means of film radiographs. Odont Sec R Soc Med Trans 1909–1910;3:87.
29. Goerig AC, Neaverth EJ. A simplified look at the buccal object rule in endodontics. JOE 1987;13:570.
30. Grady JR, Clausen H. Establishing your point. Clinic Am Assoc Endod New Orleans, LA 1975.
31. Ingle JI, Beveridge EE, Olson C. Rapid processing of endodontic "working" films. Oral Surg 1965;19:101.
32. Kaffe I, Gratt BM. E-speed dental films processed with rapid chemistry: a comparison with D-speed film. Oral Surg 1987;64:367.
33. Pestritto ST. Comparison of diagnostic quality of dental radiographs produced by five rapid processing techniques. J Am Dent Assoc 1974;89:353.
34. Maddalozzo D, et al. Performance of seven rapid radiographic processing solutions. Oral Surg 1990;69:382.
35. Benz C, Mouyen F. Evaluation of the new Radio VisioGraphy system image quality. Oral Surg 1991;72:627.
36. Nelvig P, Wing K, Welander U. Sens-A-Ray. A new system for direct digital intraoral radiography. Oral Surg 1992;74:818.
37. Molteni R. Direct digital dental x-ray imaging with Visualix/VIXA. Oral Surg 1993;76:235.
38. Pascon E, Introcaso J, Langeland K. Development of predictable periapical lesion monitoring by subtraction radiography. Endod Dent Traumatol 1988;4:253.
39. Kullendorf B, Grondahl K, Rohlin M, et al. Subtraction radiography for the diagnosis of periapical bone lesions. Endod Dent Traumatol 1987;3:192.
40. Tyndall D, Kapa S, Bagnell C. Digital subtraction radiography for detecting cortical and cancellous bone changes in the periapical region. JOE 1990;16:173.
41. Orstavik D, Farrants G, Wahl T, et al. Image analysis of endodontic radiographs: digital subtraction and quantitative densitometry. Endod Dent Traumatol 1990;6:6.
42. Sieraski S, Corcoran J. Osseous healing kinetics after apicoectomy in monkeys. I. An isodensitometric interpretation of radiographic images. JOE 1984;6:233.
43. Benn DK. Limitations of the digital image subtraction technique in assessing alveolar bone crest changes due to misalignment errors during image capture. Dentomaxillofac Radiol 1990;19:97.

44. Tahibana H, Matsumoto K. Applicability of x-ray computerized tomography in endodontics. Endod Dent Traumatol 1990;6:16.
45. Brynolf I. Improved viewing facilities for better roentgenodiagnosis. Oral Surg 1971;32:808.
46. Spiegler G. Wiesollen Rontgenufrahmen Betrachtet Werden? Forstchr Geb Roentgenstr 1937;56:662.
47. Ball KA. Endoscopic surgery. St. Louis (MO): Mosby/Year Book; 1997. p. 1.
48. Detsch S, Cunninghan W, Langloss J. Endoscopy as an aid to endodontic diagnosis. JOE 1979;5:60.
49. Held S, Kao Y, Well D. Endoscope B and endodontic application. JOE 1996;22:327.
50. Shulman B, Leung B. Endodscopic surgery: an alternative technique. Dent Today 1996;15:42.
51. Bahcall JK, DiFiore PM, Pouladakis TK. An endoscopic technique for endodontic surgery. JOE 1999;25:132.
52. Bahcall JK, Barss JT. Orascopic endodontics: changing the way we "think" about endodontics in the 21st century. Dent Today 2000;19.
53. Bahcall JK, Barss JT. Fiberoptic endoscope usage for intracanal visualization. JOE 2001;27:128.
54. Malamed SF. Beyond the basics: emergency medicine in dentistry. J Am Dent Assoc 1997;128:843.
55. Walton RE, Abbott BJ. Periodontal ligament injection: a clinical evaluation. J Am Dent Assoc 1981;103:571.
56. Malamed SF. Teeth requiring supplemental injections. Unpublished data, 1997.
57. Malamed SF. Handbook of local anesthesia. 4th ed. St. Louis (MO): Mosby; 1997.
58. Jastak JT, Yagiela JA. Local anesthesia of the oral cavity. Philadelphia: WB Saunders; 1995.
59. Gow-Gates GAE. Mandibular conduction anesthesia: a new technique using extraoral landmarks. Oral Surg 1973;36:321.
60. Malamed SF. The Gow-Gates mandibular nerve block: evaluation after 4275 cases. Oral Surg 1981;51:463.
61. Jofre J, Munzenmayer C. Design and preliminary evaluation of an extraoral Gow-Gates guiding device. Oral Surg 1998;85:661.
62. Akinosi JO. A new approach to the mandibular nerve block. Br J Oral Surg 1977;15:83.
63. Vasirani SJ. Closed mouth mandibular nerve block: a new technique. Dent Dig 1960;66:10.
64. Loetscher CA, Melton DC, Walton RE. Injection regimen for anesthesia of the maxillary first molar. J Am Dent Assoc 1988;117:337.
65. Malamed SF. The periodontal ligament (PDL) injection: an alternative to inferior alveolar nerve block. Oral Surg 1982;53:117.
66. Brannstrom M, Lindskog S, Nordenvall KJ. Enamel hypoplasia in permanent teeth induced by periodontal ligament anesthesia of primary teeth. J Am Dent Assoc 1984;109:735.
67. ADA Council on Dental Materials, Instruments, and Equipment. Status report: the periodontal ligament injection. J Am Dent Assoc 1983;106:222.
68. Leonard M. The efficacy of an intraosseous injection system of delivering local anesthesia. J Am Dent Assoc 1995;126:81.
69. Leonard M. The Stabident System of intraosseous anesthesia. Dent Econ 1997;87:51.
70. Nustein J, Reader A, Nist R, et al. Anesthetic efficacy of the supplemental intraosseous injection of 2% lidocaine with 1:100,000 epinephrine in irreversible pulpitis. JOE 1998;24:487.
71. Parente SA, Anderson RW, Herman WW, et al. Anesthetic efficacy of the supplemental intraosseous injection for teeth with irreversible pulpitis. JOE 1998;24:826.
72. Malamed SF, Weine F. Profound pulpal anesthesia [audiotape]. Chicago: American Association of Endodontics; 1988.
73. Bobotis HG, et al. A microleakage study of temporary restorative materials used in endodontics. JOE 1989;15:569.
74. Parris L, Kapsimalis P. Effect of temperature change on the sealing properties of temporary filling materials. Oral Surg 1960;13:982.
75. Anderson RW, et al. Microleakage of temporary restorations in complex endodontic access preparations. JOE 1989;15:526.
76. Goulschin J, Heling B. Accidental swallowing of an endodontic instrument. Oral Surg 1971;40:621.
77. Gouila CD. Accidental swallowing of an endodontic instrument. Oral Surg 1979;48:269.
78. Lambrainidis T, Bettes P. Accidental swallowing of endodontic instruments. Endod Dent Traumatol 1996;12: 301.
79. Friedman S, Torneck CD. In vivo model for assessing the functionally efficacy of endodontic filling materials and techniques. JOE 1997;23:557.
80. Roy A, Epstein J, Onno E. Latex allergies in dentistry: recognition and recommendations. J Can Dent Assoc 1997;63:297.
81. Fors UGH, Berg J-O, Sandberg H. Microbiological investigation of saliva leakage between rubber dam and tooth during endodontic treatment. JOE 1986;12:396.
82. Roahen JO, Lento CA. Using cyanoacrylate to facilitate rubber dam isolation of teeth. JOE 1992;18:517.
83. Bramwell JD, Hicks ML. Solving isolation problem with rubber base adhesive. JOE 1986;12:363.
84. Madison S, Jordan RD, Krell KV. The effects of rubber dam retainers on porcelain-fused-to-metal restorations. JOE 1986;12:183.
85. Zerr MA, Johnson WT, et al. Effect of rubber dam retainers on porcelain-fused-to-metal. Gen Dent 1996;44:132.
86. Sutton J, Saunders WP. Effect of various irrigant and autoclaving regimes on the fracture resistance of rubber dam clamps. Int Endod J 1996;29:333.
87. Mejia JL, Donado JE, Posada A. Accidental swallowing of a rubber dam clamp. JOE 1996;22:619.
88. Alexander RE, Delhom JJ. Rubber dam clamp ingestion, an operative risk: report of a case. J Am Dent Assoc 1971;82:1387.
89. Beemster G. Unusual position for a rubber dam clamp. Oral Surg 1978;45:979.
90. Hollist HO. Clamp usage when applying rubber dam. Br Dent J 1998;18:579.
91. Wakabayashi H, et al. A clinical technique for the retention of a rubber dam clamp. JOE 1986;12:422.

Chapter 10

ENDODONTIC CAVITY PREPARATION

John I. Ingle, Van T. Himel, Carl E. Hawrish, Gerald N. Glickman, Thomas Serene, Paul A. Rosenberg, L. Stephen Buchanan, John D. West, Clifford J. Ruddle, Joe H. Camp, James B. Roane, and Silvia C. M. Cecchini

The chapter on success and failure (chapter 13) substantiates the endodontic dogma of **careful cavity preparation and canal obturation** as the keystones to successful root canal therapy. Apical moisture-proof seal, the first essential for success, is not possible unless the space to be filled is carefully prepared and débrided to receive the restoration. **As in restorative dentistry, the final restoration is rarely better than the initial cavity preparation.**

Endodontic cavity preparation begins the instant the involved tooth is approached with a cutting instrument, and the final obturation of the canal space will depend in great measure on the care and accuracy exercised in this initial preparation.

DIVISIONS OF CAVITY PREPARATION

For descriptive convenience, endodontic cavity preparation may be separated into two anatomic divisions: **(a) coronal preparation and (b) radicular preparation.** Actually, coronal preparation is merely a means to an end, but to accurately prepare and properly fill the radicular pulp space, intracoronal preparation must be correct in size, shape, and inclination.

If one thinks of an endodontic preparation as a continuum from enamel surface to apex, Black's principles of cavity preparation—Outline, Convenience, Retention, and Resistance Forms—may be applied (Figure 10-1).[1] The entire length of the preparation is the full **outline** form. In turn, this **outline** may have to be modified for the sake of **convenience** to accommodate canal anatomy or curvature and/or instruments. In some techniques, the canal may be prepared for slight **retention** of a primary gutta-percha point. But most important, **resistance** must be developed at the apical terminus of the preparation, the so-called "apical stop," the barrier against which virtually every canal filling must be compacted.

CORONAL CAVITY PREPARATION

Basic Coronal Instruments

Preparations **on and within the crown** are completed with power-driven rotary instruments. For optimal operating efficiency, separate ranges of bur speed are needed. Although two handpieces are usually required, developments in electric handpiece engineering allow one motor to provide both low- and high-speed ranges of rpm. Handpieces are also being developed that automatically reverse on lockage of the file.[2]

The correct burs are mounted by the dental assistant prior to their use. Rarely should a bur have to be placed or changed during the operation. For initial entrance through the enamel surface or through a restoration, the ideal cutting instrument is the **round-end carbide fissure bur** such as the Maillefer Transmetal bur or Endo Access diamond stone (Dentsply/Maillefer, Tulsa, Okla.), mounted in a contra-angle handpiece operating at accelerated speed. With this instrument, enamel, resin, ceramic, or metal perforation is easily accomplished, and surface extensions may be rapidly completed.

Porcelain-fused-to-metal restorations, however, are something else. Stokes and Tidmarsh have shown the effectiveness of various bur types in cutting through different types of crowns[3] (Figure 10-2). Precious metal alloys are relatively easy to penetrate, whereas nonprecious metals present considerable difficulty. Although nonprecious alloys can be cut with tungsten carbide burs, they "chatter" severely. This vibration results in patient discomfort and tends to loosen the crown from the luting cement. "The extra coarse, dome-ended cylinder…was the only bur type that cut smoothly and remained clinically effective during the cutting of five successive access cavities in the nonprecious metal" found frequently under metal-ceramic crowns.[3] Teplitsky and Sutherland also found diamond instrumentation perfect for access

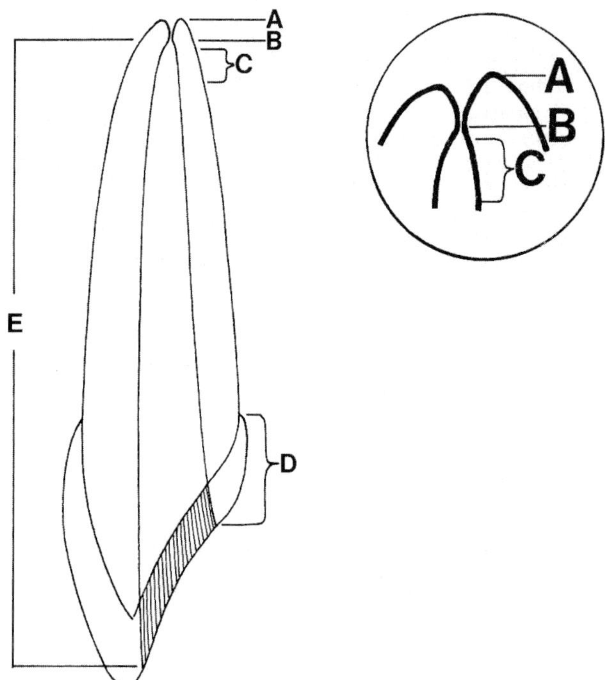

Figure 10-1 Concept of total endodontic cavity preparation, coronal and radicular as a continuum, based on Black's principles. Beginning at apex: A, Radiographic apex. B, Resistance Form, development of the "apical stop" at the cementodentinal junction against which filling is to be compacted and a stop to resist extrusion of canal debris and filling material. C, Retention Form to retain primary filling point. D, Convenience Form subject to revision as needed to accommodate larger, less flexible instruments. External modifications change the Outline Form. E, Outline Form, basic preparation throughout its length dictated by canal anatomy.

openings in Cerestone (cast ceramic) crowns,[4] as did Cohen and Wallace with Dicor crowns.[5] In Teplitsky and Sutherland's study, not a single crown fractured of 56 prepared with diamonds. Carbide burs were ineffective.[4]

Tapered instruments should never be forced but should be allowed to cut their own way with a light touch by the operator. If a tapered instrument is forced, it will act as a wedge. This causes the enamel to "check" or "craze" and will materially weaken the tooth (Figure 10-3). If a porcelain jacket crown is to be entered, a small diamond bur should be used. Again, care must be exercised not to split the jacket by forcing the action.

As soon as the enamel or restorative penetration and minor surface extensions are complete, the accelerated handpiece is put aside, and the slow-speed (3,000 to 8,000 rpm) contra-angle handpiece is used, mounted with a round bur. Three sizes of round burs, Nos. 2, 4, and 6, and two lengths, regular and surgical, are routinely used. The regular-length round bur in a conventional latch-type contra-angle handpice will "reach" 9.0 mm from the nose of the contra-angle. The surgical-length bur will "reach" 14 or 15 mm and is necessary in some deep preparations (Figure 10-4).

The round burs are for dentin removal in both anterior and posterior teeth. These burs are first used to drill through the dentin and "drop" into the pulp chamber. The same bur is then employed in the removal of the roof of the pulp chamber. The choice of the size of the round bur is made by estimating the canal width and chamber size and depth apparent in the initial radiograph.

The No. 2 round bur is generally used in preparing **mandibular** anterior teeth and most maxillary premolar teeth with narrow chambers and canals. It is also occasionally used in the incisal pulp horn area of maxillary anterior teeth. The No. 4 round bur is generally used in the maxillary anterior teeth and the mandibular premolar teeth. It is also occasionally used in "young" maxillary premolars and "adult" molars in both arches, that is, molars with extensive secondary dentin. The No. 6 round bur is used only in molars with large pulp chambers. A No. 1 round bur is also occasionally used in the floor of the pulp chamber to seek additional canal orifices. In addition, sonic and ultrasonic units, with specially designed endodontic tips, allow clinicians to more precisely remove dentin and expose orifices. In conjunction with magnification (loupes, fiber-optic endoscope, or microscope), the operator is better able to visualize the pulp chamber floor.

As soon as the bulk of the overhanging dentin is removed from the roof of the chamber, the slower operating round burs are put aside, and, once again, the high-speed fissure bur is used to finish and slope the side walls in the visible portions of the preparation. Again, the Maillefer Endo-Z carbide fissure bur (Dentsply/Maillefer, Tulsa, Okla.) is recommended. It is safe-ended and will not scar the pulpal floor. Moreover, it is longer bladed (9 mm) for sloping and funneling the access cavity.

Rotary cutting instruments, operating at greatly accelerated speeds, play a most important role in endodontic cavity preparation, especially for the patient with discomfort. At the same time, a good deal of damage may be rendered with these instruments because of the loss of tactile sense in their use. **High-speed burs should not be used to penetrate into, or initially enlarge, the pulp chamber unless the operator is skilled in endodontic preparations.** In this operation, the clinician depends almost entirely on the "feel" of the bur deep inside the tooth, against the roof and walls of the pulp chamber, to judge the extensions that are necessary. High-speed equipment is operated

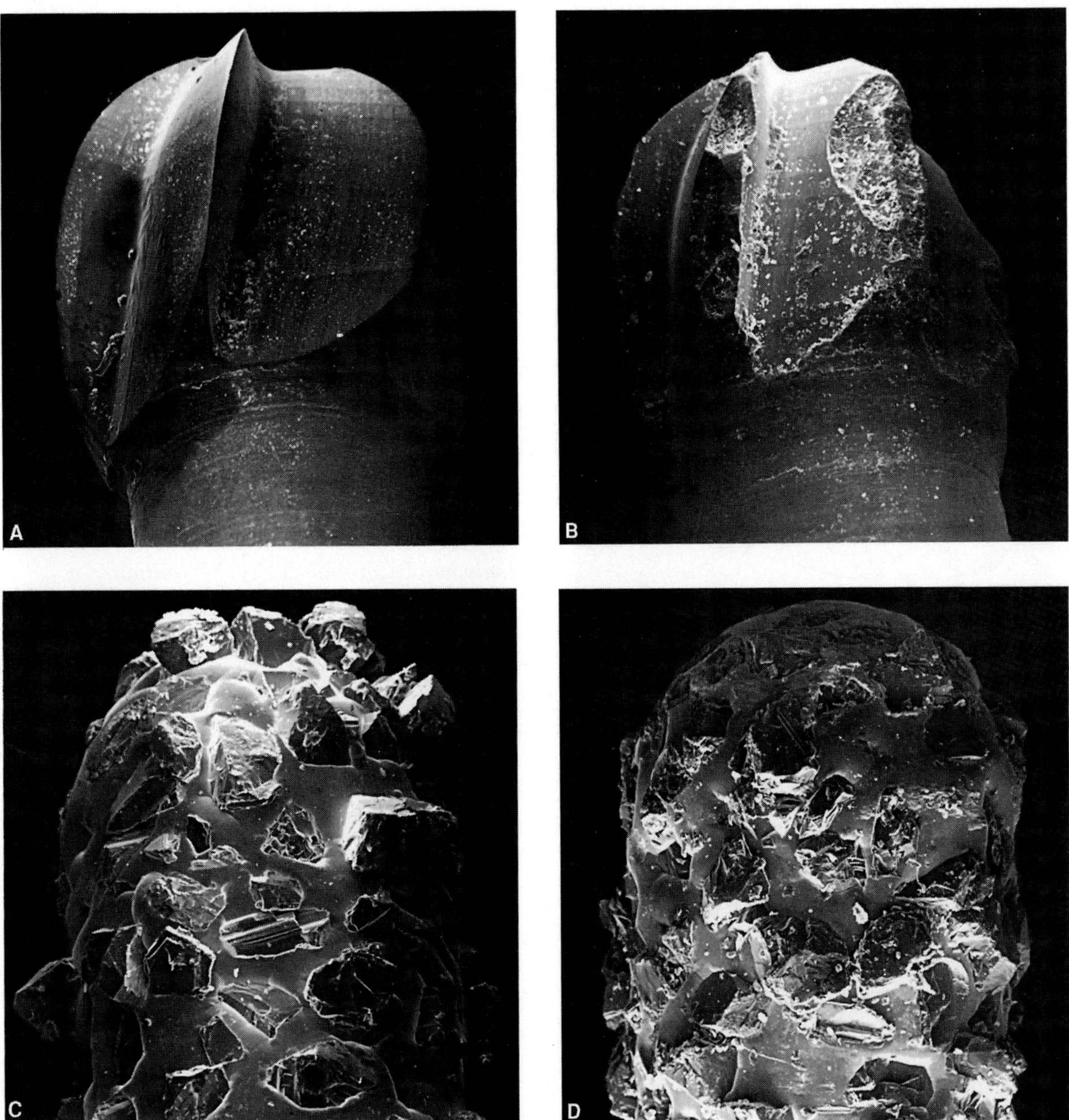

Figure 10-2 Comparison of round tungsten carbide burs versus extra-coarse dome-ended cylinder diamond burs used to cut nonprecious alloys. **A**, Tungsten carbide round bur before use. **B**, Same bur after preparing five cavities. **C**, Extra-coarse diamond bur before use. **D**, Same after preparing two cavities. Loss of abrasive on dome end. Tungsten carbide burs always "chattered." The coarse diamond bur was the only one "that cut smoothly and remained clinically effective" during five successive cavity preparations. Reproduced with permission from Stokes AN and Tidmarsh BG.[3]

by sight alone and is not generally employed in a blind area where reliance on tactile sensation is necessary.

Pulp Anatomy in Relation to Cavity Preparation

The alliance between endodontic cavity preparation and pulp anatomy is inflexible and inseparable. To master the anatomic concept of cavity preparation, the operator must develop a mental, three-dimensional image of the inside of the tooth, from pulp horn to apical foramen. Unfortunately, radiographs provide only a two-dimensional "blueprint" of pulp anatomy. It is the third dimension that the clinician must visualize, as a supplement to two-dimensional thinking, if one is to clean and shape accurately and fill the total pulp space (Plate 1, A).

Often the number or anatomy of the canals dictates modifications of the cavity preparation. If, for example, a fourth canal is found or suspected in a molar tooth, the preparation outline will have to be expanded to allow for easy, unrestrained access into the extra canal.

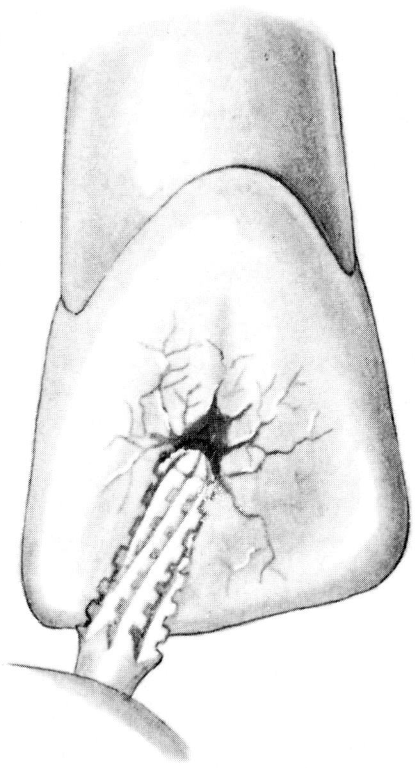

Figure 10-3 Forcing accelerated tapered bur or diamond severely crazes lingual enamel. The instrument should be allowed to cut its own way.

On the other hand, it became quite fashionable to grossly expand cavity preparations to accommodate large instruments used in canal preparation or filling. This violates the basic tenets of endodontic cavity preparation—**gross** modifications made for the sake of the clinician and the method rather than the more modest convenience modifications that may be dictated by the pulp anatomy itself.

PRINCIPLES OF ENDODONTIC CAVITY PREPARATION

Any discussion of cavity preparation must ultimately revert to the basic **Principles of Cavity Preparation** established by G. V. Black.[1] By slightly modifying Black's principles, a list of principles of endodontic cavity preparation may be established. In laying down his principles, Black dealt completely with cavity preparations limited to the crowns of teeth; however, his principles can be applied to radicular preparations as well. Endodontic preparations deal with both coronal and radicular cohorts—each prepared separately but ultimately flowing together into a single preparation. For convenience of description, **Black's principles** are therefore divided into the following:

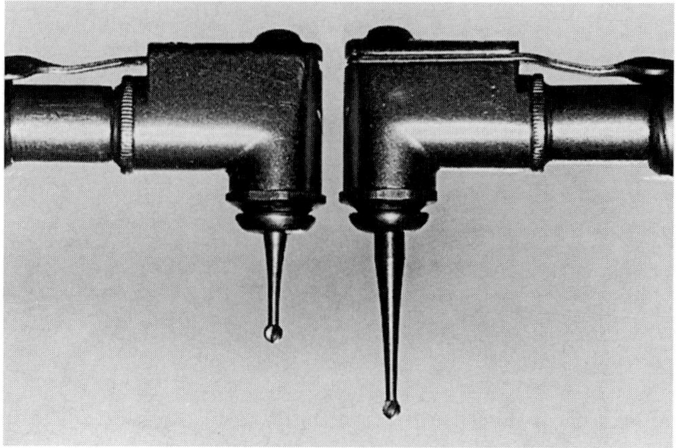

Figure 10-4 Two identical contra-angle handpieces holding No. 4 round burs. The regular-length bur on the left will reach 9 mm. The surgical-length bur on the right will reach 14 mm.

Endodontic ***Coronal*** *Cavity Preparation*

I.	Outline Form
II.	Convenience Form
III.	Removal of the remaining carious dentin (and defective restorations)
IV.	Toilet of the cavity

Endodontic ***Radicular*** *Cavity Preparation*

I and II.	Outline Form and Convenience Form (continued)
IV.	Toilet of the cavity (continued)
V.	Retention Form
VI.	Resistance Form

In the first half of this chapter, endodontic coronal cavity preparation will be discussed; the second half will be devoted to radicular preparation. A similar approach to coronal preparation was suggested by Pucci and Reig in 1944.[6]

Principle I: Outline Form

The outline form of the endodontic cavity must be correctly shaped and positioned to establish complete access for instrumentation, from cavity margin to apical foramen. Moreover, external outline form evolves from the internal anatomy of the tooth established by the pulp. Because of this internal-external relationship, endodontic preparations must of necessity be done in a reverse manner, from the inside of the tooth to the outside. That is to say, external outline form is established by mechanically projecting the internal anatomy of the pulp onto the external surface. This may be accomplished only by drilling into the open space of the pulp chamber and then working with the bur from the inside of the tooth to the outside, cutting away the dentin of the pulpal roof and walls overhanging the floor of the chamber (Plate 1, B).

This intracoronal preparation is contrasted to the extracoronal preparation of operative dentistry, in which outline form is always related to the **external anatomy** of the tooth. The tendency to establish endodontic outline form in the conventional operative manner and shape must be resisted (Plate 1, C).

To achieve optimal preparation, three factors of internal anatomy must be considered: (1) the size of the pulp chamber, (2) the shape of the pulp chamber, and (3) the number of individual root canals, their curvature, and their position.

Size of Pulp Chamber. The outline form of endodontic access cavities is materially affected by the size of the pulp chamber. In young patients, these preparations must be more extensive than in older patients, in whom the pulp has receded and the pulp chamber is smaller in all three dimensions (Plate 1, D). This becomes quite apparent in preparing the anterior teeth of youngsters, whose larger root canals require larger instruments and filling materials—materials that, in turn, will not pass through a small orifice in the crown (Plate 1, E).

Shape of Pulp Chamber. The finished outline form should accurately reflect the shape of the pulp chamber. For example, the floor of the pulp chamber in a molar tooth is usually triangular in shape, owing to the triangular position of the orifices of the canals. This triangular shape is extended up the walls of the cavity and out onto the occlusal surface; hence, the final occlusal cavity outline form is generally triangular (Plate 1, C). As another example, the coronal pulp of a maxillary **premolar** is flat mesiodistally but is elongated buccolingually. The outline form is, therefore, an elongated oval that extends buccolingually rather than mesiodistally, as does Black's operative cavity preparation (Plate 1, F).

Number, Position, and Curvature of Root Canals. The third factor regulating outline form is the number, position, and curvature or direction of the root canals. To prepare each canal efficiently without interference, the cavity walls often have to be extended to allow an unstrained instrument approach to the apical foramen. When cavity walls are extended to improve instrumentation, the outline form is materially affected (Plate 1, G). This change is for convenience in preparation; hence, convenience form partly regulates the ultimate outline form.

Principle II: Convenience Form

Convenience form was conceived by Black as a modification of the cavity outline form to establish greater convenience in the placement of intracoronal restorations. In endodontic therapy, however, convenience form makes more convenient (and accurate) the preparation and filling of the root canal. Four important benefits are gained through convenience form modifications: (1) unobstructed access to the canal orifice, (2) direct access to the apical foramen, (3) cavity expansion to accommodate filling techniques, and (4) complete authority over the enlarging instrument.

Unobstructed Access to the Canal Orifice. In endodontic cavity preparations of all teeth, enough tooth structure must be removed to allow instruments to be placed easily into the orifice of each canal without interference from overhanging walls. The clinician must be able to see each orifice and easily reach it with the instrument points. Failure to observe this principle not only endangers the successful outcome of the case but also adds materially to the duration of treatment (Plate 2, A to D).

In certain teeth, extra precautions must be taken to search for additional canals. The lower incisors are a case in point. Even more important is the high incidence of a second separate canal in the **mesiobuccal** root of maxillary molars. A second canal often is found in the distal root of mandibular molars as well. The premolars, both maxillary and mandibular, can also be counted on to have extra canals. During preparation, the operator, mindful of these variations from the norm, searches conscientiously for additional canals. In many cases, the outline form has to be modified to facilitate this search and the ultimate cleaning, shaping, and filling of the extra canals (Figure 10-5).

Luebke has made the important point that an entire wall need not be extended in the event that instrument impingement occurs owing to a severely curved root or an extra canal (personal communication, April 1983) (Plate 1, G). In extending only that portion of the wall needed to free the instrument, a cloverleaf appearance may evolve as the outline form. Hence, Luebke has termed this a "shamrock preparation" (Plate 1, H).

It is most important that as much crown structure be maintained as possible. MOD cavity preparations reduce tooth "stiffness" by more than 60%, and the "loss of marginal ridge integrity was the greatest contribution to loss of tooth strength."[7]

Direct Access to the Apical Foramen. To provide direct access to the apical foramen, enough tooth structure must be removed to allow the endodontic instruments freedom within the coronal cavity so they can extend down the canal in an unstrained position. This is especially true when the canal is severely curved or

PLATE 1

Outline Form

A. A standard radiograph (**left**) in buccolingual projection provides only a two-dimensional view of what is **actually a three-dimensional problem.** If a **mesiodistal** x-ray projection could be made (**right**), one would find the pulp of the maxillary second premolar to be flat tapering "ribbon" rather than round "thread" visualized on the initial radiograph. The final ovoid occlusal cavity preparation (F) will mirror the internal anatomy rather than the buccolingual x-ray image.

B. Coronal preparation of a maxillary first molar illustrating the major principle of endodontic cavity outline form: **the internal anatomy of the tooth (pulp) dictates the external outline form.** This is accomplished by extending preparation from inside of the tooth to the outside surface, that is, working from inside to outside.

C. Endodontic cavity preparation, mandibular first molar, superimposed on inlay, restoring proximal-occlusal surfaces. **Black's outline form** of **inlay** is related to the external anatomy and environment of the tooth, that is, the extent of carious lesions, grooves, and fissures and the position of the approximating premolar. A **triangular** or **rhomboidal outline form** of **endodontic preparation,** on the other hand, is related to the internal anatomy of the pulp. No relationship exists between the two outline forms.

D. Size and shape of endodontic coronal preparations in mandibular incisors related to **size** and **shape** of the **pulp** and **chamber.** A contrast in outline form between a "young" incisor (**left**) with a large pulp and an adult incisor (**right**) is apparent. The large triangular preparation in a youngster reflects pulpal horn extension and size of the pulp chamber, whereas ovoid preparation in an adult relates to a grossly receded pulp. Extension toward the incisal allows central-axis access for instruments.

E. Large size and shape of coronal preparation in a recently calcified incisor relate to huge pulp housing. To remove all pulp remnants and to accommodate large endodontic instruments and filling materials, coronal preparation must be an extensive, triangular, funnel-shaped opening. Actually, no more than the lingual wall of pulp chamber has been removed. In lower incisors, the outline form may well be extended into the incisal edge. This preparation allows absolutely **direct** access to apex.

F. The outline form of the **endodontic** coronal cavity in the **maxillary** first premolar is a narrow, elongated oval in buccolingual projection (**bottom**), which reflects the size and shape of a broad, flat pulp chamber of this particular tooth.

G. **Buccal** view of an **inadequate** coronal preparation in a maxillary molar with a defalcated mesiobuccal root. There has been no compensation in cavity preparation for severe curvature of the mesial canal or for the obtuse direction by which the canal leaves the chamber. The operator can no longer maintain control of the instrument, and a ledge has been produced (**arrow**). Extension of the outline form and internal preparation to the mesial (**dotted line**) would have obviated this failure.

H. **"Shamrock preparation."** Modified outline form to accommodate the instrument unrestrained in the severely curved mesial canal seen in G.

PLATE 1

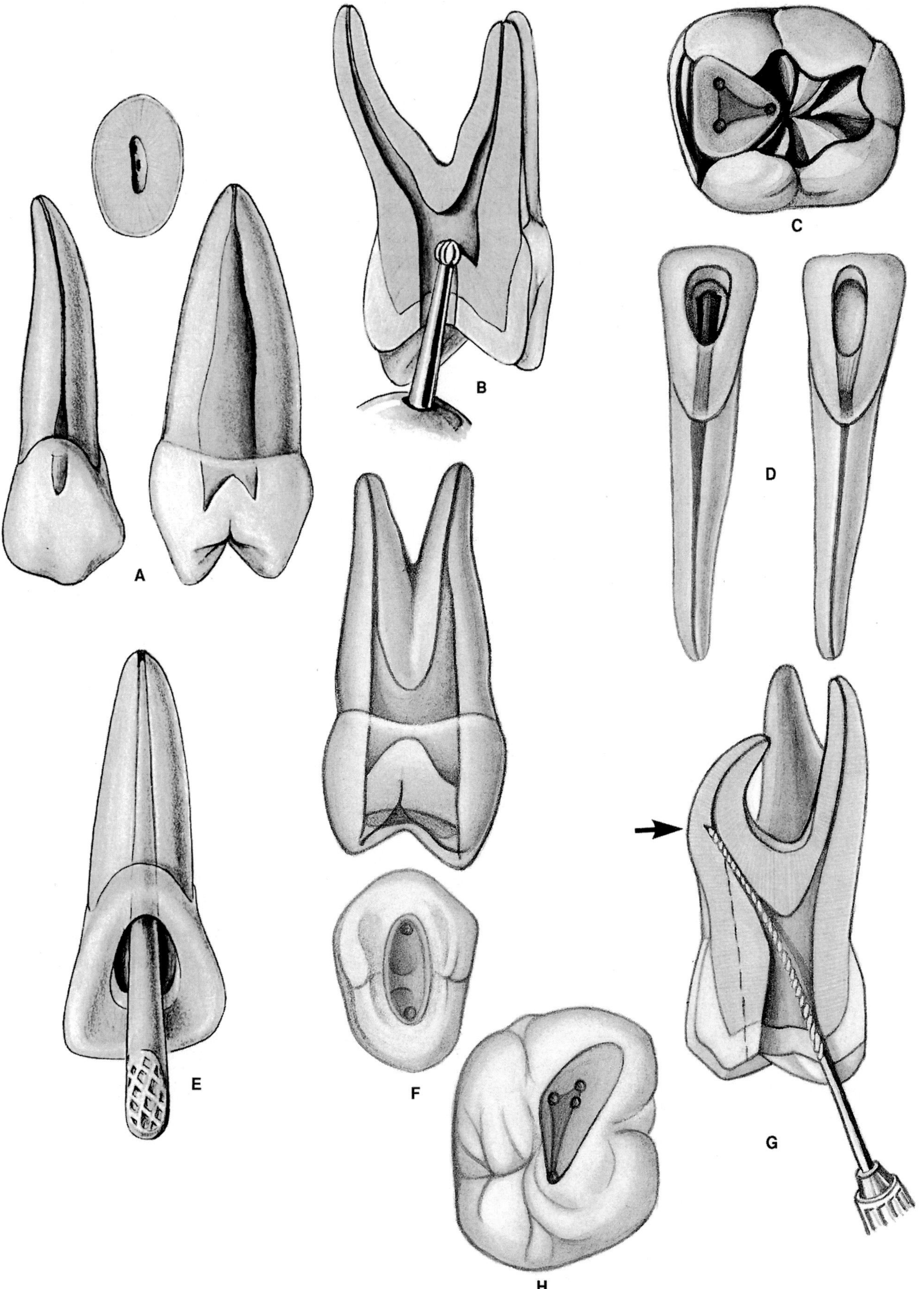

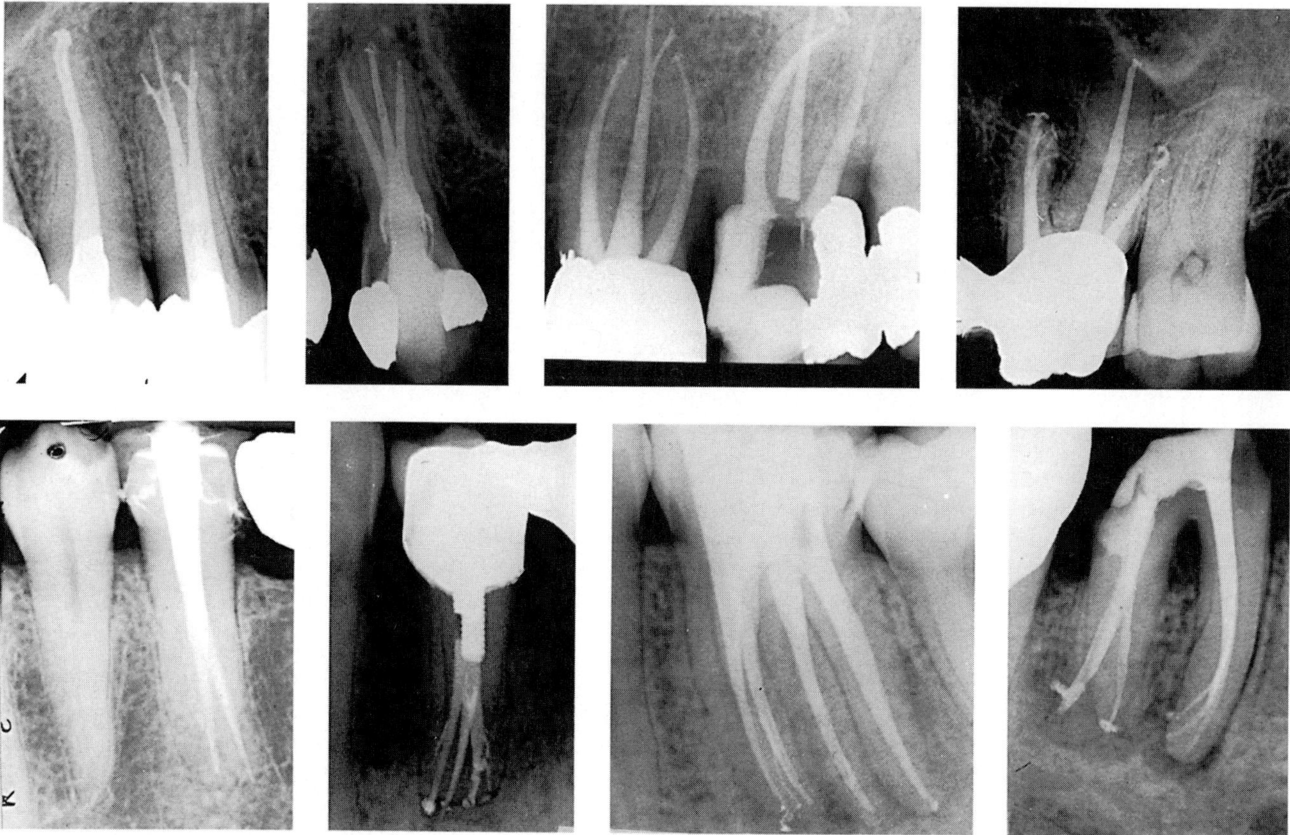

Figure 10-5 **"Rogues' Gallery"** of aberrant canals, bifurcations, and foramina, all cleaned, shaped, and obturated successfully. (Courtesy of Drs. L. Stephen Buchanan and Clifford J. Ruddle.)

leaves the chamber at an obtuse angle (Plate 2, E). Infrequently, total decuspation is necessary.

Extension to Accommodate Filling Techniques. It is often necessary to expand the outline form to make certain filling techniques more **convenient** or practical. If a softened gutta-percha technique is used for filling, wherein rather rigid pluggers are used in a vertical thrust, then the outline form may have to be widely extended to accommodate these heavier instruments.

Complete Authority over the Enlarging Instrument. It is imperative that the clinician maintain complete control over the root canal instrument. If the instrument is impinged at the canal orifice by tooth structure that should have been removed, the dentist will have lost control of the direction of the tip of the instrument, and the intervening **tooth structure** will dictate the control of the instrument (Plate 2, G).

If, on the other hand, the tooth structure is removed around the orifice so that the instrument stands free in this area of the canal (Plate 2, H), the instrument will then be controlled by only two factors: the clinician's fingers on the handle of the instrument and the walls of the canal at the tip of the instrument. Nothing is to intervene between these two points (Plate 2, F).

Failure to properly modify the access cavity outline by extending the convenience form will ultimately lead to failure by either root perforation, "ledge" or "shelf" formation within the canal, instrument breakage, or the incorrect shape of the completed canal preparation, often termed "zipping" or apical transportation.

Principle III: Removal of the Remaining Carious Dentin and Defective Restorations

Caries and defective restorations remaining in an endodontic cavity preparation must be removed for three reasons: (1) to eliminate mechanically as many bacteria as possible from the interior of the tooth, (2) to eliminate the discolored tooth structure, that may ultimately lead to staining of the crown, and (3) to eliminate the possibility of any bacteria-laden saliva leaking into the prepared cavity. The last point is especially true of proximal or buccal caries that extend into the prepared cavity.

After the caries are removed, if a carious perforation of the wall is allowing salivary leakage, the area must be repaired with cement, preferably from inside the cavity. A small piece of premixed temporary cement, Cavit or Cavit G (Premier Dental Products; Plymouth, Pa.), may be forced through the perforation and applied to the dry walls of the cavity, while care is taken to avoid forcing the cement into a canal orifice. A cotton pellet, moistened with any sterile aqueous solution such as saline or a local anesthetic, will cause the Cavit to set. Coronal perforations may also be repaired with adhesive composite resins placed by the acid-etch technique in a perfectly dry milieu.

If the caries is so extensive that the lateral walls are destroyed, or if a defective restoration is in place that is loose and leaking, then the entire wall or restoration should be removed and later restored. It is important that restoration be postponed until the radicular preparation has been completed. It is much easier to complete the radicular preparation through an open cavity than through a restored crown. As a matter of fact, the more crown that is missing, the easier the radicular preparation becomes. The ultimate in ease of operation is the molar tooth broken off at the gingival level (Figure 10-6). As long as a rubber dam can be placed on the tooth, it need not be built up with amalgam, cement, or an orthodontic band; having to work through a hole only complicates the endodontic procedures. In addition, if the band comes off, the length of tooth measurements is invalidated and must be re-established. An adequate temporary filling can always be placed in the remaining pulp chamber.

If enough tooth does not remain above the gingiva to place a rubber dam clamp and seal against saliva, and if it is imperative that the tooth be retained, a simple gingivoplasty will establish the required "crown" length. In any case, this procedure is usually necessary before the tooth can be restored. In this case, the occlusal cavity may be sealed and the incised gingiva protected with the placement of a putty-like periodontal dressing over the entire stump and gingiva. Cotton, and then a thin layer of Cavit, should first cover the canal orifices.

Principle IV: Toilet of the Cavity

All of the caries, debris, and necrotic material must be removed from the chamber before the radicular preparation is begun. If the calcified or metallic debris is left in the chamber and carried into the canal, it may act as an obstruction during canal enlargement. Soft debris carried from the chamber might increase the bacterial population in the canal. Coronal debris may also stain the crown, particularly in anterior teeth.

Round burs, of course, are most helpful in cavity toilet. The long-blade, endodontic spoon excavator is ideal for debris removal (Figure 10-7). Irrigation with sodium hypochlorite is also an excellent measure for cleansing the chamber and canals of persistent debris.

The chamber may finally be wiped out with cotton, and a **careful** flush of air will eliminate the remaining debris. However, air must never be aimed down the canals. Emphysema of the oral tissues has been pro-

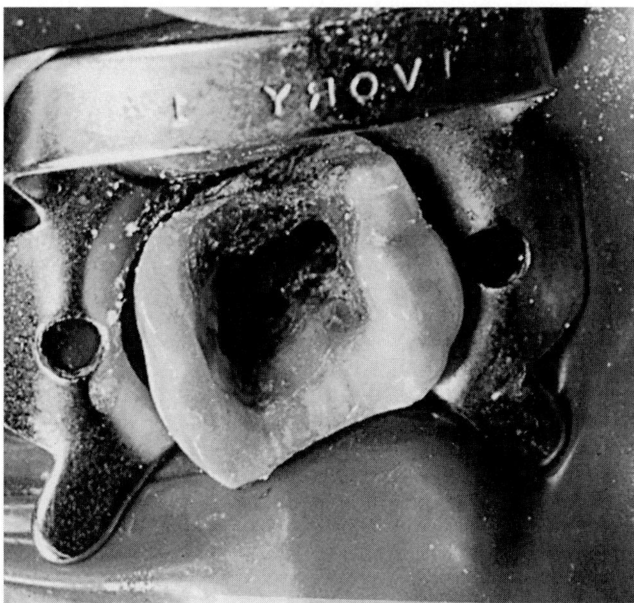

Figure 10-6 Carious involvement of the maxillary molar has destroyed most of the crown. Enough tooth structure remains to adapt the rubber dam clamp. A wide-open cavity allows greater ease of operation. If the caries extends below the gingival level, gingivectomy will expose solid tooth structure.

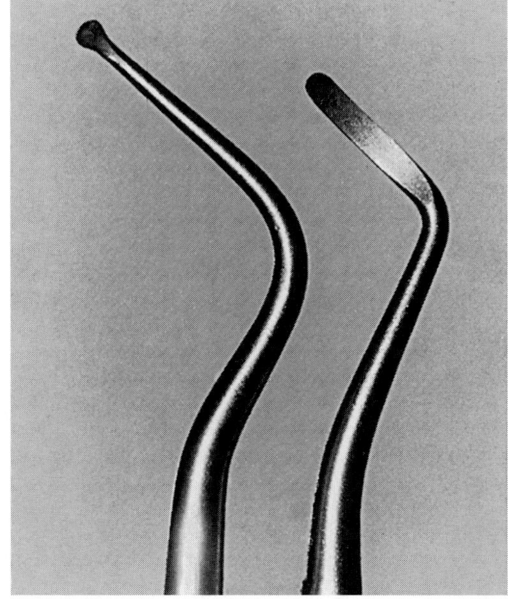

Figure 10-7 Long-blade endodontic spoon excavator compared with standard Black's spoon excavator. The long-blade instrument (**left**) is needed to reach the depths of molar preparations.

PLATE 2

Convenience Form

A. **Obstructed access** to mesial canals in a mandibular first molar. The overhanging roof of the pulp chamber misdirects the instrument mesially, with resulting ledge formation in the canal. It is virtually impossible to see and difficult to locate mesial canal orifices each time the instrument is introduced.

B. **Internal cavity preparation.** Removing the roof completely from the pulp chamber will bring canal orifices into view and allow immediate access to each orifice. Using a round bur and working from the inside out will accomplish this end.

C. **Final finish of the convenience form** is completed with a fissure bur, diamond point, or non–end-cutting batt bur. The entire cavity slopes toward the mesial direction of approach, which greatly simplifies instrument placement.

D. **Unobstructed access to canal orifices. The mesial** wall has been **sloped to mesial** for the approach to the mandibular molar is from the mesial. The tip of the instrument follows down the mesial wall at each corner of the triangular preparation and literally "falls" into orifices. After the position of each orifice has been determined, the mouth mirror may be laid aside.

The distal wall of preparation also slopes to the mesial and is easily entered from the mesial approach.

E. **Direct access to apical foramen.** Extensive removal of coronal tooth structure is necessary to allow complete freedom of endodontic instruments in the coronal cavity and **direct access to the apical canal.** This is especially true when the root is severely curved or leaves the chamber at an obtuse angle.

Walls are generally reduced with burs or long, thin diamond points (see B and C above) and with endodontic files, Gates-Glidden drills, or orifice openers. Burs are rarely used in the floor or immediate orifice area. In the event that a second canal is suspected in the mesiobuccal root of the maxillary molar, the cavity outline would be extended in both of these directions to broaden the search.

Depending on the technique used to fill the canal, the outline form may also be expanded somewhat to accommodate pluggers used in obturation.

F. **The complete authority of the enlarging instrument is maintained** when all intervening tooth structure is removed and the instrument is controlled by the clinician's fingers on the handle of the instrument and the tip of the instrument is free in the lumen of the canal.

G. **Complete authority of enlarging instrument.** If the lateral wall of the cavity has not been sufficiently extended and the pulpal horn portion of the orifice still remains in the wall, the orifice will have the appearance of a tiny "mouse hole." This **lateral wall** will then impinge on enlarging the instrument and will dictate the direction of the instrument tip. The operator will have lost control of the instrument and the situation.

H. **By extending the lateral wall** of the cavity, thus removing all intervening dentin from the orifice, the "mouse hole" in the wall will be eliminated and the **orifice** will appear **completely in the floor.** Now the enlarging instrument will stand free of the walls, and the **operator will regain control of the instrument** (see F above).

PLATE 2

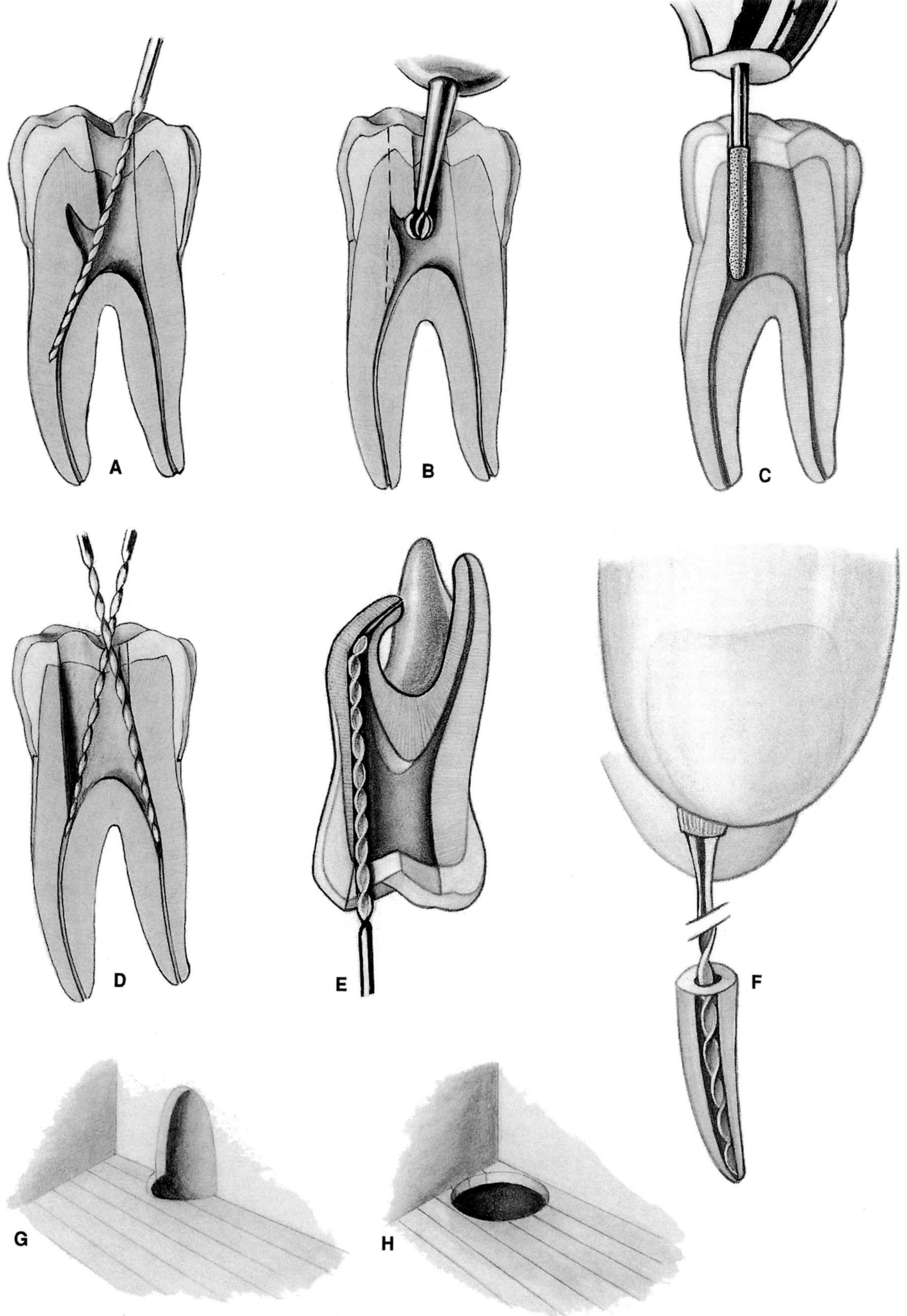

duced by a blast of air escaping out of the apex. In an *in vitro* study, Eleazer and Eleazer found a direct relation between the size of the apical foramen and the likelihood of expressing air into the periapical tissues. Addtional risks are incurred as air from these syringes is not sterile.[8] Some dental schools do not allow the use of the three-way air/water syringe once access into the chamber has been achieved.

As previously stated, **toilet of the cavity** makes up a significant portion of the radicular preparations.

DETAILED CORONAL CAVITY PREPARATION

Descriptions and Caveats

With the basic principles of endodontic cavity preparation in mind, the student is urged to study the detailed plates that follow, each dealing with coronal preparation. Again, keep in mind the importance of the intracoronal preparation to the ultimate radicular preparation and filling.

For each group of teeth—for example, maxillary anterior teeth, mandibular premolar teeth—there is a plate showing in detail the suggested cavity preparation and operative technique applicable to that particular group of teeth. The technique plate is followed by plates of the individual teeth within the group. Four separate views of each tooth are presented: (1) the facial-lingual view as seen in the radiograph; (2) the mesiodistal view, impossible to obtain radiographically but necessary to the three-dimensional mental image of the pulp anatomy; (3) a cross-sectional view at three levels; and (4) a view of the occlusal or lingual surface with cavity outline form.

Detailed variations in preparation related to each particular tooth, as well as information about tooth length, root curvature, and canal anatomy variations, are presented. These plates are followed by a plate of **errors** commonly committed in the preparation of this group of teeth.

The mandibular incisors—centrals and laterals—are so anatomically similar that they are confined to one plate.

The reader is reminded that the preparations illustrated here are **minimal** preparations, that the outline form is a direct reflection of the pulp anatomy. If the pulp is expansive, the outline form will also be expansive. Furthermore, the outline form may have to be greatly enlarged to accept heavier instruments or rigid filling materials.

Generally speaking, the length-of-tooth measurements are approximations. Nonetheless, they are helpful and should alert the dentist to what to expect as "normal." When there is a lack of agreement between authors, we have chosen the larger figures, that is, the figures furthest from normal.[9–24] We have also adapted liberally from the important work by Dempster et al. on the angulation of the teeth in the alveolar process.[25] In addition, new information on multiple canals has been brought to light.

Multiple and Extra Canals

Although it should come as no surprise, the high incidence of additional canals in molars, premolars, and mandibular incisors is significant. Hess, as early as 1925, pointed out that 54% of his 513 maxillary molar specimens had four canals.[26] For years these facts were generally ignored.

At this juncture, however, one cannot help but be struck by the magnitude of the numbers of additional versus traditional canals. For example, **maxillary molars** may have four canals rather than three canals as much as 95% of the time. Using a No. 1 round bur **and/or ultrasonic instruments** to remove secondary dentin from the pulpal floor along the mesiobuccal-palatal leg of the molar triangle will uncover an additional 31% of these orifices.[27] An earlier study found these secondary canals 69% of the time *in vitro* but only 31% *in vivo*.[23] Another *in vivo* study found two canals in the mesiobuccal roots of maxillary first molars 77% of the time, and, of these, 62% had two apical foramina.[28] Although a fourth root in maxillary molars is rare (0.4%),[29,30] single-canal taurodontism ("bull-tooth") was found in 11.3% of one patient cohort.[31]

The incidence of **accessory canals** in the **furcation** of **maxillary molars,** canals that extend all the way from the pulpal floor to the furcation area, is 48% in one study[32] and 68% in another.[33] These accessory canals are only about twice the size of a dentinal tubule and so are rarely mistaken for a canal orifice even though they are large enough to admit bacteria to the pulp from a furcal periodontal lesion. In **mandibular** molars, through-and-through furcal accessory canals are found 56% of the time in one study[32] and 48% in another.[33]

Mandibular molars also exhibit secondary root canals, over and above the traditional three. Although as many as five canals[34] and as few as one and two canals[35,36] rarely occur in mandibular molars, four canals are not unusual. Bjorndal and Skidmore reported this occurrence 29% of the time in a US cohort, a second distal canal being the usual anomaly.[23] The Chinese found four canals in 31.5% of their cases.[37] Weine et al. however, reported that only 12.5% of their second molar specimens had a second distal canal and that only one had two separate apical foramina.[35] Anomalies also occur in the mesial root.[38]

Premolar teeth are also prone to secondary canals. Maxillary first premolars, which generally have two canals, have three canals 5 to 6% of the time.[14,39] Twenty-four percent of maxillary second premolars have second root canals and occasionally three canals.[15] In Brazil, two canals were found 32.4% of the time and three canals in 0.3% of the cases.[40]

Mandibular premolars are notorious for having extra canals—26.5% in first premolars and 13.5% in second premolars.[21] A US Army group reported canal bifurcations as deep as 6 to 9 mm from the coronal orifice 74% of the time in **mandibular** first premolars.[22]

Almost one-third of all **mandibular lateral incisors** have two canals with two foramina.[11] A Turkish report lists two newly defined canal configurations, one that ends in three separate foramina.[12]

Every dentist who has done considerable root canal therapy must ask, "How many of these extra canals have I failed to find in the past?" Also, there appears to be a wide discrepancy between the figures quoted above, which are based on laboratory studies, and those found under clinical conditions. Hartwell and Bellizi found four canals in maxillary first molars only 18% of the time *in vivo* (in comparison to the figure of 85% found *in vitro*, cited above).[41] In mandibular first molars, the reverse was true: they actually filled a fourth canal 35% of the time, whereas 29% of extracted teeth had a fourth canal.[41]

How may one account for the wide discrepancy between these figures of incidence of additional canals? Ethnic variance may be one part of the equation. African Americans have more than twice as many two-canal mandibular premolars (32.8% versus 13.7%) than do Caucasian patients: "Four out of ten black patients had at least one lower premolar with two or more canals."[42] In a southern Chinese population, however, the roots of **mandibular second molars** are fused 52% of the time and only have two canals, rather than three, 55% of the time.[36] The Chinese also have two canal lower incisors 27% of the time, but only 1% terminate in two foramina,[43] compared to two foramina terminations 30% of the time in a US study.[11] A Brazilian study reports two canals with two foramina in 1.2% of **mandibular canines.**[44]

The incidence of taurodontism varies all over the world. In Saudi Arabia, 43.2% of adult molars studied were taurodonts in 11.3% of the patient cohort.[31] In Brazil, 11 cases of taurodontism in mandibular **premolars,** a very rare occurrence, were described.[45] The seminal studies of Pineda and Kuttler were done in Mexico on extracted teeth, many presumably from a native cohort.[14,18]

In any event, anomalous and multiple canals are a worldwide problem, a fact that makes imperative a careful search in every tooth for additional canals. Just as important, the facts emphasize the necessity of choosing a method of preparation and filling that will ensure the obturations of these additional canals (see Figure 10-5).

Plates 3 to 27

Folio of
CORONAL ENDODONTIC CAVITY PREPARATIONS

Originally Illustrated by
VIRGINIA E. BROOKS
Modified by
PHYLLIS WOOD

PLATE 3

Endodontic Preparation of Maxillary Anterior Teeth

A. Entrance is **always** gained through the lingual surface of **all** anterior teeth. Initial penetration is made in the exact center of the lingual surface at the position marked "X." A common error is to begin the cavity too far gingivally.

B. Initial entrance is prepared with a round-point tapering fissure bur in an **accelerated-speed** contra-angle handpiece with air coolant, operated at a **right angle** to the long axis of the tooth. **Only enamel is penetrated at this time.** Do not force the bur; allow it to cut its own way.

C. **Convenience extension** toward the incisal continues the initial penetrating cavity preparation. Maintain the point of the bur in the central cavity and rotate the handpiece toward the incisal so that the bur **parallels** the long axis of the tooth. Enamel and dentin are beveled toward the incisal. **Entrance into the pulp chamber should not be made with an accelerated-speed instrument.** Lack of tactile sensation with these instruments **precludes their use inside** the tooth.

D. The preliminary cavity outline is funneled and fanned incisally with a fissure bur. Enamel has a **short** bevel toward the incisal, and a "nest" is prepared in the dentin to receive the round bur to be used for penetration.

E. **A surgical-length** No. 2 or 4 round bur in a **slow-speed** contra-angle handpiece is used to penetrate the pulp chamber. If the pulp has greatly receded, a No. 2 round bur is used for initial penetration. Take advantage of **convenience extension** toward the incisal to allow for the shaft of the penetrating bur, operated nearly parallel to the long axis of the tooth.

F. **Working from inside the chamber to outside,** a round bur is used to remove the lingual and labial walls of the pulp chamber. The resulting cavity is smooth, continuous, and flowing from cavity margin to canal orifice.

G. After the outline form is completed, the surgical-length bur is carefully passed into the canal. **Working from inside to outside,** the lingual "shoulder" is removed to give continuous, smooth-flowing preparation. Often a long, tapering diamond point will better remove the lingual "shoulder."

H. Occasionally, a No. 1 or 2 round bur must be used laterally and incisally to eliminate pulpal horn debris and bacteria. This also prevents future discoloration.

I. Final preparation relates to the **internal anatomy** of the chamber and canal. In a "young" tooth with a large pulp, the outline form reflects a large triangular internal anatomy—an extensive cavity that allows thorough cleansing of the chamber as well as passage of large instruments and filling materials needed to prepare and fill a large canal. Cavity extension toward the incisal allows greater access to the midline of the canal.

J. Cavity preparations in "adult" teeth, with the chamber obturated with secondary dentin, are ovoid in shape. Preparation **funnels** down to the orifice of the canal. The further the pulp has receded, the more difficult it is to reach to this depth with a round bur. Therefore, when the radiograph reveals advanced pulpal recession, **convenience extension must be advanced further incisally** to allow the bur shaft and instruments to operate in the central axis.

K. Final preparation with the reamer in place. The instrument shaft **clears** the incisal **cavity margin** and **reduced** lingual "shoulder," allowing an unrestrained approach to the apical third of the canal. The instrument remains under the complete control of the clinician. An optimal, **round, tapered cavity** may be prepared in the apical third, tailored to the requirements of **round, tapered filling** materials to follow. The remaining ovoid part of the canal is cleaned and shaped by circumferential filing or Gates-Glidden drills.

PLATE 3

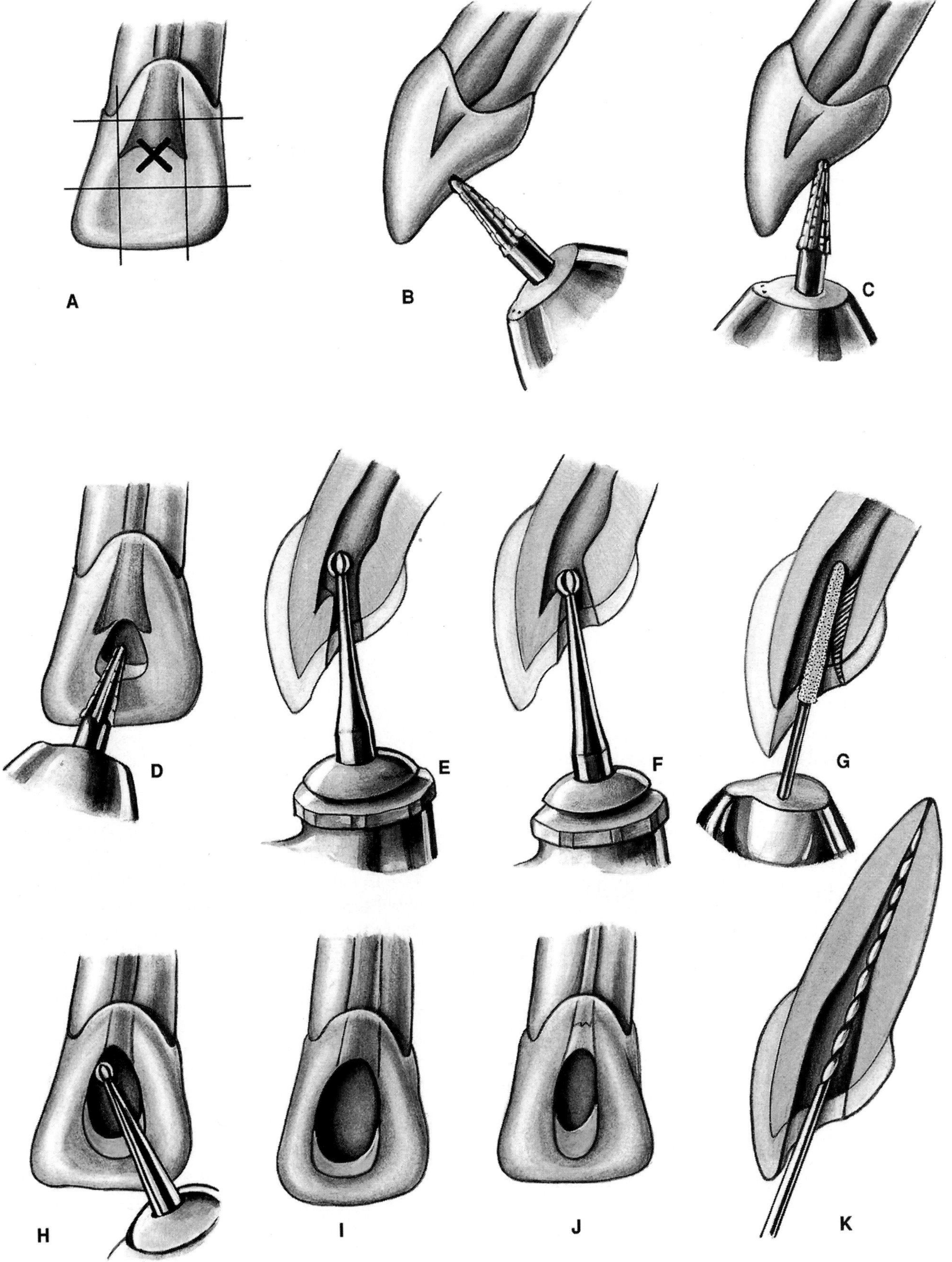

PLATE 4

Maxillary Central Incisor

Pulp Anatomy and Coronal Preparation

A. **Lingual** view of a recently calcified incisor with a large pulp. A radiograph will reveal
   1. extent of the pulp horns
   2. mesiodistal width of the pulp
   3. apical-distal curvature (8% of the time)
   4. 2-degree mesial-axial inclination of the tooth

   These factors seen in the radiograph are borne in mind when preparation is begun.

B. **Distal** view of the same tooth demonstrating details **not apparent in the radiograph:**
   1. presence of a **lingual** "shoulder" at the point where the chamber and canal join
   2. broad labiolingual extent of the pulp
   3. 29-degree lingual-axial angulation of the tooth

   The operator must recognize that
   a. the lingual "shoulder" must be removed with a tapered diamond point to allow better access to the canal.
   b. these "unseen" factors affect the **size, shape,** and **inclination** of final preparation.

C. Cross-sections at three levels: 1, cervical; 2, midroot; and 3, apical third:
   1. **Cervical** level: the pulp is enormous in a young tooth, wider in the mesiodistal dimension. Débridement in this area is accomplished by **extensive perimeter filing.**
   2. **Midroot** level: the canal continues ovoid and requires perimeter filing and multiple point filling.
   3. **Apical third** level: the canal, generally round in shape, is enlarged by reshaping the cavity into a **round tapered** preparation. Preparation terminates at the cementodentinal junction, 0.5 to 1.0 mm from the radiographic apex. An unusually large apical third canal is more ovoid in shape, must be prepared with **perimeter filing** rather than reaming, and must be obturated with multiple points or warm gutta-percha.

D. Large, triangular, funnel-shaped **coronal preparation** is necessary to adequately débride the chamber of all pulp remnants. (The pulp is "ghosted" in the background.) Note the beveled extension toward the incisal that will carry the preparation labially and thus nearer the central axis. Incisal extension allows better access for large instruments and filling materials used in the apical third canal.

E. **Lingual** view of an **adult** incisor with extensive secondary dentin formation.
   A radiograph will reveal
   1. full pulpal recession
   2. apparently straight canal
   3. 2-degree mesial-axial inclination of the tooth

F. **Distal** view of the same tooth demonstrating details **not apparent in the radiograph:**
   1. narrow labiolingual width of pulp
   2. reduced size of the lingual shoulder
   3. apical-labial curvature (9% of the time)
   4. 29-degree lingual-axial angulation of the tooth

   The operator must recognize that
   a. a small canal orifice is difficult to find.
   b. **apical**-labial curvature, **not usually seen radiographically,** can be determined by exploration with a fine curved file and mesially oriented radiographs.
   c. axial inclination of the root calls for careful orientation and alignment of the bur to prevent "gouging."

G. Cross-sections at three levels: 1, cervical; 2, midroot; and 3, apical third:
   1. **Cervical** level: the canal, only slightly ovoid, becomes progressively more round.
   2. **Midroot** level: the canal varies from slightly ovoid to round.
   3. **Apical third** level: the canal is generally round in the older patient.

H. Ovoid, funnel-shaped coronal preparation provides adequate access to the root canal. The pulp chamber, obturated by secondary dentin, need not be extended for coronal débridement. "Adult" cavity preparation is narrow in the mesiodistal width but is almost as extensive in the incisogingival direction as preparation in a young tooth. This beveled incisal extension carries preparation nearer the central axis, allowing better access to the curved apical third.

Maxillary Central Incisors

Length of tooth		*Canal*	*Lateral canals*	*Apical ramifications*	*Root curvature*	
Average Length	23.3 mm	One canal 100%	23%	13%	Straight	75%
Maximum Length	25.6 mm				Distal Curve	8%
Minimum Length	21.0 mm				Mesial Curve	4%
Range	4.6 mm				*Labial Curve	9%
					*Lingual Curve	4%

*Not apparent in radiograph

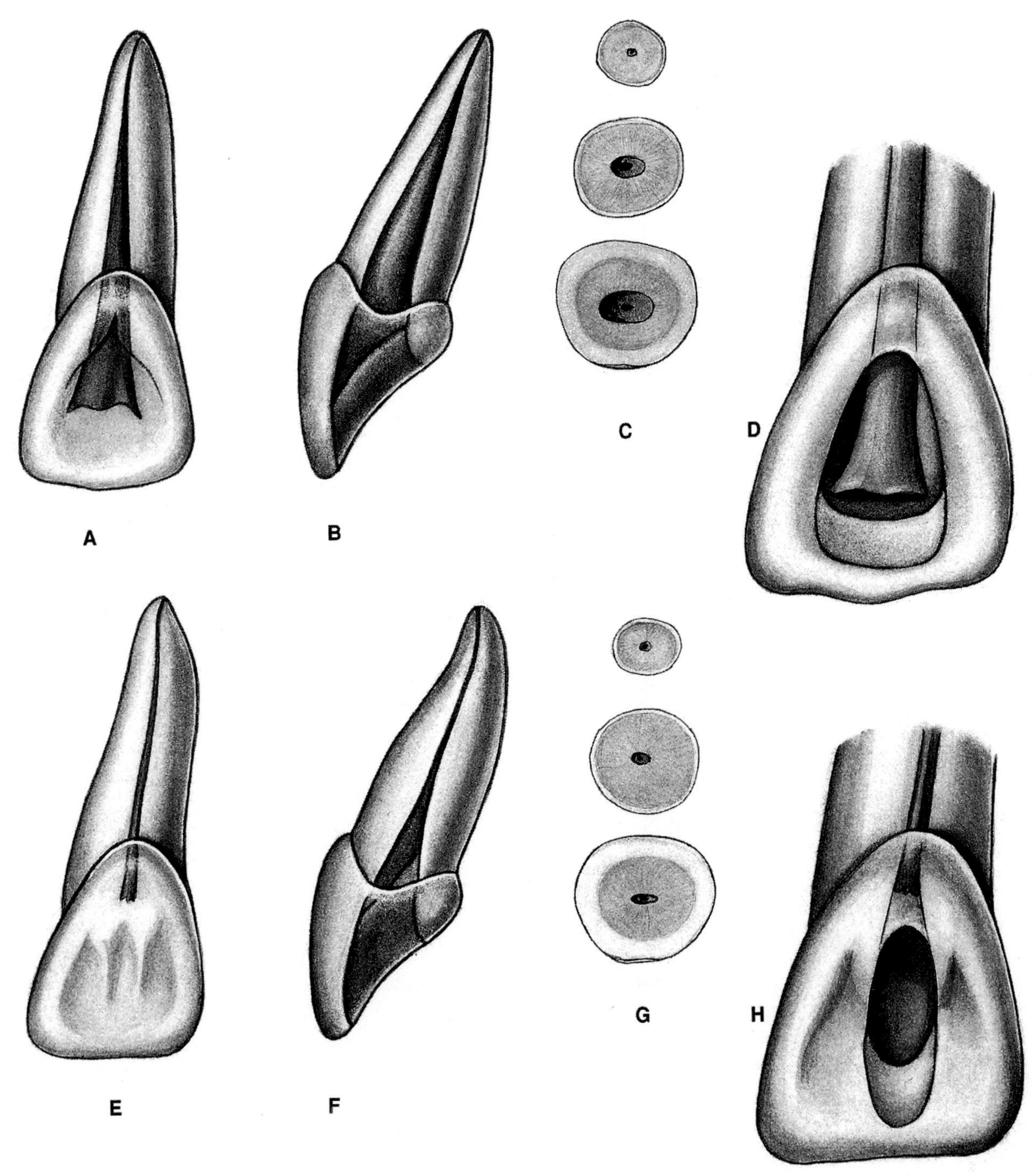

PLATE 5

Maxillary Lateral Incisor

Pulp Anatomy and Coronal Preparation

A. Lingual view of a recently calcified incisor with a large pulp. A radiograph will reveal
   1. extent of the pulp horns
   2. mesiodistal width of the pulp
   3. apical-distal curvature (53% of the time)
   4. 16-degree mesial-axial inclination of the tooth

   Factors seen in the radiograph are borne in mind when preparation is begun.

B. **Distal** view of the same tooth demonstrating details **not apparent in the radiograph:**
   1. presence of a **lingual** "shoulder" at the point where the chamber and canal join
   2. broad labiolingual extent of the pulp
   3. 29-degree lingual-axial angulation of tooth

   The operator must recognize that
   a. the lingual "shoulder" must be removed with a tapered diamond point to allow better access to the canal.
   b. these "unseen" factors will affect the **size, shape,** and **inclination** of final preparation.

C. Cross-sections at three levels: 1, cervical; 2, midroot; and 3, apical third:
   1. **Cervical** level: the pulp is large in a young tooth and wider in the labiolingual dimension. Débridement in this area is accomplished by extensive perimeter filing.
   2. **Midroot** level: the canal continues ovoid and requires additional filing to straighten the gradual curve. Multiple point filling is necessary.
   3. **Apical third** level: the canal, generally round and **gradually curved,** is enlarged by filing to a straightened trajectory. Preparation is completed by shaping the cavity into a **round, tapered** preparation. Preparation terminates at the cementodentinal junction, 0.5 to 1.0 mm from the radiographic apex.

D. Large, triangular, funnel-shaped coronal preparation is necessary to adequately débride the chamber of all pulpal remnants. (The pulp is "ghosted" in the background.) Note the beveled extension toward the incisal, which will carry the preparation labially and thus nearer the central axis. Incisal extension allows better access to the apical third of the canal.

E. **Lingual** view of an **adult** incisor with extensive secondary dentin formation.

   A radiograph will reveal
   1. full pulp recession
   2. severe apical curve to the distal
   3. 16-degree mesial-axial inclination of the tooth

F. **Distal** view of the same tooth demonstrating details **not apparent in the radiograph**
   1. narrow labiolingual width of the pulp
   2. reduced size of the lingual shoulder
   3. apical-**lingual** curvature (4% of the time)
   4. 29-degree lingual-axial angulation of the tooth

   The operator must recognize that
   a. a small canal orifice is difficult to find.
   b. apical-lingual curvature, **not usually seen radiographically,** can be determined by exploration with a fine curved file and mesially oriented radiographs.
   c. axial inclination of the root calls for careful orientation and alignment of the bur to prevent labial "gouging." A "corkscrew" curve, to the distal and lingual, complicates preparation of the apical third of the canal.

G. Cross-sections at three levels: 1, cervical; 2, midroot; and 3, apical third:
   1. **Cervical** level: the canal is only slightly ovoid and becomes progressively rounder.
   2. **Midroot** level: the canal varies from slightly ovoid to round.
   3. **Apical third** level: the canal is generally round in the older patient.

   A curved canal is enlarged by alternate reaming and filing. Ovoid preparation will require multiple point filling.

H. Ovoid, funnel-shaped coronal preparation should be only slightly **skewed** toward the mesial to present better access to the apical-distal. It is not necessary to extend preparation for coronal débridement, but an extensive bevel is necessary toward the incisal to carry preparation nearer the central axis, allowing better access to the apical third.

Maxillary Lateral Incisors

Length of tooth		*Canal*	*Lateral canals*	*Apical ramifications*	*Root curvature*	
Average Length	22.8 mm	One canal 99.9%	10%	12%	Straight	30%
Maximum Length	25.1 mm				Distal Curve	53%
Minimum Length	20.5 mm				Mesial Curve	3%
Range	4.6 mm				*Labial Curve	4%
					*Bayonet and Gradual Curve	6%

*Not apparent in radiograph

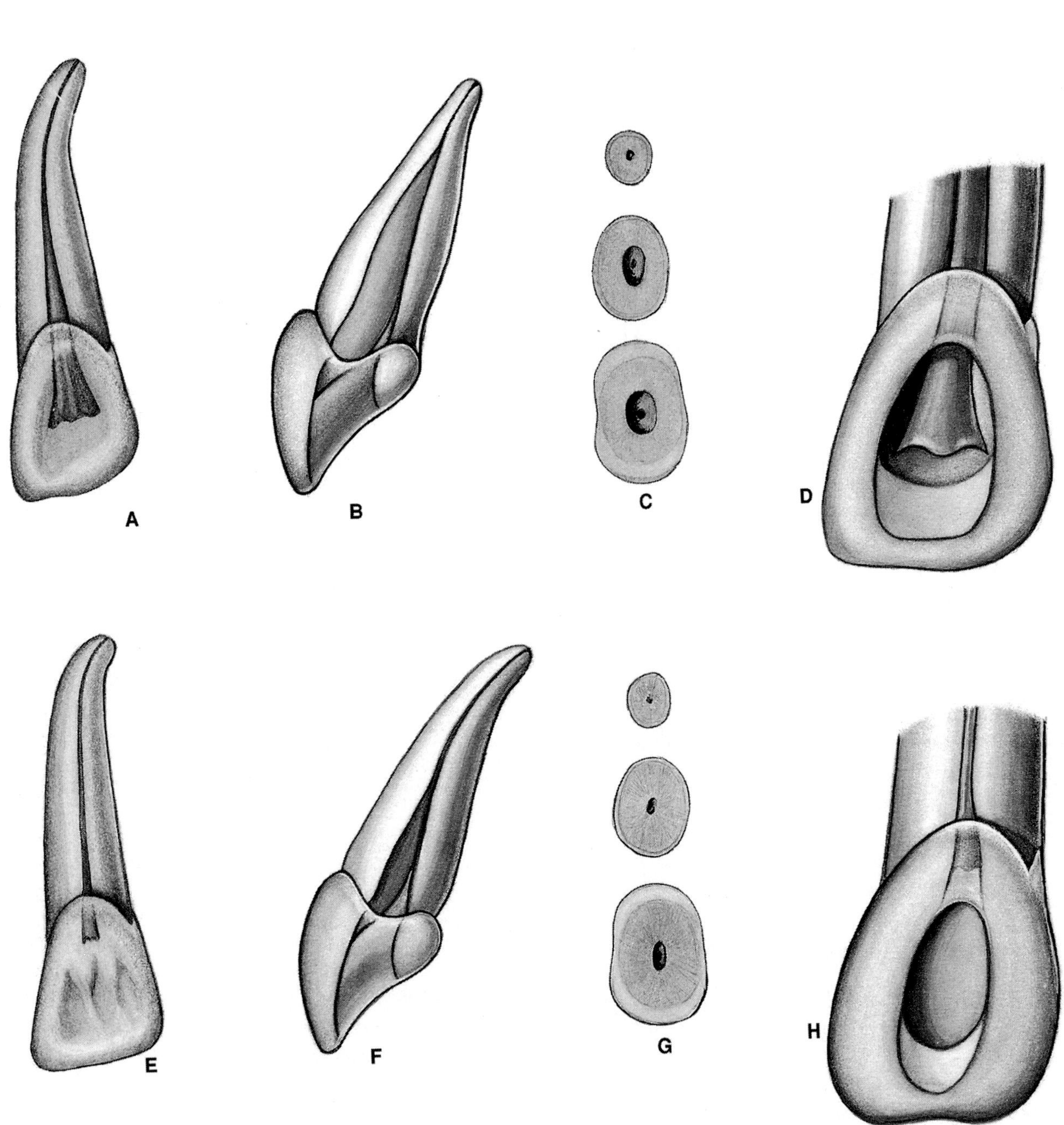

PLATE 6

Maxillary Canine

Pulp Anatomy and Coronal Preparation

A. **Lingual** view of a recently calcified canine with a large pulp. A radiograph will reveal
   1. coronal extent of the pulp
   2. **narrow** mesiodistal width of the pulp
   3. apical-distal curvature (32% of the time)
   4. 6-degree distal-axial inclination of the tooth

   These factors, **seen** in the radiograph, are borne in mind when preparation is begun, particularly the severe apical curve.

B. **Distal** view of the same tooth demonstrating details **not apparent in the radiograph:**
   1. huge ovoid pulp, larger labiolingually than the radiograph would indicate
   2. presence of a **labial** "shoulder" just below the cervical
   3. narrow canal in the apical third of the root
   4. 21-degree lingual-axial angulation of the tooth

   These "unseen" factors will affect the **size, shape,** and **inclination** of the final preparation.

C. Cross-section is at three levels: 1, cervical; 2, midroot; and 3, apical third:
   1. **Cervical** level: the pulp is enormous in a young tooth, much wider in the **labiolingual** direction. Débridement in this area is accomplished with a long, tapered diamond point and extensive perimeter filing.
   2. **Midroot** level: the canal continues ovoid in shape and requires perimeter filing and multiple point filling.
   3. **Apical third** level: the straight canal (39% of time), generally round in shape, is prepared by shaping the cavity into **round tapered** preparation. Preparation should terminate at the cementodentinal junction, 0.5 to 1.0 mm from the radiographic apex. If unusually large or curved, the apical canal requires perimeter filing and multiple point or warm gutta-percha filling.

D. Extensive, **ovoid,** funnel-shaped **coronal preparation** is necessary to adequately débride the chamber of all pulpal remnants. (The pulp is "ghosted" in the background.) Note the long, beveled extension toward the incisal, which will carry the preparation labially and thus nearer the central axis. Incisal extension allows better access for large instruments and filling materials used in the apical third of the canal.

E. **Lingual** view of an **adult** canine with extensive secondary dentin formation. A radiograph will reveal
   1. full pulp recession
   2. straight canal (39% of the time)
   3. 6-degree distal-axial inclination of tooth

F. **Distal** view of the same tooth demonstrating details **not apparent in the radiograph:**
   1. narrow labiolingual width of the pulp
   2. apical **labial** curvature (13% of the time)
   3. 21-degree lingual-axial angulation of the tooth

   The operator should recognize that
   a. a small canal orifice is difficult to find.
   b. apical **labial** curvature, not seen radiographically, can be determined only by exploration with a fine curved file and mesially oriented radiographs.
   c. distal-lingual axial inclination of the root calls for careful orientation and alignment of the bur to prevent "gouging."
   d. **apical foramen** toward the labial is a problem.

G. Cross-sections at three levels: 1, cervical; 2, midroot; and 3, apical third:
   1. **Cervical** level: the canal is slightly ovoid.
   2. **Midroot** level: the canal is smaller but remains ovoid.
   3. **Apical third** level: the canal becomes progressively rounder.

H. Extensive, ovoid, funnel-shaped preparation must be **nearly as large** as for a young tooth. A beveled incisal extension carries preparation nearer the central axis, allowing better access to the curved apical third. Discovery by exploration of an **apical-labial** curve calls for even greater incisal extension.

PLATE 6

Maxillary Canines

Length of tooth		*Canal*	*Lateral canals*	*Apical ramifications*	*Root curvature*	
Average Length	26.0 mm	One canal 100%	24%	8%	Straight	39%
Maximum Length	28.9 mm				Distal Curve	32%
Minimum Length	23.1 mm				Mesial Curve	0%
Range	5.8 mm				*Labial Curve	13%
					*Lingual Curve	7%
					Bayonet and Gradual Curve	7%

*Not apparent in radiograph

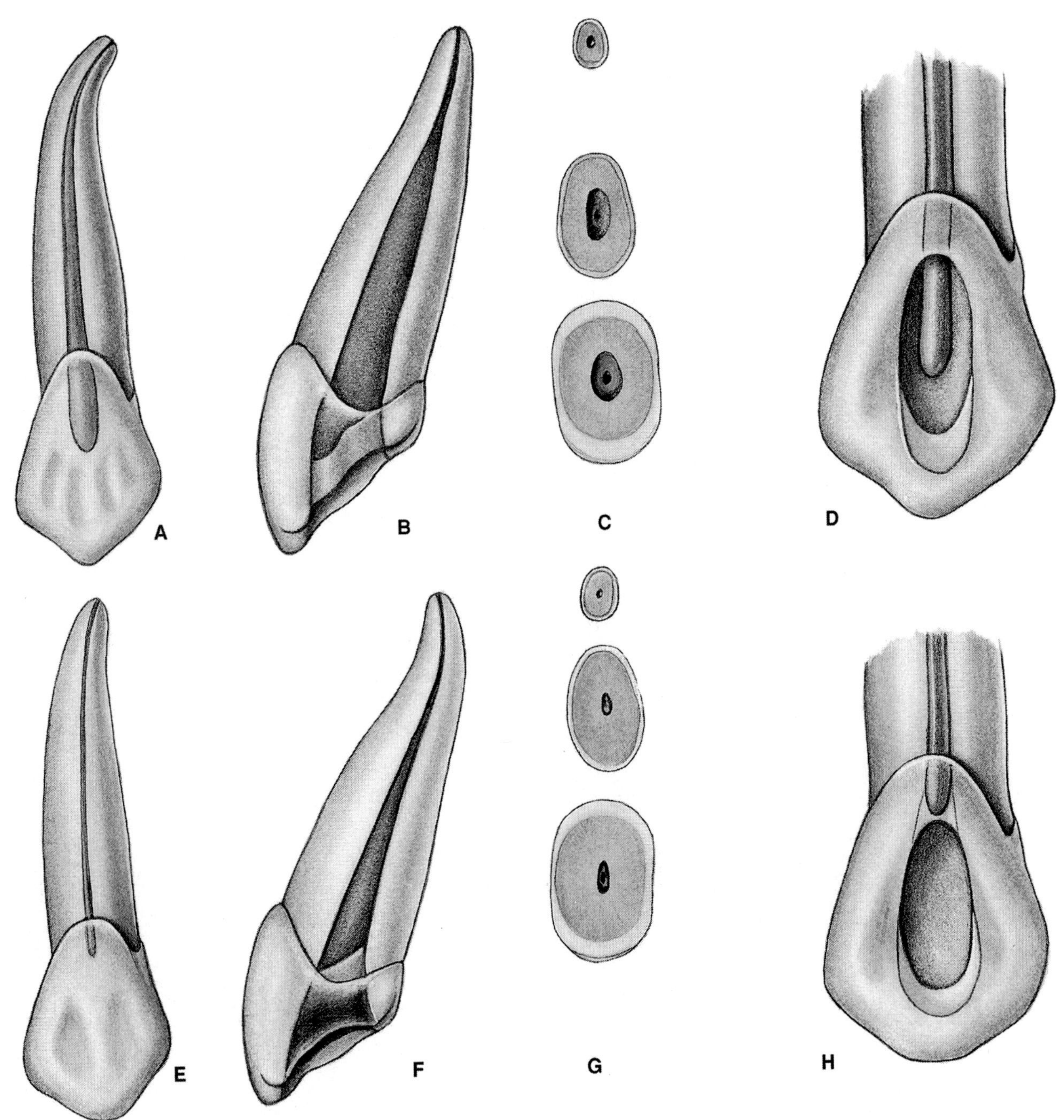

PLATE 7

Maxillary Anterior Teeth

ERRORS in Cavity Preparation

A. PERFORATION at the labiocervical caused by **failure to complete convenience extension** toward the incisal, prior to the entrance of the shaft of the bur.

B. GOUGING of the labial wall caused by **failure to recognize** the 29-degree lingual-axial angulation of the tooth.

C. GOUGING of the distal wall caused by **failure to recognize** the 16-degree mesial-axial inclination of the tooth.

D. PEAR-SHAPED PREPARATION of the apical canal caused by **failure to complete convenience extensions.** The shaft of the instrument rides on the cavity margin and lingual "shoulder." Inadequate débridement and obturation ensure failure.

E. DISCOLORATION of the crown caused by failure to remove pulp debris. The access cavity is too far to the gingival with no incisal extension.

F. LEDGE formation at the apical-distal curve caused by using an uncurved instrument too large for the canal. The cavity is adequate.

G. PERFORATION at the apical-distal curve caused by using too large an instrument through an **inadequate** preparation placed too far gingivally.

H. LEDGE formation at the apical-labial curve caused by **failure to complete the convenience extension.** The shaft of the instrument rides on the cavity margin and "shoulder."

PLATE 7

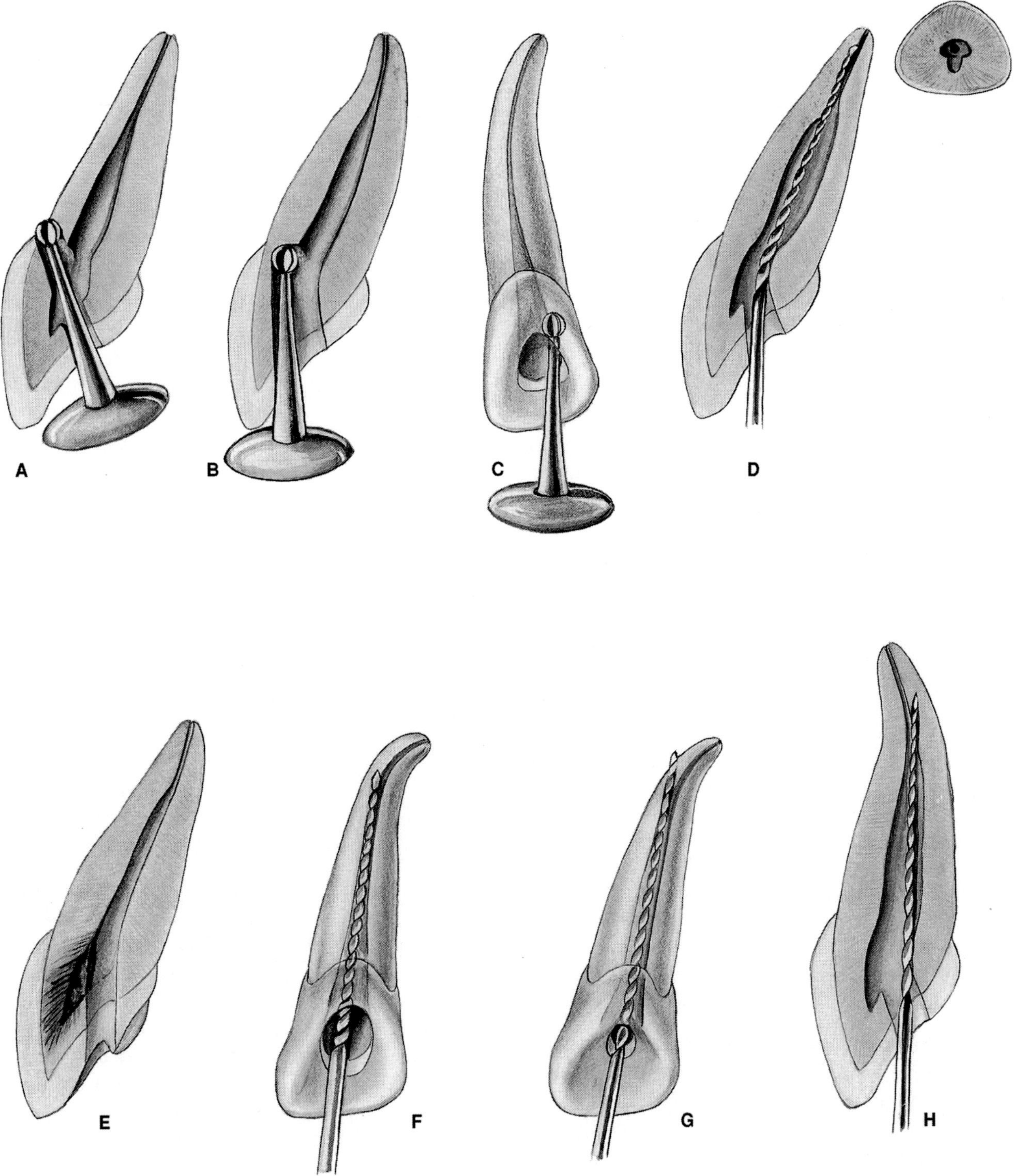

PLATE 8

Endodontic Preparation of Mandibular Anterior Teeth

A. Entrance is always gained through the lingual surface of all anterior teeth. Initial penetration is made in the exact center of the lingual surface at the position marked "X." A common error is to begin too far gingivally.

B. The initial entrance cavity is prepared with a 701 U tapering fissure bur in an **accelerated-speed** contra-angle handpiece with air coolant, operated at a **right angle** to the long axis of the tooth. **Only enamel is penetrated at this time.** Do not force the bur; allow it to cut its own way.

C. **Convenience extension** toward the incisal continues initial penetrating cavity. Maintain the point of the bur in the central cavity and rotate the handpiece toward the incisal so that the bur **parallels** the long axis of the tooth. Enamel and dentin are beveled toward the incisal. **Entrance into the pulp chamber should not be made with an accelerated-speed instrument.** Lack of tactile sensation with these instruments **precludes their use inside** the tooth.

D. The preliminary cavity outline is funneled and fanned incisally with a fissure bur. The enamel has a short bevel toward the incisal, and a "nest" is prepared in the dentin to receive the round bur to be used for penetration.

E. A **surgical-length** No. 2 round bur in a **slow-speed** contra-angle handpiece is used to penetrate into the pulp chamber. If the pulp has greatly receded, the No. 2 round bur is used for initial penetration. Take advantage of **convenience extension** toward the incisal to allow for the shaft of the penetrating bur, operated nearly parallel to the long axis of the tooth.

F. **Working from inside the chamber to the outside,** a round bur is used to remove the lingual and labial walls of the pulp chamber. The resulting cavity is smooth, continuous, and flowing from cavity margin to canal orifice.

G. After the outline form is completed, a surgical-length bur is carefully passed down into the canal. **Working from inside to outside,** the lingual "shoulder" is removed with a long, fine, tapered diamond point to give a continuous, smooth-flowing preparation.

H. Occasionally, a No. 1 round bur must be used laterally and incisally in the cavity to eliminate pulpal horn debris and bacteria. This also prevents future discoloration.

I. Final preparation related to the **internal anatomy** of the chamber and canal. In a "young" tooth with a large pulp, the outline form reflects triangular internal anatomy—an extensive cavity that allows thorough cleansing of the chamber as well as passage of large instruments and filling materials needed to prepare and fill the large canal. Note extension toward the incisal to allow better access to the central axis.

J. Cavity preparations in an "adult" tooth with the chamber obliterated with secondary dentin are ovoid. Preparation **funnels** down to the orifice of the canal. The further the pulp has receded, the more difficult it is to reach to this depth with a round bur. Therefore, when a radiograph reveals advanced pulpal recession, **convenience extension** must be advanced further incisally to allow the bur shaft to operate in the central axis. The incisal edge may even be invaded and later restored by composites.

K. Final preparation showing the reamer in place. The instrument shaft **clears** the incisal **cavity margin** and reduced lingual shoulder, allowing an unrestrained approach to the apical third of the canal. The instruments remain under the complete control of the clinician. **Great care must be taken to explore for additional canals, particularly to the lingual of the pulp chamber.** An optimal **round, tapered cavity** may be prepared in the apical third, tailored to requirements of round, tapered filling materials to follow. The remaining ovoid part of the canal is cleaned and shaped by extensive filing.

PLATE 8

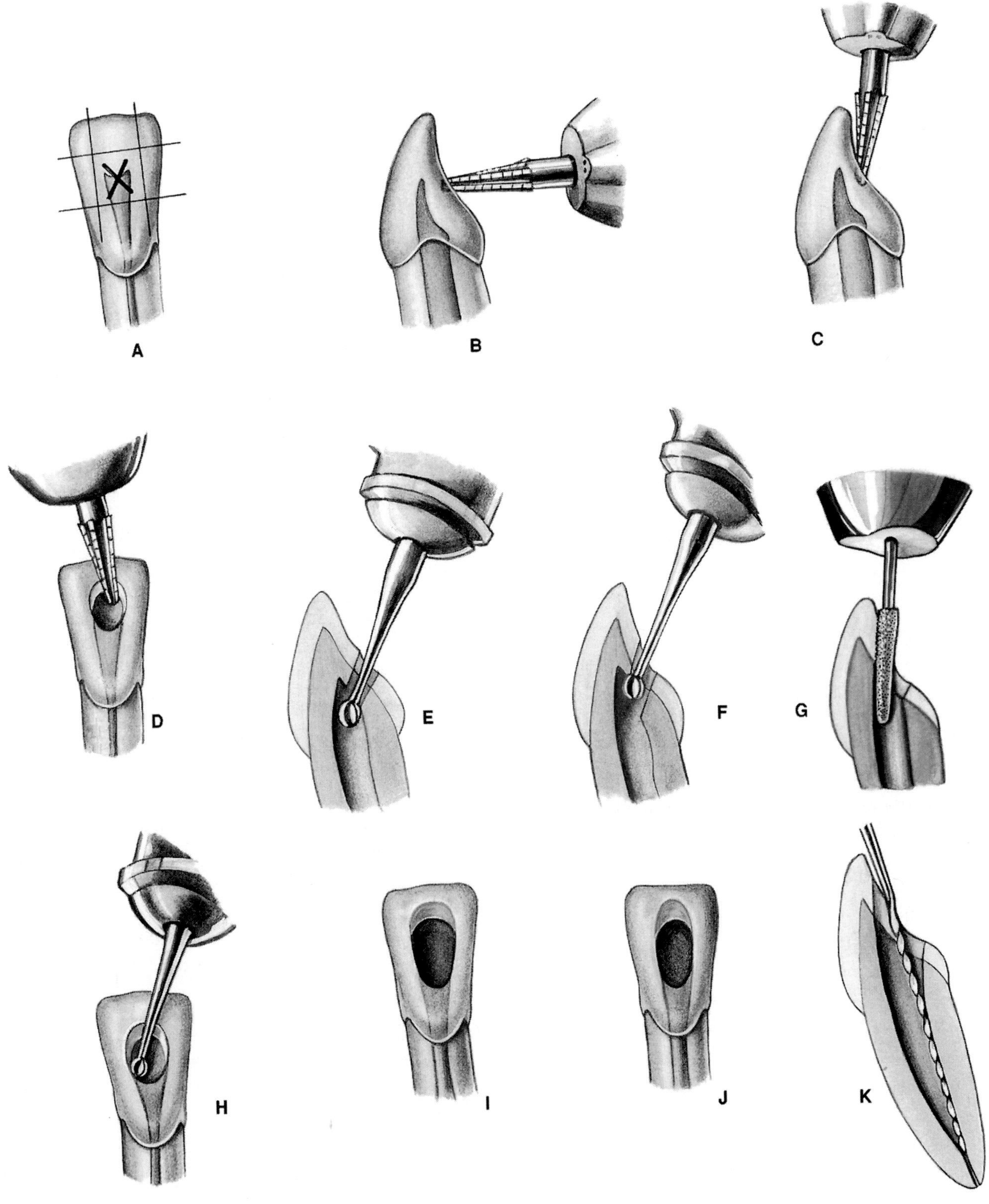

PLATE 9

Mandibular Central and Lateral Incisors

Pulp Anatomy and Coronal Preparation

A. **Lingual** view of a recently calcified incisor with a large pulp. A radiograph will reveal
   1. extent of the pulp horns
   2. mesiodistal width of the pulp
   3. slight apical-distal curvature of the canal (23% of the time)
   4. mesial-axial inclination of the tooth (central incisor 2 degrees, lateral incisor 17 degrees).

   These factors, seen in the radiograph, are borne in mind when preparation is begun.

B. **Distal** view of the same tooth demonstrating details **not apparent in the radiograph:**
   1. presence of a lingual "shoulder" at the point where the chamber and canal join
   2. broad labiolingual extent of the pulp
   3. 20-degree lingual-axial angulation of the tooth

   The operator must recognize that
   a. the lingual "shoulder" must be removed with a fine, tapered diamond point to allow better access to the canal.
   b. these "unseen" factors affect the **size, shape,** and **inclination** of the final preparation.

C. Cross-sections at three levels: 1, cervical; 2, midroot; 3, apical third:
   1. **Cervical** level: the pulp is enormous in a young tooth, wider in the labiolingual dimension. Débridement in this area is accomplished by **extensive perimeter** filing.
   2. **Midroot** level: the canal continues ovoid and requires perimeter filing and multiple point filling.
   3. **Apical third** level: the canal, generally round in shape, is enlarged by shaping the cavity into a **round, tapered** preparation. Preparation terminates at the cementodentinal junction, 0.5 to 1.0 mm from the radiographic apex.

D. Large, triangular, funnel-shaped coronal preparation is necessary to adequately débride the chamber of all pulp remnants. (The pulp is "ghosted" in the background.) Note the beveled extension toward the incisal, which will carry the preparation labially and thus nearer the central axis. Incisal extension allows better access for instruments and filling materials used in the apical third of the canal.

E. **Lingual** view of an **adult** incisor with extensive secondary dentin formation.
   A radiograph will reveal:
   1. full pulp recession
   2. an apparently straight canal
   3. mesial-axial inclination of the tooth (central incisor 2 degrees, lateral incisor 17 degrees).

F. **Distal** view of the same tooth demonstrating details **not apparent in the radiograph:**
   1. labiolingual width of the pulp
   2. reduced size of the lingual shoulder
   3. **unsuspected presence of bifurcation of pulp into the labial and lingual canals nearly 30% of the time**
   4. 20-degree lingual-axial angulation of the tooth

   The operator must recognize that
   a. smaller canal orifices are more difficult to find.
   b. **labial and lingual** canals are discovered by exploration with a fine curved file to **both labial** and **lingual.**
   c. axial inclination of the root calls for careful orientation and alignment of the bur to prevent "gouging."

G. Cross-sections at three levels: 1, cervical; 2, midroot; and 3, apical third:
   1. **Cervical** level: the canal is only slightly ovoid.
   2. **Midroot** level: the two canals are essentially round.
   3. **Apical third** level: the canals are round and curve toward the labial.

   It is important that all mandibular anterior teeth be explored to both labial and lingual for the possibility of two canals.

H. Ovoid, funnel-shaped coronal preparation provides adequate access to the root canal. An "adult" cavity is narrow in the mesiodistal width but is as extensive in the incisogingival direction as preparation in a young tooth. This beveled incisal extension carries preparation nearer to the central axis. The incisal edge may even be invaded. This will allow better access to **both canals** and the **curved apical third. Ideal lingual extension and better access will often lead to discovery of the second canal.**

PLATE 9

Mandibular Central and Lateral Incisors

Length of tooth	*Central Incisors*	*Lateral Incisors*	*Canals*	*Central Incisors*	*Lateral Incisors*	*Root curvature*	
Average Length	21.5 mm	22.4 mm	One canal One foramen	70.1%	56.9%	Straight	60%
Maximum Length	23.4 mm	24.6 mm	Two canals One foramen	23.4%	14.7%	Distal Curve	23%
Minimum Length	19.6 mm	20.2 mm	Two canals Two foramens	6.5%	29.4%	Mesial Curve	0%
Range	3.8 mm	4.4 mm	Lateral canals	5.2%	13.9%	*Labial Curve	13%
						*Lingual Curve	0%

*Not apparent in radiograph

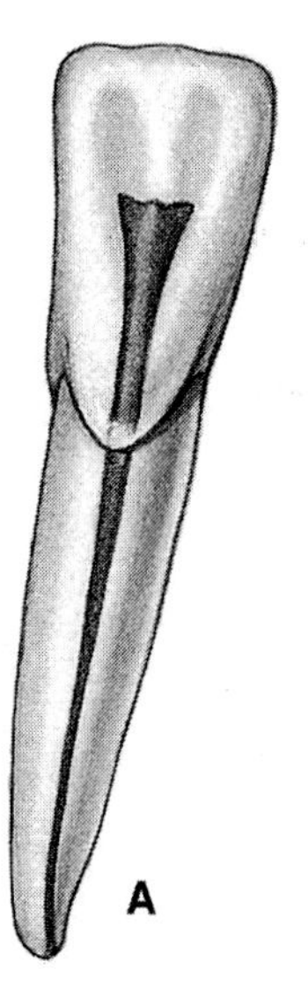

A

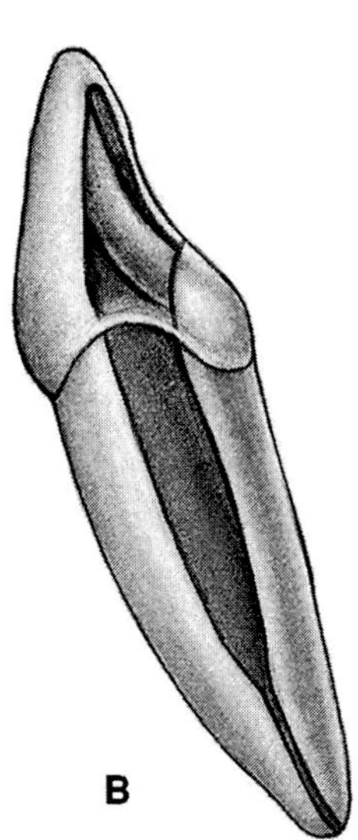

B

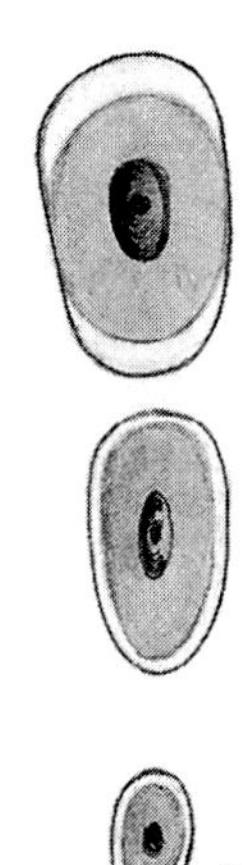

C

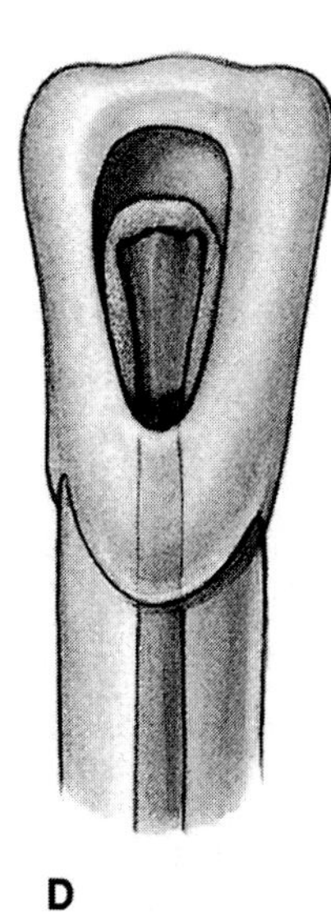

D

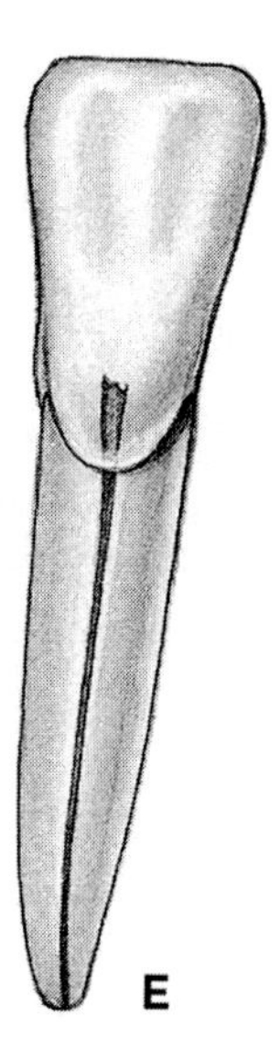

E

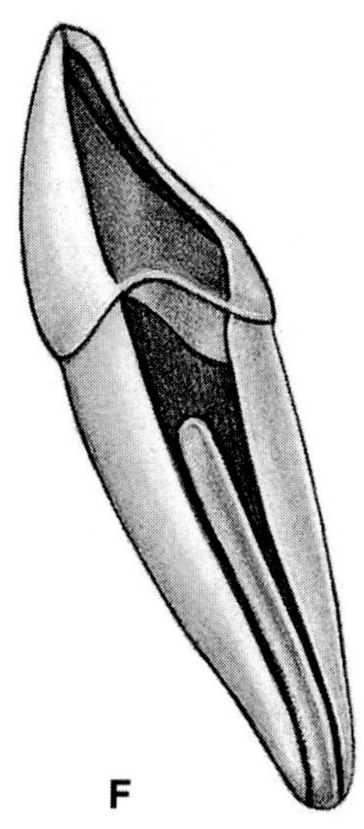

F

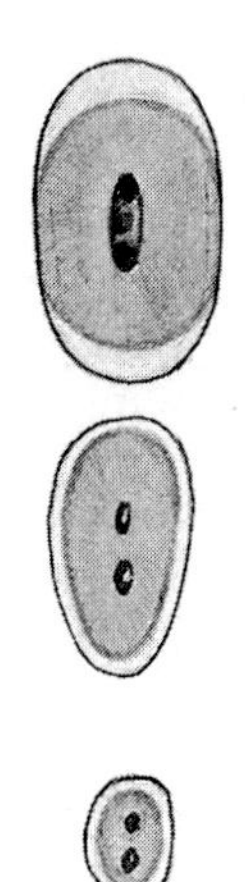

G

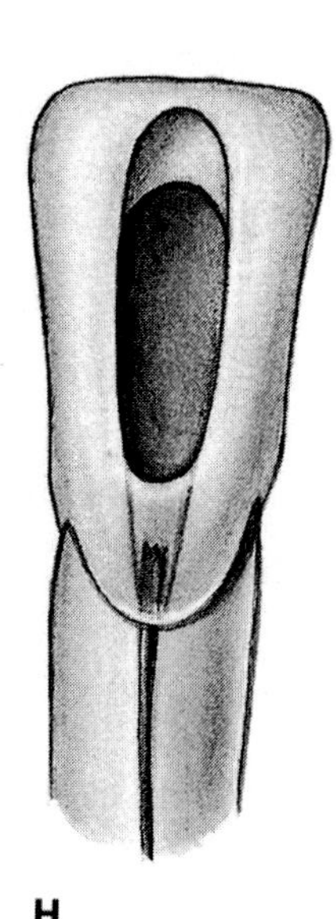

H

PLATE 10

Mandibular Canine

Pulp Anatomy and Coronal Preparation

A. **Lingual** view of a recently calcified canine with a large pulp. A radiograph will reveal
   1. coronal extent of the pulp
   2. narrow mesiodistal width of the pulp
   3. apical-distal curvature (20% of the time)
   4. 13-degree mesial-axial inclination of tooth

   These factors, **seen** in the radiograph, are borne in mind when preparation is begun.

B. **Distal** view of the same tooth demonstrating details **not apparent in the radiograph:**
   1. broad labiolingual extent of the pulp
   2. narrow canal in the apical third of the root
   3. apical-labial curvature (7% of time)
   4. 15-degree lingual-axial angulation of the tooth

   These "unseen factors" affect the **size, shape,** and **inclination** of the final preparation.

C. Cross-sections at three levels: 1, cervical; 2, midroot; and 3, apical third:
   1. **Cervical** level: the pulp is enormous in a young tooth, wider in the labiolingual direction. Débridement in this area is accomplished with **extensive perimeter filing.**
   2. Midroot level: the canal continues ovoid and requires perimeter filing and multiple gutta-percha point filling.
   3. **Apical third** level: the canal, generally round, is enlarged by filing to reduce the curve to a relatively straight canal. This canal is then completed by shaping action into **round, tapered** preparation. Preparation terminates at the cementodentinal junction, 0.5 to 1.0 mm from the radiograph apex. If unusually large or ovoid, the **apical** canal requires perimeter filing.

D. Extensive ovoid, funnel-shaped **coronal preparation** is necessary to adequately débride the chamber of all pulp remnants. (The pulp is "ghosted" in the background.) Note the beveled extension toward the incisal, which will carry the preparation labially and thus nearer the central axis. Incisal extension allows better access for large instruments and filling materials used in the apical third canal.

E. **Lingual** view of an **adult** canine with extensive secondary dentin formation. A radiograph will reveal
   1. full pulp recession
   2. slight distal curve of the canal (20% of the time)
   3. 13-degree mesial-axial inclination of the tooth

F. Distal view of the same tooth demonstrating details **not apparent in the radiograph:**
   1. labiolingual width of the pulp
   2. 15-degree lingual-axial angulation of the tooth

   The operator must recognize that
   a. a small canal orifice, positioned well to the **labial,** is difficult to find.
   b. lingual-axial angulation calls for careful orientation of the bur to prevent "gouging."
   c. apical-labial curvature (7% of the time).

G. Cross-sections at three levels: 1, cervical; 2, midroot; and 3, apical third:
   1. **Cervical** level: the canal is slightly ovoid.
   2. **Mid-root** level: the canal is smaller but remains ovoid.
   3. **Apical third** level: the canal becomes progressively rounder.

   The canal is enlarged by filing and is filled.

H. Extensive ovoid, funnel-shaped preparations must be as large as preparation for a young tooth. The cavity should be extended incisogingivally for room to find the orifice and enlarge the apical third without interference. An apical-labial curve would call for increased extension incisally.

PLATE 10

Mandibular Canines

Length of tooth		*Canals*		*Lateral canals*	*Root curvature*	
Average Length	25.2 mm	One canal	94%	9.5%	Straight	68%
Maximum Length	27.5 mm	Two canals			Distal Curve	20%
Minimum Length	22.9 mm	Two foramina	6%		Mesial Curve	1%
Range	4.6 mm				*Labial Curve	7%
					*Lingual Curve	0%
					Bayonet Curve	2%

*Not apparent in radiograph

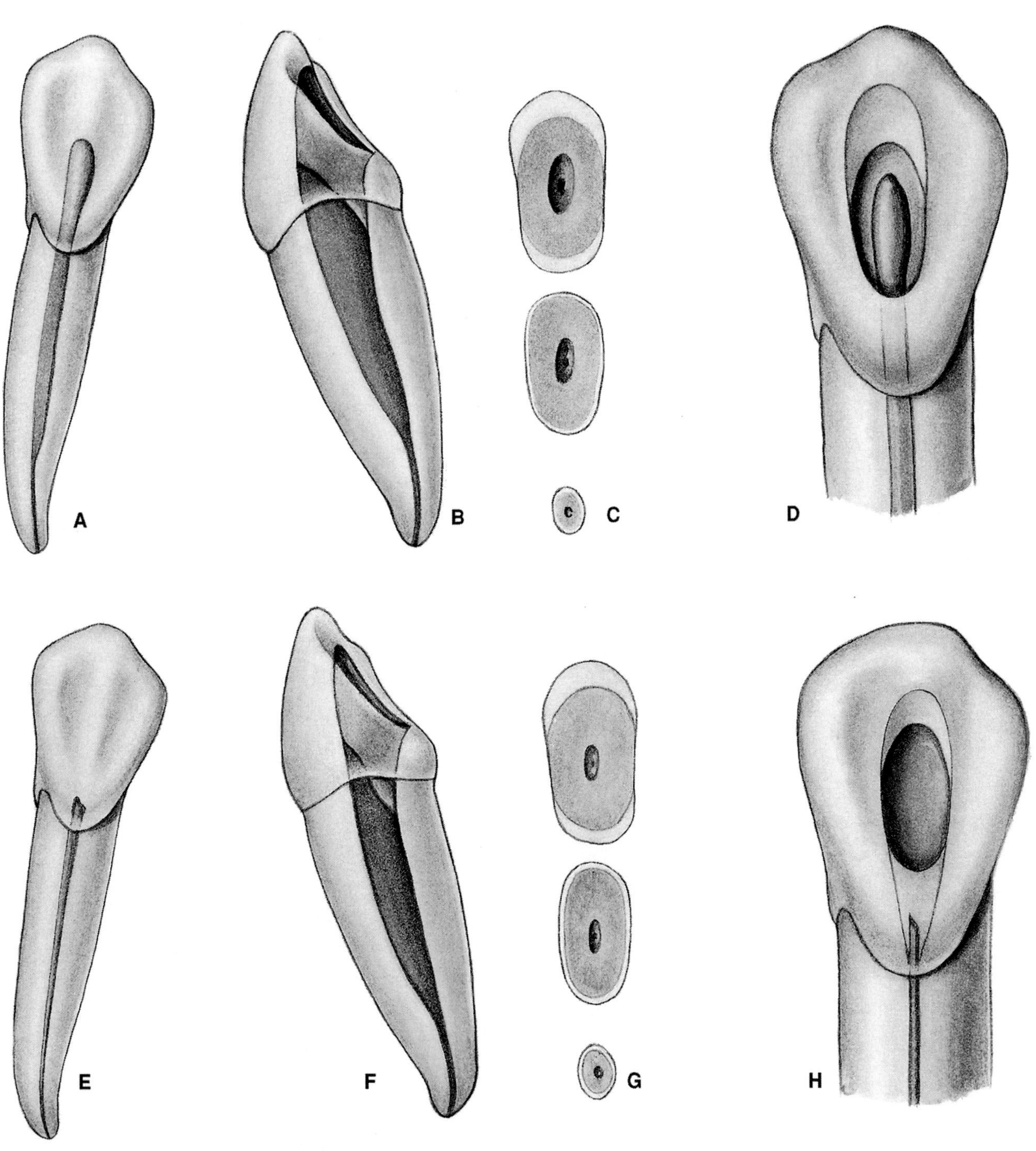

PLATE 11

Mandibular Anterior Teeth

ERRORS in Cavity Preparation

A. GOUGING at the labiocervical caused by **failure to complete convenience extension** toward the incisal prior to entrance of the shaft of the bur.

B. GOUGING of the labial wall caused by failure to recognize the 20-degree lingual-axial angulation of the tooth.

C. GOUGING of the distal wall caused by **failure** to **recognize** the 17-degree mesial-axial angulation of the tooth.

D. FAILURE to explore, débride, or fill the second canal caused by **inadequate incisogingival extension of the access cavity.**

E. DISCOLORATION of the crown caused by failure to remove pulp debris. The access cavity is too far to the gingival with no incisal extension.

F. LEDGE formation caused by complete loss of control of the instrument passing through the access cavity prepared in proximal restoration.

PLATE 11

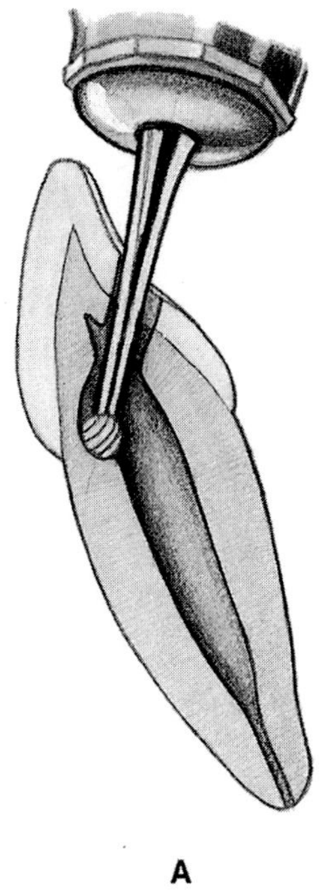

A

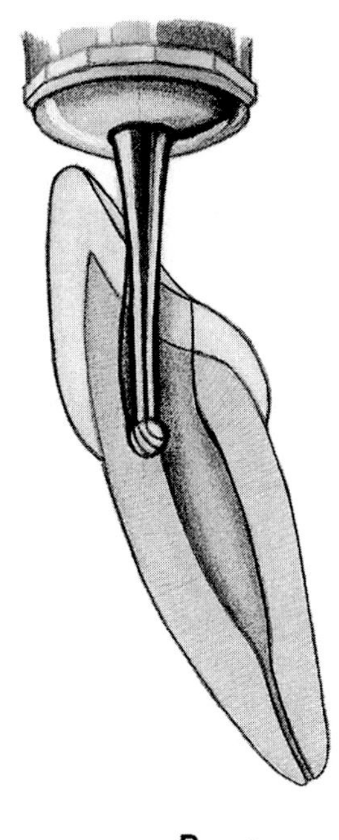

B

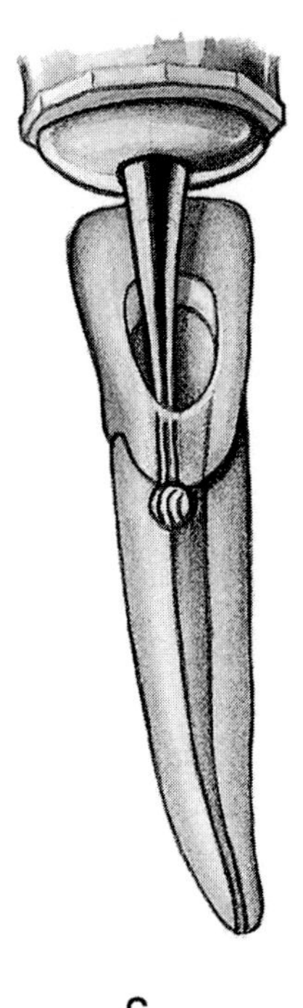

C

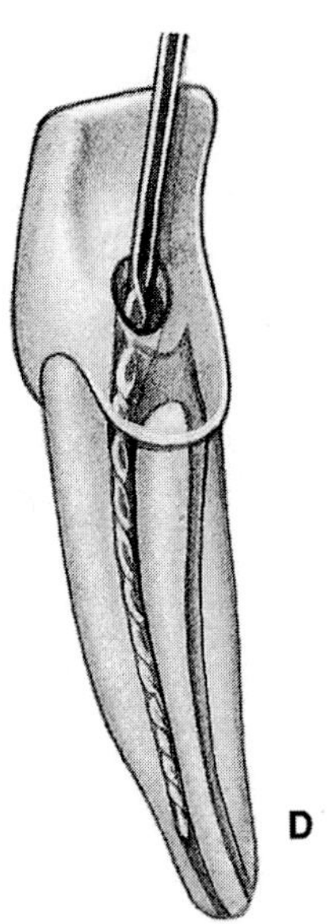

D

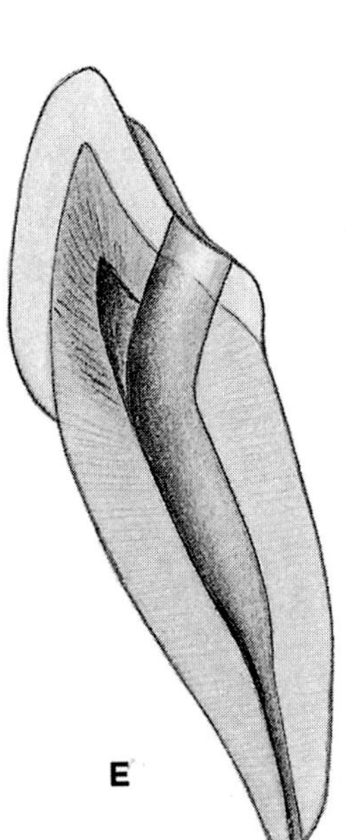

E

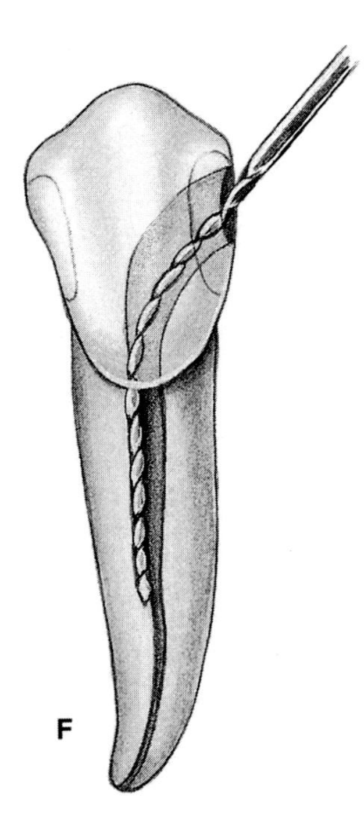

F

PLATE 12

Endodontic Preparation of Maxillary Premolar Teeth

A. Entrance is **always** gained through the **occlusal** surface of all posterior teeth. Initial penetration is made parallel to the long axis of the tooth in the exact center of the central groove of the maxillary premolars. The 701 U tapering fissure bur in an accelerated-speed contra-angle handpiece is ideal for penetrating gold casting or virgin enamel surface to the depth of the dentin. Amalgam fillings are opened with a No. 4 round bur in a slow-speed contra-angle handpiece.

B. A **regular-length** No. 2 or 4 round bur is used to open into the pulp chamber. The bur will be felt to "drop" when the pulp chamber is reached. If the chamber is well calcified and the "drop" is not felt, vertical penetration is made until the contra-angle handpiece rests against the occlusal surface. This depth is approximately 9 mm, the position of the floor of the pulp chamber that lies at the cervical level. In removing the bur, **the orifice is widened buccolingually** to twice the width of the bur to allow room for exploration for canal orifices. If a surgical-length bur is used, care must be exercised not to perforate the furca.

C. An endodontic explorer is used to locate orifices to the **buccal** and **lingual** canals in the **first premolar** or the **central canal** in the **second premolar.** Tension of the explorer shaft against the walls of preparation will indicate the amount and direction of extension necessary.

D. Working from inside the pulp chamber to outside, a round bur is used at low speed to extend the cavity buccolingually by removing the roof of the pulp chamber.

E. Buccolingual extension and finish of cavity walls are completed with a 701 U fissure bur at accelerated speed.

F. Final preparation should provide unobstructed access to canal orifices. Cavity walls should not impede complete authority over enlarging instruments.

G. **Outline form** of final preparation will be **identical for** both **newly erupted** and **"adult" teeth.** Buccolingual ovoid preparation reflects the anatomy of the pulp chamber and the position of the buccal and lingual canal orifices. The cavity must be extensive enough to allow for instruments and filling materials needed to enlarge and fill canals. **Further exploration** at this time is imperative. It may reveal the orifice to an additional canal, a **second canal** in the second premolar, or a **third canal** in the first premolar.

PLATE 12

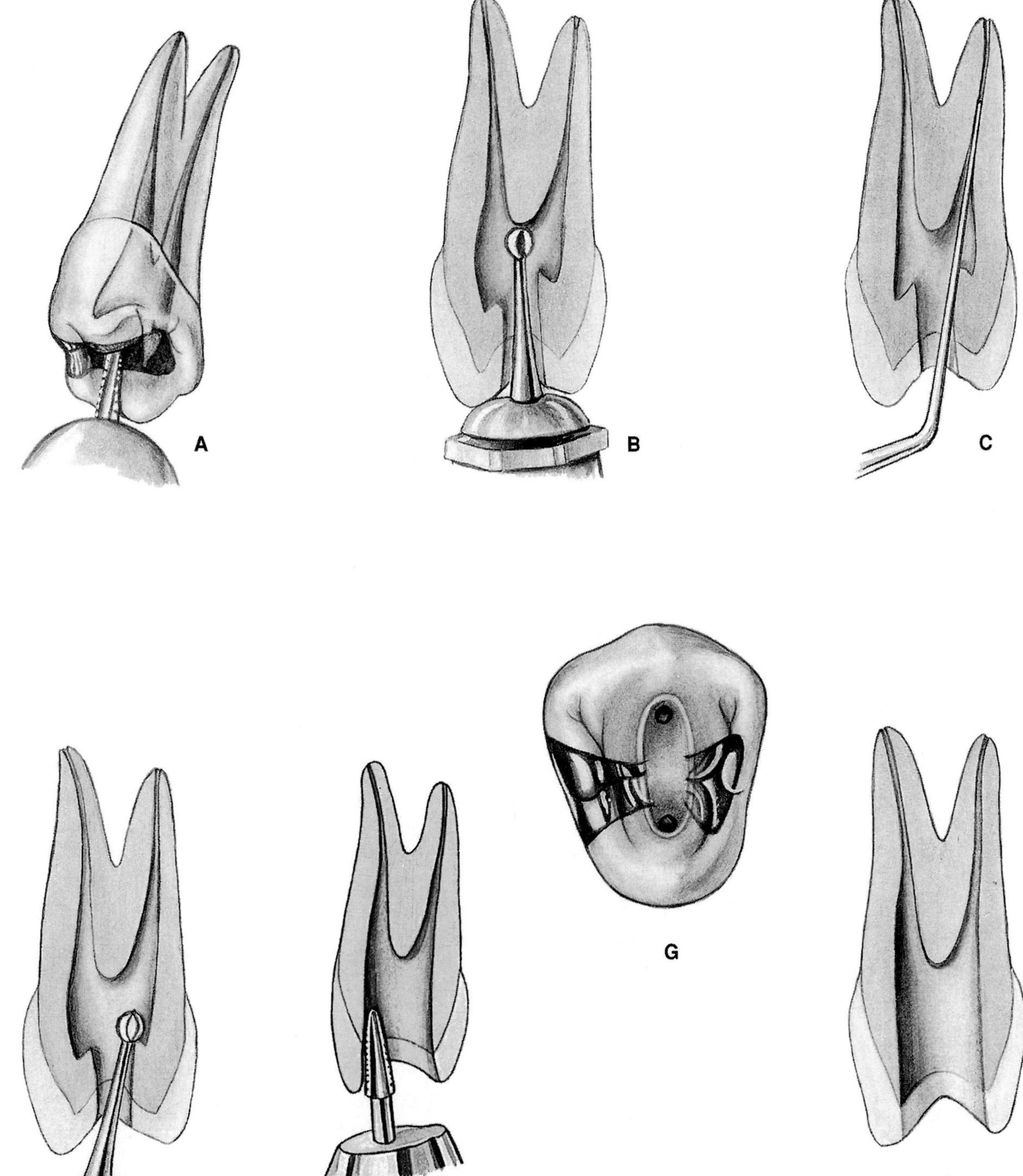

PLATE 13

Maxillary First Premolar

Pulp Anatomy and Coronal Preparation

A. **Buccal** view of a recently calcified first premolar with a large pulp.
   A radiograph, if exposed slightly from the mesial, will reveal
   1. mesiodistal width of the pulp
   2. presence of two pulp canals
   3. apparently straight canals
   4. 10-degree distal-axial inclination of the tooth

   These factors, **seen** in the radiograph, are borne in mind when preparation is begun. One should always expect two and occasionally three canals.

B. **Mesial** view of the same tooth demonstrating details **not apparent in the radiograph:**
   1. height of the pulp horns
   2. broad buccolingual dimension of the pulp
   3. two widespread and separate roots, each with a single straight canal
   4. 6-degree buccal-axial angulation of the tooth

   These "unseen" factors will affect the size and shape of the final preparation. Pulp horns in the roof of the pulp **chamber** are not to be confused with true canal orifices in the cavity floor. Verticality of the tooth simplifies orientation and bur alignment.

C. Cross-sections at three levels: 1, cervical; 2, midroot; and 3, apical third:
   1. **Cervical** level: the pulp is enormous in a young tooth, very wide in the buccolingual direction. Débridement of the chamber is completed in coronal cavity preparation with a round bur. Canal orifices are found well to the buccal and lingual.
   2. **Midroot** level: the canals are only lightly ovoid and may be enlarged to a round, tapered cavity.
   3. **Apical third** level: the canals are round and are shaped into **round, tapered** preparations. Preparations terminate at the cementodentinal junction, 0.5 to 1.0 mm from the radiographic apex.

D. **Ovoid** coronal preparation need not be as long buccolingually as the pulp chamber. However, the **outline form** must be large enough to provide two filling points at same time. Buccal and lingual walls smoothly flow to orifices.

E. **Buccal** view of an **adult** first premolar with extensive secondary dentin formation. A radiograph will reveal
   1. full pulp recession and thread-like appearance of the pulp
   2. **radiographic appearance** of only one canal
   3. 10-degree distal-axial inclination of the tooth

   Owing to misalignment of the bur, **perforation of the mesiocervical, at the point of mesial indentation, may occur.**

F. **Mesial** view of the same tooth demonstrating details **not apparent in the radiograph:**
   1. pulp recession and a greatly flattened pulp chamber
   2. buccolingual width revealing the pulp to be "ribbon shaped" rather than "thread-like"
   3. single root with **parallel canals and a single apical foramen**
   4. 6-degree buccal-axial angulation of the tooth

   The operator must recognize that
   a. small canal orifices are found well to the buccal and lingual and are difficult to locate.
   b. the direction of each canal is determined only by exploration with a fine curved instrument.
   c. a single apical foramen cannot be determined; therefore, two canals must be managed as two separate canals.
   d. virtually **always** there will be two and occasionally three canals.

G. Cross-sections at three levels: 1, cervical; 2, midroot; and 3, apical third:
   1. **Cervical** level: the chamber is very narrow ovoid, and canal orifices are at the buccal and lingual termination of the floor.
   2. **Midroot** level: the canals are round.
   3. **Apical third** level: the canals are round.

H. Ovoid coronal preparation must be more extensive in the buccolingual direction because of parallel canals. More extensive preparation allows instrumentation without interference.

Maxillary First Premolars

Length of tooth	
Average Length	21.8 mm
Maximum Length	23.8 mm
Minimum Length	18.8 mm
Range	5 mm

Canals	
One canal One foramen	9%
Two canals One foramen	13%
Two canals Two foramina	72%
Three canals Three foramina	6%

	Curvature of Roots		
		Double Roots	
Direction	*Single Root*	*Buccal*	*Palatal*
Straight	38%	28%	45%
Distal Curve	37%	14%	14%
Mesial Curve	0%	0%	0%
*Buccal Curve	15%	14%	28%
*Lingual Curve	3%	36%	9%
Bayonet Curve	0%	8%	0%

*Not apparent in radiograph

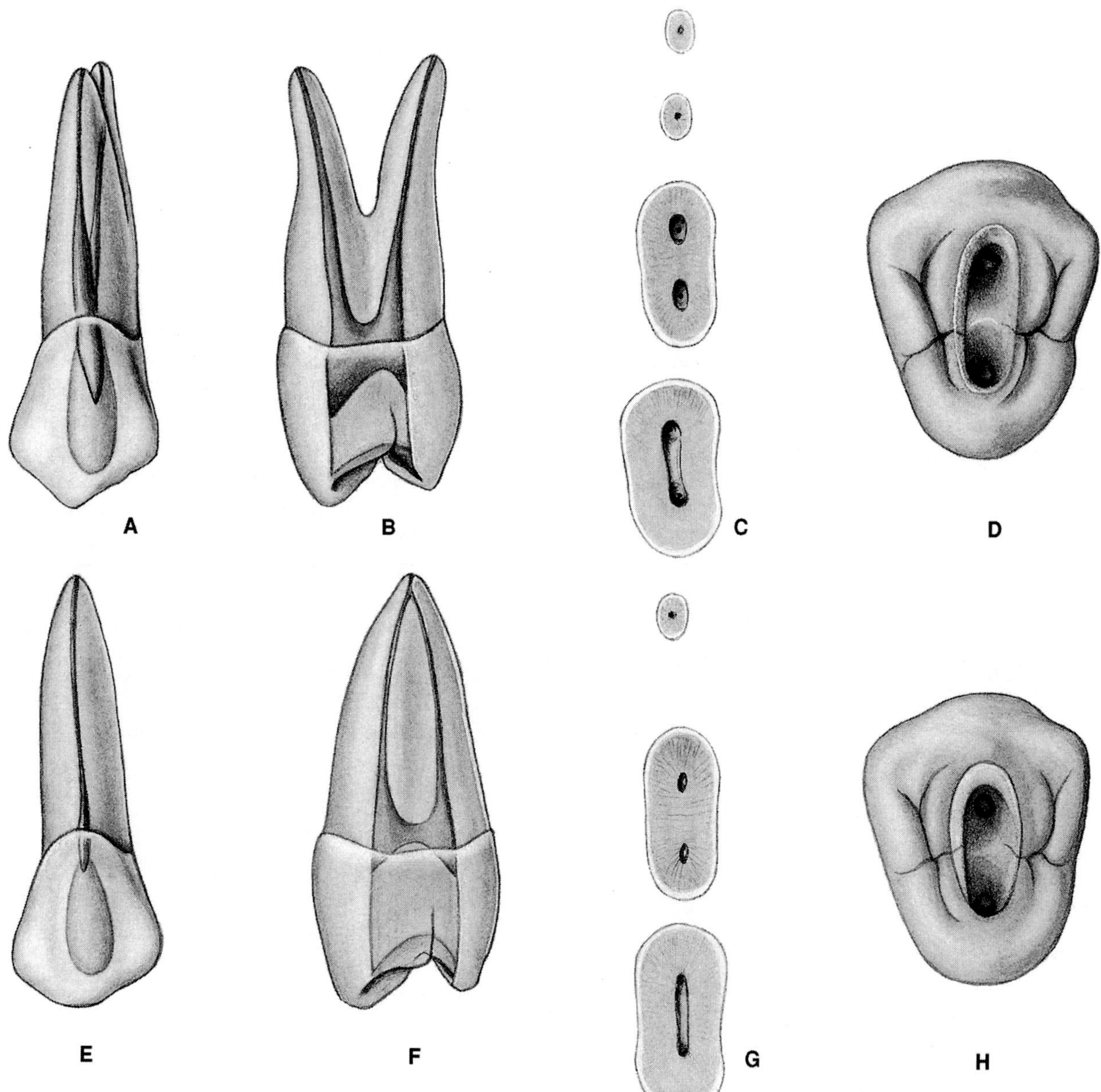

PLATE 14

Maxillary Second Premolar

Pulp Anatomy and Coronal Preparation

A. **Buccal** view of a recently calcified second premolar with a large pulp. A radiograph will reveal
   1. narrow mesiodistal width of the pulp
   2. apical-distal curvature (34% of the time)
   3. 19-degree distal-axial inclination of the tooth

   These factors, **seen** in the radiograph, are borne in mind when preparation is begun.

B. **Mesial** view of the same tooth demonstrating details **not apparent** in the radiograph:
   1. broad buccolingual width revealing the pulp to be "ribbon shaped"
   2. single root with a large single canal
   3. 9-degree lingual-axial angulation of the tooth

   The pulp is shown to be a broad "ribbon" rather than a "thread" as it appears from radiograph. These "unseen" factors affect the **size, shape,** and **inclination** of the final preparation.

C. Cross-sections at three levels: 1, cervical; 2, midroot; and 3, apical third:
   1. **Cervical** level: the pulp is enormous in a young tooth, very wide in the buccolingual direction. Débridement of the chamber is completed during coronal cavity preparation with a round bur. The canal orifice is directly in the center of the tooth.
   2. **Midroot** level: the canal remains ovoid in shape and requires perimeter filing.
   3. **Apical third** level: the canal, round in shape, is filed and then shaped into a **round, tapered** preparation. Preparation terminates at the cementodentinal junction, 0.5 to 1.0 mm from the radiographic apex.

D. Ovoid preparation allows débridement of the entire pulp chamber and funnels down to the ovoid midcanal.

E. **Buccal** view of an **adult** second premolar with extensive secondary dentin formation. A radiograph, if exposed slightly from the mesial, will reveal
   1. pulp recession and the "thread-like" appearance of the pulp
   2. roentgen appearance of two roots (2% of the time)
   3. bayonet curve of the roots (20% of the time)
   4. 19-degree distal-axial inclination of the tooth

F. **Mesial** view of the same tooth demonstrating details **not apparent in the radiograph:**
   1. buccolingual width revealing the coronal pulp to be "ribbon shaped" rather than "thread-like"
   2. high bifurcation and two separate apical third roots
   3. 9-degree lingual-axial angulation of the tooth

   The operator must recognize that
   a. small canal orifices are deeply placed in the root and will be difficult to locate.
   b. the direction of each canal is determined by exploration with a **fine curved** file carried down the wall until the orifice is engaged. Then, by half-rotation, the file is turned to match the first curve of the canal, followed by penetration until the tip again catches on the curved wall. A second half-turn and further penetration will carry the tip of the instrument to within 0.5 to 1.0 mm of the radiographic apex. Retraction will remove dentin at both curves.

G. Cross-sections at three levels: 1, cervical; 2, midroot; and 3, apical third:
   1. **Cervical** level: the chamber, very narrow ovoid, extends deeply into the root.
   2. **Midroot** level: the bayonet curve and round canal orifices are apparent.
   3. **Apical third** level: the canals are round. The severe curve at the "bayonet" is reduced by filing action into a gradual curve.

H. An ovoid coronal cavity is prepared **well to the mesial** of the occlusal surface, with a depth of penetration **skewed toward the bayonet curvature. Skewing the cavity** allows an unrestrained approach to the first curve.

PLATE 14

Maxillary Second Premolars

Length of tooth	
Average Length	21 mm
Maximum Length	23 mm
Minimum Length	19 mm
Range	4 mm

Canals	
One canal	75%
One foramen	
Two canals	24%
Two foramina	
Three canals	1%

Curvature	
Straight	9.5%
Distal Curve	27.0%
Mesial Curve	1.6%
Buccal Curve	12.7%
*Lingual Curve	4.0%
Bayonet Curve	20.6%

*Not apparent in radiograph

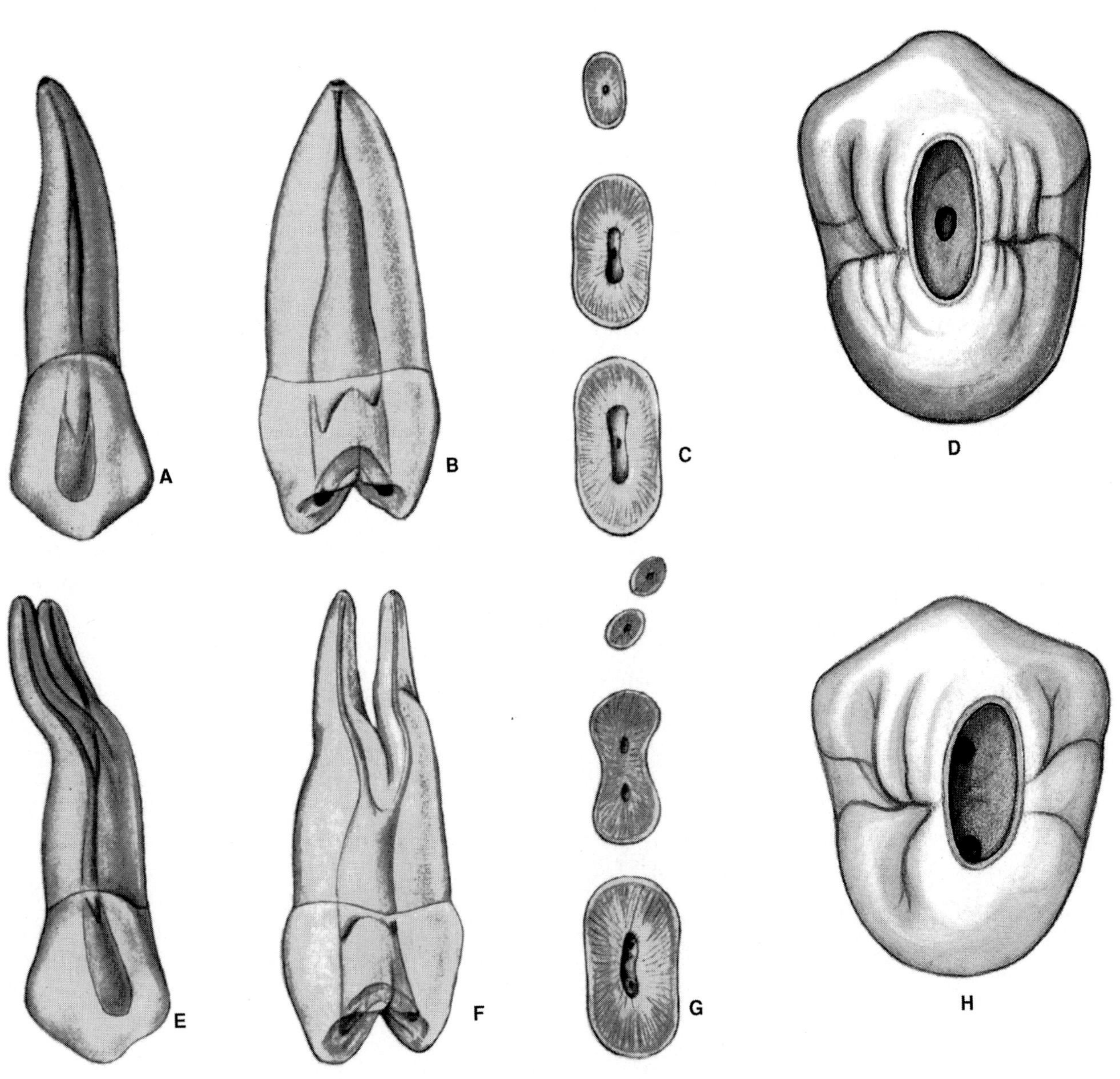

PLATE 15

Maxillary Premolar Teeth
ERRORS in Cavity Preparation

A. UNDEREXTENDED preparation exposing only pulp horns. Control of enlarging instruments is abdicated to cavity walls. The **white color** of the **roof** of the **chamber** is a clue to a shallow cavity.

B. OVEREXTENDED preparation from a fruitless search for a receded pulp. The enamel walls have been completely undermined. Gouging relates to failure to refer to the radiograph, which clearly indicates pulp recession.

C. PERFORATION at the mesiocervical indentation. Failure to observe the distal-axial inclination of the tooth led to **bypassing** receded pulp and perforation. The maxillary first premolar is one of the most commonly perforated teeth.

D. FAULTY ALIGNMENT of the access cavity through **full veneer restoration** placed to "straighten" the crown of a rotated tooth. Careful examination of the radiograph would reveal the rotated body of the tooth.

E. BROKEN INSTRUMENT twisted off in a "cross-over" canal. This frequent occurrence may be obviated by extending the internal preparation to straighten the canals (**dotted line**).

F. FAILURE to explore, débride, and obturate the third canal of the maxillary **first** premolar (6% of the time).

G. FAILURE to explore, débride, and obturate the second canal of the maxillary **second** premolar (24% of the time).

PLATE 15

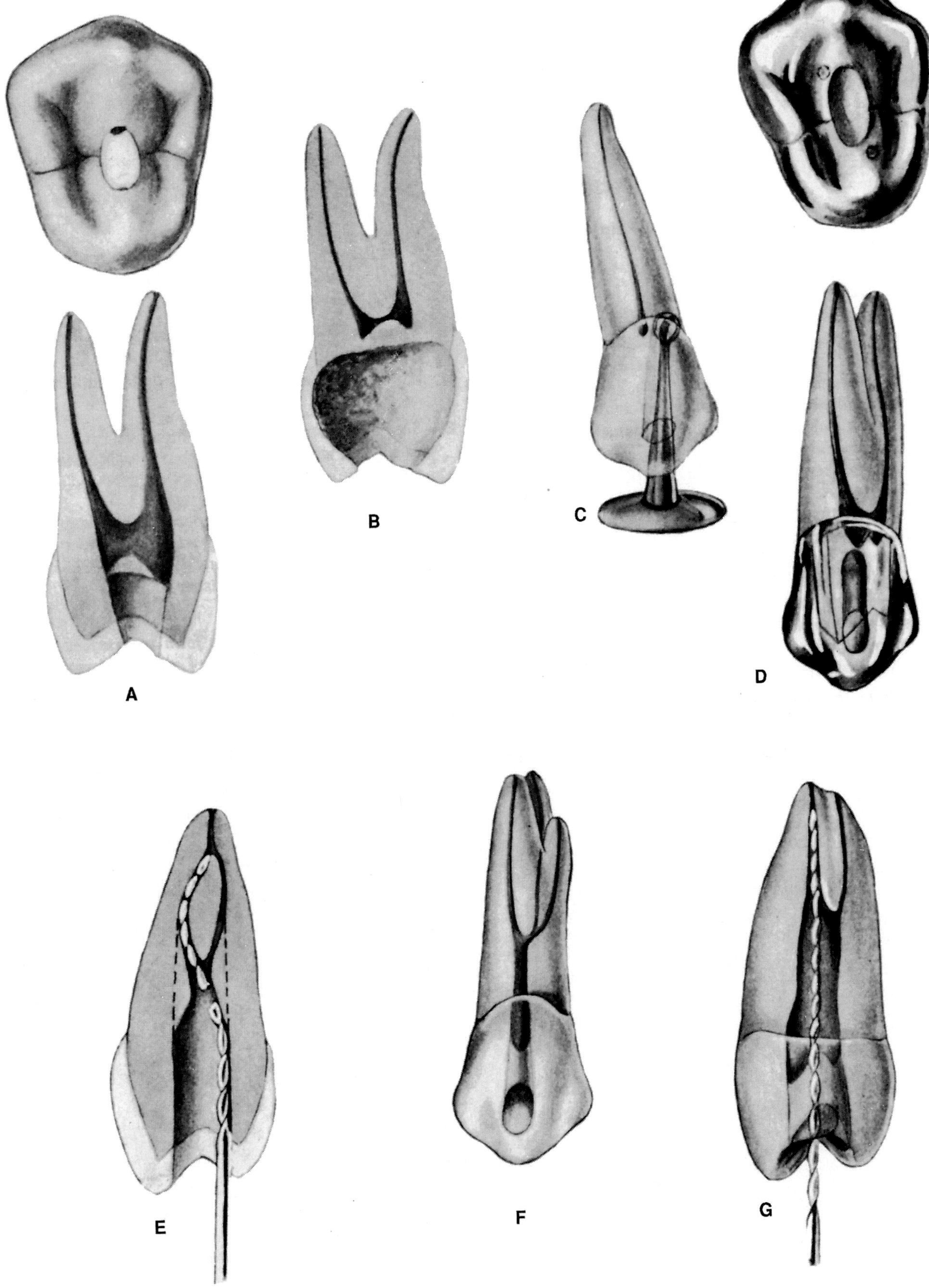

PLATE 16

Endodontic Preparation of Mandibular Premolar Teeth

Pulp Anatomy and Coronal Preparation

A. Entrance is **always** gained through the occlusal surface of **all** posterior teeth. Initial penetration is made in the exact center of the central groove of mandibular premolars. The bur is directed parallel to the long axis of the tooth. The 702 U taper fissure bur in an **accelerated-speed** contra-angle handpiece is ideal for perforating gold casting or virgin enamel surface **to the depth of the dentin.** Amalgam fillings are penetrated with a round bur in a high-speed contra-angle handpiece.

B. A regular-length No. 4 round bur is used to open vertically into the pulp chamber. The bur will be felt to "drop" when the pulp chamber is reached. If the chamber is **well calcified,** initial penetration is continued until the contra-angle handpiece rests against the occlusal surface. This depth of 9 mm is the usual position of the canal orifice that lies at the cervical level. In removing the bur, the occlusal opening is widened buccolingually to twice the width of the bur to allow room for exploration.

C. An endodontic explorer is used to locate the central canal. Tension of the explorer against the walls of preparation will indicate the amount and direction of extension necessary.

D. **Working from inside the pulp chamber to outside,** a regular-length No. 2 or 4 round bur is used to extend the cavity buccolingually by removing the roof of the pulp chamber.

E. Buccolingual extension and finish of cavity walls are completed with a 702 U fissure bur at accelerated speed.

F. Final ovoid preparation is a tapered funnel from the occlusal to the canal, providing **unobstructed access** to the canal. No overhanging tooth structure should impede complete authority over enlarging instruments.

G. Buccolingual ovoid **outline form** reflects the anatomy of the pulp chamber and position of the centrally located canal. The cavity is extensive enough to allow for instruments and filling the materials needed to enlarge and fill canals. **Further exploration** at this time **may reveal** the orifice to an **additional canal,** especially a **second canal** in the **first premolar.** The outline form of the final preparation will be identical for both newly erupted and "adult" teeth.

PLATE 16

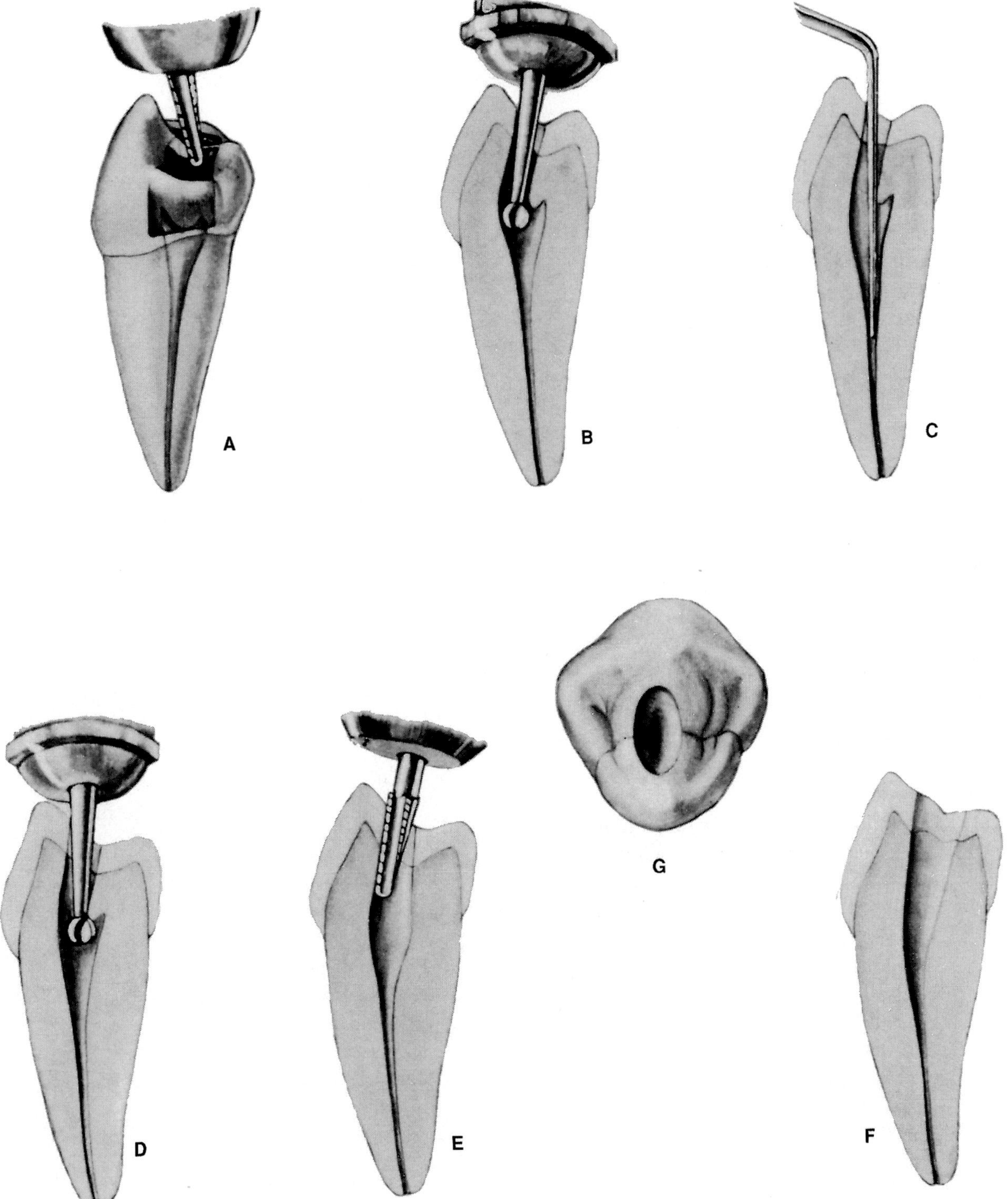

PLATE 17

Mandibular First Premolar

Pulp Anatomy and Coronal Preparation

A. **Buccal** view of a recently calcified first premolar with a large pulp. A radiograph, if exposed slightly from the mesial, will reveal:
   1. narrow mesiodistal width of the pulp
   2. presence of one pulp canal
   3. relatively straight canal
   4. 14-degree distal-axial inclination of the root

   All of these factors, **seen** in radiograph, are borne in mind when preparation is begun.

B. **Mesial** view of the same tooth demonstrating details not apparent from the radiograph:
   1. height of the pulp horn
   2. broad buccolingual extent of the pulp
   3. apical-buccal curvature (2% of the time)
   4. 10-degree lingual-axial angulation of the root

   These "unseen" factors will affect the **size, shape,** and **inclination** of the final preparation. Severe apical curvature can be detected only by exploration with a fine curved file. Near-verticality of the tooth simplifies orientation and bur alignment.

C. Cross-sections at three levels: 1, cervical; 2, midroot; and 3, apical third:
   1. **Cervical** level: the pulp is enormous in a young tooth, very wide in the buccolingual dimension. Débridement of the ovoid chamber is completed during coronal cavity preparation with a round bur.
   2. **Midroot** level: the canal continues ovoid and requires perimeter filing.
   3. **Apical third** level: the canal, generally round in shape, is enlarged by shaping into a **round, tapered** preparation. Preparation terminates at the cementodentinal junction, 0.5 to 1.0 mm from the radiographic apex.

D. **Ovoid** coronal preparation allows débridement of the entire pulp chamber, funnels down to the ovoid midcanal, and is large enough buccolingually to allow passage of instruments used to enlarge and fill the canal space.

E. **Buccal** view of an **adult** first premolar with extensive secondary dentin formation. A radiograph will reveal
   1. pulp recession and "thread-like" appearance of the pulp
   2. radiographic appearance of only one canal
   3. 14-degree distal-axial inclination of the root

F. **Mesial** view of the same tooth demonstrating details **not apparent in the radiograph:**
   1. buccolingual "ribbon-shaped" coronal pulp
   2. single-root, bifurcated canal at the midroot level and a single apical foramen
   3. 10-degree lingual-axial angulation of the root

   The operator must recognize that
   a. small orifices are difficult to locate.
   b. the presence of a bifurcated canal is determined only by exploration with a fine curved file.
   c. a single apical foramen can be determined by placing instruments in both canals at the same time. The instruments will be heard and felt to grate against each other.

G. Cross-sections at three levels: 1, cervical; 2, midroot; and 3, apical third:
   1. **Cervical** level: the chamber is very narrow ovoid.
   2. **Midroot** level: the two branches of the canal are round.
   3. **Apical third** level: the canal is round.

   Divisions of the canal are enlarged by filing. The buccal canal would be filled to the apex and the lingual canal to the point where the canals rejoin.

H. Ovoid funnel-shaped coronal preparation must be extensive enough buccolingually to allow for enlarging and filling both canals.

Mandibular First Premolar

Length of tooth

Average Length	22.1 mm
Maximum Length	24.1 mm
Minimum Length	20.1 mm
Range	4.0 mm

Canals

One canal	73.5%
One foramen	
Two canals*	6.5%
One foramen	
Two canals*	19.5%
Two foramina	
Three canals	0.5%

Curvature of root

Straight	48%	†Buccal Curve	2%
Distal Curve	35%	†Lingual Curve	7%
Mesial Curve	0%	Bayonet Curve	7%

*Incidence higher in black persons than in white persons

†Not apparent in radiograph

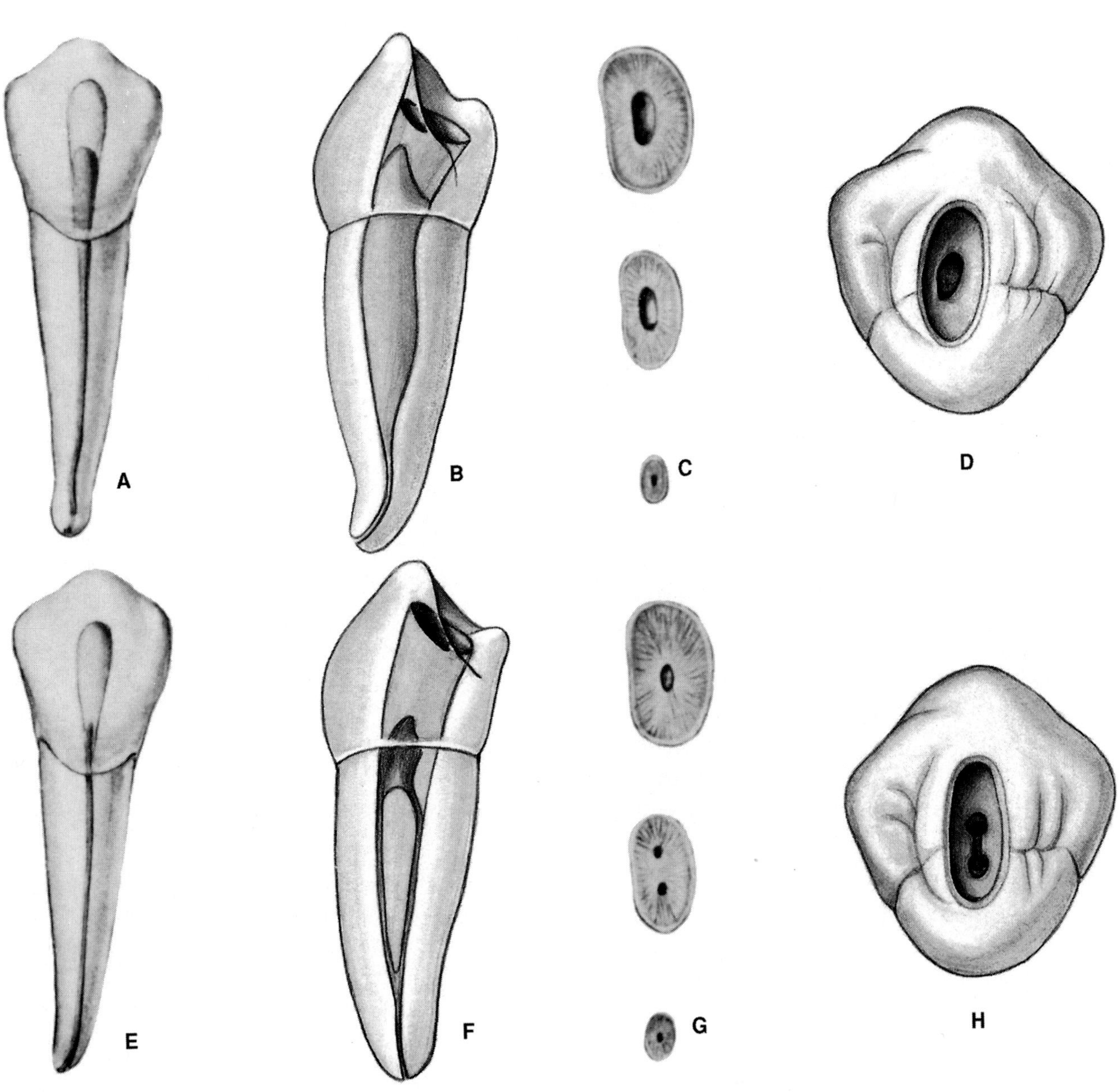

PLATE 18

Mandibular Second Premolar

Pulp Anatomy and Coronal Preparation

A. **Buccal** view of a recently calcified second premolar with a large pulp. A radiograph will reveal
   1. mesiodistal width of the pulp
   2. apical-distal curvature (40% of the time)
   3. 10-degree distal-axial inclination of the root

   These factors, **seen** in the radiograph, are borne in mind when preparation is begun.

B. **Mesial** view of the same tooth demonstrating details **not apparent in the radiograph:**
   1. broad buccolingual "ribbon-shaped" coronal pulp
   2. single root with pulpal bifurcation in the apical third
   3. 34-degree buccal-axial angulation of the root

   These "unseen" factors affect the **size, shape,** and **inclination** of the final preparation. Apical third bifurcation, **unseen in the radiograph,** emphasizes the necessity of careful canal exploration.

C. Cross-sections at three levels: 1, cervical; 2, midroot; and 3, apical third:
   1. **Cervical** level: the pulp is large in a young tooth, very wide in the buccolingual dimension. Débridement of the chamber is completed during coronal cavity preparation with a round bur.
   2. **Midroot** level: the canal continues to be long ovoid and requires perimeter filing.
   3. **Apical third** level: the canals, generally round, are shaped into **round, tapered** preparations. Preparation terminates at the cementodentinal junction, 0.5 to 1.0 mm from the radiographic apex.

D. **Ovoid,** coronal funnel-shaped preparation allows débridement of the entire pulp chamber down to the ovoid midcanal. The cavity is large enough buccolingually to allow enlarging and filling of both canals.

E. **Buccal** view of an **adult** second premolar with extensive secondary dentin formation. A radiograph, if exposed slightly from the mesial, will reveal
   1. pulp recession and "thread-like" appearance of the pulp
   2. sweeping distal curve of the apical third of the root of the tooth (40% of the time)
   3. 10-degree distal-axial angulation of the root

F. **Mesial** view of the same tooth demonstrating details **not apparent in the radiograph:**
   1. buccolingual "ribbon-shaped" pulp
   2. minus 34-degree buccal-axial angulation of the root

   The operator should recognize that
   a. a small canal orifice will be difficult to locate.
   b. the direction of the canal is best explored with a fine curved file that is carried to within 0.5 to 1.0 mm of the radiographic apex. Retraction will then remove dentin at the curve.

G. Cross-sections at three levels: 1, cervical; 2, midroot; and 3, apical third:
   1. **Cervical** level: the chamber is very narrow ovoid.
   2. **Midroot** level: the canal is less ovoid.
   3. **Apical third** level: the canal is round.

   The sweeping curve at the apical third is filed to a gradual curve.

H. **Ovoid** funnel-shaped coronal cavity is modest in size and skewed slightly to the mesial, allowing adequate room to instrument and fill the curved apical third.

PLATE 18

Mandibular Second Premolars

Length of tooth	
Average Length	21.4 mm
Maximum Length	23.7 mm
Minimum Length	19.1 mm
Range	4.6 mm

Canals	
One canal One foramen	85.5%
Two canals* One foramen	1.5%
Two canals* Two foramina	11.5%
Three canals	0.5%

Curvature of root			
Straight	39%	†Lingual Curve	3%
Distal Curve	40%	Bayonet Curve	7%
Mesial Curve	0%	Trifurcation Curve	1%
†Buccal Curve	10%		

*Incidence much higher in black persons than in white persons

†Not apparent in radiograph

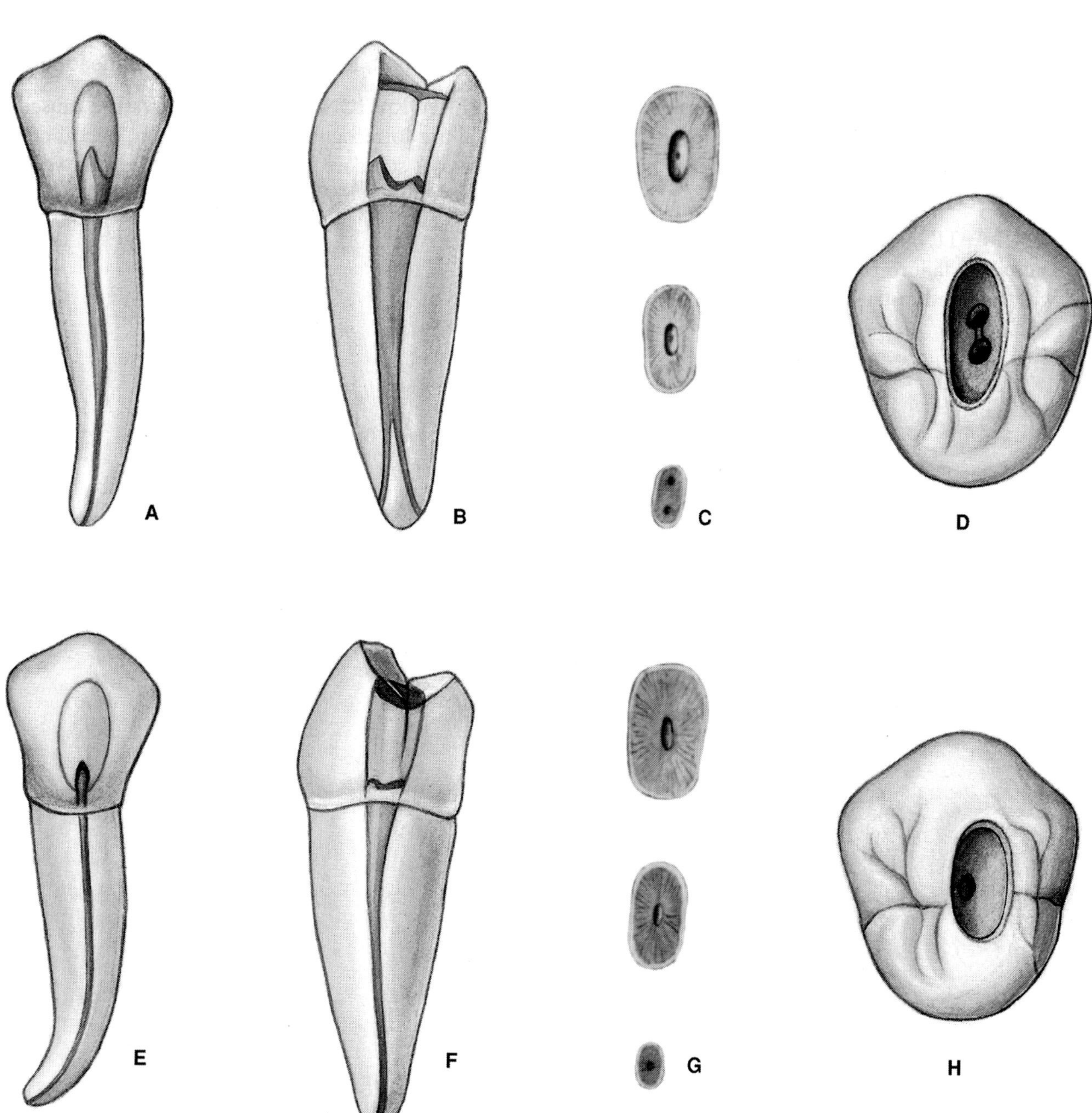

PLATE 20

Endodontic Preparation of Maxillary Molar Teeth

A. Entrance is **always** gained through the occlusal surface of all posterior teeth. Initial penetration is made in the exact center of the mesial pit, with the bur directed toward the lingual. The 702 U tapering fissure bur in an **accelerated-speed** contra-angle handpiece is ideal for perforating gold casting or virgin enamel surface **to the depth of dentin.** Amalgam fillings are penetrated with a No. 4 or 6 round bur operating in a slow-speed contra-angle handpiece.

B. According to the size of the chamber, a **regular-length** No. 4 round bur is used to open into the pulp chamber. The **bur** should be **directed toward the orifice** of the **palatal canal or toward the mesiobuccal canal orifice,** where the greatest space in the chamber exists. It will be felt to "drop" when the pulp chamber is reached. If the chamber is **well calcified,** initial penetration is continued until the contra-angle rests against the occlusal surface. This depth of 9 mm is the usual position of the floor of the pulp chamber, which lies at the cervical level. Working from inside out, back toward the buccal, the bur removes enough roof of the pulp chamber for exploration.

C. An endodontic explorer is used to locate orifices of the **palatal, mesiobuccal,** and **distobuccal** canals. Tension of the explorer against the walls of preparation will indicate the amount and direction of extension necessary. **Orifices of canals form the perimeter** of preparation. **Special care must be taken to explore for a second canal in the mesiobuccal root.**

D. Again, working at slow speed from inside to outside, a round bur is used to remove the roof of the pulp chamber. Internal walls and floor of preparation should not be cut into unless difficulty is encountered in locating orifices. In that case, **surgical-length** No. 2 round burs are necessary to explore the floor of the chamber.

E. Final finish and funneling of cavity walls are completed with a 702 U fissure bur or tapered diamond points at accelerated speed.

F. Final preparation provides unobstructed access to canal orifices and should not impede complete authority of enlarging instruments. Improve ease of access by **"leaning" the entire preparation toward the buccal,** for all instrumentation is introduced from the buccal. Notice that the preparation extends almost to the height of the buccal cusps. The walls are perfectly smooth, and the orifices are located **at the exact pulpal-axial angles** of the cavity floor.

G. Extended outline form reflects the anatomy of the pulp chamber. The base is toward the buccal and the apex is to the lingual, with the canal orifice positioned at each angle of the triangle. The cavity is entirely within the mesial half of the tooth and need not invade the transverse ridge but is extensive enough, buccal to lingual, to allow positioning of instruments and filling materials. Outline form of final preparation is identical for both a newly erupted and an "adult" tooth. **Note the orifice to the fourth canal.**

PLATE 20

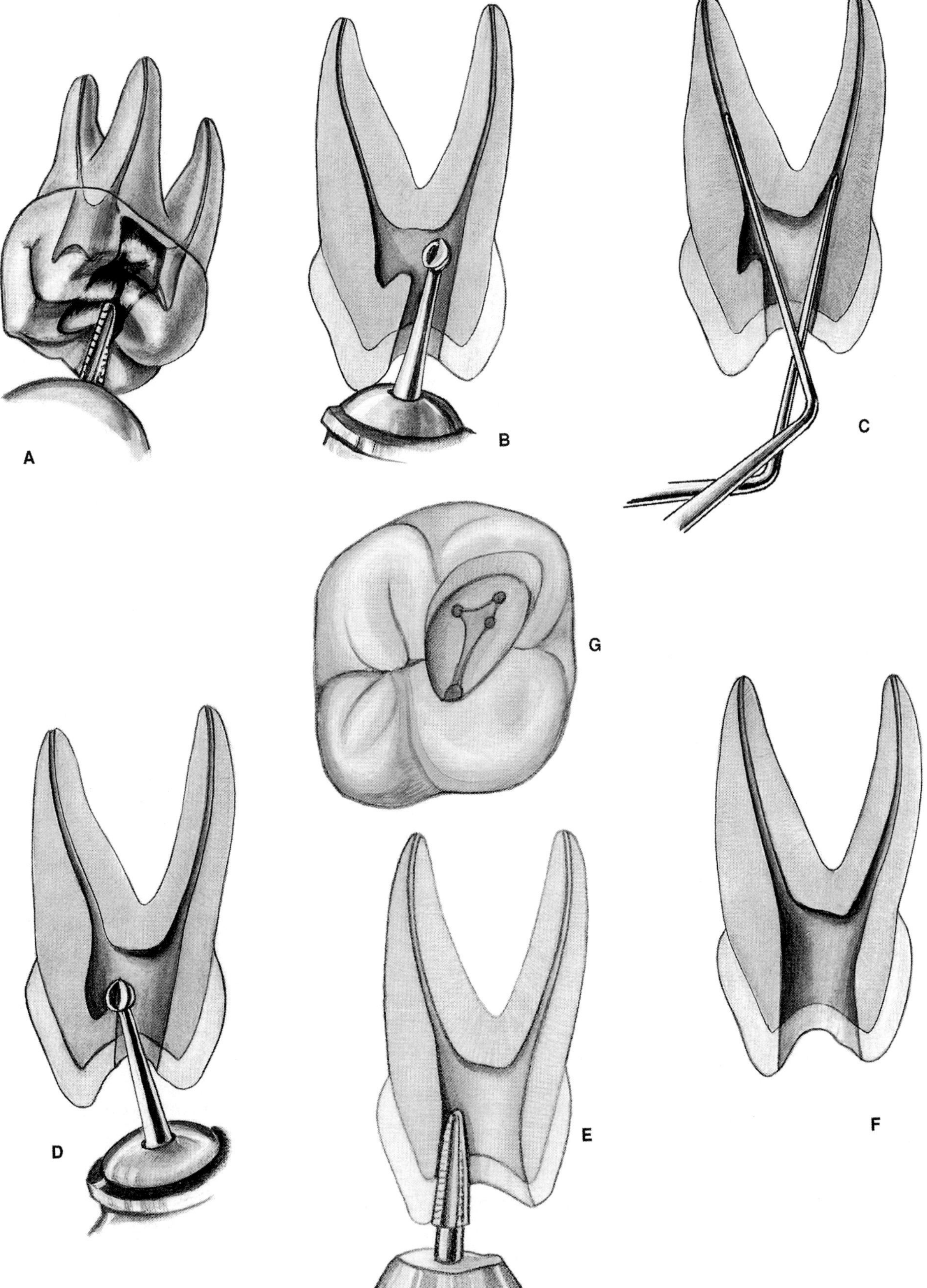

PLATE 21

Maxillary First Molar

Pulp Anatomy and Coronal Preparation

A. **Buccal** view of a recently calcified first molar with large pulp. A radiograph will reveal
   1. large pulp chamber
   2. mesiobuccal root with two separate canals, distobuccal, and palatal roots, each with one canal
   3. slightly curved buccal roots
   4. slightly curved palatal root
   5. vertical axial alignment of the **tooth**

   These factors, **seen** in radiograph, are borne in mind when preparation is begun. Care must be taken to explore for an additional mesiobuccal canal.

B. **Mesial** view of the same tooth demonstrating details **not apparent in the radiograph:**
   1. buccolingual width of the pulp chamber
   2. apical-buccal curvature of the palatal root (55% of the time)
   3. buccal inclination of buccal roots
   4. vertical axial alignment of the **tooth**

   These "unseen" factors will affect the **size, shape,** and **inclination** of the final preparation. Sharp **buccal curvature** of the **palatal canal requires great care** in exploration and instrumentation. Canals must be carefully explored with **fine curved files.** Enlargement of buccal canals is accomplished by reaming and filing and of the palatal canal by step-back filing.

C. Cross-section at two levels: 1, cervical; and 2, apical third:
   1. **Cervical** level: the pulp is enormous in a young tooth. Débridement of a **triangular** chamber is completed with a round bur. A **dark** cavity floor with **"lines"** connecting orifices is in marked contrast to white walls. A palatal canal requires perimeter filing.
   2. **Apical third** level: the canals are essentially round. Buccal canals are shaped into **round, tapered** preparations. Preparations terminate at the cementodentinal junction, 0.5 to 1.0 mm from the radiographic apex.

D. **Triangular outline form,** with the base toward the buccal and the apex toward the lingual, reflects the anatomy of the pulp chamber, with the orifice positioned at each angle of the triangle. Both **buccal** and **lingual walls slope buccally.** Mesial and distal walls **funnel** slightly **outward.** The cavity is entirely within the mesial half of the tooth and should be extensive enough to allow positioning of instruments and filling materials needed to enlarge and fill canals. The orifice to an **extra middle mesial canal** may be found in the groove near the mesiobuccal canal.

E. **Buccal** view of an **adult** first molar with extensive secondary dentin formation. A radiograph will reveal
   1. pulp recession and "thread-like" pulp
   2. mesiobuccal, distobuccal, and palatal roots, each with one canal
   3. straight palatal root, apical curve, distal root
   4. apical-distal curvature of the mesial root (78% of the time)
   5. vertical axial alignment of the **tooth**

F. **Mesial** view of the same tooth demonstrating details **not apparent in the radiograph:**
   1. pulp recession
   2. relatively straight palatal root
   3. buccal inclination of the buccal roots
   4. vertical axial alignment of the **tooth**

   The operator must recognize that
   a. careful exploration for orifices and canals is imperative.
   b. severe curvature of buccal roots will require careful enlargement with curved instruments.

G. Cross-section at two levels: 1, cervical; and 2, apical third:
   1. **Cervical** level: a triangular chamber constricted from secondary dentin formation is débrided during coronal cavity preparation with a round bur. Round palatal and distobuccal canals will be shaped to a **round, tapered** preparation.
   2. **Apical third** level: the canals are round. A curved mesiobuccal canal is enlarged by step-back filing. Preparations terminate at the cementodentinal junction, 0.5 to 1.0 mm from the radiographic apex.

H. **Triangular outline** form reflects the anatomy of the pulp chamber. Both **buccal** and **lingual** walls **slope buccally. The mesial wall slopes mesially** to allow for instrumentation of a severely curved mesiobuccal canal. If an **additional canal is found in the mesiobuccal root, its orifice will usually be in the groove leading to the palatal canal.**

Maxillary First Molars

Length of Tooth	*Mesiobuccal*	*Distobuccal*	*Palatal*	*Canal*		*Direction*	*Palatal*	*Mesial*	*Distal*	*Canals in the mesiobuccal root*	
						Curvature of roots					
Average Length	19.9 mm	19.4 mm	20.6 mm	Three canals	41.1%	Straight	40%	21%	54%	One canal	41.1%
Maximum Length	21.6 mm	21.2 mm	22.5 mm	Four canals	56.5%	Distal Curve	1%	78%	17%	One foramen	
Minimum Length	18.2 mm	17.6 mm	17.6 mm	Five canals	2.4%	Mesial Curve	4%	0%	19%	Two canals	40%
Range	3.4 mm	3.6 mm	3.8 mm			*Buccal Curve	*55%	0%	0%	One foramen	
						*Lingual Curve	0%	0%	0%	Two canals	18.9%
						Bayonet Curve	0%	1%	10%	Two foramina	

*Not apparent in radiograph

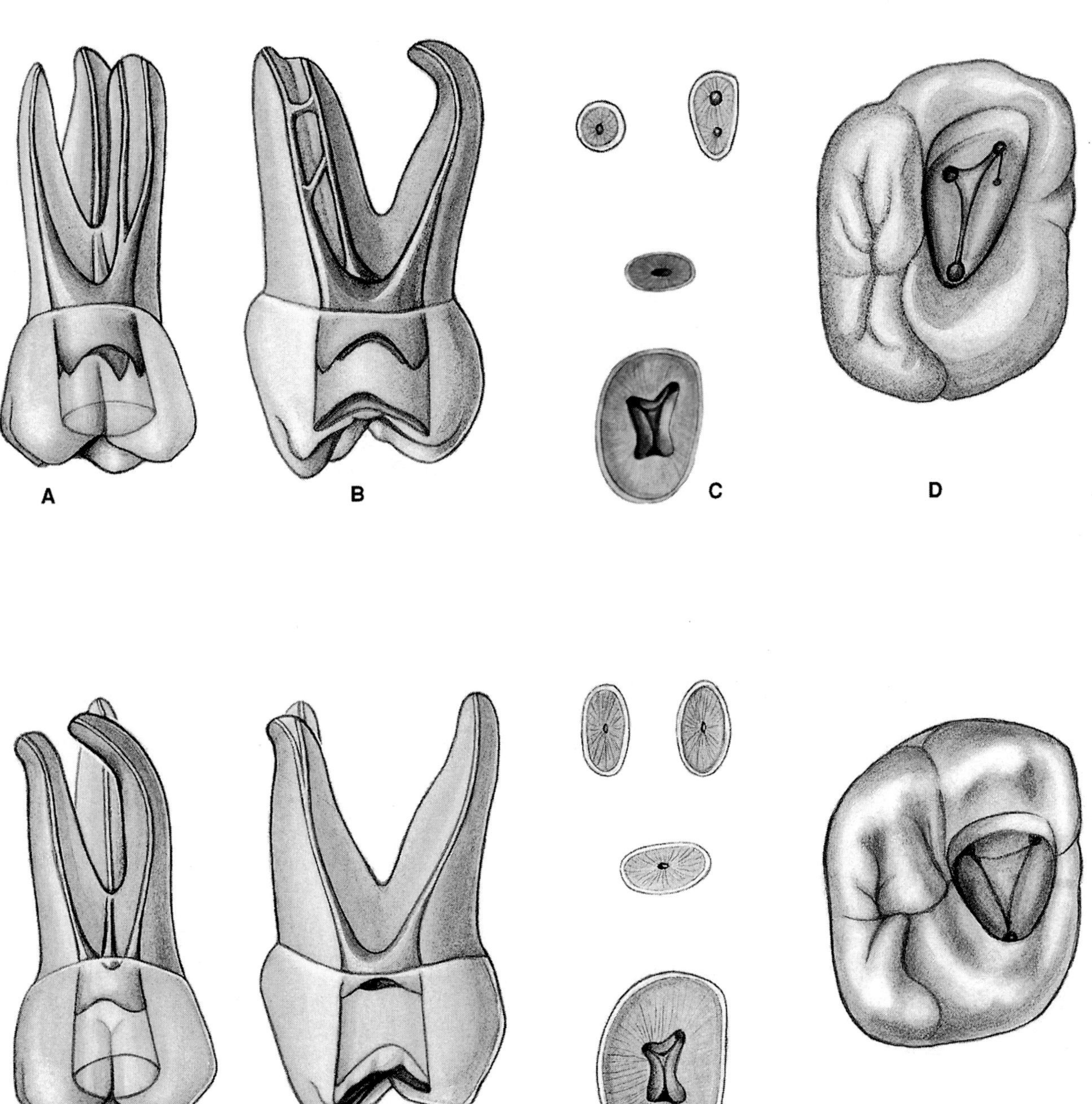

PLATE 22

Maxillary Second Molar

Pulp Anatomy and Coronal Preparation

A. **Buccal** view of a recently calcified second molar with a large pulp. A radiograph will reveal
   1. large pulp chamber
   2. mesiobuccal, distobuccal, and palatal roots, each with one canal
   3. gradual curvature of all three canals
   4. vertical axial alignment of the **tooth**

   These factors, **seen** in radiograph, are borne in mind when preparation is begun.

B. **Mesial** view of the same tooth demonstrating details **not apparent in the radiograph:**
   1. buccolingual width of the pulp chamber
   2. gradual curvature in two directions of all three canals
   3. buccal inclination of the buccal roots
   4. vertical axial alignment of the **tooth**

   These "unseen" factors will affect the **size, shape,** and **inclination** of the final preparation.

C. Cross-section at two levels: 1, cervical; and 2, apical third:
   1. **Cervical** level: the pulp is enormous in a young tooth. Débridement of a **triangular** chamber is completed with round burs. The **dark** cavity floor with **"lines"** connecting orifices is in marked contrast to white walls.
   2. **Apical third** level: the canals are essentially round and are shaped into a **round, tapered** preparation. Preparations terminate at the cementodentinal junction, 0.5 to 1.0 from the radiographic apex.

D. **Triangular outline form** is "flattened" as it reflects the internal anatomy of the chamber. Note that the distobuccal canal orifice is nearer the center of the cavity floor. The entire preparation sharply slopes to the buccal and is extensive enough to allow positioning of instruments and filling materials needed to enlarge and fill canals.

E. **Buccal** view of an adult second molar with extensive secondary dentin formation.
   A radiograph will reveal
   1. pulp recession and "thread-like" pulp
   2. **anomalous** appearance of only **one root** and **two canals**
   3. vertical axial alignment of the **tooth**

F. **Mesial** view of the same tooth demonstrating details **not apparent in the radiograph:**
   1. pulp recession
   2. **anomalous** appearance of only **one root** and **two canals**
   3. sweeping curvature of the lingual canal
   4. vertical axial alignment of the **tooth**

   The operator must recognize that
   a. canal orifices are difficult to find by exploration.
   b. a **detailed search must be made for the third canal.**

G. Cross-sections at two levels: 1, cervical; and 2, apical third.
   1. **Cervical** level: **ovoid** pulp chamber is débrided during cavity preparation with a round bur.
   2. **Apical third** level: canals are round. Preparations terminate at the cementodentinal junction, 0.5 to 1.0 mm from the radiographic apex.

H. **Ovoid** outline form reflects the internal anatomy of the pulp chamber and elongated parallelogram shape of the occlusal surface. The entire preparation slopes sharply to the buccal.

PLATE 22

Maxillary Second Molars

Length of Tooth	*Mesiobuccal*	*Distobuccal*	*Palatal*	*Number of Roots*		*Curvature of roots*				*Canals in the mesiobuccal root*	
						Direction	*Palatal*	*Mesial*	*Distal*		
Average Length	20.2 mm	19.4 mm	20.8 mm	Three	54%	Straight	63%	22%	54%	One canal	63%
Maximum Length	22.2 mm	21.3 mm	22.6 mm	Fused	46%	Distal	0%	54%	?	One foramen	
Minimum Length	18.2 mm	17.5 mm	19.0 mm			Mesial	0%	0%	17%	Two canals	13%
Range	4.0 mm	3.8 mm	3.6 mm			*Buccal	37%			One foramen	
						Lingual	0%			Two canals	24%
										Two foramina	

*Not apparent in radiograph

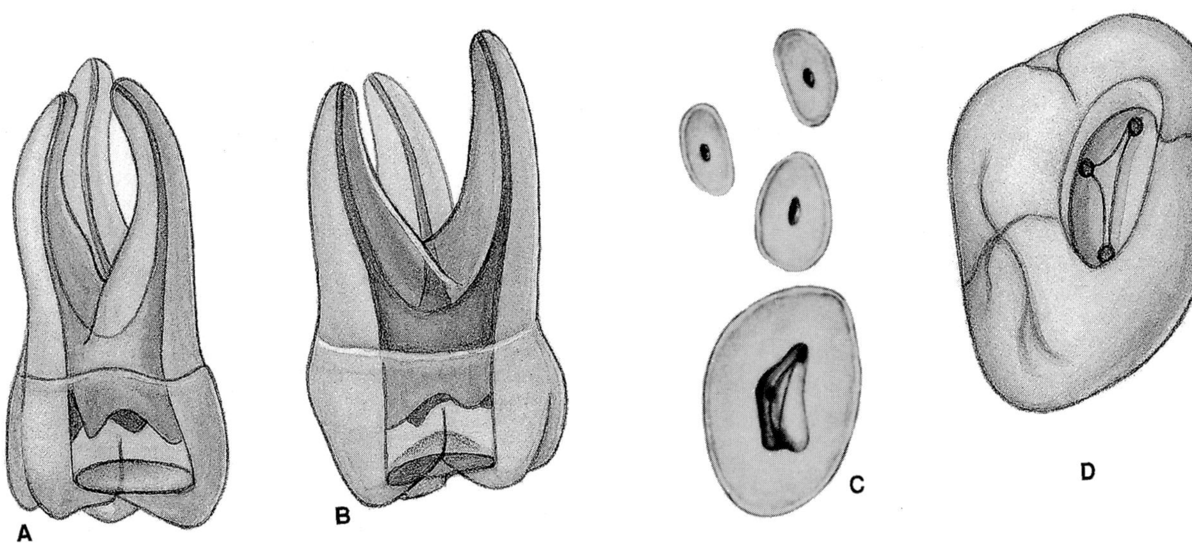

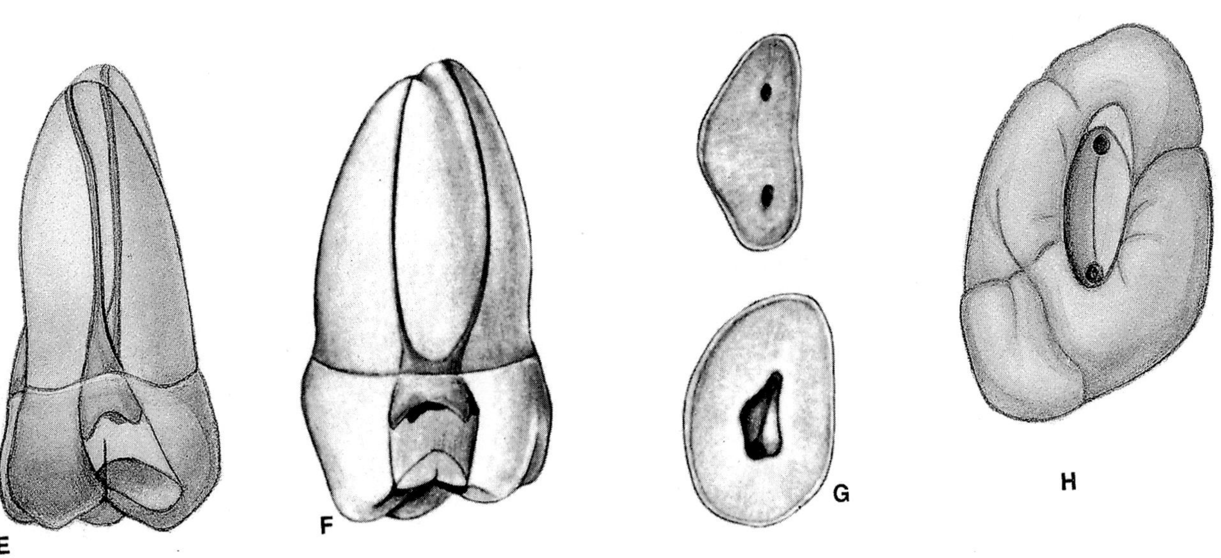

PLATE 23

Maxillary Molar Teeth

ERRORS in Cavity Preparation

A. UNDEREXTENDED preparation. Pulp horns have merely been "nicked," and the entire roof of the pulp chamber remains. "White" color dentin of the roof is a clue to underextension (A^1). Instrument control is lost.

B. OVEREXTENDED preparation undermining enamel walls. The crown is badly gouged owing to failure to observe pulp recession in the radiograph.

C. PERFORATION into furca using a **surgical-length** bur and failing to realize that the narrow pulp chamber had been passed. Operator error in failure to compare the length of the bur to the depth of the pulp canal floor. Length should be marked on the bur shank with Dycal.

D. INADEQUATE vertical preparation related to failure to recognize severe buccal inclination of an unopposed molar.

E. DISORIENTED occlusal outline form exposing only the palatal canal. A faulty cavity has been prepared in full crown, which was placed to "straighten" a **rotated molar** (E^1). Palpating for mesiobuccal root prominence would reveal the severity of the rotation.

F. LEDGE FORMATION caused by using a large straight instrument in a curved canal.

G. PERFORATION of a palatal root commonly caused by assuming the canal to be straight and failing to explore and enlarge the canal with a fine curved instrument.

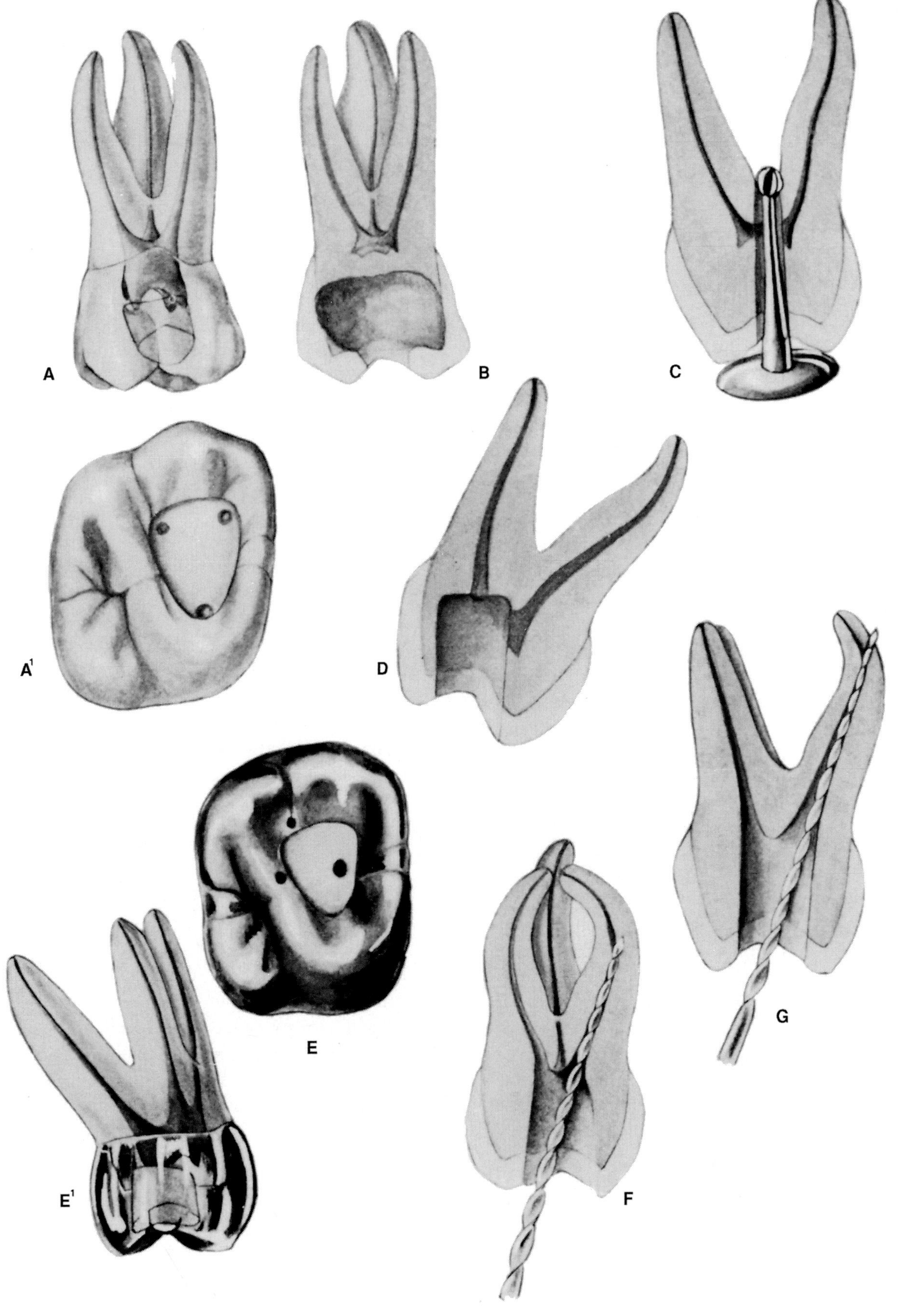
A
B
C
A¹
D
E
G
E¹
F

PLATE 24

Endodontic Preparation of Mandibular Molar Teeth

A. Entrance is **always** gained through the occlusal surface of **all** posterior teeth. Initial penetration is made in the exact center of the mesial pit, with the bur directed toward the distal. The 702 U tapering fissure bur in an **accelerated-speed** contra-angle handpiece is ideal for perforating gold casting or virgin enamel surface to the **depth of dentin.** Amalgam fillings are penetrated with a No. 4 round bur operating in a high-speed contra-angle handpiece.

B. According to the size of the chamber, a regular-length No. 4 or 6 round bur is used to open into the pulp chamber. The bur should be **directed toward the orifice** of the **mesiobuccal or distal canal,** where the greatest space in the chamber exists. It will be felt to "drop" when the pulp chamber is reached. If the chamber is well calcified, initial penetration is continued until the contra-angle handpiece rests against the occlusal surface. This depth of 9 mm is the usual position of the floor of the pulp chamber, which lies at the cervical level. Working from inside out, back toward the mesial, the bur removes enough roof of the pulp chamber for exploration.

C. An endodontic explorer is used to locate orifices of the **distal, mesiobuccal,** and **mesiolingual** canals. Tension of the explorer against the walls of preparation indicates the amount and direction of extension necessary. **Orifices of the canals form the perimeter** of preparation. **Special care must be taken to explore for an additional canal in the distal root.** The distal canal should form a triangle with two mesial canals. If it is asymmetric, always look for the fourth canal 29% of the time.

D. Again, working at slow speed from the inside to outside, a round bur is used to remove the roof of the pulp chamber. Internal walls and floor of preparation should not be cut into unless difficulty is encountered in locating orifices. In that case, **surgical-length** No. 2 or 4 round burs are necessary to explore the floor of the chamber.

E. Final finish and funneling of cavity walls are completed with a 702 U fissure bur or diamond point at accelerated speed.

F. Final preparation provides unobstructed access to canal orifices and should not impede the complete authority of enlarging instruments. Improve ease of access by **"leaning" the entire preparation toward the mesial,** for all instrumentation is introduced from the mesial. Notice that the cavity outline extends to the height of the mesial cusps. The walls are perfectly smooth and the orifices located **at the exact pulpal-axial angle** of the cavity floor.

G. "Square" outline form reflects the anatomy of the pulp chamber. Both mesial and distal walls slope mesially. The cavity is primarily within the mesial half of the tooth but is extensive enough to allow positioning of the instrument and filling materials. The outline form of the final preparation will be identical for both a newly erupted and an "adult" tooth. Further exploration should determine if a fourth canal can be found in the distal. If so, the outline is extended in that direction. In that case, an orifice will be positioned at each angle of the square.

PLATE 24

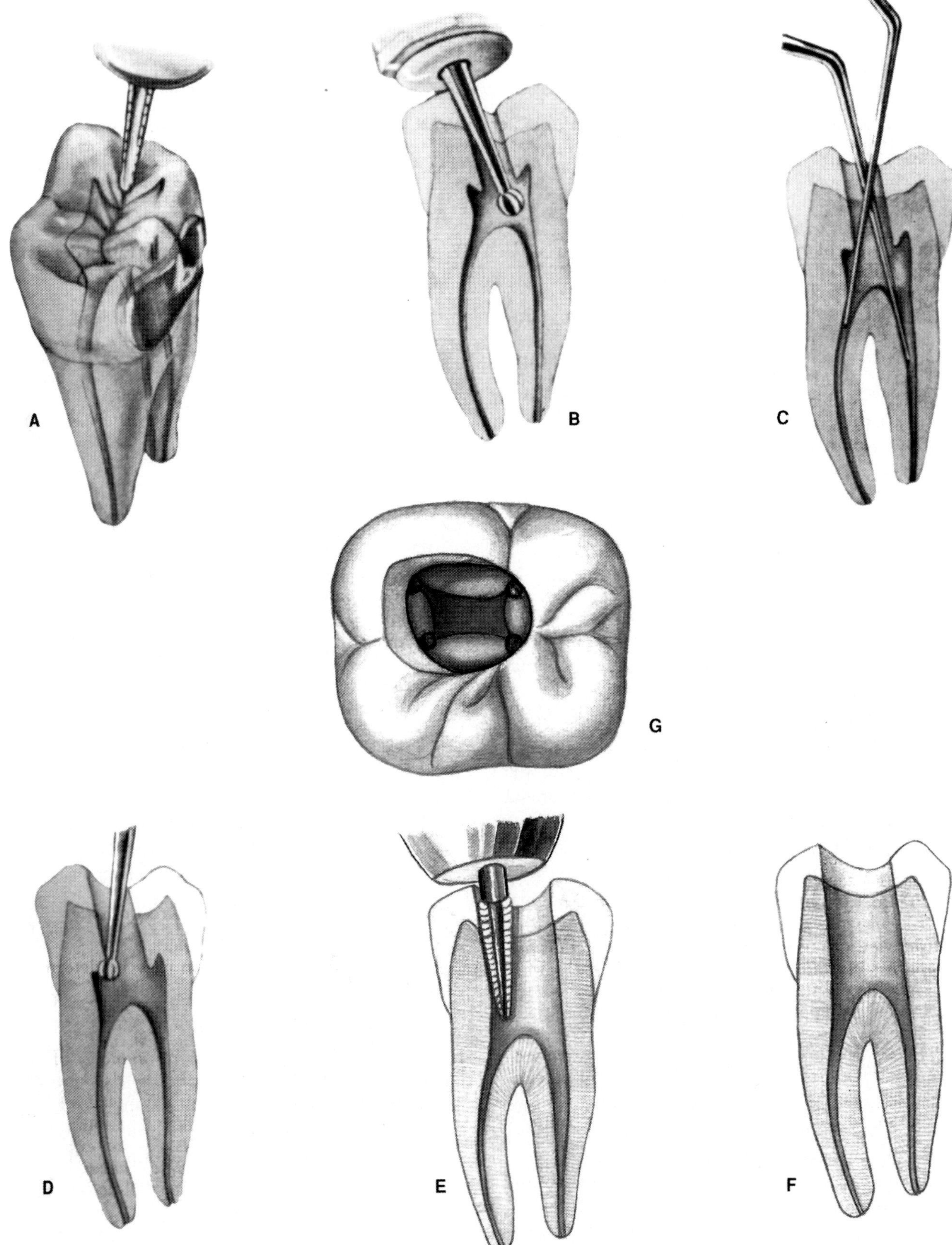

PLATE 25

Mandibular First Molar

Pulp Anatomy and Coronal Preparation

A. **Buccal** view of a recently calcified first molar with large pulp. The initial radiograph will reveal
   1. large pulp chamber
   2. mesial and distal roots, each **apparently** containing one canal
   3. vertical distal root with a severe apical curvature
   4. curvature of the mesial root (84% of the time)
   5. distal-axial inclination of the **tooth**

   These factors, **seen** in radiograph, are borne in mind when preparation is begun.

B. **Mesial** view of the same tooth demonstrating details **not apparent in the radiograph:**
   1. **single mesial root** with **two canals**
   2. minus 58-degree buccal-axial inclination of the **roots**

   All of these **unseen** factors will affect the **size, shape,** and **inclination** of the final preparation.

C. Cross-section at three levels: 1, cervical; 2, midroot; and 3, apical third:
   1. **Cervical** level: the pulp, enormous in a young tooth, is débrided during coronal cavity preparation with a round bur.
   2. **Midroot** level: the canals are ovoid. Severe indentation on the distal surface of the mesial root brings the canal within 1.5 mm of the external surface, an area frequently perforated by "stripping."
   3. **Apical third** level: the canals are round and are shaped into **round, tapered** preparations. Preparations terminate at the cementodentinal junction, 0.5 to 1.0 mm from the radiographic apex.

D. **Distal** view of the same tooth demonstrating details **not apparent in the radiograph:**
   1. height of distal pulp horns
   2. "ribbon-shaped" distal canal

E. **Buccal** view of an **adult** first molar with extensive secondary dentin formation. A radiograph will reveal
   1. pulp recession and "thread-like" pulp
   2. mesial and distal roots, each **apparently** containing one canal
   3. mesial curvature of the distal root (5% of the time) and distal curvature of the mesial root (84% of the time)
   4. distal-axial inclination of the tooth

F. **Mesial** view of the same tooth demonstrating details **not apparent in the radiograph:**
   1. pulp recession
   2. **mesial** root, **two canals**, and a single foramen
   3. minus 58-degree buccal-axial inclination of the **roots**

   The operator must recognize that
   a. careful exploration with two instruments at the same time reveals a common apical foramen.
   b. mesial canals curve in two directions.

G. Cross-section at three levels: 1, cervical; 2, midroot; and 3, apical third:
   1. **Cervical** level: the chamber is débrided during coronal cavity preparation with a round bur.
   2. **Midroot** level: the canals are nearly round and are enlarged during reaming of an apical third.
   3. **Apical third** level: the canals are round and are shaped into a **round, tapered** preparation. Preparations terminate at the cementodentinal junction, 0.5 to 1.0 mm from the radiographic apex.

H. **Distal** view of the same tooth demonstrating details **not apparent in the radiograph:**
   1. pulp recession
   2. **distal** root with **the usual single canal**
   3. buccal-axial inclination of the roots
   4. distal canal curves in two directions

   The operator should recognize that
   a. the presence of a fourth canal can be determined only by careful exploration.

I. **Triangular outline form** reflects the **anatomy** of the pulp chamber. Both mesial and distal walls slope mesially. The cavity is primarily within the mesial half of the tooth but is extensive enough to allow positioning of instruments and filling materials. **Further exploration should determine whether a fourth canal can be found in the distal.** In that case, an orifice will be positioned at each angle of the rhomboid.

PLATE 25

Mandibular First Molars

Length of Tooth	*Mesial*	*Distal*
Average Length	20.9 mm	20.9 mm
Maximum Length	22.7 mm	22.6 mm
Minimum Length	19.1 mm	19.2 mm
Range	3.6 mm	3.4 mm

Roots		*Canals*	
Two roots	97.8%	Two canals	6.7%
Three roots	2.2%	Three canals	64.4%
		Four canals	28.9%

Canals			
Mesial		*Distal*	
Two canals One foramen	40.5%	One canal	71.1%
Two canals Two foramina	59.5%	Two canals	28.9%
		Two canals One foramen	61.5%
		Two canals Two foramina	38.5%

Curvature of Roots		
Direction	*Mesial*	*Distal*
Straight	16%	74%
Distal	84%	21%
Mesial	0%	5%
Buccal	0%	0%
Lingual	0%	0%

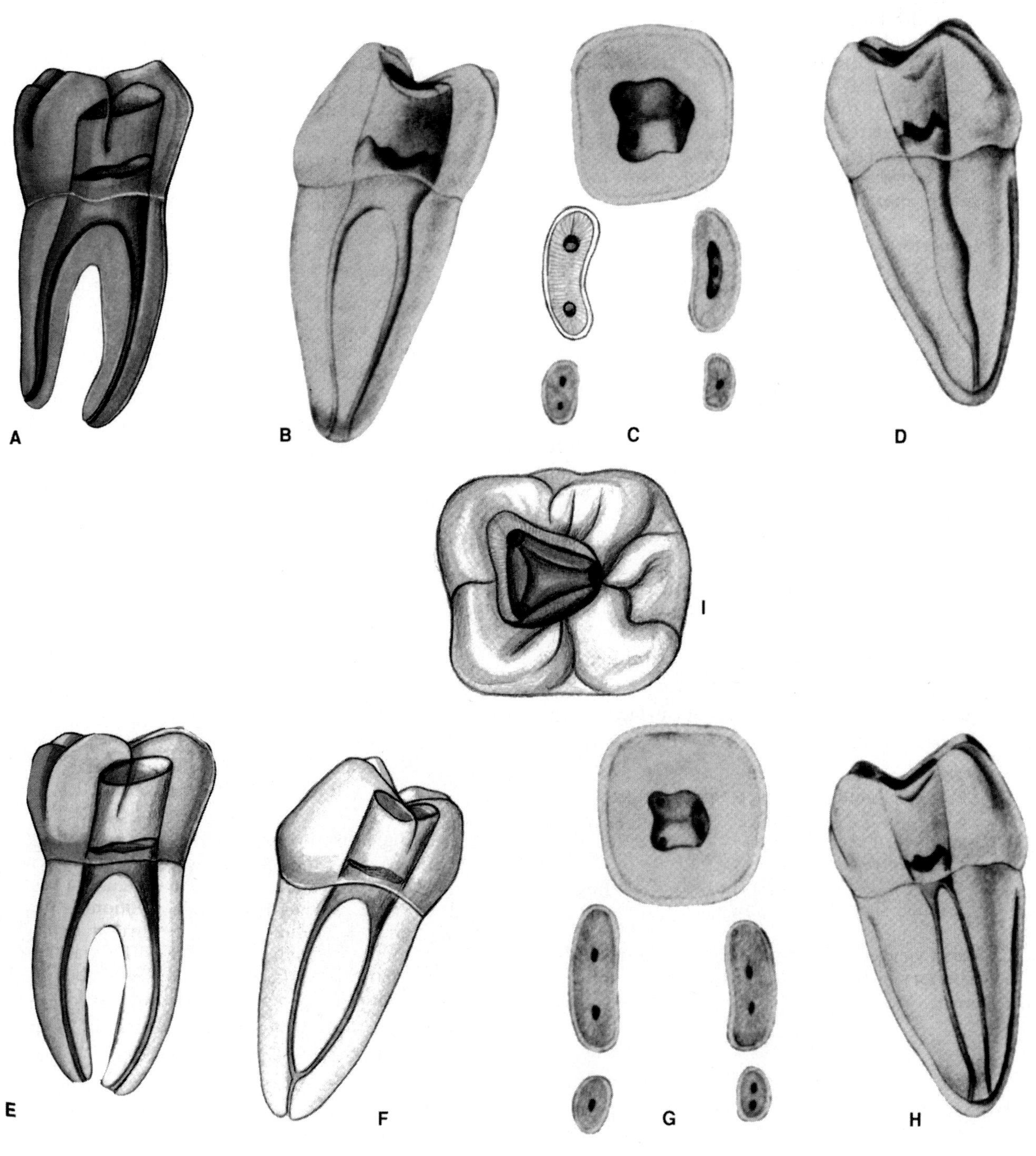

PLATE 26

Mandibular Second Molar

Pulp Anatomy and Coronal Preparation

A. **Buccal** view of a recently calcified second molar with a large pulp. A radiograph will reveal
   1. large pulp chamber
   2. mesial and distal roots, each **apparently** containing one canal
   3. mesial curvature of the distal root (10%)
   4. bayonet curvature of the mesial root (7%)
   5. distal-axial inclination of the **tooth**

   These factors, **seen** in radiograph, are borne in mind when preparation is begun.

B. **Mesial** view of the same tooth demonstrating details **not apparent in the radiograph:**
   1. **mesial** root with **two canals**
   2. lingual curvature of the mesiobuccal canal
   3. "S" curvature of the mesiolingual canal
   4. minus 52-degree buccal-axial inclination of the **roots**

   These **unseen** factors will affect the **size, shape,** and **inclination** of the final preparation. Canals must be carefully explored with a fine curved file. The **double "S" curvature** of the **mesiolingual** canal is especially challenging. All three canals are enlarged by step-back or step-down filing.

C. Cross-section at three levels: 1, cervical; 2, midroot; and 3, apical third:
   1. **Cervical** level: the pulp, enormous in a young tooth, is débrided during coronal cavity preparation with a round bur.
   2. **Midroot** level: the canals are ovoid. Carefully avoid filing against the distal surface of the mesial root, where "stripping" perforation often occurs.
   3. **Apical third** level: the canals are round and are shaped into **round, tapered** preparations. Preparations terminate at the cementodentinal junction, 0.5 to 1.0 mm from the radiographic apex.

D. **Distal** view of the same tooth demonstrating details **not apparent in the radiograph:**
   1. height of the distal pulp horns
   2. "ribbon-shaped" distal canal

E. **Buccal** view of an **adult** second molar with extensive secondary dentin formation. A radiograph will reveal:
   1. pulp recession and a "thread-like" pulp
   2. mesial and distal roots, each **apparently** containing one canal
   3. "straight" distal root (58%) and distal curvature of the mesial root (84%)
   4. distal-axial inclination of the **tooth**

F. **Mesial** view of the same tooth demonstrating details **not apparent in the original radiograph:**
   1. pulp recession
   2. **mesial** root with **two** canals that join and "cross over"
   3. minus 52-degree buccal-axial inclination of the roots

   The operator should recognize that
   a. careful exploration with curved instruments is imperative.
   b. mesial canals curve in two directions.

G. Cross-section at three levels: 1, cervical; 2, midroot; and 3, apical third:
   1. **Cervical** level: the chamber is débrided during coronal cavity preparation with a round bur.
   2. **Midroot** level: the canals, only slightly ovoid in shape, will be enlarged by step-back filing of the apical third of the canals.
   3. **Apical third** level: the canals are round and are shaped into **round, tapered** preparations. Preparations terminate at the cementodentinal junction, 0.5 to 1.0 mm from the radiographic apex.

H. **Distal** view of the same tooth demonstrating details **not apparent in the radiograph:**
   1. pulp recession
   2. single distal root with a usual single canal
   3. buccal-axial inclination of the tooth

I. Triangular outline form reflects the anatomy of the pulp chamber. Both mesial and distal walls slope mesially. The cavity is primarily within the mesial half of the tooth but is extensive enough to allow positioning of instruments and filling materials. Further exploration should determine whether a fourth canal can be found in the distal. In that case, an orifice will be found at each angle of the rhomboid.

PLATE 26

Mandibular Second Molars

Length of Tooth	*Mesial*	*Distal*
Average Length	20.9 mm	20.8 mm
Maximum Length	22.6 mm	22.6 mm
Minimum Length	19.2 mm	19.0 mm
Range	3.4 mm	3.6 mm

	Canals	
	Mesial	*Distal*
One canal	13%	92%
One foramen		
Two canals	49%	5%
One foramen		
Two canals	38%	3%
Two foramina		

	Curvature of roots		
	Single	*Double Root*	
Direction	*Root*	*Mesial*	*Distal*
Straight	53%	27%	58%
Distal Curve	26%	61%	18%
Mesial Curve	0%	0%	10%
*Buccal Curve	0%	4%	4%
*Lingual Curve	2%	0%	0%
Bayonet Curve	19%	7%	6%

*Not apparent in radiograph

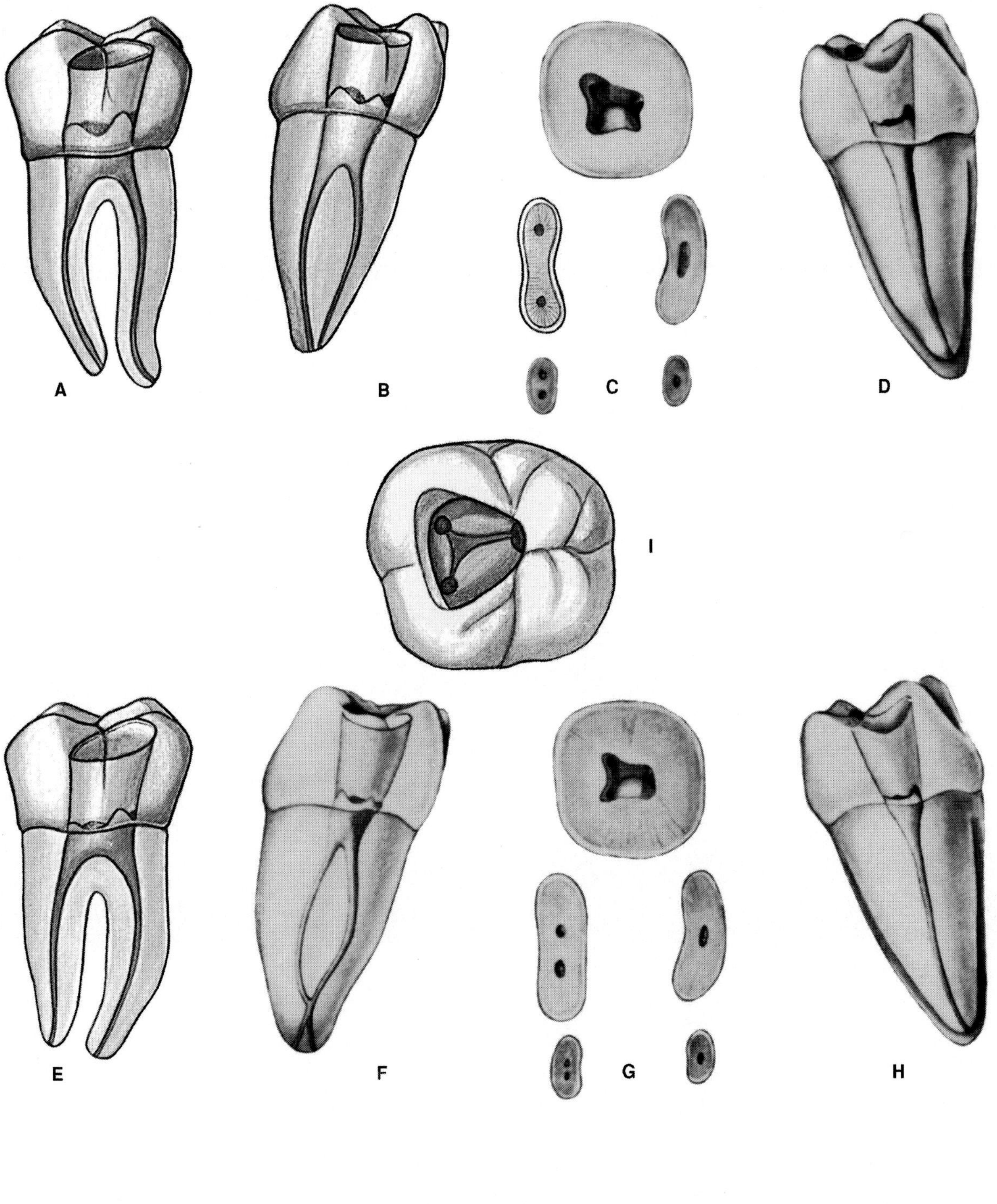

A B C D

I

E F G H

PLATE 27

Mandibular Molar Teeth

ERRORS in Cavity Preparation

A. OVEREXTENDED preparation undermining enamel walls. The crown is badly gouged owing to failure to observe pulp recession in the radiograph.

B. PERFORATION into furca caused by using a longer bur and failing to realize that the narrow pulp chamber had been passed. The bur should be measured against the radiograph and the depth to the pulpal floor marked on the shaft with Dycal.

C. PERFORATION at the mesial-cervical caused by failure to orient the bur with the long axis of the molar severely **tipped** to the mesial.

D. DISORIENTED occlusal outline form exposing only the mesiobuccal canal. A faulty cavity has been prepared in full crown, which was placed to "straighten up" a lingually tipped molar (D^1).

E. FAILURE to find a **second distal** canal owing to lack of exploration for a fourth canal.

F. LEDGE FORMATION caused by faulty exploration and using too large of an instrument.

G. PERFORATION of the curved distal root caused by using a large straight instrument in a severely curved canal.

PLATE 27

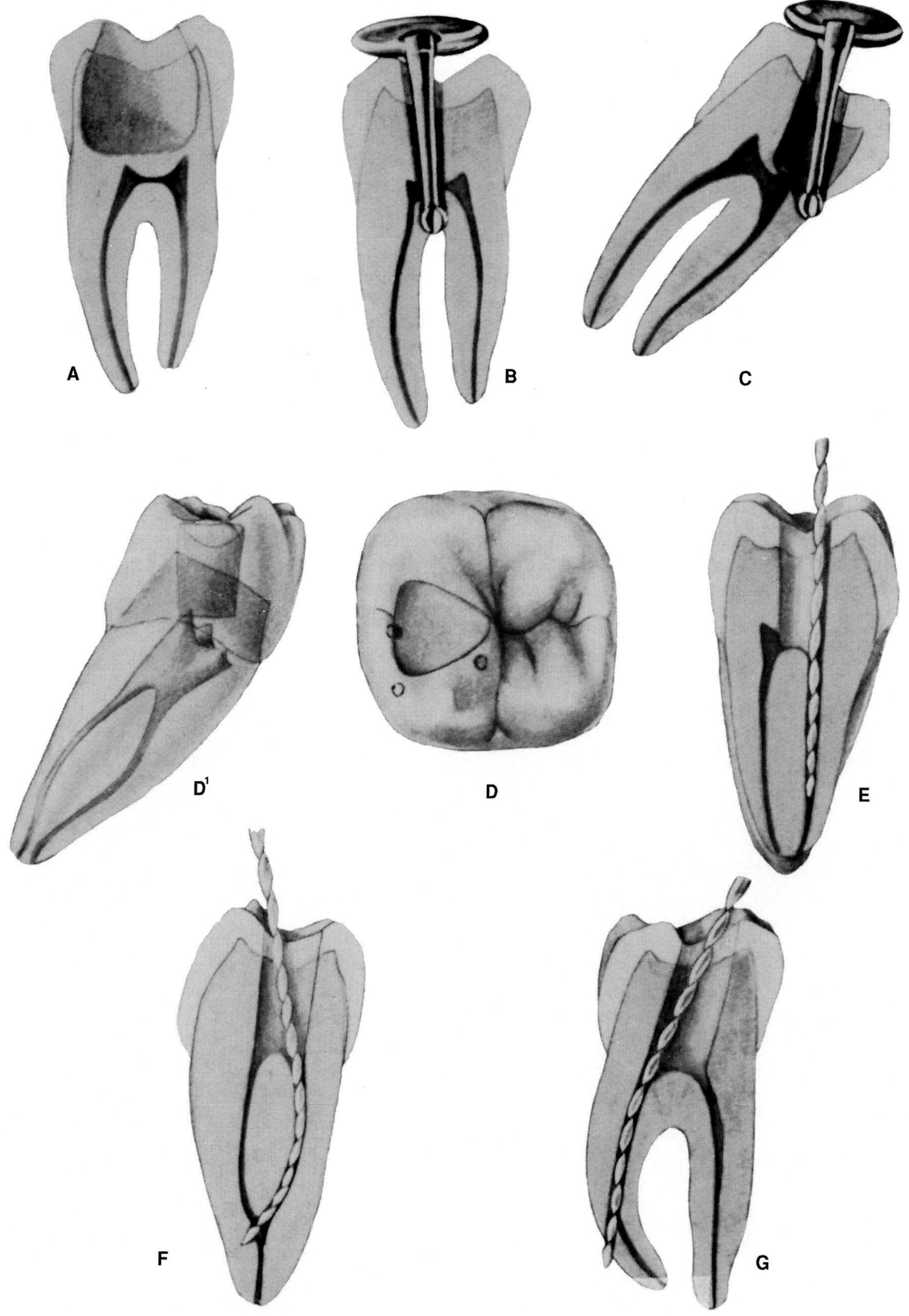

RADICULAR CAVITY PREPARATION

Objectives

With the completion of the coronal access cavity, preparation of the **radicular** cavity may be started. Root canal preparation has two objectives: thorough débridement of the root canal system and the specific shaping of the root canal preparation to receive a specific type of filling. A major objective, of course, is the **total obturation** of this designed space. The ultimate objective, however, should be to create an environment in which the body's immune system can produce healing of the apical periodontal attachment apparatus.

Cleaning and Débridement of the Root Canal

The first objective is achieved by skillful instrumentation coupled with liberal irrigation. This double-pronged attack will eliminate most of the bacterial contaminants of the canal as well as the necrotic debris and dentin.[46] In addition to débridement, remaining bacteria have long been controlled by intracanal medication. This is still true today even though many dentists, as well as endodontists, merely seal a dry cotton pellet in the chamber in multiappointment cases. This practice cannot be recommended, and the reader is urged to read chapter 2, which deals in detail with the importance of intracanal medication. Single-appointment treatment, of course, precludes interappointment medication.

Cleaning and sanitizing the root canal have been likened to the removal of carious dentin in a restorative preparation—that is, enough of the dentin wall of the canal must be removed to eliminate the attached necrotic debris and, insofar as possible, the bacteria and debris found in the dentinal tubuli (Figure 10-8). Along with repeated irrigation, the débriding instruments must be constantly cleaned. A sterile 2 × 2 gauze square soaked in alcohol is used to wipe the instruments.[47]

Preparing the Root Canal

Over the years, two different approaches to root canal cleaning and shaping have emerged: the **"step-back"** and the **"step-down"** preparations. The **step-back** preparation is based upon the traditional approach: beginning the preparation at the apex and working back up the canal coronally with larger and larger instruments. The **step-down** preparation, often called "the crown-down approach," begins coronally and the preparation is advanced apically, using smaller and smaller instruments, finally terminating at the apical stop. All of the techniques of canal cleaning and shaping, including those modified by new instruments or devices, will use variations of either a step-back or a

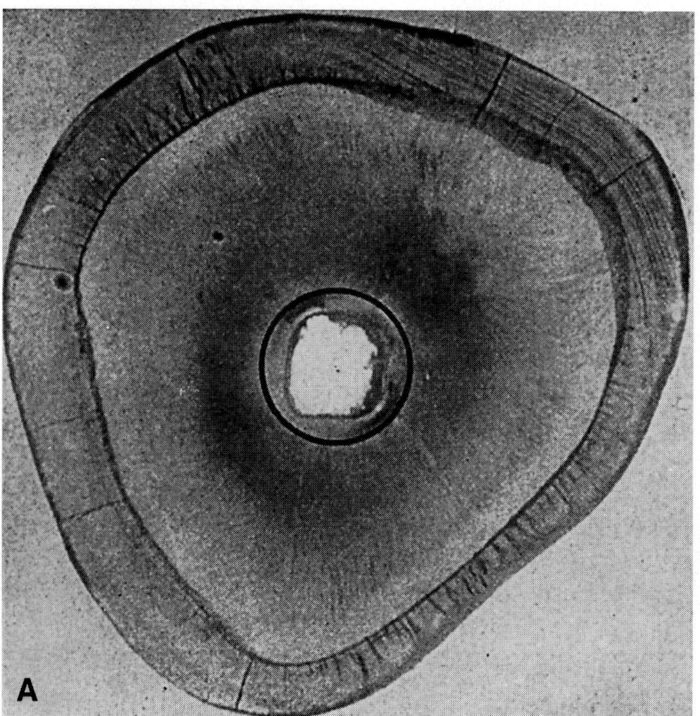

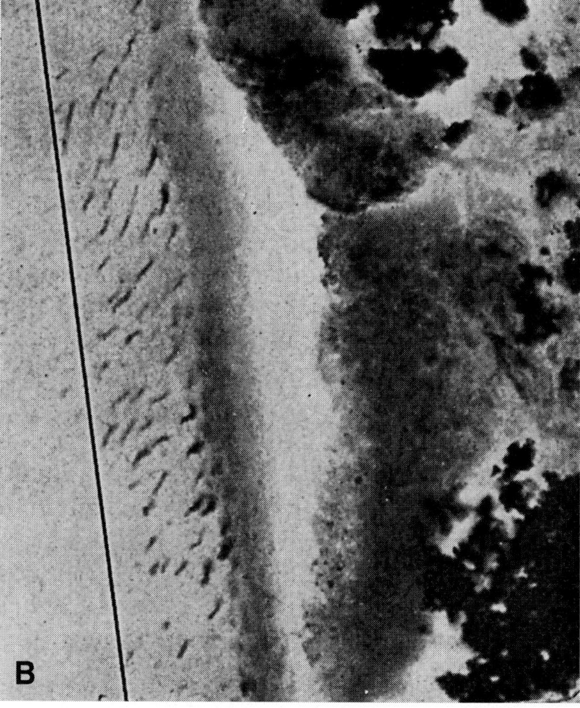

Figure 10-8 **A,** Cross-section through pulp canal showing ideal round preparation to remove canal debris and enough dentin to eliminate virtually all bacteria in the tubuli. **B,** Serial section showing necrotic canal contents and debris-saturated dentin. Débridement of necrotic mass and instrumentation of the dentin to the black line are the goals of instrumentation.

step-down approach. In either event, certain principles of cavity preparation (in this case, radicular and coronal) must be followed to ensure thorough cleaning and proper shaping for obturation.

Principles

Once again, as expounded for coronal cavity preparation, a return to Black's **Principles of Cavity Preparation** is in order.[1] The root canal "cavity" is prepared with the same principles in mind:

- Outline Form
- Convenience Form
- Toilet of the cavity
- Retention Form
- Resistance Form
- Extension for prevention

Figure 10-9 repeats the entire endodontic cavity preparation, from **Outline Form** beginning at the enamel's edge to **Resistance Form** at the apical foramen. In some preparations, **Retention Form** may be developed in the last 2 to 3 mm of the apical canal. Usually, however, the preparation is a **continuous tapered preparation** from crown to root end.

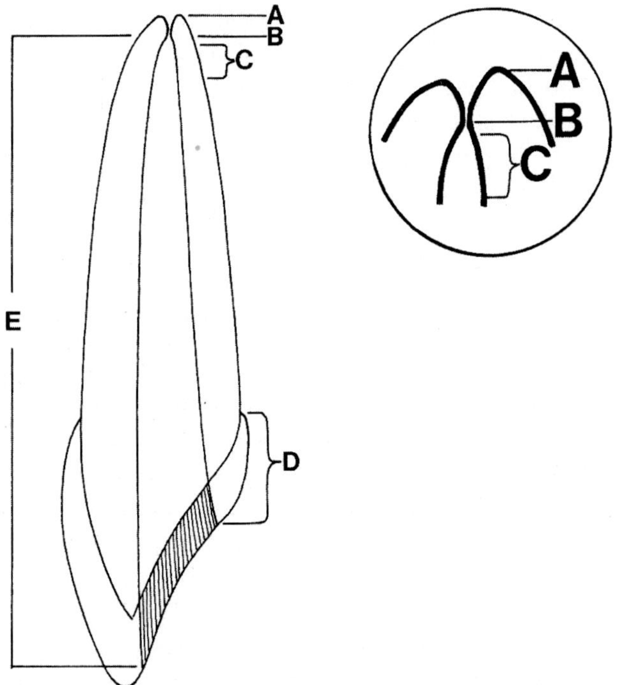

Figure 10-9 Concept of total endodontic cavity preparation, coronal and radicular as a continuum, based on **Black's principles.** Beginning at apex: A, Radiographic apex. B, **Resistance Form,** development of "apical stop" at the cementodentinal junction against which filling is to be compacted and to resist extrusion of canal debris and filling material. C, **Retention Form,** to retain primary filling point. D, **Convenience Form,** subject to revision as needed to accommodate larger, less flexible instruments. External modifications change the **Outline Form.** E, **Outline Form,** basic preparation throughout its length dictated by canal anatomy.

The entire length of the cavity falls under the rubric **Outline Form** and **toilet of the cavity.** At the coronal margin of the cavity, the **Outline Form** must be continually evaluated by monitoring the tension of the endodontic instruments against the margins of the cavity. **Remember** to retain control of the instruments; they must stand free and clear of all interference. Access may have to be expanded (**Convenience Form**) if instruments start to bind, especially as larger, less flexible instruments are used.

The size and shape of the entire preparation will be governed by the anatomy of the root canal. One attempts to retain this basic shape while thoroughly cleaning and flaring to accommodate the instruments and filling materials used in débridement and obturation.

The entire preparation, crown to apex, may be considered **extension for prevention** of future periradicular infection and inflammation.

Outline Form and Toilet of the Cavity

Meticulous cleaning of the walls of the cavity until they feel glassy-smooth, accompanied by continuous irrigation, will ensure, as far as possible, thorough débridement. One must realize, however, that total débridement is not possible in some cases, that some "nooks and crannies" of the root canal system are virtually impossible to reach with any device or system.[48] One does the best one can, recognizing that in spite of microscopic remaining debris, success is possible. Success depends to a great extent on whether unreachable debris is laden with viable bacteria that have a source of substrate (accessory canal or microleakage) to survive—hence the importance of thorough douching through irrigation, **toilet of the cavity.**[49]

Retention Form

In some filling techniques, it is recommended that the initial primary gutta-percha point fit tightly in the apical 2 to 3 mm of the canal. These nearly parallel walls (**Retention Form**) ensure the firm seating of this principal point. Other techniques strive to achieve a continuously tapering funnel from the apical foramen to the cavosurface margin. Retention Form in these cases is gained with custom-fitted cones and warm compaction techniques.

These final 2 to 3 mm of the cavity are the most crucial and call for meticulous care in preparation. This is where the sealing against future leakage or percolation into the canal takes place. This is also the region where accessory or lateral canals are most apt to be present.

Coronally, from the area of retention, the cavity walls are deliberately flared. The degree of flare will vary according to the filling technique to be used—lateral compaction with cold or warm gutta-percha or vertical compaction of heat-softened gutta-percha.

Resistance Form

Resistance to overfilling is the primary objective of **Resistance Form.** Beyond that, however, maintaining the integrity of the natural constriction of the apical foramen is a key to successful therapy. Violating this integrity by overinstrumentation leads to complications: (1) acute inflammation of the periradicular tissue from the injury inflicted by the instruments or bacteria and/or canal debris forced into the tissue, (2) chronic inflammation of this tissue caused by the presence of a foreign body—the filling material forced there during obturation, and (3) the inability to compact the root canal filling because of the loss of the limiting apical termination of the cavity—the important ***apical stop***. This could be compared to an attempt to place a Class II amalgam filling without the limiting presence of a proximal matrix band.

Establishing Apical Patency

Bearing in mind that canal preparations should terminate at the dentinocemental junction, slightly short of the apex, one is left with a tiny remaining portion of the canal that has not been properly cleaned and may contain bacteria and packed debris. It is this section of the canal that is finally cleaned, not shaped, with fine instruments—No. 10 or 15 files. This action is known as ***establishing apical patency.*** It should not be confused with overenlargement—destroying the apical foramen. Cailleteau and Mullaney surveyed all dental schools in the United States to determine the prevalence of teaching apical patency. They found that 50% of the 49 schools responding teach the concept.[50]

In some cases—youngsters, root fractures, apical root resorption—the apical foramen is open, and these cases always present difficulties in instrumentation and obturation. Special techniques, to be discussed later, have been devised to overcome the loss of resistance form.

In Mexico, Kuttler has shown that the narrowest waist of the apical foramen often lies at the dentinocemental junction (Figure 10-10).[51] He established this point at approximately 0.5 mm from the outer surface of the root in most cases. The older the patient, however, the greater this distance becomes because continued cemental formation builds up the apex. One is also reminded that the dentinocemental junction, where **Resistance Form** may be established, is the apical termination of the pulp. Beyond this point, one is dealing with the tissues of the periodontal ligament space, not the pulp.

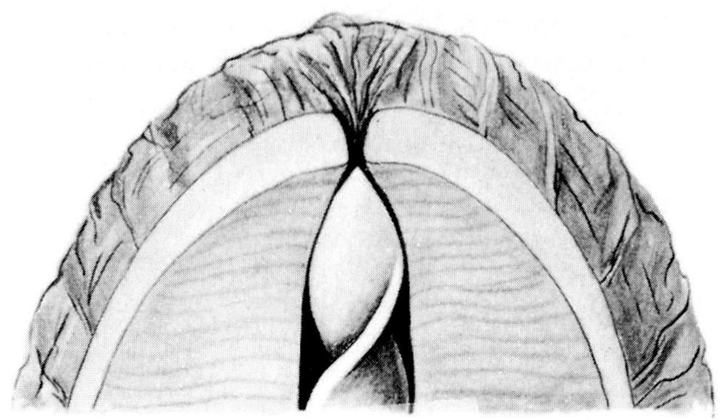

Figure 10-10 Instruments and filling material should terminate short of the cementodentinal junction, the narrowest width of the canal, and its termination at the foramen. This point is often 0.5 to 1.0 mm from the apex.

The fact must also be established that the apical **foramen** does not always lie at the exact apex of the root. Most often, canals exit laterally, short of the radiographic apex. This may be revealed by careful scrutiny of the film with a magnifying glass or by placing a curved exploratory instrument to the exact **canal** length and repeating the radiograph examination. Japanese researchers reported from a native cohort that the apical foramen exits the exact apex only 16.7% of the time in maxillary anterior teeth.[52]

Extension for Prevention

Seidler once described the **ideal** endodontic cavity as a round, evenly tapered space with a minimal opening at the foramen.[53] Because one is working with round, tapered materials, one would think that this ideal is easily achieved, particularly when one thinks of root canals as naturally round and tapered. As seen in the anatomic drawings in this chapter, however, few canals are round throughout their length. Thus, one must usually compromise from the ideal, attempting to prepare the round, tapered cavity but knowing that filling techniques must be used to make up for the variance from ideal. This is why single-point fillings, whether silver or gutta-percha, are seldom used.

The **extension** of the cavity preparation throughout its entire length and breadth is necessary, however, to ensure **prevention** of future problems. Peripheral enlargement of the canal, to remove all of the debris, followed by total obturation is the primary preventive method.

INSTRUMENTS AND METHODS FOR RADICULAR CLEANING AND SHAPING

Before launching into a detailed or even a broad discussion of the methods and shapes of canal cavity preparation, a description of the instruments and methods used in cleaning and shaping the canal is necessary. "The order of their appearance" during preparation will also be discussed: basic endodontic instruments, irrigation, exploration for canal orifices, exploration of the canal, and length of tooth determination. Then the techniques of intraradicular cavity preparation will follow in detail. Pulpectomy is discussed later.

Basic Endodontic Instruments

After years of relative inactivity, a remarkable upsurge in endodontic instrument design and refinement has recently developed. Historically, very little was done to improve the quality or standardization of instruments until the 1950s, when two research groups started reporting on the sizing, strength, and materials that went into hand instruments.[54–57] After the introduction of standardized instruments,[57] about the only changes made were the universal use of stainless rather than carbon steel and the addition of smaller (Nos. 6 and 8) and larger (No. 110 to 140) sizes as well as color coding and the re-emergence of power-driven instruments.

By 1962, a working committee on standardization had been formed including manufacturers, the American Association of Endodontists (AAE), and the American Dental Association (ADA). This group evolved into the present-day International Standards Organization (ISO). It was not until 1976, however, that the first approved specification for root canal instruments was published (ADA Specification No. 28), 18 years after Ingle and Levine first proposed standardization in 1958.[56]

Endodontic Instrument Standardization

Before 1958, endodontic instruments were manufactured without benefit of any established criteria. Although each manufacturer used what seemed to be a unified size system, the numbering (1 through 6) was entirely arbitrary. An instrument of one company rarely coincided with a comparable instrument of another company. In addition, there was little uniformity in quality control or manufacture, no uniformity existed in progression from one instrument size to the next, and there was no correlation of instruments and filling materials in terms of size and shape.

Beginning in 1955, a serious attempt was made to correct these abuses, and in 1959, a new line of standardized instruments and filling material was introduced to the profession[56]:

1. A formula for the diameter and taper in each size of instrument and filling material was agreed on.
2. A formula for a graduated increment in size from one instrument to the next was developed.
3. A new instrument numbering system based on instrument metric diameter was established.

After initial resistance by many manufacturers, who felt that the change would entail a "considerable investment in new dies and machinery to produce them," all manufacturers, worldwide, eventually accepted the new sizing.

This numbering system, last revised in 2002,[58] using numbers from 6 to 140, was not just arbitrary but was based on the diameter of the instruments in hundredths of a millimeter at the beginning of the tip of the blades, a point called D0 (diameter 1) (Figure 10-11), and extending up the blades to the most coronal part of the cutting edge at D16 (diameter 2)—16 mm in length. Additional revisions are under way to cover instruments constructed with new materials, designs, and tapers greater than 0.02 mm/mm.

At the present time, instruments with a **taper greater** than the ISO 0.02 mm/mm have become popular: **0.04,**

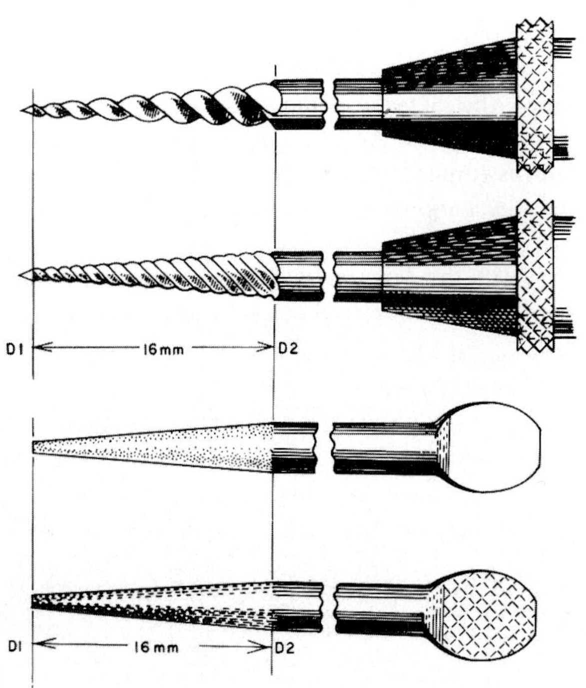

Figure 10-11 Original recommendation for **standardized instruments.** Cutting blades 16 mm in length are of the same size and numbers as standardized filling points. The number of the instrument is determined by diameter size at D_1 in hundredths of millimeters. Diameter 2 (D_2) is uniformly 0.32 mm greater than D_1. Reproduced with permission from Ingle JI. In: Grossman LI, editor. Transactions of the Second International Conference on Endodontics. Philadelphia: University of Pennsylvania; 1958. p. 123.

0.06, and 0.08. This means that for every millimeter gain in the length of the cutting blade, the width (taper) of the instrument increases in size by 0.04, 0.06, and 0.08 of a millimeter rather than the ISO standard of 0.02 mm/mm. These new instruments allow for greater coronal flaring than the 0.02 instruments.

In contrast to these widened-flare files, a number of manufacturers have issued **half sizes** in the 0.02 flare—2.5, 17.5, 22.5, 27.5, 32.5, and 37.5—to be used in shaping extremely fine canals.

The full extent of the shaft, up to the handle, comes in three lengths: standard, 25 mm; long, 31 mm; and short, 21 mm. The long instruments are often necessary when treating canines over 25 mm long. Shorter instruments are helpful in second and third molars or in the patient who cannot open widely. Other special lengths are available, such as the popular 19 mm instrument.

Ultimately, to maintain these standards, the AAE urged the ADA and the United States Bureau of Standards to appoint a committee for endodontic instrument standardization. A committee was formed and, after considerable work and several drafts, produced a specification package that slightly modified and embellished Ingle's original standardization.[57] These pioneering efforts reached international proportions when a worldwide collaborative committee was formed: the ISO, consisting of the *Fédération Dentaire International,* the World Health Organization, and the ADA Instrument Committee. The ISO has now formulated international specifications using the ADA proposal as a model.

In 1989, the American National Standards Institute (ANSI) granted approval of "ADA Specification No. 28 for endodontic files and reamers" (Figure 10-12). It established the requirements for diameter, length, resistance to fracture, stiffness, and resistance to corrosion. It also included specifications for sampling, inspection, and test procedures.[58] The revision to ADA Specification No. 28 for K-type files and reamers highlighted 30 years of work to achieve international standardization (Table 10-1). Since then, Specification No. 28 has been modified again (1996), and still another revision is in progress.

The ANSI/ADA standards have also been set for other instruments and filling materials: No. 58, Hedstroem files; No. 63, rasps and barbed broaches; No. 71, spreaders and condensers; No. 95, root canal enlargers; as well as No. 57, filling materials; No. 73, absorbent points; and No.78, obturating points. The ISO's standards are comparable with these specifications (N Luebke, personal communication, March 24, 1999).

Initially, manufacturers of endodontic instruments worldwide adhered rather closely to these specifications. Some variations have been noted, however, in size maintenance (both diameter and taper), surface debris, cutting flute character, torsional properties, stiffness, cross-sectional shape, cutting tip design, and type of metal[59–65] (Figure 10-13). More recently, Stenman and Spangberg were disappointed to note that the dimensions of root canal instruments are becoming poorly standardized and that few brands are now within acceptable dimensional standards.[66]

Cormier et al. and Seto have both warned of the importance of using only one brand of instruments because of discrepancies in instrument size among manufacturers.[61,62] Early on, Seto also noted that grinding the flutes in files rather than twisting them "does not improve the strength or ductility of the instrument…(and) may also create more undesirable fluting defects."[63] Since then, however, grinding has improved and gained importance since all nickel-titanium instruments must be machined, not twisted. Several recent studies have indicated that this type of manufacturing does not weaken instruments. In fact, most studies indicate that both manufacturing processes produce files that meet or exceed ADA standards.[67–69]

It has also been found that autoclaving has no significant deleterious effects on stainless steel or nickel-titanium endodontic instruments.[70–72]

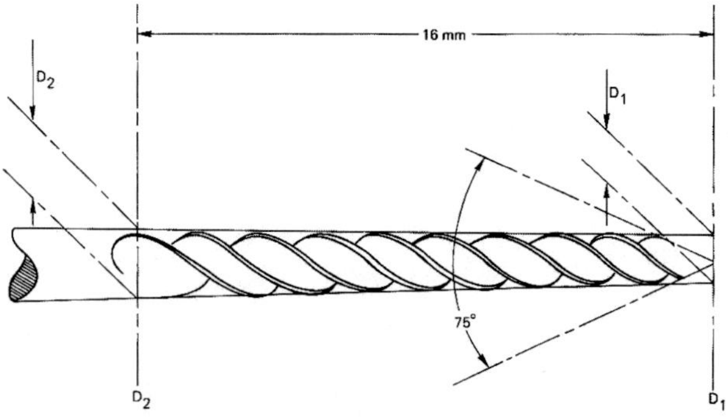

Figure 10-12 Standardized dimensions of root canal files and reamers established by the ISO. Two modifications from Ingle's original proposal are an additional measurement at D_3, 3 mm from D_1, and specification for shapes of the tip: 75 degrees, ± 15 degrees. The taper of the spiral section must be at a 0.02 mm gain for each millimeter of cutting length. Specifications for a noncutting tip are forthcoming.

ISO Grouping of Instruments

In due time, the ISO-*Fédération Dentaire International* committee grouped root canal instruments according to their method of use:

Table 10-1 Dimensions in Millimeters. Revision of ADA Specification No. 28 Added Instrument Sizes 08 and 110 to 150 to the Original Specification

Size	Diameter (Tolerance ± 0.02 mm) D_1 mm	D_2 mm	D_3 mm	Handle Color Code
08	0.08	0.40	0.14	Gray
10	0.10	0.42	0.16	Purple
15	0.15	0.47	0.21	White
20	0.20	0.52	0.26	Yellow
25	0.25	0.57	0.31	Red
30	0.30	0.62	0.36	Blue
35	0.35	0.67	0.41	Green
40	0.40	0.72	0.46	Black
45	0.45	0.77	0.51	White
50	0.50	0.82	0.56	Yellow
55	0.55	0.87	0.61	Red
60	0.60	0.92	0.66	Blue
70	0.70	1.02	0.76	Green
80	0.80	1.12	0.86	Black
90	0.90	1.22	0.96	White
100	1.00	1.32	1.06	Yellow
110	1.10	1.42	1.16	Red
120	1.20	1.52	1.26	Blue
130	1.30	1.62	1.36	Green
140	1.40	1.72	1.46	Black
150	1.50	1.82	1.56	White

*New diameter measurement point (D_3) was added 3 mm from the tip of the cutting end of the instrument. Handle color coding is official.

- **Group I: Hand use only—files,** both **K** type (Kerr) and **H** type (Hedstroem); **reamers, K** type and **U** type; and broaches, pluggers, and spreaders.
- **Group II: Engine-driven** latch type—*same design as Group I* but made to be attached to a handpiece. Also included are paste fillers.
- **Group III: Engine-driven** latch type—**drills** or reamers such as Gates-Glidden (**G** type). Peeso (**P** type), and a host of others—A-, D-, O-, KO-, T-, M-type reamers and the Kurer Root-Facer.
- **Group IV: Root canal points**—gutta-percha, silver, paper.

The ISO grouping of endodontic instruments makes convenient a discussion by group of their manufacture, use, cutting ability, strengths, and weaknesses.

ISO Group I Instruments, Reamers, or Files. First designed as early as 1904 by the Kerr Manufacturing Company (Figure 10-14), K-style files and reamers are the most widely copied and extensively manufactured endodontic instruments worldwide. Now made universally of nickel titanium and stainless steel rather than carbon steel, K-type instruments are produced using one of two techniques. The more traditional is produced by grinding graduated sizes of round "piano" wire into various shapes such as square, triangular, or rhomboid. A second grinding operation properly tapers these pieces. To give the instruments the spirals that provide the cutting edges, the square or triangular stock is then grasped by a machine that twists it counterclockwise a programmed number of times—tight spirals for files, loose spirals for reamers. The cutting blades that are produced are the sharp edges of either the square or the triangle. In any instrument, these edges are known as the "rake" of the blade. The more acute the angle of the rake, the sharper the blade. There are approximately twice the number of spirals on a file than on a reamer of a corresponding size (Figure 10-15, A, B).

The second and newer manufacturing method is to grind the spirals into the tapered wire rather than twist the wire to produce the cutting blades. Grinding is totally necessary for nickel-titanium instruments. Because of their superelasticity, they cannot be twisted.

Originally, the cross-section of the K file was square and the reamer triangular. Recently, manufacturers have started using many configurations to achieve better cutting and/or flexibility. Cross-section is now the prerogative of individual companies.

K-Style Modification. After having dominated the market for 65 years, K-style endodontic instruments came into a series of modifications beginning in the 1980s. Not wholly satisfied with the characteristics of their time-honored K-style instrument, the Kerr Manufacturing Company in 1982 introduced a new instrument design that they termed the **K-Flex File** (Sybron Endo/Kerr; Orange Calif.), a departure from the square and triangular configurations (Figure 10-15, C).

The cross-section of the K-Flex is rhombus or diamond shaped. The spirals or flutes are produced by the same twisting procedure used to produce the cutting edge of the standard K-type files; however, this new cross-section presents significant changes in instrument flexibility and cutting characteristics. The cutting edges of the high flutes are formed by the two acute angles of the rhombus and present increased sharpness and cutting efficiency. The alternating low flutes formed by the obtuse angles of the rhombus are meant to act as an auger, providing more area for increased debris removal. The decreased contact by the instrument with the canal walls provides a space reservoir that, with proper irrigation, further reduces the danger of compacting dentinal filings in the canal.

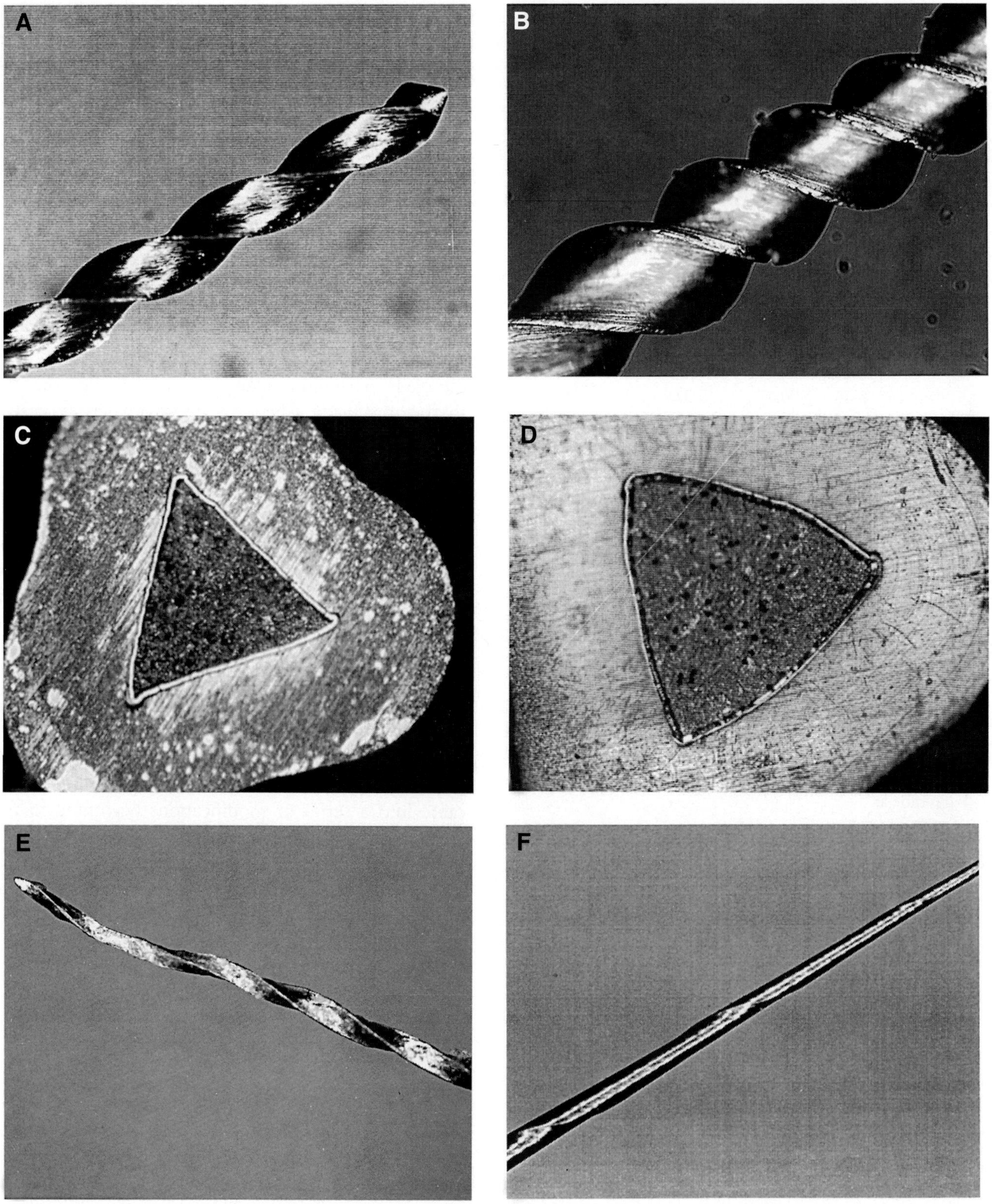

Figure 10-13 Comparisons of the condition of **unused** instruments from different manufacturers. **A**, New No. 30 K file with consistently sharp blades and point. **B**, New No. 35 K file, different brand, exhibiting dull blades. **C**, Cross-sectional profile of triangular No. 20 file showing consistency in angles. **D**, Cross-section of competing No. 20 file with dull, rounded angles of cutting blades. **E**, No. 15 file showing lack of consistency in the blade, reflecting poor quality control. **F**, New No. 08 file with no cutting blades at all.

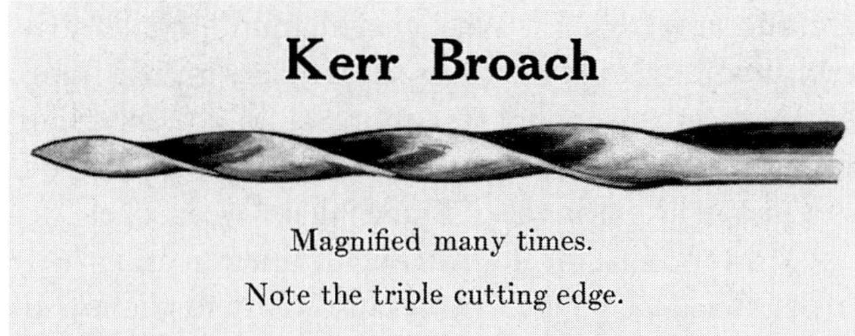

Figure 10-14 Historical illustration, **circa 1904,** of the original **Kerr reamer** (titled a broach at that time), the origin of today's **K-style** instruments. (Courtesy of Kerr Dental Manufacturing Co., 1904 catalog.)

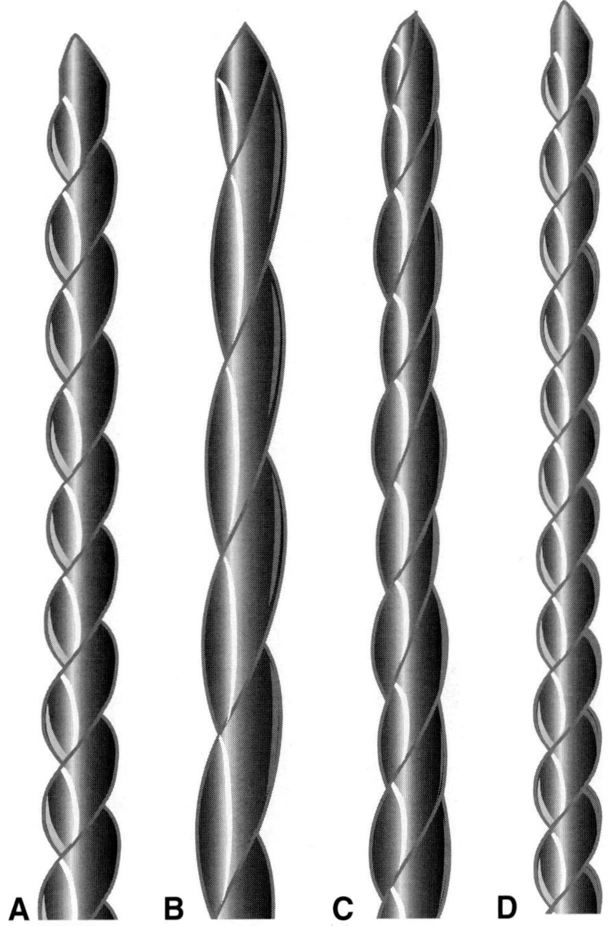

Figure 10-15 ISO Group I, K-style endodontic instruments. **A.** K-style file. **B.** K-style reamer. **C.** K-flex file. **D.** Triple-Flex file with tip modification.

Testing five brands of K-type files for stiffness, the San Antonio group found **K-Flex files** to be the most flexible. Moreover, not a single K-Flex fractured in torque testing, even when twisted twice the recommended level in the ADA specification.[73]

More recently, Kerr has introduced a hybrid instrument they call the **Triple-Flex File (Kerr; Orange, Calif.)** It has more spiral flutes than a K reamer but fewer than a K file. Made from triangular stainless steel and twisted, not ground, the company claims the instrument is more aggressive and flexible than the regular K-style instruments (see Figure 10-15, D).

Reamers. The clinician should understand the importance of differentiating endodontic files and reamers from drills. Drills are used for boring holes in solid materials such as gold, enamel, and dentin. Files, by definition, are used by rasping.

Reamers, on the other hand, are instruments that ream—specifically, a sharp-edged tool for enlarging or tapering holes (see Figure 10-15B). Traditional endodontic reamers cut by being tightly inserted into the canal, twisted clockwise one quarter- to one half-turn to engage their blades into the dentin, and then withdrawn—penetration, rotation, and retraction.[6] The cut is made during retraction. The process is then repeated, penetrating deeper and deeper into the canal. When working length is reached, the next size instrument is used, and so on.

Reaming is the only method that produces a round, tapered preparation, and this only in perfectly straight canals. In such a situation, reamers can be rotated one half-turn before retracting. In a slightly curved canal, a reamer should be rotated only one quarter-turn. More stress may cause breakage. The heavier reamers, however, size 50 and above, can almost be turned with impunity.

Files. The tighter spiral of a file (see Figure 10-15, A) establishes a cutting angle (rake) that achieves its primary action on withdrawal, although it will cut in the push motion as well. The cutting action of the file can be effected in either a filing (rasping) or reaming (drilling) motion. In a filing motion, the instrument is placed into the canal at the desired length, pressure is exerted against the canal wall, and while this pressure is maintained, the rake of the flutes rasps the wall as the instrument is withdrawn without turning. The file need not contact all walls simultaneously. For example, the entire length and circumference of large-diameter canals can be filed by inserting the instrument to the desired working distance and filing circumferentially around all of the walls.

To use a file in a reaming action, the motion is the same as for a reamer—penetration, rotation, and retraction.[6] The file tends to set in the dentin more readily than the reamer and must therefore be treated more gingerly. Withdrawing the file cuts away the engaged dentin.

The tactile sensation of an endodontic instrument "set" into the walls in the canal may be gained by pinching one index finger between the thumb and forefinger of the opposite hand and then rotating the extended finger (Figure 10-16).

To summarize the basic action of files and reamers, it may be stated that either files or reamers may be used to ream out a round, tapered apical cavity but that files are also used as push-pull instruments to enlarge by rasping certain curved canals as well as the ovoid portion of large canals. In addition, copious irrigation and constant cleansing of the instrument are necessary to clear the flutes and prevent packing debris at or through the apical foramen (Figure 10-17).

The subject addressed—how K-style files and reamers work—must logically be followed by asking how well they work. One is speaking here, primarily, about stainless steel instruments.

Oliet and Sorin evaluated endodontic reamers from four different manufacturers and found "considerable variation in the quality, sharpness of the cutting edges, cross sectional configuration, and number of flutes of the 147 different reamers tested." They further found that "triangular cross sectional reamers cut with greater efficiency than do the square cross sectional reamers," but the failure rate of the triangular instruments was considerably higher.[74] Webber et al. found that "instruments with triangular cross sections were initially more efficient but lost sharpness more rapidly than square ones of the same size."[75]

Oliet and Sorin also found that "wear does not appear to be a factor in instrument function, but rather instruments generally fail because of deformation or fracture of the blades. Once an instrument became permanently distorted, additional rotation only caused additional distortion, with minimum cutting frequently leading to fracture."[74] A more recent *in vitro* study of stainless steel files at Connecticut demonstrated that significant wear and potential loss of efficiency occurred after only one use of 300 strokes. They proposed that endodontic instruments should be available in sterile packaging for single-patient use.[76] Another study, from Brazil, concluded that stainless steel instruments, in small sizes, should be used once, and the No. 30 could be used three times. The No. 30 nickel-titanium instruments, however, "even after five times, did not show appreciable abnormalities in shape."[77] Most endodontists use the small instruments, 08 to 25 sizes only once.

Webber et al. used a linear cutting motion in moist bovine bone and found that "there was a wide range of cutting efficiency between each type of root canal instrument, both initially and after successive use."[75]

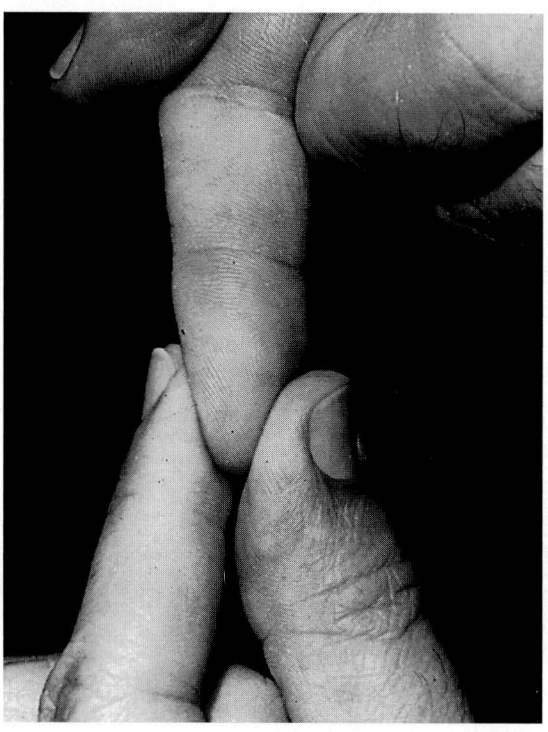

Figure 10-16 Demonstration of sensation of an endodontic instrument, which is "set" into dentin walls during reaming action.

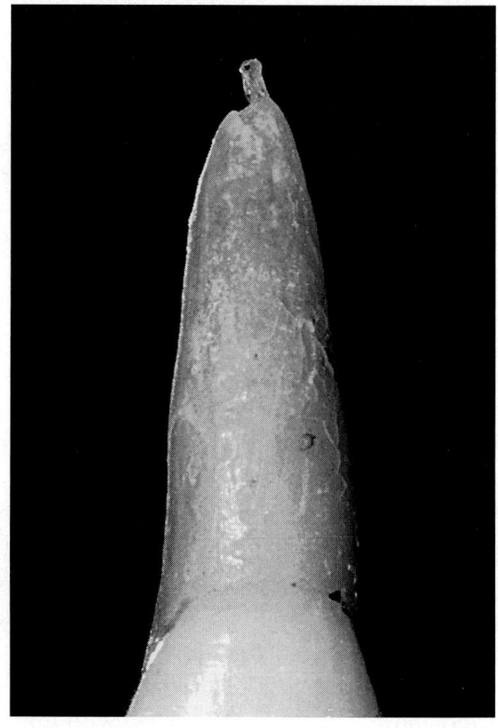

Figure 10-17 "Worm" of necrotic debris forced from the apex during canal enlargement. This mass of material could contain millions of bacteria that act as a nidus for acute apical abscess.

Similar findings were made by a group at Marquette University, who compared K-type files with five recently introduced brands in three different sizes, Nos. 20, 25, and 30.[78] Significant differences were noted in the *in vitro* cutting efficiency among the seven brands. Wear was exhibited by all instruments after three successive 3-minute test periods. Depth of groove is also a significant factor in improving cutting ability (Figure 10-18).

A group of researchers in Michigan also studied the cutting ability of K-type files.[79] They reported a wide variance in the cutting ability of individual files. This study appears to confirm what dentists have long noted—the wide variance in cutting ability among individual instruments, even from the same manufacturer. Contrary to the Marquette findings,[78] this study reported an insignificant role played by wear in decreasing the cutting ability of regular K-type stainless steel files.[79] This speaks of the strength of instruments, but what of their weaknesses?

The Oliet and Sorin,[74] Webber et al.[75] and Neal et al.[79] studies all alluded to certain weaknesses in K-style instruments. In addition, Luks has shown that the smaller reamers and files may be easily broken by twisting the blades beyond the limits of the metal until the metal separated.[80] On the other hand, Gutierrez et al. found that although the instrument did not immediately break, a progression of undesirable features occurred.[81] Locking and twisting clockwise led to unwinding and elongation as well as the loss of blade cutting edge and blunting of the tip. With continued clockwise twisting, a reverse "roll-up" occurred. Cracks in the metal eventually developed that finally resulted in breakage, with all of its attendant problems. These findings were unusual in that breakage would have normally resulted long before "roll-up" occurred. It may reflect a variance in the quality of metal used by the individual manufacturing companies. This point was borne out in a study by Lentine, in which he found a wide range of values within each brand of instrument as well as between brands.[82]

An additional study of 360-degree clockwise rotation (ISO revision of ADA Specification No. 28) found

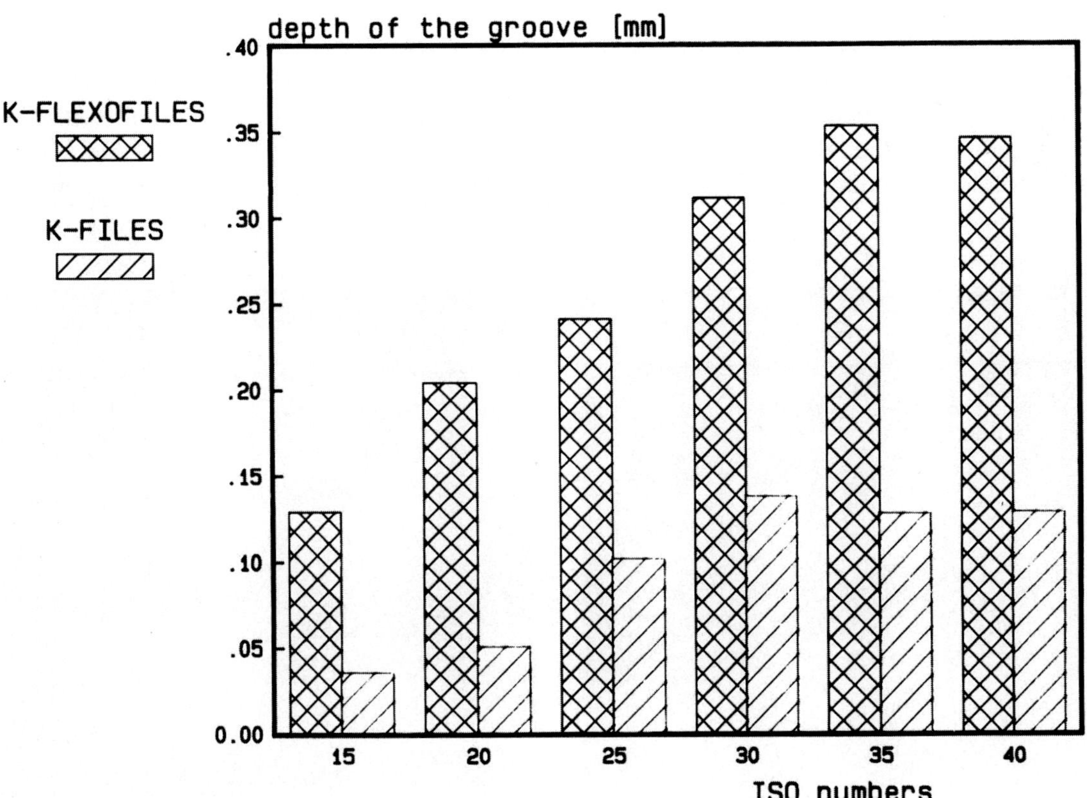

Figure 10-18 Comparison between two competing brands of endodontic instruments showing widely different cutting ability related to the depth of the blade groove.

only 5 K-style files failing of 100 instruments tested. They were sizes 30 to 50, all from one manufacturer.[73]

Attempts to "unscrew" a locked endodontic file also present a problem. Researchers at Northwestern University demonstrated that "endodontic files twisted in a counterclockwise manner were extremely brittle in comparison to those twisted in a clockwise manner."[83] They warned that dentists "should exercise caution when 'backing-off' embedded root canal instruments." This finding was strongly supported by Lautenschlager and colleagues, who found that "all commercial files and reamers showed adequate clockwise torque, but were prone to brittle fracture when placed in counterclockwise torsion."[84]

In contrast, Roane and Sabala at the University of Oklahoma found that clockwise rotation was more likely (91.5%) to produce separation and/or distortion than counterclockwise rotation (8.5%) when they examined 493 discarded instruments.[85] In laboratory tests, the Washington group also found greater rotational failure in clockwise rotation and greater failure in machined stainless steel K files over twisted K files.[63]

Sotokawa in Japan also studied discarded instruments and indicted metal fatigue as the culprit in breakage and distortion[86]: "First a starting point crack develops on the file's edge and then metal fatigue fans out from that point, spreading towards the file's axial center" (Figure 10-19). Sotokawa also classified the types of damage to instruments (Figure 10-20). He found the No. 10 file to be the most frequently discarded.[86]

Montgomery evaluated file damage and breakage from a sophomore endodontics laboratory and also found that most damage (87%) "occurred while filing canals in posterior teeth with #10 stainless files. One file separated for every 3.91 posterior teeth that were filed," and each student averaged over 5 (range 1 to 11) damaged files in the exercise.[87]

A group in France compared instrument fracture between traditional K and H files and the newer "hybrid" instruments. They found that "the instruments with triangular cross sections, in particular the Flexofile (Dentsply/Maillefer; Tulsa, Okla.), were found to be the most resistant to fracture." French researchers, like the Japanese researchers, found starting-point cracks and ductile fracture as well as plastic deformations and axial fractures[88] (Figure 10-21).

A group at the University of Washington compared rotation and torque to failure of stainless steel and nickel-titanium files of various sizes. An interesting relation was noted. Stainless steel had greater rotations to failure in a clockwise direction, and the nickel titanium was superior in a counterclockwise direction. Despite these differences, the actual force to cause failure was the same.[89]

Buchanan, among others, pointed out the importance of bending **stainless steel** files to conform to curved canals. He recommended the use of pliers to make the proper bend.[90] Yesilsoy et al. on the other hand, observed damage (flattening of the flutes) in cotton plier-bent files (Figure 10-22, A). The finger-bent files, however, although not damaged, were coated with accumulated debris-stratified squamous epithelium cells and nail keratin[91] (Figure 10-22, B). Finger-bent files should be bent while wearing washed rubber gloves or between a sterile

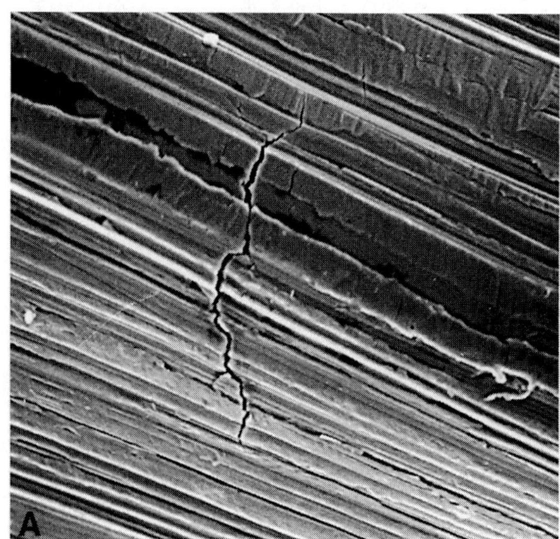

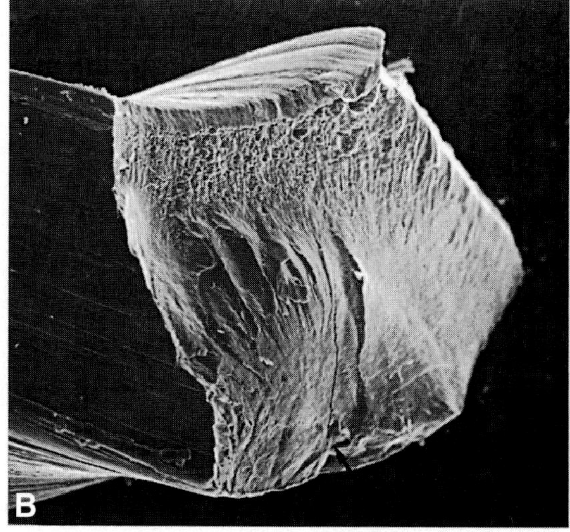

Figure 10-19 Instrument breakage. A, Initial crack across the shaft near the edge of the blade, Type V (original magnification ×1,000). B, Full fracture of file broken in a 30-degree twisting simulation, Type VI (original magnification ×230). Reproduced with permission from Sotokawa T.[86]

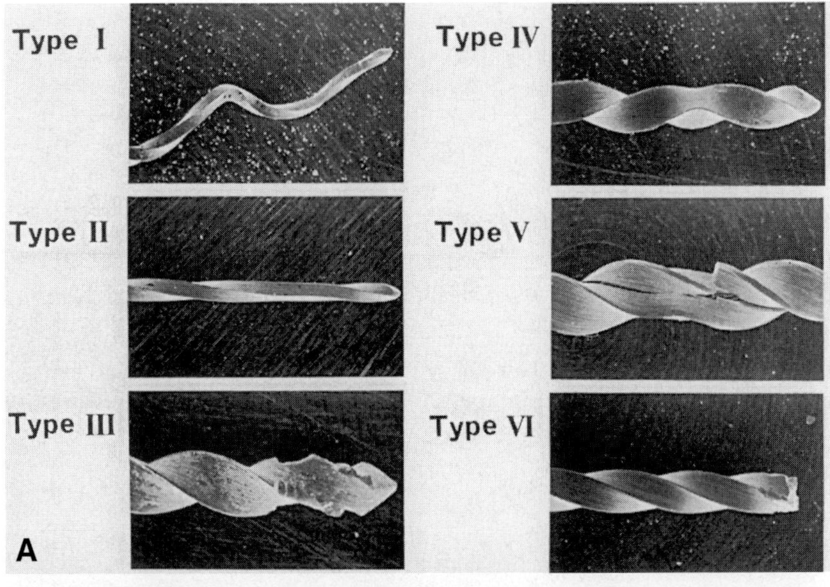

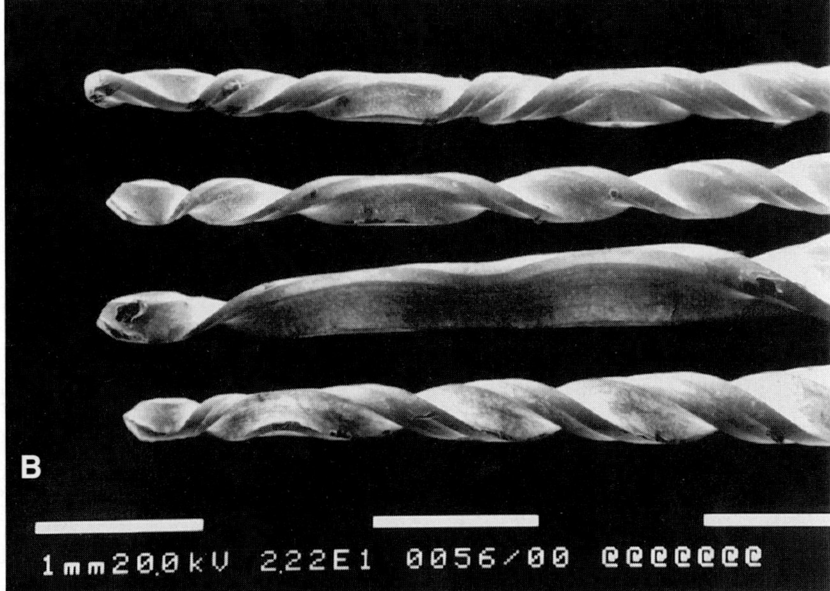

Figure 10-20 A, Sotokawa's classification of instrument damage. Type I, Bent instrument. Type II, Stretching or straightening of twist contour. Type III, Peeling-off metal at blade edges. Type IV, Partial clockwise twist. Type V, Cracking along axis. Type VI, Full fracture. B, Discarded **rotary nickel-titanium files** showing visible defects without fracture. All files show unwinding, indicating a torsional defect, and are very dangerous to be used further. A reproduced with permission from Sotokawa T.[86] B reproduced with permission from Sattapan B, Nervo GJ, Palamara JEA, Messer HH. JOE 2000;26:161.

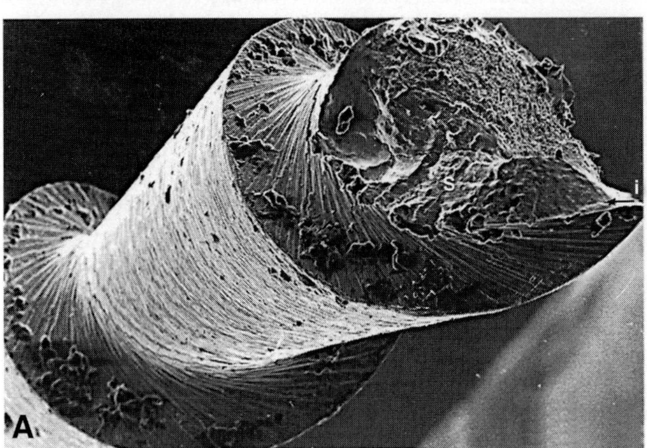

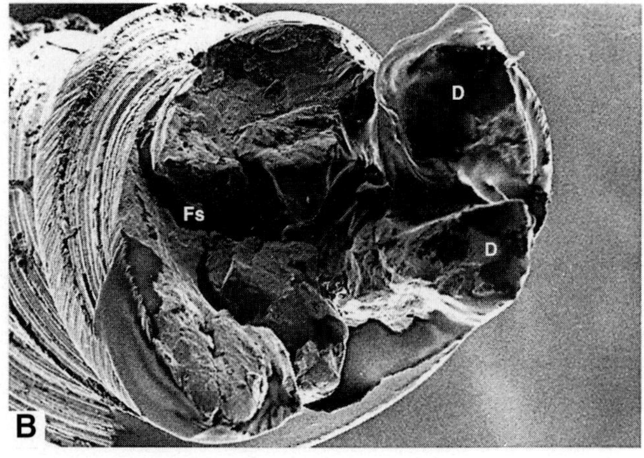

Figure 10-21 Instrument fracture by cracks and deformation. **A**, Broken Hedstroem file with starting point at i (**far right**) spreading to cracks (S) and ductile fracture (F). **B**, Broken K-Flex file with plastic deformations at D and axial fissure at Fs. Reproduced with permission from Haikel Y et al.[88]

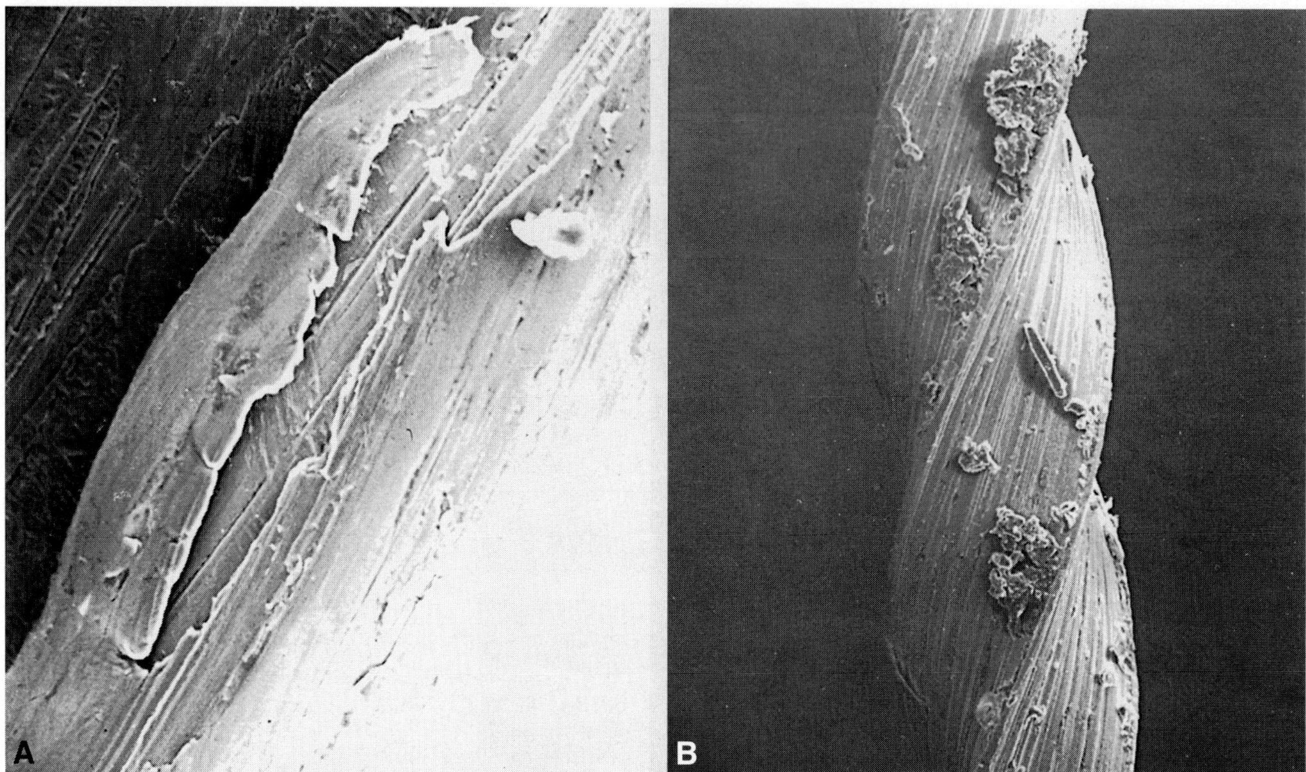

Figure 10-22 Instruments precurved with cotton pliers or fingers. **A**, Cotton plier-precurved No. 25 file with attached metal chips, **left**. Flutes are badly damaged. **B**, Finger-precurved No. 25 file with accumulated cellular debris between flutes. Reproduced with permission from Yesilsoy C et al.[91]

gauze sponge. Maillefer manufactures a hand tool called a Flexobend (Dentsply/Maillefer; Tulsa, Okla.) for properly bending files without damage.

To overcome the problems chronicled above—distortion, fracture, and precurvature—a group at Marquette University suggested that **nickel titanium,** with a very low modulus of elasticity, be substituted for stainless steel in the manufacture of endodontic instruments.[92] On the other hand, the cutting efficiency of the Nitinol #35 K files was only 60% that of matching stainless steel files.[93]

Tip Modification. Early interest in the cutting ability of endodontic instruments centered around the sharpness, pitch, and rake of the blades. By 1980, interest had also developed in the sharpness of the instrument tip and the tip's effect in penetration and cutting as well as its possible deleterious potential for ledging and/or transportation—machining the preparation away from the natural canal anatomy.

The Northwestern University group noted that tip design, as much as flute sharpness, led to improved cutting efficiency.[94] They later designed experiments to exclude tip design because the tip might "overshadow the cutting effects of flute design."[95] Somewhat later, they reported that "tips displayed better cutting efficiency than flutes" and that triangular pyramidal tips outperformed conical tips, which were least effective.[96,97]

At the same time that a pitch was being made for the importance of cutting tips, other researchers, centered around the University of Oklahoma, were redesigning tips that virtually eliminated their cutting ability. Powell et al. began modifying the tips of K files by "grinding to remove the transition angle" from tip to first blade.[98,99] This was an outgrowth of Powell's indoctrination at the University of Oklahoma by Roane et al.'s introduction of the Balanced Force concept of canal preparation.[100]

By 1988, Sabala et al. confirmed previous findings that the modified tip instruments exerted "less transportation and more **inner curvature** preparation. The modified files maintained the original canal curvature better and more frequently than did the unmodified files."[101] These findings were essentially confirmed *in vitro* by Sepic et al.[102] and *in vivo* by McKendry et al.[103]

Powell et al. noted that each stainless steel "file's **metallic memory** to return to a straight position, increases the tendency to transport or ledge and eventually to perforate curved canals."[99] This action takes place on the outer wall, the convex curvature of the canal. They pointed out that when this tip "angle is reduced, the file stays centered within the original canal and cuts all sides (circumference) more evenly." This modified-tip file has been marketed as the **Flex-R-file** (Moyco/Union Broach, Miller Dental; Bethpage, N.Y.) (Figure 10-23).

Recognizing the popularity of modified-tip instruments, other companies have introduced such instruments as **Control Safe** files (Dentsply/Maillefer; Tulsa, Okla.), the **Anti-Ledging Tip** file (Brasseler; Savannah, Ga.), and **Safety Hedstrom** file (Sybron Endo/Kerr; Orange, Calif.).

At the University of Wales, rounded-tipped files were compared with other files with triangular cross-sections and various forms of tip modification. Although the round-tipped files were the least efficient, they prepared canals more safely and with less destruction than did the other files.[104]

Hedstroem Files (aka Hedstrom). H-type files are made by cutting the spiraling flutes into the shaft of a piece of round, tapered, stainless steel wire. Actually, the machine used is similar to a screw-cutting machine. This accounts for the resemblance between the Hedstroem configuration and a wood screw (Figure 10-24, A).

It is impossible to ream or drill with this instrument. To do so locks the flutes into the dentin much as a screw is locked in wood. To continue the drilling action would fracture the instrument. Furthermore, the file is impossible to withdraw once it is locked in the dentin and can be withdrawn only by backing off until the flutes are free. This action also "separates" files.

Hedstroem files cut in one direction only—**retraction**. Because of the very positive rake of the flute design, they are also more efficient as files *per se*.[105–110] French clinicians (Yguel-Henry et al.) reported on the importance of the lubricating effect of liquids on cutting efficiency, raising this efficiency by 30% with H-style files and 200% with K-files.[108] Temple University researchers, however, reported the proclivity that H files have for packing debris at the apex.[106] On the other hand, El Deeb and Boraas found that H files tended **not** to pack debris at the apex and were the most efficient.[110]

Owing to their inherent fragility, Hedstroem files are not to be used in a torquing action. For this reason, ADA Specification No. 28 could not apply, and a new specification, No. 58, has been approved by the ADA and the American National Standards Committee.[111]

H-Style File Modification. McSpadden was the first to modify the traditional Hedstroem file. Marketed as the **Unifile** and **Dynatrak,** these files were designed with two spirals for cutting blades, a double-helix design, if you will. In cross-section, the blades presented an "S" shape rather than the single-helix teardrop cross-sectional shape of the true Hedstroem file.

Unfortunately, breakage studies revealed that the Unifile generally failed the torque twisting test (as did the four other H files tested) based on ISO Specification No. 58.[112] The authors concluded that the specification was unfair to H-style files, that they should not be twisted more than one quarter-turn.[73,112] At this time, Unifiles and Dynatraks are no longer being marketed; however, the **Hyflex file** (Coltene/Whaledent/Hygenic, Mahwah,

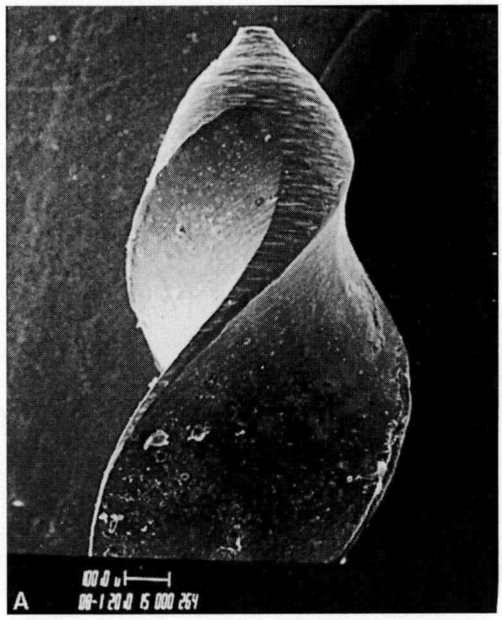

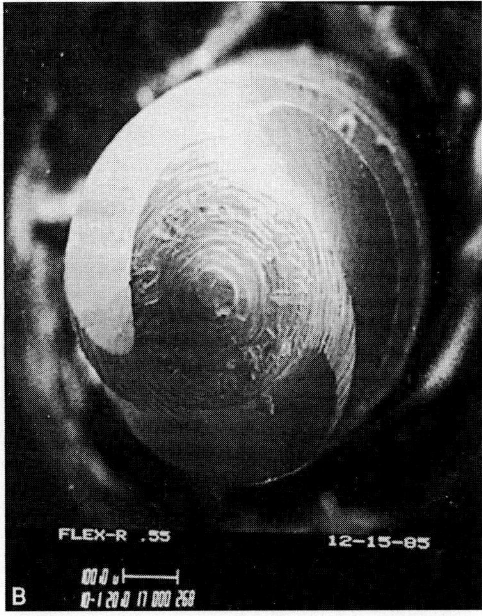

Figure 10-23 **Flex-R-file** with noncutting tip. **A**, Note rounded tip. **B**, "Nose" view of a noncutting tip ensures less gouging of the external wall and reduced cavity transport. (Courtesy of Moyco Union Broach Co.)

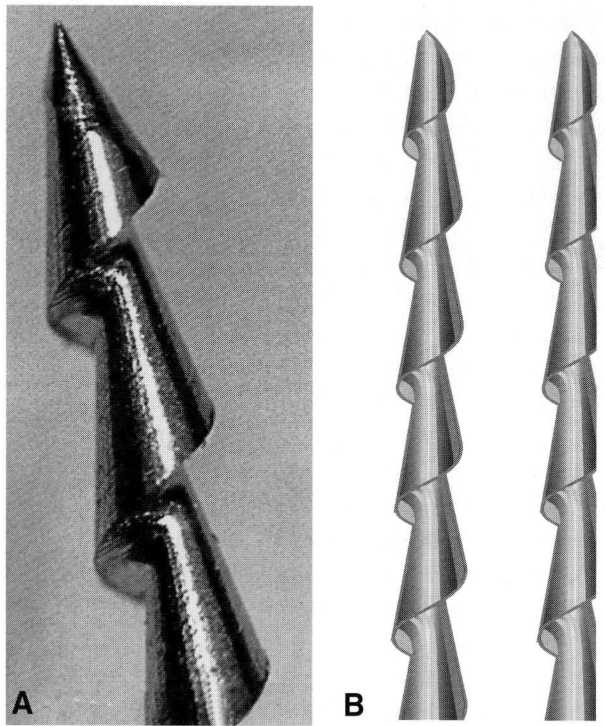

Figure 10-24 ISO Group I, H-style instruments. **A.** Maillefer Hedstroem file resembling a wood screw. **B.** Modified Hedstroem file (**left**) with non-cutting tip. "Safety" Hedstroem (**right**) with flattened non-cutting side to prevent "stripping". A. Reproduced with permission from Keate KC and Wong M.[64]

N.J.) appears to have the same cross-sectional configuration. The **"S" File** (J-S Dental; Ridgefield, Conn.) also appears to be a variation of the Unifile in its double-helix configuration. Reports on this instrument are very favorable.[109,113] Buchanan has further modified the Hedstroem file, the **Safety Hedstrom** (Sybron Endo/Kerr; Orange, Calif.), which has a noncutting side to prevent ledging in curved canals (see Figure 10-24, B right).

The U-File. A new endodontic classification of instrument, for which there is no ISO or ANSI/ADA specification as yet, is the U-File, developed by Heath (personal communication, May 3, 1988) and marketed as **ProFiles**, **GT Files** (Dentsply/Tulsa Dental; Tulsa, Okla.), **LIGHTSPEED** (LightSpeed Technology Inc; San Antonio, Tex.), and **Ultra-Flex** files (Texeed Corp., USA).

The U-File's cross-sectional configuration has two 90-degree cutting edges at each of the three points of the blade (Figure 10-25, A). The flat cutting surfaces act as a planing instrument and are referred to as radial lands. Heath pointed out that the new U shape adapts well to the curved canal, aggressively planing the external convex wall while avoiding the more dangerous internal concave wall, where perforation stripping occurs (Figure 10-25, B). A noncutting pilot tip ensures that the file remains in the lumen of the canal, thus avoiding **transportation** and "zipping" at the apex. The

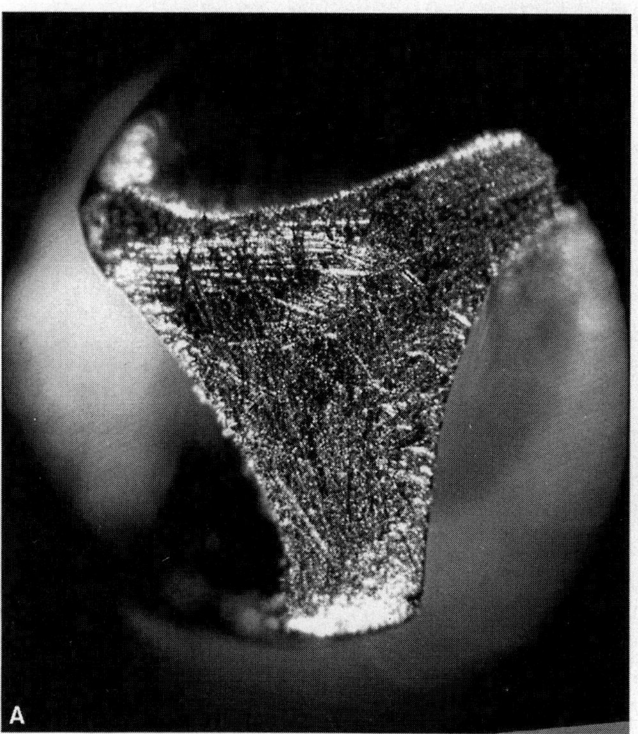

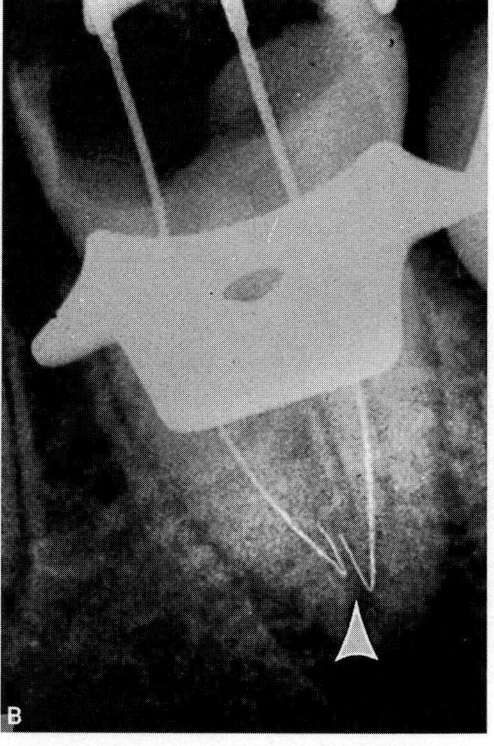

Figure 10-25 A, Cross-sectional view of a **U File** reveals six corners in cutting blades compared with four corners in square stock and three corners in triangular stock K files. **B**, Nickel-titanium U-shaped files in C-shaped molar canals. Note extreme flexibility (**arrow**) without separation. (A courtesy of Derek Heath, Quality Dental Products. **B** courtesy of Dr. John McSpadden.)

files are used in both a push-pull and rotary motion and are very adaptable to nickel-titanium rotary instruments. **ProFiles** are supplied in 0.04, 0.05, 0.06, 0.07, and 0.08 tapers and ISO tip sizes of 15 through 80.

GT ProFiles, developed by Buchanan in the U design, are unusual in that the cutting blades extend up the shaft only 6 to 8 mm rather than 16 mm, and the tapers start at 0.06 mm/mm (instead of 0.02), as well as 0.08 and 0.10, tapered instruments. They are made of nickel titanium and come as hand instruments and rotary files. GT instruments all start with a noncutting tip ISO size 20.

An unusual variation of the **U-shaped** design is the **LIGHTSPEED** instrument[114–117] (Figure 10-26). Made only in nickel titanium, it resembles a Gates-Glidden drill in that it has only a small cutting head mounted on a long, noncutting shaft. It is strictly a rotary instrument but comes with a handle that may be added to the latch-type instrument for hand use in cleaning and shaping abrupt apical curvatures where rotary instruments may be in jeopardy. The instruments come in ISO sizes beginning with No. 20 up to No. 100. Half sizes begin at ISO 22.5 and range to size 65. The heads are very short—only 0.25 mm for the size 20 and up to 1.75 mm for the size 100.

It is recommended that the LIGHTSPEED be used at 1,300 to 2,000 rpm and that the selected rpm remain constant. As with many of the new rotary instruments, this speed calls for a controlled, preferably electric handpiece. One of LIGHTSPEED's touted advantages is the ability to finish the apical-third preparation to a larger size if dictated by the canal diameter. It has been said that "canal diameter, particularly in the apical third, is a forgotten dimension in endodontics" (personal communication, Dr. Carl Hawrish, 1999).

Gates-Glidden Modification. A hand instrument also designed for apical preparation is the **Flexogates**, aka Handygates (Dentsply/Maillefer; Tulsa, Olka.). A safe-tipped variation of the traditional Gates-Glidden drill, the Flexogates is still to be tested clinically, although Briseno et al. compared Flexogates and Canal Master (Brasseler, Savannah, Ga.) *in vitro* and found Flexogates less likely to cause apical transportation (Figure 10-27).[118]

Quantec "Files." The newly designed **Quantec** instrument (Sybron-Endo/Kerr; Orange, Calif.), although called a "file," is more like a reamer—a drill, if you will. It is not designed to be used in the file's push-pull action but rather in the reamer's rotary motion. Produced as both hand- and rotary-powered instruments, the Quantec has proved to be very effective as a powered instrument. First designed by McSpadden, the instrument has undergone a number of modifications that have improved its efficiency and safety. Quantec is produced in three different tapers—0.02, 0.04, and 0.06 mm/mm—as well as safe-cutting and noncutting tips (Figure 10-28). The instruments are sized at the tip and numbered according to the ISO system—15, 20, 25, etc. The radial lands of the Quantec are slightly relieved to reduce frictional contact with the canal wall, and the helix angle is configured to efficiently remove debris.

Hand Instrument Conclusions. The literature is replete with references to the superiority of one instrument or one method of preparation over all others.[110,119–122] Quite true is the statement, "Regardless of the instrument type, none was able to reproduce ideal

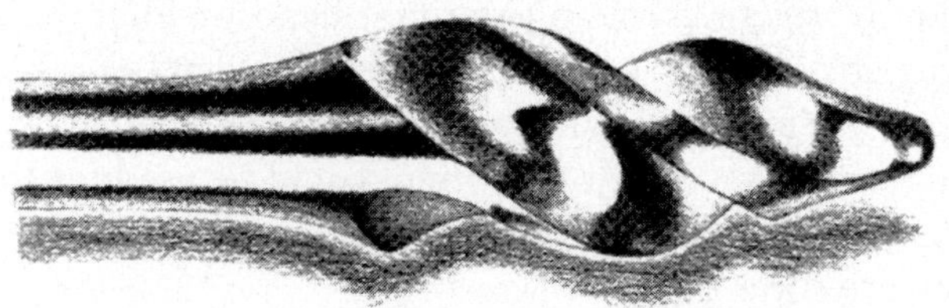

Figure 10-26 The unusual **LightSpeed instrument.** "U" shaped in design with a noncutting tip, the LightSpeed **cutting head** terminates a 16 mm noncutting shaft. Made only in nickel titanium in ISO sizes 20 to 100 and in half sizes as well, they are used in rotary preparations at 2,000 rpm. (Courtesy of LightSpeed Technology Inc.)

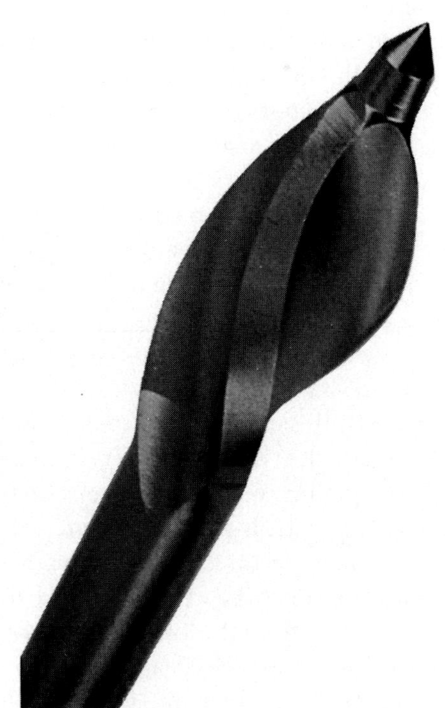

Figure 10-27 **Flexogates** (aka "Handy Gates") **hand**-powered version of a Gates-Glidden drill used to perfect apical cavity preparation. Note the safe noncutting pilot tip. (Courtesy of Dentsply/Maillefer.)

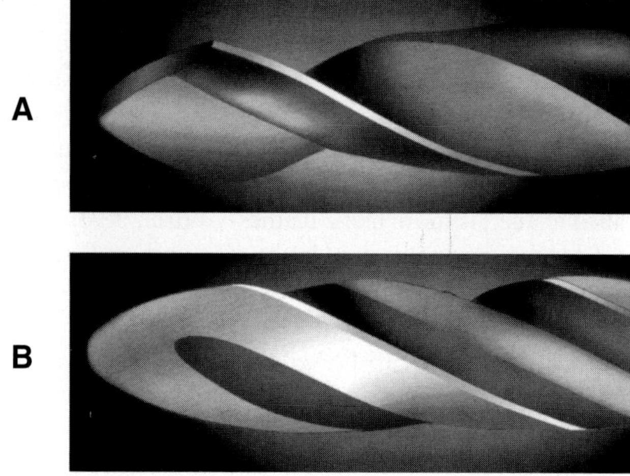

Figure 10-28 **Quantec "files"** are more like a reamer, a drill as it appears, and are used in a rotary motion, not push-pull **A**, Quantec **safe-cutting tip** file. **B**, Quantec **noncutting tip** file. The files are produced in three different tapers: 0.02, 0.04, and 0.06 mm/mm. (Courtesy of Sybron-Endo/Kerr)

results; however, clinically acceptable results could be obtained with all of them."[123] These German authors went on to say, "These observations were subjective and might differ from one operator to another."

All too often clinicians report success with the instruments and technique with which they are most comfortable. No ulterior motive is involved, but often a report reflects badly on an instrument when it is the clinician's inexperience with an unfamiliar technique that is unknowingly being reported. Stenman and Spångberg said it best: it "is difficult to assess, as results from published investigations often vary considerably."[124]

Barbed Broaches. Barbed broaches are short-handled instruments used primarily for vital pulp extirpation. They are also used to loosen debris in necrotic canals or to remove paper points or cotton pellets. ISO Specification No. 63 sets the standards for barbed broaches. Rueggeberg and Powers tested all sizes of broaches from three manufacturers and found significant differences in shape, design, and size, as well as results from torsion and deflection tests.[125] The authors warned that a "jammed broach" should be removed vertically without twisting.

Broaches are manufactured from round wire, the smooth surface of which has been notched to form barbs bent at an angle from the long axis (Figure 10-29, A). These barbs are used to engage the pulp as the broach is carefully rotated within the canal until it begins to meet resistance against the walls of the canal. The broach should never be forced into a canal beyond the length where it first begins to bind. Forcing it farther apically causes the barbs to be compressed by the canal walls. Subsequent efforts to withdraw the instrument will embed the barbs in the walls. Increased withdrawal pressure to retrieve the instrument results in breaking off the embedded barbs or the shaft of the instrument itself at the point of engagement (Figure 10-29, B). A broken barbed broach embedded in the canal wall is seldom retrievable. (Proper use of this instrument will be described in the section on pulpectomy.)

There is also a **smooth broach**, sometimes used as a pathfinder. The newly released **Pathfinder CS** (Sybron-Endo/Kerr; Orange, Calif.), made of carbon steel, is less likely to collapse when forced down a fine canal. Carbon steel will rust and cannot be left in sodium hypochlorite.

NICKEL-TITANIUM ENDODONTIC INSTRUMENTS

A new generation of endodontic instruments, made from a remarkable alloy, nickel titanium, has added a striking new dimension to the practice of endodontics. The superelasticity of nickel titanium, the property that allows it to return to its original shape following significant deformation, differentiates it from other metals, such as stainless steel, that sustain deformation and retain permanent shape change. These properties make nickel-titanium endodontic files more flexible and better able to conform to canal curvature, resist fracture, and wear less than stainless steel files.

History. In the early 1960s, the superelastic property of nickel-titanium alloy, also known as **Nitinol**, was discovered by Buehler and Wang at the US Naval Ordnance Laboratory.[126] The name Nitinol was derived from the elements that make up the alloy, nickel and titanium, and "nol" for the Naval Ordnance Laboratory. The trademark Nitinol refers specifically to the first nickel-titanium wire marketed for orthodontics.

As early as 1975, Civjan and associates[127] reported on potential applications of nickel-titanium alloys containing nickel 55% by weight (55-Nitinol) and nickel 60% by weight (60-Nitinol). They found that the characteristics of 60-Nitinol suggested its use in the fabrication of tough corrosion-resistant hand or rotary cutting instruments or files for operative dentistry, surgery, periodontics, and endodontics. Further, it was suggested that 55- or 60-Nitinol could be used for the manufacture of corrosion-resistant root canal points to replace silver points.

A first potential use of nickel titanium in endodontics was reported in 1988 by Walia and associates.[128] Number 15 files fabricated from nickel-titanium orthodontic alloy were shown to have two or three times the elastic flexibility in bending and torsion, as well as supe-

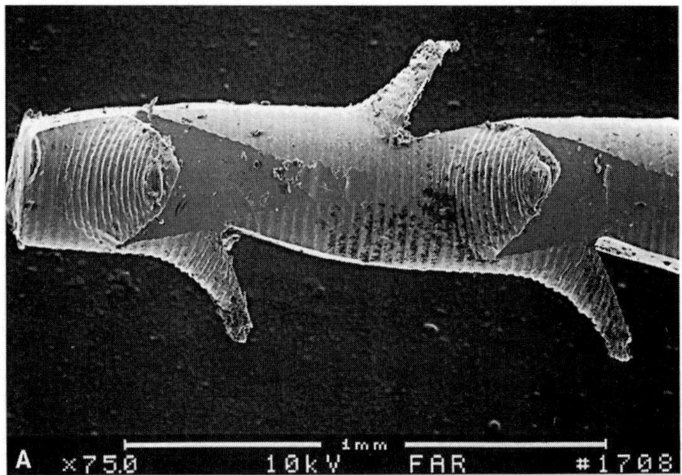

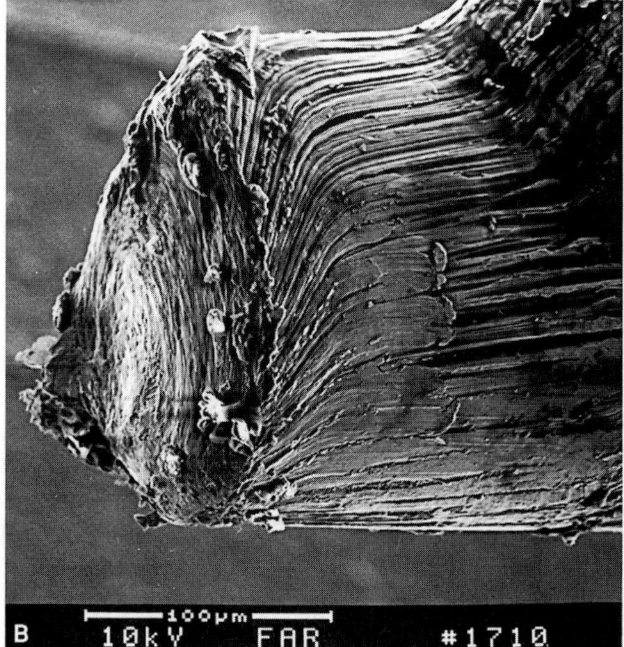

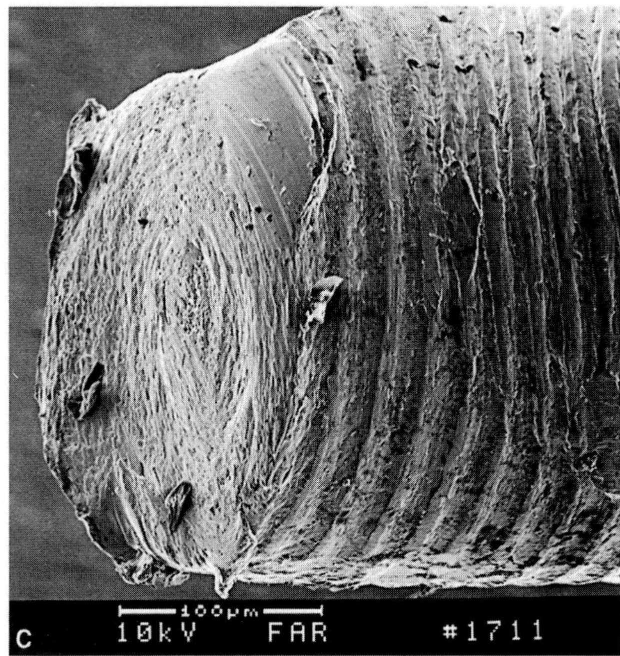

Figure 10-29 A, **Barbed broach.** As a result of a careless barbing process, the effective shaft diameter is greatly reduced. Size "coarse." **B**, Ductile failure of size "xx fine" barbed broach fractured after axial twisting greater than 130 degrees. C, Brittle failure of coarse broach caused by twisting while jammed in place. Reproduced with permission from Rueggeberg FA and Powers JM.[125]

rior resistance to torsional fractures, compared with No. 15 stainless steel files manufactured by the same process. The results suggested that Nitinol files might be promising for the instrumentation of curved canals.

In 1992, a collaborative group made a decision to examine and study the possibility of producing nickel-titanium instruments. The nickel-titanium revolution in endodontics followed, and in May 1992, Serene introduced these new files to students in the College of Dental Medicine at the Medical University of South Carolina. Later these and other similar files became available to the profession generally.

Superelasticity

Alloys such as nickel titanium, that show superelasticity, undergo a stress-induced martensitic transformation from a parent structure, which is austenite. On release of the stress, the structure reverts back to austenite, recovering its original shape in the process. Deformations involving as much as a 10% strain can be completely recovered in these materials, as compared with a maximum of 1% in conventional alloys.

In a study comparing piano wire and a nickel-titanium wire, Stoeckel and Yu found that a stress of 2500 MPa was required to stretch a piano wire to 3% strain, as compared with only 500 MPa for a nickel-titanium wire.[129] At 3% strain, the music wire breaks. On the other hand, the nickel-titanium wire can be stretched much beyond 3% and can recover most of this deformation on the release of stress.

The superelastic behavior of nickel titanium also occurs over a limited temperature window. Minimum residual deformation occurs at approximately room temperature.[129] A composition consisting of 50 atomic percent nickel and 50 atomic percent titanium seems ideal, both for instrumentation and manufacture.

Manufacture. Today, nickel-titanium instruments are precision ground into different designs (K style, Hedstrom, Flex-R, X-double fluted, S-double fluted, U files, and drills) and are made in different sizes and tapers. In addition, spreaders and pluggers are also available. Nickel-titanium instruments are as effective or better than comparable stainless steel instruments in machining dentin, and nickel-titanium instruments are more wear resistant.[130] U and drill designs make it possible to use mechanical (ie, rotary handpiece) instrumentation. Moreover, new prototype rotary motors now offer the potential for improved torque control with automatic reversal that may ultimately decrease rotary instrument breakage.

Finally, nickel-titanium files are biocompatible and appear to have excellent anticorrosive properties.[131] In addition, implantation studies have verified that nickel titanium is biocompatible and acceptable as a surgical implant.[132] In a 1997 AAE questionnaire, the endodontic membership answered the following question, "Do you think nickel-titanium instruments are here to stay and will become basic armamentaria for endodontic treatment?" The responses were quite positive: "yes," 72%; "maybe," 21%; and "no," 4%.[133]

With the ability to machine flutes, many new designs such as radial lands have become available. Radial lands allow nickel-titanium files to be used as reamers in a 360-degree motion as opposed to the traditional reamers with more acute rake angles. Although the most common use of this new design has been as a rotary file, the identical instrument is available as a hand instrument. In addition, a converter handle is available that allows the operator to use the rotary file as a hand instrument.

Torsional Strength and Separation. The clinician switching from stainless to nickel-titanium hand instruments should not confuse nickel titanium's superelastic characteristics with its torsional strength and so assume that it has super strength. This misconception has led to unnecessary file breakage when first using this new metal. Studies indicate that instruments, whether stainless steel or nickel titanium, meet or exceed ANSI/ADA Specification No. 28. However, when reviewing the literature on this subject the results seem to be mixed. Canalda and Berastequi found nickel-titanium files (Nitiflex and Naviflex) (Dentsply; Tulsa, Okla.) to be more flexible than the stainless files tested (Flexofile and Flex-R).[134] However, the stainless steel files were found to be more resistant to fracture. Both types of metal exceeded all ANSI/ADA specifications. Canalda et al., in another study, compared identical instruments: CanalMaster (aka LIGHTSPEED) stainless steel and CanalMaster nickel titanium. Within these designs, the nickel-titanium values were superior in all aspects to those of stainless steel of the same design.[135]

Tepel et al. looked at bending and torsional properties of 24 different types of nickel-titanium, titanium-aluminum, and stainless steel instruments.[136] They found the nickel-titanium K files to be the most flexible, followed in descending order by titanium aluminum, flexible stainless steel, and conventional stainless steel. When testing for resistance to fracture for 21 brands, however, they found that No. 25 stainless steel files had a higher resistance to fracture than their nickel-titanium counterpart.[136]

Wolcott and Himel, at the University of Tennessee, compared the torsional properties of stainless steel K-type and nickel-titanium U-type instruments. As in previous studies, all of the stainless steel instruments showed no significant difference between maximum torque and torque at failure, whereas the nickel-titanium instruments showed a significant difference between maximum torque and torque at failure.[137] Essentially, this means that the time between "wind-up" and fracture in nickel-titanium instruments is extended, which could lead to a false sense of security.

While studying cyclic fatigue using nickel-titanium LIGHTSPEED instruments, Pruett et al. determined that canal curvature and the number of rotations determined file breakage. Separation occurred at the point of maximum curvature of the shaft.[138] Cyclic fatigue should be considered a valid term, even for hand instrumentation, in light of the fact that many manufacturers are placing handles on files designed for rotational use.

From these studies, it seems that if the clinician is changing from a high-torque instrument, such as stainless steel, to a low-torque instrument, such as nickel titanium, it would be wise to know that nickel-titanium instruments are more efficient and safer when used passively.

Although instrument breakage should be rare, any instrument, hand or rotary, can break. It is the clinician's knowledge and experience, along with the manufacturer's quality control, that will ultimately minimize breakage. At both the University of Tennessee and University of California at Los Angeles, breakage has not increased with the routine use of nickel-titanium instruments. If breakage occurs, the fractured piece can occasionally be removed or bypassed using ultrasonics and hand instruments in conjunction with magnification. The dentist having problems with file breakage should seek help in evaluating his technique. One should practice on extracted teeth until a level of confidence is reached that will help ensure safe and efficient patient care.

The following is a list of situations that place nickel-titanium hand instruments at risk along with suggestions for avoiding problems:

Nickel-Titanium Precautions and Prevention

1. Often too much pressure is applied to the file. Never force a file! These instruments require a passive technique. If resistance is encountered, stop immediately, and before continuing, increase the coronal taper and negotiate additional length, using a smaller, 0.02 taper stainless steel hand file. Stainless steel files should be used in sizes smaller than a No. 15. If one is using more finger pressure than that required to break a No. 2 pencil lead, too much pressure is being used. Break a sharp No. 2 pencil lead and see how little pressure is required!
2. Canals that join abruptly at sharp angles are often found in roots such as the mesiobuccal root of maxillary molars, all premolars, and mandibular incisors and the mesial roots of mandibular molars. The straighter of the two canals should first be enlarged to working length and then the other canal, only to where they join. If not, a nickel-titanium file may reverse its direction at this juncture, bending back on itself and damaging the instrument.
3. Curved canals that have a high degree and small radius of curvature are dangerous.[138] Such curvatures (over 60 degrees and found 3 to 4 mm from working length) are often seen in the distal canals of mandibular molars and the palatal roots of maxillary first molars.
4. Files should not be overused! All clinicians have experienced more fracture after files have been used a number of times. Remember that all uses of a file are not equal. A calcified canal stresses the file more than an uncalcified canal. A curved canal stresses the file more than a straight canal. One must also bear in mind operator variability and the use of lubricants, which will affect stress.

   Consider discarding a file after abusive use in calcified or severely curved canals even though it has been used only in one tooth. Use new files in hard cases and older files in easier cases. No one knows the maximum or ideal number of times a file can be used. Follow manufacturers' instructions and the rule of being "better safe than sorry." **Once only** is the safest number.
5. Instrument fatigue occurs more often during the initial stages of the learning curve. The clinician changing from stainless steel to nickel titanium should take continuing education courses with experienced clinicians and educators, followed by *in vitro* practice on plastic blocks and extracted teeth. Break files in extracted teeth! Developing a level of skill and confidence allows one to use the technique clinically.
6. Ledges that develop in a canal allow space for deflection of a file. The nickel-titanium instrument can then curve back on itself. A nickel-titanium instrument should not be used to bypass ledges. **Only a small curved stainless steel** file should be used, as described, in another section of this text.
7. Teeth with "S"-type curves should be approached with caution! Adequate **flaring of the coronal third to half** of the canal, however, will decrease problems in these cases. It may also be necessary to go through a series of instruments an additional time or two in more difficult cases.
8. If the instrument is progressing easily in a canal and then feels as if it hits bottom, DO NOT APPLY ADDITIONAL PRESSURE! This will cause the instrument tip to bind. Additional pressure applied at this point may cause weakening or even breakage of the instrument. In this situation, remove the instrument and try a smaller, 0.02 taper hand instrument, either stainless steel or nickel-titanium, carefully flaring and enlarging the uninstrumented apical portion of the canal.
9. Avoid creating a canal the same size and taper of the instrument being used. The only exception is in the use of the Buchanan GT file concept (to be discussed later). On removal from the canal, the debris pattern on the file should be examined. Debris should appear on the middle portion of the file. Except for negotiating calcified canals and enlarging the apical portion of the canal, the tip and coronal section of the file should not carry debris. **Avoid cutting with the entire length of the file blade.** This total or frictional fit of the file in the canal will cause the instrument to lock.

   If this occurs, rotate the instrument in a counterclockwise direction and remove it from the canal.

The greater the distance a single file is advanced into the canal, the greater will be the chance of files "locking up." When the file feels tight throughout the length of blade, it is an indication that the orifice and coronal one-third to two-thirds of the canal need increased taper. Instruments of varying design and/or taper can be used to avoid frictional fit. Nickel-titanium instruments with tapers from 0.04, 0.06, and greater, as well as Gates-Glidden drills and sonic/ultrasonic instruments, serve this purpose well.

10. Sudden changes in the direction of an instrument caused by the operator (ie, jerky or jabbing movements) must be avoided. A smooth gentle reaming or rotary motion is most efficient.
11. As with any type of instrument, **poor access preparation** will lead to procedural errors.
12. Advancing or pushing an instrument into a canal in too large an increment causes it to act as a drill or piston and greatly increases stress on the metal. Except for the most difficult cases and the necessity of using small instruments, the tip should not be used to cut into or drill into the canal; it should act only as a guide. Regardless of the technique being used, nickel-titanium instruments should be advanced in small increments with a more passive pressure than that used with stainless steel.
13. Do not get in a hurry! **Do not get in a hurry!** Do not get greedy and try to make nickel titanium do more than it is designed to do.
14. Inspection of instruments, particularly used instruments, by staff and doctor is critical. Prior to insertion and on removal, look at the blade. Rotate the file, looking for deflections of light. This indicates a damaged instrument. Also remember that, unlike stainless steel, nickel titanium has an excellent memory. The file should be straight. If any bend is present, the instrument is fatigued and should be replaced.
15. Do not assume that the length of files is always accurate; measure each file. Some files are longer from handle to tip than others. Files may also become longer or shorter if they are unraveled or twisted.

Comparative Studies

Nickel-titanium instruments function differently than those made of stainless steel, even when the cross-sectional design, taper, flutes, and tip are identical. In an effort to compare hand nickel-titanium to stainless steel files, a series of studies were initiated at The University of Tennessee. Eighty-two second-year dental students were required to instrument two epoxy blocks containing curved canals. The only variable was the use of stainless steel files in one block and nickel-titanium files in the second block. Standardized photographs were taken of the blocks before and after instrumentation. Overlay tracings were made of these photographs, and differences in the shapes of the before and after drawings were measured.

The nickel-titanium blocks received a higher grade 67.9% of the time and the stainless steel blocks 14.8% of the time. Working length was maintained significantly more often ($p < .05$) in the nickel-titanium group than in the stainless steel group. There was **no ledging** of canals using the more flexible nickel-titanium files compared with 30.4% ledging when stainless steel files were used. When using nickel-titanium files, the students were short of working length in only 3% of the canals compared with 46% of the canals when using stainless steel files. Although the canals were instrumented beyond the intended working length in 25% of the nickel-titanium blocks, the students were able to develop an apical stop within 1 mm between working length and the end of the canal. In the stainless steel group, 6% of canals fell into this category. The degree of destruction around the foramen was significantly different ($p < .05$). Apical zipping occurred 31.7% less often with the Nitinol files.[139] Stripping of the canal walls was less with the nickel-titanium files. A second study in which the blocks were instrumented by a member of the faculty had similar findings.[140]

An observation from these studies was the creation of a smooth belly shape on the outer aspect of the apical third of the canals instrumented with nickel-titanium instruments. This seemed to replace the ledging that occurred with stainless steel. Other studies have shown that this may be attributable to the technique in which the files were used.

Are nickel-titanium hand instruments best used with a push-pull filing motion or with a reaming or rotary motion? In one study, nickel-titanium files used in a filing motion caused a significantly greater amount of the outer canal wall to be removed, between 3 and 6 mm short of working length. The stainless steel files, however, removed significantly more of the outer canal wall, at working length and in the danger zone, than did the rotary or hand nickel-titanium files. The **rotary** nickel-titanium files were significantly faster and maintained better canal shape than the other groups. The results of this study indicate that **nickel-titanium instruments should be used with a rotational or reaming motion and are effective in shaping root canal systems.**[141]

Using computed tomography, Gambill et al. reamed extracted teeth with either stainless steel or nickel-titanium files and reported that the nickel-titanium files caused less canal transportation, removed less dentin, were more efficient, and produced more centered canals.[142]

On the other hand, not all studies are in agreement concerning cutting efficiency. Tepel et al. tested 24 brands of hand instruments specifically for cutting efficiency. They found that flexible stainless steel files were more efficient than nickel titanium. However, they did not address the quality of the completed canal.[143]

Elliot et al., at Guy's Hospital in London, used resin blocks to compare stainless steel (Flexofiles) and nickel-titanium (Nitiflex) instruments used with either a balanced force or stepback technique.[144] The authors concluded that it is preferable to use nickel-titanium instruments in a balanced force technique and stainless steel in a filing technique because stainless steel files can be precurved. Considering the results from Tennessee and London, nickel-titanium instruments should be used as reamers, not files.

ISO Groups II and III

Engine-driven instruments can be used in three types of contra-angle handpieces: a full rotary handpiece, either latch or friction grip, a reciprocating/quarter-turn handpiece, or a special handpiece that imparts a vertical stroke but with an added reciprocating quarter-turn that "cuts in" when the instrument is stressed. In addition, there are battery-powered, slow-speed handpieces that are combined with an apex locator, designed to prevent apical perforations. Because the instruments used in these handpieces are generally designed for the type of action delivered, it is best to describe the handpiece before discussing their instruments.

Rotary Contra-angle Handpiece Instruments. Instrumentation with a full rotary handpiece is by straight-line drilling or side cutting. Mounted with round or tapered burs or diamond points, full rotary contra-angle handpieces can be used to develop **coronal access** to canal orifices. In addition, special reamers, listed under ISO Group II, may be used to funnel out orifices for easier access, to clean and shape canals with slow-turning nickel-titanium reamer-type instruments, and to prepare post channels for final restoration of the tooth.

Since some of these instruments (stainless) do not readily bend, they should be used in perfectly straight canals. Because they are often misdirected or forced beyond their limits, they notoriously cause perforations or break in the hands of neophytes.

One solution to these problems is to use a slower handpiece: the Medidenta/Micro Mega MM 324 reduction gear Handpieces (Medidenta/Micro Mega, Woodside, N.Y.), the Aseptico Electric Motor Handpiece (Aseptico International, Woodinville, Wash.), the Quantec ETM Electric torque control motor (Sybron-Endo; Irving, Calif.), and the Moyco/Union Broach Sprint EDM Electronic Digital Motor handpiece (Miller Dental; Bethpage, N.Y.). These electric motors are specifically designed to power the new **nickel-titanium** instruments in canal preparation. The speeds vary from 300 rpm suggested for the NiTi ProFiles (Tulsa Dental; Tulsa, Okla.)to 2,000 rpm recommended for the LightSpeed instruments.

Newer electric handpieces are available wherein not only the speed can be controlled but the torque as well, that is, the speed and torque can be set for a certain size instrument and the handpiece will "stall" and reverse if the torque limit is exceeded. Emerging as contenders in this field are the new Aseptico ITR Motor handpiece (Aseptico International; Woodinville, Wash.), the Nouvag TCM ENDO motor (Nouvag, Switzerland), the new Endo-Pro Electric (Medidenta/MicroMega; Woodside, N.Y.), and the new ProTorq motor handpiece (Micro Motors Inc; Santa Ana, Calif.).

An entirely new "wrinkle" in rotary handpieces is the Morita **Tri Auto-ZX** (J. Morita USA Inc. Irvine, CA), a cordless, battery-powered, endodontic, slow-speed (280 rpm) handpiece **with a built-in apex locator.** It uses rotary nickel-titanium instruments held by a push-button chuck. The Tri Auto-ZX has three automatic functions: The handpiece automatically starts when the file enters the canal and stops when the file is removed. If too much pressure is applied, the handpiece automatically stops and reverses rotation. It also automatically stops and reverses rotation when the file tip reaches the **apical stop**, as determined by the build-in apex locator. The Tri Auto-ZX will work in a moist canal.

Reciprocating Handpiece. A commonly used flat plane reciprocating handpiece is the **Giromatic** (Medidenta/MicroMega; Woodside, N.Y.). It accepts only latch-type instruments. In this device, the quarter-turn motion is delivered 3,000 times per minute. More recently, Kerr has introduced the **M4 Safety Handpiece** (Sybron-Kerr; Orange, Calif.), which has a 30-degree reciprocating motion and a unique chuck that locks regular hand files in place by their handles (Figure 10-30). The Kerr Company recommends that their **Safety Hedstrom** Instrument be used with the M4. Zakariasen et al. found the M4, mounted with Safety Hedstrom files, to be somewhat superior to "step-back hand preparations and a shorter time of preparation."[145,146] German researchers found much the same for both the M4 and the Giromatic.[147]

The **Endo-Gripper** (Moyco/Union Broach; Bethpage, N.Y.) is a similar handpiece, with a 10:1 gear ratio and a 45-degree turning motion. As with the Kerr M4, the Endo-Gripper also uses regular hand, not contra-angle,

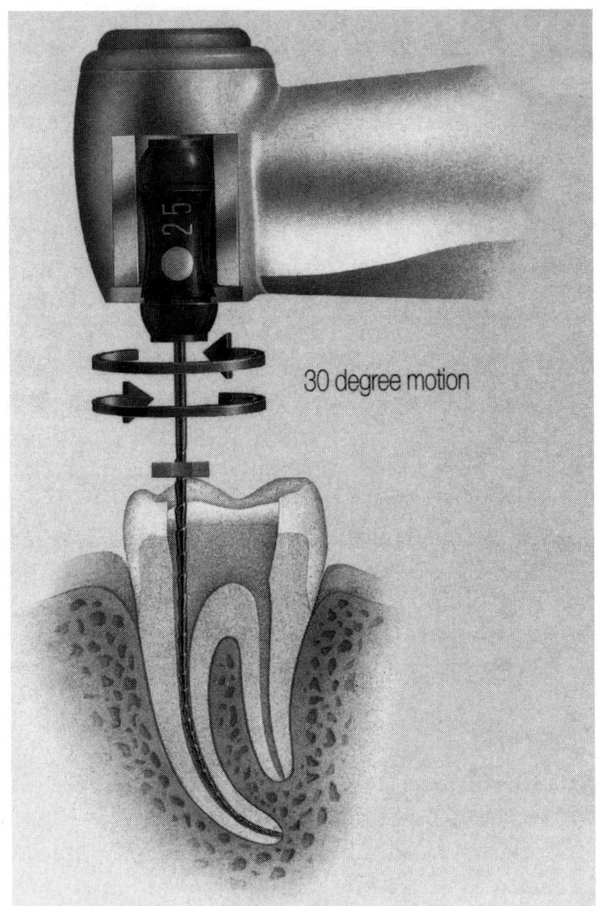

Figure 10-30 The **M4 Safety Handpiece** reciprocates in a 30-degree motion and locks regular hand files in place. The manufacturer recommends that **Safety Hedstrom files** be used. (Courtesy of Sybron-Endo/Kerr, Orange, Calif.)

instruments. Union Broach recommends their Flex-R and Onyx-R files.

The Giromatic handpiece probably got off to a bad start because of the instruments initially used. Broaches proved less than effective. Then Hedstroem-type files were introduced followed by K-style reamers.[148–152] Today, Micro Mega recommends their RispiSonic or Triocut as the instruments of choice.

In any event, as the cutting instruments improved, a number of well-known endodontists "came out of the closet," so to speak, admitting that they often used these reciprocating instruments. The reports were mixed, however, between "zipping" at the apical foramen versus round, tapered preparations.[153–156]

Vertical Stroke Handpiece. Levy introduced a handpiece that is driven either by air or electrically that delivers a vertical stroke ranging from 0.3 to 1 mm. The more freely the instrument moves in the canal, the longer the stroke. The handpiece also has a quarter-turn reciprocating motion that "kicks in," along with the vertical stroke, when the canal instrument is under bind in a tight canal. If it is too tight, the motion ceases, and the operator returns to a smaller file. Developed in France, the **Canal Finder System** (Marseille, France) uses the A file, a clever variation of the H file.

ROTARY INSTRUMENTS

Two of the most historic and popular engine-driven instruments are **Gates-Glidden** drills and **Peeso** reamers (drills) (Figure 10-31, A and B).

Gates-Glidden drills are an integral part of new instrumentation techniques for both initial opening of canal orifices and deeper penetration in both straight and curved canals. Gates-Glidden drills are designed to have a weak spot in the part of the shaft closest to the handpiece so that, if the instrument separates, the separated part can be easily removed from the canal. They come in sizes 1 through 6, although these sizes are being converted to the ISO instrument sizes and colors.

In a laboratory study, Leubke and Brantley tested two brands of Gates-Glidden drills by clamping the head of the drill and then twisting the handles either clockwise or counterclockwise. There was no specific pattern to their fracture except that some broke at the head and some high on the shaft near the shank.[157] Luebke and Brantley later repeated the experiment, allowing the drill head to turn as it would in a clinical situation. This

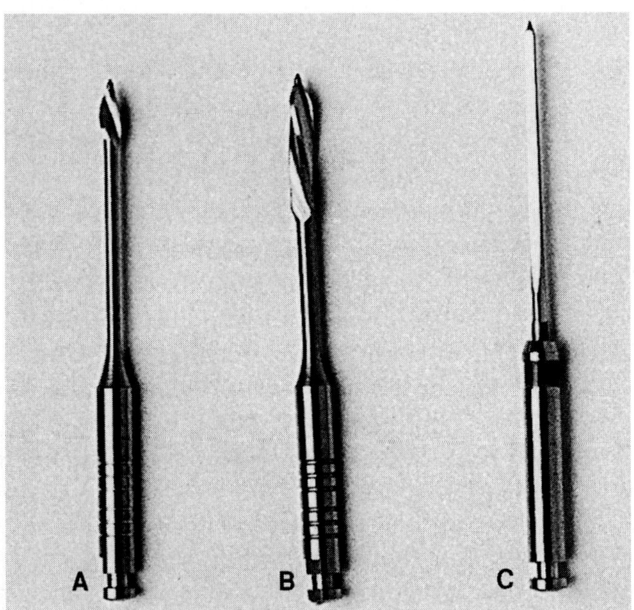

Figure 10-31 Engine-driven instruments used in a slow-speed handpiece. A, **Gates-Glidden drills** come in sizes 1 through 6, end cutting or non–end cutting, and are used extensively in enlarging the straight part of the canal. B, **Peeso reamer** (drill) used primarily for post preparation. C, New Orifice Opener, in instrument sizes 25 through 70, used in the straight part of the canal. (Courtesy of Dentsply/Maillefer.)

time, all of the drills fractured near the shank, "a major departure from the previous test."[158,159]

The **Peeso reamer** (Dentsply/Maillefer; Tulsa, Okla.) is most often used in preparing the coronal portion of the root canal for a post and core. One must be careful to use the "safe-ended" Peeso drill to prevent lateral perforation. Gutta-percha should have previously been removed to post depth with a hot plugger. Round burs should never be used.

The use of rotary instruments will be described in the instrumentation section. If used correctly, they can be a tremendous help in facilitating instrumentation.

Rotary K-Type, U-Type, H-Type, and Drill-Type Instruments

As previously stated, the same instrument designs described for hand instruments are available as rotary-powered instruments. To think this a new idea, one has only to return to a year 1912 catalog to learn that rotary instruments were being used nearly a century ago, K-style rotary "broaches" (reamers) made of carbon steel (Figure 10-32). At that early time, the probability of their breakage was precluded by the very slow speed of the treadle-type, foot-powered handpieces.

Today, at speeds that vary from 300 to 2,500 rpm, and with the growing use of nickel-titanium instruments, rotary canal preparation is once again very much in vogue. Although the K-style configuration is still widely used, the rotary U-style (ProFile) and drill style (Quantec) instruments are proving ever more popular. The use of these instruments will be described later in the chapter.

Ultrasonic and Sonic Handpieces

Instruments used in the handpieces that move near or faster than the speed of sound range from standard K-type files to special broach-like instruments. "Ultrasonic endodontics is based on a system in which sound as an energy source (at 20 to 25 kHγ) activates an endodontic file resulting in three-dimensional activation of the file in the surrounding medium."[160] The main débriding action of ultrasonics was initially thought to be by cavitation, a process by which bubbles formed from the action of the file, become unstable, collapse, and cause a vacuum-like 'implosion.' A combined shock, shear and vacuum action results."[160]

Ultrasonic handpieces use K files as a canal instrument. Before a size 15 file can fully function, however, the canal must be enlarged with hand instruments to at least a size 20.

Although Richman must be credited with the first use (1957) of ultrasonics in endodontics,[161] Martin and Cunningham were the first to develop a device, test it, and see it marketed in 1976.[162–171] Ultimately named the

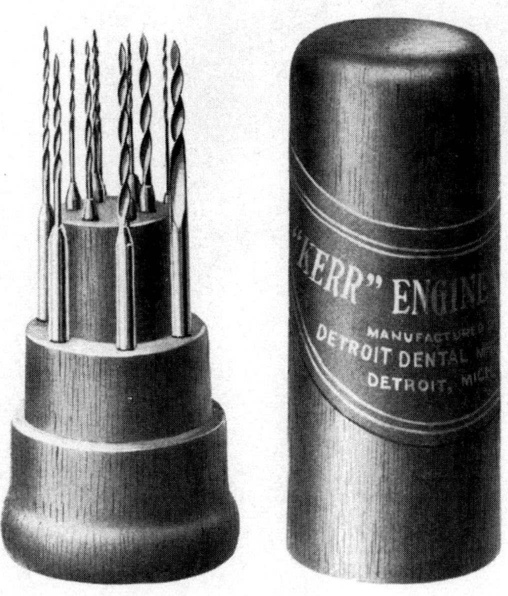
Kerr Engine Drills
These Drills are made after the plan of our well known Universal Broach, with the exception that they are provided with a SPECIAL DRILL POINT, thus giving a most rapid and clean cutting instrument for enlarging or drilling in the root canal.
They clear themselves of all cuttings while drilling and do not clog.
Made from the toughest spring steel, they can be easily sharpened.
They are put up in sets on a neat wooden block where each drill has its place.
A set comprises twelve drills, six in straight shank for use in canals of the anterior teeth and six for use in the right angle attachment.
Price, each...... $ .35
Full set as per cut 3.50

Figure 10-32 Historical illustration of **Kerr Engine Drills, circa 1912**. The shape of the drills resembles present-day K-style reamers. Made of carbon steel, they were probably safe to use in straight canals with a slow, treadle-type, foot-powered handpiece. (Courtesy of Kerr Dental Manufacturing Co., 1912 catalog.)

Cavitron Endodontic System (Dentsply/Caulk; York, Pa.), (Figure 10-33), it was followed on the market by the **Enac** unit (Osada Electric Co., Los Angeles, Calif.) and the **Piezon Master 400** (Electro Medical Systems, SA, Switzerland), as well as a number of "copycat" devices.

These instruments all deliver an irrigant/coolant, usually sodium hypochlorite, into the canal space while cleaning and shaping are carried out by a vibrating K file.

The results achieved by the ultrasonic units have ranged from outstanding[162–183] to disappointing.[184–189] Surely, there must be an explanation for such wide variance in results.

The answer seems to lie in the extensive experimentation on ultrasonic instruments carried out, principally at Guy's Hospital in London. They thoroughly studied the mechanisms involved and questioned the role that cavitation and implosion play in the cleansing process.[190–192] They believe that a different physical phenomenon, "acoustic streaming," is responsible for the débridement. They concluded that "transient cavitation does not play a role in canal cleaning with the CaviEndo unit; however, acoustic streaming does appear to be the main mechanism involved."[190] They pointed out that acoustic streaming "depends on free displacement amplitude of the file" and that the vibrating file is "dampened" in its action by the restraining walls of the canal.

The Guy's Hospital group found that the smaller files generated greater acoustic streaming and hence much cleaner canals. After canals are fully prepared, by whatever means, they recommended returning with a fully oscillating No. 15 file for 5 minutes with a free flow of 1% sodium hypochlorite.[191] In another study, the Guy's Hospital group found that **root canals had to be enlarged to the size of a No. 40 file** to permit enough

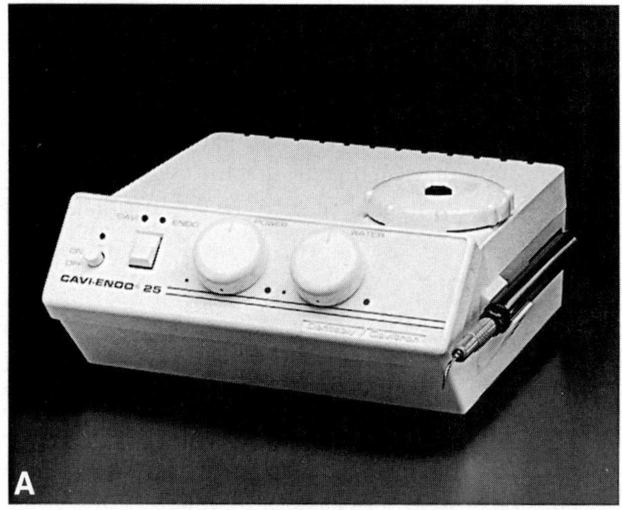

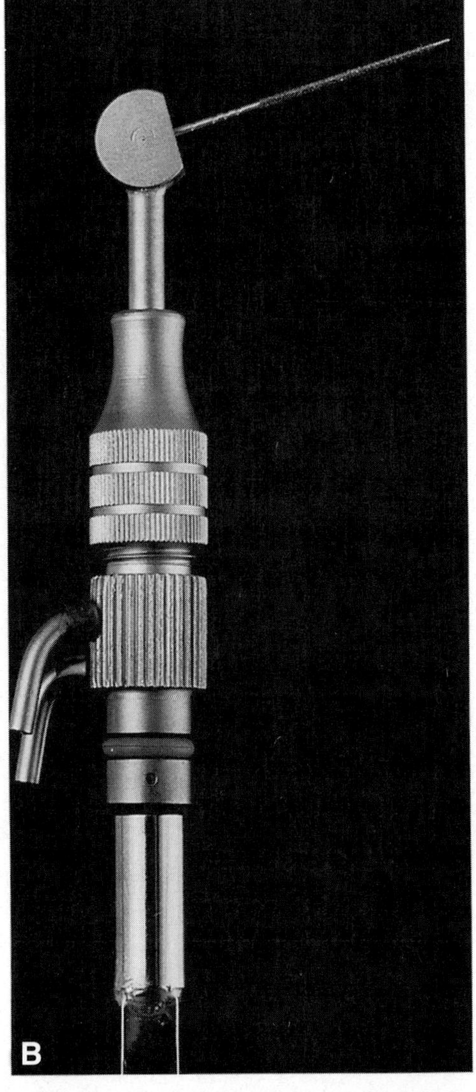

Figure 10-33 A, **CaviEndo unit** with handpiece (**right**) and reservoir hatch (**top right**). Dials (**front panel**) regulate vibratory settings. Foot control not shown. B, CaviEndo handpiece mounted with an **Endosonic** diamond file. Irrigating solution emits through a jet in the head. (Courtesy of Dentsply/Cavitron.)

clearance for the free vibration of the No. 15 file at full amplitude.[192] Others, including Martin, the developer, have recommended that the No. 15 file be used exclusively.[165,174,186] The efficacy of ultrasonography to thoroughly débride canals following step-back preparation was dramatically demonstrated by an Ohio State/US Navy group. There was an **enormous difference in cleanliness** between canals merely needle-irrigated during preparation and those canals prepared and followed by **3 minutes of ultrasonic instrumentation with a No. 15 file and 5.25% sodium** hypochlorite.[193]

Another British group reached similar conclusions about the oscillatory pattern of endosonic files.[194] These researchers pointed out that the greatest displacement amplitude occurs at the unconstrained tip and that the greatest restraint occurs when the instrument is negotiating the apical third of a curved canal. This is the damping effect noted by the Guy's Hospital group, the lack of freedom for the tip to move freely to either cut or cause acoustic streaming to cleanse.[190] Krell at The University of Iowa observed the same phenomenon, that the irrigant could not advance to the apex "until the file could freely vibrate."[195] The British researchers also reported better results if K files were precurved when used in curved canals.[196]

At Guy's Hospital, another interesting phenomenon was discovered about ultrasonic canal preparation—that, contrary to earlier reports,[170] **ultrasonics alone** actually **increased** the viable counts of bacteria in simulated root canals.[197] This was felt to be caused by the lack of cavitation and the dispersal effects of the bacteria by acoustic streaming. **On substitution of sodium hypochlorite** (2.5%) for water, however, **all of the bacteria were killed,** proving once again the importance of using an irrigating solution with bactericidal properties.[197]

Ahmad and Pitt Ford also pitted one ultrasonic unit against the other—CaviEndo versus Enac.[198] They evaluated canal shape and elbow formation: "There was no significant difference...in the amount of apical enlargement." They did find, however, that the Enac unit had a greater propensity for producing "elbows," as well as apical deviation and change of width.[198]

Ahmad, at Guy's Hospital, suggested that "the manufacturers of ultrasonic units consider different file designs." She found the K-Flex to be more efficient than the regular K style.[199]

Ultrasonic Conclusions

One can draw the conclusion that ultrasonic endodontics has added to the practice of root canal therapy. There is no question that canals are better débrided if **ultrasonic oscillation with sodium hypochlorite** is used at the conclusion of cavity preparation. But the files must be small and loose in the canal, particularly in curved canals, to achieve optimum cleansing.

Sonic Handpieces

The principal **sonic** endodontic handpiece available today is the **Micro Mega 1500 (or 1400) Sonic Air Endo System** (Medidenta/ Micro Mega) (Figure 10-34). Like the air rotor handpiece, it attaches to the regular airline at a pressure of 0.4 MPa. The air pressure may be varied with an adjustable ring on the handpiece to give an oscillatory range of 1,500 to 3,000 cycles per second.

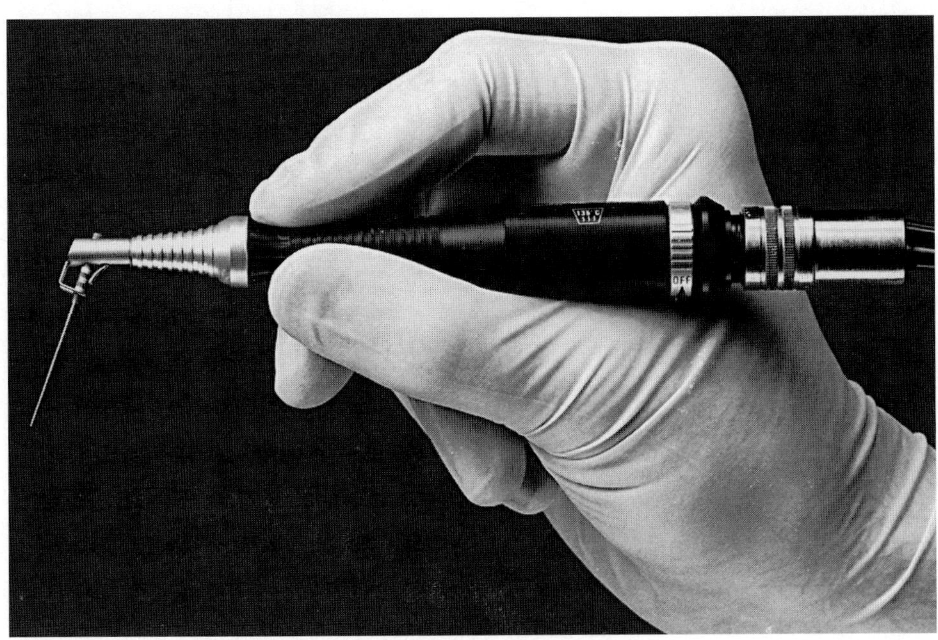

Figure 10-34 Micro Mega 1500 Sonic Air handpiece. Activated by pressure from the turbine air supply, the Micro Mega1500 can be mounted with special instruments easily adjusted to the length of the tooth. Water spray serves as an irrigant. (Courtesy of Medidenta/Micro Mega.)

Tap water irrigant/coolant is delivered into the preparation from the handpiece.

Walmsley et al., in England, studied the oscillatory pattern of **sonically** powered files. They found that out in the air, the sonic file oscillated in a large elliptical motion at the tip. When loaded, as in a canal, however, they were pleased to find that the oscillatory motion changed to a longitudinal motion, up and down, "a particularly efficient form of vibration for the preparation of root canals."[200]

The strength of the Micro Mega sonic handpiece lies in the special canal instruments used and the ability to control the air pressure and hence the oscillatory pattern.

The three choices of file that are used with the **Micro Mega 1500** are the **RispiSonic**, developed by Dr. Retano Spina in Italy, the **Shaper Sonic** (Medidenta; Woodside, N.Y.), developed by Dr. J. M. Laurichesse in France, and the **Trio Sonic** (Medidenta; Woodside, N.Y.) (also called in Europe the Heliosonic and the Triocut File) (Figure 10-35). The Rispi Sonic resembles the old rat-tail file. The ShaperSonic resembles a husky barbed broach. The TrioSonic resembles a triple-helix Hedstroem file. All of these instruments have safe-ended noncutting tips.

The RispiSonic has 8 cutting blades and the Shaper Sonic has 16. The ISO sizes range from 15 to 40. Because graduated-size instruments have varying shaft sizes, the instrument must be tuned with the unit's tuning ring to an optimum tip amplitude of 0.5 mm.

As with the ultrasonic canal preparation, these instruments must be free to oscillate in the canal, to rasp away at the walls, and to remove necrotic debris and pulp remnants. To accommodate the smallest instrument, a size 15, the canal must be enlarged to the working length with hand instruments through size No. 20. The sonic instruments, with the 1.5 to 2.0 mm safe tips, begin their rasping action this far removed from the apical stop. This is known as the "sonic length." As the instrument becomes loose in the canal, the next-size instrument is used, and then the next size, which develops a flaring preparation. The sonic instruments are primarily for step-down enlarging, not penetration.

Cohen and Burns emphasized the three objectives of **shaping** the root canal: "(a) developing a continuous tapering conical form; (b) making the canal narrow apically with the narrowest cross-sectional diameter at its terminus, and (c) leaving the apical foramen in its original position spatially."[201]

To satisfy these requirements, two of the sonic instruments have been quite successful. At the dental school in Wales, Dummer et al. found the Rispi Sonic and Shaper Sonic files to be the most successful, the Trio Sonic less so[202]: "In general, the Shaper Sonic files widened the canals more effectively than the Rispi Sonic files, whilst the Heliosonic [Trio Sonic] files were particularly ineffective…"[202]

The research group at Temple University found essentially the same results. They recommended that the Shaper Sonic files be used first and that the remaining two-thirds of the canal be finished with the Rispi Sonic.[203] Ehrlich et al. compared canal apical transport using Rispi Sonic and Trio Sonic files versus hand instrumentation with K files.[204] They found no difference in zipping among the three instruments. Even the worst transport was only 0.5 mm. Tronstad and Niemczyk also tested the Rispi and Shaper files against other instruments. They reported no complications (broken instruments, perforations, etc) with either of the Sonic instruments.[205] Miserendino et al. also found that the "Micro Mega sonic vibratory systems using Rispi Sonic and Shaper files were significantly more efficient than the other systems tested."[206]

Comparisons in Efficacy and Safety of Automated Canal Preparation Devices

Before making an investment in an automated endodontic device, one should know the comparative values of the different systems and their instruments.

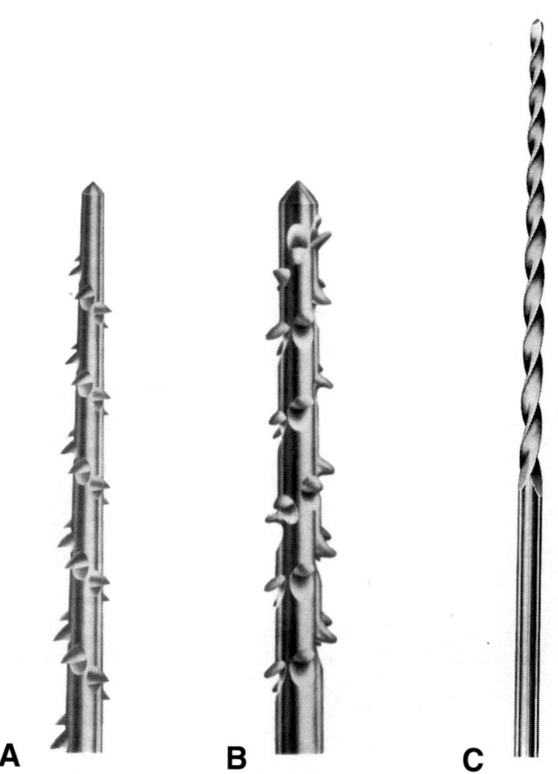

Figure 10-35 Three instruments used with the MM1500 Sonic Air handpiece. **A, RispiSonic. B, ShaperSonic. C, TrioSonic** (aka Heliosonic or Triocut). (Courtesy of Medidenta/Micro Mega.)

Unfortunately, the ultimate device and instrument has not been produced and tested as yet. Some are better in cutting efficiency, some in following narrow curved canals, some in producing smooth canals, and some in irrigating and removing smear layer, but apparently none in mechanically reducing bacterial content.

As stated above, Miserendino et al. found that the cutting varied considerably. They ranked the RispiSonic file at the top, followed by the ShaperSonic, the Enac "U" file (Osada Electric), and the CaviEndo K file.[206]

Tronstad and Niemczyk's comparative study favored the Canal Finder System in narrow, curved canals. On the other hand, the Rispi and Shaper files in the Micro Mega Sonic handpiece proved the most efficacious "in all types of root canals." The Cavitron Endo System was a disappointment in that it was so slow, blocked and ledged the canals, and fractured three files in severely curved canals. They also found the Giromatic with Rispi files to be effective in wide straight canals, less so in curved canals, where four Rispi files fractured.[205]

Bolanos et al. also tested the Giromatic with Rispi files against the Micro Mega Sonic handpiece with Rispi and Shaper files. They found the RispiSonic best in straight canals, the ShaperSonic best in curved canals, and both better than the Giromatic/Rispi and/or hand instrumentation with K-Flex files. The Shaper files left the least debris and the Giromatic/Rispi left "an extensive amount of debris."[203]

Kielt and Montgomery also tested the Micro Mega Sonic unit with TrioSonic files against the ultrasonic Cavitron Endo and Enac units with K files.[207] Even though others found the Trio Sonic files less effective (than the Rispi or Shaper files),[204] Kielt and Montgomery concluded that "overall the Medidenta unit was superior to the other endosonic systems and to the hand technique (control)."[207] The Zakariasen group at Dalhousie University reported unusual success in combining hand instrumentation with sonic enlargements using the Micro Mega 1500.[208]

Walker and del Rio also compared the efficacy of the Cavitron Endo and Enac ultrasonic units against the Micro Mega Sonic unit and found "no statistically significant difference among the groups, however, liquid extruded from the apical foramen in 84% of their test teeth. They felt that "sodium hypochlorite may improve the débridement of the canal." They also did not test the Rispi or Shaper Sonic files.[209]

At the University of Minnesota, the ultrasonic units were again tested against the sonic unit. The researchers found the Micro Mega Sonic to be the fastest in preparation time and caused the "least amount of straightening of the canals."[210] On the other hand, Reynolds et al., at Iowa, found hand preparation with the step-back technique superior to sonic and ultrasonic preparation except in the important apical area, where they were similar.[211] The Iowa group also found that ultrasonic and sonic files best cleaned ovoid canals.[212]

Lev et al. prepared the cleanest canals using the step-back technique followed by 3-minute use of a CaviEndo ultrasonic file with sodium hypochlorite.[213] **This approach has become an optimum and standard procedure for many endodontists.**

Stamos et al. also compared cleanliness following ultrasonic débridement with sodium hypochlorite or tap water. Using water alone, the Enac system was more effective, but when sodium hypochlorite was used, the CaviEndo unit (which has a built-in tank) was superior. They also reported ultrasonic preparation to be **"significantly faster"** than hand instrumentation.[214]

A US Army research group tested sonic versus ultrasonic units and concluded that they were all effective in canal preparation but judged the Micro Mega Sonic Air System, using Rispi and Shaper Sonic files, "as the best system tested."[215]

Fairbourn et al. compared four techniques according to the amount of debris extruded from the apex. **The sonic technique extruded the least** and hand instrumentation the most debris. Ultrasonic was halfway between.[216] Whether the debris discharged into the apical tissue contains bacteria was of the utmost importance. Using **sterile saline** as an irrigant, Barnett et al. found **sodium hypochlorite** to be four times more effective than sterile saline.[217] A US Navy group found essentially the same thing.[218]

Comparative Conclusion of Automated Devices. It appears safe to say that no one automated device will answer all needs in canal cleaning and shaping. Hand instrumentation is essential to prepare and cleanse the apical canal, no matter which device, sonic or ultrasonic, is used. The sonic unit Micro Mega 1500 reportedly enlarges the canal the fastest when Rispi or Shaper files are used, whereas the Canal Finder System, using A-style files, leads in instrumenting narrow curved canals. Finally, the ultrasonic CaviEndo and Enac units, using small K files and half-strength sodium hypochlorite for an extended time (3 minutes), seem to débride the canal best. **No technique without sodium hypochlorite kills bacteria, however.**

One must evaluate one's practice and decide which device, no device, or all three best suit one's needs.

ISO Group IV Filling Materials

An ADA specification has also been written for filling materials—core materials such as gutta-percha and silver points, as well as sealer cements classified by their chemical make-up and mode of delivery.

IRRIGATION

Chemomechanical Débridement

The pulp chamber and root canals of untreated nonvital teeth are filled with a gelatinous mass of necrotic pulp remnants and tissue fluid (Figure 10-36). Essential to endodontic success is the careful removal of these remnants, microbes, and dentinal filings from the root canal system. The apical portion of the root canal is especially important because of its relationship to the periradicular tissue. Although instrumentation of the root canal is the primary method of canal débridement, irrigation is a critical adjunct. Irregularities in canal systems such as narrow isthmi and apical deltas prevent complete débridement by mechanical instrumentation alone. Irrigation serves as a physical flush to remove debris as well as serving as a bactericidal agent, tissue solvent, and lubricant. Furthermore, some irrigants are effective in eliminating the smear layer.

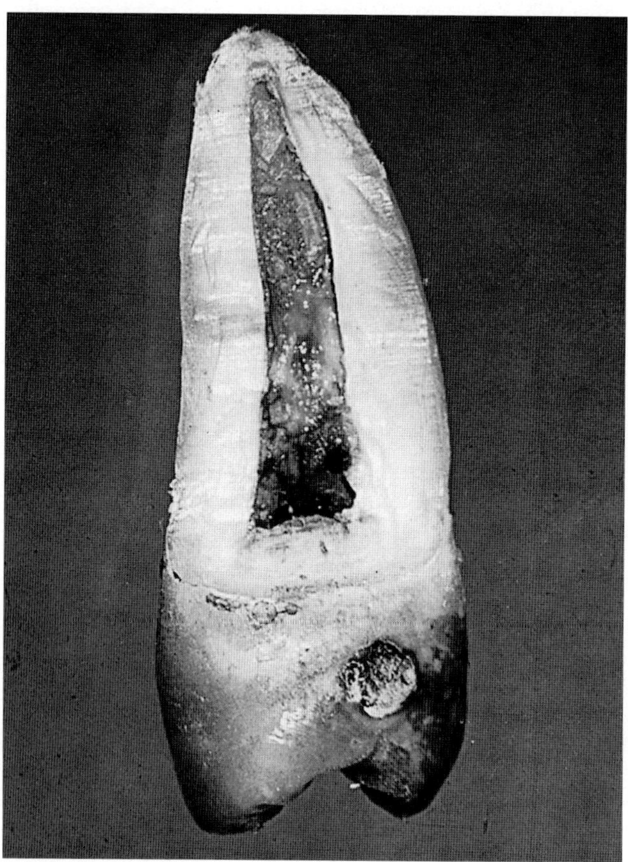

Figure 10-36 Gelatinous mass of necrotic debris should be eliminated from the pulp canal before instrumentation is started. Forcing this noxious infected material through the apical foramen might lead to an acute apical abscess.

A potential complication of irrigation is the forced extrusion of the irrigant and debris through the apex. This raises questions concerning the choice of irrigating solution, the best method of delivering the irrigant, and the volume of irrigant used. Other variables include how long the solution is left in the canal, ultrasonic activation, temperature of the irrigant, and the effect of combining different types of solutions. Although the presence of an irrigant in the canal throughout instrumentation facilitates the procedure, there are specific lubricating agents designed for that purpose: examples are **RC Prep** (Premier Dental; King of Prussia, Pa.), **GlyOxide** (Smith Kline Beecham, Pittsburgh, Pa.), **REDTAC** (Roth International, Chicago, Ill.), and **Glyde File Prep** (Dentsply/Maillefer; Tulsa, Okla.). It is highly recommended that canals always be instrumented while containing an irrigant and/or a lubricating agent. Instrumentation in this manner may prevent the complication of losing contact with the measurement control owing to an accumulation of debris in the apical segment of the canal.

Root Canal Irrigants

A wide variety of irrigating agents are available. It is recommended that the practitioner understands the potential advantages and disadvantages of the agent to be used.

Sodium Hypochlorite. Sodium hypochlorite is one of the most widely used irrigating solutions. Household bleach such as Chlorox contains 5.25% sodium hypochlorite. Some suggest that it be used at that concentration, whereas others suggest diluting it with water, and still others alternate it with other agents, such as ethylenediaminetetraacetic acid with centrimide (EDTAC) (Roydent Products; Rochester Hills, Mich.) or chlorhexidine (Proctor & Gamble, Cincinnati, Ohio). Sodium hypochlorite is an effective antimicrobial agent, serves as a lubricant during instrumentation, and dissolves vital and nonvital tissue. Questions concerning the use of sodium hypochlorite are often focused on the appropriate concentration, method of delivery, and concern with cellular damage caused by extrusion into the periradicular tissues. Researchers do not agree on the precise concentration of sodium hypochlorite that is advisable to use.

Baumgartner and Cuenin, in an *in vitro* study, found that 5.25%, 2.5%, and 1.0% solutions of sodium hypochlorite completely removed pulpal remnants and predentin from uninstrumented surfaces of single-canal premolars.[219] Although 0.5% sodium hypochlorite removed most of the pulpal remnants and predentin from uninstrumented surfaces, it left some fibrils on the surface. They commented that "It seemed probable that there would be a greater amount of organic residue present following irrigation of longer, narrower, more convoluted root canals that impede the delivery of the irrigant." This concern seems reasonable as the ability of an irrigant to be distributed to the apical portion of a canal is dependent on canal anatomy, size of instrumentation, and delivery system. Trepagnier et al. reported that either 5.25% or 2.5% sodium hypochlorite has the same effect when used in the root canal space for a period of 5 minutes.[220]

Spångberg et al. noted that 5% sodium hypochlorite may be too toxic for routine use.[221] They found that 0.5% sodium hypochlorite solution dissolves necrotic but not vital tissue and has considerably less toxicity for HeLa cells than a 5% solution. They suggested that 0.5% sodium hypochlorite be used in endodontic therapy. Bystrom and Sundquist examined the bacteriologic effect of 0.5% sodium hypochlorite solution in endodontic therapy.[222] In that *in vivo* study, using 0.5% sodium hypochlorite, no bacteria could be recovered from 12 of 15 root canals at the **fifth** appointment. This was compared with 8 of 15 root canals when saline solution was used as the irrigant. Baumgartner and Cuenin also commented that "The effectiveness of low concentrations of NaOCl may be improved by using larger volumes of irrigant or by the presence of replenished irrigant in the canals for longer periods of time."[219] On the other hand, a higher concentration of sodium hypochlorite might be equally effective in shorter periods of time.

Siqueira et al., in an *in vitro* study, evaluated the effect of endodontic irrigants against four black-pigmented gram-negative anaerobes and four facultative anaerobic bacteria by means of an agar diffusion test. A 4% sodium hypochlorite solution provided the largest average zone of bacterial inhibition and was significantly superior when compared with the other solutions, except 2.5% sodium hypochlorite ($p < .05$). Based on the averages of the diameters of the zones of bacterial growth inhibition, the antibacterial effects of the solution were ranked from strongest to weakest as follows: 4% sodium hypochlorite; 2.5% sodium hypochlorite; 2% chlorhexidine, 0.2% chlorhexidine EDTA, and citric acid; and 0.5% sodium hypochlorite.[223]

The question of whether sodium hypochlorite is equally effective in dissolving vital, nonvital, or fixed tissue is important since all three types of tissue may be encountered in the root canal system. Rosenfeld et al. demonstrated that 5.25% sodium hypochlorite dissolves vital tissue.[224] In addition, as a necrotic tissue solvent, **5.25% sodium hypochlorite** was found to be significantly better than 2.6%, 1%, or 0.5%.[225] In another study, 3% sodium hypochlorite was found to be optimal for dissolving tissue fixed with parachlorophenol or formaldehyde.[226] Clearly, the final word has not been written on this subject.

Sodium Hypochlorite Used in Combination with Other Medicaments. Whether sodium hypochlorite should be used alone or in combination with other agents is also a source of controversy. There is increasing evidence that the efficacy of sodium hypochlorite, as an antibacterial agent, is increased when it is used in combination with other solutions, such as calcium hydroxide, EDTAC, or chlorhexidine. Hasselgren et al. found that pretreatment of tissue with calcium hydroxide can enhance the tissue-dissolving effect of sodium hypochlorite.[227]

Wadachi et al., using 38 bovine freshly extracted teeth, studied the effect of calcium hydroxide on the dissolution of soft tissue on the root canal wall.[228] They found that the combination of calcium hydroxide and sodium hypochlorite was more effective than using either medicament alone.

However, Yang et al., using 81 freshly extracted human molars, examined the cleanliness of main canals and inaccessible areas (isthmi and fins) at the apical, middle, and coronal thirds.[229] Complete chemomechanical instrumentation combined with 2.5% sodium hypochlorite irrigation alone accounted for the removal of most tissue remnants in the main canal. Prolonged contact with calcium hydroxide to aid in dissolving main canal tissue remnants after complete instrumentation was ineffective. They also found that tissues in inaccessible areas (isthmi and fins) of root canals were not contacted by calcium hydroxide or sodium hypochlorite and were poorly débrided. As they noted, however, it could be that their study did not permit sufficient time (1 day or 7 days) for the tissue to be degraded. Hasselgren et al. reported that porcine muscle was completely dissolved after 12 days of exposure to calcium hydroxide.[227] The contrasting results of some investigators may be explained by their different methodologies including varied tissues studied, as well as a variety of delivery systems and the vehicle included in the calcium hydroxide mix.

Other variables to be considered include temperature as well as shelf life of the solution.[230–232] Raphael et al. tested 5.25% sodium hypochlorite on *Streptococcus faecalis, Staphylococcus aureus,* and *Pseudomonas aeruginosa* at 21°C and 37°C and found that increasing the temperature made no difference on antimicrobial efficacy and may even have decreased it.[233] *Pseudomonas aeruginosa* was particularly difficult to eliminate. Buttler and Crawford, using *Escherichia coli* and *Salmonella typhosa,* studied 0.58%, 2.7%, and 5.20% sodium hypochlorite for its ability to detoxify endotoxin.[234] All three concentrations were equally effective; however, large amounts of *E. coli* endotoxin could not be detoxified by 1 mL of 0.58% or 2.7% sodium hypochlorite. How this relates to the clinical situation is uncertain.

Against most anaerobic bacteria, Byström and Sundqvist found 5.0% and 0.5% sodium hypochlorite equally effective. By combining 5.0% sodium hypochlorite with EDTA, however, the bactericidal effect was considerably enhanced. **This could be related to the removal of the contaminated smear layer by EDTA.**[235]

Fischer and Huerta believe that it is the alkaline property (pH 11.0 to 11.5) of sodium hypochlorite that makes it effective against anaerobic microbes,[236] and a US Army group found **full-strength sodium hypochlorite to be effective in 5 minutes against obligate anaerobes.**[237]

Possibly, the bactericidal effect gained by combining sodium hypochlorite with other chemicals comes from the release of chlorine gas. This was especially true of citric acid and to some extent with EDTA, but not with peroxide.[238]

Sodium hypochlorite is a tissue irritant, and this has deterred its use, particularly at full strength. There is no question that, forced out the apex, most irrigants can be destructive. This will be discussed in detail in chapter 14 on mishaps.

Other Irrigants. **Salvizol** (Ravensberg Konstanz, Germany) is a root canal chelating irrigant, N1-decamethylene-bis-4-aminoquinaldinium-diacetate. Kaufman et al. have suggested that Salvizol, with a neutral pH, has a broad spectrum of bactericidal activity and the ability to chelate calcium. This gives the product a cleansing potency while being biologically compatible[239] (Figure 10-37). This applies to **Tublicid** (green, red, and blue) (Dental Therapeutics AB, Sweden) as well.

Chlorhexidine gluconate is an effective antimicrobial agent, and its use as a endodontic irrigant has been well documented.[240–242] It possesses a broad-spectrum antimicrobial action,[243] substantivity,[244] and a relative absence of toxicity.[241] However, chlorhexidine gluconate is not known to possess a tissue-dissolving property.[238]

The results from the individual trial of chlorhexidine gluconate and sodium hypochlorite indicate that they are equally effective antibacterial agents. However, when Kuruvilla and Kamath combined the solutions within the root canal, the antibacterial action was suggestive of being augmented.[245]

The results of their study indicate that the alternate use of sodium hypochlorite and chlorhexidine gluconate irrigants resulted in a greater reduction of microbial flora (84.6%) when compared with the individual use of sodium hypochlorite (59.4%) or chlorhexidine gluconate (70%) alone.[245]

White et al. found that chlorhexidine instills effective antimicrobial activity for many hours after instrumentation.[246] Although sodium hypochlorite is equal-

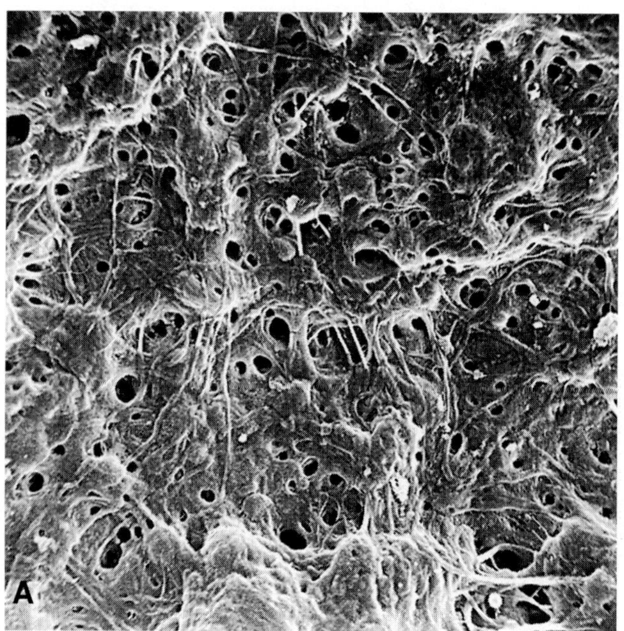

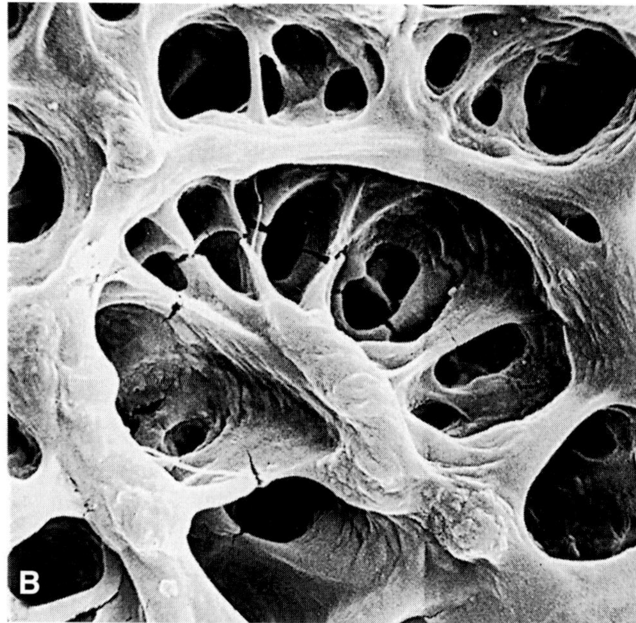

Figure 10-37 A, Coronal portion of a root canal of a tooth treated *in vivo* with **Salvizol**. The canal wall is clean, and very small pulpal tissue remnants are present; the tubules are open, and many intertubular connections with small side branches are visible. **B**, Middle portion of root canal treated with **Salvizol**. Note the tridimensional framework arrangement of tubular openings. Very little tissue debris is present. Intratubular connections are clearly seen. Reproduced with permission from Kaufman AY et al.[239]

ly effective on initial exposure, it is not a substantive antimicrobial agent.

Kaufman reported the success of several cases using ***bis-dequalinium acetate*** (BDA) as a disinfectant and chemotherapeutic agent[247] He cited its low toxicity, lubrication action, disinfecting ability, and low surface tension, as well as its chelating properties and low incidence of post-treatment pain.

Others have pointed out the efficacy of BDA. In one report, it was rated superior to sodium hypochlorite in débriding the apical third.[248] When marketed as **Solvidont** (Dentsply/DeTrey, Switzerland), the University of Malaysia reported a remarkable decrease in postoperative pain and swelling when BDA was used. They attributed these results to the chelation properties of BDA in removing the smear layer coated with bacteria and contaminants as well as the surfactant properties that allow BDA "to penetrate into areas inaccessible to instruments."[249] Bis-dequalinium acetate is recommended as an excellent substitute for sodium hypochlorite in those patients who are allergic to the latter. Outside North America, it enjoys widespread use.

A Loyola University *in vitro* study reported that full-strength Clorox (sodium hypochlorite) and Gly-Oxide (urea peroxide), used alternately, were 100% effective against *Bacteroides melaninogenicus*, which has been implicated as an endodontic pathogen. Alternating solutions of sodium hypochlorite and hydrogen peroxide cause a foaming action in the canal through the release of nascent oxygen. Hydrogen peroxide (3%) alone also effectively "bubbles" out debris and mildly disinfects the canal. In contrast, Harrison et al. have shown that using equal amounts of 3% hydrogen peroxide and 5.25% sodium hypochlorite inhibited the antibacterial action of the irrigants.[250] Because of the potential for gaseous pressure from residual hydrogen peroxide, it must always be neutralized by the sodium hypochlorite and not sealed in the canal.

It must be understood that each of the studies cited above has examined limited test results concerning the use of various irrigants or combinations of irrigants. However, there are other factors aside from the solution used. For example, Ram pointed out that the irrigational removal of root canal debris seems to be more closely related to canal diameter than to the type of solution used.[251] This, in turn, must be related to the viscosity or surface tension of the solution, the diameter and depth of penetration of the irrigating needle, the volume of the solution used, and the anatomy of the canal.

Ultrasonic Irrigation. As stated previously, the use of ultrasonic or sonic irrigation to better cleanse root canals of their filings, debris, and bacteria, **all the way to the apex**, has been well documented by Cunningham et al.[168,169] as well as others. More recently, they have been joined by a number of clinicians reporting favorable results with ultrasonic/sonic irrigation, from thoroughly cleansing the walls in necrotic open apex cases, [252] to removing the smear layer.[253] Griffiths and Stock preferred half-strength sodium hypochlorite to Solvidont in débriding canals with ultrasound.[254] Sjögren and Sundqvist found that ultrasonography was best in eliminating canal bacteria but still recommended the "use of an antibacterial dressing between appointments.[255]

Others were not as impressed.[256,257] In fact, one group found sodium hypochlorite somewhat better than tap water when used with ultrasonography but also noted that both irrigants were ineffective "in removing soft tissue from the main canal, the isthmus between canals, the canal fins, and the multiple branches or deltas."[252] However, they used ultrasonics for only 3 minutes with a No. 15 file and 1 minute with a No. 25 diamond file.[252] As Druttman and Stock pointed out, "with the ultrasonic method, results depended on irrigation time."[258] As previously noted, the cleanest canals are achieved by irrigating with ultrasonics and sodium hypochlorite for 3 minutes **after the canal has been totally prepared** (Figure 10-38). Moreover, ultrasonics proved superior to syringe irrigation alone when the canal narrowed to 0.3 mm (size 30 instrument) or less.[259] Buchanan noted that it is the irrigants alone that clean out the accessory canal. Instruments cannot reach back into these passages. Only the copious use of a tissue-dissolving irrigant left in place for 5 to 10 minutes repeatedly will ensure auxiliary canal cleaning.[260]

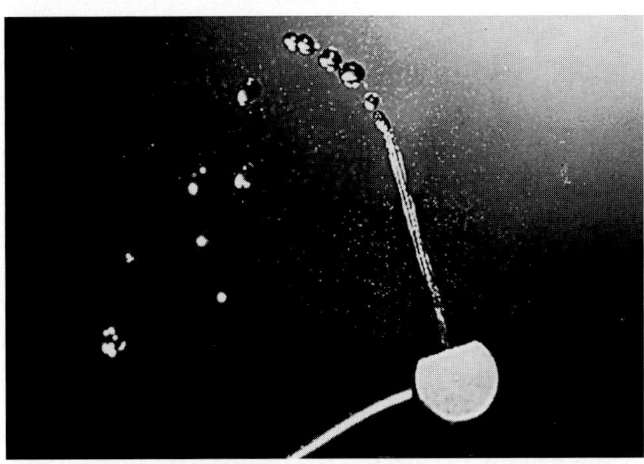

Figure 10-38 Irrigating solution climbs the shaft of a CaviEndo vibrating No. 15 file to agitate and débride unreachable spaces in the canal. (Courtesy of Dentsply/Cavitron.)

Method of Use

Although the technique for irrigation is simple, the potential for serious complications exists. Regardless of the delivery system, the solution must be introduced slowly and **the needle never wedged in the canal.** The greatest danger exists from forcing the irrigant and canal debris into the periradicular tissue owing to a piston-like effect. Several types of plastic disposable syringes are available.

Usually, the irrigating solution is kept in a dappen dish that is kept filled. The syringe is filled by immersing the hub into the solution while withdrawing the plunger. The needle, or probe in the case of the **ProRinse** (Dentsply/Tulsa Dental; Tulsa, Okla.), is then attached. Care must be taken with irrigants like sodium hypochlorite to prevent accidents. Sodium hypochlorite can be irritating to the eyes, skin, and mucous membranes. Some practioners provide protective glasses to their patients to protect their eyes. Also, it can ruin clothing.

The irrigating needle may be one of several types. It should be bent to allow easier delivery of the solution and to prevent deep penetration of the needle or probe (see Figure 10-38). A commonly used needle is the 27-gauge needle with a notched tip, allowing for solution flowback (see Figure 10-39, insert), or the blunt-end ProRinse. It is ***strongly recommended*** that the ***needle lie passively*** in the canal and not engage the walls. Severe complications have been reported from forcing irrigating solutions beyond the apex by wedging the needle in the canal and not allowing an adequate backflow.[261] This is an important point in view of results suggesting that the proximity of the irrigation needle to the apex plays an important role in removing root canal debris.[262]

Moser and Heuer reported Monoject endodontic needles (Tyco/Kendall; Mansfield, Mass.) to be the most efficient delivery system in which longer needles of a blunted, open-end system were inserted to the full length of the canal.[263] The point is that a larger volume of solution can be delivered by this method. However, the closer the needle tip is placed to the apex, the greater the potential for damage to the periradicular tissues. Druttman and Stock found much the same results, that with "conventional methods, irrigation performance varied with the size of the needle and volume of irrigant."[258]

Walton and Torabinejad stated that "**Perhaps the most important factor is the delivery system and not the irrigating solution per se.**" Furthermore, it was found that the volume of the irrigant is more important than the concentration or type of irrigant.[264] Chow found that there was little flushing beyond the depth of the needle, unless the needle was "bound" in the canal and the irrigant forcibly expressed.[265] Wedging a needle in a canal is dangerous and can cause serious sequelae.

Canal size and shape are crucial to the penetration of the irrigant. The **apical 5 mm** are not flushed until they have been **enlarged to size 30** and more often **size 40 file.**[266,267] It is reported that "In order to be effective, the needle delivering the solution must come in close proximity to the material to be removed."[262] Small-diameter needles were found to be more effective in reaching adequate depth but were more prone to problems of possible breakage and difficulty in expressing the irrigant from the narrow needles.[262] Of course, the closer the needle is to the apical foramen, the more likely it is that solution will be extended into the periradicular tissues.

Kahn, Rosenberg et al. at New York University, in an *in vitro* study, tested various methods of irrigating the canal. Evaluated were **Becton-Dickinson (BD)**, (Franklin Lake, N.J.) 22-gauge needles; **Monoject endodontic needles**, 23 and 27 gauge (Tyco/Kendall, Mansfield, Mass.) (Figure 10-39); **ProRinse** 25-, 28-, and 30-gauge probes (Dentsply/Tulsa Dental; Tulsa, Okla); **CaviEndo ultra-**

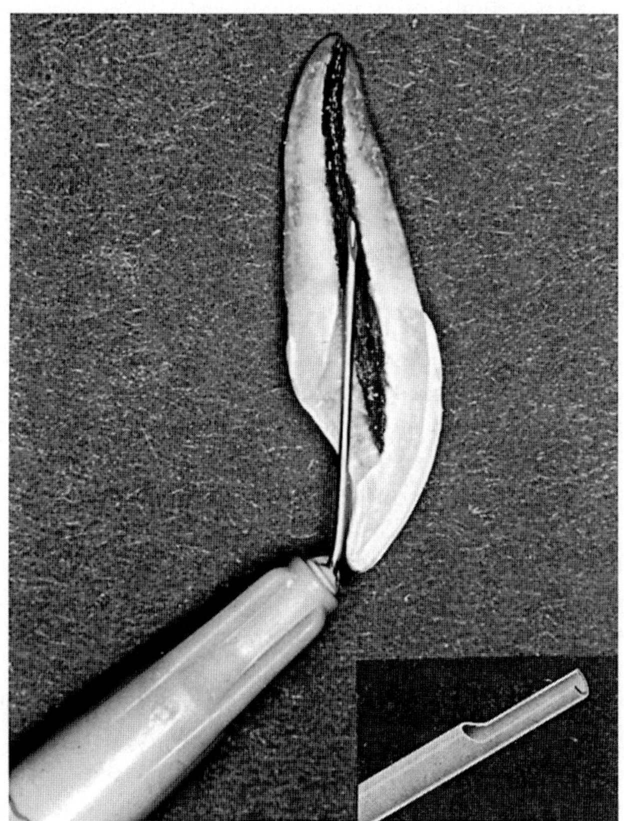

Figure 10-39 Simplest endodontic irrigating system—plastic disposable syringe and needle. Note that the needle is loose in the canal to allow backflow. Notched needle tip (**inset**) eliminates pressure (**Monoject**).

sonic handpiece (Dentsply/Caulk, York, Pa.); and the **MicroMega 1500**; Woodside, N.Y.). Canals in plastic blocks were filled with food dye and instrumented to progressively larger sizes.

ProRinse probes were highly effective in all gauges and in all sizes of canals tested. In canals instrumented to size 30 K file and size 35 K file, the smaller-lumen 27-gauge notch-tip needle was found to be highly effective. The larger 23-gauge notch-tip needle was found to be relatively ineffective, as was the standard 22-gauge beveled needle.

The **Micromega 1500** and **CaviEndo** systems were highly effective at the size 20, 25, and 30 K-file levels. Recapitulation, with smaller-sized vibrating files, completely cleared dye from the few apical millimeters.

The zones of clearance beyond the tip of the ProRinse probes were significant in that they indicated that highly effective canal clearance occurred without having to place the tip of the probes at the apical foramina. The effectiveness of the ProRinse seemed related to its design. It has a blunt tip, with the lumen 2 mm from the tip. Expression of fluid through the lumen creates turbulence around and beyond the end of the probe (Figure 10-40).

This model system was created to enable the investigators, using a Sony camcorder, to observe the differences of different irrigating systems. However, there are inherent differences in the *in vitro* test model from the *in vivo* situation. *In vivo* variables that affect delivery of the irrigant are canal length and quality of instrumentation. *In vitro* results, although potentially valuable, cannot be directly extrapolated to the *in vivo* situation.

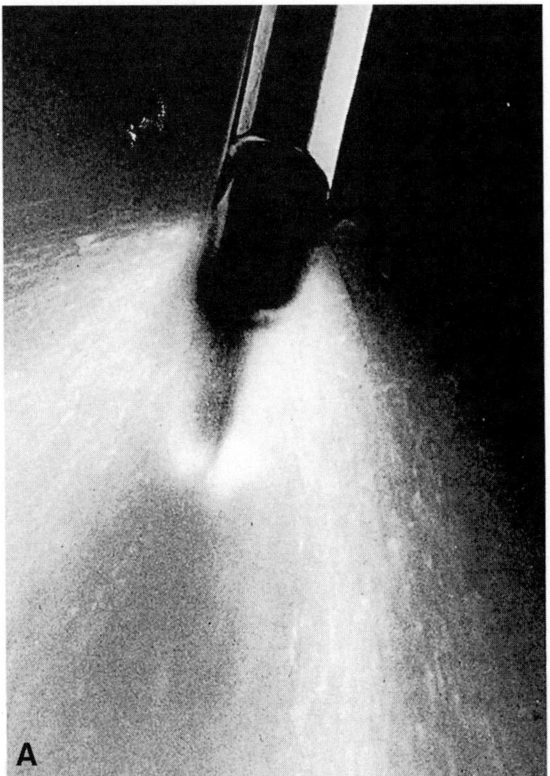

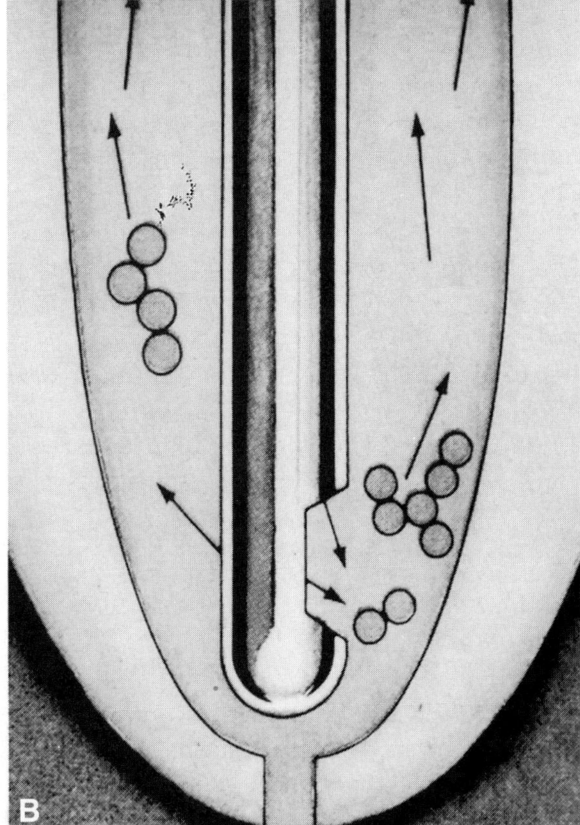

Figure 10-40 **ProRinse** needles irrigate through a side vent. **A**, Douching spray reaches all regions of the canal by rotating the needle. **B**, Closed-end needle eliminates possibilities of puncture of the apical foramen or a "water cannon" effect from open-end needles. (Courtesy of Dentsply/Tulsa Dental.)

Removal of the Smear Layer

Organic Acid Irrigants. The use of organic acids to irrigate and débride root canals is as old as root canal therapy itself. More recently, though, it has been investigated by Tidmarsh, who felt that 50% citric acid gave the cleanest dentin walls without a smear layer[268] (Figure 10-41). Wayman et al. also reported excellent filling results after preparation with citric acid (20%), followed by 2.6% sodium hypochlorite and a final flushing with 10% citric acid.[269]

In two separate studies, the US Army reported essentially the same results. Both studies, however, emphasized the importance of recapitulation—re-instrumentation with a smaller instrument following each irrigation.[270,271] Not to be outdone, the US Air Force tested both citric acid and sodium hypochlorite against anaerobic bacteria. They reported them equally effective as a bactericide in 5 to 15 minutes.[272]

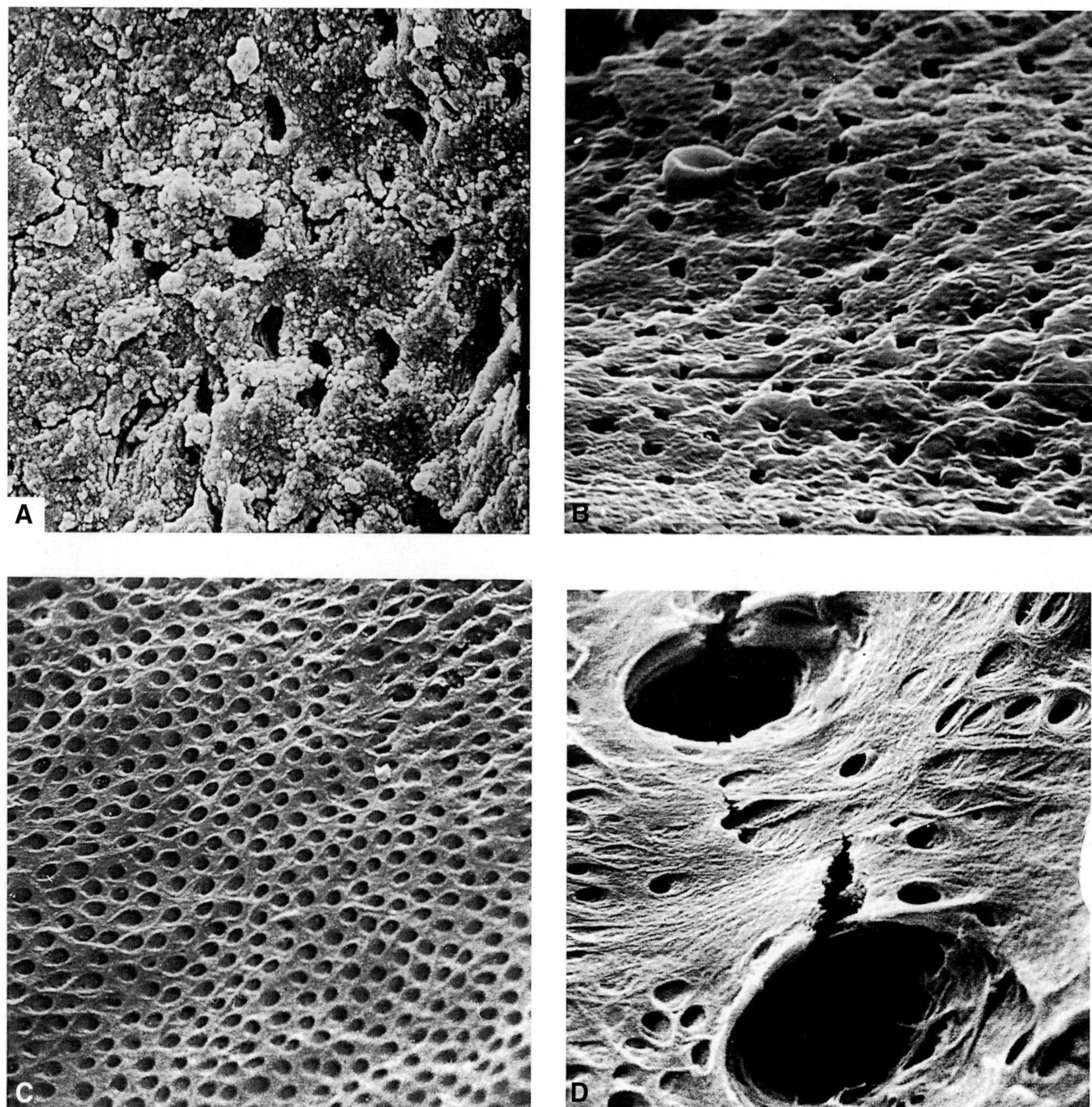

Figure 10-41 A, Canal wall **untreated** by acid. Note granular material and obstructed tubuli. B, Midroot canal wall treated with citric acid. The surface is generally free of debris. C, Midroot canal wall cleaned with phosphoric acid, showing an exceptionally clean regular surface. D, Apical area of root canal etched by phosphoric acid, revealing lateral canals. Reproduced with permission from Tidmarsh BG.[268]

Other organic acids have been used to remove the smear layer: polyacrylic acid as Durelon and Fuju II liquids, both 40% polyacrylic acid.[273]

Chelating Agents. The most common chelating solutions used for irrigation include Tublicid, EDTA, EDTAC, File-Eze, and RC Prep, in all of which EDTA is the active ingredient. Nygaard-Østby first suggested the use of EDTA for cleaning and widening canals.[274] Later, Fehr and Nygaard-Østby introduced EDTAC (N-O Therapeutics Hd, Sweden), quaternary ammonium bromide, used to reduce surface tension and increase penetration.[275] The optimal pH for the demineralizing efficacy of EDTA on dentin was shown by Valdrighi to be between 5.0 and 6.0.[276]

Goldberg and Abramovich have shown that EDTAC increases permeability into dentinal tubules, accessory canals, and apical foramina[277] (Figure 10-42). McComb and Smith found that EDTA (in its commer-

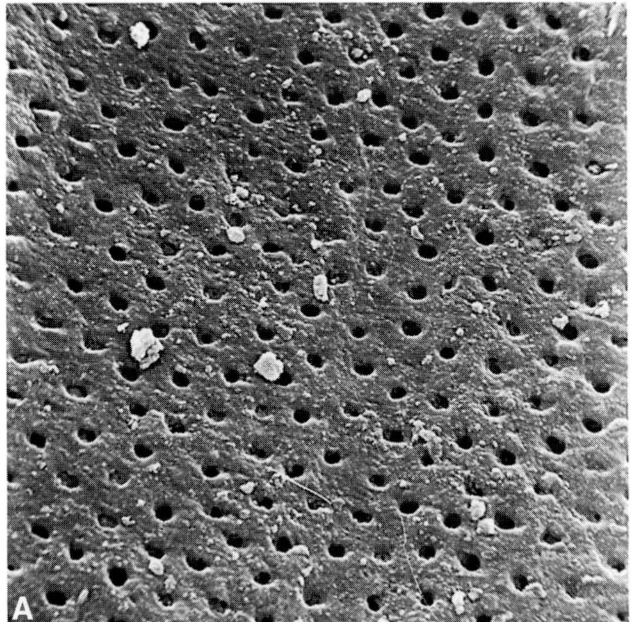

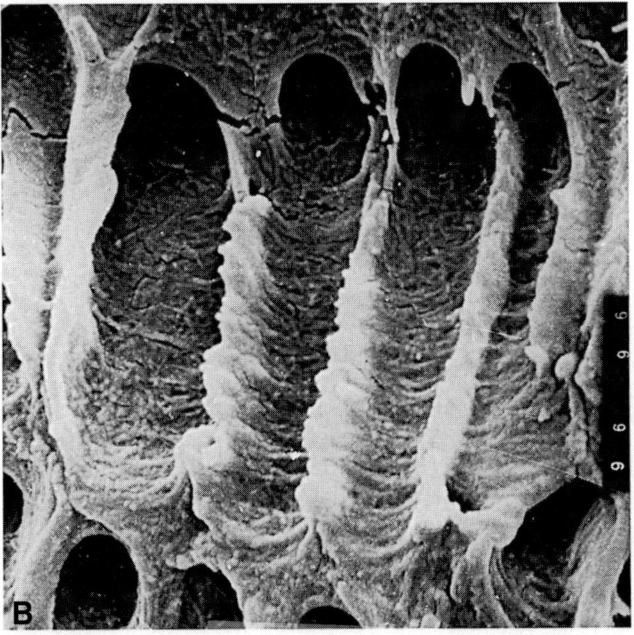

Figure 10-42 A, Coronal portion of canal of *in vivo* endodontically treated tooth with **EDTAC.** The tubules are open, and the canal is clean and free of smear. B, Filed canal treated with EDTAC. Longitudinal section of dentinal tubules shows thin intertubular matrix. A reproduced with permission from Kaufman AY et al.[239] B reproduced with permission from Goldberg F and Abramovich A.[277]

cial form, REDTA), when sealed in the canal for 24 hours, produced the cleanest dentinal walls.[278] Goldman and colleagues have shown that the smear layer is not removed by sodium hypochlorite irrigation alone but is removed with the combined use of REDTA.[279] This study helps answer the question of the composition of the smear layer since **chelating agents remove only calcified tissue**, whereas **sodium hypochlorite removes organic material.** Goldberg and Spielberg have shown that the optimal working time of EDTA is 15 minutes, after which time no more chelating action can be expected.[280] This study indicates that EDTA solutions should perhaps be renewed in the canal each 15 minutes.

Since Goldman et al.'s landmark research in 1981, reporting the efficacy of EDTA and sodium hypochlorite to remove the smear layer, a host of confirming reports have been published.[281–289] The US Army Institute of Dental Research, after first reporting the constituents, the thickness, and the layering of the smear layer,[281] followed up with two reports detailing the importance of alternate use of 15% EDTA and 5.25% sodium hypochlorite.[282–287] They introduced a total of 33 mL of irrigants into each canal, using 27 g blunt Monoject endodontic needles. The original Nygaard-Østby formula for 15% EDTA was used: disodium salt of EDTA, 17 g; distilled water, 100 mL; and 5 N sodium hydroxide, 9.25 mL.[287]

Developed by Stewart and others in 1969,[290] **RC-Prep** is composed of EDTA and urea peroxide in a base of Carbowax. **It is not water soluble.** Its popularity, in combination with sodium hypochlorite, is enhanced by the interaction of the urea peroxide in RC-Prep with sodium hypochlorite, producing a bubbling action thought to loosen and help float out dentinal debris.[291]

Zubriggen et al., however, reported that a residue of RC-Prep remains in the canals in spite of further irrigation and cleansing.[292] This led to the question of the effect of RC-Prep residue on apical seal. Cooke et al. showed that RC-Prep allowed maximum leakage into filled canals—over 2.6 times the leakage of the controls.[293]

EXPLORATION FOR THE CANAL ORIFICE

Before the canals can be entered, their orifices must be found. In older patients, finding a canal orifice may be the most difficult and time-consuming operation.

Obviously, a knowledge of pulp anatomy (knowing where to look and expect to find the orifices) is of first importance. Perseverance is the second requirement, followed by a calm resolve not to become desperate and decimate the internal tooth when the orifice does not appear.

The endodontic explorer is the greatest aid in finding a minute canal entrance (Figure 10-43), feeling along the walls and into the floor of the chamber in the area where the orifices are expected to be. Extension of the walls toward these points forms the basic perimeter of the preparation.

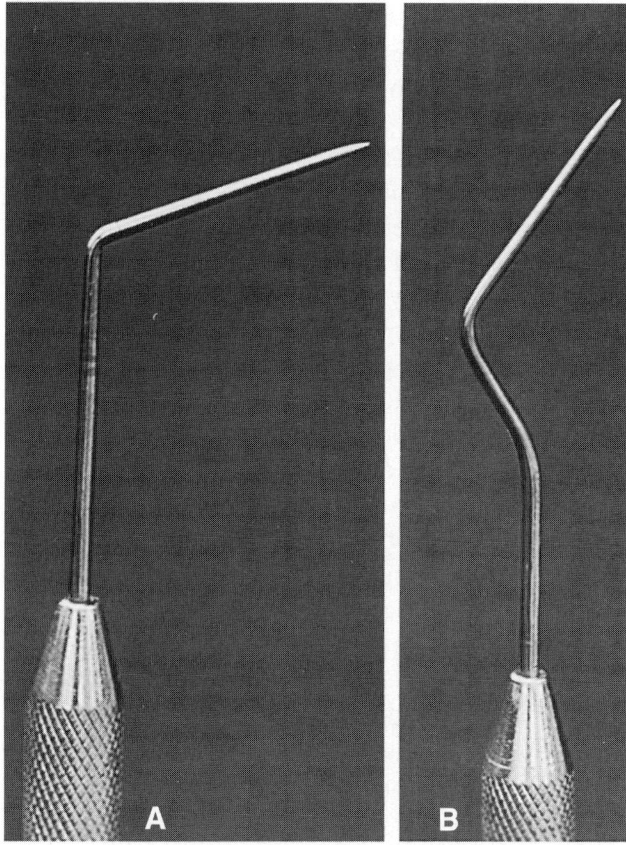

Figure 10-43 Opposite ends of an endodontic **DG explorer.** **A**, Right angle. **B**, Binangle. (Courtesy of Interdent, Inc., Culver City, Calif.)

A new addition to finding and enlarging canal orifices is the Micro-Opener (Dentsply/Maillefer; Tulsa, Okla.) (Figure 10-44, A), with K-type flutes in 0.04 and 0.06 tapers, mounted like a spreader, that can be used to uncover, enlarge, and flare orifices. This can be followed by the Micro-Debrider in ISO 0.02 taper, Hedstroem-type flutes (Figure 10-44, B) to further flare down the canal.

The radiograph is invaluable in determining just where and in which direction canals enter into the pulp chamber. This is especially true in the maxillary molars. The initial radiograph is one of the most important aids available to the clinician but, unfortunately, one of the least used during cavity preparation. A bite-wing radiograph is particularly helpful in providing an undistorted view of the pulp chamber. The handpiece and bur may be held up to the radiograph to estimate the correct depth of penetration and direction to the orifices (Figure 10-45).

Color is another invaluable aid in finding a canal orifice. The floor of the pulp chamber and the continuous anatomic line that connects the orifices (the so-called molar triangle) are dark (Figure 10-46, A)—dark gray or sometimes brown in contrast to the white or light yellow of the walls of the chamber (Figure 10-46, B). Using a No. 1 or 2 bur and "following out" the colored pathway from one orifice often leads to the elusive second, third, or even fourth orifice.

Canal orifices are often so restrictive that they need to be flared so that instruments may enter easily. Orifice openers, from hand-operated Micro-Openers to contra-angle powered reamers with a greater taper (.0.04, 0.06), and Gates-Glidden drills are *de rigueur.*

More recent is the development of endodontic ultrasonic units for surgical procedures, that has resulted in attachments for use in the pulp chamber, orifice, and canal. One of these attachments is a "cutting explorer." These tips allow the clinician not only to pick at the orifice but also to cut into the orifice without removing excessive amounts of dentin. **Using magnification** (loupes, **Orascope** [Spectrum Dental, Inc. North

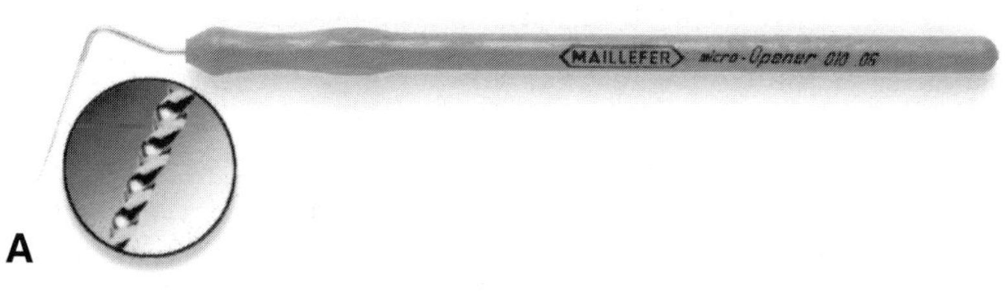

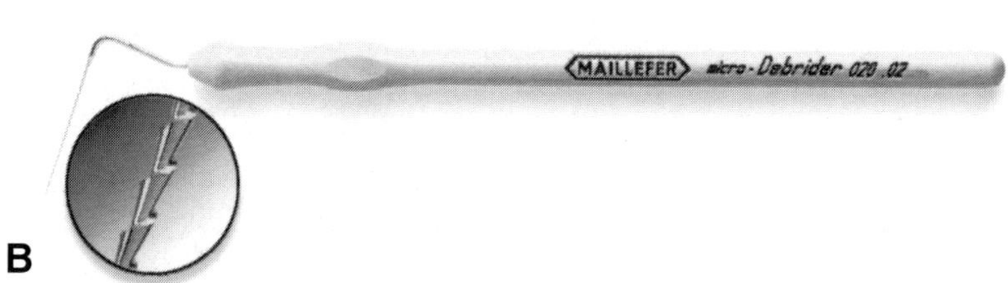

Figure 10-44 **A**, The **Micro-Opener** with K-style flutes and 0.04 and 0.06 flare is used to enlarge the orifice of the canal so that **B**, the **Micro-Debrider**, with Hedstroem-type flutes and an .02 flare, can be used to further open and widen the canal orifice. (Courtesy of Dentsply/Maillefer.)

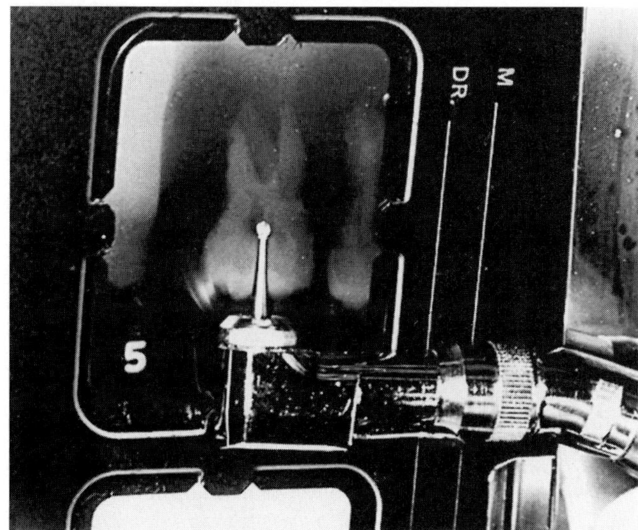

Figure 10-45 Bur held alongside radiograph to estimate the depth of penetration. (Courtesy of Dr. Thomas P. Mullaney.)

Attlebora, Mass.], or a microscope) can also be a tremendous help in finding and negotiating these canals.

Sometimes a greatly receded pulp has to be followed well down into the root to find the orifice to the remaining canal. Measurements on the radiograph indicate how many millimeters to drill before the orifice is encountered. The use of surgical-length burs, even in a miniature handpiece, will extend the depth of cut to well beyond 15 mm.

It is most important to enlarge the occlusal opening so complete authority over the direction of the instrument can be maintained (Figure 10-47). Repeated radiographs to verify the depth and direction of the cut are also invaluable.

Axioms of Pulp Anatomy

Remembering the following axioms of pulp anatomy can be most helpful:

1. The two orifices of the **maxillary** first premolar are further to the buccal and the lingual than is usually suspected (Plate 13).
2. The orifices of the mesiobuccal canals in both the maxillary and mandibular molars are well up under the mesiobuccal cusp, and the outline form must often be widely extended into the cusp (Plates 21 and 22).
3. The orifice to the lingual canal in the **maxillary** molars is **not far** to the lingual but is actually in the center of the mesial half of the tooth (Plates 21 and 22, 24 and 25).
4. The orifice to the distobuccal canal of the **maxillary** molars is **not far** to the distobuccal but is actually almost directly buccal from the lingual orifice (Plates 21 and 22).

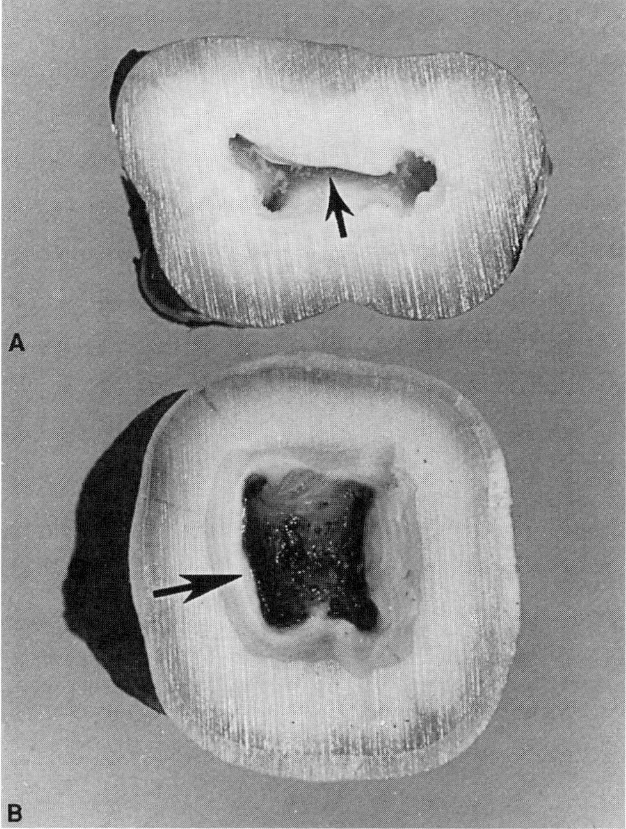

Figure 10-46 A, The dark line of the molar triangle is obvious in this cross-section of a mandibular second molar. **B,** The dark color of the floor of the pulp chamber contrasts markedly with the light color (**arrow**) of the side walls of preparation.

5. The orifice to the distal canal in **mandibular** molars is **not far** to the distal but is actually in almost the exact center of the tooth (Plates 25 and 26).
6. The orifice to the mesiolingual canal of the **mandibular** molars is **not far** to the mesiolingual but is actually almost directly mesial from the distal orifice (Plates 25 and 26).
7. Certain anatomic variations occur with enough frequency to warrant mention here:
   a. The mesiobuccal root of the **maxillary first molar** may often have an extra mesiolingual canal just lingual to the mesiobuccal orifice (Figure 10-48). It is found in the groove that comes off the mesiobuccal orifice like the tail on a comma. This entire groove should be explored for the mesiolingual canal; 62% of the time, the two mesial canals exit through two separate foramina.[28]
   b. **Mandibular second** molars frequently have a common mesial orifice that divides about 1 mm

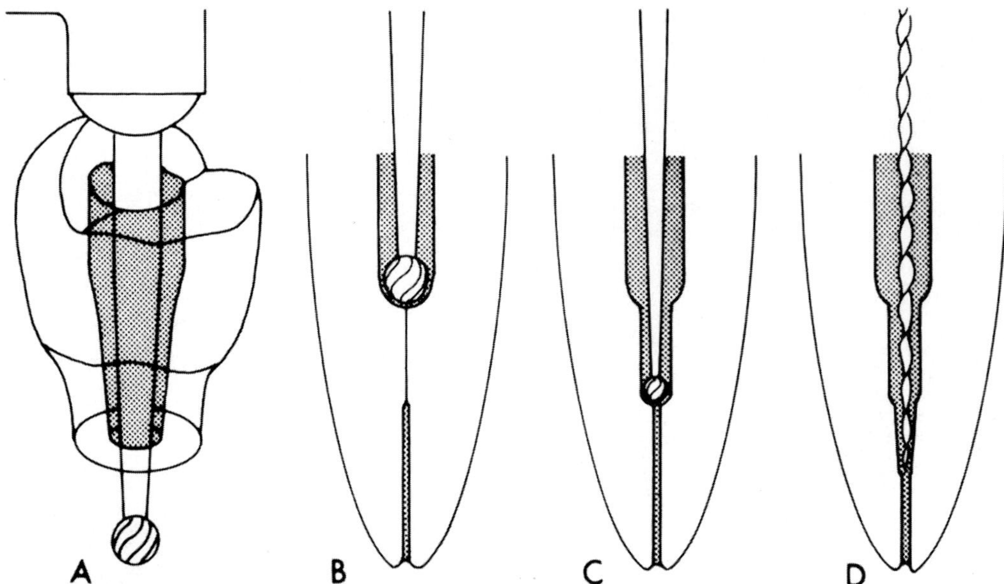

Figure 10-47 "Step-down" preparation. Necessity of maintaining control over burs and endodontic instruments in following out advanced pulpal recession. **A**, Coronal cavity is enlarged sufficiently to accommodate the shaft of a No. 4 surgical-length bur that must function without touching the cavity walls. **B**, Freely operating the No. 4 surgical-length bur following out receded pulp. **C**, A No. 2 surgical-length bur used in depths of preparation. Repeated radiographs may be necessary to judge the progress of the instrument. **D**, Fine root canal instrument used to explore and finally enlarge the patent portion of the canal.

below the floor of the pulp chamber into a mesiobuccal and a mesiolingual canal.

c. **Mandibular** first and second molars may have two **distal** canals, with either separate orifices, or a common orifice as described for the mesial.
d. **Mandibular first** premolars frequently have a second canal branching off the main canal to the buccal or lingual, several millimeters below the pulp chamber floor.

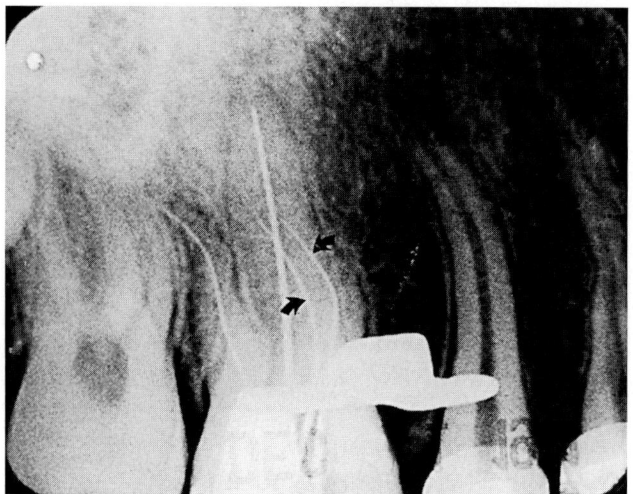

Figure 10-48 Two canals in the mesial root are clearly discernible by radiograph (**arrows**). Both canals apparently have separate apical foramina. (Courtesy of Dr. James D. Zidell.)

e. **Mandibular** incisors **frequently have two canals.** The lingual canal is hidden beneath the **internal** "shoulder" that corresponds to the lingual cingulum. This "shoulder" prominence must be removed with a No. 2 long-shank round bur or a fine tapered diamond "stone" to permit proper exploration.

In summary, **the unexpected should always be anticipated**, and the operator must be prepared to expand the access cavity for convenience in enlarging one of these canals or even just to increase visual examination of the pulp chamber floor in searching for such anatomic variance.

EXPLORATION OF THE CANAL

Besides the use of radiographs, the use of a fine curved reamer or file is a method available to determine curvature in canals. Stainless steel instruments are better suited for this purpose. The superelastic properties of nickel titanium, which make them desirous during the cleaning and shaping phase, are not helpful in the smaller sizes (6, 8, 10) when used for pathfinding. Many times, however, it cannot be determined that the canal is curved until enlargement begins and resistance develops to instrument placement above the No. 25 or No. 30 file owing to a lack of file flexibility. This will be discussed later in the chapter.

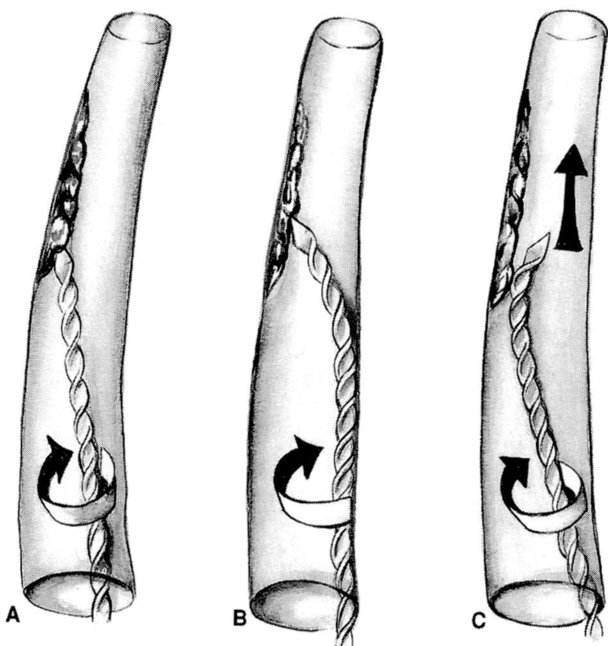

Figure 10-49 A, When a **straight** instrument catches on a canal obstruction, turning the instrument merely drives the point deeper into the obstruction. B and C, When a **curved** instrument catches on an obstruction, the rotating point of the instrument detaches it from the obstruction so that the instrument may be moved up the canal.

When tentative working length is reached with a curved pathfinder file, the operator can determine the direction of curvature by noting the direction of the tip of the file when it is withdrawn. This is a valuable clue for now the clinician knows the direction in which the canal curves and may guide the instrument accordingly. Valuable time is saved by eliminating exploration each time the instrument is placed in the canal. If a **teardrop-shaped** silicone stop is placed on the files, the pointed end indicates the direction of the file curvature.

One method to curve an instrument is to insert the tip into the end of a sterile cotton roll or gauze sponge and bend the instrument under the pressure of the thumbnail (Figure 10-51). Cotton pliers used to make this bend damage the flutes of fine instruments. The Buchanan **Endo-Bender** is better for this task (Sybron Endo/Analytic; Orange, Calif.)[90,91]

In exploring a canal with a curved instrument, the clinician should always expect the worst. One should probe with the point toward the buccal and lingual, that is, toward the direction of the x-ray beam, always searching for the unusual curvature that does not show on the radiograph. As mentioned previously, the palatal canals of **maxillary** molars, and the **maxillary** lateral

A curved pathfinder file should be used to explore the walls and direction of the canal. The argument against using a straight instrument is that it may tend to engage the wall at the curve or pivot on a catch on the walls (Figure 10-49). The curved tip of the instrument will scribe a circle when the instrument is turned on its axis, whereas the perfectly straight instrument will rotate only on the central axis of the instrument (Figure 10-50).

A curved pathfinding instrument can be rotated away from a catch or curve on the wall and advanced down the canal to the apical region (see Figure 10-49). From the initial pathfinding instrument, the length of the tooth may be established. With control of probing, poking, twisting, and turning, the fine pathfinder can almost always be penetrated to working length. The action can best be described as a "watch-winding" type of finger action.

If unable to reach the apex with reasonable effort, however, the clinician should increase the taper of the **coronal part** of the canal. Nickel-titanium files, with tapers greater than the standard ISO 0.02 mm/mm, have proved to make this process safe and more efficient. Once this has been achieved, it becomes possible to advance the pathfinder to working length.

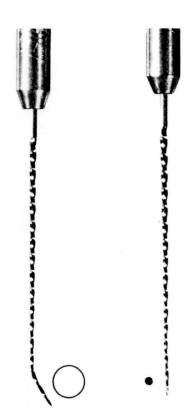

Figure 10-50 When turned on its axis, the tip of a curved instrument (**left**) scribes a circle. The tip of a straight instrument (**right**) turns on its own axis, which reduces control of the tip of the instrument.

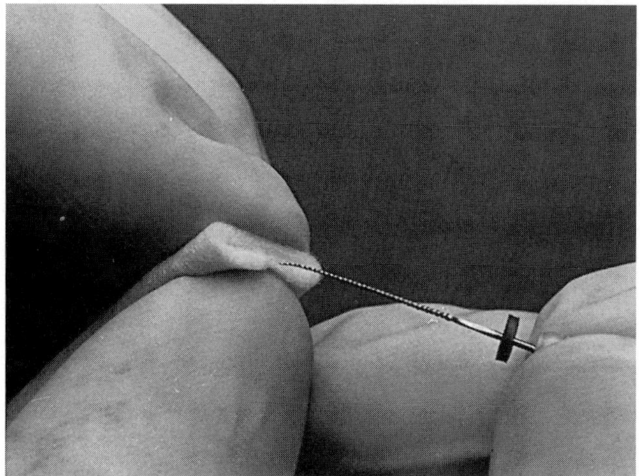

Figure 10-51 Curving point of an instrument. The tip is introduced into the end of a sterile cotton roll and is bent under a thumbnail padded by cotton.

incisors and canines, are always suspect. In mandibular **premolars,** curvature of the canal toward the buccal or lingual is a common occurrence as well (Figure 10-52). In these teeth, particularly the **mandibular** first premolar, anomalies of the canals frequently exist: double canals, bifurcated canals, and apical deltas are common. This also applies to the **mandibular** anterior teeth, where a search with the curved pathfinder should always be made for two canals, toward the labial and the lingual (Plates 9, F and 11, D).

Extra canals, such as three canals in the maxillary first premolar, two canals in the maxillary second premolar, or two canals in the mesiobuccal root of the maxillary first molar, should also be searched for (Plates 13, 14, 21). The fourth canal toward the distal in a mandibular molar is occasionally found by careful exploration, first with the endodontic explorer and then with the curved instrument. Finding the extra or unusual canal spells the difference between success and failure.

DETERMINATION OF WORKING LENGTH

The determination of an accurate working length is one of the most critical steps of endodontic therapy. The cleaning, shaping, and obturation of the root canal system cannot be accomplished accurately unless the working length is determined precisely.[294–296]

Anatomic Considerations and Terminology

Simon has stressed the need for clarification and consistency in the use of terms related to working length determination.[297] **Working length** (Figure 10-53) is defined in

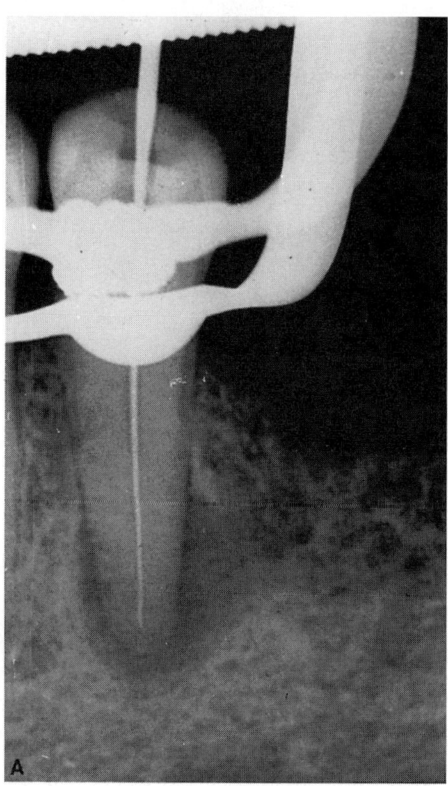

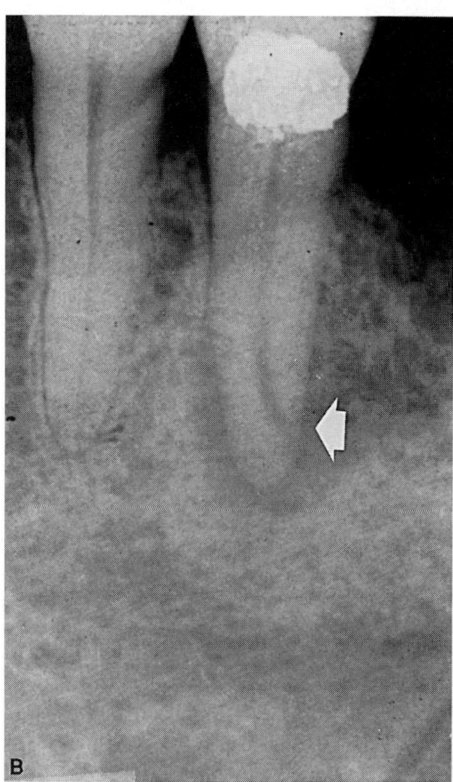

Figure 10-52 A, Working length film, mandibular premolar. The patient experienced sensitivity even though the instrument appears approximately 3 mm short of the radiographic apex. B, Preoperative **mesio-angled** radiograph of the same tooth showing canal curvature and the labial exit of the foramen (**arrow**) not evident on the working length film. (Courtesy of Dr. Thomas P. Mullaney.)

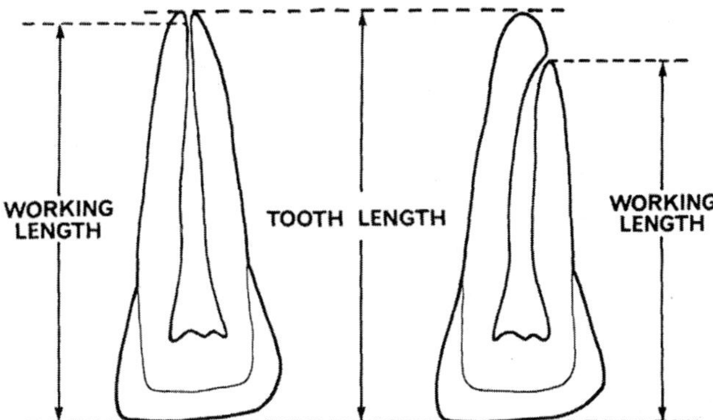

Figure 10-53 Care should be exercised to establish the position of the foramen. Hopefully, it appears at the apex, and 0.5 to 1.0 mm is simply subtracted from that tooth length as a safety factor. The lateral exit of the canal (**right**) can sometimes be seen in radiograph or discovered by instrument placement and re-examined radiographically. Even the patient's reaction to the instrument is a warning of "early exit," especially toward the labial or lingual unseen in the radiograph. Reproduced with permission from Serene T, Krasny R, Ziegler P, et al. Principles of preclinical endodontics. Dubuque (IA): Kendall/Hunt Publishing; 1974.

the endodontic *Glossary* as "the distance from a coronal reference point to the point at which canal preparation and obturation should terminate,"[298] the ideal apical reference point in the canal, the "apical stop," so to speak.

The **anatomic apex** is the tip or the end of the root determined morphologically, whereas the **radiographic apex** is the tip or end of the root determined radiographically.[298] Root morphology and radiographic distortion may cause the location of the radiographic apex to vary from the anatomic apex.

The **apical foramen** is the main apical opening of the root canal. It is frequently eccentrically located away from the anatomic or radiographic apex.[299–301] Kuttler's investigation showed that this deviation occurred in 68 to 80% of teeth in his study.[301] An **accessory foramen** is an orifice on the surface of the root communicating with a lateral or accessory canal.[298] They may exist as a single foramen or as multiple foramina.

The **apical constriction** (minor apical diameter) (Figure 10-54) is the apical portion of the root canal having the narrowest diameter. This position may vary but is usually 0.5 to 1.0 mm short of the center of the apical foramen.[298–300] The **minor diameter** widens apically to the foramen (major diameter) and assumes a funnel shape.

The apical third is the most studied region of the root canal.[299,300,302–307] Dummer and his coworkers reported many variations in the apical constriction.[300] In 6% of cases, the constriction may be blocked by cementum.[300]

The **cementodentinal junction** is the region where the dentin and cementum are united, the point at which the cemental surface terminates at or near the apex of a tooth.[298] It must be pointed out, however, that the cementodentinal junction is a histologic landmark that cannot be located clinically or radiographically. Langeland reported that the cementodentinal junction does not always coincide with the apical constriction.[308]

The location of the cementinodentinal junction also ranges from 0.5 to 3.0 mm short of the anatomic apex.[298–305,309–313] Therefore, it is generally accepted that the apical constriction is most frequently located

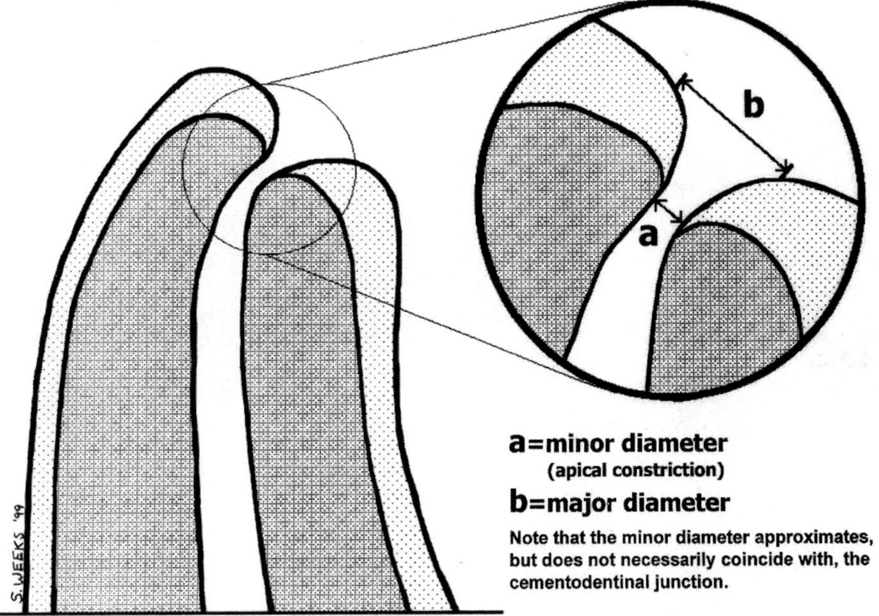

Figure 10-54 Diagrammatic view of the periapex. The importance of differentiating between the **minor diameter** (apical stop) and the **major diameter** (radiographic apex) is apparent. (Courtesy of Dr. Stephen Weeks.)

0.5 to 1.0 mm short of the radiographic apex, but with variations. Problems exist in locating apical landmarks and in interpreting their positions on radiographs.

Clinical Considerations

Before determining a definitive **working length,** the coronal access to the pulp chamber must provide a straight-line pathway into the canal orifice. Modifications in access preparation may be required to permit the instrument to penetrate, unimpeded, to the apical constriction. As stated above, a small **stainless steel** K file facilitates the process and the exploration of the canal.

Loss of working length during cleaning and shaping can be a frustrating procedural error. Once the apical restriction is established, it is extremely important to **monitor the working length** periodically since the working length may change as a curved canal is straightened ("a straight line is the shortest distance between two points").[314,315] The loss may also be related to the accumulation of dentinal and pulpal debris in the apical 2 to 3 mm of the canal or other factors such as failing to maintain foramen patency,[316] skipping instrument sizes, or failing to irrigate the apical one-third adequately. Occasionally, working length is lost owing to ledge formation or to instrument separation and blockage of the canal.

Two *in vivo* studies measured the effect of canal preparation on working length.[314–316] The mean shortening of all canals in these studies was found to range from 0.40 mm to 0.63 mm.

There has been debate as to the optimal **length** of canal preparation and the optimal level of canal obturation.[317] Most dentists agree that the desired end point is the apical constriction, which is not only the narrowest part of the canal[318] but a morphologic landmark[299,302] that can help to improve the apical seal when the canal is obturated.[319–321]

Failure to accurately determine and maintain working length may result in the length being **too long** and may lead to perforation through the apical constriction. Destruction of the constriction may lead to overfilling or overextension and an increased incidence of postoperative pain. In addition, one might expect a prolonged healing period and lower success rate owing to incomplete regeneration of cementum, periodontal ligament, and alveolar bone.[322–325]

Failure to determine and maintain working length accurately may also lead to shaping and cleaning **short** of the apical constriction. **Incomplete** cleaning and underfilling may cause persistent discomfort, often associated with an incomplete apical seal. Also, apical leakage may occur into the uncleaned and unfilled space short of the apical constriction. Such leakage supports the continued existence of viable bacteria and contributes to a continued periradicular lesion and lowered rate of success.

In this era of improved illumination and magnification, working length determination should be to the **nearest one-half millimeter**. The measurement should be made from a secure reference point on the crown, in close proximity to the straight-line path of the instrument, a point that can be identified and monitored accurately.

Stop Attachments. A variety of stop attachments are available. Among the least expensive and simplest to use are silicone rubber stops. Several brands of instruments are now supplied with the stop attachments already in place on the shaft. Special **tear-shaped** or marked rubber stops can be positioned to align with the direction of the curve placed in a precurved stainless steel instrument.

The length adjustment of the stop attachments should be made against the edge of a sterile metric ruler or a gauge made specifically for endodontics. Devices have been developed that assist in adjusting rubber stops on instruments[326] (Figure 10-55). It is critical that the stop attachment be perpendicular and not oblique to the shaft of the instrument (Figure 10-56).

There are several disadvantages to using rubber stops. Not only is it time consuming, but rubber stops may move up or down the shaft, which may lead to preparations short or past the apical constriction.

The clinician should develop a mental image of the position of the rubber stop on the instrument shaft in relation to the base of the handle. Any movement from that position should be immediately detected and corrected. One should also develop a habit of looking directly at the rubber stop where it meets the reference

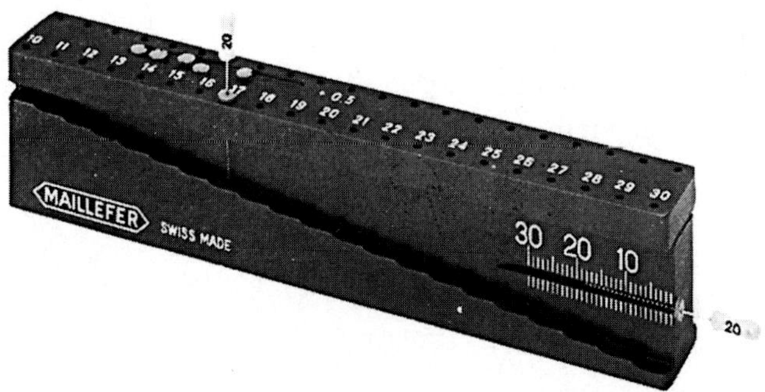

Figure 10-55 Guldener **Endo-M-Bloc** has 32 depth guides in two rows. Front row indicators from 10 to 30 mm in 1 mm increments. Back row indicators are 0.5 mm deeper. Helpful ruler at end. The device is invaluable in step-back or step-down techniques. (Courtesy of Dentsply/Maillefer).

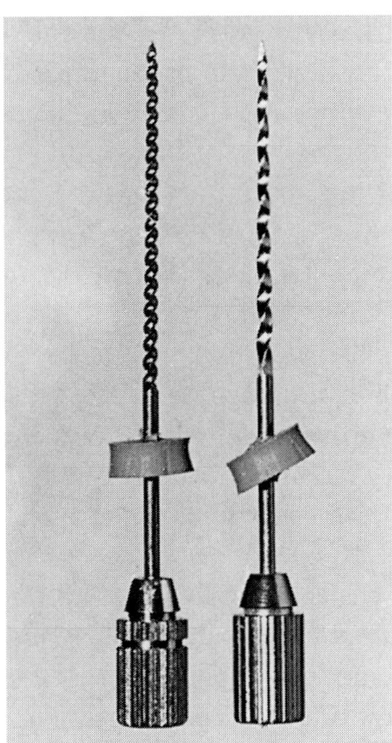

Figure 10-56 **Left**, Stop attachment should be placed perpendicular to the long axis of the instrument. **Right**, Obliquely placed stop attachment varies the length of tooth measurement by over 1 mm.

point on the tooth. It is also essential to record the reference point and the working length of each instrument in the patient's chart.

Instruments have been developed with millimeter marking rings etched or grooved into the shaft of the instrument. These act as a built-in ruler with the markings placed at 18, 19, 20, 22, and 24 mm. With these marking rings, the best coronal reference point on the tooth is at the **cavo-incisal** or **cavo-occlusal** angle. These marking rings are necessary when **rotary** nickel-titanium instruments are used.

METHODS OF DETERMINING WORKING LENGTH

Ideal Method

The requirements of an ideal method for determining working length might include rapid location of the apical constriction in all pulpal conditions and all canal contents; easy measurement, even when the relationship between the apical constriction and the radiographic apex is unusual; rapid periodic monitoring and confirmation; patient and clinician comfort; minimal radiation to the patient; ease of use in special patients such as those with severe gag reflex, reduced mouth opening, pregnancy etc; and cost effectiveness.[327,328]

To achieve the highest degree of accuracy in working length determination, a combination of several methods should be used. This is most important in canals for which working length determination is difficult. The most common methods are radiographic methods, digital tactile sense, and electronic methods. Apical periodontal sensitivity and paper point measurements have also been used.

Determination of Working Length by Radiographic Methods

Methods **requiring formulas** to determine working length have been abandoned. Bramante and Berbert reported great variability in formulaic determination of working length, with only a small percentage of successful measurements.[295]

The radiographic method known as the Ingle Method[329] has been compared with three other methods of determining working length.[295] The Ingle Method proved to be "superior to others" in the study. It showed a high percentage of success with a smaller variability. This method, first proposed more than 40 years ago, has withstood the test of time and has become the standard as the most commonly used method of radiographic working length estimation.

Radiographic Apex Location. *Materials and Conditions.* The following items are essential to perform this procedure:

1. Good, undistorted, preoperative radiographs showing the total length and all roots of the involved tooth.
2. Adequate coronal access to all canals.
3. An endodontic millimeter ruler.
4. Working knowledge of the average length of all of the teeth.
5. A definite, repeatable plane of reference to an anatomic landmark on the tooth, a fact that should be noted on the patient's record.

It is imperative that teeth with fractured cusps or cusps severely weakened by caries or restoration be reduced to a flattened surface, supported by dentin. Failure to do so may result in cusps or weak enamel walls being fractured between appointments (Figure 10-57). Thus, the original site of reference is lost. If this fracture goes unobserved, there is the probability of overinstrumentation and overfilling, particularly when anesthesia is used.

To establish the length of the tooth, a stainless steel reamer or file with an instrument stop on the shaft is needed. The exploring instrument size must be small enough to negotiate the total length of the canal but large enough not to be loose in the canal. A loose instrument may move in or out of the canal after the radi-

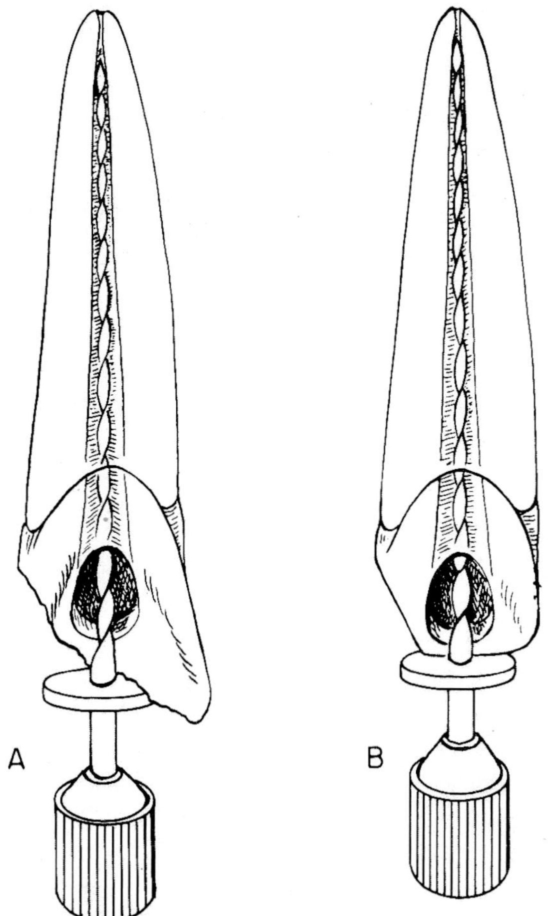

Figure 10-57 **A,** Do not use weakened enamel walls or diagonal lines of fracture as a reference site for length-of-tooth measurement. **B,** Weakened cusps or incisal edges are reduced to a well-supported tooth structure. Diagonal surfaces should be flattened to give an accurate site of reference.

ograph and cause serious error in determining the length of tooth. Moreover, fine instruments (Nos. 08 and 10) are often difficult to see in their entirety in a radiograph,[330] as are nickel-titanium instruments. Once again, in a curved canal, a **curved instrument** is essential.

Method

1. Measure the tooth on the preoperative radiograph (Figure 10-58, A).
2. Subtract at least 1.0 mm "safety allowance" for possible image distortion or magnification.[331]
3. Set the endodontic ruler at this tentative working length and adjust the stop on the instrument at that level (Figure 10-58, B).
4. Place the instrument in the canal until the stop is at the plane of reference unless pain is felt (if anesthesia has not been used), in which case, the instrument is left at that level and the rubber stop readjusted to this new point of reference.
5. Expose, develop, and clear the radiograph.
6. On the radiograph, measure the difference between the end of the instrument and the end of the root and add this amount to the original measured length the instrument extended into the tooth (Figure 10-58, C). If, through some oversight, the exploring instrument has gone beyond the apex, subtract this difference.
7. From this adjusted length of tooth, subtract a 1.0 mm "safety factor" to conform with the apical termination of the root canal at the apical constriction (see Figure 10-58, C).[332]

   Weine has made a sensible improvement in this determination: If, radiographically, there is no resorption of the root end or bone, shorten the length by the standard 1.0 mm.[332] If periapical bone resorption is apparent, shorten by 1.5 mm, and if both root and bone resorption are apparent, shorten by 2.0 mm (Figure 10-59). The reasoning behind this suggestion is thoughtful. If there is root resorption, the apical constriction is probably destroyed—hence the shorter move back up the canal. Also, when bone resorption is apparent, there probably is also root resorption, even though it may not be apparent radiographically.
8. Set the endodontic ruler at this new corrected length and readjust the stop on the exploring instrument (Figure 10-58, D).
9. Because of the possibility of radiographic distortion, sharply curving roots, and operator measuring error, a confirmatory radiograph of the adjusted length is highly desirable. In many instances, an added investment of a few minutes will prevent the discomfort and failure that stem from inaccuracy.
10. When the length of the tooth has been accurately confirmed, reset the endodontic ruler at this measurement.
11. Record this final working length and the coronal point of reference on the patient's record.
12. Once again, it is important to emphasize that the final working length may shorten by as much as 1 mm as a curved canal is straightened out by instrumentation.[314,315] It is therefore recommended that the "length of the tooth" in a curved canal be reconfirmed after instrumentation is completed.

Variations. When the two canals of a maxillary first premolar appear to be superimposed, much confusion and lost time may be saved by several simple means. Occasionally, it is advantageous to take individual radiographs of each canal with its length-of-tooth

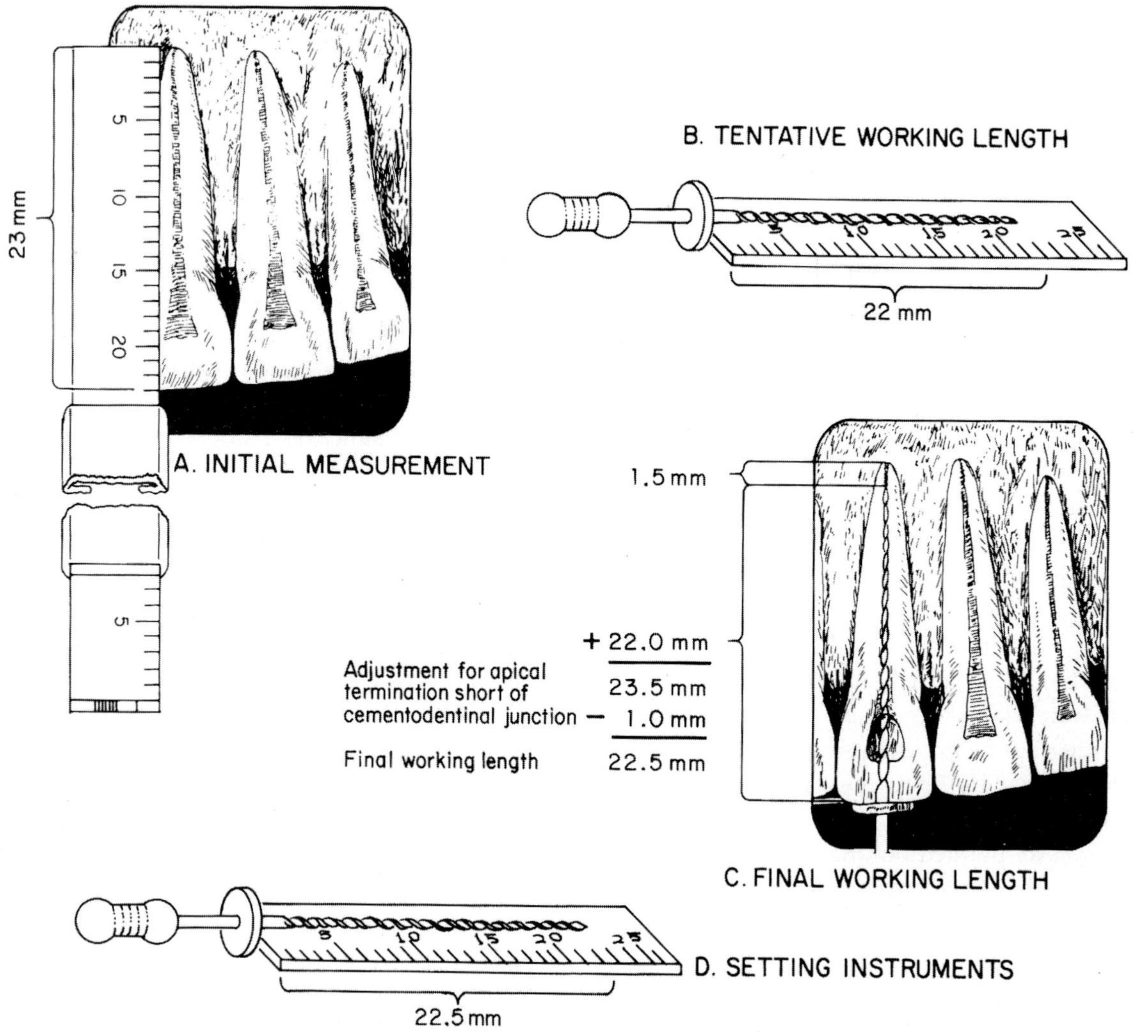

23 mm

A. INITIAL MEASUREMENT

B. TENTATIVE WORKING LENGTH

22 mm

1.5 mm

+ 22.0 mm

23.5 mm

Adjustment for apical termination short of cementodentinal junction − 1.0 mm

Final working length 22.5 mm

C. FINAL WORKING LENGTH

D. SETTING INSTRUMENTS

22.5 mm

Figure 10-58 A, Initial measurement. The tooth is measured on a good preoperative radiograph using the long cone technique. In this case, the tooth appears to be 23 mm long on the radiograph. **B**, Tentative working length. As a safety factor, allowing for image distortion or magnification, subtract at least 1 mm from the initial measurement for a tentative working length of 22 mm. The instrument is set with a stop at this length. **C**, Final working length. The instrument is inserted into the tooth to this length and a radiograph is taken. Radiograph shows that the image of the instrument appears to be 1.5 mm from the radiographic end of the root. This is added to the tentative working length, giving a total length of 23.5 mm. From this, subtract 1.0 mm as adjustment for apical termination short of the cementodentinal junction (see Anatomic Considerations). The final working length is 22.5 mm. **D**, Setting instruments. The final working length of 22.5 mm is used to set stops on instruments used to enlarge the root canal.

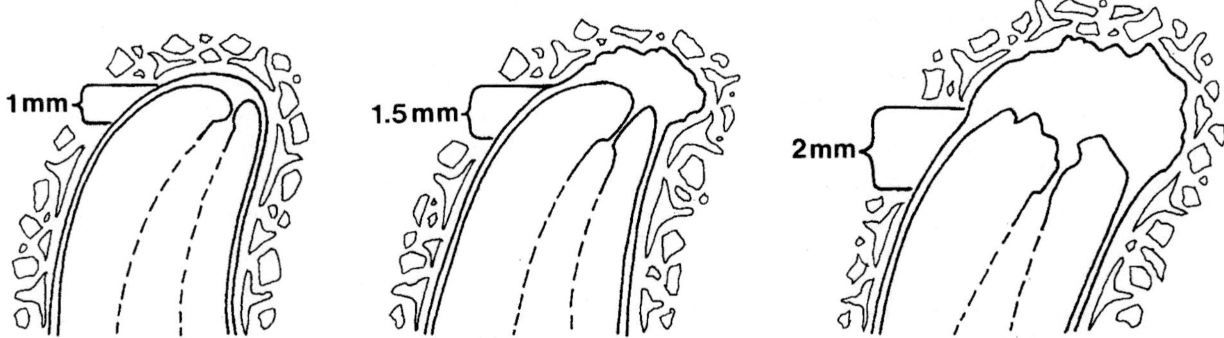

Figure 10-59 Weine's recommendations for determining working length based on radiographic evidence of root/bone resorption. **A**, If no root or bone resorption is evident, preparation should terminate 1.0 mm from the apical foramen. **B**, If bone resorption is apparent but there is no root resorption, shorten the length by 1.5 mm. **C**, If both root and bone resorption are apparent, shorten the length by 2.0 mm. (Courtesy of Dr. Franklin Weine.)

instrument in place. A preferable method is to expose the radiograph from a **mesial**-horizontal angle. This causes the lingual canal to always be the more mesial one in the image (MLM, Clark's rule) or, alternatively, **MBD**—when the x-ray beam is directed from the Mesial, the Buccal canal is projected toward the Distal on the film.

When a mandibular molar appears to have two mesial roots or apices of different lengths or positions, two mesial instruments can be used, and again the tooth can be examined radiographically from the mesial and Clark's or Ingle's rule (MLM or MBD) applied.

Accuracy. Just how accurate is this radiographic measurement method? For one thing, accuracy depends on the radiographic technique used. Forsberg, in Norway, demonstrated that paralleling technique was "significantly more reliable" than the bisecting-angle technique.[333] A US Army group, however, found that the paralleling technique was absolutely accurate only 82% of the time.[334] Von der Lehr and Marsh were accurate in anterior teeth 89% of the time.[335] Paralleling still magnifies actual tooth length by 5.4%.[331]

As Olson et al. pointed out, 82 to 89% accuracy is not 100%, so they recommended back-up methods such as tactile feel, moisture on the tip of a paper point, or electronic apex locators.[334] Similar results and recommendations have been reported worldwide.[336–341] A British group, for example, recommended the use of radiovisiography with image enhancement to improve the quality of length-of-tooth radiographs.[341]

Accuracy of Working Length Estimation by Direct Digital Radiography or Xeroradiography

Several studies have evaluated the advantages of using direct digital radiography or xeroradiography for the estimation of working length.[342–355]

The results of the studies indicate that there is no statistically significant difference in working length estimation accuracy between conventional film, direct digital radiography, and xeroradiography. On the other hand, **rapid imaging and reduction in radiation** by these techniques represent a significant advancement in dental radiography (see Chapter 9).

Determination of Working Length by Digital Tactile Sense

If the **coronal portion** of the canal is not constricted, an experienced clinician may detect an increase in resistance as the file approaches the apical 2 to 3 mm. This detection is by tactile sense. In this region, the canal frequently constricts (minor diameter) before exiting the root. There is also a tendency for the canal to deviate from the radiographic apex in this region.[299,301,302,339,356]

Seidberg et al. reported an accuracy of just 64% using digital tactile sense.[296] Another *in vivo* study found that the exact position of the apical constriction could be located accurately by tactile sense in only 25% of canals in their study.[357]

If the canals were preflared, it was possible for an expert to detect the apical constriction in about 75% of the cases.[358] If the canals were **not preflared**, determination of the apical constriction by tactile sensation was possible in only about **one-third** of the cases.[359]

All clinicians should be aware that this method, by itself, is often inexact. It is ineffective in root canals with an immature apex and is highly inaccurate if the canal is constricted throughout its entire length or if the canal has excessive curvature. This method should be considered as **supplementary** to high-quality, carefully aligned, parallel, working length radiographs and/or an apex locator.

A survey found that few general practice dentists and no endodontists trust the digital tactile sense method of determining working length by itself.[360] Even the most experienced specialist would be prudent to use two or more methods to determine accurate working lengths in every canal.

Determination of Working Length by Apical Periodontal Sensitivity

Any method of working length determination, based on the patient's response to pain, does not meet the ideal method of determining working length. Working length determination should be painless. Endodontic therapy has gained a notorious reputation for being painful, and it is incumbent on dentists to avoid perpetuating the fear of endodontics by inserting an endodontic instrument and using the patient's pain reaction to determine working length.

If an instrument is advanced in the canal toward **inflamed tissue**, the hydrostatic pressure developed inside the canal may cause moderate to severe, instantaneous pain. At the onset of the pain, the instrument tip may still be several millimeters short of the apical constriction. When pain is inflicted in this manner, little useful information is gained by the clinician, and considerable damage is done to the patient's trust.

When the canal contents are **totally necrotic**, however, the passage of an instrument into the canal and past the apical constriction may evoke only a mild awareness or possibly no reaction at all. The latter is common when a periradicular lesion is present because the tissue is not richly innervated. On the other hand, Langeland and associates reported that vital pulp tissue with nerves and vessels may remain in the most apical part of the main canal even in the presence of a large periapical lesion.[361–363] This suggests that a painful response may be obtained inside the canal even though the canal contents are "necrotic" and there is a periapical lesion.

It would appear that any response from the patient, even an eye squint or wrinkling of the forehead, calls for reconfirmation of working length by other methods available and/or profound supplementary anesthesia.

Determination of Working Length by Paper Point Measurement

In a root canal with an immature (wide open) apex, the most reliable means of determining working length is to gently pass the **blunt end** of a paper point into the canal after profound anesthesia has been achieved. The moisture or blood on the portion of the paper point that passes beyond the apex may be an estimation of working length or the junction between the root apex and the bone. In cases in which the apical constriction has been lost owing to resorption or perforation, and in which there is no free bleeding or suppuration into the canal, the moisture or blood on the paper point is an estimate of the amount the preparation is overextended. This paper point measurement method is a **supplementary** one.

A new dimension has recently been added to paper points by the addition of millimeter markings (Figure 10-60). These paper points have markings at 18, 19, 20, 22, and 24 mm from the tip and can be used to estimate the point at which the paper point passes out of the apex. These paper points were designed to ensure that they be inserted fully to the apical constriction. The accuracy of these markings should be checked on a millimeter ruler.

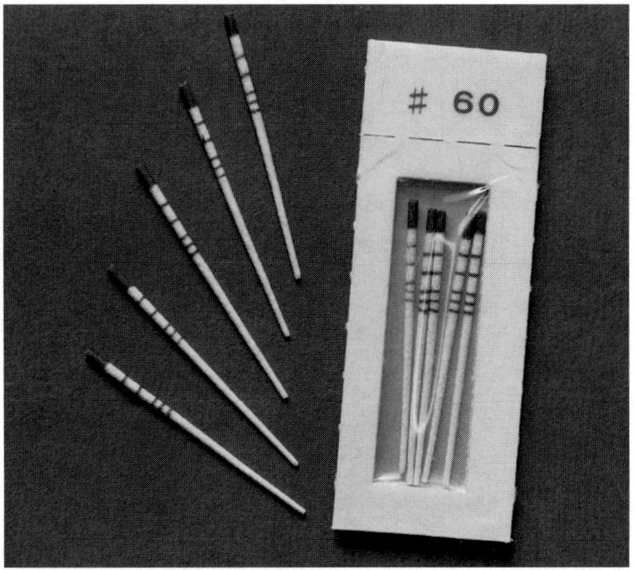

Figure 10-60 Absorbent paper points, sterilized, color coded, and marked with millimeter markings. (Courtesy of Diadent Group, Burnaby, BC, Canada)

Determination of Working Length by Electronics

Evolution of Apex Locators. Although the term "apex locator" is commonly used and has become accepted terminology,[298] it is a misnomer.[364] Some authors have used other terms to be more precise.[365–372] These devices all attempt to locate the apical constriction, the cementodentinal junction, or the apical foramen. They are not capable of routinely locating the radiographic apex. In 1918, Custer was the first to report the use of electric current to determine working length.[373] The scientific basis for apex locators originated with research conducted by Suzuki in 1942.[374] His *in vivo* research on dogs using direct current discovered that the electrical resistance between the periodontal ligament and the oral mucosa was a constant value of 6.5 kilo-ohms. In 1960, Gordon was the second to report the use of a clinical device for electrical measurement of root canals.[375] Sunada adopted the principle reported by Suzuki and was the first to describe the detail of a simple clinical device to measure working length in patients.[376] He used a simple direct current ohmmeter to measure a constant resistance of 6.5 kilo-ohms between oral mucous membrane and the periodontum regardless of the size or shape of the teeth. The device used by Sunada in his research became the basis for most apex locators.

Inoue made significant contributions to the evolution of apex locators in North America with his reports on the Sono-Explorer.[294,377–380] In recent years, several advancements and modification in the electronic design of apex locators have been reported.[381–388]

All apex locators function by using the human body to complete an electrical circuit. One side of the apex locator's circuitry is connected to an endodontic instrument. The other side is connected to the patient's body, either by a contact to the patient's lip or by an electrode held in the patient's hand. The electrical circuit is complete when the endodontic instrument is advanced apically inside the root canal until it touches periodontal tissue (Figure 10-61). The display on the apex locator indicates that the apical area has been reached.

This simple and commonly accepted explanation for the electronic phenomenon has been challenged.[382,383,389]

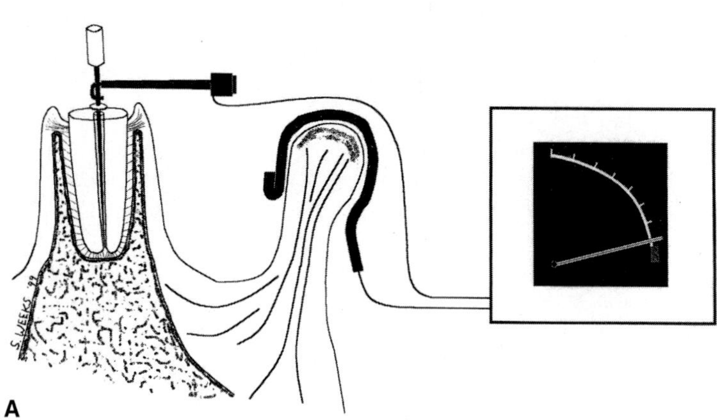

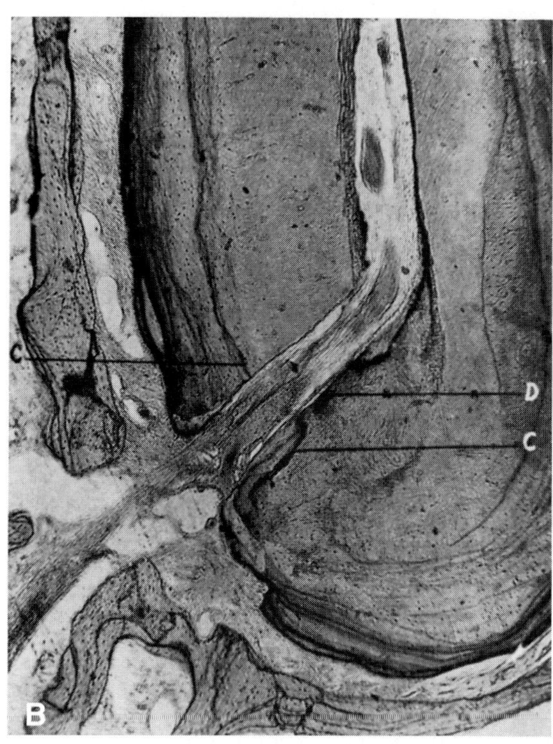

Figure 10-61 **A**, Typical circuit for electronic determination of working length. Current flows from Electronic apex locator (EAL) to the file, to the cementoenamel junction and back to the EAL, where the position of the tips is illustrated. The circuit is completed through lip attachment. **B**, The apical foramen some distance from the radiographic apex stresses the importance of finding the actual orifice by EAL. D = dentin; C = cementum. **A** courtesy of Dr. Stephen Weeks. **B** reproduced with permission from Skillen WG. J Am Dent Assoc 1930;17:2082.

There is evidence that electronic devices measure mainly the impedance of the probing electrode (contact impedance with the tissue fluid) rather than tissue impedance itself. Huang reported that the principle of electronic root canal measurement can be explained by physical principles of electricity alone.[389] Ushiyama and colleagues presented this as the "voltage gradient method" that could accurately measure working length in root canals filled with electrolyte.[381–383] A major disadvantage with this method was that it used a special bipolar electrode that was too large to pass into narrow root canals.

Experimental Design and Parameters of Accuracy Studies. *In vitro* accuracy studies may be conducted on models using an extracted tooth in an electrolyte to simulate clinical conditions.[366,368–370,390–394] The ideal conditions in *in vitro* testing may give accuracy results higher than those obtainable in clinical practice. Alternatively, in the fabrication of the *in vitro* model, electrolyte may be inadvertently forced into the canal space and give rise to an inaccuracy.

In vivo accuracy studies more closely reflect the reality of conditions in clinical practice. The best studies are those that use an apex locator to determine the working length of a canal followed by "locking" the measuring instrument at the electronic length. The tooth is extracted, and the exact relationship between the electronic length and the apical constriction is determined. Unfortunately, this design is not a viable alternative in most studies. Even when the design is used, the studies might be improved by prior shaping and cleaning of the canal followed by multiple electronic working length determinations.

In *in vivo* comparative studies in which the electronic file tip to apical constriction is also assessed by radiographs, the validity of the results is open to question. The comparisons are only as accurate as the accuracy of the radiographic method of estimating working length. Current information places this accuracy in the 39 to 86% range.[301,340,356,365,395–398]

Using cadavers, Pratten and McDonald compared the accuracy of three parallel radiographs of each canal at three horizontal angles with the accuracy of the Endex apex locator.[399] Even in these ideal conditions, radiographic estimation was no more accurate than electronic determination.

Another important point in accuracy studies is the **error tolerance** that is accepted in the experimental design. There appears to be a growing concern that either a +0.5 error or a –0.5 error may give rise to clinical problems and that the **±0.5 tolerance may be unacceptable.**[400]

It would be useful clinically to use the apical constriction as the ideal apical reference point in the canal rather than the apical foramen.[401,402] Consideration should also be given to using –0.5 to 0.0 mm as the most **clinically ideal** error tolerance.

Classification and Accuracy of Apex Locators. The classification of apex locators presented here is a modification of the classification presented by

McDonald.[403] This classification is based on the type of current flow and the opposition to the current flow, as well as the number of frequencies involved.

First-Generation Apex Locators. First-generation apex location devices, also known as resistance apex locators,[403] measure opposition to the flow of direct current or resistance. When the tip of the reamer reaches the apex in the canal, the resistance value is 6.5 kilo-ohms (current 40 mA). Although it had some problems, the original device was reported to be most accurate in palatal canals of maxillary molars and premolars.[295] Initially, the Sono-Explorer (Satalec, Inc, Mount Laurel, N.J.) was imported from Japan by Amadent. Today, most first-generation apex location devices are off the market.

Second-Generation Apex Locators. Second-generation apex locators, also known as impedance apex locators,[403] measure opposition to the flow of alternating current or impedance. Inoue developed the **Sono-Explorer**,[377–380] one of the earliest of the second-generation apex locators. Several other second-generation apex locators then became available, including a number of improvements in the Sono-Explorer.

The major disadvantage of second-generation apex locators is that the root canal has to be reasonably free of electroconductive materials to obtain accurate readings. The presence of tissue and electroconductive irrigants in the canal changes the electrical characteristics and leads to inaccurate, usually shorter measurements.[390] This created a "catch-22" situation. Should canals be cleaned and dried to measure working length, or should working length be measured to clean and dry canals?[404]

There is another issue: not all apex locators incorporate the same degree of sophistication in electronic circuitry that adjusts its sensitivity to compensate for the intracanal environment[405] or indicates on its display that it should be switched from a "wet" to a "dry" mode or vice versa. Pilot and Pitts reported that 5.25% sodium hypochlorite solution, 14.45% EDTA solution, and normal saline were conductive, whereas RC Prep and isopropyl alcohol were not.[406]

The Apex Finder (Sybron Endo/Analytic; Orange, Calif.) has a visual digital LED indicator and is self-calibrating. The **Endo Analyzer (Analytic/Endo; Orange, Calif.)** is a combined apex locator and pulp tester. The Apex Finder has been subjected to several in vivo studies.[365,397,407,408] Compared to radiographic working length estimations, one study placed the accuracy at 67% (± 0.5 mm from the radiographic apex).[365] In a study in which Apex Finder working length determinations were compared with direct anatomic working length measurements, only 20% of the determinations were "coincident," and 53% were short.[397]

The **Digipex** (Mada Equipment Co., Carlstadt, N.J.) has a visual LED digital indicator and an audible indicator.[404] It requires calibration. The **Digipex II** is a combination apex locator and pulp vitality tester.

The **Exact-A-Pex** (Ellman International, Hewlett, N.Y.) has an LED bar graph display and an audio indicator.[404] An *in vivo* study reported an accuracy of 55% (± 0.5 mm from the apical foramen).

The **Foramatron IV** (Parkell Dental, Farmingdale, N.Y.) has a flashing LED light and a digital LED display and does not require calibration. Two *in vivo* studies were reported on the Foramatron IV (Figure 10-62).[408,409] Electronic determinations in one study were found to be accurate (± 0.5 mm from the radiographic apex) in 65% of the cases.[408] In the other study, 32% of the cases were "coincident" with the radiographic apex and 36% were short.[409] None were long. This device is small, lightweight, and inexpensive.

The **Pio** (Denterials Ltd., St. Louis, Mo.) apex locator has an analog meter display and an audio indicator. It has an adjusting knob for calibration.

Third-Generation Apex Locators. The principle on which "third-generation" apex locators are based requires a short introduction. In biologic settings, the reactive component facilitates the flow of alternating current, more for higher than for lower frequencies. Thus, a **tissue** through which two alternating currents of differing frequencies are flowing **will impede** the lower-frequency current more than the higher-frequency current. The reactive component of the circuit may change, for example, as the position of a file changes in a canal. When this occurs, the impedances offered by the circuit to currents of differing frequencies will change relative to each other. This is the principle on which the operation of the "third-generation" apex locators is based (SM Weeks, personal communication, 1999).

Since the impedance of a given circuit may be substantially influenced by the frequency of the current flow, these devices have been called "**frequency dependent**" (SM Weeks, personal communication, 1999). Since it is impedance, not frequency, that is measured by these devices, and since the relative magnitudes of the impedances are converted into "length" information, the term "**comparative impedance**" may be more appropriate (SM Weeks, personal communication, 1999).

Endex (Osada Electric Co., Los Angeles, Calif. and Japan), the original third-generation apex locator, was described by Yamaoka et al.[410] (Figure 10-63). In Europe and Asia, this device is available as the APIT. It uses a very low alternating current.[411] The signals of

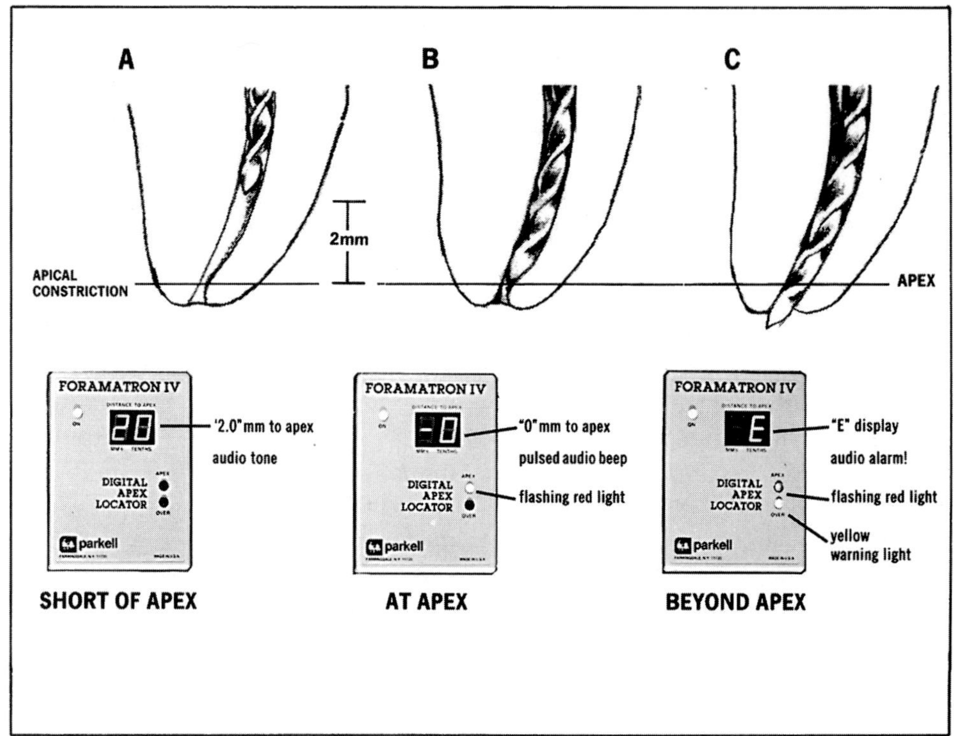

Figure 10-62 Modern electrical apex locator that displays **A**, by digital readout, distance of the file tip to the cementodentinal junction in tenths of millimeters; **B**, "O" reading, flashing red light, and pulsing tone when the cementodentinal junction is reached. **C**, If the apical constriction is penetrated, a yellow warning light flashes, a visual "E" (error) is displayed, and an audio alarm warns the dentist. (Courtesy of Formatron/Parkell Products, Inc., Farmingdale, N.Y.)

two frequencies (5 and 1 kHz) are applied as a composite waveform of both frequencies. As the attached endodontic reamer enters the coronal part of the canal, the difference in the impedances at the two frequencies is small. As the instrument is advanced apically, the difference in impedance values begins to change. As the apical constriction is reached, the impedance values are at their maximum difference, and these differences are indicated on the analog meter and audio alarm. This impedance difference is the basis of the "difference method."[380] The unit must then be "reset" (calibrated) for each canal.

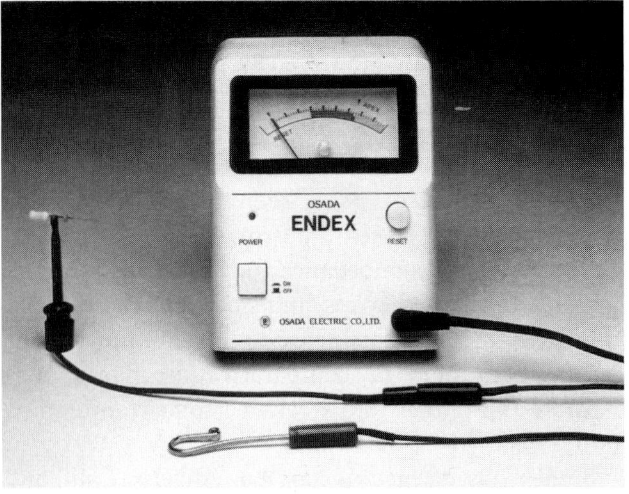

Figure 10-63 Endex (aka APIT), the original third-generation apex locator. It measures the impedance between two currents and works in a "wet" canal with sodium hypochlorite. (Courtesy of Osada Electric Co.)

The device operates most accurately when the canal is filled with electrolyte (ie, normal saline or sodium hypochlorite). Gutta-percha must be removed from the canals in re-treatment cases before electronic working length determination is made with this device. The manufacturer indicates that the size of the endodontic instrument does not affect the measurement.[411]

The Endex has been the subject of several accuracy studies.[358,364,397,399,412–420] One *in vitro* study reported that the Endex was superior to second-generation devices when there was conductive fluid in the canals and when the apical foramen was widened.[413] Other *in vitro* studies compared the Endex electronic working length determination with direct anatomic working length measurement. One study reported an accuracy of 96.5% (–0.5 to 0.0 mm from the apical foramen).[414] Another study reported an accuracy of 85% (± 0.5 mm from the apical foramen).[358]

The Pratten and McDonald *in vitro* study of teeth in human cadavers compared Endex determinations to radiograph estimations and to direct anatomic working length measurements. The Endex was slightly more reliable than the radiographic technique: 81% of the Endex determinations were –0.5 to 0.0 mm from the **apical constriction** in the study.[399]

Two *in vivo* studies compared the Endex determinations to radiographic working length estimations. One study reported that 63% of the determinations were –1.0 to 0.0 mm from the radiographic apex,[409] whereas the other study reported an accuracy of 89.6% (± 0.5 mm from the apical constriction) in moist canals.[415] One *in vivo* study reported that the Endex could be used to determine working length under various conditions, such as bleeding, exudate, and hypochlorite in the canals.[420] Four studies reported on the comparison of Endex determinations and direct anatomic measurements. Two of the studies reported an accuracy of 72% and 93%, respectively (± 0.5 mm from the apical foramen).[364,418] A third study reported that about 66% of the determinations were –0.75 to 0.0 mm from the apical constriction and the determinations were unaffected by pulp status.[417] The fourth study reported that the determinations were "coincident" with the minor foramen in 37% of the canals and short in 47%.[397]

The **Neosono Ultima Ez** Apex Locator (Satelec Inc; Mount Laurel, N.J.) is a third-generation device that supersedes the second-generation Sono-Explorer line. To circumvent the Japanese patents of two alternating current frequencies, Amadent developed a device with multiple frequences and implanted a microchip that sorts out two of the many frequencies to give an accurate reading in either wet or dry canals. It works best in the presence of sodium hypochlorite. The Ultima-Ez is mounted with a root canal graphic showing file position as well as an audible signal. The ability to "set" the digital readout at 0.5 or 1.0 mm allows measurements of wide open canals as well. The Ultima-Ez also comes with an **attached pulp tester**, called the **Co-Pilot** (Amadent; Cherry Hill, N.J.). To date, the **Dental Advisor** (Ogden, Utah) has had five consultants who used the device 26 times and reported its reliability to be better in wet canals than in dry. They also stated that it was "Quick and easy to use."

The **Mark V Plus** (Moyco/Union Broach, Miller Dental, Bethpage, N.Y.) is identical in circuitry and performance to the Neosono Ultima Ez. To date, no evaluations of the device have been published.

The **JUSTWO** or **JUSTY II** (Toesco Toei Engineering Co./Medidenta, Woodside, N.Y. and Japan) is another third-generation apex locator. The device uses frequencies of 500 and 2,000 Hz in a "relative value method."[421] Two electric potentials are obtained that correspond to two impedances of the root canal. These two potentials are converted to logarithmic values, and one is subtracted from the other. The result drives the meter. The rationale of the JUSTWO resembles that of the Root ZX.[422] The analog meter and audio indicator display the position of the instrument tip inside the canal. The unit determines working length in the presence of electrolytes. Although no calibration is required, a calibration check is recommended.

Two *in vitro* studies have been reported on this device. In one, in which electronic measurements were compared to radiographic working length, the mean distance from the radiographic apex was 0.98 ± 0.44 mm. In the other study, the device showed an average deviation of 0.04 ± 0.05 mm from the direct anatomic working length measurement.[423]

The **APEX FINDER A.F.A.** ("All Fluids Allowed"—Model 7005, Sybron Endo/Analytic; Orange, Calif.) uses multiple frequencies and comparative impedance principles in its electronic circuitry (Figure 10-64). It is reported to be accurate regardless of irrigants or fluids in the canals being measured. It has a liquid crystal display (LCD) panel that indicates the distance of the instrument tip from the apical foramen in 0.1 mm increments. It also has an audio chime indicator. The display has a bar graph "canal condition indicator" that reflects canal wetness/dryness and allows the user to

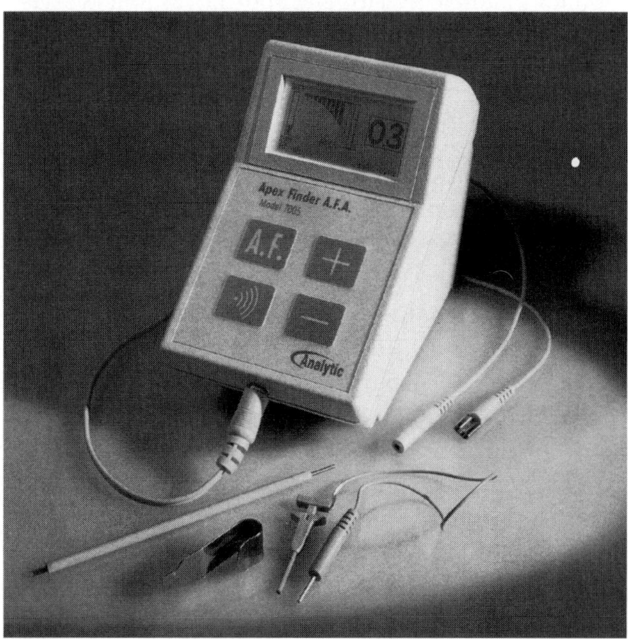

Figure 10-64 The Apex Finder A.F.A. (All Fluids Allowed) third-generation apex locator. It functions best with an electrolyte present and displays, on an LCD panel, the distance of the file tip from the apex in 0.1 mm increments. (Courtesy of Sybron Endo/Analytic.)

improve canal conditions for electronic working length determination.[424] The **Endo Analyzer 8005** combines electronic apex location and pulp testing in one unit.

McDonald et al. reported an *in vitro* study of the Apex Finder A.F.A.[425] The device was able to locate the **cementodentinal junction** or a point 0.5 mm coronal to it **with 95% accuracy.**

The **ROOT ZX** (J. Morita Mfg. Co.; Irvine, Calif. and Japan), a third-generation apex locator that uses dual-frequency and comparative impedance principles, was described by Kobayashi (Figure 10-65)[387,388] The electronic method employed was the "ratio method" or "division method." The Root ZX simultaneously measures the two impedances at two frequencies (8 and 0.4 kHz) inside the canal. A microprocessor in the device calculates the ratio of the two impedances. The quotient of the impedances is displayed on an LCD meter panel and represents the position of the instrument tip inside the canal. The quotient "was hardly influenced by the electrical conditions of the canal but changed considerably near the apical foramen."[388]

The Root ZX is mainly based on detecting the change in electrical capacitance that occurs near the apical constriction.[388] Some of the advantages of the **Root ZX** are that it **requires no adjustment or calibration** and can be used when the canal is filled with strong electrolyte or when the canal is "empty" and **moist.** The meter is an easy-to-read LCD. The position of the instrument tip inside the canal is indicated on the LCD meter and by the monitor's audible signals. The Root ZX, as well as several other apex locators, allows shaping and cleaning of the root canal with simultaneous, continuous monitoring of the working length.[371,387,388,419,426–429]

Several studies have reported on the accuracy and reliability of the Root ZX.[392,403,412,430–432] In these studies, electronic working length determinations made by the Root ZX were compared with direct anatomic working length mesurements. Three studies reported an accuracy for the device that ranged from 84 to 100% (± 0.5 mm from the apical foramen).[392,412,430] Murphy et al. used the **apical constriction** as the ideal apical reference point in the canal and reported an accuracy of 44% in the narrow tolerance range of 0.0 to + 0.5 mm from the apical constriction.[402] One study reported that the Root ZX showed less average deviation than a second-generation device (Sono-Explorer Mark III) tested.[432]

Studies on the Root ZX "display increment marks" reiterate that the Root ZX display is a relative scale and does not indicate absolute intracanal distances from the apical constriction. In clinical practice, the 0.5-increment mark is often taken to correspond to the apical constriction, but, according to the manufacturer, the 0.5-increment mark is an average of –0.2 to 0.3 mm beyond the apical constriction.[428] The operating instructions for the Root ZX state, "The working length of the canal used to calculate the length of the filling material is actually somewhat shorter. Find the length of the apical seat (i.e., the end point of the filling material) by subtracting –0.5-1.0 mm from the working length indicated by the 0.5 reading on the meter."[428] They suggested that the Root ZX should be used with the 0.0 or "APEX" increment mark as the most accurate apical reference point. The clinician should then adjust the working length on the endodontic instrument for the margin of safety that is desired (ie, 1 mm short).

A number of *in vitro* and *in vivo* studies on the accuracy and reliability of the Root ZX have been reported.[397,401,433–438] Electronic working length determinations made with the Root ZX were compared with direct anatomic working length measurements after extraction of the teeth in the study. Four studies indicated an accuracy for the Root ZX in the range of 82 to 100% (± 0.5 mm from the apical foramen).[433–438] One study reported an accuracy of 82% (± 0.5 mm from the apical constriction).[401] McDonald et al. reported that the Root ZX demonstrated 95% accuracy in their study when the parameters were –0.5 to 0.0 mm from the cementodentinal junction.[425]

Combination Apex Locator and Endodontic Handpiece. The **Tri Auto ZX** (J. Morita Mfg. Corp. USA; Irvine, Calif.) is a cordless electric **endodontic handpiece with a built-in Root ZX apex locator** (Figure 10-66).[439] The handpiece uses nickel-titanium rotary instruments that rotate at 280 ± 50 rpm.[440] The position of the tip of the rotary instrument is continuously monitored on the LED control panel of the handpiece during the shaping and cleaning of the canal.

The Tri Auto ZX has three automatic safety mechanisms. The handpiece automatically starts rotation when the instrument enters the canal and stops when the instrument is removed (**auto-start-stop mechanism**). The handpiece also automatically stops and reverses the rotation of the instrument when the torque threshold (30 grams/centimeter) is exceeded (**auto-torque-reverse mechanism**), a mechanism developed to prevent instrument breakage. In addition, the handpiece automatically stops and reverses rotation when the instrument tip reaches a distance from the apical constriction that has been preset by the clinician (**auto-apical-reverse mechanism**), a mechanism controlled by the built-in Root ZX apex locator and developed to prevent instrumentation beyond the apical constriction.

The Tri Auto ZX has four modes. In the Electronic Measurement of Root (**EMR**) mode, a lip clip, hand file, and file holder are used with the apex locator in the handpiece to determine working length. The handpiece motor does not operate in this mode. In **LOW** mode, the torque threshold is lower than in the HIGH mode. The LOW mode is used with small to mid-sized instruments for shaping and cleaning the apical and mid-third sections of the root canal. All three automatic safety mechanisms are functional in this mode. In **HIGH** mode, the torque threshold is higher than the LOW mode but lower than the MANUAL mode. The HIGH mode is used with mid-size to large instruments for shaping and cleaning in the mid-third and coronal-third sections of the root canal. All three automatic safety mechanisms are functional in this mode. **MANUAL** mode offers the highest threshold of torque. In MANUAL mode, the auto-start-stop and the auto-torque-reverse mechanisms do not function. The auto-apical-reverse mechanism does function. MANUAL mode is generally used with large instruments for coronal flaring.

Kobayashi et al. suggested that "to get the best results, it may be necessary to use some hand instrumentation" in combination with the Tri Auto ZX, depending on the difficulty and morphology of the root canal being treated.[439]

In vitro, the accuracy of the EMR mode of the Tri Auto ZX to determine working length to the apical constriction has been reported at 0.02 ± 0.06 mm.[441] Another *in vitro* study reported that about half of the canals studied were short (-0.48 ± 0.10 mm) and half were long ($+ 0.56 \pm 0.05$).[431] A second study concluded that shaping and cleaning with the Tri Auto ZX (AAR mechanism set at 1.0) consistently approximated

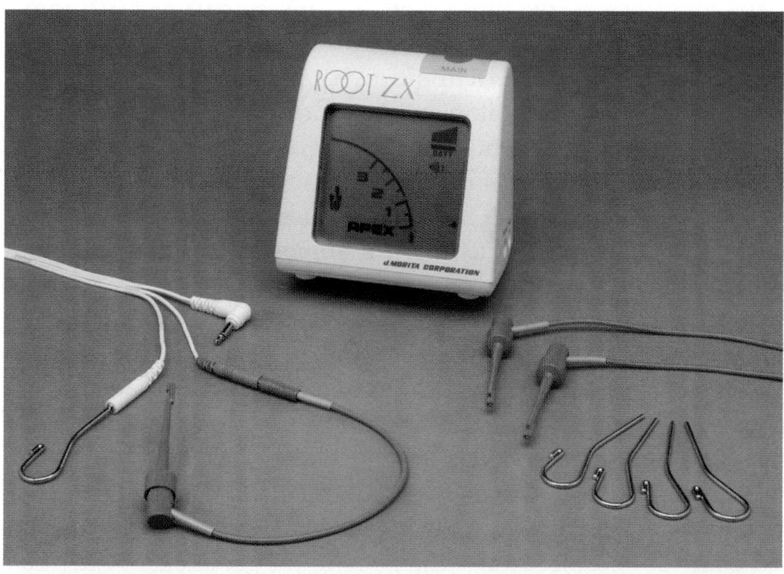

Figure 10-65 **Root ZX** third-generation apex locator with accessories (**left**) and extra accessories (**right**). The Root ZX microprocessor calculates the ratio of two impedances and displays a file's approach to the apex on a liquid crystal display. It functions in both a "dry" or canal "wet" with electrolyte. (Courtesy of J. Morita Mfg. Co.)

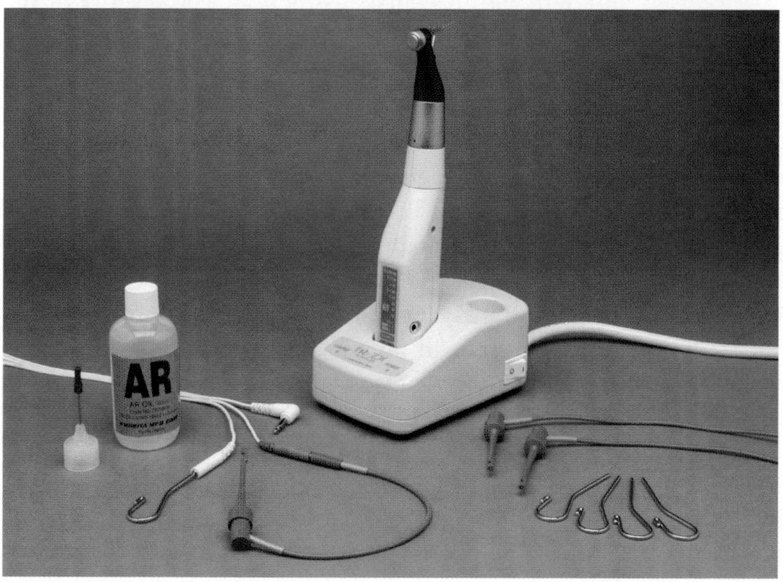

Figure 10-66 The **Tri-Auto ZX** is primarily a cordless, automatic, endodontic handpiece with a built-in **Root ZX** apex locator. The position of the nickel-titanium rotary instrument tip is constantly being monitored and displayed on the LED control panel. A built-in safety feature stops and reverses the motor when the apex is approached by the tip of the file. Accessories include (**left**) an **AR** contra-angle lubricant with a dispensing cap and apex locator attachments. Additional accessories (**right**). (Courtesy of J. Morita Mfg. Co.)

the apical constriction.[442] The accuracy was reported to have 95% "acceptable" measurements (± 0.5 mm) in a study that compared the direct anatomic working length with the electronic working length.[443]

The accuracy of the level of instrumentation with the Tri Auto ZX (J. Morita Mfg. Corp. USA; Irvine, Calif.) was reported in an *in vivo* study.[444] The canals were shaped and cleaned with the Tri Auto ZX (low mode) with the auto-apical-reverse mechanism set at 1.0. In all cases, radiographs showed that the preinstrumentation working length was within 0.5 mm of the final instrument working length and without overextension of gutta-percha, instrument breakage, or canal transportation.

Other Apex-Locating Handpieces. Kobayashi et al. reported the development of a new ultrasonic root canal system called the **SOFY ZX** (J. Morita Mfg. Corp.; Irvine, Calif.), which uses the Root ZX to electronically monitor the location of the file tip during all instrumentation procedures.[445,446] The device minimizes the danger of overinstrumentation.

The **Endy 7000** (Ionyx SA, Blanquefort Cedex, France) is available in Europe. It is an endodontic handpiece connected to an Endy apex locator that reverses the rotation of the endodontic instrument when it reaches a point in the apical region preset by the clinician.

Other Uses of Apex Locators. Sunada suggested the possibility of using apex locators to detect **root perforations.**[376] It was later reported that Electronic Apex Locators (EALs) could accurately determine the location of root or pulpal floor perforations.[447,448] The method also aided in the diagnosis of **external resorption** that had invaded the dental pulp space or **internal resorption** that had perforated to the external root surface.[367] A method for conservative treatment of root perforations using an apex locator and thermal compaction has been reported.[449]

An *in vitro* study to test the accuracy of the Root ZX to detect root perforations compared with other types of apex locators reported that all of the apex locators tested were acceptable for detection of root perforations.[450] No statistical significance was found between large perforations and small perforations. **Prepared pin holes** can be checked by apex locators to detect perforation into the pulp or into the periodontal ligament.[451] Horizontal or vertical **root fractures** could also be detected as well as **post perforations.**

In this latter case, the EAL file holder is connected to a large file, and the file then contacts the top of the post. The Root ZX will sound a single sustained beep, and the word "APEX" will begin flashing.

An *in vivo* study has evaluated the usefulness of an apex locator in endodontic treatment of teeth with **incomplete root formation** requiring **apexification.**[452] They reported that in all cases, the EAL was 2 to 3 mm short of the radiographic apex at the beginning of apexification therapy. When the apical closure was complete, the apex locator was then 100% accurate. In cases of **immature teeth with open apices**, a study reported that apex locators were **inaccurate.**[453] In contrast, an *in vivo* study using absorbent paper points for estimating the working lengths of immature teeth has been described.[454] They reported that in 95% of the cases for which the working length was estimated by paper points, they were within 1 mm of the working length estimated by radiographs.

An *in vitro* study evaluated the accuracy of the **Root ZX** in determining working length in **primary teeth.**[455] Electronic determinations were compared with direct anatomic and radiographic working lengths. They reported that the electronic determinations were similar to the direct anatomic measurements (–0.5 mm). Radiographic measurements were longer (0.4 to 0.7 mm) than electronic determinations.

Apex locators can be very useful in management of inpatients and outpatients. For example, they can be an important tool in endodontic treatment in the **operating room.** They also **reduce the number of radiographs,** which may be important for those who are very concerned about radiation hygiene. In some patients, such concern is so strong that dental radiographs are refused. An apex locator can be of enormous value in such situations.

Contraindications. The use of apex locators, and other **electrical devices** such as pulp testers, electrosurgical instruments, and desensitizing equipment, is **contraindicated for patients who have cardiac pacemakers.** Electrical stimulation to the pacemaker patient can interfere with pacemaker function. The severity of the interference depends on the specific type of pacemaker and the patient's dependence on it.[456] In special cases, an apex locator may be used on a patient with a pacemaker when it is done in close consultation with the patient's cardiologist.[457]

The Future. The future of apex locators is very bright. Significant improvement in the reliability and accuracy of apex locators took place with the development of third-generation models. It is probable that more dentists will now use apex locators in the management of endodontic cases. At this time, however, the conclusions of **studies have not demonstrated** that apex locators are clearly superior to radiographic techniques, nor can they **routinely** replace radiographs in working length determination. It has been demonstrated that they are at least equally accurate.[399]

Studies have concluded that when apex locators are used in conjunction with radiographs, there is a reduction in the number of radiographs required[365,408,458] and that some of the problems associated with radiographic working length estimation can be eliminated.[459]

An understanding of the morphology in the apical one-third of the canal is essential.[299–308,311,312] Consideration should be given to adopting the parameter of 0.5 to 0.0 mm (from the apical constriction) as the most ideal apical reference point in the canal. Electronic working length determinations should be accomplished with multiple measurements and should be done in conjunction with the shaping and cleaning procedure. Consideration should be given to the evaluation of the accuracy of obturation as an indicator of the accuracy of the working length determination. Future apex locators should be able to determine working length in all electric conditions of the root canal without calibration. The meter display on future apex locators should accurately indicate how many millimeters the endodontic instrument tip is from the apical constriction.[371]

TECHNIQUES OF RADICULAR CAVITY PREPARATION

Over the years, there has been a gradual change in the ideal configuration of a prepared root canal. At one time, the suggested shape was round and tapered, almost parallel, resembling in silhouette an obelisk like the Washington Monument, ending in a pyramid matching the 75-degree point of the preparatory instruments. After Schilder's classic description of "cleaning and shaping," the more accepted shape for the finished canal has become a **gradually increasing taper**, with the smallest diameter at the apical constricture, terminating larger at the coronal orifice.[460]

This gradually increasing taper is effective in final filling for as Buchanan pointed out, the "apical movement of the cone into a tapered apical preparation...only tightens the apical seal."[461] But, as Buchanan further noted, "overzealous canal shaping to achieve this taper has been at the expense of tooth structure in the coronal two-thirds of the preparation leading to perforations" and, one might add, materially weakening the tooth.[461] Grossly tapered preparations may well go back to Berg, an early Boston endodontist, who enlarged canals to enormous size to accommodate large heated pluggers used to condense warm sectional gutta-percha.[462]

Step-Back or Step-Down?

As previously stated, two approaches to débriding and shaping the canal have finally emerged: either starting at the apex with fine instruments and working one's way back up (or down) the canal with progressively larger instruments—the **"step-back"** or serial technique—or the opposite, starting at the cervical orifice with larger instruments and gradually progressing toward the apex with smaller and smaller instruments—the **"step-down"** technique, also called **"crown-down"** filing.

Hybrid approaches have also developed out of the two methods. Starting coronally with larger instruments, often power driven, one works down the straight coronal portion of the canal with progressively smaller instruments—the step-down approach. Then, at this point, the procedure is reversed, starting at the apex with small instruments and gradually increasing in size as one works back up the canal—the step-back approach. This hybrid approach could be called, quite clumsily, the step-down-step-back technique or "modified double-flared technique." [463]

Any one of these methods of preparing the root canal will ensure staying within the confines of the canal and delivering a continuously tapered preparation and, as Buchanan noted, eliminate blocking, "apical ledging, transportation, ripping, zipping and perforation."[464]

Step-Back Preparation. Weine, Martin, Walton, and Mullaney were early advocates of step-back, also called telescopic or serial root canal preparation.[465–468] Designed to overcome instrument transportation in the apical-third canal, as described earlier (Figure 10-67), it has proved quite successful. When Weine coined the term "zip" to describe this error of commission, it became a "buzz word," directing attention to apical aberrant preparations, principally in curved canals. Walton has depicted these variations, ranging from ledge to perforation to zip (Figure 10-68). The damage not only destroys the apical constriction, so important to the compaction of the root canal filling, but also produces an hourglass-shaped canal.[469] In this, the narrowest width of the canal is transported far away from the apex and prevents the proper cleansing and filling of the apical region (see Figure 10-68). In the case of severely curved canals, perforation at the curve's elbow leads to disastrous results (Figure 10-69).

Step-Back Preparation and Curved Canals. This method of preparation has been well described by Mullaney.[468] His approach has been modified, however, to deliver a continuing tapered preparation.[461] Mullaney divided the step-back preparation into two phases. Phase I is the apical preparation starting at the apical constriction. Phase II is the preparation of the remainder of the canal, gradually stepping back while increasing in size. The completion of the preparation is the Refining Phase IIA and IIB to produce the continuing taper from apex to cervical (Figure 10-70).

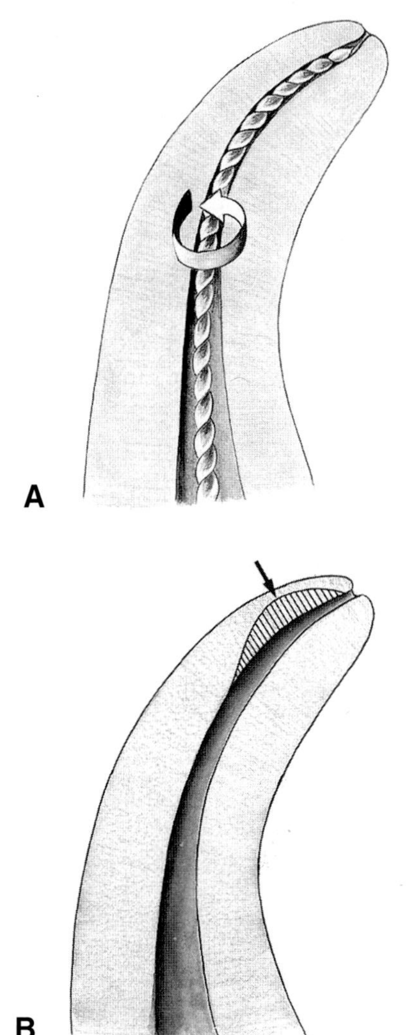

Figure 10-67 A, Incorrect enlargement of the apical curve leads to cavitation. Larger, stiffer instruments transport preparation at the external wall. B, Ovoid cavitation (arrow) developed by incorrect cleaning and shaping.

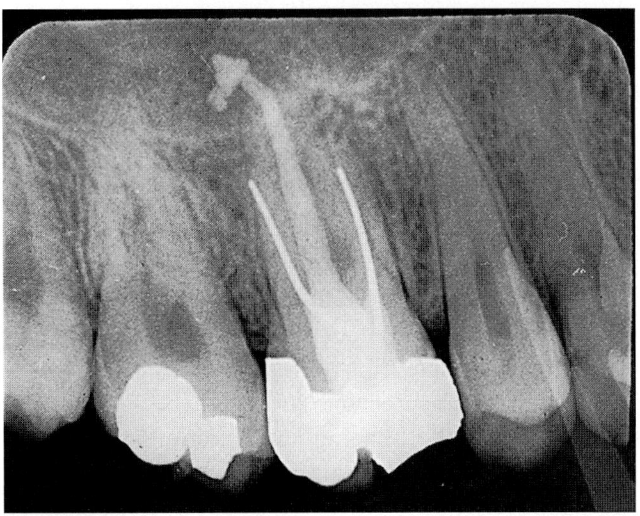

Figure 10-69 Apical curve to the buccal of the palatal root went undetected and was perforated by heavy instruments and then overfilled. Right-angle radiographs failed to reveal buccal or lingual curves. Step-back preparation could have prevented perforation. (Courtesy of Dr. Richard E. Walton.)

Although the step-back technique was designed to avoid zipping the apical area in curved canals, it applies as well to straight canal preparation. As Buchanan noted, "all root canals have some curvature. Even apparently straight canals are usually curved to some degree."[461] Canals that appear to curve in one direction often curve in other directions as well (Figure 10-71).

Prior to the introduction of nickel-titanium files, one of the first axioms of endodontics has been to "always use a curved instrument in a curved canal." The degree and direction of the curve are determined by the canal shadow in the radiograph. Buchanan has made an art of properly curving instruments to match the

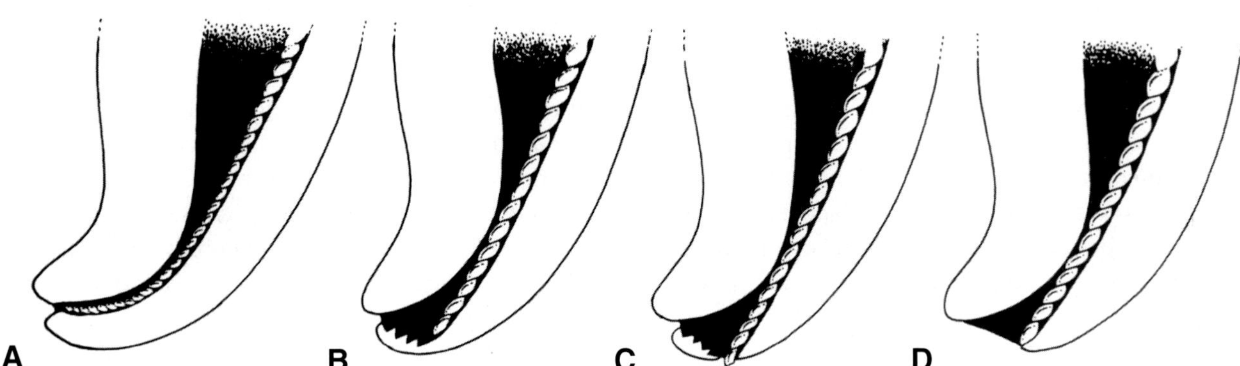

Figure 10-68 Hazards of overenlarging the apical curve. A, Small flexible instruments (No. 10 to No. 25) readily negotiate the curve. B, Larger instruments (No. 30 and above) markedly increase in stiffness and cutting efficiency, causing ledge formation. C, Persistent enlargement with larger instruments results in perforation. D, A "zip" is formed when the working length is fully maintained and larger instruments are used. (Courtesy of Dr. Richard E. Walton.)

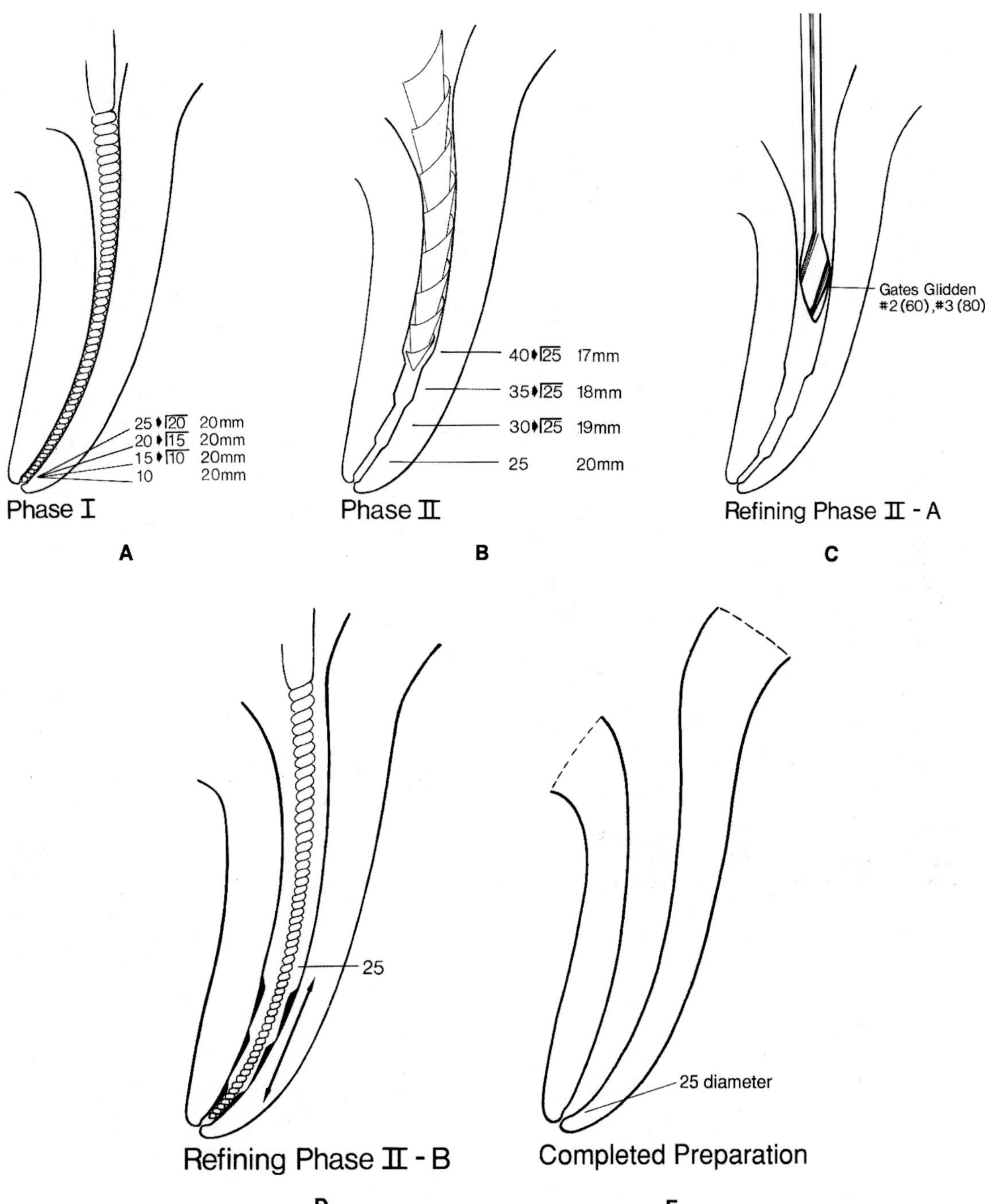

Figure 10-70 Step-back preparation. **A,** Phase I—Apical preparation up to file No. 25 with recapitulation using prior size files. **B,** Phase II—Stepping-back procedure in 1 mm increments, Nos. 25 through 45. Recapitulation with a No. 25 file to full working length. **C,** Refining Phase II-A—Gates-Glidden drills Nos. 2, 3, and 4 used to create coronal and midroot preparations. **D,** Refining Phase II-B—No. 25 file, circumferential filing smooths step-back. **E,** Completed preparation—a continuous flowing flared preparation from the cementodentinoenamel junction to the crown. Adapted with permission from Mullaney TP.[468]

canal silhouette in the film.[461,464] He made the point that the bladed part of the file must be bent all the way, even up to the last half millimeter, remembering "that canals curve most in the apical one-third"[470] (Figure 10-72). One must also remember that the most difficult curves to deal with are to the buccal and/or the lingual for they are directly in line with the x-ray beam. Their apical orifices appear on the film well short of the root apex. So, curving the file to match the canal is paramount to success in the step-back maneuver unless nickel-titanium files are used. Attempting to curve nickel-titanium files can introduce metal fatigue.

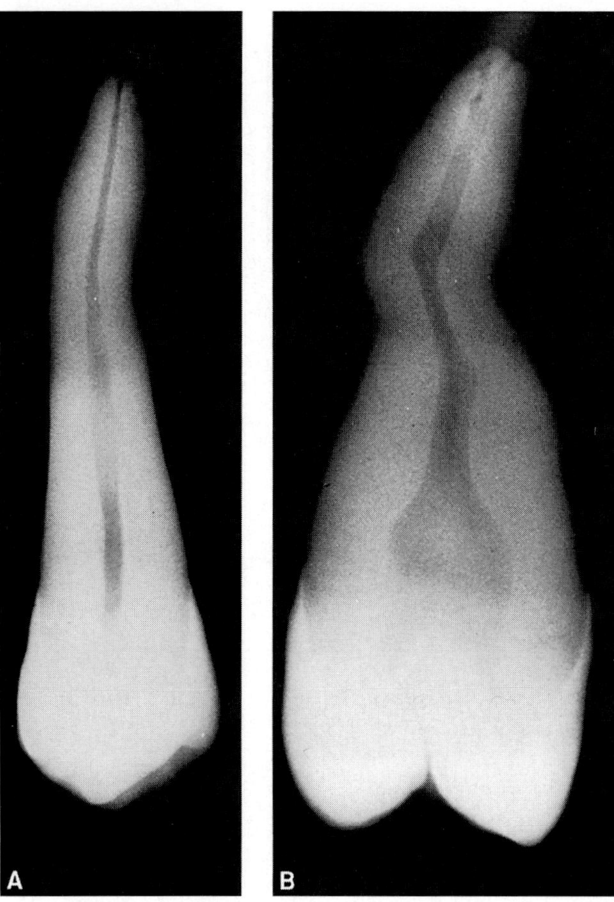

Figure 10-71 A, Unsuspected aberration in canal anatomy is not apparent in a standard buccolingual radiograph. B, The severe bayonet shape of a canal seen in a mesiodistal radiograph should be determined by careful exploration. Also note the apical delta.

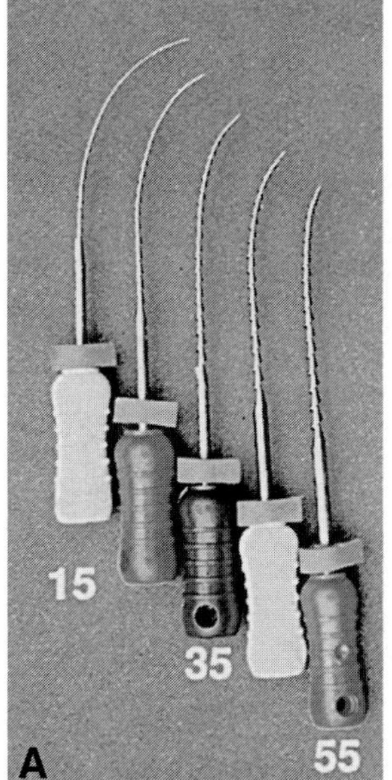

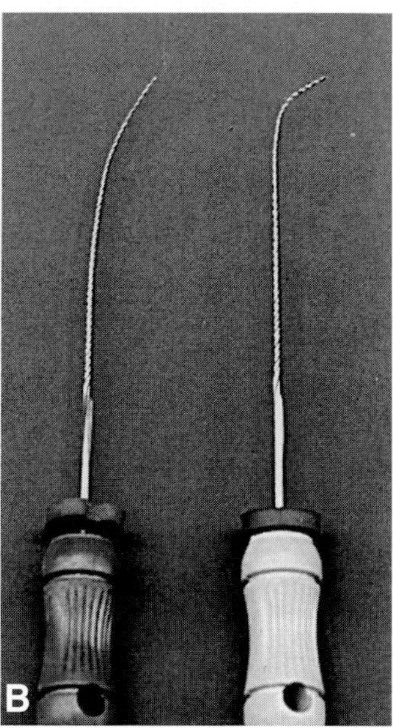

Figure 10-72 A, Stainless steel file series appropriately bent for continuously tapering preparation. Note that the instrument shaft straightens more and more with size increase. B, The file on the left is bent for straight or slightly curved canals. The file on the right is bent to initially explore and negotiate abrupt apical canal curvatures. Reproduced with permission from Buchanan LS.[464]

Step-Back, Step-by-Step—Hand Instrumentation. *Phase I.* To start Phase I instrumentation, it must be assumed that the canal has been explored with a fine pathfinder or instrument and that the working length has been established—that is, the **apical constriction identified.** The first active instrument to be inserted should be a fine (No. 08, 10, or 15) 0.02, tapered, stainless steel file, curved and coated with a lubricant, such as Gly-Oxide, R.C. Prep, File-Eze, Glyde, K-Y Jelly, or liquid soap. The flexibilty of nickel titanium does not lend itself to this pathfinding function in sizes smaller than No. 15.

The motion of the instrument is **"watch winding,"** two or three quarter-turns clockwise-counterclockwise and then retraction. On removal, the instrument is wiped clean, **recurved,** relubricated, and repositioned. "Watch winding" is then repeated. Remember that the instrument must be to full depth when the cutting action is made. This procedure is repeated until the instrument is loose in position. Then the next size K file is used—length established, precurved, lubricated, and positioned. Again, the watch-winding action and retraction are repeated. Very short (1.0 mm) filing strokes can also be used at the apex. At the University of Tennessee, nickel-titanium 0.02 tapered instruments were shown to be effective when used with this technique. Nickel-titanium files were not curved and maintained the canal shape better than stainless steel.

It is most important that a lubricant be used in this area. As Berg[462] and Buchanan[461] pointed out, it is often fibrous pulp stumps, compacted into the constricture, that cause apical blockage. In very fine canals, the irrigant that will reach this area will be insufficient to dissolve tissue. Lubrication, on the other hand, emulsifies tissue, allowing instrument tips to macerate and remove this tissue. It is only later in canal filing that dentin chips pack apically, blocking the constriction. By then the apical area has been enlarged enough that sodium hypochlorite can reach the debris to douche it clear.

By the time a size 25 K file has been used to full working length, Phase I is complete. The 1.0 to 2.0 mm space back from the apical constriction should be clean of debris (Figure 10-73) unless this area of the canal was large to begin with, as in a youngster. Then, of course, larger instruments are used to start with.

Using a number 25 file here as an example is not to imply that all canals should be shaped at the apical

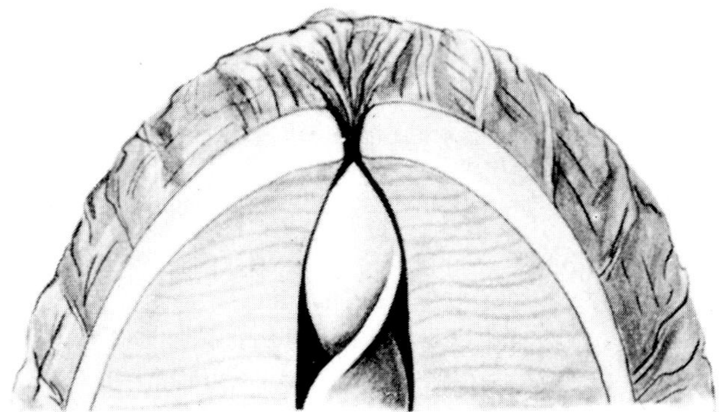

Figure 10-73 Apical limitations of instrumentation should be at the apical constriction, which is about 0.5 to 1.0 mm from the anatomic (radiographic) end of the root.

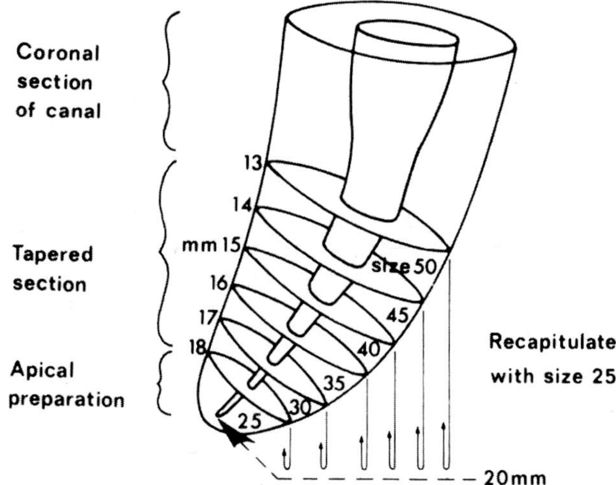

Figure 10-74 A stylized step-back (telescopic) preparation. A working length of 20 mm is used as an example. The apical 2 to 3 mm are prepared to size 25. The next 5 mm are prepared with successively larger instruments. Recapitulation with No. 25 to full length between each step. The coronal part of the canal is enlarged with circumferential filing or Gates-Glidden drills. Reproduced with permission from Tidmarsh BG. Int Endod J 1982;15:53.

restriction only to size 25. Hawrish pointed out the apparent **lack of interest in canal diameter** versus the great interest in the proper canal length (personal communication, 1999). Many, in fact most, canals should be enlarged beyond size 25 at the apical constriction in order to round out the preparation at this point and remove as much of the extraneous tissue, debris, and lateral canals as possible. A size 25 file is used here as an example and as a danger point **for beyond No. 25 lies danger!**

As stainless steel instruments become larger, they become stiffer. Metal "memory" plus stress on the instrument starts its straightening. It will no longer stay curved and starts to dig, to zip the outside (convex) wall of the canal.

It must be emphasized here that irrigation between each instrument use is now in order, as well as **recapitulation** with the previous smaller instrument carried to full depth and watch wound. This breaks up the apical debris so that it may be washed away by the sodium hypochlorite. All of these maneuvers (curved instruments, lubrication, cleaning debris from the used instrument, copious irrigation, and recapitulation) will ensure patency of the canal to the apical constriction.

Phase II. In a **fine canal** (and in this example), the step-back process begins with a No. 30 K-style file. Its **working length is set 1 mm short** of the full working length. It is precurved, lubricated, carried down the canal to the new shortened depth, watch wound, and retracted. The same process is repeated until the No. 30 is loose at this adjusted length (Figure 10-74). Recapitulation to **full length** with a No. 25 file follows to ensure patency to the constriction. This is followed by copious irrigation before the next curved instrument is introduced. In this case, it is a No. 35, again shortened by 1.0 mm from the No. 30 (2.0 mm from the apical No. 25). It is curved, lubricated, inserted, watch wound, and retracted followed by recapitulation and irrigation.

Thus, the preparation steps back up the canal **1 mm** and **one larger** instrument at a time. When that portion of the canal is reached, usually the straight midcanal, where the instruments no longer fit tightly, then perimeter filing may begin, along with plenty of irrigation (Figure 10-75).

It is at this point that Hedstroem files are most effective. They are much more aggressive rasps than the K files. The canal is shaped into the continuous taper so conducive to optimum obturation. Care must be taken to recapitulate between each instrument with the original No. 25 file along with ample irrigation.

This midcanal area is the region where reshaping can also be done with power-driven instruments: Gates-Glidden drills, starting with the smaller drills (Nos. 1 and 2) and gradually increasing in size to No. 4, 5, or 6. Proper continuing taper is developed to finish Phase IIA preparation. Gates-Glidden drills must be used with great care because they tend to "screw" themselves into the canal, binding and then breaking. To avoid this, it has been recommended that the larger sizes be run in reverse. But, unfortunately, they do not cut as well when reversed. A better suggestion is to lubricate the drill heavily with RC-Prep or Glyde, which "will prevent binding and the rapid advance problem." Lubrication also suspends the chips and allows for a better "feel" of the cutting as well as the first canal curvature. Used Gates-Glidden drills are also less aggressive than new ones.

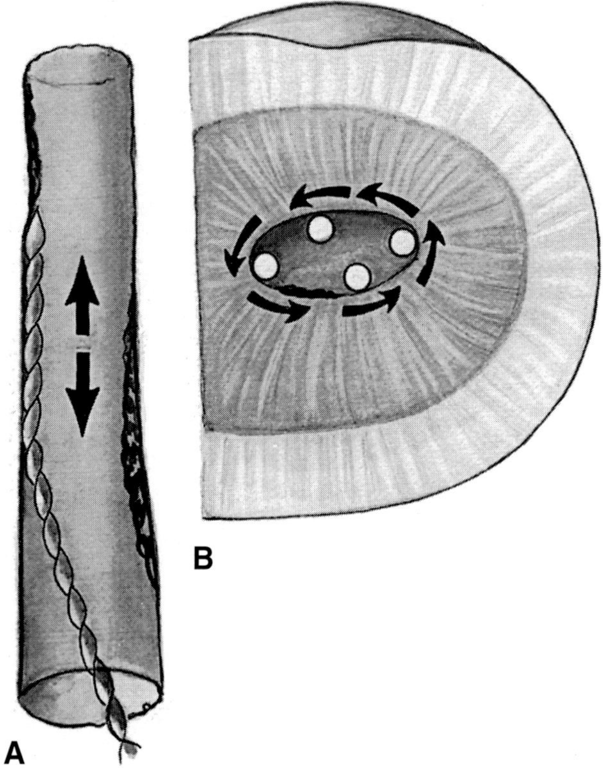

Figure 10-75 A, Perimeter filing action used to débride and shape larger ovoid portions of the canal. The file is used in an up-and-down rasping action with pressure exerted cross-canal against all walls. B, Cross-section showing shaping of an ovoid canal. This "multiple exposure" illustration shows how the file is used as a rasp against walls around the entire perimeter of the canal. Only a small area remains to be cleaned and shaped. A stainless steel Hedstroem file is best suited for this purpose.

Newer instruments with various tapers from 0.04 to 0.08 mm/mm of taper are now available for this purpose as well and can be used as power-driven or hand instruments. With any of the power-driven instruments, using them in a passive pecking motion will decrease the chances of binding or screwing into the canal.

Refining Phase IIB is a return to a size No. 25 (or the last apical instrument used), smoothing all around the walls with vertical push-pull strokes, to perfect the taper from the apical constriction to the cervical canal orifice. In this case, a safe-ended, noncutting-tip Hedstroem file is the most efficient. It produces a good deal of dentin chips, however, that must be broken up at the apex with a cutting-tip K file and then flushed out with abundant sodium hypochlorite.

At this point, Buchanan recommended that sodium hypochlorite be left in place to the apex for 5 to 10 minutes. This is the only way in which the auxiliary canals can be cleaned.[461] Hand-powered Gates-Glidden drills (Handy Gates) or LIGHTSPEED instruments may be used for this final finish, as well as the new handpiece Orifice Openers or Gates-Glidden drills. Gutmann and Rakusin pointed out that the "final preparation should be an exact replica of the original canal configuration—shape, taper, and flow, only larger"[471] (Figure 10-76, A). So-called "Coke-bottle" preparations should be avoided at all cost (Figure 10-76, B).

This completes the chemomechanical step-back preparation of the continuing taper canal. It is now ready to be filled or medicated and sealed at the coronal cavity until the next appointment. If it is to be filled, the smear layer should first be removed. This procedure is detailed in chapter 11.

Modified Step-Back Technique. One variation of the step-back technique is more traditional. The preparation is completed in the apical area, and then the step-back procedure begins 2 to 3 mm up the canal. This gives a short, almost parallel retention form to receive the primary gutta-percha point when lateral condensation is being used to fill the canal. The gutta-percha trial point should go fully to the constriction, and a slight tug-back should be felt when the point is removed (retention form). This shows that it fits tightly into the last 2 to 3 mm of the prepared canal.

Efficacy of the Step-Back Technique. Three research groups tested the efficacy of the step-back maneuver. Using the techniques detailed here (precurving, watch winding, and step-back), a Swiss group stated that the "step back shapings consistently presented the best taper and apical stop design..."[472] In marked contrast, two groups from Great Britain used straight, not precurved, instruments in "simple in/out filing...with no attempt at rotation or twisting."[473] Both British groups reported preparations that were hourglass in shape, and one had a deformation and instrument breakage as well as severe zipping in the apical area[473–475] (Figure 10-77).

These findings, using stainless steel files, emphasize the necessity of precurving instruments and using limited rotation for enlargement in the apical region. Vessey found that a limited reaming action (as recommended above) produced a circular preparation, whereas files used vertically as files (rasps) produced ovoid preparations.[476] Others found essentially the same[477,478] (Figure 10-78). In Scotland, W. P. and E. M. Saunders achieved better results using a step-down/step-back approach rather than straight step-back instrumentation. On the other hand, they broke a number of files using the modified approach.[463] Positive findings have been noted using nickel-titanium instruments. They seem to maintain canal shape better and improved cutting efficiency when used as a reamer.

Figure 10-76 Preparation configurations. **A**, Original canal shape, taper and flow, only larger. **B** (**right**), "Coke bottle" preparation from overuse of Gates-Glidden drills or Peeso reamers negates the efficient flow of gutta-percha. Reproduced with permission from Gutmann JL and Rakusin H.[471]

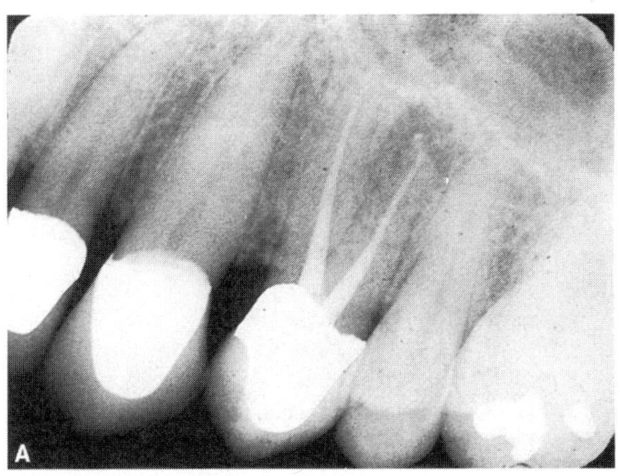

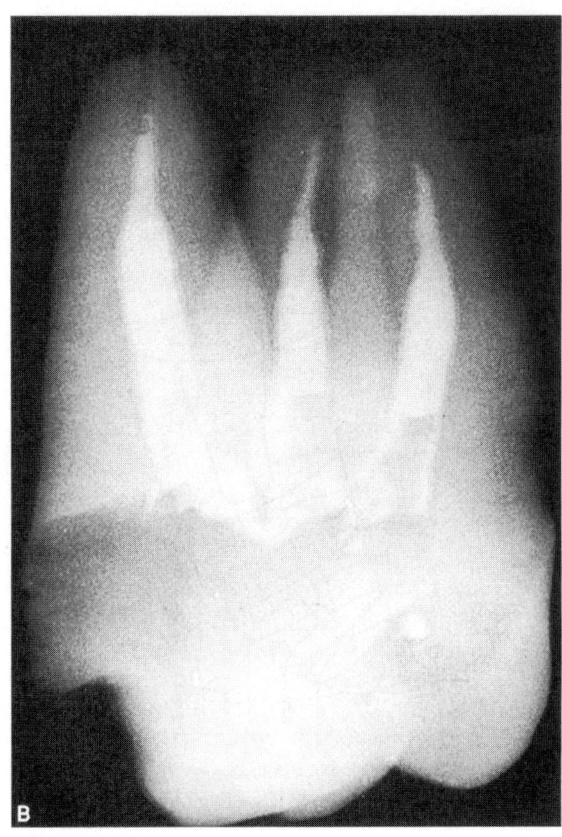

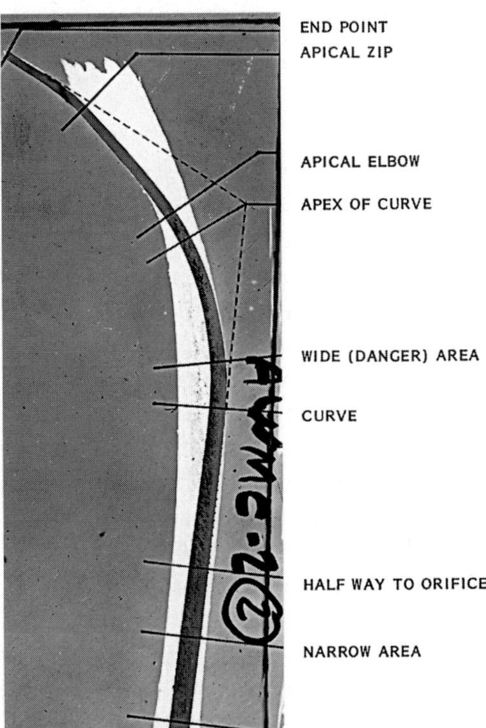

Figure 10-77 Composite print of an original curved canal (**dark**). Overlay details areas of instrument divergence (**white**). Note the hourglass shape, apical zip, and apical elbow as a result of straight filing with straight instruments. Reproduced with permission from Alodeh MHA et al.[475]

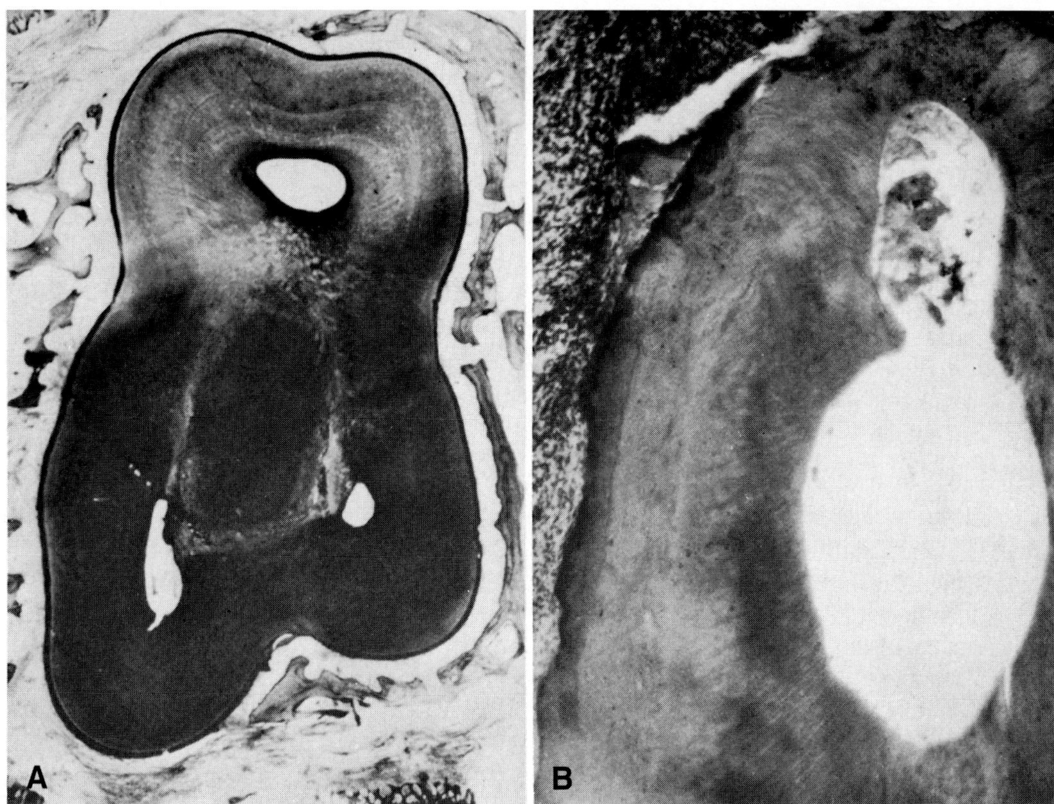

Figure 10-78 A, Ovoid canal shape in a "young" mandibular molar sectioned just below the floor of the pulp chamber. The distal canal (**top**) and the mesiobuccal canal (**lower left**) both require perimeter filing to complete their preparation. Watch-winding or reaming action alone would accurately shape mesiolingual canal (**lower right**) into a round tapered preparation. **B**, "Dumbbell"-shaped canal that could not accurately be enlarged into a round tapered preparation. Perimeter filing action and multiple gutta-percha point filling would be required to accurately shape and obturate this shape of a canal. Tactile sensation with a curved exploring instrument should inform the operator that he is not dealing with a round tapered canal. (Note related abscess, **upper left.**)

Chelation and Enlargement. A number of canals, particularly fine curved canals, will appear to be almost calcified or blocked by attached pulp stones. They may still be negotiated if the clinician uses a chelating agent and the utmost patience.

Ethylenediaminetetraacetic acid buffered to a pH of 7.3 was long ago advocated by Nygaard-Østby to "dissolve" a pathway for exploring instruments.[275,479] When the mineral salts have been removed from the obstructing dentin by chelation, only the softened matrix remains.[480] This may be removed by careful watch-winding action to "drill" past the obstruction. This maneuver may be improved if the coronal portion of the canal is widened so that only the instrument tip is cutting.

Files with tapers greater than the traditional 0.02 mm/mm have made negotiating these "calcified" canals more predictable. Calcification occurs nearest the irritant to which the pulp is reacting. Since most irritants are in the coronal region of the pulp, the farther apical one goes into the canal, the more unlikely it is to be calcified. When files bind in these canals, it may be from small constrictions in the coronal part of the canal. If working length is estimated to be 20 mm but the clinician can negotiate only 10 mm of canal, **increasing the taper** of the canal to the 10 mm level often removes the constrictions and allows a small file to negotiate farther into the canal. This is one of the strengths of following the step-down or crown-down technique.

Fraser has shown that, contrary to popular belief, chelating agents "do not soften dentin in the narrow parts of the canal," although softening can occur in the cervical and middle portions.[481,482] Ethylenediaminetetraacetic acid must be concentrated enough in an area to be effective.

R C Prep, File-Eze, and Glyde, which contain EDTA, act more as lubricating agents since the concentration of EDTA contained therein is very modest. The Canal Finder System, using No. 08 files, has been very effective in opening curved calcified canals in the presence of an EDTA lubricant.

Selden and McSpadden have recommended the use of a dental operating microscope for peering down "calcified" canals.[483,484] More recently, the fiber-optic endoscope, such as used in abdominal and brain surgery, has given dentists a whole new look at the pulpal floor and the root canal. The **OraScope** (Spectrum Dental Inc; North Attlebora, Mass.), for example, has a 0.9 mm fiber-optic probe that will penetrate down the root canal, displaying its view, enormously magnified, on a computer screen. Incidentally, there is recent evidence that root canal calcification may be associated with long-term prednisone therapy (60 mg per day over 8 years to treat lupus erythematosus).[485]

Step-Down Technique—Hand Instrumentation

Initially, Marshall and Pappin advocated a "Crown-Down Pressureless Preparation" in which Gates-Glidden drills and larger files are first used in the coronal two-thirds of the canals and then progressively smaller files are used from the "crown down" until the desired length is reached[486] This has become known as the **step-down** or crown-down technique of cleaning and shaping. It has risen in popularity, especially among those using nickel-titanium instruments with varying tapers.

A primary purpose of this technique is to minimize or eliminate the amount of necrotic debris that could be extruded through the apical foramen during instrumentation. This would help prevent post-treatment discomfort, incomplete cleansing, and difficulty in achieving a biocompatible seal at the apical constriction.[486]

One of the major advantages of step-down preparation is the freedom from constraint of the apical enlarging instruments. By first flaring the coronal two-thirds of the canal, the final apical instruments are unencumbered through most of their length. This increased access allows greater control and less chance of zipping near the apical constriction.[487] In addition, it "provides a coronal escapeway that reduces the "piston in a cylinder effect" responsible for debris extrusion from the apex.[488]

Step-Down, Step-by-Step. In this method, the access cavity is filled with sodium hypochlorite, and the first instrument is introduced into the canal. At this point, there is a divergence in technique dictated by the instrument design and the protocol for proceeding recommended by each instrument manufacturer. All of the directions, however, start with exploration of the canal with a fine, stainless steel, .02 taper (No. 8, 10, 15, or 20 file, determined by the canal width), **curved instrument**. It is important that the canal be patent to the apical constriction before cleaning and shaping begin. Sometimes the chosen file will not reach the apical constriction, and one assumes that the file is binding at the apex. But, more often than not, the file is **binding in the coronal canal.** In this case, one should start with a wider (0.04 or 0.06 taper) instrument or a Gates-Glidden drill to free up the canal so that a fine instrument may reach the mid- and apical canal. This would be the beginning of step-down preparation. Buchanan has also emphasized the importance of removing all pulp remnants before shaping begins to ensure that this tissue does not "pile up" at the constriction and impede full cleaning and shaping to that point.[461]

K-File Series Step-Down Technique. As stated above, the initial penetrating instrument is a small, curved, stainless steel K file, exploring to the apical constriction and **establishing working length**. To ensure this penetration, one may have to enlarge the coronal third of the canal with progressively smaller Gates-Glidden drills or with instruments of larger taper such as the .04 or the .06 instruments. At this point, and in the presence of sodium hypochlorite and/or a lubricant such as Glyde, step-down cleaning and shaping begins with **K-Flex, Triple-Flex, or Safety Hedstrom** (Sybron Endo/Kerr; Orange, Calif.) instruments in either the 0.02, 0.04, or 0.06 taper configuration depending on the canal size to begin with. Starting with a No. 50 instrument (for example) and working down the canal to, say, a size No. 15, the instruments are used in a watch-winding motion until the apical constriction (or working length) is reached. When resistance is met to further penetration, the next smallest size is used. Irrigation should follow the use of each instrument and recapitulation after every other instrument. To properly enlarge the apical third, and to round out ovoid shape and lateral canal orifices, a reverse order of instruments may be used starting with a No. 20 (for example) and enlarging this region to a No. 40 or 50 (for example). The tapered shape can be improved by stepping back up the canal with ever larger instruments, bearing in mind all the time the importance of lubrication, irrigation, and recapitulation. At this point, the canal should be ready for smear layer removal, drying, and either medication or obturation.

Modified Technique. There have been a number of modifications of the step-down technique since it was first promulgated. One of the most recent was by Ruddle (personal communication, 2001). Following complete access, he suggested that clinicians "face-off" the orifices with an appropriately sized Gates-Glidden drill. This creates a smooth guide path to facilitate the placement of subsequent instruments. Certain canal systems contain deep divisions and may be initially opened at their coronal ends with **Micro Openers** (Dentsply Maillefer; Tulsa, Okla.).

If the pulp is vital, a broach may be selected to quickly extirpate it if space permits. At this stage of treatment, the coronal two-thirds of any canal should be "scouted" with a No. 10 or 15 curved, stainless steel K file in the presence of a lubricant and/or sodium hypochlorite. Exploration of this portion of the canal will confirm straight-line access, cross-sectional diameter, and root canal system anatomy. Files are used serially to flare the canal until sufficient space is generated to safely introduce either Gates-Gliddens or nickel-titanium rotary shaping files. Frequent irrigation with sodium hypochlorite and recapitulation with a No. 10 file will discourage canal blockage and move debris into solution, where it can be liberated from the root canal system. One way to accomplish pre-enlargement of the canal is with Gates-Glidden drills that are used at approximately 800 rpm, serially, passively, and like a brush to remove restrictive dentin. Initially, one should start with a Gates-Glidden drill No. 1 and carry each larger instrument short of the previous instrument to promote a smooth, flowing, tapered preparation. Frequent irrigation with sodium hypochlorite and recapitulation with a small clearing file to prevent blockage are in order.

Following pre-enlargement, Ruddle believes in negotiating the apical one-third last, establishing patency, and confirming working length. He then recommends finishing the apical zone so that there is a smooth uniform taper from the orifice level to the radiographic terminus. He emphasized that a variety of instruments may be used to create the "deep shape." If the clinician chooses 0.02 tapered files to "finish" the apical one-third, Ruddle uses a concept he calls "Gauging and Tuning." "Gauging" is knowing the cross-sectional diameter of the foramen that is confirmed by the size of instrument that "snugs in" at working length. "Tuning" is ensuring that each sequentially larger instrument uniformly backs out of the canal ½ mm.

After removing the sodium hypochlorite, the canal is rinsed with 17% aqueous EDTA to remove the smear layer in preparation for obturation. Dentsply Maillefer has developed a "Clean & Shape" Kit that contains all of the instruments necessary for this technique.

PROFILE GT (Greater Taper) Technique. If these instruments (Dentsply/Tulsa Dental; Tulsa, Okla.) are used, Buchanan, the developer, recommends that one start with a 0.10 GT instrument to flare out the coronal third of the canal. This means that this instrument is an ISO size 20 at the tip, but the taper is 0.10 mm/mm, that establishes a wider freedom for those instruments to follow. The instrument is used in a twisting motion, first counterclockwise and then clockwise with apical pressure, before retraction. The instrument is cleaned and the operation repeated until the instrument is loose. A lubricant such as RC PREP or GLYDE should be used. At this point, the canal should be flooded with EDTA and the next smaller-size GT file is used, number 0.08, in the same manner—counterclockwise, engage, twist clockwise, and retract. One continues down the canal using the 0.08, and 0.06 taper instruments until the apical restriction is reached. Constant irrigation with sodium hypochlorite is most important! This constitutes what Buchanan terms the "Second Shaping Wave," and it should be completed in a matter of minutes.

The second wave is followed by the "Third Shaping Wave," in which regular ISO instruments are used to the constriction to enlarge the apical canal diameter beyond size 20, the tip diameter of the GT files. Beginning with fine instruments, and then stepping back 1 or 2 mm with instruments, up to size 35 or 40, the apical region is "rounded out." The final shaping is a return of the last GT file used in the canal.

Buchanan pointed out that the GT instruments are sized to fit certain size canals. The 0.06 file, for instance, is recommended for "extremely thin or curved roots." The 0.08 file is best for lower anterior teeth, multirooted premolars, and the buccal roots of maxillary molars. The 0.10 file better matches the distal canal of mandibular molars, the palatal roots of maxillary molars, single-canal premolars, mandibular canines, and maxillary anterior teeth. The 0.12 instrument is for larger canals.

Buchanan is a great believer in the necessity of cleaning what he terms the "patency zone," that tiny space between the apical constriction and the apical terminus. For this, in the presence of sodium hypochlorite, he carefully instruments this space with a regular No. 10 file. He also believes that sodium hypochlorite should be present in this region for a total of 30 minutes. If preparation time has been less than 30 minutes, he recommends that a final lavage should remain in the canal until 30 minutes have passed. This, in his view, dissolves the final debris and tissue packed there, even in the accessory canals (personal communication, 2001).

Quantec Instrument Technique. Using **Quantec instruments** (Sybron Endo/Analytic; Orange, Calif.), which are more reamer like than files, the recommended technique for **hand instrumentation** is divided into three phases: **negotiation, shaping, and apical preparation.**

NEGOTIATION: As is standard with virtually all cleaning and shaping techniques, the canal, in the presence of sodium hypochlorite, is first explored with a standard No. 10 or 15 0.02 taper, curved, stainless steel K file and working length is established (Figure 10-79, A). Exploration is followed by a **Quantec No. 25, 0.06**

taper, nickel-titanium instrument, advanced in a reaming action, from the canal orifice to just short of the apical third, and followed by irrigation with sodium hypochlorite (Figure 10-79, B and C).

With a standard ISO **0.02, stainless steel, No. 10 or 15** file, a **"Glide Path"** for the instruments to follow is developed to working length (Figure 10-79, D). The canal is then irrigated with EDTA (Figure 10-79, E), and the No. **20 and 25 stainless steel, 0.02** instruments are used to clean and shape the apical third to the apical constriction. This is followed again by copious irrigation (Figure 10-79, F).

SHAPING: Using lubricants and sodium hypochlorite, one returns to the Quantec instruments, all with an ISO size No. 25 tip. Returning to the **No. 25, 0.06** taper instrument, it is used in a reaming action, as far down the canal as it will comfortably go (Figure 10-79, G). It is followed in succession by the **No. 0.05 taper Quantec** and then the **0.04 and 0.03 tapers** until the apical stop is reached (Figure 10-79, H to J). Copious irrigation follows the use of each instrument.

QUANTEC APICAL PREPARATION: To ensure accuracy, the working length should be rechecked. If an apical preparation larger in diameter than a No. 25 is desired, one may return to the **0.02 taper Quantec instruments** (which will now be quite loose in the midcanal), and the diameter of the apical third can then be enlarged up to a size No. 40, 45, or 50, depending on the original size of the canal (Figure 10-79, K). Final irrigation to remove the smear layer with EDTA and sodium hypochlorite prepares the tapered canal for medication or filling (Figure 10-79, L).

Efficacy of the Step-Down Technique. Compared to the step-back "circumferential filing technique with precurved files as described by Weine,"[488] Morgan and Montgomery found the step-down technique significantly better in shape and terminus.[489]

Another *in vitro* study found significantly less debris extruded from the apical orifice when step-down procedures were used compared to step-back procedures. Neither technique was totally effective, however, in preventing total debris extrusion.[490]

Variation of the Three Basic Preparations

A variety of techniques have been developed, all based on the step-down, step-back, or hybrid approach to preparation. Most are inspired by new canal instruments and/or vibratory devices.

Balanced Force Concept Using Flex-R Files. After many years of experimentation, Roane et al. introduced their **Balanced Force concept** of canal preparaton in 1985.[100] The concept came to fruition, they claimed, with the development and introduction of a new K-type file design, the **Flex-R File**[100,101] (Moyco Union Broach). The technique can be described as "positioning and pre-loading an instrument through a clockwise rotation and then shaping the canal with a counterclockwise rotation."[100] The authors evaluated damaged instruments produced by the use of this technique. They discovered that a greater risk of instrument damage was associated with clockwise movement.[85]

For the best results, preparation is completed in a **step-down** approach. The coronal and mid-thirds of a canal are flared with Gates-Glidden drills, sizes 2 through 6, and then instrument shaping is carried into the apical areas. This approach is less difficult than the conventional step-back technique. Increasing the diameter of the coronal and mid-thirds of a canal removes most of the contamination and provides access for a more passive movement of hand instruments into the apical third. Shaping becomes less difficult: the radius of curvature is increased as the arc is decreased. In other words, the canal becomes straighter and the apex accessible with less flexing of the shaping instruments (Figure 10-80).

After mechanical shaping with Gates-Glidden drills, balanced force hand instrumentation begins: placing, cutting, and removing instruments using only rotary motions (Figure 10-80, C). Insertion is done with a quarter-turn clockwise rotation while slight apical pressure is applied (Figure 10-81, 1). Cutting is accomplished by making a **counterclockwise rotation,** "again while applying a light apical pressure (Figure 10-81, 2). The amount of apical pressure must be adjusted to match the file size (ie, very light for fine instruments to fairly heavy for large instruments)."[100] Pressure should maintain the instrument at or near its clockwise insertion depth. Then counterclockwise rotation and apical pressure act together to enlarge and shape the canal to the diameter of the instrument. Counterclockwise motion must be 120 degrees or greater. It must rotate the instrument sufficiently to move the next larger cutting edge into the location of the blade that preceded it, in order to shape the full circumference of a canal. A greater degree of rotation is preferred and will more completely shape the canal to provide a diameter equal to or greater than that established by the counterclockwise instrument twisting during manufacture.

It is important to understand that clockwise rotation "sets" the instrument, and this motion should not exceed 90 degrees. If excess clockwise rotation is used, the instrument tip can become locked into place and the file may unwind. If continued, when twisted counterclockwise, the file may fail unexpectedly. The process

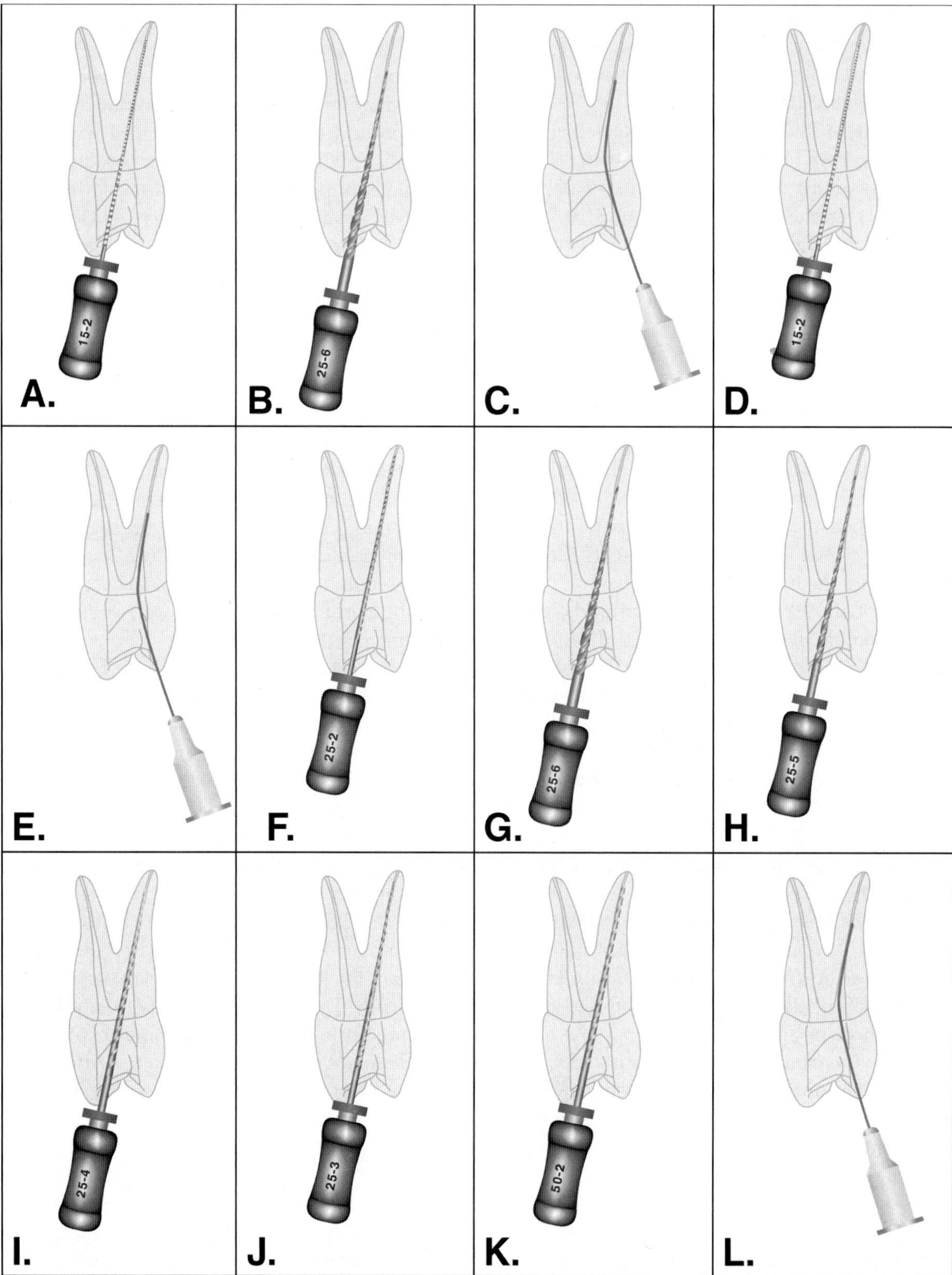

Figure 10-79 **Step-down technique**, with Quantec hand instruments, cleaning and shaping. **A**, Explore to the apex and establish working length (WL) with a stainless steel (SS) No. 10 or 15 **0.02** taper file. **B**, Enlarge the orifices and two-thirds of the way down the canal with a nickel-titanium (NiTi) No. 25 **0.06** taper file. **C**, Irrigate all of the canals with sodium hypochlorite (NaOCl). **D**, Establish a "glide path" to WL with SS No. 15, 0.02 taper file. **E**, Irrigate with ethylenediaminetetraacetic acid (EDTA). **F**, Enlarge to WL with SS No. 20 and 25 **0.02** files. Irrigate with NaOCl. **G**, With Glyde and NaOCl, enlarge down the canal as far as possible with NiTi No. 25 **0.06** file. Irrigate. **H**, Continue further down the canal with a NiTi No. 25 **0.05** file. **I**, Continue further with a No. 25 **0.04** file. **J**, Continue to WL with a NiTi No. 25 **0.03** file. **K**, Enlarge apical one-third up to size Nos. 40, 45, or 50 with **0.02** taper files. **L**, Final irrigation with EDTA and NaOCl to remove smear layer. Dry.

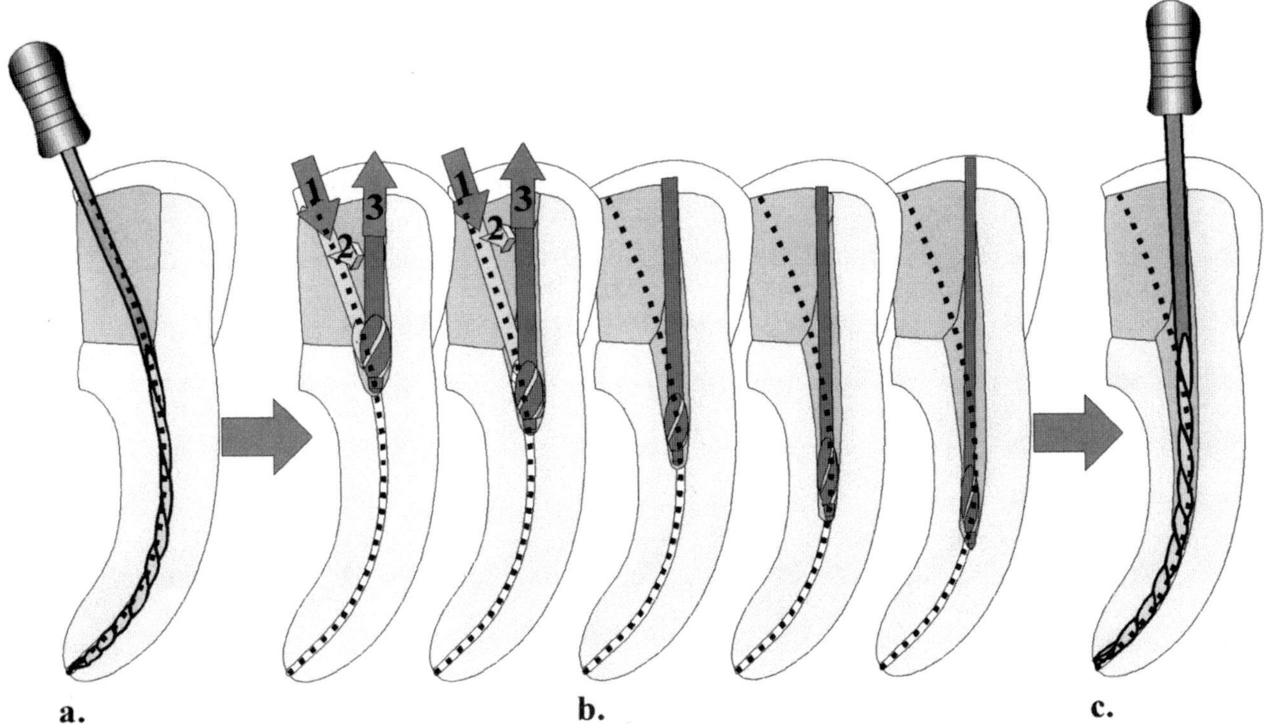

Figure 10-80 a, File displays full curvature of the canal before **radicular** access is modified. b, Radicular access is completed with a descending series of **Gates-Glidden drills** progressing toward the apex in 2.0 mm or less increments. c, The **dotted line** indicates the original curvature, whereas the file displays the affective curvature after radicular access is improved. This modification materially reduces the difficulty of apical shaping. (Courtesy of Dr. James B. Roane.)

is repeated (clockwise insertion and counterclockwise cutting), and the **instrument is advanced toward the apex in shallow steps.** After the working depth is obtained, the instrument is freed by one or more counterclockwise rotations made while the depth is held constant. The file is then removed from the canal with a slow clockwise rotation that loads debris into the

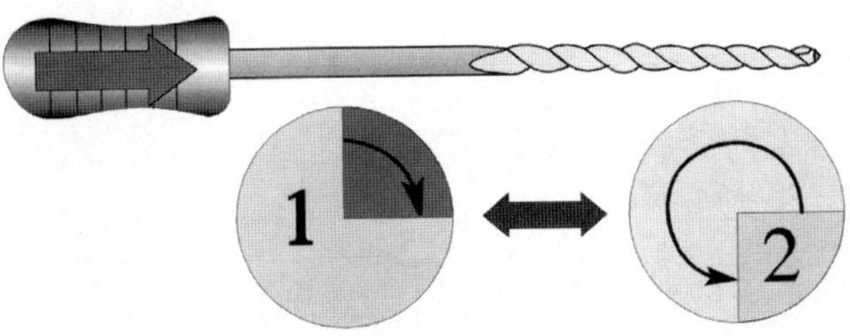

Figure 10-81 1. For a **balanced force** motion, the file is pushed inwardly and rotated one quarter-turn clockwise. 2. It is then rotated more than one half-turn counterclockwise. The inward pressure must be enough to cause the instrument to maintain depth and strip away dentin as it rotates counterclockwise. These alternate motions are repeated until the file reaches working length. (Courtesy of Dr. James B. Roane.)

flutes and elevates it away from the apical foramen.[100] **Generous irrigation** follows each shaping instrument since residual debris will cause transportation of the shape. Debris applies supplemental pressures against the next shaping instrument and tends to cause straightening of the curvature.

Repeating the previously described steps, the clinician gradually enlarges the apical third of the canal by advancing to larger and larger instruments. Working depths are changed between instruments to produce an apical taper. The working loads can and should be kept **very** light by limiting the clockwise motion and thereby reducing the amount of tooth structure removed by each counterclockwise shaping movement. **This technique can and should be used with minimal force.**

The balanced force technique can be used with any K-type file[491]; however, the shaping and transportation control are maximum when a Flex-R file is used.[492] The Flex-R file design incorporates a guiding plane and removes the transition angles inherent on the tip of standard K-type files (see Figure 10-23). Those angles, if present, enable the tip to cut in an outward direction and give it the ability to cut a ledge into the canal wall. **Lacking a**

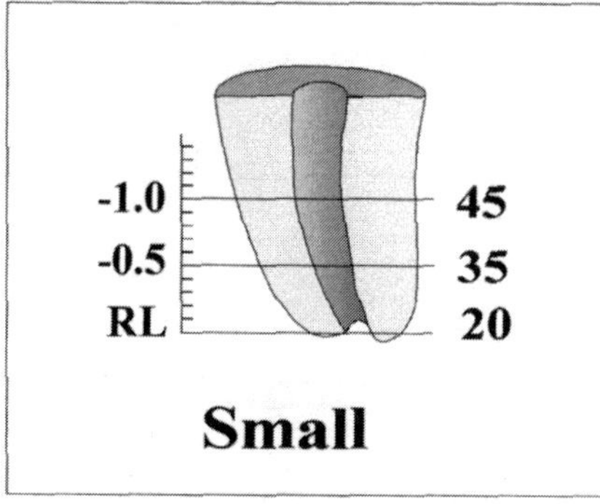

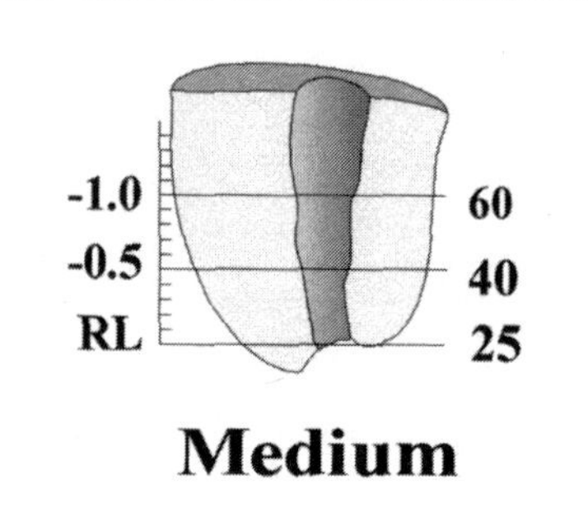

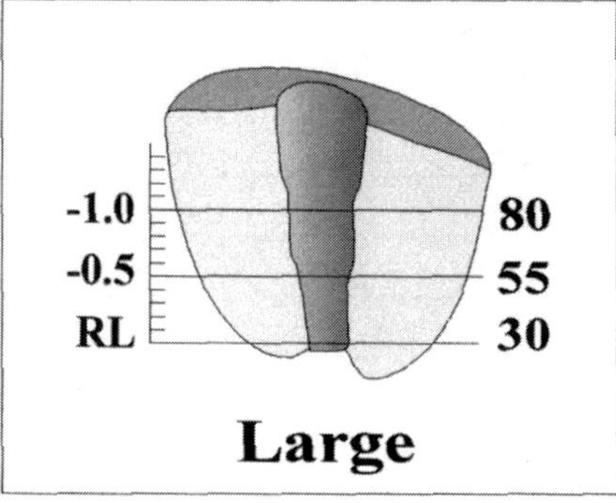

Figure 10-82 Details of the final balanced force step-back preparation in the apical control zone. Apical constriction is formed at a measured depth for small, medium, or large canals. Root length (**RL**) and millimeters of step-back are shown **left**. Instrument size is shown **right**. (Courtesy of Dr. James B. Roane.)

sharp transition angle, Flex-R files follow the canal and are prevented from gouging into the walls. The tip design causes a Flex-R file to hug the inside of a curve and prevents tip transport into the external wall of that curve.[493]

Balanced force instrumentation was born out of necessity because Roane firmly believes in enlarging the apical area to sizes larger than generally practiced. He expects a minimum enlargement of size 45, 1.5 mm short of the foramen in curved canals, and size 80 in larger single-rooted teeth (Figure 10-82). These sizes, of course, depend on root bulk, fragility, and the extent of curvature. Sabala and Roane also believe in carrying the preparation through to "full length," the **radiographic apex** of the root. They "purposely" shape the foraminal area, and yet patients rarely experience flareups.[494] A step-back in ½-mm increments is used with at least two groups of instruments to form an apical control zone. This shaping provides a minimum diameter at a known depth within the canal. A size 45 control zone is shaped by first expending a size 15 and 20 file to the periodontal ligament and then reducing the working depth by 0.5 mm for sizes 25, 30, and 35 and completing the apical shape 1 mm short using sizes 40 and 45. It goes without saying that sodium hypochlorite irrigation is used. Single-appointment preparation and obturation are *de rigeur* and also play an important role in the formation of these shaping concepts.

The success of this shaping technique and enlarging scheme has been closely evaluated in both clinical practice and student clinics. Clinical responsiveness is impressive, and the efficiency has been unmatched until rotary shaping (Figure 10-83).

Efficacy of Balanced Force Preparation. Sabala and Roane reported that, using the balanced force concept,

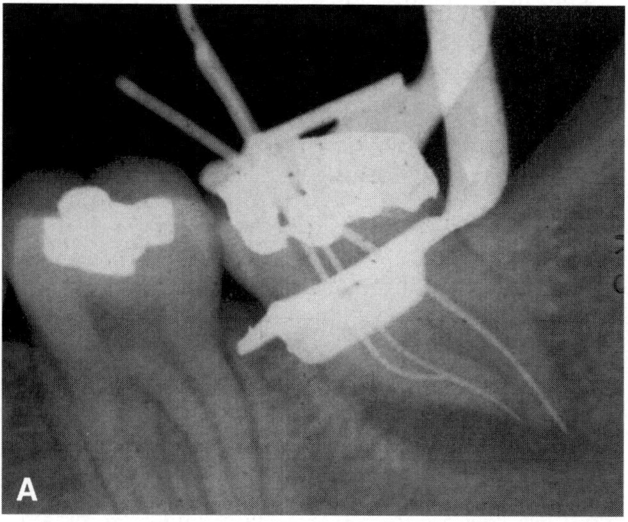

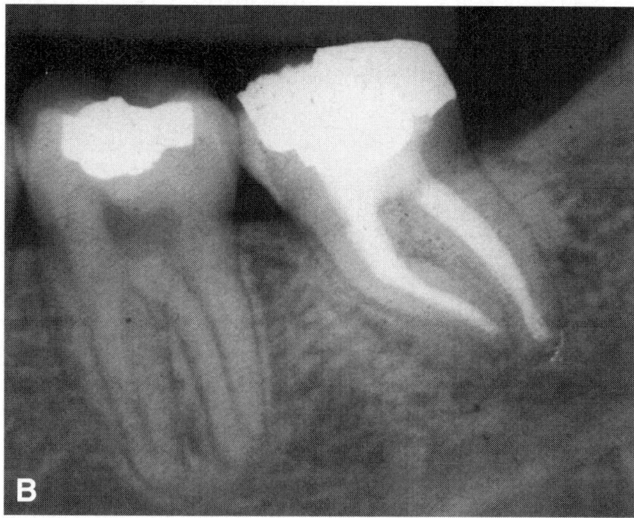

Figure 10-83 Impressive result of balanced force canal preparation and obturation. **A**, Instruments in place demonstrating canal curvature. **B**, Final obturation to extended sizes is more assurance that the canals have been thoroughly débrided. (Courtesy of Dr. James B. Roane.)

students at the University of Oklahoma could enlarge canals (in a laboratory exercise) with no measurable apical transportation.[494] Moreover, the modified-tip instrument (**Flex-R file**) developed a nontransported preparation more frequently and predictably. Procedural accidents occurred in 16.7% of the samples.[493] In a previous publication, the authors concluded that most instruments damaged by students (91.5%) using balanced force technique were damaged by overzealous clockwise rotation.[85]

A University of Washington balanced force study, using standard K-type files, concluded that "effective instrumentation of curved root canals may be accomplished with straight instruments of fairly large size without significant deviation from the original canal position." The original canal position was maintained 80% of the time after shaping with a No. 40 file. Original position was maintained in only 40% when a size 45 file was the final apical instrument.[491] A second University of Washington study compared balanced force and step-back techniques. This study disclosed that Balanced Force using Flex-R prototype files produced significantly less deviation from the center of the original canal than did the step-back method using conventional K-type and Hedstroem files.[492] The authors noted that **no instrument separations** were experienced in this study.

McKendry at the University of Iowa reported that the Balanced Force technique débrided the apical canal at least as adequately as the step-back filing technique and as well as the CaviEndo ultrasonic method. Furthermore, significantly less debris was extruded apically using balanced force compared to sonic or step-back preparations.[495,496] While testing the Balanced Force method at Georgia, the investigators found that early radicular flaring (step-back) made instrumentation much easier but did not necessarily improve the quality of the apical shape.[497]

It has been well established that the Balanced Force technique using guiding-tip files is fast and efficient. However, Balanced Force, like any new technique, should be practiced before it is used clinically. If excessive pressure is used, instrument separation may result. The large radicular shaping provided by use of Gates-Glidden drills, if improperly guided, might cause a strip perforation into the furcation. Use in undergraduate clinics has proven this technique reliable and safe for routine use. Once mastered, Balanced Force technique expands the shaping possibilities and extends one's operative abilities.

Ultrasonic and Sonic Preparations. *Ultrasonic.* As stated before, ultrasonic instrumentation today is used primarily in final canal débridement. For canal cleanliness, ultrasonic activation with a No. 15 file for 3 full minutes in the presence of 5% sodium hypochlorite produced "smooth, clean canals, free of the smear layer and superficial debris along their entire length."[498] This is exactly the technique used by a number of dentists seeking the cleanest canals in spite of which clean and shape technique they might have used. This should be done after the smear layer has been removed to ensure that all of the detritus, including bacteria, is all flushed out.

Concern over the possible harmful effects of sodium hypochlorite spilling out of the apical foramen was dealt with at the State University of Louisiana. Investigators intentionally overinstrumented past the apex in a monkey study and then evaluated the tissue response when sodium hypochlorite was used with conventional filing versus ultrasonic filing/irrigation. They were pleased to find no significant difference between the two methods and a low to moderate inflammatory response.[499]

Sonic. Sonic canal preparation and débridement with the **Micro Mega 1500 Sonic Air** (Micro Mega/MediDenta, France/USA) handpiece has been quite popular, particularly with the military. Camp has considerable experience with the **Sonic handpiece** and instruments and recommended that stainless steel hand files size 10 or 15 first be used to establish a pathway down the canals until resistance is met, usually about two-thirds of the canal length. He then begins the **step-down approach** with the sonic instruments—the No. 15 Shaper or Rispisonic file (see Figure 10-34), their length set 2 mm shy of the length reached with the previous instrument. About 30 seconds are spent in each canal using a quick up and down, 2 to 3 mm stroke and circumferentially filing under water irrigation supplied by the handpiece. This is the time to remove any isthmus or fins between canals. The use of each instrument is followed by copious sodium hypochlorite irrigation. The water from the handpiece is turned off and the irrigant is agitated in the canal with the fine Sonic file.

At this point, **working length is established** by a radiograph or an electric apex locator, and the extension to the apical constriction is carried out with stainless steel hand files to full working length—Nos. 15, 20, 25, and 30. Following sodium hypochlorite irrigation, Camp returns to the Sonic No. 15 (or a 20 or 25 in larger canals) Shaper or Rispisonic file for 30 seconds in each canal. After irrigation, No. 30, 35, and 40 hand files are again used followed by a larger Sonic instrument, and then No. 50 to 60 hand files are used to step-back up the canal to ensure a tapered preparation. Final use of the small Sonic file, with copious sodium hypochlorite to the constriction, removes the remaining debris and filings. Recapitulation with a No. 20 hand file will check the correct length of tooth and the apical stop at the constriction. After final irrigation, the canal is dried with paper points and is ready for medication or filling as the case may be (personal communication, 2001).

Efficacy and Safety of Ultrasonic/Sonic Preparations. The Iowa faculty tested step-back versus step-down approach with ultrasonic and sonic devices. They found that the **ultrasonic** instruments produced a better preparation when the **step-back** approach was used. The **step-down** preparation was preferred for **sonic** preparation.[500]

Another group of clinicians compared step-down, step-back hand instrumentation versus ultrasonic and sonic preparations. Both hand methods, as well as sonic enlargement, caused the extrusion of debris apically. In ranking from least to worst extrusion, Sonic was 1, best; step-down was 2; ultrasonic was 3; and conventional, circumferential, step-back preparation was 4, worst.[216]

Finally, a French group evaluated the degree of leakage following obturation of canals prepared with the Sonic Air unit using Shaper Sonic files versus hand preparation. The researchers found that the highest degree of leakage occurred overall with the manual method; however, both methods leaked apically. They felt that the smear layer present might have been responsible.[501]

ROTARY INSTRUMENTATION USING NICKEL TITANIUM

Over the past few years, the movement toward using rotary nickel-titanium instruments for root canal preparation has resulted in a multitude of instrumentation systems in the marketplace. The manufacture of variably tapered and "Gates-Glidden-like," flexible nickel-titanium instruments, for use in gear-reduction, slow-speed handpieces, either air driven or electric, has enabled the skilled clinician to deliver predictable canal shapes (Figure 10-84) with enhanced speed and increased efficiency.[502–510]

Problems associated with hand and rotary instrumentation with **stainless steel** have plagued both generalists and endodontists for years; these include (1) too many instruments and steps needed to generate the desired shape, thus increasing the time of canal preparation; (2) each resultant shape will be different, making obturation less predictable; (3) canal transportation naturally results as instruments increase in diameter and stiffness; and (4) the use of traditional coronal enlargement burs such as Gates-Glidden drills can cause excessive dentin removal.

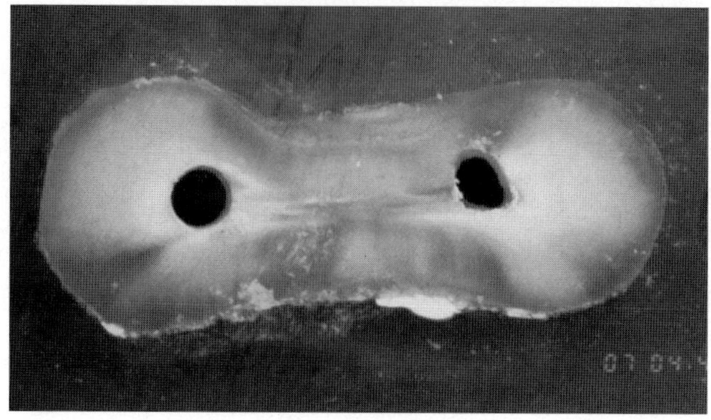

Figure 10-84 Comparison in the efficacy of two different methods of cleaning and shaping. **Left**, Preparation using nickel-titanium rotary instrumentation leaves a perfectly round canal thoroughly débrided. **Right**, Preparation using stainless steel K-type files in a step-back sequence. Note the uneven shape and possible debris. (Courtesy of Dr. Sergio Kuttler.)

Although nickel-titanium endodontic rotary instruments do overcome some of these shortcomings associated with stainless steel instruments, the clinician must also understand that nickel-titanium is not completely "fail-safe"; one must be aware of the fact that although nickel-titanium files are flexible, nickel-titanium metal, like any other metal, will eventually fatigue and fail when it becomes overstressed, especially during rotation in curved root canals[511–514] or if improperly used or abused (see Figure 10-20, B). In turn, strict monitoring of instrument use in all systems should be maintained so that nickel-titanium files can be periodically disposed of prior to failure.[512] In fact, **single use** (ie, use one time per case) in **severely curved or calcified canals** should be the rule. In addition, care must be taken to use these systems as per the manufacturer's instructions (eg, **a step-down approach with light pressure** is essential when using nickel-titanium rotary instruments).

It is also important to understand that these systems require a **significant learning curve** to achieve mastery and are not deemed to be a panacea.

ProFile 0.04 and 0.06 Taper Rotary Instruments and ProFile Orifice Shapers

ProFile 0.04 and 0.06 Taper Rotary Instruments and ProFile Orifice Shapers (Dentsply/Tulsa Dental; Tulsa, Okla.) are proportionately sized nickel-titanium U-shaped instruments (Figure 10-85) designed for use in a controlled, slow-speed, high-torque, rotary handpiece.[504,509,510,515] Although a study by Gabel et al. demonstrated four times more file separation/distortion at 333 rpm than at 166 rpm, the preferred speed

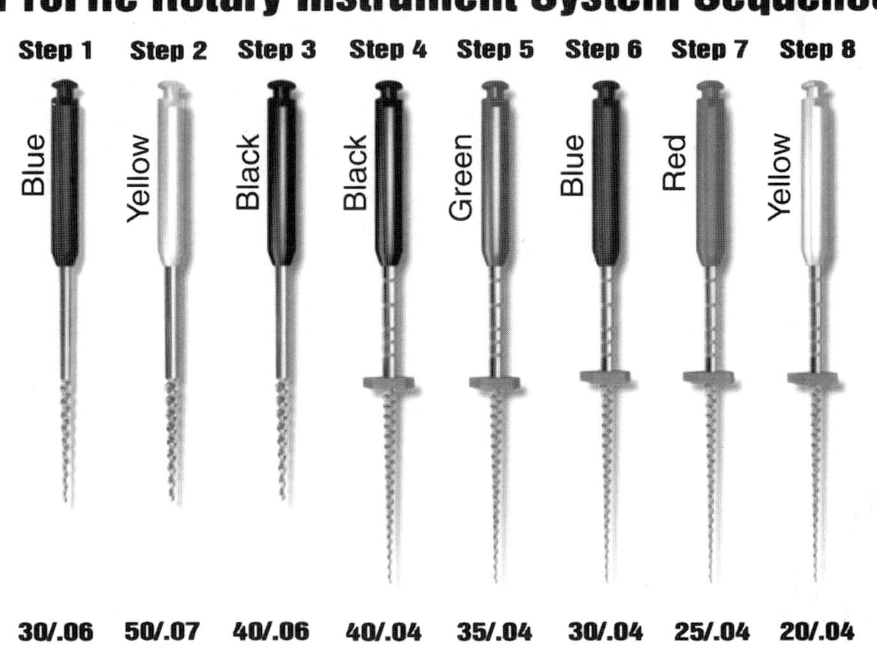

Figure 10-85 **ProFile** instrument sequence showing **Orifice shapers** and **0.04 tapers.** (Courtesy of Dentsply/Tulsa Dental.)

range is still from 275 to 325 rpm.[516] As these more tapered instruments are rotated, they produce an accelerated step-down preparation, resulting in a funnel-form taper from orifice to apex. As these "reamers" rotate clockwise, pulp tissue and dentinal debris are removed and **travel counterclockwise back up the shaft.** As a result, these instruments require periodic removal of dentin "mud" that has filled the "U" portion of the file.

The **U-blade design**, similar in cross-section to the LightSpeed, has flat outer edges that cut with a planing action, allowing it to remain more centered in the canal compared to conventional instruments (Figure 10-86).[504–506,509,510,515] The ProFile tapers also have a built-in safety feature, in which, by patented design, they purportedly unwind and then wind up backward prior to breaking. These **Profile Variable Taper** instruments are manufactured in standard ISO sizing as well as Series 29 standards (ie, every instrument increases 29% in diameter).

The **Orifice Shapers**, in 0.06 and 0.07 mm/mm tapers, are designed to **replace Gates-Glidden drills** for shaping the coronal portion of the canal. Because of their tapered, radial-landed flutes and U-file design, these instruments remain centered in the canal while creating a tapering preparation. In turn, this **preflaring** allows for more effective cleaning and shaping of the **apical half of the canal with the Profile Series 0.04 Tapers.**

In contrast to Profile Tapers, however, the total length of the **Orifice Openers** is 19 mm, with a cutting length of approximately 9 mm. Besides reducing file separation, this shorter length also makes them easier to manipulate in difficult access areas. **ISO tip sizes** of 30, 40, and 50 are built into these files with tapers of 0.06 and 0.07. These instruments serve the same function as the Quantec Flares.

The ProFile Variable Taper has a 60-degree bullet-nose tip that smoothly joins the flat radial lands.

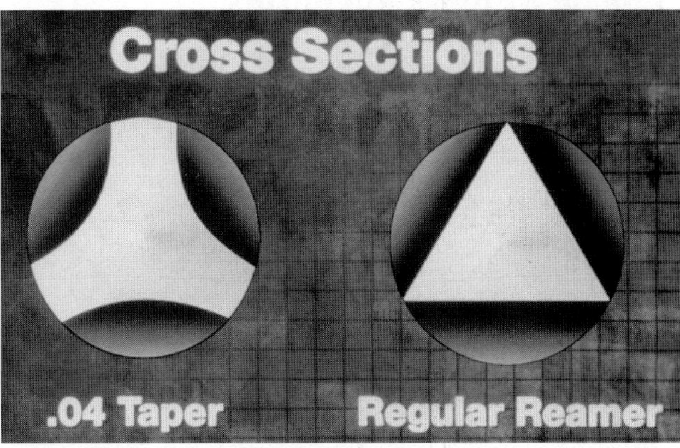

Figure 10-86 Comparative cross-sectional shapes between a U-shaped **Profile 0.04 taper** with a 90-degree rake angle and the conventional triangular reamer with a 60-degree cutting angle. (Courtesy of Dentsply/Tulsa Dental.)

Although these tapers have a 90-degree cutting angle (Figure 10-87), the nonaggressive radial landed flutes gently plane the walls without gouging and self-threading; in addition, they are cut deeper to add flexibility and help create a parallel inner core of metal. Thus, when the Profile Taper is rotated, stresses become more evenly distributed along the entire instrument in contrast to a nonparallel core or tapered shaft of a conventional instrument in which stresses are more concentrated toward the tip of its narrow end. An investigation by Blum, Mactou et al., however, demonstrated that torque can still develop at the apical 3 mm of the ProFiles even when used in a step-down procedure.[517]

ProFile instruments are available in either 0.04 (double taper) or 0.06 (triple taper) over the ISO 0.02 taper. Kavanaugh and Lumley found no significant differences between the 0.04 and 0.06 tapers with respect to canal transportation. On the other hand, the use of 0.06 tapers improved canal shape.[515] The 0.04 is more suitable for small canals and apical regions of most canals, including the mesial roots of mandibular molars and buccal roots of maxillary molars. The 0.06 is recommended for the midroot portions of most canals, distal roots of mandibular molars, and palatal roots of maxillary molars. Similar to the graduating taper technique of the Quantec Series, the clinician has the option of using alternating tapers within a single canal (ie, combinations of 0.04, 0.06, and 0.07 taper ProFile instruments).

Since the development of the ProFile tapers, a number of methods for use have been espoused. As such, there is currently no recommended "stand-alone" technique. In fact, a number of clinicians incorporate the Profile System near the end of the canal preparation to blend the apical preparation with coronal preflare.

Canal Preparation

A basic technique that primarily uses Orifice Shapers and Profile tapers is as follows: Once access, canal patency, and an estimated working length have been determined, the **No. 30 0.06 taper Orifice Shaper** is taken several millimeters into the canal, thus creating a pathway for the next instruments. The **No. 50 0.07 Orifice Shaper** is then used to create more coronal flare followed by the **No. 40 0.06 taper Orifice Shaper.** This last instrument should be advanced about **halfway down the canal** using minimal pressure. Constant irrigation and recapitulation must be followed throughout the entire sequence.

A working length radiograph is then taken with a **stainless steel hand file** to determine the precise length. The tip of all subsequent tapers becomes a guide as the instrument cuts higher up the shaft, mostly with the middle blades. In all cases, **a ProFile taper file should never be used in the canal longer than 4 to 6 seconds.** The clinician must now **passively** advance the 0.04 or 0.06 taper instruments, or combinations thereof, to or near the working length. As the rotary reamers move closer to length, a funnel shape is imparted to the canal walls. In most cases, a No. 30 or an equivalent 29 Series 0.04 taper eventually reaches at or near the working length with minimal resistance. In more constricted cases, however, a No. 25 or 20 0.04 taper may be the first to reach the working length. If the tapers are not taken to full working length, hand files, either stainless steel or nickel-titanium, can be used to complete the apical 1 to 2 mm.

ProFile GT Non-Cutting Tips

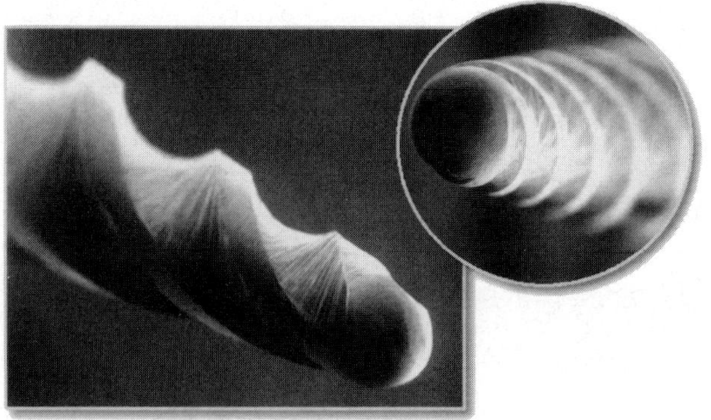

Figure 10-87 Scanning electron micrograph of a **Profile GT** depicting a 60-degree bullet-nosed tip. The tip allows for a smooth transition angle where the tip meets the flat radial lands. (Courtesy of Dentsply/ Tulsa Dental.)

ProFile GT Rotary Instrumentation

ProFile GT (Greater Taper) Rotary Files (Dentsply/Tulsa Dental; Tulsa, Okla.) are made of nickel-titanium alloy, and their intended purpose is to create a predefined shape in a single canal. Designed by Dr. Steven Buchanan and also available as hand files, these uniquely engineered files are manufactured in 0.06, 0.08, 0.10, and 0.12 tapers, all having a constant ISO **noncutting tip** diameter of 0.20 mm (ISO size 20) to ensure maintenance of a small apical preparation (Figure 10-88). They have variably pitched, radial-landed, clockwise cut **U-blade flutes** that provide reamer-like efficiency at the shank with K-file strength at their tips (ie, they have closed flute angles at their tips and more open flute angles at their shank ends). The open flute angles at the shank end also tend to reduce the file's ability to thread into the canal, a typical problem that occurs with other rotary designs. The maxi-

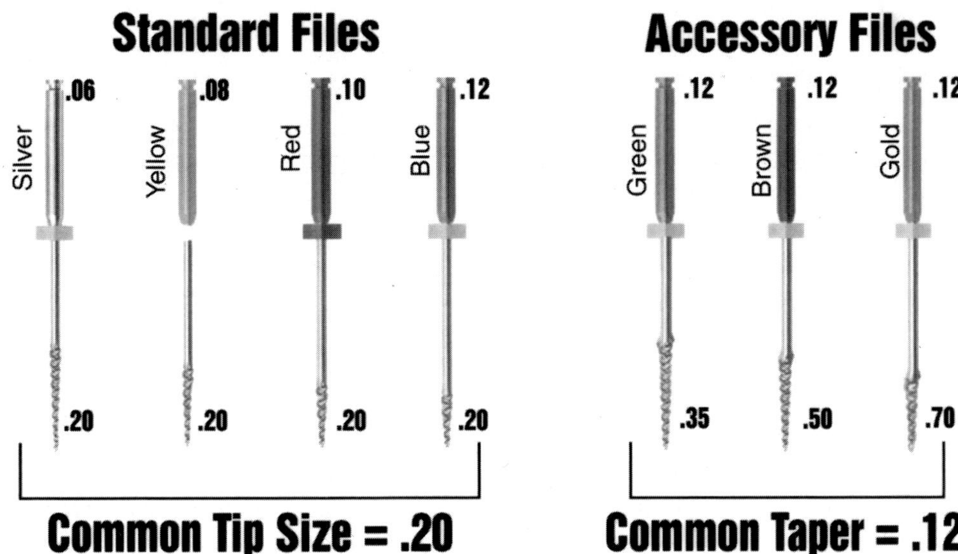

Figure 10-88 **Profile GT** Rotary sizes and tapers of the **standard GT:** 0.06, 0.08, 0.10, and 0.12 mm/mm tapers with a common ISO size 20 tip and the **Accessory** files with a common 0.12 mm/mm taper but variable tips of ISO sizes 35, 50, and 70. (Courtesy of Dentsply/Tulsa Dental.)

mum flute diameter is also set at 1.0 mm, safely limiting coronal enlargement.

Because the GT files **vary by taper** but have the same tip diameters and maximum flute diameters, the flute lengths become shorter as the tapers increase. The 0.06 taper is designed for moderate to severely curved canals in small roots, the 0.08 taper for straight to moderately curved canals in small roots, and the 0.10 taper for straight to moderately curved canals in large roots. A set of three accessory GT files (see Figure 10-88) is available for unusually large root canals having apical diameters greater than 0.3 mm. These instruments have a taper of 0.12 mm per mm, a larger maximum flute diameter of 1.5 mm, and varying tip diameters of 0.35, 0.50, and 0.70 mm. When used in canals with **large apical diameters,** they are typically able to complete the whole shape with one file. The ProFile GT files are thus designed so that the final taper of the preparation is essentially equivalent to the respective GT file used.

A recent study (unpublished, 2000) conducted at the University of Pacific found that undergraduate dental students, who were trained in the GT rotary technique, completed shapes in 75% less time than with standard K files and Gates-Glidden drills. Shapes were also rounder throughout their lengths, and coronal canal shaping was more conservative.

Canal Preparation. According to the manufacturer, the **ProFile GT technique** can be broken down into three steps: **step-down** with ProFile GTs and then **step back** with ProFile 0.04 taper files and a GT file to create final canal shape. As in all rotary techniques, a step-down approach is used once initial negotiation is completed with hand files and lubricant. Standard GT files (0.12, 0.10, 0.08, and 0.06 tapers) are then used in a step-down manner at 150 to 300 rpm, allowing each to cut to their passive lengths.

Working length should be determined once the GT file has reached two-thirds of the estimated length of the canal. In some cases, the 0.06 taper will reach full length. Since the standard GT files all have a 0.20 mm tip diameter, the 0.08 and 0.10 taper files should easily go to length if a 0.08 or 0.10 taper is desired for that particular canal.

Rather than using the GT file to the apical terminus, **a variation of the technique** involves the creation of an apical taper. **ProFile 0.04 taper** instruments, usually sizes 25 to 35, can be used in a **step-back** fashion, **starting about 2 mm short of working length.** The standard **GT files** can then be used in a **step-down fashion again** to create the final canal shape right to working length, or, if preferred, hand instruments may be used to shape the apical 2 mm of the canal. If additional coronal flare is needed, an appropriate **GT accessory file** can be used.

With the ProFile GT rotary instrumentation technique, as with most other nickel-titanium rotary techniques, basic rules need to be adhered to. **Speeds must**

be kept constant, a light touch must be used, the GT files should not be used in a canal more than 4 to 6 seconds, and **irrigation and lubrication** must be continually used throughout the procedure.

ProTaper Rotary System

According to the developers, **ProTaper** (Progressively Tapered), nickel-titanium rotary files substantially simplify root canal preparation, particularly in curved and restricted canals. The claim is made that they consistently produce proper canal shaping that enables predictable obturation by any vertical obturation method. This new instrument system, consisting of three "shaping" and three "finishing" files, was co-developed by Drs. Clifford Ruddle, John West, Pierre Mactou, and Ben Johnson and was designed by François Aeby and Gilbert Rota of Dentsply/Maillefer in Switzerland.

The distinguishing feature of the **ProTaper System** (Dentsply/Tulsa Dental) is the **progressively variable tapers** of each instrument that develop a "progressive preparation" in both vertical and horizontal directions. Under use, the file blades engage a smaller area of dentin, thus reducing torsional load that leads to instrument fatigue and file separation. During rotation, there is also an increased tactile sense when compared with traditionally shaped rotary instruments. "Taper lock" is reportedly reduced, extending a newly found freedom from concern about breakage. As with any new system, however, the ProTaper beginner is advised to first practice on extracted teeth with restricted curved canals.

ProTaper Configurations. As previously stated, the ProTaper System consists of only six instrument sizes: three shaping files and three finishing files.

Shaping Files. The Shaping Files are labeled **S-X, S-1, and S-2.** The **S-X Shaper** (Figure 10-89, A) is an auxiliary instrument used in canals of teeth with shorter roots or to extend and expand the coronal aspects of the preparation, similar to the use of Gates-Glidden drills or orifice openers. The S-X has a much increased rate of taper from D_0 (tip diameter) to D_9 (9.0 mm point on the blades) than do the other two shapers, S-1 and S-2. At the tip (D_0), the S-X shaper has an ISO diameter of 0.19 mm. This rises to 1.1 mm at D_9 (comparable to the **tip size** of a size 110 ISO instrument). After D_9, the **rate of taper** drops off up to D_{14}, which thins and increases the flexibility of the instrument.

The **S-1** and **S-2 files** start at tip sizes of 0.17 mm and 0.20 mm, respectively, and each file gains in taper up to 1.2 mm (Figure 10-89, B). But unlike the consistent increase of taper per millimeter in the ISO instruments, the **ProTaper Shapers have increasingly larger tapers** each millimeter over the 14 mm length of their cutting blades. This is what makes the instruments unique.

Shaping File S-1 is designed to prepare the coronal one-third of the canal, whereas **Shaping File S-2** enlarges and prepares the middle third in addition to the critical coronal region of the apical third. Eventually, both size instruments may also help enlarge the apical third of the canal as well.

Finishing Files. The three finishing files have been designed to plane away the variations in canal diameter in the **apical one-third. Finishing Files F-1, F-2,** and **F-3** have tip diameters (D_0) of ISO sizes 20, 25, and 30, respectively. Their tapers differ as well (Figure 10-89, C). Between D_0 nd D_3, they taper at rates of 0.07, 0.08, and 0.09 mm/mm, respectively. From D_4 to D_{14}, each instrument shows a decreased taper that improves its flexibility.

Although primarily designed to finish the apical third of the canal, finishers do progressively expand the middle third as well. Generally, only one instrument is needed to prepare the apical third to working length, and tip sizes (0.20, 0.25, or 0.30) will be selected based on the canal's curvature and cross-sectional diameter. **Finisher F-3** has been further engineered to increase its flexibility in spite of its size (Figure 10-89, D).

ProTaper Benefits.

1. The progressive (multiple) taper design improves flexibility and "carving" efficiency, an important asset in curved and restrictive canals (Figure 10-89, E).
2. The balanced pitch and helical angles of the instrument optimize cutting action while effectively augering debris coronally, as well as preventing the instrument from screwing into the canal.
3. Both the "shapers" and the "finishers" remove the debris and soft tissue from the canal and finish the preparation with a smooth continuous taper.
4. The triangular cross-section of the instruments increases safety, cutting action, and tactile sense while reducing the lateral contact area between the file and the dentin (Figure 10-89, F).
5. The modified guiding instrument tip can easily follow a prepared glide path without gouging side walls.

Canal Preparation.
ProTaper System: Guidelines for Use

1. Prepare a straight-line access cavity with no restrictions in the entry path into the chamber.
2. Fill the access cavity brimful with sodium hypochlorite and/or **ProLube**.

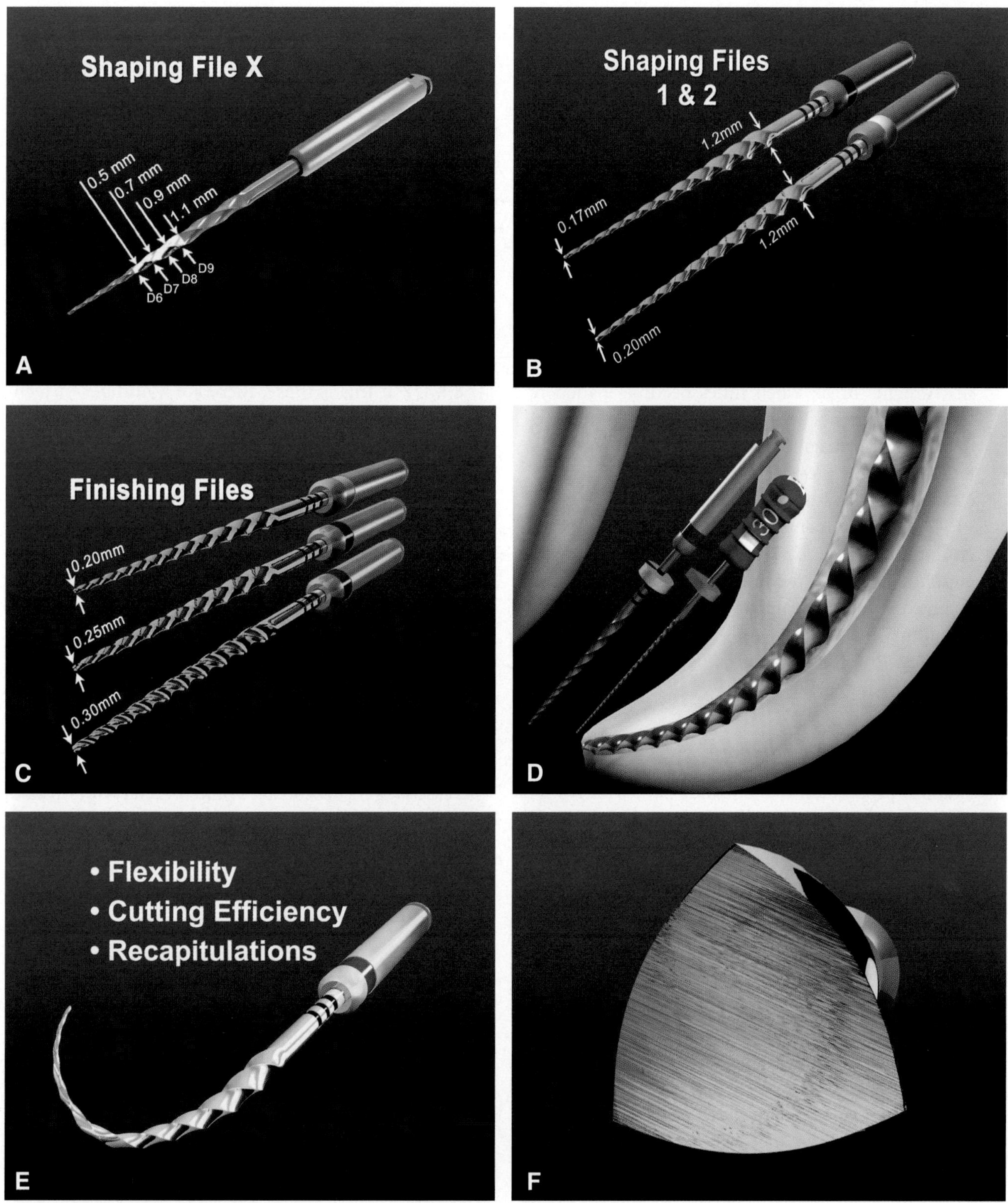

Figure 10-89 **The ProTaper File Rotary System. A, Shaping File X,** an auxiliary instrument used primarily to extend canal orifices and widen access as well as create coronal two-thirds shaping in short teeth. **B, Shaping Files 1 and 2,** used primarily to open and expand the coronal and middle thirds of the canal. C, **Finishing Files 1, 2, and 3,** used to expand and finish the apical third of progressively larger canals. D, **Finishing File 3** is used to finish the apical third of larger canals. A No. 30 file is used to gauge the apical opening. Recapitulation with a regular No. 30 instrument, followed by liberal irrigation, is most important. **E,** The flexibility and cutting ability of nickel-titanium ProTaper Rotary Files are assets in preparing curved constricted canals. **F,** Triangular cross-section presents three sharp blade edges that improve cutting ability and tactile sense. Reproduced with permission from ADVANCED ENDODONTICS video and Drs. John West and Clifford Ruddle. (**Color reproduction courtesy of Dentsply Tulsa Dental**)

3. Establish a smooth glide path with No. 10 and No. 15 stainless steel hand files.
4. Use maximum magnification to observe the movement of the rotary instrument. "Seeing" rotary apical movement is safer than simply "feeling" such movement.
5. Use a torque- and speed-controlled electric motor, powering the handpiece at **200 to 300 rpm.**
6. Be much gentler than with hand instruments. Always treat in a moist canal. Irrigate frequently!
7. **Slow down!** Each instrument should do minimal shaping. Only two, three, or four passes may be required for the file to engage restrictive dentin and carve the shape to the proper depth.
8. Instruments break when flutes become loaded or when instruments are forced. Check the flutes frequently under magnification and clean them. Cyclic fatigue from overuse, or if the glide path is not well established, also leads to breakage.
9. ProTaper instruments are disposable and, like all endodontic files and reamers, are designed for single-patient use. Sometimes instruments are even changed within the same treatment (eg, in the case of a four-canal molar).
10. Irrigate with 17% EDTA or a viscous chelator during the ProTaper shaping.

ProTaper System: Directions for Use

1. Establish proper access and a glide path with No. 10 and No. 15 stainless steel files to the working length or the apical constriction exit.
2. Flood the canal and chamber with sodium hypochlorite and begin shaping with the **Shaper S-1** using multiple, passive-pressure passes. Go no deeper than three-quarters of the estimated canal length. Irrigate and recapitulate with a No. 10 hand file, establishing patency to full working length. Now, with **S-1**, extend the preparation to full working length. Again irrigate and recapitulate.
3. "Brush" with the **Shaper S-X** to improve the straight-line access in short teeth or to relocate canal access away from furcations in posterior teeth.
4. **Shaping file S-2** is now used to full working length. Irrigate, recapitulate, and reirrigate.
5. Confirm and maintain working length with a hand file. (Remember, as curves are straightened, canals are shortened.)
6. With **Finisher F-1,** passively extend the preparation to within 0.5 mm of the working length. **Withdraw after one second! And only one second!** The F-1 has a tip size of 0.20 mm, and if a No. 20 hand instrument is found to be snug, the preparation is finished. With the instrument in place, radiographically verify the exact length before final irrigation.
7. If the **F-1** and the No. 20 hand file are **loose**, continue the preparation with the **Finisher F-2,** which is 0.25 mm diameter at the tip. Confirm with a No. 25 hand instrument and, if snug, confirm the length radiographically, irrigate, and complete.
8. If the **F-2** instrument and the No. 25 hand file are **loose**, continue the preparation to just short of the working length with the **Finisher F-3 file,** which has a 0.30 mm tip diameter, and follow with the confirming No. 30 instrument. If the No. 30 is found to be snug, the preparation is finished (see Figure 10-89, D). If this is loose, there are a number of techniques to enlarge the apical third to larger sizes.
9. Frequent irrigation and file cleansing are imperative—**irrigation and recapitulation!**

Now that the perfectly tapered preparation is complete, smear layer removal with EDTA and sodium hypochlorite is in order, followed by either medication and/or obturation.

Quantec System and Graduating Taper Technique

The Quantec Series (Sybron Endo/Analytic; Orange, Calif.) consists of a series of 10 graduated nickel-titanium tapers from 0.02 through 0.06 with ISO tip sizing[507,518] (Figure 10-90). The Quantec **Flare Series,** with increased tapers of 0.08, 0.10, and 0.12, all with **tip sizes of ISO 25,** are designed to quickly and safely **shape the coronal third** of the canal. In contrast to the basic principles of other rotary instrument techniques, this system incorporates a built-in **"graduated tapers technique,"** whereby a **series of varying tapers** are used to prepare a single canal. The instruments are used at **300 to 350 rpm** in a high-torque, gear-reduction, slow-speed handpiece.

Proponents of the **graduating tapers** technique claim that, theoretically, using a series of files of a **single taper,** whether it is a conventional 0.02 taper or a greater taper, will result in decreased efficiency as larger instruments are used, that is, more of the file comes into contact with the dentinal walls, making it more difficult to remove dentin as forces are generated over a larger area.[518] Ultimately, each instrument will become fully engaged along the canal wall, potentially inhibiting proper cleaning and shaping of the apical canal.

In contrast and in accordance with the graduating tapers technique, by **restricting the surface contact** between instrument and wall, an instrument's efficiency is increased since the forces used are concentrated on a smaller area. In this technique, for example, once a

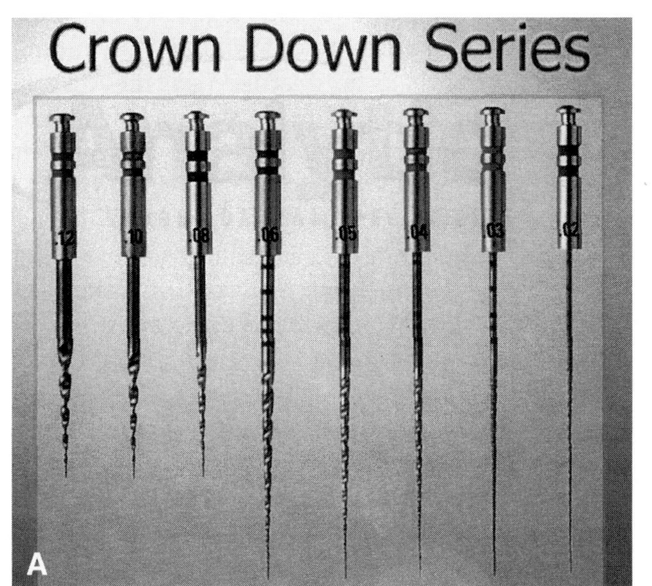
Crown Down Series
A

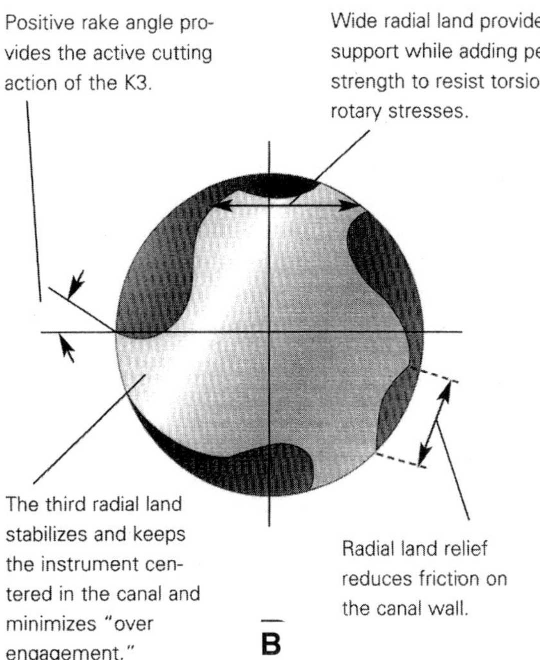
ENGINEERED FOR EFFICIENCY
Positive rake angle provides the active cutting action of the K3.
Wide radial land provides blade support while adding peripheral strength to resist torsional and rotary stresses.
The third radial land stabilizes and keeps the instrument centered in the canal and minimizes "over engagement."
Radial land relief reduces friction on the canal wall.
B

Figure 10-90 A, The **Quantec** series of variably tapered instruments comes in both safe-cutting (**SC**) and noncutting (**LX**) tips and three lengths: 17, 21, and 25 mm (see Figure 10-28). Quantec files are 30% shorter in the rotary "handle," and when used in the **Axxess Minihead** handpiece, over 5 mm of length are saved. **B**, Cross-section of the newest **Sybronendo** rotary file-**K3**. Note that three cutting blades have positive rakes that materially increase the cutting ability. Also note that the radial land relief reduces friction and provides debris collection space. The nickel-titanium files come in 0.04 and 0.06 tapers, tip sizes ISO 10 to 60, and increasing variable helical flute angle from D_1 to D_{16}. (Courtesy of **SybronEndo.**)

0.02 taper has shaped the canal, a 0.03 taper with the same apical diameter would engage the canal more coronally; by altering the taper from 0.02, to 0.03, and up the scale to 0.06, the efficiency of canal preparation is maximized by restricting surface contact.

The Quantec rotary instruments are uniquely engineered with slightly positive rake or blade angles on each of their twin flutes; these are designed to shave rather than scrape dentin (negative rake angle), which most conventional files do. Flute design also includes a 30-degree helical angle with flute space that becomes progressively larger distal to the cutting blade, helping channel the debris coronally. More peripheral mass has been added to these files rather than depending on core strength alone as in other rotary systems.

Quantec's wide radial lands are purported to **prevent crack formation** in the blades and aid in deflecting the instrument around curvatures. By recessing the wide radial lands behind the blade, there is a concomitant reduction in frictional resistance while maintaining canal centering.

With respect to tip geometry, the clinician has a choice of two designs. The SC safe-cutting tip (see Figure 10-28, A) is specifically designed for small, tight canals, narrow curvatures, and calcified canal systems. This faceted 60-degree tip cuts as it moves apically; as the tip approaches a curve, conceptually, a balance takes place between file deflection and cutting. The LX noncutting tip, on the other hand, is a nonfaceted bullet-nosed tip, acting as a pilot in the canal and deflecting around severe curvatures in less constricted canals (see Figure 10-28, B). These LX Quantec instruments are also recommended for enlarging the body and coronal segments and managing delicate apical regions.

Canal Preparation. The Graduating Tapers technique involves a modified step-down sequence, **starting with a larger tapered file first and progressing with files of lesser taper** until working length is achieved. The technique involves canal **negotiation**, canal **shaping**, and, finally, **apical preparation.** As in all instrumentation techniques, straight-line access to the canal orifices must be made first, followed by passive negotiation of the canal using No. 10 and No. 15 0.02 taper hand files. A Quantec No. 25, 0.06 taper, 17 mm in length, is passively used. In most cases, this instrument should approach the apical third of the canal; at this point, the working length must be established.

A "Glide Path" is now established for all subsequent Quantec files by working No. 10 and No. 15 0.02 taper hand files along with sodium hypochlorite to the established working length. During the shaping phase, each Quantec file, **progressing sequentially from a 0.12 taper down to a 0.03 taper**, is passively carried into the canal as far as possible. In all cases, **light apical pressure** must be applied, using a **light pecking motion** and never advancing more than 1 mm per second into the canal. Each instrument should be used for no more than 3 to 5 seconds. The sequence is repeated until a 0.06 or 0.05 taper reaches the working length. The **apical preparation** can then be deemed complete or **further enlarged** by using the Quantec standard 0.02 taper No. 40 or No. 45 rotary instruments or hand files.

With the Quantec series, the correct amount of apical pressure must be maintained at all times; the continuously rotating instrument should either be inserted or withdrawn from the canal while allowing for its slow apical progression. The instrument, however, **should be withdrawn** after the desired depth has been reached and not left in the canal for an extended period of time, potentially causing canal transportation, ledge formation, and instrument separation. Thus, to reduce procedural problems, there should always be a **continuous apical/coronal movement** of the instrument, and, if the rotating file begins to make a **clicking sound** (file binding), one should withdraw the file and observe for instrument distortion.

LightSpeed Endodontic Instruments

The LightSpeed rotary instrumentation system (LightSpeed Technology; San Antonio, Tex.), so named because of the "light" touch needed as the "speed" of instrumentation" is increased, involves the use of specially engineered nickel-titanium "Gates-Glidden-like" reamers (see Figure 10-90) that allow for enhanced tactile control and apical preparations larger than those created via conventional techniques and other nickel-titanium rotary systems.[502,508,514,519–521] The set of instruments consists of ISO-sized rotary files from size 20 through 100, including nine half-sizes ranging from 22.5 through 65. The half sizes help reduce stress on both the instrument and root during preparation and decrease the amount of cutting that each instrument must accomplish. In most clinical cases, about 8 to 14 instruments are needed. They are used in a continuous, 360-degree clockwise rotation with very light apical pressure in a slow-speed handpiece. The recommended rpm is between **750 and 2,000**, with preference toward the 1,300 to 2,000 range.

Owing to the flexible, slender, parallel shaft (Figure 10-91) that makes up the body of the instrument, the clinician can prepare the apical portion of the canal with the "head" of the LightSpeed to a size larger than what could normally be produced using tapered instruments. Since taper adds metal and decreases both flexibility and tactile feel toward the more apical regions of the canal, the LightSpeed instrument head, with its short cutting blades, only binds at its tip, thus increasing the accuracy of the tactile feedback. This results in **rounder and centered apical preparations.**[502,508,514,519–521] Success with the LightSpeed, however, is predicated on straight-line access, an adequate coronal preflare, and establishment of **working length** prior to its introduction into a canal.

The LightSpeed instrument has a short cutting blade with three flat radial lands, which keeps the instrument from screwing into the canal, a noncutting pilot tip (see Figures 10-90 inset, and Figure 10-26), and a small-diameter **noncutting flexible shaft**, which is smaller than the blade and eliminates contact with the canal wall. Laser-etched length control rings on the shaft eliminate the need for silicone stops (see Figure 10-90). The LightSpeed instrument has a cross-sectional **U-blade design** in which flat radial lands with neutral rake angles enhance planing of the canal walls and centering of the instrument within the canal. The helical blade angle and narrow shaft diameter facilitate debris removal coronally.

Canal Preparation. Following proper coronal access, **preflaring** with Gates-Glidden drills or another method is highly recommended. The working length must first be established with at least a No. 15 stainless steel K file. Prior to using the LightSpeed in the handpiece, the clinician should first select and hand-fit a No. 20 LightSpeed instrument that binds short of the working length. Once

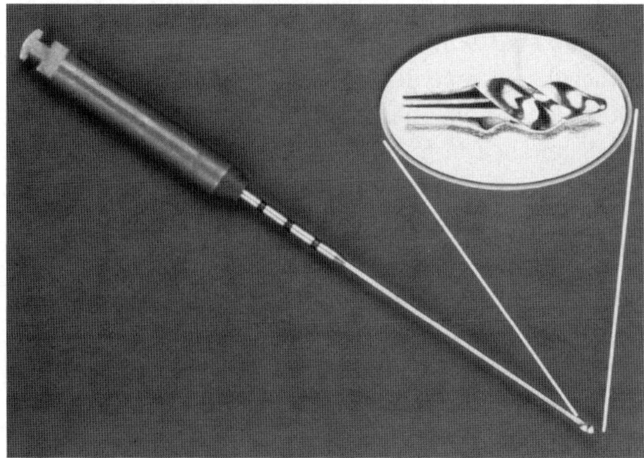

Figure 10-91 **LightSpeed** instrument. The head has a noncutting tip and is the U-style design. Note the small cutting head and the long noncontacting shaft, making the LightSpeed a unique instrument, much like a Gates-Glidden in configuration. (Courtesy of LightSpeed Technology.)

fitted, that LightSpeed instrument is now inserted in the gear-reduction, slow-speed handpiece. The LightSpeed must **enter and exit the canal at the proper rpm**, preferably 1,300 to 2,000 rpm for smoother and faster instrumentation.[520] As with other systems, the rpm must be kept constant to avoid abrupt changes that may result in loss of tactile feedback and instrument breakage.

There are two recommended motions with LightSpeed: (1) if no resistance is felt, the LightSpeed is gently advanced to the desired length and withdrawn, or (2) **if resistance is felt, a very light apical pecking motion** (advance and withdraw motion) should be used until **working length is attained.** In either case, the instrument should **never stay in one place** as this increases transportation and enhances separation. This gentle pecking motion prevents blade locking, removes debris coronally, and aids in keeping the blades clean.

Increasingly larger LightSpeed instruments are used to the working length, **never skipping sizes, including the half-sizes.** Irrigation should occur at least once after every three instruments. Once the apical stop has been established, the LightSpeed should never be forced beyond this point. If forced, buckling along the shaft may occur, potentially leading to fatigue and instrument separation.

The **MAR**, or Master Apical Rotary (the smallest LightSpeed size to reach the working length, yet large enough to clean the apical part of the canal), becomes the subsequent instrument that first binds 3 to 4 mm short of the working length. This instrument will require 12 to 16 pecks (ie, 4 pecks per millimeter advancement) to reach the working length. This MAR, typically larger than the size achieved with most other methods, has been shown to clean the sides of the canal while remaining centered and creating a round preparation.[502,508,519–521]

The apical 4 mm of the canal are shaped using sequentially larger instruments in **step-back sequence** with 1 mm intervals. The remainder of the step-back is done by feel. Finally, the last instrument taken to full working length is used for recapitulation. The taper of a canal prepared with LightSpeed is approximately 0.025 mm/mm to preserve tooth structure. To prevent instrument separation from torsional overload or from buckling along the shaft (cyclic or bending fatigue), LightSpeed instruments must always be **used with light apical pressure—never forced.**[514] If the blade breaks off, it frequently can be bypassed.

Rapid Body Shapers, Rotary Reamers, and Pow-R Rotary Files

Rapid Body Shaper (RBS) (Moyco/Union Broach; Bethpage, N.Y.) consists of a series of four nickel-titanium rotary engine reamers (Figure 10-92). These

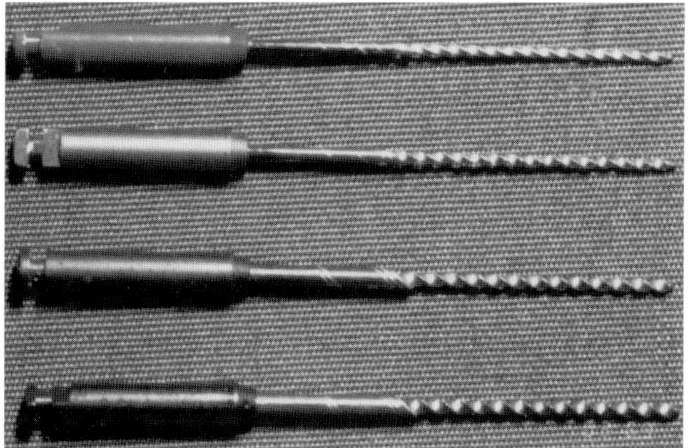

Figure 10-92 Series of four **Rapid Body Shapers.** From the top to the bottom, Nos. 1, 2, 3, and 4. (Courtesy of Moyco/Union Broach.)

instruments feature the patented nonledging Roane bullet tip and allow the practitioner to rapidly **shape the body of the canal** without the problems that can occur using Gates-Glidden drills. The RBS instruments develop a **parallel-walled canal shape.** The RBS series consists of four instruments: No. 1 (0.61 mm at the tip), No. 2 (0.66 mm at the tip), No. 3 (0.76 mm at the tip), and No. 4 (0.86 mm at the tip).

Canal Preparation. Prior to using RBS, the apical region of the canal must be prepared with a minimum No. 35 ISO instrument to within 0.5 mm of the apex. The **No. 1 RBS** is then placed in a gear-reduction, slow-speed handpiece at **275 to 300 rpm** and allowed to track down the canal **2 to 3 mm.** Constant and **copious irrigation** is necessary at all times. The RBS is removed to clean the fluting and is reinserted to track another 2 to 3 mm down the canal. This sequence is repeated until the **No. 1 RBS is within 4 mm of the apex.** The **No. 2 RBS** is then used like the No. 1, also to within 4 mm or shorter from the apex. The **No. 3 RBS,** followed by the **No. 4 RBS,** is used to within 7 mm of the apex, completing the body shaping. The No. 1 RBS will feel very aggressive, whereas the No. 2 through 4 RBS feel almost passive in comparison. Apical refinement is subsequently completed by hand instruments or via Pow-R nickel-titanium rotary instruments.

Pow-R Nickel-Titanium Rotary Files (Moyco/Union Broach; Bethpage, N.Y.), also with a nonledging Roane bullet tip, are available in both 0.02 and 0.04 tapers and, owing to their taper design, allow the practitioner to clean and shape the middle and apical regions of the canal in a conservative manner. These instruments come in standard ISO instrument sizes as well as in **half sizes** 17.5, 22.5, 27.5, 32.5, and 37.5 for more precise apical refinement. They follow standard ISO color codes as well.

Canal Preparation. Once Gates-Glidden drills are used to prepare and shape the coronal region of the canal in a step-down manner, and the canal has been at least partially negotiated with hand files, Pow-R files can be used. The clinician should select a file that binds at its tip in the middle third and begin to gradually move and push that file as it is rotating, slightly withdrawing it every 0.25 mm penetration until no more than 2 mm of depth are achieved or until resistance is felt. Like any other nickel-titanium file, these instruments must be **used passively** and with a **light touch or pecking motion**. The working length should now be determined using a hand file. Constant recapitulation with hand files is the rule along with constant irrigation. **The next smaller Pow-R file** is used to continue shaping an additional 1 to 2 mm deeper. Rotary instrumentation continues, **decreasing sizes in sequence** until the shaping is about 1.5 mm short of the apical foramen. The remaining portion of the canal can be finished with hand instruments or with Pow-R files. If more flare is needed, particularly if an obturation technique that requires deep condenser penetration is considered, a rotary incremental step-back can be used to generate additional space in the apical and middle portions of the canal.

Both the RBS files and Pow-R instruments are used in high-torque, gear-reduction handpieces with rpm ranging from 300 to 400.

Principles of Nickel-Titanium Rotary Instrumentation

Irrespective of the nickel-titanium system used, nickel-titanium instruments are **not designed** for pathfinding, negotiating small calcified or curved canals, or bypassing ledges. Placing undue pressure on these extremely flexible instruments may lead to file breakage. This is attributable to the fact that nickel-titanium has less longitudinal strength and may deflect at a point where pressure is off the file. As mentioned throughout this section, stainless steel instruments should be used initially for pathfinding owing to their enhanced stiffness. Once the canal has been negotiated with at least a stainless steel No. 15 K-type file or a ledge has been bypassed and removed, then rotary nickel-titanium instruments can be used. Stainless steel instruments are also more radiopaque than nickel-titanium and "show up" better in tooth length measurements.

When using a gear-reduction, slow-speed, nickel-titanium rotary handpiece, the clinician must always keep the handpiece head **aligned with the long axis of each canal** as good straight-line access decreases excessive bending on the instrument. Nickel-titanium rotary instruments must be used with **light apical pressure** and never be forced and **must always be used in a lubricated canal system** to reduce frictional resistance, preferably with RC-Prep or Glyde or another acceptable lubricant.

Abrupt curvatures, S-shaped canal systems, and canals that join must be avoided with any nickel-titanium rotary file; use of rotary files in these cases may also lead to breakage. When a nickel-titanium file rotates inside any canal system, it becomes stressed and may subsequently "wobble" in the handpiece once the instrument is removed; the file should be disposed of. As the nickel-titanium file experiences any undue stress, including cyclic fatigue,[514] the metal undergoes a crystalline (microscopic) phase transformation and can become structurally weaker. In many cases, there is usually no visible or macroscopic indication that the metal has fatigued. With repeated sterilization, Rapisarda et al. demonstrated decreased cutting efficiency and alteration of the superficial structure of **Nickel-titanium ProFiles**, thus indicating a weakened structure, possibly prone to fracture.[522] Essentially, a nickel-titanium file may disarticulate without any warning, especially if not properly used. Thus, it behooves the astute clinician to develop a systematic method for recognizing potential problems (grabbing or frictional locking of files into the canal, unwinding, twisting, cyclic fatigue, etc) and disposing of these nickel-titanium instruments. No one knows the maximum or ideal number of times that a nickel-titanium file can be used.

There is no doubt that the evolution of mechanized or rotary instrumentation using specially designed nickel-titanium files in gear-reduction, high-torque handpieces has revolutionized endodontics owing to their speed and efficacy in canal shaping and maintaining canal curvature. There is also no doubt that the development of the shape-memory alloy, **nickel titanium,** for use in endodontics has elevated the practice of endodontics to a higher level. With the evolution of torque-control electric motors and the continual engineering of more sophisticated instrument designs, cleaning and shaping with rotary instruments, made with shape-memory alloys, may eventually become the standard of care.

LASER-ASSISTED CANAL PREPARATION

After the development of the ruby laser by Maiman in 1960, Stern and Sognnaes (1964) were the first investigators to look at the effects of ruby laser irradiation on hard dental tissues.[523] Early studies of the effects of lasers on hard dental tissues were based simply on the empirical use of available lasers and an examination of the tissue modified by various techniques.

Laser stands for Light Amplification by Stimulated Emission of Radiation, and it is characterized by being monochromatic (one color/one wavelength), coherent, and unidirectional. These are specific qualities that differentiate the laser light from, say, an incandescent light bulb.

For any procedures using lasers, the optical interactions between the laser and the tissue must be thoroughly understood to ensure safe and effective treatment. The laser-light interaction is controlled by the irradiation parameters, that is, the wavelength, the repetition rate, the pulse energy of the laser, as well as the optical properties of the tissue. Typically, optical properties are characterized by the refraction index, scattering (μs), and absorption coefficients (μa). However, the ultimate effects of laser irradiation on dental tissue depend on the distribution of energy deposited inside the tooth. Laser energy must be absorbed by tissue to produce an effect. The **temperature rise** is the fundamental effect determining the extent of changes in the morphology and chemical structure of the irradiated tissue.[524]

Lasers emitting in the ultraviolet, visible (ie, **argon laser**—488 and 514 nm), and near infrared (ie, neodymium:yttrium-aluminum-garnet [**Nd:YAG**] laser—1.064 μm) are weakly absorbed by dental hard tissue, such as enamel and dentin, and light scattering plays a very important role in determining the energy distribution in the tissue. Nd:YAG laser energy, on the other hand, interacts well with dark tissues and is transmitted by water. Argon lasers are more effective on pigmented or highly vascular tissues.

Excimer lasers (193, 248, and 308 nm) and the **erbium laser** (~3.0 μm) are strongly absorbed by dental hard tissues. Neev et al. have shown that the excimer at 308 nm is efficiently absorbed by dentin since it overlaps protein absorption bands.[525,526] The erbium laser emits in the mid-infrared, which coincides with one of the peaks of absorption of water and the OH- of **hydroxyapatite**. Because of that, this laser is strongly absorbed by water, the absorbed energy induces a rapid rise in temperature and pressure, and the heated material is explosively removed.

The **carbon-dioxide** lasers emitting in the far infrared (10.6 μm) were among the first used experimentally for the **ablation** of dental hard tissues. The **carbon-dioxide laser** is the most effective on tissues with high water content and is also well absorbed by hydroxyapatite.

Studies have been conducted evaluating the effects of laser irradiation inside root canals. The authors have discussed laser-endodontic therapy, some as supplementary and others as a purely laser-assisted method.[527] Although the **erbium:YAG** (May 1997) and **erbium:YSGG** (October 1998) lasers were approved for dental hard tissues, **lasers still need to be approved** by the US Food and Drug Administration (FDA) Committee on Devices **for intracanal irradiation.** The FDA's clearance for these devices includes caries removal and cavity preparation, as well as roughening enamel. Other countries, such as Germany, Japan, and Brazil, have been conducting basic research and laser clinical trials, and some of the devices have been used there for treatment.

Laser Endodontics

In 1971, at the University of Southern California, Weichman and Johnson were probably the first researchers to suggest the use of lasers in endodontics.[528] A preliminary study was undertaken to attempt to retroseal the apical orifice of the root canal using an **Nd:YAG** and a **carbon-dioxide laser.** Although the goal was not achieved, relevant data were obtained. In 1972, Weichman et al. suggested the occurrence of chemical and physical changes of irradiated dentin.[529] The same laser wavelengths were then used, with different materials, in an attempt to seal internally the apical constriction.

Applications of lasers in endodontic therapy have been aggressively investigated over the last two decades. According to Stabholz of Israel, there are three main areas in endodontics for the use of lasers: (1) the periapex, (2) the root canal system, and (3) hard tissue, mainly the dentin.[530] One of the major concerns of endodontic therapy is to extensively clean the root canal to achieve necrotic tissue débridement and disinfection. In this sense, lasers are being used as a coadjuvant tool in endodontic therapy, for bacterial reduction, and to modify the root canal surface. The action of different types of laser irradiation on dental root canals—the carbon-dioxide laser,[531] the Nd:YAG laser,[532] the argon laser,[533] the excimer laser,[534] the holmium:YAG laser,[535] the diode laser,[536] and, more recently, the erbium:YAG laser[537]—has been investigated.

Unlike the carbon-dioxide laser, the **Nd:YAG** (Figure 10-93, A), argon, excimer, holmium, and erbium laser beams can be delivered through an **optical fiber** (Figure 10-93, B) that allows for better accessibility to different areas and structures in the oral cavity,[530] including root canals. The technique requires widening the root canal by conventional methods before the laser probe can be placed in the canal. The fiber's diameter, used inside the canal space, ranges from 200 to 400 μm, equivalent to a No. 20-40 file (Figure 10-93, C).

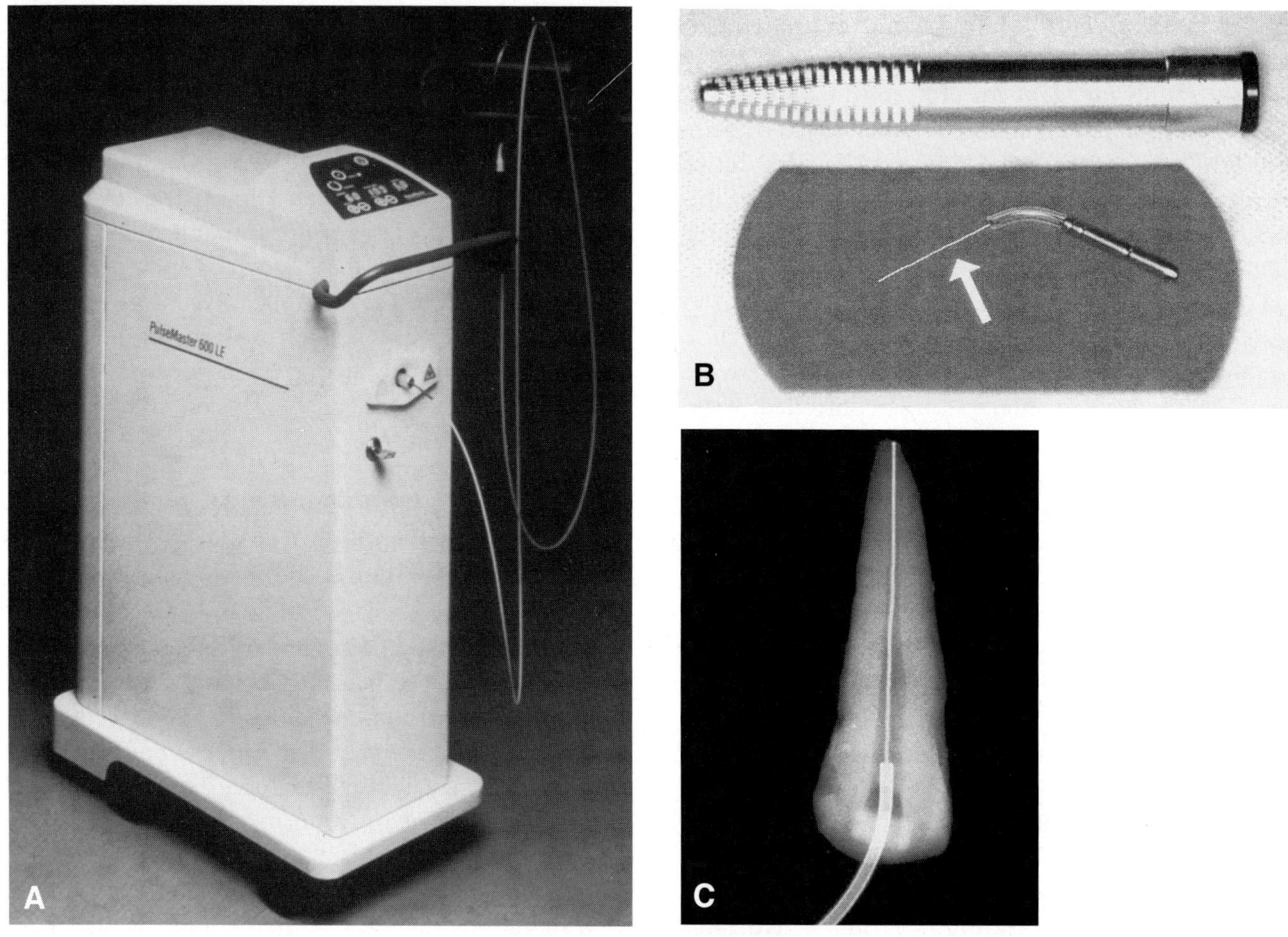

Figure 10-93 A, Nd:YAG (1.06 μm) laser device delivered by a quartz fiber optic—200, 300, 320, and 400 μm diameter fiber available. **B**, Endo fiber (**arrow**) (285 and 375 μm fiber available) and handpiece for the erbium:YAG laser. **C**, Radiograph of canine tooth with Erbium:YAG fiber introduced into the root canal. (Courtesy of American Dental Technologies; Corpus Christi, Tex.)

Dederich et al., in 1984, used an Nd:YAG laser to irradiate the root canal walls and showed melted, recrystalized, and glazed surfaces.[527] Bahcall et al., in 1992, investigated the use of the pulsed Nd:YAG laser to cleanse root canals.[538] Their results showed that the Nd:YAG laser may cause harm to the bone and periodontal tissues—a good example that laser parameters should constitute one of the factors for safety and efficacy of laser treatment.

According to Levy[532] and Goodis et al.,[539] the **Nd:YAG**, in combination with hand filing, is able to produce a **cleaner root canal** with a general absence of smear layer. The sealing depth of 4 μm produced by the Nd:YAG laser was reported by Liu et al.[540]

One concern for laser safety is the heat produced at the irradiated root surface that may cause damage to surrounding supporting tissue. Studies evaluating changes at the apical constriction and histopathologic analysis of the periapical tissues were presented by Koba and associates.[541,542] They maintained the fiber optic at a stationary point, 1 mm from the apical foramen, for 2 to 3 seconds. Infiltration of inflammatory cells was observed in all groups in 2 weeks, including the control group. Indeed, the degree of inflammation reported in the laser-irradiated group at 2 weeks, 30 Hz (0.67 mJ/p) for 2 seconds, was significantly less than in the control group at 4 and 8 weeks. However, the same authors have shown[542] that carbonization was observed in irradiated root canals depending on the parameter used. A technique considered optimal by Gutknecht et al. would be the irradiation from apical to coronal surface in a continuous, circling fashion.[543]

Different laser **"initiators"** (dyes to increase absorption) with the **Nd:YAG laser** were tested by Zhang et al.[544] Black ink was an effective initiator for this laser, but the root canal was inconsistently changed. It might be a consequence of the lack of uniformity in the distribution of the ink or laser irradiation inside the canals.

Under the scanning electron microscope (SEM), lased dentin showed different levels of canal débridement, including smear layer removal and morphologic changes, related to the energy level and repetition rate used.[545] There was no indication of cracking in all of the SEM samples at these laser parameters. The **erbium:YAG laser**, at 80 mJ, 10 Hz, **was more effective for debris removal** (Figure 10-94, A), producing a cleaner surface with a higher number of open tubules when compared with the other laser treatment and the control—without laser treatment (Figure 10-94, B). A decreased level was observed **when the energy was reduced** from 80 to 40 mJ. **Nd:YAG laser**-irradiated samples presented melted and recrystalized dentin and smear layer removal (Figure 10-94, C).

The root canal walls irradiated by the **erbium:YAG laser** were free of debris, the smear layer was removed, and the dentinal tubules were opened, as recently reported by Takeda et al.[546,547] and Harashima et al.,[548] although areas covered by residual debris could be found where the laser light did not enter into contact with the root canal surface.[548] Scanning electron microscopic evaluation showed different patterns as a result of the different mechanisms of laser-tissue interaction by these two wavelengths.[546–548]

According to Hibst et al., the use of a highly absorbed laser light, like the **erbium laser,** tends to localize heating to a thin layer at the sample surface, thus minimizing the absorption depth.[549] There follows a decrease in the risk of subsurface thermal damage since less energy is necessary to heat the surface.

The efficacy of **argon laser** irradiation in removing debris from the root canal system was evaluated by Moshonov et al.[533] After cleaning and shaping, a 300 μm fiber optic was introduced into the root canals of single-rooted teeth to their working length. During irradiation, the fiber was then retrieved, from the apex to the orifice. Scanning electron microscopic analysis revealed that significantly more debris was removed from the lased group than from the control (Figure 10-95).

Although it appears that **argon laser** irradiation of the root canal system efficiently removes intracanal debris, its use as a treatment modality in endodontics requires further investigation. This is partially true because this laser is emitted in a continuous mode—like the carbon-dioxide laser—in the range of milliseconds. This means that a longer period of interaction with the intracanal surface is required and, consequently, a great increase in temperature.

One of the limitations of the laser treatment was demonstrated by Harashima et al.[550] Where the **(argon) laser optic fiber** had not touched or reached the canal walls, areas with clean root canal surfaces were interspersed with areas **covered by residual debris.** Access into severely curved roots and the cost of the equipment are other limitations.

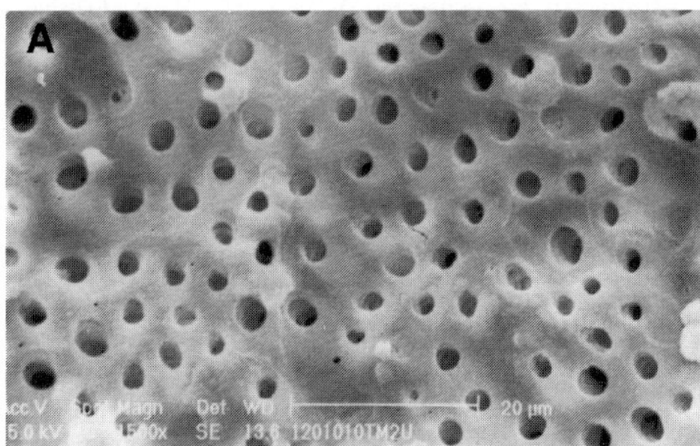

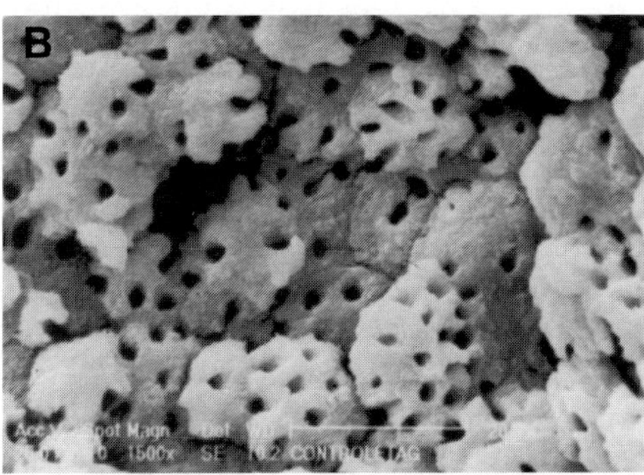

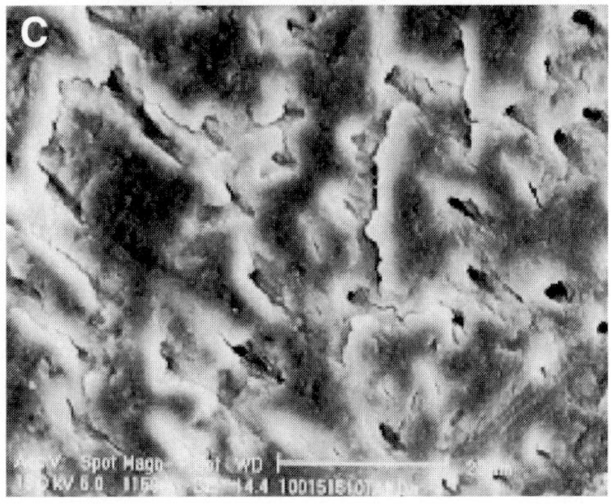

Figure 10-94 Intracanal dentin surfaces (apical third) under SEM–1500X- laser parameters: **A**, Dentin surface lased with **erbium:YAG** 100 mJ and 15 Hz. Effective debris removal. **B**, **Control**; unlased dentin surface. **C**, **Nd:YAG reduced** to 80 mJ and 10 Hz. Note melted and recrystalized dentin surface. Reproduced with permission from Cecchini SCM et al.[545]

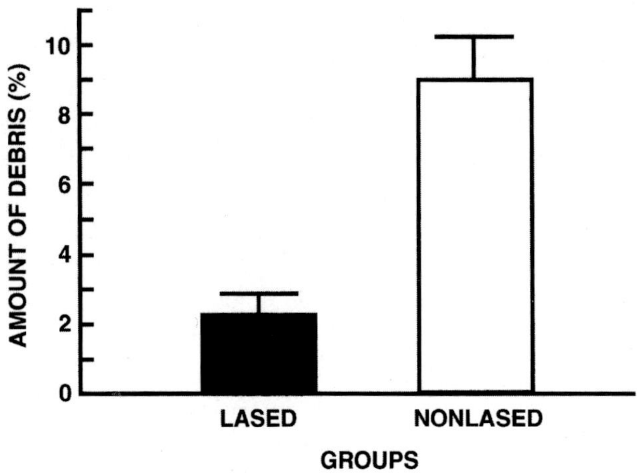

Figure 10-95 Effect of argon laser on intracanal debris. Mean and standard deviation of overall cleanliness of root canal wall surfaces in lased and nonlased specimens. Reproduced with permission from Moshonov J et al.[533]

The Future

Wavelengths emitted at the **ultraviolet** portion of the electromagnetic spectrum appear to be promising in endodontics. **ArF excimer laser at 193 nm** is well suited to slow selective removal of necrotic debris from the root canal, leaving behind smooth, crack-free and fissure-free, melted dentin walls (P Wilder-Smith, personal communication, July 26, 1993). The **XeCl (308 nm) excimer laser** was capable of melting and closing dentinal tubules in a study performed by Stabholz and colleagues.[551]

Very short pulses (15 ns) will avoid significant heat accumulation in the irradiated tooth. When higher-energy densities were used (4 J/cm^2), however, rupture of the molten materials and exposure of the tubules were noted. No clinical results are presently available. The **second harmonic alexandrite laser (377 nm/ultraviolet)**, in development by Hennig and colleagues in Germany, has been shown to selectively remove dental calculus and caries and appears to be very promising for bacterial reduction, as well as for future application in periodontics and endodontics.[552]

Indeed, the ability of certain lasers to **ablate** necrotic organic materials and tissue remnants and reduce microorganisms seems highly promising in endodontics. A significant reason for using laser intracanal irradiation is the microbial reduction, usually achieved by temperature rise. Several studies have evaluated the effectiveness of lasers in sterilizing root canals and have reported significant in vitro decreases in number of bacteria.[537,553–557] However, the performance of this equipment, concerning safe and effective wavelength and energy levels related to temperature rise, morphologic changes, and microbial reduction, should be well documented before it becomes a current method of treatment.

It is important to realize that different types of lasers have different effects on the same tissue, and the same laser will interact differently depending on the types of tissue. Safety precautions used during laser irradiation include safety glasses specific for each wavelength (compatible optical density to filtrate that wavelength), warning signs, and high-volume evacuation close to the treated area (used in soft tissue procedures, cavity preparation, etc).

Noninstrumentation Root Canal Cleansing

Based on the premise that "[O]ptimal cleansing of the root canal system is a prime prerequisite for long term success in endodontics," Lussi and his associates at the University of Bern, Switzerland, introduced devices to cleanse the root canal "without the need of endodontic instrumentation."[558] The first device, reported in 1993, consisted of a "pump" that inserted an irrigant into the canal, creating "bubbles" and cavitation that loosened the debris. This pressure action was followed by a negative pressure (suction) that removed the debris: "The irrigant fluid was injected through the outer tube while the reflux occurred through the inner tube." More recently, they have improved the device and reported that the "smaller new machine produced equivalent or better cleanliness results in the root canal system using significantly less irrigant (NaOCl)."[559] This cleanses the canal but, of course, does nothing to shape the canal (Figure 10-96).

PULPECTOMY

Rather than break into the flow of detailing the methods of cleaning and shaping the root canal, we have reserved until now the often necessary task of removing a vital pulp, diseased though it may be. This is termed pulp **extirpation** or **pulpectomy. Total pulpectomy,** extirpation of the pulp to or near the apical foramen, is indicated when the root apex is fully formed and the foramen sufficiently closed to permit obturation with conventional filling materials. If the pulp must be removed from a tooth with an incompletely formed root and an open apex, **partial pulpectomy** is preferred. This technique leaves the apical portion of pulp intact with the hope that the remaining stump will encourage completion of the apex (Figure 10-97). The necrotic or "mummified" tissue remaining in the pulp cavity of a pulpless tooth has lost its identify as an organ; hence, its removal is called **pulp cavity débridement.**

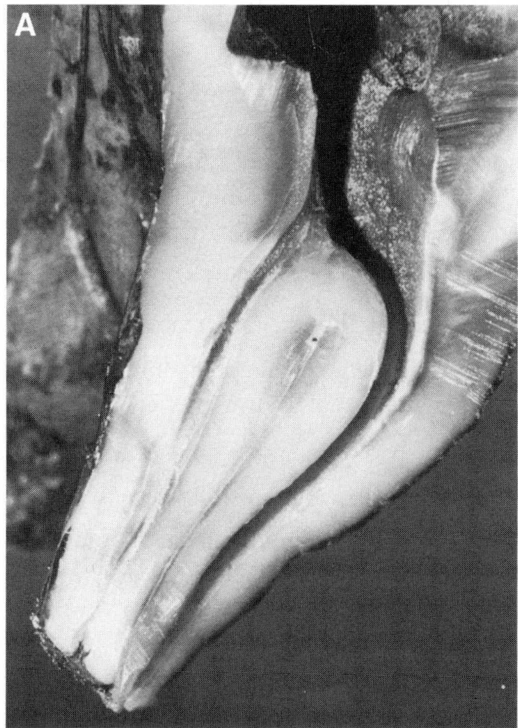

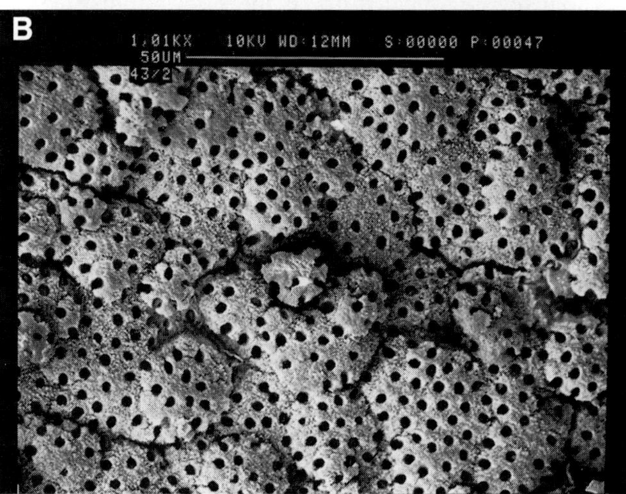

Figure 10-96 A, Root canal cleansed for 10 minutes with the new miniaturized hydrodynamic turbulence device using 3% sodium hypochlorite. Tiny residual fragment of pulp tissue remains at the apex of one canal. B, Photomicrograph shows calcospherites and open dentinal tubules, but no smear layer that develops with instrumentation. Reproduced with permission from Lussi A et al.[559]

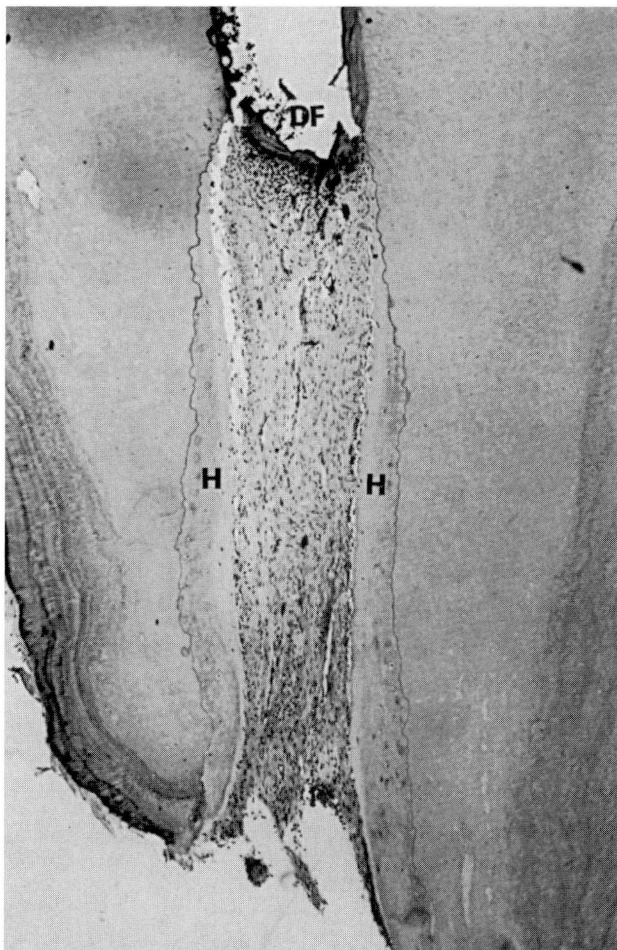

Figure 10-97 Partial pulpectomy. Observation period of 6 months. Only slight accumulation of lymphocytes adjacent to a plug of dentin particles and remnants of Kloropercha (DF at top). Cell-rich fibrous connective tissue occupies the residual pulp canal. Large deposits of hard tissue (H) along walls. Reproduced with permission from Horstad P, Nygaard-Østby B. Oral Surg 1978;46:275.

Indications

Pulp "mummification" with arsenic trioxide, formaldehyde, or other destructive compounds was at one time preferable to extirpation.[560] With the advent of effective local anesthetics, pulpectomy has become a relatively painless process and superseded "mummification," with its attendant hazards of bone necrosis and prolonged postoperative pain.

Pulpectomy is indicated in all cases of irreversible pulp disease. With pulpectomy, dramatic relief is obtained in cases of acute pulpitis resulting from infection, injury, or operative trauma. Pulpectomy is usually the treatment of choice when carious or mechanical exposure has occurred. In a number of instances, restorative and fixed prosthetic procedures require intentional extirpation.[561]

Technique

The following are the steps in the performance of a well-executed pulpectomy:

1. Obtain regional anesthesia.
2. Prepare a **minimal coronal opening** and, with a sharp explorer, test the pulp for depth of anesthesia.
3. If necessary, inject anesthetic intrapulpally.

4. Complete the access cavity.
5. Excavate the coronal pulp.
6. Extirpate the radicular pulp.
7. Control bleeding and débride and shape the canal.
8. Place medication or the final filling.

Each of these steps must be completed carefully before the next is begun, and each requires some explanation.

Profound Anesthesia

Methods for obtaining profound infiltration and conduction anesthesia have been considered earlier (chapter 9). One aspect of the subject deserves repetition: its unusual importance in endodontics! From the era when pulps were extirpated by driving wooden pegs, red-hot wires, or crude broaches into the living tissues without benefit of anesthesia,[562] there has persisted a profound and widespread dread of "having a 'nerve' taken out of a tooth." The popular misconception that endodontic treatment invariably involves suffering will not be completely dispelled until all practitioners employ effective anesthesia techniques while completing procedures as potentially painful as pulpectomy.

Minimal Coronal Opening and Intrapulpal Anesthesia

It is wise to anticipate that, in spite of apparently profound anesthesia, an intraligamentary or intrapulpal injection may be required to obtain total anesthesia, particularly with an inflamed pulp. If the patient experiences pain during the initial stage of access preparation, there is no question that manipulation of the pulp will be a painful process. The success of the **intrapulpal injection** will be ensured if the initial penetration of the pulp chamber is made with a sharp explorer close to the size of the injection needle. Since the needle fits the small opening tightly, the anesthetic can be forced into the pulp under pressure. Total anesthesia follows immediately (for greater detail, see chapter 9).

Completion of the Access Preparation

Coronal access must be adequate and complete to allow thorough excavation of the tissue from the pulp chamber. Because intrapulpal injection with 2% lidocaine with 1:50,000 epinephrine promotes excellent hemostasis, it can be used during the completion of the access cavity to prevent interference from hemorrhaging tissue.

Excavation of the Coronal Pulp

All of the tissue in the pulp chamber should be removed before extirpation of the radicular pulp is begun. All pulp tissue that has not been removed by the round bur should be eliminated with a sharp spoon excavator. The tissue is carefully curetted from the pulp horns and other ramifications of the chamber. Failure to remove all tissue fragments from the pulp chamber may result in later discoloration of the tooth. At this point, the chamber should be irrigated well to remove blood and debris.

Extirpation of Radicular Pulp

The instrument used for this procedure is determined by the size of the canal and/or the level at which the pulp is to be excised.

Large Canal, Total Pulpectomy

If the canal is large enough to admit a barbed broach (Figure 10-98, A) and a total pulpectomy is desired, the approach is as follows:

1. A pathway for the broach to follow is created by sliding a reamer, file, or pathfinder along the wall of the canal to the apical third. If the pulp is sensitive or bleeding, the anesthetic syringe needle may be used as the "pathfinder." A drop of anesthetic deposited

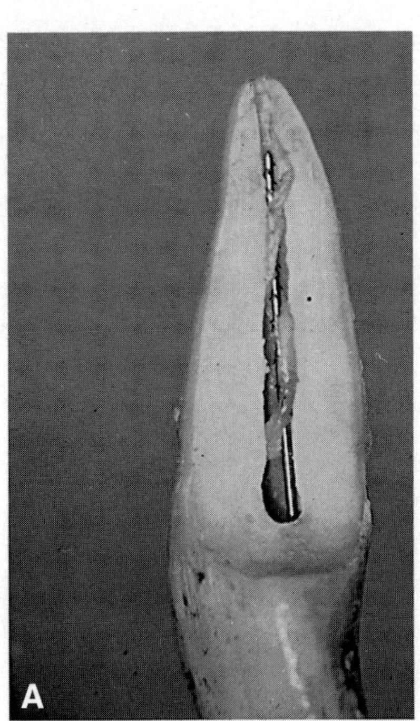

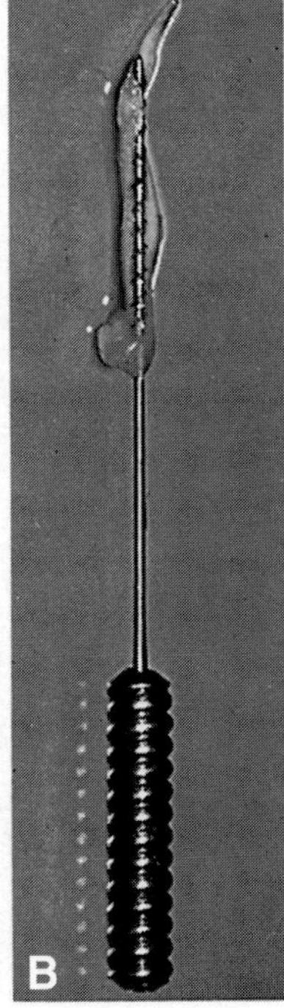

Figure 10-98 A, Total pulpectomy accomplished with a large barbed broach that fits loosely in the canal. With careful rotation of the broach, the pulp has become entwined and will be removed on retraction. B, Total pulpectomy by a barbed broach. Young, huge pulps may require two or three broaches inserted simultaneously to successfully entwine pulp.

near the apical foramen will stop the flow of blood and all pain sensations. At the same time, the needle displaces the pulp tissue and creates the desired pathway for a broach.

2. A broach, small enough not to bind in the canal, is passed to a point just short of the apex. The instrument is rotated **slowly**, to engage the fibrous tissue in the barbs of the broach, and then slowly withdrawn. Hopefully, the entire pulp will be removed with the broach (Figure 10-98, B). If not, the process is repeated. If the canal is large, it may be necessary to insert two or three broaches simultaneously to entwine the pulp on a sufficient number of barbs to ensure its intact removal.
3. If the pulp is not removed intact, small broaches are used to "scrub" the canal walls from the apex outward to remove adherent fragments. A word of caution: The barbed broach is a friable instrument and must never be locked into the canal. Handle with care!

Small Canal, Total Pulpectomy

If the canal is slender, and a total pulpectomy is indicated, extirpation becomes part of canal preparation. A broach need not be used. Small files are preferred for the initial instrumentation because they cut more quickly than reamers. In such a canal, Phase I instrumentation to a No. 25 file is usually minimal to remove the apical pulp tissue (Figure 10-99). New rotary increased-tapered instruments open up the coronal third of the canal, allowing for more efficient removal of the pulp.

Partial Pulpectomy

When a partial pulpectomy is planned, a technique described by Nygaard-Østby (personal communication, 1963) is employed. From a good radiograph, the width of the canal at the desired level of extirpation is determined. A Hedstroem file of correct size is blunted so that the flattened tip will bind in the canal at the predetermined point of severance. The Hedstroem file has deep fluting and makes a cleaner incision than other intracanal instruments. Enlargement of the canal coronal portion is then carried out with a series of larger instruments trimmed to the same length.

Neither Stromberg[563] nor Pitt Ford[564] was particularly enthusiastic about healing following pulpectomy, either total or partial. Working with dogs, both were troubled by postoperative periradicular infections possibly induced by coronal microleakage. Pitt Ford considered anachoresis the route of bacterial contamination. Others have found, however, that intracanal infections by anachoresis do not occur unless the periradicular tissues were traumatized with a file and bleeding was induced into the canal.[565]

Control of Bleeding and Débridement of Canal

Incomplete pulpectomy will leave in the canal fragments of tissue that may remain vital if their blood

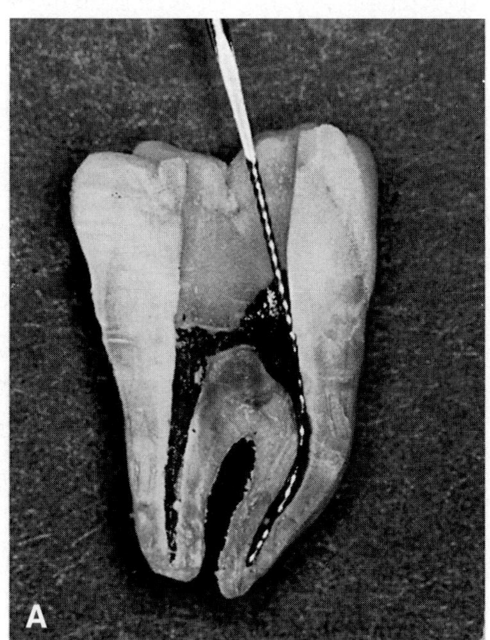

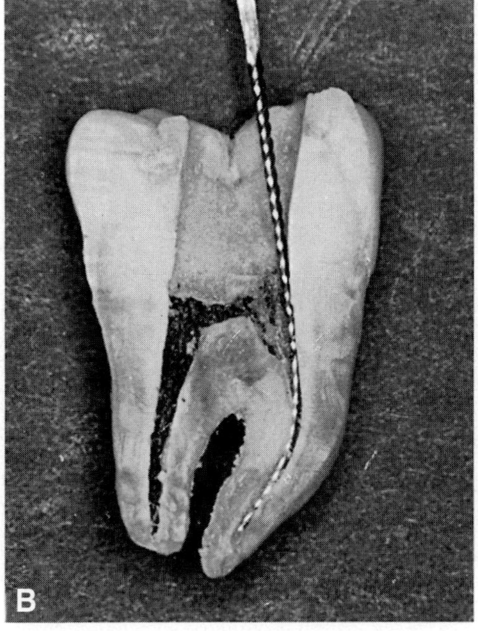

Figure 10-99 **A**, Space between canal walls and No. 10 file demonstrates need to instrument the canal to at least file size No. 25 for total pulpectomy. **B**, No. 25 instrument engaging walls and removing pulp. (Courtesy of Dr. Thomas P. Mullaney.)

supply is maintained through accessory foramina or along deep fissures in the canal walls (Figure 10-100). **These remnants of the pulp may be a source of severe pain** to the patient, who will return seeking relief as soon as the anesthesia wears off. This is a desperately painful condition and requires immediate reanesthetization and extirpation of all tissue shreds. Any overlooked tissue will also interfere with proper obturation during immediate filling procedures.

Persistent bleeding following extirpation is usually a sign that "tags" of pulp tissue remain. If the flow of blood is not stopped by scrubbing the canal walls with a broach, as described above, it may originate in the periradicular area. In these cases, it is best to dry the canal as much as possible after irrigating with anesthetic. A dry cotton pellet is then **sealed in** until a subsequent appointment.

Emergency Pulpotomy

Although complete pulpectomy is the ideal treatment for an irreversibly inflamed vital pulp requiring endodontic therapy, a temporary pulpotomy can be performed in a relatively short period of time. In a busy practice, where it may not be practical to complete instrumentation at the emergency visit, a pulpotomy can be done. First, anesthetic solution is used to irrigate the pulp chamber. The coronal pulp is then amputated with a sharp excavator. A **well-blotted** Formocresol pellet may be sealed in with a suitable temporary. Some advocate sealing in cotton alone, with no medication. The temporary pulpotomy will normally provide the patient with relief until complete instrumentation can be carried out at a subsequent appointment. Swedish dentists used this technique in 73 teeth with irreversible pulpitis and arrested toothache 96% of the time. Three patients, however, had to return for total pulpectomy for pain relief.[566]

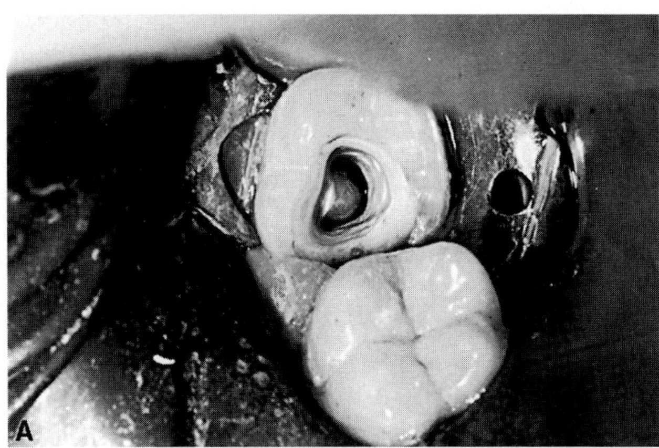

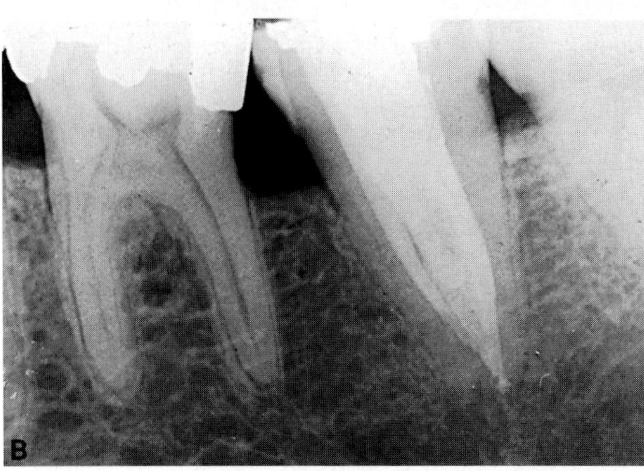

Figure 10-100 **A**, C-shaped canal in mandibular molar. **B**, One can imagine the severe difficulty encountered in attempting to totally remove all pulp tissue from such an aberrant canal system. (Courtesy of Dr. L. Stephen Buchanan.)

Placement of Medication or Root Canal Filling

If pulpectomy was necessitated by pulpitis resulting from operative or accidental trauma, or planned extirpation of a normal pulp for restorative purposes was done, cleaning and shaping and obturation of the canal can be completed immediately. If a delay is necessary, a drug of choice or dry cotton should be sealed in the chamber. The final canal filling should never be placed, however, unless all pulpal shreds are removed and hemorrhage has stopped. Immediate filling is contraindicated if the possibility of pulpal infection exists.

INTRACANAL MEDICATION

Antibacterial agents such as calcium hydroxide are recommended for use in the root canal between appointments. While recognizing the fact that most irrigating agents destroy significant numbers of bacteria during canal débridement, it is still thought good form to further attempt canal sterilization between appointments. The drugs recommended and technique used are thoroughly explored in chapter 3.

IATRAL ERRORS IN ENDODONTIC CAVITY PREPARATION

For a description of the prevention and correction of mishaps in endodontic cavity preparations, see chapter 15.

REFERENCES

1. Black GV. Operative dentistry. 7th ed. Vol II. Chicago: Medico-Dental Publishing; 1936.
2. Kobayashi C, Yoshioka T, Suda H. A new engine-driven canal preparation system with electronic canal measuring capability. JOE 1997;23:75.
3. Stokes AN, Tidmarsh BG. A comparison of diamond and

tungsten carbide burs for preparing endodontic access cavities through crowns. JOE 1988;14:550.

4. Teplitsky PE, Sutherland JK. Endodontic access openings through Cerestore crowns [abstract]. JOE 1985;10.
5. Cohen BD, Wallace JA. Castable glass ceramic crowns and their reaction to endodontic therapy. Oral Surg 1991;72:108.
6. Pucci FM, Reig R. Conductos radiculares. Vol II. Buenos Aires: Editorial Medico-Quirurgica; 1944.
7. Reeh ES, et al. Reduction in tooth stiffness as a result of endodontic and restorative procedures. JOE 1989;15:512.
8. Eleazer PD, Eleazer K R. Air pressures developed beyond the apex from drying root canals with pressurized air. JOE 1998;24:833.
9. Shillinburg H Jr, et al. Root dimensions and dowel sizes. J Calif Dent Assoc 1982;10:43.
10. Vargo JW, Hartwell GR. Modified endodontics for lengthy canals. JOE 1992;18:512.
11. Leuck M. Root canal morphology of mandibular incisors and canines [thesis]. Iowa City (IA): Univ. of Iowa; 1973.
12. Kartal N, Yanikoglu FC. Root canal morphology of mandibular incisors. JOE 1992;18:562.
13. Fahid A. Root canal morphology of human maxillary incisors and canines [thesis]. Iowa City (IA): Univ. of Iowa.
14. Pineda F, Kuttler Y. Mesiodistal and buccolingual roentgenographic investigation of 7275 root canals. Oral Surg 1972;33:101.
15. Vertucci FJ, Selig A, Gillis R. Root canal morphology of the human maxillary second premolar. Oral Surg 1974;38:456.
16. Grey R. Root canal morphology of maxillary first molar [thesis]. Univ. of Iowa City (IA); 1974.
17. Seidberg BH, et al. Frequency of two mesiobuccal root canals in maxillary permanent first molars. J Am Dent Assoc 1973;87:852.
18. Pineda F. Roentgenographic investigation of the mesiobuccal root of the maxillary first molar. Oral Surg 1973;36:253.
19. Pomeranz HH, Fishelberg G. The second mesiobuccal canal of maxillary molars. J Am Dent Assoc 1974;88:119.
20. Fahid A, et al. Coronal root canal preparation. Dent Stud J 1983;61:S46.
21. Zillich R, Dowson J. Root canal morphology of mandibular first and second premolars. Oral Surg 1973;36:783.
22. Baisden MK, et al. Root canal configuration of the mandibular first premolar. JOE 1992;18:505.
23. Bjorndal AM, Skidmore AE. Anatomy and morphology of human teeth. Iowa City (IA): Univ. of Iowa; 1983.
24. Green D. Double canals in single roots. Oral Surg 1973;35:689.
25. Dempster WT, Adams WJ, Duddles RS. Arrangements in the jaws of the roots of teeth. J Am Dent Assoc 1963;67:779.
26. Hess W. The anatomy of the root canals of the teeth of the permanent dentition. London: John Bale and Sons and Danielson; 1925.
27. Kulild JC, Peters DD. Incidence and configuration of canal systems in the mesiobuccal root of maxillary first and second molars. JOE 1990;16:311.
28. Neaverth EJ, et al. Clinical investigation (in vivo) of endodontically treated maxillary first molars. JOE 1987;10:506.
29. Fahid A. Maxillary second molar with three buccal roots. JOE 1988;14:181.
30. Libfeld H, Rolstein I. Incidence of four-rooted maxillary second molars: Literature review and radiographic survey of 1200 teeth. JOE 1989;15:129.
31. Ruprecht A, et al. The incidence of taurodontism in dental patients. Oral Surg 1987;63:743.
32. Vertucci FJ, Anthony RL. A scanning electron microscopic investigation of accessary foramina in the furcation and pulp chamber floor of molar teeth. Oral Surg 1986;62:319.
33. Niemann RW, et al. Dye ingress in molars: furcation to chamber floor. JOE 1993;19:293.
34. Beatty RG, Krell K. Mandibular molars with five canals: report of two cases. J Am Dent Assoc 1987;114:802.
35. Weine FS, et al. Canal configuration of the mandibular second molar using a clinically oriented *in vitro* method. JOE 1988;14:207.
36. Walker RT. Root form and canal anatomy of mandibular second molars in a southern Chinese population. JOE 1988;14:325.
37. Yew S-C, Chan K. A retrospective study of endodontically treated mandibular first molars in a Chinese population. JOE 1993;19:471.
38. Pomeranz HH, et al. Treatment considerations of the middle mesial canal of mandibular first and second molars. JOE 1981;7:565.
39. Sierashi SM. Identification and endodontic management of three-canaled maxillary premolars. JOE 1989;15:29.
40. Pecora JD, et al. In vitro study of root canal anatomy of maxillary second premolars. Braz Dent J 1992;3:81.
41. Hartwell G, Bellizi R. Clinical investigation of *in vivo* endodontically treated mandibular and maxillary molars. JOE 1982;8:555.
42. Trope M, et al. Mandibular premolars with more than one root canal in different race groups. JOE 1986;12:343.
43. Walker RT. The root canal anatomy of mandibular incisors in a southern Chinese population. Int Endod J 1988;21:218.
44. Pecora JD, et al. Internal anatomy, direction and number of roots and size of human mandibular canines. Braz Dent J 1993;4:53.
45. Madeina MC, et al. Prevalence of taurodontism in premolars. Oral Surg 1986;61:158.
46. Ingle JI, Zeldow BJ. An evaluation of mechanical instrumentation and the negative culture in endodontic therapy. J Am Dent Assoc 1958;57:471.
47. Murgel C, Walton R, et al. A quantitative evaluation of three different cleaning techniques for endodontic files: an SEM examination [abstract 24]. JOE 1989;15:175
48. Mandel E, et al. Scanning electron microscope observation of canal cleanliness. JOE 1990;16:279.
49. Lin L, et al. Histopathologic and histobacteriologic study of endodontic failure [abstract]. JOE 1986;12.
50. Cailleteau JG, Mullaney TP. Prevalence of teaching apical patency and various instrumentation and obturation techniques in United States dental schools. JOE 1997;3:394.
51. Kuttler Y. Microscopic investigation of root apexes. J Am Dent Assoc 1955;50:544.
52. Mizutani T, et al. Anatomical study of the root apex in maxillary anterior teeth. JOE 1992;18:344.
53. Seidler B. Root canal filling: an evaluation and method. J Am Dent Assoc 1956;53:567.
54. Ingle JI. The need for endodontic instrument standardization. Oral Surg 1955;8:1211.
55. Green EN. Microscopic investigation of root canal file and reamer width. Oral Surg 1956;10:532.
56. Ingle JI, Levine M. The need for uniformity of endodontic instruments, equipment and filling materials. In: Transactions of the 2nd International Conference of Endodontics. Philadelphia: Univ. of Pennsylvania Press; 1958. p. 123.

57. Ingle JI. A standardized endodontic technique using newly designed instruments and filling materials. Oral Surg 1961;14:83.
58. American Dental Association Council on Dental Materials, Instruments and Equipment. Revised ANSI/ADA specification no. 28 for root canal files and reamers, type-K, and no. Chicago. J Am Dent Assoc Press 2002.
59. Kerekes K. Evaluation of standardized root canal instruments and obturating points. JOE 1979;5:145.
60. Serene TP, Loadholt C. Variations in same-size endodontic files. Oral Surg 1984;57:200.
61. Cormier CJ, et al. A comparison of endodontic file quality and file dimensions. JOE 1988;14:138.
62. Seto BG. Criteria for selection of endodontic files [thesis]. Seattle: Univ. of Washington School of Dentistry; 1989.
63. Seto BG, et al. Torsional properties of twisted and machined endodontic files. JOE 1990;16:355.
64. Keate KC, Wong M. A comparison of endodontic file tip quality. JOE 1990;16:488.
65. Stenman E, Spangberg L. Machining efficiency of endodontic K-files and Hedstroem files. JOE 1990;16:375.
66. Stenman E, Spangberg L. Root canal instruments are poorly standardized. JOE 1993;19:327.
67. Canalda S, Berastegui J. A comparison of bending and torsional properties of K-files manufactured with different metallic alloys. Int Endod J 1996;29:185.
68. Tepel A, Schafer E, Hoppe W. Properties of endodontic hand instruments used in rotary motion. Part 3: resistance to bending and fracture. JOE 1997;23:141.
69. Wolcott J, Himel VT. Torsional properties of nickel-titanium versus stainless steel endodontic files. JOE 1997;23:843.
70. Mitchell BF, et al. The effect of autoclave sterilization on endodontic files. Oral Surg 1983;55:204.
71. Morrison S, et al. Effects of sterilization and usage on cutting efficiency of endodontic instruments [abstract 26]. JOE 1989;15:175
72. Mize SB, et al.Effect of sterilization on cyclic fatigue of rotary nickel-titanium endodontic instruments. JOE 1998;24:843.
73. Roth WC, et al. A study of the strength of endodontic files. JOE 1983;9:228.
74. Oliet S, Sorin SM. Cutting efficiency of endodontic reamers. Oral Surg 1973;36:243.
75. Webber J, Moser JB, Heuer MA. A method to determine the cutting efficiency of root canal instruments in linear motion. JOE 1980;6:829.
76. Kazemi RB, Stenman E, Larz SW. The endodontic file as a disposal instrument. JOE 1995;21:451.
77. Filho IB, Esberard M, Leonardo R D. Microscopic evaluation of three endodontic files, pre- and postinstrumentation. JOE 1998;24:461.
78. Newman JG, Brantley WA, Gerstein H. A study of the cutting efficiency of seven brands of endodontic files in linear motion. JOE 1983;9:316.
79. Neal RG, et al. Cutting ability of K-type endodontic files. JOE 1983;9:52.
80. Luks S. An analysis of root canal instruments. J Am Dent Assoc 1959;58:85.
81. Gutierrez JH, Gigoux C, Sanhueza I. Physical and chemical deterioration of endodontic reamers during mechanical preparation. Oral Surg 1969;28:394.
82. Lentine FN. A study of torsional and angular deflection of endodontic files and reamers. JOE 1979;5:181.
83. Chernick LB, Jacobs JJ, Lautenschlauger EP, Heuer MA. Torsional failures of endodontic files. JOE 1976;2:94.
84. Lautenschlager EP, Jacobs JJ, Marshall GW, Heuer MA. Brittle and ductile torsional failures of endodontic instruments. JOE 1977;3:175.
85. Roane JB, Sabala C. Clockwise or counterclockwise? JOE 1984;10:349.
86. Sotokawa T. An analysis of clinical breakage of root canal instruments. JOE 1988;14:75.
87. Montgomery S, et al. File damage during root canal preparation. JOE 1984;10:45.
88. Haikel Y, et al. Dynamic fracture of hybrid endodontic hand instruments compared with traditional files. JOE 1991;17:217.
89. Rowan MB, Nicholls JI, Steiner J. Torsional properties of stainless steel and nickel-titanium endodontic files. JOE 1996;32:341.
90. Buchanan LS. File bending: essential for management of curved canals. Endod Rep 1987;Spring/Summer:16.
91. Yesilsoy C, et al. A scanning electron microscopic examination of surface changes obtained from two variable methods of precurving files: a clinical observation. JOE 1986;12:408.
92. Walia H, et al. An initial investigation of the bending and torsional properties of Nitinol root canal files. JOE 1988;14:346.
93. Walia H, et al. Torsional ductility and cutting efficiency of the Nitinol file [abstract 22]. JOE 1989;150:174.
94. Villalobos RL, et al. A method to determine the cutting efficiency of root canal instruments in rotary motion. JOE 1980;6:667.
95. Felt RA, et al. Flute design of endodontic instruments: Its influence on cutting efficiency. JOE 1982;8:253.
96. Miserendino LJ, et al. Cutting efficiency of endodontic instruments. Part II: analysis of tip design. JOE 1986;12:8.
97. Miserendino LJ, et al. Cutting efficiency of endodontic instruments. Part I: a quantitative comparison of the tip and fluted regions. JOE 1985;11:435.
98. Powell SE, Simon JHS, et al. A comparison of the effect of modified and nonmodified instrument tips on apical configuration. JOE 1986;12:293.
99. Powell SE, et al. A comparison of the effect of modified and nonmodified tips on apical canal configuration. Part II. JOE 1988;14:224.
100. Roane JB, Sabala CL, et al. The "balanced force" concept for instrumentation of curved canals. JOE 1985;11:203.
101. Sabala CL, Roane JB, et al. Instrumentation of curved canals using a modified tipped instrument: a comparison study. JOE 1988;14:59.
102. Sepic AO, et al. Comparison of Flex-R-files and K-files in curved canals [abstract]. JOE 1988;14:194.
103. McKendry DJ, et al. Clinical incidence of canal ledging with a new endodontic file [abstract]. JOE 1988;14:194.
104. Dummer PMH, Alomari MAO, Bryant S. Comparison of performance of four files with rounded tips during shaping of simulated root canals. JOE 1998;24:363.
105. Machian GR, et al. The comparative efficiency of four types of endodontic instruments. JOE 1982;8:398.
106. Mizrahi SJ, Tucker JW, Seltzer S. A scanning electron microscopic study of the efficacy of various endodontic instruments. JOE 1975;1:324.
107. Miserendino LJ, et al. Cutting efficiency of endodontic hand instruments. Part IV. Comparison of hybrid and traditional designs. JOE 1988;14:451.

108. Yguel-Henry S, et al. High precision, simulated cutting efficiency measurement of endodontic root canal instruments: influence of file configuration and lubrication. JOE 1990;16:418.
109. Newsletter: Endodontic "S" file found to be fast and efficient. Clin Res Assoc 1985;9:10.
110. El Deeb ME, Boraas JC. The effect of different files on the preparation shape of curved canals. Int Endod J 1985;18:1.
111. American National Standards Institute/ADA specification no. 58 for root canal files, Type H (Hedstroem). J Am Dent Assoc 1989;118:239.
112. Bolger WL, et al. A comparison of the potential for breakage: the Burns Unifile versus Hedstroem files. JOE 1985;11:110.
113. Stenman E, Spangberg LSW. Machining efficiency of Flex-R, K-Flex, Trio-Cut and S-Files. JOE 1990;16:575.
114. Wildey WL, Senia S. A new root canal instrument and instrumentation technique: a preliminary report. Oral Surg 1989;67:198.
115. Leseberg DA, Montgomery S. The effects of Canal Master, Flex-R, and K-Flex instrumentation on root canal configuration. JOE 1991;17:59.
116. Wildey WL, Senia ES, Montgomery S. Another look at root canal instrumentation. Oral Surg 1992;74:499.
117. Baumgartner JC, et al. Histomorphometric comparison of canals prepared by four techniques. JOE 1992;18:530.
118. Briseno BM, et al. Comparison by means of a computer-supported device of the enlarging characteristics of two different instruments. JOE 1993;19:281.
119. Cirnis GJ, et al. Effect of three file types on the apical preparations of moderately curved canals. JOE 1988;14:441.
120. Sepic AO, et al. A comparison of Flex-R files and K-type files for enlargement of severely curved molar root canals. JOE 1989;15:240.
121. Calhoun G, Montgomery S. The effects of four instrumentation techniques on root canal shape. JOE 1988;14:273.
122. Alodeh MHA, Dummer PMH. The comparison of the ability of K-files and Hedstroem files to shape simulated root canals in resin blocks. Int Endod J 1989;22:226.
123. Briseño BM, Sonnabend E. The influence of different root canal instruments on root canal preparation: an *in vitro* study. Int Endod J 1991;24:15.
124. Stenman E, Spångberg LSW. Machining efficiency of endodontic files: a new methodology. JOE 1990;16:151.
125. Rueggenberg FA, Powers JM. Mechanical properties of endodontic broaches and effects of bead sterilization. JOE 1988;14:133.
126. Buehler WJ, Wang E. Effect of low temperature phase on the mechanical properties of alloy near composition NiTi. J Appl Physio 1963;34:1475.
127. Civjan S, Huget EF, DeSimon LB. Potential applications of certain nickel-titanium (nitinol) alloys. J Dent Res 1975;54:1.
128. Walia H, Brantley WA, Gerstein H. An initial investigation of the bending and torsional properties of nitinol root canal files. JOE 1988;14:346.
129. StoeckelD, Yu W. Superelastic Ni-Ti wire. Wire J Int 1991; March:45–50.
130. Kazemi RB, Stenman E, Spångberg LSW. Machining efficiency and wear resistance of nickel-titanium endodontic files. Oral Surg 1996;81:596.
131. Serene TP, Adams JD, Saxena A. Physical tests, in nickel-titanium instruments: application in endodontics. St. Louis: Ishiyaku EuroAmerica; 1995.
132. Hsich M, Yu F. The basic research on NiTi shape-memory alloy-anti-corrosive test and corrosive test and histological observation. Chin Med J 1982;1:105–20.
133. Glickman GN, Himel VT, Serene TP. Point-counterpoint: the nickel-titanium paradigm in endodontics. Presented at the American Association of Endodontics 54th Annual Session, 1997. Seattle, WA.
134. Canalda S, Berastequi J. A comparison of bending and torsional properties of K files manufactured with different metallic alloys. Int Endod J 1996;29:185.
135. Canalda SC, Brau AE, Berastegui JE. Torsional and bending properties of stainless steel and nickel-titanium CanalMaster U and Flexogate instruments. Endod Dent Traumatol 1996;12:141.
136. Tepel J, Schafer E, Hoppe W. Properties of endodontic hand instruments used in rotary motion. Part 3. Resistance to bending and fracture. JOE 1997;23:141.
137. Wolcott J, Himel VT. Torsional properties of nickel-titanium versus stainless steel endodontic files. JOE 1997;23:217.
138. Pruett JP, et al. Cyclic fatigue testing of NiTi endodontic instruments. JOE 1997;27:77.
139. Himel VT, Ahmed KM, Wood DM, Alhadainy HA. An evaluation of Nitinol and stainless steel files used by dental students in a laboratory proficiency exam. Oral Surg 1995;79:232.
140. Ahmed K, Himel VT. Instrumentation effects of endodontic files on canal shape and apical foramen [abstract 19]. JOE 1993;19:208
141. Himel VT, Moore RE, Hicks VE. The effects that 3 endodontic files have on canal shape [abstract]. JOE 1994;20.
142. Gambill JM, Alder M, Del Rio CE. Comparison of nickel-titanium and stainless steel hand file instrumentation using computed tomography. JOE 1996;22:369.
143. Tepel J, Schafer E, Hoope W. Properties of endodontic hand instrumentation used in rotary motion. Part 1. Cutting efficiency. JOE 1995;21:418.
144. Elliot LM, CurtisRV, Pitt Ford TR. Cutting pattern of nickel-titanium files using two preparation techniques. Endod Dent Traumatol 1998;14:10.
145. Zakariasen KA, Zakariasen KL. Comparison of hand, hand/sonic, and hand/mechanical instrumentation methods. J Dent Res 1994;73:215.
146. Zakariasen KL, Buerschen GH, Zakariasen KA. A comparison of traditional and experimental instruments for endodontic instrumentation. J Dent Res 1994;73:20.
147. Hulsman M, Stryga F. Comparison of root canal preparation using different automated devices and hand instrumentation. JOE 1993;19:141.
148. Dihn Q. An *in-vitro* evaluation of the Giromatic instrument in the mechanical preparation of root canals [thesis]. Univ. of Minnesota; Minn. 1972.
149. Molven O. A comparison of the dentin removing ability of five root canal instruments. Scand J Dent Res 1970;78:500.
150. O'Connell DT, Brayton SM. Evaluation of root canal preparation with two automated endodontic handpieces. Oral Surg 1975;39:298.
151. Klayman S, Brilliant J. A comparison of the efficacy of serial preparation versus Giromatic preparation. JOE 1974;1:334.
152. Sargenti A. Engine powered canal preparation. Addendum to Endodontics. Locarno (Switzerland): AGSA Publication Scientifiques; 1974.
153. Weine F, et al. Effect of preparation with endodontic handpieces on original canal shape. JOE 1976;2:298.

154. Harty F, Stock C. The Giromatic system compared with hand instrumentation in endodontics. Br Dent J 1974;6:233.
155. Felt RA, Moser JB, Heuer MA. Flute design of endodontic instruments: its influence on cutting efficiency. JOE 1982;8:253.
156. Spyropoulos S, et al. The effect of Giromatic files on the preparation shape of severely curved canals. Int Endod J 1987;20:133.
157. Luebke NH, Brantley WA. Physical dimensions and torsional properties of rotary endodontic instruments. I. Gates-Glidden drills. JOE 1990;16:438.
158. Luebke NH. Performance of Gates-Glidden drill with an applied deflection load. JOE 1989;15:175.
159. Luebke NH, Brantley WA. Torsional and metallurgical properties of rotary endodontic instruments. II Stainless steel Gates-Glidden drills. JOE 1991;17:319.
160. Johnson TA, Zelikow R. Ultrasonic endodontics: a clinical review. J Am Dent Assoc 1987;114:655.
161. Richman MJ. The use of ultrasonics in root canal therapy and root resection. J Dent Med 1957;12:12.
162. Cunningham WT, Martin H. A scanning electron microscope evaluation of root canal debridement with the endosonic ultrasonic synergistic system. Oral Surg 1975;53:527.
163. Martin H. Ultrasonic disinfection of the root canal. Oral Surg 1976;42:92.
164. Martin H, Cunningham WT, et al. Ultrasonic versus hand filing of dentin: a quantitative study. Oral Surg 1980;49:79.
165. Martin H, Cunningham WT, Norris JP. A quantitative comparison of the ability of diamond and K-type files to remove dentin. Oral Surg 1980;50:566.
166. Martin H, Cunningham WT. The effect of Endosonic and hand manipulation on the amount of root canal material extruded. Oral Surg 1982;53:611.
167. Martin H, Cunningham WT. An evaluation of postoperative pain incidence following Endosonic and conventional root canal therapy. Oral Surg 1982;54:74.
168. Cunningham WT, Martin H, Forrest WR. Evaluation of root canal debridement with the Endosonic ultrasonic synergistic system. Oral Surg 1982;53:401.
169. Cunningham WT, Martin H. A scanning electron microscope evaluation of root canal debridement with the Endosonic ultrasonic synergistic system. Oral Surg 1982;53:527.
170. Cunningham WT, Martin H, et al. A comparison of antimicrobial effectiveness of Endosonic and hand root canal therapy. Oral Surg 1982;54:238.
171. Martin H. High tech root canal preparation and obturation and new instrumentation. Alpha Omegan 1990;83:55.
172. Cameron JA. The use of ultrasonics in the removal of the smear layer: a scanning electron microscope study. JOE 1983;9:289.
173. Goodman A, et al. The efficacy of serialization technique versus a serialization/ultrasonic technique [abstract]. JOE 1984;10:118.
174. Chenail B, Teplitsky PE. Performance of endosonics in curved root canals [abstract]. JOE 1985;11:369.
175. Barnett F, et al. Bacteriological status of the root canal after sonic, ultrasonic and hand instrumentation [abstract]. JOE 1985;11:148.
176. Collinson DM, et al. Microbiological assessment of ultrasonics in root canal therapy [abstract]. JOE 1986;12:131.
177. Lev R, et al. Efficacy of the step-back versus a step-back/ultrasonic technique [abstract]. JOE 1986;12:128.
178. Scott GL, Walton RE. Ultrasonic endodontics: the wear of instruments with usage. JOE 1986;12:279.
179. Krell KV, Neo J. The use of ultrasonic endodontic instrumentation in the retreatment of a paste-filled endodontic tooth. Oral Surg 1985;60:100.
180. Yamaguchi M, et al. The use of ultrasonic instrumentation in the cleansing and enlargement of the root canal. Oral Surg 1988;65:349.
181. Cameron JA. The effect of ultrasonic endodontics on the temperature of the root canal wall. JOE 1988;14:554.
182. Haidet J, et al. An *in vivo* comparison of the step-back technique versus a step-back/ultrasonic technique in human mandibular molars. JOE 1989;15:195.
183. Briggs PFA, et al. The dentine-removing characteristics of an ultrasonically energized K-file. Int Endod J 1989;22:259.
184. Baker MC, et al. SEM comparison of ultrasonic versus hand instrumentation of root canals [abstract]. JOE 1985;110:138.
185. Pedicord D, et al. Hand versus ultrasonic instrumentation: its effect on canal shape and instrumentation time. JOE 1986;12:375.
186. Chenail BL, Teplitsky PE. Endosonics in curved root canals. Part II. JOE 1988;14:214.
187. Baker MC, et al. Ultrasonic compared with hand instrumentation: a scanning electron microscope study. JOE 1988;14:435.
188. Krell KV, Johnson RJ. Irrigation patterns of ultrasonic files. Part II. Diamond coated files. JOE 1988;14:535.
189. Walsh CL, et al. The effect of varying the ultrasonic power setting on canal preparation. JOE 1990;16:273.
190. Ahmad M, Pitt Ford TR, Crum LA. Ultrasonic debridement of root canals: an insight into the mechanisms involved. JOE 1987;13:93.
191. Ahmad M, et al. Ultrasonic debridement of root canals: acoustic streaming and its possible role. JOE 1987;13:490.
192. Ahmad M, et al. Ultrasonic debridement of root canals: acoustic cavitation and its relevance. JOE 1988;14:486.
193. Archer R, et al. An *in vivo* evaluation of the efficacy of ultrasound after step-back preparation in mandibular molars. JOE 1992;18:549.
194. Walmsley AD, Williams AR. Effects of constraint on the oscillatory pattern of Endosonic files. JOE 1989;15:189.
195. Krell KV, et al. Irrigation patterns during ultrasonic canal instrumentation. Part I. K-type files. JOE 1988;14:65.
196. Lumley PJ, Walmsley AD. Effect of precurving on the performance of Endosonic K-files. JOE 1992;18:232.
197. Ahmad M, et al. Effectiveness of ultrasonic files in the disruption of root canal bacteria. Oral Surg 1990;70:328.
198. Ahmad M, Pitt Ford TR. Comparison of two ultrasonic units in shaping curved canals. JOE 1989;15:457.
199. Ahmad M. Shape of the root canal after ultrasonic instrumentation with K-Flex files. Endod Dent Traumatol 1990;6:104.
200. Walmsley AD, et al. The oscillatory pattern of sonically powered endodontic files. Int Endod J 1989;22:125.
201. Cohen S, Burns RC. Pathways of the pulp. 3rd ed. St. Louis: CV Mosby; 1984.
202. Dummer PMH, et al. Shaping of simulated root canals in resin blocks using files activated by a sonic handpiece. Int Endod J 1989;22:211.
203. Bolanos OR, et al. A comparison of engine and air-driven instrumentation methods with hand instrumentation. JOE 1988;14:392.

204. Ehrlich AD, et al. Effect of sonic instrumentation on the apical preparation of curved canals. JOE 1989;15:200.
205. Tronstad L, Niemczyk SP. Efficacy and safety tests of six automated devices for root canal instrumentation. Endod Dent Traumatol 1986;2:270.
206. Miserendino LJ, et al. Cutting efficiency of endodontic instruments. Part III. Comparison of sonic and ultrasonic instrument systems. JOE 1988;14:24.
207. Kielt LW, Montgomery S. The effect of Endosonic instrumentation in simulated root canals. JOE 1987;13:215.
208. Zakariasen KL, et al. Today's sonics: using the combined hand/sonic endodontic technique. J Am Dent Assoc 1992;123:67.
209. Walker TL, del Rio CE. Histological evaluation of ultrasonic and sonic instrumentation of curved root canals. JOE 1989;15:49.
210. Yahya AS, El Deeb ME. Effect of sonic versus ultrasonic instrumentation on canal preparation. JOE 1989;15:235.
211. Reynolds MA, et al. An *in vitro* histological comparison of the step-back, sonic and ultrasonic instrumentation techniques in small curved canals. JOE 1987;13:307.
212. Lumley PJ, et al. Cleaning of oval canals using ultrasonic or sonic instrumentation. JOE 1993;19:453.
213. Lev R, et al. An *in vitro* comparison of the step-back technique versus a step-back/ultrasonic technique for 1 and 3 minutes. JOE 1987;11:523.
214. Stamos DE, et al. An *in vitro* comparison study to quantitate the debridement ability of hand, sonic and ultrasonic instrumentation. JOE 1987;13:434.
215. Goldman M, et al. A silicone model method to compare three methods of preparing the root canal. Oral Surg 1989;68:457.
216. Pugh RJ, Goerig AC, et al. A comparison of four endodontic vibration systems. Gen Dent 1989;37:296.
217. Barnett F, et al. Bacteriologic status of the root canal after sonic, ultrasonic and hand instrumentation. Endod Dent Traumatol 1985;1:228.
218. Fairbourn DR, et al. The effect of four preparation techniques on the amount of apically extruded debris. JOE 1987;13:102.
219. Baumgartner JC, Cuenin PR. Efficacy of several concentrations of sodium hypochlorite for root canal irrigation. JOE 1992;18:605.
220. Trepagnier CM, Madden RM, Lazzari EP. Quantitative study of sodium hypochlorite as an in vitro endodontic irrigant. JOE 1977;3:194.
221. Spångberg L, Engstrom B, Langeland K. Biological effects of dental materials: III. Toxicity and antimicrobial effects of endodontic antiseptics *in vitro*. Oral Surg 1974;55:856.
222. Bystrom A, Sundquist G. Bacteriological evaluation of the effect of 0.5 percent sodium hypochlorite in endodontic therapy. Oral Surg 1983;55:307.
223. Siqueira JF Jr, Batista MM, Fraga RC, de Uzeda M. Antibacterial effects of endodontic irrigants on black-pigmented gram-negative anaerobes and facultative bacteria. JOE 1998;24:414.
224. Rosenfeld EF, James GA, Burch BS. Vital pulp tissue response to sodium hypochlorite. JOE 1978;4:140.
225. Hand RE, Smith ML, Harrison JW. Analysis of the effect of dilution on the necrotic tissue dissolution property of sodium hypochlorite. JOE 1978;4:60.
226. Thé SD. The solvent action of sodium hypochlorite on fixed and unfixed necrotic tissue. Oral Surg 1979;47:558.
227. Hasselgren G, et al. Effects of calcium hydroxide and sodium hypochlorite on the dissolution of necrotic porcine muscle tissue. JOE 1988;14:125.
228. Wadachi R, Araki K, Suda H. Effect of calcium hydroxide on the dissolution of soft tissue on the root canal wall. JOE 1998;24:326.
229. Yang SF, Riveria EM, Walton RE, Baumgartner KR. Canal debridement: effectiveness of sodium hypochlorite and calcium hydroxide as medicaments. JOE 1998;20:276.
230. Johnson BR, Remeikis NA. Effective shelf-life of prepared sodium hypochlorite solution. JOE 1993;19:40.
231. Cunningham WT, Balekjian AY. Effect of temperature on collagen-dissolving ability of sodium hypochlorite endodontic irrigant. Oral Surg 1980;49:175.
232. Cunningham WT, Joseph SW. Effect of temperature on the bactericidal action of sodium hypochlorite endodontic irrigant. Oral Surg 1980;50:569.
233. Raphael D, Wong TA, Moodnick R, Borden BG. The effect of temperature on the bactericidal efficiency of sodium hypochlorite. JOE 1981;7:330.
234. Buttler TK, Crawford JJ. The detoxifying effect of varying concentrations of sodium hypochlorite on endotoxins. JOE 1982;8:59.
235. Byström A, Sundqvist G. The antibacterial action of sodium hypochlorite and EDTA in 60 cases of endodontic therapy. Int Endod J 1985;18:35.
236. Fischer R, Huerta J. Effects of pH on microbial flora of necrotic root canals. JOE 1984;10:153.
237. Nicholaus BE, et al. The bactericidal effect of citric acid and sodium hypochlorite on anaerobic bacteria. JOE 1988;14:31.
238. Baumgartner JC, Ibay AC. The chemical reactions of irrigants used for root canal debridement. JOE 1987;13:47.
239. Kaufman AY, et al. New chemotherapeutic agent for root canal treatment. Oral Surg 1978;46:283.
240. Jeansonne MJ, White RR. A comparison of 2% chlorhexidine gluconate and 5.25% sodium hypochlorite as antimicrobial endodontic irrigants. JOE 1994;20;276.
241. Validaty A, Pitt Ford TR, Wilson RF. Efficacy of chlorhexidine in disinfecting dentinal tubules *in vitro*. Endod Dent Traumatol 1993;9:243.
242. Yesiloy C, Whittaker E, Cleveland E, et al. Antimicrobial and toxic effects of established and potential root canal irrigants. JOE 1995;21:513.
243. Lee LW, Lan WH, Wang GY. An evaluation of chlorhexidine as an endosonic irrigant. J Formos Med Assoc 1990;89:491.
244. Parson GJ, Patterson SS, Newton CW, et al. Uptake and release of chlorhexidine by bovine pulp and dentin specimens and their subsequent acquisition of antibacterial properties. Oral Surg 1980;49:455.
245. Kuruvilla JR, Kamath MP. Antimicrobial effect of 2.5% sodium hypochlorite and 0.2% chlorhexidine gluconate separately and combined as endodontic irrigants. JOE 1998;24:472.
246. White RR, Hays GL, Janer LR. Residual antimicrobial activity after canal irrigation with chlorhexidine. JOE 1997;23:231.
247. Kaufman AY. The use of dequalinium acetate as a disinfectant and chemotherapeutic agent in endodontics. Oral Surg 1981;51:434.
248. Kaufman AY, Greenberg I. Comparative study of the configuration and the cleanliness level of root canals prepared with the aid of sodium hypochlorite and bis-dequalinium-acetate solutions. Oral Surg 1986;62:191.

249. Mohd Sulong MZA. The incidence of postoperative pain after canal preparation of open teeth using two irrigation regimens. Int Endod J 1989;22:248.
250. Harrison JW, Svec TA, Baumgartner JC. Analysis of clinical toxicity of endodontic irrigants. JOE 1978;4:6.
251. Ram A. Effectiveness of root canal irrigation. Oral Surg 1977;44:306.
252. Cameron JA. The use of sodium hypochlorite activated by ultrasound for the debridement of infected, immature root canals. JOE 1986;12:550.
253. Cameron JA. The synergistic relationship between ultrasound and sodium hypochlorite: a scanning electron microscopic study. JOE 1987;13:541.
254. Griffiths BM, Stock CJR. The efficiency of irrigants in removing root canal debris when used with an ultrasonic preparation technique. Int Endod J 1986;19:277.
255. Sjögren U, Sundqvist G. Bacteriologic evaluation of ultrasonic root canal instrumentation. Oral Surg 1987;63:366.
256. Krell KV, McKendry DJ. The use of a chelating agent and 2.5% NaOCl with sonic and ultrasonic endodontic instrumentation [abstract]. JOE 1988;14:199.
257. Walker TL, del Rio CE. Histological evaluation of ultrasonic debridement comparing sodium hypochlorite and water. JOE 1991;17:66.
258. Druttman ACS, Stock CJR. An *in vitro* comparison of ultrasonic and conventional methods of irrigant replacement. Int Endod J 1989;22:174.
259. Teplitsky PE, et al. Endodontic irrigation—a comparison of endosonic and syringe delivery systems. Int Endod J 1987;20:233.
260. Buchanan LS. Endodontics Palm Springs Seminar, Palm Springs, California, April 8, 1989.
261. Kaufman AY. Facial emphysema caused by hydrogen peroxide irrigation: report of case. JOE 1981;7:470.
262. Abou-Rass M, Piccinino MU. The effectiveness of four clinical irrigation methods on the removal of root canal debris. Oral Surg 1982;54:323.
263. Moser JB, Heuer MA. Forces and efficiency in endodontic irrigation systems. Oral Surg 1982;53:425.
264. Walton RE, Torabinejad M. Principles and practice of endodontics. Philadelphia: WB Saunders; 1989.
265. Chow TW. Mechanical effectiveness of root canal irrigation. JOE 1983;9:475.
266. Salzgeber RM, Brilliant JD. An *in vitro* study of the penetration of a root canal irrigating solution in root canals. JOE 1977;3:394.
267. Senia ES, Marshall FJ, Rosen S. The solvent action of sodium hypochlorite on the pulp tissue of extracted teeth. Oral Surg 1971;31:96.
268. Tidmarsh BG. Acid-cleansed and resin-sealed root canals. JOE 1978;4:117.
269. Wayman BE, Kopp WM, Pinero GJ. Citric and lactic acids as root canal irrigants *in vitro*. JOE 1979;5:258.
270. Baumgartner JC, et al. A scanning electron microscopic evaluation of root canal debridement using saline, sodium hypochlorite, and citric acid. JOE 1984;10:525.
271. Cecic PA, et al. The comparative efficiency of final endodontic cleansing procedures in removing a radioactive albumin from root canal systems. Oral Surg 1984;58:336.
272. Kaufman AY, et al. New chemotherapeutic agent for root canal treatment. Oral Surg 1978;46:283.
273. Berry EA, et al. Dentin surface treatments for the removal of the smear layer: an SEM study. J Am Dent Assoc 1987;115:65.
274. Nygaard Østby B. Chelation in root canal therapy. Odontol Tidskr 1957;65:3.
275. Fehr F, Nygaard Østby B. Effect of EDTAC and sulfuric acid on root canal dentin. Oral Surg 1963;16:199.
276. Valdrighi L. The demineralizing efficiency of EDTA solutions on dentin. Oral Surg 1981;52:446.
277. Goldberg F, Abramovich A. Analysis of the effect of EDTAC on the dentinal walls of the root canal. JOE 1977;3:101.
278. McComb D, Smith DC. A preliminary electron microscopic study of root canals after endodontic procedures. JOE 1975;1:238.
279. Goldman LB, Goldman M, Kronman JH, Sun Lin P. The efficacy of several irrigating solutions for endodontics: a scanning electron microscopic study. Oral Surg 1981;52:197.
280. Goldberg F, Spielberg C. The effect of EDTAC and the variation of its working time analyzed with scanning electron microscopy. Oral Surg 1982;53:74.
281. Mader CL, et al. Scanning electron microscopic investigation of the smeared layer on root canal walls. JOE 1984;10:477.
282. Baumgartner J, Mader CL. A SEM survey of root canal debridement using three irrigants [abstract]. JOE 1985;11:144
283. Berg MS, et al. A comparison of five irrigating solutions: a sem study [abstract]. JOE 1984;10.
284. Goldberg F, et al. Effect of irrigation solutions on the filling of lateral root canals. Endod Dent Traumatol 1986;2:65.
285. Goldberg F, Massone EJ. Instrumetacion manual y ultrasonica. Rev Esp Endod 1985;3:61.
286. Berg MS, et al. A comparison of five irrigating solutions: a scanning electron microscopic study. JOE 1986;12:192.
287. Baumgartner JC, Mader CL. A scanning electron microscopic evaluation of four root canal irrigation regimens. JOE 1987;13:147.
288. El-Tagouri H, et al. The effectiveness of the Canal Finder System. JOE 1988;14:194.
289. Cengiz T, et al. The effect of dentinal tubule orientation on the removal of smear layer by root canal irritants. A scanning electron microscopic study. Int Endod J 1990;23:163.
290. Stewart GG, et al. EDTA and urea peroxide for root canal preparation. J Am Dent Assoc 1969;78:335.
291. Brown JI, Doran JE. An *in vitro* evaluation of the particle flotation capability of various irrigating solutions. Calif Dent J 1975;3:60.
292. Zubriggen T, del Rio C, Brady JM. Post-debridement retention of endodontic reagents: a quantitative measurement with radioiostope. JOE 1975;1:298.
293. Cooke HG, Grower MF, del Rio C. Effects of instrumentation with a chelating agent on the periradicular seal of obturated root canals. JOE 1976;2:312.
294. Inoue N, Skinner DH. A simple and accurate way of measuring root canal length. JOE 1985;11:421.
295. Bramante CM, Berbert A. A critical evaluation of some methods of determining tooth length. Oral Surg 1974;37:463.
296. Seidberg BH, Alibrandi BU, Fine H, Logue B. Clinical investigation of measuring working length of root canals with an electronic device and with digital-tactile sense. J Am Dent Assoc 1975;90:379.
297. Simon JHS. The apex: how critical is it? Gen Dent 1994;42:330.

298. Glossary: contemporary terminology for endodontics. 6th ed. Chicago: American Association of Endodontists; 1998.
299. Kuttler Y. Microscopic investigation of root apexes. J Am Dent Assoc 1955;50:544.
300. Dummer PMH, McGinn JH, Ree DG. The position and topography of the apical constriction and apical foramen. Int Endod J 1984;17:192.
301. Palmer MJ, Weine FS, Healey HJ. Position of the apical foramen in relation to endodontic therapy. J Can Dent Assoc 1971;8:305.
302. Green D. A stereomicroscopic study of the root apicies of 400 maxillary and mandibular teeth. Oral Surg 1956;9:249.
303. Green FN. Microscopic investigation of root canal diameters. J Am Dent Assoc 1958;57:636.
304. Green D. Stereomicroscopic study of 700 root apices of maxillary and mandibular teeth. Oral Surg 1960;13:728.
305. Chapman CE. A microscopic study of the apical region of human anterior teeth. J Br Endod Soc 1969;3:52.
306. Morfis A, et al. Study of the apices of human permanent teeth with the use of a scanning electronic microscope. Oral Surg 1994;77:172.
307. Guiterrez G, Aguayo P. Apical foraminal openings in human teeth. Number and location. Oral Surg 1995;79:769.
308. Langeland K, cited in Riccuci D. Apical limit of root canal instrumentation and obturation. Int Endod J 1998;31:384.
309. Kuttler Y. A precision and biologic root canal filling technique. J Am Dent Assoc 1958;58:38.
310. Storms JL. Factors that influence success of endodontic treatment. J Can Dent Assoc 1969;35:83.
311. Levy AB, Glatt L. Deviation of the apical foramen from the radiographic apex. J NJ State Dent Soc 1970;41:12.
312. Burch JG, Hulen S. The relationship of the apical foramen to the anatomic apex of the tooth root. Oral Surg 1972;34:262.
313. Tamse A, Kaffe I, Fishel D. Zygomatic bone and interference with correct radiographic diagnosis in maxillary molar endodontics. Oral Surg 1980;50:563.
314. Farber JP, Bernstein M. The effect of instrumentation on root canal length as measured with an electronic device. JOE 1983;9:114.
315. Caldwell JJ. Change in working length following instrumentation of molar canals. Oral Surg 1976;11:114.
316. Rivera EM, Seraji MK. Effect of recapitulation on accuracy of electronically determined canal length. Oral Surg 1993;76:225.
317. Hasselgren G. Where shall the root filling end? N Y State Dent J 1994;June/July:34.
318. Calleteau JG, Mullaney TP. Prevalence of teaching apical patency and various instrumentation and obturation techniques in United States dental schools. JOE 1997;23:394.
319. Schilder H. Cleaning and shaping the root canal. Dent Clin North Am 1971;18:269.
320. Allison CA, Weber CR, Walton RE. The influence of the method of canal preparation on the quality of apical and coronal seal. JOE 1979;5:298.
321. George JW, Michanowicz AE, Michanowicz JR. A method of canal preparation to control apical extrusion of low-temperature gutta-percha. JOE 1987;13:18.
322. Bhaskar SN, Rappaport HM. Histologic evaluation of endodontic procedures in dogs. Oral Surg 1971;31:526.
323. Seltzer S, Soltanoff W, Smith J. Biologic aspects of endodontics. Part V. Peripical tissue reactions to root canal instrumentation beyond the apex and root canal fillings short of and beyond the apex. Oral Surg 1973;36:725.
324. Oguntebi B, Slee AM, Tanker JM, Langeland K. Predominant microflora associated with human dental periapical abscesses. J Clin Microbiol 1982;15:964.
325. Pascon EA, Introcaso JH, Langeland K. Development of predictable periapical lesion monitored by subtraction radiography. Endod Dent Traumatol 1987;3:192.
326. Guldener P, Imobersteg C. Neu Methode zur exakten Langeneinstellung von Wurkzelkand - Instrument. Schweiz Mschr Zahneheilk 1972;82:280.
327. Katz A, Tamse A, Kaufman AY. Tooth length determination: a review. Oral Surg 1991;72:238.
328. Steffen H, Splieth CH, Behr K. Comparison of measurements obtained with hand files or the Canal Leader attached to electronic apex locators: an *in vitro* study. Int Endod J 1999;32:103.
329. Ingle JI. Endodontic instruments and instrumentation. Dent Clin North Am 1957;11:805.
330. Dummer PMH, Lewis JM. An evaluation of the endometric probe in root canal length estimation. Int Endod J 1987;20:25.
331. Vande Voorde H, Bjorndahl A. Estimating endodontic "working length" with paralleling radiographs. Oral Surg 1969;27:106.
332. Weine F. Endodontic therapy. St. Louis: CV Mosby; 1982.
333. Forsberg J. Radiographic reproduction of endodontic "working length" comparing the paralleling and bisecting-angle techniques. Oral Surg 1987;64:353.
334. Olson AK, Goerig AC, et al. The ability of the radiograph to determine the location of the apical foramen. Int Endod J 1991;24:28.
335. Von der Lehr WN, Marsh RA. A radiographic study of the point of endodontic egress. Oral Surg 1973;35:105.
336. Cox VS, Brown CE, Bricker SL. Radiographic interpretation of endodontic file length. Oral Surg 1972;72:340.
337. Eckerboom M, Magnusson T. Evaluation of technical quality of endodontic treatment—reliability of intra-oral radiographs. Endod Dent Traumatol 1997;13:259.
338. Bhakdinarenk A, Manson-Hing LR. Effect of radiographic technique upon the prediction of tooth length in intraoral radiography. Oral Surg 1981;51:100.
339. Teo CS, Chan NC, Loh HS. The position of the apical foramen of the permanent incisors. Aust Dent J 1988;33:51.
340. Mandel E. Obturation canalaire et position du foramen apical. Rev Franc Endod 1983;31:49.
341. Shearer AC, Horner K, Wilson NHF. Radiovisiography for length estimation in root canal treatment: an *in vitro* comparison with conventional radiography. Int Endod J 1991;24:233.
342. Shearer AC, Horner K, Wilson NHF. Radiography for imaging root canals: an in vitro comparison with conventional radiography. Quintessence Int 1990;21:789.
343. Horner K, Shearer AC, Walker A, Wilson NHT. Radiovisiography: initial evaluation. Br Dent J 1990;168:244.
344. Griffiths BM, Brown JA, Hyatt AT, Linney AD. Comparison of three imaging techniques for assessing endodontic working length. Int Endod J 1992;25:279.
345. Sanderink GCG, Huiskens R, van der Stelt PF, et al. Image quality of direct digital intraoral sensors in assessing root canal length. The RadioVisioGraphy, Visualix/VIXA, Sens-a-Ray and Flash Dent Systems compared with Ektaspeed films. Oral Surg 1994;78:125.

346. Hedrick RT, Dove SB, Peters DP, McDavid WD. Radiographic determination of canal length: direct digital radiography versus conventional radiography. JOE 1994;20:320.
347. Leddy BJ, Miles DA, Newton CW, Brown CE. Interpretation of endodontic file lengths using RadioVisioGraphy. JOE 1994;20:542.
348. Ong EY, Pitt Ford TR. Comparison of Radiovisiography with radiographic film in root length determination. Int Endod J 1995;28:25.
349. Ellingsen MA, Harrington GW, Hollender LG. Radiovisiography versus conventional radiography for detection of small instruments in endodontic length determination. Part 1. In vitro evaluation. JOE 1995;21:326.
350. Garcia AA, Navarro LF, Castelló VU, Laliga RM. Evaluation of digital radiography to estimate working length. JOE 1997;23:363.
351. Cederberg RA, Tidwell E, Frederiksen NL, Benson BW. Endodontic working length assessment. Comparison of storage phosphor digital imaging and radiographic film. Oral Surg 1998;85:325.
352. San Marco S, Montgomery S. Use of xeroradiography for length determination in endodontics. Oral Surg 1984;57:308.
353. Alexander JB, Andrews JD. A comparison between xeroradiographs and conventional radiographs as an aid in root canal therapy for maxillary molars. Oral Surg 1989;67:443.
354. Barkhordar RA, Nicholson RJ, Nguyen NT, Abbasi J. An evaluation of xeroradiographs and radiographs in length determination in endodontics. Oral Surg 1987;65:747.
355. White S, Gratt BM. Clinical trials of intra-oral dental xeroradiography. J Am Dent Assoc 1979;99:810.
356. Berman LH, Fleischman SB. Evaluation of the accuracy of the Neosono-D electronic apex locator. J Endod 1984;10:164.
357. Bal CS, Chaudhary M. Evaluation of accuracy of an electric device (Neosono-D/SE) for measurement of tooth length. I JDR 1989;1:58.
358. Stabholz A, Rotstein I, Torabinejad M. Effect of preflaring on tactile detection of the apical constriction. JOE 1995;21:92.
359. Ounsi HF, Haddad G. *In vitro* evaluation of the reliability of the Endex electronic apex locator. JOE 1998;24:120.
360. Clouse HR. Electronic methods of root canal treatment. Gen Dent 1991;39:132.
361. Anderson DM, Langeland K, Clark GE, Galich JW. Diagnostic criteria for the treatment of caries-induced pulpitis. Bethesda (MD): Department of the Navy, Navy Dental Research Institute; 1980. NDERI-PR 81-03.
362. Lin L, Shovlin F, Skribner J, Langeland K. Pulp biopsies from the teeth associated with periapical radiolucencies. JOE 1984;10:436.
363. Langeland K. Tissue response to dental caries. Endod Dent Traumatol 1987;3:149.
364. Lauper R, Lutz F, Barbakow F. An *in vivo* comparison of gradient and absolute impedance electronic apex locators. JOE 1996;22:260.
365. Fouad AF, Krell KV, McKendry DJ, et al. A clinical evaluation of five electronic root canal length measuring instruments. JOE 1990;16:446.
366. Aurelio JA, Nahmias Y, Gerstein H. A model for demonstrating an electronic canal length measuring device. JOE 1983;9:568.
367. Nahmias Y, Aurelio JA, Gerstein H. Expanded use of electronic canal length measuring devices. J Endod 1983;9:347.
368. Nahmias Y, Aurelio JA, Gerstein H. An *in vitro* model for evaluation of electronic root canal measuring devices. JOE 1987;13:209.
369. Donnelly JC. A simplified model to demonstrate the operation of electronic root canal measuring devices. JOE 1993;19:579.
370. Czerw RJ, Fulkerson MS, Donnelly JC. An *in vitro* test of a simplified model to demonstrate the operation of an electronic root canal measuring device. JOE 1994;20:605.
371. Kobayashi C. Electronic canal length measurement. Oral Surg 1995;79:226.
372. Kovacevic M, Tamarut T. Influence of the concentration of ions and foramen diameter on the accuracy of electronic root canal length measurement—an experimental study. JOE 1998;24:346.
373. Custer LE. Exact methods of locating the apical foramen. J Natl Dent Assoc 1918;5:815.
374. Suzuki K. Experimental study on ionophoresis. J Jpn Stomatol 1942;16:411.
375. Gordon E. An instrument for measuring the length of root canals. Dent Pract XI 1960;3:86.
376. Sunada I. New method for measuring the length of the root canals. J Dent Res 1962;41:375.
377. Inoue N. Dental stethoscope measures root canal. Dent Surv 1972;48:38.
378. Inoue N. An audiometric method for determining the length of root canals. J Can Dent Assoc 1973;39:630.
379. Inoue N. Dental stethoscope audiometric method for determining root canal length. Medicon Neserland 1975;11:27.
380. Inoue N. A clinico-anatomical study for the determining root canal length by use of a novelty low-frequency oscillation device. Bull Tokyo Dent Coll 1977;18:71.
381. Ushiyama J. New principle and method for measuring the root canal length. JOE 1983;9:97.
382. Ushiyama J. Reliability and safety of the voltage gradient method of root canal measurement. JOE 1984;10:532.
383. Ushiyama J, Nakamura M, Nakamura Y. A clinical evaluation of voltage gradient method of measuring root canal length. JOE 1988;14:283.
384. Hasegawa K, Iitsuka M, Nihei M, Ohashi M. A new method and apparatus for measuring root canal length. J Nihon Univ Sch Dent 1986;28:117.
385. Saito T, Yamashita Y. Electronic determination of root canal length by a newly developed measuring device: influence of the diameter of apical foramen, the size of K-file and the root canal irrigants. Dent Jpn 1990;27:65.
386. Yamashita Y. A study of a new electronic root canal measuring device using relative values of frequency response—influences of the diameter of apical foramen, the size of electrode and the concentration of sodium hypochlorite. Jpn J Conserv Dent 1990;33:547.
387. Kobayashi C, Okiji T, Kawashima N, et al. A basic study on the electronic root canal length measurement. Part 3. Newly designed electronic root canal length measuring device using division method. Jpn J Conserv Dent 1991;34:1442.
388. Kobayashi C, Suda H. New electronic canal measuring device based on the ratio method. JOE 1994;20:111.
389. Huang L. An experimental study of the principle of electronic root canal measurement. JOE 1987;13:60.
390. Fouad AF, Krell KV. An *in vitro* comparison of five root canal length measuring instruments. JOE 1989;15:577.
391. Kaufman AY, Katz A. Reliability of Root ZX apex locator tested by an *in vitro* model [abstract]. JOE 1993;19:201.
392. Falchetta M, Castellucci A. *In vitro* evaluation and clinical impressions of the electronic apex locator Root ZX. G Ital Endod 1993;4:173.

393. Kaufman AY, Fuchs M, Freidman S, et al. An *in vitro* model for practicing the use of nickel titanium files with combined automated engine devices using a built-in apex locator. [In preparation].
394. Olson AK, Goerig AC, Cavataio RE, Luciano J. The ability of the radiograph to determine the location of the apical foramen. Int Endod J 1991;24:28.
395. Chunn CB, Zardiackas LD, Menke RA. *In vivo* root canal length determination using the Forameter. JOE 1981;7:515.
396. Kaufman AY, Szajkis S, Niv D. The efficiency and reliability of the Dentometer for detecting root canal length. Oral Surg 1989;67:573.
397. Walia HD, White PW, Kniaz A, Austin BP. *In vivo* evaluation of five apex locators [abstract]. JOE 1997;23:271.
398. Hemborough JH, Weine FS, Pisano JV, Eskoz N. Accuracy of an electronic apex locator: a clinical evaluation in maxillary molars. JOE 1993;19:242.
399. Pratten DH, McDonald NJ. Comparison of radiographic and electronic working lengths. JOE 1996;22:173.
400. Kaufman AY, et al. Internat Endodon J 1997;30:403.
401. Dunlap GA, Remeikis NA, BeGole EA, Rauschenberger CR. An *in vivo* evaluation of the electronic apex locator that uses the ratio method in vital and non-vital canals. JOE 1998;24:48.
402. Murphy PM, Johnson JD, Hutter JW, Nicoll BK. Intracanal calibration of the Root ZX electronic apex locator. [Unpublished].
403. McDonald NJ. The electronic determination of working length. Dent Clin North Amer. 1992;36:293.
404. Clinical Research Associates Newsletter. 1984;8.
405. Kolnick J. Locating the elusive apex. NY Acad Gen Dent, March, 1989.
406. Pilot TF, Pitts DL. Determination of impedance changes at varying frequencies in relation to root canal file position and instrument. JOE 1997;23:719.
407. Ramil-Diwo M, Gerhardt T, Bremer M, Heidemann D. Clinical application of three electronic apex locators compared with determining working length by radiographs [abstract]. Workshop on Measurement Techniques in Endodontics and Pulp Biology, Cumbria, England, June 1992.
408. Himel VT, Cain C. An evaluation of two electronic apex locators in a dental student clinic. Quintessence Int 1993;24:803.
409. Cavelleri G, Menegazzi G, Gersosa R, et al. Electronic measurement of root canal length. G Ital Endod 1993;1:13.
410. Yamaoka M, Yamashita Y, Saito T. Electrical root canal measuring instrument based on a new principle [thesis]. Tokyo: Nihon Univ. School of Dentistry; 1989.
411. Osada Electric Co. Endex—electronic apex sensor, operator's manual. Los Angeles: Osada Electric Co.; 1990.
412. White PW, Austin BP, Walia HD, Dhuru VB. Comparison of accuracy of four apex locators [abstract]. JOE 1996;22:216.
413. Fouad AF, Rivera EM, Krell KV. Accuracy of the Endex with variations in canal irrigants and foramen size. JOE 1993;19:63.
414. Felippe MCS, Soares IJ. *In vitro* evaluation of an audiometric device in locating the apical foramen of teeth. Endod Dent Traumatol 1994;10:220.
415. Forsberg J. Radiographic distortion in endodontics [thesis]. Bergen: Univ. of Bergen; 1987.
416. Frank AL, Torabinejad M. An *in vivo* evaluation of Endex electronic apex locators. JOE 1993;19:177.
417. Mayeda DL, Simon JHS, Aimar DF, Finley K. *In vivo* measurement accuracy in vital and necrotic canals with Endex apex locator. JOE 1993;19:545.
418. Arora RK, Gulabivala K. An *in vivo* evaluation of the Endex and RCM Mark II electronic apex locators in root canals with different contents. Oral Surg 1995;79:497.
419. Kobayashi C, Matoba K, Suda H, Sunada I. New practical model of the division method electronic root canal length measuring device. J Jpn Endod Assoc 1991;12:143.
420. Mezawa S, Komori S, Saito T. Clinical evaluation in electronic measuring of root canal length using several devices [abstract]. JOE 1992;18:184.
421. TOESCO Toei Electric Co. user's manual—full auto root apex locator JUSTWO TME-601. Tokyo: Toei Electric Co.,2002.
422. Kobayashi C. A basic study on electronic root canal length measurement. Part 6. A basic evaluation of the Sono-Explorer MK II Junior, Neosono MC and Justy. J Jpn Endo Assoc 1994;15:137.
423. Igarashi Y, Nii K, Jou YT, Kim S. Comparison of four electronic apex locators in determining canal length [abstract]. JOE 1997;23:256.
424. Instruction Manual : Apex Finder A.F.A. (All Fluids Allowed) Model #7005: Orange (CA): Sybron Endo/Analytic Technology; 1997.
425. McDonald NJ, Pileggi R, Glickman GN, Varella C. An in vivo evaluation of third generation apex locators [abstract]. J Dent Res 1999;219:136.
426. Kobayashi C, Suda H. A basic study on the electronic root canal length measurement. Part 4. A comparison of six apex locators. Jpn J Conserv Dent 1993;36:185.
427. Christie WH, Peikoff MD, Hawrish CE. Clinical observation on a newly designed electronic apex locator. J Can Dent Assoc 1993;59:765.
428. J. Morita Manufacturing Corp. Fully automatic root canal length measuring device, Root ZX, operation instructions. Kyoto: J. Morita Manufacturing Corp.; 1996.
429. Kobayashi C. The evolution of apex locating devices. Alpha Omegan 1997;90:21.
430. Czerw RJ, Fulkerson MS, Donnelly JC, Walmann JO. *In vitro* evaluation of the accuracy of several electronic apex locators. JOE 1995;21:572.
431. Igarashi Y, Jabev J, Jou YT, Kim S. The effect of foramen morphology on apex locators [abstract]. JOE 1997;23:273.
432. Voss A, Markula-Liegau A. Accuracy of the ROOT ZX reading the apical constriction *in vivo* [abstract]. Int Endod J 1998;31:189.
433. Ounsi HF, Naaman A. *In vitro* evaluation of the reliability of the Root ZX electronic apex locator. Int Endod J 1999;32:120.
434. Weiger R, John C, Geigle H, Lost C. Evaluation of two apex locators—an *in vitro* study [abstract]. Int Endod J 1998;31:189.
435. Shabahang S, Goon WWY, Gluskin A. An in vivo evaluation of the Root ZX electronic apex locator. JOE 1996;22:616.
436. Vajrabhaya L, Tepmongkol P. Accuracy of an apex locator. Endod Dent Traumatol 1997;13:180.
437. Ambu E, Barboni MG, Vanelli M. Clinical and *in vivo* evaluation of the Root ZX electronic apex locator and its reliability. G Ital Endod 1997;4:192.
438. Pagavino G, Pale R, Baccetti T. A SEM study of *in vivo* accuracy of the Root ZX electronic apex locator. JOE 1998;24:438.
439. Kobayashi C, Yoshioka T, Suda H. A new engine-driven canal preparation system with electronic measuring capability. JOE 1997;23:751.

440. User's guide for the Tri Auto ZX. Tustin (CA): J. Morita USA Inc; Irvine, Ca.
441. Weathers AK, Wahl P. New endodontic handpiece takes guesswork out of endodontic preparation. Oral Health 1998; 88:31.
442. Campbell D, Friedman S, Nguyen HQ, Kaufman A, Kelia S. Apical extent of rotary canal instrumentation with an apex-locating handpiece *in vitro*. Oral Surg 1998;85:319.
443. Grimberg F, Banegas G, Zmener O. Analisis preliminar del Tri Auto ZX: una experiencia *in vitro*. Rev Asoc Odontol Argent 1998;86:533.
444. Campbell D, Friedman S. Clinical assessment of rotary canal instrumentation with an apex locating handpiece [abstract]. JOE 1997;23:273.
445. Kobayashi C, Yoshioka T, Suda H. A new ultrasonic canal preparation system with electronic monitoring of file tip position. JOE 1996;22:489.
446. Kobayashi C, Yoshioka T, Aramaki S, et al. A basic study of the electronic root canal length measurement. Part 5. Development of an ultrasonic canal preparation system with electronic canal length measurement. J Jpn Endod Assoc 1994;15:129.
447. Kaufman A. The Sono-Explorer as an auxillary device in endodontics. Isr J Dent Med 1976;25:27.
448. Fuss Z, Assoline LS, Kaufman AY. Determination of location of root perforations by electronic apex locators. Oral Surg 1996;82:324.
449. Kaufman AY, Keila S. Conservative treatment of root perforation using apex locator and thermatic compactor: case study of a new method. JOE 1989;15:267.
450. Kaufman AY, Fuss Z, Keila S, Waxenberg S. Reliability of different electronic apex locators to detect root perforations *in vitro*. Int Endod J 1997;30:403.
451. Knibbs PJ, Foreman PC, Smart ER. The use of an analog type apex locator to assess the position of dentine pins. Clin Prev Dent 1989;11:22.
452. Hülsmann M, Pieper K. Use of an electronic apex locator in the treatment of teeth with incomplete root formation. Endod Dent Traumatol 1989;5:238.
453. Wu NY, Shi JN, Huang LZ, Xu YY. Variables affecting electronic root canal measurement. Int Endod J 1992;25:88.
454. Baggett FJ, Mackie IC, Worthington HV. An investigation into the measurement of working length of immature incisor teeth requiring endodontic treatment in children. Brit Dent J. 1996;181:96.
455. Katz A, Mass E, Kaufman AY. Electronic apex locator: a useful tool for root canal treatment in the primary dentition. J Dent Child 1996;63:414.
456. Wooley LH, Woodworth J, Dobbs JL. A prelminary evaluation of the effects of electric pulp testers on dogs with artificial pacemakers. J Am Dent Assoc 1974;89:1099.
457. Beach CW, Bramwell JD, Hutter JW. Use of an electronic apex locator on a cardiac pacemaker patient. JOE 1996;22:182.
458. Fouad AC, Reid LC. Effects of using apex locators on selected endodontic treatment parameters [abstract]. JOE 1998;24:271.
459. Stein TJ, Corcoran JF. Radiographic "working length" revisited. Oral Surg 1992;74:796.
460. Schilder H. Cleaning and shaping the root canal. Dent Clin North Am 1974;18:269.
461. Buchanan LS. Paradigm shifts in cleaning and shaping. Calif Dent Assoc J 1991;19:23.
462. Berg B. The endodontic management of multirooted teeth. Oral Surg 1953;6:399.
463. Saunders WP, Saunders EM. Effect of noncutting tipped instruments on the quality of root canal preparation using a modified double-flared technique. JOE 1992;18:32.
464. Buchanan LS. Management of the curved root canal. Calif Dent Assoc J 1989;17:40.
465. Weine F. Endodontic therapy. St. Louis: CV Mosby; 1972.
466. Martin H. A telescopic technique for endodontics. J District Columbia Dent Soc 1974;49:12.
467. Walton R. Histologic evaluation of different methods of enlarging the pulp canal space. JOE 1976;2:304.
468. Mullaney T. Instrument of finely curved canals. Dent Clin North Am 1979;4:575.
469. Weine FS, et al. The effect of preparation procedures on original canal shape and on apical foramen shape. JOE 1975;8:255.
470. Buchanan LS. File bending: essential for management of curved canals. Endodont Rep Spring/Summer, 1987. p.16.
471. Gutmann JL, Rakusin H. Perspectives on root canal obturation with thermoplasticized injectable gutta-percha. Int Endod J 1987;20:261.
472. Cuicchi B, et al. Comparison of curved canal shape using filing and rotational instrumentation techniques. Int Endod J 1990;23:139.
473. Lim KC, Webber J. The effect of root canal preparation on the shape of the curved root canal. Int Endod J 1985;18:233.
474. Lim KC, Webber J. The validity of simulated root canals for the investigation of prepared root canal shape. Int Endod J 1985;18:240.
475. Alodeh MHA, et al. Shaping of simulated root canals in resin blocks using the step-back technique with K-files manipulated in a simple in/out filing motion. Int Endod J 1989;22:107.
476. Vessey RA. The effect of filing vs. reaming on the shape of the prepared root canal. Oral Surg 1969;27:543.
477. Jungmann CL, Uchin RA, Bucher JF. Effect of instrumentation on the shape of the root canal. JOE 1975;1:66.
478. Haga CS. Microscopic measurements of root canal preparations following instrumentation. J Br Endod Soc 1969;2:41.
479. Nygaard-Østby B. Chelation in root canal therapy. Sartryck Odontol Tidsk 1957;65:1.
480. Patterson SS. *In vitro* and *in vivo* studies of the effect of the disodium salt of ethylenediamine tetraacetate on human dentin and its endodontic implications. Oral Surg 1963;16:83.
481. Fraser JG. Chelating agents: their softening effect on root canal dentin. Oral Surg 1974;37:803.
482. Fraser JG, Laws AL. Chelating agents: their effect on permeability of root canal dentin. Oral Surg 1976;41:534.
483. Selden HS. The role of a dental microscope in improving nonsurgical treatment of "calcified" canals. Oral Surg 1989;68:93.
484. McSpadden J. Use of the Infinity Scope. Advanced Endodontic Concepts; 1991.
485. Gold SI. Root canal calcification associated with prednisone therapy: a case report. J Am Dent Assoc 1989;119:523.
486. Marshall FJ, Pappin J. A crown-down pressureless-preparation root canal enlargement technique. Technique manual. Portland (OR): Oregon Health Sciences Univ.; 1980.
487. Leeb JI. Canal orifice enlargement as related to biomechanical preparation. JOE 1983;9:463.

488. Weine FS. Endodontic therapy. 3rd ed. St. Louis: CV Mosby; 1981.
489. Morgan LF, Montgomery S. An evaluation of the crown-down pressureless technique. JOE 1984;10:491.
490. Ruiz-Hubard EE, et al. A quantitative assessment of canal debris forced periradicularly during root canal instrumentation using two different techniques. JOE 1987;12:554.
491. Southard DW, et al. Instrumentation of curved molar root canals with the Roane technique. JOE 1987;10:479.
492. Bachman CA, et al. A radiographic comparison of two root canal instrumentation techniques. JOE 1992;18:19.
493. Roane JB. Presentation, American Association of Endodontics Annual Meeting, Las Vegas, Nevada April 1990.
494. Sabala CL, Roane JB, et al. Instrumentation of curved canals using a modified typed instrument: a comparison study. JOE 1988;14:59.
495. McKendry DJ. A histologic evaluation of apical root canal debridement comparing two endodontic instrument techniques [abstract]. JOE 1988;14:198.
496. McKendry DJ. Comparison of balanced forces, endosonic and step-back filing instrumentation techniques: quantification of extruded apical debris. JOE 1990;16:24.
497. Swindle RB, et al. Effect of coronal-radicular flaring on apical transportation. JOE 1991;17:147.
498. Charles TJ, Charles JE. The balanced force concept of instrumentation of curved canals revisited. Int Endod J 1998;31:166.
499. Alacam T. Scanning electron microscope study comparing the efficacy of endodontic irrigating systems. Int Endod J 1987;20:287.
500. Jahde EM, et al. A comparison of short-term periradicular responses to hand and ultrasonic overextension during root canal instrumentation in the *Macaca fascicularis* monkey. JOE 1987;13:388.
501. Mungel C, et al. The efficacy of step-down procedures during endosonic instrumentation. JOE 1991;17:111.
502. Glosson CR, Haller RH, Dove SB, del Rio CE. A comparison of root canal preparations using NiTi engine-driven, and K-Flex endodontic instruments. JOE 1995;21:146.
503. Luiten D, Morgan L, Baumgartner C, Marshall JG. Comparison of four instrumentation techniques on apical canal transportation. JOE 1995;21:26.
504. Weine FS. The use of non-ISO-tapered instruments for canal flaring. Compend Dent Educ 1996;17:651.
505. Bryant ST, Dummer PMH, Pitoni C, et al. Shaping ability of .04 and .06 taper ProFile rotary nickel-titanium instruments in simulated root canals. Int Endod J 1999;32:155.
506. Bryant ST, Thompson SA, Al-Omari MA, Dummer PMH. Shaping ability of Profile rotary nickel titanium instruments with ISO sized tips in simulated root canals. Part 1. Int Endod J 1998;31:275.
507. Thompson SA, Dummer PMH. Shaping ability of Quantec Series 2000 rotary nickel-titanium instruments in simulated root canals: part 1. Int Endod J 1998;31:259.
508. Thompson SA, Dummer PMH. Shaping ability of LightSpeed rotary nickel-titanium instruments in simulated root canals: part 1, Int Endod J 1997;23:698.
509. Thompson SA, Dummer PMH. Shaping ability of Profile .04 taper Series 29 rotary nickel-titanium instruments in simulated root canals. Part 1. Int Endod J 1997;30:1.
510. Thompson SA, Dummer PMH. Shaping ability of Profile .04 taper Series 29 rotary nickel-titanium instruments in simulated root canals. Part II. Int Endod J 1997;30:8.
511. Serene TP, Adams JD, Saxena A. Nickel-titanium instruments: applications in endodontics. St. Louis: Ishiyaku EuroAmerica; 1994.
512. Zuolo ML, Walton RE. Instrument deterioration with usage: nickel-titanium versus stainless steel. Quintessence Int 1997;28:397.
513. Rowan M, Nicholls J, Steiner J. Torsional properties of stainless steel and nickel-titanium files. JOE 1996;22:341.
514. Pruett JP, Clement DJ, Carnes DL Jr. Cyclic fatigue testing of nickel-titanium endodontic instruments. JOE 1997;23:77.
515. Kavanaugh D, Lumley PJ. An *in vitro* evaluation of canal preparation using Profile .04 and .06 taper instruments. Endod Dent Traumatol 1988;14:16.
516. Gabel WP, Hoen M, Steinman HR, et al. Effect of rotational speed on nickel-titanium file distortion. JOE 1999;25:752.
517. Blum JY, Machtou P, Micallef JP. Location of contact areas on rotary Profile instruments in relationship to the forces developed during mechanical preparation on extracted teeth. Int Endod J 1999;32:108.
518. Schwartz FS, McSpadden JT. The Quantec rotary nickel titanium instrumentation system. Endod Pract 1999;2:14.
519. Tharuni SL, Parameswaran A, Sukumaran VG. A comparison of canal preparation using the K-file and LightSpeed in resin blocks. JOE 1996;22:474.
520. Knowles KI, Ibarolla JL, Christiansen RK. Assessing apical deformation and transportation following the use of LightSpeed root-canal instruments. Int Endod J 1996;29:113.
521. Poulsen WB, Dove SG, del Rio CE. Effect of nickel-titanium engine-driven instrument rotational speed on root canal morphology. JOE 1995;21:609.
522. Rapisarda E, Bonaccorso A, Tripi TR, Guido G. Effect of sterilization on the cutting efficiency of rotary nickel-titanium endodontic files. Oral Surg 1999;88:343.
523. Stern RH, Sognnaes RF. Laser beam effect on dental hard tissues [abstract]. J Dent Res 1964;43:873.
524. Wigdor HA, Walsh JT, Featherstone JDB, et al. Lasers in dentistry. Laser Surg Med 1995;16:103.
525. Neev J, Liaw LL, Stabholz A, et al. Tissue alteration and thermal characteristics of excimer laser interaction with dentin. SPIE Proc 1992;1643:386.
526. Neev J, Stabholz A, Liaw LL, et al. Scanning electron microscopy and thermal characteristics of dentin ablated by a short pulsed XeCl excimer laser: Laser Surg Med 1993;12:353.
527. Dederich DN, Zakariasen KL, Tulip J. Scanning electron microscopic analysis of canal wall dentin. JOE 1984;10:428.
528. Weichman JA, Johnson FM. Laser use in endodontics. A preliminary investigation. Oral Surg 1971;31:416.
529. Weichman JA, Johnson FM, Nitta LK. Laser use in endodontics. Part II. Oral Surg 1972;34:828.
530. Stabholz A. Lasers in endodontics. In: Proceedings 6th International Congress on Lasers in Dentistry, Maui, Hawaii, July 28–31, 1998. p. 7.
531. Zackariasen KL, Dederich DN, Tulip J, et al. Bacterial action of carbon dioxide laser irradiation in experimental dental root canals. Can J Microbiol 1986;32:942.
532. Levy G. Cleaning and shaping the root canal with a Nd:YAG laser beam: a comparative study. JOE 1992;18:123.
533. Moshonov J, Sion A, Kasirer J, et al. Efficacy of argon laser irradiation in removing intracanal debris. Oral Surg 1995;79:221.

534. Pini R, Salimbeni R, Vannini M, Barone R. Laser dentistry: a new application of excimer in root canal therapy. Laser Surg Med 1989;9:352.
535. Nuebler-Moritz M, Gutknecht N, Sailer HF, Hering P, Prettl W. Laboratory investigation of the efficacy of holmium:YAG laser irradiation in removing intracanal debris. In: Wigdor HA, Featherstone JDB, Rechmann P, editors. Lasers in dentistry III. Proc SPIE 1997;2973:150.
536. Moritz A, Gutknecht N, Goharkhay K, et al. In vitro irradiation of infected root canals with a diode laser: results of microbiologic, infrared spectrometric, and stain penetration examinations. Quintessence Int 1997;28:205.
537. Mehl A, Folwaczny M, Haffner C, Hickel R. Bactericidal effects of 2.94 μm Er:YAG laser radiation in dental root canals. JOE 1999;25:490.
538. Bahcall J, Howard HA, Miserendino L, Walia H. Preliminary investigation of the histological effects of laser endodontic treatment on the periradicular tissues in dogs. JOE 1992;18:47.
539. Goodis HE, White JM, Marshall SJ, Marshall GW. Scanning electron microscopic examination of intracanal wall dentin: versus laser treatment. Scanning Microsc 1993;7:979.
540. Liu HC, Lin CP, Lan WH. Sealing depth of Nd:YAG laser on human dentinal tubules. JOE 1997;23:691.
541. Koba K, Kimura Y, Matsumoto K, et al. A histopathological study of the morphological changes at the apical seat and in the periapical region after irradiation with a pulsed Nd:YAG laser. Int Endod J 1998;31:415.
542. Koba K, Kimura Y, Matsumoto K, et al. A histological study of the effects of pulsed Nd:YAG laser irradiation on infected root canal in dogs. JOE 1999;25:151.
543. Gutknecht N, Kaiser F, Hassan A, Lampert F. Long-term clinical evaluation of endodontically treated teeth by Nd:YAG lasers. J Clin Laser Med Surg 1996;14(1):7.
544. Zhang C, Kimura Y, Matsumoto K, et al. Effects of pulsed lased Nd:YAG laser irradiation on root canal wall dentin with different lasers initiators. JOE 1998;24:352.
545. Cecchini SCM, Zezell DM, Bachmann L, et al. Evaluation of two laser systems for intracanal irradiation. In: Featherstone JDB, Rechmann P, Fried D, editors. Lasers in dentistry V. Proc SPIE 1999;3593:31.
546. Takeda FH, Harashima T, Kimura Y, Matsumoto K. The morphological study of root canal walls with Er:YAG laser irradiation in removing debris and smear layer on root canal walls. JOE 1998;24:548.
547. Takeda FH, Harashima T, Eto JN, et al. Effect of Er:YAG laser treatment on the root canal walls of human teeth: an SEM study. Endod Dent Traumatol 1998;14:270.
548. Harashima T, Takeda FH, Kimura EJN, Matsumoto K. Effect of Nd: YAG laser irradiation for removal of intercanal debris and smear layer extracted human teeth. Jour of Clin Laser Med and Surg. 1997;15:131.
549. Hibst R, Stock K, Gall R, Keller U. ErYAG laser for endodontics efficiency and safety. In: Wigdor H, Featherstone JDB, Rechmann P, editors. Lasers in dentistry II. Proc SPIE 1997;3192:14.
550. Harashima T, Takeda FH, Kimura EJN, Matsumoto K. Effect of argon laser irradiation on instrumented root canal walls. Endod Dent Traumatol 1998;14:26.
551. Stabholz A, Neev J, Liaw LHL, et al. Sealing of human dentinal tubules by Xe-Cl 308-nm excimer laser. JOE 1993;19:267.
552. Hennig T, Rechmann P, Hadding U. Influences of 2nd harmonic alexandrite laser radiation on bacteria. In: Proceedings 6th International Congress on Lasers in Dentistry, Maui, Hawaii, July 28–31, 1998. p. 225.
553. White JM, Goodis HE, Cohen JN. Bacterial reduction of contaminated dentin by Nd:YAG laser [abstract]. J Dent Res 1991;70:412.
554. Stabholz A, Kettering J, Neev J, Torabinejad M. Effects of the XeCl excimer laser on *Streptococcus mutans*. JOE 1993;19:232.
555. Gutknecht N, Moritz A, Conrads G, et al. Bacterial effect of Nd:YAG laser in *in vitro* root canals. J Clin Laser Med Surg 1996;14:77.
556. Gutknecht N, Nuebler-Moritz M, Burghardt SF, Lampert F. The efficiency of root canal disinfection using a holmium:yttrium-alumimium-garnet laser *in vitro*. J Clin Laser Med Surg 1997;15:75.
557. Gouw-Soares SC. Avaliacao bacteriana em dentina radicular contaminada irradiada com laser de Ho:YAG. Estudo *in vitro* [thesis]. Sao Paulo (Brazil): Faculdade de Odontologia da Universidade de Sao Paulo; 1998.
558. Lussi A, Nussbacher U, Grosrey J. A novel non-instrumented technique of cleansing the root canal system. JOE 1993;19:549.
559. Lussi A, Portman P, Nussbacher U, et al. Comparison of two devices for root canal cleansing by the noninstrumentation technology. JOE 1999;25:9.
560. McQuillen JH. Dr. Maynard's method of extirpating the pulp. Dent Cosmos 1860;1:312.
561. Bohannan HM, Abrams L. Intentional vital pulp extirpation for prosthesis. J Prosthet Dent 1961;11:781.
562. McQuillen JH. Review of dental literature and art: "Who first filled nerve cavities?" Dent Cosmos 1862;3:556.
563. Stromberg T. Wound healing after total pulpectomy in dogs. Odontol Revy 1969;20:147.
564. Pitt Ford TR. Vital pulpectomy—an unpredictable procedure. Int Endod J 1982;15:121.
565. Delivarris PD, Fan VSC. The localization of blood-borne bacteria in instrumented unfilled and overinstrumented canals. JOE 1984;10:521.
566. Hasselgren G, Reit C. Emergency pulpotomy: pain relieving effect with and without the use of sedative dressing. JOE 1989;15:254.

Chapter 11

OBTURATION OF THE RADICULAR SPACE

John I. Ingle, Carl W. Newton, John D. West, James L. Gutmann, Gerald N. Glickman, Barry H. Korzon, and Howard Martin

The Washington Study of endodontic success and failure suggests percolation of periradicular exudate into the incompletely filled canal as the greatest cause of endodontic failure. Nearly 60% of the failures in the study were apparently caused by incomplete obliteration of the radicular space (see chapter 13).

Dow and Ingle demonstrated *in vitro* the possibility of apical percolation using a radioactive isotope.[1] After filling the root canals of extracted teeth, they placed the teeth in radioactive iodine (^{131}I). In teeth with a fluid-tight seal of the apical foramen and a well-obliterated canal space, there was no penetration of the radioactive iodine (Figure 11-1, A). In the poorly filled canals—filled so by design—a deep penetration into the canal by ^{131}I was apparent in the radioautographs (Figure 11-1, B).

On the basis of this study, one might hypothesize that the penetration of radioactive iodine into a poorly filled root canal *in vitro* is analogous to fluid percolation into the canal of *in situ* pulpless teeth with incomplete canal obliteration (Figure 11-2). Apical percolation may be considered a logical hypothesis. However, the role of the end products of microleakage in the production of periradicular inflammation is open to speculation. It would seem safe to assume that the noxious products leaking from the apical foramen act as an inflammatory irritant. The unanswered question concerns the production of irritants in the canal. It is presently speculated that the transudate constantly leaking into the unfilled or partially filled canal arises indirectly from the blood serum and consists of a number of water-soluble proteins, enzymes, and salts. It is further speculated that the serum is trapped in the *cul-de-sac* of the poorly filled canal, away from the influences of the bloodstream, and undergoes degradation there. Later, when the degraded serum slowly diffuses out to the periradicular tissue, it acts as a physiochemical irritant to produce the periradicular inflammation of apical periodontitis.

Such a sequence of events might well explain the paradox of the periradicular lesion associated with a noninfected pulpless tooth. Periradicular inflamma-

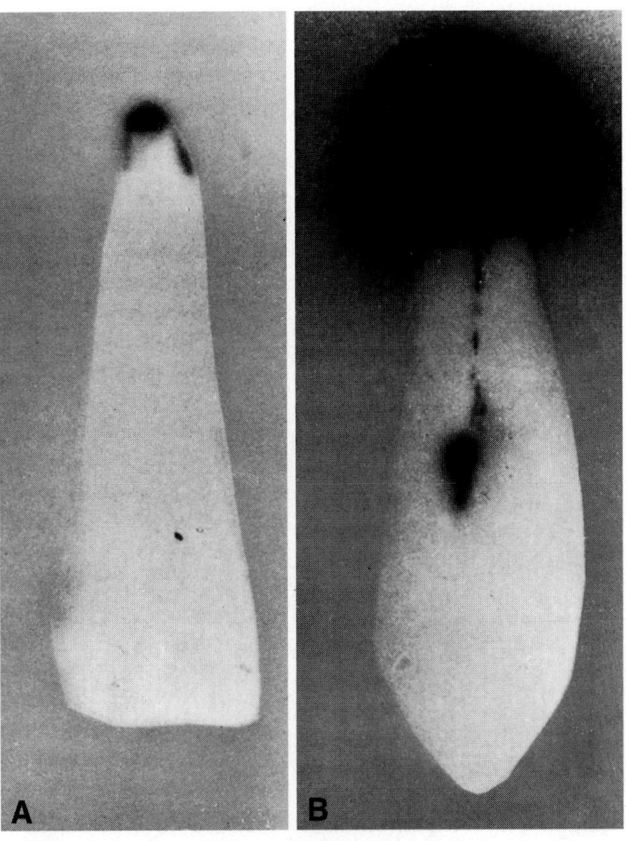

Figure 11-1 A, Failure of radioactive iodine (^{131}I) to penetrate into well-filled canal. Only periradicular cementum that was not coated with sticky wax has absorbed isotope. **B**, Massive reaction to penetration of radioactive iodine (^{131}I) into poorly filled canal. Violent response at periapex is comparable to *in vivo* response to toxic canal products. Reproduced with permission from Dow PR and Ingle JI.[1]

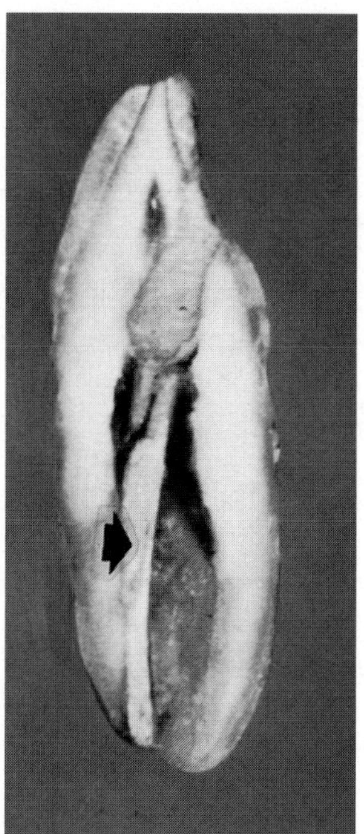

Figure 11-2 Lateral section of endodontic failure. Gutta-percha point (**arrow**) in no way obliterates foramen. Unfilled canal space contains necrotic and/or bacterial debris, a severe irritant.

tion is presumed to persist under the influence of any noxious substance. **Bacteria** certainly play a major role in the production of toxic products in the root canal. However, in the absence of bacteria, degraded serum *per se* may well assume the role of the primary tissue irritant. The persistence of periradicular inflammation, in the absence of bacterial infection, might thus be attributed to the continuing apical percolation of serum and its breakdown products.

Add a bacterial factor to this picture and the situation worsens. It is embarrassing to note that Prinz stated this thought nearly 90 years ago. Speaking before the St. Louis Dental Society on September 2, 1912, Dr. Prinz stated, "If the canal is not filled perfectly, serum will seep into it from the apical tissues. The serum furnishes nutrient material for the microorganisms present in the tubulii of a primarily infected root canal."[2] As the Scandinavians have repeatedly pointed out, bacteria are the primary source of persistent periradicular inflammation and endodontic failure.

OBJECTIVES

From this discussion, it is apparent that the preliminary objectives of operative endodontics are total débridement of the pulpal space, development of a fluid-tight seal[1*] at the apical foramen, and total obliteration of the root canal. By the same token, one must not overlook the importance of a coronal seal. **Microleakage around coronal restorations**, down through the root canal filling, and out the apical foramen into the periradicular tissues is also a potential source of bacterial infestation.

Many studies on the preparation[3] and obturation[4–6] of root canals, however, indicate that most fillings do not completely fill the root canal system. The permeability of the dentin-filling interface has been demonstrated by

*The commonly used term "hermetic seal" is not accurate. "Hermetic" is defined as "airtight by fusion or sealing." Air is not the problem at the periapex—**fluid** is the problem. "**Impermeable**" is a more accurate term. Ramsey, WD. Hermetic sealing of root canals. JOE 1982;198:100.

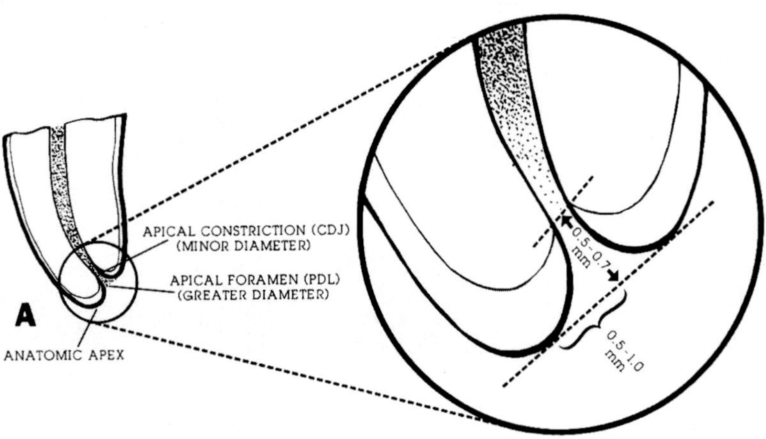

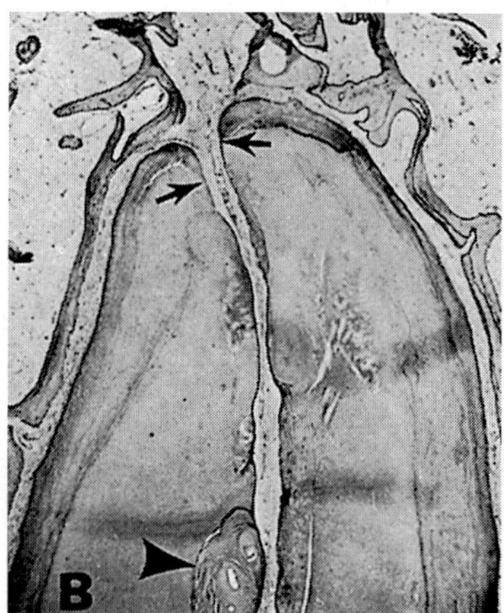

Figure 11-3 Ideal termination of canal preparation and obturation. **A**, Apical constriction at cementodentinal junction marks end of root canal. From this point to anatomic apex (0.5 to 0.7 mm), tissue is periodontal. **B**, Photomicrograph of periapex. **Small arrows** at cementodentinal junction. **Large arrow** (**bottom**) at denticle inclusion. **A** reproduced with permission from Goerig AC. In: Besner E, et al, editors. Practical endodontics. St. Louis: CV Mosby; 1993. p. 46. **B** reproduced with permission from Brynolf I. Odontol Revy 1967;18 Suppl. 11.

dye,[7–14] radioisotope,[1,15–19] electrochemical,[20–22] fluorometric,[23,24] and scanning electron microscopic examination.[25,26] This is only a partial listing of the vast number of microleakage studies that have been done as endodontic research continues to seek improved sealing efficiency of new materials and techniques.

EXTENSION OF THE ROOT CANAL FILLING

The **anatomic limits** of the pulp space are the **dentinocemental junction** apically, and the pulp chamber coronally. Debate persists, however, as to the ideal **apical** limit of the root canal filling.

Canals filled to the apical dentinocemental junction are filled to the anatomic limit of the canal. Beyond this point, the periodontal structures begin (Figure 11-3). Under the rubric "Why Root Canals Should Be Filled to the Dentinocemental Junction," three early endodontic advocates prescribed this limitation over 70 years ago.[27–29] Two of them, Orban and Skillen, were world-renowned dental scientists.

The dentinocemental junction is an average of about 0.5 to 0.7 mm from the external surface of the apical foramen, as clearly demonstrated by Kuttler,[30] and is the major factor in limiting filling material to the canal (Figure 11-4). A clarification in terminology is in order. Two terms, **overfilling** and **overextension,** are often used interchangeably. This is not correct. **Overfilling** denotes "total obturation of the root canal space with excess material extruding beyond the apical foramen."[31] Note the emphasis on "total obturation." **Overextension,** on the other hand, may also denote extrusion of filling material beyond the apical foramen but with the *caveat* that the canal **has not** been adequately filled and the apex has not been sealed.[31] It has been said facetiously that "overfilling happens to you, whereas overextension happens to the other guy."

With these definitions in mind, let it be said that a number of dentists disagree with the contention that the terminus of the filling should be at the dentinocemental junction. They prefer instead to fill to the radiographic external surface of the root or just beyond. They seek to develop a small "puff" of overfilling (Figure 11-5).

Filling to the radiographic end of the root is actually overfilling, for, as Figure 11-3 shows, the apical flare of the foramen is filled with periodontal tissue. Purposely overfilling to produce a periradicular "puff" is advocated primarily by the proponents of the diffusion technique or the softened gutta-percha technique. Ostensibly, the "puff" or "button" is designed to compensate for shrinkage of the filling by pulling down tightly against the apex. Although no proof exists that this is true, the advocates of softened gutta-percha fillings interpret the apical "puff" as an indicator that the gutta-percha has been densely packed into the apical

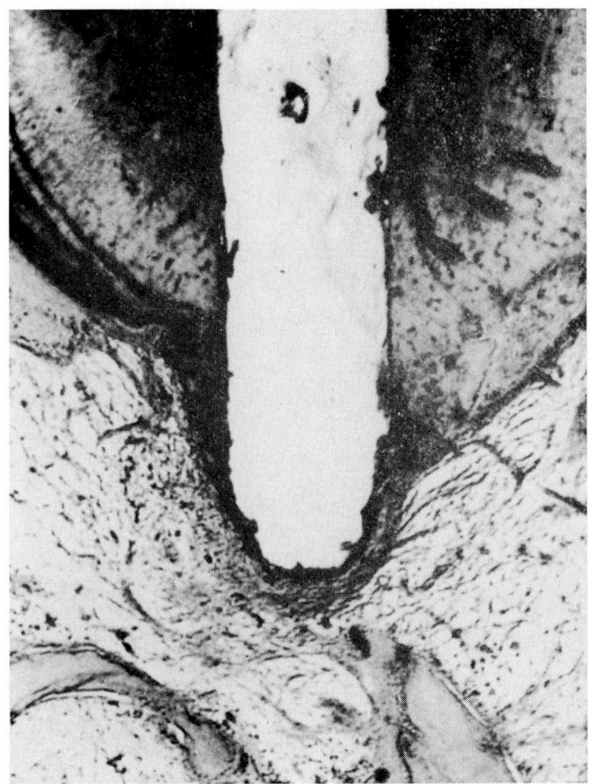

Figure 11-4 Instrumentation and root canal filling beyond apical limitation. Minor inflammatory and foreign body reaction has developed in response to irritant. (Courtesy of Dr. Seiichi Matsumiya.)

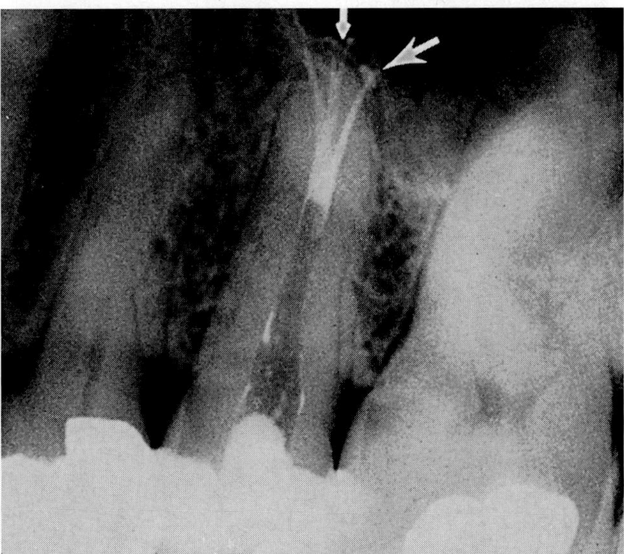

Figure 11-5 Periradicular "puff" (**arrows**) at four portals of exit, maxillary premolar, provides assurance that canals are filled.

preparation and that all of the aberrations, as well as the lateral and accessory canals of the root canal system, have been cleansed and filled. No accounting is given of postoperative discomfort. In any case, overfilled canals tend to cause more postoperative discomfort than do those filled to the dentinocemental junction.

Many authors believe that filling just short of the radiographic apex is greatly preferred to overfilling. Filling short of the apex following pulpectomy is especially recommended by Nygaard-Østby,[32] Blayney,[33] and most recently Strindberg.[34] Horsted and Nygaard-Østby reported on pulpectomies of 20 vital human teeth, stating that the space between the gutta-percha-Kloropercha fillings and the tissue surface was filled by new connective tissue within a few months.[35] They claimed the same results with clinically healthy and chronically inflamed pulps (Figure 11-6). The University of Washington study also found no failures among those **well-obliterated** cases in which the filling terminated slightly short of the apex, whereas 3.85% of the failures were caused by overfilling.

Despite all of this, a high degree of success is still achieved if overfilling occurs. Fortunately, most of the root canal sealers currently used, as well as the solid-core filling materials, are **eventually** tolerated by the periradicular tissues once the cements have set. The tissue reaction that does occur can be a fibrous walling off of the foreign body (Figure 11-7). On the other hand, fewer stormy postoperative reactions can be expected if canal instrumentation and filling are limited by the narrowest waist of the apical foramen.

WHEN TO OBTURATE THE CANAL

The root canal is ready to be filled when the canal is cleaned and shaped to an optimum size and dryness. Many feel that the smear layer lining the canal walls should also be removed. The tooth should be comfortable. Dry canals may be obtained with absorbent points except in cases of apical periodontitis or apical cyst, in which "weeping" into the canal persists.

The exception to the aforementioned criteria is the case in which mild discomfort persists. Experience has shown that filling the root canal in such cases usually alleviates the symptoms. However, **filling a root canal known to be infected is risky**. Ingle and Zeldow have described the increase in postoperative discomfort from filling infected root canals.[36] They also have shown that the degree of success in a group of infected cases was 11.2% less than that in an *a priori* group of cases with negative bacteriologic cultures.[37] More

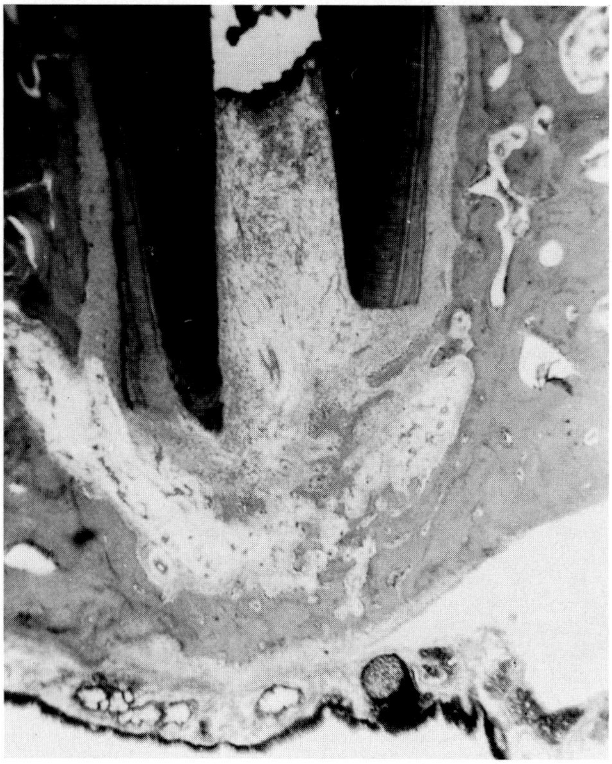

Figure 11-6 Partial pulpectomy adequately obliterated to point of amputation. Even though root canal filling is short of apex, perfect healing has developed, as evidenced by normal pulp and periradicular tissue. (Courtesy of Dr. Seiichi Matsumiya.)

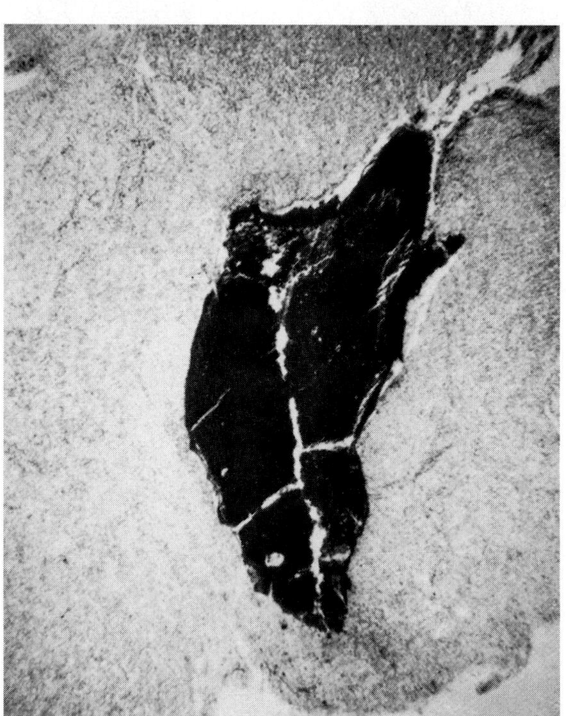

Figure 11-7 Tissue reaction to foreign body such as gutta-percha. (Courtesy of Dr. S.N. Bhaskar and US Army Institute of Pathology.)

recently, Sjögren and his associates in Sweden found that, after 5 years, **94%** of those cases exhibiting **negative cultures** at the time they were filled were completely successful. In marked contrast, only **68%** of the cases filled with **positive cultures** were successful after 5 years, a 26% difference in success rate.[38]

MATERIALS USED IN OBTURATION

The materials used to fill root canals have been legion, running the gamut from gold to feathers. Grossman grouped acceptable filling materials into plastics, solids, cements, and pastes.[39] He also delineated 10 requirements for an ideal root canal filling material that apply equally to metals, plastics, and cements:

1. It should be easily introduced into a root canal.
2. It should seal the canal laterally as well as apically.
3. It should not shrink after being inserted.
4. It should be impervious to moisture.
5. It should be bacteriostatic or at least not encourage bacterial growth.
6. It should be radiopaque.
7. It should not stain tooth structure.
8. It should not irritate periradicular tissue.
9. It should be sterile or easily and quickly sterilized immediately before insertion.
10. It should be removed easily from the root canal if necessary.

Both gutta-percha and silver points meet these requirements. If the gutta-percha point has a fault, it lies in its inherent plasticity, for it requires special handling to position it. The major fault with the silver point is its **lack** of plasticity—its inability to be compacted. Both must be cemented into place, however, to be effective.

Solid-Core Materials

Gutta-percha is by far the most universally used solid-core root canal filling material and may be classified as a plastic. To date, modern plastics have been disappointing as solid-core endodontic filling materials. However, new plastics are on the horizon. Silver amalgam, used in the retrosurgical technique wherein the canal is filled from the apex, must also be considered a "plastic" filling material.

Gutta-percha

Because modern petrochemical plastics have proved so disappointing for canal obturation, a new interest has developed in old-fashioned gutta-percha. First shown as a curiosity in the mid-seventeenth century, gutta-percha escaped notice as a practical product for nearly 200 years. The first successful use of the curious material seems to have been as insulation for undersea cables. This was in 1848, and patents followed for its use in the manufacture of corks, cement thread, surgical instruments, garments, pipes, and sheathing for ships. Some boats were made entirely of gutta-percha. Gutta-percha golf balls were introduced by the latter part of the nineteenth century; until 1920, golf balls were called "gutties." Gutta-percha has been known to dentistry for over 100 years.[40]

Actually, true gutta-percha may not be the product presently supplied to the dental profession. Manufacturers privately admit they have long used **balata,** which is the dried juice of the Brazilian trees *Manilkara bidentata,* of the sapodilla family. Gutta-percha also comes from the sapodilla family, but from Malaysian trees, genera *Payena* or *Palaquium.* Chemically and physically, balata and gutta-percha appear to be essentially identical; investigators in this field may have been given balata to test and told it was gutta-percha. In any event, the point appears to be moot, and either product is here called "gutta-percha."

Chemically pure gutta-percha (or balata) exists in two distinctly different crystalline forms (alpha and beta) that can be converted into each other. The alpha form comes directly from the tree. Most commercial gutta-percha, however, is the beta crystalline form.[40] There are few differences in physical properties between the two forms, merely a difference in the crystalline lattice depending on the annealing and/or drawing process used when manufacturing the final product.[41]

Traditionally, the beta form of gutta-percha was used to manufacture endodontic gutta-percha points to achieve an improved stability and hardness and reduce stickiness. However, through special processing and/or modifications to the formulation of the gutta-percha compound, more alpha-like forms of gutta-percha have been introduced, resulting in changes in the melting point, viscosity, and tackiness of the gutta-percha point. Gutta-percha with low viscosity will flow with less pressure or stress,[42] while an increase in tackiness will help create a more homogeneous filling. Various manufacturers have introduced products to take advantage of these properties (eg, Thermafil, Densfil, Microseal).

The effect of heating on the volumetric change of gutta-percha is most important to dentistry. Gutta-percha expands slightly on heating, a desirable trait for an endodontic filling material.[43] This physical property manifests itself as an increased volume of material that may be compacted into a root canal cavity. Volumetric studies show that it is possible to "overfill" a root canal preparation when heat and vertical condensation are applied because the volume of the gutta-percha filling is greater than the space it occupies.[44]

Although the material is thought to be compressed with force that would reduce its volume, studies have shown that it is actually **compacted,** not compressed,[45] and increased volumetric changes are due to heating.

Unfortunately, warmed gutta-percha also **shrinks** as it returns to body temperature. Schilder et al. therefore recommend "that vertical pressure be applied in all warm gutta-percha techniques to compensate for volume changes that occur as cooling takes place."[46] Camps et al. found that, even though warm gutta-percha is easily compacted, the plugger must be introduced apically since permanent deformation is undergone only after a 50% reduction in volume.[47] This contrasts with the use of cold gutta-percha in which an important pressure must be applied to obtain permanent deformation, but the spreaders do not have to be introduced apically since a 6% deformation is already permanent. Although techniques of gutta-percha placement involving heating in the root canal caused reversible physical changes, no apparent changes in chemical composition take place.[48]

Studies of pure gutta-percha are actually rather meaningless because endodontic gutta-percha contains only a fraction of gutta-percha *per se*. A study at Northwestern University[49] of the chemistry of gutta-percha filling points supplied by five manufacturers found only about 20% of the chemical composition to be gutta-percha, whereas the 60 to 75% of the composition is zinc oxide filler (Table 11-1). The remaining constituents are wax or resin to make the point more pliable and/or compactible and metal salts to lend radiopacity. On an organic versus inorganic basis, gutta-percha points are only 23.1% organic (gutta-percha and wax) and 76.4% inorganic fillers (zinc oxide and barium sulfate).[49] High zinc oxide levels were found to increase brittleness in the points and decrease tensile strength. These percentages of composition essentially have been confirmed by a French group. However, they found that it is the high content of **gutta-percha** in the points that results in their brittleness.[50]

Gutta-percha points also become brittle as they age, probably through oxidation.[51] Storage under artificial light also speeds their rate of deterioration.[52] On the other hand, they can be rejuvenated somewhat by alternate heating and cooling.[53]

Evidence of slight antibacterial activity from gutta-percha points exists[54]; however, it is too weak to be an effective microbiocide. As the destruction of bacteria is key to endodontic success, a new formulation of gutta-percha that contains iodoform, Medicated Gutta-Percha (**MGP**) (Medidenta, Woodside, N.Y.), has been developed by Martin and Martin.[55] Within the filled root canal, the iodine/iodoform depot in the MGP cone is a biologically active source for inhibiting microbial growth. The iodoform is centrally located within the gutta-percha and takes about 24 hours to leach to the surface. "The iodoform remains inert until it comes in contact with tissue fluids that activate the free iodine."[55] A canal filled with MGP gutta-percha could serve as a protection against bacterial contamination from coronal microleakage reaching the apical tissue. The use of heat during obturation does not affect either the release of the iodoform or its chemical composition.

Gutta-percha cones have also been introduced that contain a high percentage of calcium hydroxide (40–60%) (Roeko) to permit simple placement of the medicament within the canal space between appointments. Once the calcium hydroxide has leached out, the point is no longer useful as a filling material and must be removed. Holland et al. have reported on the use of

Table 11-1 Mean ($\bar{x}$) and Standard Deviation (SD) of Percentage Weights from Chemical Assay of the Gutta-percha Endodontic Filling Materials

	Gutta-percha	Wax and/or Resin	Metal Sulfates	Zinc Oxide
Brand	$\bar{x} \pm$ SD	$\bar{x} \pm$ SD	$\bar{x} \pm$ SD	$\bar{x} \pm$ SD
Premier	18.9 ± 0.1	4.1 ± 0.2	14.5 ± 0.4	61.5 ± 0.5
Mynol	19.9 ± 0.1	3.9 ± 0.2	16.2 ± 1.8	59.1 ± 2.0
Indian Head	21.8 ± 0.2	1.0 ± 0.2	17.3 ± 0.3*	59.6 ± 0.1
Dent-O-Lux	19.9 ± 0.2	2.8 ± 0.2	1.5 ± 0.3*	75.3 ± 0.5
Tempryte	20.6 ± 1.4	2.9 ± 0.2	3.4 ± 2.1*	73.4 ± 2.0

*Colored residue found with metal sulfate.

Reproduced with permission from Friedman CE, Sandrik JL, Heuer MA, Rapp GW. JOE 1977;8:305.

an experimental calcium hydroxide containing gutta-percha cone that can be used for root canal filling. Their results indicated that these points produced an improvement in the apical sealing quality of the root canal filling.[56]

Beyond these biocide qualities, gutta-percha also exhibits a degree of tissue irritation, the latter probably related to the high content of zinc oxide, which is known to be an irritant.[57] Wolfson and Seltzer found early on a severe tissue reaction to all eight brands of gutta-percha points injected into rat skin.[58]

Configuration

Gutta-percha points (or cones) are supplied in two shapes. The **traditional form** is cone shaped to conform to the perceived shape of the root canal. Today these **cones** are preferred by dentists who use the warm gutta-percha/vertical compaction technique of filling. Also, because the original spreaders used in the lateral compaction technique were shaped to match these cone shapes and sizes, traditional cones have long been used as the accessory cones in the lateral compaction technique.

The other shape of gutta-percha **points** is standardized to the same size and shape as the **standardized** (ISO) endodontic instruments. These points are available in the standardized .02 taper as well as in increased taper sizes (.04, .06, etc) to correspond to the newer tapered instrument sizes. Color coding the numbered points to match ISO instrument color has become routine and it is now rare to find the standardized points without these convenient markings (N. Lenz, personal communication). Although gutta-percha points are supposed to be standardized according to instrument size, a startling lack of uniformity has been found,[59] as well as an alarming degree of deformation of the points in their apical third[60] (Figure 11-8).

Before being used for root canal filling, gutta-percha points should be free of pathogenic microorganisms. Siqueira et al. studied four commonly used disinfectants and found that only 5.25% sodium hypochlorite was effective in eliminating *Bacillus subtilis* spores from gutta-percha cones after 1 minute of contact. Glutaraldehyde, chlorhexidine, and ethyl alcohol did not decontaminate the gutta-percha points even after 10 minutes of contact.[61]

Silver

Silver points are the most widely used solid-core metallic filling material, although points of gold, iridioplatinum, and tantalum are also available. Silver points may be indicated in **mature teeth** with small or

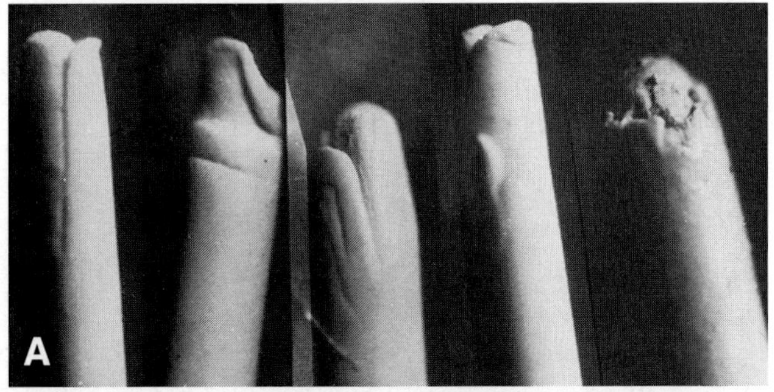

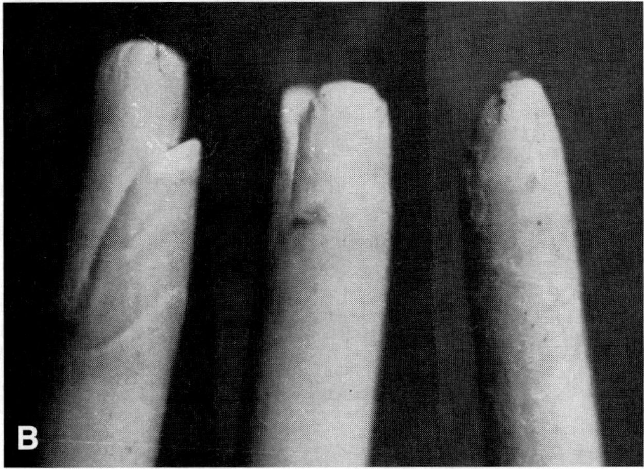

Figure 11-8 A, Five different brands of standardized gutta-percha points showing irregularities in apical one third of tip. B, Three different brands of standardized gutta-percha points of same size showing irregularities that produce variations in tip caliber. Reproduced with permission from Goldberg F et al.[60]

well-calcified round tapered canals: maxillary first premolars with two or three canals, or the buccal roots of mature maxillary molars and mesial roots of mandibular molars if they are straight. In youngsters, even these canals are too large and too ovoid for single silver point use. Silver points are also not indicated for filling anterior teeth, single canal premolars, or large single canals in molars.

Silver points often fail when used outside these situations (Figure 11-9). These failures in judgment have given silver points a bad name. Seltzer and colleagues have dramatically shown that **failed** silver points are always black and corroded when removed from the canal.[62] Goldberg has further noted that corrosion may be observed microscopically in cases previously judged to be successful by clinical and radiographic criteria.[63] Kehoe reported a case of localized argyia of the buccal gingiva, a dark-blue pigmented "tattoo" surrounded by a gray halo (Figure 11-9, C), related to severe corrosion of a failing silver point[64] (Figure 11-9, D).

Gutierrez and his associates in Chile found that canal irrigants corrode silver points.[65] Brady and del Rio reported that sulfur and chlorides were detected by

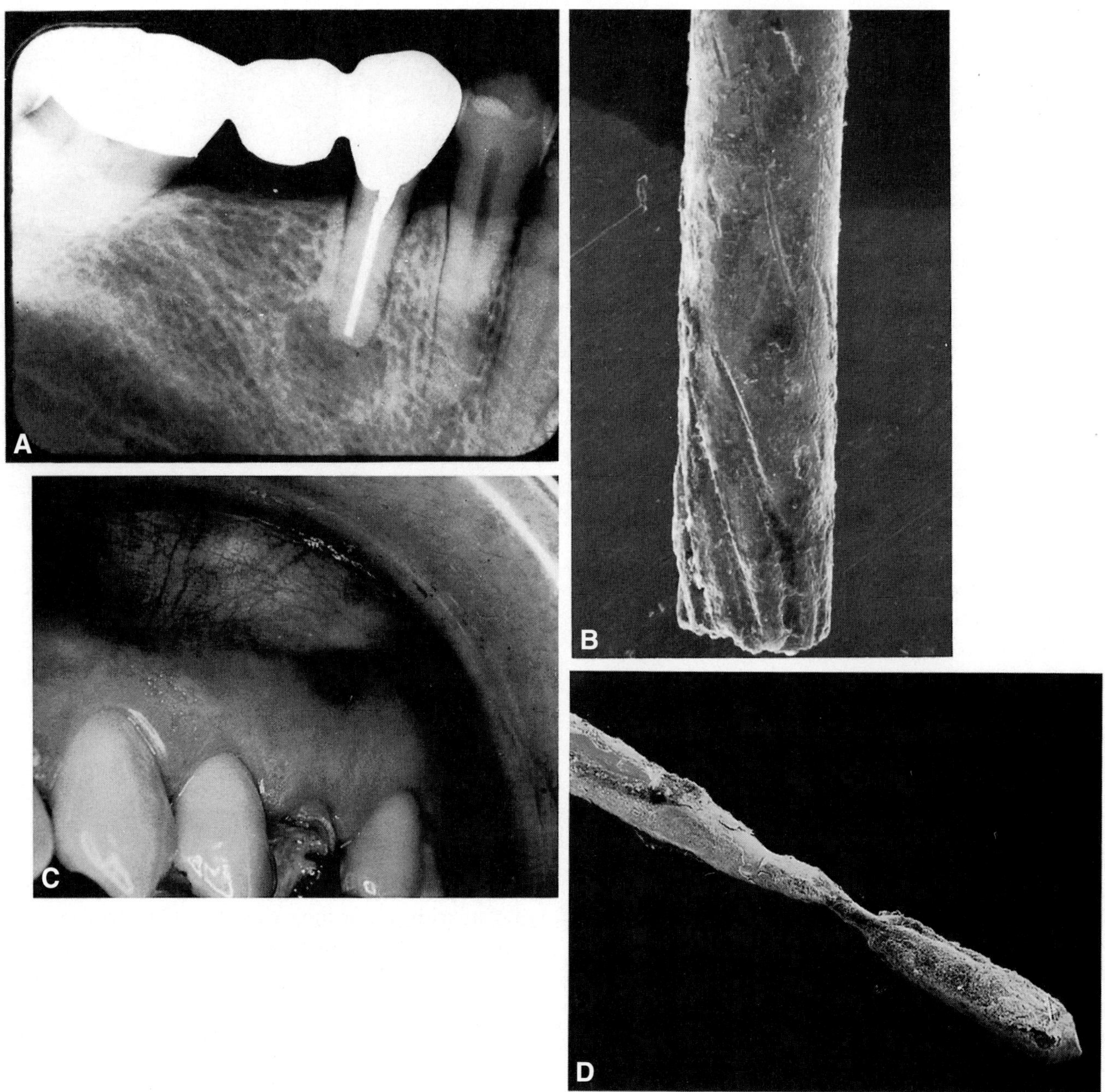

Figure 11-9 Root canal filling failure after 20 years. **A**, Silver point incorrectly used in mandibular premolar. Pain and swelling were first indications of periradicular inflammation. **B**, Electron photomicrograph (×300 original magnification) of corroded silver point removed from canal seen in **A**. Moisture and decomposed cement were found in canal as well. **C**, Dark blue-pigmented lesion (argyria) surrounded by gray halo caused by leakage from silver point corrosion. **D**, Corroded silver point removed from lingual canal in **C** 10 years after insertion. (Electron photomicrograph, **B**, courtesy of Samuel Seltzer). C and D reproduced with permission from Kehoe JC.[64]

microanalysis of failed corroded points.[66] Possibly the corrosion begins from within the canal, an aftermath of apical microleakage.

From such studies and a good deal of clinical evidence, the assumption has developed that silver points always corrode. This need not be true if the round tapered point truly fits the round tapered cavity, sealing the foramen as a cork seals a bottle (Figure 11-10). The only cement depended on is a "flashing" between the silver and the dentin wall. Silver has more rigidity than gutta-percha and hence can be pushed into tightly fitting canals and around curves where it is difficult to force gutta-percha. In an effort to avoid the problems inherent in silver points, yet make use of their versatility, Messing suggested that points be made of titanium.[67] After 3 years, Messing, using titanium, reported

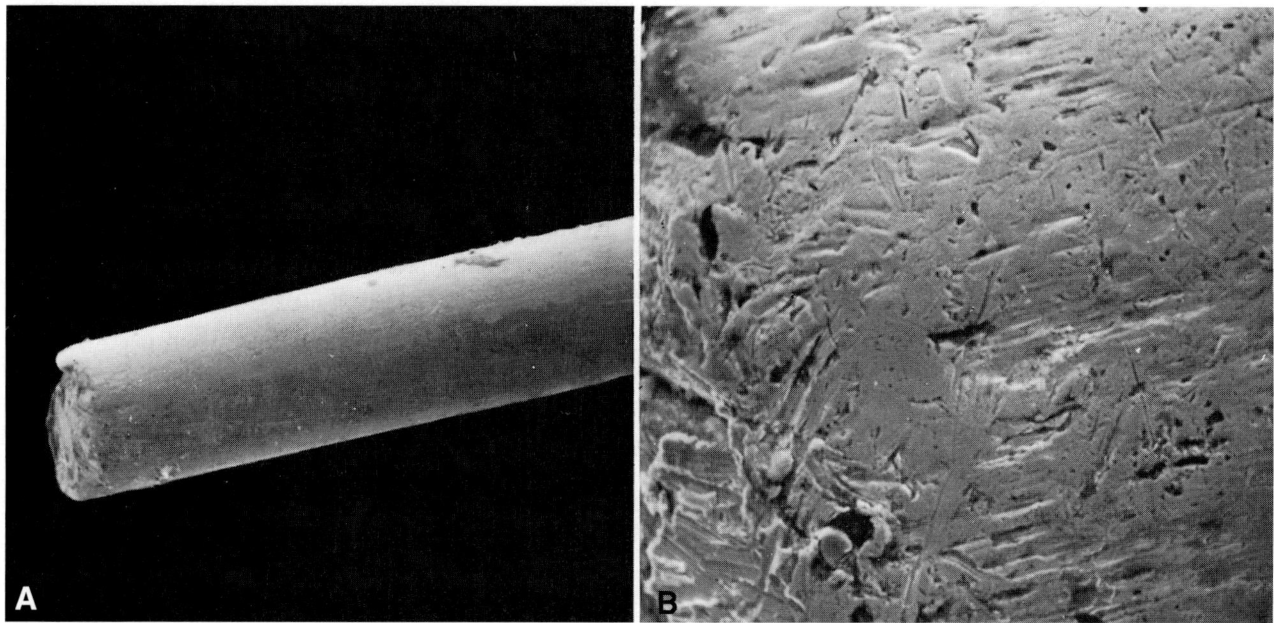

Figure 11-10 Silver point removed from palatal canal of successfully treated molar, 7 years after treatment. No corrosive deposits are apparent. **A**, ×60 original magnification; **B**, ×600 original magnification. Reproduced with permission from Seltzer S et al.[62]

three failures caused by excessive canal curvature and "tear-drop" ("zip") perforations with leakage, cases contraindicated for either titanium or silver.[67]

Sealers

In addition to the basic requirements for a solid filling material, Grossman listed 11 requirements and characteristics of a good root canal sealer[68]:

1. It should be tacky when mixed to provide good adhesion between it and the canal wall when set.
2. It should make a hermetic [sic] seal.
3. It should be radiopaque so that it can be visualized in the radiograph.
4. The particles of powder should be very fine so that they can mix easily with the liquid.
5. It should not shrink upon setting.
6. It should not stain tooth structure.
7. It should be bacteriostatic or at least not encourage bacterial growth.
8. It should set slowly.
9. It should be insoluble in tissue fluids.
10. It should be tissue tolerant, that is, nonirritating to periradicular tissue.
11. It should be soluble in a common solvent if it is necessary to remove the root canal filling.

One might add the following to Grossman's 11 basic requirements:

12. It should not provoke an immune response in periradicular tissue.[69–72]
13. It should be neither mutagenic nor carcinogenic.[73,74]

Unfortunately, zinc oxide–eugenol (ZOE) paste and ZOE paste modified with paraformaldehyde have been found to alter dog pulp tissue, making it antigenetically active.[75] Epoxy resin sealer (AH-26), on the other hand, "does not produce any systemic antibody formation or delayed hypersensitivity reaction."[72]

As far as mutagenicity and carcinogenicity are concerned, Harnden[73] reported that eugenol and its metabolites, although suspect, were uniformly negative in a bacterial mutagenicity test; hence the probability that eugenol is a carcinogen is relatively low.

Formaldehyde, formalin, and paraformaldehyde, on the other hand, are highly suspect. The US Consumer Product Safety Commission has issued warnings about the hazards of formaldehyde[75] following a study on the subject by the National Academy of Sciences.[76]

In regard to some of the other 11 requirements originally elucidated by Grossman,[68] it can be said that only polycarboxylates and glass ionomers satisfy requirement No. 1, good adhesion to dentin.[77] Newer adhesives are being tested at this time, however, and some appear promising.

As far as requirement No. 2, the hermetic sic seal, is concerned, the literature is replete with evaluations of sealing effectiveness, many of them contradictory, and virtually all questionable as to their validity.[78–80] This is discussed later in the chapter.

Radiopacity, requirement No. 3, is provided by salts of heavy metals and a halogen: lead, silver, barium, bismuth, or iodine. Beyer-Olsen and Orstavik measured the radiopacity of 409 root canal sealers and concluded that it would be difficult to compare radiographically the quality of root filling when such a variance exists in radiopacifiers.[81]

Requirement No. 4, dealing with particle size, was also investigated by Orstavik, who found sealer film thicknesses, after mixing, ranging from 49 to 180 μm.[82] There was no apparent correlation, however, between particle size and film thickness. He did point out the problems encountered with a thick film and proper sealing of the primary gutta-percha point. He found that some "sealers may prevent reinsertion of a gutta-percha point to its correct prefitted position."[82]

Requirement No. 5, "It should not shrink upon setting," is notoriously violated if a canal is filled with gutta-percha dissolved in chloroform. Whatever the volume of the chloroform in the mixture, that will be the percentage of shrinkage as the chloroform gradually evaporates.[83] Moreover, all of the sealers shrink slightly on setting, and gutta-percha also shrinks when returning from a warmed or plasticized state. At the University of Connecticut Kazemi et al. found that ZOE sealers begin shrinking "within hours after mixing" but that AH-26…first expanded and showed no shrinkage for 30 days." They concluded that "significant dimensional change and continued volume loss can occur in some endodontic sealers."[84]

The admonition that sealers and filling materials "should not stain tooth structure," Grossman's requirement No. 6, is evidently being violated by a number of sealers. Van der Burgt from Holland and her associates reported that "Grossman's cement, zinc oxide–eugenol, Endomethasone, and N2 induced a moderate orange-red stain" to the crowns of upper premolar teeth.[85] She further found that "Diaket and Tubli-Seal caused a mild pink discoloration," whereas "AH-26 gave a distinct color shift toward grey." On the other hand, "Riebler's paste caused a severe dark red stain." Diaket caused the least discoloration.[86] As far as the staining ability of other materials is concerned, Van der Burgt found that Cavit produced "a light to moderate yellowish/green stain," that "gutta-percha caused a mild pinkish tooth discoloration," that "AH-26 Silver-Free and Duo Percha induced a distinct color shift towards grey" and that crowns filled with IRM and Dycal became somewhat darker. "No discolorations were recorded for teeth filled with Durelon, Fuji glass ionomer, Fletcher's cement, or zinc phosphate cement."[87] Sealers that contain silver as a radiopacifier, such as Kerr's Root Canal Sealer (Rickert's Formula) or the original AH-26, are notorious as tooth stainers. All in all, it seems wise to avoid leaving any sealers or staining cements in the tooth crown.

Grossman himself investigated the significance of his requirement No. 7, bacteriostatic effect of sealers.[88] After testing 11 root canal cements, he concluded that they all "exerted antimicrobial activity to a varying degree," those containing paraformaldehyde to a greater degree initially. With time, however, this latter activity diminished, so that after 7 to 10 days the formaldehyde cements were no more bactericidal than the other cements.

A British group studying the antibacterial activity of four restorative materials reached much the same conclusion regarding ZOE and glass ionomer cements.[89] Another study found that 10 sealers **inhibited** growth of *Streptococcus sanguis* and *Streptococcus mutans*.[90] A Temple University study found that Grossman's Sealer had the greatest overall antibacterial activity, but that AH-26 was the most active against *Bacteroides endodontalis,* an anaerobe.[91] Heling and Chandler, at Hebrew University, also found AH26, within dentinal tubules, to have the strongest antimicrobial effect over three other well-known sealers.[92] The Dundee University group, working with anaerobes, found, in descending order of antimicrobial activity, Roth Sealer (Grossman's) to be the best, followed by Ketac-Endo, Tubliseal, Apexit, and Sealapex.[93] Mickel and Wright also found Roth Sealer to be more bactericidal than the calcium hydroxide sealers and attributed the effect to the concentration of eugenol.[94] From Germany, Schafer and Bossman reported on the efficacy of a new liquid antimicrobial, camphorated chloroxylenol (ED 84), as a good "temporary root canal dressing for a duration of 2 days." For a longer term dressing, they recommended calcium hydroxide.[95]

Grossman stated in requirement No. 9 that sealers should not be soluble in tissue fluids. Smith[96] and McComb and Smith[97] found a wide variance in sealer solubility after 7 days in distilled water, ranging from 4% for Kerr's Pulp Canal Sealer to much less than 1% for Diaket (Figure 11-11). Peters found after 2 years that virtually all of the sealer was dissolved out of test teeth filled by lateral or vertical compaction.[98] Therefore most sealers are soluble to some extent.

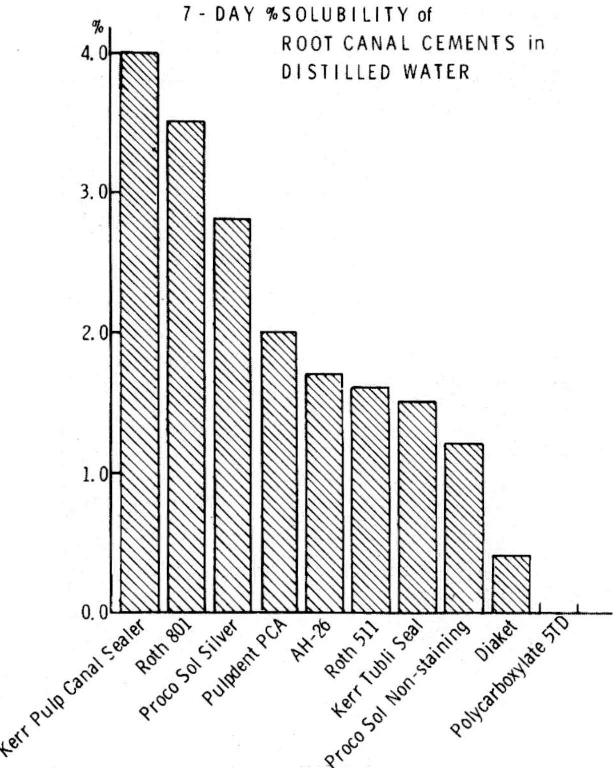

Figure 11-11 Solubility of root canal cements. Zinc oxide–eugenol cements were most soluble, and polyketones and polycarboxylates were least soluble. Reproduced with permission from McComb D and Smith D.[97]

The very important requirement No. 10, **tissue tolerance**, will be dealt with at length later in the chapter. Suffice it to say at this time that the paraformaldehyde-containing sealers appear to be the most toxic and irritating to tissue. A case in point is reported from Israel: necrosis of the soft tissue and sequestration of crestal alveolar bone from the leakage of paraformaldehyde paste from a gingival-level perforation.[99]

Cements, Plastics, and Pastes

The **cements**, which have wide American acceptance, are primarily ZOE cements, the polyketones, and epoxy. The **pastes** currently in worldwide vogue are chloropercha and eucapercha, as well as the iodoform pastes, which include both the rapidly absorbable and the slowly absorbable types. Despite their disadvantages, pastes are applicable in certain cases. The plastics show promise, as do the calcium phosphate products. At present the methods most frequently used in filling root canals involve the use of solid-core points, that are inserted in conjunction with cementing materials. Gutta-percha and silver *per se* are not considered adequate filling material **unless** they are cemented in place in the canal. The sealers are to form a fluid-tight seal at the apex by filling the minor interstices between the solid material and the wall of the canal, and also by filling patent accessory canals and multiple foramina. Dye-immersion studies have shown the necessity of cementation, without which dye penetrates back into the canal after compaction; this occurs with all known solid-core root canal–filling techniques.

Cements

Zinc Oxide–Eugenol. An early ZOE cement, developed by Rickert (**Kerr Pulp Canal Sealer;** Kerr Dental; Orange, Calif.), has been the standard of the profession for years. It admirably met the requirements set down by Grossman except for severe staining. The silver, added for radiopacity, causes discoloration of the teeth, thus creating an undesirable public image for endodontics. Removing all cement from the crowns of teeth would prevent these unfortunate incidents.[100]

Pulp Canal Sealer (PCS) has more recently emerged as the favorite sealer of the warm gutta-percha, vertical condensation adherents. However, one of its disadvantages was the rapid setting time in high heat/humidity regions of the world. To solve this problem, Kerr reconfigured the formula into Pulp Canal Sealer **EWT** (Extended Working Time) (Sybron Endo/Kerr; Orange, Calif.) that now has a "6 hour working time." The regular-set cement is also still available. Recent apical microleakage studies have shown the regular **Pulp Canal Sealer (PCS)** to be "significantly better than Roth 801 and AH26 at 24 weeks."[101]Additional research, comparing sealing ability between regular **Pulp Canal Sealer** and the new **EWT** sealer, found no significant difference between the two.[102]

In 1958 Grossman recommended a **nonstaining** ZOE cement as a substitute for Rickert's formula.[103] Now available as Roth's Sealer, it has become the standard by which other cements are measured because it reasonably meets most of Grossman's requirements for cement. The formula is as follows[68]:

Powder	
Zinc oxide, reagent	42 parts
Staybelite resin	27 parts
Bismuth subcarbonate	15 parts
Barium sulfate	15 parts
Sodium borate, anhydrous	1 part
Liquid	
Eugenol	

This cement is available commercially as **Roth's 801** (Roth's Pharmacy, USA) or **U/P Root Canal Sealer** (Sultan, USA).

All ZOE cements have an extended working time but set faster in the tooth than on the slab because of increased body temperature and humidity. If the eugenol used in the preceding nonstaining cement becomes oxidized and brown, the cement sets too rapidly for ease of handling. If too much sodium borate has been added, the setting time is overextended.

The main virtues of such a cement are its plasticity and slow setting time in the absence of moisture, together with good sealing potential because of the small volumetric change on setting. Zinc eugenate has the disadvantage, however, of being decomposed by water through a continuous loss of the eugenol. This makes ZOE a weak, unstable material and precludes its use in bulk, such as for retrofillings placed apically through a surgical approach.[96] Other zinc oxide–type cements in use are **Tubliseal** (Sybron Endo/Kerr; Orange, Calif.), **Wach's Cement** (Roth's Pharmacy, Chicago Ill.), and **Nogenol** (G-C America; Alsip, Ill. and Japan).

As Kerr's PCS fell into some disfavor because of staining, the company developed a nonstaining sealer, **TubliSeal.** Marketed as a two-paste system, it is quick and easy to mix. It differs from Richert's cement in that its zinc oxide–base paste also contains barium sulfate as a radiopacifier as well as mineral oil, cornstarch, and lecithin. The catalyst is made up of a polypale resin, eugenol, and thymol iodide. If the advantage of TubliSeal is its ease of preparation, its disadvantage has been its rapid set, especially in the presence of moisture. The company has reformulated the sealer to extend working time, and it is now available as Sealapex Regular or Sealapex **EWT** (Extended Working Time).

Wach's Cement. Meanwhile, in the Chicago area, Wach's cement became popular. A much more complicated formula, its powder base consists of zinc oxide, with bismuth subnitrate and bismuth subiodide as radiopacifiers, as well as magnesium oxide and calcium phosphate. The liquid consists of oil of clove along with eucalyptol, Canada balsam, and beechwood creosote.

The advantage of Wach's is a smooth consistency without a heavy body. The Canada balsam makes the sealer tacky. A disadvantage is the odor of the liquid—like that of an old-time dental office.

At one time, medicated variations of ZOE cements were very popular and, to some extent, remain so today. **N2** and its American counterpart, **RC2B**, are the best examples, along with **Spad** and **Endomethasone** in Europe. There is no evidence that these products seal canals better than or as well as other sealers. However, there is evidence that they dissolve in fluid and thus break the seal.

The one common denominator of these medicated sealers is **formaldehyde** in one form or another. Since formalin is such a tissue-destructive chemical, it is no wonder that every cytotoxic test lists these sealers as the number one irritant.

It is the claim of their advocates that these sealers constantly release antimicrobial formalin. This appears to be true, but it is this dissolution that breaks the seal and leads to their destructive behavior (see "Tissue Tolerance of Root Canal Sealers, Cements, and Pastes").

Nogenol was developed to overcome the irritating quality of eugenol.[103] The product is an outgrowth of a noneugenol periodontal pack. The base is zinc oxide, with barium sulfate as the radiopacifier along with a vegetable oil. Set is accelerated by hydrogenated rosin, methyl abietate, lauric acid, chlorothymol, and salicylic acid. Removing eugenol from Nogenol evidently does exert the sought-after effect of reducing toxicity.

It seems quite obvious that "...all these root canal cements differ widely in setting times, plasticity and physical properties. None of the materials show hermetic [sic] sealing in the literal sense."[96]

Calcium Hydroxide Sealers. In the second edition of *Endodontics* (1976), Luebke and Ingle first forecast a new paradigm for endodontics: a broader use of calcium hydroxide in medicating and sealing the root canal. This is coming to pass, particularly with the introduction of the calcium hydroxide sealers.

CRCS (Calciobiotic Root Canal Sealer, Coltene/Whaledent/Hygenic; Mahwah, N.J.) is essentially a ZOE/eucalyptol sealer to which calcium hydroxide has been added for its so-called osteogenic effect. CRCS takes 3 days to set fully in either dry or humid environments. It also shows very little water sorption.[104] This means it is quite stable, which improves its sealant qualities, but brings into question its ability to actually stimulate cementum and/or bone formation. If the calcium hydroxide is not released from the cement, it cannot exert an osteogenic effect, and thus its intended role is negated.

SealApex (Sybron Endo/Kerr; Orange, Calif.) is also a calcium hydroxide–containing sealer delivered as paste to paste in collapsible tubes. Its base is again zinc oxide, with calcium hydroxide as well as butyl benzene, sulfonamide, and zinc stearate. The catalyst tube contains barium sulfate and titanium dioxide as radiopacifiers as well as a proprietary resin, isobutyl salicylate, and aerocil R972. In 100% humidity, it takes up to 3 weeks to reach a final set. In a dry atmosphere, it never sets. It is also the only sealer that expands while setting.[105] As with CRCS, the question remains: Is SealApex soluble in tissue fluids to release the calcium hydroxide for its osteogenic effect? And if so, does this dissolution lead to an inadequate seal?

At Creighton University it was established that, in a limited surface area, such as in a minimal apical opening, "a negligible amount of dissolution occurred."[106] At Baylor University, however, Gutmann and Fava found *in vivo* that extruded SealApex disappeared from the periapex in 4 months.[107] This dissolution did not appear to delay healing. However, the authors suspected sealer dissolution may continue within the canal system as well, thus eventually breaking the apical seal.

If water sorption is an indicator of possible dissolution, SealApex showed a weight gain of 1.6% over 21 days in water. In contrast, CRCS gained less than 0.4%.[104] The fluid sorption characteristics of SealApex may be due to its porosity, which allows marked ingress of water.

LIFE (Sybron Endo/Kerr; Orange, Calif.), a calcium hydroxide liner and pulp-capping material similar in formulation to SealApex, has also been suggested as a sealer.[108]

From Liechtenstein comes an experimental calcium hydroxide sealer called **Apexit** (Vivadent; Schaan, Liechtenstein). Australians found that it sealed better than SealApex and **ImbiSeal.**[109]

Japanese researchers have introduced a calcium hydroxide sealer that also contains 40% **iodoform.** It is named **Vitapex** (NEO Dental, Japan), and its other component appears to be silicone oil.[110] Iodoform, a known bactericide, is released from the sealer to suppress any lingering bacteria in the canal or periapex. One week following deposits in rats, Vitapex, containing ^{45}Ca-labeled calcium hydroxide, was found throughout the skeletal system. This attests to the dissolution and uptake of the iodoform material. No evidence is given about the sealing or osteogenic capabilities of Vitapex.[110] NEO Dental has also produced another ZOE-type sealer that contains not only iodoform but calcium hydroxide as well. It is called **Dentalis** and is distributed in North America by DiaDent, Canada. It sets rapidly (5 to 7 minutes) and is very tacky.

Martin has also introduced a US Food and Drug Administration (FDA)-approved ZOE sealer, **MCS,** Medicated Canal Sealer (Medidenta, Woodside, N.Y.), that **contains iodoform,** to go along with **MGP** gutta-percha points that also contain 10% iodoforml.[55] Testing of MCS *in vitro* showed that it developed a **bacterial zone of inhibition twice the size of regular ZOE sealer.**

Researchers in Germany have also developed an experimental calcium hydroxide sealer that was reported on favorably by Pitt-Ford and Rowe.[111]

Plastics and Resins

Other sealers that enjoy favor worldwide are based more on resin chemistry than on essential oil catalysts. **Diaket** (3M/Espe; Minneapolis, Minn.), an early one first reported in 1951, is a resin-reinforced chelate formed between zinc oxide and a small amount of plastic dissolved in the liquid B-diketone. A very tacky material, it contracts slightly while setting, which is subsequently negated by uptake of water. In a recent dye-penetration study, the sealing ability of Diaket was similar to Apexit but significantly better than Ketac-Endo[112] (3M/Espe; Minneapolis, Minn.).

AH-26 (Dentsply/Maillefer, Tulsa, Okla), an epoxy resin, on the other hand, is very different. It is a glue, and its base is biphenol A-epoxy. The catalyst is hexamethylene–tetramine. It also contains 60% bismuth oxide for radiographic contrast. As AH-26 sets, traces of formaldehyde are temporarily released, which initially makes it antibacterial. AH-26 is not sensitive to moisture and will even set under water. It will not set, however, if hydrogen peroxide is present. It sets slowly, in 24 to 36 hours. The Swiss manufacturers of AH-26 recommend that mixed AH-26 be warmed on a glass slab over an alcohol flame, which renders it less viscous. AH-26 is also sold worldwide as **ThermaSeal** (Dentsply/Tulsa; Tulsa, Okla.).

Recognizing the advantages of AH-26 (high radiopacity, low solubility, slight shrinkage, and tissue compatibility), as well as some of its disadvantages (formaldehyde release, extended setting time [24 hours], and staining), the producers of AH26 set out to develop an improved product they renamed **AH PLUS** (Dentsply International). They retained the epoxy resin **"glue"** of AH26 but added new amines to maintain the natural color of the tooth. AH Plus comes in a paste–paste system, has a working time of 4 hours and a setting time of 8 hours, half the film thickness and half the solubility of regular AH26, and may be removed from the canal if necessary. In a comparative toxicity study, AH Plus was found to be less toxic than regular AH-26.[113] AH Plus is also sold worldwide as **ThermaSeal Plus** (Dentsply/Tulsa; Tulsa, Okla.).

Glass ionomer cements have also been developed for endodontics. One of these is presently marketed as **Ketac-Endo** (3M/Espe; Minneapolis, Minn.). Saito appears to have been an early proponent of endodontic glass ionomers. He suggested using Fuji Type I luting cement to fill the entire canal.[114] Pitt-Ford in England recommended endodontic glass ionomers as early as 1976.[115] However, he found the setting time too rapid. Stewart was combining Ketac-Bond and Ketac-Fil before these glass ionomers were specifically formulated for endodontics. He was pleased with the result in six cases.[116]

At Temple University, eight different formulations of Ketac cement were researched for ease of manipulation, radiopacity, adaptation of the dentin–sealer interface, and flow.[117] Ray and Seltzer chose the sealer with the best physical qualities: the best bond to dentin, the fewest voids, the lowest surface tension, and the best flow. A method of triturating and injecting the cement into the canal was also developed. **Ketac-Endo** was the outcome.

In a follow-up study, the Temple group evaluated the efficacy of Ketac-Endo as a sealer in obturating 254 teeth *in vivo*. At the end of 6 months, they reported a success and failure rate comparable to that of other studies using other sealers.[118]

Their greatest concern was the problem of removal in the event of re-treatment since there is no known solvent for glass ionomers. A Toronto/Israel group reported, however, that Ketac-Endo sealer "can be effectively removed by hand instruments and chloroform solvent followed by one minute with an ultrasonic No. 25 file."[119]

More recently, leakage studies compared Ketac-Endo with AH26[120,121] and Roth's 801E and AH26.[122] US Navy researchers found "Ketac-Endo allowed **greater** dye penetration than Roth's 801E and AH26."[122] On the other hand, the Amsterdam group found **AH26** "leaked more than Ketac-Endo." They related the difference to film thickness: 39 microns for AH26 and 22 microns for Ketac-Endo.[120] In addition, the new AH product, **AH Plus**, has half the film thickness of regular AH26. Conversely, a Turkish group found "no statistical differences" in leakage between Ketac-Endo and AH26.[121]

As far as toxicity is concerned, two Greek studies found "Ketac-Endo to be a very biocompatible material." The first study compared Ketac-Endo to **Endion**, which they found to be "highly toxic,"[123] and the second study found only mild inflammation with Ketac-Endo, whereas **TubliSeal** (Sybron Endo/Kerr; Orange, Calif.) caused necrosis and inflammation as long as 4 months later.[124] A study from Mexico, however, found that **Ketac Silver,** the precursor to Ketac-Endo, "induces irreversible **pulpal** damage."[125]

Experimental Sealers

In the never-ending search for the perfect root canal sealers, new fields have been invaded, including resin chemistry, which is proving so successful in restorative dentistry, and calcium phosphate cements, which are a return to nature.

Early on, at Tufts University, a group experimented with a **Bis GMA** unfilled resin as a sealer.[126] The new material was found to be biocompatible but impossible to remove.

Low-viscosity resins such as **pit and fissure sealants** have also been tried as sealers but "would not seem suitable as root canal filling materials."[127] Close adaptation depends on smear-layer removal, which is difficult to achieve in the apical third of the canal.

At Loma Linda University, **isopropyl cyanoacrylate** was found to be more adequate in sealing canals than were three other commercial sealers.[128] However, further research was discontinued because of a lack of acceptance by the FDA (M. Torabinejad, personal communication, August 1997).

A polyamide varnish, **Barrier** (Interdent, Inc; Culver City, Calif.), has also been tried as a sealer but was found to be not as effective as ZOE.[129]

At the University of Minnesota, the efficacy of four different **dentin bonding agents** used as root canal sealers was tested. "No leakage was measurable in 75% of the canals sealed with **Scotchbond** (3-M Corporation; South El Monte, Calif.), in 70% of canals sealed with **Restodent** (Lee Pharmaceuticals; St. Paul, Minn.), in 60% of canals sealed with **DentinAdhesit** (Ivoclar; Schaan, Leichtenstein), and in only 30% of canals sealed with **GLUMA**[130] (Bayer Dental; Laver Kusan, Germany). The same researchers reported the "dramatic improvement in the quality of sealing root canals using dentin bonding agents."[131]

It seems quite probable that dentin bonding agents will play a major role in sealant endodontics. Their ability to halt microleakage is a superb requisite for future investigation. The Minnesota study[130] returned to single-cone gutta-percha filling with the adhesives, the cone inserted undoubtedly to spread the adhesive laterally and to occupy space to reduce shrinkage. One might even visualize a rebirth of the silver point combined with one of the adhesives such as **Amalgambond** (Parkell Co., Farmingdale, N.Y.), which adheres to dentin as well as to metals.

From Zagreb, Croatia, a group used two different compaction methods, vertical and lateral, to condense **composite resin with a bonding agent** as a total filling material. They first developed an apical plug with bonding agent **Clearfil** (Morita Co.; Irvine, Calif. and Japan) and then photopolymerized layer on layer of composite resin with an argon laser as they compacted the composite with pluggers. They found fewer voids in their final filling than with lateral condensation[132] (Figure 11-12).

From Siena, Italy, another group used **dentin bonding agents**, along with AH26 sealer and gutta-percha laterally condensed, to obturate canals for leakage tests. They found less leakage in those cases in which the bonding agents were used **along with AH26** versus AH26 alone.[133]

Problems

Some obvious obstacles must be overcome, however, before these bonding agents become commercial

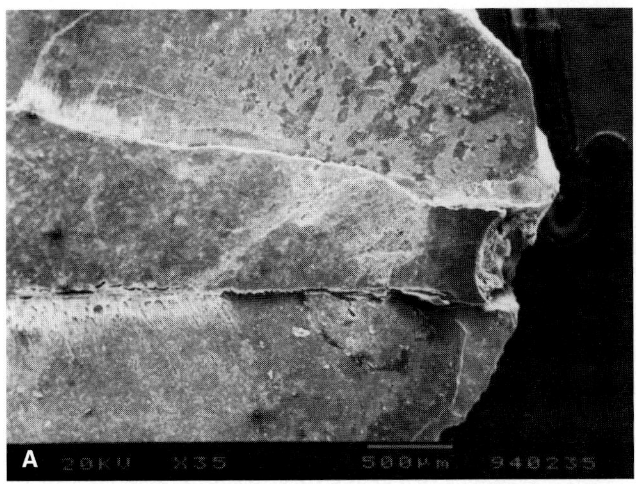

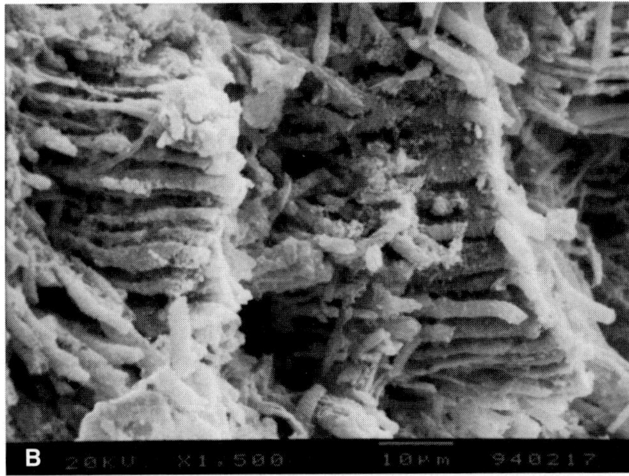

Figure 11-12 A, Apical bonding plug of **Clearfil.** Margin between bonding plug and composite filling can be seen clearly. **B,** Bundles of the resin tags remaining at the composite replica after the dentin was dissolved *in vitro*. Reproduced with permission from Anic I et al.[132]

endodontic sealants. First is preparation of the dentin to remove all of the smear layer. As Rawlinson pointed out, it is very difficult to remove all of the smear from the apical third canal, even if sodium hypochlorite and citric acid are used with ultrasonic débridement.[127]

A second obstacle is radiopacity. Radiopaquing metal salts must be added to the adhesive, and this is sure to upset the delicate chemical balance that leads to polymerization.[134] All of the bonding agents are very technique sensitive, and many do not polymerize in the presence of moisture or hydrogen peroxide.[135] The third problem is placement: Which delivery system will best ensure a total, porosity-free placement?[136] A final obstacle is removal in the event of failure. These resins polymerize very hard, all the more reason to place a gutta-percha core allowing future entry down the canal.

Calcium Phosphate Obturation

The possibility that one could mix two dry powders with water, inject the mixture into a root canal, and have it set up as hard as enamel within 5 minutes is exciting, to say the least. And yet just such a possibility may be emerging.

Developed and patented at the American Dental Association (ADA) Paffenbarger Research Center at the National Institute of Standards and Technology by Drs. W. E. Brown and L. C. Chow and their associates, calcium phosphate cements might well be the future ideal root canal sealer, long sought but never achieved.[137,138] In mixing two variations of calcium phosphate with water, Brown and Chow demonstrated that hydroxyapatite would form.The pros and cons of calcium phosphate (hydroxyapatite) obturation is discussed in greater detail at the end of this chapter (see "A New Endodontic Paradigm").

Sealer Efficacy

Hovland and Dumsha probably summarized it best: "Although all root canal sealers leak to some extent—there is probably a critical level of leakage that is unacceptable for healing, and therefore results in endodontic failure. This leakage may occur at the interface of the dentine and sealer, at the interface of the solid core and sealer, through the sealer itself, or by dissolution of the sealer."[139] And one might add, "microleakage from the crown down alongside even a well-compacted root filling." The authors went on to find that Sealapex was no different after 30 days than TubliSeal or Grossman's Sealer when it comes to leakage.[139]

No question, there **is** a variance in the impermeability of the many sealers on the market. The literature is replete with test after test, most done without prejudice but some done to promote a product. Microleakage research can be "rigged" to prove a point. "Should I use radioisotopes, or should I use India ink with its large particle size? Should I use methylene blue or should I use bacteria larger than the tubuli? Should I allow the sealer to set on the bench top or in 100% humidity? Should I test immediately, at 24 hours, 1 week, 1 month? Should the tests be done under normal atmospheric pressure or under vacuum? Should I centrifuge the test pieces? Should I remove the smear layer?" All of these factors have been shown to affect sealability results materially, to favor one product over another.

In choosing a sealer, factors other than adhesion must be considered: setting time, ease of manipulation, antimicrobial effect, particle size, radiopacity, proclivity to staining, dissolvability, chemical contaminants (hydrogen peroxide, sodium hypochlorite), cytotoxicity, cementogenesis, and osteogenesis.

Therefore, rather than quoting from the endless list of reports, each one suppressing or refuting another, a resumé will be presented and a long list of references provided for perusal by the interested student.

Resumé of Adhesion. All presently available sealers leak; they are not impermeable. That is the first caveat. The second is that some leak more than others, mostly through dissolution. The greater the sealer/periradicular tissue interface, that is, apical perforations or blunderbuss open apices, the faster dissolution takes place. It goes without saying that readily dissolving sealers are not indicated in these cases.

Zinc Oxide, Calcium Hydroxide-Type Sealers. In a 2-year solubility study, Peters found that ZOE sealer was completely dissolved away.[98] This fact alone should cause one to question the advisability of totally filling the canal with ZOE cement.

One might think that first lining the canal with varnishes such as Barrier[129] or Copalite[140] might improve the seal, but neither does.

On the basis of **leakage studies alone** one would be hard pressed to favor one of the ZOE or zinc oxide-calcium hydroxide sealers over the others. Kerr's Pulp Canal Sealer (Rickert's), Nonstaining Root Canal Sealer (Grossman's), Wach's Sealer, TubliSeal, Nogenol, CRCS, SealApex, Vitapex, Apexit, or even Dycal or Life, all appear to "be a wash" when numerous studies are examined.[104,112,120–122,132,133,141–147] A study comparing the newer **Kerr Pulp Canal Sealer EWT** (Extended Working Time) versus the original Pulp Canal Sealer found no significant difference in microleakage.[102] Moreover, recent studies comparing Pulp Canal Sealer (**PCS**) with **Roth 801** and **AH26** found **PCS** a "significantly better" sealant.[101]

The reports are not as favorable, however, for the paraformaldehyde-containing sealers N2, RC2B, Spad, and Endomethasone. Sargenti has asserted that **obliteration,** along with disinfection, is important for success.[148] On the other hand, he has stated that it is "not mandatory to have a compact root canal filling."[149] He also claims that N2 is not resorbed from the canal but is slowly absorbed from the periradicular tissues, an action he calls "semi-resorbable."[149] At another time and place, he modifies the statement by saying that N2 is "practically nonresorbable from the canal."[148] Yates and Hembree found N2 to be the least effective sealer when compared with TubliSeal or Diaket after 1 year.[143] Block and Langeland reported 50 failed cases treated with N2 or RC2B.[150]

More recent studies relating to zinc oxide-base sealers (and those previously referenced) have found essentially the same results for ZOE and calcium hydroxide sealer solubility,[96,98,105,106,110] leakage,[104,108,109,127,139,141,153–159] and **bacterial inhibition.**[88,91,151,160,161]

Despite their deficiencies, ZOE cements and their variations continue to be the most popular root canal sealers worldwide. But they are just that, sealers, and any attempt to depend on them wholly or in great part materially reduces long-term success. That is the principal reason why silver points failed—too little solid core and too much cement in an ovoid canal (see Figure 11-9, A).

If the apical orifice can be blocked principally by solid-core material, success is immeasurably improved over the long term, if not for a lifetime.[162] On the other hand, in every study in which obturation **without** sealers is attempted, the leakage results are enormously greater. **Sealers are necessary!** Researchers agree, however, that thorough cleaning and shaping of the canal space are the key to perfect obturation.

Plastic and Resin-Type Sealers. It seems reasonable to assume that plastics, resins, and glues should be more adhesive to dentin and less resorbable than the mineral oxide cements. But they have not proved to be dramatically so. In one study, AH-26 was found comparable to ZOE sealer but better than six others.[141]

In another study, AH-26 and Diaket were "found satisfactory as sealers" along with all the ZOE products.[142] Another study found Diaket less effective than TubliSeal but better than N2.[143]

In a recent Australian study, however, AH-26 was found to have better sealing capabilities than were three other cements: Apexit, Sealapex, and TubliSeal.[108,109] In New Zealand, however, Sealapex outperformed AH-26 up to the twelfth week, but there was no significant difference after that time.[158]

As far as the new glass ionomer cement, Ketac-Endo, is concerned, Ray and Seltzer found it superior to Grossman's Sealer,[117] but others found it difficult to remove in re-treatment.[118] More recently, Dutch researchers found Ketac superior in sealing to AH26.[120] On the other hand, US Navy researchers found Roth's 801E and AH26 superior to Ketac Endo.[122] Moreover, one Turkish group found Apexit and Diaket superior to Ketac,[112] but a second Turkish group found no difference.[121] It would appear the "jury is still out" on the sealing ability of Ketac Endo.

The early leakage reports on the **adhesives** used experimentally as root canal sealers are most encouraging. A 1987 report, when adhesives were in their infancy, placed Scotchbond first, with "no leakage measurable in 75% of the canals" and GLUMA last, with 30% showing no leakage.[130,131] Adhesives today are in their third and fourth generations, far superior to the initial resins. Also, there are adhesives such as **C & B Metabond** (Parkell Co., USA) or **All Bond** (Bisco Products, USA) that actually polymerize best in a moist environment. Canals obturated for leakage studies with laterally condensed gutta-percha sealed with a combination of dentin **bonding agents plus AH26** versus AH26 alone were to be found to be superior.[133]

A thoroughly modern approach of sealing the apical foramen with a resin bond called **Clearfil** (Morita Co.; Irvine, Calif.), followed by obturation with a composite resin condensed laterally as it was being photopolymerized in the canal with an argon laser, layer by layer, shows promise for the future (see Figure 11-12).[132]

With any use of dentin adhesives and/or composite resin, it is imperative that the smear layer be removed so that the hybrid layer may form against the dentin and the adhesive is able to flow into the dentinal tubuli (see Figure 11-12, B). Once again, the difficulty of removing the smear layer in the apical region must be emphasized.[127]

Experimental Calcium Phosphate Sealers (CPC). Already, the early reports on Japanese apatite sealers find them comparable to Sealapex but better sealants than two other ZOE cements.[163]

Studies emanating from the A.D.A. Paffenbarger Center find calcium phosphate cements very praiseworthy for their sealing properties as well as for their tissue compatibility. In one study, they proved better sealants than a ZOE/gutta-percha filling.[164] In another study, researchers found that the apatite injectable material "demonstrated a uniform and tight adaptation to the dentinal surfaces of the chambers and root canal walls." CPC also infiltrated the dentinal tubules.[165] Since these sealers set as hydroxyapatite, one must be aware that they are very difficult, but not impossible, to remove from the canal.

Tissue Tolerance of Root Canal Sealers, Cements, and Pastes

Without question, all of the materials used at this juncture to seal root canals—gutta-percha, silver, the sealers, cements, pastes, and plastics—irritate periradicular tissue if allowed to escape from the canal. And, if placed against a pulp stump, as in partial pulpectomy, they irritate the pulp tissue as well. The argument seems to be not whether the tissue is irritated when this happens but rather to what degree and for how long it is irritated, as well as which materials are tolerable or which are intolerable irritants.

At present, four approaches are being used to evaluate scientifically (as opposed to empirically) the toxic effects of endodontic materials: (1) cytotoxic evaluation, (2) subcutaneous implants, (3) intraosseous implants, and (4) *in vivo* periradicular reactions. The studies done on the toxicity of the materials in question are categorized into these four evaluative methods.

Cytotoxic Evaluation. Cytotoxic studies are done by measuring leukocyte migration in a Boyden chamber; by measuring the effect that suspect materials or their extracts have on fibroblasts or HeLa cells in culture; or by using radioactively labeled tissue culture cells, or tissue culture–agar overlay, or a fibroblast monolayer on a millipore filter disk. The results are quite similar.

The numerous cytotoxic evaluations may be summarized by stating that a disappointing number of today's sealers are toxic to the very cells they have been compounded to protect. Some of them are toxic when first mixed, while they are setting over hours, days, or weeks, and some continue to ooze noxious elements for years. This is, of course, caused by dissolution of the cement, thus releasing the irritants. All of the zinc oxide-type sealers, for example, gradually dissolve in fluid, releasing eugenol, which Grossman, in 1981, pointed out "is a phenolic compound and is irritating" (L.I. Grossman, personal communication, August 1981). More recently, this has been confirmed by the group in Verona, Italy.[166]

Chisolm introduced zinc oxide and oil of clove (unrefined eugenol) cement to dentistry in 1873.[167] One would think that after 125 years something less toxic would be the favorite root canal sealer.[167] Eugenol is not only cytotoxic but neurotoxic as well.[168]

Zinc oxide and eugenol, even when calcium hydroxide is added to the mixture, has been found universally to be a leading cytotoxic agent.[168–181] Removing eugenol (or any of the essential oils) from the mixture greatly reduces the toxicity. Witness the spectacular differences in cytotoxicity when unsaturated fatty acids are substituted for eugenol and/or eucalyptol in sealers such as **Nogenol** or experimental Japanese sealers.[105,182,183]

Eugenol alone is not the only culprit in ZOE irritation. **Zinc oxide itself must also be indicted.** Early on, Das found zinc oxide to be quite toxic.[57] More recently, Meryon reported that the cytotoxicity of ZOE cement may be based more on the possible toxic effect of zinc ions.[184] Maseki et al. also indicated that zinc might be a major offender when they found that dilutions of eugenol released from set cement allowed viability of 75% of their test cells.[185]

Toxicity from zinc ions may well extend beyond that found in sealers. In testing the toxicity of **gutta-percha**

points, Pascon and Spångberg concluded that all brands of points were "highly cytotoxic" and further that although "...pure raw gutta-percha was nontoxic, zinc oxide...showed high toxicity." The toxicity of gutta-percha points was attributed to leakage of zinc ions into the fluids."[186] Adding calcium hydroxide to ZOE-type cements mollifies their toxicity somewhat.[178,179]

If one were forced to classify **popular ZOE**-type sealers from worst to best as far as cytotoxicity studies are concerned, one would have to rank the pure ZOE sealers as worst: Grossman's and Rickert's, followed by Wach's and TubliSeal, Sealapex, CRCS, and finally Nogenol,[183] although there is not universal agreement on this total ranking. At Loma Linda University, for example, TubliSeal was found the least toxic followed by Wach's and Grossman's,[175] whereas at Connecticut, Wach's ranked ahead of TubliSeal.[174] Later at the University of Connecticut, however, researchers reporting *in vitro* studies found TubliSeal to be "virtually non-toxic at all experimental levels."[177] In marked contrast, a Greek group reported *in vivo* studies showing TubliSeal exhibited "severe inflammation and necrosis" as long as 4 months later.[124] The same group also found **Apexit** (a calcium hydroxide additive sealer) and Kerr's classic **Pulp Canal Sealer** (ZOE) remained as irritants over a 4-month period.[187] Researchers in India also found TubliSeal severely toxic at 48 hours and 7 days but not so at 3 months.[188]

An extensive study in Venezuela found that **CRCS** (ZOE-calcium hydroxide additive) was the least cytotoxic against human gingival fibroblasts, followed by **Endomet** and **AH26.** They also reported that **MTA** (Dentsply/Tulsa; Tulsa, Okla.) root-end filling material was not cytotoxic.[189] Another study of calcium hydroxide-containing sealers found that, with **Sealapex**, "no inflammatory infiltrate occurred," whereas with **CRCS,** a "moderate inflammatory infiltrate occurred." Inflammation "of the severe type" accompanied **Apexit.**[190]

Paraformaldehyde-containing sealers "are something else." Not only do they generally contain zinc oxide and eugenol, but they also boast 4.78 to 6.5% highly toxic paraformaldehyde. Virtually every cytotoxic study on N2, RC2B, Traitment SPAD, Endomethasone, Triolon, Oxpara, Riebler's paste, and so forth finds these materials to be the most toxic of all the sealers on the market, bar none.[171,172,191] This is discussed further later in the chapter.

Once again one must bear in mind that the resorbability, the dissolvability of all of the zinc oxide sealers, allows them to continue to release their toxic elements and to "break their seal." Augsburger and Peters followed 92 cases for up to 6½ years after the canals had been overfilled with standard ZOE (Grossman's-type sealer). "In no recall 50 months or longer did material remain in the periradicular tissues" was their conclusion. In 12 cases, "...careful evaluation of the radiographs of these cases convinced the authors that sealer had also been absorbed from **within the canal.**"[192]

Cytotoxic studies on the **plastics and resins** reveal much the same results as with the zinc oxide-type cements. For example, some have found **AH-26,** the epoxy resin, the most toxic of the resins tested,[183] and some found it the least toxic. In the latter study, Diaket (and TubliSeal) showed moderate cytotoxic effect.[193] In contrast, both studies found that formaldehyde-containing sealers were highly toxic.[183,193]

Early on, a US Navy study found AH-26 the least toxic, as did a study at Tennessee.[169,172] Again, Diaket was in between. Swedish dentists reported a "mild response using AH-26."[194] In Buenos Aires, AH-26 was found to have a moderate effect and Diaket a markedly toxic effect, both at the **end of 1 hour.**[195] AH-26, remember, releases formaldehyde as it sets. Both of these resin sealers were much less toxic, however, than the ZOE control. Statistically significant were the very mild effects of glass ionomer endodontic sealer.[195]

Newer formulations—**AH Plus** and **Ketac Endo**—have had cytotoxic and genotoxic studies done.[113,123] **AH Plus** was compared with its original product, **AH 26,** and in an *in vitro* test "caused only slight or no cellular injuries" and did not cause any genotoxicity or mutagenicity.[113] In a study done in Greece, **Ketac Endo** "proved to be a very biocompatible material, whereas **Endion** was highly cytotoxic."[123]

Subcutaneous Implants. Subcutaneous implants of root canal sealers, to test their toxic effects, are done either by needle injection under the skin of animals, or by incision and actual insertion of the product, either alone or in Teflon tubes or cups. Freshly mixed material may be implanted, allowing it to set *in situ*, or completely set material may be inserted to judge long-term effects.

The results are what one would expect from the cytotoxicity studies. Eugenol, as all of the essential oils, is a tissue irritant,[196–198] particularly during initial set.[104]

The long-term results are also not promising.[199,200] As Tagger and Tagger observed after 2 months, "...the more severe subcutaneous tissue reaction to the zinc oxide-eugenol sealer was probably due to the instability of the material, which slowly disintegrated in contact with tissue moisture."[201,202]

At Northwestern University Nogenol proved to be better tolerated initially than TubliSeal or Richert's sealer, but at 6 months the effects of TubliSeal were worse and the effects of Richert's (Kerr's RCS) and Nogenol were the same.[104] Both contain zinc oxide.

Initial inflammation surrounding implants of SealApex and CRCS, the calcium hydroxide sealers, appears to be resolved at 90 days.[203] Yesilsoy found SealApex caused a less severe inflammation reaction than did CRCS. "Both Grossman's ZOE sealer and CRCS did not have overall favorable histologic reactions."[203] Japanese researchers, announcing a new calcium hydroxide sealer, **Vitapex**, which also contains iodoform and silicone oil, stated that granulation tissue formed around the implanted material and a **nidus of calcification** then developed within this tissue.[204]

AH-26 elicited "no response at 35 days" in one study[205] and was "well tolerated" at 60 days in another.[126] Without question, N2 and other paraformaldehyde/ZOE cements are consistently the most toxic.[205,206]

Tissue-implantation ranking of endodontic sealers would again have to list Nogenol, then AH-26, SealApex, and TubliSeal. CRCS, along with the ZOE sealers, would rank higher in toxicity, and the **formaldehyde cements rank as unacceptable.** A recent comparative study found the formalin-containing cements caused faster and more prolonged nerve inhibition and paresthesia.[207]

Osseous Implant. Surprisingly, sealers implanted directly into bone evoke less inflammatory response than these same cements evoke in soft tissue. From Marseille comes a report of two ZOE sealers implanted into rabbits' mandibles. At 4 weeks, both sealer implants showed "slight to moderate reactions—no bone formation or bone resorption." At 12 weeks, there were "slight to very slight reactions—**bone formation** in direct contact with the sealers—and bone ingrowth into the implant tubes." Part of the implanted sealer was absorbed, and **macrophages were loaded with the sealer.**[208]

A US Army group found essentially the same as the French group.[209] When Deemer and Tsaknis overfilled the tubes, "the overfillings did not significantly compromise the healing of the rat intraosseous tissue." However, they noted "the irritating properties of unset Grossman's sealer."[210]

In Argentina, Zmener and Dominguez tested glass ionomer cements in dog tibias and stated that at 90 days "the inflammatory picture had resolved with progressive new bone formation."[211]

Again, the paraformaldehyde-containing cements came off second best.[212–214]

There is not enough evidence to rank cements implanted into bone. However, one must be impressed with the mild-to-stimulating reactions that are reported in bone.

***In Vivo* Tissue Tolerance Evaluations.** There is no question that the ideal method of testing a drug, a substance, or a technique is *in vivo* in a human subject. Unfortunately, human experimentation is often dangerous, costly, and unethical, and therefore, for the most part, animals are substituted. It can also be said that the closer one rises up the phylum tree to *Homo sapiens,* the more valid the experiment: Monkeys are better than dogs, and pigs, believe it or not, are better than cats.

In any event, many of the earlier studies were done on rats. This was tiny meticulous root canal therapy compared with the treatment of human beings. Erausquin and Muruzabal, working in Buenos Aires, performed the seminal *in vivo* research on tissue tolerance to sealers with hundreds of tests on techniques and materials.[215] They concluded that all of the commercial root canal sealers were toxic, causing extensive to moderate tissue damage as soon as they escape through the foramen (Figure 11-13). In all honesty, however, the authors did believe that periradicular necrosis may be due in part to an infarct caused by pressure obstruction of the region's vessels.[216] Necrosis of the periodontal ligament provoked necrosis in the adjacent cementum and alveolar bone as well (Figure 11-14). In the rat, the periodontal ligament regenerated within 7 days if toxic irritation did not continue.

In comparing the various sealers, Erausquin and Muruzabal found that straight ZOE cement was "highly irritating to the periradicular tissues and caused necrosis of the bone and cementum."[217] Inflammation persisted for 2 weeks or more. Finally, the ZOE became encapsulated. Much the same inflammatory reaction was observed at the US National Bureau of Standards when monkey teeth were overfilled with ZOE cement[218] (Figure 11-15).

In a further study, Erausquin and Muruzabel studied other ZOE-based cements. All of the cements, if the canal was overfilled, "showed a tendency to be resorbed" by phagocytes. Grossman's Sealer and N2 both provoked severe inflammatory reactions, and Rickert's sealer caused moderate infiltration. **The most severe destruction of the alveolar bone, however, was caused by poor débridement and poor filling of the canals.** The least reaction was found when the canal was **not** overfilled.[215]

The tissue reactions to overinstrumentation and overfilling noted by Erausquin and Muruzabal were confirmed by Seltzer and colleagues.[219] In all cases, they found immediate periradicular inflammation in response to overinstrumentation. When the root canals were **filled short** of the foramen, the reactions tended to subside

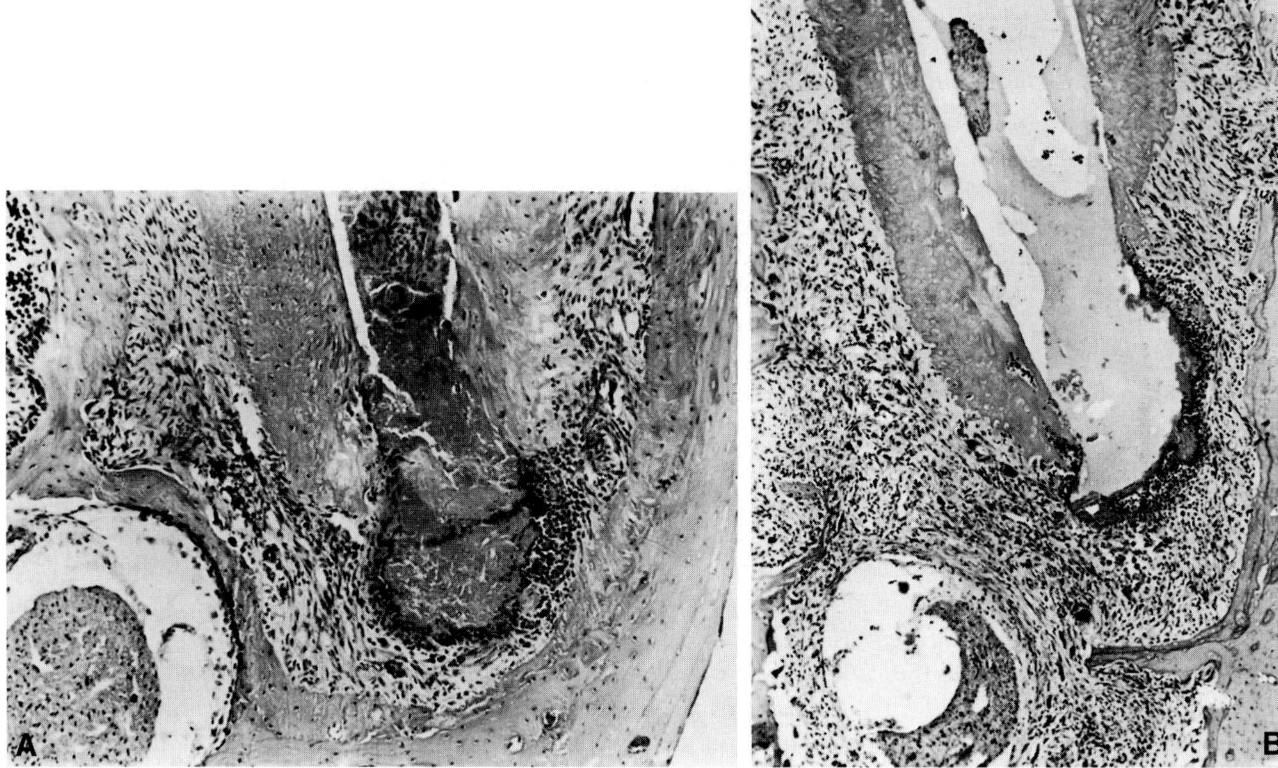

Figure 11-13 Periradicular tissue reaction to overfilling of rat's teeth. **A**, Filling with Procosol Nonstaining Sealer (zinc oxide–eugenol) 1 day postoperatively. Polymorphonuclear leukocytes have invaded even crack in cement. **B**, Filling with zinc oxide–eugenol cement 4 days postoperatively. Early polymorphonuclear leukocyte infiltration in reaction to material is apparent. Reproduced with permission from Erausquin J, Muruzabal M. Arch Oral Biol 1966;11:373.

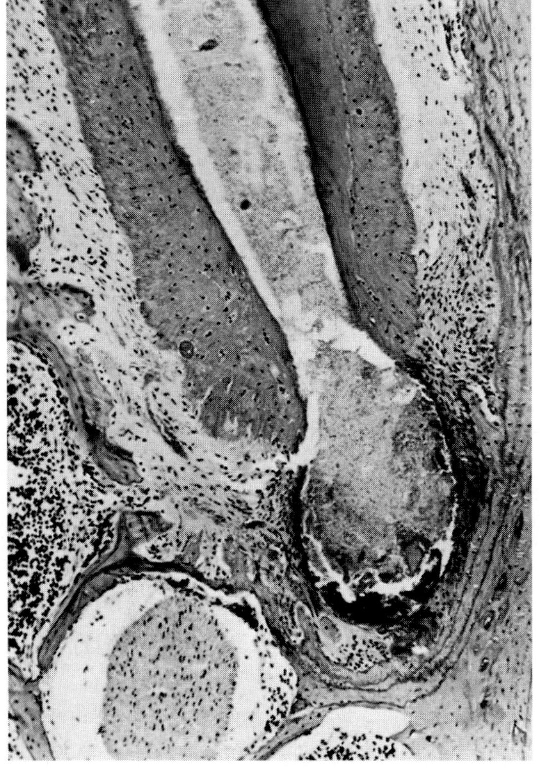

Figure 11-14 Periradicular tissue reaction to overfilling with N2 formalin cement, 1 day postoperatively. N2 protruding beyond apical foramen has caused compression of periodontal ligament. Reproduced with permission from Erausquin J, Muruzabal M. Arch Oral Biol 1966;1:373.

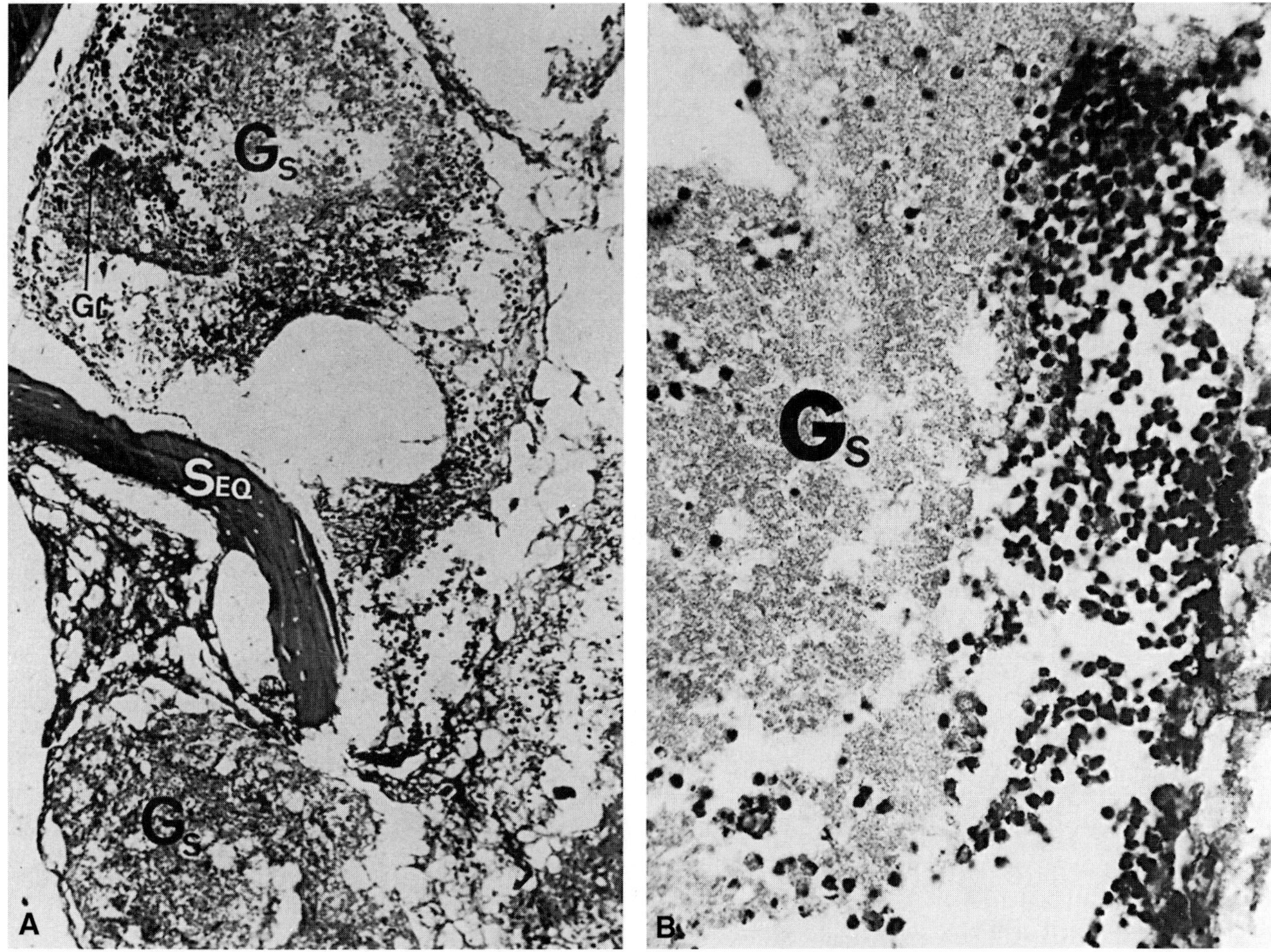

Figure 11-15 Monkey study, periradicular area, 2 months after ZOE Grossman Sealer overfill (**Gs**). **A**, Acute inflammation with giant cells (Gc) and necrotic bone sequestration (**SEQ**). **B**, Marked acute inflammation. Polymorphonuclear leukocytes predominate. Reproduced with permission from Hong YC et al.[218]

within 3 months and complete repair eventually took place. In contrast, the teeth with **overfilled** root canals exhibited persistent chronic inflammatory responses. There was also a greater tendency toward epithelial proliferation and cyst formation in the overfilled group. Another South American group reported on dog periradicular specimens overfilled with SealApex, CRCS, and ZOE. All responded with chronic inflammation.[220]

The least irritating of the cements tested by Erausquin and Muruzabal were Diaket and AH-26. Following overfilling with these sealers, the "inflammation was generally very mild." Diaket, which showed a marked tendency to be projected beyond the apex, became readily encapsulated (Figure 11-16). AH-26, on the other hand, was resorbed instead (Figure 11-17). The researchers observed, "when a foreign body is not too irritating, it becomes either resorbed or encapsulated by the body" (see Figure 11-17). Both of these processes occurred in teeth filled with Diaket and AH-26.[221]

More recently, Norwegian researchers tested AH26 against Endomethasone, Kloropercha, and ZOE. At 6 months they concluded that "the periradicular reaction to the endodontic procedures and to the materials was limited."[222] On the other hand, the University of Connecticut group found long-term (2 or 3 years) differences, ranking AH26 as a mild irritant, ZOE as moderate, and Kloropercha as severe.[223]

One must remember that gutta-percha points themselves can be a periradicular tissue irritant,[186,224,225] as well as an allergen.[226] Moreover, solvents such as chloroform, eucalyptol, and xylol can also act as irritants.[227]

One must conclude that periradicular tissue reaction to all of the cements will at first be inflammatory, but as the cements reach their final set, cellular repair takes place unless the cement continues to break down, releasing one or more of its toxic components.

In retrospect, one must not overlook the casual observation made by the group at Tufts University: "There

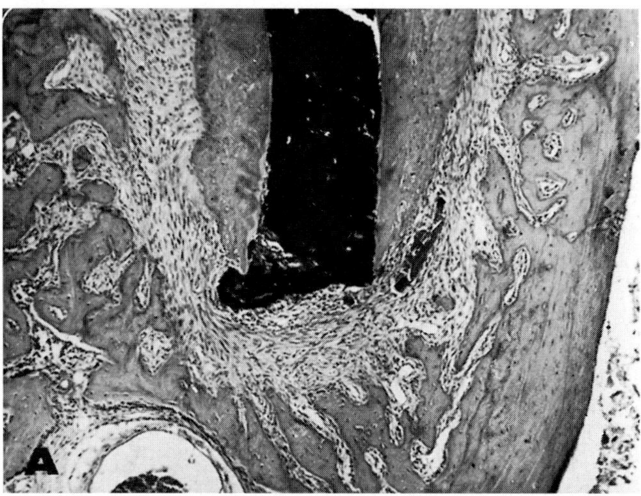

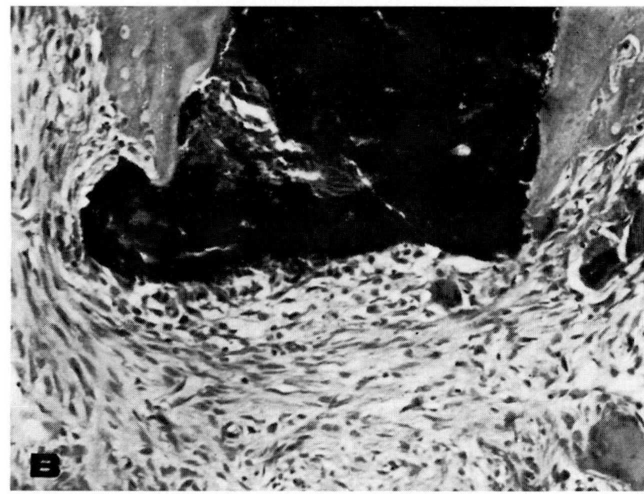

Figure 11-16 **A**, Moderate overfilling with **Diaket** 15 days postoperatively. Debris from instrumentation is to right of apex and black filling. **B**, High-power (×22 original magnification) view of Diaket and periapex. Loose connective tissue, abundance of fibroblasts, and some macrophages and giant cells are apparent. Dentinal debris (right border) is also being attacked by macrophages. Reproduced with permission from Erausquin J and Muruzabal M.[221]

were several small well-encapsulated areas of mild inflammation that seemed to be associated with apical ramifications that were not cleaned and that contained necrotic debris."[224] Although arborization of the pulp at the periapex is more apt to happen in dogs and monkeys than in humans, one cannot blink away the fact that a final filling is no better than its preparation, and if necrotic and infected dentin and debris are left in place, the case stands a greater chance of eventual failure.

One can summarize the discussion on root canal sealers by repeating a statement made more than 100 years ago by Dr. A. E. Webster of Toronto: "**It would seem that the dental profession has not yet decided upon a universal root canal filling material.**"[228]

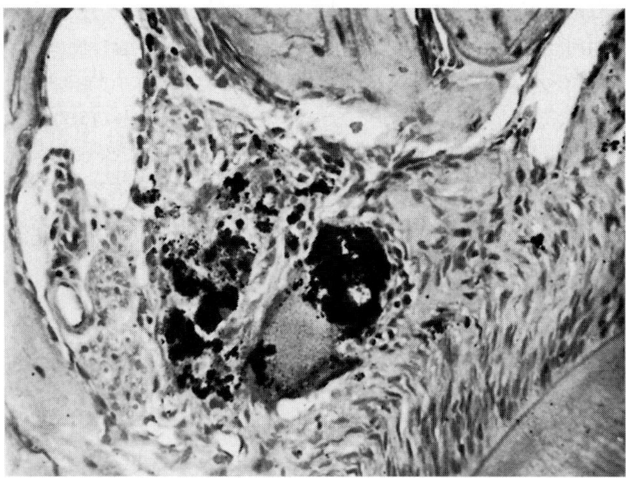

Figure 11-17 Fragments of **AH-26** scattered throughout periradicular tissue 30 days postoperatively, indicating resorption of sealer. Giant cells surrounded large fragment of AH-26. Reproduced with permission from Erausquin J and Muruzabal M.[221]

The N2/Sargenti Controversy. The term **N2,** as used here, is a code word for formaldehyde-containing endodontic cements. Actually, formaldehyde is a gas, whereas the forms used in dentistry are variations of formalin, the aqueous solution, or paraformaldehyde, a white crystalline polymer.

N2 itself contains 6.5% paraformaldehyde, as does its US counterpart, **RC2B.** Other paraformaldehyde/formalin-containing cements, popular in Europe, such as Endomethasone, Riebler's Paste, or the SPAD products, may contain more or less than 6.5% formaldehyde. All of them are toxic.

Legal Status in the United States. The controversy swirling around N2 and RC2B deserves special discussion. The use of these cements, recommended primarily by members of the American Endodontic Society (a group of general dentists), has become a *cause célèbre,* pitting endodontist against generalist, academician against practitioner. Along with these cements comes a method of practice—the so-called "Sargenti Method."

The method and Sargenti have been imported from Switzerland, but the N2 cement was barred at the borders by the FDA in about 1980. To evade the importation ban, disciples of Sargenti developed their own (and very similar) cement powder, RC2B. This was also banned under an FDA order that stated that the Agency "will take immediate regulatory action to stop the commercial manufacture and distribution of N2 type drugs" (R. J. Crout, personal communication, June 19, 1980).

The FDA pointed out, however, that they do not regulate the practice of dentistry and that "an endodontist or a 'general dentist' may use the N2 product themselves or arrange to have a supply obtained by prescription for **that individual patient.**" The dentist, however, should recognize that he is responsible for the consequences of the use of N2 within his practice (R. J. Crout, personal communication, June 19, 1980).

The basis for these actions and this warning is the statement, "The Food and Drug Administration has long held, and still does, that N2 has **not** been demonstrated to be safe and effective for use in root canal therapy" (R. J. Crout, personal communication, June 19, 1980).

As late as 1992, the FDA was still warning dentists that "...the N2 material is considered to be an unapproved new drug—and may not legally be imported or distributed in interstate commerce...,"[229] and in 1993 an advisory panel to the FDA rejected new drug application No. 19-182 submitted by N2 Products Corporation of Levittown, Pennsylvania.[230]

This action follows on the heels of jury awards of $250,000 in one case and $280,000 in another to patients injured by overextension of N2 into the periradicular tissues of two female patients.[229,231]

Paralegally, the Council on Dental Therapeutics of the American Dental Association reissued a resolution against paraformaldelyde sealers that concluded "that the FDA has not approved any products with this formulation, [so] the Council cannot recommend the use of these products at this time."[232] This report buttressed two previous negative pronouncements by Council in 1977 and 1987.[233,234]

At the state level, the Florida Board of Dentistry has banned "Sargenti cement, charging that use of the filling material falls short of the minimum standard of (dental) care in Florida."[235] This action was precipitated by a number of lawsuits, including an out-of-court settlement for $1,000,000 to a woman horribly disfigured after paraformaldehyde paste was misused (R. Uchin, personal communication, September 22, 1992).

The American Association of Endodontists has also issued a position statement condemning the use of paraformaldehyde sealers.[236]

Paraformaldehyde Toxicity. As initially compounded, N2 was a ZOE cement containing 6.5% paraformaldehyde as well as some lead and mercury salts. Concern over lead and mercury transport via the bloodstream to vital organs[237–247] forced the American producers of the N2 lookalike, RC2B, to drop the heavy metals. However, in no way would they reduce the toxic paraformaldehyde from the formula. A myriad of damaging research papers—*in vitro, in vivo,* clinical—denouncing these products, has been published in the last 25 years from all over the world.[248–256] Pitt-Ford found, for example, that N2 and Endomethasone caused a universal ankylosis and root resorption of dogs' teeth filled, but not overfilled, with these toxic products.[250]

The two most definitive *in vivo* studies on the effects of paraformaldehyde were done at Indiana University.[257,258] In a 1-month study using monkeys, researchers found apical periodontitis around 7 of 9 apices and "a granuloma with considerable loss of bone around another" when RC2B was applied to 10 inflamed pulps, as recommended by Sargenti. The "treated" pulps were in no better shape than the untreated inflamed controls.[257]

At 6 months and 1 year, severe periradicular inflammation with liquefaction necrosis developed after RC2B was applied to coronal pulps with pulpitis. None of the control teeth had periradicular inflammation.[258] When RC2B was used to fill well-prepared root canals, previously allowed to become necrotic, the results were even more overwhelming: osteomyelitis at 6 months and abscess formation, even cyst formation, within massive periradicular lesions at 1 year (Figure 11-18). The cases "treated" with RC2B were no better, or were worse, than the necrotic canal cases **left open** to salivary bacteria (Figure 11-19). Around a fragment of RC2B found in the tissue, advanced inflammation, necrosis, and even osteomyelitis were present (Figure 11-20). At the National Bureau of Standards, much the same destruction was found (Figure 11-21).[218]

The most important constituent in any of these cements (N2, RC2B, Endomethasone, SPAD) is the paraformaldehyde, according to their proponents. As a matter of fact, Sargenti allows for the removal of any ingredient from the powder **except** paraformaldehyde.[148] Unfortunately, it is this toxic product, unique to these cements, that causes the destruction. It is its release, as the sealers are resorbed, that allows for their destructive behavior. Neiburger reported a case showing radiographic disappearance of RC2B from the periapex within 5 weeks.[259] The Indiana group noted resorption of RC2B within 1 month.[257]

Nerve Damage from Paraformaldehyde. It has long been recommended by its proponents that N2 be placed in the canal with a fast-spinning Lentulo spiral. This is a perfectly reasonable approach, but one has to know when enough is enough. Sargenti warns that, without great care, overfilling is likely with this technique. He does not say, however, how very damaging such overextension will be.[148] Periradicular destruction was shown in the Indiana studies.[257,258] Also, "the ADA Council on Dental Therapeutics and Devices has

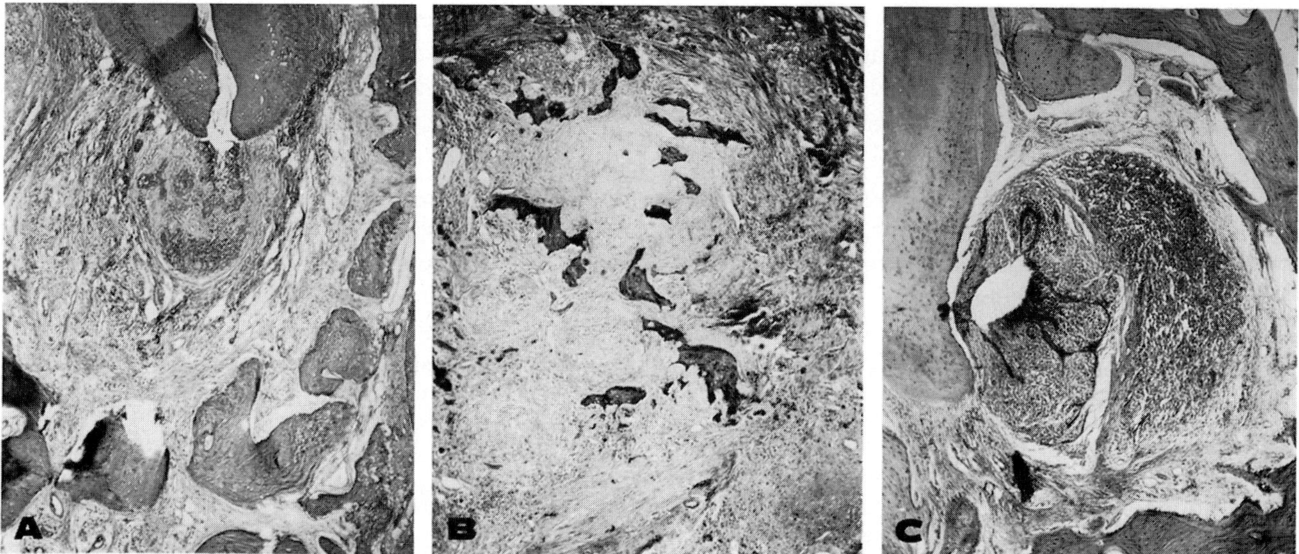

Figure 11-18 N2/RC2B formalin cement study. **A**, **Control** specimen, pulp necrosis 3 months standing. Apical granuloma with epithelial proliferation. **B**, Osteomyelitis 6 months after treatment of necrotic canal with RC2B. Areas of necrotic bone within dense inflammatory infiltrate. **C**, Apical cyst developing 6 months after treatment of necrotic canal with RC2B. Note epithelial lining within dense inflammatory infiltrate. Reproduced with permission from Newton CW et al.[258]

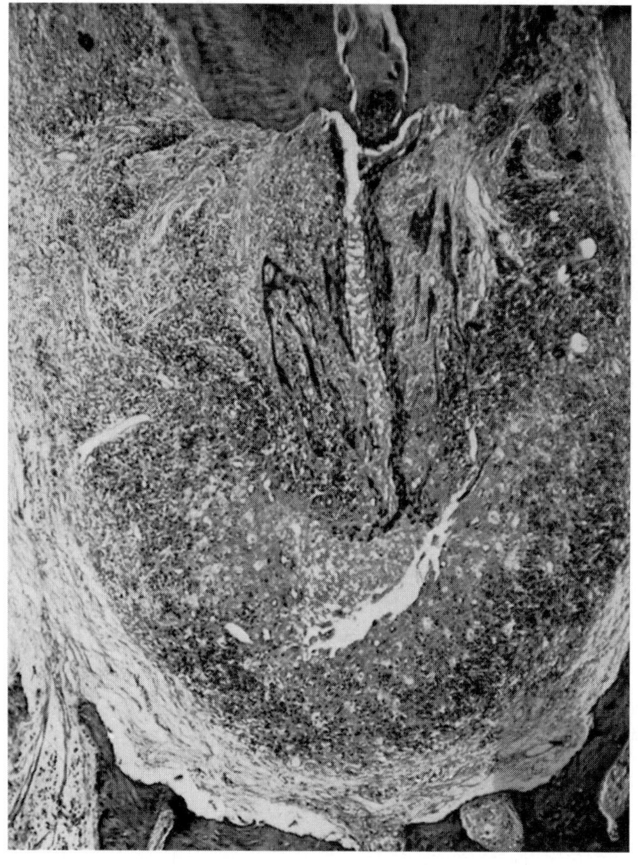

Figure 11-19 One year after treatment of necrotic canal with RC2B, large granuloma and strands of proliferating epithelium are apparent. Reproduced with permission from Newton CW et al.[258]

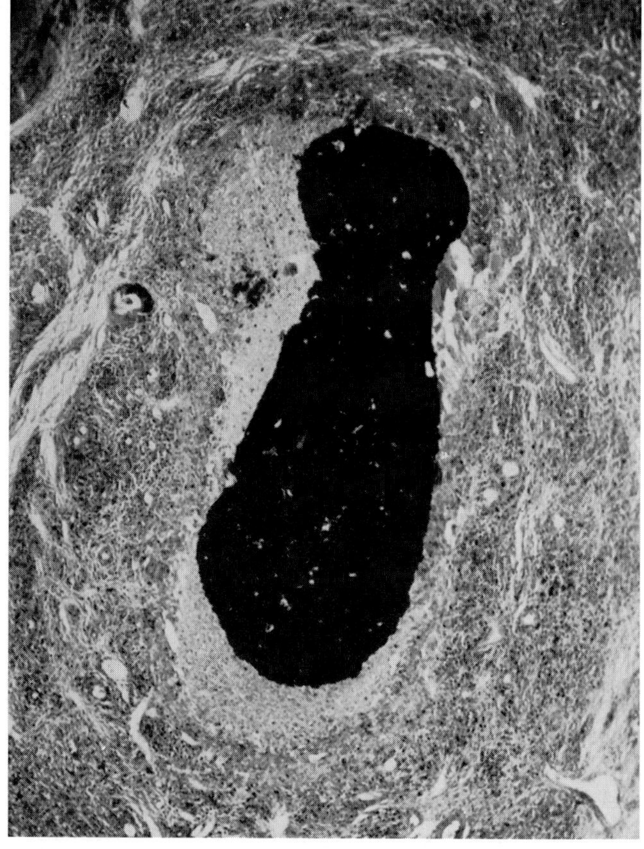

Figure 11-20 Overfill with **RC2B**. After 1 year, severe inflammation with necrosis is apparent. Adjacent bone was osteomyelitic. Reproduced with permission from Newton CW et al.[258]

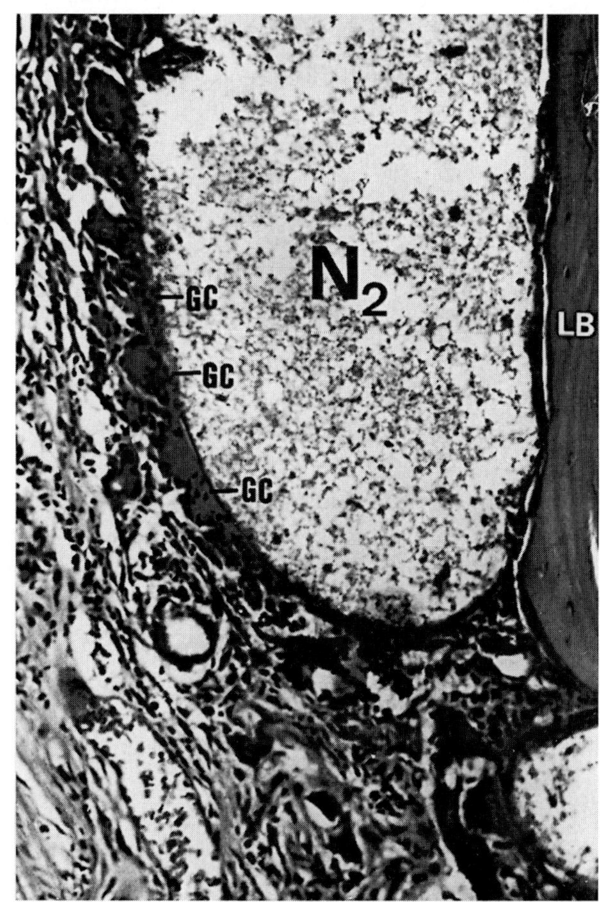

Figure 11-21 Monkey study, periradicular area, 2 months after **N2** overfill (N_2). Giant cells (GC) separating N_2 from connective tissue (**left**) and lamellar bone (LB) (**right**). Reproduced with permission from Hong YC et al.[218]

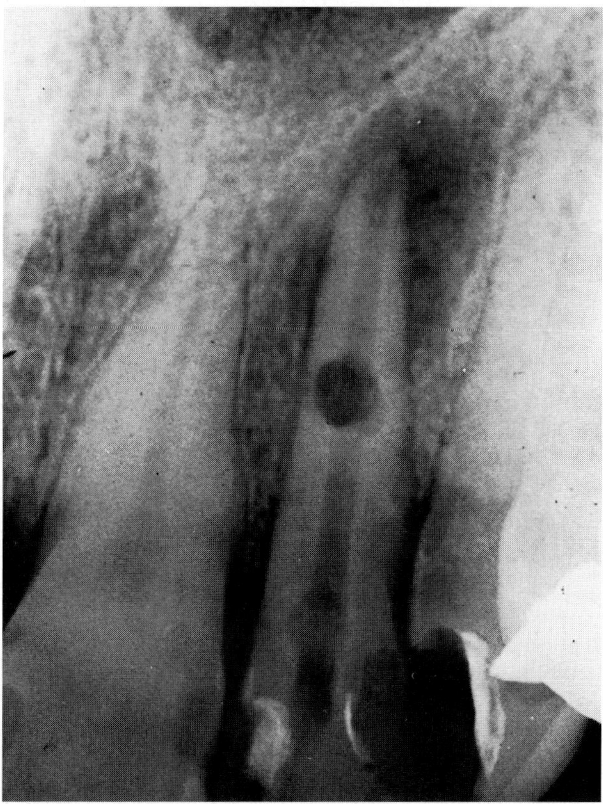

Figure 11-22 Perforation of maxillary incisor through incorrect use of **Fistulator**. (Courtesy of Dr. Alfred L. Frank.)

specifically cautioned dentists regarding severe postoperative complications that not infrequently accompany these [Sargenti] pastes when inadvertently extruded past the apex."[260]

Endodontic overfillings are no surprise to anyone who does root canal therapy. But, despite Sargenti's warning to his followers not to overfill, 15% of the 806 cases submitted for "Fellowship" status in the American Endodontic Society demonstrated overfilling.[261]

Reaction to the physical and chemical trauma of paraformaldehyde periradicularly can be so severe that immediate apical trephination is highly recommended by the Sargenti proponents. For this exigency, the dentist is supplied with a "Fistulator" to trephine to the periapex to relieve the pressure and pain that might follow treatment with N2 (Figure 11-22). A survey conducted by the American Endodontic Society of 48,134 cases treated by 411 dentists shows 9,910 cases of trephination.[148] This figure indicates that the method was necessary 20.5% of the time when N2 or RC2B was used.

An even greater problem occurs when N2 or RC2B is forced into the maxillary sinus or the mandibular canal. A number of cases of persisting paresthesia, primarily of the inferior alveolar nerve, have been reported following the misuse of paraformaldehyde cements.[262–268] That this accident can happen with any root canal sealer cannot be denied.[269–273] However, as Weichman, a lawyer-endodontist, points out, paresthesia from other cements gradually fades away (J. Weichman, personal communication, June 2, 1982). Paresthesia from paraformaldehyde, on the other hand (since the nerve is literally embalmed), may remain forever (Figure 11-23). From Ankara, Turkey, a comparative study of the neurotoxic effects of sealers revealed that formalin cements caused a faster and more prolonged inhibitory effect on nerve transmission, as well as paresthesia, than did other tested sealers.[207]

After reviewing the literature in 1988, Brodin noted that more than 40 cases of neurotoxicity caused by overfilling had been reported and that "sealers containing formaldehyde were irreversible unless surgical treatment was performed (22 of 25 cases)."[274] Since then, a number of cases involving N2, RC2B, SPAD, and Endomethasone have been reported.[275–278]

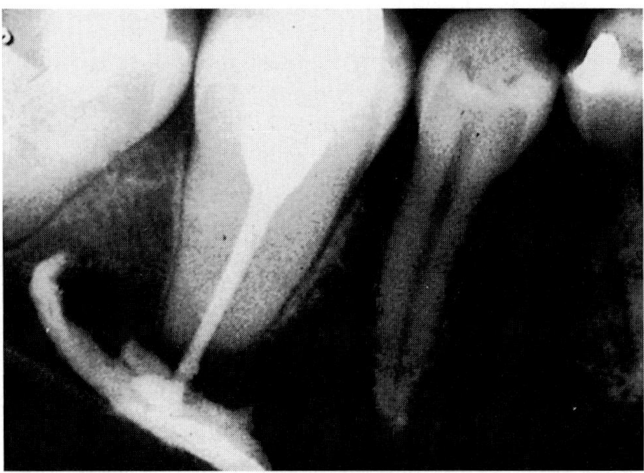

Figure 11-23 Massive overextension of **RC2B** into inferior alveolar canal. Patient suffered permanent paresthesia. Lawsuit settled out of court against dentist and in favor of 26-year-old female secretary in Pennsylvania. (Courtesy of Edwin J. Zinman, DDS, JD)

The tragedy of overfilling into the mandibular canal, especially with such toxic materials, relates to a misconception of the size of the pulp. Dentists spin more and more material into the canal, far more than it takes to fill the space. Fanibunda points out that the average pulp space of a maxillary central incisor is the size of a drop of water. This is the **entire** pulpal space, crown and root. The root canal is only a small portion of this volume. A mandibular molar pulp space would hold only four drops, pulp chamber included.[279] Enough is enough!

In summation, one might ask, "Why isn't the Sargenti method taught in American dental schools?"[280] and "Why does the Sargenti method raise so many troublesome questions?"[281] The answer to both questions is rather simple. The Sargenti method has become a cult and, like most cults, is based more on testimonials than on facts. The second reason, of course, relates to the toxic components of the material that the cult insists are necessary to success.

These reasons, along with the countless lawsuits and out-of-court settlements centering around the technique and cements, keep many from joining while many desert the ranks. Pitt-Ford reports the same turnaround in Britain. "N2 is now seldom used—probably because of the numerous reports of its adverse effects and the fact that it is not recommended by dental schools."[250]

Sargenti himself indicated a double standard of endodontic treatment when he publicly stated, "If I had endodontic problems myself, and if I wished to have an exact endodontic treatment, I should certainly ask Dr. Herbert Schilder to treat me."[282]

PREPARATION FOR OBTURATION

To this point, a good deal has been said about the materials that go into the canal: their efficacy, their toxicity, their resorbability. But as the old adage goes, "What comes out of the canal is much more important than what goes into it." For this reason, great emphasis has been placed on radicular preparation and débridement—"biochemical preparation" à la Grossman or "cleaning and shaping" per Schilder.

Even if the canal space is perfectly débrided and is free of all debris and bacteria, what of the dentin walls left? Are they free of bacteria? Are they prepared to adhere to the obturating material or will the sealants chemically adhere to them? One look at these so-called "glassy smooth" walls in an electron micrograph leaves one in doubt (Figure 11-24, A). The smear layer may also be loaded with bacteria that penetrate out of the layer into the dentinal tubules (Figure 11-24, B).

The Dentin Interface

"Many of our currently accepted methods of chemomechanical preparation are inadequate in producing a debris-free canal."[283] In addition to the pulp tissue debris and bacteria, several papers have described a sludge or a "smeared layer" left attached to the inner canal walls, obstructing the dentinal tubules.[283–289] Goldman and colleagues have demonstrated that the smear layer, created by instrumentation, is primarily calcific (inorganic) in nature.[290]

However, there is also an organic component, undoubtedly reflecting the chemical composition of dentin: the greater inorganic and lesser organic component of the smear layer,[291] as well as necrotic tissue and bacteria. Remember that the smear layer is subject to early dissolution, and if apical leakage occurs, the loss of the smear layer will provide an easy ingress for fluid and bacteria.

There is no direct evidence that the smear layer must be removed. On the other hand, Yamada et al. state that a case can be made for its removal: "For instance, it may interfere with the adaptation of filling materials to the canal wall by imposing an additional interface."[283] At Aristotle University in Greece, researchers reported that "smear layer removal resulted in a statistically significant reduction in microleakage when AH26 was used as a sealer. However, the presence or absence of the smear layer had no significant effect on the sealing ability of Roth 811."[292] In another vein, Yamada et al. went on to state, "In addition, opening all the tubules can perhaps provide a better seal by allowing sealer or filling material to penetrate" the dentin.[283]

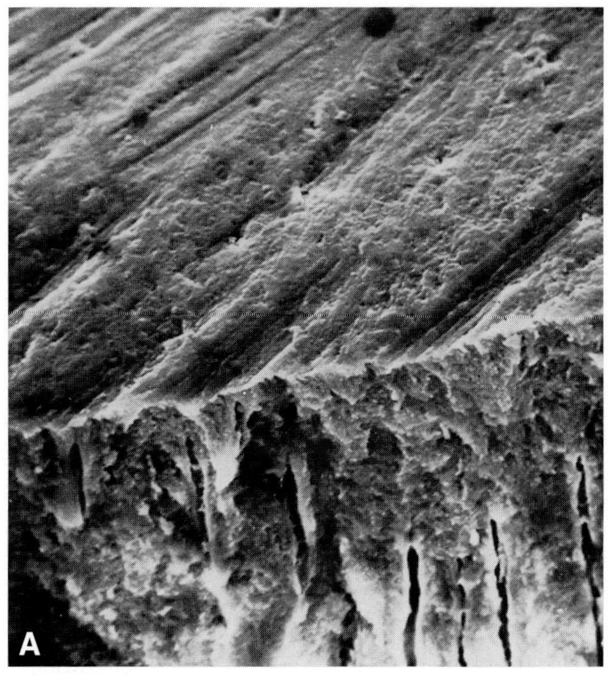

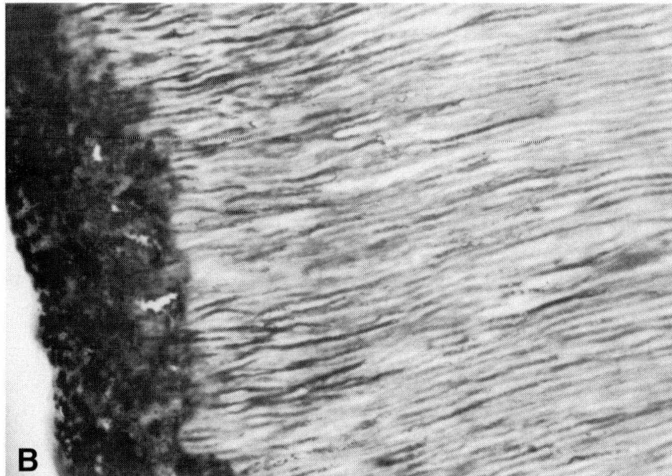

Figure 11-24 A, Scanning electron micrograph view of dentin smear layer. **Top half** of photo is smear. **Lower half** of cut surface shows occluded tubuli. B, Smear layer (**left**) after canal preparation. Note packed debris and extensions into tubuli. (Courtesy of Drs. Martin Brännström and James L. Gutmann.)

Gutmann, for example, has noted that thermoplasticized gutta-percha, and of course sealer, penetrates well into patent tubules freed of the smear layer.[284] An Athens research group also pointed out the importance of using ethylenediaminetetraacetic acid (EDTA) to remove any calcium hydroxide clinging to the dentin walls and thus blocking the tubuli.[293]

Opening the tubuli makes great sense. If chemical adhesion between the dentin and sealers, pastes, cements, or plastics cannot be achieved, then why not a mechanical lock? The material will flow or be forced back into the empty dentin tubules, gripping like tentacles and forever resisting displacement (see Figure 11-12, B).

Opening the orifices of the dental tubules can be achieved with acids as shown by Loel,[294] Tidmarsh,[295] Waymen and colleagues,[296] and Pashley and colleagues,[297] using various strengths of citric, phosphoric, or lactic acid (Figure 11-25), or by others using EDTA as chelators.[288,298–308] Calt and Serper, using EDTA, also pointed out the importance of removing calcium hydroxide dressing from the dentinal walls to open the tubuli.[309]

More recently, workers at Tufts University found that "...the combined use of 10 cc of 17% EDTA (pH.7.5) followed by 10 cc of 5.25% sodium hypochlorite (NaOCl) produced the best overall results in removing both superficial debris and the smeared

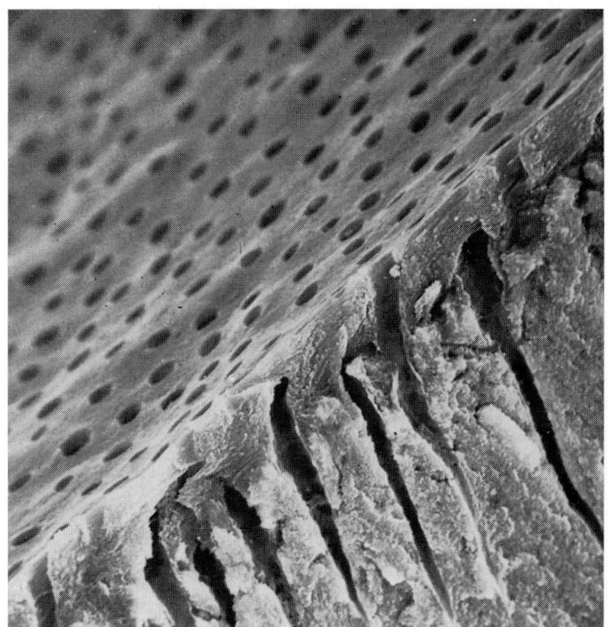

Figure 11-25 Scanning electron microscope view of smear layer etched away and tubuli opened by a 2-minute application of 37% phosphoric acid. A similar effect can be achieved in 5 to 15 seconds. (Courtesy of Dr. Martin Brännström.)

layer"[283] (Figure 11-26). A group in Turkey achieved a similar result using 17% EDTA combined with 5% ethylenediamine, an organic solvent.[285] In arriving at these conclusions, they had tested saline, citric acid (25%), and various combinations of sodium hypochlorite and EDTA. The chelator (EDTA) was very efficient in removing the inorganic (calcium salts) from the smear layer all the way to the apical third. But the sodium hypochlorite was needed to dissolve and douche away the organic (dentin matrix, pulp remnants, necrotic and bacterial debris) constituents of the smear. It goes without saying that sodium hypochlorite irrigation was used between instrument sizes during canal preparation.

Recent research reinforces the evidence that smear removal is efficacious. One must bear in mind Rawlinson's findings, however, that 1 minute of ultrasonic irrigation with citric acid and sodium hypochlorite did not remove all of the smear layer in the important apical third.[127] The Minnesota group recommended 3 minutes of irrigation, each with EDTA and sodium hypochlorite. This improved the bond with AH-26.[302] The original group at Tufts used 10 cc each of EDTA and sodium hypochlorite[306,307] to improve the bond with Bis GMA resin.[126] Others reported improved bonding with ZOE, SealApex, AH-26, TubliSeal, and Diaket.[302–309]

With this final smear layer removal, the dentin interface needs only thorough drying to be ready to receive the obturating materials.

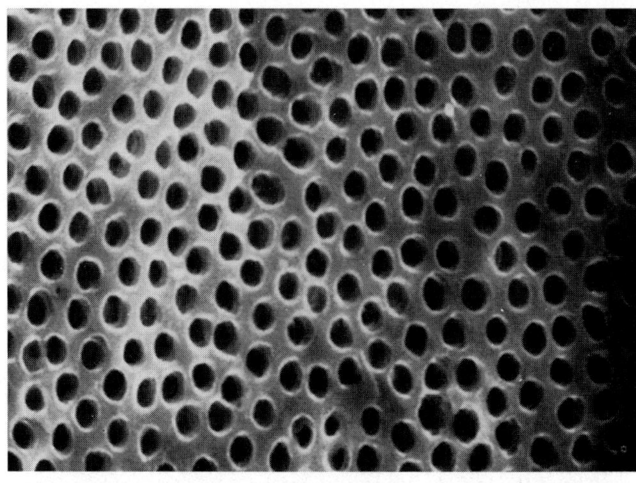

Figure 11-26 Dentinal tubuli cleaned of smear layer and opened following combined use of ethylenediaminetetraacetic acid and sodium hypochlorite. Reproduced with permission from Yamada RS et al.[283]

METHODS OF OBTURATING THE ROOT CANAL SPACE

Over the years, countless ways and materials have been developed to fill prepared canals. Again, Webster noted over 100 years ago, "...it would seem that the dental profession has not yet decided upon a universal root canal filling material."[228] At least today's attempts seem a bit more sophisticated than the "cotton, raw cotton, and cotton and gutta-percha," noted by Webster. On the other hand, he favorably recommended warm gutta-percha and vertical compaction, but also noted that warmed gutta-percha shrinks when it cools.[228]

Today, most root canals are being filled with gutta-percha and sealers. The methods vary by the direction of the compaction (lateral or vertical) and/or the temperature of the gutta-percha, either cold or warm (plasticized).

These are the two basic procedures: lateral compaction of cold gutta-percha or vertical compaction of warmed gutta-percha. Other methods are variations of warmed gutta-percha.

The methods are listed as follows:

I. Solid Core Gutta-Percha with Sealants
  A. Cold gutta-percha points
    1. Lateral compaction
    2. Variations of lateral compaction
  B. Chemically plasticized cold gutta-percha
    1. Essential oils and solvents
      a. Eucalyptol
      b. Chloroform
      c. Halothane
  C. Canal-warmed gutta-percha
    1. Vertical compaction
    2. System B compaction
    3. Sectional compaction
    4. Lateral/vertical compaction
      a. Endotec II
    5. Thermomechanical compaction
      a. Microseal System, TLC, Engine-Plugger, and Maillefer Condenser
      b. Hybrid Technique
      c. J.S.-Quick-Fill
      d. Ultrasonic plasticizing
  D. Thermoplasticized gutta-percha
    1. Syringe insertion
      a. Obtura
      b. Inject-R-Fill, backfill
    2. Solid-core carrier insertion
      a. Thermafil and Densfil,
      b. Soft Core and Three Dee GP
      c. Silver points

II. Apical-Third Filling
  A. Lightspeed Simplifill

Figure 11-27 ISO standardized spreaders and matching gutta-percha points. A, Size #25 hand spreader and matching gutta-percha point. B, Size #25 finger spreader and matching gutta-percha point. Instruments and points are color-coded the same. (Spreaders courtesy of Dentsply/Maillefer Co. Points courtesy of Coltene Whaledent/Hygenic Co.)

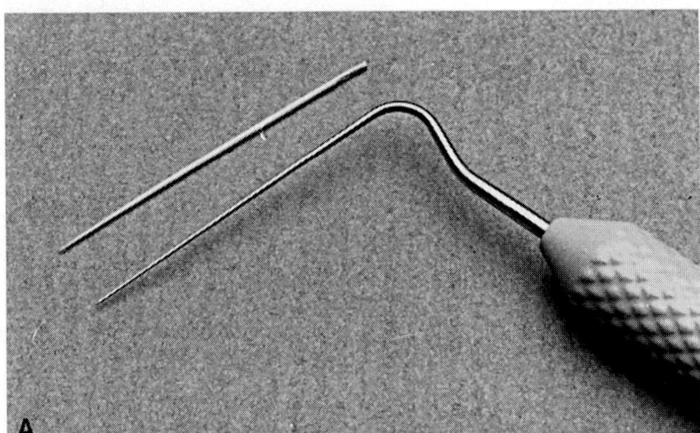

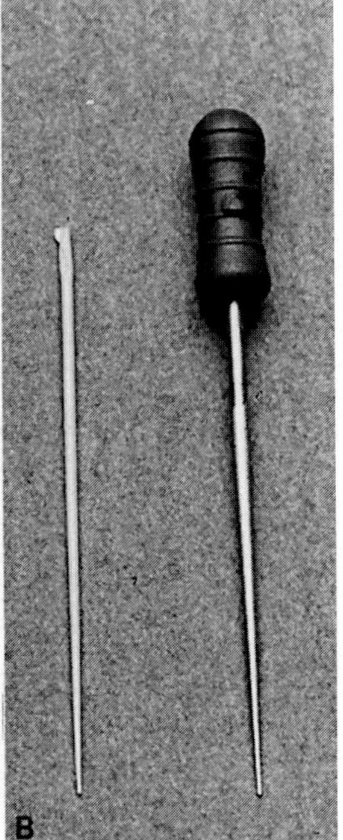

   B. Dentin-chip
   C. Calcium hydroxide

III. Injection or "Spiral" Filling
   A. Cements
   B. Pastes
   C. Plastics
   D. Calcium phosphate

The "compleat" clinician will master many, if not all, of these techniques. The rigidity of being "married" to one particular method or material limits not only case acceptance but success as well.

Lateral Compaction of Cold Gutta-percha

The lateral compaction of cold gutta-percha points with sealer is the technique most commonly taught in dental schools and used by practitioners and has long been the standard against which other methods of canal obturation have been judged. This technique encompasses first placing a sealer lining in the canal, followed by a measured primary point, that in turn is compacted laterally by a plugger-like tapering spreader used with vertical pressure, to make room for additional accessory points (Figure 11-27). The final mass of points is severed at the canal's coronal orifice with a hot instrument, and final vertical compaction is done with a large plugger. If executed correctly, solid canal obturation will totally reflect the shape and diversions of the properly prepared canal network (Figure 11-28).

Lateral condensation can only be achieved if certain criteria are fulfilled in canal preparation and instrument selection. The final canal shape should be a **continuous taper**, approaching parallel in the apical area, that matches the taper of the spreader/plugger. The

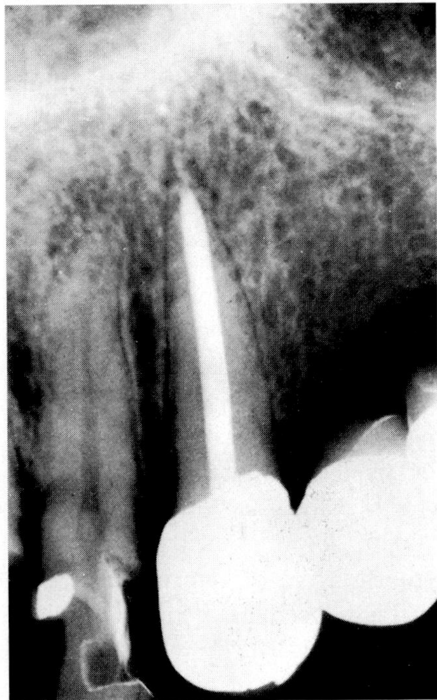

Figure 11-28 Complete root canal obliteration using multiple point technique. Notice density of gutta-percha mass. Filling conforms exactly to size and shape of last endodontic instrument used.

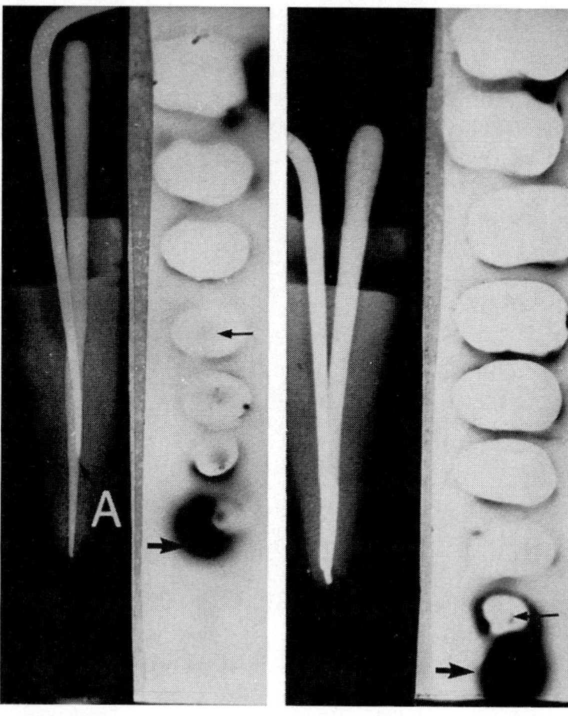

Figure 11-29 Microleakage into obturated canals related to flare of cavity preparation and depth of spreader penetration. **Left**, Final depth of spreader, A, is 5 mm short of prepared length of canal. Radioisotope leakage is 4.8 mm (**between arrows**) into canal. **Right**, Canal with flared preparation allows spreader depth to within 1 mm of primary point length. Radioisotope leakage (**between arrows**) only 0.8 mm into canal. Reproduced with permission from Allison DA et al.[310]

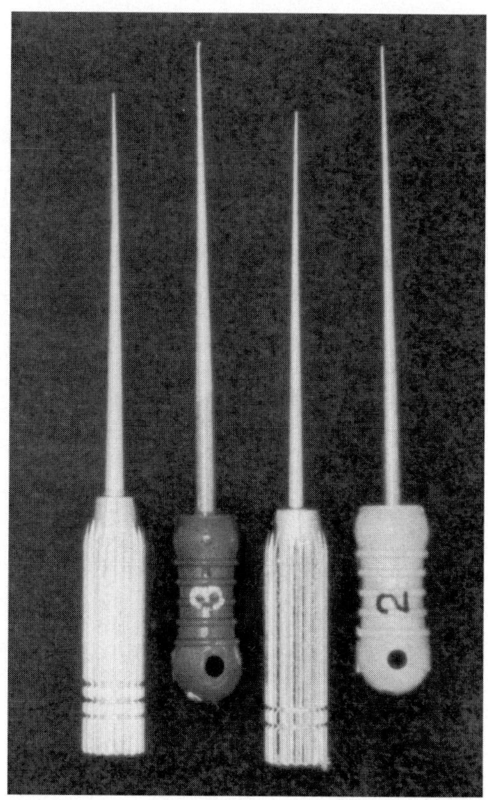

Figure 11-30 **Luks finger pluggers** are available in four different sizes and two lengths. The apical diameter is the same for all—a little less than 0.20 mm—and they vary in increasing diameters of their taper. (Courtesy of Dr. Carl W. Newton.)

spreader must reach within 1.0 to 2.0 mm of the working length (Figure 11-29), an apical stop must be created to resist apically directed condensation, and the accessory gutta-percha cones must be smaller in diameter than the spreader/plugger (see Figure 11-27). Lateral condensation is not the technique of choice in preparations that cannot meet these criteria and not all canals can be shaped to meet these criteria. Before embarking on the filling process, however, several important steps in preparation must first be completed: **spreader size determination, primary point and accessory point size determination, drying the canal, and mixing and placement of the sealer.**

Spreader Size Determination. Before trying in the trial point, it is mandatory to fit the spreader to reach to within 1.0 to 2.0 mm of the true working length and to match the taper of the preparation. Spreaders are available that have been numbered to match the instrument size (Figure 11-30). Therefore, a spreader of the same apical instrument size or one size larger is chosen so that it reaches to within 1.0 to 2.0 mm but will not penetrate the apical orifice. Not all canals can be shaped to fit the variety of lengths and tapers of available spreaders. This technique requires a knowledge and understanding of the size and shapes created by different cleaning and shaping instruments, as well as of the spreaders. If the spreader taper is greater than the canal taper, there will be an apically directed force during condensation that can result in overfill. If the taper of the canal is greater than that of the spreader, there is a tendency to displace the master cone coronally during condensation.

Allison and his colleagues at the University of Georgia vividly demonstrated the importance of deep spreader penetration. They also pointed out that "the most important factor affecting the quality of the apical seal is the shape of the canal," a true tapered preparation that would allow the spreader to nearly reach the apical terminus. Canals so treated had virtually no apical percolation[310] (Figure 11-31). Spreaders should always be fit into an empty canal (Figure 11-32) to ensure that the force is absorbed by the gutta-percha and not the canal walls, which could result in root fracture. After the gutta-percha is placed, and the spreader is inserted but does not reach the premeasured depth, condensation of the gutta-percha will occur laterally

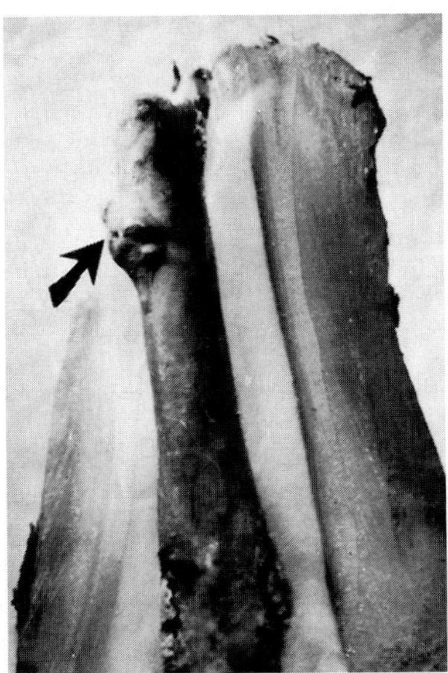

Figure 11-31 Prepared root canal obturated by lateral condensation of gutta-percha and sealer. Note extension of gutta-percha into depression in canal (**arrow**). (Courtesy of Dr. J. H. Gutiérrez and Dr. C. Gigoux, Concepcion, Chile.)

from a force directed from the canal walls toward the gutta-percha.

A rubber stop should be placed on the shaft of the spreader to mark true working length **minus 1 mm.** It is then set aside for immediate use.

Primary Point Size Determination. Gutta-percha **points** have been **standardized** in size and shape to match the standardized instrument sizes. They have even been color-coded to match the instrument's color. **Conventional sized cones** are too tapered with a bulk of material in the coronal area that would resist penetration of the spreader. However, nothing should be left to chance; the primary point should be selected to match the size of the last instrument used at the apex and should be tested in place and confirmed radiographically.

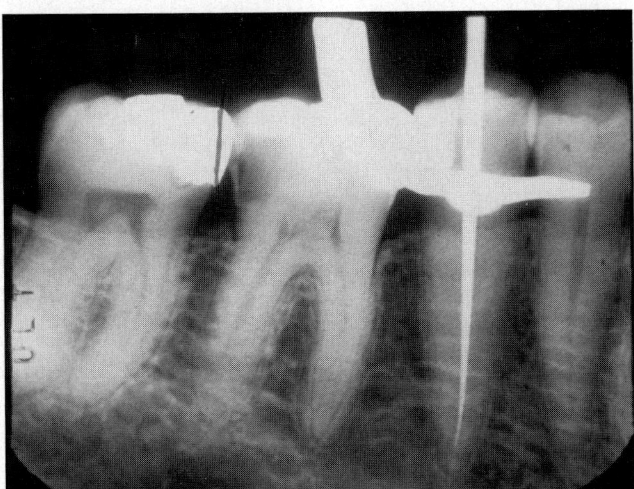

Figure 11-32 The **Luks plugger** is premeasured and placed in the empty canal to verify penetration into the apical 1.0 to 2.0 mm. Condensation at this depth can be achieved with the assurance that the gutta-percha will absorb the pressure and not the canal walls. (Courtesy of Dr. Carl W. Newton.)

Gutta-percha comes sterilized from the package or it may be sterilized with a germicide for 5 minutes in sodium hypochlorite (5.25%), hydrogen peroxide (3%), or chlorhexidine (2%).[311,313] Gutta-percha itself does not readily support bacterial growth.[313]

The four methods used to determine the proper fit of the primary point are as follows: (1) visual test, (2) tactile test, (3) patient response, and (4) radiographic test.

Visual Test. To test the point visually, it should be measured and grasped with cotton pliers at a position within **1 mm short** of the prepared length of the canal. The point is then carried into the canal until the cotton pliers touch the external reference point of the tooth. This master point should always be tried in a **wet canal** to simulate the lubrication of the sealer. If the working length of the tooth is correct and the point goes completely to position, the visual test has been passed unless the point can be pushed beyond this position. This can be determined by grasping **1 mm farther back** on the point and attempting to push it apically. If the point can be pushed to the root end, it might well be pushed beyond into the tissue. Either the foramen was originally large or it has been perforated. If the point can be extended beyond the apex, the next larger size point should be tried. If this larger point does not go into place, the original point may be used by cutting pieces off the tip. Each time the tip is cut back 1 mm, the diameter becomes larger by approximately .02 mm. By trial and error, the point is retried in the canal until it goes to the correct position.

Jacobsen has shown the distortion in the point that ensues if scissors are used to "snip" off the tip. He shows that distortion can be avoided by "rolling the point back and forth on a sterile glass plate and applying gentle pressure with a No. 15 scalpel blade"[314] (Figure 11-33). The main reason for trial point testing is to be sure the point extends far enough for total obturation but will not extend beyond the apical foramen. The termination of the point within 1 mm short of the prepared length provides for **apical movement from the vertical forces** of compaction aided by lubrication from the sealant. One cannot predictably rely on the spreader to seat the master point if it has not been confirmed to the desired position. If everything is right, the solid-core material is sealed exactly into the prepared space, not pushed beyond into an overfill.

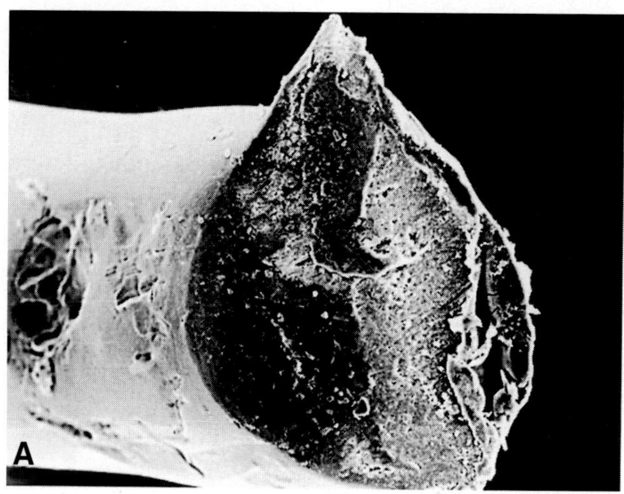

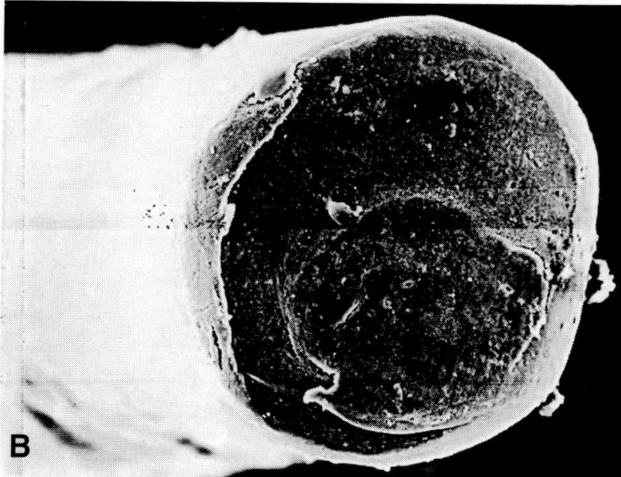

Figure 11-33 Length-adjusted gutta-percha points. A, Size 30 gutta-percha point shortened with scissors. Distortion prevents proper placement at apical seal. B, Size 30 gutta-percha point trimmed with scalpel, allowing more perfect apical fit. Reproduced with permission from Jacobsen EL.[314]

Tactile Test. The second method of testing the trial point is by **tactile sensation** and will determine whether the point tightly fits the canal. In the event the apical 3 to 4 mm of the canal have been prepared with near **parallel walls** (in contrast to a continuous taper), some degree of force should be required to seat the point, and, once it is in position, a pulling force should be required to dislodge it. This is known as "**tugback.**" Allison and the Georgia group have shown, however, that significant tugback in primary gutta-percha point placement is not essential to ensure a proper root canal seal.[315]

Again, if the point is **loose** in the canal, the next larger size point should be tried, or the method of cutting segments from the tip of the initial point, followed by trial and error positioning, should be used. Care must be taken not to force the sharp tip of a point through the foramen.

Patient Response. Patients who are not anesthetized during the treatment of a nonvital pulp or at the second appointment of a vital pulp may feel the gutta-percha penetrate the foramen. Adjustments can then be made until it is completely comfortable. This is a good test when the position of the foramen does not appear to be accurately determined by the radiograph or by tactile sensation. Pulp remnants from a short preparation will cause a sensation of much greater intensity than periapical tissue. Granulation tissue may not produce any sensation at all.

Radiograph Test. After the visual and tactile tests for the trial point have been completed, its position must be checked by the final test—the **radiograph** (Figure 11-34). The film must show the point extending to within 1 mm from the tip of the preparation. **Radiographic** adaptation is a better criterion of success than either the visual or tactile method.[315]

The trial point radiograph presents the final opportunity to check all of the operative steps of therapy completed to date. It will show whether the **working length** of the tooth was correct, whether instrumentation followed the **curve of the canal**, and whether a **perforation developed.** It will also, of course, show the relationship of the initial filling point to the preparation.

Occasionally the radiograph shows the point forced well beyond the apex. If this is the case, an incorrect working length has been used during instrumentation, and the operator may have wondered why the patient complained of discomfort. The overextended point

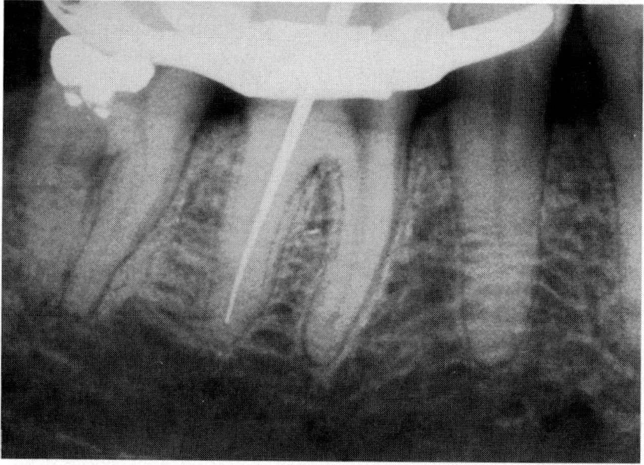

Figure 11-34 Trial point radiograph. Confirmation film indicates the primary point should be advanced by another 2.0 mm by either enlarging one more size or trying the next smaller point. (Courtesy of Dr. Carl W. Newton.)

should always be shortened from the fine end and then carefully returned to proper position. It should **never be just pulled back** to a new working length, in which case it would be loose in the canal. In this new position, it should again pass the tactile and radiographic tests of trial points. It should never be manipulated so that it just **appears** to fit in the film. **It must fit tightly and come to a dead stop.**

Sometimes the initial point will not go completely into place even though it is the same number as the last enlarging instrument. This condition may arise because (1) the enlarging instrument was not used to its fullest extent, (2) there was a larger than standard deviation between the sizes of instruments and gutta-percha, (3) debris remains or was dislodged into the canal, or (4) a ledge exists in the canal on which the point is catching.

In any case, the problem can be solved by one of two methods: selecting a new file of the same number and re-instrumenting the canal to full working length until the file is loose in the canal, or selecting a smaller size gutta-percha point. Trial and error will determine when the point is seated. If a ledge has been developed in the canal wall, it must be removed by the method suggested in chapter 10.

Preparation of the Initial Point. After the initial point has passed the trial point tests, it should be removed with cotton pliers that scar the soft point or snipped with the scissors at the reference point (Figure 11-35).

Drying the Canal. While preparations are being made to cement the filling point, an absorbent paper point should be placed in the canal to absorb moisture or blood that might accumulate. Larger paper points are followed by smaller paper points until full length is achieved. To determine the presence of moisture in the canal, one must remove the absorbent point and draw the tip along the surface of the rubber dam. If the point is moist, it will leave a mark as it removes the powder from the dam. When this procedure has been repeated with fresh points that no longer streak the dam, the final paper point is left in place to be removed just as the sealer is to be introduced. Any bleeding should be stopped, the blood irrigated from the canal, and care taken to avoid penetrating beyond the apex with the final paper point. Excess moisture or blood may affect the properties of the sealer, although fluids may be completely displaced during condensation and not affect the seal.[316]

Mixing and Placement of the Sealer. *Mixing.* A sterile slab and spatula are removed from the instrument case or are sterilized by wiping with a gauze sponge soaked in germicide and dried with a sterile sponge. One or two drops of liquid are used and the cement is mixed according to the manufacturer's directions. The cement should be creamy in consistency but quite heavy, and should string out at least an inch when the spatula is lifted from the mix (Figure 11-36).

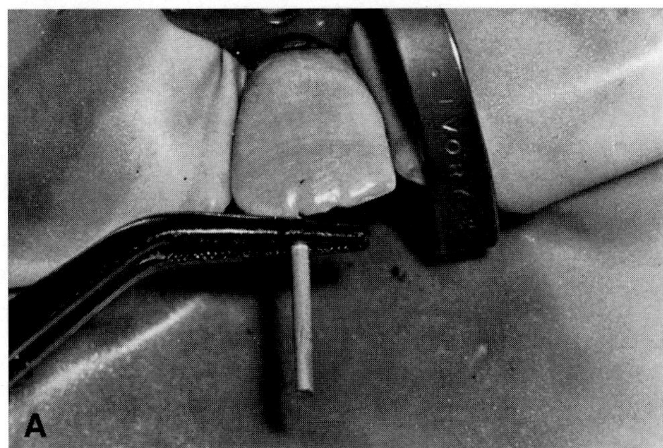

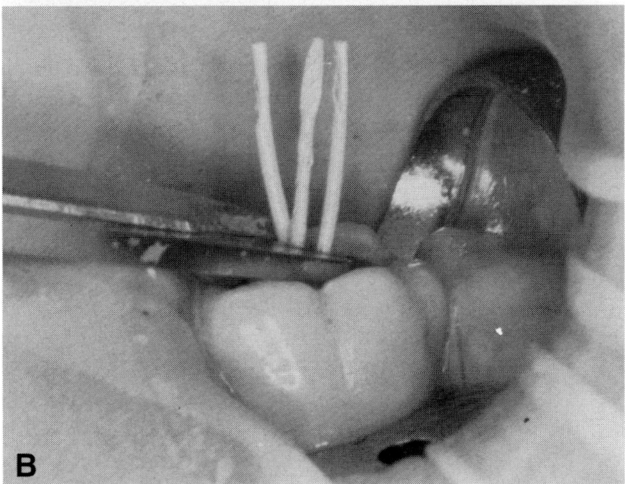

Figure 11-35 A, Removal of measured and tested initial gutta-percha point. Cotton pliers mark gutta-percha at incisal edge. B, Standardized points are seated at the working length and trimmed at the occlusal reference point with scissors. The master points should reach to within 1.0 mm of the working length. (Courtesy of Dr. Carl W. Newton.)

Benatti and colleagues tested five commercially available sealers and concluded that ideal consistency is achieved when the mixture can be held for 10 seconds on an inverted spatula without dropping off and will stretch between the slab and spatula 2 cm before breaking. Ideal consistency permits ample clinical working time and minimal dimensional change.[317]

Sealer should not be mixed too thin, but on the other hand, it must not be so viscous that it will not flow between the gutta-percha points or penetrate accessory and lateral canals or the dentin tubules.[318]

Placement. Sealer can be place in abundance to ensure thorough canal wall contact because the tech-

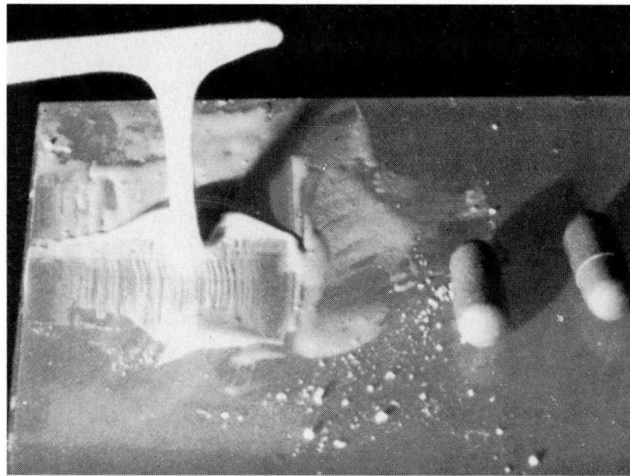

Figure 11-36 Root canal cement should be mixed to thick, creamy consistency, which may be strung off slab for 1 inch.

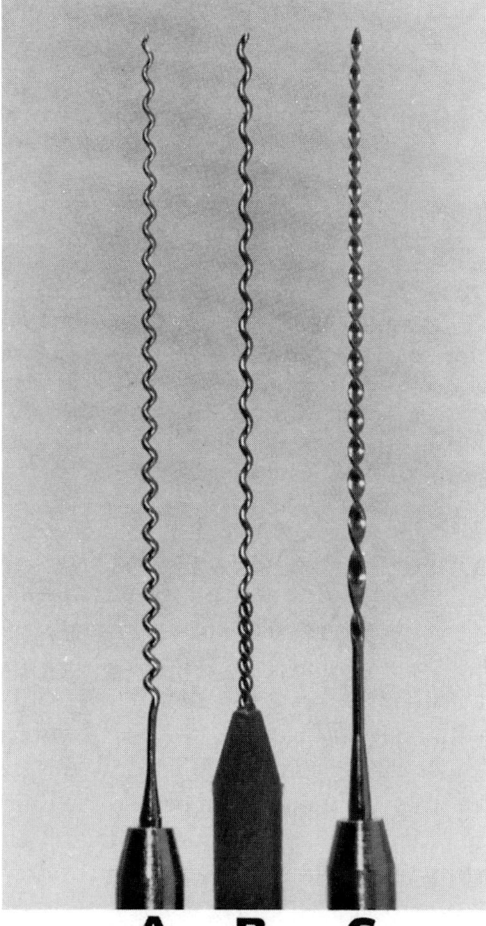

Figure 11-37 Rotary paste fillers made for contra-angle handpiece can also be rotated **clockwise** by finger action. Used for placing initial sealer with solid core root fillings or completely filling the canal with paste filling. **A**, Produits Dentaires, Switzerland. **B**, Micro Mega, France. **C**, Hawes-Neos, Switzerland. The Hawes-Neos type is preferred because of its stronger rectangular blade. (Courtesy of Dr. Frederick Harty, London.)

nique will displace all excess sealer coronally. Root canal cement/sealer may be placed in a number of ways. Some clinicians "pump" the sealer into the canal with a gutta-percha point. Some carry it in on a file or reamer, which is twirled counterclockwise, pumped up and down, and wiped against all the walls. Some use rotary or spiral paste fillers turned clockwise in one's fingers or very slowly in a handpiece (Figure 11-37).

Using rotary or spiral paste fillers is not without danger. If powered by a handpiece, they can be easily locked in the canal and snapped off (Figure 11-38). Twirling them in the fingers is safer, and Lentulo spirals are now being made with regular instrument handles (Dentsply/Maillefer; Tulsa, Okla. and Switzerland).

Another problem encountered in using rotary-powered Lentulo spirals comes from "whipping up" the cement in the canal and causing it to set prematurely. The primary point will then not go into place. Investigators in Scotland also found that the powered Lentulo spiral consistently caused sealer extrusion.[319]

A more recent method is to place the cement with an ultrasonic file—run without fluid coolant, of course.[319] A US Army group found **ultrasonic** endodontic sealer placement significantly superior (p = .001) to hand reamer placement. They were pleased to see proper coverage **to the apical orifice** but not beyond. Lateral and accessory canals were filled as well. As with the Lentulo spiral-placement, they found that ZOE cement set within a few seconds when ultrasonically spatulated in the canal. Heat generated by ultrasonics can acceler-

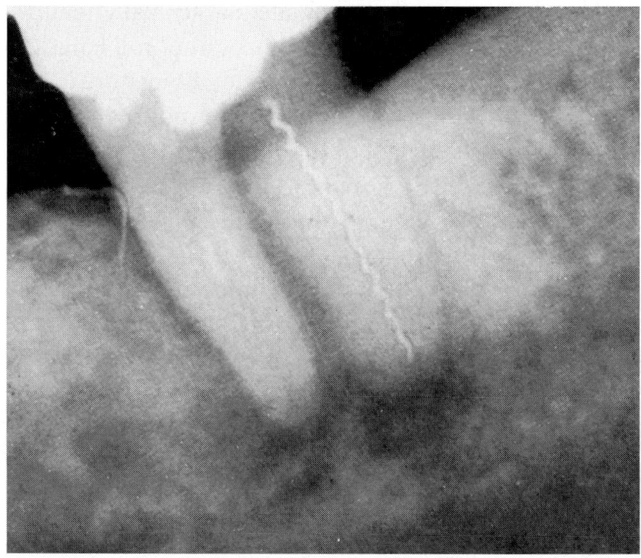

Figure 11-38 **Lentulo spiral** fractured in distal canal of lower molar. Careful observation reveals spiral also fractured in mesial canal and a cervical perforation and a broken reamer in mesial gingiva. (Retouched for clarity.)

ate ZOE sealers. However, they used AH-26 successfully.[320,321] A San Antonio group also found the Lentulo to be the most efficient in coating the walls: 90.2%, compared with using a K-file at 76.4% or using a gutta-percha point at 56.4%. They suggested that **complete** coverage may not be possible.[322]

Placement of the Master Point. The premeasured **primary** (or master, or initial) point is now coated with cement (Figure 11-39) and **slowly** moved to full working length. The sealer acts as a lubricant. The patient may experience some minor discomfort from this procedure as **air or sealer is evacuated** from the canal through the foramen. If the resistance form has been correctly prepared so that a "minimal opening" exists at the foramen, no more than, and usually not as much as, a **tiny puff** of cement will be forced from the apex.

It is frequently asked why the well-fitting initial point does not force a great quantity of cement through the apical foramen. The answer lies in the tapered shape of the point and corresponding shape of the canal. One should not think of the point as a plunger, for a plunger has straight walls. The tapered point does not actually touch the walls of the prepared canal until just that moment when it reaches its final seat. It will thus not force quantities of cement ahead of it, but will rather displace cement coronally as it is slowly moved into position. Thus one need not fear that there is an excessive amount of cement in the canal prior to placement of the point.

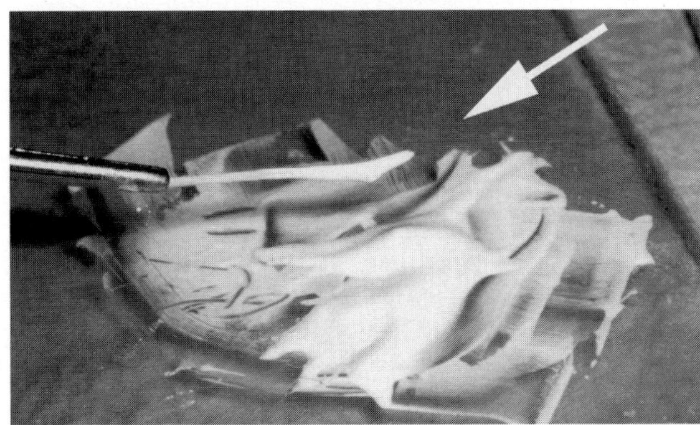

Figure 11-39 Primary point (**arrow**) coated with cement. Sealer may be used in abundance to ensure thorough coating since excess sealer will be displaced coronally in a properly shaped canal. (Courtesy of Dr. Carl W. Newton.)

Multiple-Point Obturation with Lateral Compaction

When the fit of the **cemented primary point** is ensured (Figure 11-40, A), the butt end, extending into the coronal cavity, should be removed with a hot instrument or scissors to allow room for visualization and the spreader that is to follow.

The **premeasured** spreader is then introduced into the canal alongside the primary point, and with a **rotary vertical motion** is slowly moved apically **to full penetration**, marked on the shaft with a silicone stop. (Figure 11-40, B). It is the wedging force that occurs between the canal walls toward the gutta-percha that results in deformation and molding of the gutta-percha to the opposite canal walls (Figure 11-41). There is no need to apply a lateral force to the spreader. Weine recommends that the initial spreader be left in place a full minute to allow the primary gutta-percha time to reconform to this pressure.[323] One must know that, along with the lateral force of spreading, a vertical force, albeit less, is also exerted.[315,324] If the spreader does not reach the premeasured length within the apical 1 mm, firm apical pressure can be applied with the knowledge that the gutta-percha, and not the tooth, is absorbing the force that could result in fracture (Figure 11-42). If full penetration is still not achieved, a spreader that is a size smaller can be used, which will bind apically to the previous spreader. The master point may appear to elongate slightly coronally as it stretches to plasticity at the point of condensation. Remember, adequate condensation does not occur unless the initial spreader reaches length.

The spreader is then removed with the same reciprocating motion and is immediately followed by the first auxiliary point inserted to the full depth of the space left by the spreader (Figure 11-40, C). Selecting auxiliary cones that are the same size or smaller in diameter or taper than the spreader requires a knowledge of ISO Standards for conventional gutta-percha cones and manufacturer's specifications for the chosen spreaders. Spreader penetration that is limited by a **bulk** of gutta-percha **in the midroot** area does not result in adequate condensation in the important apical area. Some clinicians use heat at this point to soften the bulk of gutta-percha and allow easier penetration through the coronal area. This point is followed by more spreading (Figure 11-40, D) and more points (Figure 11-40, E), more spreading and more points, until the entire root cavity is filled.

To ensure a cohesive filling, **additional sealer** should be added with each point as a lubricant to facilitate full penetration. Obturation is considered complete when the spreader can no longer penetrate the filling mass beyond the cervical line.

At this time the protruding points are severed at the orifice of the canal with a hot instrument (Figure 11-40, F). Vertical compaction with a large plugger will then ensure the tightest possible compression of the

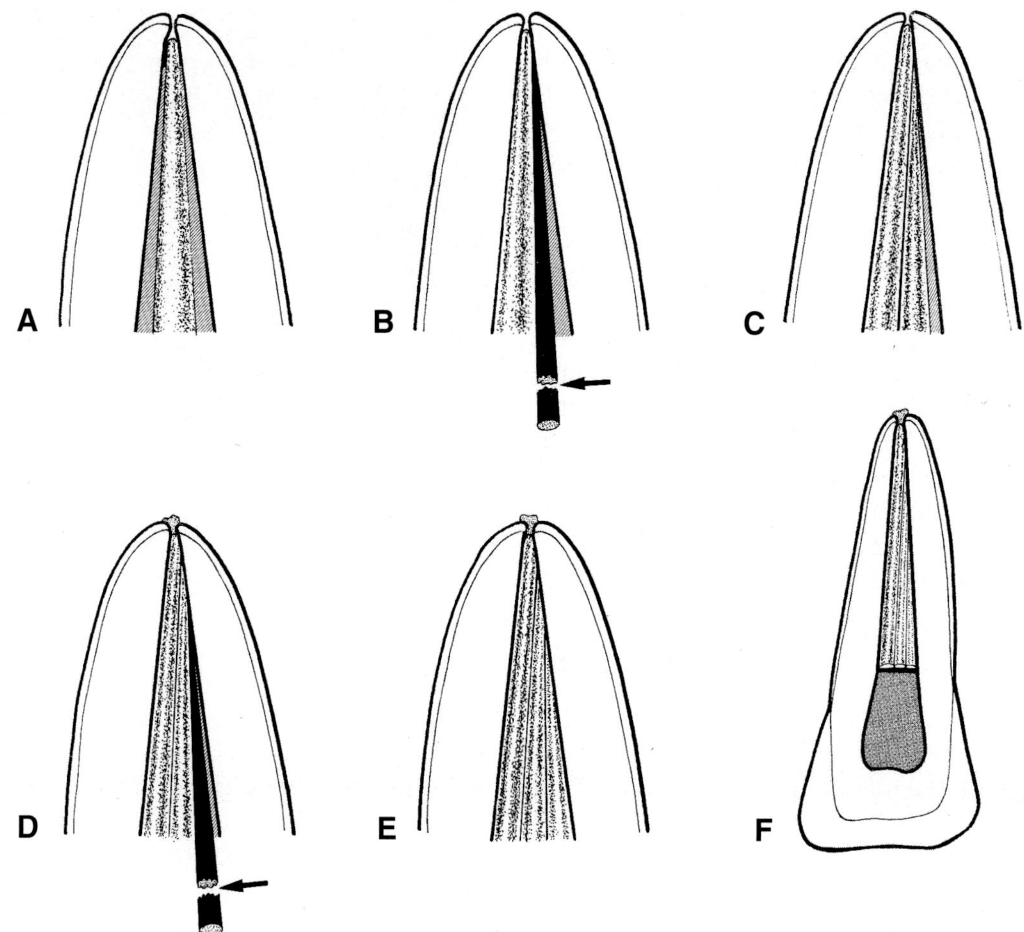

Figure 11-40 Lateral compaction, multiple-point filling procedure. Spreader has previously been tested to reach to within 1.0 mm of apical constriction. Thin layer of sealer lines canal walls, tip of point is coated with cement. **A**, Primary point is carried fully to place, to within 1.0 mm of "apical stop." Excess in crown is severed at cervical with hot instrument. **B**, Spreader (**arrow**) is inserted to full depth, allowed to remain 1 full minute as gutta-percha is compacted laterally and somewhat apically. **C**, Spreader is removed by rotation and immediately replaced by first auxiliary point previously dipped in sealer. **D**, Spreader (**arrow**) is returned to canal to laterally compact mass of filling. Secondary vertical compaction seals apical foramen. **E**, Spreader is again removed, followed by matching auxiliary point. Process continues until canal is totally obturated. **F**, All excess gutta-percha and sealer are removed from crown to below free gingival level. Vertical compaction completes root filling. After an intraorifice barrier is placed, a permanent restoration with adhesives is placed in crown.

gutta-percha mass and provide a more effective seal against coronal leakage.[325] All of the sealer and gutta-percha should then be removed from the pulp chamber and a final radiograph taken (Figure 11-43). After an intraorifice barrier is placed, either a final or temporary coronal filling should follow.

If one follows this technique—lateral compaction of cold gutta-percha points—a number of questions may arise: What size and style of spreader should be used? Which accessory gutta-percha points match the spreaders in size and taper? How much force should be used with a spreader? Can vertical fractures occur?

Spreader Size and Taper. Spreaders are supplied in multiple shapes, sizes, lengths, and tapers, including hand spreaders with a bent binangle shaft, and small straight finger spreaders. Nickel titanium has also improved flexibility and has been shown to penetrate to significantly greater depths than does stainless steel in curved canals.[326]

In 1955 Ingle drew attention to the discrepancy in spreader sizes as well as matching gutta-percha points.[327] After 35 years of confusion, the ISO/ADA endodontic standardization committee, in 1990, recommended that spreaders and pluggers be modeled after the accepted standardized instruments and gutta-percha points, No. 15-45 for spreaders and No. 15-140 for pluggers.

This new attempt to bring order out of chaos would abandon the old confusing numbering systems (1-10, D-11, D-11T, ABCD, XF, FF, MF, F, FM, M, etc) and recommend that all spreaders, pluggers, and auxiliary

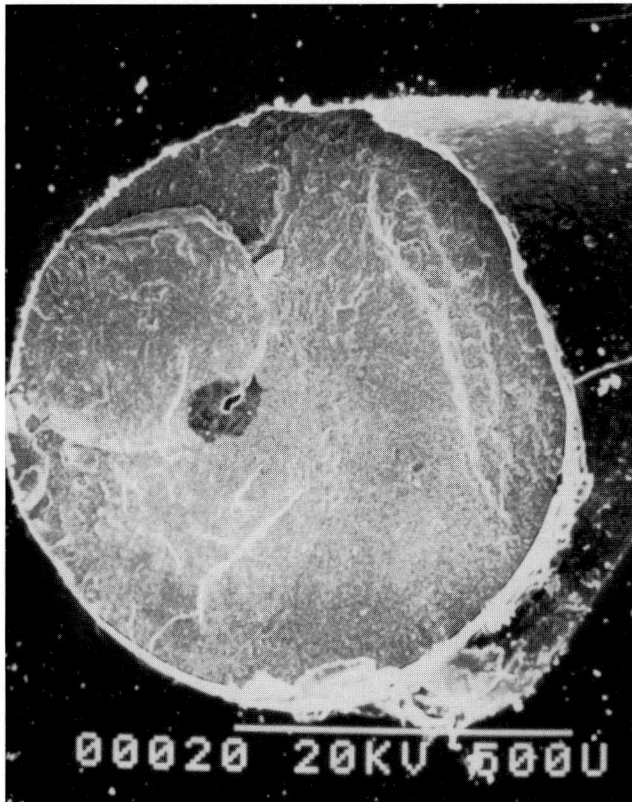

Figure 11-41 SEM cross-sections of lateral compaction illustrates how the gutta-percha is condensed in the apical area with the placement of the initial spreader. Note how all the spreader tracts occur from the canal wall into the gutta-percha in a "wedging" fashion and adapt the gutta-percha to the opposite walls. (Courtesy of Dr. Carl W. Newton.)

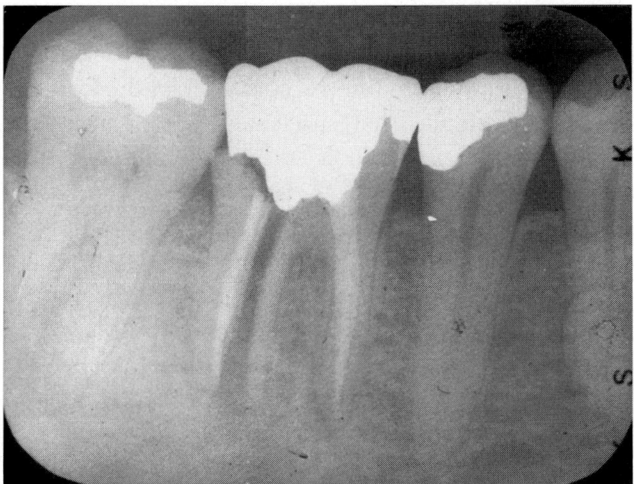

Figure 11-42 Root fracture occurs when the wedging force is absorbed by the canal walls. Premeasuring the spreader depth can reduce risk of fracture. (Courtesy of Dr. Carl W. Newton.)

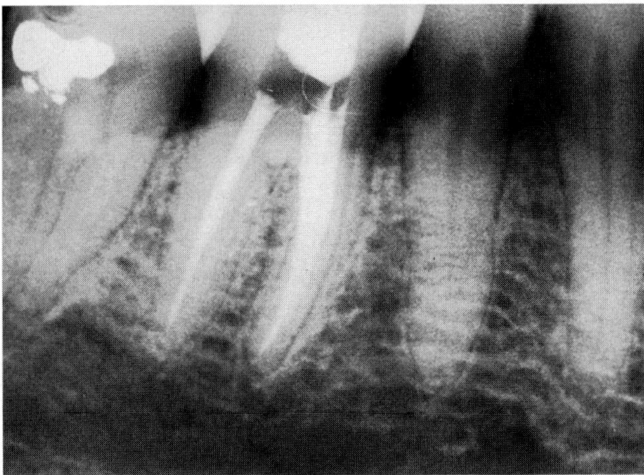

Figure 11-43 Final compaction of three canals reflects proper preparation, premeasured spreader depth, full adaptation of primary point, and careful addition of accessory points. (Courtesy of Dr. Carl W. Newton.)

gutta-percha points meet the ISO/ADA specification. More recent developments in non-ISO/ADA specification for the variable taper (.04/.06 taper instruments) will require more understanding of the final dimensions of the preparation for spreader selection. Rotary instrumentation with these instruments offers the possibility of a very standardized preparation with known diameter and taper at every level of the canal.

A number of investigations that attempted to untangle the problem would become moot if standardization went into effect.[328–331] In 1991, Hartwell and his associates[331] forwarded the same opinion regarding standardization that was voiced by Ingle 36 years before.[327]

In keeping with the trend toward standardization, Martin has introduced a set of calibrated hand spreaders and pluggers to match in size and taper the ISO/ADA instrument standardization. The instruments, with color-coded handles, range in size from No. 20 through No. 60 M Series (Figure 11-44) (Dentsply/Maillefer; Tulsa, Okla.). The space made by these spreaders may be filled with gutta-percha points (again color-coded) of the same number.

Stress and Fractures from Lateral Compaction. Hatton and his associates found they could adequately seal root canals with as little as 1 kg of spreader pressure. They applied up to 2.5 kg and suggested that excessive forces could produce fractures.[332] The Iowa group found 3 kg to be the average lateral condensation pressure exerted by six endodontists. Although they found the incidence of immediate vertical root fractures to be low at 3 kg, they speculated that a buildup of root distortion, "stored" in the root, could well be released later as a fracture. They produced more frac-

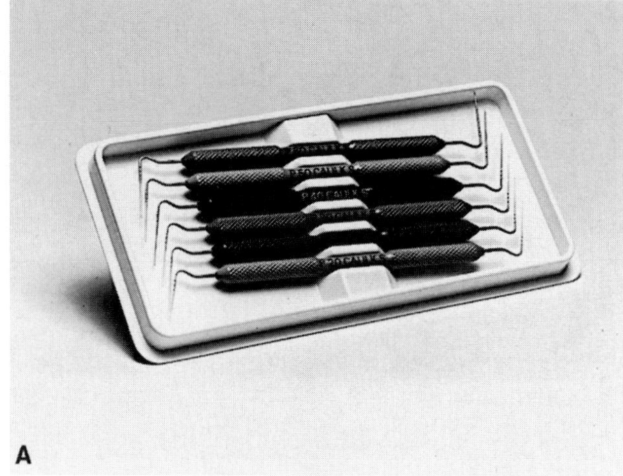

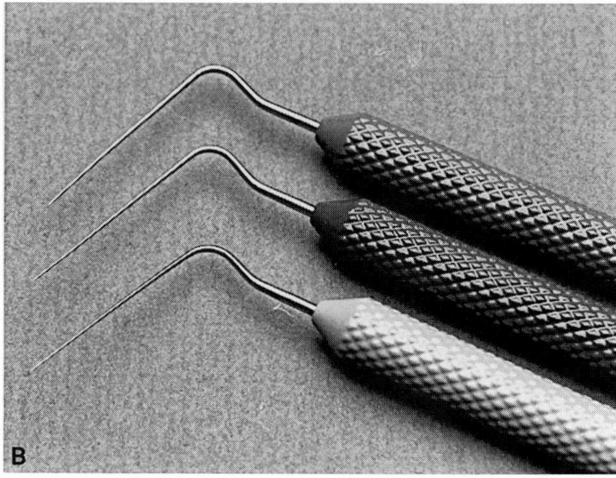

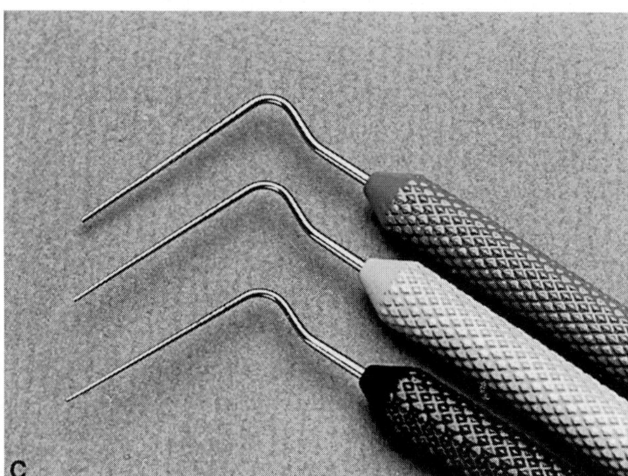

Figure 11-44 **A**, Standardized, double-ended, spreader/pluggers, sized and color coded to match ISO instrument sizes. **B**, Spreader—note sharp point. **C**, Plugger—note blunted point. (Courtesy of Dentsply/Maillefer-M-Series.)

tures with the D-11 hand spreader than with the less tapered B-finger spreader.[333]

At Melbourne University researchers compared load and **strain** using hand versus finger spreaders and found "that strains generated by finger spreaders were significantly lower than hand spreaders." They also concurred with the Iowa group when they noted that lateral condensation may lead to **incomplete** root fractures and that these fractures may later lead to **full vertical fractures** under the stresses of restoration or mastication.[334] Blum described the intracanal pressure developed during condensation as the "wedging effect" and measurements graphed from a force analyzer device showed that gutta-percha deformation occurs at only 0.8 kg for lateral condensation.[335]

Researchers at the University of Washington found it took 7.2 kg (15.8 lbs) to fracture a **maxillary** central incisor. However, 16% of their maxillary anterior teeth fractured at loads under 10 kg. They felt that 5 kg (11 lbs) were a "safe load" for these **husky** teeth.[336] When this same group tested **mandibular incisors**, they produced fractures with only 1.5 kg (3.3 lbs) of load, and 22% of their lower incisors fractured at loads less than 5 kg, in marked contrast to the maxillary incisors and canines. In the lower incisor sample, fractures occurred when only three accessory points were compacted. Like the Iowa and Melbourne groups, they speculated that "vertical root fractures might not be detected clinically until long after the fracture was initiated."[337] Again at Iowa, the relationship between tooth reduction and vertical fracture was studied to show that vertical root fracture did not occur in maxillary anterior teeth under a constant force of 3.3 kg for 15 seconds until 40% of the total canal width was reduced and was always preceded by visible craze lines.[338]

From Greece, Morfis condemned lateral condensation and long post placement as responsible for root fractures. He reported 17 (3.69%) vertical fractures of 480 endodontically treated teeth.[339]

Using engineering models, a US Air Force group found that "lateral condensation required a smaller amount of force than vertical condensation to produce the same amount of stress near the apex..." whereas "the average stress throughout the entire canal was higher for vertical condensation...." They felt that the "term lateral condensation may be somewhat of a misnomer," and that "lateral condensation may be more likely to produce undesirable stress concentrations than is vertical condensation."[340] This was noted earlier at the University of Georgia, when it was stated that "the force of the spreader is apparently transmitted 1 to 2 mm beyond the spreader tip and molds the points and sealer against the walls as it forces them apically."[315] Essentially the same thing was noted at the University of North Carolina.[341]

Nickel-Titanium Spreaders

Studying the distribution of forces in lateral condensation, a US Army group used photoelastic models to demonstrate that nickel-titanium spreaders induced stress patterns distributed along the surface of curved canals compared to concentrated spikes of stress when stainless steel spreaders were used.[342] They also pointed out that, because of their flexibility, nickel-titanium "spreaders penetrated to a significantly greater depth than the stainless steel spreaders in curved canals."[343]

Variations of Lateral Compaction. The preceding illustration of obturating a straight canal by lateral compaction applies with modifications for filling curved canals, immature open apices, or tubular canals.

Curved Canals. Virtually all canals exhibit some curvature. Over 40% of maxillary lateral incisors have a "breaking curve" in the apical third. Over 50% of the palatal roots of maxillary first molars curve back to the buccal. These are examples of the apical curves. General root curvature is apparent radiographically in most of the posterior teeth. Many "hidden" curves to the buccal or lingual cannot be seen radiographically in anterior teeth.

Lateral compaction of curved canals can be very effective in most cases. However, it may be difficult if not impossible in severely curved, dilacerated, or bayonet canals. If smaller, more flexible spreaders cannot reach within the apical 1 mm, or the taper of the preparation is less than that of the spreader, then lateral condensation is not the technique of choice. Teasing a flexible primary point smaller than size 30 to place at the apex, or expecting a stiff spreader to reach within 1 mm of the working length precludes the use of proper lateral compaction. There are other techniques that use warmed or thermoplasticized gutta-percha that are more applicable. They will be discussed subsequently.

In the vast majority of curved canals, where lateral compaction is applicable, the routine is exactly the same: sealer placement and primary point placement, followed by spreaders and auxiliary points. Alternating spreader sizes is usually required to reach the premeasured depth in narrowly prepared canals. One must know, however, that more vertical force will be exerted against the primary point as the spreader will tend to catch in the gutta-percha and force it apically (Figure 11-45). Overfills occur with greater frequency when the vertical force is greater. This also occurs when the spreader taper is greater than the canal preparation. Nickel-titanium spreaders will penetrate to greater depths and distribute forces more evenly than will stainless steel spreaders in curved canals (Figure 11-46).

Immature Canals and Apices. The immature canal is complicated by a gaping foramen. The apical opening is either a nonconstrictive terminus of a tubular canal or a flaring foramen of a "blunderbuss" shape.

Every effort should be made to attain the genetically programmed closure of the foramen that remains open because of early pulp death. This can be accomplished by **apexification,** a method of recharging the growth potential and restoring root growth and foramen closure. Apexification is discussed thoroughly in chapter 15.

If apexification fails or is inappropriate, special methods must be used to obturate the canals without benefit of the constrictive foramen serving as a confining matrix against which to condense. Fortunately, in

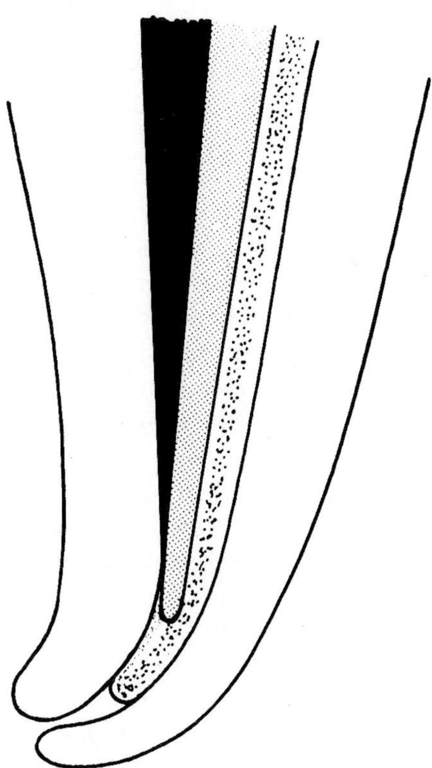

Figure 11-45 Lateral compaction of primary gutta-percha point in curved canal. Spreader catches into point, forcing it apically. Extra vertical compaction must be compensated for.

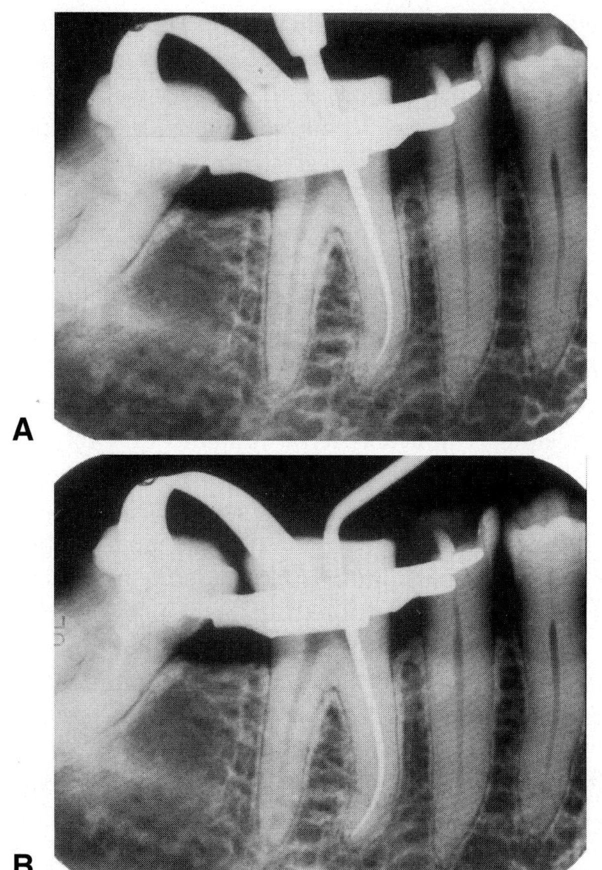

Figure 11-46 Note the difference in ability of same-size spreaders to reach to within 1.0 mm of working length in a curved canal. **A**, Stainless spreader 2.0 mm shy of goal. **B**, Nickel-titanium spreader reaches fully to apical stop. (Courtesy of Dr. Carl W. Newton.)

most of these cases, pulps of straight-root maxillary incisors have been devitalized by impact trauma. In other cases, the foramen has been either trephined to allow for abscess drainage or destroyed by the erosion of external root resorption. Occasionally an immature first molar with pulp necrosis from early caries is a candidate. In either case, calcium hydroxide apexification should be first tried.

Complete obturation requires the use of the largest gutta-percha points customized ("tailor made") to fit the irregular apical stop or barrier. Lateral compaction is not the technique of choice because the resistance of the canal walls for lateral pressure is reduced in immature teeth and the greater bulk of gutta-percha requires an even greater force to deform. Remember that compaction occurs from the canal wall into the mass of gutta-percha. Gutta-percha, in seldom-used sizes, can become brittle in storage and requires even greater pressure to deform. **Warm gutta-percha techniques** are best suited for filling immature canals and apices.

Tubular Canals. The large tubular canal with little constriction at the foramen may best be filled with a "**coarse**" primary gutta-percha cone that has been **blunted** by cutting off the tip. Sometimes the canal is such that a large "tailor-made" point must be used. In either case, the "trial point" should pass the tests of proper fit.

The objective of the primary point is to block the foramen, insofar as possible, while auxiliary points are condensed to complete the filling (Figure 11-47). The length of tooth must be marked on the spreader so that it will not be forced out the apex. With care, a well-compacted filling may be placed without gross overfilling of either cement or gutta-percha. Warm gutta-percha techniques should be considered in larger canals after the apical seal has been achieved by customizing or lateral compaction.

Tailor-Made Gutta-Percha Roll. If the tubular canal is so large that the largest gutta-percha point is still loose in the canal, a tailor-made point must be used as a primary point. This point may be prepared by heating a number of large gutta-percha cones and combining them, butt to tip, until a roll has been developed much the size and shape of the canal (Figure 11-48).

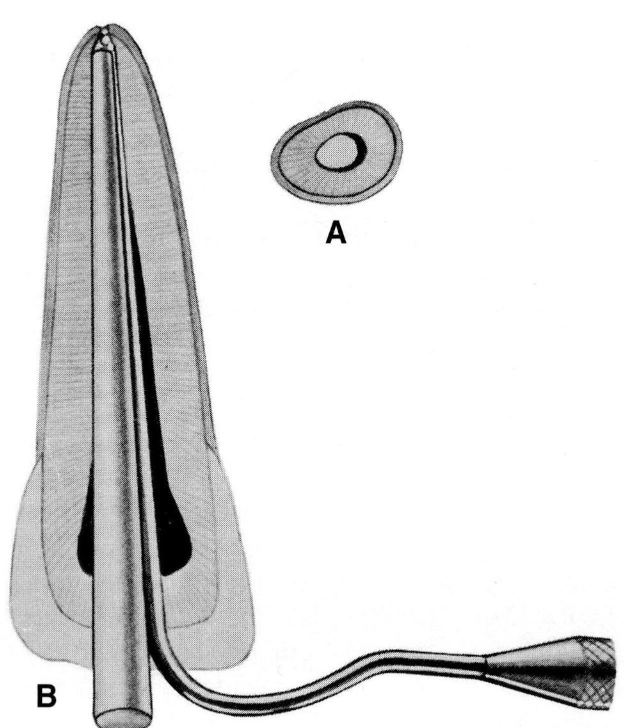

Figure 11-47 **A**, Cross-section of tubular canal in "young" tooth, ovoid in shape. **B**, Blunted, "coarse" gutta-percha cone or tailor-made cone used as primary point, followed by spreading and additional points to totally obturate ovoid space. Final vertical compaction with large plugger.

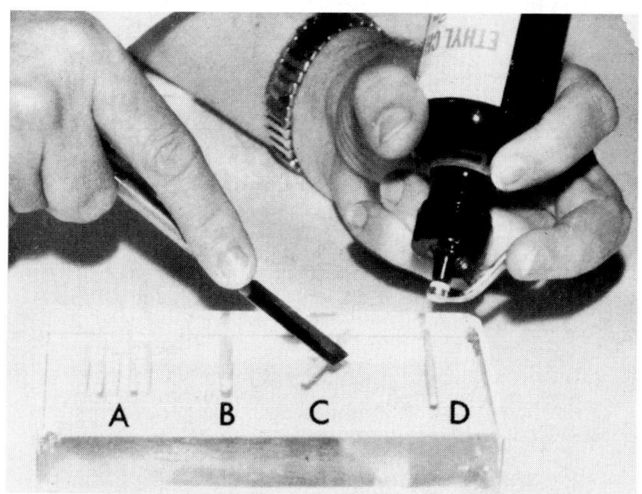

Figure 11-48 Preparation of "tailor-made" gutta-percha roll. A, Number of heated, coarse, gutta-percha points are arranged butt to tip, butt to tip on sterile glass slab. B, Points are rolled with spatula into rod-shaped mass. C, By repeated heating and rolling, the roll of gutta-percha is formed to approximate size of canal to be filled. No voids should exist in mass. D, Before trial point testing of tailor-made roll, gutta-percha should be chilled with ethyl chloride spray.

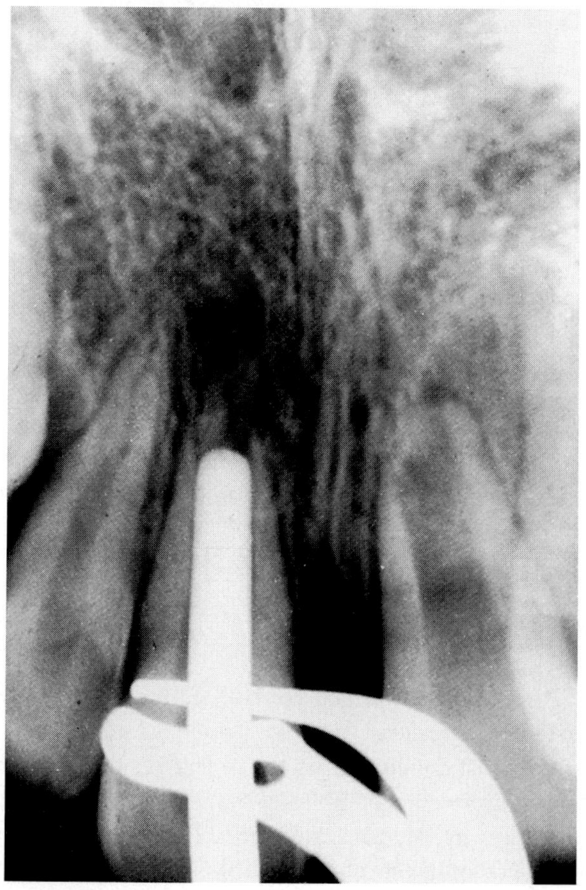

Figure 11-49 Trial point radiograph of tailor-made gutta-percha point. Space exists alongside this roll, which indicates it should be enlarged and retested.

The roll must be chilled with a spray of ethyl chloride or ice water to stiffen the gutta-percha before it is fitted in the canal. If it goes to full depth easily but is too loose, more gutta-percha must be added. If it is only slightly too large, the outside of the gutta-percha can be flash-heated over the flame and the roll forced to proper position. By this method, an impression of the canal is secured (Figure 11-49).

The outer surface of the stiffened point may also be softened by heat or "flash"-dipping the point in chloroform, eucalyptol, or halothane (Figure 11-50, A). By repeating this exercise, one can essentially take an

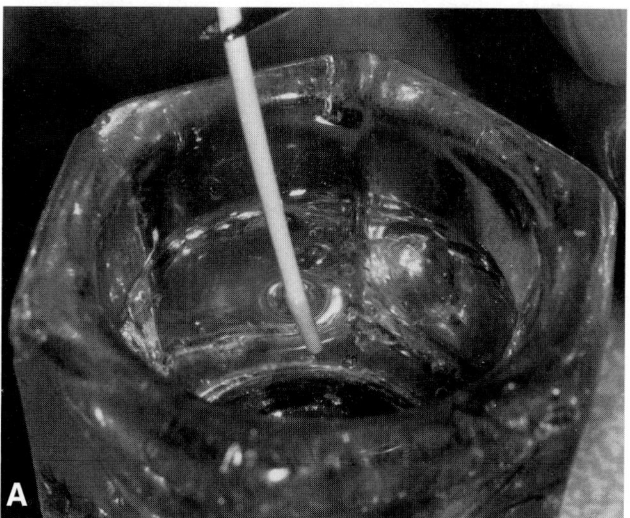

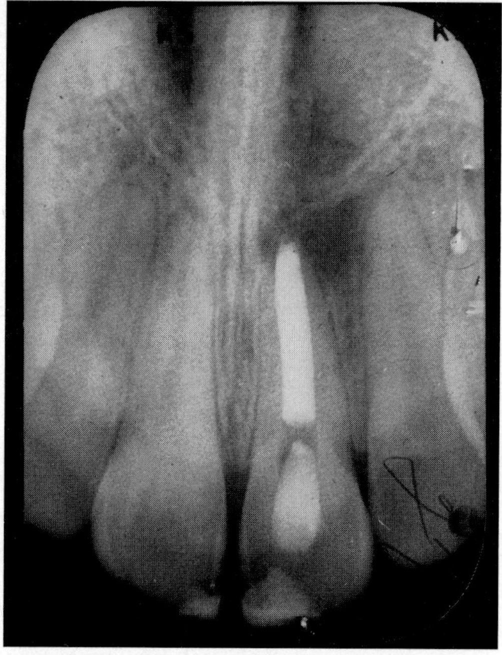

Figure 11-50 Chloroform dip technique. A, Note that just the tip is immersed and for **only 1 second.** B, Final compaction of tubular canal. Warm gutta-percha/vertical compaction is preferred technique for cases with such thin walls. (Courtesy of Dr. Carl W. Newton.)

internal impression of the canal. A mark is made on the buccal surface of the cone and it is dipped in alcohol to stop the action of this solvent. Alcohol can also be used to assist in drying the canal prior to filling. Some shrinkage may alter the final impression and any compaction before the solvent has evaporated will permit the point to continue to flow under pressure.

Simpson and Natkin have suggested a specialized filling technique for those teeth with tubular canals **but closed apices.**[344] These are the roots that were originally blunderbuss in shape but have been induced to complete their growth by the introduction into the root canal of a biologically active chemical, such as calcium hydroxide.

Efficacy of Lateral Compaction. As previously stated, lateral compaction of gutta-percha with sealer is the obturation technique against which other techniques are measured. In some cases, it has been **proved better** than other methods.[345–351] In other reports, it was found to be **as effective** as other techniques.[352–370] But in other citings, it proved **not as adequate.**[371–380]

Weine, a longtime advocate of lateral compaction, and his associates have shown that lateral compaction, done correctly, provides an optimum obturation of the entire canal.[323] The Loyola research was prompted by Schilder's characterization of lateral compaction as ineffective, that "...gutta-percha cones never merge into a homogeneous mass, but they slip and glide and are frozen in a sea of cement"[381] (Figure 11-51).

The Weine group enlarged curved canals in plastic blocks to size 30 apically and flared to size 45 coronally. They then cemented into place a pink No. 30 gutta-percha point and followed it with a No. A finger plugger (with a rounded tip) used as a spreader. Each No. 20 auxiliary gutta-percha point that followed was specially colored a **different color.**

As Figure 11-52 shows, the primary and accessory points more than adequately fill the canal and illustrate how the spreader uses the wall opposite to provide the compressive force of the gutta-percha against the opposite canal wall. And far from "being frozen in a sea of cement," the points dominate the space with only two small flashes of cement showing.[382]

The Indiana research group also showed the efficacy of lateral compaction as well as the paramount importance of thoroughly débriding the canal.[345] Fifteen days following obturation, they found healing already under way. After 45 days, only slight inflammation remained. At the end of 1 year, even though one canal was overfilled (Figure 11-53, A), the tissue was remarkedly healthy. In marked contrast, a **poorly filled canal** exhibited chronic apical periodontitis at 75 days (Figure 11-53, B). All of the unfilled control teeth suffered severe periradicular lesions.[345]

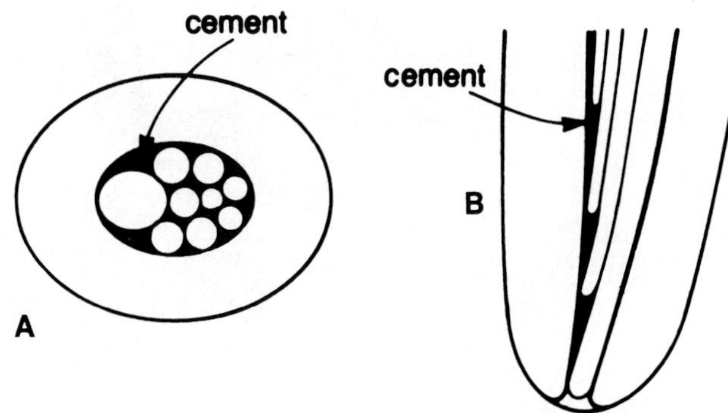

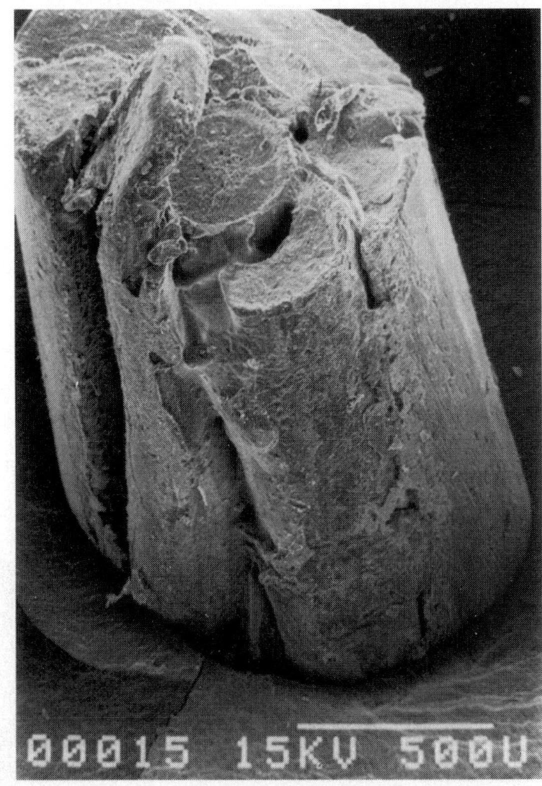

Figure 11-51 **Top,** Schilder's concept of obturation by lateral compaction. A, "Cross-section of middle third of root demonstrating primary and auxiliary cones. Gutta-percha cones frozen in a sea of cement." B, "Gutta-percha cones never merge into homogeneous mass." **Bottom,** Example of truly inadequate lateral compaction caused by paucity of sealer and poor spreading. **Top** reproduced with permission from Schilder H.[381] (**Bottom** courtesy of Dr. Carl W. Newton.)

One must conclude that the objectives of root canal therapy are well met by total canal débridement and obturation by lateral compaction. Failures will be due to neglect of these objectives plus overzealous compaction leading to fracture.

Chemically Plasticized Cold Gutta-percha. A modification of the lateral compaction technique involves

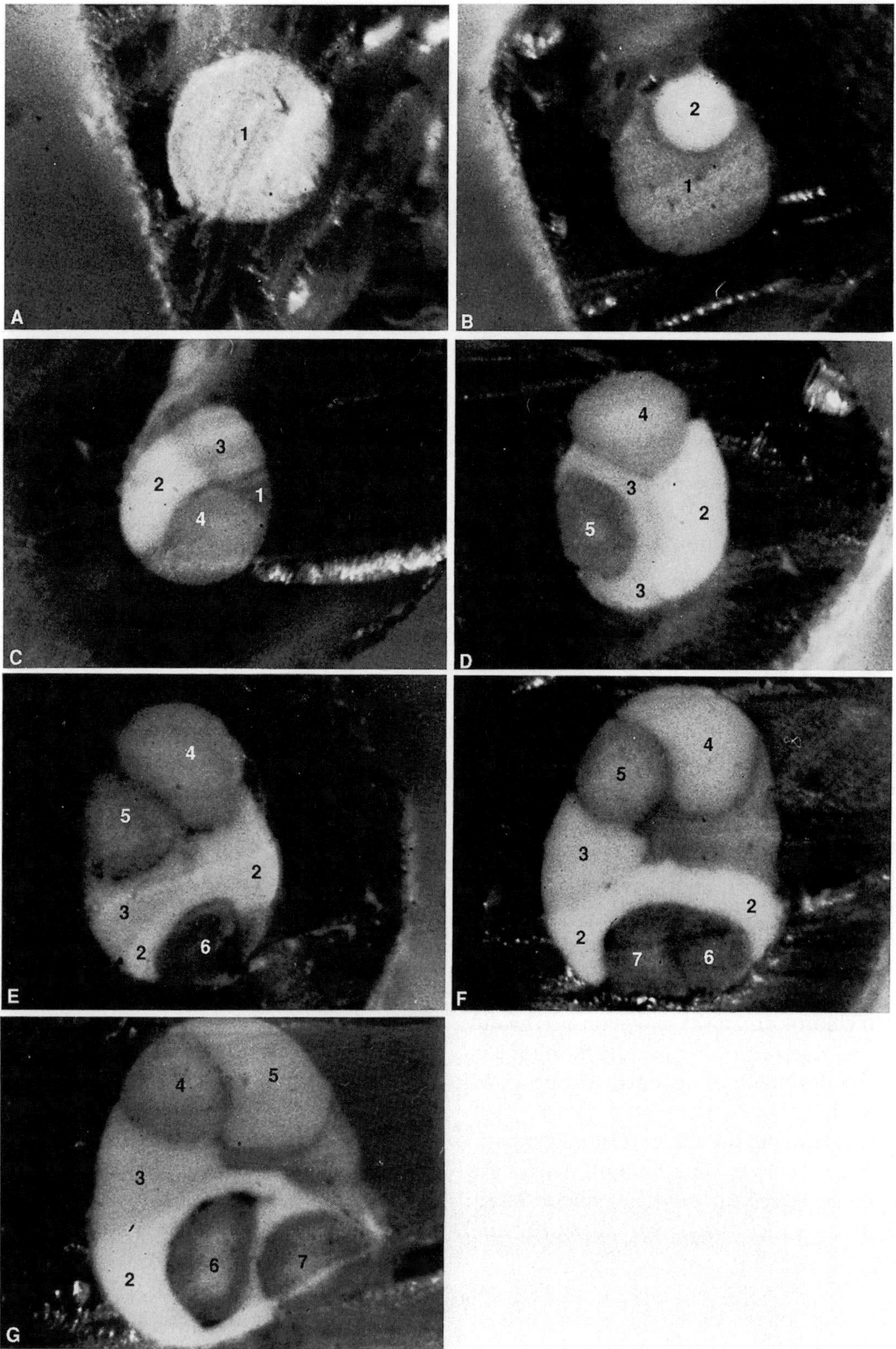

Figure 11-52 Cross-sections of an in vitro study, demonstrating the efficacy of lateral compaction of cold gutta-percha points, each point a different color. A, Single primary point **1.0 mm** from apex apparently fills canal. B, First auxiliary point added following distortion of master point, **2.0 mm** from apex. C, Second and third auxiliary points **3.0 mm** from apex. Canal still totally obturated. D, Second, third, and fourth points fill canal. Primary point not visible. Small amount of sealer at 4 o'clock and 7 o'clock positions **4.0 mm** from apex. E, Fifth point joins other; master point does not show. Small amount of sealer at 5 o'clock and 7 o'clock **5.0 mm** from apex. F, Sixth point added; master point "reappears" **6.0 mm** from apex. G, Seventh point in place, no sealer apparent, canal totally obturated, **7.0 mm** from apex. Reproduced with permission from Sakhal S et al.[382]

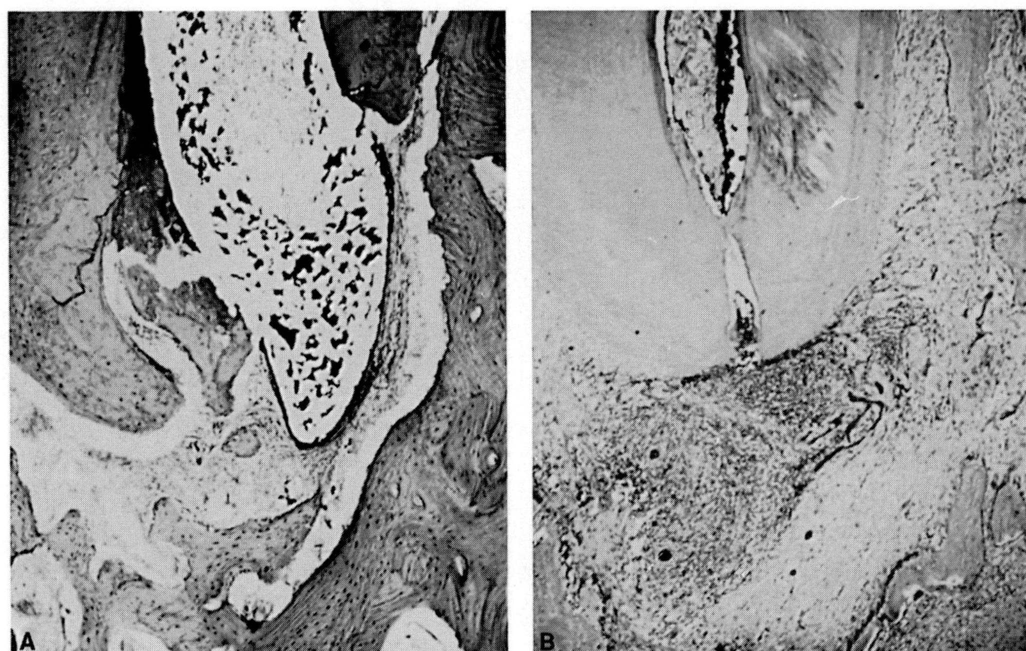

Figure 11-53 Comparative results of lateral compaction following well-compacted versus poorly compacted root canal fillings. **A**, Complete healing 1 year after treatment despite overfilling with gutta-percha. (Spaces are artifacts). **B**, Periradicular granuloma developing 75 days following **poorly compacted** root filling. Bacteria and necrotic debris left in canal. Reproduced with permission from Malooley J et al.[345]

the use of a solvent to soften the primary gutta-percha point in an effort to ensure that it will better conform to the aberrations in apical canal anatomy. This is a variation of a very old obturation method, the so-called Callahan-Johnston technique first promulgated by Callahan in July of 1911.[383] The problem with the original technique centered around the use of too much of the chloroform solvent. Price, a foe of Callahan, set out to prove how ineffective the Callahan root fillings were.[384] Although Callahan claimed that the mixture of chloroform, rosin, and gutta-percha did not shrink, Price observed a 24% decrease in volume *in vitro*. The chloroform had evaporated leaving powdered gutta-percha.

Today's use of solvents is quite modest in comparison with the older methods. Usually only the tip of the point is dipped in the solvent and then only for **1 second** (see Figure 11-50, A). Two or three dips will cause serious leakage.[385]

In this technique the primary point is blunted and fitted **2.0 mm short** of the working length. It is then dipped in the solvent for 1 second and set aside while sealer is placed in the canal. This allows the solvent to partially evaporate. Too much solvent, as with a two- or three-dip method, will materially increase leakage. Not only does the gutta-percha volume shrink as the solvent evaporates in the canal, the **sealer** leaks as well, probably because of solvent dissolution.[385]

To begin the **obturation by lateral compaction**, one must immediately position the customized master point to its full measured length and then spread it aside to allow the softened gutta-percha to flow. The spreader is rotated out and is followed by additional points, spreader and points. Because 2.0 mm of the master tip have been solvent softened, it will flow to place to produce "smooth, homogeneous, well-condensed gutta-percha fills closely adapted to the internal canal configuration in the apical third, including the filling of lateral canals, fins, and irregularities."[385] An Israeli group warns, however, that the point should be positioned and spread within 15 seconds of being softened; otherwise, it will have lost its plasticity. After 30 seconds of air drying, it changes shape.[386]

The principal solvent used in this technique is chloroform. At one time there was concern that it was carcinogenic, but it has recently been cleared for clinical use in dentistry by the FDA, Occupational Safety and Health Administration, and ADA.[387] In any event, other solvents such as eucalyptol, halothane, xylene, and rectified turpentine have been evaluated as substitutes for chloroform.[388]

In addition to the popular dip technique, sealers are prepared by dissolving gutta-percha in these solvents as well as in rosin and balsam. These mixtures have long been popular as sealers and dips for gutta-percha points. Such mixtures are called chloropercha, Kloropercha, or

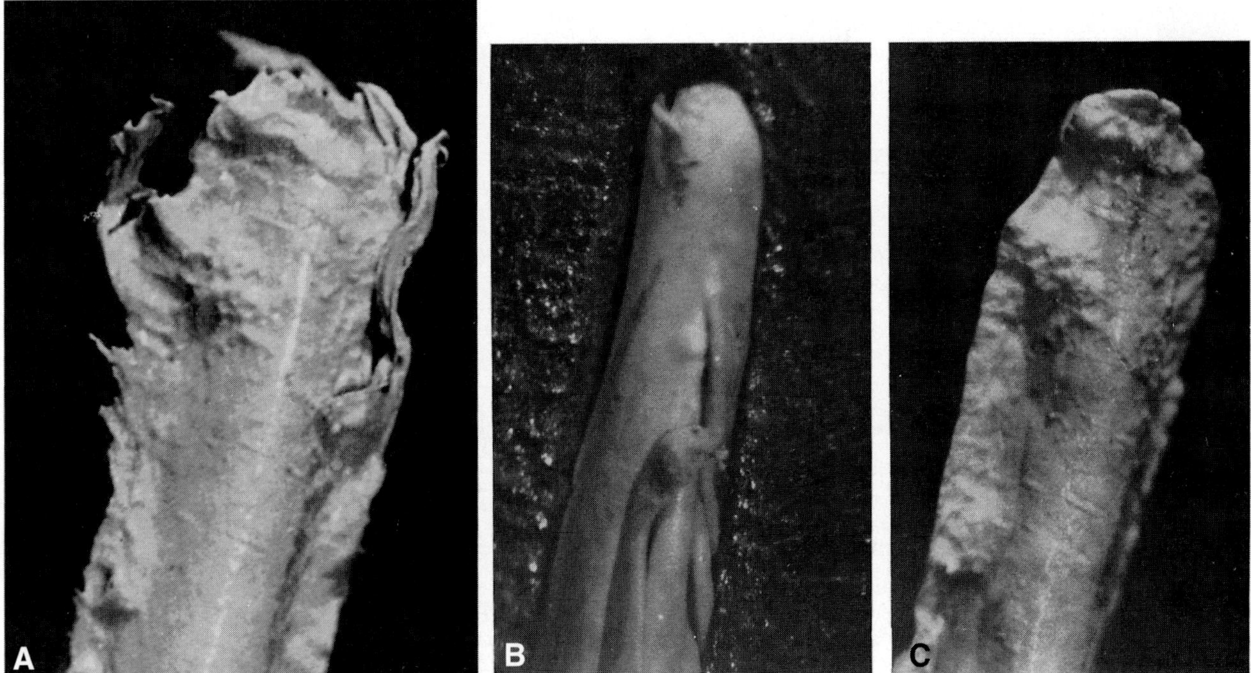

Figure 11-54 Compaction results from three methods of obturation purposely done without sealer. **A**, Chloropercha filling presents best **immediate** appearance. Unfortunately, a **12.4% shrinkage** follows, leading to massive leakage. **B**, Lateral compaction—cold gutta-percha showing coalescence of primary and accessory points at apex but separating midcanal. **C**, Warm gutta-percha/vertical compaction. Filling is homogeneous; replication is excellent. Reproduced with permission from Wong M et al.[409]

eucapercha. Sealers such as CRCS (Calciobiotic Root Canal Sealer) and Wach's Sealer, respectively, contain the solvents oil of eucalyptol and Canada balsam.

Efficacy of Solvent-Customized Gutta-percha Master Points. As the University of Washington group noted, customizing master points with solvents improves the seal of gutta-percha.[385] At the University of Iowa, researchers found essentially the same thing.[389] Peters found virtually no solubility in distilled water after 2 years when the chloroform dip method was used with lateral compaction.[389a]

Goldman found Kloropercha as a sealer superior to chloropercha or lateral compaction with ZOE sealer.[390] Kloropercha contains balsam, rosin, and zinc oxide in addition to gutta-percha and chloroform, which makes it more homogeneous. The US Army Research Institute also tested chloropercha and Kloropercha. Initially, with the solvent/gutta-percha filling, they achieved dramatic results (Figure 11-54, A). After 2 weeks, however, chloropercha shrank 12.42% and the Kloropercha 4.68%, whereas the **simple chloroform dip shrank only 1.4%.** The comparative results versus lateral and vertical compaction were dramatic[391] (Figure 11-54, B and C).

Morse and Wilcko recommend eucalyptol as a solvent to form euchapercha. It shrinks 10% less than chloropercha.[392,393] Others found the quick-dip technique superior to euchapercha as a sealer.[394]

Halothane and eucalyptol, as alternatives to chloroform, were found to be no better in dissolving or sealing ability.[395–397] However, Morse and the Temple University group used eucapercha as a sealer and noted that it shrinks less than warm gutta-percha or gutta-percha/chloropercha.[398]

A Tel Aviv group summarized best the value of customized master points softened by solvents. They found that chloroform-dipped points provided a significantly better seal than standardized points when obturating "flat" canals.[399] Few canals are perfectly round in shape.

Vertical Compaction of Warm Gutta-percha*

Over 30 years ago, Schilder introduced a concept of cleaning and shaping root canals in a conical shape and then obturating the space "three-dimensionally" with gutta-percha, warmed in the canal and compacted vertically with pluggers.[400] It was his contention that all the "portals of exit" were clinically significant and would be obturated with a maximum amount of gutta-percha and a minimum amount of sealer (Figure 11-55).

*John West gratefully acknowledges the assistance of Herbert Schilder and James Clark in preparing this section.

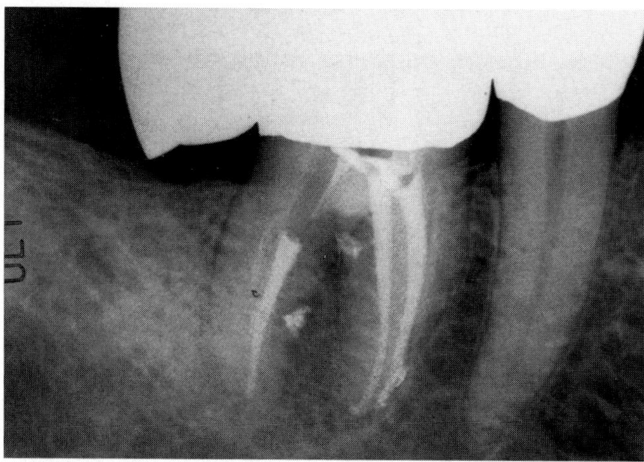

Figure 11-55 Warm gutta-percha/vertical compaction. Root canal system anatomy is "discovered" during compaction; see multiple portals of exit. (Courtesy of Dr. John D. West.)

Fitting the Master Gutta-percha Cone. Following the preparation of a thoroughly cleansed and continuously tapering canal,[401] the critical step of fitting the master cone is the next important feature of this technique. For this, the **conventional cone-shaped** gutta-percha points are used, not the standardized numbered points. The cone-shaped gutta-percha more closely mirrors the tapered canal shape (Figure 11-56). The primary cone is virtually tailor fit, particularly in the apical third (Figure 11-57).

The cone is placed to reach the radiographic terminus and then cut back slightly short (0.5–1.0 mm) of this length (see Figure 11-57). This allows heat molding of the round cone into the **nonround** portal of exit and minimizes sealer/tissue contact (Figure 11-58). Under cone-fit guidelines, the shorter, wider, and straighter the canal, the farther the cone should be cut back from the radiographic terminus. Conversely, the longer, more curved, and narrower the canal, the closer the cone should fit to the radiographic terminus. Beginners often cut back the cone too much.

Occasionally the cone fit does not reach the apex. In this event, one should attempt a smaller cone or, better yet, improve the shape of the canal. In short, fit the cone **0.5 to 1 mm short** of the radiographic terminus and it should possess good tugback.

As stated earlier, fit of the master cone is the key to success in this technique—a successful relationship between the radicular preparation and the master cone. Cleaning and shaping and obturation are clinically inseparable. When the gutta-percha is subsequently warmed and compacted, it fills not only the critical parts of the canal but the cleaned portals of exit as well (see Figure 11-57, C). When compacted, the primary cone provides **the body** of the warm "wave of compaction" moving apically and then a warm wave of compaction moving coronally. The cone must fit tightly in the apical third, that is, have "tugback," and have diminished taper toward the middle and coronal thirds as well.

It is typical of vertical compaction that more than one portal of exit per canal will be filled—two portals of exit per canal in one sampling.[402] In the graduate endodontic clinic at Boston University, more than one foramen is filled over 40% of the time.[381] Similar results are reported at the University of Washington (Figure 11-59).[403] There is virtually no risk of compacting too short or too long if the first cone fits properly.[404]

Prefitting the Vertical Pluggers. Practitioners of warm gutta-percha vertical compaction prefer using a set of pluggers designed by Schilder (Dentsply/Maillefer; Tulsa, Okla.), a wider plugger for the coronal third of the canal, a narrower plugger for the middle third, and the narrowest plugger for the apical third of the canal. The objective is for the widest appropriate

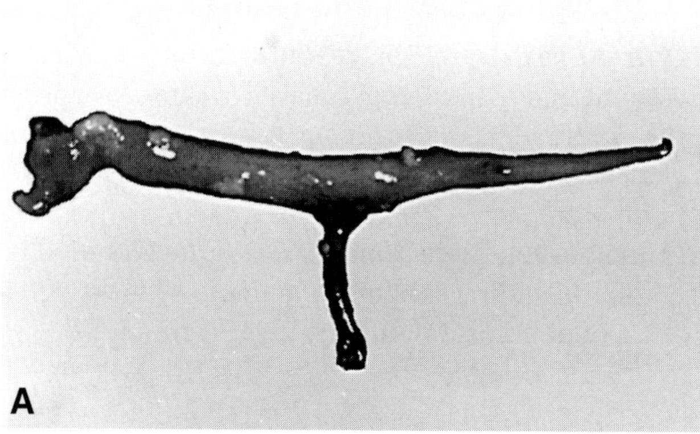

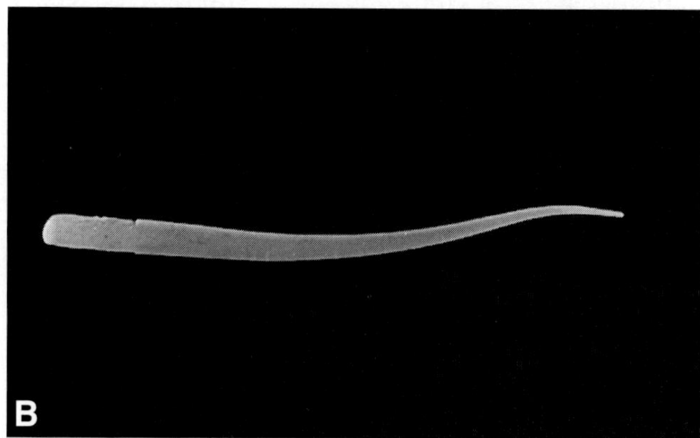

Figure 11-56 Comparison in shape and size between pulp and **traditional** gutta-percha cones. **A**, Conical pulp extirpated from 10-year-old boy. Note enormous lateral canal. **B**, Traditional (nonstandardized) gutta-percha cone similar in taper and bulk to pulp anatomy. (Courtesy of Dr. John D. West.)

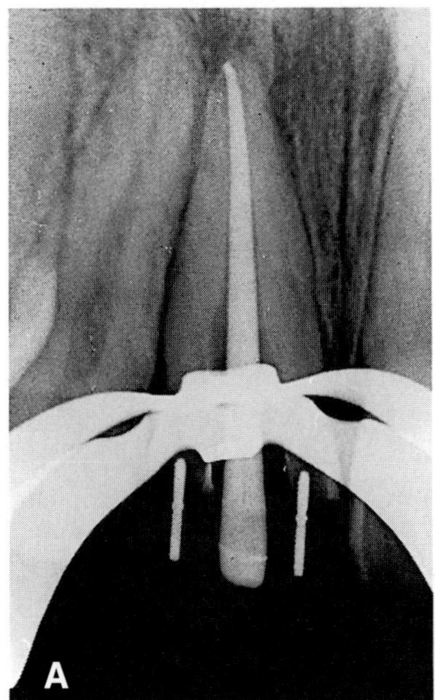

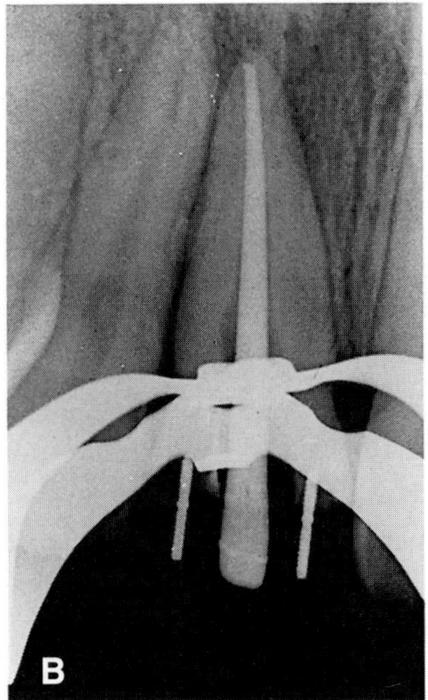

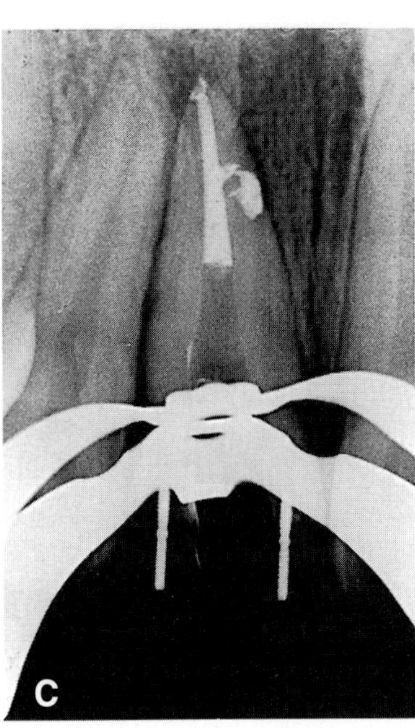

Figure 11-57 Fitting the master gutta-percha cone. **A**, Cone fit to radiographic terminus. **B**, Cone is cut back 0.5 mm. When placed to depth, the incisal reference remains the same. **C**, Compaction film reveals two apical foramina as well as large lateral canal opposite lateral lesion. (Courtesy of Dr. John D. West.)

plugger to capture the maximum cushion of warm gutta-percha as the heat wave is carried apically.[405] Only one or two pluggers may be needed for shorter teeth, whereas three or four are used in longer canals. Most cases require three graduated sizes.

Schilder pluggers are marked with serrations every 5 mm, so that the depth that each instrument penetrates should be recorded by plugger number and depth of penetration. The pluggers are then set aside for immediate use.

Heat Transfer Instrument. Initially, an instrument designed much like a spreader was used to transfer heat from a Bunsen burner to the gutta-percha. It was heated "cherry-red," immediately carried into the canal, sub-

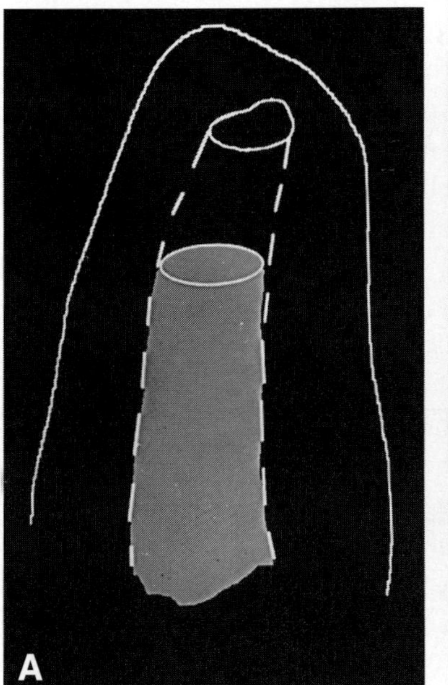

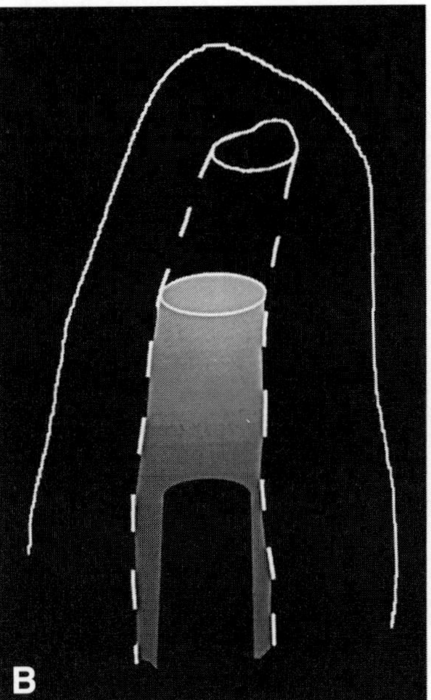

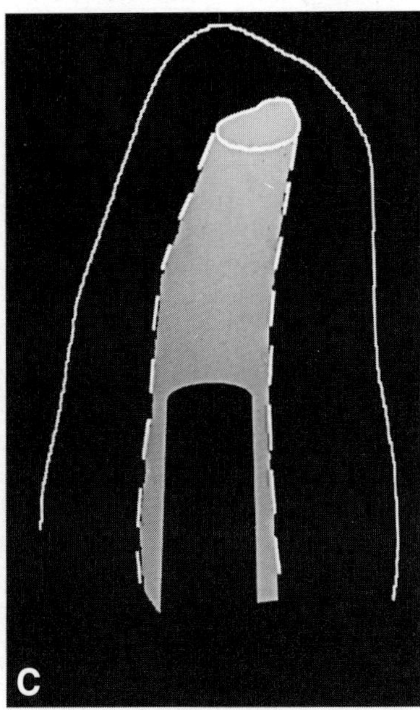

Figure 11-58 Warm gutta-percha conforming to "egg-shaped" canal. **A**, Primary gutta-percha cone fits 0.5 to 1.0 mm short of radiographic apex. **B**, Cold plugger advances the thermoplasticized gutta-percha into apical constricture. **C**, Vertical pressure compacts warmed gutta-percha into nonround foramen. (Courtesy of Dr. John D. West.)

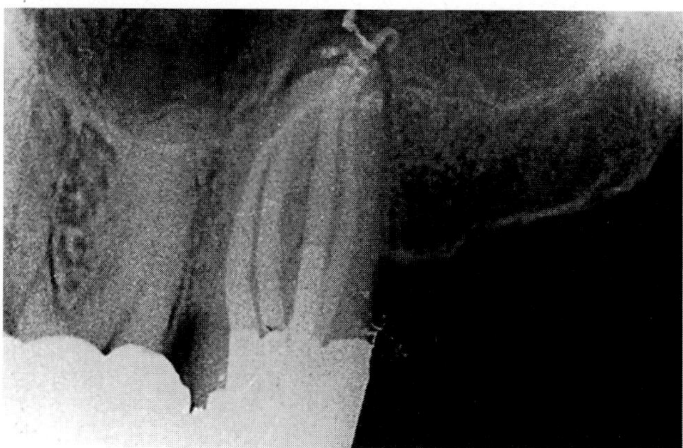

Figure 11-59 Four-canal maxillary second molar. Second mesiobuccal canal in mesiobuccal root has separate portal of exit. (Courtesy of Dr. John D. West.)

merged into the mass of gutta-percha, and drawn through the gutta-percha for 2 or 3 seconds to allow the heat to transfer from the heat carrier. It was then withdrawn in a slightly circular wiping motion, "freezing" some of the gutta-percha onto the heat carrier. Successive waves of vertical compaction immediately followed.

The Schilder heat carrier has been essentially superseded by the **Touch 'n Heat 5004** (SybronEndo/Analytic; Irvine, Calif.), an electronic device specially developed for the warm gutta-percha technique (Figure 11-60). It exhibits the same thermal profile as the original heat carrier but has the advantage of generating heat automatically at the tip of the instrument. Battery or AC models are available.

Root Canal Sealer. Practitioners of this technique generally prefer using **Kerr Pulp Canal Sealer,** Richert's

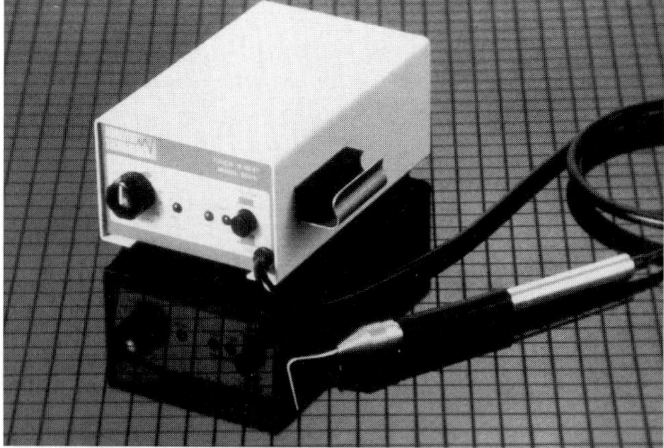

Figure 11-60 **"Touch 'n Heat" 5004,** battery-powered (rechargeable) heat source. Heat carrier heats to glowing within seconds to plasticize gutta-percha in canal. Also used in removal of gutta-percha for postpreparation or re-treatment. (Courtesy of Sybron Endo/Analytic Tech., Irvine, Calif.)

original ZOE cement that contains rosin as well as precipitated silver used as a radiopaquing medium. The advantages, they feel, are the short setting time and low resorbability.[406] Recently, Kerr introduced Pulp Canal Sealer EWT, which allows for Extended Working Time.

Step-by-Step Procedure of Vertical Compaction of Warm Gutta-percha

1. Dry the canal! This is best achieved by using 100% alcohol irrigated deep within the root canal system using thin, safe-tipped irrigating "needles." The canal is then dried with paper points and air dried with the Stropko irrigator (SybronEndo/Analytic Tech; Irvine, Calif.). Confirm the patency of the foramen with an instrument smaller than the last size instrument used to develop the apical preparation.
2. Fit the appropriate gutta-percha cone to the patent radiographic terminus. It should visually go to full working length and exhibit tug-back. Confirm the position radiographically. Cut off the butt end of the cone at the incisal or occlusal reference point (Figure 11-61, A).
3. Remove the cone and cut back **0.5 to 1.0 mm** of the tip, reinsert, and check the length and tug-back. The cone's apical diameter should be the same diameter as the last apical instrument to reach the radiographic terminus of the preparation (Figure 11-61, B). Remove the cone, dip it in alcohol, and curve it slightly by drawing it through a folded 2 × 2 gauze so that it will more easily follow the probable curved shape of the canal. Set the cone aside.
4. Prefit the three pluggers to the canal preparation: first the widest plugger to a 10 mm depth (Figure 11-61, C); next, the middle plugger to a 15 mm depth (Figure 11-61, D); finally, the narrowest plugger to within 3 to 4 mm of the terminus (Figure 11-61, E). Record the lengths of the desired plugger depth.
5. Deposit a small amount of root canal sealer in the canal with a **Handy Lentulo** spiral. (Dentsply/Maillefer; Tulsa, Okla.). Lightly coat all of the walls.
6. Coat the apical third of the gutta-percha cone with a thin film of sealer.
7. Grasp the butt-end of the cone with cotton pliers and slide the cone approximately halfway down the canal. Then gently follow it fully into place with the closed tip of the cotton pliers (Figure 11-61, F). In a curved canal, the cone will rotate as it responds to the curvature.
8. Using the Touch 'n Heat 5004 heat carrier, sear off the cone surplus in the pulp chamber down to the cervical level (Figure 11-61, G). This transfers heat to the **coronal third** of the gutta-percha cone

and creates a platform to begin the first wave of compaction.

9. Using the **widest vertical plugger** that has previously been coated with cement powder as a separating medium, the gutta-percha is folded into a mass and compacted in an apical direction with sustained 5- to 10-second pressure (Figure 11-61, H). This is the first heat wave. The temperature of the gutta-percha has been raised 5 to 8°C above body temperature, which allows deformation from compaction. At this temperature (42 to 45°C), the gutta-percha retains its same crystalline beta form with minimal shrinkage as it cools back to body temperature.
10. The second heat wave begins by introducing the heat carrier back into the gutta-percha, where it remains for 2 to 3 seconds (Figure 11-61, I) and, when retrieved, carries with it the first selective gutta-percha removal (Figure 11-61, J).
11. Immediately, the **midsized** coated plugger is submerged into the warm gutta-percha. The vertical pressure also exerts lateral pressure. This filling mass is shepherded apically in 3 to 4 mm waves created by **repeated heat** and compaction cycles (Figure 11-61, K).
12. The second heating of the heat carrier warms the next 3 to 4 mm of gutta-percha and again an amount is removed on the end of the heat carrier (Figure 11-61, L).
13. The narrowest plugger is immediately inserted in the canal and the surplus material along the walls is folded centrally into the apical mass so that the heat wave begins from a flat plateau. The warmed gutta-percha is then compacted vertically, and the material flows into and seals the apical portals of exit (Figure 11-61, M).
14. The **apical** "down-pack" is now completed, and if a **post** is to be placed at this depth, no more gutta-percha need be used (Figure 11-61, N).
15. "Backpacking" the remainder of the canal completes the obturation. The classic method of backpacking consists of placing **5 mm precut segments** of gutta-percha in the canal, cold welding them with the appropriate plugger to the apical material (Figure 11-61, O), warming them with the heat-carrier (Figure 11-61, P), and then compacting. It should be noted that no selective removal of gutta-percha is attempted in the backpacking (Figure 11-61, Q). This sectional procedure is continued with heat and the next wider plugger until the entire canal is obturated (Figure 11-61, R).
16. An alternative method of backpacking may be done by injecting plasticized gutta-percha from one of the syringes, such as Obtura II (Obtura/Spartan, USA). In any event, the plasticized gutta-percha must be compacted with vertical pluggers to ensure its flow against canal walls, to weld it to the apical materials, and to minimize shrinkage (Figure 11-61, S).
17. The final act involves the thorough cleansing of the pulp chamber below the CE junction, the addition of an appropriate barrier, and the placement of a permanent restoration (Figure 11-61, T). In molar teeth, extra sealer should be placed in the chamber area, warm gutta-percha is syringed into the chamber flow, and the gutta-percha is compacted with large amalgam pluggers to ensure that any furcal portals of exit will be filled prior to final restoration (Figure 11-62).

Like all dental techniques, vertical compaction of warm gutta-percha is technique sensitive. It is imperative, therefore, to seek professional training in this special obturation method.[407]

Efficacy of Vertical Compaction of Warm Gutta-percha. Warm gutta-percha, vertically compacted, has proved most effective in filling the canals of severely curved roots and roots with accessory, auxiliary, or lateral canals, or with multiple foramina. Since the first indication of such anatomic variations may be observed during the filling procedure, it behooves the dentist to use a filling technique that ensures obturation in case such unusual canals are open and patent.

The chief proponents of the warm gutta-percha technique at Boston University point out that consistent success in obturation will be achieved only when the canal is properly cleaned and shaped, and when copious amounts of sodium hypochlorite are used to flush away the debris, bacteria, and dentinal filings.[408] After this proper preparation, predictable three-dimensional obturation with vertical compaction is easily accomplished. In this technique, the two concepts, cleaning and shaping and three-dimensional obturation, are inseparable.

As previously stated, very few microleakage studies have been done comparing warm gutta-percha/vertical compaction with other techniques. Lateral compaction is usually used as a control in these studies. The few that do exist, however, speak favorably for warm/vertical compaction.

Brothman compared lateral and vertical techniques and found "no statistically significant difference in filling efficiency."[356] He reported, however, a significantly greater incidence of accessory canal filling with **sealer** by vertical compaction. He concluded that ribbon-shaped canals were better filled by lateral compaction, whereas "for centric canals, vertical condensation appears better."[356] Reader and Himel reported "significantly more **gutta-percha** in the lateral canals" when compared with cold lateral or warm lateral/vertical compaction.[357] Torabinejad et al. compared a number of obturation techniques and concluded that comparable results were achieved with all four methods, but reported close adaptation in the middle and apical thirds by the vertical method.[358] Wong et al. reported a homogeneous filling with excellent replication.[409] At Dalhousie University, three obturation methods were compared and all three "techniques proved equally satisfactory," although the researchers did note "cold-welds" with vertical compaction.[352] Lugassey and Yee also noted the cold welds as well as "microscopic voids, folds and inclusions scattered randomly throughout the root canal."[410] A US Army group tested three different methods and found the differences in radioactive microleakage to ^{45}Ca were not significant.[353]

A tendency to **overfill the canal** while using the warm gutta-percha/vertical compaction technique was noted by a Lebanese group who reported that "apical cone displacement was greater with vertical compaction." Clinically, they observed that "overextension is more likely to occur...when the master cone is adapted only 0.5 mm short." There were no overextensions with lateral compaction.[411]

Schilder has twice reported to meetings of the American Association of Endodontists his evaluations

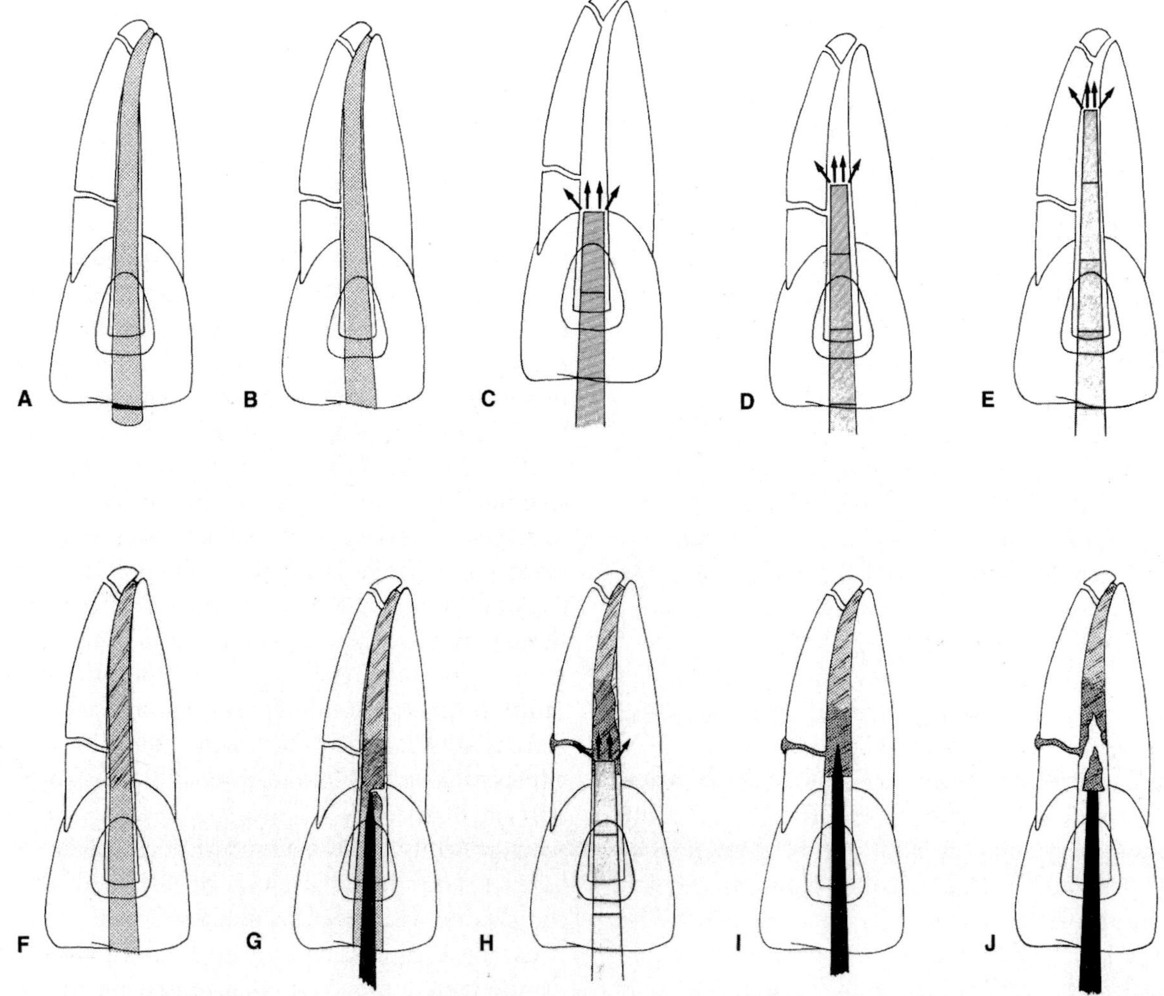

Figure 11-61 Technique of **warm gutta-percha/vertical compaction. A,** Master gutta-percha cone fits tightly to radiographic apex. Marked at incisal edge to establish length reference. **B,** Master cone cut back 0.5 to 1.0 mm at tip and retried in canal. Trimmed incisal reference remains same. **C,** Largest plugger prefit to coronal third of canal. **D,** Midsize plugger prefit to midcanal without touching walls. **E,** Smallest plugger prefit to within 3 to 4 mm of radiographic apex. Remains free in canal. **F,** Kerr Sealer deposited in midcanal with Handy Lentulo spiral. Apical third of master cone is lightly coated with sealer and gently teased to place. Incisal reference checked. **G,** Surplus gutta-percha removed with heat carrier down to canal orifice. **H,** Largest plugger compacts warmed gutta-percha into bolus. Midroot lateral canal being obturated. **I,** Heat carrier transfers heat 3 to 4 mm into middle third of mass. Wiping carrier against walls softens excess gutta-percha. **J,** First selective gutta-percha removal.

of success and failure when his recommendations of cleaning and shaping and obturation with warm gutta-percha and vertical compaction were followed. The cases were done by endodontic graduate students at Boston University.

The first was a radiographic study, treatment of 100 maxillary anterior teeth with periradicular lesions.[412] The lesions ranged in size from 8 to 35 mm. The age range was 14 to 84 years and involved both sexes. Radiographic observations were made at 6, 12, 18, and 24 months. Healing was judged as totally healed (90%), partially healed (75%), no healing (50%), or worse. Total healing or 90% healing was noted in 56% of the cases within the first 6 months. At 24 months, 99% of the 100 cases "were fully healed."[412] The one failed case (an 84-year-old woman) was subsequently revealed by surgery to have an apical bifurcation. Apicoectomy below the bifurcation allowed normal healing within 1 year.

On the basis of this radiographic study of **maxillary anterior teeth**, Schilder reported 100% success after 2 years for cleaning and shaping and three-dimensional obturation by warm gutta-percha/vertical compaction.[412]

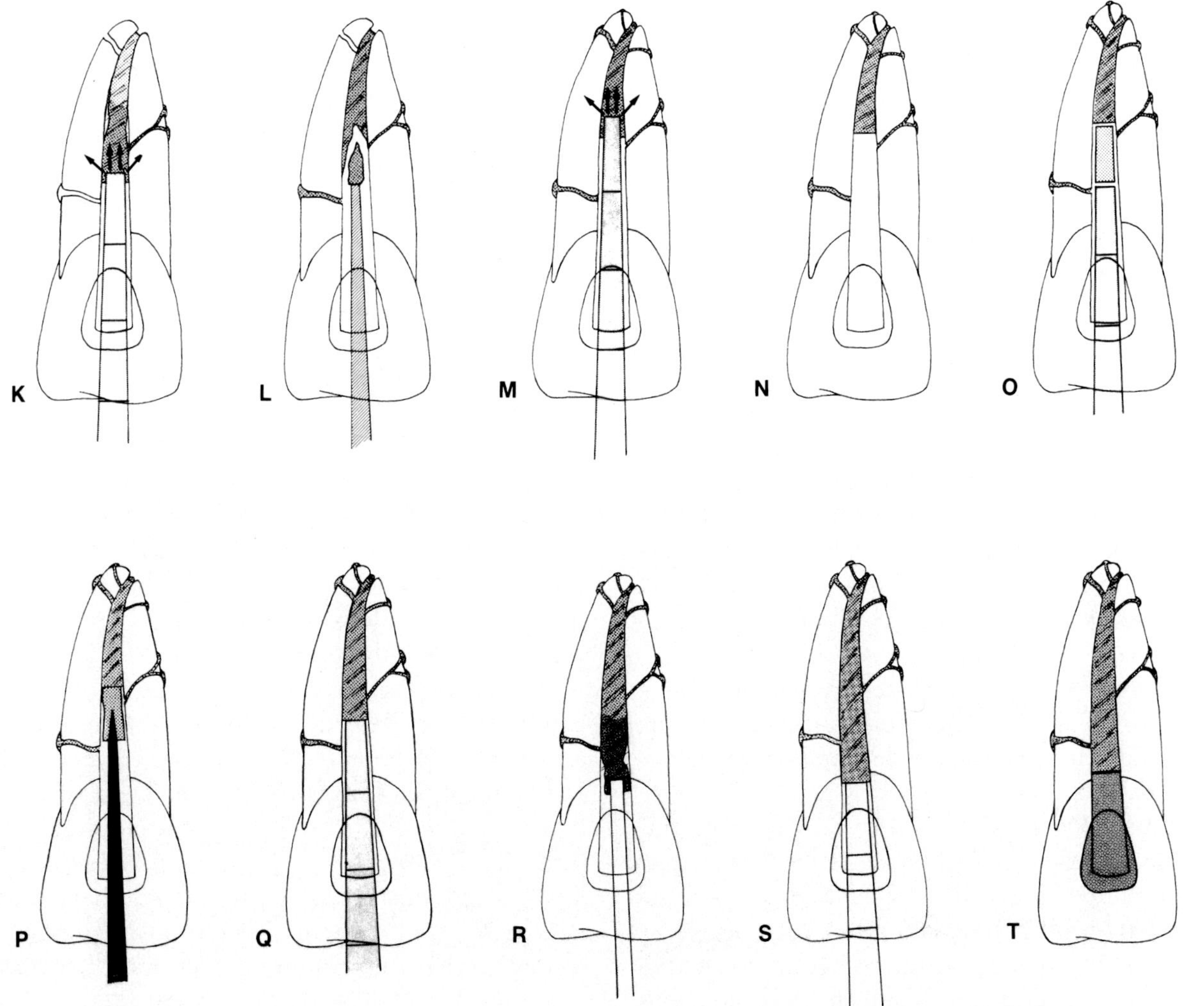

Figure 11-61 (Continued) K, Midsize plugger compacts heat-softened gutta-percha apically. Second lateral canal appears as obturated. **L**, Heat transfer instrument warms apical gutta-percha. Second selective removal of material. **M**, Smallest plugger compacts apical mass into apical preparation and accessory canals now appear obturated as well. **N**, Plugger folds surplus gutta-percha around walls into flattened central mass. Radiograph confirms total obturation of apical third of canal. If a post is to be placed, obturation is complete. **O**, To complete obturation by segmented gutta-percha, a 3 mm blunted section is placed and "cold-welded" with the medium plugger to the apical mass. **P**, Heat carrier warms first backpack piece. **Q**, Warmed backpack piece married by compaction to apical filling. Process is continued to fill entire canal. **R**, If gutta-percha gun (Obtura II) is used for backfill, the needle is inserted to the apical segment and then backed out, leaving deposit. Plasticized gutta-percha is compacted to complete obturation to canal orifice. **S**, Final compaction of backpack done with largest plugger. **T**, Gutta-percha and sealer are removed to below free gingival level, crown is thoroughly cleansed, and final restoration is placed in the coronal cavity. (Courtesy of Dr. John D. West.)

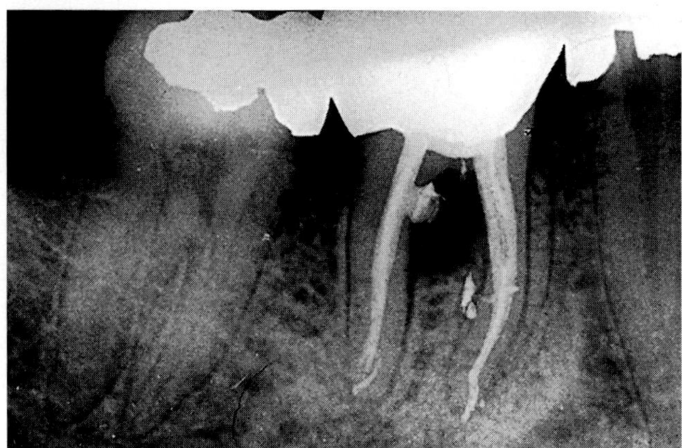

Figure 11-62 Furcal accessory canal and lateral canal, mesial root filled by vertical compaction of warm gutta-percha. (Courtesy of Dr. John D. West.)

As a follow-up to the preceding report, Schilder presented in 1977 a histologic study of 25 lesions of endodontic origin.[413] Intentional surgical biopsy was scheduled from 1 to 25 months following obturation. The study, however, was terminated at 15 months when all of the remaining cases appeared healed.

Some interesting histologic observations were made by Schilder. Within 1 week of canal débridement and even **before** obturation, new bone formation was noted at the periphery of a large lesion. Healing always occurred from the periphery toward the apex. The presence or absence of excess sealer, or occasionally gutta-percha, had no observable influence on the inexorable resolution of the lesions and their replacement with normal bone. By 12 months, all of the lesions in the study were fully healed.[413]

Schilder concluded these two reports with the observation that "failure is the result of inadequate cleaning and shaping of the root canal system and/or inadequate obturation."[413]

Quite possibly, the success to be achieved with this technique, as with any technique, is highly operator sensitive. As Kerekes and Rowe so aptly stated, "success of treatment [will] be influenced to a high degree by the technical skill of the practitioners: practitioners less experienced in endodontic treatment have problems carrying out root fillings to a satisfactory technical standard."[354]

Finally, something should be said about some of the concerns voiced about this technique. One is that too much stress is introduced into the tooth through vertical compaction. Early on, researchers at Temple University observed that "when canals were filled by the vertical condensation method, more cracks in the dentin were discernible than were seen in the teeth filled by lateral condensation."[414] Schilder replied that the cracks seen in the Temple University microphotographs were laboratory artifacts (H. Schilder, personal communication, August 1977). More recently, a US Army study done with mathematical models and "finite element analysis" suggested "that lateral condensation may be more likely to produce undesirable stress concentrations than is vertical condensation." These researchers also said that the term "lateral condensation may be somewhat of a misnomer," that it produced more stress with less force near the apex (where a root is finer and more likely to fracture) than did vertical compaction. However, "the average stress throughout the entire canal was higher for vertical condensation..."[324] A group at the University of Iowa tested both lateral and vertical compaction techniques for stresses induced and concluded that "the highest stress concentrations occurred in the apical third of the root...and progressed incisally." Both lateral and vertical stresses were culpable.[340]

Another concern relates to the temperatures generated within the canal from the warming process. The Boston University group found the maximum temperature in the body of the canal to be 80°C (176°F), whereas in the apical region the temperature peaked at 45°C (113°F).[415] A US army group reported that "the use of hot instruments for the condensation of filling material did not appear to endanger the integrity of the lateral periodontium."[416] In later research, an Army group again studied intracanal temperatures, produced this time with the Touch 'n Heat unit. They felt the operator should restrict the use of the unit to lower power settings of #2 or #3 and increase the length of time the heated tip is activated. They warned that at the top setting of #6 the unit could increase the intracanal temperature to as high as 114.51°C, a potentially damaging temperature.[417] Lee et al., at the University of Illinois, remarked that "the critical level of root surface heat required to produce irreversible bone damage is believed to be >10° C." In this context, they noted that "caution should be used with the Touch 'n Heat and flame heated carriers on mandibular incisors."[418]

System B: Continuous Wave of Obturation

Buchanan, long an impressive advocate of the warm gutta-percha vertical compaction technique, has developed a variation of the method that he perceives as faster and more accurate. Concerned with the complexity and time consumed in completing an obturation, he retained the principles of vertical compaction but improved the methodology. Working with Analytic Technology, which had developed the Touch 'n Heat device for warming gutta-percha in the canal, Buchanan and Analytic perfected the **System-B Heat Source** and associated pluggers (SybronEndo/Analytic; Irvine, Calif.). This new heat source monitors the temperature at the tip of the heat-carrier pluggers, thus "delivering a precise amount of heat for an indefinite time."[419]

System B obturation is predicated on a precise preparation, perfectly tapered to match as closely as possible the shape of the nonstandardized gutta-percha cones-fine, fine-medium, medium, and medium-large (F, FM, M, and ML). Another Buchanan/Analytic development is gutta-percha cones that match the shape produced during canal preparation using **Greater Taper** instruments.

Downpack Technique. An appropriate size gutta-percha cone, matching the completed preparation shape, is tested in the canal to be sure it goes fully to place. This is confirmed radiographically. "Continuous Wave Technique requires good canal shape and meticulous gutta-percha cone fitting. The cone must fit in its last 1 mm, and fit to full length before minimal cutback (less than 0.5 mm)."[419] The cone is then removed and the corresponding **plugger** is tried for size in the canal. It should stop at its **"binding-point,"** about **5 to 7 mm short** of the working length. The stop attachment is then adjusted at the coronal reference point and the plugger is removed and attached to the **Heat Source**. The canal is dried.

The primary point is coated with sealer and pushed into place, all the way to the apical stop. The Heat Source is activated, set for "use" and "touch," and the temperature is set for 200°C and the power dial at 10. The cone is then seared at the orifice with the preheated plugger tip, and the preheated plugger is then "driven" smoothly through the gutta-percha to within 3 to 4 mm of its **binding point** in the canal. This will take about 2 seconds. Maintaining apical pressure, the plugger will continue to move apically, and at this time the heat switch is released. The plugger is held there, **cold,** under sustained pressure, for an additional 10 seconds. It is during this period the gutta-percha flows to the apical matrix and into accessory canals. The pressure also compensates for the shrinkage that might occur as the mass cools.

To remove the plugger: while still maintaining apical pressure, the heat switch is activated for **only 1 second** followed by a 1-second pause. The "cold" plugger is then quickly withdrawn. Following radiographic confirmation, the remainder of the canal is now ready for backfill.

Backfill Technique. Using the same size gutta-percha cone and plugger, the cone is coated with sealer and positioned in the backfill space in the canal. The System B temperature is now set at 100°C. Preheat the plugger out of the canal for only ¼ second, cut the heat, but immediately plunge the plugger into the backfill cone and hold it in place for 3 to 5 seconds as the gutta-percha cools. Another cone is added in the backfill space and heat is again applied. The final plugging is done with a large cold regular plugger. Another method of backfilling is to use the Obtura II gutta-percha gun.

To date there have been few reports on the success of the System B Technique. On the other hand, concern has been expressed about the 200°C heated plugger so near the thin root at the apex. The short period of time this high heat is delivered, however, seems to preclude any periodontal damage.

Warm/Sectional Gutta-percha Obturation. The use of small warmed pieces of gutta-percha, the so-called sectional obturation technique, is one of the earliest modifications of the vertical compaction method described earlier. Webster might well have been describing this procedure in 1911 when he spoke about filling "with gutta-percha, using points heated and well packed in with hot instruments."[228] Eventually this became known as the "Chicago" technique since it was widely promoted by Coolidge, Blayney, and Lundquist, all of Chicago. It was also the favorite technique of Berg of Boston.[420]

The method begins like other methods: fitting the plugger to the prepared tapered canal (Figure 11-63, A). It should fit loosely and extend to within 3 mm of the working length. A silicone stop is then set on the shaft marking this length (Figure 11-63, B). Next, the primary gutta-percha point is blunted and carried to place. It should be fitted 1 mm short of the working length and confirmed radiographically (Figure 11-63, C). Upon removal, 3 mm of the tip of the point are cleanly excised with a scalpel (Figure 11-63, D) and this small piece is then luted to the end of the warmed plugger (Figure 11-63, E). Sealer is placed, lining the canal, the gutta-percha tip is warmed by passing it through an alcohol flame, and it is then carried to place. Under apical pressure, the plugger is rotated to separate the gutta-percha (Figure 11-63, F) and it is thoroughly packed in place. At this point, it is best to expose a radiograph to be sure the initial piece is in position (Figure 11-63, G). If so, the remainder of the canal is filled in a like manner, compacting additional pieces of warmed gutta-percha until the canal is filled to the coronal orifice[421] (Figure 11-63, H).

If a post is planned, the compaction can stop after the second piece, leaving 5 to 6 mm of apical canal filled. Another variation of heat-softening the gutta-percha is

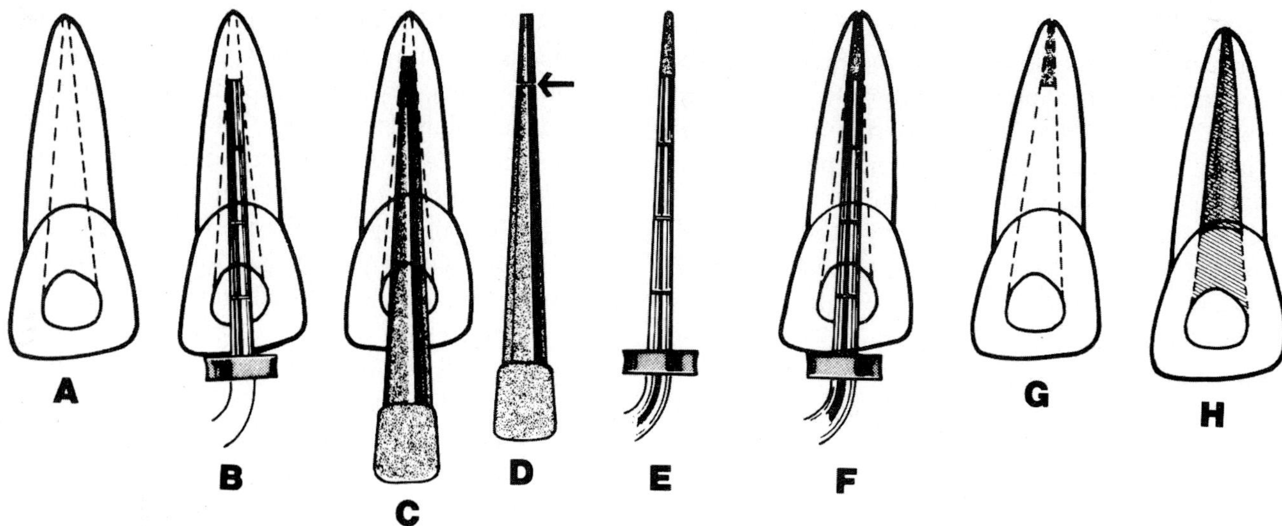

Figure 11-63 Sectional gutta-percha obturation. **A**, Canal prepared with flare. **B**, Plugger preselected to fit loosely in canal and extend to within 3 mm of working length. **C**, Master gutta-percha point fitted to within 1.0 mm of working length. Confirm by radiograph. **D**, Gutta-percha is removed and 3 mm of apical point are excised (**arrow**). **E**, Plugger is warmed in alcohol flame and point is luted to plugger. Gutta-percha is warmed by passing through alcohol flame and quickly coated with cement. **F**, Warm gutta-percha is carried to place; plugger is rotated to loosen and then used for compaction. **G**, Radiograph should confirm well-condensed apical filling. **H**, Remainder of canal is filled by lateral or vertical condensation, by Compactor or Obtura. (Courtesy of Dr. Ahmad Fahid.)

to soften each piece in chloroform or halothane in a quick "dip."

Rather than laboriously adding sections of gutta-percha, backfilling may be done with thermoplasticized gutta-percha from one of the gutta-percha "guns." In evaluating such backfill, Johnson and Bond noted that "it may be clinically acceptable to backfill canals up to 10 mm in a single increment using sealer and the Obtura II gutta-percha system."[422]

Lateral/Vertical Compaction of Warm Gutta-percha. Considering the ease and speed of lateral compaction as well as the superior density gained by vertical compaction of warm gutta-percha, Martin developed a device that appears to achieve the best qualities of both techniques. Called **Endotec II** (Medidenta Inc; Woodside, N.Y.), the newly designed device is a battery-powered, heat-controlled spreader/plugger that ensures complete thermo-softening of any type of gutta-percha. It is supplied with two AA batteries that provide the energy to heat the attached plugger/spreader tips (Figure 11-64). The quick-change, heated tips are sized equivalent to a No. 30 instrument, are autoclavable, and may be adjusted to any access angulation. Martin claims that the "Endotec combines the best of the two most popular obturation techniques: warm/vertical and the relative simplicity of lateral compaction" (H. Martin, personal communication, December 1999).

Canal cleaning and shaping for this technique is a continuous taper design with a definite apical stop. After the primary point is fitted to full working length, the hand spreader and the Endotec plugger/spreader are fitted as well. At this point, silicone stops are placed to mark the length of canal.

After drying of the canal, a limited amount of sealer is applied. The primary point is then firmly positioned and gently adapted with a hand or finger spreader. It has also been recommended that one or two additional gutta-percha points be placed to reduce the possibility that the warm plugger will loosen the point when the tip is retracted.

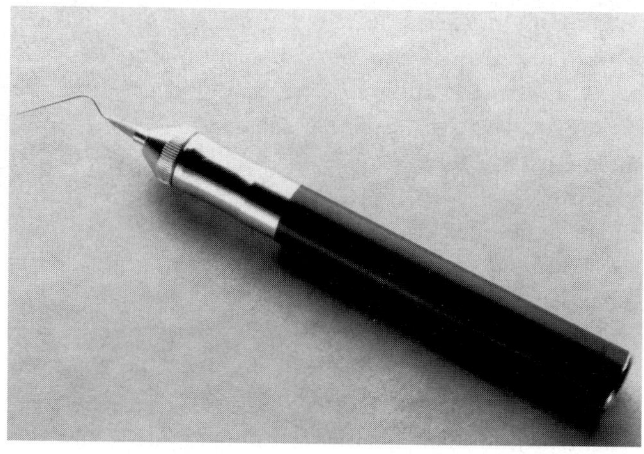

Figure 11-64 **Endotec II** handpiece contains battery power pack. Button initiates heat in attached plugger. (Courtesy of Medidenta, Inc.)

At this juncture the Endotec plugger is placed in the canal to full depth. The activator button is pressed and the heating plugger is moved in a **clockwise motion**. The heat button is then released and the plugger cools immediately. It is now removed from the gutta-percha with a **counterclockwise motion**. This lateral compaction has formed a space for an additional point to be added, after which the plugger is again placed, heated, moved clockwise for 10 to 15 seconds, cooled, and retracted counterclockwise (Figure 11-65). Now the plugger can be used cold to compact the softened gutta-percha, followed again by warming and lateral space preparation for additional points.

In this manner (lateral compaction with the heated plugger to provide space for additional gutta-percha, and the vertical compaction with the cooled plugger to condense the heat-softened gutta-percha) the canal is entirely obturated. Finally, a cold hand plugger can be used to firmly condense the fused gutta-percha bolus.

The Endotec can also be used to soften and remove gutta-percha for post preparation or in the event of retreatment. An Air Force group also found they could measurably improve compaction while obturating a mandibular molar with a C-shaped canal by using the EndoTec in what they termed a "zap and tap" maneuver: preheating the Endotec plugger for 4 to 5 seconds before insertion (zap) and then moving the hot instrument in and out in short continuous strokes (taps) 10 to 15 times. The plugger was removed while still hot, followed by a "cold spreader with insertion of additional accessory points."[423]

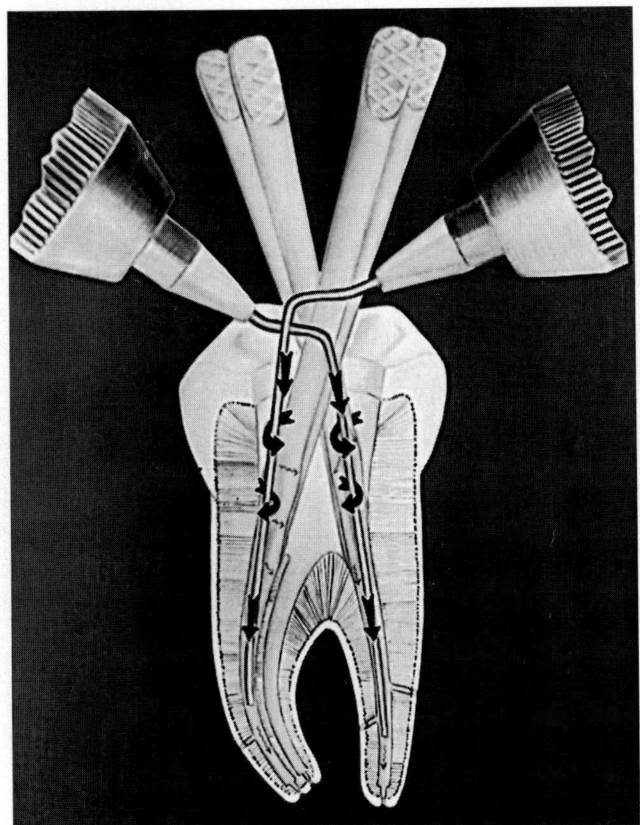

Figure 11-65 Motion for using **Endotec II**- plugger/spreader—vertical pressure with sweeping lateral pressure. Additional gutta-percha points will be added. (Courtesy of Dr. Howard Martin.)

Concern has been voiced that heat from the tip will damage the periodontium, and that the lateral/vertical pressure exerted will be too stressful. In the first instance, it was found there was "no heat related damage to periodontal tissues from either of the two methods employed": Endotec and warm/vertical compaction.[424] A US Army group also tested for heat damage from the **Touch 'n Heat** unit, which produces more heat (816°C) than the Endotec. They pointed out that even though the internal gutta-percha mass reached 102°C, gutta-percha and dentin are poor heat conductors, and this temperature "would not be of sufficient magnitude to cause damage in the periodontal tissues."[425]

In the second instance, that of stress development, Martin and Fischer have shown, in a photoelastic stress test, that "warm lateral condensation (Endotec) created less stress during obturation than did cold lateral condensation."[373]

Efficacy of the Warm/Lateral Technique. Because gutta-percha is heated with this technique, there must be a commensurate shrinkage when it cools. This fact alone would bring into question the density of the final filling. However, Martin point out that the Schilder compaction method leads to 0.45% shrinkage, and since Endotec temperatures are lower than with the other technique, shrinkage following Endotec usage should be lower as well.[426]

A US Army group evaluated the quality of the apical seal produced by lateral versus warm lateral compaction and found no significant difference in leakage.[359] In contrast, Kersten, in Amsterdam, reported that "Endotec had significantly less leakage than any of four other methods."[372] Ewart and Saunders, in Glasgow, found much the same.[427]

Himel and Cain, at Tennessee, achieved the best result with the Endotec if they condensed the gutta-percha bolus five times with the **cold** plugger after each warming with the plugger heated. This practice filled lateral and accessory canals as well: "the gutta-percha was not melted but soft enough it would flow into fins and ramifications."[428] A US Army group reported they could improve the density (by weight) of laterally compacted canals by 14.63% by a follow-up use of the Endotec. A second use added another 2.43% of gutta-percha.[429]

As far as tissue reactions to the technique are concerned, Castelli et al. found that "some Endotec specimens generated small restrictive inflammatory infiltrates restricted to the root canal opening," whereas the warm gutta-percha "vertical condensation inflammatory reactions, because of their extensive nature, were probably the source of maintaining discomfort and pain."[424]

Thermomechanical Compaction of Gutta-percha. A totally new concept of heat softening and compacting gutta-percha was introduced by McSpadden in 1979. Initially called the **McSpadden Compactor**, the device resembled a reverse Hedstroem file, or a reverse screw design. It fit into a latch-type handpiece and was spun in the canal at speeds between 8,000 and 20,000 rpm. At these speeds, the heat generated by friction softened the gutta-percha and the design of the blades forced the material apically. In experienced hands, canals could be filled in seconds.

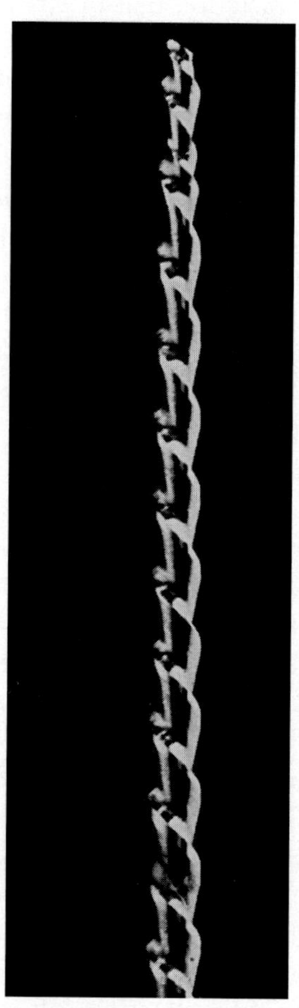

Figure 11-66 **Micro-Seal Gutta-percha Condenser** is operated at slow speed. The **reverse-screw action** compacts plasticized gutta-percha apically and laterally. (Courtesy of SybronEndo/Analytic-Quantec.)

However, problems developed and the Compactor fell into disfavor. Fragility and fracture of the instruments, along with overfilling because of the difficulty in mastering the technique, led to its demise. However, phoenix-like, it rose again in different shapes and forms. In Europe, Maillefer modified the Hedstroem-type instrument as the **Gutta-Condenser,** and Zipperer (Germany) called its modification the **Engine Plugger**. The latter more closely resembles an inverted K-file.

McSpadden, in the meantime, modified his original patent and brought out a newer, gentler, slower-speed model. It is now supplied as an engine-driven instrument made of nickel titanium (see Figure 11-66) and presented as part of the **Microseal System** (Analytic/Quantec, USA). Because of their flexibility, the NiTi condensers may be used in curved canals.

The Microseal Condenser is used in conjunction with heat-softened, alpha phase-like gutta-percha as well as regular gutta-percha points. Of course, sealer is always used. To obturate a canal, the clinician is advised to place the primary gutta-percha point, followed by the appropriate size Condenser (one that will reach near the working length), which has been coated with the heat-softened gutta-percha (Figure 11-67). The Condenser is spun in the canal with a controlled speed handpiece at 1,000 to 4,000 rpm to form a firmer core. This "flings" the gutta-percha laterally and vertically (Figure 11-68).

McSpadden has developed a technique to fill open-apex cases as well by initially depositing a bolus of low-heat gutta-percha at the apex with a large condenser. This is allowed to cool and harden to form an apical plug against which the remaining canal is obturated with gutta-percha points and additional heat-softened gutta-percha.[430]

To date, this particular technique—combining the reverse screw-type condenser with warmed alpha gutta-percha—has not been widely reported in US literature; however, the technique is popular in Europe, with some reporting from there.

Efficacy of the Thermomechanical Compaction Method. The original McSpadden compactor was well studied in the 1990s, and these findings are not totally moot because a modification is being distributed as the Brasseler TLC (Thermal Lateral Condensation) as well as the aforementioned European models, the Maillefer **Gutta-Condensor** and the Zipperer **Engine Plugger**. These instruments have enjoyed a good deal of use, particularly for "backfilling" after the initial vertical or lateral compaction is complete.

This latter method has been termed the **hybrid technique** by Tagger et al. of Tel Aviv.[375] They first coat their

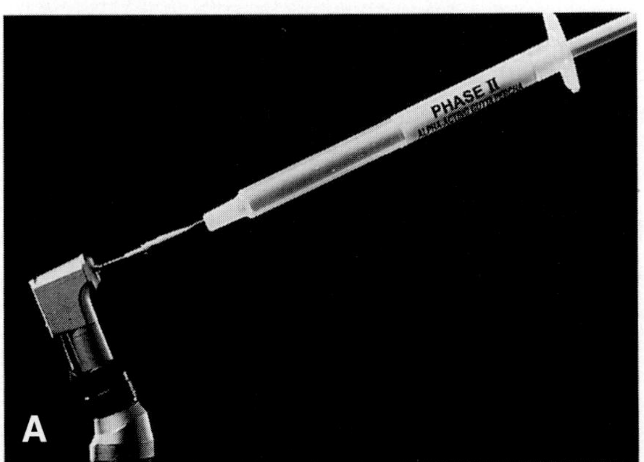

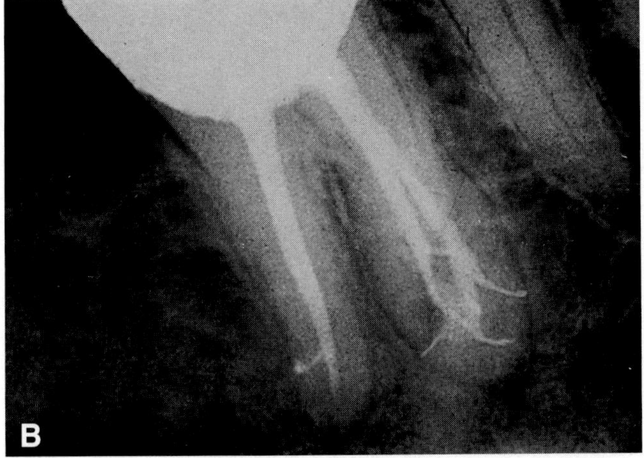

Figure 11-67 A, Loading plasticized Phase II gutta-percha onto Micro-Seal Condenser already coated with Phase I gutta-percha. B, Obturation of curved and accessory canals using **Condenser** and Phase I and II gutta-percha. (Courtesy of Analytic/Quantec Endodontics.)

regular primary point with sealer, move it to place, and spread it aside with a finger spreader followed by an accessory point. They then place an Engine Plugger, size 45 or 50, 4 or 5 mm into the canal and rotate it at 15,000 rpm. After 1 second, it is advanced into the canal until resistance is met and then slowly backed out while still rotating. Only 2 or 3 seconds are involved to completely fill the canal.

Comparing the hybrid technique with lateral condensation, Tagger et al. reported **significantly less apical leakage** with the hybrid technique.[375] They previously had reported no significant difference in leakage when they used thermomechanical compaction alone (not the hybrid technique) versus lateral compaction.[361] Some agreed,[360,374,431] whereas others found thermomechanical compaction **improved** the apical seal.[371,376]

Saunders at the University of Dundee found that "the Hybrid method would be the technique of choice." He found that it was "quicker to complete than conventional lateral condensation, should carry a reduced risk of fracture to slender roots and is relatively easy to master." Overfilling is also less likely.[432]

Concern has been expressed about the intracanal heat generated during thermomechanical compaction. Could it be damaging to the periodontium? Hardie at the University of Dundee recorded *in vitro* "rises in temperature up to 27°C" on the **external** midsection of roots. She voiced a need for caution if a 4-second appli-

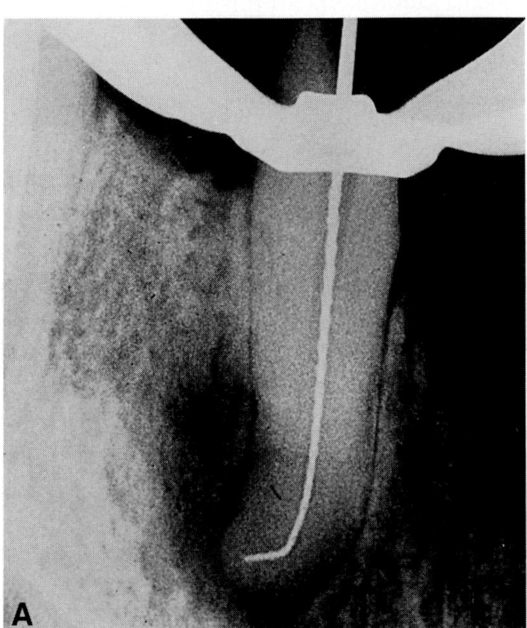

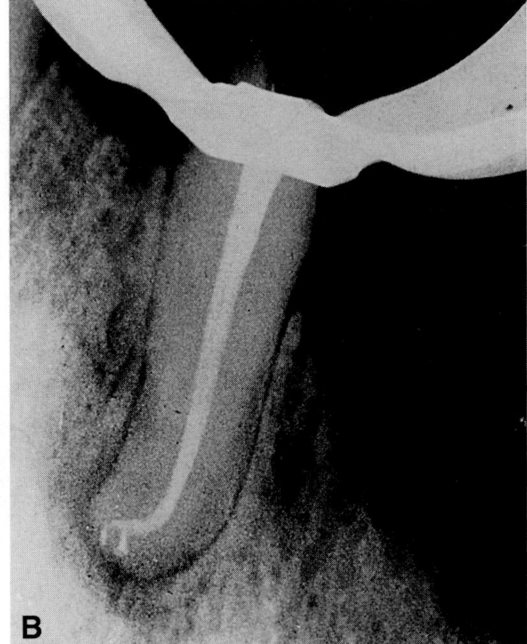

Figure 11-68 A, Remarkable flexibility of nickel-titanium condenser allows careful rotation in curved canals at very slow speed. B, Final filling by Condenser. (Courtesy of Dr. John McSpadden.)

cation of a spinning compactor could produce this much rise in temperature.[433] Saunders, also at Dundee, performed *in vivo* hyperthermia studies on ferrets using an Engine Plugger at 10,000 rpm. He found a median 18.31°C temperature rise during use, which then dropped to a 1.25°C rise in 1 minute.[434] He also examined these specimens histologically 20 days after testing and found resorption of cementum in 20% of the specimens. At 40 days he found about 25% exhibited resorption as well as **ankylosis of bone to cementum** and sounded a note of caution.[435]

In Sweden, with workers using the compactor for 8 seconds, temperature increases as much as 50°C (35°C mean) were recorded. They, too, felt that "periodontal complications from thermomechanical condensation are possible."[436] At the University of Florida, a group stated that higher speeds or longer duration than recommended could "cause an adverse temperature rise…and a detrimental effect upon the quality of the seal."[437]

These "outer-limit" studies lead one to conclude that care must be used, "kinder and gentler," in any of these mechanical, heat-generating methods. On the other hand, they make a case for the less aggressive method: **slower-speed, lower-temperature** plasticized gutta-percha that can be placed with less stress to the tooth, yet provide optimal obturation.

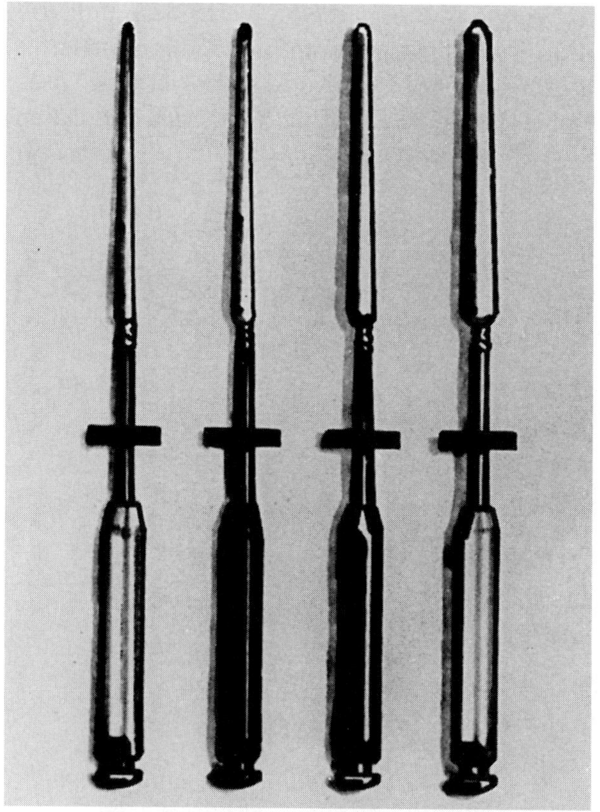

Figure 11-69 **J.S. Quick-Fill** titanium carriers coated with alpha-phase gutta-percha comes in four sizes and operates in regular slow-speed handpiece. Friction plasticizes gutta-percha. Titanium core may be severed and left or removed while still spinning. (Courtesy of J.S. Dental Mfg. Co.)

Thermomechanical Solid-Core Gutta-percha Obturation. One other innovation using the thermomechanical principle to compact gutta-percha in the root canal has been introduced as the **J.S. Quick-Fill** (J.S. Dental Co., Sweden/USA). This system consists of titanium core devices that come in ISO sizes 15 to 60, resemble latch-type endodontic drills, coated with alpha-phase gutta-percha (Figure 11-69). These devices are fitted to the prepared root canal and then, following the sealer, are spun in the canal with a regular low-speed, latch-type handpiece. Friction heat plasticizes the gutta-percha and it is compacted to place by the design of the Quick-Fill core. After compaction, there are two choices: either the compactor may be removed while it is spinning and final compaction completed with a hand plugger or the titanium solid core may be left in place and separated in the coronal cavity with an inverted cone bur.

Pallares and Faus, from Valencia, Spain, conducted an apical leakage dye study comparing J.S. Quick-Fill against lateral condensation. They found no significant difference in efficacy; however, they did find with the J.S. Quick-Fill that the sealer (AH26) adapted more peripherally against the dentin walls and the gutta-percha was more centrally located. The cement had also penetrated the dentinal tubules and the lateral and accessory canals.[438] Canalda-Sahli and his coworkers, also from Spain, found that J.S. Quick-Fill could be used successfully to seal root canals in teeth with large straight canals.[439]

Ultrasonic Plasticizing. The technique of plasticizing gutta-percha in the canal with an ultrasonic instrument was first suggested by Moreno from Mexico.[440] He used a **Cavitron ultrasonic scaler** (Dentsply/Caulk; Milford, Dela.) with a PR30 insert, but because of its design it could be used only in the anterior mouth. Moreno placed gutta-percha points to virtually fill the canal. He then inserted the attached endodontic instrument into the mass, activated the ultrasonic instrument (without the liquid coolant), and as it plasticized the gutta-percha by friction, advanced it to the measured root length. Final vertical compaction could be done with hand or finger pluggers.[440]

At San Antonio, workers questioned the heat generated by this technique. Would it be damaging? Using the Cavitron PR30, they found very little heat rise: 6.35°C in 6.3 seconds. Using an **Enac ultrasonic unit** (Osada Co.; Los Angeles, Calif. and Japan), however, they recorded a

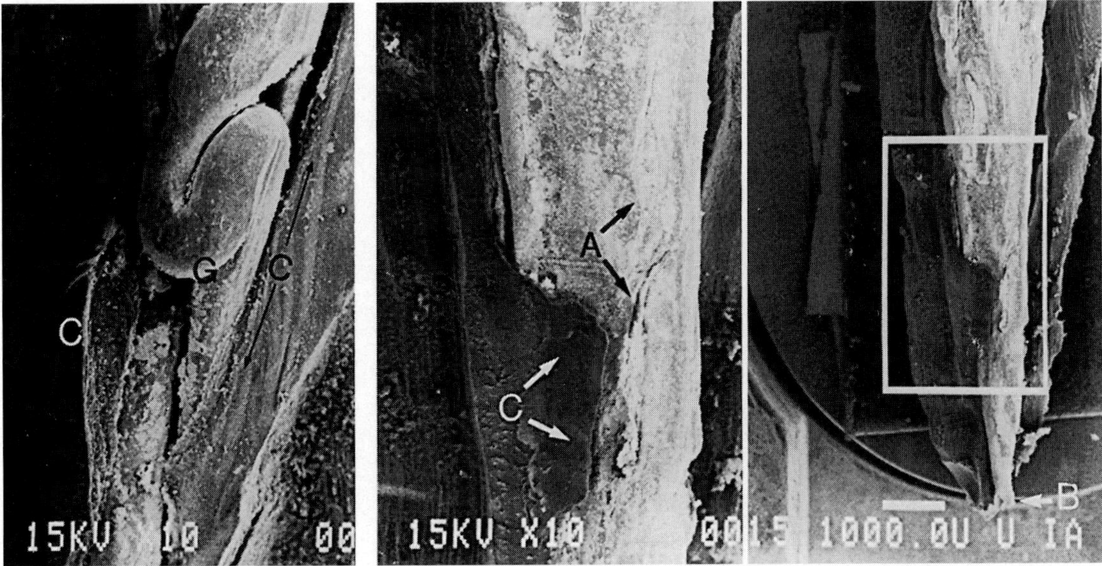

Figure 11-70 Comparison in obturation between hand-lateral compaction and **ultrasonic compaction. Left,** Accessory point folded in canal during lateral compaction following finger spreading. G, individual gutta-percha points. C, canal wall. High power (×320 original magnification). **Center,** Gutta-percha compacted by **Enac ultrasonic** spreader tips (no fluid coolant.) Note uniformity of gutta-percha mass with only two "crevice marks" (A). C denotes canal walls. High power (×320 original magnification). **Right,** Low power (×10 original magnification) of apical third obturation by ultrasonic. B marks well-filled foramen. Rectangular area is seen at high power in center panel. Reproduced with permission from Baumgardner KR and Krell KV.[442]

19.1°C rise in temperature because it took 141 seconds to plasticize the mass. They felt the heat generated by the Cavitron would not be harmful.[441]

At the University of Iowa, on the other hand, a group was quite impressed with a technique using an **Enac ultrasonic unit (Osada) with an attached spreader.** Unlike the University of Texas group, however, they did not attempt to plasticize the gutta-percha. They felt the spreader more easily penetrated the mass of gutta-percha than did the finger spreaders, and that in the end, the **energized spreading technique** led to a more homogeneous compaction of gutta-percha with less stress and less apical microleakage[442] (Figure 11-70).

Thermoplasticized Injectable Gutta-percha Obturation. An innovative device, introduced to the profession in 1977, immediately caught the fancy of dentists interested in the compaction of warm gutta-percha. Developed by a group at Harvard/Forsyth Institute, gutta-percha was ejected out of a prototype pressure syringe that had warmed it to 160°C. At this temperature, the gutta-percha would flow through an 18-gauge needle.[443] From this early model, a more efficient system was developed and patented.[444,445] Today, through further improvements, the device is marketed as the **Obtura II Heated Gutta-Percha System** (Obtura-Spartan Corp., Fulton; Mo.) (Figure 11-71), with digitally controlled temperatures ranging from 160°C to 200°C while the needle size has been reduced to either 20 gauge (equal to a size 60 file) or 23 gauge (equal to a size 40 file) (Figure 11-72).

Although regular **beta-phase gutta-percha** is still used, the clinician can now choose a less viscous, higher flow form of gutta-percha known as **Easy Flow** (Charles B. Schwed Co.; Kew Gardens, N.Y.).

Gutmann and Rakusin, leading proponents of thermoplasticized gutta-percha obturation, have emphasized the importance of properly preparing the canal to receive the injection needle and compacting the warm gutta-percha. They point out the importance of preparing a "continuously tapering funnel from the apical matrix to the canal orifice."[446] They especially note the significance of properly shaping the transitional area from the apical third to the middle third, particularly in curved canals (Figure 11-73), and warn against the development of the "coke-bottle" canals so frequently seen following Gates-Glidden canal preparations (Figure 11-74). The tapered preparation enhances the flow of the plasticized material, whereas the Coke-bottle preparation negates the flow.[446]

A definitive **apical matrix** is also important. This constriction prevents the extrusion of filling material into the periapex (see Figure 11-73). Preparations to size 25 or 30 files at the apical terminus, tapered to a size 60 file at the coronal orifice, have proven perfectly

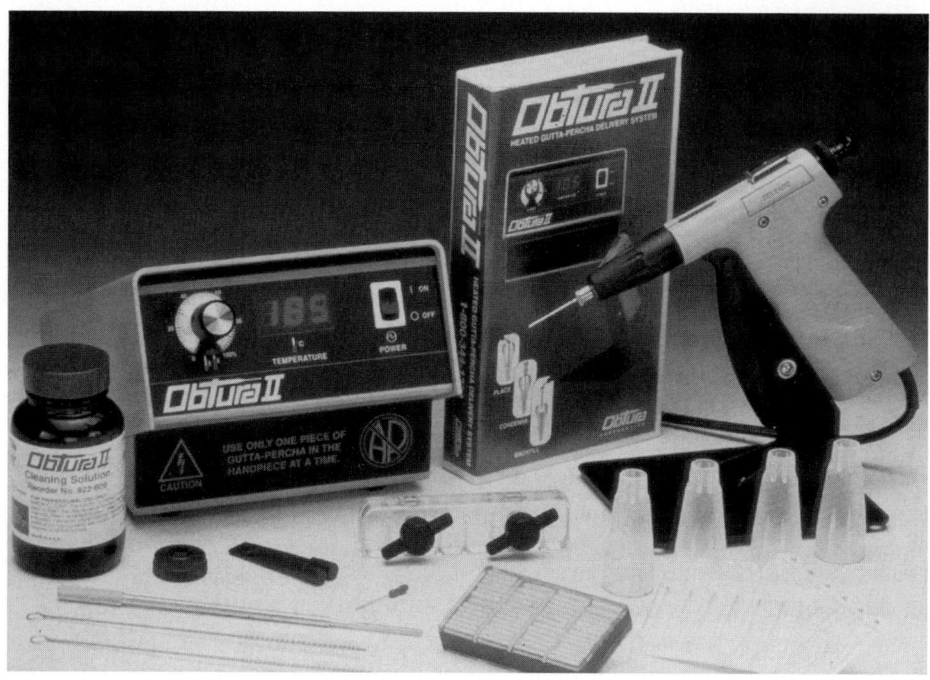

Figure 11-71 Obtura II delivery system. Panel has temperature control and digital temperature display in degrees Celsius. The pistol-grip syringe (**right**) extrudes plasticized beta-phase gutta-percha through flexible needle. Technique VHS is included. (Courtesy of Obtura/Spartan USA.)

adequate as long as there is sufficient blending of the coronal preparation with the apical preparation.

Methods of Use. Although initially it was hoped that the "gutta-percha gun" could be used to totally obturate the canal, it soon became apparent that sealer and further compaction were necessary. Sealer serves its usual role of filling the microscopic interface between the dentin and gutta-percha as well as acting as a lubricant. Compaction became necessary to close spaces and gaps while forcing the gutta-percha laterally and vertically. It also compensates for shrinkage as the gutta-percha cools. Furthermore, the smallest injection needle, 23 gauge, was too large to reach the apex in most cases.

Initially, a technique was developed of depositing the warm plasticized gutta-percha well down into the canal and then compacting it with hand or finger pluggers to the apical terminus. In using this method, however, one must be prepared to act as soon as the gutta-percha is placed because it cools rapidly and hardens, often within 1 minute; however, the **Easy Flow** gutta-percha does afford at least 10 to 15 more seconds of working time.

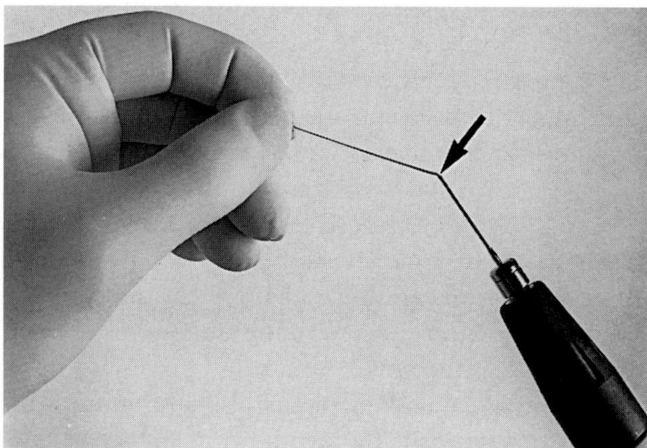

Figure 11-72 Warm plasticized gutta-percha stream extruded through needle tip (**arrow**) of Obtura II. (Courtesy of Obtura/Spartan USA.)

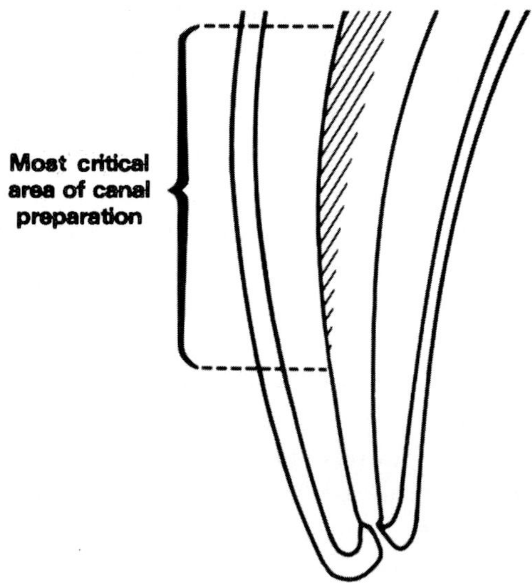

Figure 11-73 Gutmann insists that the most critical area of canal preparation is the transition from the apical third to the middle third of the canal. Reproduced with permission from Gutmann JL and Rakusin H.[446]

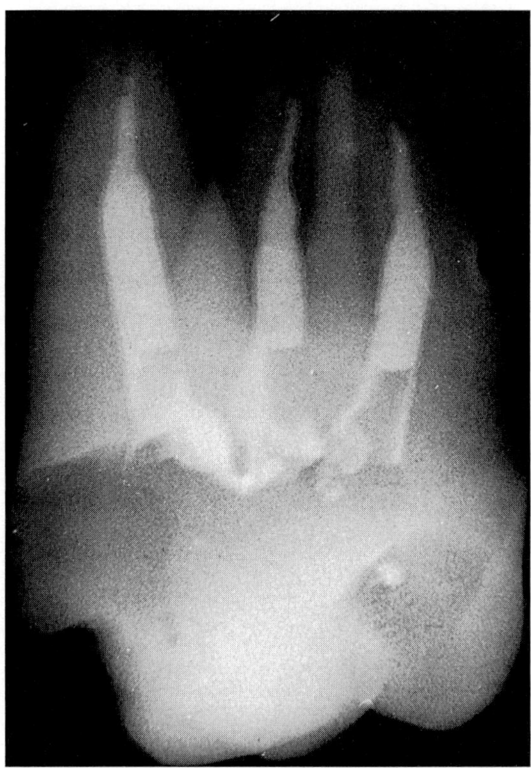

Figure 11-74 Excessive preparation with Gates-Glidden burs or Peeso reamers creates rapid tapering. The "Coke-bottle effect" of the canal negates efficient flow of plasticized gutta-percha. Reproduced with permission from Gutmann JL and Rakusin H.[446]

The injection needle and pluggers must have been previously tried for size in the canal. Although the manufacturer recommends that they should reach within 3.5 to 5 mm of the terminus and fit loosely at that point, sufficient compaction can still occur as long as the needle reaches halfway between the canal orifice and apical terminus in a well-prepared canal. In fact, Lambrianidis and coworkers in 1990 demonstrated that there was no statistically significant difference in linear dye leakage in **Obtura-filled** canals in which there were varying distances of the needle tip from the apical foramen during obturation.[447] Regardless of whether a sectional technique is used or a complete filling method is used, silicone stops are placed on **pluggers of adequate diameter** to ensure they will move and compact the softened material and not just "pierce" through it.

A light liner of a slow-setting sealer is placed into the dried canal to the prechosen depth short of the apex. Excessive sealer causes pooling and should be avoided. Sealers such as **Roth's 801, AH Plus, or Sealapex** are recommended. This is followed by the Obtura needle, and a **deposit of gutta-percha is made**. The canal may be totally filled as the needle is withdrawn, or a small deposit may be made and compacted with the intention of filling the canal segmentally.

Research by Johnson and Bond at Louisiana State University showed no difference in dye penetration in canals that were backfilled with 1 mm, 4 to 5 mm, or 10 mm increments irrespective of whether Roth's 801 or AH26 sealer was used.[448] However, the clinician probably has better control of moving and compacting gutta-percha when segmental filling is done.

Once the deposit is placed, the premeasured plugger is rapidly used to move the gutta-percha apically and laterally. A drop of sealer on the tip of the plugger will prevent its adhering to the gutta-percha. When one is satisfied that the apical third is obturated, a quick radiograph or digital image can be made to ensure the placement. Once viewed, the obturation may be completed.

If the filling is short, gutta-percha, if now firm, may be warmed with a hot instrument and then further compacted; the bolus may also be completely removed and the canal refilled. In this event, one may warm the tip of a Hedstroem file, insert it into the gutta-percha, let it cool for 1 minute, and then remove the bolus of gutta-percha. Refilling of the canal can then be done, this time inserting the pluggers to a **greater depth**, using Easy Flow gutta-percha and/or **re**preparing the canal first. The radiograph of the final result should show a thoroughly compacted, totally obturated reflection of the tapered canal preparation (Figure 11-75).

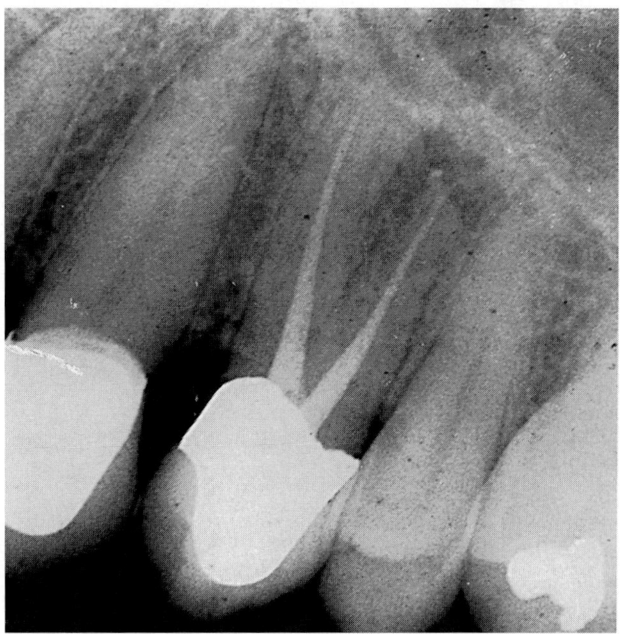

Figure 11-75 Ideal tapered preparation for any obturation technique, particularly syringe delivery of plasticized gutta-percha. Reproduced with permission from Gutmann JL and Rakusin H.[446]

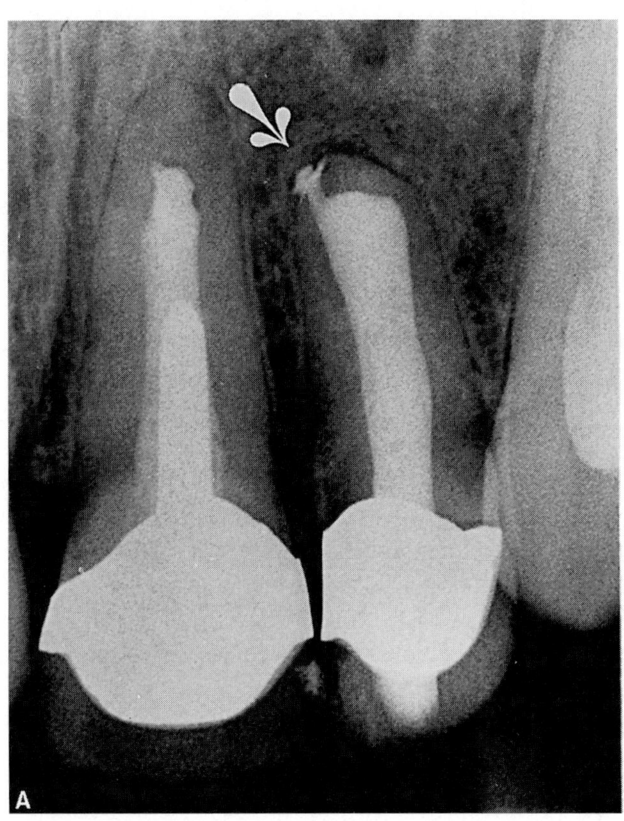

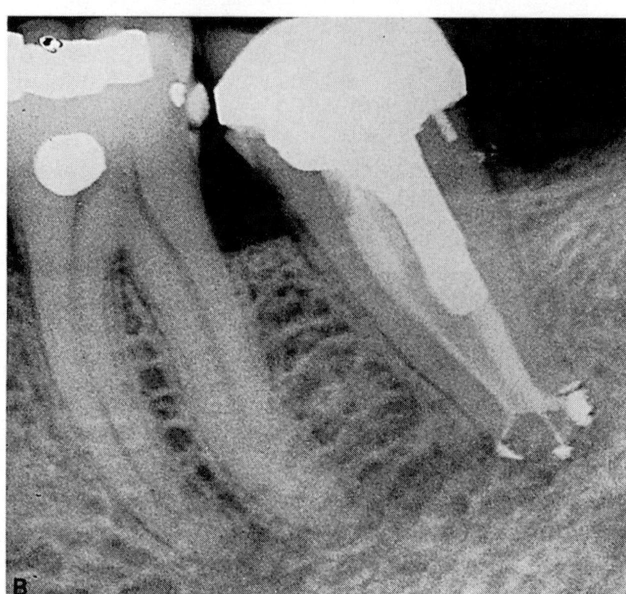

Figure 11-76 Use of the **Obtura II** in obturating enormous canals. **A**, Filling following apexification. Open foramen denotes necessity of obturation. **B**, C-shaped canal with trident foramina (**arrow**). (**A** courtesy of John G. Schoeffel.) **B** reproduced with permission from Serota KS. Oral Health 1989;79:35.

Another popular obturation method used by many endodontists is to initially place a fitted master point to the apical terminus and follow this with the Obtura needle-tip, depositing a bolus of warm gutta-percha around the point. This is immediately compacted vertically and laterally. More plasticized gutta-percha is then added and compacted. This technique will better ensure **apical closure without overfilling.**

Success with any of these techniques is operator dependent. Repeated practice on plastic-block canals as well as extracted teeth is imperative. To gain intraoral experience, one might start by using the device to **backfill** other methods before tackling full-treatment cases and by initially using the system on large, relatively straight canals. As a matter of interest, the Obtura II is probably being used more frequently as a backfilling device than for primary obturation.

Efficacy and Safety of the Thermaplastic Injectable Gutta-Percha Technique. A number of studies on the heat generated by this method have been done. Gutmann et al. found *in vitro* that the gutta-percha emerged from the needle at 71.2°C in a body temperature environment.[449]

In an *in vivo* study on dogs, the mean intracanal temperature of the gutta-percha was 63.7°C. Maximum temperature elevation on the bone overlying these test teeth was only 1.1°C over 60 seconds. This appears to be a safe temperature level.[450]

Others recorded much higher (137.81°C) intracanal recordings.[451] Hardie recorded a temperature rise of 9.65°C on the external surface of a tooth.[452] This dropped to 4.75°C in 3 minutes and compared with a 15.38°C rise in temperature generated by an Engine Plugger compactor spinning at 8,000 rpm.[452] Bone injury has been reported with external root temperature rises of 10°C if maintained for 1 minute.[453] Hardie's reported 9.65°C increase (dropping to 8.20°C in 1 minute) appears to fall within safe limits.[452] Weller and Koch evaluated external root temperatures *in vitro* when using gutta-percha thermoplasticized at 200°C and additionally found that the rise in temperature was well below the critical level of 10°C.[454]

The efficacy of thermoplasticized gutta-percha in filling fins and *cul-de-sacs*,[455] internal resorption cavities,[456,457] "C"-shaped canals, accessory canals, and arborized foramina is well documented (Figure 11-76). All researchers insist, however, that sealer is necessary to prevent microleakage.[347,458] Clinical success rates with the injection technique have been reported at 93.1%.[459]

Compared with other techniques, the thermoplasticized, regular beta-phase (higher heat) gutta-percha proved equal to laterally compacted cold gutta-percha in a number of studies of microleakage[362–364] and significantly poorer in others.[347,348] Virtually all of the studies reported some overfilling and apical extrusions.[347,348,362,363] At least one author admitted, however, that his group's results "confirmed the opinion of Gutmann and Rakusin that clinicians should take time to master the technique before employing it in the treatment of their patients."[347] As with any obturation technique, the efficacy and long-term success of the method are highly dependent on the cleaning and shaping of the canal and the resultant degree of retention and resistance form that is developed.

Inject-R Fill–Backfilling Technique. As stated earlier, the Obtura II is frequently used in "backfilling," a method for completing total canal obturation after the apical third of the canal has been filled. Another method of **backfilling** has been developed by **Roane** at the University of Oklahoma and is marketed as **Inject-R Fill** (Moyco-Union Broach; Bethpage, N.Y.).

Inject-R Fill, a miniature-sized metal tube containing conventional gutta-percha and plunger, simplifies warmed vertical compaction by altering the backfilling process. The technique allows for delivery of a **single backfill injection** of gutta-percha once the apical segment of a canal has been obturated (Figure 11-77).

The apical segment of the canal can be obturated using any technique including lateral compaction, traditional warm vertical compaction, or System B. If a cold lateral technique is used, the cones of gutta-percha extruding from the canal must first be heat severed at a sufficient depth so a plugger can be used to compact the remaining heat-softened segment in the apical third of the canal. If the System B or vertical compaction is used, the method already results in an apically compacted segment.

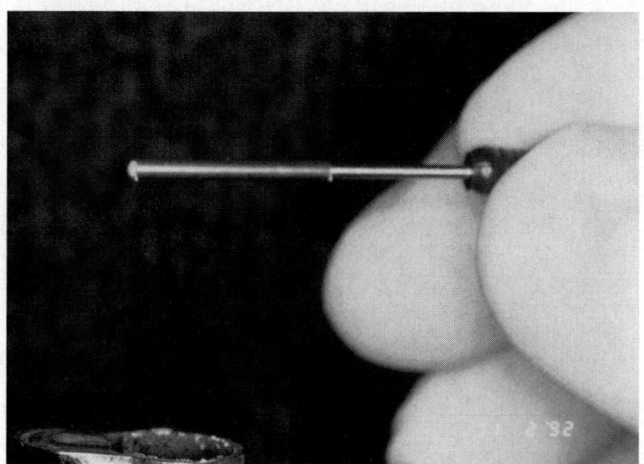

Figure 11-77 **Inject-R-Fill** shows protrusion of heat-softened gutta-percha prior to its insertion into the canal. (Courtesy of Moyco/Union Broach Co.)

According to the **Inject-R Fill technique**, the coronal walls must be resealed with sealer prior to filling the region with gutta-percha from the device.[460] The Inject-R Fill must first be heated in a flame or an electronic heater and the coronal surface of the gutta-percha already in the canal should be warmed using a heated instrument. When a burner is used, the stainless steel gutta-percha filled sleeve is waved through the flame until gutta-percha **begins to extrude** from the open end. The warmed unit is then placed into the orifice of the canal. For the device to fit, the **canal orifice must be at least 2 mm in diameter**. A push of the handle toward the canal injects the heated gutta-percha into the canal. The carrier is then rotated to break it free from the access.

Prefitted hand or finger pluggers are subsequently used to compact the gutta-percha and push the injected mass into contact with the apical segment. The plugger must be positioned in the center of the mass and pressed firmly toward the apex. Pressure is sustained for a few seconds before the plugger is rocked from side to side and rotated to break it free. As the plugger is removed, a small void is left in the center of the mass. The void is closed by folding over remaining gutta-percha from the sides and packing it apically. This process is repeated until a larger plugger can be used without creating a void and the gutta-percha mass is firm. Coating the tip of each Inject-R Fill with sealer before placing it in the canal will prevent sticking of the gutta-percha and should enhance the gutta-percha/sealer/canal interface. According to Roane, the technique is rapid and produces a result similar to that of warm vertical compaction (personal communicaton, April 2000).

An important caveat must be issued, warning anyone using a system of injection, thermoplasticized gutta-percha—**be very careful not to force or overinject the heat-softened material.**[461] Disastrous results may develop if, for example, the softened gutta-percha is injected into the maxillary sinus or the inferior alveolar canal (Figure 11-78).

SOLID-CORE CARRIER: MANUAL INSERTION

ThermaFil (Dentsply/Tulsa)
Densfil (Dentsply/Maillefer),
Soft-Core (Soft-Core System, Inc.), and
Three Dee GP (Deproco UK Ltd.)

In 1978, Johnson described a unique yet simple method of canal obturation with thermoplasticized

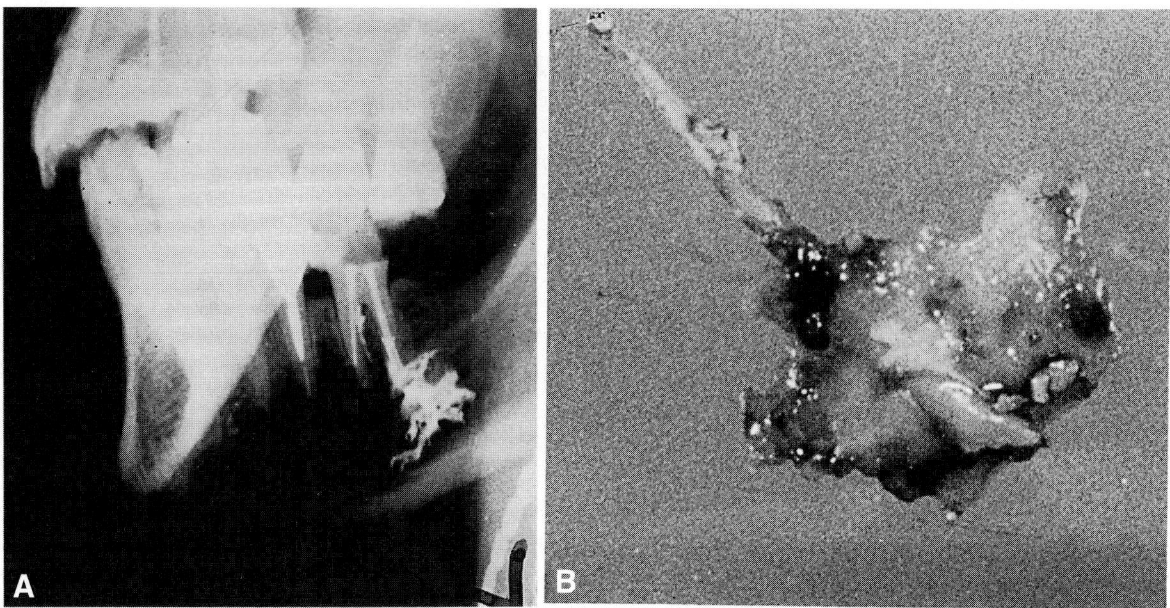

Figure 11-78 A, Plasticized gutta-percha extruded from syringe overfills enormous area of mandible. **B**, Pathologic specimen of osteomyelitic bone and chronic inflammation attached to extruded gutta-percha. Reproduced with permission from Gatot A et al.[461]

alpha-phase gutta-percha carried into the canal on an endodontic file.[462] What was a curiosity in 1978 has become today a popular and respected technique of canal obturation (Figure 11-79). ThermaFil is considered the major core-carrier technique, and through a licensing agreement with Dentsply, a duplicate product, Densfil was created. Recently, two similar products were introduced: **Soft-Core**, and its European version, **Three Dee GP**.

"ThermaFil is a patented endodontic obturator consisting of a flexible central carrier, sized and tapered to match variable tapered files (.04/.06) endodontic files. The central carrier is uniformly coated with a layer of refined and tested alpha-phase gutta-percha."[463] The use of the variable tapered files in canal preparation has enhanced the fit, placement, movement, and compaction of the gutta-percha delivered by the ThermaFil core carrier. Likewise, the ThermaFil system now

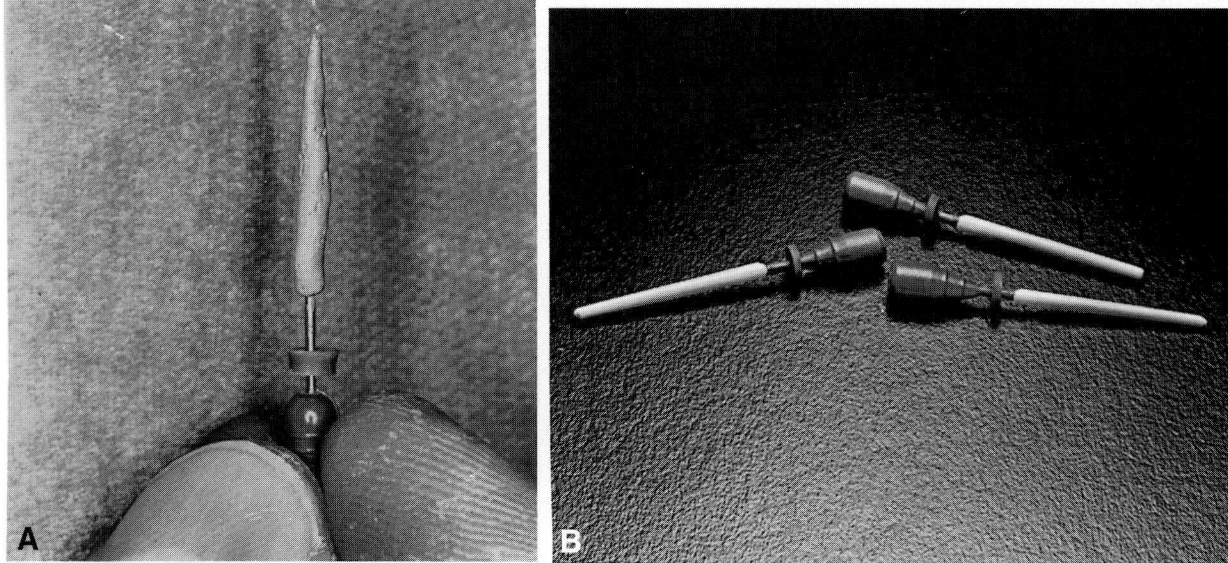

Figure 11-79 A, Original handmade gutta-percha obturator mounted on regular endodontic file. **B**, Modern manufactured **Thermafil Obturators**—alpha-phase gutta-percha mounted on radiopaque, flexible, plastic carriers. Note silicone stop attachments. **A** reproduced with permission from Johnson WB.[462] (**B** courtesy of Dentsply/Tulsa Dental Products.)

comes with metallic **size verifiers** that are used to determine, with greater precision, the size and shape of the prepared canal prior to choosing the correct ThermaFil carrier.

Initially, the **central carrier** was a newly designed stainless steel device. Contemporary carriers are made of radiopaque plastic that is grooved along 60 degrees of their circumference (Figure 11-80). While the gutta-percha covering the original carriers was heated in a flame, the new plastic core carriers are heated in a controlled oven environment called the **ThermaPrep Plus heating system** (Dentsply/Tulsa; Tulsa, Okla.) (Figure 11-81). The heating time is well delineated and is dependent on the size of the core carrier. The use of the oven, according to the manufacturer's directions, is essential for success with this technique.

Soft-Core, or its counterpart, **Three Dee GP**, is similar to ThermaFil; however, it contains a bipolymer compound and a tungsten core that is radiopaque. It has an easily detachable handle, referred to as a metallic insertion pin, that is removed with a slight twisting action. This leaves the coronal portion of the plastic core hollow, thus facilitating postspace preparation. The presence of the metallic insertion pin also allows a curving of the coronal portion of the carrier, thus facilitating the angle of core insertion. It is supplied in a sterile blister pack that also contains a matching size verifier. The carriers are thinner in taper than the ThermaFil carriers but are ISO sized at the apex. This was done to facilitate their use in small canals that are difficult to shape. Heating of the gutta-percha on the Soft-Core carrier is done in a halogen oven that is thermostatically controlled.

Method of Use. The detailed use of the core carrier obturation technique has evolved after years of development and clinical use.[464] Careful cleaning and shaping of the canal are essential, as is the development of a **continuously tapering preparation.** Contemporary dictates favor the use of the **variable tapered endodontic files** to achieve this goal and to enhance the obturation afforded by the ThermaFil technique.

Prior to obturation, it is recommended that the smear layer be removed with the appropriate agents. This will promote the movement of the softened material into the dentinal tubules and enhance the seal.[465] After the canal is dried, a **very light** coat of sealer is applied to all of the walls. It acts as an adhesive as well as a lubricant. Preferred sealers include **Thermaseal** (Dentsply/Tulsa; Tulsa, Okla), **AH-Plus** (Dentsply/Maillefer; Tulsa, Okla.), **Sealapex** (Kerr/Analytic; Orange, Calif.), or ZOE cements. Quick-setting cements such as Tubliseal, or cements that contain natural gutta-percha softeners, such as Sealex or CRCS, **should be avoided** with this technique. In the case of the former, the sealer sets up too rapidly when warmed. In the case of the latter, the chemical softening of the gutta-percha makes it too tacky and adherent to the dentin walls, thereby reducing its flow apically and into the canal irregularities.

Immediately after the sealer is applied, the warmed obturator is removed from the ThermaPrep Plus heater and carried slowly to full working length in the canal.

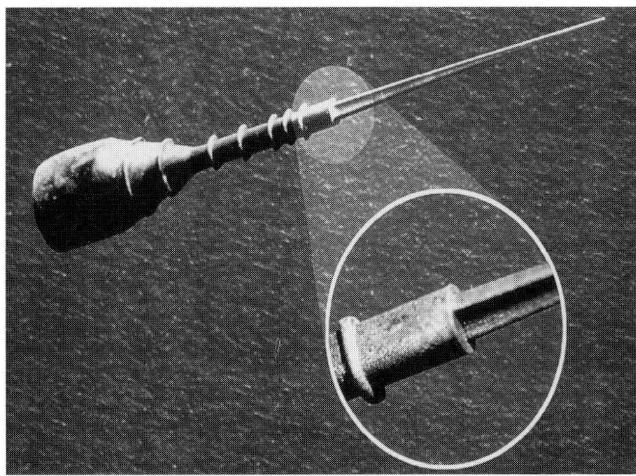

Figure 11-80 Details of the anatomy of the Thermafil plastic **Carrier.** The core is grooved to allow for the release of trapped air during the placement of the carrier. Note also the circular millimeter markings above the grooved area that facilitate length placement of the carrier. (Courtesy of Dentsply/Tulsa Dental Products.)

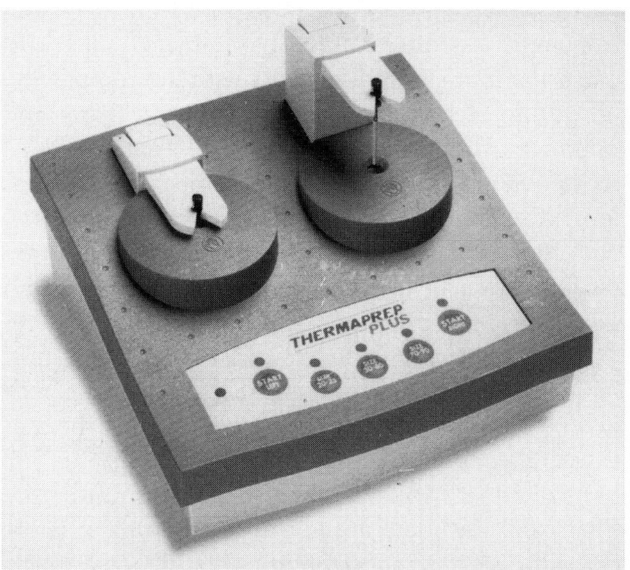

Figure 11-81 **ThermaPrep Plus** oven ensures proper softening of Thermafil Obturators within seconds. (Courtesy of Dentsply/Tulsa Dental Products.)

Previously, the **built-in rubber stop**, on the calibrated shaft, had been set at the proper length position. The carrier is not twisted during placement, and attempts to reposition the carrier should be avoided to prevent disruption of the gutta-percha that was initially positioned through the compacting action of the core carrier.

Once it is ensured radiographically that the canal has been filled to the desired position, the shaft is severed in the coronal cavity. While the handle is firmly held aside, a No. 37 inverted cone bur is used to trim off the shaft **2 mm above** the coronal orifice. Specific burs have also been developed for this task: **Prepi Bur** (**Pre**post **P**reparation **I**nstrument) (Dentsply/Tulsa; Tulsa, Okla.). The Prepi Bur, a noncutting metal ball, is run in a handpiece and is also used to create postspace safely and efficiently when needed. This space can be created immediately or on a delayed basis without altering the apical seal.[466]

Johnson has suggested that the final compaction can be improved if a 4 to 5 mm piece of a regular gutta-percha cone is inserted into the softened gutta-percha and compacted apically and laterally with a large plugger.[464] Gutta-percha accessory points can also be used in a similar fashion to achieve a greater depth of material delivery if the canal is very wide buccolingually. In this case, an appropriately sized spreader would be used to compact the cones into the softened mass. The use of warm injected gutta-percha by **Obtura** (Obtura/ Spartan, USA) is also an accepted technique to add sufficient bulk to the obturating material. The gutta-percha reaches its final set in 2 to 4 minutes.

THERMAFIL SAFETY

Saw and Messer from Australia evaluated and compared the root strains associated with the compaction of gutta-percha delivered from the Obtura and ThermaFil with lateral compaction.[467] The **ThermaFil technique** required only minimal compaction that was limited to the coronal end of the carrier. Therefore, with this technique there was **significantly less strain** during delivery and compaction than there was with the other tested techniques.

An **apical stop** or definitive apical constriction must be present to prevent movement of the gutta-percha and/or the plastic core from extending beyond the root canal. Often, a small puff of sealer or gutta-percha will be extruded.[464] A US Army group found that ThermaFil was more apt to extrude through a patent apical foramen than was Obtura, Ultrafil, or warm lateral compaction (Endotec). On the other hand, if a dentin "plug" was present at the apical orifice, ThermaFil was less apt to extrude than were the others.[468] The use of the size verifiers in choosing the correctly sized core carrier has also reduced the incidence of material overextension.

The precurving of ThermaFil obturators is usually not necessary if the canal is prepared properly, as the flexible carrier will easily move around curves. With this technique, gutta-percha will flow easily into canal irregularities such as fins, anastomoses, lateral canals, and resorptive cavities[464,469] (Figure 11-82).

Efficacy of ThermaFil Obturation. A nationally recognized evaluator of materials, devices, and techniques, **Clinical Research Associates (CRA),** headed by Christensen, has indicated that "ThermaFil allows simple, fast, predictable filling of root canals. It was found to be especially useful for small or very curved canals."[470] Radiographic assessment of this gutta-percha delivery technique has been quite favorable,[468] and recent adaptation studies that have looked at the contemporary use of the technique have found it comparable to, if not better than, lateral compaction.[469,471]

Gutmann et al. and W. P. and E. M. Saunders from Glasgow evaluated ThermaFil versus lateral compaction in a series of studies.[469,471] They reported that "ThermaFil resulted in more dense and well adapted root canal fillings throughout the entire canal system than lateral condensation with standard gutta-percha." Both techniques "demonstrated acceptable root canal fillings in the apical one-third of the canal." Similar excellent adaptation was observed when comparing ThermaFil with the System B technique.[472] However, the gutta-percha from the ThermaFil carrier did show a greater propensity to extrude beyond the apex.[469,472]

Wolcott and coworkers, in an *in vitro* study at Tennessee, found that the movement of ThermaFil gutta-percha and sealer into lateral canals was comparable to lateral compaction; however, the ThermaFil was more effective in the main canal.[473] Weller et al. at Georgia used a split-tooth model to assess gutta-percha adaptation using Obtura, three types of ThermaFil core carriers, and lateral compaction.[474] No root canal sealer was used. The best adaptation was with Obtura obturations, followed by ThermaFil plastic, ThermaFil titanium, ThermaFil stainless steel, and lateral compaction. Of interest in this study was the lack of apical extrusion noted with the ThermaFil obturations.

In assessing leakage patterns with the **contemporary** ThermaFil technique, Gutmann and W. P. and E. M. Saunders found initially "no significant differences in leakage between the techniques."[469] At 3 to 5 months, however, both techniques revealed apical microleakage. On the other hand, "ThermaFil obturations demonstrated greater adaptation to the intricacies of the canal

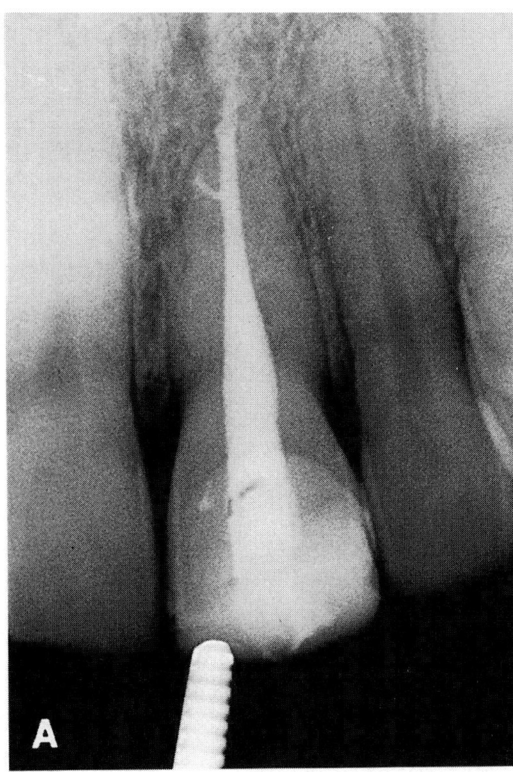

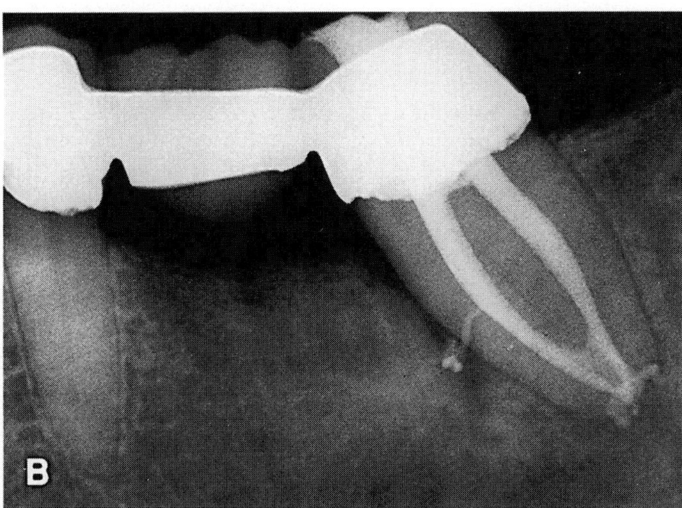

Figure 11-82 Obturation with **Thermafil. A**, Central incisor filled with size 60 Thermafil Obturator—plastic carrier. Note lateral canal near apex. **B**, Both mesial and distal canals filled with size 45 Thermafil Obturators—plastic carrier. Note apical fill and lateral canal. (Courtesy of Dr. W. Ben Johnson.)

system."[469] Fabra-Campos reported much the same from Spain.[475] Using plastic-carrier ThermaFil and lateral compaction, Pathomvanich and Edmunds from Wales used four different leakage methods and found no difference in the leakage patterns with any of the evaluative techniques, nor was there any difference between lateral compaction and ThermaFil.[476] Valli and coworkers compared Densfil (Thermafil look-a-like) **obturations** with lateral compaction in canals that were prepared with hand instruments.[477] While the Densfil obturations showed less mean apical leakage (1.39 mm) than lateral compaction (2.76 mm), the data were not significant. Similarily, they also compared the **coronal leakage** with both techniques, with the mean **coronal leakage** for Densfil being 2.87 mm and the mean coronal leakage for the lateral compaction being 4.028 mm, but no statistically significant differences were noted.

Most recently, both short- and long-term leakage comparing **ThermaFil with System B** in the absence of the smear layer was reported by Kytridou et al.[472] There were no significant differences in the short-term leakage patterns (10 and 24 days); however, leakage at 67 days was greater in the ThermaFil group. Unlike other studies, however, these specimens were stored in Hanks Balanced Salt Solution to better simulate the periradicular tissue fluid environment.

Silver Point Technique. Another solid-core material of long standing (but not in good standing) is the silver point technique. Despite nearly universal disapprobation, there are uses for silver points.

The fault lies not in the point but in the execution. The cavity prepared to receive the point must be as perfectly rounded and tapered as the point itself. "It must fit like a cork in a bottle." Too often, **round** silver points are cemented into **ovoid** canals. Over the years, as the sealer surrounding the point gradually dissolves away, microleakage and a subsequent periradicular lesion develop.

With all of the other techniques available, why use silver points at all? They are very easy to use in narrow canals. They are rigid, yet flexible, and can be positioned rapidly. Ingle has pointed out that "...When properly cemented to place, they provide a perfectly adequate filling for the **geriatric patient** at a real time saving."[478] He further noted that the very elderly have a limited life expectancy, and that silver points, even improperly done, have been known to last over 20 years. Treatment for a 75-year-old patient may be somewhat different than that for a 25-year-old patient.

Furthermore, secondary dentin formation narrows the canal lumen in "ancient" teeth, lending them to **preparation by reaming.** "Good candidates would be the straight round canals in upper central incisors, or the two canals in upper first premolars, or a straight palatal canal in an upper first molar, or a straight distal canal of a lower first molar. Occasionally, even buccal canals in upper molars, upper canines, or mesial canals in lower molars qualify if they are straight."[478]

These might well be cases in which the final apical preparation can best be done with one of the new reamer-type instruments: the **Handy-Gates** (Dentsply/Maillefer; Tulsa, Okla. and Switzerland) or the **LightSpeed** (LightSpeed Tech., Inc.; San Antonio, Tex.). In any event, "the silver point baby need not be thrown out with the bath."

APICAL THIRD FILLING

SimpliFill Obturation Technique

SimpliFill is a relatively new, two-phased obturation method that advocates the use of a stainless steel carrier to place and compact a 5 mm segment of gutta-percha into the **apical portion** of a canal (Figure 11-83). Once placed, the carrier is removed, leaving a plug of gutta-percha. If a post is not desired, the **second phase** uses a specially designed syringe to backfill the remainder of the canal with Ketac-Endo sealer along with accessory cones of gutta-percha. The clinician can also choose any other method to backfill the remaining portion of the canal. According to the manufacturer, the overall advantages of SimpliFill are that its use helps conserves dentin because of the Lightspeed instrumentation technique (less flaring); it eliminates additional internal forces since no spreader or plugger is used to compact the apical plug; it is simple to master; and, in contrast to other core-carrier systems, no carrier is left in the canal.

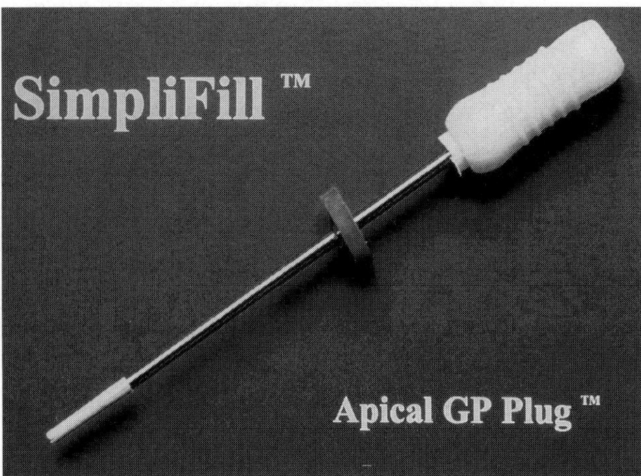

Figure 11-83 **SimpliFill** apical gutta-percha plug. Point is lightly heated and used as primary apical fill. Carrier is twisted for removal and used as plugger. (Courtesy of LightSpeed Technol.)

SimpliFill was originally developed by Senia at Lightspeed Technology to complement the canal shape created using Lightspeed instruments. The **Apical GP Plug size** is the same ISO size as the **Lightspeed "Master Apical Rotary"** (**MAR**) (see Chapter 10).

Following the completion of canal preparation using rotary Lightspeed, the specially designed **Apical GP Plug Carrier** corresponding to the MAR is **trial fitted without sealer** into the dry canal. Before insertion, however, the rubber stopper on the carrier, with its attached gutta-percha, is set **2 mm short** of the working length. The carrier is then inserted into the canal and slowly advanced, until it should start to bind at the length indicated by the rubber stop (ie, 2 mm short of the working length). Once the fit has been verified, the Apical Plug carrier is removed and the canal is coated with an appropriate sealer using the MAR or a sealer saturated paper point. The rubber stopper on the carrier is **now advanced 2 mm to the working length.** The GP Plug is subsequently coated with sealer, inserted in the canal, and advanced until resistance is felt, about 2 mm short of the working length. Using the carrier, the GP Plug is now vertically compacted to the working length with firm apical pressure. The **carrier must not be rotated** during insertion or compaction. Once the GP Plug is snugly fit, the **GP Plug is released by rotating the carrier handle counterclockwise.** During this rotation, the carrier must not be pushed or pulled. If the GP Plug does not release, the carrier sleeve is grasped with cotton pliers and, while pushing apically on the sleeve, the handle of the carrier is rotated counterclockwise and withdrawn.

Phase two consists of backfilling the remaining canal if no post is desired. The clinician has a number of options for backfilling, including the method advocated by the manufacturer described as follows. A **SimpliFill syringe** is loaded with a sealer such as **Ketac-Endo** and the sealer is slowly injected into the canal space as the tip of the needle, equivalent to size #40 file, contacts the GP Plug and is slowly withdrawn. Inserting the needle all the way to the top of the plug will help eliminate formation of air bubbles during the backfill. An ISO standardized gutta-percha cone, equivalent in size to the Apical GP Plug used to fill the apical segment, is then coated with sealer and placed into the sealer-filled canal until it contacts the compacted GP Plug. Accessory gutta-percha cones can be added as space fillers. As stated earlier, the clinician can also backfill using traditional warm-vertical compaction or may simply backfill using the **Obtura II.**

Since the technique is so new, there was only one published study. In 1999, Santos and coworkers at the

University of Texas at San Antonio evaluated the prototype sectional method (**SimpliFill**) and compared it to laterally compacted gutta-percha.[479] In their study, single canal teeth were **prepared using Lightspeed** and were subsequently obturated using three methods: lateral gutta-percho compaction with Ketac-Endo sealer, lateral compaction with Roth's 801 sealer, or the SimpliFill sectional method with Ketac-Endo sealer followed by a single cone of gutta-percha in Ketac-Endo sealer as backfill. Using India ink to measure leakage, they found **no statistically significant difference** in apical microleakage among the three groups. In addition, it was noted that the **sectional method was significantly faster than lateral compaction.**[479] Although the technique appears promising, further studies will be necessary along with clinical trials to determine the long-term efficacy of **the SimpliFill system**.

Dentin Chip Apical Filling. A method finding increasing favor, and one that inadvertently happens more often than not, is the apical **dentin chip plug**, against which other materials are then compacted. Quite probably, some of the so-called "miraculous cures" occur apically, to prepared but **unfilled** canals, because the apical foramens have actually been obturated by dentin chips from the preparation.[480] To do this deliberately constitutes the "new technique," a "biologic seal" rather than a mechanochemical seal.

The premise that dentin filings will stimulate osteo or cementogenesis is well founded. Gottlieb and Orban noted cementum forming around dentin chips in the PDL as early as 1921. The German literature is replete with this method. Mayer and Ketterl filled 1,300 canals with apical dentin chips and reported 91% success.[481] Ketterl later reported 95% success with cementum-like closure at the apex.[482] Waechter and Pritz also reported "osteocementum" apical closing in 20 human cases.[483] Baume et al. described "osteodentin" closings but incomplete calcification across all of their histologic serial sections.[484]

More often than not, dentin chip obturation undoubtedly prevents overfilling. El Deeb et al. found exactly that: "The presence of the apical dentinal plug," they stated, "was significantly effective in confining the irrigating solutions and filling materials to the canal space."[485]

This same conclusion was reached by Oswald et al., who observed that dentin chips lead to quicker healing, minimal inflammation, and apical cementum deposition, even when the apex is perforated[486] (Figure 11-84). Holland et al., from Sao Paulo, found, however, that dentin chips, **if infected**, are a serious deterrent to

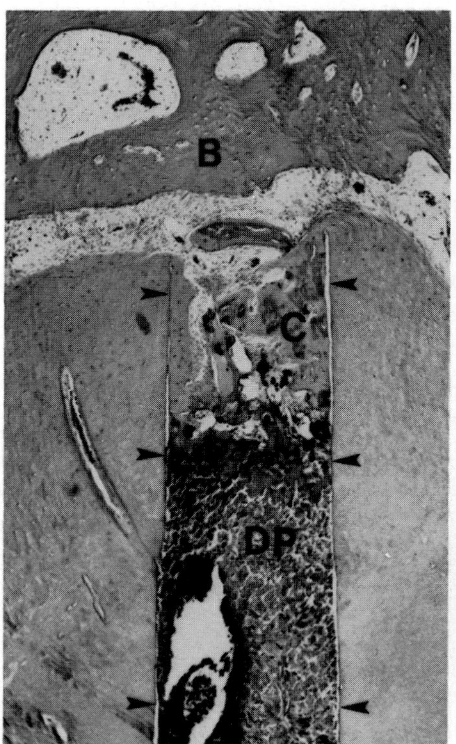

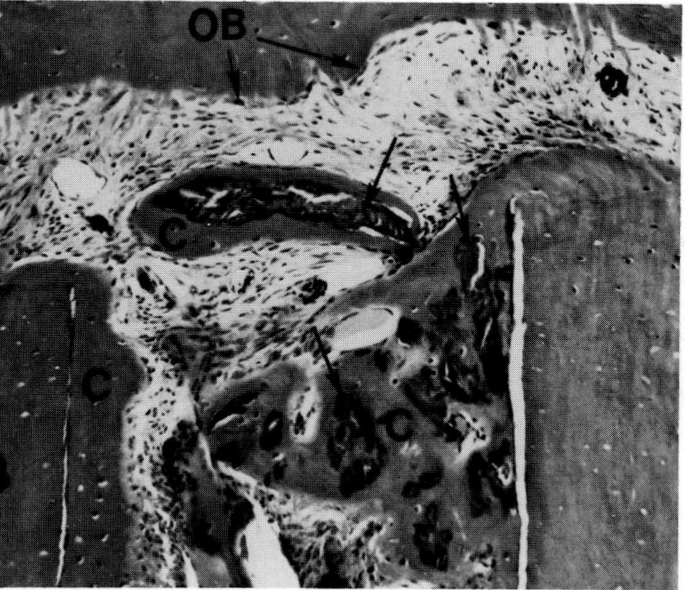

Figure 11-84 Dentin chip root canal plug after 3 months. **Left,** Periradicular area. B, bone, C, cementum, DP, dentin plug. **Arrows** indicate canal wall. **Right,** High-power view of same periradicular area. C, cementum within canal around dentin chips (**arrows**). OB, new bone cells. Reproduced with permission from Oswald RJ and Friedman CE.[486]

healing,[487] and Torneck et al. found that some dentin chips may actually irritate and hinder repair.[488]

Method of Use. The dentin chip technique has been used and taught at the Universities of Oregon and Washington (J. Marshall, personal communication, July 26, 1981; G. Harrington, personal communication, August 13, 1982). After the canal is totally débrided and shaped and the **dentin no longer "contaminated,"** a Gates-Glidden drill or Hedstroem file is used to produce dentin powder in the central position of the canal (Figure 11-85, A). These dentin chips may then be pushed apically with the butt end (Figure 11-85, B) and then the blunted tip of a paper point (Figure 11-85, C). They are finally packed into place at the apex using a premeasured file one size larger than the last apical enlarging instrument[489](Figure 11-85, D). One to 2 mm of chips should block the foramen (G. Harrington, personal communication, August 13, 1982). Completeness of density is tested by resistance to perforation by a No. 15 or 20 file. The final gutta-percha obturation is then compacted against the plug (Figure 11-86).

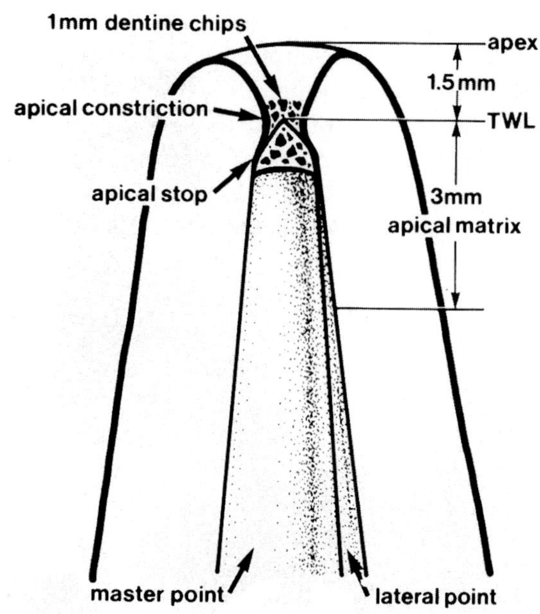

Figure 11-86 Dentin chips compacted into last 2 mm of preparation, spilling over from true working length (TWL) to stimulate cementogenesis. Gutta-percha and sealer complete obturation. Redrawn from Oregon Health Sciences University. Laboratory manual. Portland (OR): Oregon Health Sciences University; 1980.

Japanese researchers found they could totally prevent apical microleakage if they injected 0.02 mL of **Clearfil New Bond** dentin adhesive (J. Morita, Japan) into the **coronal half of the dentinal apical plug.**[490]

Harrington points out that a dentin plug is *de rigueur* if the apical foramen is perforated or open for any reason (G. Harrington, personal communication, August 13, 1982). In flaring the wall to produce dentin chips, care must be taken not to thin the walls excessively.

Efficacy of Dentin Chip Apical Obturation. As stated earlier, one of the positive effects of a dentin plug filling is the elimination of extrusion of sealer or gutta-percha through the apex. This reduces periradicular inflammation.[486] It also provides an apical matrix against which gutta-percha is compacted.[442,491] The group at the University of Connecticut found, however, that they could not totally block the apical foramen with chips following vital pulpectomy in baboons.[492] On the other hand, they did report "...hard tissue formation was common but no total closure occurred," and that "...tissue response to dentin chips was generally favorable."[492]

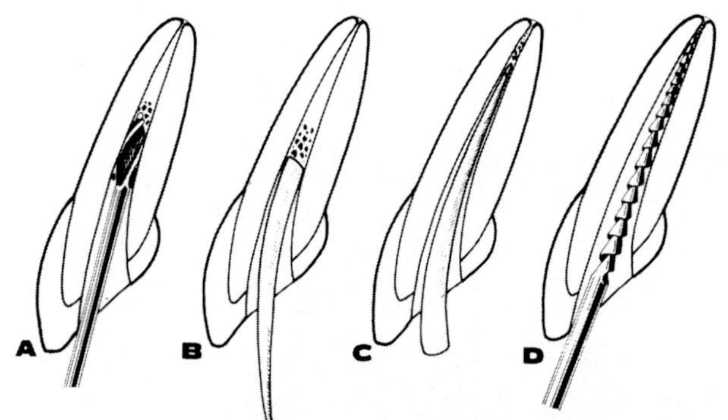

Figure 11-85 Dentin chip–apical plug filling. **A**, Clean dentin chips produced in midcanal with Gates-Glidden drill. **B**, Loose chips collected and moved apically with butt end of paper point. **C**, Dentin chips compacted at apical foramen with blunted paper point. **D**, Final compaction with file, one size larger than last enlarging instrument. Redrawn from Oregon Health Sciences University. Laboratory manual. Portland (OR): Oregon Health Sciences University; 1980.

In a monkey study at Indiana University, no attempt was made either to form or avoid forming a dentin plug. It was found, however, that 77% **of 43 cases had demonstrable plugs.** It was further reported that teeth with plugs "had a significantly lower frequency of [periradicular] inflammation than teeth without plugs ($p = 0.02$)." Although not a consistent finding, "new cementum was observed adjacent to dentin filings"[493] (Figure 11-87). However, in this experiment, the dentin plugs were not purposely produced. Also, residual pulp tissue was sometimes present.

Another monkey study done at Loma Linda University indicated that the inorganic component of dentin, **hydroxyapatite,** is evidently the principal stimulant in producing more hard tissue formation and less inflammation than are fresh dentin chips or demineralized dentin.[494]

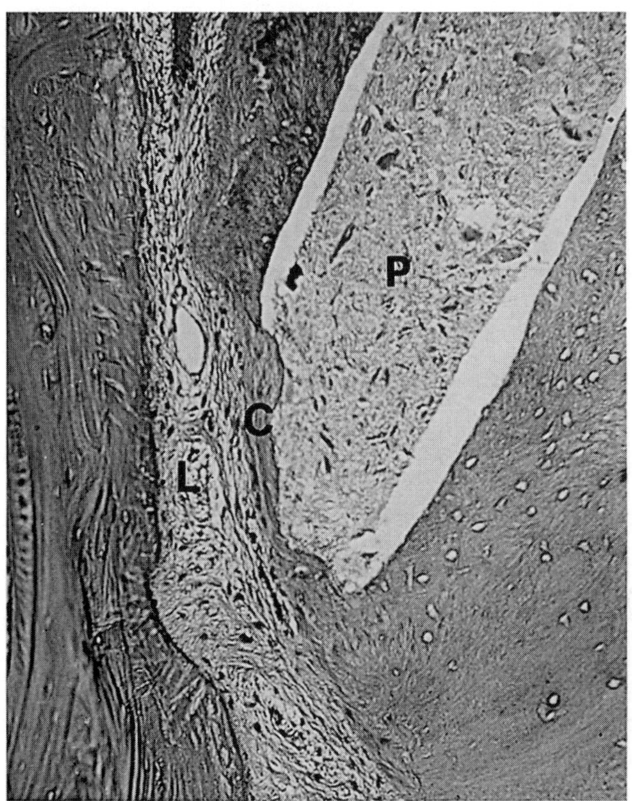

Figure 11-87 Dentin plug-induced cemental formation. Band of cementum (C) is seen adjacent to dentin plug (P). Periodontal ligament (L) is normal. Reproduced with permission from Patterson SM et al.[493]

After previously noting that **infected** dentin chips hindered periradicular healing,[487] Holland et al. compared the cementogenesis and inflammation between dentin chips and calcium hydroxide. They found that dentin chips were responsible for thicker cementum formation but that overall there was no discernible difference between the two materials in ferrets.[495]

The group at the University of Washington, in a smaller study, found that "the dentin plugs were more complete than those observed with calcium hydroxide." No inflammation was present after 1 month. Both materials worked equally well to **control the extrusion of the filling material;** however, the calcium hydroxide tended to wash out quickly.[496]

Returning to the original German studies,[423–425] through the reports by Erasquin in 1972[497] and Tronstad in 1978,[498] and including more recent reports,[490–496] one must conclude that the **dentin chip apical plug is a valuable contribution** to endodontic success and deserves to be more widely used.

Calcium Hydroxide Apical Filling. Cementogenesis, which is stimulated by dentin filings, appears to be replicated by **calcium hydroxide** as well[499–506] (Figure 11-88). Dentists have long observed the dramatic repair that occurs at the apex of a wide open canal of a tooth whose pulp was destroyed by trauma. Removing the necrotic canal contents and bacterial flora, thoroughly débriding

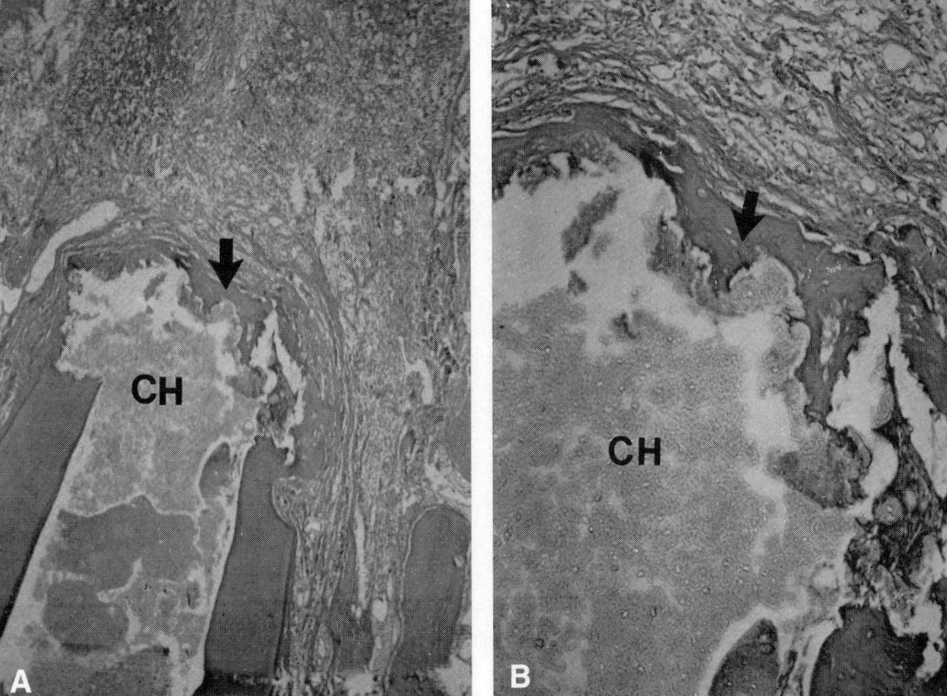

Figure 11-88 Periradicular repair following intracanal application of calcium hydroxide. **A**, Low-power view of periapex. Acute inflammatory resorption of dentin and cementum following pulpectomy. Canal filled with calcium hydroxide mixture (CH). New hard tissue forming across apex in response to $Ca(OH)_2$. **B**, Higher-power view of repair leading to apical "cap" (**arrow**). (Courtesy of Dr. Billie Gail Jeansonne.)

the dentin walls, disinfecting the space, and totally filling the canal with calcium hydroxide, will practically ensure apexification (Figure 11-89). The same phenomenon applies to the **closed** apex—cementification reacting to the placement of a plug of calcium hydroxide. This is also the theory behind the calcium hydroxide–containing sealers that appear to be better in theory than in practice.[507]

As noted previously, calcium hydroxide resorbs away from the apex faster than do dentin chips.[496] However, Pissiotis and Spångberg noted that calcium hydroxide mixed with saline resorbed but was replaced by bone in mandible implant studies.[508]

Method of Use. Calcium hydroxide can be placed as an apical plug in either a dry or moist state. Dry calcium hydroxide powder may be deposited in the coro-

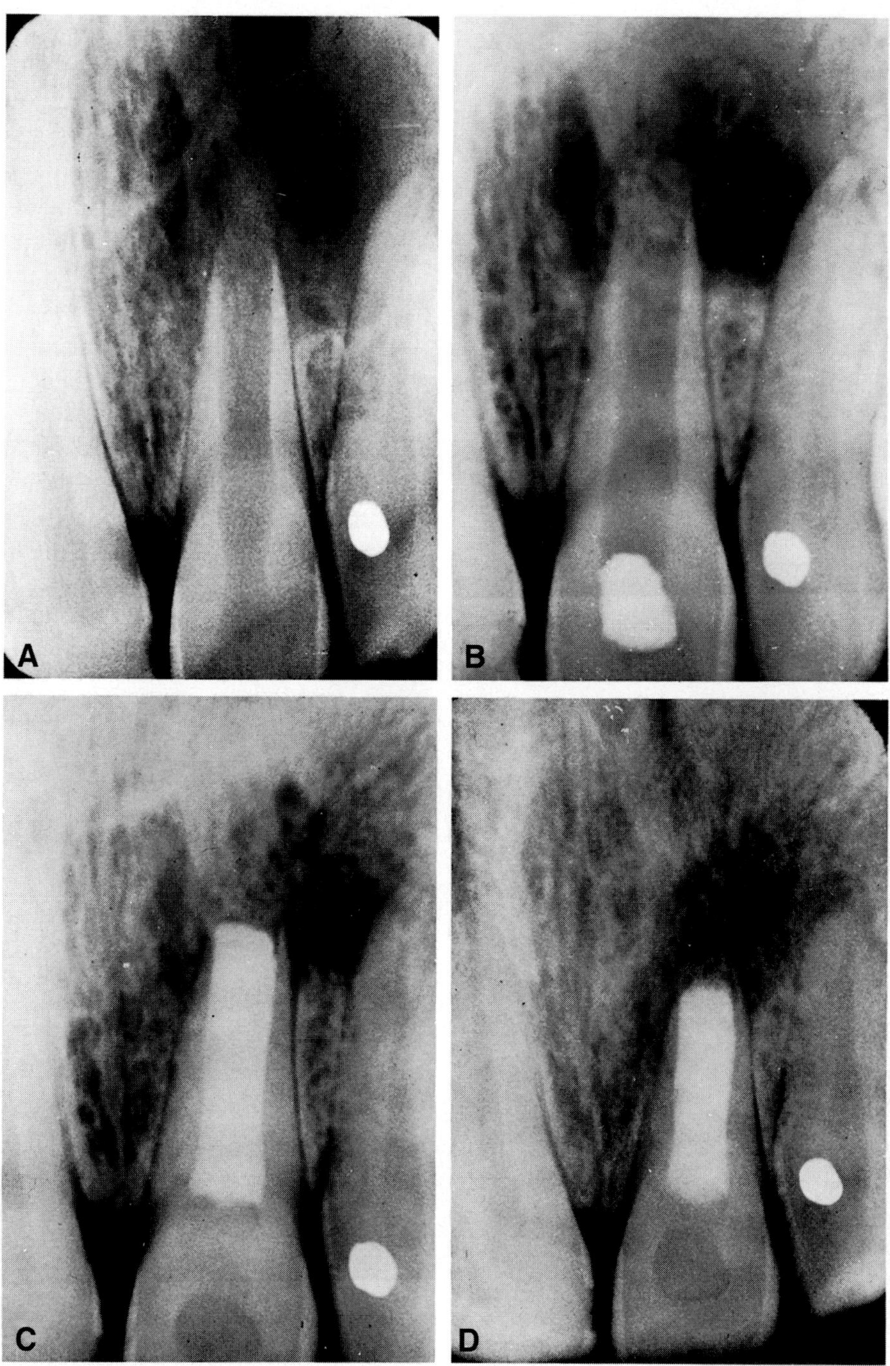

Figure 11-89 Apexification of pulpless incisor with periradicular lesion. **A**, Preoperative film. **B**, Calcium hydroxide and camphorated monochlorophenol filling canal and extruding through apex. **C**, Nine months later, canal filled with sealer, softened gutta-percha, and heavy vertical compaction. No overfilling. **D**, Two-year recall. (Courtesy of Dr. Raymond G. Luebke.)

nal orifice from a sterilized amalgam carrier. The bolus may then be forced apically with a premeasured plugger and tapped to place with the last size apical file that was used. **One to 2 mm** must be well condensed to block the foramen. Blockage should be tested with a file that is one size smaller.

Moist calcium hydroxide can be placed in a number of ways: as described earlier with amalgam carrier and plugger, with a Lentulo spiral, or by injection from one of the commercial syringes loaded with calcium hydroxide: **Calasept** (J.S. Dental Prod., Sweden/USA) or **TempCanal** (Pulpdent Corp.; Boston Mass.). In the latter method, the calcium hydroxide paste is deposited directly at the apical foramen from a 27-gauge needle and is then "tamped" to place with a premeasured plugger. If some escapes, no great damage occurs. Because of time constraints in military dentistry, a US Air Force group recommended compacting a plug of dry calcium hydroxide powder at the open apex and immediately placing the final root canal filling.[509]

In a comparison of techniques for filling entire small curved canals with calcium hydroxide, the University of North Carolina group found the Lentulo spiral the most effective, followed by the injection system. Counterclockwise rotation of a No. 25 file was the least effective.[510] If the calcium hydroxide deposit is thick enough and well condensed, it should serve not only as a stimulant to cemental growth but also as a **barrier to extrusion** of well-compacted gutta-percha obturation.

Efficacy of Calcium Hydroxide Apical Obturation. The University of Washington group reported good results with calcium hydroxide plugs. Both calcium hydroxide and dentin chips worked equally well controlling extrusion of filling materials. Although "...both plugs resulted in significant calcification at the foramen...the dentin plugs were complete..." No significant difference in periradicular inflammation was noted.[496] However, Holland noted persisting chronic inflammation and a wide variance in hard tissue deposition.[495] One would suspect contamination by oral bacteria compromised his results.

A University of Alabama group tested for microleakage canals filled by lateral compaction but blocked at the apex with three forms of calcium hydroxide: calcium hydroxide-USP, **Calasept,** or **Vitapex** (DiaDent Group International; Burnaby, B.C., Canada). There was no significant difference in leakage among the three forms of calcium hydroxide.[511] Weisenseel et al. confirmed much the same, stating that "...teeth with apical plugs of calcium hydroxide demonstrated significantly less leakage than teeth without apical plugs." All were filled with laterally compacted gutta-percha.[512]

INJECTION OR "SPIRAL" OBTURATION

By all accounts, filling the entire root canal by injection, or pumping, or spiraling material into place has great appeal. Unfortunately, the methods fall short, either because the technique is inappropriate or the materials used are inadequate.

Already discussed are the deficiencies encountered when warm gutta-percha is injected from one of the syringes to fill the entire canal. These inadequacies are caused by shrinkage from the heated to the cooled state, by failure to compact and eliminate voids, or by extrusion—serious overfilling.

An earlier favorite method of filling the canal with chloropercha and pumping it into place with gutta-percha points failed because of the severe shrinkage from chloroform evaporation.[383] This method was followed by totally filling the canal with injected ZOE cement, which will provide an immediate seal, but is often subject to dissolution and leakage over the years, leading to eventual failure.

Fogel tested five sealers placed in canals with a pressure syringe. After 30 days, he found that AH-26, Cavit, Durelon, and ZOE cement all exhibited microleakage, although AH-26 had the least marginal leakage and was the easiest to manage.[513]

The fate of totally obturating canals with cements alone using a Lentulo spiral was sealed when a number of disasters of gross overfilling with N2 or RC2B were reported. The material itself could hardly be blamed, even though it is quite toxic. Rather, the blame falls on the dentist misusing the device in a spinning handpiece (Figure 11-90). The Lentulo spiral will also cause **underfilling** if not carefully monitored (Figure 11-91).

One possible exception to the dangers and foibles of injecting filling material into the root canal may lie with the emerging hydroxyapatite as an obturant. In this case, the calcium phosphate powders are mixed with glycerine and the paste is injected into the canal. The moisture left in the canal and the apical moisture cause the paste to set to hydroxyapatite. If the material is extruded, it resorbs and will be replaced by bone. Admittedly, neither the technique nor the product have been thoroughly researched to date.[137,138,163,164]

DOWEL OR POST PREPARATION: POSSIBLE LEAKAGE

Once again, what comes out of the canal may be more important than what goes in. In this case, it is the removal of a coronal portion of the root canal filling to accommodate post or dowel placements.

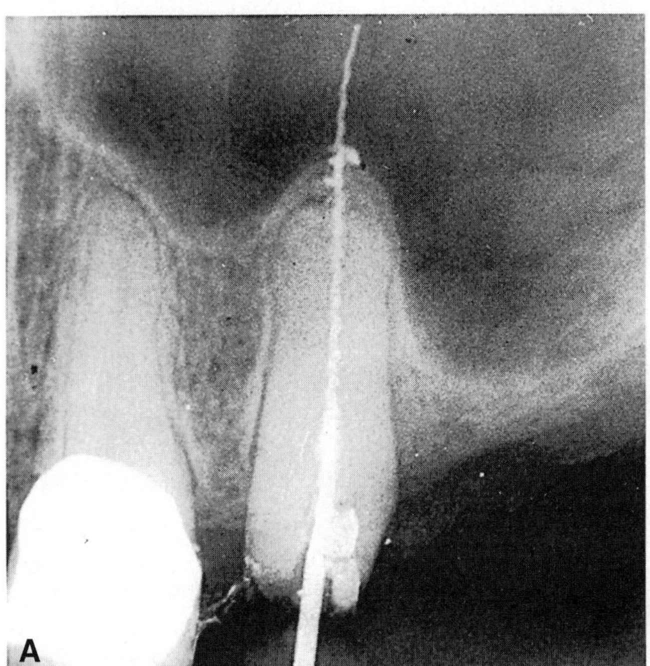

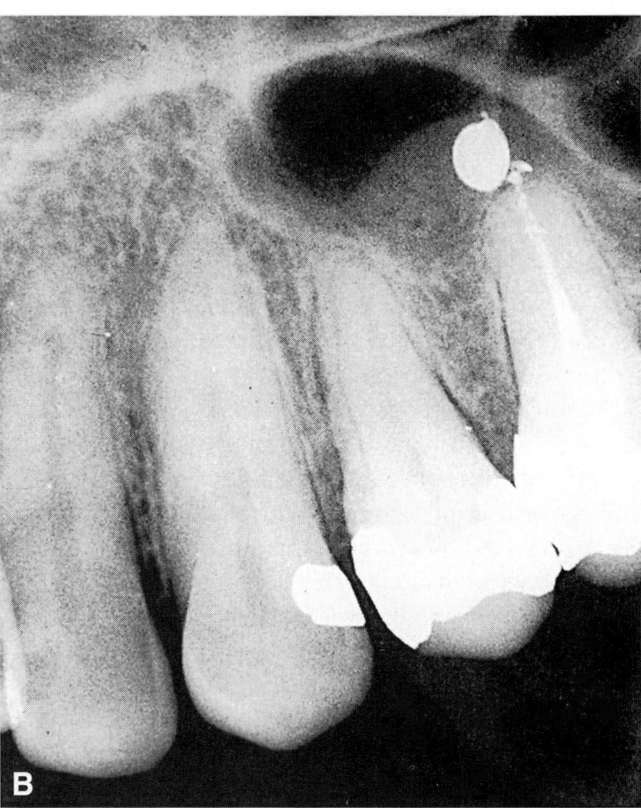

Figure 11-90 Gross negligence in canal instrumentation and obturation. **A**, Apical perforation into maxillary sinus. **B**, Gross overfilling by syringe leads to chronic sinusitis. Dentist was found guilty of negligence.

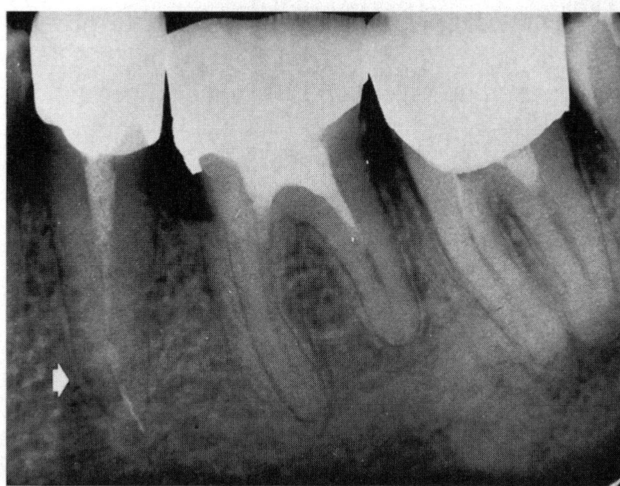

Figure 11-91 Three failures of teeth with paste-filled canals. **Right to Left**, Second molar shows periradicular lesion and root resorption as well as osteosclerosis indicating chronic inflammation. First molar has distal root resorption indicative of chronic inflammation. Premolar has broken Lentulo spiral at apex and mesial lateral periradicular lesion associated with porous root canal filling. (Courtesy of Dr. Worth Gregory.)

At Louisiana State University, two studies have been carried out examining the method of gutta-percha removal, the sealant used for obturation, and the length of the interval between obturation and the removal of gutta-percha to form the "posthole."[514,515]

The three removal methods were as follows:

1. Use of a hot plugger
2. Use of Peeso reamers
3. Use of chloroform and K-files

The results are very interesting: the **method** of removal did not seem to particularly affect the leakage results, whereas the **time** of removal was quite significant. If a hot plugger is used, the best results are achieved if the posthole gutta-percha is removed immediately after obturation.[514] If Peeso reamers or chloroform and K-files are used, however, the removal should be delayed 1 week to allow for the final set of the cement sealer.[515] Conjecture is that the hot plugger served immediately as a form of vertical condensation, improving the seal.

Other studies have essentially confirmed these findings. A US Army group found no significant difference in microleakage when they removed all but 4 mm of laterally condensed gutta-percha and sealer with four different methods of removal: a flame-heated endodontic plugger, an electrically heated Touch 'n Heat spreader, Peeso reamers, and GPX burs.[516] **GPX burs** (Brasseler; Savannah, Ga.) are designed specifically to remove gutta-percha and will not engage the dentin walls (Figure 11-92). Others have evaluated the efficacy of the methods used in filling canals prior to post preparation. In a Belgian leakage study, researchers found "no significant difference between obturation techniques": silver points, lateral compaction, warm/vertical compaction, Ultrafil injected, or Obtura technique.[517]

At Loma Linda University, lateral and vertical obturation was followed by gutta-percha removal with hot pluggers down to 5 to 6 mm from the apex. **Coronal leakage** studies in these specimens were then compared with Thermafil obturation in which the metal-core carrier was notched 5 to 6 mm from the tip and then twisted off after the obturator was fully into place. "The apical plugs in the Thermafil group had the highest degree of coronal dye penetration." The reason behind a **coronal leakage** study was based on the fact that cemented posts have an inherently weak seal and that oral fluids (with bacteria) penetrate apically alongside the post and may reach the periapex if the apical gutta-percha plug fails.[518]

Saunders et al. found in **apical leakage** studies that when **Thermafil plastic core** carriers were used, the seal was not adversely affected by either immediate or delayed post preparation.[519] Mattison found little difference between Thermafil plastic and metal carriers.[520] A significant Swedish report of periradicular radiolucencies found that 15% of the failure cases had posts in place. The important findings, however, were the relationships to the length of the remaining apical plug and the ineffective cemented seal of the post. A significantly higher percentage of **failures** was related to apical fillings **under 3 mm** (Figure 11-93), and 24% of the posts with improper cement seal were associated with periradicular radiolucencies.[521]

REMOVAL OF DEFECTIVE ROOT CANAL FILLINGS AND OBJECTS AND RE-TREATMENT

Endodontists have long complained that their specialty has regressed from primary care into "re-treatodontics." Many specialists note that 30 to 50% of their practice is **re-treatment.** That includes having to take over a partially treated case, or worse yet, having to remove defective root canal fillings and entirely redo the treatment.

Chenail and Teplitsky reviewed the iatral as well as patient-placed objects that block root canals. Among the iatral obstructions, they listed paper points, burs, files, glass beads, amalgam, and gold filings (and, one might add, plugger and spreader tips, and of course gutta-percha, cements and sealers, broaches, silver points, and posts). Among the objects placed by patients in teeth left open to drain, they listed nails, pencil lead, toothpicks, tomato seeds, hatpins, needles, pins, and other metal objects.[522] Numerous methods and devices have been developed to retrieve and remove these obstructions.

Gutta-percha and Sealer Removal. Compared with other filling materials, gutta-percha and sealer are

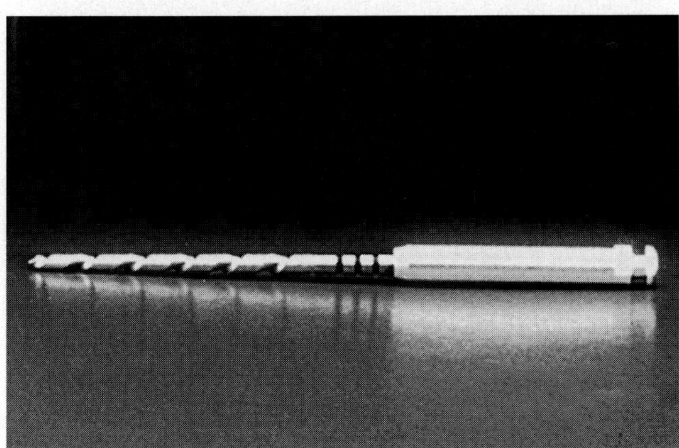

Figure 11-92 Brasseler GPX gutta-percha remover fits low-speed handpiece and features spiraled vents through which gutta-percha extrudes coronally as it is plasticized by frictional heat. (Courtesy of Brasseler, USA, Inc.)

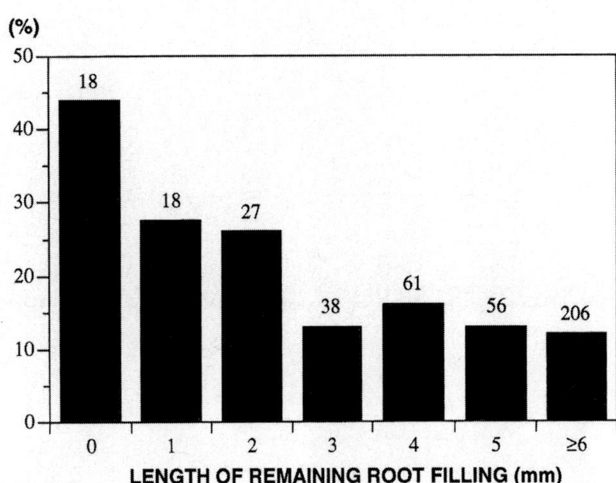

Figure 11-93 Frequency of periradicular lesions related to the length of the remaining gutta-percha root canal filling in 424 endodontically treated roots with posts. Note the much lower failure rate with 3 mm or more remaining filling. Reproduced with permission from Kvist T et al.[521]

relatively easy to remove. After the canal orifice of the defective filling is uncovered, the adhesion of the gutta-percha is tested with a **fine Hedstroem file.** That is, an attempt is made to pass the file alongside the filling to the apical stop. If the filling is really defective, it may be lifted out by blades of the file, or possibly, with two fine files, one on either side of the gutta-percha.

If the gutta-percha is solid but the filling failed because it is well short of the apex, a hot plugger may be repeatedly plunged into the mass, bringing out gutta-percha each time. As much of the filling as possible should be removed by heat before instruments are used to complete the job. Pieces of filling in the canal have been known to divert the file, and with persistence, a perforation may be developed (Figure 11-94). Peeso reamers, Gates-Glidden drills, and round burs **should not be used** because they are easily diverted. A GPX gutta-percha remover is less dangerous in a low-speed handpiece because it **coronally** extrudes the frictionally heated gutta-percha without contacting the dentin walls (see Figure 11-92).

Occasionally, gutta-percha solvents will need to be used. Again, a "well" is made in the center of the defective filling and one or two drops of solvent are introduced from a syringe or the beaks of cotton pliers. The reaming and filing actions are much improved as the gutta-percha dissolves. One must be careful, however, not to pump the liquified mixture out through the apical foramen. Larger files are used high in the canal, decreasing markedly in size toward the apex.[523]

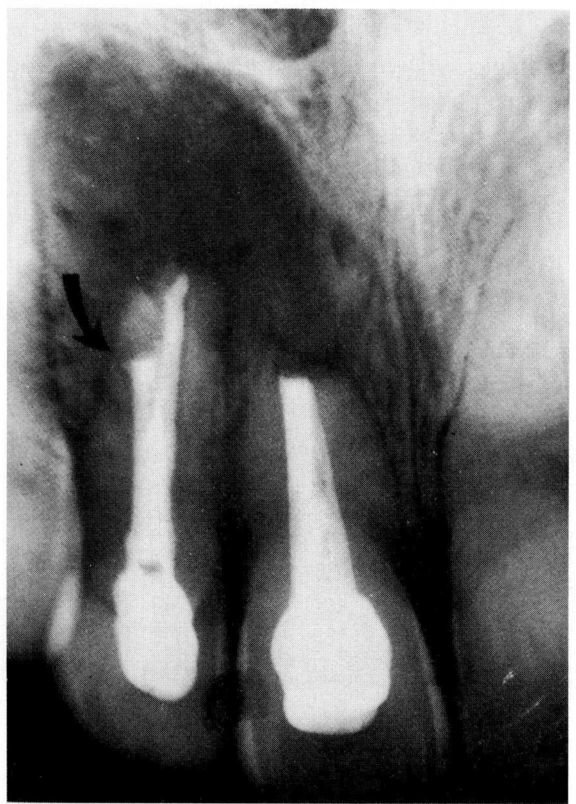

Figure 11-94 Perforation (**arrow**) developed during attempt to remove old gutta-percha filling. Small pieces of gutta-percha will divert endodontic instruments leading to perforation.

After the bulk of the old filling is removed, aggressive filing is done in an attempt to remove all of the gutta-percha and sealer from the walls. Plaques of smear layer, debris, and bacteria must be uncovered to ensure future success.

The solvents commonly used to liquefy gutta-percha are chloroform, xylol, eucalyptol, and halothane. Chloroform has been the favorite but fell into disfavor from a carcinogenic scare. Halothane was recommended as a substitute even though it is harder to obtain. With the **lifting of the FDA ban on chloroform**, fear of it waned and it is still widely used.

A number of studies evaluated solvents plus mechanical means of filling, namely, removal and reinstrumentation. Chloroform was used successfully in bypassing gutta-percha in well-sealed canals using a Canal Finder System with K-files. The vertical stroke of the Canal Finder handpiece served well to carry the files to the apical stop in an average of 32 seconds in the *in vivo* cases.[524]

Wilcox et al. found that no technique or solvent removed all of the debris, although it appears that initially using heated pluggers, followed by chloroform with ultrasonic instrumentation, had a slight edge.[525] Wilcox later found canals were no cleaner when either chloroform or sodium hypochlorite was used.[526]

Others have compared chloroform with other solvents, and each time chloroform comes out ahead as the most rapid and complete solvent.[527–531] Chloroform dissolves gutta-percha nearly three times faster than halothane.[528] A US Navy group found "halothane to be an acceptable alternative to chloroform," particularly when used with ultrasonic instrumentation.[530] At Creighton University, a group found both chloroform and halothane effective in removing Thermafil gutta-percha fillings with plastic cone carriers.[531]

Re-treatment Success Following Gutta-percha and Sealer Removal. Bergenholtz et al. examined 660 teeth after **re-treatment** for failures and reported a 94% success rate 2 years later. Of the cohort with periradicular radiolucencies, however, 48% completely healed, 30% appeared to be healing, and 22% remained as failures.[531] They later reported that, when teeth with periradicular lesions had overextensions during retreatment, success was significantly reduced.[532]

Block and Langeland reported re-treatment of 50 endodontic failures that had been filled with N2. They too stated that "...paste placed beyond the foramen caused tissue damage and reduced prognosis."[533]

Hard Paste Filling Removal. Gutta-percha and soft sealer removal is one thing, but removing hard pastes and cements such as N2, zinc phosphates, and silicates, that have no known solvents, is quite another. Krell and Neo reported the successful yet laborious removal of hard pastes using a **Cavi-Endo** ultrasonic unit.[534] At the University of Minnesota, using an **Enac** ultrasonic device with continuous water irrigation and a No. 30 file, they were able to remove hard paste fillings in 3 minutes in one case and 10 minutes in another. The Enac unit vibrates at 30,000 Hz and had to be operated at the full setting of "8" to be effective. The Cavi-Endo vibrates at 25,000 Hz.[535]

Silver Point, Post, and Obstruction Removal. The removal of a cemented silver point is usually more difficult than the removal of gutta-percha. If the point is broken off down in the canal, a method suggested by Feldman[536] in 1914 and modified by Glick (D. Glick, personal communication, February, 1965) may be used. Glick forces three fine Hedstroem files down alongside the point as far as they will go (Figure 11-95, A). The three files are then twisted around one another, thus entangling the soft silver point in a grip much like that exerted by a broach holder (Figure 11-95, B). This method has also been compared with the grip exerted by the trick Mexican straw "finger-cot" that becomes tighter the harder one pulls. The gradual pull on the files often loosens the silver point. This procedure may be repeated a number of times, each time loosening the silver point a bit more.

Getting down alongside the point to get a purchase with the files may be difficult. Using a **No. 1/2 round bur** in a slow handpiece, removing sealer and dentin but not nicking the point, is a start. After this, small files, chloroform, and/or EDTA may extend the distance alongside the point to allow deeper penetration with the very fine Hedstroem files.

If the point has fortunately been left protruding into the pulp chamber, a sharp spoon excavator or curette also may be used to pry the point from its seat. A more efficient spoon excavator has been marketed by Stardent with a triangular notch cut out in the tip of the blade. With this modification, the blade grips the silver from two sides rather than just by the curve of the blade, (Figure 11-95, C). Silver points may sometimes be grasped with an alligator ear forceps or an ophthalmic suture holder (**Castroviejo curved**) (Hu-Friedy; Chicago, Ill.), broken loose from the cement by twisting, and removed.

Rowe has devised another technique using cyanoacrylate glue (Permabond or Superglue #3) and hypodermic needles (A. H. R. Rowe, personal communication, 1981). From an assortment of different gauge needles, one is selected that fits **snugly,** like a sleeve, over the protruding silver point. The bevel is removed, blunting the needle, which is then cemented over the silver point. After 5 minutes of setting time, the needle is grasped with pliers or heavy hemostat and the silver point "worried" from place (Figure 11-95, D). A variation of this method uses a larger-gauge needle and a small Hedstroem file. The piece of blunted needle is placed over the butt of the silver point. The file is then inserted down the inside of the needle and wedged tightly into the space between (Figure 11-95, E).

Another unique approach uses orthodontic ligature wire and plastic tubing. First, a groove is cut around the protruding butt end of the silver point with a half round or wheel bur. The ligature wire is then doubled over, and the two free ends are passed through the tubing to form a loop at the end. The groove in the silver point is then "lassoed" with the wire loop (Figure 11-95, F), which is cinched up tight with the plastic sleeve. Adding a drop of cyanoacrylate cement may improve the grip. The tubing is tightly grasped with pliers or a hemostat and the point is worked loose.[537]

Acknowledging the source (see Figure 11-95, D), Johnson and Beatty developed a commercial version of this tube/cyanoacrylate device. It may be used to remove silver points, broken files, cemented posts, or metal carriers of Thermafil.[538] The **EndoExtractor** (Brasseler, USA) consists of tubular, trepan-end cutting burs described by Masseram,[539] along with a variety of sizes of tubes with handles attached. The different-sized **trepan** burs fit over the point/post and are used to cut a trench around it, thus freeing a few millimeters of the point that may be grasped. An appropriate-sized hollow-tube extractor is chosen that will **snugly** fit the **extruding point.**The extractor is then cemented to at least 2 mm of the point with cyanoacrylate glue, and 5 minutes are allowed for it to set. The handle on the tube may then be used to twist and lift the point from its seat. At the University of Minnesota, researchers have reported the successful use of the EndoExtractor to remove posts, silver points, and broken files when all else failed.[540]

An improved version of the **Endo Extractor** (Roydent Dent. Prod., USA) uses the same principle, except that a "Jacobs chuck," activated by a twist of the handle, grasps the point/post, so that it may be pulled from the canal. Ruddle has also developed a post puller, the Ruddle Instrument Removal System **(IRS)**

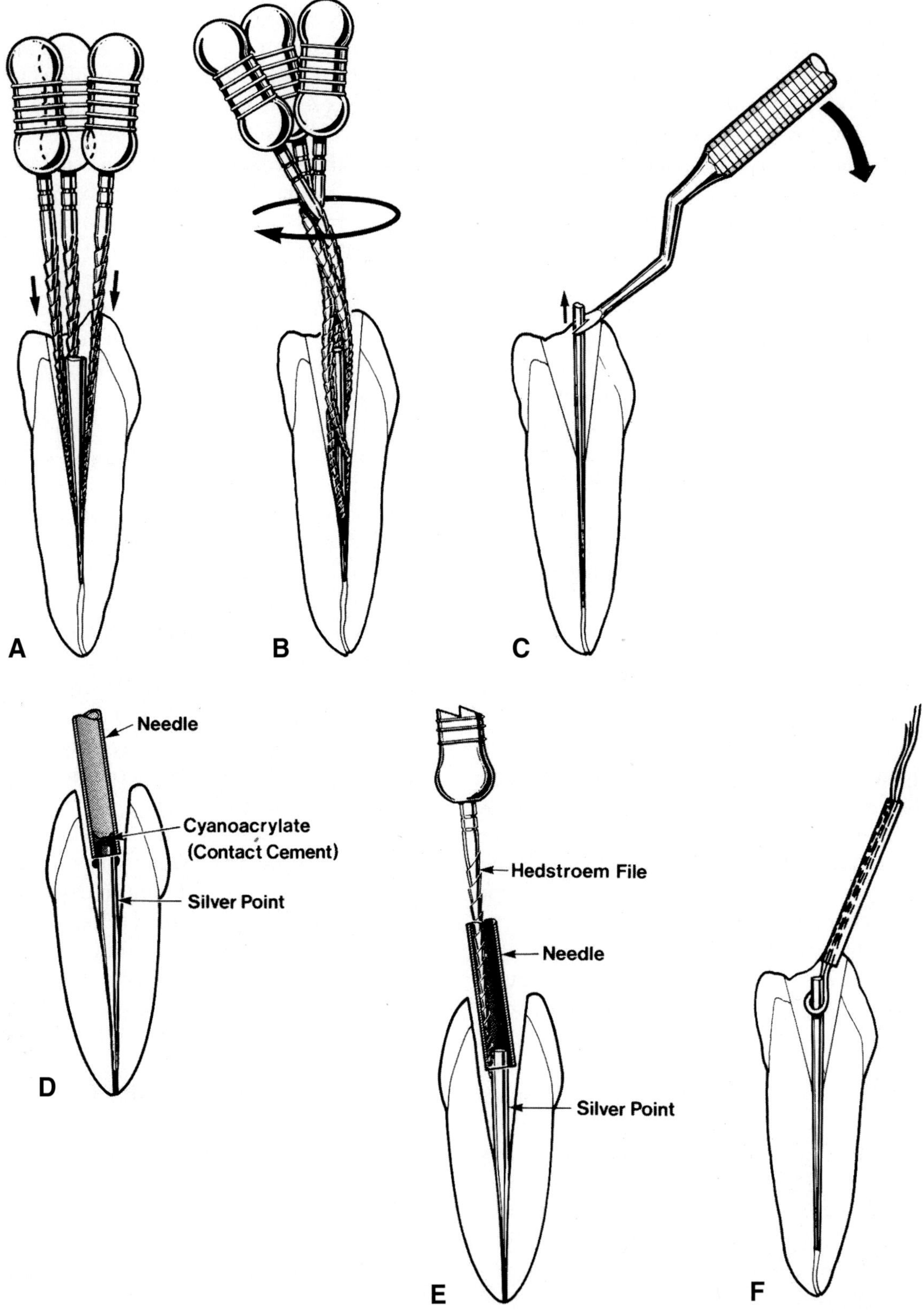

Figure 11-95 Methods of removing silver points. **A**, Three fine Hedstroem files are worked down alongside silver point. **B**, By clockwise motion, three files are twisted around each other, forming vise-like grip on soft silver that can then be dislodged. **C**, Special "split-tongue" excavator used to pry point from place. **D**, Blunted hypodermic needle that fits tightly over silver point attached by cyanoacrylate. When adhesive sets, needle is grasped with pliers or heavy hemostat. **E**, Loose-fitting blunted hypodermic needle is placed over silver point. Hedstroem file is wedged alongside and used to "worry" point loose. **F**, Loop of orthodontic wire in plastic sleeve used to "lasso" groove cut in silver point. Cyanoacrylate may be used to improve attachment.

(Dentsply/Tulsa Dental; Tulsa, Okla.), that trephines around the post by ultrasonics, then screws onto it and levers the post from the canal.

Ultrasonic/Sonic Removal of Canal Obstructions. "The tightly fitted, well-cemented silver point that is flush with the canal orifice is a challenge to remove."[541] In these cases, and in the case of cemented posts, removal is enhanced through the use of sonic or ultrasonic devices. At the University of Iowa, researchers placed a fine Hedstroem file down into the canal alongside the defective silver point. The file was then enervated by a **Cavitron scaler** and slowly withdrawn (Figure 11-96). A number of tries were usually necessary before the silver point loosened and could be retrieved.

At UCLA, Kuttler activated posts with a **Cavitron** scaler until the cement seal was broken and the post could be either extracted or unscrewed.

Deeper in the canal, the ultrasonic **CaviEndo endodontic unit**, mounted with a No. 15 file, can be used to loosen obstructions and often "float" them out.[523] At the University of Saskatchewan, it was reported that copious water irrigation was necessary and that "gentle up and down strokes were used until the fragments floated out..." They removed not only silver points and broken files, but spreader and bur tips as well. They warn that patience is needed.[522]

In Germany, the use of the Canal Finder System vertical stroke handpiece retrieved 50% of the defective silver points and fractured instruments. Alternate use of an ultrasonic activated file was also recommended.[542]

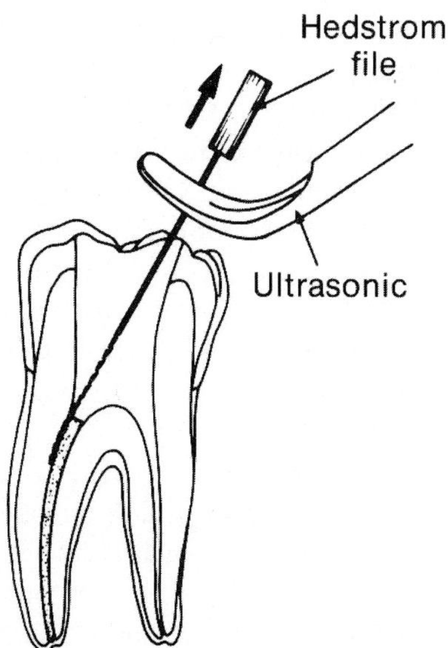

Figure 11-96 Removal of silver point flush with canal orifice being removed with ultrasonic aid. Hedstroem file is placed alongside point and **ultrasonic scaler** is activated as file is withdrawn. Reproduced with permission from Krell KV et al.[541]

One must conclude that the ultrasonic and sonic handpieces have added a whole new dimension to **clearing obstructed canals**, whether soft gutta-percha and sealer, hard setting cements, or metallic objects that must be removed for re-treatment.

TEMPORARY CORONAL FILLING MATERIALS

An unusual amount of research time and effort has been expended in testing the efficacy of various intermediate coronal filling materials. At the outset, it is safe to say that neither gutta-percha nor temporary stopping is presently used. Since those days, quickly placed, yet apparently adequate, cements such as **Cavit** (Premier Dental, King of Prussia, Pa.) have dominated the field.

To properly select a temporary, one should know the criteria for selection. "The role of these cements is to prevent the root canal system from becoming contaminated during treatment by food debris, buccal fluids and microorganisms."[543] Torabinejad et al. have pointed out that, during or after treatment, root canals can be contaminated under several circumstances: (1) if the temporary seal has broken down, (2) if the filling materials and/or tooth structure have fractured or been lost, and (3) if the patient delays final restoration too long.[544]

The properties that a good temporary material must possess have been well delineated by French researchers: good sealing to tooth structure against marginal microleakage, lack of porosity, dimensional variations to hot and cold close to the tooth itself, good abrasion and compression resistance, ease of insertion and removal, compatibility with intracanal medicaments, and good esthetic appearance.[543]

This same French group has produced the definitive study on the leading temporary cements presently on the market: Cavit and **IRM** and **TERM** (Dentsply/Caulk, USA). They note that Cavit is a premixed paste supplied in collapsible tubes, that IRM is a ZOE cement reinforced by a polymethylemethacrylate resin, and that TERM is a light-cure composite (urethane dimethacrylate polymer resin).[543]

Others have learned that Cavit can cause discomfort in vital teeth, probably through dessication. Also, it is a moisture-initiated, autopolymerizing premixed calcium sulfate polyvinyl chloride acetate cement, and it expands while setting.[545] IRM must be mixed on a slab, and thus porosity may be incorporated; TERM is injected into the cavity and light cured for 40 seconds.

French researchers used bacteria in their microleakage study because bacteria are the principal problem. *Streptococcus sanguis*, an oral pathogen, is 500 times greater in size than blue aniline dye. Therefore, any leakage indicates "wide" gaps or high porosity. The French group placed temporary fillings **4 mm thick** and tested leakage after 4 days of immersion in bacteria, and then after thermocycling from 4 to 57°C.

They found that **Cavit and TERM did not allow bacteria to penetrate** before or after thermocycling, whereas 30% of the IRM fillings let *S. sanguis* pass before thermocycling and 60% of the IRMs leaked after thermocycling. They believe that IRM was leaking through the filling material itself because of mixing porosity, as well as marginally.[543] There is no question that, for short-duration, intermediate fillings, **Cavit and TERM are preferred.**

Seven years later, the French group again tested the efficacy of Cavit, IRM, TERM, and a new adhesive, **Fermit** (Vivadent, France/USA), via leakage studies.[546] They concluded that "Cavit was more leakproof than the other cements at day 2...and at day 7." Cement thickness averaged 4.1 mm.[546]

In Taiwan, a new temporary material, **Caviton** (G-C Dental, Japan/USA), was tested against Cavit and IRM. The Chinese reported that Caviton provided the best seal, followed by Cavit. IRM was a poor last.[547]

Others have tested these materials (Cavit, IRM, and TERM) and other temporary cements as well. The results are confusing, probably because of the indicator dyes used, the significant temperature changes,[548–550] the stresses of mastication,[551] the softening effect of medicaments,[552,553] and the length of time the fillings withstand the variables.[554]

Some found that Cavit must be at least 3.5 mm thick,[554] and that one should not plan an "intervisit period for longer than 1 week.[553,555] Most found Cavit, Cavit-G, and Cavit-W (hardness variations) as good as, if not the best of, the temporaries.[543,555–563, 567] Others found Cavit less adequate than IRM and ZOE cements.[550,551,564,568–570]

Many studies agreed with the Deveaux group in Lille, France, that **TERM was superior** or equal to all of the other temporary coronal sealants.[543,558,561–564,571] At the Universities of Iowa, Saskatchewan, and California, workers disagreed with the value of TERM as a sealant.[556,559,560] Most others also agreed with Deveaux that the use of **IRM is ill-advised**, and that it leaks badly before and after thermocycling.[543,558,559,562–564]

More recently, a Berlin group found it efficacious to **add glass-ionomer** cement to temporary replacements.[572] They reported "that only glass-ionomer cement and IRM combined with glass-ionomer cement may prevent bacterial penetration to the periapex of root filled teeth over a 1 month period."[572]

Some research groups found zinc phosphate and polycarboxylate cements most **inadequate,**[562,563] but the **glass ionomer Ketac Fil** to be quite **adequate** if the cavity is first acid etched. This rather time-consuming approach gave a similar result to **Kalzinol** (Dentsply/DeTrey, Switzerland/USA), a reinforced ZOE cement.[555]

There are other factors that might affect the temporary seal, one being the intracanal medicaments that could dissolve and loosen the seal from below. Rutledge and Montgomery found, however, that neither eugenol, formocresol, nor CMCP broke the seal of TERM, although the "walking bleach" paste of sodium perborate and superoxol did so.[573] Another group suggested that a pellet of cotton soaked in a medicament (CMCP) would act as a barrier if bacteria leaked through the temporary filling.[574]

Does a filling **already in place** that is penetrated by the access cavity have any effect on microleakage? The answer is yes on two counts. First, the filling itself may be faulty and leaking, and second, the **temporary filling-in-the-filling** may not adhere, and leakage will ensue.

If one suspects that the filling to be perforated for access is already faulty, it should be totally removed.[560] If this happens, a temporary filling will have to withstand the trauma and abuse suffered by a two- or three-surface filling. In this event, a temporary material must be chosen to withstand these stresses. At the University of Georgia, researchers determined that "TERM restorations provided excellent seals and were statistically superior to Cavit and IRM for restoring **complex** endodontic access preparations." IRM leaked immediately from "thermal stress." Cavit has a setting expansion of 14%, so that it literally "grew" right out of Class II cavities and severely cracked. Its low compressive strength and high solubility made it unacceptable for long-term use.[564]

At the University of Georgia, workers prepared endodontic access cavities **in Class I amalgam fillings** and then restored the access cavities with various temporary materials. Glass ionomer, TERM, Cavit-G, and IRM "all provided excellent seals" **for up to 2 weeks**, whereas zinc phosphate and polycarboxylate cements proved inadequate. No thermocycling was done. It tends to break the seal of all of these materials placed in amalgam cavities.[565]

At Indiana University, they tested ZOE and Cavit in cavities prepared **in amalgam and composite.** They found that "ZOE seals against marginal leakage better than Cavit when the access opening is placed through composite resin, and that Cavit seals better than ZOE when the access opening is placed through amalgam." Thermocycling apparently broke the bond with amalgam.[566]

Torabinejad et al. pointed out the importance of the temporary seal lasting even after root canal therapy is completed, emphasizing the importance of **early final restoration** of the tooth. It took only 19 days for *Staphylococcus* placed in the crown to reach the apex in 50% of the test cases and 42 days for 50% of the *Proteus* samples to do the same.[544] The Torabinejad team later reported that bacteria in natural saliva will contaminate root canals obturated by either lateral or vertical compaction, from crown to apex, in just 30 days if left open to the saliva.[575]

At Temple University, it was found that bacterial **endotoxin** could penetrate the full length of an obturated canal in just 20 days.[576] More recently, the Iowa group found that endotoxin, " a potent inflammatory agent, may be able to penetrate obturating materials faster than bacteria."[577] They also extended the caveat: "the need for an immediate and proper coronal restoration after root canal treatment is therefore reinforced."[577]

One must conclude from this full discussion that temporary fillings are most important in multiple-appointment treatment to prevent recontamination between appointments and, further, that the material must be tough enough to withstand mastication. Between-appointment intervals should **not exceed 1 week,** and the temporaries must be thick enough to prevent leakage. Finally, **long-term temporization is inadvisable.**

TERM and glass-ionomer cement appear to be the most acceptable **temporaries,** followed by Cavit in Class I cavities. ZOE, zinc phosphate, polycarboxylate cements, and IRM, *per se*, are much less acceptable, and, of course, temporary stopping is totally unacceptable.

FINAL CORONAL RESTORATION: MICROLEAKAGE

It might be that as many root canal fillings fail because of bacterial entry from leaking **coronal** restorations as fail from periradicular leakage. As stated earlier, Torabinejad et al. demonstrated an inordinate (50%) bacterial contamination from the crown clear through to the apex, around and through well-compacted gutta-percha fillings.[544]

After bacteria pass permanent occlusal fillings, there appears to be a clear track right past the bases placed over the root canal filling—either zinc phosphate cement or temporary stopping.[578]

Melton et al. recommended that leaking permanent restorations "should be removed in their entirety before endodontic treatment"[560]; it makes even more sense to remove any suspicious restorations **after** treatment as well, not try simply to restore the access cavity.

There is a terrifying body of literature, for example, that testifies to microleakage all the way to the pulp under full crowns.[579–583] One must assume that, along these pathways, bacteria could reach the pulp space occupied by root canal fillings and then down the root canal filling to the apex.[544] "None of the current luting agents routinely prevent marginal leakage of cast restorations."[582] Furthermore, "...all crowns leaked gingivally regardless of the type of crown margin preparation."[583]

Therefore, it goes without saying that so-called "permanent" restorations of endodontic access cavities suffer microleakage as well. At the University of Iowa, Wilcox and Diaz-Arnold restored lingual access cavities with either Ketac-Fil glass ionomer cement or **Herculite** composite resin (Sybron Endo/Kerr Dental Orange, Calif.). Acid etch was used as well as GLUMA dentin-bonding agent. After thermocycling, **all of the specimens leaked** and they leaked right past the zinc phosphate and/or temporary-stopping bases underneath. One specimen even leaked all the way to the apical foramen.[578]

A series of experiments at the University of Iowa found that coronal microleakage, in the presence of saliva, was inevitable up to 85% of the time.[584] At Indiana University, researchers also noted the penetrating effect of saliva and recommended "**re-treatment** of obturated root canals that have been exposed to the oral cavity for at least 3 months."[585]

To confirm *in vivo* the penetrating effects of saliva from leaking coronal restorations seen in vitro,[586] the Iowa group did coronal microleakage studies on monkeys. They reported dye penetration down the filled root canals no matter which sealer was used: Sealapex, AH-26, or ZOE.[587]

Undoubtedly, one of the causes of microleakage under cemented restorations relates to the dissolution of the cement. Phillips et al., in a human *in vivo* study, found that zinc phosphate cement was much more likely to disintegrate than were polycarboxylate or glass ionomer cements.[588] This is particularly important because zinc phosphate is still the most widely used luting agent.

If all of these standard luting cements are faulty in their sealing ability, what is one to do to prevent microleakage? The answer appears to lie in the use of the new adhesive resins, or glue that will adhere to all tooth structures, as well as metals, other resins, and porcelain.

Tjan, Tan, and Li, at Loma Linda University, have shown that when the 4-META adhesive **Amalgambond** (Parkell Dental, Farmingdale, N.Y.) is used to line both the prepared dentin and enamel, the newly placed amalgam filling is virtually leakproof (Figure 11-97, A).

In contrast, a cavity lined with Copalite allowed leakage around the amalgam as far as the pulp[589,590] (Figure 11-97, B). Amalgambond can also be used to bond new amalgam to old amalgam, or composite to amalgam, gold, or other composite. Another 4-META product, **C & B Metabond** (Parkell Dental, USA), will lute gold or porcelain restorations to tooth without future leakage.

Wilcox attempted to use **GLUMA** (Miles Laboratories, USA), the dentin-bonding agent, to adhere a composite resin to the tooth structure of endodontic access cavities in anterior teeth. After thermocycling, it failed.[578]

At this juncture, the solution to the problem of microleakage appears to be the resin-adhesive agents, particularly those that will adhere to more than just other resins, and possibly another approach—placing an **intraorifice barrier base**, medicated or nonmedicated, over the coronal root canal filling.

At the University of Tennessee, the Himel group placed pigmented glass-ionomer cements over the coronal termination of the root canal filling. They reported that "the teeth without an **intraorifice barrier** leaked significantly more than the teeth with the [glass-ionomer] barriers ($p < .05$)."[591] Similar research at Northwestern University revealed much the same results—the root canals that received an **intraorifice barrier leaked significantly less** than the unsealed controls, all of which leaked in < 49 days.[592]

At the University of Toronto a different approach was tried—sealing the canals with two experimental **glass-ionomer sealers**, one containing an antimicrobial substance. The first sealer proved effective in preventing the "penetration of *E. faecalis*" probably because of the natural release of fluoride. The experimental sealer with the added antibacterial "needs more study."[593]

Martin has recently introduced gutta-perch points and an accompanying ZOE sealer, both of which contain **iodoform**, a well-known bacterial suppressant. *In vitro* results appear promising; however, long-term *in vivo* efficacy has yet to be shown. The products are marketed as **MPG** gutta-percha points and **MCS** root canal sealer (Medidenta Products, Woodside, N.Y.).

A NEW ENDODONTIC PARADIGM

It has been recognized for decades that the ideal end result of root canal therapy would be the closure of the apical and all lateral foramina with reparative cementum.[594,595] This permits re-establishment of a complete

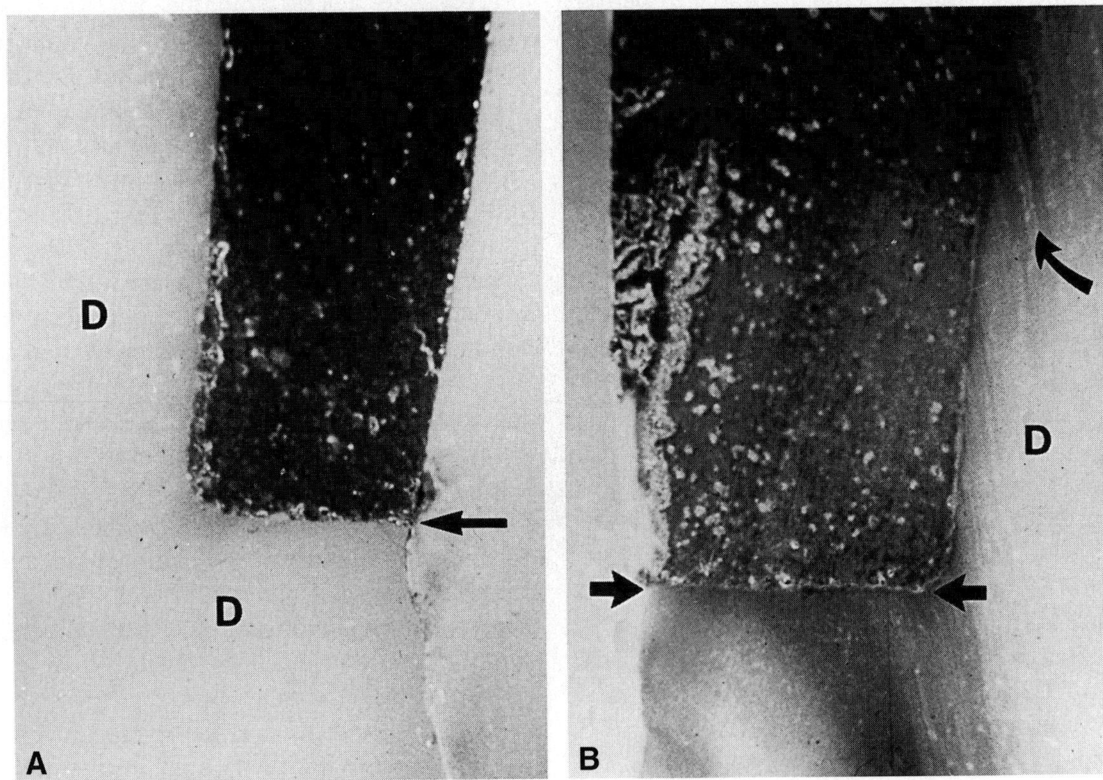

Figure 11-97 Comparative study in microleakage between resin adhesive and copal varnish. **A**, Amalgam filling bonded to dentin (D) and cementum (**arrow**) with **Amalgambond** and no microleakage. **B**, Amalgam filling lined with **Copalite.** Gross microleakage at gingival floor (**arrows**) as well as from upper margin (**curved arrow**). (Courtesy of Drs. A. H. L. Tjan and D. E. Tan.)

attachment apparatus and precludes future failure caused by pulpoperidontal fluid exchange and retroinvasion of bacteria.

Following well-executed treatment, wherein infection and irritation are terminated, cementoblasts and periodontal ligament slowly resurface the damaged root and even close minor foramina that no longer contain neurovascular bundles.

But well-obturated major foramina that present a surface of sealers and/or gutta-percha to the periradicular tissue will not be closed over. Cementum will not grow across mildly irritating sealer surfaces. This leaves these foramina vulnerable to leakage as cement sealers dissolve away over the years. How can this dilemma be resolved?

Cementification. In the last two editions of this text, Ingle and Luebke made a case for the wider use of calcium hydroxide as a stimulating and healing agent (Figure 11-98). The same thought occurred to others—to use calcium hydroxide in filling the canal as well as an interappointment canal medicament.[595–597]

Today, these speculations have become a reality. Calcium hydroxide is frequently being used as an apical plug before total obturation.[499–526,598] Furthermore, calcium hydroxide is being incorporated into root canal sealers in such commercial products as CRCS and Sealapex. Although the reviews have been mixed on these latter products, there have been some favorable reports, but not without unfavorable side effects from overfilling.[105–111,153–160,599–601]

A Turkish group found "hard tissue formation more pronounced after root filling with Sealapex than with calcium hydroxide..."[600] However, a Tel Aviv group reported that the "...disintegration of Sealapex indicated that solubility may be the price for increased activity."[601] In other words, these sealers must dissolve to release their calcium hydroxide. It then becomes a question of which will happen first—cementification across the apex or leakage into the exposed canal with its attendant problems? Is there a substitute for calcium hydroxide that may have its stimulating effects but not its drawbacks? The answer may be **hydroxyapatite!**

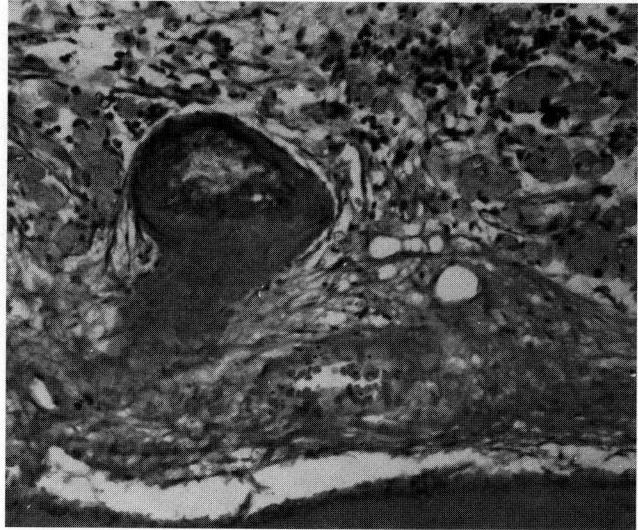

Figure 11-98 Calcification forming around nidus of calcium hydroxide in tissue (**arrow**). (Courtesy of Dr. Raymond G. Luebke.)

Calcium-Phosphate Cement Obturation. Years ago, Nevins and his associates were using cross-linked collagen–calcium phosphate gels to induce hard tissue formation.[602] More recently, Harbert has suggested using tricalcium phosphate as an apical plug, much like dentin shavings and calcium hydroxide have been used.[603] Even more recently, calcium phosphate cement (CPC) has been suggested as a total root canal filling material.[138]

The ADA-Paffenbarger Dental Research Center at the US National Institute of Standards and Technology has developed a simple mixture of calcium phosphates that sets to become **hydroxyapatite.** "Two calcium phosphate compounds, one acidic and one basic, are unique in that when mixed with water they set into a hardened mass"—**hydroxyapatite—the principal mineral in teeth and bones.**[137] Tetracalcium phosphate is the **basic** constituent, and the **acidic** component is either dicalcium phosphate dihydrate or anhydrous dicalcium phosphate. "Water is neither a reactant nor an important product in the reaction, but merely a vehicle for dissolution of the reactants."[137] Setting time may be extended by adding glycerin to the mixture. Using a mild phosphoric acid solution speeds the dissolution of the components. Even aliquots of blood from a surgical site may be substituted for water.

The final set, **calcium phosphate cement (CPC),** consists of nearly all crystalline material, and porosity is in direct ratio to the amount of solvent (water) used. It is as radiopaque as bone. It is nearly insoluble in water and **is insoluble** in saliva and blood, but is readily soluble in strong acids, which may be considered in the event it must be removed.[137]

In testing the sealing ability of CPC when used as a root canal sealer-filler, the Paffenbarger group reported that in most of the specimens there was "no dye penetration into the filler-canal wall interface" (Figure 11-99). The mean depth of penetration was only 0.15 mm overall.

Glycerin was used in mixing the CPC to improve its extrudability from a 19-gauge needle. A funnel-shaped needle is being considered (L. C. Chow, personal communication, August 1992). As far as tissue response to

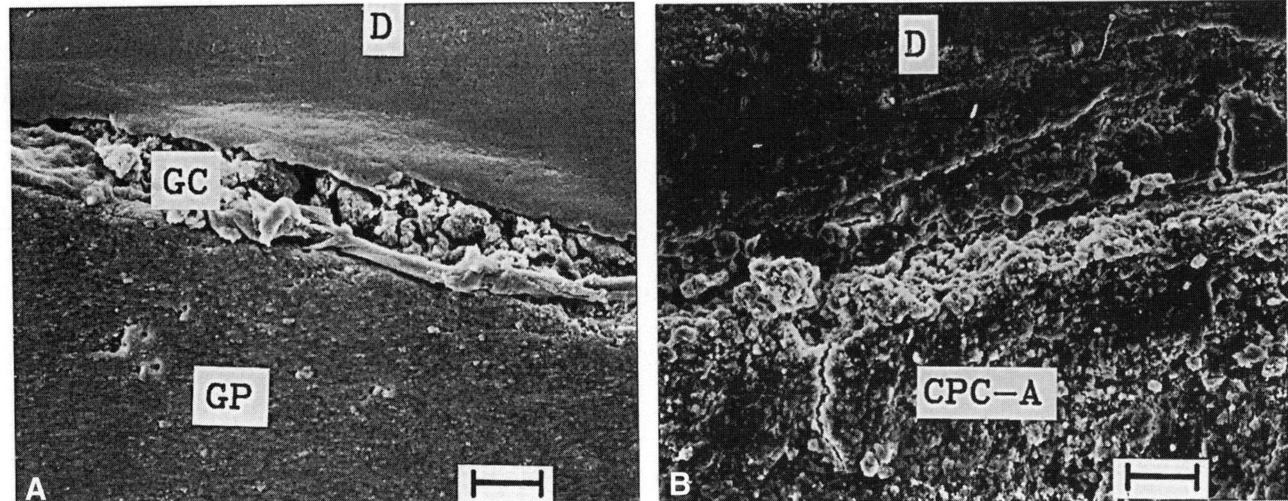

Figure 11-99 Noticeable difference in density of interface between filling materials and dentin wall (D). **A**, Canal filled with gutta-percha (GP) and **Grossman's cement** (GC). Note discrepancies in sealer interface. **B**, Canal filled with **calcium phosphate cement (CPC-A)**. Dense interface explains superiority in apical leakage pattern. Reproduced with permission from Sugawara A, et al. JOE 1990;16:162.

CPC is concerned, the "calcium phosphate treated animals showed mild irritation after 1 month, but thereafter the adverse tissue reactions were minimal. New bone formation adjacent to the cement was also observed."[137] In another study, 63% of the specimens "showed no evidence of inflammatory response to the CPC."[604] Still another study, done on monkeys, in which canals were deliberately overfilled, new bone formation developed immediately adjacent to the cement[218] (Figures 11-100, 11-101). Exhaustive tests of CPC by Chinese researchers in Shanghai found that "CPC had no toxicity and all tests for mutagenicity and potential carcinogenicity of CPC extracts are negative." They also noted that "the implant tightly joined with the surrounding bone...."[605]

Krell and Wefel also found that, as a sealer, CPC adheres well to the canal wall.[606] In marked contrast to

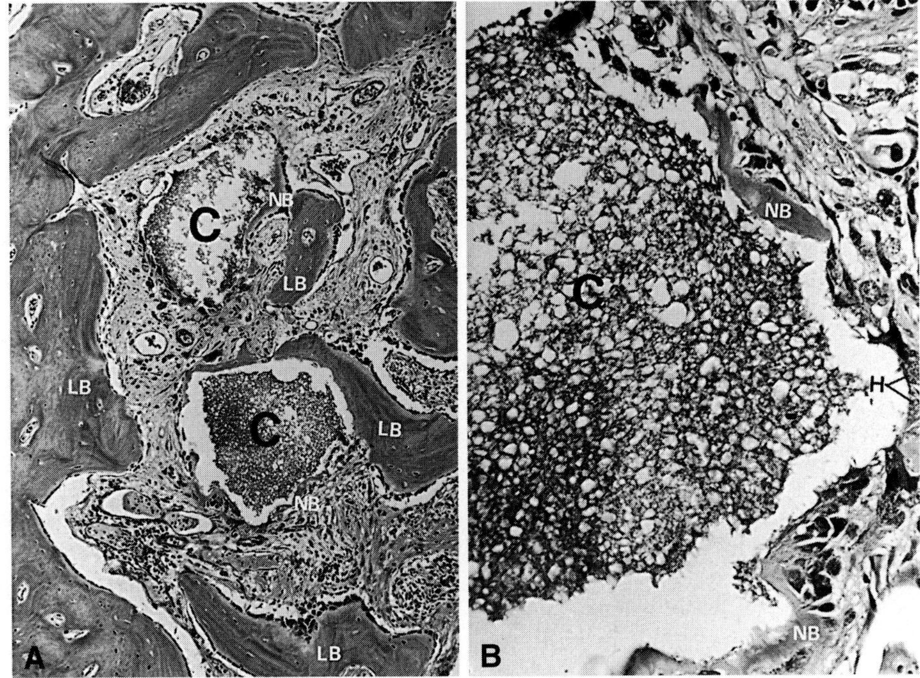

Figure 11-100 Periradicular area 3 months after purposeful overfill of canal with calcium phosphate cement **CPC**. The CPC (C) is bordered by slender new bone trabeculae (NB) at the periphery where foam histocytes (H) are frequently present **(right)**. LB, lamellar bone. **A**, ×75 original magnification. **B**, ×300 original magnification. Reproduced with permission from Hong YC et al.[218]

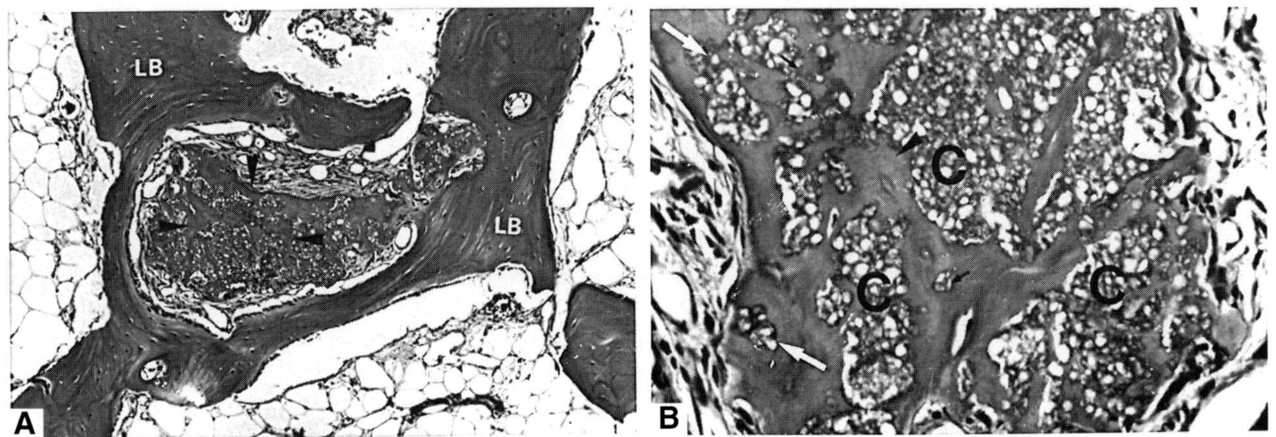

Figure 11-101 Periradicular area 6 months after **CPC** overfill. **A,** Numerous ossification nidi (**arrowheads**) extend in various directions to communicate with one another. Surrounding calcium phosphate cement (C), better seen in **B**, high power (×300 original magnification). LB, lamellar bone. Reproduced with permission from Hong YC et al.[218]

CPC, leakage was observed in the gutta-percha/ZOE controls[138] (see Figure 11-99). And at the US Naval Dental School, CPC was used as an apical barrier to facilitate obturation much as dentin chips and calcium hydroxide have been used. "The teeth receiving apical CPC barriers...had significantly less dye penetration than teeth without apical barriers." They recommended CPC as a replacement for calcium hydroxide in apexification cases.[607]

Japanese researchers have already marketed **apatite sealers.** Two of them, G-5 and G-6, were tested at Indiana University against Super-EBA for biocompatability.[608] While finding Super-EBA and G-5 biocompatable, the researchers found G-6 "promoted moderate inflammation and foreign body giant cell response." In addition to CPC, both G-5 and G-6 contain radiopacifiers, potassium fluoride, and citric acid, except G-6 contained more of the latter.[608]

A Japanese group at Osaka tested another commercial apatite sealer, ARS (Apatite Root Sealer), and found that it "caused severe inflammatory reactions."[609] In the same test, the Osaka group added 2.5% chondroitin sulfate to CP cement (TMD-5) and reported that it "has excellent histocompatability and potential as a root canal sealer."[609]

An Italian company has added hydroxyapatite to ZOE sealer, Bioseal (Ogna Lab. Farma., Italy), much as calcium hydroxide has been added to CRCS sealer. Whereas Gambarini and Tagger reported that Bioseal "did not adversely affect the sealing properties" of the cement, its beneficial effects were "not within the scope of the study."[610]

In an entirely different direction in the development of **apical barrier materials**, Japanese researchers have tested the use of freeze-dried allogenic dentin powder as well as True Bone Ceramics (TBC), the latter derived from the incineration of bovine bone.[611] Initially, with both products, multinucleate giant cells and bone resorption appeared. Within 3 months, however, new bone had formed and "the apex had been closed completely with new hard tissue."[611]

If a delivery system can be perfected for CPC, it could well be the sealer/barrier/filler of future endodontics. The Paffenbarger Center did find that their material provided better sealant qualities than did ZOE and gutta-percha.[165] The fact that hydroxyapatite is a naturally occurring product, and that bone grows into and eventually replaces extruded material, makes it very acceptable biologically.[612] Moreover, it may replace calcium hydroxide in treating open-apex cases and fractured roots.

Another possibility of using hydroxyapatite relates to the **laser.** A cross-linked collagen-hydroxyapatite mixture has been placed in the root canal and "melted" to place with a laser beam through a fiber optic.

To date, none of these uses of calcium phosphate cements have been approved by the US Food and Drug Administration, although clinical trials have been applied for. This long, slow, and costly process must be undertaken before the products can be released for use by the profession. More recently, an experimental material, **mineral trioxide aggregate** (**MTA**), has been suggested as a root-end filling material.[613] This may also turn out to be a promising material for use as an orthograde filling of the apical end of the root canal prior to filling the remainder of the canal with gutta-percha. It is presently being used primarily as a retrofilling material.

Adhesive Resins. Very little has been published on the use of adhesives in filling root canals.[126,130,131] It stands to reason that adhesive resins could serve to seal dentin walls after smear removal. If it can be made to adhere to other filling materials such as gutta-percha, and if it can be made radiopaque without ruining its setting and adhesive qualities, one would think that adhesives may have a bright future in endodontics. **Amalgambond** already has been used to seal amalgam retrofillings against microleakage.

At the University of Minnesota, Zidan and El Deeb found that **Scotchbond**, which bonds chemically to calcium, provided a significantly better seal than Tubliseal.[130,131] In Australia, Gee found that he could only achieve a result comparable to lateral compaction with AH-26 as a sealer by falling back on a complex system involving GLUMA as a bonding agent, followed by Concise composite, plus AH-26 and gutta-percha. GLUMA and Concise alone gave a poor leakage result.[614] This hardly speaks well for GLUMA or Concise.

Kanca has shown that certain "bonding" agents will not adhere to moist dentin. GLUMA is one of these, as well as Scotchbond II, Clearfil, Photobond, and Tenure. Since it is almost impossible to totally dry a root canal, an adhesive must be selected that bonds to both wet and dry dentin. Kanca recommended **All Bond 2** (Bisco Dental, USA),[615] although Amalgambond and C & B Metabond are just as effective.

SUMMARY

All in all, one must be aware that on the horizon, there are a number of possible methods of obturating root canals that will be "kinder and gentler." More laboratory and clinical research is needed, along with FDA approval, before **a new endodontic paradigm** is fulfilled. Endodontics is moving from nineteenth-century gutta-percha and calcium hydroxide into the twenty-first century of chemistry and lasers. The transition is slow, but exciting.

REFERENCES

1. Dow PR, Ingle JI. Isotope determination of root canal failure. Oral Surg 1955;8:1100.
2. Prinz, H. Paper delivered before the St. Louis, Missouri Dental Society; Sept 2, 1912.
3. Gutierrez JH, Garcia J. Microscopic and macroscopic investigation on results of mechanical preparation of root canals. Oral Surg 1968;25:108.
4. Brayton SM, Davis SR, Goldman M. Gutta-percha root canal fillings. Oral Surg 1973;35:226.
5. Seltzer S. Endodontology: biologic considerations. In: Endodontic procedures. New York: McGraw-Hill; 1971. p. 381.
6. Kapsimalis P, Evans R. Sealing properties of endodontic filling materials using radioactivity polar and nonpolar isotopes. Oral Surg 1966;22:386.
7. Antoniazzi JH, Mjor IA, Nygaard-Østby B. Assessment of the sealing properties of root filling materials. Odontol Tidskr 1968;76:261.
8. Zakariasen KL, Stadem PS. Microleakage associated with modified eucapercha and chloropercha root canal filling techniques. Int Endod J 1982;15:67.
9. Keane KM, Harrington GW. The use of chloroform-softened gutta-percha master cone and its effect on the apical seal. JOE 1984;10:57.
10. Holland, GR. Periradicular response to apical plugs of dentin and calcium hydroxide in ferret canines. JOE 1984;10:71.
11. El Deeb ME, Zucker KJ, Messer H. Apical leakage in relation to radiographic density of gutta-percha using different obturation techniques. JOE 1985;11:25.
12. El Deeb ME. The sealing ability of injection-molded thermoplasticized gutta-percha. JOE 1985;11:84.
13. Kennedy WA, Walker WA III, Gough RW. Smear layer removal effects on apical leakage. JOE 1986;12:21.
14. Kersten HW, et al. Thermomechanical compaction of gutta-percha. I. A comparison of several compaction procedures. Int Endod J 1986;19:125. Also II. 1986;19:134.
15. Marshall FJ, Massler M. Sealing pulpless teeth evaluated with radioisotopes. J Dent Med 1961;16:172.
16. Yee FS, Lugassy AA, Peterson JN. Filling of the root canals with adhesive materials. JOE 1975;1:145.
17. Czonstkowsky M, Michanowicz A, Varques JA. Evaluation of an injection of thermoplasticized low-temperature gutta-percha using radioactive isotopes. JOE 1985;11:71.
18. Fuss Z, et al. Comparative sealing quality of gutta-percha following the use of the McSpadden compactor and the engine plugger. JOE 1985;11:117.
19. Hopkins, JH, et al. McSpadden versus lateral condensation: the extent of apical microleakage. JOE 1986;12:198.
20. Jacobson SM, Von Fraunhofer JA. The investigation of microleakage in root canal therapy. Oral Surg 1976;42:817.
21. Delivanis PD, Chapman KA. Comparison and reliability of techniques for measuring leakage and marginal penetration. Oral Surg 1982;53:410.
22. Cohen T, Gutmann JL, Wagner M. An assessment in vitro of the sealing properties of Calciobiotic root canal sealer. Int Endod J 1985;18:172.
23. Ainley JE. Fluorometric assay of the apical seal of root canal fillings. Oral Surg 1970;29:753.
24. Hovland EJ, Dumsha TC. Leakage evaluation in vitro of the root canal sealer cement Sealapex. Int Endod J 1985;18:179.
25. Wollard RR, Brough SO, Maggio J, Seltzer S. Scanning electron microscopic examination of root canal filling materials. JOE 1976;2:98.
26. White RR, Goldman M, Lin PC. The influence of the smeared layer upon dentinal tubule penetration by plastic filling materials. JOE 1984;10:558.
27. Grove CJ. Why root canals should be filled to the dentinocemental junction. J Am Dent Assoc 1930;17:293.
28. Orban B. Why root canals should be filled to the dentinocemental junction. J Am Dent Assoc 1930;17:1086.
29. Skillen WG. Why root canals should be filled to the dentinocemental junction. J Am Dent Assoc 1930;17:2082.
30. Kuttler Y. Microscopic investigation of root apexes. J Am Dent Assoc 1955;50:544.
31. American Association of Endodontists. Glossary of terms used in endodontics. 4th ed. Chicago (IL): American Association Endodontists; 1984. p. 10.

32. Nygaard-Østby B. The role of the blood clot in endodontic therapy. Acta Odontol Scand 1961;19:323.
33. Blayney JR. The medicinal treatment and the filling of root canals. J Am Dent Assoc 1928;15:239.
34. Strindberg LZ. The difference in the results of pulp therapy on certain factors. Acta Odontol Scand 1956;14 Suppl 21.
35. Horsted P, Nygaard-Østby BN. Tissue formation in the root canal after total pulpectomy and partial root filling. Oral Surg 1978;46:275.
36. Ingle JI, Zeldow BJ. An evaluation of mechanical instrumentation and the negative culture in endodontic therapy. J Am Dent Assoc 1958;57:471.
37. Zeldow BJ, Ingle JI. Correlation of the positive culture to the prognosis of endodontically treated teeth: a clinical study. J Am Dent Assoc 1963;66:23.
38. Sjögren U, et al. Influence of infection at the time of root filling on the outcome of the endodontic treatment of teeth with apical periodontitis. Int Endod J 1996;30:297.
39. Grossman LI. Endodontic practice. 10th ed. Philadelphia: Lea & Febiger; 1982. p. 279.
40. Goodman A, Schilder H, Aldrich W. The thermomechanical properties of gutta percha. II. The history and molecular chemistry of gutta-percha. Oral Surg 1974;37:954.
41. Arvanitoyannis I, Kolokuris I, Blanshard JMV, Robinson C. Study of the effect of annealing, draw ratio, and moisture upon the crystallinity of native and commercial gutta-percha (transpolyisoprene) with DSC, DMTA, and x-rays: determination of the activation energies of T. Appl Polymer Sci 1993;48:987.
42. Gibbs M, Maddox L, Ricketson E. Flow and temperature characteristics of gutta-percha. Unpublished.
43. Gurney BF, et al. Physical measurements of gutta-percha. Oral Surg 1971;32:260.
44. Marlin J, Schilder H. Physical properties of gutta-percha when subjected to heat and vertical condensation. Oral Surg 1973;36:872.
45. Schilder H, Goodman A, Aldrich W. The thermomechanical properties of gutta-percha. I. The compressibility of gutta-percha. Oral Surg 1974;37:916.
46. Schilder H, et al. The thermomechanical properties of gutta-percha. Part V. Volume changes in bulk gutta-percha as a function of temperature and its relationship to molecular phase transformation [sic]. Oral Surg 1985;59:285.
47. Camps JJ, Pertot WJ, Escavy JY, Pravaz M. Young's modulud of warm and cold gutta-percha. Endod Dent Traumatol 1996;12:50.
48. Cohen BD, Combie ED, Lilley JD. Effect of thermal placement techniques on some physical properties of gutta-percha. Int Endod J 1992;25:292.
49. Friedman CE, Sandrik JL, Heuer MA, Rapp GW. Composition and physical properites of gutta-percha endodontic filling materials. JOE 1977;3:304.
50. Marciano J, Michailesco PM. Dental gutta-percha chemical composition, x-ray identification, enthalpic studies and clinical implications. JOE 1989;15:149.
51. Oliet S, Sorin SM. Effect of aging on the mechanical properties of handrolled gutta-percha endodontic cones. Oral Surg 1977;43:954.
52. Johansson BI. A methodological study of the mechanical properties of endodontic gutta-percha. JOE 1980;6:781.
53. Solomon SM, Oliet S. Rejuvenation of aged (brittle) endodontic gutta-percha cones. JOE 1979;5:233.
54. Moorer WR, Genet JM. Evidence for antibacterial activity of endodontic gutta-percha cones. Oral Surg 1982;53:503.
55. Martin H, Martin TR. Iodoform gutta-percha: MGP a new endodontic paradigm. Dent Today 1999;18:76.
56. Holland R, Murata SS, Dezan E, Garlipp O. Apical leakage after root canal filling with an experimental calcium hydroxide gutta-percha point. JOE 1996;22:71.
57. Das S. Effect of certain dental materials on human pulp in tissue culture. Oral Surg 1981;52:76.
58. Wolfson EM, Seltzer S. Reaction of rat connective tissue to some gutta-percha formulations. JOE 1975;12:395.
59. Mayne JR, Shapiro S, Abramson II. An evaluation of standardized gutta-percha points. Oral Surg 1971;31:250.
60. Goldberg F, Gurfinkel J, Spielberg C. Microscopic study of standardized gutta-percha points. Oral Surg 1979;47:275.
61. Siqueira JF Jr, da Silva CH, Cerqueira MD, et al. Efectiveness of four chemical solutions in eliminating *Bacillus subtilis* spores on gutta-percha cones. Endod Dent Traumatol 1998;14:124.
62. Seltzer S, Green DB, Weiner N, DeRenzis F. A scanning EM examination of silver cones removed from endodontically treated teeth. Oral Surg 1972;33:589.
63. Goldberg F. Relationship between corroded silver points and endodontic failure. JOE 1981;7:224.
64. Kehoe JC. Intracanal corrosion of a silver cone producing localized argyria. JOE 1984;10:199.
65. Gutierrez JH, Villena F, Gigoux C, Mujica F. Microscope and scanning electron microscope examination of silver points corrosion caused by endodontic materials. JOE 1982;8:301.
66. Brady JM, Del Rio CE. Corrosion of endodontic silver cones in humans: a scanning electron microscope and x-ray microprobe study. JOE 1975;6:205.
67. Messing, JJ. The use of titanium cones and apical tips as root filling materials. Br Dent J 1980;148:41.
68. Grossman LI. Endodontic practice. 10th ed. Philadelphia: Lea & Febiger; 1982. p. 297.
69. Block RM, Lewis RD, Sheats JB, Burke SH. Antibody formation to dog pulp tissue altered by N2-type paste within the root canal. JOE 1977;8:309.
70. Block RM, et al. Cell-mediated response to dog pulp tissue altered by N2 paste within the root canal. Oral Surg 1978;45:131.
71. Block RM, et al. Cell-mediated immune response to dog pulp tissue altered by Kerr (Rickert's) sealer via the root canal. JOE 1978;4:110.
72. Torabinejad M, Kettering JD, Bakland LK. Evaluation of systemic immunological reactions to AH-26 root canal sealer. JOE 1979;5:196.
73. Harnden DG. Tests for carcinogenicity and mutagenicity. Int Endod J 1981;14:35.
74. Lewis BB, Chestner SB. Formaldehyde in dentistry: a review of the mutagenic and carcinogenic potential. J Am Dent Assoc 1981;103:429.
75. U.S. Consumer Product Safety Commission. The hazards of formaldehyde. Alert Sheet. U.S. Consumer Product Safety Commission (Bulletin); Mar 1980.
76. National Academy of Science. Formaldehyde—an assessment of its health effect. National Academy of Science; Mar 1980.
77. Council on Dental Materials, Instruments, and Equipment. Council update on 'adhesion' and 'adhesive' materials. J Am Dent Assoc 1981;102:252.
78. Antoniazzi HJ, Mjor IA, Nygaard-Østby B. Assessment of the sealing properties of root filling materials. Sattrykk Odontol Tidskr 1968;76:261.

79. Zakariasen KL, et al. JDR Abstract. 59th Annual Session; Mar 19, 1981; Philadelphia, Pa.
80. Nielsen TH. Sealing ability of chelate root filling cements: capillary physical concepts applied to leakage in root-filled teeth. JOE 1980;6(Pt 2):777.
81. Beyer-Olsen EM, Orstavik D. Radiopacity of root canal sealers. Oral Surg 1981;51:320.
82. Orstavik D. Seating of gutta-percha points: effect of sealers with varying film thickness. JOE 1982; 8:213.
83. Wong M, Peters DD, Lorton L, Bernier WE. Comparison of gutta-percha filling techniques: three chloroform gutta-percha filling techniques. JOE 1982;8(Pt 2):4.
84. Kazemi RB, Safavi KE, Spångberg LSW. Dimensional changes of endodontic sealers. Oral Surg 1993;76:766.
85. van der Burgt TP, et al. Staining patterns in teeth discolored by endodontic sealers. JOE 1986;12:187.
86. van der Burgt TP, Mullaney TP, Plasschaert AJM. Tooth discoloration induced by endodontic sealers. Oral Surg 1986;61:84.
87. van der Burgt TP, Plasschaert AJM. Tooth discoloration induced by dental materials. Oral Surg 1985;60:666.
88. Grossman LI. Antimicrobial effect of root canal cements. JOE 1980;6:594.
89. Tobias RS, Browne RM, Wilson CA. Antibacterial activity of dental restorative materials. Int Endod J 1985;18:161.
90. Barkhordar RA. Evaluation of antimicrobial activity in vitro of ten root canal sealers on *S. sanguis* and *S. mutans.* Oral Surg 1989;68:770.
91. Al-Khatib ZZ, et al. The antimicrobial effect of various endodontic sealers. Oral Surg 1990;70:784.
92. Heling I, Chandler NP. The antimicrobial effect within dentinal tubules of four root canal sealers. JOE 1996;22:257.
93. Abdulkader A, Duguid R, Saunders EM. The antimicrobial activity of endodontic sealers to anaerobic bacteria. Int Endod J 1996;29:280.
94. Mickel AK, Wright ER. Growth inhibition of *Streptococcus anginosus (milleri)* by three calcium hydroxide sealers and one zinc oxide-eugenol sealer. JOE 1999;25:34.
95. Schafer E, Bossman K. Antimicrobial effect of camphorated chloroxylenol (ED 84) in the treatment of infected root canals. JOE 1999;25:547.
96. Smith DC. Some observations on endodontic cements. Presented at meeting of Canadian and American Association of Endodontists Montreal, PQ; Apr 1972.
97. McComb D, Smith DC. Comparison of the physical properties of polycarboxylate-based and conventional root canal sealers. JOE 1976;2:228.
98. Peters DP. Two-year in vitro solubility evaluation of four gutta-percha sealer obstruction techniques. JOE 1986;12:139.
99. Heling B, Ram Z, Heling I. The root treatment of teeth with Toxavit. Oral Surg 1977;43:306.
100. Rickert UG, Dixon CM. The control of root surgery. Transactions 8th International Dental Congress, Sec. IIIA. No. 9, p. 15, 1931. J Am Dent Assoc 1933;20:1458.
101. Yared GM, Bou Dagher F. Sealing ability of the vertical condensation with different root canal sealers. JOE 1996;22:6.
102. Bou Dagher F, Yared GM, Machtou P. Microleakage of new and old Kerr root canal sealers. JOE 1997;23:442.
103. Grossman LI. An improved root canal cement. J Am Dent Assoc 1958;56:381.
104. Caicedo R, von Fraunhofer JA. The properties of endodontic sealers. JOE 1988;14:527.
105. Crane DL, Heuer MA, Kaminski EJ, Moser JB. Biological and physical properties of an experimental root canal sealer without eugenol. JOE 1980;6:438.
106. Sleder FS, et al. Long-term sealing ability of a calcium hydroxide sealer. JOE 1991;11:541.
107. Gutmann JL, Fava LRG. Perspectives on periradicular healing using SealApex: a case report. Int Endod J 1991;24:135.
108. Limkangwalmongkol S, et al. Apical dye penetration with four root canal sealers and gutta-percha using longitudinal sectioning. JOE 1992;18:535.
109. Limkangwalmongkol S, et al. A comparative study of the apical leakage of four root canal sealers and laterally condensed gutta-percha. JOE 1991;17:495.
110. Kawakami T, et al. Fate of ^{45}Ca-labeled calcium hydroxide in a canal filling paste embedded in rat subcutaneous tissues. JOE 1987;13:220.
111. Pitt-Ford TR, Rowe AHR. A new root canal sealer based on calcium hydroxide. JOE 1989;15:286.
112. Ozata F, Onai B, Erdilek N, Turkun SL. A comparative study of apical leakage of Apexit, Ketac-Endo, and Diaket root canal sealers. JOE 1999;25:603.
113. Leyhausen G, Heil J, Reifferscheid G, et al. Genotoxicity and cytotoxicity of the epoxy resin based root canal sealer AH Plus. JOE 1999;25:109.
114. Saito S. Characteristics of glass ionomer cements and clinical application. J Dent Med 1979;10:1.
115. Pitt-Ford TR. The leakage of root canal fillings using glass ionomer cement and other materials. Br Dent J 1979;146:273.
116. Stewart GG. Clinical application of glass ionomer cements in endodontics: case reports. Int Endod J 1990;23:172.
117. Ray H, Seltzer S. A new glass ionomer root canal sealer. JOE 1991;17:598.
118. Loest C, Trope M, Friedman S. Followup of root canals obturated with a glass ionomer root canal sealer [abstract]. JOE 1993;19:201.
119. Friedman S, et al. Efficacy of removing glass ionomer cement, zinc oxide eugenol, and epoxy resin sealers from retreated root canals. Oral Surg 1992;73:609.
120. Wu M-K, De Gee A, Wesselink PR. Leakage of AH26 and Keto-Endo used with injected gutta-percha. JOE 1997;23:331.
121. Dalat DM, Onai B. Apical leakage of a new glass ionomer root canal sealer. JOE 1998;24:161.
122. Rohde TR, Bramwell JD, Hutter JW, Roahen JO. An in vitro evaluation of microleakage of a new root canal sealer. JOE 1996;22:365.
123. Beltes P, Koulaouzidou E, Kolokuris I, Kortsaris AH. *In vitro* evaluation of the cytotoxicity of two glass-ionomer root canal sealers. JOE 1997;23:572.
124. Kolokuris I, Beltes P, Economides N, Viemmas L. Experimental study of the biocompatibility of a new glass-ionomer root canal sealer (Ketac-Endo). JOE 1996;22:395.
125. Garces-Ortiz M, Ledesma-Montes C. Cytotoxicity of Ketac silver cement. JOE 1997;23:371.
126. Molloy D, et al. Comparative tissue tolerance of a new endodontic sealer. Oral Surg 1992;73:490.
127. Rawlinson A. Sealing root canals with low-viscosity resins in vitro: scanning electron microscopy study of canal cleansing and resin adaptation. Oral Surg 1989;68:330.
128. Torabinejad M, et al. Isopropyl cyanoacrylate as a root canal sealer. JOE 1984;10:304.
129. Smith DW, Wong M. Comparison in apical leakage in teeth obturated with a polyamide varnish or zinc oxide and eugenol cement using lateral condensation. JOE 1992;18:25.

130. Zidan O, et al. Obturation of root canals using the single cone gutta-percha technique and dentinal bonding agents. Int Endod J 1987;20:128.
131. Zidan O, El Deeb ME. The use of a dentinal bonding agent as a root canal sealer. JOE 1985;11:176.
132. Anic I, Shirasuka T, Matsumoto K. Scanning electron microscopic evaluation of two compaction techniques using a composite resin as a root canal filling material. JOE 1995;21:594.
133. Mannocci F, Ferrari M. Apical seal of roots obturated with laterally condensed gutta-percha, epoxy resin cement, and dentin bonding agent. JOE 1998;24:81.
134. Leinfelder KF. Current status of dentin adhesive systems. Alpha Omegan 1998;91:17.
135. Torneck CK, et al. The influence of time of hydrogen peroxide exposure on the adhesion of composite resin to bleached bovine enamel. JOE 1990;16:123.
136. Wiemann AH, Wilcox LR. *In vitro* evaluation of four methods of sealer placement. JOE 1991;17:444.
137. Brown WE, Chow LC. A new calcium phosphate setting cement [abstract]. J Dent Res 1983;62:672.
138. Brown WE, Chow LC. Dental restoration cement pastes. US patent 4, 518, 430. 1985.
139. Hovland EJ, Dumsha TC. Leakage evaluation *in vitro* of the root canal sealer cement SealApex. Int Endod J 1985;18:179.
140. Jacobsen EL, Shugars KA. The sealing efficacy of a zinc oxide-eugenol cement, a cyanoacrylate, and a cavity varnish used as root canal cements. JOE 1990;16:516.
141. Kapsimalis P, Evans R. Sealing properties of endodontic filling materials using radioactive isotopes. Oral Surg 1966;22:386.
142. Curson I, Kirk EEJ. An assessment of root canal sealing cements. Oral Surg 1968;26:229.
143. Yates J, Hembree J. Microleakage of three root canal cements. JOE 1980;6:591.
144. von Fraunhofer JA, Branstetter J. The physical properties of four endodontic sealer cements. JOE 1982;8:126.
145. Goldberg F, Gurfinkel J. Analysis of the use of Dycal with gutta-percha points as an endodontic filling technique. Oral Surg 1979;47:78.
146. Wollard R, Brough S, Maggio J, Seltzer S. Scanning and electron microscopic examination of root canal filling materials. JOE 1976;2:98.
147. Shively J, et al. An in vitro autoradiographic study comparing the apical seal of uncatalyzed Dycal to Grossman's Sealer. JOE 1985;11:62.
148. Sargenti AG. Fifth International Conference on Endodontics; 1973; Philadelphia.
149. Sargenti A. Cassette tape that accompanies Sargenti endodontics. Locarno (Switzerland): Angelo G. Sargenti; 1973.
150. Block RM, Langeland K, et al. Paste technique re-treatment study: a clinical, histopathologic, and radiographic evaluation of 50 cases. Oral Surg 1985;60:76.
151. Pupo J, Langeland K, et al. Antimicrobial effects of endodontic filling cements on microorganisms from root canal. Oral Surg 1983;55:622.
152. Delivanis PD, Mattison GC, Mendel RW. The survivability of F-43 strain of *Streptococcus sanguis* in root canals filled with gutta-percha and Procosol cement. JOE 1983;9:407.
153. Zmener O. Evaluation of the apical seal obtained with two calcium hydroxide based endodontic sealers. Int Endod J 1987;20:87.
154. Jacobsen EL, et al. An evaluation of two newly formulated calcium hydroxide cements: a leakage study. JOE 1987;13:164.
155. Rothier A, et al. Leakage evaluation in vitro of two calcium hydroxide and two zinc oxide-eugenol-based sealers. JOE 1987;13:336.
156. Barkhordar RA, et al. An evaluation of sealing ability of calcium hydroxide sealers. Oral Surg 1989;68:88.
157. Cohen T, Gutmann JL, et al. An assessment in vitro of the sealing properties of Calciobiotic Root Canal Sealer. Int Endod J 1985;18:172.
158. Lim KIC, Tidmarsh BG. The sealing ability of SealApex compared to AH-26. JOE 1986;12:564.
159. Rice RT, et al. The choice of a root canal sealer. Compend Contin Educ Dent 1988;9:184.
160. Canalda C, Pumarola J. Bacterial growth inhibition produced by root canal sealer cements with a calcium hydroxide base. Oral Surg 1989;68:99.
161. Pumarola J, et al. Antimicrobial activity of seven root canal sealers. Oral Surg 1992;74:216.
162. Branstetter J, von Fraunhafer SA. The physical properties and sealing action of endodontic sealer cements: a review of the literature. JOE 1982;8:312.
163. Sugawara A, Chow LC, et al. *In vitro* evaluation of the sealing ability of a calcium phosphate cement when used as a root canal sealer-filler. JOE 1990;16:162.
164. Barkhordar RA, et al. Evaluation of the apical sealing ability of apatite root canal sealer. Quintessence Int 1992;23:515.
165. Chohayeb AA, Chow LC, et al. Evaluations of calcium phosphate as a root canal sealer-filler material. JOE 1987;13:384.
166. Gerosa R, Borin M, et al. In vitro evaluation of the cytotoxicity of pure eugenol. JOE 1998;22:532.
167. Chisolm EC. Proceedings of the Tennessee Dental Association, 7th Annual Meeting. Dent Reg 1873;27:517.
168. Hume WR. The pharmacologic and toxicological properties of zinc oxide-eugenol. J Am Dent Assoc 1986;113:789.
169. Doblecki W, Turner DW, Osetek EM, Pellen GB. Leukocyte migration response to dental materials using Boyden chambers. JOE 1980;6:636.
170. Spångberg L, Langeland K. Toxicity of root canal filling materials on HeLa cells in vitro. Oral Surg 1973;35:402.
171. Munaco FS, et al. A study of long-term toxicity of endodontic materials with use of an *in vitro* model. JOE 1978;4:151.
172. Antrim DD. Evaluation of the cytotoxicity of root canal sealing agents on tissue culture cells *in vitro*. Grossman's sealer, N2 (permanent). Rickert's sealer and Cavit. JOE 1976;2:111.
173. Mohammad AR, et al. Cytotoxicity evaluation of root canal sealers by the tissue culture-agar overlay technique. Oral Surg 1978;45:768.
174. Spångberg L, Pascon EA. The importance of material preparation for the expression of cytotoxicity during *in vitro* evalaution of biomaterials. JOE 1988;14:247.
175. Kettering JD, Torabinejad M. Cytotoxicity of root canal sealers: a study using HeLa cells and fibroblasts. Int Endod J 1984;17:60.
176. Meryon SD, Brook AM. *In vitro* comparison of the cytotoxicity of twelve endodontic materials using a new technique. Int Endod J 1990;23:203.
177. Safavi KE, Spångberg LS, et al. An *in vitro* method for longitudinal evaluation of toxicity of endodontic sealers. JOE 1989;15:484.
178. Feiglin B. Effect of some endodontic sealers on cell migration experimental gramulomas. Oral Surg 1987;63:371.

179. Briseno BM, Willerhausen B. Root canal sealer cytotoxicity with human gingival fibroblasts. III. Calcium hydroxide-based sealers. JOE 1992;18:110.
180. Guimaraes SAC, Percinoto C. Effect of some endodontic material on the influx of macrophages and multinucleated giant cell development in experimental granulomas. JOE 1984;10:101.
181. Biggs JT, et al. Rat macrophage response to implanted sealer cements. JOE 1985;11:30.
182. Matsumoto K, et al. The effect of newly developed root canal sealers on rat dental pulp cells in primary culture. JOE 1989;15:60.
183. Nakamura H, et al. Study on the cytotoxicity of root canal filling materials. JOE 1986;12:156.
184. Meryon SD, et al. Eugenol release and the cytotoxicity of different zinc oxide-eugenol combinations. J Dent 1988;16:66.
185. Maseki T, et al. Lack of correlation between the amount of eugenol released from zinc oxide-eugenol sealer and cytotoxicity of the sealer. JOE 1991;17:76.
186. Pascon EA, Spångberg LSW. In vitro cytotoxicity of root canal filling materials: 1. Gutta-percha. JOE 1990;16:429.
187. Kolokouris I, Economides N, Beltes P, Vlemmas I. In vivo comparison of the biocompatabilty of two root canal sealers implanted into the subcutaneous connective tissue of dogs. JOE 1998;24:82.
188. Mittal M, Chandra S, Chandra S. Comparative tissue evaluation of four endodontic sealers. JOE 1995;21:622.
189. Osorio RM, Hefti A, Vertucci FJ, Shawley AL. Cytotoxicity of endodontic materials. JOE 1998;24:91.
190. Leonardo MR, Silva LAB, Ether SS. Calcium hydroxide root canal sealers–histopathologic evaluation of apical and periapical repair after endodontic treatment. JOE 1997;23:428.
191. Spångberg L. Studies on root canal medicaments. Swed Dent J 1971;64:1.
192. Angsburger RA, Peters DD. Radiographic evaluation of extruded obturation materials. JOE 1990;16:492.
193. Yesilsoy C, Feigal J. Effects of endodontic materials on cell viability across standard pore size filters. JOE 1985;11:401.
194. Wennberg A. Biological evaluation of root canal sealers using in vitro and in vivo methods. JOE 1980;6:784.
195. Zmener O, Cabrini RL. Adhesion of human blood monocytes and lymphocytes to different endodontic cements. A methodological *in vitro* study. JOE 1986;12:150.
196. Grossman LI, Lally ET. Assessment of irritating potential of essential oils for a root canal cement. JOE 1982;8:208.
197. Grossman LI. Setting time of selected essential oils with a standard root canal cement powder. JOE 1982;8:277.
198. Morse DR, Wilcko JM, et al. A comparative tissue toxicity evaluation of the liquid components of gutta-percha root canal sealers. JOE 1981;7:545.
199. Olsson B, Sliwkowski A, Langeland K. Subcutaneous implantation for the biologic evaluation of endodontic materials. JOE 1981;7:355.
200. Ørstavik D, Mjor IA. Histopathology and x-ray micro-analysis of the subcutaneous tissue response to endodontic sealers. JOE 1988;14:13.
201. Tagger M, Tagger E. Effect of implantation of AH-26 silver-free in subcutaneous tissue of guinea-pigs. Int Endod J 1986;99:90.
202. Tagger M, Tagger E. Subcutaneous reactions to implantation of tubes with AH-26 and Grossman's sealer. Oral Surg 1986;62:434.
203. Yesilsoy C, et al. A comparative tissue toxicity evaluation of established and newer root canal sealers. Oral Surg 1988;65:459.
204. Kawakami T, et al. Ultrastructural study of initial calcification in the rat subcutaneous tissues elicited by a root canal filling material. Oral Surg 1987;63:360.
205. Rappaport HM, Lilly GE, Kapsimalis P. Toxicity of endodontic filling materials. Oral Surg 1964;18:785.
206. Guttuso J. Histopathologic study of rat connective tissue response to endodontic materials. Oral Surg 1963;16:7.
207. Serper A, Ucer O, Oner R, Etikan I. Comparative neurotoxic effects of root canal filling materials on rat sciatic nerve. JOE 1998;24:592.
208. Pertot WJ, et al. *In vivo* comparison to two root canal sealers implanted into the mandibular bone of rabbits. Oral Surg 1992;73:613.
209. Wenger JS, et al. The effects of partially filled polyethylene tube intraosseous implants in rats. Oral Surg 1978;46:88.
210. Deemer JP, Tsaknis PJ. The effects of overfilled polyethylene tube intraosseous implants in rats. Oral Surg 1979;48:358.
211. Zmener O, Dominguez FV. Tissue response to a glass ionomer used as an endodontic cement. Oral Surg 1983;56:198.
212. Hoover J, et al. The effect of endodontic sealers on bone. JOE 1980;6:586.
213. Spångberg L. Biologic effects of root canal filling materials. Oral Surg 1974;38:934.
214. Friend LA, Browne RM. Tissue reactions to some root canal filling materials implanted in the bone of rabbits. Arch Oral Biol 1969;14:629.
215. Erausquin J, Muruzabal M. Tissue reactions to root canal cements in the rat molar. Oral Surg 1968;26:360.
216. Erausquin J, Muruzabal M. Necrosis of the periodontal ligament in root canal overfilling. J Dent Res 1966;45:1084.
217. Erausquin J, Muruzabal M. Root canal filling with zinc oxide-eugenol cement in rat molars. Oral Surg 1967;24:548.
218. Hong YC, et al. The periradicular tissue reactions to a calcium phosphate cement in the teeth of monkeys. J Biomed Mater Res 1991;25:485.
219. Seltzer S, et al. Periradicular tissue reactions to root canal instrumentation beyond the apex and root canal fillings short of and beyond the apex. Oral Surg 1973;36:725.
220. Soares I, Goldberg F, et al. Periradicular tissue response to two calcium hydroxide-containing endodontic sealers. JOE 1990;16:166.
221. Erausquin J, Muruzabal M. Response to periradicular tissues in the rat molar to root canal fillings with Diaket and AH-26. Oral Surg 1966;21:786.
222. Orstavik D, Mjor IA. Usage test of four endodontic sealers in Maca fasicularis monkeys. Oral Surg 1992;73:337.
223. Pascon EA, et al. Tissue reaction to endodontic materials: methods, criteria, assessment, and observations. Oral Surg 1991;72:222.
224. Rising DW, et al. Histologic appraisal of three experimental root canal filling materials. JOE 1975;1:172.
225. Leonardo MR, et al. A comparison of subcutaneous connective tissue responses among three formulations of gutta-percha used in thermatic techniques. Int Endod J 1990;23:211.
226. Gezelius B, et al. Unexpected symptoms to root filling with gutta-percha. A case report. Int Endod J 1986;19:202.
227. Morse DR, et al. A comparative tissue toxicity evaluation of gutta-percha root canal sealers. Part II. Forty-eight hour findings. JOE 1984;10:484.

228. Webster AE. Some experimental root canal fillings. Dominion Dent J 1900;12:109.
229. The courts: FDA explains status of N2 material. J Am Dent Assoc 1992;123:236.
230. Notice: Agency panel scrutinizes N2 data. ADA News 1993.
231. Notice: Jury finds N2 sealant defective. Cal Dent Assoc Update 1992;4:5.
232. Notice: CDT resoluation on paraformaldehyde pastes. ADA News 1991;22:17.
233. Council on Dental Therapeutics. Status report on the use of root canal filling materials containing paraformaldehyde. J Am Dent Assoc 1977; 94:924.
234. Council on Dental Therapeutics. The use of root canal filling materials containing paraformaldehyde: a status report. J Am Dent Assoc 1987;114:95.
235. Notice: Board bans cement in Florida. ADA News 1992;23:15.
236. American Association of Endodontists. Position statement: paraformaldehyde-containing endodontic filling materials and sealers. American Association of Endodontists; April 1991.
237. Spångberg L, Langeland K. Biological effects of dental materials. Oral Surg 1973;35:402.
238. Grossman LI, et al. Lead blood levels after use of N2. Presented at meeting of the American Association of Endodontists; San Diego, Calif. Apr 18, 1974.
239. Shapiro IM, et al. Blood-lead levels of monkeys treated with lead-containing N2 root canal cement: a preliminiary report. JOE 1975;1:294.
240. Oswald RJ, Cohn SA. Systemic distribution of lead from root canal fillings. JOE 1975;1:159.
241. Garry JF, et al. Lead health hazards in root canal filling material. Pharmacol Ther Dent 1975;2:217.
242. Chong R, Senzer J. Systemic distribution of ^{210}PbO from root canal fillings. JOE 1976;2:381.
243. Peron LC, Toffaletti JG. Concentration of lead in various endodontic filling materials. JOE 1976;2:21.
244. West NM, et al. Level of lead in blood of dogs with RC2B root canal fillings. JOE 1980;6:598.
245. England MC, et al. Tissue level in dogs with RC2B root canal fillings. JOE 1980;6:728.
246. Horsted P, et al. Studies on N2 cement in man and monkey-cement lead content, lead blood level, and histologic findings. JOE 1982;8:341.
247. Block RM, et al. Systemic distribution of N2 paste containing ^{141}C paraformaldehyde following root canal therapy in dogs. Oral Surg 1980;50:350.
248. Langeland K, et al. Methods in the study of biologic responses to endodontic materials. Tissue responses to N2. Oral Surg 1969;27:522.
249. Frankl Z. Treatment of vital exposed pulps in molars with N2 normal. Quintessence Int 1978;4:17.
250. Pitt-Ford TR. Tissue reactions to two root canal sealers containing formaldehyde. Oral Surg 1985;60:661.
251. Lambjerg-Hansen H. Vital pulpectomy and root filling with N2 or Endomethasone. Int Endod J 1987;20:194.
252. Woodhouse BM, et al. Radiographic evaluation of intra-osseous implants of endodontic materials. Oral Surg 1991;71:218.
253. Pissiotis E, Spångberg LSW. Toxicity of Pulpi-Spad using four different cell types. Int Endod J 1991;24:249.
254. Negm MM, Sherif SH. Biologic evaluation of SPAD. Oral Surg 1987;63(Pt I):478.
255. Negm MM. Biologic evaluation of SPAD. Oral Surg 1987;63(Pt 2):487.
256. Tziafas D, Pantelidou O. Treatment of periradicular lesions on dog's teeth using periradicularly extruded SPAD. Int Endod J 1988;21:361.
257. Cohler CM, et al. Studies of Sargenti's technique of endodontic treatment: short term response in monkeys. JOE 1980;6:473.
258. Newton CW, et al. Studies of Sargenti's technique of endodontic treatment: six-month and one-year responses. JOE 1980;6:509.
259. Neiburger EJ. Rapid RC-2B resorption. Report of a case. Oral Surg 1980;50:350.
260. Cohen S. Letter. Cal Dent Assoc J 1981;9:6.
261. Am. Endodont. Soc. Newsletter. 1981;33:Winter.
262. Ehrman EH. Treatment with N2 root canal sealer. Br Dent J 1964;117:409.
263. Orlay H. Overfilling in root canal treatment. Two accidents with N2. Br Dent J 1966;120:376.
264. Grossman LI. Paresthesia from N2 or N2 substitute. Oral Surg 1978;45:114.
265. Grossman LI, Tatoian G. Paresthesia from N2. Report of a case. Oral Surg 1978;46:700.
266. Montgomery S. Paresthesia following endodontic treatment. JOE 1976;2:345.
267. Kaufman A, Rosenberg L. Paresthesia caused by Endomethasone. JOE 1960;6:529.
268. Foreman PC. Adverse tissue reactions following the use of SPAD. Int Endod J 1982;15:184.
269. Tamse A, et al. Paresthesia following over-extension of AH-26. Report of 2 cases and review of the literature. JOE 1982;8:88.
270. Speilman A, et al. Anesthesia following endodontic overfilling with AH-26. Oral Surg 1981;52:554.
271. Orstavik D, et al. Paresthesia following endodontic treatment: survey of the literature and report on a case. Int Endod J 1983;16:167.
272. Nitzan DW, et al. Concepts of accidental overfilling and overinstrumentation in the mandibular canal during root canal treatment. JOE 1983;9:81.
273. Neaverth EJ. Disabling complications following inadvertent overextension of a root canal filling material. JOE 1989;15:135.
274. Brodin P. Neurotoxic and analgesic effects of root canal cements and pulp protecting materials. Endod Dent Traumatol 1988;4:1.
275. Klier DJ, Averbach RE. Painful dysesthesia of the inferior alveolar nerve following use of paraformaldehyde containing root canal sealer. Endod Dent Traumatol 1988;4:46.
276. LaBanc JP, Epker BN. Serious inferior alveolar dysesthesia after endodontic procedure: report of 3 cases. J Am Dent Assoc 1984;108:665.
277. Erisen R, et al. Endomethasone root canal filling material in the mandibular canal. Oral Surg 1989;68:343.
278. Allard KUB. Paraesthesia—a consequence of controversial root-filling material? A case report. Int Endod J 1986;19:205.
279. Fanibunda KB. A method of measuring the volume of human dental pulp cavities. Int Endod J 1986;19:194.
280. Weine FS. Why isn't the Sargenti method taught in dental schools? Dent Stud 1976;55:30.
281. Searls FJ. Sargenti method raises troublesome questions. Dent Stud 1976;55:26.
282. Sargenti A. Endodontic sealing techniques [transcript of panel discussion]. Annual Meeting of the American Dental Association, Washington DC; Nov 10, 1974.

283. Yamada RS, et al. A scanning electron microscopic comparison of a high volume final flush with several irrigating solutions. JOE 1983;9(Pt III):137.
284. Gutmann JL. Adaptation of injected thermoplasticized gutta-percha in the absence of the dentinal smear layer. Int Endod J 1993;26:87.
285. Aktener BO, Bilkay U. Smear layer removal with different concentrations of EDTA-ethylenediamine mixture. JOE 1993;19:278.
286. Moodnik RM, et al. Efficacy of biochemical instrumentation: a scanning electron microscopic study. JOE 1976;2:261.
287. Bolanos OR, Jensen JR. Scanning electron microscope comparisons of the efficacy of various methods of root canal preparation. JOE 1980;6:815.
288. McComb D, Smith DC. A preliminary scanning electron microscope study of root canals after endodontic procedures. JOE 1975;1:238.
289. Lester KS, Boyd A. Scanning electron microscopy of instrumented, irrigated and filled canal. Br Dent J 1977;143:359.
290. Goldman LB, et al. The efficacy of several endodontic irrigating solutions: a scanning electron microscopic study. Oral Surg 1981;52:199.
291. Goldman M, et al. The efficacy of several endodontic irrigating solutions: a scanning electron microscopic study. JOE 1982;8:487.
292. Economides N, Liolios E, Kolokurise I, Beltes P. Long-term evaluation of the influence of smear layer removal on the sealing ability of different sealers. JOE 1999;25:123.
293. Margelos J, Eliades G, Verdelis C, Poalaghias G. Interaction of calcium hydroxide with zinc oxide-eugenol type sealers: a potential clinical problem. JOE 1997;23:43
294. Loel DA. Use of acid cleanser in endodontic therapy. J Am Dent Assoc 1975;90:148.
295. Tidmarsh BG. Acid-cleansed and resin-sealed canals. JOE 1978;4:117.
296. Wayman BE, et al. Citric and lactic acids as root canal irrigants in vivo. JOE 1979;5:258.
297. Pashley DH, et al. Dentin permeability: effects of smear layer removal. J Prosthet Dent 1981;46:531.
298. McComb D, et al. The results of in vivo endodontic chemomechanical instrumentation—a scanning electron microscope study. J Br Endod Soc 1976;9:11.
299. Goldberg F, Abramovich A. Analysis of the effect of EDTAC on the dentin walls of the root canal. JOE 1977;3:101.
300. Cury JA, et al. The demineralizing efficiency of EDTA solutions on dentin. Oral Surg 1981;52:446.
301. Goldberg F, Speilberg C. The effect of EDTAC and the variation of its working time analyzed with scanning electron microscopy. Oral Surg 1982;53:74.
302. Gettleman BH, et al. Adhesion of sealer cements to dentin with and without the smear layer. JOE 1991;17:15.
303. Wennberg A, Orstavik D. Adhesion of root canal sealers to bovine dentin and gutta-percha. Int Endod J 1990;23:13.
304. Civechi B, et al. The effectiveness of different endodontic irrigation procedures on the removal of the smear layer: a scanning electron microscopic study. Int Endod J 1989;22:21.
305. Cergneux M, et al. The influence of the smear layer on the sealing ability of canal obturation. Int Endod J 1987;20:228.
306. White RR, et al. The influence of the smeared layer upon dentinal tubule penetration by plastic filling materials. JOE 1984;10:558.
307. White RR, et al. The influence of the smeared layer upon dentinal tubule penetration by endodontic filling materials. JOE 1987;13:369.
308. Kennedy WA, et al. Smear layer removal effects on apical leakage. JOE 1986;12:21.
309. Calt S, Serper A. Dentinal tubule penetration of root canal sealers after root canal dressing with calcium hydroxide. JOE 1999;25:431.
310. Allison DA, et al. The influence of the method of canal preparation on the quality of apical and coronal obturation. JOE 1979;5:298.
311. Linke HAB, Chohayeb AA. Effective surface sterilization of gutta-percha points. Oral Surg 1983;55:73.
312. Stabholz A, et al. Efficiency of different chemical agents in decontamination of gutta-percha cones. Int Endod J 1987;20:211.
313. Cleary PT, Newton CW, Morrison SW, Kafrawy AH. Histologic examination of gutta-percha exposed to paraformaldehyde implanted in rats. JOE 1992;18:63.
314. Jacobsen EL. Clinical aid: adapting the master gutta-percha cone for apical snugness. JOE 1984;10:274.
315. Allison DA, et al. The influence of master cone adaptation on the quality of the apical seal. JOE 1981;7:61.
316. Kuhre AN, Kessler JR. Effects of moisture on the apical seal of laterally condensed gutta-percha. JOE 1993;19:277.
317. Benatti O, et al. Verification of the consistency, setting time and dimensional changes of root canal filling materials. Oral Surg 1978;46:107.
318. Vermilyea S, et al. The rheologic properties of endodontic sealers. Oral Surg 1978;46:711.
319. Jeffrey IWM. An investigation into the movement of sealer during placement of gutta-percha points. Int Endod J 1986;19:21.
320. Hoen MM, et al. Ultrasonic endodontic sealer placement. JOE 1988;14:169.
321. West LA, et al. Obturation quality utilizing ultrasonic cleaning and sealer placement followed by lateral condensation with gutta-percha. JOE 1989;15:507.
322. Hall MC, Clement DJ, Dove SB, Walker WA. A comparison of sealer placement techniques in curved canals. JOE 1996;22:638.
323. Sakhal S, Weine FS, et al. Lateral condensation: inside view. Compend Contin Educ Dent 1991;12:796.
324. Simlin DR, et al. A comparison of stresses produced during lateral and vertical condensation using engineering models. JOE 1986;12:235.
325. Baumgardner KR, Taylor J, Walton R. Canal adaptation and coronal leakage: lateral condensation compared to Thermafil. J Am Dent Assoc 1995;126:351.
326. Berry KA, Loushine RJ, Primack PD, Runyun DA. Nickel-titanium versus stainless steel finger spreaders in curved canals. JOE 1998;24:752.
327. Ingle JI. The need for endodontic instrument standardization. Oral Surg 1955;8:1211.
328. Simons J, et al. Leakage after lateral condensation with finger spreaders and D-11-T spreaders. JOE 1991;17:101.
329. Jerome CE, et al. Compatability of accessory gutta-percha cones used with two types of spreaders. JOE 1988;14:428.
330. Balbachan L, et al. A study of compatibility between gutta-percha points and finger spreaders. J Assoc Odont Argentina 1990;14:48.
331. Hartwell GR, et al. Evaluation of size variation between endodontic finger spreaders and accessory gutta-percha cones. JOE 1991;17:8.

332. Hatton JF, et al. The effect of condensation pressure on the apical seal. JOE 1988;14:305.
333. Dang DA, Walton RE. Vertical root fracture and root distortion: effect of spreader design. JOE 1989;15:294.
334. Lertchirakarn V, Palamara JEA, Messer H. Load and strain during lateral condensation and vertical root fracture. JOE 1999;25:99.
335. Blum J, Machtou P, Micallef J. Analysis of forces developed during obturation. JOE 1998;24:223.
336. Pitts DL, et al. An *in vitro* study of spreader loads required to cause vertical root fracture during lateral condensation. JOE 1983;9:544.
337. Holcomb JQ, et al. Further investigation of spreader loads required to cause vertical root fracture during lateral condensation. JOE 1987;13:277.
338. Wilcox LR, Roskelley C, Sutton T. The relationship of root canal enlargement to finger spreader induced vertical root fracture. JOE 1997;23:533.
339. Morfis AS. Vertical root fractures. Oral Surg 1990;69:631.
340. Ricks L, et al. 3-D finite element analysis of endodontic condensation stresses. JOE 1993;19:206.
341. Harvey TF, et al. Lateral condensation stress in root canals. JOE 1981;7:151.
342. Joyce AP, Loushine PD, West LA, et al. Photoelastic comparison of stress induced by using stainless steel versus nickel-titanium spreaders. JOE 1998;24:714.
343. Berry KA, Loushine RJ, Primack PD, Runyun DA. Nickel-titanium versus stainless steel finger spreaders in curved canals. JOE 1998;24:752.
344. Simpson TH, Natkin E. Gutta-percha techniques for filling canals of younger permanent teeth after induction of apical root formation. J Br Endod Soc 1972;3:59.
345. Malooley J, et al. Response of periradicular pathosis to endodontic treatment in monkeys. Oral Surg 1979;47:545.
346. Hopkins JH, et al. McSpadden versus lateral condensation: the extent of apical microleakage. JOE 1986;12:198.
347. Bradshaw GB, et al. The sealing ability of injection-moulded thermoplasticized gutta-percha. Int Endod J 1989;22:17.
348. LaCombe JS, et al. A comparison of the apical seal produced by two thermoplasticized injectable gutta-percha techniques. JOE 1988;14:445.
349. Lares C, El Deeb ME. The sealing ability of the Thermafil obturation technique. JOE 1990;16:474.
350. Chohayeb AA. Comparison of conventional root canal obturation techniques with Thermafil obturators. JOE 1992; 18:10.
351. Barkins W, Montgomery S. Evaluation of Thermafil obturation of curved canals prepared by the Canal Master-U system. JOE 1992;18:285.
352. Larder TC, et al. Gutta-percha: a comparative study of three methods of obturation. JOE 1976;2:289.
353. Benner MD, et al. Evaluation of a new thermoplastic gutta-percha obturation technique using ^{45}Ca. JOE 1981;7:500.
354. Kerekes K, Rowe AHR. Thermomechanical compaction of gutta-percha root filling. Int Endod J 1982;15:27.
355. Ishley DJ, El Deeb ME. An *in vitro* assessment of the quality of apical seal of thermomechanically obturated canals with and without sealer. JOE 1983;9:242.
356. Brothman P. A comparative study of the vertical and the lateral condensation of gutta-percha. JOE 1981;7:27.
357. Reader CM, Himel V, et al. Effect of three obturation techniques on the filling of lateral canals and the main canal. JOE 1993;19:404.
358. Torabinejad M, et al. Scanning electron microscopic study of root canal obturation using thermoplasticized gutta-percha. JOE 1978;4:245.
359. Luccy CT, et al. An evaluation of the apical seal produced by lateral and warm lateral condensation techniques. JOE 1990;10:170.
360. Fuss Z, et al. Comparative sealing quality of gutta-percha following the use of the McSpadden Compactor and the Engine Plugger. JOE 1985;11:117.
361. Tagger M, et al. Efficacy of apical seal of Engine Plugger condensed root canal fillings: leakage to dyes. Oral Surg 1983;56:641.
362. El Deeb ME. The sealing ability of injection-molded thermoplasticized gutta-percha. JOE 1985;11:84.
363. Mann SR, McWalter GM. Evaluation of apical seal and placement control in straight and curved canals obturated by laterally condensed and thermoplasticized gutta-percha. JOE 1987;13:10.
364. Olson AK, et al. Evaluation of the controlled placement of injected thermoplasticized gutta-percha. JOE 1989;15:306.
365. Jensen MR, et al. An evaluation of Ultrafil obturation [abstract]. JOE 1989;15:181.
366. Michanowicz AE, et al. Low-temperature (70°C) injection gutta-percha: a scanning electron microscopic investigation. JOE 1986;12:64.
367. Michanowicz AE, et al. Clinical evaluation of low temperature thermoplasticized injectable gutta-percha: a preliminary report. JOE 1989;15:602.
368. Lares-Ortiz C, El Deeb ME. Sealing ability of the Thermafil obturation technique [abstract]. JOE 1989;15:177.
369. McMurtey LG, et al. A comparison between Thermafil and lateral condensation in highly curved canals. JOE 1992;18:68.
370. Scott AC, et al. An evaluation of the Thermafil obturation technique. JOE 1992;18:340.
371. El Deeb ME, et al. Apical leakage in relation to radiographic density of gutta-percha using different obturation techniques. JOE 1985;11:25.
372. Kersten HW. Evaluation of three thermoplasticized gutta-percha filling techniques using a leakage model *in vitro*. Int Endod J 1988;21:353.
373. Martin H, Fischer E. Photoelastic stress comparison of warm (Endotec) *versus* cold lateral condensation techniques. Oral Surg 1990;70:325.
374. Kersten HW, et al. Thermomechanical compaction of gutta-percha. II. A comparison with lateral condensation in curved canals. Int Endod J 1986;19:134.
375. Tagger M, et al. Evaluation of the apical seal produced by a hybrid root canal filling method, combining lateral condensation and thermatic compaction. JOE 1984;10:299.
376. Budd CS, et al. A comparison of thermoplasticized injectable gutta-percha obturation techniques. JOE 1991;17:260.
377. Czonstkowsky M, et al. Evaluation of an injection thermoplasticized low temperature gutta-percha using radioactive isotopes. JOE 1985;11:71.
378. Michanowicz AE, Czonstkowsky M. Sealing properties of an injection-thermoplasticized low-temperature (70°C) gutta-percha: a preliminary study. JOE 1984;10:563.
379. Beatty RG, et al. The efficacy of four root canal obturation techniques in preventing apical dye penetration. J Am Dent Assoc 1989;119:633.

380. Hata G, et al. Sealing ability of Thermafil with and without sealer. JOE 1992;18:322.
381. Schilder H. Vertical compaction of warm gutta-percha. In: Gerstein H, editor. Techniques in clinical endodontics. Philadelphia: WB Saunders; 1983. p. 76.
382. Sakhal S, Weine FS, et al. Lateral condensation: an inside view. Compend Contin Educ Dent 1991;12:796.
383. Callahan JR. Rosin solution for the sealing of the dentinal tubuli and as an adjuvant in filling the root canals. J Allied Dent Soc 1914;9:53.
384. Price WA. Report of laboratory investigations on the physical properties of root filling materials and the efficiency of root fillings for blocking infection from sterile tooth structure. J Natl Dent Assoc 1918;5:1260.
385. Keane KM, Harrington GW. The use of chloroform-softened gutta-percha master cone and its effect on the apical seal. JOE 1984;10:57.
386. Metzger Z, et al. Residual chloroform and plasticity in customized gutta-percha master cones. JOE 1988;14:546.
387 McDonald MN, Vire DE. Chloroform in the endodontic operatory. JOE 1992;18:301.
388. Kaplowitz GJ. Evaluation of gutta-percha solvents. JOE 1990;6:539.
389. Beatty RG, Zakariasen KL. Apical leakage associated with three obturation techniques in large and small canals. Int Endod J 1984;17:67.
389a. Peters DD. Two-year in vitro solubility evaluation of four gutta-percha sealer obturation techniques. JOE 1986;12:139.
390. Goldman M. Evaluation of two filling methods for root canals. JOE 1975;1:69.
391. Wong M, Peters DD, Lorton L. Comparison of gutta-percha filling techniques: three chloroform-gutta-percha filling techniques. JOE 1982;8(Pt 2):4.
392. Morse DR, Wilcko JM. Gutta-percha-eucapercha: a new look at an old technique. Gen Dent 1978;26:58.
393. Morse DR, Wilcko JM. Gutta-percha-eucapercha: a pilot clinical study. Gen Dent 1980;28:24.
394. Haas SB, et al. A comparison of four root canal filling techniques. JOE 1989;15:596.
395. Hunter KR, et al. Halothane and eucalyptol as alternative to chloroform for softening gutta-percha. JOE 1991;17:310.
396. Yancich PP, et al. A comparison of apical seal: chloroform versus eucalyptol-dipped gutta-percha obturation. JOE 1989;15:257.
397. Smith JJ, Montgomery S. A comparison of apical seal: chloroform versus halothane-dipped gutta-percha cones. JOE 1992;18:156.
398. Morse DR, et al. Gutta-percha/eucapercha: characteristics and an update on the technique. Compend Contin Educ Dent 1987;8:708.
399. Metzger Z, et al. Apical seal by customized versus standardized master cones: a comparative study in flat and round canals. JOE 1988;14:381.
400. Schilder H. Filling root canals in three dimensions. Dent Clin North Am 1967.
401. Schilder H. Cleaning and shaping the root canal. Dent Clin North Am 1974:269.
402. Broweleit D, Casanova F, Coppola S, et al. An unpublished, one month patient sampling to determine the frequency of demonstratively filled portals of exit per root canal; 1992.
403. McKinley B, West J. Participation courses in the vertical compaction of warm gutta-percha. University of Washington, Department of Continuing Education; 1976–1992.
404. West J. The relationship between the three-dimensional endodontic seal and endodontic failures [thesis]. Boston: Boston Univ. Goldman School Grad. Dent.; 1975.
405. Blum JY, Parahy E, Machtou P. Warm vertical compaction sequences in relation to gutta-percha temperature. JOE 1997;23:307.
406. Casanova F. Understanding of some clinically significant physical properties of Kerr sealer through investigation [thesis]. Boston: Boston Univ. Goldman School of Grad. Dent.; 1975
407 Dagher FB, Yared GM. Influence of operator proficience on sealing ability of the vertical condensation. JOE 1995;21:335.
408. Lifshitz J, et al. Scanning electron microscope study of the warm gutta-percha technique. JOE 1983;9:17.
409. Wong J, et al. Comparison of gutta-percha filling techniques, compaction (mechanical, vertical (warm), and lateral) condensation techniques. JOE 1981;7(Pt I):551.
410. Lugassey AA, Yee F. Root canal obturation with gutta-percha: a scanning electron microscope comparison of vertical compaction and automated thermatic condensation. JOE 1982;8:120.
411. Yared GM, et al. Master cone apical behavior under in vitro compaction. JOE 1992;18:318.
412. Schilder H. Clinical correlation: biology of the apical and periradicular tissue. A radiographic study. Presented at 19th Annual Meeting American Association Endodontists; 1962; Miami, Florida.
413. Schilder H. Evaluation of healing of human endodontic lesions: a histologic study. Presented at 34th Ann. Meeting, American Association Endodontists; 1977; Atlanta, Georgia.
414. Wollard RR, et al. Scanning electron microscopic examination of root canal filling materials. JOE 1976;2:98.
415. Goodman A, et al. The thermomechanical properties of gutta-percha. Part IV. A thermal profile of the warm gutta-percha packing procedure. Oral Surg 1981;51:544.
416. Hand RE, et al. Effects of a warm gutta-percha technique on the lateral periodontium. Oral Surg 1976;42:395.
417. Jurcak JJ, et al. In vitro intracanal temperatures produced during warm lateral condensation of gutta-percha. JOE 1992;18:1.
418. Lee FS, Van Cura JE, BeGole E. A comparison of root surface temperatures using different obturation heat sources. JOE 1998;24:617.
419. Buchanan LS. The continuous wave of obturation. Dent Today 1996.
420. Berg B. The endodontic management of multirooted teeth. Oral Surg 1953;6:399.
421. Fahid A, et al. Sectional warm gutta percha technique. Gen Dent 1985;33:440.
422. Johnson BT, Bond MS. Leakage associated with single or multiple increment backfill with the Obtura II gutta-percha system. JOE 1999;25:613.
423. Liewehr FR, et al. Obturation of a C-shaped canal using an improved method of warm lateral condensation. JOE 1993;19:474.
424. Castelli WA, et al. Periodontium response to a root canal condensing device (Endotec). Oral Surg 1991;71:333.
425. Jurcak JJ, et al. In vitro intracanal temperature produced during warm lateral condensation of gutta-percha. JOE 1992;18:1.
426. Martin H. Endodontics Palm Springs seminar; Jan 18, 1992.

427. Ewart A, Saunders EM. An investigation into the apical leakage of root-filled teeth prepared for a post crown. Int Endod J 1990;23:239.
428. Himel VT, Cain CW. An evaluation of the number of condenser insertions needed with warm lateral condensation of gutta percha. JOE 1993;19:79.
429. Liewehr FR, et al. Improved density of gutta-percha after warm lateral condensation. JOE 1993;19:489.
430. McSpadden J. Endodontics Palm Springs seminar; Jan 18, 1992.
431. Kersten HW, et al. Thermomechanical compaction of gutta-percha. I. A comparison of several compaction procedures. Int Endod J 1986;19:125.
432. Saunders EM. The effect of variation in thermomechanical compaction techniques upon the quality of apical seal. Int Endod J 1989;22:163.
433. Hardie EM. Heat transmission to the outer surface of the tooth during the thermomechanical compaction technique of root canal obturation. Int Endod J 1986;19:73.
434. Saunders E.M. *In vivo* findings associated with heat generation during thermomechanical compaction of gutta-percha. Part I. Temperature levels at the external surface of the root. Int Endod J 1990;23:263.
435. Saunders EM. *In vivo* findings associated with heat generation during thermomechanical compaction of gutta-percha. Part II. Histological response to temperature elevation on the external surface of the root. Int Endod J 1990;23:268.
436. Fors U, et al. Measurements of the root surface temperature during thermomechanical root canal filling in vitro. Int Endod J 1985;18:199.
437. Beatty RG, et al. Thermomechanical compaction of gutta-percha: effect of speed and duration. Int Endod J 1988;21:367.
438. Pallares A, Faus V. A comparative study of the sealing ability of two root canal obturation techniques. JOE 1995;21:449.
439. Canalda-Sahli C, Berastegui E, Brau-Aguade E. Apical sealing using two thermoplasticized gutta-percha techniques compared with lateral condensation. JOE 1997;23:636.
440. Moreno A. Thermomechanically softened gutta-percha root canal filling. JOE 1977; 3:186.
441. Joiner HL, et al. Temperature changes in thermoplasticized gutta-percha: a comparison of two ultrasonic units. Oral Surg 1989;68:764.
442. Baumgardner KR, Krell KV. Ultrasonic condensation of gutta-percha. An in vivo dye penetration and scanning electron microscope study. JOE 1990;16:253.
443. Yee FS, et al. Three-dimensional obturation of the root canal using injection-molded, thermoplasticized gutta-percha. JOE 1977;3:168.
444. Herschowitz SB, et al. Patent 831714.
445. Marlin J, et al. Clinical use of injection-molded thermoplasticized gutta-percha for obturation of the root canal system: a preliminary report. JOE 1981;7:277.
446. Gutmann JL, Rakusin H. Perspectives on root canal obturation with thermoplasticized injectable gutta-percha. Int Endod J 1987;20:261.
447. Lambrianidis T, Veis A, Zervas P, Molyvdas I. Apical placement of the needle tip with an injection thermoplasticized gutta-percha technique for root canal obturation. Endod Dent Traumatol 1990;6:56.
448. Johnson BT, Bond MS. Leakage associated with single or multiple increment backfill with the Obtura II gutta-percha system. JOE 1999;25:613.
449. Gutmann JL, et al. Evaluation of heat transfer during root canal obturation with thermoplasticized gutta-percha. Part I. *In vitro* heat levels during extrusion. JOE 1987;13:378.
450. Gutmann JL, et al. Evaluation of heat transfer during root canal obturation with thermoplasticized gutta-percha. Part II. *In vivo* response to heat levels generated. JOE 1987;13:441.
451. Donley DL, et al. *In vitro* intracanal temperatures produced by low and high temperature thermoplasticized injectable gutta-percha. JOE 1991;17:307.
452. Hardie EM. Further studies on heat generation during obturation techniques involving thermally softened gutta-percha. Int Endod J 1987;20:122.
453. Eriksson AR, Alberktson T. Temperature threshold levels for heat-induced bone tissue injury. J Prosthet Dent 1983;50:101.
454. Weller RN, Koch KA. *In vitro* radicular temperatures produced by injectable thermoplasticized gutta-percha. Int Endod J 1995;28:86.
455. Marlin J. Injectable standard gutta-percha as a method of filling the root canal. JOE 1986;12:354.
456. Stamos DE, Stamos DG. A new treatment modality for internal resorption. JOE 1986;12:315.
457. Wilson PR, Banes IE. Treatment of internal resorption with thermoplasticized gutta-percha. Int Endod J 1987;20:94.
458. Roane JB. Balanced Force, crown-down preparation, and Inject-R Fill obturation. Compend Contin Educ Dent 1998;19:1137.
459. Skinner RL, Himel VT. The sealing ability of injection-molded thermoplasticized gutta-percha with and without sealers. JOE 1987;13:315.
460. Sobarzo-Navarro V. Clinical experience in root canal obturation by an injection thermoplasticized gutta-percha technique. JOE 1991;17:389.
461. Gatot A, et al. Endodontic overextension produced by injected thermoplasticized gutta-pestuddayrcha. JOE 1989;15:273.
462. Johnson WB. A new gutta-percha technique. JOE 1978;4:184.
463. Thermafil Endodontic Obturators—Instruction Manual. Tulsa (OK): Thermafil/Tulsa Dental Products; 1991.
464. Johnson WB. Thermafil Technique Palm Springs seminar; Jan 18, 1992.
465. Behrend GD, Cutler CW, Gutmann JL. An *in vitro* study of smear layer removal and microbial leakage along root canal fillings, Int Endod J 1996;29:99.
466. Saunders WP, Saunders EM, Gutmann JL, Gutmann ML. An assessment of the plastic Thermafil obturation technique. Part 3: The effect of post space preparation of the apical seal. Int Endod J 1993;26:184.
467. Saw L-H, Messer HH. Root strains associated with different obturation techniques. JOE 1995;21:314.
468. Scott AC, Vire DF. An evaluation of the ability of a dentin plug to control extrusion of thermoplasticized gutta-percha. JOE 1992;18:52.
469. Gutmann JL, Saunders WP, Saunders EM. An assessment of the plastic Thermafil obturation technique. Part 2. Material adaptation and sealability. Int Endod J 1993;26:179.
470. Clinical Research Associates Newsletter. Clinical Research Associates; Provo (UT): Vol 13; Issue 9. 1989.
471. Gutmann JL, Saunders WP, Saunders EM. An assessment of the plastic Thermafil obturation technique. Part I. Radiographic evaluation of adaptation and placement. Int Endod J 1993;26:173.
472. Kytridou V, Gutmann JL, Nunn MH. Adaptation and sealability of two contemporary obturation techniques in the absence of the dentinal smear layer. Int Endod J 1999;32:464.

473. Wolcott J, Himel VT, Powell W, Penney J. Effect of two obturation techniques on the filling of lateral canals and the main canal. JOE 1997;23:636.
474. Weller RN, Kimbrought WF, Anderson RW. A comparison of thermoplastic obturation techniques: adaptation to the canal walls. JOE 1997;23:703.
475. Fabra-Campos H. Experimental apical seal with a new canal obturation system. JOE 1993;19:71.
476. Pathomvanich S, Edmonds DH. The sealing ability of Thermafil obturators assessed by four different microleakage techniques. Int Endod J 1996;29:327.
477. Valli KS, Rafeed RN, Walker RT. Sealing capacity *in vitro* of thermoplasticized gutta-percha with a solid core endodontic filling technique. Endod Dent Traumatol 1998;14:68.
478. Ingle JI. Geriatric endodontics. Alpha Omegan 1986;79:47.
479. Santos MD, Walker WA, Carnes DL. Evaluation of apical seal in straight canals after obturation using the Lightspeed sectional method. JOE 1999;25:609.
480. Dubrow H. Silver points and gutta-percha and the role of the root canal fillings. J Am Dent Assoc 1976;93:976.
481. Mayer A, Ketterl W. Dauerofolae bei der Pulpitis-behandlung. Dtsch Zahnaeztl Z 1958;13:883.
482. Ketterl W. Kriterion fur den Erfolg der Vitalexstirpation. Dtsch Zahnaerztl Z 1965;20:407.
483. Waechter R, Pritz W. Hartsubstanzbildung nach Vitalexstirpation. Dtsch Zahnaerztl Z 1966;21:719.
484. Baume L, et al. Radicular pulpotomy for Category III pulps. J Prosthet Dent 1971;25(Pts I–III):418.
485. El Deeb ME, et al. The dentinal plug: its effect on confining substances to the canal and on the apical seal. JOE 1983;9:355.
486. Oswald RJ, et al. Periradicular response to dentin filings. Oral Surg 1980;49:344.
487. Holland R, et al. Tissue reaction following apical plugging of the root canal with infected dentin chips. Oral Surg 1980;49:366.
488. Torneck CD, et al. Biologic effects of procedures on developing incisor teeth. II. Effect of pulp injury and oral contamination. Oral Surg 1973;35:378.
489. University of Oregon. Clinical syllabus. University of Oregon; 1981.
490. Hasegawa M, et al. An experimental study of the sealing ability of a dentinal apical plug treated with a bonding agent. JOE 1993;19:570.
491. George JW, et al. A method of canal preparation to control apical extrusion of low temperature thermoplasticized gutta-percha. JOE 1988;13:128.
492. Safavi K, et al. Biological evaluation of the apical dentin chip plug. JOE 1985;11:18.
493. Patterson SM, et al. The effect of an apical dentin plug in root canal preparation. JOE 1988;14:1.
494. Brandell DW, et al. Demineralized dentin, hydroxylapatite and dentin chips as apical plugs. Endod Dent Traumatol 1986;2:210.
495. Holland GR. Periradicular response to apical plugs of dentin and calcium hydroxide in ferret canines. JOE 1984;10:71.
496. Pitts DL, et al. A histological comparison of calcium hydroxide plugs and dentin plugs used for the control of gutta-percha root canal filling material. JOE 1984;10:283.
497. Erausquin J. Periradicular tissue response to the apical plug in root canal treatment. J Dent Res 1972;51:483.
498. Tronstad L. Tissue reactions following apical plugging of the root canal with dentin chips in monkey teeth subjected to pulpectomy. Oral Surg 1978;45:297.
499. Holland R, et al. Reaction of human periradicular tissue to pulp extirpation and immediate root canal filling with calcium hydroxide. JOE 1977;3:63.
500. Holland R, et al. Root canal treatment with calcium hydroxide. I. Effect of overfilling and refilling. Oral Surg 1979;47:87.
501. Holland R, et al. Root canal treatment with calcium hydroxide. II. Effect of instrumentation beyond the apices. Oral Surg 1979;47:93.
502. Holland R, et al. Root canal treatment with calcium hydroxide. III. Effect of debris and pressure filling. Oral Surg 1979;47:185.
503. Leonardo MR, et al. Pulpectomy: immediate root canal filling with calcium hydroxide. Oral Surg 1980;49:441.
504. Holland R, et al. Overfilling and refilling monkey's pulpless teeth. J Can Dent Assoc 1980;6:387.
505. Holland R, et al. Apical hard tissue deposition in adult teeth of monkeys with use of calcium hydroxide. Aust Dent J 1980;25:189.
506. Manhart JJ. The calcium hydroxide method of endodontic sealing. Oral Surg 1982;54:219.
507. Guglielmoth MB, et al. A radiographic, histological, and histometric study of endodontic materials. JOE 1989;15:1.
508. Pissiotis E, Spångberg LSW. Biological evaluation of collagen gels containing calcium hydroxide and hydroxyapatite. JOE 1990;16:468.
509. Schumacher JW, Rutledge RE. An alternative to apexification. JOE 1993;19:529.
510. Sigurdsson A, et al. Intracanal placement of $Ca(OH)_2$: a comparison of techniques. JOE 1992; 18:367.
511. Porkaew P, et al. Effects of calcium hydroxide paste as an intracanal medicament on apical seal. JOE 1990;16:369.
512. Weisenseel JA, et al. Calcium hydroxide as an apical barrier. JOE 1987;13:1.
513. Fogel BA. A comparative study of five materials for use in filling root canal spaces. Oral Surg 1977;43:284.
514. Bourgeois RS, Lemon RR. Dowel space preparation and apical leakage. JOE 1981;7:66.
515. Dickey DJ, et al. Effect of post space preparation on apical seal using solvent techniques and Peeso reamers. JOE 1982;8:351.
516. Hiltner RS, et al. Effect of mechanical versus thermal removal of gutta-percha on the quality of the apical seal following post space preparation. JOE 1992;18:451.
517. DeNys M, et al. Evaluation of dowel space preparation on the apical seal using an image processing system. Int Endod J 1989;22:240.
518. Ravanshad S, Torabinejad M. Coronal dye penetration of the apical filling materials after post space preparation. Oral Surg 1992;74:644.
519. Saunders WP, et al. Assessment of Thermafil obturated teeth prepared for a post [abstract]. IADR meeting; 1992 July 1–4, Glasgow, Scotland.
520. Mattison G, et al. The effect of post preparation on the apical seal in teeth filled with Thermafil: a volumetric analysis [abstract]. IADR meeting; 1992 July 1–4, Glasgow, Scotland.
521. Kvist T, et al. The relative frequency of periradicular lesions in teeth with root canal-retained posts. JOE 1989;15:578.
522. Chenail BL, Teplitsky PE. Orthograde ultrasonic retrieval of root canal obstructions. JOE 1987;13:186.

523. Gilbert BO, Rice RT. Re-treatment in endodontics. Oral Surg 1987;64:333.
524. Friedman S, et al. Bypassing gutta-percha root fillings with automated device. JOE 1989;15:432.
525. Wilcox LR, et al. Endodontic retreatment: evaluation of gutta-percha and sealer removal and canal reinstrumentation. JOE 1987;13:453.
526. Wilcox LR. Endodontic retreatment: ultrasonics and chloroform as the final step in reinstrumentation. JOE 1989;15:125.
527. Kaplowitz GJ. Evaluation of gutta-percha solvents. JOE 1990;16:539.
528. Wourms DJ, et al. Alternative solvents to chloroform for gutta-percha removal. JOE 1990;16:224.
529. Ibarrola JL, et al. Retrievability of Thermafil plastic cores using organic solvents. JOE 1993;19:417.
530. Ladley RW, et al. Effectiveness of halothane used with ultrasonic or hand instrumentation to remove gutta-percha from the root canal. JOE 1991;17:221.
531. Bergenholtz G, et al. Retreatment of endodontic fillings. Scand J Dent Res 1979;87:217.
532. Bergenholtz G, et al. Influence of apical overinstrumentation and overfilling on retreated root canals. JOE 1979;5:310.
533. Block RM, Langeland K, et al. Paste technique retreatment study: a clinical, histopathologic, and radiographic evaluation of 50 cases. Oral Surg 1985;60:76.
534. Krell KV, Neo J. The use of ultrasonic endodontic instrumentation in the retreatment of endodontic teeth. Oral Surg 1985;60:100.
535. Jeng H-W, El Deeb ME. Removal of hard paste fillings from the root canal by ultrasonic instrumentation. JOE 1987;13:295.
536. Feldman HJ. To remove broken reamer or bur from a root. Outlook 1914;1:254.
537. Roig-Greene JL. The retrieval of foreign objects from root canals: a simple aid. JOE 1983;9:394.
538. Johnson WB, Beatty RG. Clinical technique for the removal of root canal obstructions. J Am Dent Assoc 1988;117:473.
539. Masserann J. Entfernen metallischer fragment a us wurzelkanalen [translation]. J Br Endod Soc 1971;2:5.
540. Gettleman BH, et al. Removal of canal obstructions with the Endo Extractor. JOE 1991;17:608.
541. Krell KV, et al. The conservative retrieval of silver cones in difficult cases. JOE 1984;10:269.
542. Hulsmann M. The removal of silver cones and fractured instruments using the Canal Finder System. JOE 1990;16:596.
543. Deveaux E, et al. Bacterial microleakage of Cavit, IRM, and TERM. Oral Surg 1992;74:634.
544. Torabinejad M, et al. In vitro bacterial penetration of coronally unsealed endontically treated teeth. JOE 1990;16:566.
545. Widerman FH, et al. The physical and biologic properties of Cavit. J Am Dent Assoc 1971;82:378.
546. Deveaux E, Hildebert P, Neut C, Romond C. Bacterial microleakage of Cavit, IRM, TERM, and Fermit: a 21 day in vitro study. JOE 1999;25:653.
547. Lee Y-C, et al. Microleakage of endodontic temporary restorative materials. JOE 1993;19:516.
548. Oppenheimer S, Rosenberg PA. Effect of temperature change on the sealing properties of Cavit and Cavit G. Oral Surg 1979;48:250.
549. Gilles JA, et al. Dimensional stability of temporary restoratives. Oral Surg 1975;40:796.
550. Maerki HS, et al. Stress relation of interim restoratives. Oral Surg 1979;47:479.
551. Blaney TD, et al. Marginal sealing quality of IRM and Cavit as assessed by microbial penetration. JOE 1981;7:453.
552. Olmstead JS, et al. Surface softening of temporary cement after contact with endodontic medicaments. JOE 1977;3:342.
553. Lamers AC, et al. Microleakage of Cavit temporary filling material in endodontic access cavities in monkey teeth. Oral Surg 1980;49:541.
554. Webber RT, et al. Sealing quality of a temporary filling material. Oral Surg 1978;46:123.
555. Lim KC. Microleakage of intermediate restorative materials. JOE 1990;16:116.
556. Teplitsky PE, Meimans IT. Sealing ability of Cavit and TERM as intermediate restorative materials. JOE 1988;14:278.
557. McInerney ST, Zillich R. Evaluation of internal sealing ability of three materials. JOE 1992;18:376.
558. Noguera AP, McDonald NJ. A comparative in vitro coronal microleakage study of new endodontic restorative materials. JOE 1990;16:523.
559. Barkhordar RA, Stark MM. Sealing ability of intermediate restorations and cavity design used in endodontics. Oral Surg 1990;69:99.
560. Melton D, et al. A comparison of two temporary restorations: light-cured resin versus a self-polymerizing temporary restoration. Oral Surg 1990;70:221.
561. Anderson B, et al. Microleakage of temporary endodontic restorations [abstract]. JOE 1987;13:133.
562. Anderson B, et al. Microleakage of three temporary endodontic restorations. JOE 1988;14:497.
563. Bobotis HG, et al. A microleakage study of temporary restorative materials used in endodontics. JOE 1989;15:569.
564. Anderson RW, et al. Microleakage of temporary restorations in complex endodontic access preparations. JOE 1989;15:526.
565. Turner JE, et al. Microleakage of temporary restorations in teeth restored with amalgam. JOE 1990;16:1.
566. Orahood JP, et al. *In vitro* study of marginal leakage between temporary sealing materials and recently placed restorative materials. JOE 1986;12:523.
567. Marosky JE, et al. Marginal leakage of temporary sealing materials used between endodontic appointments and assessed by ^{45}Ca—an in vivo study. JOE 1977;3:110.
568. Krakow AA, et al. In vivo study of temporary filling materials used in endodontics in anterior teeth. Oral Surg 1977;43:615.
569. Todd MJ, Harrison JW. An evaluation of the immediate and early sealing properties of Cavit. JOE 1979;5:362.
570. Friedman S, et al. Comparative sealing ability of temporary filling materials evaluated by leakage of radiosodium. Int Endod J 1986;19:187.
571. Herman KP, Ludlow MO. An *in vitro* investigation comparing the marginal leakage of Cavit. Cavit G, and TERM. Gen Dent 1989;37:214.
572. Barthel CR, Strobach A, Briedigkeit H, et al. Leakage in roots coronally sealed with different temporary fillings. JOE 1999;25:731.
573. Rutledge RE, Montgomery S. Effect of intracanal medicaments on the sealing ability of TERM. JOE 1990;16:260.
574. Simon M, et al. A root canal disinfectant with reduced formaldehyde concentration. Int Endod J 1982;15:71.
575. Khayat A, Lee S-J, Torabinejad M. Human saliva penetration of coronally unsealed root canals. JOE 1993;19:458.

576. Chow E, Trope M, Nissan R. In vitro endotoxin penetration of coronally unsealed endodontically treated teeth [abstract]. JOE 1993;19:187.
577. Alves J, Walton R, Drake D. Coronal leakage: Endotoxin penetration from mixed bacterial communities through obturated post-prepared root canals. JOE 1998;24:587.
578. Wilcox LR, Diaz-Arnold A. Coronal microleakage of permanent lingual access restorations in endodontically treated anterior teeth. JOE 1989;15:584.
579. Mondelli J, et al. Marginal microleakage in cemented complete crowns. J Prosthet Dent 1978;40:632.
580. Larsen TD, Jensen JR. Microleakage of composite resin and amalgam core material under complete cast core crowns. J Prosthet Dent 1980;44:40.
581. Tjan AHL, et al. The effect of thermal stress on the marginal seal of cast gold full crowns. J Am Dent Assoc 1980;100:48.
582. Kawamura RM, et al. Marginal seal of cast full crowns: an in vitro study. Gen Dent 1983;31:282.
583. Goldman M, et al. Microleakage—full crowns and the dental pulp. JOE 1992;18:473.
584. Swanson K, Madison S. An evaluation of coronal microleakage in endodontically treated teeth. Part I. Time periods. JOE 1987;13:56.
585. Magura ME, et al. Human saliva coronal microleakage in obturated root canals: an in vitro study. JOE 1991;17:324.
586. Madison S, Swanson K, et al. An evaluation of coronal microleakage in endodontically treated teeth. Part II. Sealer types. JOE 1987;13:109.
587. Madison S, Wilcox LR. An evaluation of coronal microleakage in endodontically treated teeth. Part III. In vivo study. JOE 1988;14:455.
588. Phillips RW, et al. In vivo disintegration of luting cements. J Am Dent Assoc 1987;114:339.
589. Tjan AHL, Tan DE. Microleakage of combined amalgam/compostie resin restorations with Amalgambond [abstract]. JDR 1992;71:210.
590. Tjan AHL, Li T. Microleakage of amalgam restorations lined with Amalgambond or All-Bond liner [abstract]. JDR 1991;71:660.
591. Wolcott JF, Hicks ML, Himel VT. Evaluation of pigmented intraorifice barriers in endodontically treated teeth. JOE 1999;25:589.
592. Pisano DM, DiFiore PM, McClanahan SB, et al. Intraorifice sealing of gutta-percha obturated root canals to prevent coronal microleakage. JOE 1998;24:659.
593. McDougall IG, Patel V, Santerre P, Friedman S. Resistance of experimental glass ionomer sealers to bacterial penetration in vitro. JOE 1998;25:739.
594. Grove CJ. Nature's method of making perfect root fillings following pulp removal. Dent Cosmos 1921;63:969.
595. Coolidge ED, Kesel RG. Endodontology, 2nd ed. Philadelphia: Lea & Febiger; 1956.
596. Laws A. Calcium hydroxide as a possible root filling material. N Z Dent J 1962;58:199.
597. Cvek J. Treatment of nonvital permanent incisors with calcium hydroxide. I. Followup of periradicular repair and apical closure of immature roots. Odont Rev 1972;23:27.
598. Hendry JA, et al. Comparison of calcium hydroxide and zinc oxide and eugenol pulpectomies in primary teeth of dogs. Oral Surg 1982;54:445.
599. Holland R, DeSouza V. Ability of a new calcium hydroxide root filling material to induce hard tissue formation. JOE 1985;11:535.
600. Sonat B, et al. Periradicular tissue reaction to root fillings with Sealapex. Int Endod J 1990;23:46.
601. Tagger M, Tagger E, et al. Release of calcium and hydroxyl ions from set endodontic sealers containing calcium hydroxide. JOE 1988;14:588.
602. Nevins AJ, et al. Pulpotomy and partial pulpectomy procedures in monkey teeth using cross-linked collagen-calcium phosphate gel. Oral Surg 1980;49:360.
603. Harbert H. Generic tricalcium phosphate plugs: an adjunct in endodontics. JOE 1991;17:131.
604. Chohayeb AA, Chow LC, et al. Evaluation of calcium phosphate as a root canal sealer-filler material. JOE 1987;13:384.
605. Changsheng L, Wang W, Shen W, et al. Evaluation of the biocompatability of a nonceramic hydroxyapatite. JOE 1997;23:490.
606. Krell KV, Wefel JS. Calcium phosphate cement root canal sealer—scanning electron microscopic examination. JOE 1984;10:571.
607. Goodell GG, Mork TO, Hutter JW, Nicoll BK. Linear dye penetration of a calcium phosphate cement apical barrier. JOE 1997;23:174.
608. Steinbrunner RL, Brown CE Jr, Legan JJ, Kafrawy AH. Biocompatability of two apatite cements. JOE 1998;24:325.
609. Yoshikawa M, Hayami S, Tsuji I, Toda T. Histopathological study of a newly developed root canal sealer containing tetracalcium-dicalcium phosphates and 1.0% chondroitin sulfate. JOE 1997;23:162.
610. Gambarini G, Tagger M. Sealing ability of a new hydroxyapatite-containing sealer using lateral condensation and thermatic compaction of gutta-percha, in vitro. JOE 1996;22:165.
611. Yoshida T, Itoh T, Saitoh T, Sekine I. Hisopathological study of the use of freeze-dried allogenic dentin powder and tru bone ceramic as apical barrier materials. JOE 1998;24:581.
612. Friedman CD, et al. Hydroxyapatite cement. II. obliteration and reconstruction of the cat frontal sinus. Arch Otolaryngol Head Neck Surg 1991;117:385.
613. Torabinejad M, Watson TF, Pitt Ford TR. Sealing ability of a mineral trioxide aggregate when used as a root-end filling material. JOE 1993;19:591.
614. Gee JY. A comparison of five methods of root canal obturation by means of dye penetration. Aust Dent J 1987;32:279.
615. Kanca J III. Improving bond strength through acid etching of dentin and bonding to wet dentin surfaces. J Am Dent Assoc 1992;123:35.

Chapter 12

ENDODONTIC SURGERY

Steven G. Morrow and Richard A. Rubinstein

HISTORICAL PERSPECTIVE

Contrary to what many dentists think, endodontic surgery is not a concept developed in the twentieth century. The first recorded endodontic surgical procedure was the incision and drainage of an acute endodontic abscess performed by Aetius, a Greek physician–dentist, over 1,500 years ago.[1] Since then, endodontic surgery and endodontic surgical procedures have been developed and refined, a result of the valuable contributions of many pioneers in dentistry including Abulcasis, Fauchard, Hullihan, Martin, Partisch, and Black.[2]

William Hunter's classic presentation "An Address on the Role of Sepsis and Antisepsis in Medicine," which was delivered to the Faculty of Medicine of McGill University in Montreal in 1910, had a major impact on dentistry and initiated the conflict of "focal infection," whose embers still smolder. As a result, the development of endodontics and endodontic surgery can best be characterized as both progressive and regressive. Tremendous strides were made in the development and application of endodontic surgical techniques, but the concepts involved in endodontic surgery were being severely attacked by the medical profession.[2]

Although Hunter's presentation initiated a major conflict, it turned out to be a blessing in the development of endodontics and endodontic surgery. The stimulus to form the American Association of Endodontists was in part the result of endodontic pioneers joining in mutual support to develop scientific evidence for their concepts.

The results of scientific investigation and the clinical application of the techniques and concepts developed during the second half of the twentieth century represent the basis of what is known and will be practiced into the twenty-first century. However, endodontic surgery is dynamic, and it is imperative that scientific investigation continue; concepts, techniques, and material used in endodontic surgery must be continually evaluated and modified, and more emphasis must be placed on the assessment of long-term clinical outcomes.

CURRENT APPLICATION

During the last 20 years, endodontics has seen a dramatic shift in the application of periradicular surgery and the part it plays in the delivery of endodontic services. Previously, periradicular surgery was commonly considered the treatment of choice when nonsurgical treatment had failed or if existing restorative or prosthetic treatment would be endangered by orthograde treatment.[3] Grossman et al included in a list of indications for endodontic surgery the presence of large and intruding periapical lesions, overfilled canals, incomplete apical root formation, and destruction of the apical constriction by overinstrumentation.[4]

The dental literature contains an abundance of clinical articles, scientific reports, and textbook chapters that provide extensive lists of indications for periradicular surgery. However, many of the previously accepted indications are no longer valid in light of current concepts of the biologic basis for endodontic treatment (Figure 12-1). Therefore, it must be recognized that periradicular surgery has become very selective in contemporary dental practice (Figures 12-2, 12-3, and 12-4). Moreover, it must be emphasized that the application of surgery must always be in the best interest of the patient and also within the realm of the expertise of the practitioner.

INDICATIONS

Several factors have resulted in a significant impact on the indications for and the application of endodontic surgery. According to the American Association of Endodontists, more than 14 million root canal treatments are done annually in the United States.[5] Even though the success rate of nonsurgical endodontic

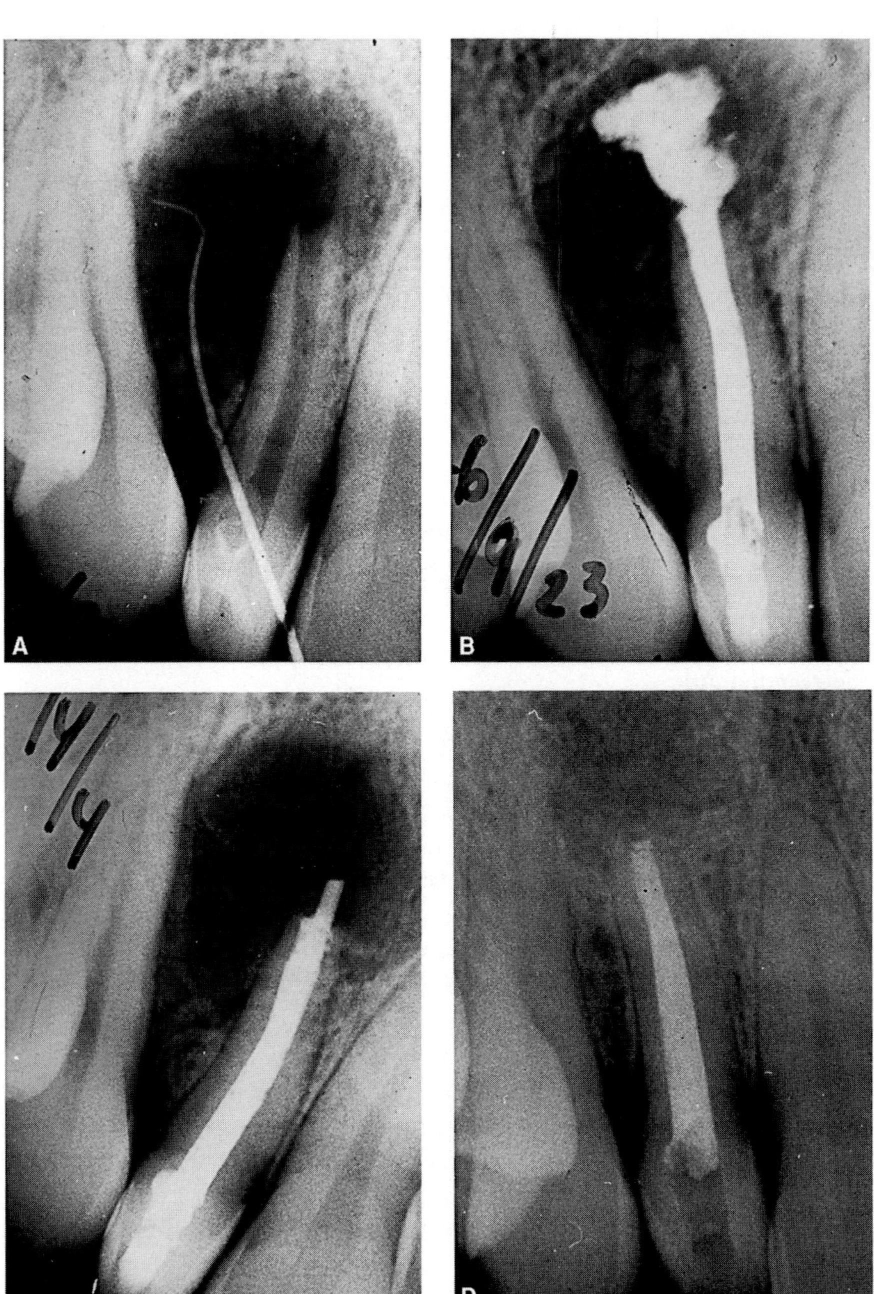

Figure 12-1 A, *Dens invaginatus* (*dens in dente*), with accompanying apical/lateral cyst. Patient is a 16-year-old girl. Gutta-percha sound placed through draining stoma. **B,** Calcium hydroxide [$Ca(OH)_2$] and iodoform (for contrast) paste fills débrided canal. **C,** Drainage ceased and $Ca(OH)_2$ resorbed away in 8 months. At this appointment, the canal was filled with gutta-percha and AH26 sealer. **D,** Follow-up radiograph 15 years after obturation. **No surgery** was done. (Courtesy of Dr. César C. Mexia de Almeida, Lisbon, Portugal.)

treatments is high, failures do occur. Many retrospective studies have established endodontic success rates, ranging from a high of 96% to a low of 53%.[6–13] Additionally, in recent years, there has been an increasing interest in endodontic **re-treatment procedures** (see chapter 13). Studies reporting the success rate for **nonsurgical re-treatment** indicate successes as low as 62% to as high as 98%.[14–18] This emphasis on nonsurgical re-treatment of endodontic failures has probably had the single greatest impact on the indications for surgical intervention in the treatment of endodontic pathosis.

A classic categorization of specific indications and contraindications was developed by Luebke, Glick, and Ingle and has been modified for this chapter[19] (Table 12-1). Even though these indications describe specific situations, they should not be considered "automatic" indications but should be applied as judgment and circumstances dictate.

CONTRAINDICATIONS

Few absolute contraindications to endodontic surgery exist. Most contraindications are relative, and they are usually limited to three areas: (1) the patient's medical status, (2) anatomic considerations, and (3) the dentist's skills and experience.

Advances in medicine have dramatically increased life expectancy and the survival rate from most of today's diseases. Dentists are, with increasing frequen-

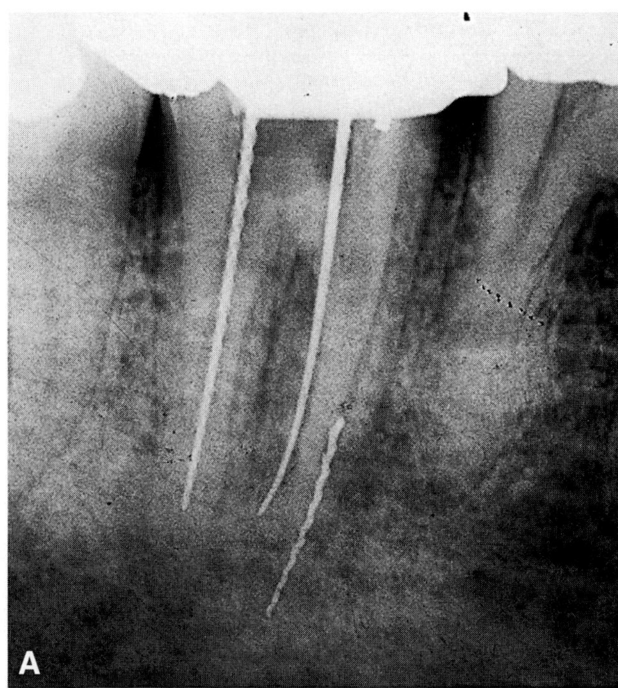

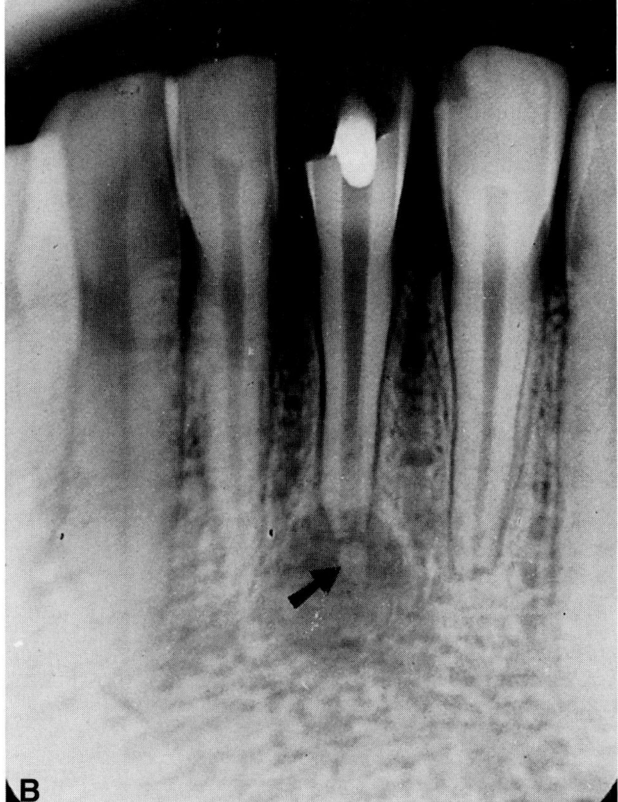

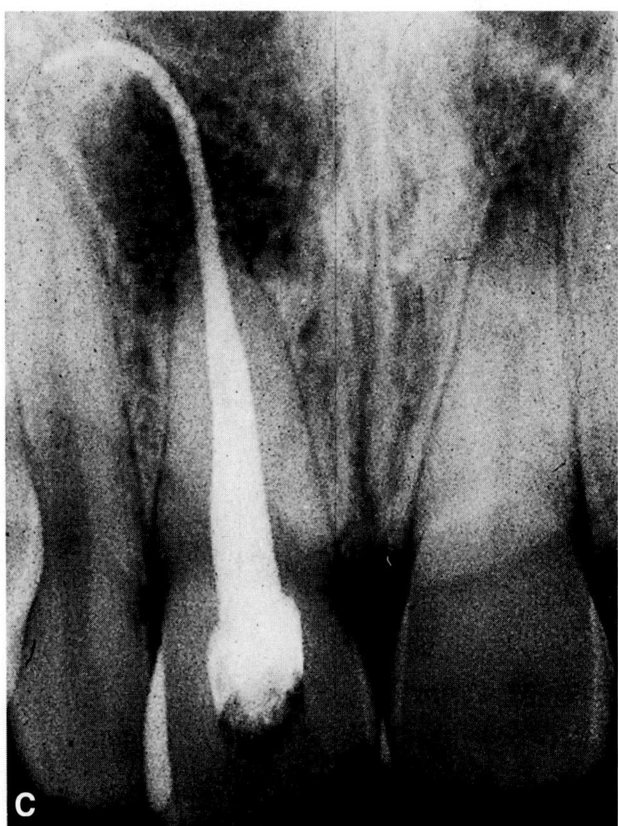

Figure 12-2 A, Fractured instrument protrudes past apical foramen of mesiolingual canal. B, Overinstrumentation has led to apical perforation and fracture of root tip (**arrow**) that must be removed surgically. C, Overextended gutta-percha filling caused physical irritation with pain and inflammation.

cy, being asked to treat medically compromised patients. When considering performing any surgical procedure on a patient who reports a major systems disorder (cardiovascular, respiratory, digestive, hepatic, renal, immune, or skeletomuscular), a thorough medical history is mandatory. Following the identification of all potential medical complications and a review of the patient's current drug regimen, a consultation with the primary care physician or specialist may be in order. The dentist should explain to the physician the needed endodontic surgical treatment, including a brief description of the procedure, anesthetic agents

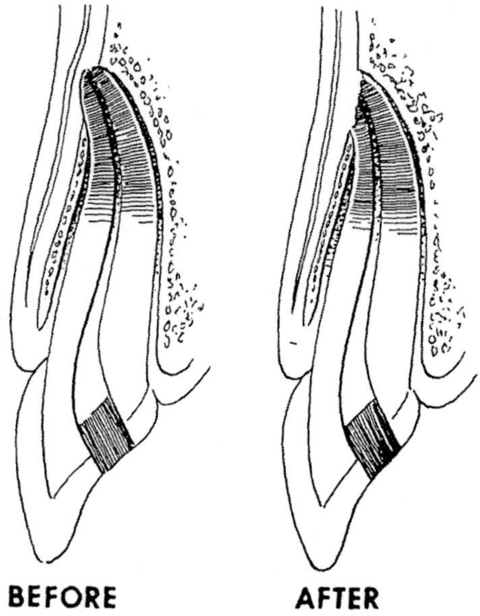

Figure 12-3 Beveling of the root apex to subcortical level relieves facial periradicular tenderness.

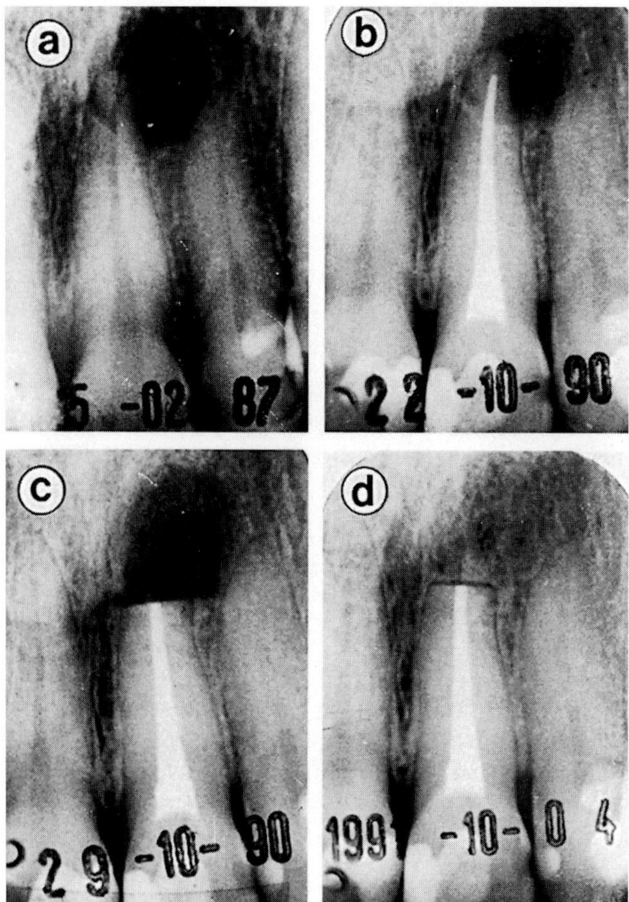

Figure 12-4 Cyst enucleation necessary to achieve healing. Longitudinal radiographs over 4 years and 9 months. **a,** Pretreatment. **b,** No healing 44 months after root filling. **c,** Apicoectomy and cyst enucleation. **d,** Complete healing 1 year later. Reproduced with permission from Nair PNR et al. Radicalar cyst affecting aroot-filled human tooth. Int Endod J 1993;26:225.

Table 12-1 Indications for Endodontic Surgery

1. Need for surgical drainage
2. Failed nonsurgical endodontic treatment
    1. Irretrievable root canal filling material
    2. Irretrievable intraradicular post
3. Calcific metamorphosis of the pulp space
4. Procedural errors
    1. Instrument fragmentation
    2. Non-negotiable ledging
    3. Root perforation
    4. Symptomatic overfilling
5. Anatomic variations
    A. Root dilaceration
    B. Apical root fenestration
6. Biopsy
7. Corrective surgery
    1. Root resorptive defects
    2. Root caries
    3. Root resection
    4. Hemisection
    5. Bicuspidization
8. Replacement surgery
    1. Replacement surgery
        1. Intentional replantation (extraction/replantation)
        2. Post-traumatic
    2. Implant surgery
        1. Endodontic
        2. Osseointegrated

and other drugs to be used, the approximate length of time required for the procedure, and the expected length of recovery. In this way, the physician can more adequately assess the medical risks involved and can assist the dentist in determining appropriate treatment modifications. These modifications may be preoperative (alteration of drug therapy, sedative or hypnotic, systemic antibiotics), intraoperative (nitrous oxide, intravenous sedation), or postoperative (reinstatement of drug therapy, sedatives, and analgesics).

Anatomic considerations are addressed in more detail later in this chapter. However, it should be emphasized that the majority of these anatomic considerations present contraindications that must be addressed for each individual patient. The major anatomic considerations of importance to endodontic surgery involve (1) the nasal floor, (2) the maxillary sinus, (3) the mandibular canal and its neurovascular bundle, (4) the mental foramen and its neurovascular bundle, and (5) anatomic limitations to adequate visual and mechanical access to the surgical site. A skilled surgeon with the needed armamentarium is usually able to circumvent these anatomic limitations and accomplish successful endodontic surgery.

It is imperative that dental professionals keep in mind that all treatment rendered by them to their patients must be in the patients' best interest and at the highest quality possible. As a professional, one has an obligation to know one's limitations of clinical skills and to confine treatment efforts to be consistent with those limitations. Unless the general practitioner has had extensive surgical training and experience, the majority of endodontic surgical procedures should be done by trained endodontic specialists. When receiving care of a specialized nature, patients need and deserve treatment that meets the standard of care delivered by competent practitioners who are trained as specialists.[19] The standard of care in dentistry is that practiced by the specialist in any given dental discipline.[20]

CLASSIFICATION OF ENDODONTIC SURGICAL PROCEDURES

Endodontic surgery encompasses surgical procedures performed to remove the causative agents of periradicular pathosis and to restore the periodontium to a state of biologic and functional health. These procedures may be classified as follows:

1. Surgical drainage
   1. Incision and drainage (I & D)
   2. Cortical trephination (fistulative surgery)
2. Periradicular surgery
   1. Curettage
   2. Biopsy
   3. Root-end resection
   4. Root-end preparation and filling
   5. Corrective surgery
      1. Perforation repair
         a. Mechanical (iatrogenic)
         b. Resorptive (internal and external)
      2. Root resection
      3. Hemisection
3. Replacement surgery (extraction/replantation)
4. Implant surgery
   1. Endodontic implants
   2. Root-form osseointegrated implants

SURGICAL DRAINAGE

Surgical drainage is indicated when purulent and/or hemorrhagic exudate forms within the soft tissue or the alveolar bone as a result of a symptomatic periradicular abscess. A significant reduction of pain and a decrease in the length of morbidity will follow the release of pressure and the evacuation of the by-products of inflammation and infection.[21] Surgical drainage may be accomplished by (1) incision and drainage (I & D) of the soft tissue or (2) trephination of the alveolar cortical plate.

Incision and Drainage

Fluctuant soft-tissue swelling occurs when periradicular inflammatory exudate exits through the medullary bone and the cortical plate. Once through the cortical plate, the exudate spreads into the surrounding soft tissues. When this occurs, an incision should be made through the focal point of the localized swelling to relieve pressure, eliminate exudate and toxins, and stimulate healing. If the swelling is intraoral and localized, the infection may be managed by surgical drainage alone. However, if the swelling is diffuse or has spread into extraoral musculofascial tissues or spaces, surgical drainage should be supplemented with appropriate systemic antibiotic therapy.[22] (Figure 12-5) (also see chapter 18, "Pharmacology for Endodontics").

Learning the correct timing for I & D takes experience. The patient often presents with a generalized, diffuse facial swelling that is indurated. Caution should always be exercised with hard swellings of this nature, especially when accompanied by a fever. Such an infection can extend into fascial planes and anatomic spaces and become life threatening. Consultation with, or referral to, an appropriate specialist may be indicated.

Unfortunately, incision into a diffuse or indurated swelling before its localization is often unsuccessful in affording immediate relief or reduction of the swelling. When this situation exists, it has been suggested that the patient be placed on appropriate systemic antibiotic therapy and instructed to use hot salt water "mouth holds" (¼–½ tsp of salt in a 10–12-oz glass of hot water) in the swollen area to assist in the localization of the swelling to a more fluctuant state. The clinical situation should be monitored every 24 hours. As soon as the swelling has localized and a fluctuant area has developed, surgical drainage should be performed.[3]

Incision and Drainage Tray Setup. The tray setup should be simple and uncluttered. The instruments and supplies needed for the procedure should be laid out in the order of their use (Figure 12-6).

Local Anesthesia. Whenever possible, nerve block injection is the preferable method for obtaining local anesthesia. In some cases, block injections must be supplemented with local infiltration to obtain adequate local anesthesia. In other clinical situations, block injections are either impossible or impractical and

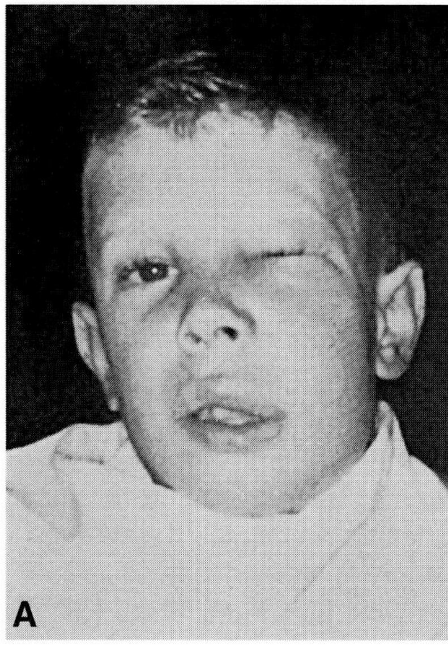

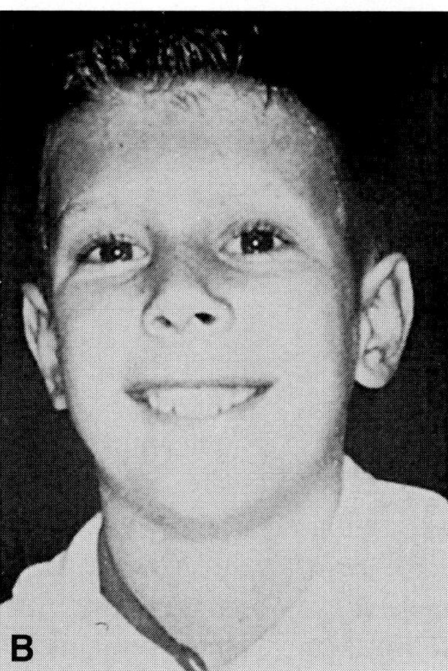

Figure 12-5 Rapid dissolution of massive cellulitis following incision and drainage and antibiotic therapy. **A,** Unilateral facial asymmetry and eye closure indicate severity of inflammatory edema from abscess, apical to maxillary lateral incisor. **B,** Five days later all signs of inflammation have vanished and patient is ready for root canal therapy. (Courtesy of Dr. Bertram L. Wolfshon.)

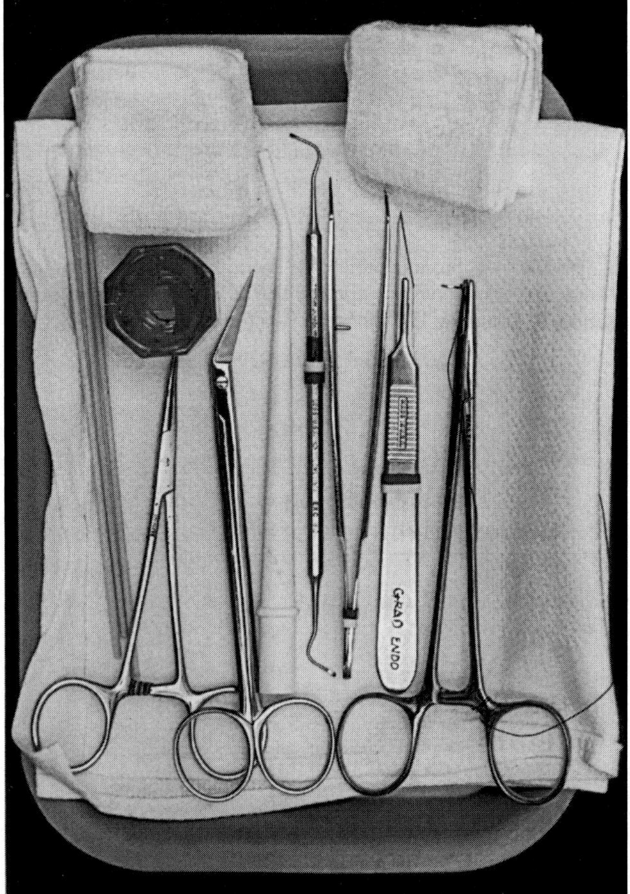

Figure 12-6 A well-organized incision and drainage ("I & D") kit is essential for efficient accomplishment of drainage procedures. (Courtesy of Graduate Endodontics, Loma Linda University.)

anesthesia will be limited to local infiltration. When local infiltration is used, the oral mucosa in the area to be injected should be dried with 2 × 2 gauze and **a topical anesthetic** placed. Local anesthetic should be deposited peripheral to the swollen mucoperiosteal tissues. Injection directly into the swollen tissues should be avoided because it is painful, may cause spread of infection, and does not produce effective anesthesia.[2]

Inflammation results in the lowering of tissue pH, which effects alteration of the equilibrium of the injected anesthetic and a significant reduction in tissue concentration of the non-ionized form. Local anesthetics with low pKa values, such as mepivacaine, are the most effective in this clinical situation.[23] Patients should be warned that, as a result of the effects of inflammation and infection, local anesthesia may not eliminate all discomfort associated with this procedure. The discomfort, however, is usually minimal and transient in nature. The reduced effectiveness of local anesthetic agents to block pain transmissions in a site of inflammation has been well documented.[24–26] Najjar has also demonstrated that inflammation in dental tissues can produce neurologic changes at distant sites along the nerve trunk, rendering local anesthetic less effective.[27] The use of nitrous oxide analgesia may be useful in reducing patient anxiety and lowering the pain threshold.

Incision. Following the administration of the appropriate block and/or infiltration anesthesia, the surgical area should be isolated with sterile 2 × 2 gauze sponges. The incision should be horizontal and placed at the dependent base of the fluctuant area. This will allow the greatest release (flow) of exudate. The incision should be made using a scalpel blade that is pointed, such as a No. 11 or No. 12, rather than a rounded No. 15 blade. The exudate should be aspirated and, if indicated, a sample collected for bacteriologic culturing. Probing with a curette or hemostat into the incisional wound to release exudate entrapped in tissue compartments will facilitate a more effective result[2] (Figure 12-7).

Placement of a Drain. The use of drains following an I & D procedure is controversial. Frank et al. recommended the use of a rubber dam drain to maintain the patency of the surgical opening.[3] McDonald and Hovland have stated that the incision alone will usually provide the needed drainage.[28] However, if initial drainage is limited, placement of a drain may be indicated. The drain may be made of either iodoform gauze or rubber dam material cut in an "H" or "Christmas tree" shape. It may be sutured in place for added retention and should be removed after 2 to 3 days. Bellizzi and Loushine recommended the use of a ¼-inch Penrose drain, which should be sutured in place and removed in 24 to 48 hours.[29]

Gutmann and Harrison stated that the use of drains following I & D procedures has been greatly abused.[2] Patients with localized or diffuse intraoral swellings, even if mild extraoral swelling is present, do not usually require drains following I & D procedures. Healing will progress much more rapidly without insertion of an artificial barrier in the incisional wound site. The tissues should be allowed to close the incisional wound at their normal wound-healing pace, which is about 24 to 48 hours. When sufficient drainage has occurred, epithelial closure of the incisional wound will follow. The insertion of a drain is only indicated in cases presenting with moderate to severe cellulitis and other positive signs of an aggressive infective process.

Cortical Trephination

Cortical trephination is a procedure involving the perforation of the cortical plate to accomplish the release of pressure from the accumulation of exudate within the alveolar bone. This is a limited-use procedure and is fraught with peril and potential negative complications. Patients who present with moderate to severe pain but with no intraoral or extraoral swelling may require drainage of periradicular exudate to alleviate the acute symptoms. Literature pertaining to this procedure is very limited and consists primarily of case reports, opinions, and clinical experiences.[2] Two clinical studies have been reported on trephination procedures. However, they were both designed to investigate the efficacy of trephination in avoiding postobturation pain rather than in treating existing acute conditions.[30,31] The treatment of choice for these patients is drainage through the root canal system (apical trephination) whenever possible. This may involve the removal of intraradicular posts and/or existing root canal obturation material. Apical trephination involves penetration of the apical foramen with a small endodontic file and enlarging the apical opening to a size No. 20 or No. 25 file to allow drainage from the periradicular lesion into the canal space. The decision about whether to perform apical or cortical trephination is based primarily on clinical judgment regarding the urgency of obtaining drainage.

Cortical trephination involves making an incision through mucoperiosteal tissues and perforating through the cortical plate with a rotary instrument (Figure 12-8). Some practitioners prefer to lay a mucoperiosteal flap to expose the buccal/labial cortical plate before the trephination procedure. The objective is to create a pathway through the cancellous bone to the vicinity of the involved periradicular tissues. It is often difficult to identify the appropriate site for cortical trephination. Good quality diagnostic radiographs and careful clinical examination will aid in determining the appropriate trephination site. The site most often recommended is at or near the root apex.[3,32–34] Gutmann and Harrison[2] suggest, however, that the trephination site should be at or about midroot level in the interdental bone, either mesial or distal to the affected tooth. Cortical trephination should always be initiated from a buccal approach, never from the lingual or palatal. Gutmann and Harrison recommend using either a No. 6 or No. 8 round bur in a high-speed handpiece to penetrate the **cortical plate**. A reamer or K-type file is then passed through the **cancellous bone** into the vicinity of the periradicular tissues. It is not necessary to pass the instrument directly to the root apex to achieve effective results.[2] The clinician must exercise good judgment to avoid anatomic structures such as the maxillary sinus and the neurovascular contents of the mandibular canal and the mental foramen, as well as the tooth itself.

PERIRADICULAR SURGERY

As previously discussed, the indications for, and the application of, periradicular endodontic surgery have undergone dramatic changes in the last two decades. These changes have been especially evident when dealing with the treatment of failed nonsurgical endodontic treatments. A widely held principle of endodontic diagnosis and treatment planning is that the primary modality for endodontic treatment failure should be **nonsurgical endodontic re-treatment** whenever possible[2,3,28,35–39] (see chapter 13, "Outcome of Endodontic Treatment and Re-treatment").

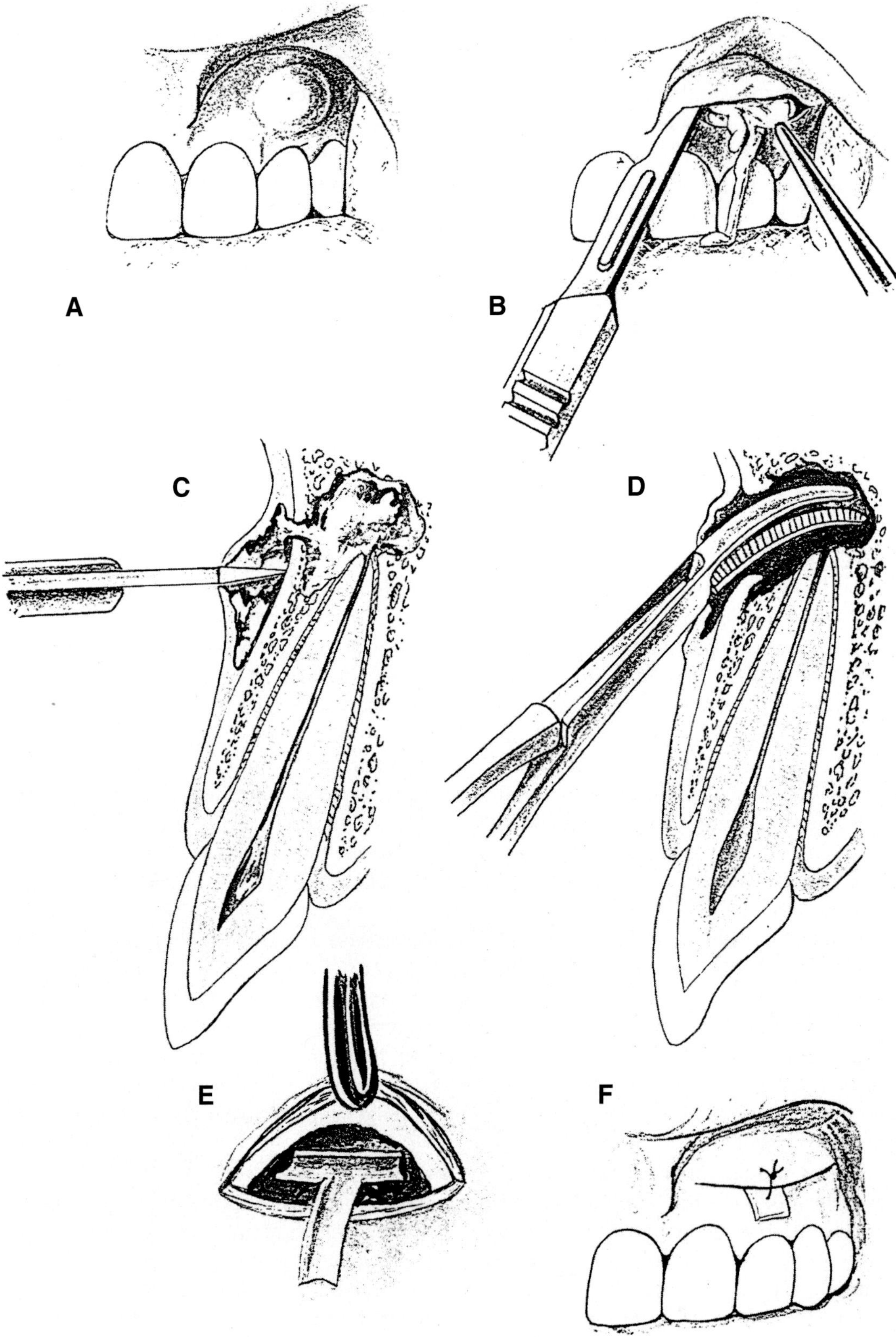

Figure 12-7 Incision and drainage of acute apical abscess. **A,** Good level of anesthesia is established and region is packed with gauze sponges. **B,** Sweeping incision is made through core of lesion with No. 11 or 12 scalpel. Drainage is aspirated by assistant. **C,** Profile view of incision showing scalpel carried through to bone. **D,** In some cases a small curved hemostat through defect of bony plate into body of infection. By spreading beaks, adequate drainage is established and may be maintained by suturing T-drain through incision. Patient requires antibiotics for bacteremia and analgesics to control discomfort. **E,** T-drain is positioned to ensure patency of incision until all drainage ceases. **F,** If drain will not remain in place, it may be sutured.

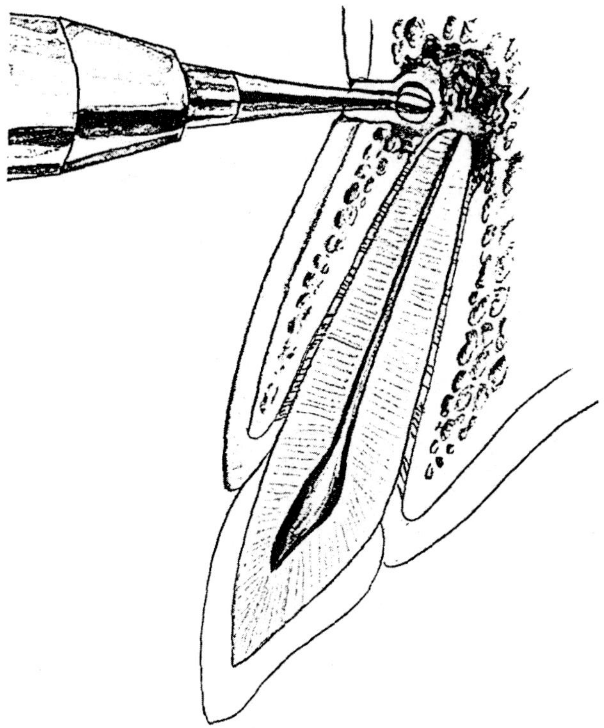

Figure 12-8 Surgical trephination of intact labial cortical plate to relieve liquid and gas pressure of acute apical abscess. Accurate pinpointing of lesion is done by radiography.

The importance of thorough and meticulous presurgical planning cannot be overemphasized. Not only must the dental practitioner and staff be thoroughly trained, but, in addition, all necessary instruments, equipment, and supplies must be readily available in the treatment room (Figure 12-9). This requires that every step of the procedure be carefully planned and analyzed. The potential for possible complications must be anticipated and incorporated into the presurgical planning.

Good patient communication is essential for thorough surgical preparation. It is important that the patient understands the reason surgery is needed as well as other treatment options available. The patient must be informed of the prognosis for a successful outcome and the risks involved in the surgical procedure, in addition to the benefits. It is also important that the patient be informed of the possible short-term effects of the surgery, such as pain, swelling, discoloration, and infection. **Signed** consent forms are advised. It is recommended that patients not be allowed to watch the procedure in a mirror, even if they so request.

A presurgical mouth rinse will improve the surgical environment by decreasing the tissue surface bacterial

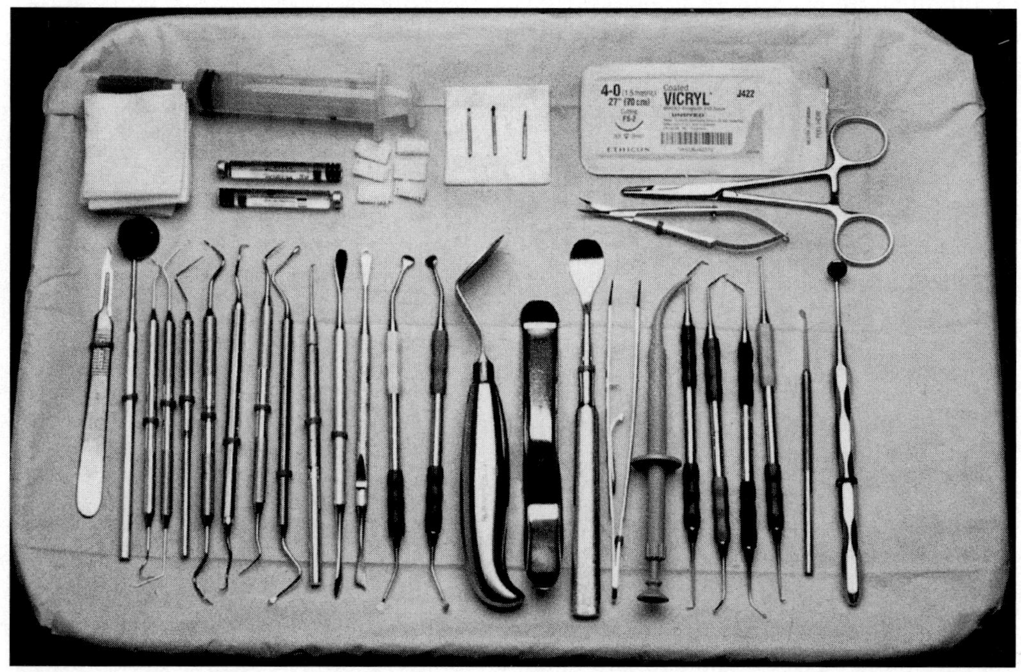

Figure 12-9 Suggested surgical instrument setup. **Top Row:** Extra 2-inch × 2-inch gauze; irrigating syringe with sterile saline, (Monoject); two extra carpules lidocaine 1/50,000 epinephrine; Teflon gauze cut in small squares; surgical length FG carbide burs No. 6, No. 8, and No. H267 (Brassler); 4-0 Vicryl (Polyglactin 910) suture; needle holder; scissors. **Bottom Row:** Scalpel handle with No. 15C Bard-Parker blade; mouth mirror, front surface No. 4; cow horn DE explorer; No. 16 DE endodontic explorer; periodontal probe; perio curettes; bone curettes; Morse No. 00 scaler (Ransom and Randolph); periosteal elevators; flap retractors; locking cotton pliers; root-end filling material carrier; root-end filling condenser; front surface micro mirrors. Instruments required for endodontic surgery are prearranged on the surgical tray with logical placement in order of their use from left to right. Instruments are sterilized and packaged in readiness for use.

contamination and thereby reducing the inoculation of microorganisms into the surgical wound. Chlorhexidine gluconate (Peridex) has been shown to decrease salivary bacterial counts by 80 to 90% with a return to normal within 48 hours.[40] Gutmann and Harrison recommend that chlorhexidine gluconate oral rinses should be started the day before surgery, given immediately before surgery, and continued for 4 to 5 days following surgery.[2] The reduction in numbers of oral bacteria before and during the early postsurgical period and the inhibition of plaque formation produce a markedly improved environment for wound healing.[2]

Most periradicular surgical procedures, regardless of their indication, share a number of concepts and principles: (1) the need for profound local anesthesia and hemostasis, (2) management of soft tissues, (3) management of hard tissues, (4) surgical access, both visual and operative, (5) access to root structure, (6) periradicular curettage, (7) root-end resection, (8) root-end preparation, (9) root-end filling, (10) soft-tissue repositioning and suturing, and (11) postsurgical care. All of these concepts and principles may not be used in any given surgery. However, an in-depth knowledge and understanding of these principles, and the manner in which they relate to the biology and physiology of the tissues involved, is of major importance. The strict adherence to and application of these principles will greatly influence the success of the surgical treatment and will minimize patient morbidity.

Anesthesia and Hemostasis

The injection of a local anesthetic agent that contains a vasoconstrictor has two equally important objectives: (1) to obtain profound and prolonged anesthesia and (2) to provide good hemostasis both during and after the surgical procedure. To sacrifice one for the other is shortsighted and unnecessary. Failure to obtain profound surgical anesthesia will result in needless pain and anxiety for the patient. Inadequate hemostasis will result in poor visibility of the surgical site, thus prolonging the procedure and resulting in increased patient morbidity. With the proper handling of any medical condition with which the patient may present, and the selection of an appropriate anesthetic agent and vasoconstrictor, it is possible to accomplish both objectives.

Selection of Anesthetic Agent. The selection of an appropriate anesthetic agent should always be based on the medical status of the patient and the desired duration of anesthesia needed (see chapter 9, "Preparation for Endodontic Treatment"). The two major groups of local anesthetic agents are the esters and amides. The important difference between these groups lies not in their ability to produce profound anesthesia but in the manner in which they are metabolized and the potential for allergic reactions. Esters have a much higher allergic potential than do amides.[41] The only ester local anesthetic available in dental cartridges in the United States is a combination of propoxycaine and procaine (Ravocaine).

The amide group of local anesthetics, which include lidocaine (Xylocaine), mepivacaine (Carbocaine), prilocaine (Citanest), bupivacaine (Marcaine), etidocaine (Duranest), and articaine (Ultracaine), undergo a complex metabolic breakdown in the liver. Patients with a known **liver dysfunction** should be administered amide local anesthetic agents with caution because of the potential for a high systemic blood concentration of the drug. Also, patients with severe **renal impairment** may be unable to remove the anesthetic agent from the blood, which may result in an increased potential for toxicity as a result of elevated blood levels of the drug. Therefore, significant renal dysfunction presents a relative contraindication, and dosage limits should be lowered.[23,41]

The high clinical success rate in producing profound and prolonged local anesthesia along with its low potential for allergic reactions makes **lidocaine (Xylocaine) the anesthetic agent of choice** for periradicular surgery. Selection of another anesthetic agent is indicated only in the presence of a true documented contraindication. If the use of an amide anesthetic agent (lidocaine) is absolutely contraindicated, the ester agent, procaine-propoxycaine with levonordefrin (Ravocaine with Neo-Cobefrin), is the only choice at present.[2]

Selection of Vasoconstrictor Agent. The choice of vasoconstrictor in the local anesthetic will have an effect on both the duration of anesthesia and the quality of hemorrhage control at the surgical site.[23,42–44] Vasopressor agents used in dentistry are direct-acting, sympathomimetic (adrenergic) amines that exert their action by stimulating special receptors (alpha- and beta-adrenergic receptors) on the smooth muscle cells in the microcirculation of various tissues. These agents include **epinephrine** (Adrenalin), **levonordefrin** (Neo-Cobefrin), and **levarterenol** (Levophed, noradrenaline, norepinephrine).[41,42] For the purpose of **hemostasis**, there is little or **no justification for the use of levarterenol.** The degree of hemostasis required for most periradicular surgical procedures cannot be produced safely by levarterenol.[41]

Ahlquist was the first to determine the existence of two types of adrenergic receptors.[45] He termed them alpha and beta. He documented that each produces different responses when stimulated. Many tissues have both alpha and beta receptors; however, one will usually predominate. Gage demonstrated that the action of a vasopressor drug on the microvasculature depends on (1) the predominant receptor type and (2) the receptor selectivity of the vasopressor drug.[46] **Alpha receptors predominate in the oral mucosa and gingival tissues, whereas beta receptors predominate in skeletal muscle.**[23,47] Epinephrine receptor selectivity is approximately equal for alpha and beta receptors. Levonordefrin receptor selectivity, however, is primarily for alpha-adrenergic receptors.

Stimulation of the **alpha-adrenergic receptors** will result in **contraction** of the smooth muscle cells in the microvasculature with a subsequent reduction of blood flow through the vascular bed. Stimulation of the **beta-adrenergic receptors** will result in a **relaxation** of the smooth muscle cells in the microvasculature with a subsequent **increased blood flow through the vascular bed.** Since epinephrine receptor selectivity is equal for alpha and beta receptors, and beta receptors predominate in skeletal muscle, **it is important not to inject epinephrine into skeletal muscles** in the area of endodontic surgery or a **vasodilation with increased blood flow will result.**[23,46]

Epinephrine is the most effective and most widely used vasoconstrictor agent used in dental anesthetics.[41,48–50] The other vasopressors available are less effective. Even though they are used in higher concentrations in an effort to compensate for their lower effectiveness, the difference in the degree of clinical effect is readily observable. Many studies have been reported measuring the plasma catecholamine levels and the clinical effects of the injection of epinephrine containing local anesthetics for dental treatment.[51–55] The results of these studies indicate that even though the plasma level of catecholamines increases following the injection, this increase does not generally appear to be associated with any significant cardiovascular effects in healthy patients or those with mild to moderate heart disease. Pallasch stated that the hemodynamic alterations seen with elevated plasma epinephrine are usually quite short in duration, probably because of the very short plasma half-life of epinephrine, usually less than 1 minute. He also stated that the good achieved by the inclusion of vasoconstrictors in dental local anesthetics greatly outweighs any potential deleterious effects of these agents.[56]

Injection Sites and Technique. For periradicular surgery, it is imperative that profound prolonged anesthesia and maximum hemostasis be achieved. In addition to the choice of anesthetic and vasopressor agents, the sites and technique of injection are important factors as well. Nerve block anesthesia involves injection in close proximity to a main nerve trunk that is usually located some distance from the surgical site. Thus, the vasopressor agent in the anesthetic preparation used in nerve block anesthesia will not significantly affect the blood flow at the surgical site. Profound nerve block anesthesia can be achieved with a local anesthetic containing dilute (1:100,000 or 1:200,000) epinephrine.[23,24]

Hemostasis, unlike anesthesia, however, cannot be achieved by injecting into distant sites.[48] Only the small vessels of the microvasculature are affected by the injected vasopressor; larger vascular channels are not. An inferior alveolar nerve block injection effectively blocks pain transmission from the surgical site; however, the vasopressor injected has no effect on the inferior alveolar artery and normal blood flow continues to the peripheral surgical site. Therefore, **additional injections** must be administered in the soft tissue in the **immediate area of the surgery.** This is accomplished by local infiltration using a higher concentration (1:50,000 epinephrine) of vasopressor in the anesthetic solution. In the maxilla, infiltration anesthesia can simultaneously achieve anesthesia and hemostasis. It is important to note that, whatever technique is used to obtain anesthesia, **infiltration in the surgical site is always required to obtain hemostasis.** [2,57]

The infiltration sites of injection for periradicular surgery are always multiple and involve deposition of anesthetic throughout the entire surgical field in the alveolar mucosa just superficial to the periosteum at the level of the root apices (Figure 12-10). **Following block anesthesia**, using a 30-gauge needle with the bevel toward bone, a small amount of solution (0.25–0.50 mL) should be slowly deposited. The needle tip is then moved peripherally (mesially and distally) and similar small amounts are slowly injected in adjacent areas.[2,48]

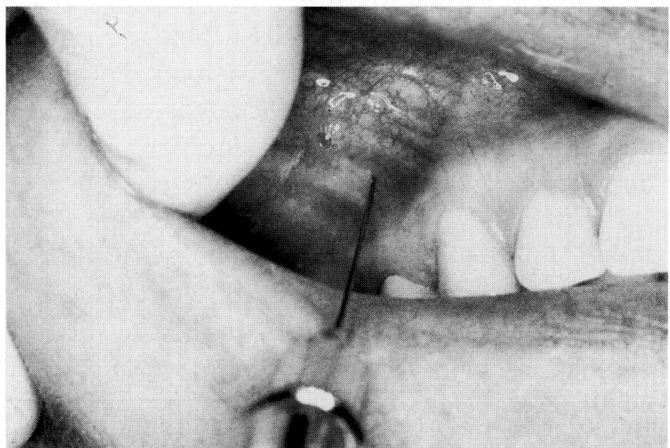

Figure 12-10 Proper placement of needle for infiltration anesthesia to obtain maximum surgical hemostasis is in the alveolar mucosa just superficial to the periosteum at the level of the root apices.

The **rate of injection** in the target sites directly affects the degree of hemostasis.[2] The recommended injection rate is 1 mL/minute, with a maximum safe rate of 2 mL/minute.[41,58] Rapid injection produces localized pooling of solution in the injected tissues, resulting in delayed and limited diffusion into adjacent tissues. This results in minimal surface contact with the microvascular bed and less than optimal hemostasis.

The amount of anesthetic solution needed varies and depends on the size of the surgical site. In a small surgical site involving only a few teeth, one cartridge (1.8 cc) of solution containing 1:50,000 epinephrine is usually sufficient to obtain adequate hemostasis. For more extensive surgery involving multiple teeth, it is rarely necessary to inject more than two cartridges (3.6 cc) of anesthetic (1:50,000 epinephrine) to achieve both anesthesia and hemostasis.

Reactive Hyperemia: The Rebound Phenomenon. It is important that the endodontic surgeon be aware of the delayed beta-adrenergic effect that follows the hemostasis produced by the injection of vasopressor amines. A rebound occurs from an alpha (vasoconstriction) to a beta (vasodilation) response and is termed **reactive hyperemia** or the **rebound phenomenon.** [59]

Following the injection of a vasopressor amine, tissue concentration of the vasopressor gradually decreases to a level that no longer produces an alpha-adrenergic vasoconstriction. The restricted blood flow slowly returns to normal but then rapidly increases far beyond normal, as a beta-adrenergic dilatation occurs.[23,59,60] This rebound phenomenon is not the result of beta receptor activity but results from localized tissue hypoxia and acidosis caused by the prolonged vasoconstriction.[47,61] Once this reactive hyperemia occurs, it is usually impossible to re-establish hemostasis by additional injections. Therefore, if a long surgical procedure is planned (multiple roots or procedures), **the more complicated** and hemostasis-dependent procedures (root-end resection, root-end preparation and filling) **should be done first**. The less hemostasis-dependent procedures, such as periradicular curettage, biopsy, or root amputation, should be reserved for last.

The rebound phenomenon has another important clinical implication: postsurgical hemorrhage and hematoma. These possible postsurgical sequelae are best minimized by proper soft-tissue repositioning and postsurgical care, described in more detail later in this chapter.

Soft-Tissue Management

The establishment of good surgical access, both visual and operative, is a requirement for all surgical procedures. Visual access enables the endodontic surgeon to see the entire surgical field. Operative access allows the surgeon to perform the needed surgical procedure(s) with the highest quality and in the shortest amount of time. This will result in the least amount of surgical trauma and a reduction in postsurgical morbidity.

All surgical procedures require the **intentional wounding** of specific tissues, and the subsequent **wound healing** depends on the type of tissues wounded and the type of wound inflicted. The surgeon's goal must always be to minimize trauma to both the soft and hard tissues involved in the surgical procedure. Most periradicular surgical procedures require the raising of a mucoperiosteal flap.

Flap Designs and Incisions. Good surgical access is fundamentally dependent on the selection of an appropriate flap design. Numerous flap designs have been proposed for periradicular surgery (Figure 12-11). It must be noted, however, that no one flap design is suitable for all surgical situations. It is necessary to know the advantages and disadvantages of each flap design.

Principles and Guidelines for Flap Design. Regardless of the design of the surgical flap, there are a number of principles and guidelines that apply to the location and extent of incisions. The adherence to these principles and guidelines will ensure that the flapped soft tissues will fit snugly in their original position and will properly cover the osseous wound site and provide an adequate vascular bed for healing:

1. **Avoid horizontal and severely angled vertical incisions.**

   The gingival blood supply is primarily from the same vessels supplying the alveolar mucosa. As these vessels enter into the gingiva, they assume a vertical course parallel to the long axis of the teeth and are positioned in the reticular layer superficial to the periosteum. They are known as the supraperiosteal vessels.[62,63]

   They are arterioles with a diameter of about 100 μm and are the terminal branches of the buccal, lingual, greater palatine, inferior alveolar, and superior alveolar arteries.[64]

   The collagen fibers of the gingiva and alveolar mucosa provide structural strength to these tissues. Collectively, these fibers are termed the gingival ligament. This ligament consists of a number of fiber groups that form attachments from crestal bone and supracrestal cementum to the gingiva and the periosteum on the buccal and lingual radicular bone. The collagen fibers that attach to the periosteum course over the crestal radicular bone in a direction parallel to the long axis of the teeth.[65]

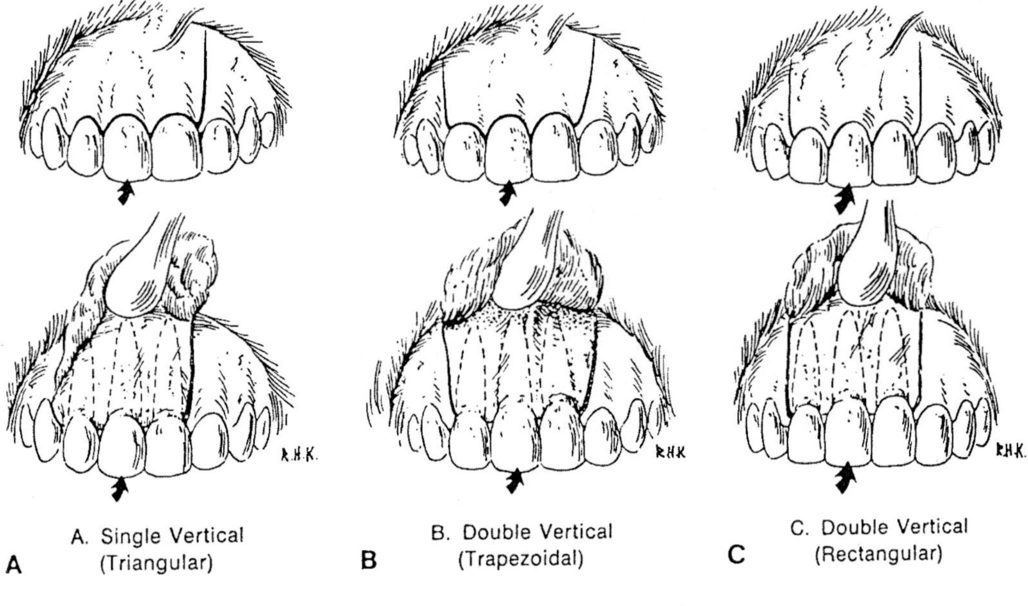

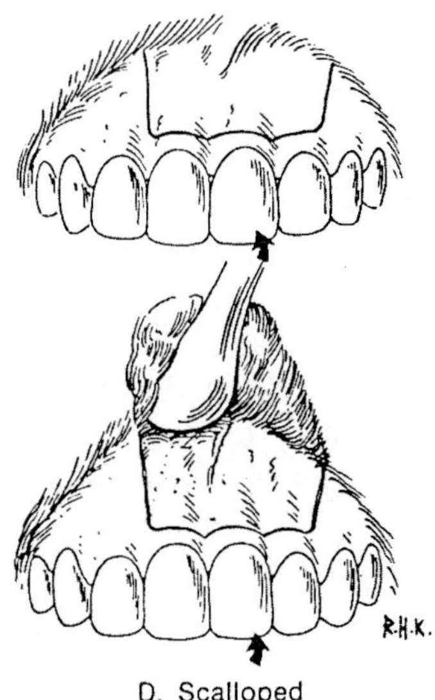

Figure 12-11 Surgical flap design and nomenclature for flaps. **A,** Single vertical (triangular). **Above,** Relaxing incision is vertical and placed over interdental bone. Horizontal incision is in the gingival sulcus and releases the papillae as it extends laterally. **Below,** Adequate access reaches periapical region of tooth involved in surgery (**arrow**). More retraction may be gained by extending both vertical and horizontal incision. **B,** Double vertical (trapezoidal). **Above,** Oblique vertical incisions provide for a broader base of the flap. They may cross, however, over radicular bone. **Below,** Trapezoidal flap when fully reflected provides excellent access to the apices of teeth in the surgical area. **C,** Double vertical (rectangular). **Above,** Recommended if bony fenestration is expected. Vertical relaxing incisions are placed over interdental bone and not over radicular surfaces to avoid fenestrated root surfaces. **Below,** Excellent surgical access is achieved to all periradicular areas of the teeth involved in the surgical area. This flap design is recommended for maximum apical extension when needed. **D,** Scalloped (Luebke-Ochsenbein). **Above,** This flap avoids interference with the architecture of the gingival sulcus and the interdental papillae. The horizontal incision is placed parallel and just apical to the free gingival grove. A vertical relaxing incision is placed at each of the terminal ends of the horizontal incision. **Below,** Surgical access is good to the middle and apical periradicular areas but limited to the incisal one-third. It is critical that solid bone support the incision when repositioning the flap.

Horizontal and severely angled incisions, such as used in semilunar flaps and in broad-based rectangular flaps, shrink excessively during surgery as a result of contraction of the cut collagen fibers that run perpendicular to the line of incision. As a result of this shrinkage, it is often difficult to return the flap edges to their original position without placing excessive tension on the soft tissues. This often results in tearing out of the sutures and subsequent scar formation from healing by secondary intention (Figure 12-12). Horizontal or severely angled incisions may also result in interference of the blood supply to the unflapped gingival tissues because of severance of the gingival blood vessels that run perpendicular to the line of incision.

2. **Avoid incisions over radicular eminences.**
   Radicular eminences, such as the canine, maxillary first premolar, and first molar mesiobuccal root prominences, often fenestrate through the cortical bone or are covered by very thin bone with a poor blood supply. These bony defects may lead to soft-tissue fenestrations if incisions are made over them. Vertical (releasing) incisions should be made parallel to the long axis of the teeth and placed between the adjacent teeth over solid interdental bone, never over radicular bone (Figure 12-13).

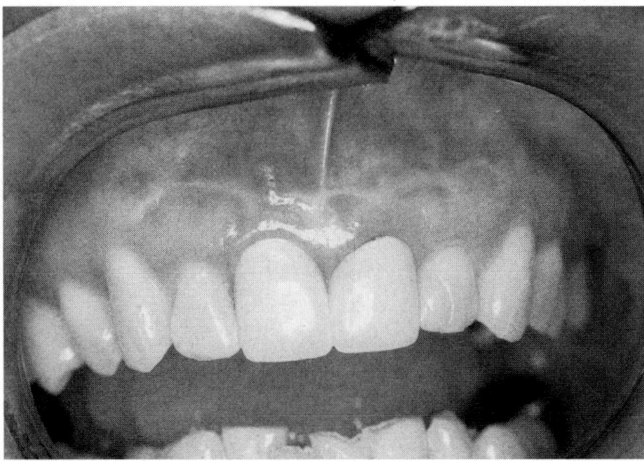

Figure 12-12 Shrinkage of the gingival tissue resulting from cut collagen fibers may result in postsurgical scarring as a result of healing by secondary intention.

3. **Incisions should be placed and flaps repositioned over solid bone.**
   Incisions should never be placed over areas of periodontal bone loss or periradicular lesions. Without good solid bone to support the repositioned edges of the mucoperiosteal flap, inadequate blood supply results in necrosis and sloughing of the soft tissue. The endodontic surgeon must take into consideration the extent of osseous bone removal necessary to accomplish the intended periradicular surgery when designing the flap so that the repositioned flap margins will be supported by solid bone. Hooley and Whitacre suggest that a minimum of 5 mm of bone should exist between the edge of a bony defect and the incision line.[66]
4. **Avoid incisions across major muscle attachments.**
   Incisions across major muscle attachments (frena) make repositioning of the flap and subsequent healing much more difficult. Healing and scar tissue formation by secondary intention healing often results. This can be circumvented by laterally extending the horizontal incision so that the vertical incision bypasses the muscle attachment and it is included within the flap.
5. **Tissue retractor should rest on solid bone.**
   The extension of the vertical incision should be sufficient to allow the tissue retractor to seat on solid bone, thereby leaving the root apex well exposed (Figure 12-14). If the vertical incisions are not adequately extended, there will be a tendency for the retractor to traumatize the mucosal tissue in the fold at the base of the flap. This may affect the blood supply to these tissues and will result in increased postsurgical morbidity.
6. **Extent of the horizontal incision should be adequate to provide visual and operative access with minimal soft-tissue trauma.**
   In general, the horizontal incision for mucoperiosteal flaps in periradicular surgery should extend at least one to two teeth lateral to the tooth to be treated (Figure 12-15). This will allow for adequate surgical access and minimize tension and stretching of the soft tissue. A time-tested axiom regarding the length of an incision is that more trauma results from too short an incision rather than too long, and incisions heal from side to side, not from end to end.

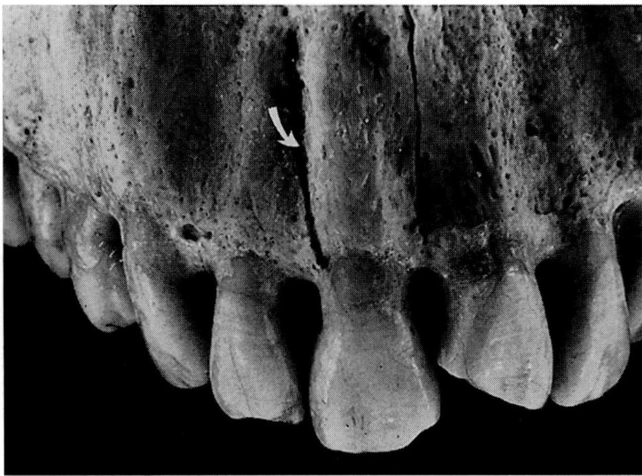

Figure 12-13 Vertical incisions should be made over the thick bone that lies in the "trough" (**arrow**) between the radicular eminences.

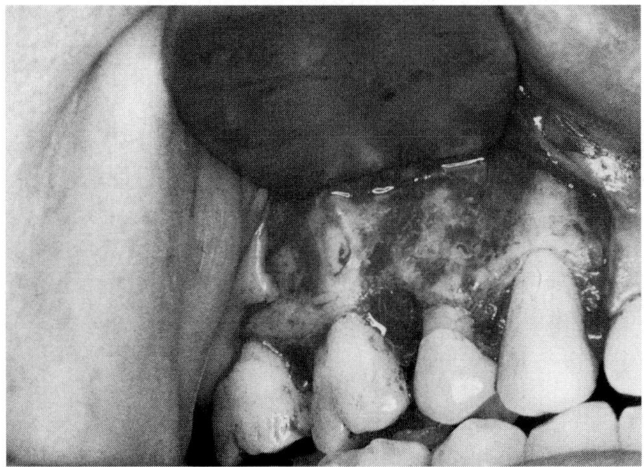

Figure 12-14 The flap retractor should be broad enough to provide visual access to the surgical site and also rest on solid bone without impinging soft tissue.

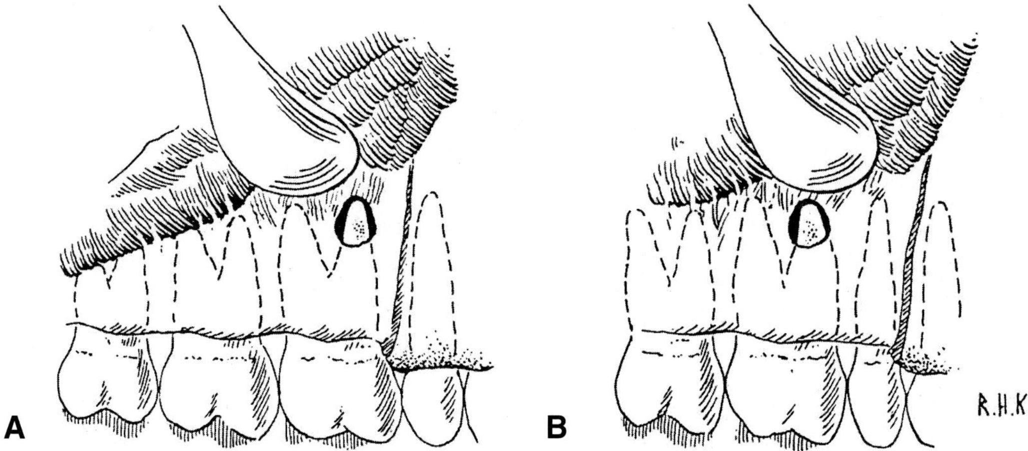

Figure 12-15 An incision should be no closer than 5 mm to a bony defect. **A,** Vertical incision is **too close** to bony defect. **B,** Incision placed one tooth mesially allows for better visual access and solid bony support for the incision.

7. **The junction of the horizontal sulcular and vertical incisions should either include or exclude the involved interdental papilla.**
Vertical releasing incisions should be made parallel to the long axis of the teeth and placed between the adjacent teeth over solid interdental bone, **never over radicular bone.** The vertical incision should intersect the horizontal incision and terminate in the intrasulcular area at the mesial or distal line angle of the tooth. The involved interdental papilla should never be split by the vertical incision or intersect the horizontal incision in the midroot area (Figure 12-16).

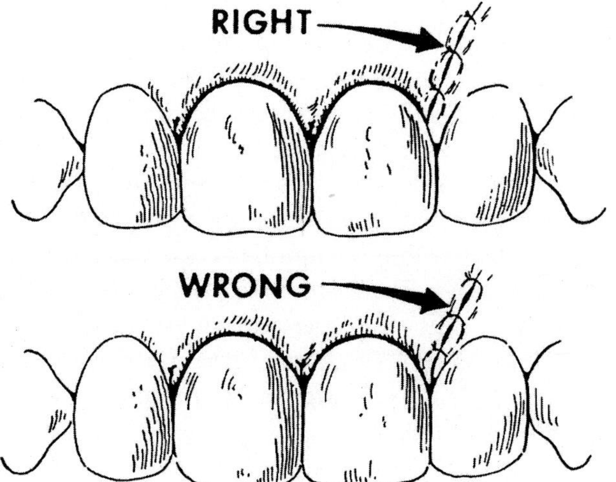

Figure 12-16 Incisions that split the papillae do not heal as well and may leave a periodontal defect following suture removal.

8. **The flap should include the complete mucoperiosteum (full thickness).**
The flap should include the entire mucoperiosteum (marginal, interdental and attached gingiva, alveolar mucosa, and periosteum). Full-thickness flaps result in less surgical trauma to the soft tissues and better surgical hemostasis than do split-thickness flaps. The major advantages of full-thickness flaps are derived from the maintenance of the supraperiosteal blood vessels that supply these tissues.

According to Gutmann and Harrison, the two major categories of periradicular surgical flaps are the **full mucoperiosteal flaps** and the **limited mucoperiosteal flaps.**[2] The location of the horizontal component of the incision is the distinguishing characteristic between the two categories of surgical flaps. All **full** mucoperiosteal flaps involve an intrasulcular horizontal incision with reflection of the marginal and interdental (papillary) gingival tissues as part of the flap. **Limited** mucoperiosteal flaps have a submarginal (subsulcular) horizontal or horizontally oriented incision, and the flap does not include the marginal or interdental tissues.[2] The addition of plane geometric terms to describe flap designs, as suggested by Luebke and Ingle, provides for an easily identifiable classification of periradicular surgical flap designs.[67] The classification of periradicular surgical flaps is found in Table 12-2, and a description of these flaps and their application in endodontic surgery follows.

Full Mucoperiosteal Flaps. *Triangular Flap.* The triangular flap is formed by a horizontal, intrasulcular incision and one vertical releasing incision (Figure 12-11, A). The primary advantages of this flap design are

Table 12-2 Classification of Surgical Flaps

1. Full mucoperiosteal flaps
   (a) Triangular (one vertical releasing incision)
   (b) Rectangular (two vertical releasing incisions)
   (c) Trapezoidal (broad-based rectangular)
   (d) Horizontal (no vertical releasing incision)
2. Limited mucoperiosteal flaps
   (a) Submarginal curved (semilunar)
   (b) Submarginal scalloped rectangular (Luebke-Ochsenbein)

that it affords good wound healing, which is a result of a minimal disruption of the vascular supply to the flapped tissue, and ease of flap reapproximation, with a minimal number of sutures required. The major disadvantage of this flap design is the somewhat limited surgical access it provides because of the single vertical releasing incision. This limited surgical access often makes it difficult to expose the root apexes of long teeth (eg, maxillary cuspids) and mandibular anterior teeth.

In posterior surgery, both maxillary and mandibular, the vertical releasing incision is always placed at the **mesial extent** of the horizontal incision, never the distal. This affords the surgeon maximum visual and operative access with minimum soft-tissue trauma. For **anterior surgery**, the vertical releasing incision should be placed at the extent of the horizontal incision that is closest to the surgeon and is therefore **dependent on the surgeon's position** to the right or left of the patient.

After reflecting a triangular flap, sometimes the surgeon may find it necessary to obtain additional access. This can be easily obtained by placement of a **distal relaxing incision.** A relaxing incision is a short vertical incision placed in the marginal and attached gingiva and located at the extent of the horizontal incision opposite the vertical releasing incision. This incision is also good for relieving flap retraction tension while achieving adequate surgical access.

As a result of the excellent wound-healing potential of this flap design and the generally favorable surgical access it provides, use of the triangular mucoperiosteal flap is recommended whenever possible. It is recommended for **maxillary incisors and posterior teeth.** It is the only recommended flap design for **mandibular posterior teeth** because of anatomic structures contraindicating other flap designs.[2]

Rectangular Flap. The rectangular flap is formed by an intrasulcular, horizontal incision and two vertical releasing incisions (see Figure 12-11, C). The major advantage of this flap design is increased surgical access to the root apex. This flap design is especially useful for **mandibular anterior teeth**, multiple teeth, and teeth with long roots, such as **maxillary canines.**

The major disadvantage of the rectangular flap design is the difficulty in reapproximation of the flap margins and wound closure. Postsurgical stabilization is also more difficult with this design than with the triangular flap. This is primarily due to the fact that the flapped tissues are held in position solely by the sutures. This results in a greater potential for postsurgical flap dislodgment. This flap design is not recommended for posterior teeth.

Trapezoidal Flap. The trapezoidal flap is similar to the rectangular flap with the exception that the two vertical releasing incisions intersect the horizontal, intrasulcular incision at an obtuse angle (see Figure 12-11, B). The angled vertical releasing incisions are designed to create a broad-based flap with the vestibular portion being wider than the sulcular portion. The desirability of this flap design is predicated on the assumption that it will provide a better blood supply to the flapped tissues. Although this concept is valid in other tissues, such as the skin, its application is unfounded in periradicular surgery.[68]

Since the blood vessels and collagen fibers in the mucoperiosteal tissues are oriented in a vertical direction, the angled vertical releasing incisions will sever more of these vital structures. This will result in more bleeding, a disruption of the vascular supply to the unflapped tissues, and shrinkage of the flapped tissues. **The trapezoidal flap is contraindicated in periradicular surgery.** [32,68]

Horizontal Flap. The horizontal, or envelope, flap is created by a horizontal, intrasulcular incision with no vertical releasing incision(s). This flap design has very limited application in periradicular surgery because of the limited surgical access it provides. Its major applications in endodontic surgery are limited to repair of cervical defects (root perforations, resorption, caries, etc) and hemisections and root amputations.

Limited Mucoperiosteal Flaps. *Submarginal Curved (Semilunar) Flap.* The submarginal or semilunar flap is formed by a curved incision in the alveolar mucosa and the attached gingiva (see Figure 12-11, E). The incision begins in the alveolar mucosa extending into the attached gingiva and then curves back into the alveolar mucosa. There are no advantages to this flap design and its disadvantages are many, including poor surgical access and poor wound healing, which results in scarring. **This flap design is not recommended for periradicular surgery.**

Submarginal Scalloped Rectangular (Luebke-Ochsenbein) Flap. The submarginal scalloped rectangular flap is a modification of the rectangular flap in that the horizontal incision is not placed in the gingival sulcus but in the buccal or labial attached gingiva. The horizontal incision is scalloped and follows the contour of the marginal gingiva **above the free gingival groove** (Figure 12-11, D). The major advantages of this flap design are that it does not involve the marginal or interdental gingiva and the crestal bone is not exposed. The primary disadvantages are that the vertically oriented blood vessels and collagen fibers are severed, resulting in more bleeding and a greater potential for flap shrinkage, delayed healing, and scar formation.

When considering the use of this flap design, the endodontic surgeon must keep in mind that the horizontal, scalloped incision must be placed and the flap repositioned over solid bone. Careful evaluation of any buccal or labial periodontal pockets must also be made to minimize the possibility of leaving unflapped gingival tissue without bony support.

The importance of properly angled diagnostic radiographs cannot be overemphasized when considering the use of this flap design. The size and position of any periradicular inflammatory bone loss must also be considered when placing the horizontal incision to ensure that the margins of the flap, when reapproximated, will be adequately supported by solid bone.

Proponents of this flap design stress the importance of not involving the marginal gingiva and the gingival sulcus in the horizontal incision, which may result in an alteration of the soft-tissue attachment and crestal bone levels. It has been reported, however, that, with proper reapproximation of the reflected tissues and good soft-tissue management, the gingival attachment level is minimally altered or unchanged when full mucoperiosteal flaps are used.

The key element in preventing loss of the soft-tissue attachment level is ensuring that the root-attached tissues are not damaged or removed during surgery.[68–70] It has also been reported that crestal bone loss is minimal (about 0.5 mm) when full mucoperiosteal flaps are used in periodontic surgery. These procedures may involve apical positioning of flaps, excision of marginal gingiva, and root planing that must rely on new attachment of soft tissue to cementum. Unlike periodontal surgery, endodontic surgery can accomplish reattachment that results in little or no crestal bone loss.[71] Harrison and Jurosky reported that crestal bone showed complete osseous repair of resorptive defects and no alteration of crestal height following periradicular surgery using a triangular (full mucoperiosteal) flap.[70] In the absence of periodontal disease, a complete return to anatomic and functional normalcy can be expected, following periradicular surgery using triangular or rectangular flap designs.[2]

Flap Design for Palatal Surgery. Periradicular surgery from a palatal approach is difficult due to the surgeon's limited visual and operative access to this area. The only flap designs indicated for palatal approach surgery are the horizontal (envelope) and the triangular, with the latter being preferred. The palatal surgical approach should be limited to the posterior teeth. Anterior teeth should be approached from the labial aspect, except when radicular pathosis dictates a palatal approach, for example, curettement of a cyst located toward the palate.

The **horizontal intrasulcular incision** for the triangular flap should extend anteriorly to the mesial side of the first premolar or, for the horizontal (envelope) flap, to the midline. It should extend distally as far as needed to afford access to the involved palatal root. A distal relaxing incision extending a few millimeters from the marginal gingiva toward the midline or over the tuberosity area can be added to achieve better access and to relieve tension on the distal extent of the flap.

The **vertical releasing incision** for the triangular flap should extend from a point near the midline and join the anterior extent of the horizontal incision mesial to the first premolar. There is no validity to concerns regarding a potential hemorrhage problem with vertical incisions in the palatal mucosa in the premolar area. The greater palatine artery branches rapidly as it courses anteriorly and an incision in the premolar area results in a minimal disruption to the vascular supply.

The palatal mucosa is tough and fibrous, and flap reflection and retraction can be difficult in this area. Placement of a sling suture in the flapped tissue attached to a tooth or a bite block on the opposite side of the maxillary arch may aid the surgeon in improving visual and operative access by eliminating the need to manually retract the flap while performing this potentially difficult surgical procedure (Figure 12-17).

Incisions. Following the selection of the flap design, it is important to select the proper scalpel blade to accomplish the delicate task of making smooth, clean, atraumatic incisions. Incisions for the majority of mucoperiosteal flaps for periradicular surgery can be accomplished by using one or more of four scalpel blades: No. 11, No. 12, No. 15, and No. 15C (Figure 12-18). The horizontal incision should be made first, followed by the vertical releasing incisions to complete the perimeters of the flap design.

The horizontal incision for a **full mucoperiosteal flap** begins in the gingival sulcus and should extend through the fibers of the gingival attachment to the crestal bone. Care should be exercised to ensure that the interdental papilla be incised through the **midcol area,**

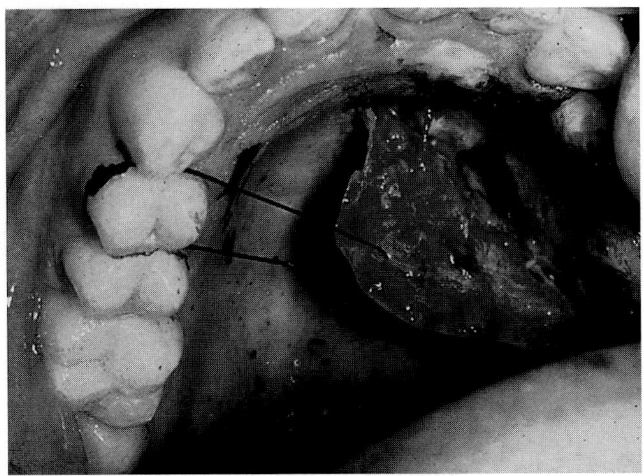

Figure 12-17 Single sling suture retracts palatal flap, giving surgical access and freeing hands of surgeon to hold mouth mirror and handpiece. (Courtesy of Dr. Donald D. Antrim.)

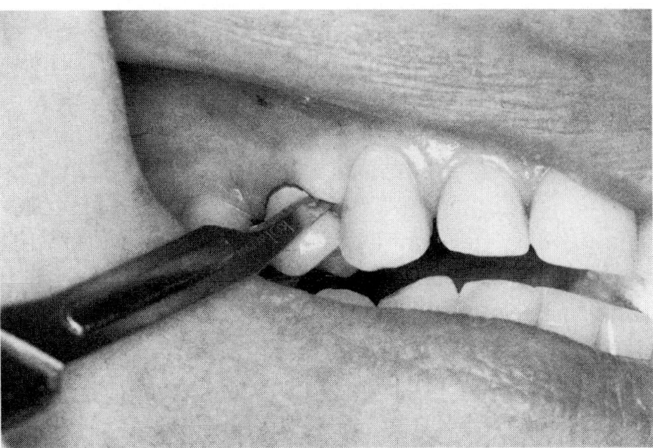

Figure 12-19 No. 15C scalpel blade placed in the gingival sulcus for horizontal incision.

separating the buccal and lingual papilla and incising the fibers of the epithelial attachment to crestal bone. Because these tissues are extremely delicate and space is very limited, this important incision is best made with a small scalpel blade, such as No. 11 or No. 15C (Figure 12-19). By holding the scalpel handle in a pen grasp and using finger rests on the teeth, the surgeon can achieve maximum control and stability when performing these delicate incision strokes. An attempt should be made to accomplish the horizontal incision using as few incision strokes as necessary to minimize trauma to the marginal gingiva.

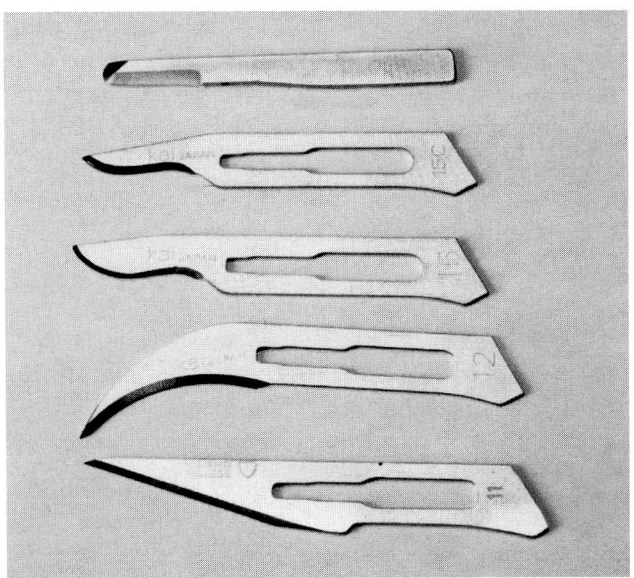

Figure 12-18 Scalpel blades for surgical incisions. **From top:** Microsurgical blade, No. 15C, No. 15, No. 12, No. 11.

The horizontal incision for a **limited mucoperiosteal flap** should begin in the attached gingiva and be placed about 2 mm coronal to the mucogingival junction (Figure 12-20). The incision should be **scalloped** following the contour of the marginal gingiva. It is important that the horizontal incision **never be placed** coronal to the depth of the gingival sulcus. The depth of the gingival sulcus must be measured before placement of this flap design. The No. 15 or No. 15C scalpel blade is recommended for this incision. An attempt should be made to incise through the gingiva and periosteum to the cortical bone using firm pressure and a single, smooth stroke. Multiple incision strokes will result in increased trauma to the gingival tissue, which, in turn, may contribute to retarded healing and scar formation.

Vertical releasing incisions, whether for full or limited mucoperiosteal flaps, should always be vertical and placed between adjacent teeth over interdental bone. **They should never be placed over radicular bone.** The incision should penetrate through the periosteum so that it can be included in the flap. The incision stroke should begin in the alveolar mucosa and proceed in a coronal direction until it intersects the horizontal incision (Figure 12-21). Contrary to a well-ingrained surgical axiom, it is not necessary to accomplish this incision in a single stroke.[2] It is often difficult to accomplish penetration completely through the gingiva, mucosa, submucosa, and periosteum in a single stroke of the scalpel. An initial incision stroke that penetrates the mucosa and gingiva can be followed by a second that penetrates through the periosteum to the surface of the cortical bone. More accurate placement of the vertical releasing incision will often result from this two-stroke

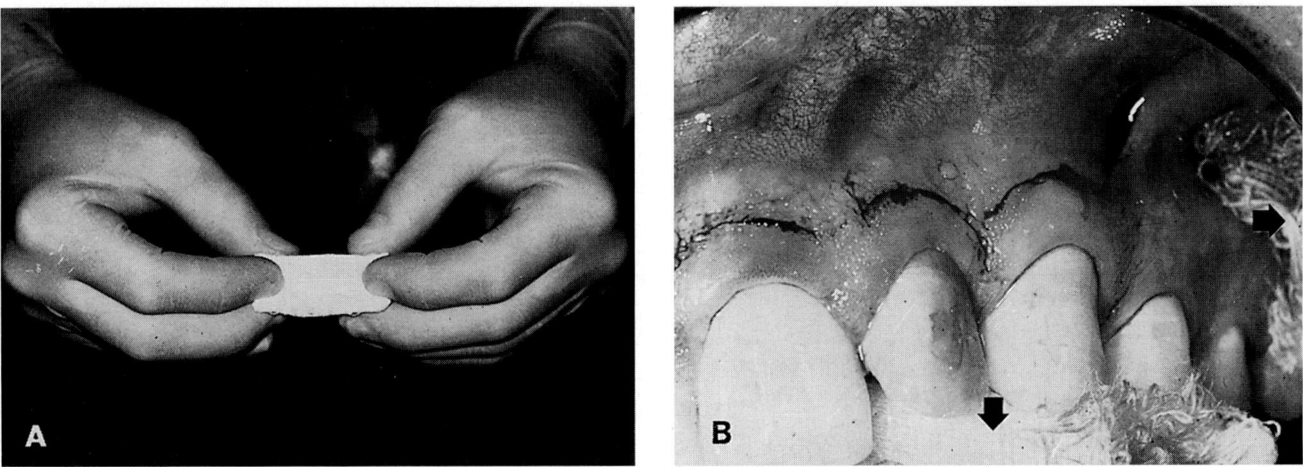

Figure 12-20 Horizontal incision for submarginal scalloped rectangular flap is placed in the attached gingiva just apical to the free gingival groove and follows the contour of the marginal gingiva. Patient biting on gauze can swallow more easily and prevents seepage of hemorrhage. (Courtesy of Dr. Donald D. Antrim.)

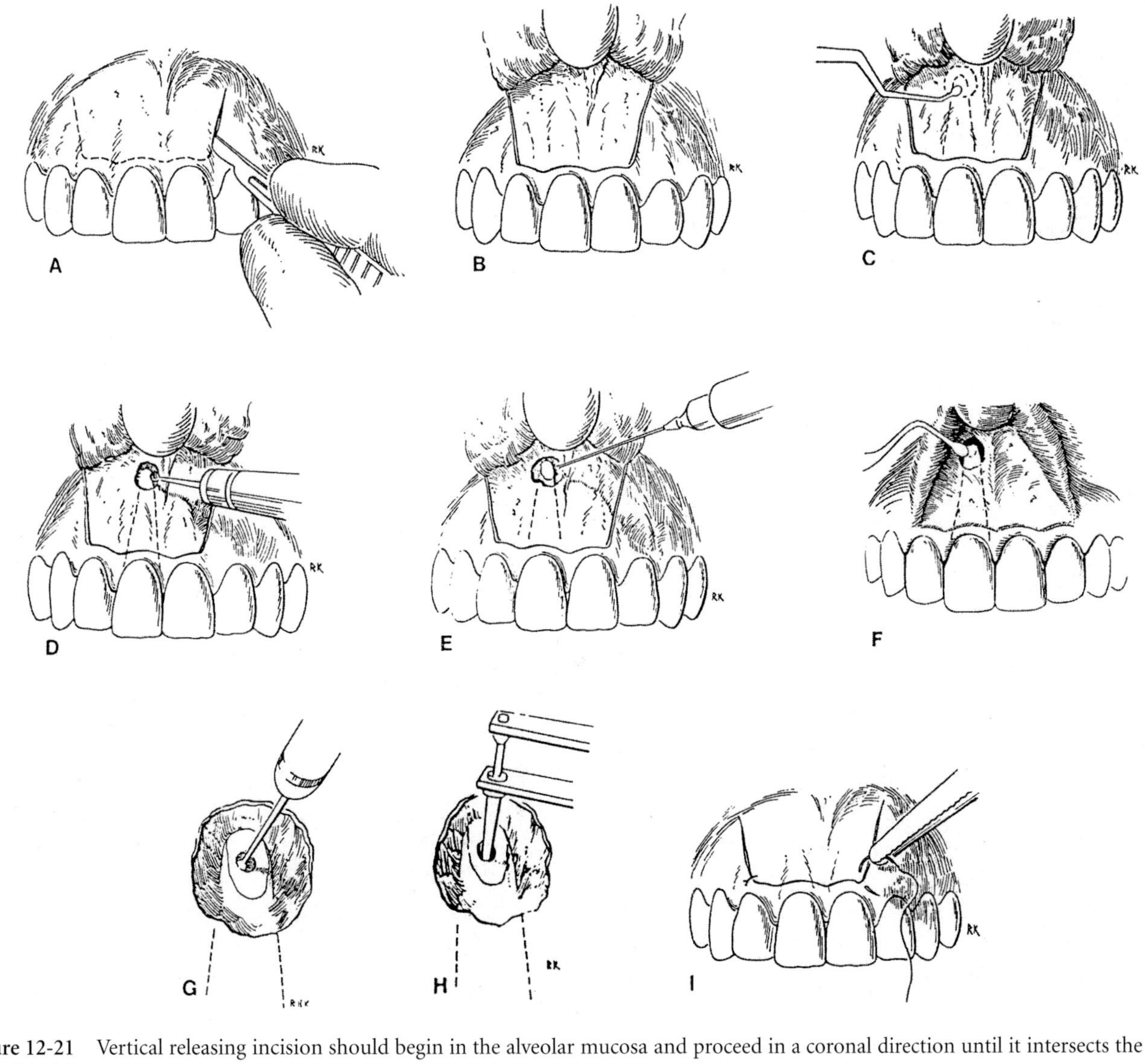

Figure 12-21 Vertical releasing incision should begin in the alveolar mucosa and proceed in a coronal direction until it intersects the horizontal incision.

incision technique because less pressure is required on the initial stroke, affording the surgeon more control over the direction of the scalpel blade. It may be necessary to replace the scalpel blade with a fresh, sharp blade to produce clean, sharp incision lines.

Flap Reflection. Reflection of soft tissues for full or limited mucoperiosteal flaps is a very critical process in the effort to reduce surgical trauma and postsurgical morbidity. Marginal gingiva is very delicate and easily injured. It is, therefore, not appropriate to begin the reflective process in the horizontal incision for full mucoperiosteal flaps. The supracrestal root-attachment fibers are of even greater clinical significance than is the marginal gingiva. These root-attachment fibers are easily damaged or destroyed by direct reflective forces. Damage to these tissues may result in the loss of their viability, allowing for apical epithelial downgrowth along the root surface. This epithelial downgrowth will result in increased sulcular depth and loss of soft-tissue attachment level.[2,72] Maintenance of the viability of these root-attachment fibers will likely result in the soft-tissue attachment levels being unaltered following surgery.[69,72]

Initiating the flap reflective process in the horizontal incision for submarginal flaps is not as injurious to the soft tissues as in the full-flap design since the horizontal incision for the former is placed in attached gingiva. This will, however, result in damaging forces being applied to a critical wound edge and should be avoided whenever possible. The horizontal incision is more subject to delayed wound healing than are the vertical incisions in this flap design. Additional trauma to the attached gingival tissues during flap reflection may result in tissue shrinkage and healing by secondary intention, which will result in increased scar-tissue formation. The reflective procedure for the limited mucoperiosteal flap should begin in the attached gingiva of the vertical incision whenever possible.

Flap reflection is the process of separating the soft tissues (gingiva, mucosa, and periosteum) from the surface of the alveolar bone. This process should begin in the **vertical incision** a few millimeters apical to the junction of the horizontal and vertical incisions (Figure 12-22). A number of periosteal elevators and curettes are available for mucoperiosteal flap elevation (Figure 12-23). The periosteal elevator of choice should be used to gently elevate the periosteum and its superficial tissues from the cortical plate.

Once these tissues have been lifted from the cortical plate and the periosteal elevator can be inserted between them and the bone, the elevator is then directed coronally. This allows the marginal and interdental

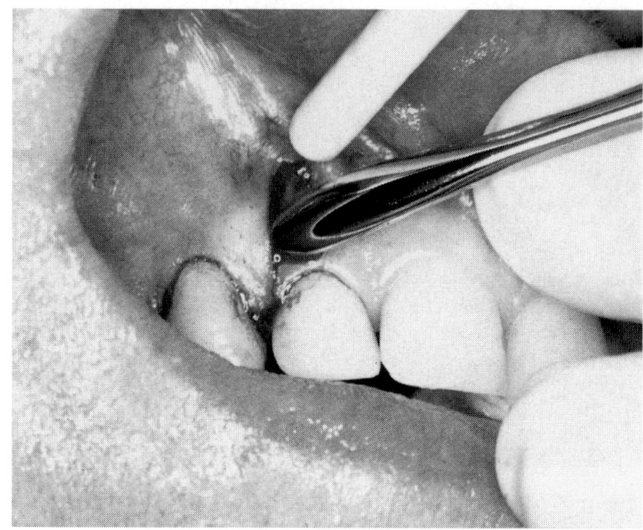

Figure 12-22 Flap reflection begins with the periosteal elevator placed in the attached gingiva a few millimeters apical to the junction of the vertical and horizontal incisions.

gingiva to be separated from the underlying bone and the opposing incisional wound edge without direct application of dissectional forces. This technique allows for all of the direct reflective forces to be applied to the periosteum and the bone. This approach to flap reflection is referred to as **"undermining elevation."**[63]

This "undermining elevation" should continue until the attached gingival tissues (marginal and interdental) have been lifted from the underlying bone to the full extent of the horizontal incision. After reflection of these tissues, soft-tissue elevation is continued in an apical direction, lifting the alveolar mucosa, along **with the underlying periosteum**, from the cortical bone until adequate surgical access to the intended surgical area has been achieved (Figure 12-24).

After the flap has been fully reflected, small bleeding tissue tags will be noted on the exposed surface of the

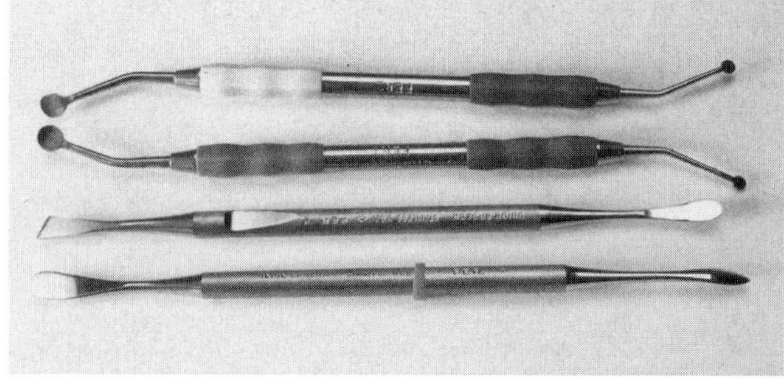

Figure 12-23 Periosteal elevators for flap reflection. **From top:** No. 1 and No. 2 (Thompson Dental Mfg. Co.); No. 2 (Union Broach Co.); No. 9 (Union Broach Co.).

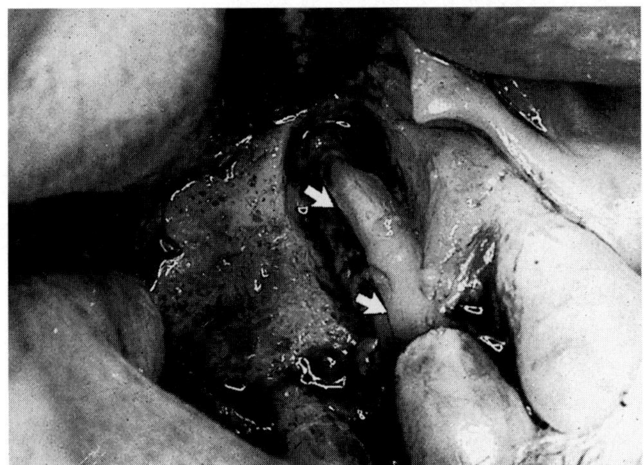

Figure 12-24 Flap fully reflected achieves visual and surgical access to all periradicular surfaces. **Arrows** indicate vertical root fracture.

cortical bone, especially in the interradicular depressed areas. Bleeding from these tissue tags will stop in a few minutes and they should not be damaged or removed. Research evidence strongly suggests that **these bleeding tissue tags are cortical retained periosteal tissues** and may play an important role in healing and reattachment of the flap to the cortical bone.[70,73]

In **posterior mandibular** surgery, it is important to be aware of the presence of the **mental foramen** and its associated neurovascular bundle. The most common location of the mental foramen is directly inferior to the crown of the second premolar and mesial to and inferior to its root apex (Figure 12-25). The mental foramen is visible approximately 75% of the time on periapical radiographs. When it is not visible on the radiograph, it is usually below the border of the film.[74,75] During flap reflection in the mandibular premolar area, the surgeon must be alert to subtle changes in the resistance of the periosteum to separation from the cortical bone. The resistance of Sharpey's fibers, which attach the periosteum to the bone, to separation results in a thin, white band at the junction of the flapped soft tissues and the cortical bone. Since there are no Sharpey's fibers attaching the periosteum to the border of the mental foramen, this thin, white band will disappear when the border of the mental foramen has been reached. Further reflection of the soft tissues in this area will result in the identification of the neurovascular bundle as it exits from the foramen. Maximum protection to the neurovascular bundle will be best achieved by its early identification during the flap reflective process. This will allow the surgeon to avoid injury to these important anatomic structures during the remainder of the surgical procedure.

Flap Retraction. Flap retraction is the process of holding in position the reflected soft tissues. Proper retraction depends on adequate extension of the flap incisions and proper reflection of the mucoperiosteum. It is necessary to provide both visual and operative access to the periradicular and radicular tissues. The tissue retractor must always rest on **solid cortical bone** with light but firm pressure. In this way, it acts as a passive mechanical barrier to the reflected soft tissues. If the retractor inadvertently rests on the soft tissue at the

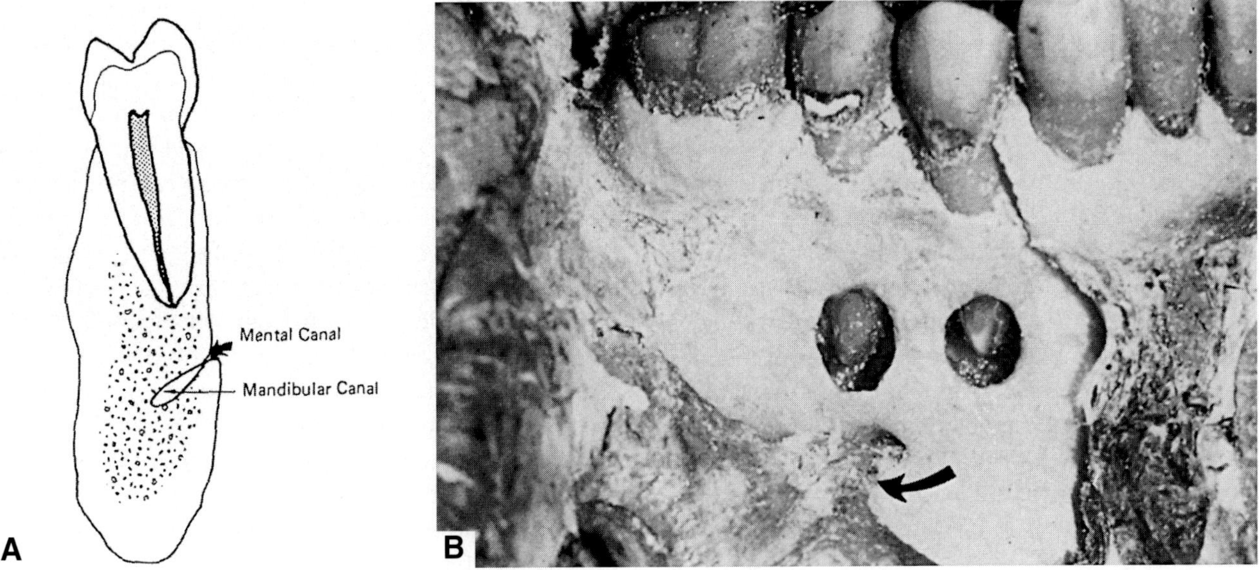

Figure 12-25 Neurovascular bundle is seen in cadaver dissection exiting through the mental foramen (**arrow**). Notice its relationship to the apices of both mandibular premolars.

base of the flap, mechanical trauma to the alveolar mucosa may result in delayed healing and increased postsurgical morbidity.

There are a number of tissue retractors available for use in endodontic surgery (Figure 12-26). Selection of the proper size and shape of the retractor is important in minimizing soft-tissue trauma. If the retractor is too large, it may traumatize the surrounding tissue. If the retractor is too small, flapped tissue falls over the retractor and impairs the surgeon's access. This results not only in increased soft-tissue trauma but also in extending the length of the surgical procedure. An axiomatic principle of endodontic surgery is that the longer the flap is retracted, the greater the postsurgical morbidity. This is a logical conclusion based on the probability that blood flow to the flapped tissues is impeded during flap retraction. In time, this will result in hypoxia and acidosis with a resulting delay in wound healing.[2,23,59]

Regardless of whether the retraction time is short or long, the periosteal surface of the flap should be irrigated frequently with physiologic saline (0.9% sodium chloride) solution. Saline should be used rather than water because the latter is hypotonic to tissue fluids. It is not necessary to irrigate the superficial surface of the flap because the stratified squamous epithelium prevents dehydration from this surface. Limited mucoperiosteal flaps are more susceptible to dehydration and may require more frequent irrigation than would full mucoperiosteal flaps.[2]

Hard-Tissue Management

Following reflection and retraction of the mucoperiosteal flap, surgical access must be made through the cortical bone to the roots of the teeth. Where cortical bone is thin, as in the maxilla, a large periradicular lesion may result in the loss of buccal or labial cortical plate, or if a natural root fenestration is present, the tooth root may be visible through the cortical plate. In other cases, the cortical bone may be very thin, and probing with a small sharp curette will allow penetration of the cortical plate.

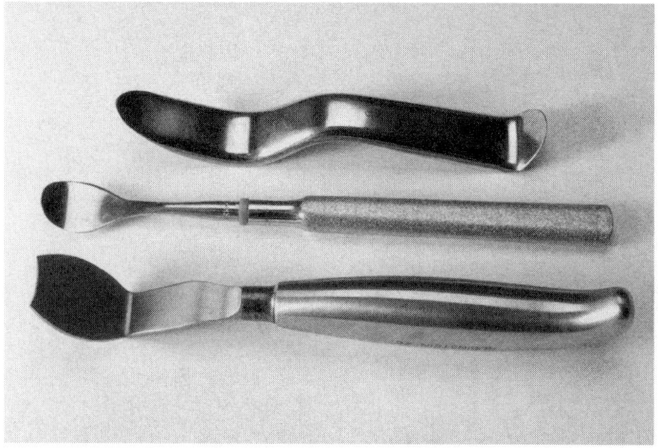

Figure 12-26 Flap retractors. **Top:** No. G3 (Hu-Friedy); **Middle:** No. 3 (Hu-Friedy); **Bottom:** Rubinstein (JedMed Co., St. Louis, MO).

The most difficult and challenging situation for the endodontic surgeon occurs when several millimeters of cortical and cancellous bone must be removed to gain access to the tooth root, especially when no periradicular radiolucent lesion is present. A number of factors should be considered to determine the location of the bony window in this clinical situation. The angle of the crown of the tooth to the root should be assessed. Often the long axis of the crown and its root are not the same, especially when a prosthetic crown has been placed. When a root prominence or eminence in the cortical plate is present, the root angulation and position are more easily determined. Measurement of the entire tooth length can be obtained from a well-angled radiograph and transferred to the surgical site by the use of a sterile millimeter ruler. After a small defect has been created on the surface of the cortical plate, a radiopaque marker, such as a small piece of lead foil from a radiographic film packet or a small piece of gutta percha, can be placed in the bony defect and a direct (not angled) radiograph exposed. The radiopaque object will provide guidance for the position of the root apex.[76–79]

When the cortical plate is intact, another method to locate the root apex is to first locate the body of the root substantially coronal to the apex where the bone covering the root is thinner. Once the root has been located and identified, the bone covering the root is slowly and carefully removed with light brush strokes, working in an apical direction until the root apex is identified (Figure 12-27). Barnes identified four ways in which the root surface can be distinguished from the surrounding osseous tissue: (1) root structure generally has a yellowish color, (2) roots do not bleed when probed, (3) root texture is smooth and hard as opposed to the granular and porous nature of bone, and (4) the root is surrounded by the periodontal ligament.[80]

Under some clinical conditions, however, the root may be very difficult to distinguish from the surrounding osseous tissue. Some authors advocate the use of methylene blue dye to aid in the identification of the periodontal ligament. A small amount of the dye is painted on the area in question and left for 1 to 2 minutes. When the dye is washed off with saline, the periodontal ligament will be stained with the dye, making it easier to identify the location of the root.[32,77,81,82]

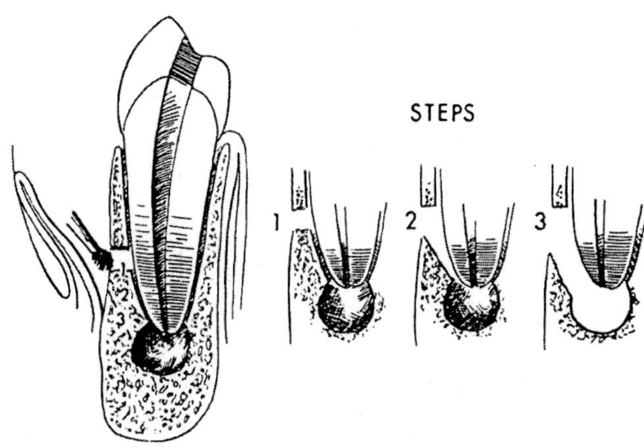

Figure 12-27 Stepwise removal of bone to the apex, after the root has been identified, prevents gouging adjacent roots or structures. (Courtesy of Dr. Merrill E. Schmidt.)

Osseous tissue response to surgical removal is complicated and depends on a number of variables. One important factor is that bone in the surgical site has a temporary decrease in vascular supply because of the local anesthetic vasoconstrictor. This results in the osseous tissue being more heat sensitive and less resistant to injury. Of major importance in osseous tissue removal by burs is the generation of heat. Variables, such as bur sharpness, rotary speed, flute design, and pressure applied, will all have a direct influence on heat generation.

The use of a **liquid coolant** is indispensable in controlling temperature increase during bone removal by dissipating the heat generated and by keeping the cutting flutes of the instruments free of debris. Osseous temperatures higher than 100°C have been recorded during bone removal with burs even when a liquid coolant was used.[83] Animal studies have shown that vascular changes occur in bone when temperatures exceed 40°C. Heating bone tissue in excess of 60°C results in inactivation of alkaline phosphatase, interruption of blood flow, and tissue necrosis.[84–87] For the coolant to be effective, it must be directed on the head of the bur enough to prevent tissue debris from clogging the flutes.

The shape of the bur used for bone removal and the design of its flutes play a significant role in postsurgical healing. Cutting of osseous tissue with **a No. 6 or No. 8 round bur** produces less inflammation and results in a smoother cut surface and a shorter healing time than when a fissure or diamond bur is used.[88–90] Burs with the ability to cut sharply and cleanly, with the largest space between cutting flutes, regardless of the speed of rotation, leave defects that heal in the shortest postsurgical time.[91]

The amount of pressure applied to the bone by burs during osseous tissue removal will have a direct effect on the frictional heat generated during the cutting process. Light "brush strokes" with short, multiple periods of osseous cutting will maximize cutting efficiency and minimize the generation of frictional heat.

Several authors have stated that because of a potential for contamination from high-speed turbines, insufficient coolant directed at the bur head and problems of obstructed vision at the surgical site, a low-speed surgical handpiece should be used for osseous removal rather than a high-speed handpiece.[32,78,92] No studies presently exist that support a biologic basis for the use of a low-speed handpiece rather than the proper use of a high-speed handpiece for bone removal.[2] In most areas of the mouth, visual access is adequate while using a high-speed handpiece and surgical-length burs. In areas of restricted visibility, the use of a high-speed handpiece with a 45-degree angled head significantly increases visibility.

The Impact Air 45-degree high-speed handpiece offers the added advantage that the air is exhausted to the rear of the turbine rather than toward the bur and the surgical site (Figure 12-28). Several case reports have been published of surgical emphysema resulting in subcutaneous emphysema of the face, intrathoracic complications including pneumomediastinum, fatal descending necrotizing mediastinitis, and Lemierre syndrome from the use of a high-speed dental handpiece.[93–95] Clinicians should be aware of the spectrum of this potential problem and, specifically, of the potential hazards of pressurized nonsterile air blown into open surgical sites by the dental drill.[96]

When performing periradicular surgery, inexperienced endodontic surgeons, in their attempt to be conservative in the removal of osseous tissue, often create too small a window through the cortical plate to expose the tooth root. As a result, both visual and operative access is impaired for the most delicate and critical part

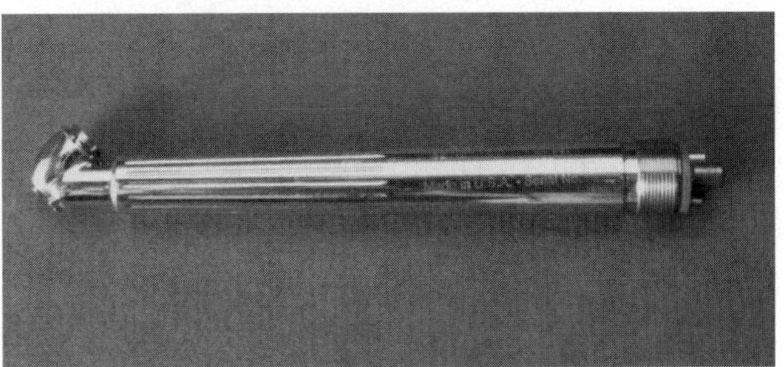

Figure 12-28 Impact Air 45-degree handpiece. Air is exhausted to the rear of the turbine rather than toward the surgical site.

of the surgery: root-end resection and root-end filling. Although it is advisable to limit osseous tissue removal to no more than is necessary, failure to achieve sufficient visual and operative access results in extending the time required for the surgical procedure, increasing the stress level of the surgeon, trauma to adjacent tissues, and postsurgical patient morbidity.

Periradicular Curettage

Once the root and the root apex have been identified and the surgical window through the cortical and medullary bone has been properly established, any diseased tissue should be removed from the periradicular bony lesion. This removal of periradicular inflammatory tissue is best accomplished by using the various sizes and shapes of sharp surgical bone curettes and angled periodontal curettes (Figure 12-29). Several instrument manufacturers provide a wide assortment of curettes that can be used for débridement of the soft tissue located adjacent to the root. The choice of specific curettes is very subjective, and endodontic surgeons will develop a preference for curettes that work best for them. It is advisable, however, to have a wide assortment of curettes available in the sterile surgery pack to use should the need arise.

Before proceeding with periradicular curettage, it is advisable to inject a local anesthetic solution containing a vasoconstrictor into the soft-tissue mass. This will reduce the possibility of discomfort to the patient during the débridement process and will also serve as hemorrhage control at the surgical site. Additional injections of local anesthetic solution may be necessary if the amount of soft tissue needing to be removed is extensive and hemorrhage control is a problem.

Curettement of the inflammatory soft tissue will be facilitated if the tissue mass can be removed in one piece. Penetration of the soft-tissue mass with a curette will result in increased hemorrhage and shredding the tissue will result in more difficult removal. To accomplish removal of the entire tissue mass, the largest bone curette, consistent with the size of the lesion, is placed between the soft-tissue mass and the lateral wall of the bony crypt with the **concave surface** of the curette facing the bone. Pressure should be applied against the bone as the curette is inserted between the soft-tissue mass and the bone around the lateral margins of the lesion. Once the soft tissue has been freed along the periphery of the lesion, the bone curette should be turned with the **concave portion toward the soft tissue** and used in a scraping fashion to free the tissue from the deep walls of the bony crypt. Again, care should be taken not to penetrate the soft-tissue mass with the curette.

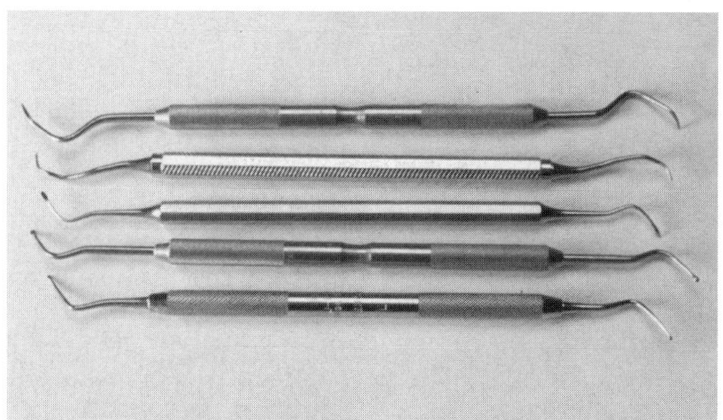

Figure 12-29 Assorted curettes for removing periradicular inflammatory soft tissue.

Once the tissue has been detached from the walls of the crypt, its removal can be facilitated by grasping it with a pair of tissue forceps. The tissue should be immediately placed in a bottle containing 10% buffered formalin solution for transportation to the pathology laboratory. Although the majority of periradicular lesions of pulpal origin are granulomas, radicular cysts, or abscesses, a multitude of benign and neoplastic lesions have been recovered from periradicular areas.[97] All soft tissue removed during periradicular curettage should be sent for histopathologic examination to ensure that no potentially serious pathologic condition exists.[98]

When the periradicular inflammatory soft tissue cannot be removed as a total mass, débridement is much more difficult and time consuming. As demonstrated by Fish, there is a considerable amount of reparative tissue in periradicular lesions.[99] Although it has been advocated for many years that all the soft tissue adjacent to the root be removed during periradicular surgery, in theory and practice this may not be necessary. This is especially true in cases where the lesion invades critical anatomic areas and structures such as the maxillary sinus, nasal cavity, mandibular canal, or adjacent vital teeth. Curettement of soft tissue in these and other critical anatomic areas should be avoided.[2]

Root-End Resection

Root-end resection is a common yet controversial component of endodontic surgery. Historically, many authors have advocated periradicular curettage as the definitive treatment in endodontic surgery **without root-end resection**. Their rationale for this approach centered primarily around the perceived need to maintain a cemental covering on the root surface and to maintain as much root length as possible for tooth stability.[100–102] According to Gutmann and Harrison, no studies are available to support either of these concerns. The rationale for periradicular curettage as a terminal procedure to protect root length and to ensure the presence of cementum is, therefore, highly questionable, especially if the source of periradicular irritant is still within the root canal system.[2] Other authors have stated that periradicular curettage per se, without root-end resection and root-end filling, should never be considered a terminal treatment in periradicular surgery unless it is associated with concurrent orthograde root canal treatment.[103,104]

Indications. There are many stated indications in the literature for **root-end resection** as part of endodontic periradicular surgery. These indications may be classified as either biologic or technical. el-Swiah and Walker reported on a retrospective study that evaluated the clinical factors involved in deciding to perform root-end resections on 517 teeth from 392 patients. They reported that biologic factors constituted 60% of the total, whereas technical factors constituted 40%. The most common biologic factors were persistent symptoms and continued presence of a periradicular lesion. The most common technical factors contributing to the need for root-end resections were interradicular posts, crowned teeth without posts, irretrievable root canal filling materials, and procedural accidents.[105]

There are three important factors for the endodontic surgeon to consider before performing a root-end resection: (1) instrumentation, (2) extent of the root-end resection, and (3) angle of the resection.

Instrumentation. The choice of bur type and the use of either a low- or high-speed handpiece for root-end resection deserve some consideration (Figure 12-30). Ingle et al. recommended that root-end resection is best accomplished by use of a No. 702 tapered fissure bur or a No. 6 or No. 8 round bur in a low-speed straight handpiece. They stated that a large round bur was excellent for this procedure because it was easily controlled and prevented gouging and the formation of sharp line angles.[106] Gutmann and Harrison, however, have stated that the use of a low-speed handpiece for root-end resection can be very difficult to control unless a good finger rest is obtained and a sharp bur is used. They have suggested the use of a high-speed handpiece and a surgical-length plain fissure bur.[2,104] Gutmann and Pitt Ford stated that, even though various types of burs have been recommended for root-end resections, there is no evidence to support an advantage of one type of bur over another with regard to tissue-healing response. For years, however, clinical practice has favored a smooth, flat, resected root surface.[103]

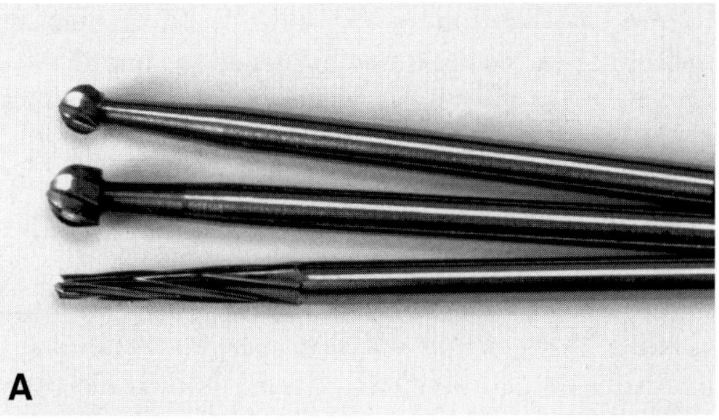

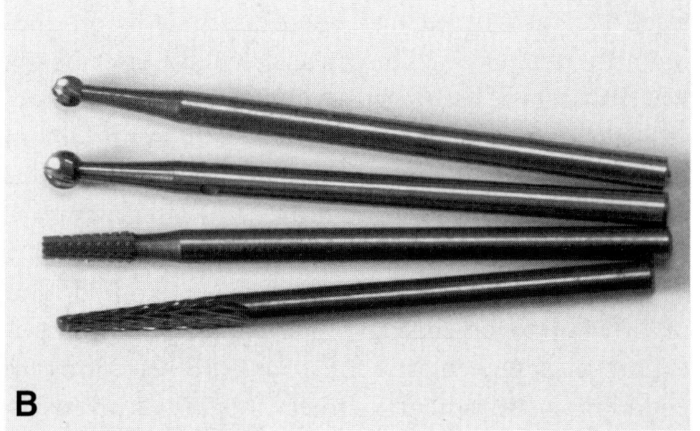

Figure 12-30 Burs for hard tissue removal. **A,** FG No. 6, No. 8, No. H267 (Brassler). **B,** SHP No. 6, No. 8, cross-cut fissure bur, plain fissure bur. Burs with larger spaces between cutting flutes result in less clogging of the bur with debris, thus reducing development of frictional heat.

Nedderman et al. used the scanning electron microscope (SEM) to evaluate the resected root face and gutta-percha fillings following root-end resection with various types of burs using both high- and low-speed handpieces. They reported that the use of round burs at both speeds resulted in scooping or ditching of the root surface. Cross-cut fissure burs at both speeds produced the roughest resected root surfaces with the gutta-percha being smeared across the root face. **Plain fissure burs**, both high- and low speed, produced the **smoothest** resected root surface, with plain fissure burs and a low-speed handpiece resulting in the **least gutta-percha distortion.**[107]

Morgan and Marshall reported on a study that compared the topography of resected root surfaces using No. 57, Lindeman, or Multi-purpose burs. Further comparisons were made after refinements with either a multi-fluted carbide or an ultra-fine diamond finishing bur. The resected root surfaces were examined by light microscopy at 20× magnification for smoothness and irregularities. Their results indicated that the **Multi-purpose bur** produced a smoother and more uniplanar surface than did the No. 57 bur and caused less damage to the root than either the No. 57 or the Lindeman bur. The multifluted carbide finishing bur tended to improve the smoothness of the resected root face, whereas the ultrafine diamond tended to roughen the surface.[108]

Since Theodore H. Maiman produced light amplification by stimulated emission of radiation (LASER) in 1960, lasers have found application in many areas of industry and medicine. Laser technology has been developed very rapidly and is now being used in various fields of dentistry. Most lasers used in dentistry operate either in the infrared or visible regions of the electromagnetic spectrum. These lasers act by producing a thermal effect. This means that the laser beam, when absorbed, has the capability to coagulate, vaporize, or carbonize the target tissue. It is important to note that different types of lasers may have different effects on the same tissue and the same laser may have different effects on different tissues.

Recently, many investigators have studied and reported on the in vitro and in vivo effects of the application of laser energy for root-end resections in endodontic periradicular surgery. A team of investigators from the Tokyo Medical and Dental University in Japan reported on an in vitro study using the Er:YAG laser for root-end resections. They reported that there was no smear layer or debris left on the resected root surfaces prepared by the use of the Er:YAG laser. Smear layer and debris, however, were left on the root surfaces prepared with a fissure bur.[109]

Komori and associates reported on an in vitro study evaluating the use of the Er:YAG laser and the Ho:YAG laser for root-end resections. They reported that the Er:YAG laser produced smooth, clean, resected root surfaces free of any signs of thermal damage. The Ho:YAG laser, however, produced signs of thermal damage and large voids between the gutta-percha root canal fillings and the root canal walls.[110]

Moritz and associates reported on an in vitro study evaluating the use of the carbon-dioxide (CO_2) laser as an aid in performing root-end resections. They chose the laser because it had previously been shown to have a sealing effect on the dentinal tubules. Their results indicated that the use of the CO_2 laser as an adjunct following root-end resection with a fissure bur resulted in decreased dentin permeability, as measured by dye penetration and sealing of dentinal tubules determined by SEM examination. Their conclusion was that CO_2 laser treatment optimally prepares the resected root-end surface to receive a root-end filling because it seals the dentinal tubules, eliminates niches for bacterial growth, and sterilizes the root surface.[111]

Maillet and associates evaluated the connective-tissue response to healing adjacent to the surface of dentin cut by a Nd:YAG laser versus dentin cut by a fissure bur. Disks of human roots 3.5 mm thick were implanted in the dorsal subcutaneous tissue of rats for 90 days. The disks were then recovered, with the surrounding tissue, at various times. The tissue against the cut dentin surfaces was assessed for extent of inflammation and fibrous capsule thickness by light microscopy. Their results showed a statistically significant increase in inflammation and fibrous capsule thickness adjacent to the dentin surfaces cut with the Nd:YAG laser compared with the bur-cut surfaces.[112]

Miserendino submitted a case report in which the CO_2 laser was used to perform a root-end resection and to sterilize the unfilled apical portion of the root canal space. He stated that the rationale for laser use in endodontic periradicular surgery includes (1) improved hemostasis and concurrent visualization of the operative field, (2) potential sterilization of the contaminated root apex, (3) potential reduction in permeability of root-surface dentin, (4) reduction of postoperative pain, and (5) reduced risk of contamination of the surgical site through elimination of the use of aerosol-producing air turbine handpieces. He concluded that the initial results of the clinical use of the CO_2 laser for endodontic periradicular surgery confirms the previous in vitro laboratory findings and indicates that further study of the application of lasers for microsurgical procedures in endodontics is in order.[113]

Komori and associates recently reported on eight patients (13 teeth) in whom the Er:YAG laser was used for root-end resections in periradicular endodontic surgery. They reported that all procedures were performed without the use of a high- or low-speed dental handpiece. Although the cutting speed of the laser was slightly slower than with the use of burs, the advantages of the laser included the absence of discomfort and vibrations, less chance for contamination of the surgical site, and reduced risk of trauma to adjacent tissue[114] (Figure 12-31).

Extent of the Root-End Resection. William Hunter's classic presentation on the role of sepsis and antisepsis in medicine had an impact that lasted for many years on the extent of root-end resections in periradicular surgery. Historically, it was believed that failure to remove all foci of infection could result in a persistence of the disease process. Since the portion of the root that extended into the diseased tissue was "infected," and the cementum was "necrotic," it was necessary to resect the root to the level of healthy bone. Andreasen and Rud, in 1972, were unable to demon-

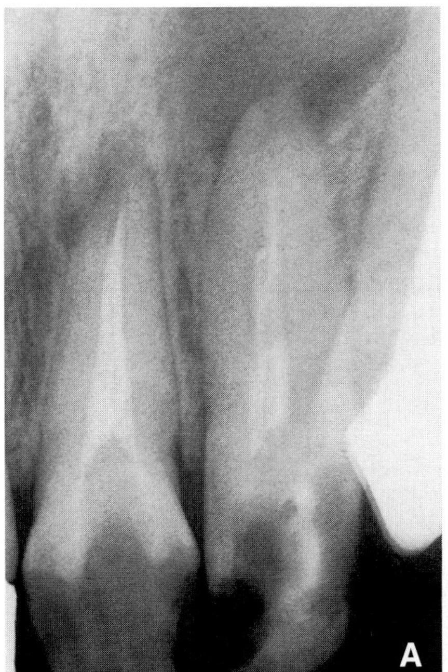

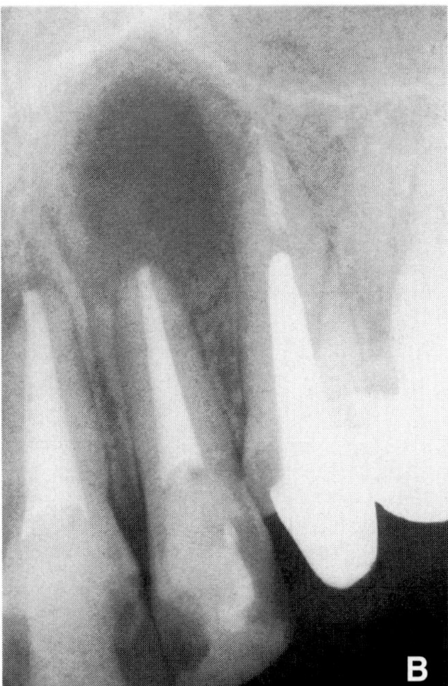

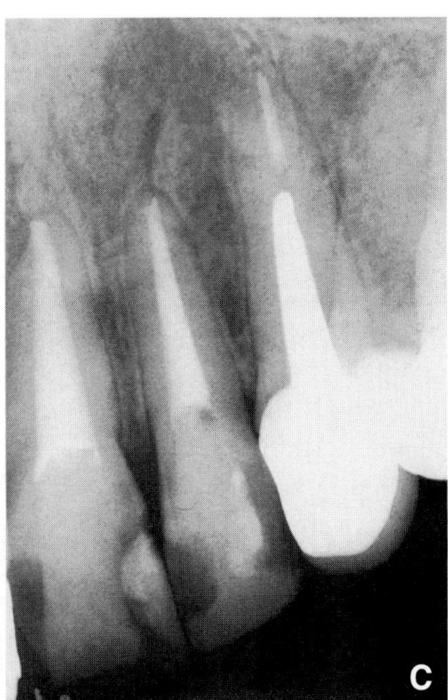

Figure 12-31 Root-end resection using LASER energy. **A,** Pretreatment radiograph revealing failing endodontic treatments with periradicular inflammatory lesions. **B,** Radiograph following endodontic retreatment and root-end resection of teeth No. 9 and No. 10 using Er:YAG laser. C, Twenty-six-month postsurgical radiograph revealing good periradicular healing. (Courtesy of Dr. Silvia Cecchini.)

strate the validity of this concept. Their findings indicated that there was no correlation between the presence of microorganisms in the dentinal tubules and the degree of periradicular inflammation.[115]

The extent of root-end resection will be determined by a number of variable factors that a dental surgeon must evaluate on an individual, case-by-case basis. It is not clinically applicable to set a predetermined amount of root-end removal that will be appropriate for all clinical situations. The following factors should be considered when determining the appropriate extent of root-end resection in periradicular surgery:

1. Visual and operative access to the surgical site (example: resection of buccal root of maxillary first premolar to gain access to the lingual root).
2. Anatomy of the root (shape, length, curvature).
3. Number of canals and their position in the root (example: mesial buccal root of maxillary molars, mesial roots of mandibular molars, two canal mandibular incisors).
4. Need to place a root-end filling surrounded by solid dentin (because most roots are conical shaped, as the extent of root-end resection increases, the surface area of the resected root face increases).
5. Presence and location of procedural error (example: perforation, ledge, separated instrument, apical extent of orthograde root canal filling).
6. Presence and extent of periodontal defects.
7. Level of remaining crestal bone.

The endodontic surgeon must constantly be aware that conservation of tooth structure during root-end resection is desirable; however, root conservation should not compromise the goals of the surgical procedure (Figure 12-32).

Angle of Root-End Resection. Historically, endodontic textbooks and other literature have recommended that the angle of root-end resections, when used in periradicular surgery, should be 30 degrees to 45 degrees from the long axis of the root facing toward the buccal or facial aspect of the root. The purpose for the angled root-end resections was to provide enhanced visibility to the resected root end and operative access to enable the surgeon to accomplish a root-end preparation with a bur in a low-speed handpiece.[2,3,29,32,63,76–78,103]

More recently, several authors have presented evidence indicating that beveling of the root end results in opening of dentinal tubules on the resected root surface that may communicate with the root canal space and result in apical leakage, even when a root end filling has been placed. Ichesco and associates, using a spectrophotometric analysis of dye penetration, concluded that the resected root end of an endodontically treated tooth exhibited more apical leakage than one

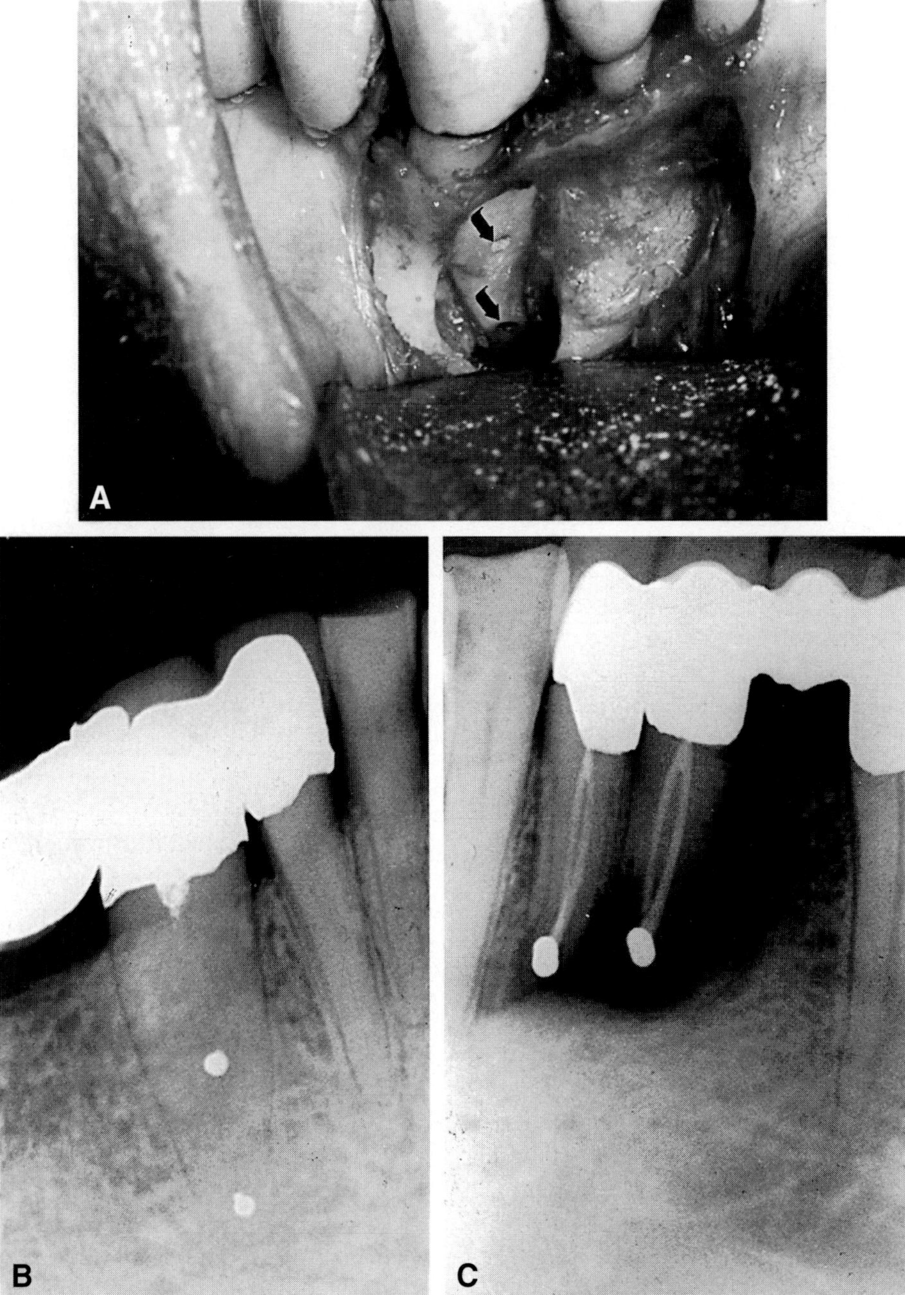

Figure 12-32 A, Mandibular canine abutment found to have two canals (**arrows**) on surgical exposure. **B,** One-year recall of **A,** with complete healing. **C,** Two-canal mandibular incisors serving as double abutments. Larger retrofillings obturate two foramina to rescue case. (Courtesy of Dr. L. Stephen Buchanan.)

without root-end resection.[116] Beatty, using a similar method of dye penetration analysis, examined apical leakage at different root-end resection angles and reported that significantly more leakage occurred in those roots where the root-end filling did not extend to the height of the bevel.[117] Vertucci and Beatty proposed that exposed dentinal tubules may constitute a potential pathway for apical leakage.[118]

Tidmarsh and Arrowsmith examined the cut root surface following root-end resections at angles between 45 degrees and 60 degrees approximately 3 mm from the root apex. Using scanning electron microscopy, they reported the presence of an average of 27,000 dentinal tubules per mm^2 on the face of the root-end resection midway between the root canal and the dentine–cementum junction.[119]

Gagliani and associates assessed the apical leakage measured by dye penetration in extracted teeth with root-end resections at 45-degree and 90-degree angles from the long axis of the root. Their findings indicated a statistically significant increase in leakage extending to the root canal space through dentinal tubules in those teeth with 45-degree angled root-end resections. They concluded that, by increasing the angle of the root-end resection from the long axis of the root, the number of exposed dentinal tubules increases. If infection persists within the root canal system coronal to the root-end filling, the likelihood of bacteria and/or bacterial by-products spreading outside of the root canal is high.[120]

Regardless of the angle or the extent of the root-end resection, it is extremely important that the resection be complete and that no segment of root is left unresected. The potential for incomplete root-end resection is especially high in cases where the root is broad in its labial–lingual dimension and where surgical access and visibility are impaired. Carr and Bentkover stated that failure to cut completely through the root in a buccal–lingual direction is one of the most common errors in periradicular surgery.[82] Once the desired extent and bevel of root-end resection have been achieved, the face of the resected root surface should be carefully examined to verify that complete circumferential resection has been accomplished. This can be accomplished by using a fine, sharp explorer or the tip of a Morse scaler guided around the periphery of the resected root surface. If complete resection is in doubt, a small amount of methylene blue dye can be applied to the root surface for 5 to 10 seconds. After the area has been irrigated with sterile saline, the periodontal ligament will appear dark blue, thereby highlighting the root outline.

Root-End Preparation

The purpose of a root-end preparation in periradicular surgery is to create a cavity to receive a root-end filling. Historically, root-end preparations have been performed by the use of small round or inverted cone burs in a miniature or straight low-speed handpiece. One major objective of a root-end preparation is that it be placed parallel to the long axis of the root. It is rare that sufficient access is present to allow a bur in a contra angle or straight handpiece to be inserted down the **long axis** of the root. These preparations are almost always placed obliquely into the root with a high risk of perforation to the lingual.

It is important for proper root-end preparation that the endodontic surgeon have a thorough knowledge of the root canal morphology of the tooth being treated. Incisor teeth with single roots and single canals most often have a straightforward, uncomplicated root canal system, except for lateral or accessory canals, usually located in the apical one-third of the root.

Roots with multiple canals, however, have the potential to have more complicated root canal systems. An isthmus or anastomosis may exist between two root canals in the same root.[121] This isthmus connection, when it occurs, becomes an important factor in the ability to thoroughly clean and débride these root canal systems (Figure 12-33). They also become a significant factor in the design and placement of the root-end preparation. If an isthmus exists and is not included in the root-end preparation, the remaining necrotic pulp tissue and debris may be a nidus for recurrent infection and subsequent treatment failure. The use of methylene blue dye placed on the resected root surface can also aid in the detection of an existing root canal isthmus.

Several authors have reported on studies investigating the actual incidence of an isthmus being present between two root canals in the same root. These reports indicate that the mesial root of the mandibular first molar has the highest incidence, at 89%, followed by the mesiobuccal root of the maxillary first molar, at 52%.[122–127] In the past, the existence of a canal isthmus was often overlooked, and when identified, it was difficult to prepare with the traditional bur preparation. The recognition and proper management of a canal isthmus is an important factor that may affect the success of periradicular surgery involving roots with two or more canals.

Importance of Surgical Hemostasis. Good visualization of the surgical field and of the resected root surface is essential in determining the optimum placement of the root-end preparation. The ability to visualize the fine detail of the anatomy on the resected root surface depends on excellent surgical hemostasis to provide a clean, dry, surgical site. Presurgical hemostasis was discussed earlier in this chapter and its importance cannot be overemphasized. Frequently, however, the need for additional hemostasis at the surgical site becomes evident. This surgical hemostasis is best achieved by the use of various topical or local hemostatic agents. Ideally, these hemostatic agents should be placed subsequent to the root-end resection and before the root-end preparation and filling.[2] These topical and local hemostatic agents have been broadly classified by their mechanism of action[128] (see Table 12-3).

Bone Wax. The recommended use of bone wax dates back more than 100 years.[128] In 1972, Selden reported bone wax to be an effective hemostatic agent in periradicular surgery.[129] Bone wax contains mostly highly purified beeswax with the addition of small

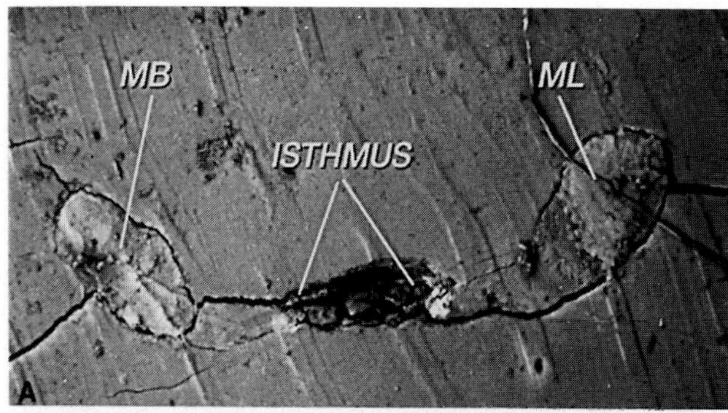

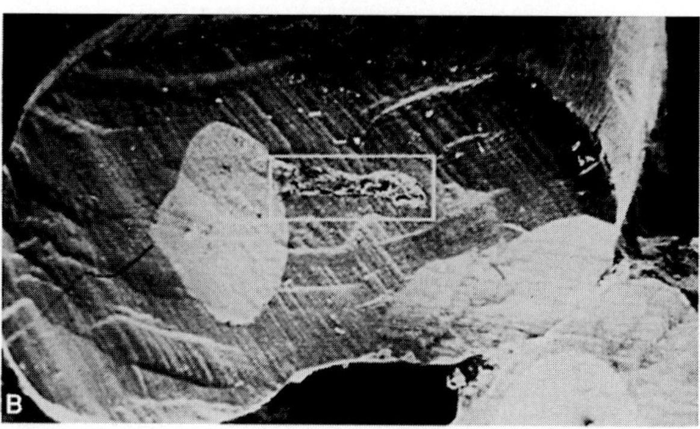

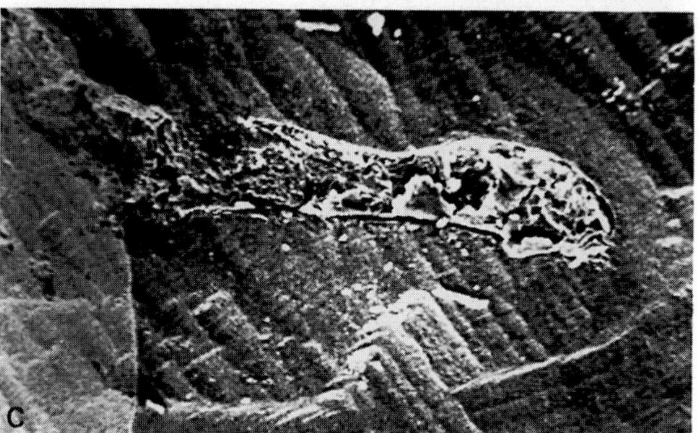

Figure 12-33 Cause of two endodontic failures revealed under dental operating microscope following root-end amputation. **A,** Nondébrided unfilled isthmus connecting mesiobuccal and mesiolingual canals. **B,** Low-power magnification reveals nondébrided unfilled portion of otherwise well-filled canal. **C,** Higher magnification of box area in **B.** (Courtesy of Dr. Gary Carr and Pacific Endodontic Research Foundation.)

Table 12-3 Classification of Topical Hemostatic Agents

1. Mechanical agents (Nonresorbable)
   a. Bone wax (Ethicon, Somerville, NJ)
2. Chemical agents
   a. Vasoconstrictors: epinephrine (Racellets, Epidri, Radri) (Pascal Co, Bellevue, WA)
   b. Ferric sulfate: Stasis (Cut-Trol, Mobile, AL); Viscostat; Astringedent (Ultradent Products, Inc, UT)
3. Biologic agents
   a. Thrombin USP: Thrombostat (Parke-Davis, Morris Plains, NJ); Thrombogen (Johnson & Johnson Medical, New Brunswick, NJ)
4. Absorbable hemostatic agents
   a. Mechanical agents
      i. Calcium sulfate USP
   b. Intrinsic action agents
      i. Gelatin: Gelfoam (Upjohn Co, Kalamazoo, MI); Spongostan (Ferrostan, Copenhagen, Denmark)
      ii. Absorbable collagen: Collatape (Colla-tec Inc, Plainsboro, NJ); Actifoam (Med-Chem Products Inc, Boston, MA)
      iii. Microfibrillar collagen hemostats: Avitene (Johnson & Johnson, New Brunswick, NJ)
   c. Extrinsic action agents
      i. Surgicel (Johnson & Johnson, New Brunswick, NJ)

USP = United States Pharmacopeia.

amounts of softening and conditioning agents. Its hemostatic mechanism of action is purely mechanical in that the wax, when placed under moderate pressure, plugs the vascular openings. **It has no effect on the blood-clotting mechanism.**

When using bone wax for surgical hemostasis, it should first be packed firmly into the entire bony cavity. The excess should then be carefully removed with a curette until only the root apex is exposed. When the root-end surgical procedure is completed, **all remaining bone wax should be thoroughly removed before surgical closure.** Numerous authors, however, have reported the presence of persistent inflammation, foreign-body giant cell reactions, and delayed healing at the surgical site following the use of bone wax.[130–133] With the availability of more biocompatible and biodegradable products for local hemostasis, **bone wax can no longer be recommended for use in periradicular surgery.** [2,134]

Vasoconstrictors. Vasoconstrictors, such as epinephrine, phenylephrine, and nordefrin, have been recommended as topical agents for hemorrhage control during periradicular surgery. Of these agents, epinephrine has been shown to be the most effective and the most often recommended.[2,128,135,136] Cotton pellets containing racemic epinephrine in varying amounts (Epidri, Racellete, Radri) are available (Figure 12-34). For example, each Epidri pellet contains 1.9 mg of

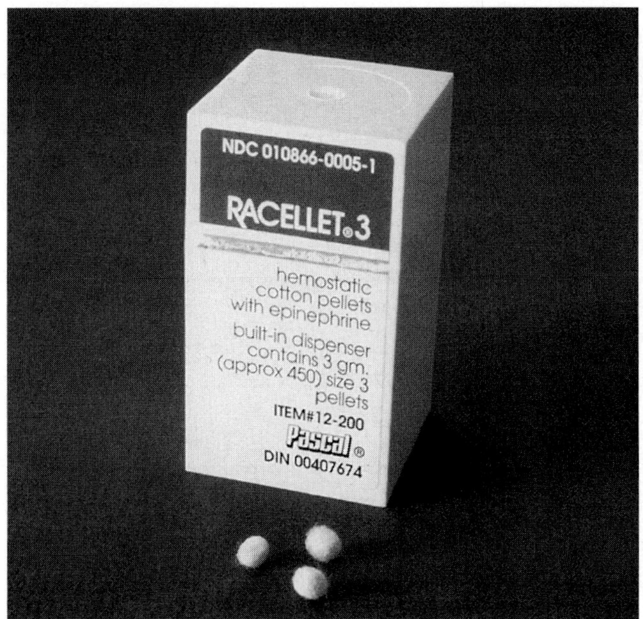

Figure 12-34 Racellet Pellets (Pascal Co, Bellevue, WA). Each pellet contains 0.55 mg of racemic epinephrine. Epidri pellets (Pascal Co) contain 1.9 mg racemic epinephrine.

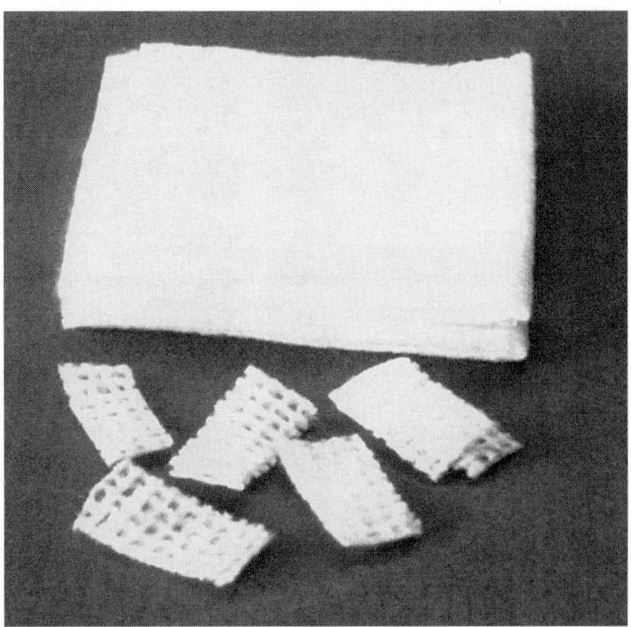

Figure 12-35 Telfa pads contain no cotton fibers and can be cut into small squares that are easily adapted to the surgical site.

racemic epinephrine. Each Racellete No. 2 pellet contains 1.15 mg and each Racellete No. 3 pellet contains 0.55 mg of epinephrine. Radri pellets contain a combination of vasoconstrictor and astringent. Each Radri pellet contains 0.45 mg of epinephrine and 1.85 mg of zinc phenolsulfonate.

Two areas of concern when using cotton pellets containing epinephrine need to be addressed. The first is the potential for leaving cotton fibers in the surgical site and the second is the possible hemodynamic effect of epinephrine on the vascular system. Gutmann and Harrison stated that cotton fibers that are left at the surgical site may impair the actual root-end seal by being trapped along the margins of the root-end filling material.[2] They also stated that cotton fibers may serve as foreign bodies in the surgical site and result in impaired would healing. Cotton pellets and gauze products containing cotton should, therefore, be considered the least desirable materials to be used for root-end isolation or hemostasis. Sterile Telfa pads (Kendall Co., Mansfield, Mass.) are useful adjuncts as they contain no cotton fibers. They can be cut into small squares that are easily adapted to the surgical site (Figure 12-35).

Weine and Gerstein and Selden have cautioned against the use of vasoconstrictors as topical agents for hemostasis during periradicular surgery because their use may result in systemic vascular change.[76,129] Besner, however, has shown that when a Racellete No. 2 pellet containing 1.15 mg of epinephrine was used during periradicular surgery, the pulse rate of the patient did not change.[137] Pallasch has stated that, although the use of vasoconstrictors in topical hemostatic agents and gingival retraction cord remains controversial, data exist from which to formulate reasonable guidelines. Elevated blood levels of epinephrine can occur with their use but do not generally appear to be associated with any significant cardiovascular effects in healthy patients or those with mild to moderate heart disease. In patients with more severe heart disease, epinephrine-impregnated cotton pellets or gauze, or gingival retraction cord, should be used with caution or avoided.[138] Kim and Rethnam, however, have stated that, because epinephrine used topically causes immediate local vasoconstriction, there is little absorption into the systemic circulation and thus a reduced chance of a systemic effect.[128]

Ferric Sulfate. Ferric sulfate is a chemical agent that has been used as a hemostatic agent for over 100 years. It was first introduced as Monsel's solution (20% ferric sulfate) in 1857. Its mechanism of action results from the agglutination of blood proteins and the acidic pH (0.21) of the solution. In contrast to vasoconstrictors, ferric sulfate effects hemostasis through a chemical reaction with the blood rather than an alpha-adrenergic effect.[128]

Ferric sulfate is easy to apply, requires no application of pressure, and hemostasis is achieved almost immediately (Figure 12-36). Ferric sulfate, however, is

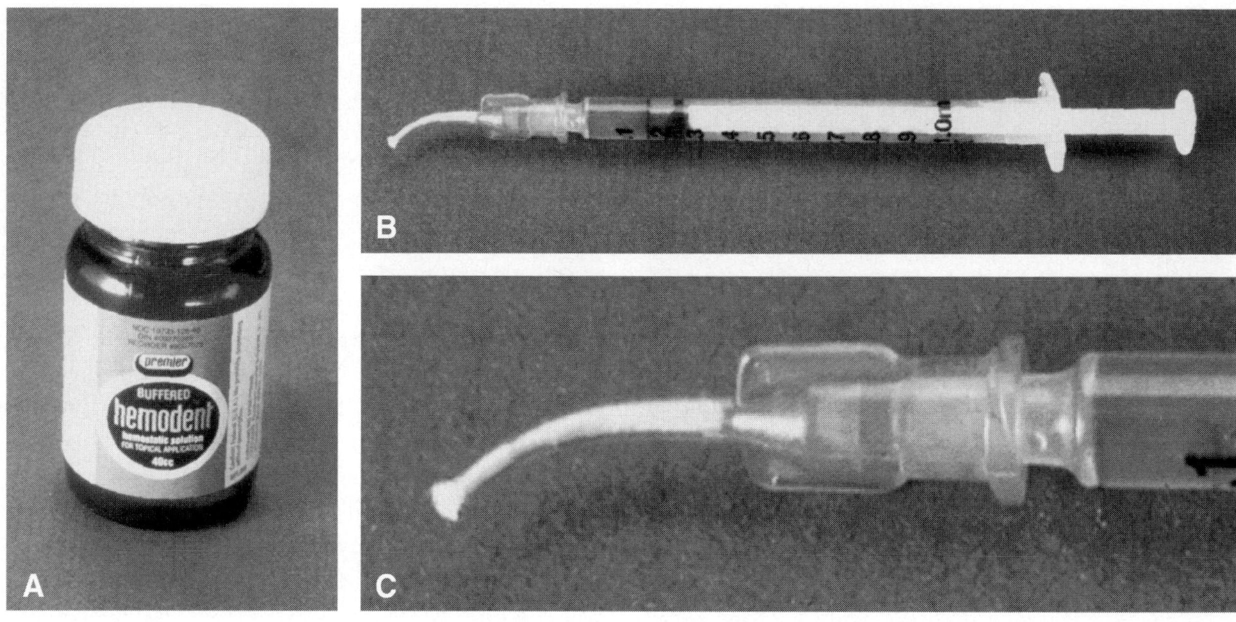

Figure 12-36 Hemodent (Premier Dental; King of Prussia, Pa.). **A,** Ferric sulfate achieves hemostasis as a result of agglutination of blood proteins rather than from an alpha-adrenergic effect like epinephrine. **B,** An Infusion Tip (Ultradent Products Inc., Utah) placed on a 1.0 cc syringe (Monoject) containing a small amount of ferric sulfate solution. The infusion tip allows for controlled placement of the hemostatic agent. C, Close-up of infusion tip.

known to be cytotoxic and may cause tissue **necrosis and tattooing**. Systemic absorption is unlikely because the agglutinated protein plugs that occlude the blood-vessel orifices isolate it from the vascular supply.[128] Lemon and associates, using rabbit mandibles, reported a significant adverse effect on osseous healing when ferric sulfate was left in the surgical site following creation of experimental surgical bony defects.[139] Jeansonne and associates, however, using a similar rabbit model, reported that when ferric sulfate was placed only until hemostasis was obtained and the surgical site was thoroughly curetted and irrigated with sterile saline 5 minutes later, there was no significant difference in osseous repair, as compared with the untreated controls.[140] Ferric sulfate appears to be a safe hemostatic agent when used in limited quantities and care is taken to **thoroughly curette and irrigate** the agglutinated protein material before surgical closure.[128]

Thrombin. Topical thrombin has been developed for hemostasis wherever wounds are oozing blood from small capillaries and venules. Thrombin acts to initiate the extrinsic and intrinsic clotting pathways. It is designed for topical application only and may be life threatening if injected. Topical thrombin has been investigated as a hemostatic agent in abating bleeding in cancellous bone. Although there was less bleeding than in the control, thrombin was **not as effective** as other available topical hemostatic agents.[134] In a report of a study by Codben and associates, no impedance of bone healing was evident 3 months following the use of topical thrombin.[141] Topical thrombin has been used successfully in neurosurgery, cardiovascular surgery, and burn surgery; however, its use in periradicular surgery has not been adequately investigated at this time. The main disadvantages of topical thrombin are its difficulty of handling and high cost.

Calcium Sulfate. Calcium sulfate (plaster of Paris) is a resorbable material used in surgery for over 100 years. It has gained popularity, in recent years, as a barrier material in guided tissue-regeneration procedures.[142,143] Calcium sulfate can also be used as a hemostatic agent during periradicular surgery. It consists of a powder and liquid component that can be mixed into a thick putty-like consistency and placed in the bony crypt using wet cotton pellets to press it against the walls. The hemostatic mechanism of calcium sulfate is similar to bone wax in that it acts as a mechanical barrier, plugging the vascular channels. In contrast to bone wax however, calcium sulfate is biocompatible, resorbs completely in 2 to 4 weeks, and does not cause an increase in inflammation. It is porous, which allows for fluid exchange so that flap necrosis does not occur when left in place following surgery. Calcium sulfate also has the advantage of being relatively inexpensive.[128]

Gelfoam and Spongostan. Gelfoam and Spongostan are hard, gelatin-based sponges that are water insoluble and resorbable. They are made of animal-skin gelatin and become soft on contact with blood. Gelatin sponges are thought to act intrinsically by promoting the disintegration of platelets, causing a subsequent release of thromboplastin. This, in turn, stimulates the formation of thrombin in the interstices of the sponge.[128]

The main indication for the use of gelatin-based sponges is to control bleeding in surgical sites by leaving it in situ, such as in extraction sockets, where hemostasis cannot be achieved by the application of pressure. During periradicular surgery, hemostasis is needed for improved visualization to accomplish the delicate task of root-end resection and filling. Once the gelatin sponge contacts blood, it swells and forms a soft, gelatinous mass. This swollen, soft, gelatinous mass tends to visually obscure the surgical site. Because it is soft, pressure cannot be applied to the severed microvasculature without dislodging the gelatin sponge, which will result in a continuation of bleeding. The major use for gelatin-based sponges in periradicular surgery is placement in the bony crypt, after root-end resection and root-end filling have been completed just before wound closure. Because gelatin-based sponges promote disintegration of platelets, release of thromboplastin, and the formation of thrombin, they may be beneficial in reducing postsurgical bleeding from the "rebound phenomenon."

The initial reaction to gelatin-based sponge material in the surgical site is a **reduction in the rate of osseous healing.** Boyes-Varley and associates examined early healing in the extraction sockets of monkeys. Histologically, the sockets containing gelatin-based sponge material displayed a greater inflammatory cell infiltrate, marked reduction in bone in-growth, and a foreign-body reaction at 8 days.[144] Olson and associates, however, reported that there was no distinguishable difference in healing rate or inflammatory cell infiltrate between extraction sockets in which Gelfoam was placed and the controls after 90 days.[145]

Collagen. Collagen-based products have been used extensively as surgical hemostatic agents. It is believed that four principal mechanisms of action are involved in hemostasis enhanced by collagen-based products: (1) stimulation of platelet adhesion, aggregation, and release reaction[146]; (2) activation of Factor VIII (Hageman Factor)[147]; (3) mechanical tamponade action[148]; and (4) the release of serotonin.[149] The collagen used for surgical hemostasis is obtained from bovine sources and is supplied in sheets (Collatape) and sponge pads (Actifoam). Both forms are applied dry, directly to the bleeding site, while using pressure. Hemostasis is usually achieved in 2 to 5 minutes.[128]

Microfibrillar Collagen Hemostat. Avitene and Instat are two popular forms of microfibrillar collagen. It is derived from purified bovine dermal collagen, shredded into fibrils, and converted into an insoluble partial hydrochloric acid salt. It functions through topical hemostasis, providing a collagen framework for platelet adhesion. This initiates the process of platelet aggregation and adhesion and formation of a platelet plug.[150] Avitene has been recommended as a viable means of controlling hemorrhage in periodontal surgery, resulting in a minimal interference in the osseous wound-healing process.[151,152,] Haasch and associates have demonstrated its potential use in periradicular surgery.[153] In a study designed to examine osseous regeneration in the presence of Avitene, Finn and associates found that bone formation proceeded uneventfully without a foreign-body reaction.[154]

The application of microfibrillar collagen products may be difficult and tedious, at times, because of their affinity for wet surfaces, such as instruments and gloves. To overcome these problems, it has been recommended that they be applied to the surgical site by use of a spray technique. This allows direct application of the hemostatic agent to the bleeding points.[155] Other disadvantages of microfibrillar collagen products: they are inactivated by autoclaving, their use in contaminated wounds may enhance infection, and they are expensive compared with other topical hemostatic agents.[128]

Surgicel. Surgicel is a chemically sterilized substance resembling surgical gauze and is prepared by the oxidation of regenerated cellulose (oxycellulose), which is spun into threads, then woven into a gauze that is sterilized with formaldehyde. Its mode of action is principally physical since it does not affect the clotting cascade through aggregation or adhesion of platelets, such as the collagen-based products. Surgicel initially acts as a barrier to blood and then as a sticky mass that acts as an artificial coagulum or plug.[134]

Surgicel left in bone following surgery has been shown to markedly **reduce the rate of repair and increase inflammation.** Difficulty in completely removing Surgicel from bony wounds has been described, with even minimally retained fragments resulting in inflammation and a foreign-body reaction.[130] The manufacturer, Johnson and Johnson, **does not recommend implantation of Surgicel** in bony defects.[156]

Instrumentation. Root-end preparation techniques have historically involved a recommendation that the endodontic surgeon, following the root-end resection, examine the root canal filling to determine the quality of the seal. Adequately evaluating the quality of seal of a root canal filling requires measurements in the area of microns, and we currently do not possess these capabilities at a clinical level. SEM studies have shown that the act of **root-end resection disturbs the gutta-percha seal.**[157,158] The preparation for, and the placement of, **a root-end filling is therefore recommended** whenever root-end resection has been performed.[82]

Root-end preparations should accept filling materials that predictably seal off the root canal system from the periradicular tissues. Carr and Bentkover have defined an ideal root-end preparation as a class I preparation at least 3.0 mm into root dentin with walls parallel to and coincident with the anatomic outline of the pulp space.[82] They also identified five requirements that a root-end preparation must fulfill:

1. The apical 3 mm of the root canal must be freshly cleaned and shaped.
2. The preparation must be parallel to and coincident with the anatomic outline of the pulp space.
3. Adequate retention form must be created.
4. All isthmus tissue, when present, must be removed.
5. Remaining dentin walls must not be weakened.

For successful root-end preparations, the endodontic surgeon must be well versed in both root morphology and root canal system anatomy. The teeth that require periradicular surgery are often those in which the anatomy is unusual or complex.[82]

Bur Preparation. The traditional root-end cavity preparation technique involved the use of either a miniature contra angle or straight handpiece and a small round or inverted cone bur. The objective was to prepare a class I cavity preparation down the long axis of the root within the confines of the root canal. The recommended depth of the preparation ranged from 1 to 5 mm, with 2 to 3 mm being the most commonly advocated.[76,78,104]

The ability of the endodontic surgeon to prepare a class I cavity parallel to the long axis of the root with a miniature contra angle handpiece may be difficult and depends on the physical access available around the root apex. According to Arens et al., this requires a minimum of 10 mm above or below the point of entry.[32] Accomplishing this with a straight handpiece is virtually impossible. These preparations are most often placed obliquely into the root, resulting in a risk of perforation and/or weakening of the dentin walls, and predisposing to a possible root fracture (Figure 12-37, A).

Ultrasonic Root-End Preparation. Ultrasonic root-end preparation techniques have been developed in an attempt to solve the major inadequacies and shortcomings of the traditional bur-type preparation. The use of ultrasonic instrumentation during periradicular surgery was first reported by Richman in 1957 when he used an ultrasonic chisel to remove bone and

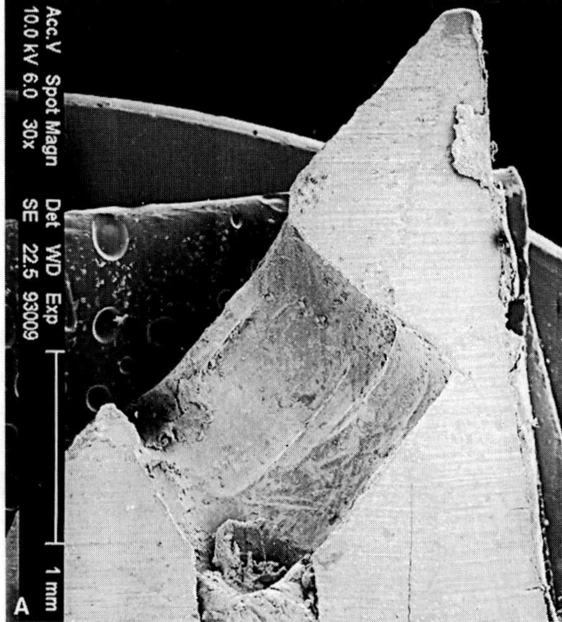

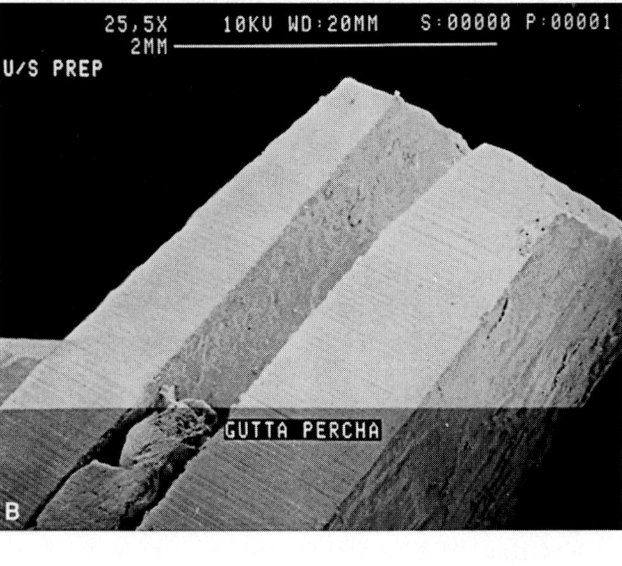

Figure 12-37 Comparison between bur and ultrasonic root-end preparations. **A,** Bur preparation shows large cavity prepared obliquely to the canal with a No. 33½ inverted cone bur. **B,** Ultrasonic preparation shows clean preparation parallel to the canal. Scanning electron micrograph. (Courtesy of Dr. Gary Wuchenich and Dr. Debra Meadows.)

root apices.[159] This concept was further developed by Bertrand and colleagues in 1957 when they reported on the use of modified ultrasonic periodontal scaling tips for root-end preparations in periradicular surgery.[160] Recently, specially designed ultrasonic root-end preparation instruments have been developed and are available from a number of instrument manufacturers (Figure 12-38). Their use has become very popular and they appear to have many advantages over the traditional bur-type preparation, such as smaller preparation size, less need for root-end beveling, a deeper preparation, and more parallel walls for better retention of the root-end filling material (Figure 12-37, B).

After the root-end resection has been completed, all soft tissue that needs to be removed has been curetted from the lesion, and proper hemostasis achieved, the resected root face should be thoroughly examined. The use of **magnification** and staining with methylene blue dye will aid in the identification of additional portals of exit, aberrant anatomy, and/or isthmuses not readily apparent. An appropriate cavity design should be planned and its outline identified by lightly etching it on the dentin of the resected root face with the sharp point of a CT-5 ultrasonic tip without irrigation to enhance vision.

After the outline of the root-end preparation has been established, the preparation should be deepened with an appropriately sized and angled ultrasonic tip, with irrigation, on the lowest power setting possible to accomplish dentin and root canal filling material removal. A light touch with a brush-type motion should be used, which will facilitate the maximum cutting efficiency and reduce pressure against the root surface. Special attention and care should be taken regarding removal of all root canal filling material on the lateral walls of the root-end cavity preparation, **especially the labial or facial wall.** This is a vulnerable area **in which root canal filling material or debris is often left**, resulting in a compromised root-end seal.

At the completion of the root-end preparation, it should be thoroughly irrigated with sterile saline, dried, and examined, preferably with **magnification**, for quality and cleanliness. Small, front-surface micromirrors are a beneficial adjunct to this examination process (Figure 12-39). Properly performed, ultrasonic root-end cavity instrumentation produces conservative, smooth, nearly parallel walled preparations (Figure 12-40). In a study involving SEM examination, root-end preparations using ultrasonic instrumentation have been reported to be contaminated with less debris and smear layer than those prepared using a bur. Ultrasonic instrumentation also resulted in root-end

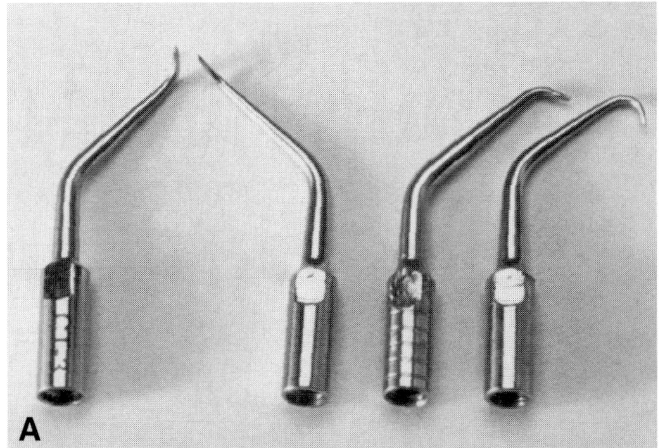

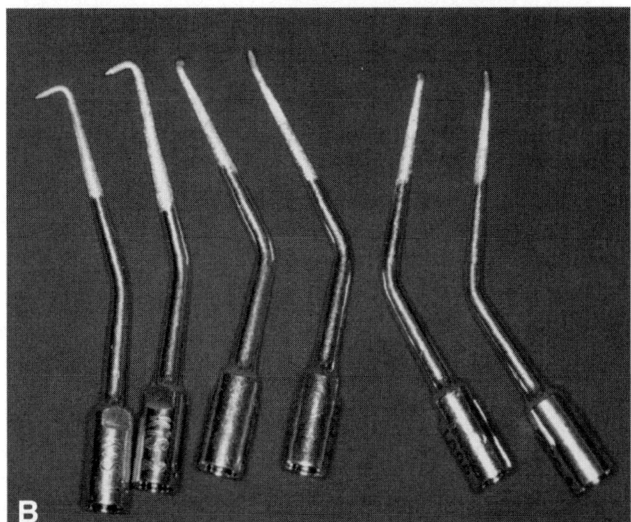

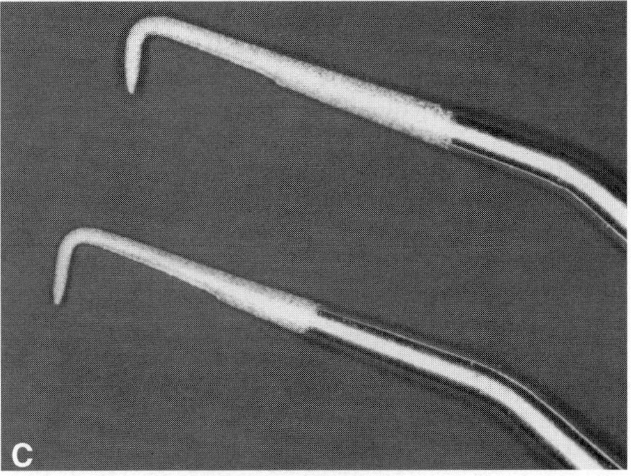

Figure 12-38 Ultrasonic tips. **A,** Ultrasonic tips developed by Dr. Gary Carr (Excellence in Endodontics, San Diego, CA). Available with plain or diamond-coated tips. **B,** KiS Microsurgical Ultrasonic Instruments (Obtura Spartan, Fenton, MO). The tips are coated with zirconium nitride for faster dentin cutting with less ultrasonic energy. **C,** Close-up of KiS Microsurgical Ultrasonic Instruments.

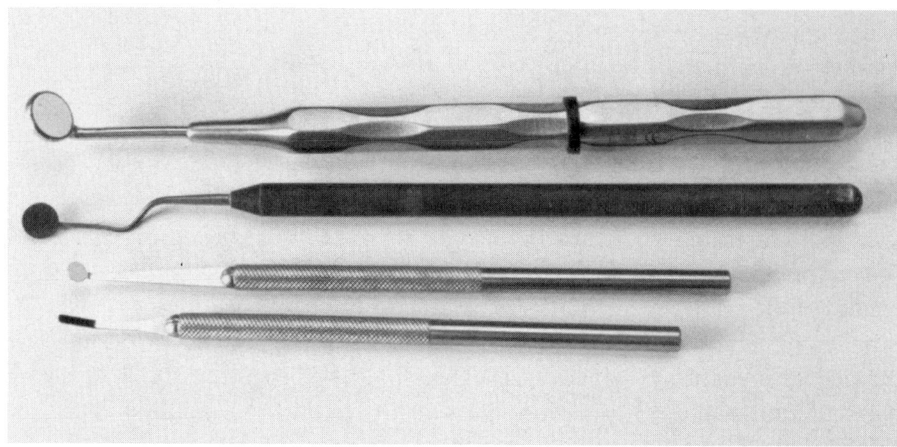

Figure 12-39 Variety of small front surface micro-mirrors for viewing root-end resection and root-end preparation through the microscope.

cavities that followed the direction or the root canal more closely than those prepared with a bur [161,162] (see Figure 12-37, B).

A recent controversy has developed regarding the potential for ultrasonic energy in root-end cavity preparation to result in the **formation of cracks** in the dentin surrounding the root-end preparation. Some authors have reported that the use of ultrasonic instrumentation resulted in an increased number and extent of dentin crack formation.[163,164] Others have reported no difference in the incidence of dentin crack formation between bur and ultrasonic root-end cavity preparation in extracted teeth.[165,166]

Layton and associates reported an in vitro study evaluating the integrity of the resected root-end surfaces, following root-end resection and after root-end preparation, with ultrasonic instrumentation at low and high frequencies. The results indicated that root-end resection alone may result in dentin crack formation regardless of the type of root-end preparation. Their data also indicated that **more dentin cracks** occurred when the ultrasonic tip was used on the **high-frequency setting** than on the low-frequency setting and that more cracks resulted following ultrasonic root-end cavity preparation, regardless of the frequency setting, than after root-end resection alone.[167]

Calzonetti and associates used a polyvinylsiloxane replication technique to study cracking after root-end resection and ultrasonic root-end preparation in cadavers' teeth. They found **no cracks** in 52 prepared root-ends examined under scanning electron microscopy.[168] Their results indicate that there is a possibility that the **intact periodontal ligament** adds a protective function by **absorbing the shock** of ultrasonic vibrations to prevent cracking in the clinical setting, a possibility that was not observed in extracted human teeth studies.

Morgan and Marshall reported on an in vivo study using electron microscopy to examine resin casts made from polyvinylsiloxane impressions taken following

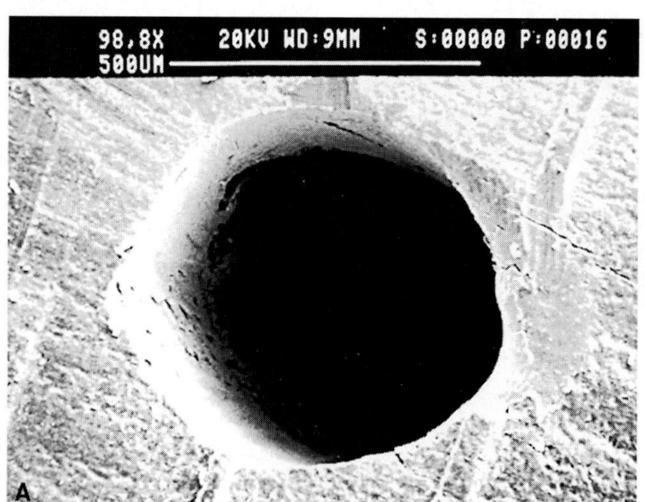

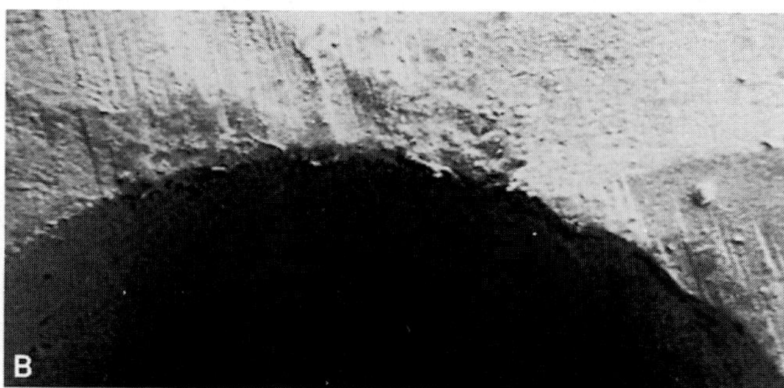

Figure 12-40 **A,** Eight-power dental operating microscope view of root-end preparation using Carr ultrasonic tips. Preparation is 0.5 mm in diameter. **B,** Higher magnification shows smoothness of walls. (Courtesy of Dr. Gary Carr.)

root-end resection and root-end preparation with ultrasonic instrumentation at **low power setting.** Their results **revealed that no cracks were evident** on any of the roots **following root-end resection alone** and **only one small**, shallow, incomplete **crack** was detected from **25 roots following ultrasonic root-end preparation.**[169]

Sumi and associates reported on a human clinical outcomes assessment study that evaluated the success/failure rate of periradicular surgeries performed on 157 teeth involving root-end cavity preparations using ultrasonic instrumentation. Observation periods ranged from 6 months to 3 years. Outcome assessment was based on clinical and radiographic findings. A success rate of 92.4% was reported. It was concluded that ultrasonic root-end preparation provides excellent clinical results.[170] **Available evidence indicates that root-end cavity preparation using ultrasonic instrumentation provides a convenient, effective, and clinically acceptable method for preparing the resected root end to receive a root-end filling.**

Root-End Filling

The purpose of a root-end filling is to establish a seal between the root canal space and the periapical tissues. According to Gartner and Dorn, a suitable root-end filling material should be (1) able to prevent leakage of bacteria and their by-products into the periradicular tissues, (2) nontoxic, (3) noncarcinogenic, (4) biocompatible with the host tissues, (5) insoluble in tissue fluids, (6) dimensionally stable, (7) unaffected by moisture during setting, (8) easy to use, and (9) radiopaque.[171] One might add, it should not stain tissue (tattoo).

Root-End Filling Materials. Numerous materials have been suggested for use as root-end fillings, including gutta-percha, amalgam, Cavit, intermediate restorative material (IRM), Super EBA, glass ionomers, composite resins, carboxylate cements, zinc phosphate cements, zinc oxide–eugenol cements, and mineral trioxide aggregate (MTA). The suitability of these various materials has been tested by evaluating their microleakage (dye, radioisotope, bacterial penetration, fluid filtration), marginal adaptation, and cytotoxicity and clinically testing them in experimental animals and humans.

A large number of in vitro studies dealing with the marginal adaptation and sealing ability (leakage) of various root-end filling material have been published. The results of these studies have often been inconsistent, contradictory, and confusing and have been questioned as to their clinical relevance. Factors such as the choice of storage solutions and the molecular size of the dye particles, and many other variables, can crucially influence the outcome of these in vitro studies.[172]

In vitro cytotoxicity and biocompatibility studies using cell cultures have also been published. Owadally and associates reported on an in vitro antibacterial and cytotoxicity study comparing IRM and amalgam. Their results indicated that IRM was significantly more antibacterial than amalgam at all time periods of exposure, and amalgam was significantly more cytotoxic than IRM.[173] Makkawy and associates evaluated the cytotoxicity of resin-reinforced glass ionomer cements compared with amalgam using human periodontal ligament cells. Their results indicated that, at 24 hours, amalgam significantly inhibited cell viability compared with resin-reinforced glass ionomer cement and the controls. At 48 and 72 hours, however, all materials tested exhibited a similar slightly inhibitory effect on cell viability.[174]

Chong and associates compared the cytotoxicity of a glass ionomer cement (Vitrebond; 3M Dental; St Paul, Minn.), Kalzinol, IRM and EBA cements, and amalgam. Their results indicated that fresh IRM cement exhibited the most pronounced cytotoxic effect of all materials tested. Aged Kalzinol was the second most cytotoxic material, with no significant difference being reported between Vitrebond EBA cement and amalgam.[175]

Zhu, Safavi, and Spangberg evaluated the cytotoxicity of amalgam, IRM cement, and Super-EBA cement in cultures of human periodontal ligament cells and human osteoblast-like cells. Their results indicated that amalgam was the most cytotoxic of the materials tested and showed a reduction in total cell numbers for both cell types. IRM and Super-EBA, however, were significantly less cytotoxic than amalgam and demonstrated no reduction in total cell numbers for both periodontal ligament and osteoblast-like cells.[176]

Several authors have published results of in vivo tissue compatibility studies of various root-end filling materials using an experimental animal model. Harrison and Johnson reported on a study designed to determine the excisional wound-healing responses of the periradicular tissues to IRM, amalgam, and gutta-percha using a dog model. Healing responses were evaluated microscopically and radiographically at 10 and 45 days postsurgically. They reported **no evidence of inhibition** of dentoalveolar or osseous wound healing associated with amalgam, gutta-percha, or IRM. Statistical analysis showed no difference in wound healing among the three materials tested.[177]

Pitt Ford and associates examined the effects of IRM, Super-EBA, and amalgam as root-end filling materials in the roots of mandibular molars of monkeys. They reported that the tissue response to IRM and Super-EBA was less severe than that to amalgam. No inflammation was evident in the bone marrow spaces adjacent to root-end fillings of IRM and Super-EBA. In contrast, however, inflammation was present in the alveolar bone marrow spaces with every root end filled with amalgam.[178,179]

A research group at Kyushu University in Japan reported the results of a histologic study comparing the effects of various root-end filling materials, including a 4-META-TBB resin (C&B Metabond, Parkell, Farmingdale, N.Y.), using a rat model. The materials tested were amalgam, light-cured glass ionomer cement, IRM, a 4-META-TBB resin, and light-cured composite resin. The 4-META-TBB resin and light-cured composite resin root-end fillings showed the most favorable histologic response among the materials tested. These materials did not provoke inflammation and did not appear to inhibit new bone formation, as seen with the other materials.[180]

Torabinejad and associates reported on a study designed to examine and compare the tissue reaction to several commonly used root-end filling material and a newly developed material, MTA (ProRoot, Tulsa Dental/Dentsply International; Tulsa, Okla.). Their study involved the implantation of amalgam, IRM, Super-EBA, and MTA in the tibias and mandibles of guinea pigs. The presence of inflammation, predominant cell type, and thickness of fibrous connective tissue adjacent to each implanted material was evaluated. The tissue reaction to implanted **MTA was the most favorable** observed at both implantation sites; in every specimen, it was **free of inflammation.** Mineral trioxide aggregate was also the material most often observed with direct bone apposition.[181]

Mineral trioxide aggregate was developed by Torabinejad and his associates at Loma Linda University. The main molecules present in MTA are calcium and phosphorous ions, derived primarily from tricalcium silicate, tricalcium aluminate, tricalcium oxide, and silicate oxide. Its pH, when set, is 12.5 and its setting time is 2 hours and 45 minutes. The compressive strength of MTA is reported to be 40 MPa immediately after setting and increases to 70 MPa after 21 days. The result of solubility testing of MTA (ADA specification #30) indicated an insignificant weight loss following testing.[182]

Mineral trioxide aggregate has been extensively evaluated for microleakage (dye penetration, fluid filtration, bacterial leakage), marginal adaptation (SEM), and biocompatibility (cytotoxicity, tissue implantation, and in vivo animal histology). The **sealing ability of MTA** has been shown to be **superior to that of Super-EBA** and was not adversely affected by blood contamination. Its marginal adaptation was shown to be better than amalgam, IRM, or Super-EBA. Mineral trioxide aggregate has also been shown to be **less cytotoxic than amalgam, IRM, or Super-EBA.** Animal usage tests in which MTA and other commonly used root-end filling material were compared have resulted in less observed inflammation and better healing with MTA. In addition, **with MTA, new cementum was observed being deposited on the surface of the material**[183–194] (Figure 12-41).

Many prospective and retrospective human clinical usage studies have been reported that assess the outcome of periradicular surgery involving the placement of various root-end filling materials. It is difficult to compare the results of these studies because the authors have used differing evaluation criteria and observations periods. It is important, however, to consider some of the more significant of these clinical usage reports.

Oynick and Oynick, in 1978, reported on the clinical use of a resin and silicone-reinforced zinc oxide and eugenol cement (Stailine, Staines, England) as a root-end filling material in 200 cases over a period of 14 years. Radiographic evaluations following periradicular surgical procedures using Stailine indicated favorable healing. Histologic and SEM evaluations of the root apex and adjacent periradicular bone, taken by block section, revealed newly formed bone in areas of previous resorption and collagen fibers growing into the filling material.[195]

Dorn and Gartner reported on a retrospective study of 488 periradicular surgical treatments in which three different root-end filling materials were used, IRM, Super-EBA, and amalgam. The evaluation period was from 6 months to 10 years. Outcome assessment was conducted by evaluation of the most recent recall radi-

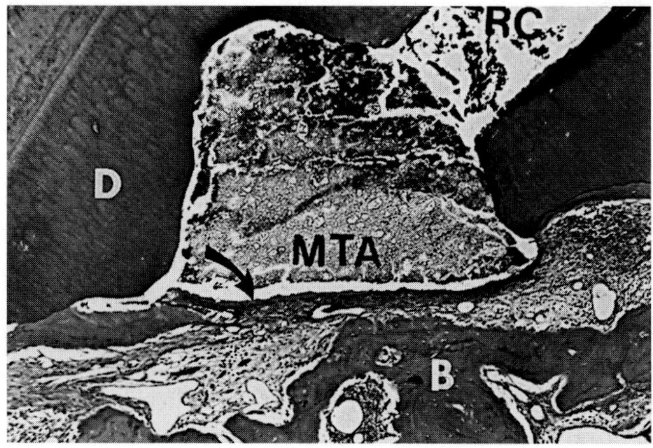

Figure 12-41 Mineral trioxide aggregate (MTA) retrofilling. Cementum (**arrow**) formed subjacent to the filling material (separated from the material during slide preparation). B = bone; D = dentin; RC = root canal. (Courtesy of Dr. M. Torabinejad.)

ograph as compared with the immediate postsurgical radiograph. Analysis of the data indicated there was no significant difference in the outcome of healing rates between IRM and Super-EBA. There was a significant difference, however, in the outcome between IRM, Super-EBA, and amalgam, the latter being the worst.[196] Pantschev and associates, however, reported on a prospective clinical study that evaluated the outcome of periradicular surgical procedures using either EBA cement or amalgam. The minimum evaluation period was 3 years and healing was based on clinical and radiographic analysis. Their data indicated no significant difference in the outcome between the two materials evaluated.[197]

Rud and associates have reported on several prospective and retrospective human usage studies in an attempt to evaluate the acceptability of a composite resin, combined **with a dentin bonding agent**, as a root-end filling material. The placement is different from other root-end fillings in that no root-end preparation, other than root-end resection, is made. The material covers the entire resected root-end surface. They have shown that the creation of a leak-resistant seal is possible with this material; however, **the process is very technique sensitive** as a result of the need for **strict moisture control**. They have reported complete bone healing in 80 to 92% of cases using this technique. Their observation periods ranged from 1 to 9 years.[198–202]

Smear Layer Removal. Instrumentation of dentin results in the accumulation of a smear layer covering the dentinal surface and occluding the dentinal tubules. It has been shown that bacteria may colonize in the smear layer and penetrate the dentinal tubules.[203] **Removal of this smear layer** seems desirable in the situation of root-end fillings that are placed in a bacterially contaminated root apex. Irrigation with tetracycline has been shown to remove the smear layer.[204] Smear layer removal from resected root ends and dentin demineralization by citric acid has been shown to be associated with more rapid healing and deposition of cementum on the resected root-end.[205]

Tetracyclines have a number of properties of interest to endodontists; they are antimicrobial agents, effective against periodontal pathogens; they bind strongly to dentin; and when released they are still biologically active.[206] Root surfaces exposed to anaerobic bacteria accumulate endotoxin and exhibit collagen loss, which may suppress fibroblast migration and proliferation, thus interfering with healing.[207] Root surface conditioning with acidic agents, such as **tetracycline**, not only **removes the smear layer**, it also **removes endotoxin** from contaminated root surfaces.[208]

Barkhordar and Russel reported on an in vitro study that examined the effect of irrigation with doxycycline hydrochloride, a hydroxy derivative of tetracycline, on the sealing ability of IRM and amalgam, when used as root-end fillings. Their results indicated significantly less microleakage following irrigation with doxycycline involving both IRM and amalgam, compared with the control irrigation with saline. They also suggested that, because of the long-lasting sustentative of **doxycycline** on root surfaces and its slow release in a biologically active state, their results support **its use for dentin conditioning** before placement of a root-end filling in periradicular surgery.[209]

Based on a review of the currently available literature, there does not appear to be an "ideal" root-end filling material. Intermediate restorative material, Super-EBA, and MTA appear to be the currently available materials that most closely meet the requirements, both physical and biologic, for a root-end filling material. MTA is a relatively new material, compared with IRM and Super-EBA, and long-term human usage studies are as yet not available for any of these materials. Final judgment on their use will need to be reserved until such clinical usage studies are available.

Placement and Finishing of Root-end Fillings. The method for placement of the root-end filling material will vary depending on the type of filling material used. Amalgam may be carried to the root-end preparation with a small K-G carrier that is sized for root-end preparations. Deeper lying apices may be more easily reached by using a Messing gun (Figure 12-42). Zinc oxide–eugenol cements (IRM and Super-EBA) are best mixed to a thick clay-like consistency, shaped into a small cone, and attached to the back side of a spoon excavator or the tip of a plastic instrument or Hollenback carver and placed into the root-end preparation.

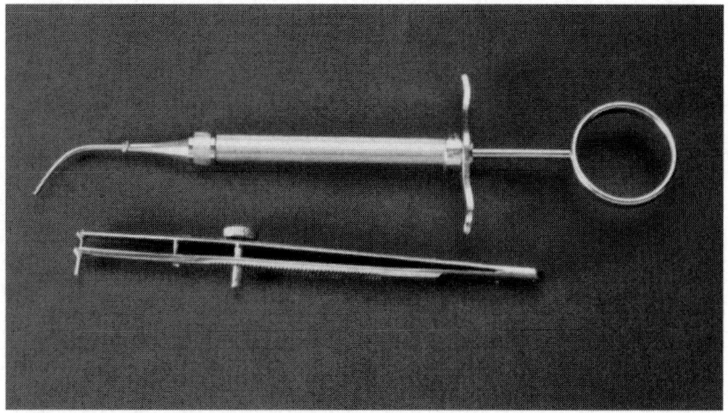

Figure 12-42 Root-end filling material carriers. **Top,** Messing gun with a curved tip. **Bottom,** Small K-G carrier.

Mineral trioxide aggregate is a unique root-end filling material with physical properties much different from other materials. It is a very fine, gray-colored powder that is mixed with a sterile liquid, such as saline or local anesthetic solution, on a sterile glass slab. It cannot be mixed to a clay-like consistency as can IRM or Super-EBA because as more powder is added to the liquid, the mix becomes dry and crumbly. If the mix is too wet, it is runny and very difficult to handle because of its lack of form. The surgical area must be kept very dry during its placement, and care must be taken not to wash out the filling material by irrigation before closure of the soft tissue. The setting time of MTA is 2.5 to 3 hours. Properly mixed, MTA should be free of excess moisture, **firm, but not crumbly**. It can be delivered to the root-end preparation by placing a small amount on the back side of a small spoon excavator or by using a small amalgam-type carrier (Figure 12-43).

Root-end preparations using ultrasonic tips tend to be smaller in diameter and extend deeper into the root canal than those prepared with a bur. As a result, the need for specially designed **root-end filling condensers** has resulted in their availability from many different manufacturers in various styles and shapes (Figure 12-44). It is important that the endodontic surgeon become familiar with the different shapes and styles of condensers to enable the surgeon to properly condense the root-end filling material to the full extent of the root-end preparation. The condenser should be small enough in diameter that it does not bind on the walls of the root-end preparation during condensation, thus resulting in the possibility of root-end fractures. It is also important that the condenser is long enough to properly condense the filling material into the deepest part of the root-end preparation.

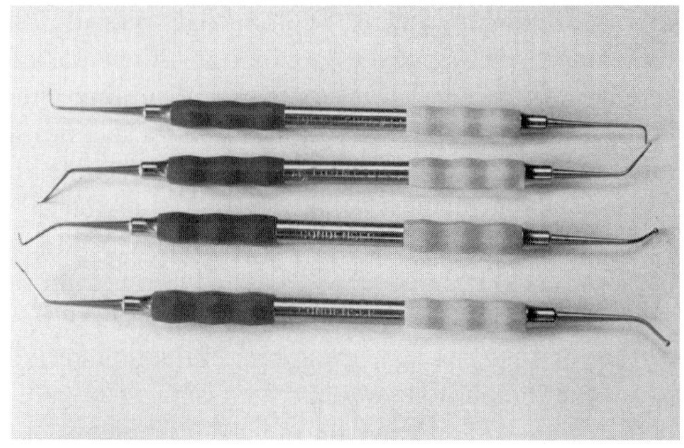

Figure 12-44 Small condensers for placing root-end filling material into ultrasonic preparations (Thompson Dental Mfg. Co).

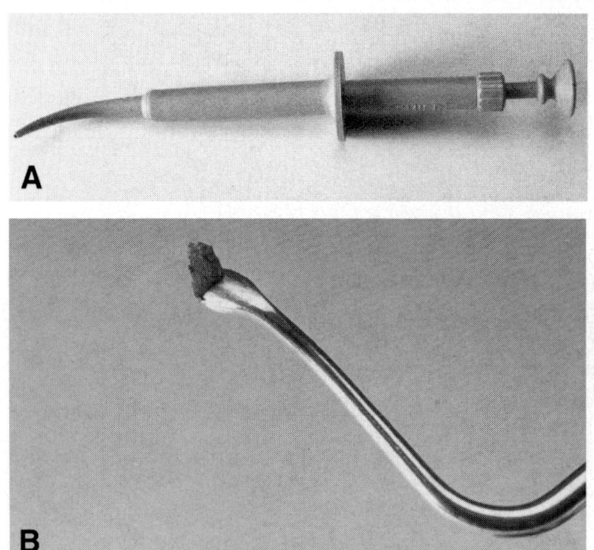

Figure 12-43 Carriers for mineral trioxide aggregate (MTA). **A,** Small plastic amalgam-type carrier (Premier Dental, King of Prussia, Pa.). **B,** A small amount of MTA can be carried and placed into the root-end preparation on the back side of a spoon excavator.

Various techniques have been advocated for finishing root-end fillings in periradicular surgery. Fitzpatrick and Steiman reported on an in vitro study designed to evaluate the marginal interfaces between the dentin and root-end fillings of IRM and Super-EBA. Following placement of the root-end fillings, they were finished by burnishing with a ball burnisher, a moistened cotton pellet, or with a carbide finishing bur in a high-speed handpiece with air/water spray. Their results indicated that **root-end fillings finished with a finishing bur** displayed significantly **better marginal adaptation**, with little evidence of flash, when compared with the other methods. There was no significant difference between the other finishing techniques or between the materials tested.[210]

Forte and associates reported on an in vitro study designed to compare microleakage, by the fluid filtration method, of root-end fillings of Super-EBA either unfinished or finished with a 30-flute high-speed finishing bur. Their results indicated **no significant difference** in microleakage, after 180 days, between root-end fillings of Super-EBA, finished or unfinished.[211]

Soft-Tissue Repositioning and Suturing

After final inspection of the root-end filling and removal of all visible excess filling material and surgical packing, a radiograph should be taken to evaluate the placement of the root-end filling and to check for the presence of any root fragments or excess root-end filling material (Figure 12-45). If ferric sulfate was used as a hemostatic

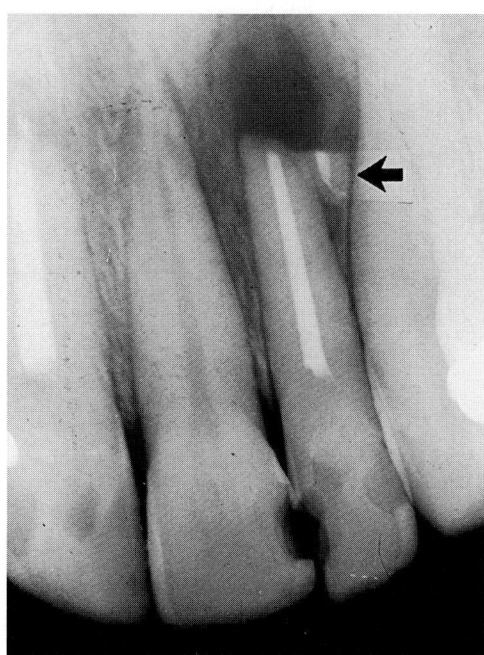

Figure 12-45 Radiograph taken **after** suturing and developed after patient left the office. The patient had to return for removal of root tip.

agent during surgery, the coagulated protein material should be thoroughly curetted and hemorrhage induced so that healing is not impaired.[128] Thorough examination of the underside of the flap, in the depth of the fold between the mucoperiosteum and the alveolar bone, should be done before repositioning the flap to remove any debris or foreign material that may be present. The final steps in the periradicular surgical procedure are wound closure and soft-tissue stabilization.

Repositioning and Compression. The elevated mucoperiosteal tissue should be gently replaced to its original position with the incision lines approximated as closely as possible. The type of flap design will affect the ease of repositioning, with full mucoperiosteal flaps generally providing less resistance to repositioning than would limited mucoperiosteal flaps. Using a surgical gauze, slightly moistened with sterile saline, gentle but firm pressure should be applied to the flapped tissue for 2 to 3 minutes (5 minutes for palatal tissue) before suturing. **Tissue compression**, both before and after suturing, not only enhances intravascular clotting in the severed blood vessels but also approximates the wound edges, especially the dissectional wound. This reduces the possibility of a blood clot forming between the flap and the alveolar bone.[2]

Suturing. It is important to stabilize the reflected tissue to prevent dislodgment until initial wound healing has taken place. Several authors have reported on studies in animals and humans designed to evaluate the effectiveness of medical grade adhesives, such as cyanoacrylate, for surgical wound closure and to compare them with sutures. Results of these studies have been mixed, and, at this time, their use has not replaced that of sutures for wound closure in endodontic surgery.[212–218]

The purpose of suturing is to approximate the incised tissues and stabilize the flapped mucoperiosteum until reattachment occurs. The placement of sutures in oral tissues, however, creates unique problems. It is evident that incisional wounds in oral tissues heal more rapidly than in skin. However, sutures are better tolerated and interfere less with postsurgical healing in the skin. "The major problem in oral tissues is the constant bathing of the suture material and suture tract with saliva containing a high concentration of microorganisms, that may gain entrance to underlying tissues."[2]

Sutures are available in many different materials, the most common being synthetic fibers (nylon, polyester, polyglactin, and polyglycolic acid), collagen, gut, and silk (Figure 12-46). Sutures are classified by absorbency (absorbable or nonabsorbable), by size according to the manufacturer's minimum diameter, and by physical design as monofilament, multifilament, twisted, or braided. The classification of suture size is complicated by the existence of two standards, the United States Pharmacopeia (USP) and the European Pharmacopeia (EP). The USP size is designated by two Arabic numbers, one a 0, separated by a hyphen (3-0, 4-0, 5-0, etc). **The higher the first number, the smaller the diameter** of the suture material. The EP system is a number that represents the manufacturer's minimum diameter tolerance of the suture in millimeters (1 = 0.10 mm, 1.5 = 0.15 mm, etc).

Silk. Silk sutures are made of protein fibers (fibroin) bound together with a biologic glue (sericin), similar to fibronectin, produced by silkworms. Silk sutures are nonabsorbable, multifilamentous, and braided. They have a high capillary action effect that enhances the movement of fluids between the fibers ("wicking" action), resulting in severe oral tissue reactions.[219–221] This tissue reaction results from the accumulation of plaque on the fibers that occurs within a few hours following insertion into the tissues.[222] Silk's advantage is limited to its ease of manipulation. Because of the severe tissue reaction to silk, it is not the suture material of choice for endodontic surgery today.[2] If silk sutures are used, however, the patient should rinse postoperatively with chlorhexidine.

Gut. Collagen is the basic component of plain gut suture material and is derived from sheep or bovine intestines. The collagen is treated with diluted

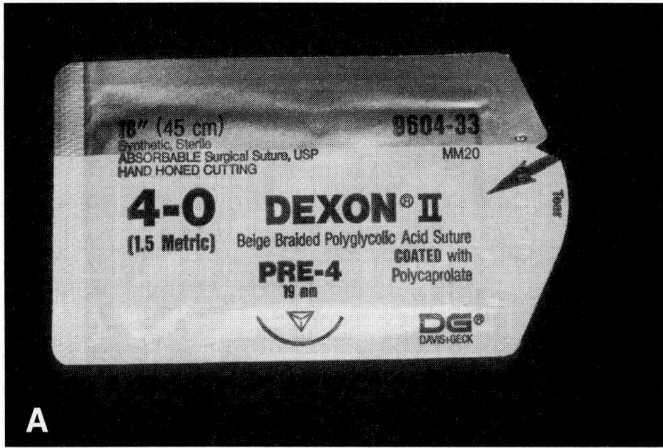

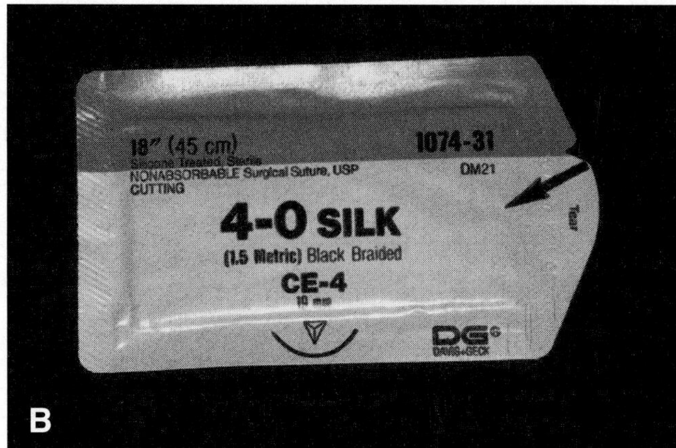

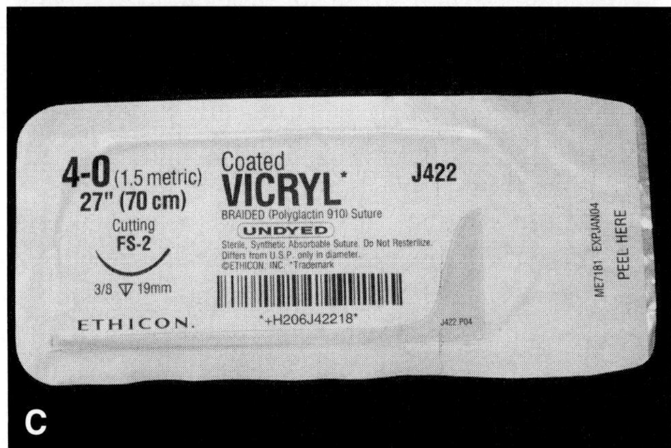

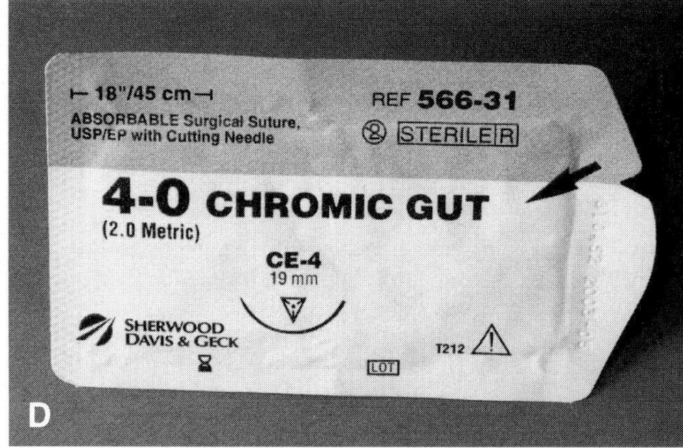

Figure 12-46 Various suture materials. **A,** Dexon II (braided absorbable polyglycolic acid) suture. **B,** Silk (braided nonabsorbable) suture. **C,** Vicryl (braided absorbable polyglactin 910) suture. **D,** API (absorbable chromic gut) suture.

formaldehyde to increase its strength and is then shaped into the appropriate monofilament size. Gut sutures are absorbable; however, the absorption rate is variable and can take up to 10 days. Because of the unpredictability of gut suture absorption in oral tissues, a scheduled suture removal appointment should be made.

Chromic gut sutures consist of plain gut that has been treated with chromium trioxide. This results in a delay in the absorption rate. Because retention of sutures beyond a few days is not recommended in endodontic surgery, the use of chromic gut sutures offers no advantage. Also, evidence indicates that plain gut is more biocompatible with oral soft tissues than is chromic gut.[2,219–221]

Gut suture material is marketed in sterile packets containing isopropyl alcohol. When removed from the packet, the suture is hard and nonpliable because of its dehydration. Before using, gut sutures should be hydrated by placing them into sterile, distilled water for 3 to 5 minutes. After hydration, the gut suture material will be smooth and pliable with manipulative properties similar to silk.[223]

Collagen. Reconstituted collagen sutures are made from bovine tendon after it has been treated with cyanoacetic acid and then coagulated with acetone and dried. Collagen sutures offer no advantage over gut for endodontic surgery since their absorption rate and tissue response are similar. They are available only in small sizes and used almost exclusively in microsurgery.

Polyglycolic Acid (PGA). Suture material made from fibers of polymerized glycolic acid is absorbable in mammalian tissue. The rate of absorption is about 16 to 20 days. Polyglycolic acid sutures consist of multiple filaments that are braided and share handling characteristics similar to silk. Polyglycolic acid was the first synthetic absorbable suture and it is manufactured as Dexon.

Polyglactin (PG). In 1975, Craig and coworkers reported the development of a copolymer of lactic acid and glycolic acid called polyglactin 910 (90 parts glycolic acid and 10 parts lactic acid).[224] Sutures of polyglactin are absorbable and consist of braided multiple filaments. Their absorption rate is similar to that of polyglycolic acid. They are commercially available as Vicryl.

Many studies have been reported evaluating the response of the oral soft tissues to gut, collagen, polyglycolic acid, and polyglactin sutures, with conflicting results. As a result, there is insufficient evidence, at this time, to make a strong recommendation among these materials. The important factor to remember about sutures, regardless of what material is used, is that they should be removed as early as the clinical situation will permit.

Needle Selection. Surgical needles are designed to carry the suture material through the tissues with minimal trauma. For that reason, a needle with a reverse cutting edge (the cutting edge is on the outside of the curve) is preferable. The arc of the surgical needle selected should match the optimum curvature needed to penetrate the tissues in and out on both sides of the incision, 2 to 3 mm from the wound margins. Suture needles are available in arcs of one-fourth, three-eighths, one-half, and five-eighths of a circle, with the most useful being the three-eighths and one-half circle. The radius of the arch of the needle is also an important consideration. The smaller the radius of the arch, the more conducive the needle is to quick turnout. For vertical incision lines and anterior embrasure suturing, a relatively tight arc is necessary to allow for quick needle turnout. Suturing in posterior areas, however, requires less curvature and a longer needle to reach through the embrasure (Figure 12-47). The final selection of an appropriate surgical needle is based on a combination of factors, including the location of the incision, the size and shape of the interdental embrasure, the flap design, and the suture technique planned.

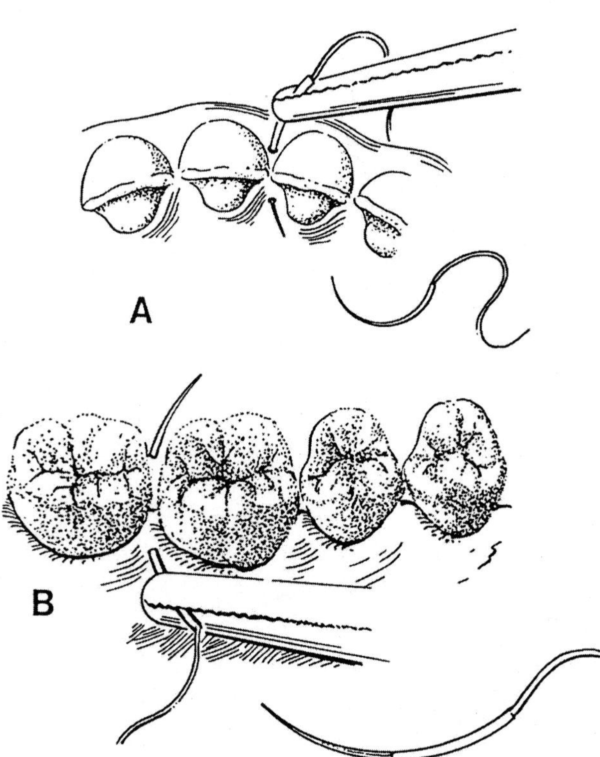

Figure 12-47 **A,** More tightly curved needle such as a half-circle is best for suturing incision lines and anterior embrasures. **B,** Straighter and longer curved needle is necessary for suturing in areas such as posterior embrasures.

Suture Techniques. There is a wide variety of suture techniques designed to accomplish the goals of closure and stabilization of flaps involving oral mucoperiosteal tissues. All suturing techniques should be evaluated on the basis of their ability to accomplish these goals.[2] Several authors have compared the effects of continuous and interrupted suture techniques. Their findings indicate that the **interrupted suturing** technique provides for **better flap adaptation** than does the continuous technique and, therefore, is the recommended technique, and the most commonly used, for endodontic surgery.[225,226] Sutures are holding mechanisms and should not pull or stretch the tissue as a tear in the flap margin may result. Sutures that close an incision too tightly compromise circulation and increase chances for the sutures to tear loose on swelling. Before placing sutures, bleeding should be controlled to prevent the formation of a hematoma under the flap. This will prevent the direct apposition of the flap to the bone and can act as a culture medium for bacterial growth. The suturing techniques that are most conducive to rapid surgical wound healing are the single interrupted suture, the interrupted loop (interdental) suture, the vertical mattress suture, and the single sling suture.

Single Interrupted Suture. The single interrupted suture is used primarily for closure and stabilization of vertical releasing and relaxing incisions in full mucoperiosteal flaps and horizontal incisions in limited mucoperiosteal flap designs (Figure 12-48). The initial needle penetration should be through the independent (movable) tissue. The point of needle entry should be from the buccal or facial side and 2 to 3 mm from the incision margin to provide sufficient tissue to minimize suture tear-out. The needle should then enter the **under surface** of the mucoperiosteum of the dependent (immovable) tissue and penetrate through the mucoperiosteum at a point 2 to 3 mm from the incision margin. To accomplish this, it is often necessary to **elevate** the attached mucoperiosteum from the underlying bone for a distance of a few millimeters at the point of needle insertion. It is important that the periosteum is included with the tissue bite—otherwise the suture will most likely tear out of the fragile attached gingiva.

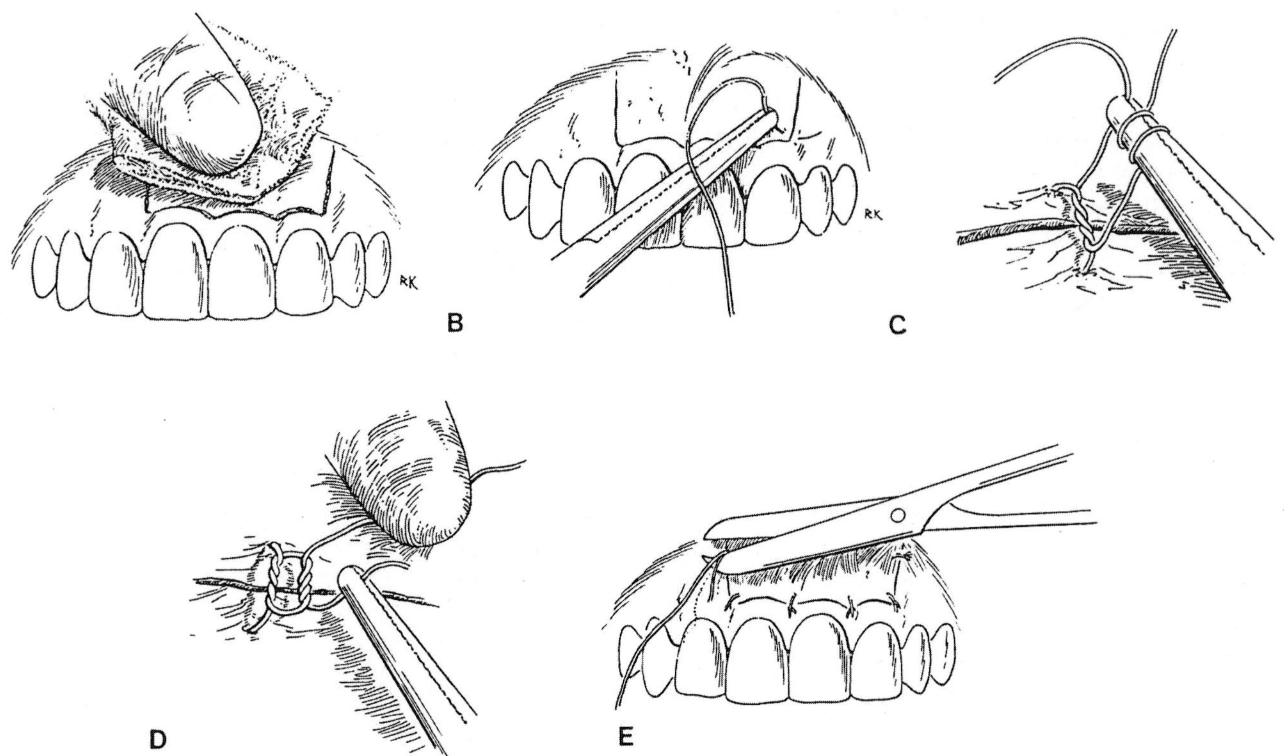

Figure 12-48 Suturing technique. **A,** Damp 2-inch × 2-inch gauze is used to smooth tissue flap into place. **B,** Most unattached portion of the flap is sutured to attached tissue. Two- to three-millimeter margin should be present between puncture points and incision lines. **C,** Wound edges are approximated with the first tie. **D,** Surgeon's knot is used to tie suture in place. **E,** Interrupted sutures are used to secure remainder of flap.

After the suture needle has been passed through the mucoperiosteum on both sides of the incision, the suture material should be drawn through the tissue until the end opposite the needle is approximately 1 to 2 inches from the tissue. The suture should be tied with a secure knot. A surgical knot is the most effective and least likely to slip. The surgeon's knot is best tied by wrapping double loops or throws of the long end (the end with the needle attached) of the suture around the needle holder. By then grasping the short end of the suture with the needle holder and slipping the throws off, the first half of the surgical knot is tied. After adjusting the tissue tension, the second half of the knot is tied by repeating the same process, except wrapping the loops of suture around the needle holder **in the opposite direction** from the first tie, like a square knot. Suture knots should be placed to the side of the incision. Suture knots collect food, plaque, and bacteria, thus resulting in localized infection and a delay in healing when placed directly over the incision (Figure 12-48, C **and** D).

Interrupted Loop (Interdental) Suture. The interrupted loop, or interdental suture, is used primarily to secure and stabilize the horizontal component of full mucoperiosteal flaps. The surgical needle is inserted through the buccal or facial interdental papillae, then through the lingual interdental papillae, and then back through the interdental embrasure. It is tied on the buccal or facial surface of the attached gingiva (Figure 12-49, A). This suture technique highly predisposes the fragile interdental tissue and col to inflammation and retarded healing, resulting in a loss of the outer gingival epithelium, with possible blunting or formation of a double papillae.

A modification of this interrupted loop suture is described as follows. After the surgical needle has been passed through the buccal and lingual papillary gingiva, the suture is passed over the interdental contact and secured with a surgeon's knot. This modification eliminates the presence of suture material in the interdental embrasure, thus reducing postsurgical inflammation to this delicate tissue. In clinical situations in which the horizontal component of a full mucoperiosteal flap involves a tooth or teeth with full-coverage crowns, this modification allows for a slight incisal or occlusal repositioning of the mucoperiosteal flap. This can be

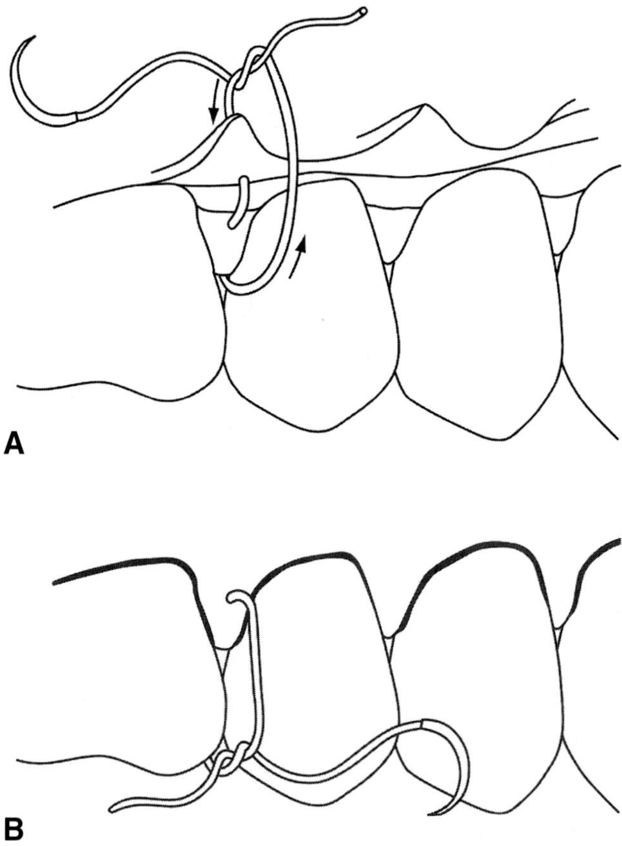

Figure 12-49 A, Interrupted loop suture. Suture is passed gingival to the interproximal contact. B, Modified interrupted loop suture. Suture is passed incisal to the interproximal contact.

accomplished by placing slight tension on the suture over the interdental contact and may compensate for a loss of gingival height resulting from the sulcular incision (Figure 12-49, B).

Vertical Mattress Suture. The vertical mattress suture has the advantage of not requiring needle penetration or suture material being passed through tissue involved in the incisional wound. The surgical needle enters and exits the flapped mucoperiosteum some distance apical from the incision line. The suture is then passed through the **interdental embrasure**, directed to the lingual gingiva of the adjacent tooth and passed back through the opposite interdental embrasure. The needle then enters and exits the flapped mucoperiosteum again, is passed through the embrasure, and, again, lingual to the tooth and through the opposite interdental embrasure to be tied on the buccal surface with a surgeon's knot (Figure 12-50). This suture technique also provides for the opportunity to return the flapped tissue to a slightly incisal or occlusal position from its original to compensate for a loss of gingival height.

Single Sling Suture. The single sling suture is similar to the vertical mattress suture. The surgical needle is passed through the attached gingiva of the flap, through the interdental embrasure, but not through the lingual soft tissue. It is then directed lingual to the tooth and passed through the opposite interdental embrasure and over the incisal or occlusal margin of the flap. The needle is then passed through the attached gingiva of the flap, from the buccal or facial side, back through the embrasure, passed lingual to the tooth, through the opposite embrasure, passed over the flap margin, and tied with a surgeon's knot (Figure 12-51). This suture technique is particularly effective for achieving the maximum incisal or occlusal level when repositioning the flap. Because the lingual anchor is the lingual surface of the tooth and not of the fragile lingual tissue, tension can be placed on the flapped tissue to adjust the height of the flap margin.

Postsurgical Care

Postsurgical management of the patient is equally as important as the surgical procedure itself. An important component of postsurgical care is a genuine expression of concern and reassurance to the patient regarding both their physical and emotional experience. It is well known that the emotional state of a patient has a direct relationship on the level of morbidity following a surgical procedure. The patient's **awareness that the surgeon cares** and is **readily available**, should the patient have a problem, is a priceless adjunct to healing. A telephone call to the patient, the evening following or the morning after endodontic surgery, is very reassuring and helps to build a strong doctor–patient relationship. This also allows any patient anxieties to be dealt with before they become major concerns.

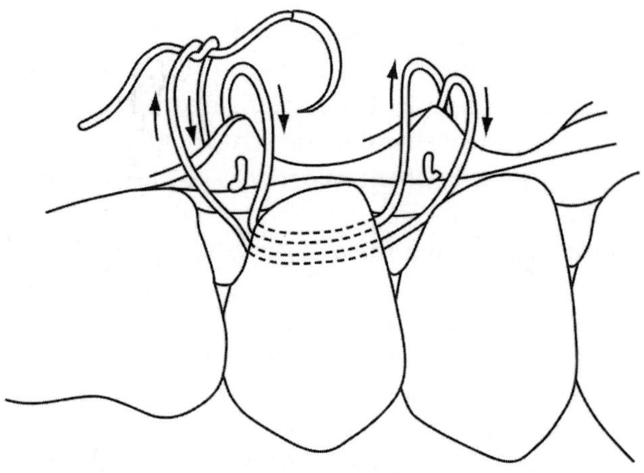

Figure 12-50 Vertical mattress suture.

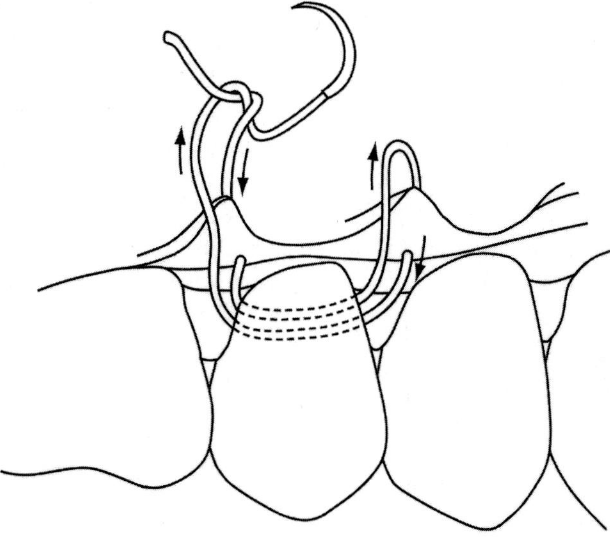

Figure 12-51 Single sling suture.

Another important component of postsurgical care is good patient communication. It is the endodontic surgeon's responsibility to properly communicate to the patient the expected and normal postsurgical sequelae as well as detailed home care instructions. These instructions are best conveyed both verbally and in writing. Alexander stated that without written reinforcement, the understanding and retention of verbal instructions cannot be ensured. He also advised that written materials should be presented after oral instructions have been given rather than the other way around. Since up to 20% of Americans are functionally illiterate, written instructions should use simple words (preferably 1 to 2 syllables) and short sentences of no more than 10 words.[227] Normal postsurgical sequelae include the possibility of slight bleeding from the surgical area for a few hours, pain that may persist for a few days, and swelling and soft-tissue discoloration (ecchymosis) in the surgical area that may be evident for as many as 8 to 10 days. An example of written postsurgical instructions, which should be reviewed verbally with the patient before he is dismissed, is provided in Table 12-4.

Table 12-4 Instructions for Postoperative Care Following Endodontic Surgery. (May Be Copied)

1. Do not do any difficult activity for the rest of the day. Easy activity is okay, but be careful and do not bump your face where the surgery was done. You should not drink any alcohol or use any tobacco (smoke or chew) for the next 3 days.
2. It is important that you have a good diet and drink lots of liquids for the first few days after surgery. Juices, soups, and other soft foods such as yogurt and puddings are suggested. Liquid meals, such as Sego, Slender, and Carnation Instant Breakfast, can be used. You can buy these at most food stores.
3. Do not lift up your lip or pull back your cheek to look at where the surgery was done. This may pull the stitches loose and cause bleeding.
4. A little bleeding from where the surgery was done is normal. This should only last for a few hours. You may also have a little swelling and bruising of your face. This should only last for a few days.
5. You may place an ice bag (cold) on your face where the surgery was done. You should leave it on for 20 minutes and take it off for 20 minutes. You can do this for 6 to 8 hours. **After 8 hours, the ice bag (cold) should not be used.** The next day after surgery, you can put a soft, wet, hot towel on your face where the surgery was done. Do this as often as you can for the next 2 to 3 days.
6. Discomfort after the surgery should not be bad, but the area will be sore. You should use the pain medicine you were given, or recommended to you, as needed.
7. Rinse your mouth with 1 tablespoon of the chlorhexidine mouthwash (Peridex) you were given or prescribed. This should be done two times a day (once in the morning and once at night before going to bed). You should do this for 5 days.
8. The stitches that were placed need to be taken out in a few days. You will be told when to return. **It is important that you come in to have this done!!**
9. You will be coming back to the office several times during the next few months so that we can evaluate how you are healing. These are very important visits and you should come in even if everything feels okay.
10. If you have any problems or if you have any questions, you should call the office. The office phone number is xxx-xxxx. If you call after regular office hours or on the weekend, you will be given instructions on how to page the doctor on call.

Bleeding, swelling, discoloration, pain, and infection are the most likely untoward sequelae following endodontic surgery. These should be thoroughly discussed with the patient during the presurgical consultation and should be reinforced at the time of surgery, before dismissal of the patient.

Bleeding and Swelling. Slight oozing of blood from severed microvessels may be evident for several hours following surgery. When a little blood is mixed with saliva, it often appears to the patient as a lot of blood. If the patient is forewarned of this possibility, it goes a long way to reducing their anxiety. Slight swelling of the intraoral and extraoral tissues is a normal consequence of surgical trauma and leakage of blood from the severed microvessels. Proper compression of the surgical flap, both before and after suturing, greatly reduces postoperative bleeding and swelling.

Additional supportive therapy is the application of an ice pack, with firm pressure, to the facial area over the surgical site. Pressure and reduction of temperature slow the flow of blood and help to counteract the rebound phenomenon, which occurs following the use of a vasoconstrictor in the local anesthetic. Application of cold also acts as an effective analgesic as a result of its reduction in sensitivity of the peripheral nerve endings. The ice pack should be applied in a 20 minutes on and 20 minutes off cycle. This regimen should be repeated for 6 to 8 hours and should preferably be started in the surgeon's office with the use of a disposable instant chemical cold pack (Figure 12-52). Continuous application of cold should be avoided. This will initiate a physiologic mechanism that will result in an increase in blood flow to the site of cold application.[228]

If minor bleeding should persist for more than 12 hours following surgery, it can usually be managed by the patient with proper home care. At the time of surgery, the patient should be given several 2-inch × 2-inch gauze pads in a sterile pack (Figure 12-53). The patient should be instructed to slightly moisten one of the sterile gauze pads and to place it over the bleeding site while applying firm pressure. Pressure should be applied to the area for 10 to 15 minutes. Should the bleeding problem persist, the patient should be instructed to place a moist tea bag, or one of the gauze pads soaked in tea, over the bleeding area and to apply pressure in the same manner as before. Tannic acid, contained in tea, is known to be an effective hemostatic agent. If home treatment fails, the patient should be seen in the dental office, where the

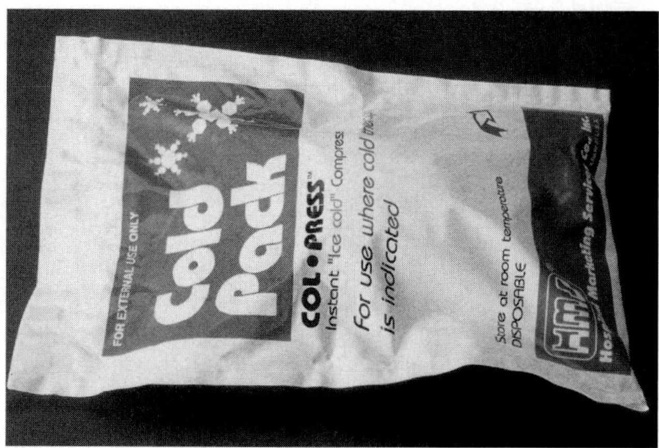

Figure 12-52 Col-Press (instant chemical cold pack), Hospital Marketing Service Co. Inc.

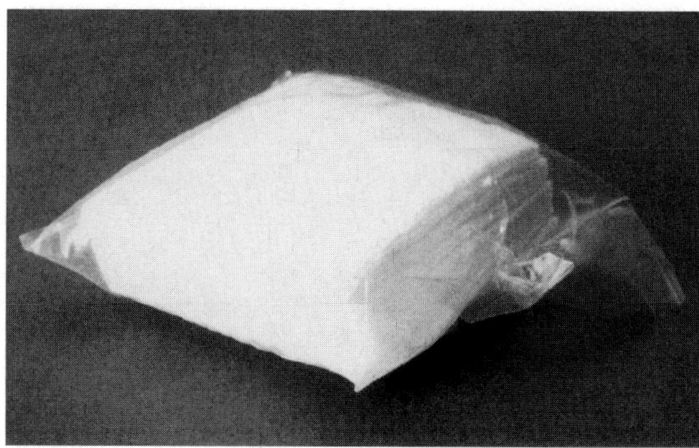

Figure 12-53 Several 2-inch × 2-inch sterile gauze pads sealed in plastic.

dentist can inject a local anesthetic agent containing 1:50,000 epinephrine and apply tissue compression to the bleeding area. Unless there is an undisclosed or undiagnosed bleeding disorder, this should resolve the problem.[2] The patient should be warned **not to take aspirin** for pain before surgery or afterward, but rather to take acetaminophen or ibuprofen.

Application of moist heat over the surgical site is recommended; **however, it should not begin until 24 hours following the surgery.** Heat promotes blood flow and enhances the inflammatory and healing processes. The application of moist heat is best accomplished by the use of a small cotton towel that has been moistened with hot tap water. The hot, moist towel should be applied to the surface of the face over the surgical area for about 30 minutes. The towel should be reheated with hot tap water every 5 to 10 minutes to maintain the temperature.

Discoloration. Discoloration of the mucoperiosteal and/or facial tissues following surgery is the result of the breakdown of blood that has leaked into the surrounding tissues. Again, patients should be made aware of the potential for postsurgical discoloration at the presurgical consultation visit and the information should be reinforced at the time of surgery (Figure 12-54). This ecchymosis can last for up to 2 weeks and is observed more in the elderly and in fair-complexioned patients. This is an esthetic problem only and requires no special treatment. In patients with ecchymosis, applications of moist heat may be beneficial for up to 2 weeks following surgery. Heat promotes fluid exchange and speeds resorption of discoloring agents from the tissues.[2]

Pain. In the majority of patients, pain following periradicular surgery is surprisingly minimal. Postsurgical pain is usually of short duration and most

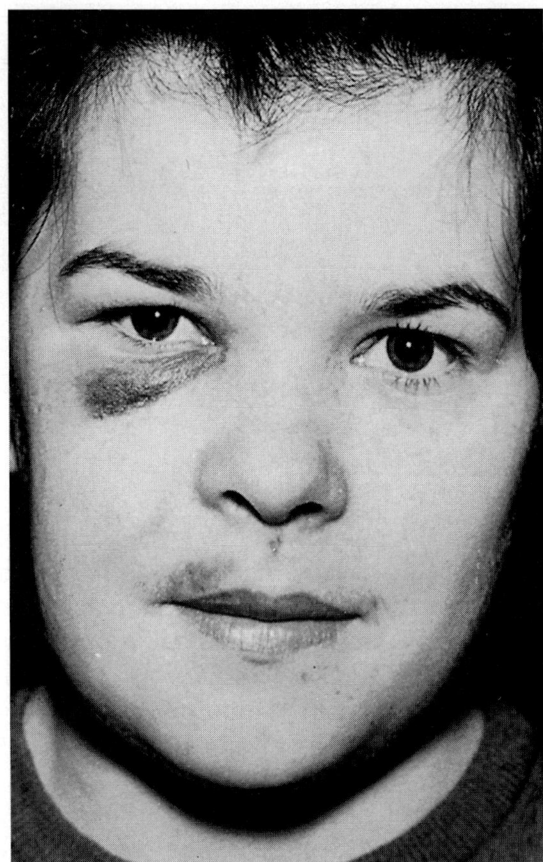

Figure 12-54 "Black eye" ecchymosis following periradicular surgery. Also note discoloration of upper lip.

often reaches its maximum intensity about 6 to 8 hours following surgery. A significant reduction in pain can usually be expected on the first postoperative day followed by a steady decrease in discomfort each day following surgery. It is unusual for a patient to experience pain that cannot be managed by mild to moderate analgesics.[229]

Another method of postsurgical pain control is the use of long-acting local anesthetic agents, such as bupivacaine (Marcaine) or etidocaine (Duranest), which provide 6 to 8 hours of local anesthesia and up to 10 hours of local analgesia.[230,231] Since these long-acting anesthetic agents contain a low concentration of vasoconstrictor (1:200,000), they are not suitable to be used alone in periradicular surgery. They can either be used before surgery, in conjunction with lidocaine 1:50,000 epinephrine, or at the conclusion of the surgical procedure before dismissal of the patient. The return of sensation is more gradual with the long-acting anesthetics than with the short-acting anesthetics; therefore, the onset of discomfort is less sudden.

Infection. Although endodontic surgery is performed in an area that is heavily populated with bacteria, postsurgical infections are rare. For this reason, peritreatment systemic antibiotic therapy is seldom required and is not considered part of routine postsurgical care in healthy patients. The most common causes of postsurgical infections following periradicular surgery are the result of inadequate aseptic techniques and improper soft-tissue reapproximation and stabilization. **These factors are under the direct control of the endodontic surgeon.**[2]

The clinical signs and symptoms of a postsurgical infection are usually evident 36 to 48 hours after surgery. The most common indications are progressively increasing pain and swelling. Suppuration, elevated temperature, and lymphadenopathy may or may not be present. Systemic antibiotic therapy should be initiated promptly, when indicated. The antibiotic of choice is penicillin V and the recommended dosage is 1.0 g as an initial dose, followed by a maintenance dose of 500 mg. The dosing interval should be every 3 to 4 hours, preferably without food. In patients allergic to penicillin, the antibiotic of choice is clindamycin with an initial dose of 600 mg, followed by a maintenance dose of 150 to 300 mg, depending on the age and weight of the patient. The dosing interval should be every 8 hours, preferably without food. The patient should be monitored every 24 hours and antibiotic therapy withdrawn as soon as the clinical condition indicates that the patient's host defenses have regained control of the infection and that the infection is resolving or has resolved. (For additional information see Chapter 18, "Pharmacology for Endodontics.")

Oral Hygiene. Oral hygiene often presents a postsurgical problem for many patients. A toothbrush should not be used as an aid to oral hygiene in the area of surgery until the day following surgery, and then only on the occlusal or incisal surfaces of the teeth. Use of a toothbrush in the surgical area may dislodge the mucoperiosteal flap and lead to serious postsurgical complications. A cotton swab soaked with chlorhexidine oral rinse (Peridex) or 3% hydrogen peroxide may be used to gently remove oral debris from the surgical area. A regimen of twice daily (morning and evening) rinsing with chlorhexidine oral rinse will provide an effective means for reduction of debris, decreasing the population of the oral microbial flora and inhibiting plaque formation. Chlorhexidine oral rinses should continue for 4 to 6 days following surgery (2 to 3 days following suture removal).

Suture Removal. According to Gutmann and Harrison, the key to preventing sutures from having a negative effect on wound healing following surgery is their early removal.[2] The primary purpose for placing sutures following endodontic surgery is to approximate the edges of the incisional wound and to provide stabilization until the epithelium and myofibroblast–fibronectin network provides a sufficient barrier to dislodgment of the flapped tissues. This usually occurs within 48 hours following surgery. It has been recommended that sutures should not be allowed to remain longer than 96 hours.

A suture removal kit should contain a cotton swab, 2-inch × 2-inch gauze sponges, suture scissors, cotton pliers, and a mouth mirror (Figure 12-55). The sutures and surrounding mucosa should be cleaned with a cotton swab containing a mild disinfectant followed by hydrogen peroxide. This helps to destroy bacteria and remove plaque and debris that have accumulated on the sutures, thus reducing the inoculation of bacteria into the underlying tissues as the suture is pulled through. **A topical anesthetic** should also be applied with a swab at the surgical site. This greatly reduces the discomfort associated with the placement of the scissors blade under the suture, a procedure that is particularly painful in areas of persistent swelling and edema, commonly seen in the mucobuccal fold.

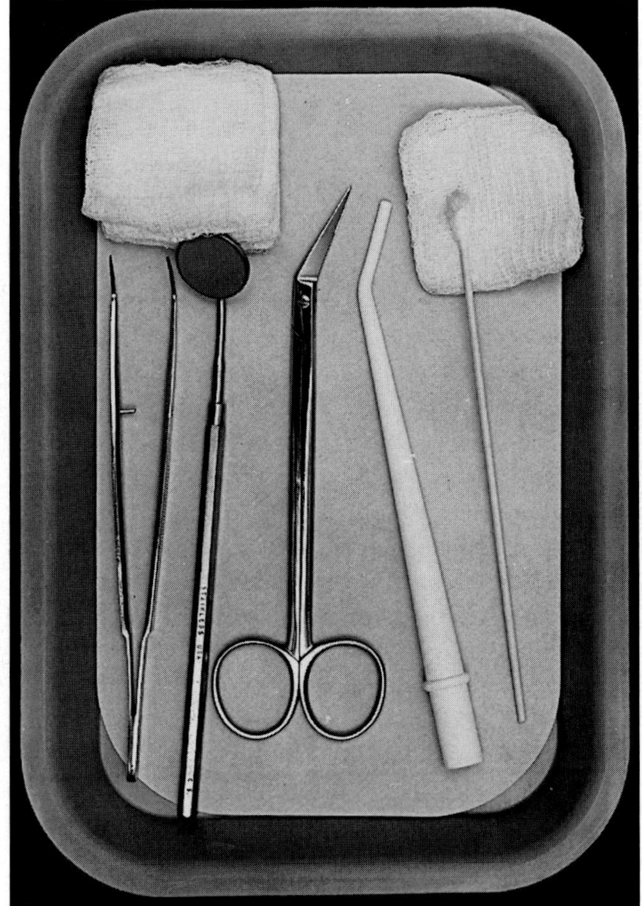

Figure 12-55 Suture removal kit should be presterilized and packaged, and it should contain all necessary instruments and auxiliary supplies needed for the procedure.

Sharp-pointed scissors are used to cut the suture material, followed by grasping the knotted portion with cotton pliers and removing the suture. Various designs of scissors are available and can be selected according to specific access needs in different areas of the mouth. It has been suggested that a No. 12 scalpel blade be used to sever the suture. The advantages are stated to be a predictably sharp cutting edge and less "tug" on the suture.[232]

Corrective Surgery

Corrective surgery is categorized as surgery involving the correction of defects in the body of the root other than the apex. When the coronal and middle thirds of the root are involved, it is imperative to physically observe, diagnose, and repair the defect. A full sulcular mucoperiosteal flap, such as the triangular or rectangular design, must be used to gain adequate visual and surgical access. Corrective surgical procedures may be necessary as a result of procedural accidents, resorption (internal or external), root caries, root fracture, and periodontal disease. Corrective surgery may involve periradicular surgery, root resection (removal of an entire root from a multirooted tooth leaving the clinical crown intact), hemisection (the separation of a multirooted tooth and the removal of a root and the associated portion of the clinical crown), or intentional replantation (extraction and replantation of the tooth into its alveolus after the corrective procedure has been done). Reparative defects of the root and associated procedures are classified as follows:

I. Perforation repair
   A. Mechanical
   B. Resorptive/caries

II. Periodontal repair
   A. Guided tissue regeneration
   B. Root resection/hemisection
   C. Surgical correction of the radicular lingual groove

Perforation Repair. *Mechanical.* Perforations are procedural accidents that can occur during root canal or postspace preparation. High potential areas for perforations are the pulp chamber floor of molars and the distal aspect of the mesial root of mandibular molars and the mesial buccal root of maxillary molars (strip perforations). When a perforation has occurred, the initial

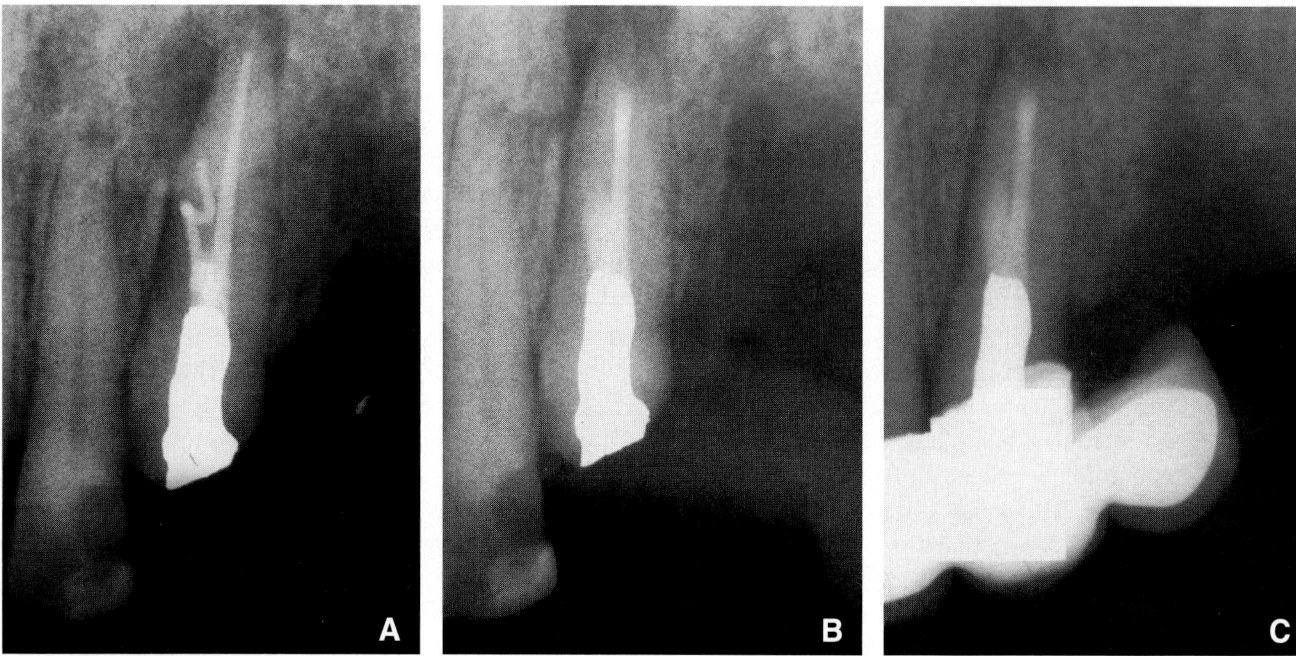

Figure 12-56 **A,** Lateral midroot perforation with extruded filling material. **B,** Radiograph following surgical removal of extruded filling material, root-end resection, root-end fill, and repair of perforation defect with mineral trioxide aggregate (MTA). **C,** Radiograph 2 years following surgery.

attempt at correction should be an internal repair (see chapter 14, "Endodontic Mishaps: Their Detection, Correction, and Prevention"). Corrective surgery should be reserved for those teeth when internal repair is not a treatment option or when internal repair has failed.

"Strip perforations" that occur on the distal aspect of the mesial roots of maxillary and mandibular molars are usually inaccessible and extremely difficult to repair surgically. Visual and surgical access is limited, and bone removal necessary to obtain access to the site of the perforation usually results in a major periodontal defect. This type of clinical situation may be better managed by intentional replantation, root resection, or hemisection.

Midroot perforations, such as those resulting from postspace preparations, should be immediately sealed internally, if possible, or calcium hydroxide should be placed as an intracanal dressing and sealed at a subsequent appointment. If the perforation is excessively large or long-standing, a full mucoperiosteal flap should be reflected, the perforation site identified, and the repair made with an appropriate repair material (Figure 12-56). If the perforation is located in the apical third of the root, a root-end resection, extending to

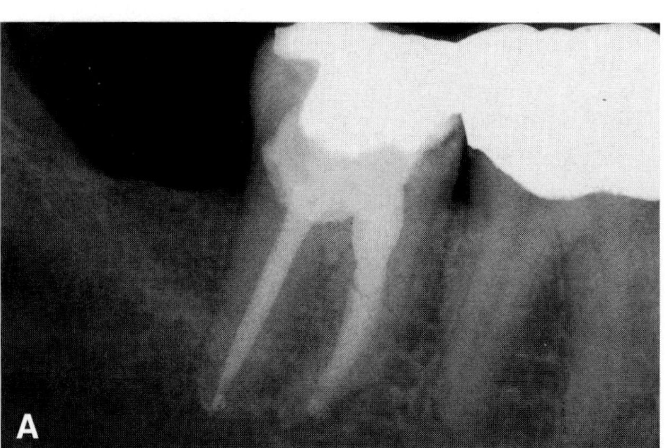

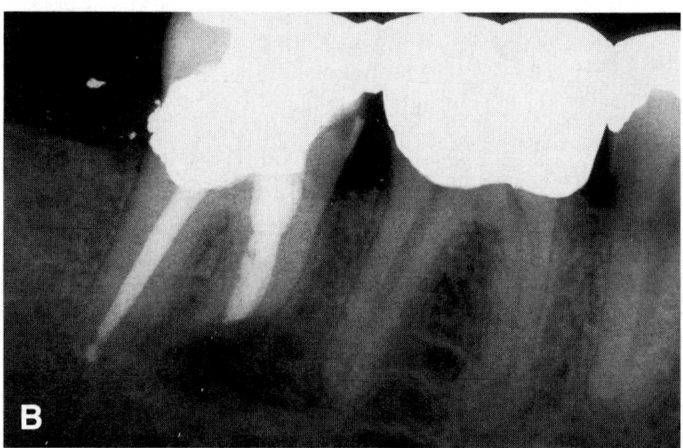

Figure 12-57 **A,** Lateral perforation of the apical one-third of the mesial root of tooth No. 31. **B,** Root-end resection of mesial root. Root canal was obturated with mineral trioxide aggregate (MTA).

the point of the perforation, and a root-end filling should be considered as a more effective and efficient way of handling this clinical situation (Figure 12-57).

Resorption (External or Internal) and Root Caries. Repair of a defect on the root surface, from either internal or external resorption, depends to a large extent on whether there is communication between the resorptive defect and the oral cavity and/or the pulp space. When communication between the defect and the oral cavity exists, a corrective surgical procedure is usually necessary. When the resorptive defect has also communicated with the pulp space, excessive and persistent hemorrhage into the pulp space is usually evident during root canal instrumentation. This makes cleaning, shaping, and obturation of the pulp space very difficult, unless surgical repair of the resorptive defect is done first. If the decision is made to repair the root defect before filling the pulp space, after the pulp tissue has been removed, a **temporary, easily removable filling** should be placed in the root canal space. A large gutta-percha point may be used for this purpose; no sealer is used. This will serve as an internal matrix to prevent the repair material from obstructing the root canal. Depending on the setting time of the repair material used, the pulp space may be prepared and obturated at the same appointment. Otherwise, an intracanal dressing of calcium hydroxide should be placed, the access cavity sealed from oral contamination, and the pulp space prepared and obturated at a subsequent appointment (Figure 12-58).

In the case of a resorptive defect that opens into the gingival sulcus, the approach depends to a great extent on the location and the extent of the defect. If it is approachable from the buccal or facial side, a full mucoperiosteal flap should be raised, and the extent of the defect established. If the resorptive **defect has not extended into the pulp space**, it should be restored with a suitable material, such as amalgam, composite resin, or glass ionomer cement. If the **defect has extended into the pulp space**, the flap should be repositioned and stabilized with a suture. A rubber dam should be placed and a conventional coronal access preparation followed by removal of the pulp tissue and placement of **a temporary internal matrix** should be done. Following this, the rubber dam should be removed, the flap elevated, the resorptive defect repaired, and the flap repositioned and stabilized with sutures. The temporary internal canal matrix should be removed and the root canal preparation and obturation completed or a calcium hydroxide intracanal dressing placed and the endodontic treatment completed at a subsequent appointment.

If the resorptive defect opens into the gingival sulcus on the lingual or palatal surface of the tooth, surgical and visual access are much more difficult. A sulcular lingual or palatal flap can be raised to explore the extent of the defect. **Vertical incisions on the lingual side of the mandible should be avoided whenever possible** because of the fragile nature of this tissue. If the resorptive defect is surgically accessible, treatment can proceed as described earlier. If it is not accessible, then intentional replantation or extraction should be considered.

Some cases of resorption or root caries are so extensive that nothing can be done to save the entire tooth. Extraction may be the solution for some cases, or total root amputation or hemisection may apply to others. A case in point calling for hemisection is illustrated in Figure 12-59. Internal–external resorption has destroyed virtually one half of a lower first molar, a terminal tooth in the arch, with opposing occlusion. Probing with a cowhorn explorer and viewing the radiograph reveals the massive lesion and defect (Figure 12-59, A and B). The crown of the tooth is sectioned buccolingually with a high-speed fissure bur (Figure 12-59, C–E). The mesial crown and root are then extracted, and immediate root canal therapy is completed in the remaining distal root (Figure 12-59, F and G). A premolar rubber dam clamp may be used on the remaining "bicuspidized" distal root of the molar. The remaining tooth structure and edentulous space should be restored with a fixed partial denture as soon as possible to prevent mesial drift of the distal root (Figure 12-59, H). This provides for function against the maxillary opponent(s), thereby preventing continual eruption.

Periodontal Repair. *Guided Tissue (Bone) Regeneration.* In the past, extensive periodontal defects required extraction or root amputation. Today, with techniques of guided bone regeneration and demineralized freeze-dried bone allografts, many teeth that were previously untreatable can be saved. Several authors have published reports on the effectiveness of the use calcium sulfate, alone and as a composite with an allograft material, and resorbable and nonresorbable barrier membranes, with and without allografts, on the quality and quantity of alveolar bone regeneration in endodontic and periodontic defects. Many of these case reports have had mixed results.[233–238]

Few controlled clinical studies comparing the results of the use of guided bone regeneration techniques have been reported. Santamaria and associates reported on a controlled clinical study to determine the degree of bone regeneration following radicular cyst enucleation. Thirty patients were involved in the study. The control group consisted of enucleation of the cyst only and the

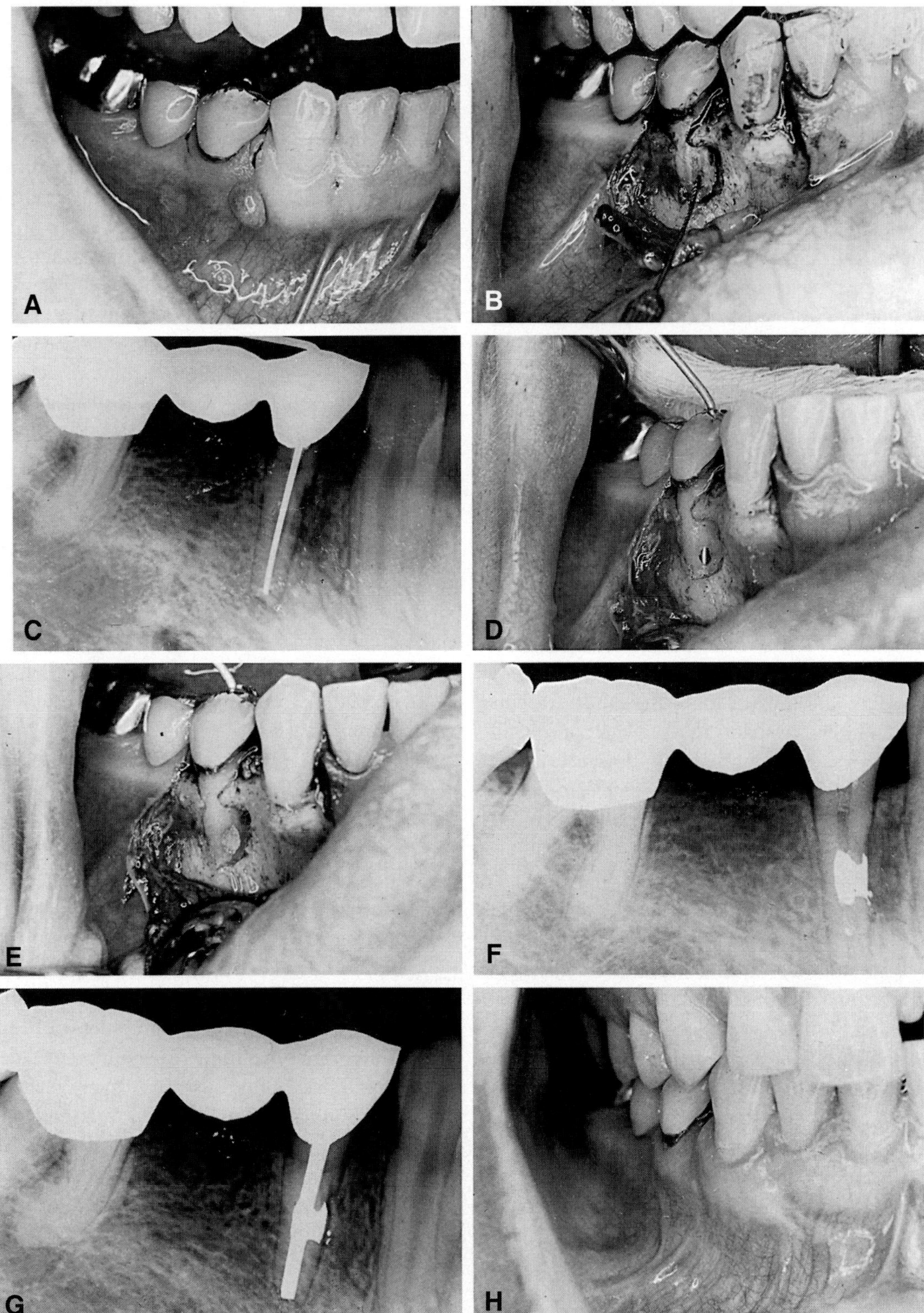

Figure 12-58 Corrective surgical repair of root-resorptive defect. **A,** Constant drainage mesial to first premolar bridge abutment. Internal and external resorption revealed in radiograph. **B,** Elevating rectangular flap uncovers huge dehiscence and resorptive defect Instrument placed into defect proves connection with pulp lesion. **C,** Conventional occlusal endodontic cavity is prepared and pulpectomy is performed. Internal matrix of endodontic silver point is placed. **D,** Internal matrix in place and hemorrhage controlled. **E,** Amalgam filling inserted into external resorptive defect. Non-zinc alloy is used. **F,** Silver point is immediately removed and flap repositioned and sutured. Because of time constraints in this particular case, canal enlargement and obliteration are completed at subsequent appointment. **G,** Radiograph 9 months following therapy. Repair of bone is apparent. **H,** Photograph 9 months following therapy. Note complete repair of draining stoma and incisions. (Courtesy of Dr. David Yankowitz.)

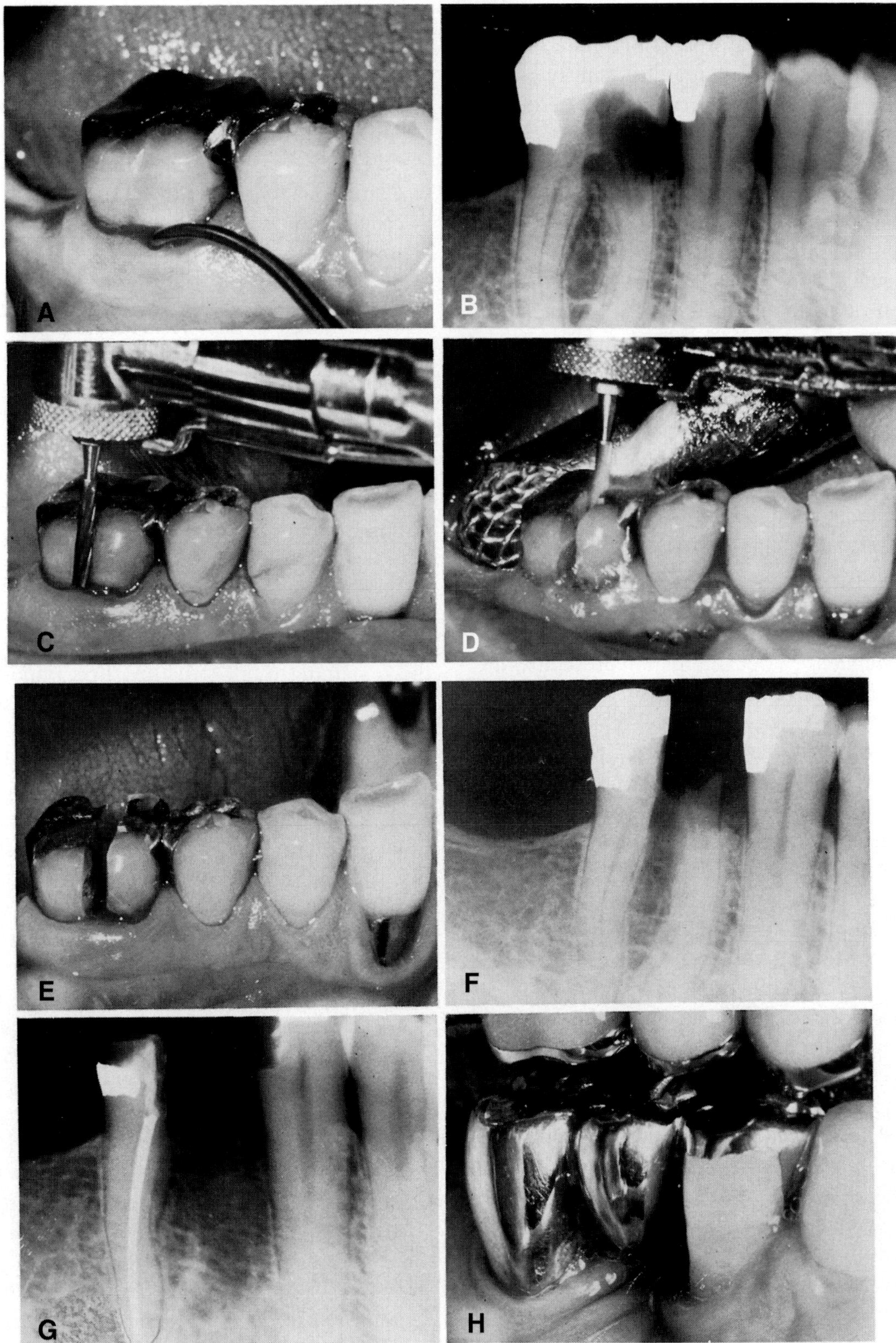

Figure 12-59 Technique for hemisecting and restoring mandibular molar. A, Using cowhorn explorer, resorptive lesion and relation to crest of alveolar process are established. B, Huge area of internal resorption involving mesial half of molar. C, Extra long #559-XL fissure bur has length or reach necessary to cut entirely through crown to furca. D, Tooth is sectioned from buccal to lingual with copious water and aspiration. E, Sectioning completed. Base of cut must terminate at alveolar crest. F, Hemisected mandibular molar. Pathologic mesial half is ready for extraction. Accuracy of sectioning is shown by radiograph. G, Care must be exercised not to gouge remaining distal portion. Root canal therapy is completed at same dental appointment. Teeth are ready for immediate restoration. H, Importance of restoration for contact with opposite arch is here demonstrated. (Restoration by Dr. Milan V. Starks.)

experimental groups involved enucleation of the cyst plus the use of either a resorbable or nonresorbable membrane. The residual volume and density of the newly formed tissue were measured by computer-assisted tomography and computer-assisted digital image analysis before and after enucleation. No statistically significant difference was noted in the volume or density of the newly formed tissue between the three treatment groups 6 months postsurgically. The results suggested that guided bone regeneration using membranes does not contribute to increased quality or quantity of bone regeneration in this clinical situation.[239]

Pecora and associates reported on a controlled clinical study involving 20 patients with large endodontic bony lesions that failed to respond to nonsurgical endodontic treatment. Following curettement of the lesions, 10 sites were covered with Gortex membranes before repositioning the flap, and 10 were left uncovered. The investigators reported that radiographic analysis of the lesions 12 months postsurgically revealed that the quality and quantity of the regenerated bone were superior when the **Gortex membranes** were used.[240]

Root Amputation. Root amputation procedures are a logical way to eliminate a weak, diseased root to allow the stronger root(s) to survive when, if retained together, they would collectively fail. Selected root removal allows improved access for home care and plaque control with resultant bone formation and reduced pocket depth. The incorporation of one half or two-thirds of a tooth can be instrumental in obviating the need for a long-span fixed partial or a removable partial denture. Quite often, amputation of a hopelessly involved root of an abutment tooth saves an entire fixed prosthesis, even one that is full arch in extent.

As always, case selection is an important factor in success. Proper diagnosis, treatment planning, case presentation, and good restorative procedures are all critical factors equally important to the resective procedure itself. The strategic value of the tooth involved must be convincing.

Evaluation of the involved tooth requires thorough periodontal evaluation of the root or roots to be retained. Remaining structures need continuing periodontal care, and this should be pointed out to the patient. Bony support, the crown–root ratio, occlusal relations, and restorability of the remaining segment all determine the case outcome.

INDICATIONS FOR ROOT AMPUTATION:

1. Existence of periodontal bone loss to the extent that periodontal therapy and patient maintenance do not sufficiently improve the condition.
2. Destruction of a root through resorptive processes, caries, or mechanical perforations.
3. Surgically inoperable roots that are calcified, contain separated instruments, or are grossly curved.
4. The fracture of one root that does not involve the other.
5. Conditions that indicate the surgery will be technically feasible to perform and the prognosis is reasonable.

CONTRAINDICATIONS FOR ROOT AMPUTATIONS:

1. Lack of necessary osseous support for the remaining root or roots.
2. Fused roots or roots in unfavorable proximity to each other.
3. Remaining root or roots endodontically inoperable.
4. Lack of patient motivation to properly perform home-care procedures.

MORPHOLOGIC FACTORS: The length, width, and contour of the roots are important factors in determining where the resective cut is made and the strength of the remaining tooth structure. It is important to be aware of the normal and varied anatomy that may be encountered as these factors will materially affect the procedures of root separation and removal. A careful check of the radiograph and probing of periodontal pockets will help to reveal tooth-to-tooth and root-to-root proximities, as well as morphologic characteristics, such as root size and curvature, furcal location, and fused roots (Figure 12-60).

Two different approaches to resection are available. One approach is to amputate horizontally or obliquely the involved root at the point where it joins the crown, a process termed **root amputation** (Figure 12-61). The other approach is to cut vertically the entire tooth in half—from mesial to distal of the crown in the maxillary molars, and from buccal to lingual of the crown in the mandibular molars—removing in either case the pathologic root and its associated portion of the crown. This procedure is termed **hemisection** (Figure 12-62).

Bisection or **"bicuspidization"** refers to a division of the crown that **leaves the two halves** and their respective roots. This bisection is designed to form a more favorable position for the remaining segments that leaves them easier to clean and maintain (Figure 12-63). If the remaining roots are too close to each other, minor orthodontic movement may be necessary to properly align them. The careful preparation and restoration of the remaining portions of the tooth to minimize food entrapment and plaque accumulation are critical to the long-term success in this situation.

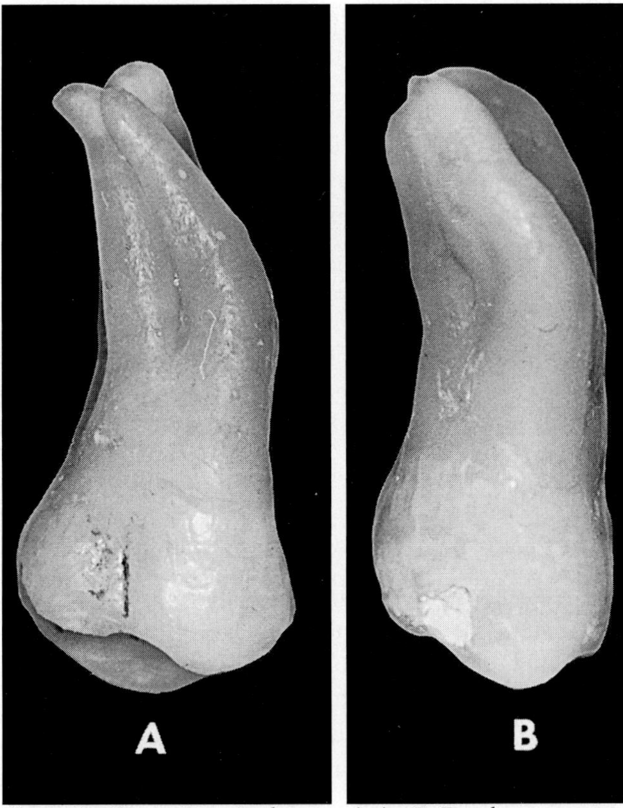

Figure 12-60 A, Roots in close proximity. B, Fused roots are very difficult to resect. Extraction must be considered.

PROCEDURAL SEQUENCE: Following diagnosis and treatment planning, but before resection, endodontic therapy should be done on the roots to be retained. The occlusion should be adjusted to eliminate the trauma of lateral excursions. After the canals of the roots to be retained have been filled, a post (or posts) should be placed when indicated and/or a core should be placed in the pulp chamber and the access cavity. Following the set of the core material, the resection procedure may be done.

AMPUTATION TECHNIQUE FOR MAXILLARY MOLARS: Maxillary molars typically have mesiobuccal roots that are relatively broad buccolingually, narrow mesiodistally, and extend about two-thirds of the distance to the palatal root. Distobuccal roots, however, are much more conical in shape and extend about one half the distance to the palatal root. The length of the palatal root and its considerable thickness impart great stability to this tooth. If occlusal alignment and periodontal factors are favorable, the palatal root can be restored successfully on its own.

The amputation procedure itself is best performed with a surgical-length smooth fissure bur. Length of the cutting portion of the fissure bur is important and especially critical in mesiobuccal roots of maxillary molars

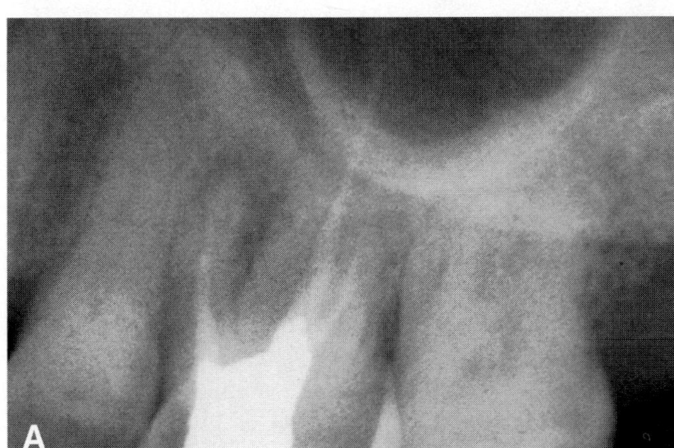

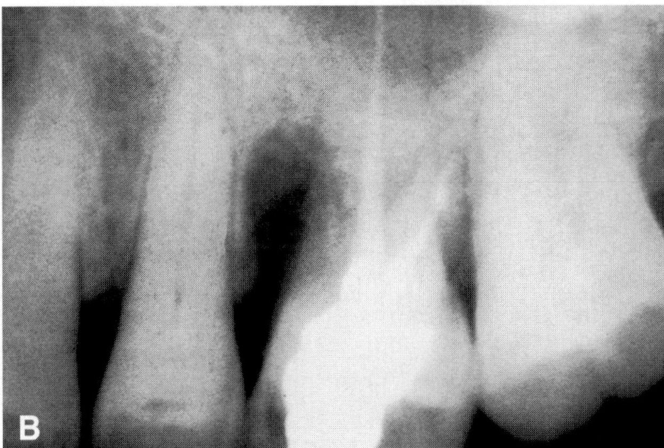

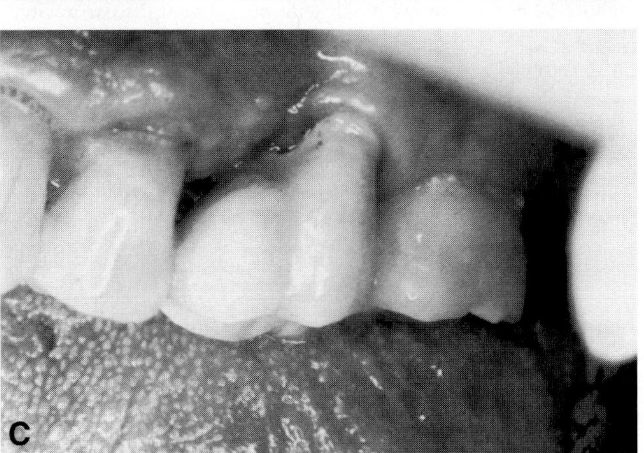

Figure 12-61 A, Periradicular lesion consistent with possible vertical root fracture. B, Mesiobuccal root amputation due to vertical root fracture. C, Clinical crown restored with porcelain-fused-to-metal prosthetic crown.

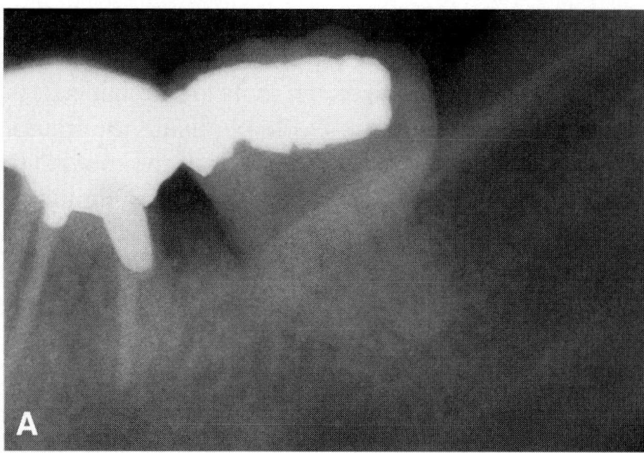

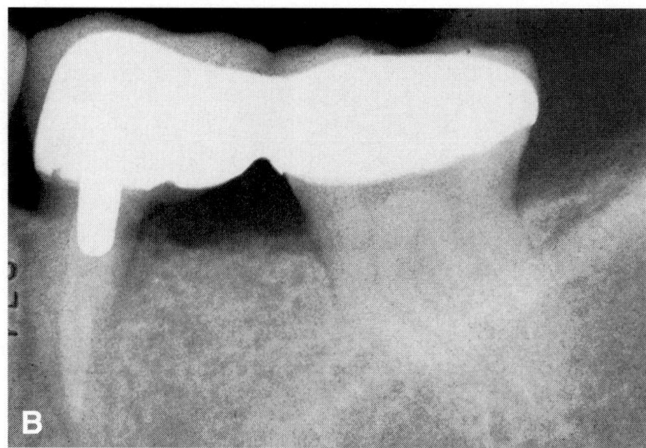

Figure 12-62 **A,** Postspace perforation on distal aspect of mandibular first molar resulting in a periodontal defect. **B,** Hemisection and distal root amputation. Note the molars have been splinted together.

and vertical resections through the crown and the furcation. Kirchoff and Gerstein suggested reshaping the crown with a bur so that the crown structure over the root to be removed is resected along with the root. This simplifies the task by making the root-furcation junction more visible for separation and extraction.[241]

To resect a root involving a tooth that is an abutment for a fixed partial denture or has previously been crowned and a new restoration has not been planned, the endodontic surgeon must do the resection horizontally or at an oblique angle. The more vertical the resective cut, the greater the ease of maintaining cleanliness.

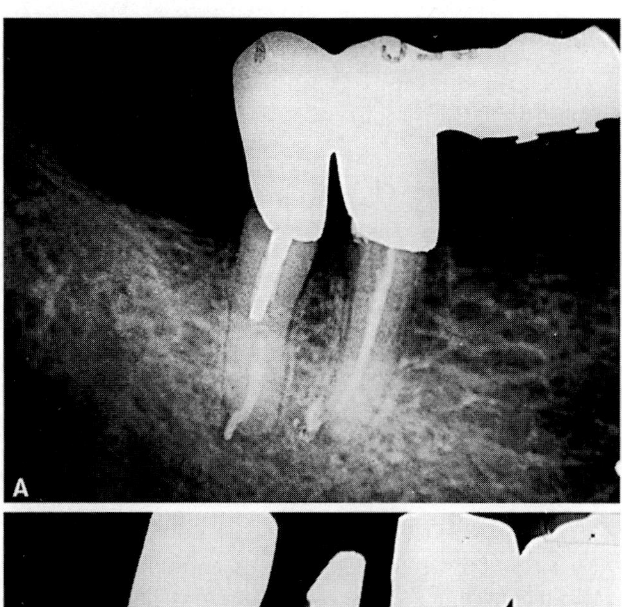

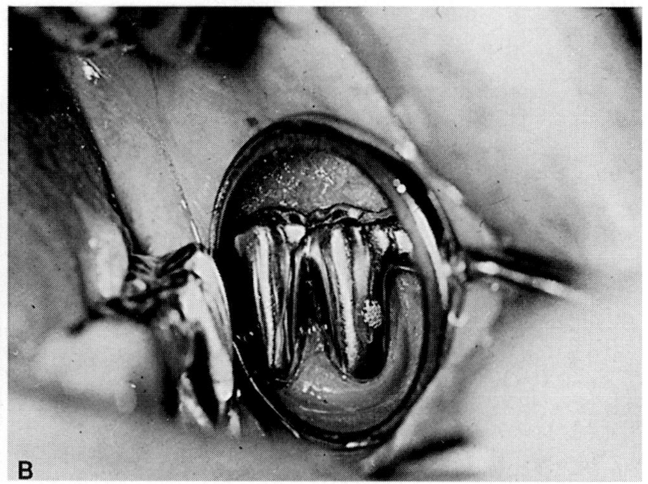

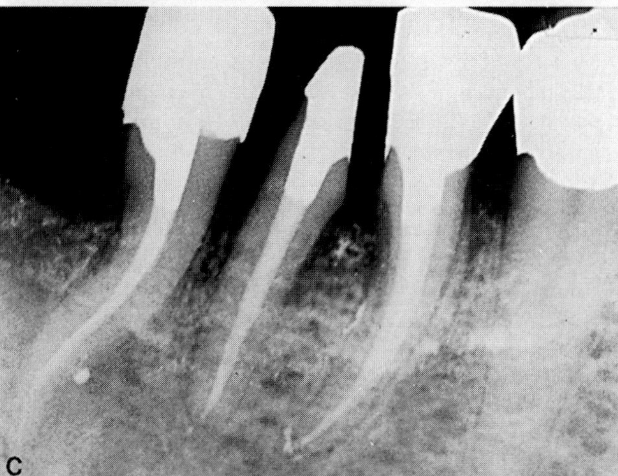

Figure 12-63 Terminal molar with periodontal disease involving furca, to be used as bridge abutment. **A,** Canals obturated with softened gutta-percha and tooth bisected. **B,** Mirror view of buccal shows how tissue may now be maintained as interdental papilla. *C,* Different case; hemisection of second molar and bisection of first molar provides three sturdy abutments for terminal bridge. (**A** and **B** courtesy of Dr. James D. Zidell; **C** courtesy of Dr. L. Stephen Buchanan.)

Care must be exercised in maintaining the correct angulation of the bur to avoid gouging the remaining root or crown.

When the root to be removed has been completely resected, there may be enough loss of periradicular bone to permit it to be lifted or elevated from the socket (Figure 12-64). It is possible, however, that sufficient periradicular bone and cortical plate remain such that reflecting a mucoperiosteal flap is necessary so that sufficient bone can be removed to facilitate root removal. Elevation of a flap also allows for osseous recontouring.

Recontouring of the crown at the point of resection is very important. Plain fissure burs and tapered diamond stones are ideal for this reshaping process. The junction of the crown with the furcation should be smooth, with a gradual taper toward the interdental embrasure. There should not be any semblance of a stump left, and enough clearance between the undersurface of the crown and the tissue should be established to facilitate good oral hygiene. Following root amputation, oral hygiene can be enhanced by the use of a small round brush (Figure 12-65). The patient should be instructed in its use and monitored postsurgically for proper effectiveness.

AMPUTATION TECHNIQUE FOR MANDIBULAR MOLARS: Treatment planning is critical when evaluating mandibular molars for root amputation. If the tooth is not a terminal tooth in the arch or an abutment for a fixed partial denture, extraction and replacement may be a preferred treatment. Some outstanding successes, however, are seen involving hemisection and placement of a three-unit fixed partial denture (see Figure 12-68).

The most common method of root amputation involving **mandibular molar teeth** is a **hemisection.** A terminal second mandibular molar is ideally suited for hemisection, provided there is opposing occlusion and adequate bone support for the remaining root (Figure 12-66). The remaining root and crown structure is restored as a premolar.

The root to be retained undergoes endodontic therapy. A post is placed in the retained root, if indicated, or a coronal–radicular core is placed. Following set of

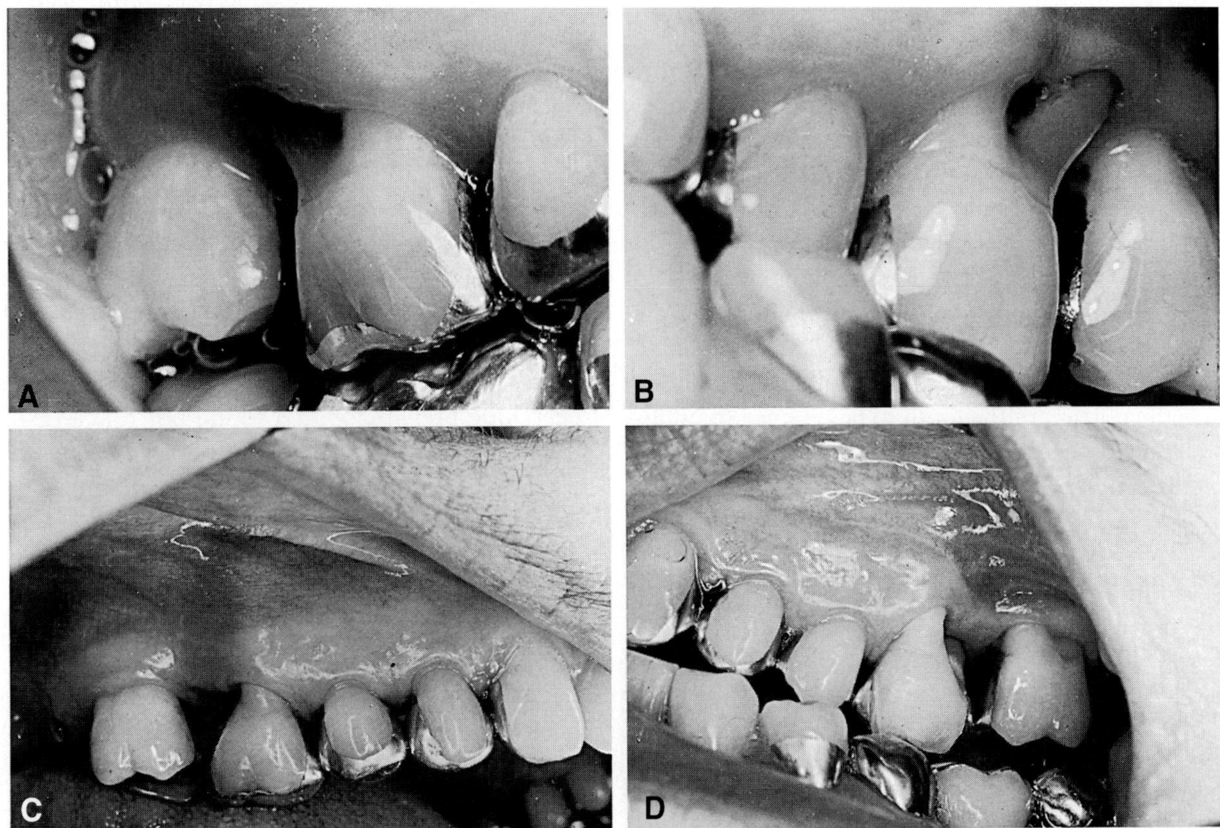

Figure 12-64 Excellent example of bilateral oblique root amputation on the same patient. **A,** Right maxillary first molar before root canal therapy and root amputation. Distobuccal root has lost its entire bony support. Because furca is exposed, flap need not be raised to amputate this root. **B,** Result 6 years after amputation. Occlusal table has been narrowed considerably. **C,** Left maxillary first molar in same patient with bony housing of distobuccal root completely destroyed. **D,** Result 6 years following root canal therapy and amputation; patient is meticulous in home care.

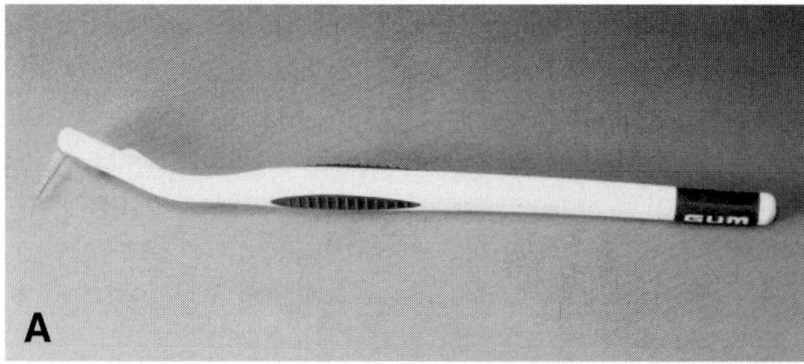

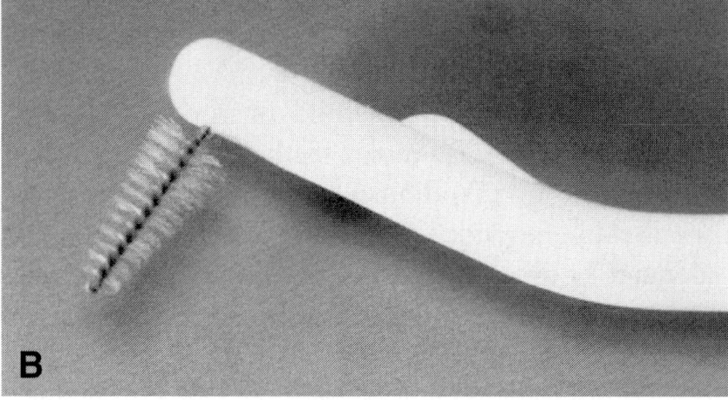

Figure 12-65 **A,** Cleaning aids such as the Butler Proxabrush (John O. Butler Co., Chicago, Il.) are important to good maintenance care. **B,** Close-up of Proxabrush head.

the core material, a sharp cowhorn explorer is used to identify the location of the buccal and lingual furcations (see Figure 12-59, A). Depending on the degree of periodontal bone loss and the thickness of the trunk of the tooth, a mucoperiosteal flap may or may not need to be raised. The coronal sectioning should be done with a fissure bur or a small tapered diamond stone in a high-speed handpiece. The cut should be initiated on the buccal surface and should section the tooth at the expense of the portion of the crown that is scheduled to be removed. Sufficient proximal furcal floor should be left on the portion of the tooth to be retained to establish a restorative finish line as well as sufficient crown for retention.

An elevator should be placed between the two halves of the crown and gently rotated to determine if the separation is complete. Once this has been verified, the pathologic root is gently removed with forceps or eased out with an elevator. Sterile gauze should be **packed into the socket** while the final contouring of the remaining coronal tooth structure is completed. This will prevent particles of tooth and restorative material from gaining entrance into the open socket. After all coronal contouring is completed, the gauze packing should be removed and, if a flap was elevated, it should be repositioned and stabilized with sutures.

Bisection or "bicuspidization" should be considered in mandibular molars in which periodontal disease has invaded the bifurcation and when repair of internal furcation perforations has been unsuccessful. The type of coronal section is similar to that used for hemisection except the location of the cut is centered in the furcation so as to evenly divide the crown. The furca is then turned into an interproximal space where the tissue is more manageable by the patient (see Figure 12-63).

Single root amputation of mandibular molar teeth (leaving the crown intact) may, on occasion, be indicated where a splint or fixed partial denture is in place. For the most part, however, an uneven exertion of occlusal forces tends to exert an unnatural force on the remaining root, thereby resulting in root fracture. Some teeth are treated successfully by single root amputation, but the length of tooth retention is unpredictable (Figure 12-67).

A tooth that is hopelessly involved, yet is a nonterminal member of a fixed partial denture, may be converted into a pontic by total amputation of its root or roots. Premolars are the most commonly involved teeth in this situation. Following pulpectomy, the canal orifice(s) are prepared with a round bur to a level below the gingival margin. The entire access cavity is filled with amalgam or composite resin following dentin

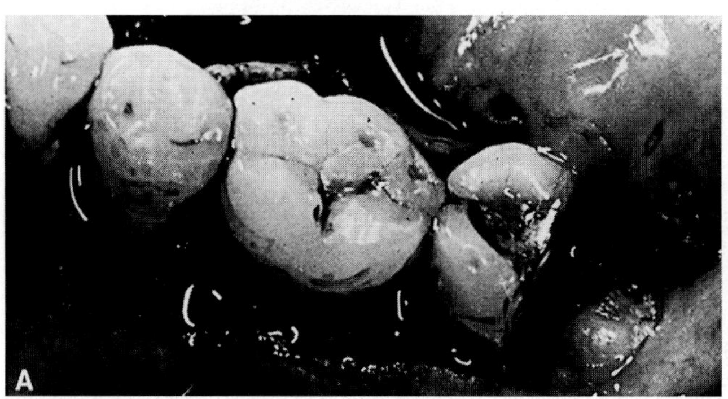

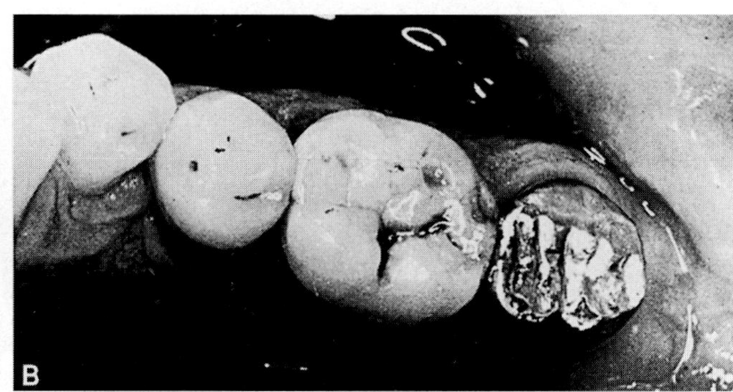

Figure 12-66 Terminal molar, hemisected and bicuspidized. **A,** Distal half of tooth removed. **B,** Final full crown restoration contacts both adjacent and opposing molars.

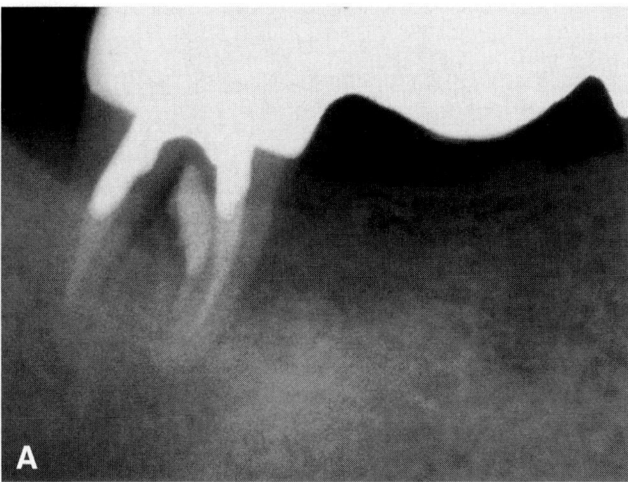

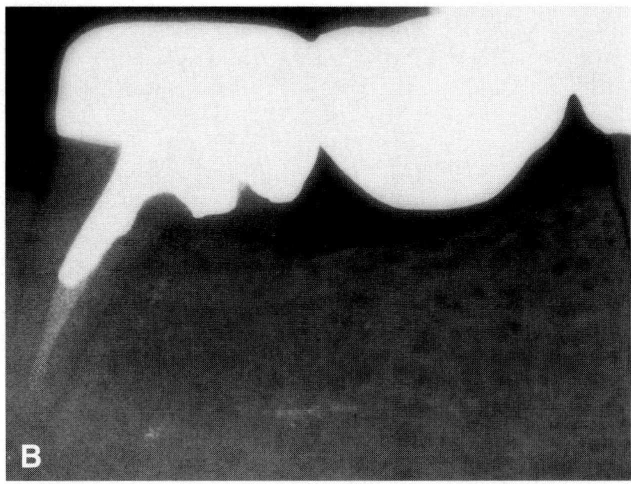

Figure 12-67 Mesial root amputation of a mandibular molar involving the distal abutment of a fixed partial denture. **A,** Root perforation with root canal filling material and bone loss in the furcation. **B,** Radiograph taken 5 years following mesial root amputation.

bonding. A buccal/facial marginal mucoperiosteal flap is raised, and the entire root is resected at a level well below the gingival margin. The remaining tooth structure should be contoured in a convex shape to resemble a pontic. The severed root should be removed to the buccal side of the alveolar bone and the flap repositioned and stabilized with appropriate sutures.

Several studies have evaluated the long-term success of root-resected and hemisected teeth. The results range from a success rate of 62 to 100% occurring over times ranging from 1 to 23 years. Combining the data from these studies indicates an overall success rate of 88% for the time periods followed.[242–251] Long-term prognosis of teeth with roots totally amputated or hemisected depends on the quality of the original surgery and recontouring of the remaining tooth structure, on the quality of the root canal treatment in the remaining root or roots, on the quality of the final restoration, on the quality and quantity of the remaining supporting bone, and on the status of periodontal care. Any one, or combination, of these factors may cause failure of the case. When all of these elements are well executed, a superb and long-lasting result may be achieved (Figure 12-68).

Surgical Correction of the Radicular Lingual Groove. Another serious periodontal defect that can sometimes be corrected surgically is the radicular lingual groove (palatogingival groove). Found almost exclusively in maxillary lateral and central incisors, this developmental defect in root formation precludes the deposition of cementum in the groove; hence it prevents periodontal ligament (PDL) attachment. The groove then causes a narrow periodontal pocket, a bacterial pathway, often to the root apex, that can lead to retroinfection of the pulp.[92]

Prevalence of these grooves may be higher than previously suspected. After examining 921 maxillary incisors, Pecora and his associates in Sao Paulo reported a 2% incidence in central incisors and a 2.6% incidence in lateral incisors. Most of the central incisor grooves, however, were found on the facial surface.[252] Goon and his associates at the University of the Pacific in San Francisco reported on an unusual **facial** radicular groove in a maxillary lateral incisor.[253]

Robinson and Cooley have suggested a surgical intervention that may, in a number of cases, correct the defect and allow healing.[254] Following a palatal surgical exposure of the defect, the groove is eliminated by grinding it away with round burs or diamond points. Shallow grooves are handled differently from deep grooves (Figure 12-69). If the lingual groove, however, is so deep that it communicates with the pulp space, the case is hopeless and extraction of the tooth is indicated.[92]

REPLACEMENT SURGERY (EXTRACTION/REPLANTATION)

Grossman, in 1982, defined intentional replantation as "the act of deliberately removing a tooth and—following examination, diagnosis, endodontic manipulation, and repair—returning the tooth to its original socket."[255] Extraction/replantation is by no means a recently developed procedure. Abulcasis, an Arabian physician practicing in the eleventh century, is the first credited with recording the principle of extraction/replantation.[256] Over the years since then, many authors have published reports of studies and case reports dealing with the technique and results of extraction/replantation.[257–261]

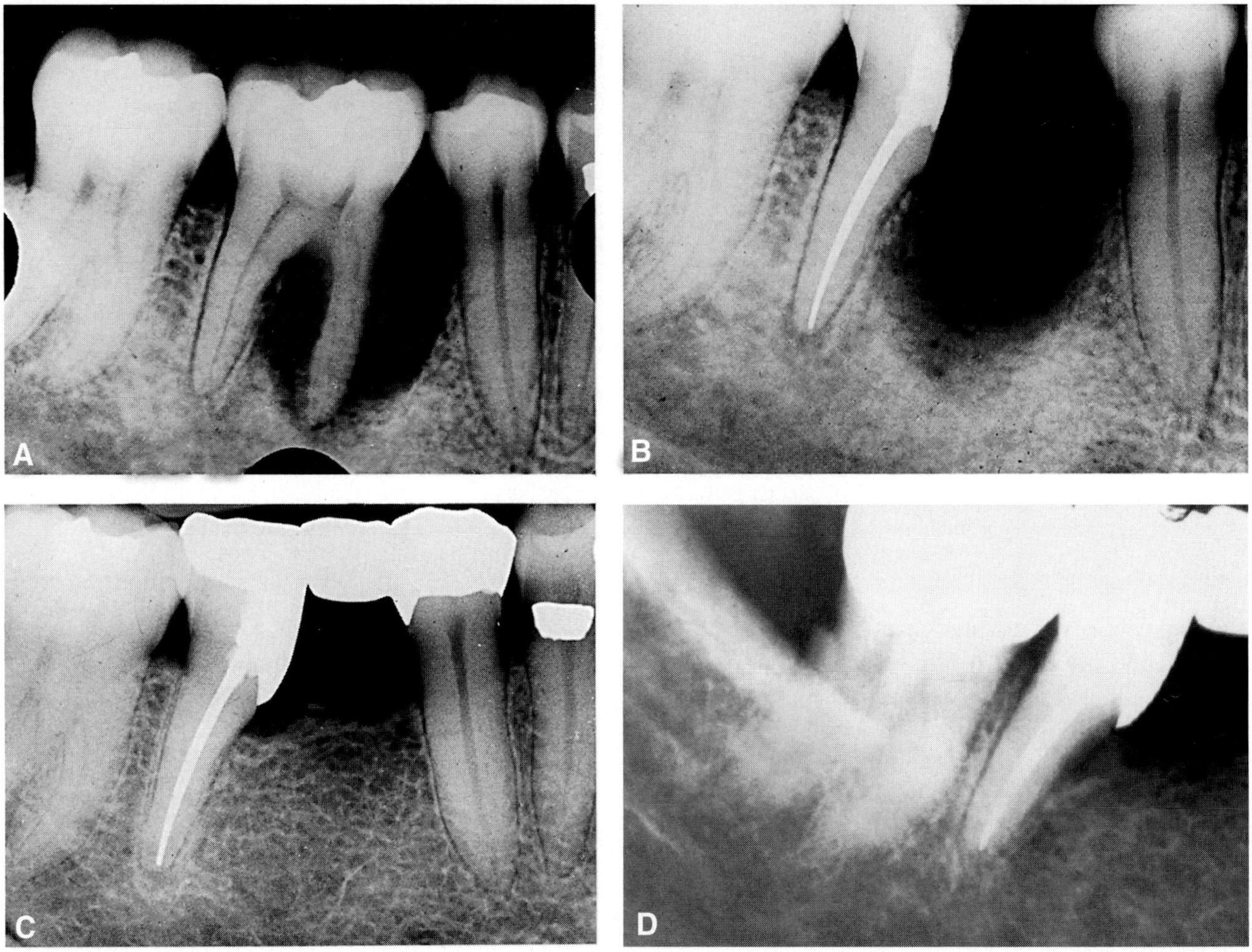

Figure 12-68 Hemisection of mandibular molar. A, Decision to hemisect molar and restore space relates to open contacts and future drifting. B, Tooth is hemisected through furca, and pathologic root removed. Root canal filling of remaining distal root is done at the same appointment through exposed pulp chamber. C, Final restoration of space converts first molar into a premolar. D, Forty-seven-year recall film attests to the meticulous therapy and long-range efficacy of this case. (Endodontic therapy by Dr. Dudley Glick and restoration by Dr. James McPherson.)

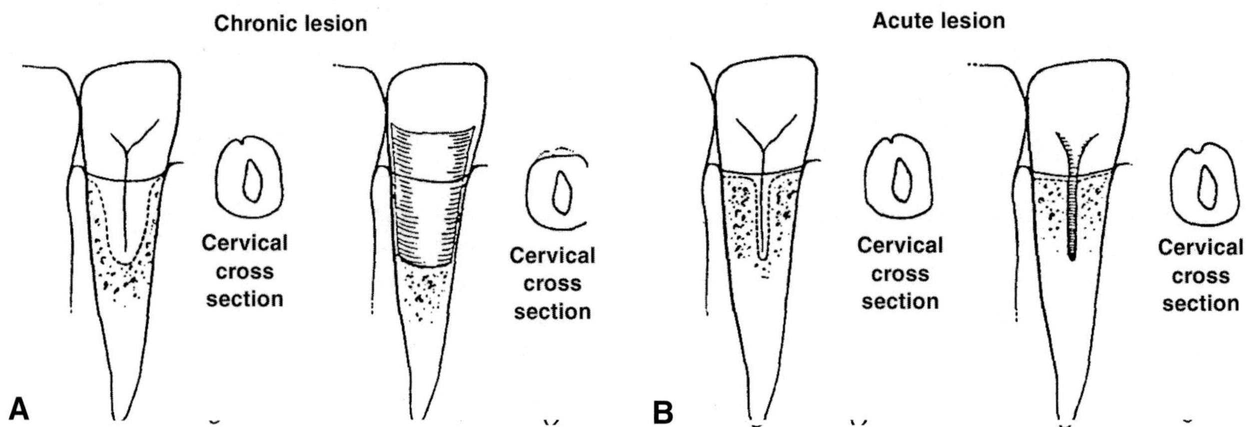

Figure 12-69 Surgical exposure of palatogingival groove allows "saucerization" with diamond stones or burs to remove pathologic groove. A, Illustration of the chronic lesion (**left**) and saucerization to eliminate the lingual groove (**right**). The cross-section shows the contour of the lingual surface with the groove (**left**) and after it has been removed. B, An acute lesion may result in less bone loss than a chronic lesion. In this situation, it may be possible to eliminate the groove without flattening the entire lingual surface. The cross-section illustrates the contour of the lingual surface as it might appear with the groove (**left**) and its contour after removal (**right**). Reproduced with permission from Robison SF, Cooley RL. Gen Dent 1988;36:340.

Indications

It is generally accepted that extraction/replantation is an acceptable treatment alternative when nonsurgical endodontic treatment is either impossible or has not been successful and periradicular surgery is inadvisable because of poor visual and/or surgical access or the danger of surgical damage to adjacent anatomic structures (mandibular canal, mental foramen). Dryden and Arens have stated that extraction/replantation should not be suggested as a routine treatment but should be considered only as a treatment of last resort. They also suggested the following as **indications for extraction/replantation**[262]:

1. Inadequate interocclusal space to perform nonsurgical endodontic treatment caused by the patient's limited range of motion of the temporomandibular joint and associated muscles.
2. Nonsurgical treatment and/or re-treatment are not feasible because of canal obstructions (ie, calcification of the pulp space, posts, separated instruments, impassable ledges).
3. Surgical approach for periradicular surgery is not practical because of limiting anatomic factors (ie, risk of paresthesia because of proximity of root apices to the mandibular canal or mental foramen).
4. Nonsurgical and surgical treatment have failed and symptoms and/or pathosis persist.
5. Visual access is inadequate to perform root-end resection and root-end filling.
6. Root defects (resorption, perforation) exist in areas that are not accessible through a periradicular surgical approach without excessive alveolar bone loss.
7. To thoroughly examine the root or roots on all surfaces to identify or rule out the presence of a root defect, such as a crack or root perforation.

Rationale and Outcome

The replantation of traumatically (accidentally) avulsed teeth is universally accepted as the treatment of choice whenever possible (see Chapter 15, "Endodontic Considerations in Dental Trauma"). If replantation has become the standard of care for teeth that have been traumatically avulsed, why would it not be justifiable to **intentionally "avulse"** a tooth under the controlled trauma of extraction and replant the tooth under aseptic conditions? Dryden and Arens state that, in a personal communication, Andreasen claims 90% success when avulsed teeth are replanted within 30 minutes.[262]

There are three factors that directly affect the outcome of extraction/replantation procedures:

1. Keeping the out-of-socket time as short as possible.
2. Keeping the periodontal ligament cells on the root surface moist with saline or Hanks Balanced Salt Solution during the time the tooth is out of the socket.
3. Minimizing damage to the cementum and periodontal ligament cells by gentle elevation and extraction of the tooth. The forcep beaks should not touch the cementum if at all possible.

It is obvious that success depends on the ability to remove the involved tooth without fracture of the root or roots. The patient should always be advised that fracture of the tooth is possible and if this occurs, the tooth must be removed and discarded.

Kingsbury and Wiesenbaugh reported on 151 mandibular premolar and molar teeth that were extracted, treated, and replanted. They evaluated these teeth over a 3-year period and reported a success rate of 95%.[263] Koenig and associates reported on a study involving 192 extracted and replanted teeth. Following an evaluation period of between 6 and 51 months, they reported a success rate of 82%.[264] More recently, Bender and Rossman reported on 31 cases of extraction/replantation. They reported a success rate of 80.6% with an observation period of up to 22 years.[265] Raghoebar and Vissink reported on 29 cases involving extraction/replantation of mandibular molar teeth. One (3%) had to be removed 4 weeks postsurgically because of pain and mobility, 3 (11%) had to be removed during the first year because of periodontal problems, 4 (14%) showed periodontal problems or root resorption but continued to be functional, and 21 (72%) were considered successful after a 5-year observation period.[266] Kratchman stated, "With increased understanding of the periodontium and improved techniques, intentional replantation should no longer be viewed as a treatment of last resort, but rather a successful treatment alternative.[267]

Steps in Extraction/Replantation

Once extraction/replantation has been determined and accepted as the treatment of choice, orthograde endodontic treatment should be completed to the best degree possible, and the pulp chamber and coronal access restored to help stabilize and reinforce the coronal tooth structure:

1. Following incision of the periodontal fibers with a No. 15 scalpel blade, the tooth to be extracted should be slowly and gently elevated with an appropriate size and style of surgical elevator until a class III

mobility is achieved. This is a very crucial step in the extraction process as it helps to accomplish extraction with the least chance of root fracture.

2. The appropriate forceps are chosen and preferably the beaks are wrapped with a sterile gauze sponge that is saturated with normal saline or Hanks Balanced Salt Solution. Every attempt should be made to minimize damage to the cementum during the extraction process.
3. Following extraction, the tooth should be held with the forceps, protected by saturated gauze or by hand at the coronal portion using a saturated gauze. The roots of the tooth should be thoroughly examined with fiber-optic illumination and magnification to evaluate for the presence of root fractures or radicular defects, such as perforations or resorptions. The application of methylene blue dye to the root surfaces may enhance visualization of otherwise nonvisible root defects. It is extremely important that the root surfaces be constantly bathed with either normal saline or Hanks Balanced Salt Solution during the time the tooth is out of its socket. Intentional replantation is best done as a team effort with each member of the team trained and skilled in their specific function.
4. If no root fractures are evident and the prognosis for replantation appears positive, any root defects should be repaired with an appropriate material. If root end resection is indicated, it should be done with a plain fissure bur in a high-speed handpiece under constant irrigation. Two to three millimeters of root-end should be resected. A small class I root-end preparation should be done with either a bur or an ultrasonic tip extending at least 3 mm into the root and an appropriate root-end filling placed.
5. Following repair of any root defects and/or root-end resection and root-end filling, the extraction socket should be irrigated with normal saline and gently suctioned to remove any blood clot that may have formed. The tooth is then carefully returned to its socket. Reinsertion of the tooth into the socket may be difficult at times, especially if there is a critical path of insertion. Care must also be taken that the tooth is returned to the socket in its proper orientation.
6. After the tooth has been inserted into the socket, a rolled gauze sponge should be placed on the occlusal aspect of the tooth and the patient instructed to bite down so that the interocclusal force will seat the tooth into its socket. The patient should be instructed to maintain interocclusal pressure for approximately 5 minutes.
7. In most cases, posterior teeth are well retained in their sockets and stabilization is usually not required. If excessive mobility is evident, splinting is suggested. The recommended splinting type and length of time are the same as those for replantation following traumatic avulsion and are discussed in chapter 15, "Endodontic Considerations in Dental Trauma." In the case of a posterior tooth, stabilization may be achieved by placing a figure-8 suture over the occlusal surface of the tooth. The suture may be secured on the occlusal surface of the tooth by placing a shallow groove on the buccal-lingual aspect of the crown (Figure 12-70). Stabilization may also be achieved by the use of a flexible wire with acid etching and bonding with composite resin to an adjacent tooth (Figure 12-71).
8. The patient should be seen 7 to 14 days following intentional replantation surgery to remove any stabilization that was placed and to evaluate tooth mobility. Postsurgical evaluation is recommended at 2, 6, and 12 months following surgery (Figure 12-72).

Intentional replantation is not a completely predictable procedure. Under favorable conditions, however, some authors have reported success rates in excess of 20 years.[262–268]

IMPLANT SURGERY

Two types of endosteal implants fall under the purview of endodontics: **endodontic implants and osseointegrated implants**, also called endosseous implants.[92] This is not to say that every dentist, or endodontist for that matter, should be placing endosteal implants, especially when the supporting alveolar bone is compromised. Only those who are specially trained and have extensive experience in periradicular and periodontal surgery should be involved in implant place-

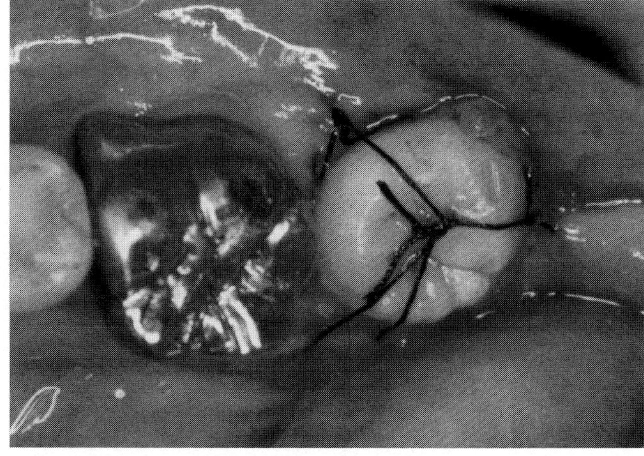

Figure 12-70 Stabilization of the replanted tooth has been achieved by placing a suture over the occlusal surface.

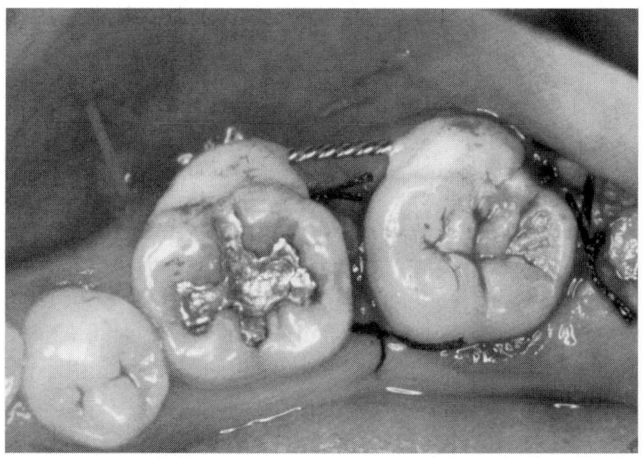

Figure 12-71 Stabilization of the replanted tooth has been achieved by bonding a flexible wire to the adjacent tooth with composite resin.

ment. Jansen has stated that many practitioners have found implant procedures to be too difficult, the learning curve long, and office support staff unsure of their role in the procedure. Restorative dentists who place implants do so only on the average of two to three a year. This is insufficient to acquire the necessary diagnostic and treatment skills to perform successful implant procedures.[269]

Endodontic Implants

It makes great sense that, if a rigid implant can safely extend beyond the apex of the tooth into sound bone, and by so doing stabilize a tooth with weakened support, the patient is well served and perhaps has avoided replacement for some time. Such is the reasoning behind the concept of the endodontic implant, many of

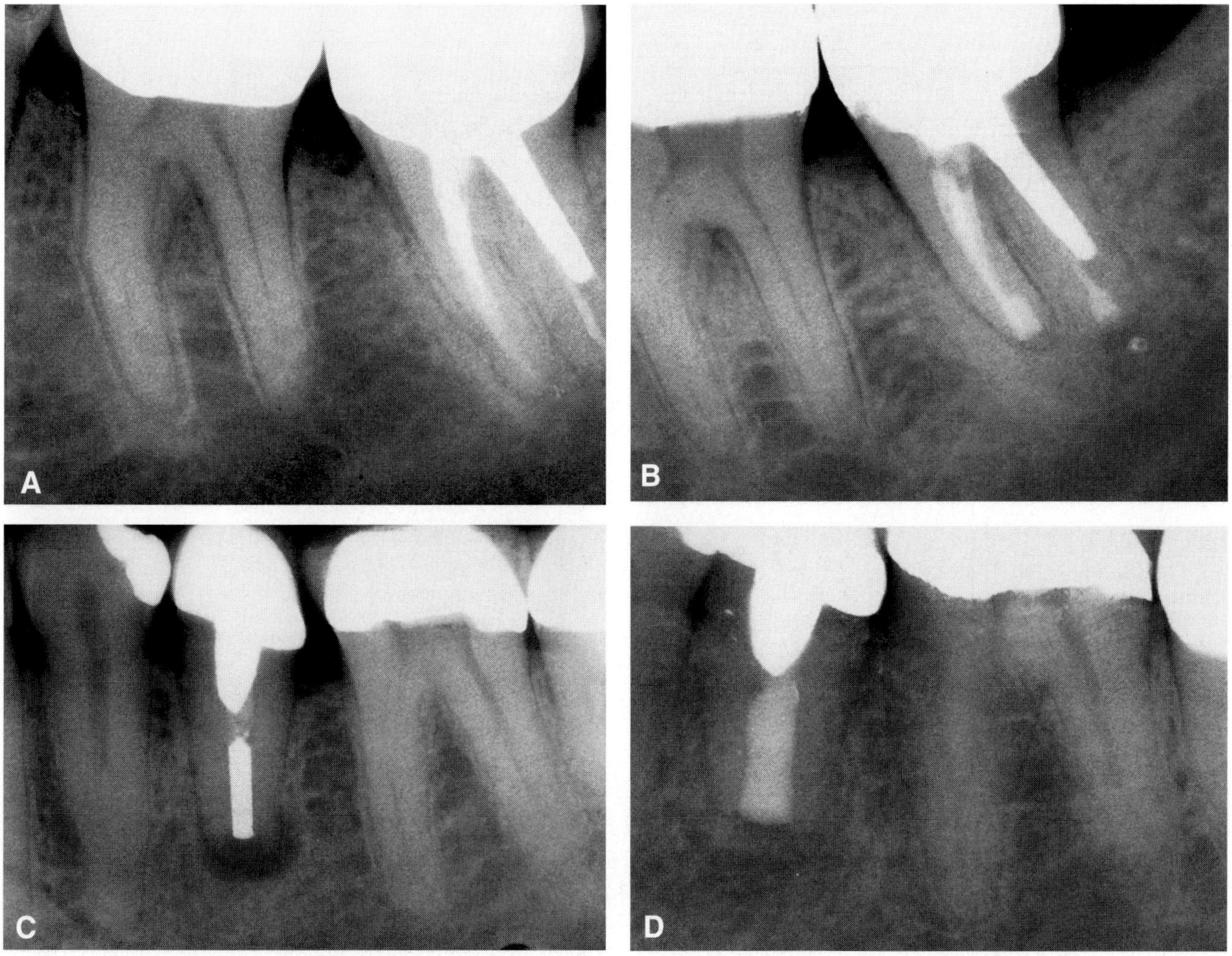

Figure 12-72 **A,** Patient reported pain to pressure 1 year following root canal therapy, post and crown. Extraction/replantation chosen due to proximity of mandibular canal. **B,** Radiograph 4 years following extraction/replantation procedure with intermediate restorative material (IRM) for root-end fillings. Patient is asymptomatic. **C,** Patient presented with pain and localized intraoral swelling, root canal therapy and crown 20 years. **D,** Three years following extraction/replantation procedure. Silver point removed and root canal space filled with gutta percha and sealer through retrograde approach.

which have proven quite successful (Figure 12-73). On the other hand, when too high a failure rate of endodontic implants developed, the profession backed off from their use. Weine and Frank, however, retrospectively "revisited" their endodontic implant cases placed over a 10-year period. While admitting to "many which did fail," they "noted some remarkable long-term successes with the technique."[270] Their recommendation was that endodontic implants not be discarded totally but used only in carefully selected cases.

Orlay may have been among the first to use and advocate endodontic implants.[271] Frank is credited, however, with standardizing the technique, developing the proper instruments, and matching implants.[272, 273] Frank and Abrams were also able to show that a properly placed endodontic implant was accepted by the periradicular tissue and that a narrow "collar" of healthy fibrous connective tissue, much like a circular periodontal ligament, surrounded the metal implant and separated it from the alveolar bone[274] (Figure 12-74).

Placing endodontic implants is a technique-sensitive procedure. A **perfectly round preparation** must be reamed through the root apex and into the alveolar bone. Failure to accomplish this task results in leakage around the implant–dentin interface and eventual failure of the implant (Figure 12-75). Another critical area is structural weakening of the walls of the root as a result of dentin removal in an attempt to create a round apical orifice. This structural weakness may result in root fracture either at the time of implant placement or as a result of functional stresses on the tooth. It is also important that the periodontal condition that has led to the periradicular bone loss has been stabilized before endodontic implant placement. If not, the case will fail as a result of continued progression of the periodontal disease.

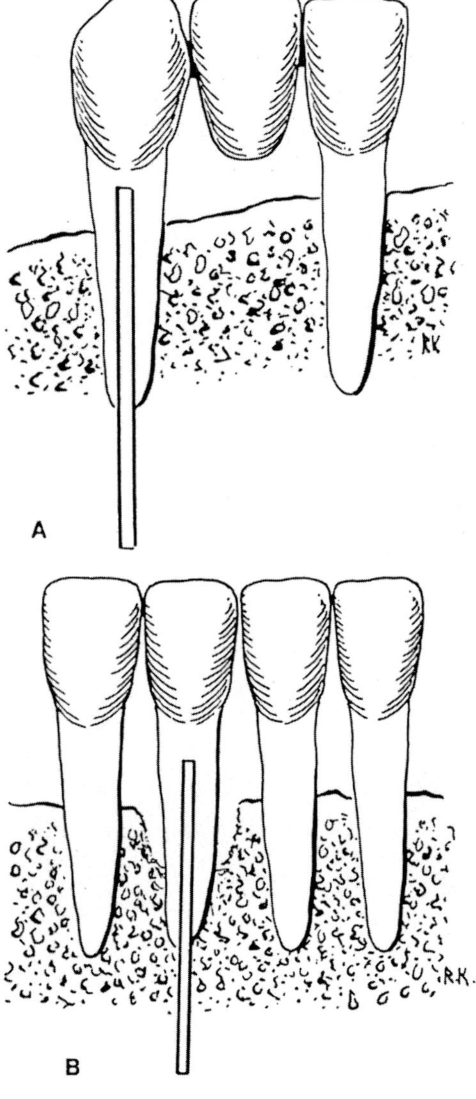

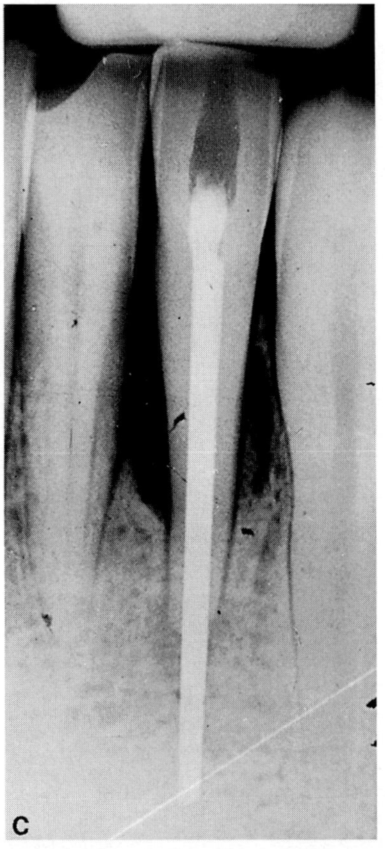

Figure 12-73 Indications for endodontic implants. A, Stabilizing periodontally weakened bridge abutment. B, Considerable restorative effort to replace tooth, and adjacent teeth would be poor abutments. C, Implant in hard-to-restore incisor. Periodontal condition must be treated and controlled. Reproduced with permission from Frank AL. Dent Clin North Am 1967;Nov:675.

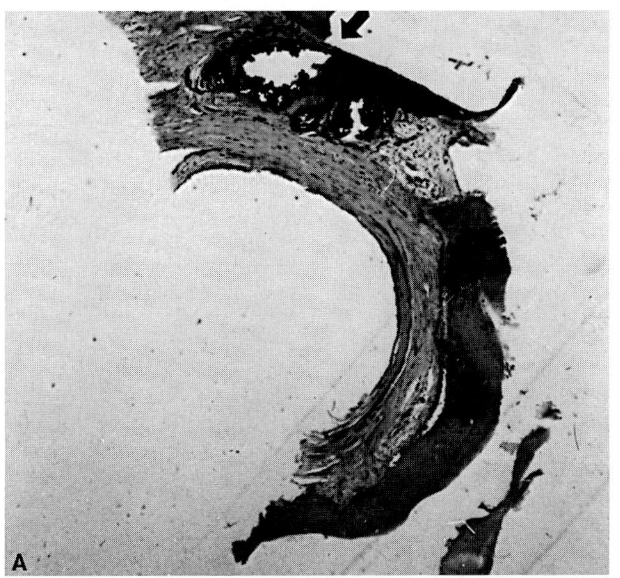
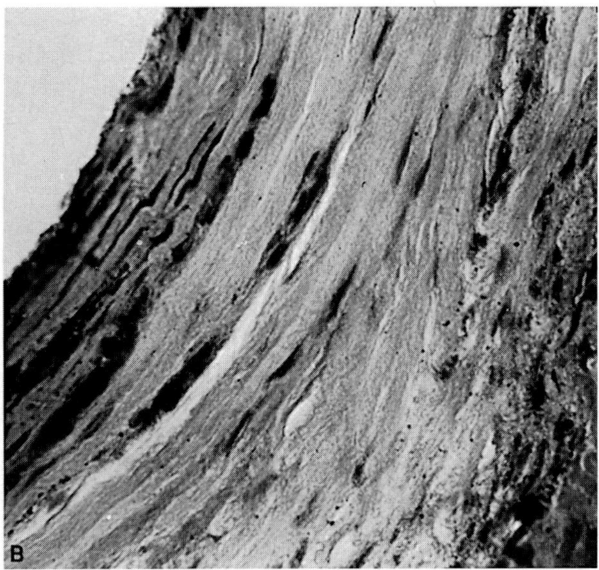

Figure 12-74 A, Low-power photomicrograph of transverse section through subapical region of endodontic implant. Dark material at top (**arrow**) is excess sealer. **B,** Higher power reveals connective tissue circular "ligament" configuration, without inflammation. Dark specks are excess sealer being scavenged and resorbed. Reproduced with permission from Frank AL. J Am Dent Assoc 1969;78:520.

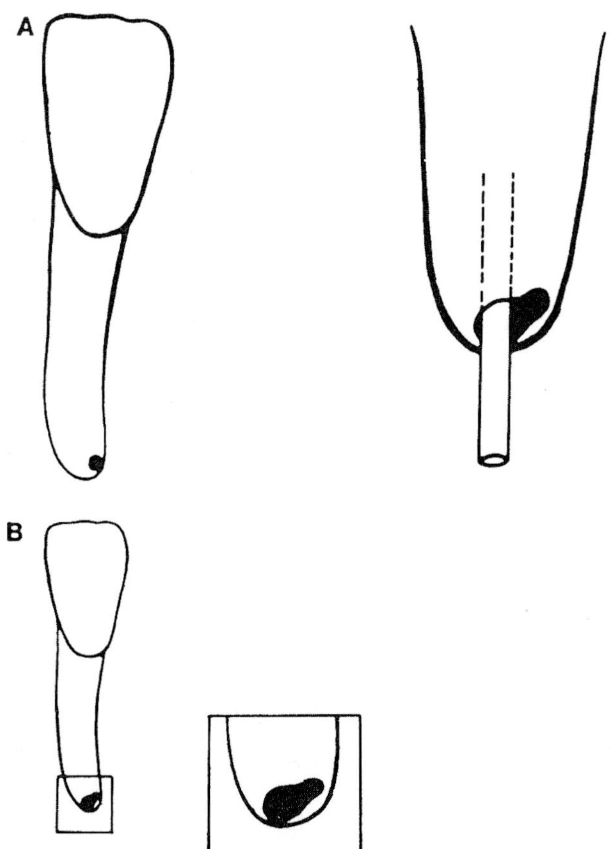

Figure 12-75 A, Portal of exit at a site not exactly at tip of root. **B,** Pear-shaped preparation is developed by large, stiff instruments. Endodontic implant only partially seals apical preparation leading to microleakage and failure. Reproduced with permission from Weine FS and Frank AL.[270]

Root-Form Osseointegrated Implants

Osseointegration is defined as "the direct structural and functional connection between ordered, living bone and the surface of a load-carrying implant."[275] Biomechanical as well as bacterial factors have long been recognized to play a substantial role in osseointegration maintenance.[276,277] Since Brånemark first introduced osseointegration, many alterations and enhancements of his original protocol have been published. In the earlier years, most attention was directed toward successful surgical placement of an implant body, with minimal regard to the implant restoration. **Preexisting bone volume was allowed to direct and guide implant position.** This treatment philosophy resulted in restorative difficulties and created biomechanical concerns as well as hygienic compromise.

Prosthetically directed implant placement involves preplanning the implant restoration before implant placement. This concept emphasizes the importance of a team approach in the overall care of the dental implant patient. This shift from site-directed to prosthetically directed implant placement has been facilitated by the success of current bone regenerative techniques using bone-grafting materials and guided tissue membranes.

Immediate Implant Placement. Of the recent advancements in implant surgery, the most applicable to the practice of endodontics is **immediate implant placement** (Figure 12-76). Implant placement immediately following tooth extraction offers several advantages over

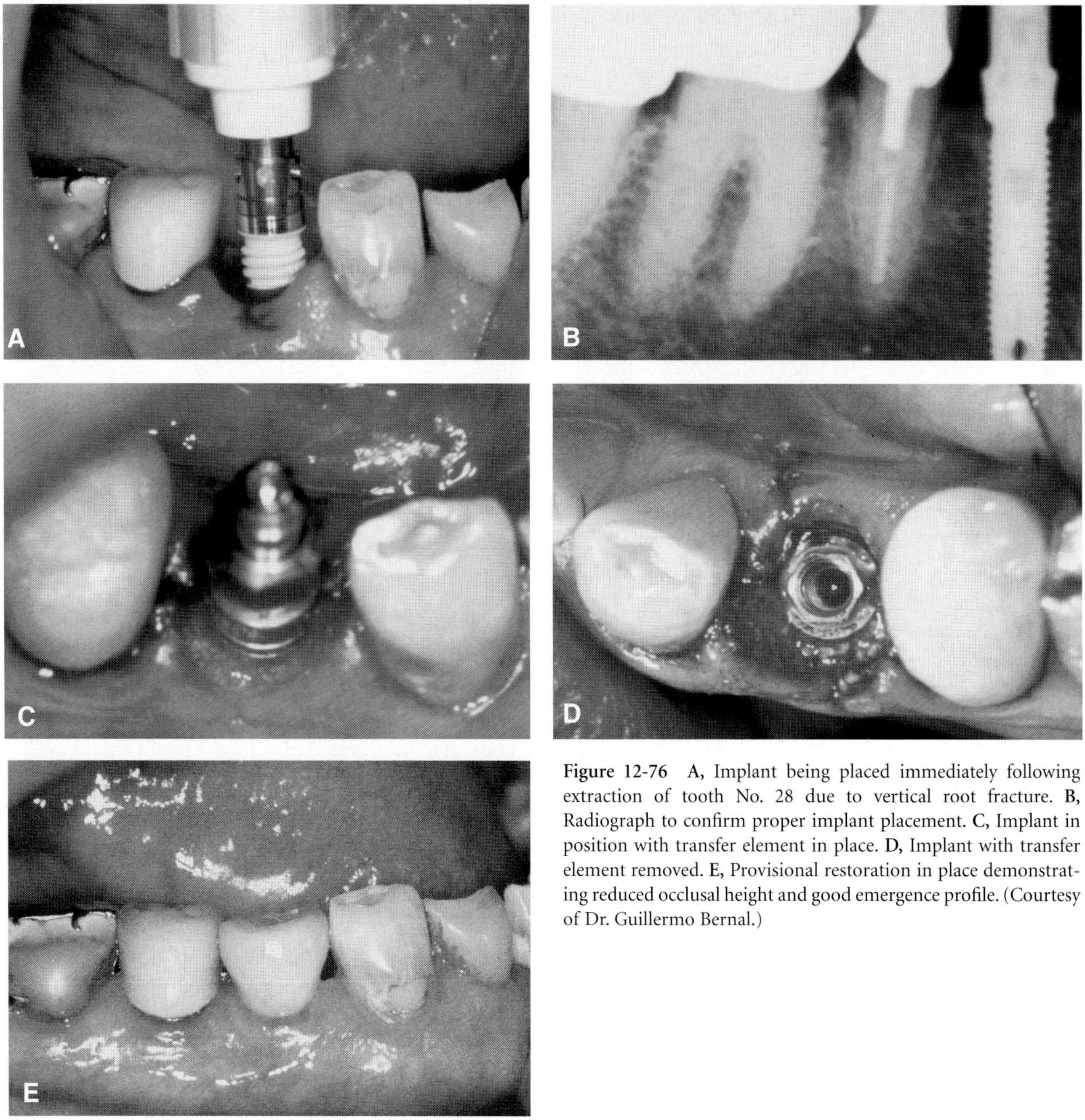

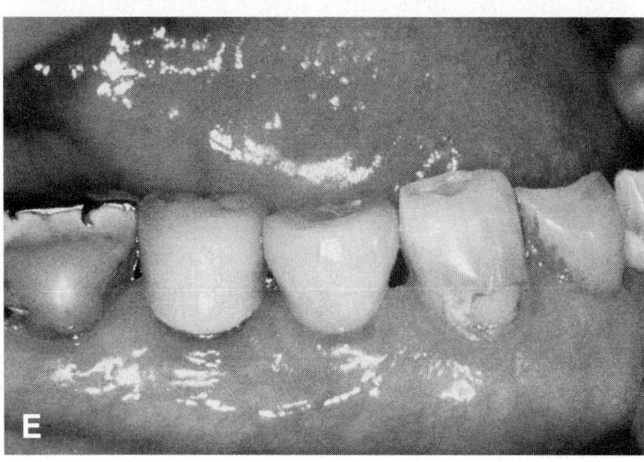

Figure 12-76 **A**, Implant being placed immediately following extraction of tooth No. 28 due to vertical root fracture. **B**, Radiograph to confirm proper implant placement. **C**, Implant in position with transfer element in place. **D**, Implant with transfer element removed. **E**, Provisional restoration in place demonstrating reduced occlusal height and good emergence profile. (Courtesy of Dr. Guillermo Bernal.)

the conventional protocol: (1) the incorporation of two procedures into one appointment, (2) the expediency of total treatment time, and (3) the minimization of osseous collapse as well as resorption and maintenance of soft-tissue architecture. Immediate implant placement, however, is not a universally applicable procedure. The presenting clinical situations may vary significantly. According to Gelb, the variables that may affect the regenerative protocol include the following:

1. Severity of the initial infection
2. Location of the root relative to the alveolus
3. Residual bone buccolingually and coronal apically
4. Vascularity of residual bone
5. Density of residual bone
6. Quality of cancellous marrow spaces
7. Availability of bony walls to contain the bone-graft material
8. Volume of bone regeneration necessary

9. Soft tissue available for closure
10. Experience of the operator[278]

Gelb also stated, "Despite these challenges, immediate implant surgery has been reported to have high predictability, which compares favorably to outcome reported in intact sites."[278] In a study by Rosenquist and associates, 109 titanium threaded implants were placed **immediately following extraction** in 51 patients and evaluated over a mean observation time of 30 months. They reported a 92% survival rate for implants that replaced teeth extracted for periodontal reasons and a 96% survival rate for implants that replaced teeth that were extracted for other reasons including endodontic treatment failure, root fracture, and extensive caries.[279]

Appropriate clinical situations for immediate implant placement should have adequate bone apical to the extraction socket and/or adequate bone buccolingually to secure initial stability of the implant. The apical dimension of bone should be a minimum of 3 to 4 mm in height and the buccolingual bone must be evaluated on the basis of both quality and quantity. The presence of a localized infection does not generally preclude immediate implant placement. Tooth removal and débridement of the area is usually sufficient to control the infection. Immediate implant placement is contraindicated in the posterior mandible when insufficient buccolingual bone exists for initial implant stability and apical extension of the implant beyond the floor of the socket will result in damage to the mandibular nerve.[278]

Extraction and Curettement Procedure. The tooth should be extracted with as little trauma as possible. It is extremely important to retain the cortical bone buccal and lingual to the extraction socket. In the case of multirooted teeth, it may be advantageous to section the crown and roots so that the roots may be individually extracted. This may save trauma to a thin cortical plate. All soft tissue should be removed from the bony crypt with curettes until a solid bone foundation is achieved.

Implant Placement. After tooth extraction and thorough débridement of the area, the major considerations for implant placement should be the specific functional and esthetic needs of the case. The drilling sequence may be altered from that of implant placement in an intact site as tapping and countersinking may not be necessary. The implant apex should be stabilized in at least 3 to 4 mm of bone and the implant head should be positioned to conform to either the central fossa, in posterior teeth, or the cingulum, in anterior teeth, for screw-retained prosthesis. For cement-retained anterior prostheses, the implant head should be placed in line with the incisal edges of the adjacent teeth. For cement-retained posterior prostheses, the implant head should be placed slightly buccal to the central fossa of the planned restoration. Placement of the implant approximately 3 mm apical to the cementoenamel junction of the adjacent teeth will ensure the maximum flexibility in the emergence profile of the restoration.[278]

Bone Graft and Membrane Placement. Preserving and/or regenerating buccal or labial bone are important to support soft-tissue dimensions and to give the appearance of a root eminence. The use of bone-grafting materials and membranes, resorbable and nonresorbable, may be used to promote bone growth around the implant and to preserve or restore labial dimensions. Demineralized freeze-dried bone allograft is a commonly used bone-graft material for this purpose.[278]

The bone-graft material is hydrated with sterile saline and packed into the void. Bone-graft material and a membrane are both used when there is a significant defect or when narrowing of the labial dimension is of major concern. When the bony walls of the defect are well defined and both cortical and cancellous anatomy are good, placement of bone-graft material alone is usually sufficient.[278]

Soft-Tissue Closure and Supportive Therapy. **Primary closure** is the closure of choice whenever possible. Care should be taken to maintain and preserve the soft tissue during incision and tooth extraction. The soft tissue should be repositioned as close as possible to its original position. When primary closure is not possible, the site should be covered with a nonresorbable membrane. Nonresorbable membranes serve as a scaffold for soft-tissue growth and migration resulting in closure over time. An alternative to placement of a nonresorbable membrane when primary closure is not possible is the use of a connective-tissue graft.[278]

Supportive therapy following immediate implant placement should include a bactericidal broad-spectrum antibiotic such as amoxicillin, cephalexin (Keflex), or clindamycin for a period of 7 to 14 days. Nonsteroidal anti-inflammatory drugs have been shown to be effective in promoting healing following implant placement.[278] Chlorhexidine oral rinses should be used routinely following implant-placement surgery. When primary closure is not possible and a connective-tissue graft is not done, débridement of the surgical area should be done with a cotton swab soaked in chlorhexidine. The patient should be instructed to continue this regimen twice daily until closure has been achieved. Gelb recommends that the sutures remain in place for 2 weeks and those cases that contain a membrane be monitored every 2 weeks until the membrane is removed.[278]

It is important to emphasize that, although implant surgery is within the scope of endodontics, it is a very technique-sensitive procedure that requires a relatively long learning curve. It is recommended that the dental practitioner participate in advanced training programs and gain considerable knowledge and experience in diagnosis, treatment planning, and placement of osseointegrated implants before implementing their use in clinical practice.

MICROSURGERY

For years, many dental practitioners have benefited from the use of vision-enhancement devices, such as loupes, surgical telescopes, and head-mounted surgical fiber-optic lamps (Figure 12-77). It is generally accepted that the better the visual access to the operating field, the higher the quality of treatment that can be accomplished.

Perhaps one of the most important recent developments in surgical endodontics has been the introduction of the surgical operating microscope (Figure 12-78). Otologists were the first medical specialists to introduce the operating microscope in the early 1940s. Slowly, the use of the operating microscope was introduced to the fields of ophthalmology, neurosurgery, urology, and other medical fields. Pioneers in the use of the operating microscope in surgical endodontics have been Buchanan,[280] Carr,[281,282] Rubinstein,[283,284] Pecora and Adreana,[285] Ruddle,[286] Selden,[287] Bellizzi and Loushine,[288] Reuben and Apotheker,[289] and others.

Surgical telescopes usually magnify in the range of ×2.5 to ×6.0, whereas the surgical operating microscope has a range of magnification of up to ×40. The obvious question is "How much magnification is enough?" As the level of magnification increases, the field of vision and the depth of field (focal depth) decrease, as does the aperture of the microscope, therefore limiting the amount of light that reaches the surgeon's eyes. This makes use of **magnification in excess of ×30 very impractical.** The slightest movement of the patient or of the operating microscope will result in the loss of visual field or focus. This can be very frustrating and result in the time-consuming need to readjust the microscope.

Magnifications in the range of ×2.5 to ×8.0 are recommended for orientation to the surgical field and to provide a wide field of view and a good depth of field. Midrange magnifications in the ×10 to ×16 are best for performing procedures such as root-end resections and root-end preparations. Higher range magnification in the area of ×18 to ×30 should be reserved for observing and evaluating fine detail.

Rubinstein has identified several advantages of the surgical operating microscope.[290] They include

1. Visualizing the surgical field.
2. Evaluating the surgical technique.
3. Reducing the number of radiographs needed.
4. Expanding patient education through video use.

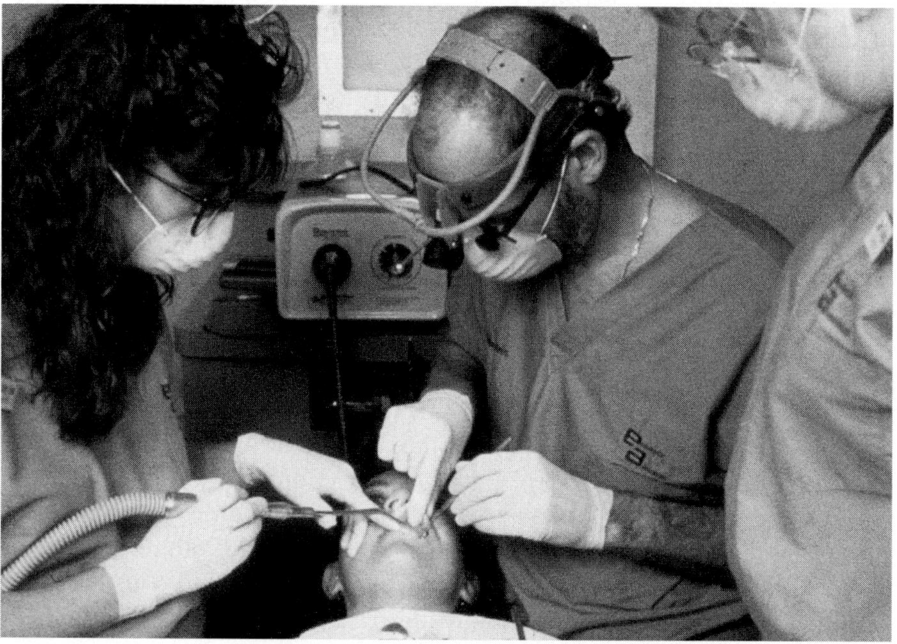

Figure 12-77 Operator using a fiber-optic headlamp system and ×2.5 surgical telescopes.

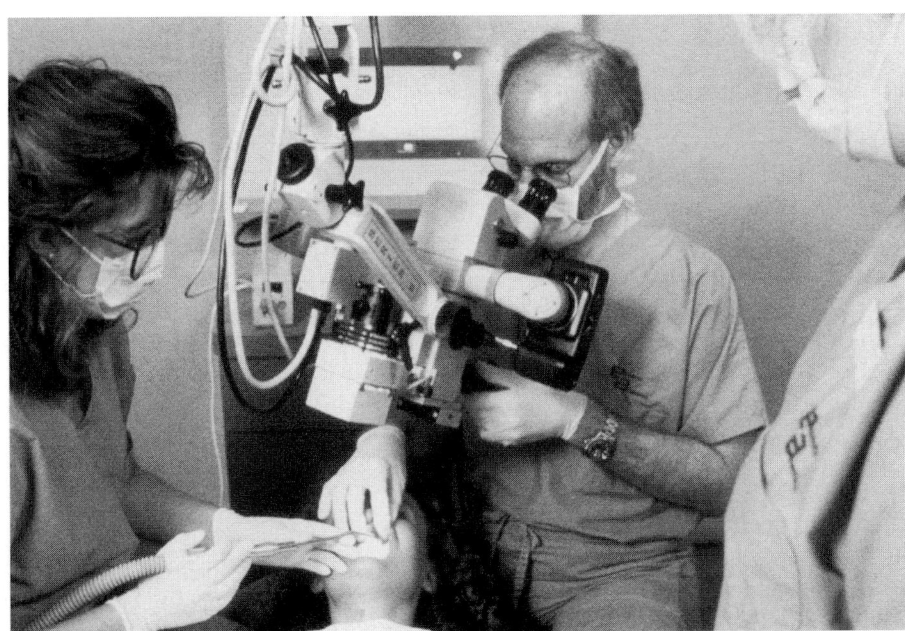

Figure 12-78 Operator using a surgical operating microscope with a 35 mm camera attached.

5. Providing reports to referring dentists and insurance companies.
6. Creating documentation for legal purposes.

The most significant of these advantages is the enhanced ability to visualize the surgical field and to evaluate the surgical technique (Figures 12-79 to 12-82). Incomplete root-end resection and failure to identify and properly include an interconnecting isthmus between multiple canals in a single root during root-end preparation have been stated as among the major causes of failure in endodontic surgery [82,121] (Figure 12-83; also see Figure 12-33). The use of good illumination and magnification will aid the surgeon in reducing these factors and should result in an increased success rate for endodontic surgery. It must be pointed out that the use of the surgical operating microscope requires a relatively long learning curve and, therefore, it is recommended that the endodontic surgeon participate in advanced training programs and gain considerable experience in surgical microscopy before implementing its use in clinical practice.

An important question that must be addressed is "Does the use of a surgical operating microscope really make a difference in the long-term outcome of endodontic surgery?" A recent report of a prospective study involving endodontic surgery performed under the surgical operating microscope and using ultrasonic root-end preparation techniques with Super EBA as the root-end filling material showed an overall success rate of 96.8%.[291] This report consisted of 94 root-end surgery

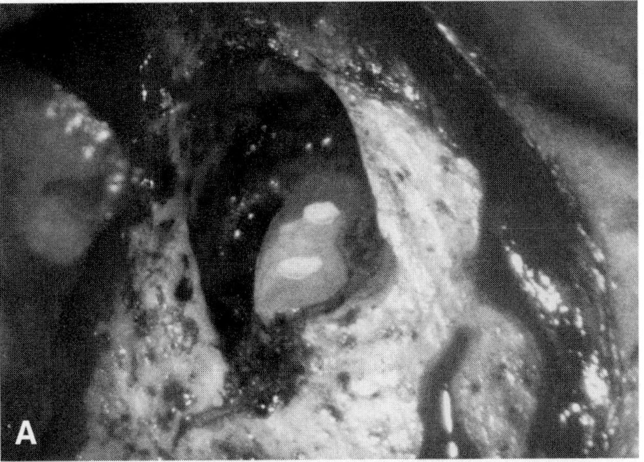

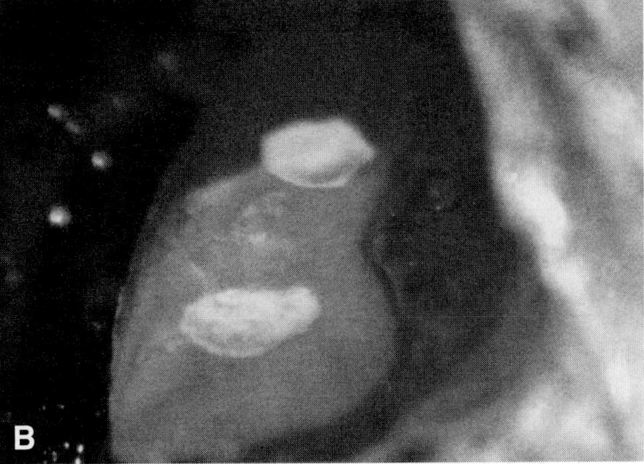

Figure 12-79 Final root-end fillings with Super EBA. A, ×8 original magnification. B, ×26 original magnification.

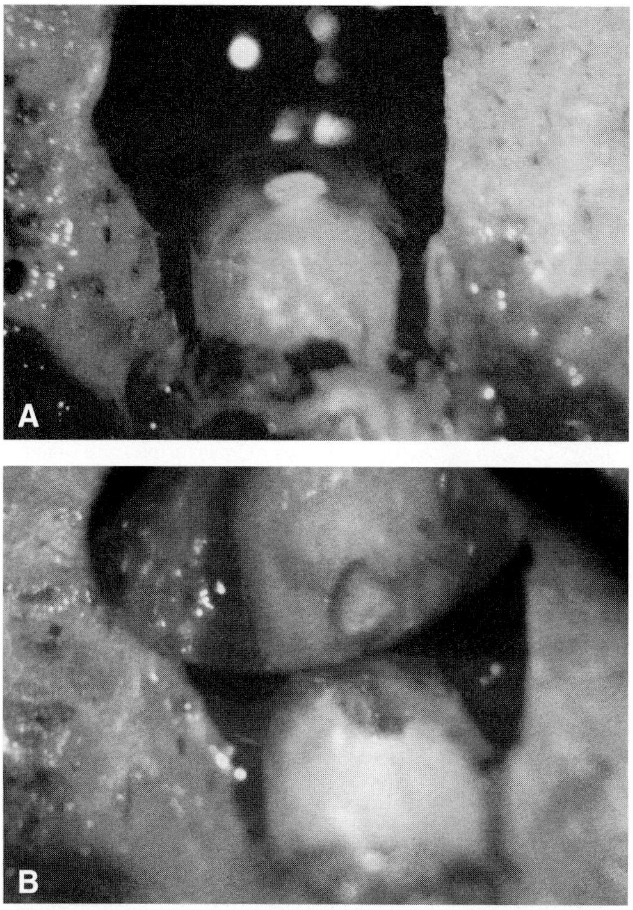

Figure 12-80 A, Beveled surface of the root of a maxillary lateral incisor following root-end resection (×16 original magnification). B, Root-end preparation following use of ultrasonic tips. Note use of microsurgical mirror (×16 original magnification).

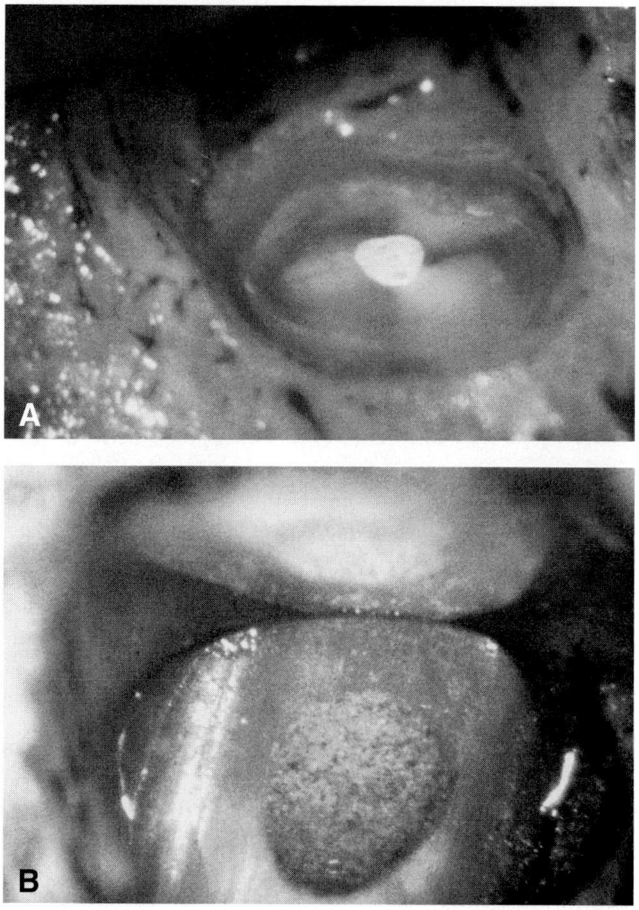

Figure 12-81 A, Finished root-end filling of a maxillary canine after use of a 30 fluted finishing bur (×16 original magnification). B, Mineral trioxide aggregate (MTA) root filling (×26 original magnification).

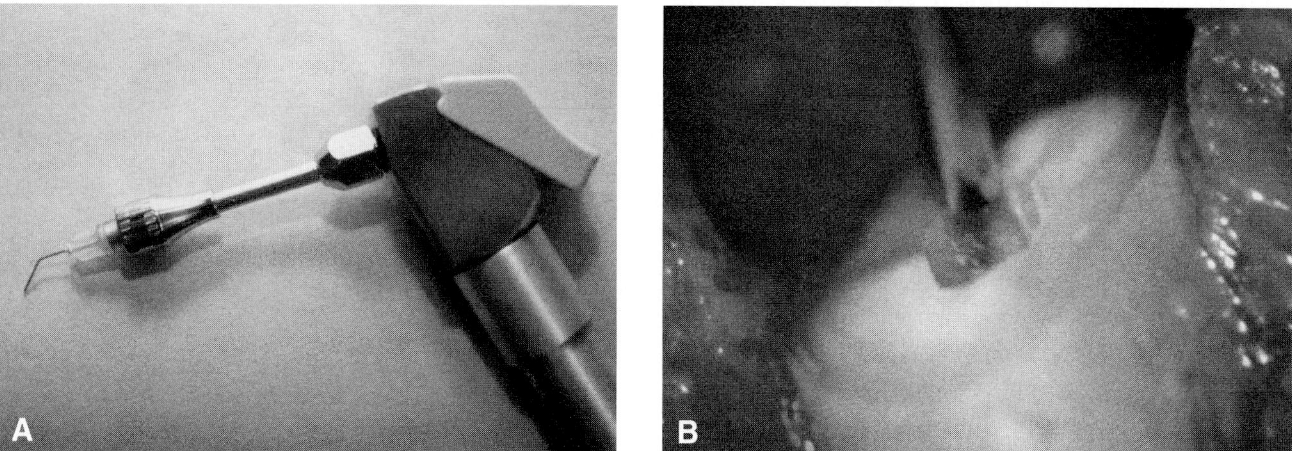

Figure 12-82 A, One-half millimeter blunt Blue Micro Tip mounted in a Stropko Irrigator on a triflow syringe. B, Blue Micro Tip drying the root-end preparation of a maxillary lateral incisor (×20 original magnification).

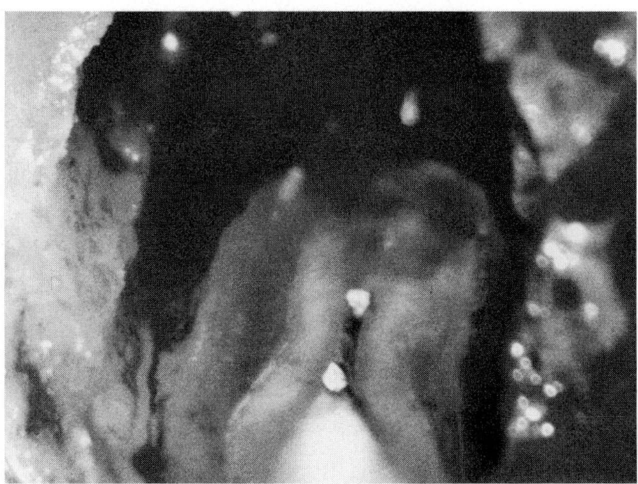

Figure 12-83 Isthmus evident connecting two canals of the mesiobuccal root of a maxillary first molar following root-end resection (×16 original magnification).

cases (31 molars, 31 premolars, 32 anterior teeth) treated by a single clinician. The evaluation period was 14 months. A case was considered successful when the lamina dura was restored or the case had healed by scar formation. Very strict case-selection criteria were used when selecting cases to be included in this study. **It also must be emphasized that this study had no control group.** The authors attribute the healing success primarily to the use of microsurgical techniques. They do state, however, that because of the short postsurgical evaluation time, their optimism regarding the outcomes of this study is tempered by the realization that cases sometimes fail following a preliminary healing phase. At the present time, there are no long-term (> 5 years) studies evaluating the outcomes of endodontic microsurgery procedures. **Time will be the judge!**

REFERENCES

1. Guerini V. A history of dentistry. Philadelphia: Lea & Febiger; 1909. p. 117.
2. Gutmann J, Harrison J. Surgical endodontics. St. Louis (MO): Ishiyaku EuroAmerica; 1994.
3. Frank A, Simon J, Abou-Rass M, Glick D. Clinical and surgical endodontics: concepts in practice. Philadelphia: JB Lippincott; 1983.
4. Grossman L, Oliet S, Del Rio C. Endodontic practice. 11th ed. Philadelphia: Lea & Febiger; 1988.
5. American Association of Endodontists Web page. For the patient. www.aae.org (accessed July 1999).
6. Sjögren U, Hagglund B, Sundquist G, Wing K. Factors affecting the long-term results of endodontic treatment. J Endod 1990;16:498.
7. Stabholtz A, Walton R. In: Principles and practice of endodontics. 2nd ed. Philadelphia: WB Saunders; 1996.
8. Eriksen H. Endodontology—epidemiologic considerations. Endod Dent Traumatol 1991;7:189.
9. Pekruhn RB. The incidence of failure following single-visit endodontic therapy. J Endod 1986;12:68.
10. Jokinen MA, Kotilainen R, Pockkeus P. Clinical and radiographic study of pulpectomy and root canal therapy. Scand J Dent Res 1978;86:366.
11. Odesjo B, Hellden L, Salonen L, Langeland K. Prevalence of previous endodontic treatment, technical standard and occurrence of periapical lesions in a randomly selected adult, general population. Endod Dent Traumatol 1990;6:265.
12. Murphy WK, Kaugars GE, Collett WK, Dodds RN. Healing of periapical radiolucencies after nonsurgical endodontic therapy Oral Surg 19091;71:620.
13. Jaoui L, Machtou P, Ouhayoun JP. Long-term evaluation of endodontic and periodontal treatment. Int Endod J 1995;28:249.
14. Friedman S. Retreatment of failures. In: Principles and practice of endodontics. 2nd ed. Philadelphia: WB Saunders; 1996.
15. Bergenholtz G, Lekholm U, Milthon R. Retreatment of endodontic fillings. Scand J Dent Res 1979;87:217.
16. Allen RK, Newton CW, Brown CE. A statistical analysis of surgical and nonsurgical retreatment cases. J Endod 1989; 15:261.
17. Van Nieuwenhuysen JP, Aouar M, D'Hoore W. Retreatment or radiographic monitoring in endodontics. Int Endod J 1994;27:75.
18. Hepworth MJ, Friedman S. Treatment outcome of surgical and nonsurgical management of endodontic failures. J Can Dent Assoc 1997;63:364.
19. Luebke RG, Glick DH, Ingle JI. Indications and contraindications for endodontic surgery. Oral Surg 1964;18:97.
20. American Association of Endodontists. Appropriateness of care and quality assurance guidelines. 3rd ed. Chicago: American Association of Endodontists; 1998.
21. Cohen S, Schwartz S. J Calif Dent Assoc 1985;13:97.
22. AAE Endodontics, Colleagues for Excellence. Chicago, Spring/Summer, 1999.
23. Milam SB, Giovannitti JA. Local anesthetics in dental practice. Dent Clin North Am 1984;28:493.
24. Holroyd SV, Requa-Clark B. Local anesthetics. In: Holroyd SV, Wynn RL, Requa-Clark B, editors. Clinical pharmacology in dental practice. 4th ed. St. Louis (MO): Mosby; 1988.
25. Ritchie JM, Ritchie B, Greengard P. The active structure of local anesthetics. J Pharmacol Exp Ther 1965;150:152.
26. Wallace JA, Mechanowicz AE, Mundell RD, Wilson EG. A pilot study of the clinical problem of regionally anesthetizing the pulp of an acutely inflamed mandibular molar. Oral Surg 1985;59:517.
27. Najjar TA. Why can't you achieve adequate regional anesthesia in the presence of infection? Oral Surg 1977;4:7.
28. McDonald NJ, Hovland EJ. Surgical endodontics. In: Walton R, Torabinejad M, editors. Principles and practice of endodontics. 2nd ed. Philadelphia: W. B. Saunders; 1996.
29. Bellizzi R, Loushine R. A clinical atlas of endodontic surgery. Quintessence Publishing; 1991.
30. Peters DD. Evaluation of prophylactic alveolar trephination to avoid pain. J Endod 1980;6:518.
31. Elliott JA, Holcomb JB. Evaluation of a minimally traumatic alveolar trephination procedure to avoid pain. J Endod 1988;14:405.
32. Arens DE, Adams WR, DeCastro RA, editors. Endodontic surgery. Philadelphia: Harper and Row; 1981.

33. Morse DR. Clinical endodontology. Springfield (IL): Charles C. Thomas; 1974.
34. Bence R. Trephination technique. J Endod 1980;6:657.
35. Lovdahl PE. Endodontic retreatment. Dent Clin North Am 1992;36:473.
36. Van Nieuwenhuysen JP, Aaouar M, D'Hoore W. Retreatment of radiographic monitoring in endodontics. Int Endod J 1994;27:75.
37. Weine FS. Nonsurgical retreatment of endodontic failures. Compend Contin Educ Dent 1995;16:324.
38. Cheung GS. Endodontic failures—changing the approach. Int Dent J 1996;46:131.
39. Moiseiwitsch JR, Trope M. Nonsurgical root canal therapy with apparent indications for root-end surgery. Oral Surg 1998;3:335.
40. Schiott CR, Loe H, Borglum-Jensen S, et al. The effects of chlorhexidine mouth rinses on the human oral flora. J Periodontal Res 1970;5:84.
41. Malamed SF. Handbook of local anesthetics. 2nd ed. St. Louis (MO): Mosby; 1986.
42. Jastak JT, Yagiela JA. Regional anesthesia of the oral cavity. St. Louis (MO): Mosby; 1981.
43. Simard-Savoie S. New method for comparing the activity of local anesthetics used in dentistry. J Dent Res 1975;54:978.
44. Sisk AL. Vasoconstrictors in local anesthesia for dentistry. Anesth Prog 1993;39:187.
45. Ahlquist RP. A study of the adrenotrophic receptors. Am J Physiol 1948;153:586.
46. Gage TW. Pharmacology of the autonomic nervous system. In: Holroyd SV, Wynn RL, Requa-Clark B. Clinical pharmacology in dental practice. 4th ed. St. Louis (MO): Mosby; 1988.
47. Weiner N. Norepinephrine, epinephrine, and the sympathomimetic amines. In: Gilman AF, Goodman LS, Gilman A, editors. Goodman and Gilman's the pharmacologic basis of therapeutics. 6th ed. New York: Macmillan Publishing; 1980.
48. Bennett CR. Monheim's local anesthesia and pain control in dental practice. 7th ed. St. Louis (MO): Mosby; 1984.
49. Council on Dental Therapeutics of the American Dental Association. Accepted dental therapeutics. 40th ed. Chicago: American Dental Association; 1984.
50. Neidle EA. Introduction to autonomic nervous system drugs. In: Neidle EA, Kroeger DC, Yageila JA, editors. Pharmacology and therapeutics for dentistry. 2nd ed. St. Louis (MO): Mosby; 1985.
51. Tolas AG, Pflug AD, Halter JB. Arterial plasma epinephrine concentrations and hemodynamic response after dental injection of local anesthetic with epinephrine. J Am Dent Assoc 1982;104:41.
52. Chernow B, Balestrieri F, Ferguson DD, et al. Local anesthesia with epinephrine: minimal effects on the sympathetic nervous system or on hemodynamic variables. Arch Intern Med 1983;143:2141.
53. Davenport RE, Porcelli RJ, Iaacono VJ, et al. Effects of anesthetics containing epinephrine on catecholamine levels during periodontal surgery. J Periodontol 1990;61:553.
54. Lipp M, Dick W, Daublander M, et al. Exogenous and endogenous plasma levels of epinephrine during dental treatment under local anesthesia. Reg Anesth 1993;18:6.
55. Replogle K, Reader A, Nist R, et al. Cardiovascular effects of intraosseous injections of 2 percent lidocaine with 1:100,000 epinephrine and 3 percent mepivacaine. J Am Dent Assoc 1999;130:649.
56. Pallasch TJ. Vasoconstrictors and the heart. Calif Dent Assoc J 1998;
57. Hecht A, App GR. Blood volume loss during gingivectomy using two different anesthetic techniques. J Periodontol 1974;45:9.
58. Roberts DH, Sowray JH. Local anesthesia in dentistry. 2nd ed. Bristol: John Wright & Sons; 1987.
59. Lindorf HH. Investigation of the vascular effects of newer local anesthetics and vasoconstrictors. Oral Surg 1979;48:292.
60. Allen GD. Dental anesthesia and analgesia. 3rd ed. Baltimore (MD): Williams and Wilkins; 1984. p. 64.
61. Yagiela JA. Local anesthetics. In: Neidle EA, Kroeger DC, Yagiela JA, editors. Pharmacology and therapeutics for dentistry 2nd ed. St. Louis (MO): Mosby; 1985; p. 256.
62. Cutright DE, Hansuck EE. Microcirculation of the perioral regions of the *Macaca rhesus*. Oral Surg 1970;29:776.
63. Gutmann JL, Harrison JW. Posterior endodontic surgery: anatomical considerations and clinical techniques. Int Endod J 1985;18:8.
64. Castelli WA, Huelke DF. The arterial system of the head and neck of the rhesus monkey with emphasis on the external carotid system. Am J Anat 1965;116:149.
65. Davis WL. Oral histology: cell structure and function. Philadelphia: WB Saunders; 1986; p. 154.
66. Hooley JR, Whitacre RJ. A self-instructional guide to oral surgery in general dentistry. 2nd ed. Seattle: Stoma Press; 1980.
67. Luebke RG, Ingle JI. Geometric nomenclature for mucoperiosteal flaps. Periodontics 1964;2:301.
68. Macphee R, Cowley G. Essentials of periodontology and periodontics. 3rd ed. Oxford: Blackwell Scientific Publications; 1981.
69. Harrison JW, Jurosky KA. Wound healing in the tissues of the periodontium following periradicular surgery. 1. The incisional wound. J Endod 1991;17:425.
70. Harrison JE, Jurosky KA. Wound healing in the tissues of the periodontium following periradicular surgery. 2. The dissectional wound. J Endod 1991;17:544.
71. Kohler CA, Ramfjord SP. Healing in gingival mucoperiosteal flaps. Oral Surg 1960;13:89.
72. Levine LH. Periodontal flap surgery with gingival fiber retention. J Periodontol 1972;43:91.
73. Ruben MP, Smukler H, Schulman SM, et al. Healing of periodontal surgical wounds. In: Goldman HM, Cohen DW, editors. Periodontal therapy. 6th ed. St. Louis (MO): Mosby; 1980.
74. Phillips JL, Weller RN, Kulild JC. The mental foramen. 1. Size, orientation, and positional relationship to the mandibular second premolar. J Endod 1990;16:221.
75. Phillips JL, Weller RN, Kulild JC. The mental foramen. 2. Radiographic position in relation to the mandibular second premolar. J Endod 1992;19:271.
76. Weine FS, Gerstein H. Periapical surgery. In: Weine FS, editor. Endodontic therapy. 4th ed. St. Louis (MO): Mosby; 1982.
77. Arens DE. Surgical endodontics. In: Cohen S, Burns R, editors. Pathways of the pulp. 4th ed. St. Louis (MO): Mosby; 1987.
78. Gerstein H. Surgical endodontics. In: Laskin DN, editor. Oral and maxillofacial surgery. Vol 2. St. Louis (MO): Mosby; 1985.
79. Gutmann JL. Principles of endodontic surgery for the general practitioner. Dent Clin North Am 1984;28:895.
80. Barnes IE. Surgical endodontics. A colour manual. Littleton (MA): PSG Publishing; 1984.

81. Cambruzzi JV, Marshall FJ. Molar endodontic surgery. J Can Dent Assoc 1983;49:61.
82. Carr GB, Bentkover SK. Surgical endodontics. In: Cohen S, Burnes R, editors. Pathways of the pulp. 7th ed. St. Louis (MO): Mosby; 1997; p. 619.
83. Tetsch P. Development of raised temperatures after osteotomies. J Maxillofac Surg 1974;21:141.
84. Eriksson AR, Albrektsson T. Heat induced bone tissue injury. Swed Dent J 1982;6:262.
85. Eriksson AR, Albrektsson T, Grane B, McQueen D. Thermal injury to bone. A vital-microscopic description of heat effects. Int J Oral Surg 1982;11:115.
86. Eriksson AR, Albrektsson T. Temperature threshold levels for heat-induced bone tissue injury: a vital-microscopic study in the rabbit. J Prosthet Dent 1984;50:101.
87. Eriksson AR, Albrektsson T. The effect of heat on bone regeneration: an experimental study in the rabbit. J Oral Maxillofac Surg 1984;42:705.
88. Boyne P. Histologic response of bone to sectioning by high-speed rotary instruments. J Dent Res 1966;45:270.
89. Moss R. Histopathologic reaction of bone to surgical cutting. Oral Surg 1964;17:405.
90. Argen E, Arwill T. High-speed or conventional dental equipment for the removal of bone in oral surgery. III: A histologic and micro radiographic study on bone repair in the rabbit. Acta Odontol Scand 1968;26:223.
91. Calderwood RG, Hera SS, Davis JR, Waite DE. A comparison of the cutting effect on bone after the production of defects by various rotary instruments. J Dent Res 1964;43:207.
92. Ingle JI, Cummings RR, Frank AL, et al. Endodontic surgery. In: Ingle JI, Bakland LK, editors. Endodontics. 4th ed. Philadelphia: Lea & Febiger; 1994.
93. Falomo OO. Surgical emphysema following root canal therapy: report of a case. Oral Surg 1984;58:101.
94. Ely EW, Stump TE, Hudspeth AS, Haponik EF. Thoracic complications of dental surgical procedures: hazards of the dental drill. Am J Med 1993;95:456.
95. Bekiroglu F, Rout PG. Surgical emphysema following dental treatment: two cases. Dent Update 1997;24:412.
96. Battrum DE, Gutmann JL. Implications, prevention and management of subcutaneous emphysema during endodontic treatment. Endod Dent Traumatol 1995;11:109.
97. Stockdale CR, Chandler NP. The nature of the periapical lesion—a review of 1108 cases. J Dent 1988;16:123.
98. McDonald NJ, Hovland ER. Surgical endodontics. In: Walton R, Torabinejad M, editors. Principles and practice of endodontics. 2nd ed. Philadelphia: WB Saunders; 1996.
99. Fish EW. Bone infection. J Am Dent Assoc 1939;26:691.
100. Barron SL, Gottliev B, Crook JH. Periapical curettage or apicoectomy. Texas Dent J 1947;65:37.
101. Pearson HH. Curette or resect? J Can Dent Assoc 1949;14:508.
102. Wakely JW, Simon WJ. Apical curettage or apicoectomy? Dent Assist 1977;46:29.
103. Gutmann JL, Pitt Ford TR. Management of the resected root end: a clinical review. Int Endod J 1993;26:273.
104. Gutmann JL, Harrison JW. Posterior endodontic surgery: anatomical considerations and clinical techniques. Int Endod J 1985;18:8.
105. el-Swiah JM, Walker RT. Reasons for apicectomies: a retrospective study. Endod Dent Traumatol 1996;12:185.
106. Ingle JI, Cummings RR, Frank AL, et al. Endodontic surgery. In: Ingle JI, Bakland LK, editors. Endodontics. 4th ed. Baltimore: Williams and Wilkins; 1994. p. 723.
107. Nedderman TA, Hartwell GR, Portell FR. A comparison of root surfaces following apical root resection with various burs: scanning electron microscopic evaluation. J Endod 1988;14:423.
108. Morgan LA, Marshall JG. The topography of root ends resected with fissure burs and refined with two types of finishing burs. Oral Surg 1998;85:585.
109. Ebihara A, Wadachi R, Sekine Y, et al. Application of Er:YAG laser to apicoectomy. 6th International Congress on Lasers in Dentistry; 1998.
110. Komori T, Yokoyama K, Matsumoto Y, Matsumoto, K. Erbium:YAG and holmium:YAG laser root resection of extracted human teeth. J Clin Laser Med Surg 1997;15:9.
111. Moritz A, Gutknecht N, Goharkhay K, et al. The carbon dioxide laser as an aid in apicoectomy: an in vitro study. J Clin Laser Med Surg 1997;15:185.
112. Maillet WA, Torneck CD, Friedman S. Connective tissue response to root surfaces resected with Nd:YAG laser or burs. Oral Surg 1996;82:681.
113. Miserendino LJ. The laser apicoectomy: endodontic application of the CO_2 laser for periapical surgery. Oral Surg 1988;66:615.
114. Komori T, Yokoyama K, Takato T, Matsumoto K. Clinical application of the erbium:YAG laser for apicoectomy. J Endod 1997;23:748.
115. Andreasen JO, Rud J. A histological study of dental and periapical structures after endodontic surgery. Int J Oral Surg 1972;1:272.
116. Ichesco WR, Ellison RL, Corcoran JR, Krause DC. A spectrophotometric analysis of dentinal leakage in the resected root [abstract]. J Endod 1986;12:129.
117. Beatty R. The effect of reverse filling preparation design on apical leakage [abstract]. J Dent Res 1986;65:259.
118. Vertucci RJ, Beatty RG. Apical leakage associated with retrofillings techniques: a dye study. J Endod 1986;12:331.
119. Tidmarsh BG, Arrowsmith MG. Dentinal tubules at the root ends of apicected teeth: a scanning electron microscopic study. Int Endod J 1989;22:184.
120. Gagliani M, Tusker S, Molinari R. Ultrasonic root-end preparation: influence of cutting angle on the apical seal. J Endod 1998;24:726.
121. Hu Young-Yi, Kim S. The resected root surface. Dent Clin North Am 1997;41:529.
122. Skidmore AE, Bjornal AM. Root morphology of the human mandibular first molar. Oral Surg 1971;33:778.
123. Pineda F, Kuttler Y. Mesiodistal and buccolingual roentgenographic investigation of 7,275 root canals. Oral Surg 1972;33:101.
124. Green D. Double canals in single roots. Oral Surg 1973;35:698.
125. Cambruzzi JV, Marshall FJ. Molar endodontic surgery. J Can Dent Assoc 1983;1:61.
126. Vertucci FJ. Root canal anatomy of the human permanent teeth. Oral Surg 1984;58:589.
127. Weller RN, Niemczyk SP, Kim S. Incidence and position of the canal isthmus. Part I. Mesiobuccal root of the maxillary first molar. J Endod 1995;21:380.
128. Kim S, Rethnam S. Hemostasis in endodontic microsurgery. Dent Clin North Am 1997;41:499.
129. Selden HS. Bone wax as an effective hemostat in periapical surgery. Oral Surg 1970;29:262.
130. Ibarrola JL, Bjorenson JE, Austin BP, Gerstein H. Osseous reactions to three hemostatic agents. J Endod 1985;11:75.

131. Aurelio J, Chenail B, Gerstein H. Foreign-body reaction to bone wax. Oral Surg 1984;58:98.
132. Finn MD, Schow SR, Schneiderman ED. Osseous regeneration in the presence of four hemostatic agents. J Oral Maxillofac Surg 1992;50:608.
133. Solheim E, Pinholt EM, Bang G, Sudmann E. Effect of local hemostatics on bone induction in rats: a comparative study of bone wax, fibrin-collagen paste and bioerodible polyorthoester with and without gentamicin. J Biomed Mater Res 1992;26:791.
134. Witherspoon DE, Gutmann JL. Haemostasis in periradicular surgery. Int Endod J 1996;29:135.
135. Grossman LI. Endodontic practice. 7th ed. Philadelphia: Lea & Febiger; 1970.
136. Sommer R, Ostrander R, Crowley M. Clinical endodontics. 2nd ed., Philadelphia: WB Saunders; 1962.
137. Besner E. Systemic effects of racemic epinephrine when applied to the bony cavity during periapical surgery. Va Dent J 1972;49:9.
138. Pallasch TJ. Vasoconstrictors and the heart. J Calif Dent Assoc 1998;26:668.
139. Lemon RR, Steele PJ, Jeansonne BG. Ferric sulfate hemostasis: effect on osseous wound healing left in situ for maximum exposure. J Endod 1933;19:170.
140. Jeansonne BG, Boggs WS, Lemon RR. Ferric sulfate hemostasis: effect on osseous wound healing. II. With curettage and irrigation. J Endod 1993;19:174.
141. Codben RH, Thrasher EL, Harris WH. Topical hemostatic agents to reduce bleeding from cancellous bone. J Bone Joint Surg 1976;58(A):70.
142. Sottosanti J. Calcium sulfate: a biodegradable and biocompatible barrier for guided tissue regeneration. Compend Contin Educ Dent 1992;13:226.
143. Pecora G, Adreana S, Margarone JE, et al. Bone regeneration with a calcium sulfate barrier. Oral Surg 1997;84:424.
144. Boyes-Varley JG, Cleaton-Jones PE, Lownie JR. Effects of a topical drug combination on the early healing of extraction sockets in the vervet monkey. Int J Oral Maxillofac Surg 1988;17:138.
145. Olson RAJ, Roberts DL, Osbon DB. A comparative study of polylactic acid, Gelfoam, and Surgicel in healing extraction sites. Oral Surg 1982;53:441.
146. Caen JP, Legrand Y, Sultan Y. Platelets: collagen interactions. Thromb Haemost 1970;40:181.
147. Mason RG, Read MS. Some effects of microcrystalline collagen preparations on blood. Haemostasis 1974;3:31.
148. Mattsson T, Anneroth G, Kondell PA, Nordenram A. ACP and Surgicel in bone hemostasis. Swed Dent J 1990;14:57.
149. Swan N. Textured collagen, a hemostatic agent. Oral Surg 1991;72:642.
150. Mason R. Hemostatic mechanisms of microfibrillar collagen. In: Proceedings of a symposium on Avitene (Microfibrillar Collagen Hemostat). Ft Worth (TX): Alcon Laboratories; 1975. p. 32.
151. Kramer GM, Pollack R. Clinical application and histological evaluation of microfibrillar collagen hemostat (Avitene) in periodontal surgery. Int J Periodontics Restorative Dent 1982;2:8.
152. Baumhammers A. Control of excessive bleeding following periodontal surgery. Gen Dent 1983;31:384.
153. Haasch GC, Gerstein H, Austin BP. Effect of two hemostatic agents on osseous healing. J Endod 1989;15:310.
154. Finn MD, Schow SR, Schneiderman ED. Osseous regeneration in the presence of four common hemostatic agents. J Oral Maxillofac Surg 1992;50:608.
155. Takeuchi H, Konaga E, Kashitani M. The usefulness of Avitene for the control of oozing in laparoscopic cholecystectomy. Surg Gynecol Obstet 1993;176:495.
156. Johnson and Johnson. Surgicel product information. New Brunswick, NJ: 1989.
157. Tanzilli JP, Raphael D, Moodnik RM. A comparison of the marginal adaptation of retrograde techniques: a scanning electron microscope study. Oral Surg 1980;50:74.
158. Nedderman TA, Hartwell GR, Portell FR. A comparison of root surfaces following apical root resection with various burs: scanning electron microscopic evaluation. J Endod 1988;14:423.
159. Richman MJ. The use of ultrasonics in root canal therapy and root resection. J Dent Med 1957;12:12.
160. Bertrand G, Festal F, Barailly R. Use of ultrasound in apicoectomy. Quintessence Int 1976;7:9.
161. Wuchenich G, Meadows D, Torabinejad M. A comparison between two root-end preparation techniques in human cadavers. J Endod 1994;20:279.
162. Gutmann JL, Saunders WP, Nguyen L, et al. Ultrasonic root-end preparation. Part 1. SEM analysis. Int Endod J 1994;27:318.
163. Abedi HR, Van Mierlo BL, Wilder-Smith P, Torabinejad M. Effects of ultrasonic root-end cavity preparation on the root apex. Oral Surg 1995;80:207.
164. Min MM, Brown CE Jr, Legan JJ, Kafrawy AH. In vitro evaluation of the effects of ultrasonic root-end preparation on resected root surfaces. J Endod 1997;23:624.
165. Beling KL, Marshall JG, Morgan LA, Baumgartner JC. Evaluation of cracks associated with ultrasonic root-end preparation of gutta-percha filled canals. J Endod 1997;23: May.
166. Waplington M, Lumley P, Walmsley AD. Incidence of root face alteration after ultrasonic retrograde cavity preparation. Oral Surg 1997;83:387.
167. Layton CA, Marshall JG, Morgan LA, Baumgartner JC. Evaluation of cracks associated with ultrasonic root-end preparation. J Endod 1996;22:157.
168. Calzonetti KJ, Iwanowski T, Komorowski R, Friedman S. Ultrasonic root-end cavity preparation assessed by an in situ impression technique. Oral Surg 1998;85:210.
169. Morgan LA, Marshall JG. A scanning electron microscopic study of in vivo ultrasonic root-end preparations. J Endod 1999;25:567.
170. Sumi Y, Hattori H, Hayashi K, Ueda M. Ultrasonic root-end preparation: clinical and radiographic results. J Oral Maxillofac Surg 1996;54:590.
171. Gartner AH, Dorn SO. Advances in endodontic surgery. Dent Clin North Am 1992;36:357.
172. Jou YT, Pertl C. Is there a best retrograde filling material. Dent Clin North Am 1997;41:555.
173. Owadally ID, Chong BS, Pitt Ford TR, Wilson RF. Biological properties of IRM with the addition of hydroxyapatite as a retrograde root filling material. Endod Dent Traumatol 1994;10:228.
174. Makkawy HM, Koka S, Lavin MT, Ewoldsen NO. Cytotoxicity of root perforation materials. J Endod 1998;24:477.
175. Chong BS, Owadally ID, Pitt Ford TR, Wilson RF. Cytotoxicity of potential retrograde root-filling materials. Endod Dent Traumatol 1994;10:129.

176. Zhu Q, Safavi E, Spangberg LSW. Cytotoxic evaluation of root-end filling materials in cultures of human osteoblast-like cells and periodontal ligament cells. J Endod 1999;25:410.
177. Harrison JW, Johnson SA. Excisional wound healing following the use of IRM as a root-end filling material. J Endod 1997;23:19.
178. Pitt Ford TR, Andreasen JO, Dorn SO, Kariyawasam SP. Effect of IRM root-end fillings on healing after replantation. J Endod 1994;20:381
179. Pitt Ford TR, Andreasen JO, Dorn SO, Kariyawasam SP. Effect of Super-EBA as a root-end filling on healing after replantation.J Endod 1995;21:13.
180. Maeda H, Hashiguchi I, Nakamuta H, et al. Histological study of periapical tissue healing in the rat molar after retrofillings with various materials. J Endod 1999;25:38.
181. Torabinejad M, Pitt Ford TR, Abedi HR, et al. Tissue reaction to implanted root-end filling materials.J Endod 1998;24:468.
182. Torabinejad M, Hong CU, McDonald F, Pitt Ford T. Physical and chemical properties of a new root-end filling material. J Endod 1995;21:349.
183. Torabinejad M, Watson TF, Pitt Ford TR. Sealing ability of a mineral trioxide aggregate when used as a root-end filling material. J Endod 1993;19:591.
184. Torabinejad M, Higa RK, McKendry DJ, Pitt Ford TR. Dye leakage of four root-end filling materials: effects of blood contamination. J Endod 1994;20:159.
185. Bates CF, Carnes DL, del Rio CE. Longitudinal sealing ability of mineral trioxide aggregate as a root-end filling material. J Endod 1996;22:575.
186. Fischer EJ, Arens DE, Miller CH. Bacterial leakage of mineral trioxide aggregate as compared with zinc-free amalgam, intermediate restorative material, and Super-EBA as a root-end filling material. J Endod 1998;24:176.
187. Torabinejad M, Rastegar AF, Kettering JD, Pitt Ford TR. Bacterial leakage of mineral trioxide aggregate as a root-end filling material. J Endod 1995;21:109.
188. Torabinejad M, Smith PW, Kettering JD, Pitt Ford TR. Comparative investigation of marginal adaptation of mineral trioxide aggregate and other commonly used root-end filling materials. J Endod 1995;21:295.
189. Koh ET, McDonald R, Pitt Ford TR, Torabinejad M. Cellular response to mineral trioxide aggregate. J Endod 1998;24.
190. Torabinejad M, Hong CU, Pitt Ford TR, Kettering JD. Cytotoxicity of four root end filling material. J Endod 1995;21:489.
191. Kettering JD, Torabinejad M. Investigation of mutagenicity of mineral trioxide aggregate and other commonly used root end filling materials. J Endod 1995;21:537.
192. Torabinejad M, Hong CU, Pitt Ford TR. Tissue reaction to implanted Super-EBA and mineral trioxide aggregate in the mandibles of guinea pigs: a preliminary report. J Endod 1995;21:569.
193. Torabinejad M, Hong CU, Lee SJ, et al. Investigation of mineral trioxide aggregate for root end filling in dogs. J Endod 1995;21:603.
194. Torabinejad M, Pitt Ford TR, McKendry DJ, et al. Histologic assessment of mineral trioxide aggregate as a root-end filling in monkeys. J Endod 1997;23:225.
195. Oynick J, Oynick T. A study of a new material for retrograde fillings. J Endod 1978;4:203.
196. Dorn SO, Gartner AH. Retrograde filling materials: a retrospective success-failure study of amalgam, EBA, and IRM. J Endod 1990;16:391.
197. Pantschev A, Carlsson AP, Andersson L. Retrograde root filling with EBA cement or amalgam. A comparative clinical study. Oral Surg 1994;78:101.
198. Rud J, Munksgaard EC, Andreasen JO, et al. Retrograde root fillings with composite and a dentin-bonding agent. Endod Dent Traumatol 1991;7(Pt 1):118.
199. Rud J, Munksgaard EC, Andreasen JO, Rud V. Retrograde root fillings with composite and a dentin-bonding agent. Endod Dent Traumatol 1991;7:126.
200. Rud J, Rud V, Munksgaard EC. Long-term evaluation of retrograde root fillings with dentin-bonded resin composite. J Endod 1996;22:90.
201. Rud J, Rud V, Munksgaard EC. Retrograde root filling with dentin-bonded modified resin composite. J Endod 1996;22:477.
202. Rud J, Rud V, Munksgaard EC. Effect of root canal contents on healing of teeth with dentin-bonded resin composite retrograde seal. J Endod 1997;23:535.
203. Michelich VJ, Schuster GS, Pashley DH. Bacterial penetration of human dentin in-vivo. J Dent Res 1980;59:1398.
204. Barkhordar RA, Watanabe LG, Marshall GW, Hussain MZ. Removal of intracanal smear layer by Doxycycline in vitro. Oral Surg 1997;84:420.
205. Craig KR, Harrison JW. Wound healing following demineralization of resected root ends in periradicular surgery. J Endod 1993;19:339.
206. Rifkin BR, Vernillo AT, Golub LM. Blocking periodontal disease progression by inhibiting tissue-destructive enzymes: a potential therapeutic role for tetracyclines and their chemically-modified analogs. J Periodontol 1993;64:819.
207. Aleo JJ, De Renzis FA, Farbet PA. In vitro attachment of human fibroblasts to root surfaces. J Periodontol 1975;46:639.
208. Minabe M, Takeuchi K, Kumada H, Umemoto T. The effect of root conditioning with minocycline HCl in removing endotoxin from the roots of periodontally involved teeth. J Periodontol 1994;65:387.
209. Barkhordar RA, Russel T. Effect of Doxycycline on the apical seal of retrograde filling materials. J Calif Dent Assoc 1998.
210. Fitzpatrick EL, Steiman HR. Scanning electron microscopic evaluation of finishing techniques on IRM and EBA retrofillings. J Endod 1997;23:423.
211. Forte SG, Hauser MJ, Hahn C, Hartwell GR. Microleakage of Super-EBA with and without finishing as determined by the fluid filtration method. J Endod 1998;24: 799.
212. Eriksson L. Cyanoacrylate for closure of wounds in the oral mucosa in dogs. Odontol Revy 1976;27:19.
213. Javelet J, Torabinejad M, Danforth R. Isobutyl cyanoacrylate: a clinical and histological comparison with sutures in closing mucosal incisions in monkeys. Oral Surg 1985;59:91.
214. Vanholder R, Misotten A, Roels H, Matton G. Cyanoacrylate tissue adhesive for closing skin wounds: a double blind randomized comparison with sutures. Biomaterials 1993;14:737.
215. Simon HK, McLario KJ, Bruns TB, et al. Long-term appearance of lacerations repaired using a tissue adhesive. Pediatrics 1997;99:193.
216. Samuel PR, Roberts AC, Nigam A. The use of Indermil (n-butyl cyanoacrylate) in otorhinolaryngology and head and neck surgery. A preliminary report on the first 33 patients. J Laryngol Otol 1997;111:536.

217. Giray CB, Atasever A, Durgun B, Araz K. Clinical and electron microscopic comparison of silk sutures and n-butyl-2-cyanoacrylate in human mucosa. Aust Dent J 1997;42:255.
218. Grisdale J. The use of cyanoacrylate in periodontal therapy. J Can Dent Assoc 1998;64:632.
219. Lilly GE, Armstrong JH, Salem JE, Cutcher JL. Reaction of oral tissues to suture materials. Oral Surg 1968;26(Pt 2):592.
220. Lilly GE, Armstrong JH, Cutcher JL. Reaction of oral tissues to suture materials. Oral Surg 26(Pt 3):432.
221. Lilly GE, Cutcher JL, Nones TC, Armstrong JH. Reaction of oral tissues to suture materials. Oral Surg 1972;33:152.
222. Ebert JR. Method for scanning electron microscopic study of plaque on periodontal suture material. J Dent Res 1974;53:1298.
223. Rakusin H, Harrison JW, Marker VA. Alteration of the manipulative properties of plain gut suture material by hydration. J Endod 1988;14:121.
224. Craig PH, Williams JA, Davis KW. A biologic comparison of polyglactin 910 and polyglycolic acid synthetic sutures. Surg Gynecol Obstet 1975;141:1.
225. Nelson EH, Junakoshi E, O'Leary TJ. A comparison of the continuous and interrupted suturing technique. J Periodontol 1977;48:273.
226. Ramfjord SP, Nissle RR. The modified Widman flap. J Periodontol 1974;45:601.
227. Alexander RE. Patient understanding of postsurgical instruction forms. Oral Surg 1999;87:153.
228. Guyton AC. Textbook of medical physiology. 7th ed. St Louis (MO): Mosby; 1986. p. 860.
229. Seymour RA, Meedhan JG, Blair GS. Postoperative pain after apicoectomy. Int Endod J 1986;19:242.
230. Davis W, Oakley J, Smith E. Comparison of the effectiveness of etidocaine and lidocaine as local anesthetic agents during oral surgery. Anesth Prog 1984;31:159.
231. Dunsky J, Moore P. Long-acting local anesthetics: a comparison of bupivacaine and etidocaine in endodontics. J Endod 1984;10:6.
232. Weisman MI. Comfortable suture removal. J Endod 1981;7:186.
233. Anson D. Calcium sulfate: a 4-year observation of its use as a resorbable barrier in guided tissue regeneration of periodontal defects. Compend Contin Educ Dent 1996;17:895.
234. Pecora G, Baek SH, Rethman S, Kim S. Barrier membrane techniques in endodontic microsurgery. Dent Clin North Am 1997;41:585.
235. Bier SJ, Sininsky MC. The versatility of calcium sulfate: resolving periodontal challenges. Compend Contin Educ Dent 1999;20:655.
236. Kellert M, Chalfin H, Solomon C. Guided tissue regeneration: an adjunct to endodontic surgery. J Am Dent Assoc 1994;125:1229.
237. Uchin RA. Use of a bioresorbable guided tissue membranes as an adjunct to bony regeneration in cases requiring endodontic surgical intervention. J Endod 1996;22:94.
238. Tseng CC, Harn WM, Chen YH, et al. A new approach to the treatment of true-combined endodontic-periodontic lesions by the guided tissue regeneration technique. J Endod 1996;22:693.
239. Santamaria J, Garcia AM, de Vincente JC, et al. Bone regeneration after radicular cyst removal with and without guided bone regeneration. Int J Oral Maxillofac Surg 1998;27:118.
240. Pecora G, Kim S, Celletti R, Davarpanah M. The guided tissue regeneration principle in endodontic surgery: one-year postoperative results of large periapical lesions. Int Endod J 1995;28:41.
241. Kirchoff DA, Gerstein H. Presurgical crown contouring for root amputation procedures. Oral Surg 1969;27:379.
242. Bergenholtz A. Radectomy of multirooted teeth. J Am Dent Assoc 1972;85:870.
243. Klanan B. Clinical observations following root amputation in maxillary molar teeth. J Periodontol 1975;46:1.
244. Hamp SE, Nyman S, Lindhe J. Periodontal treatment of multirooted teeth. Results after 5 years. J Clin Periodontol 1975;2:126.
245. Langer B, Stein SD, Wagenberg B. An evaluation of root resections. A ten-year study. J Periodontol 1981;52:719.
246. Erpenstein H. A 3-year study of hemisected molars. J Clin Periodontol 1983;10:1.
247. Buhler H. Evaluation of root-resected teeth. Results after 10 years. J Periodontol 1988;59:805.
248. Carnevale G, Febo GD, Tonelli MP, et al. A retrospective analysis of the periodontal-prosthetic treatment of molars with interradicular lesions. Int J Periodontics Restorative Dent 1991;11:189.
249. Basten CHJ, Ammons WF Jr, Persson R. Long-term evaluation of root-resected molars. A retrospective study. Int J Periodontics Restorative Dent 1996;16:207.
250. Blomlof L, Jansson L, Appelgren R, et al. Prognosis and mortality of root-resected molars. Int J Periodontics Restorative Dent 1997;17:191.
251. Carnevale G, Pontoriero R, di Fego G. Long-term effects of root-resective therapy in furcation-involved molars. A 10-year longitudinal study. J Clin Periodontol 1998;25:209.
252. Pecora JD, et al. In vitro study of the incidence of radicular grooves in maxillary incisors. Braz Dent J 1991;2:69.
253. Goon WWY, et al. Complex facial radicular groove in a maxillary lateral incisor. J Endod 1991;17:244.
254. Robinson SF, Cooley RL. Palatogingival groove lesions: recognition and treatment. Gen Dent 1988;36:340.
255. Grossman L. Intentional replantation of teeth. J Am Dent Assoc 1982;104:633.
256. Weinberger B. Introduction to the history of dentistry. Vol. 1. St. Louis (MO): Mosby; 1948. p. 105.
257. Fauchard P. Le Chirurgien Dentiste Ou Traite des'Dents. Paris: Chez Pierre-Jean Mariette; 1746. p. 375.
258. Berdmore T. A treatise on the disorders and deformities of the teeth and gums. London: White, Dodsley, Beckett, and deHondt; 1768. p. 96.
259. Hammer H. Replantation and implantation of teeth. Int Dent J 1955;5:439.
260. Deeb E, Prietto P, Mckenna R. Reimplantation of luxated teeth in humans. J South Calif State Dent Assoc 1965;33:194.
261. Grossman L, Chacker F. Clinical evaluation and histologic study of intentionally replanted teeth. In: Grossman L, editor. Transactions of the Fourth International Conference on Endodontics. Philadelphia: University of Pennsylvania; 1968. p. 127.
262. Dryden JA, Arens DE. Intentional replantation: A viable alternative for selected cases. Dent Clin North Am 1994;38:325.
263. Kingsbury B, Weisenbaugh J. Intentional replantation of mandibular premolars and molars. J Am Dent Assoc 1971;83:1053.

264. Koenig K, Nguyen N, Barkholder. Intentional replantation: a report of 192 cases. Gen Dent 1988;36:327.
265. Bender IB, Rossman LE. Intentional replantation of endodontically treated teeth. Oral Surg 1993;76:623.
266. Raghoebar GM, Vissink A. Results of intentional replantation of molars. J Oral Maxillofac Surg 1999;57:240.
267. Kratchman S. Intentional replantation. Dent Clin North Am 1997;41:603.
268. Nosonowitz D, Stanley H. Intentional replantation to prevent predictable endodontic failures. Oral Surg 1984;57:423.
269. Jansen CE. Implant procedures 101. J Calif Dent Assoc 2000;28:277.
270. Weine FS, Frank AL. Survival of the endodontic endosseous implant. J Endod 1993;19:524.
271. Orlay JG. Endodontic splinting treatment in periodontal disease. Br Dent J 1960;108:118.
272. Frank AL. Improvement in the crown:root ratio by endodontic endosseous implants. J Am Dent Assoc 1967;74:451.
273. Frank AL. Endodontic endosseous implants and treatment of the wide-open apex. Dent Clin North Am 1967;Nov:675.
274. Frank AL, Abrams AM. Histologic evaluation of endodontic implants. J Am Dent Assoc 1969;78:520.
275. Branemark PI, Zarb GA, Albektsson T. Tissue-integrated prosthesis. Chicago: Quintessence Publishing; 1985. p. 11.
276. Brunski JB, Moccaia FF, et al. The influence of functional use of endosseous dental implants on the tissue-implant interface. I. Histological aspects. J Dent Res 1979;58:1953.
277. Mombelli A, Van Ossten MAC, et al. The microbiota associated with successful or failing osseointegrated titanium implants. Oral Microbiol Immunonol 1987;2:145.
278. Gelb DA. Immediate implant surgery: ten-year clinical overview. Compend Contin Educ Dent 1999;20:1185.
279. Rosenquist B, Grenthe B, et al. Immediate placement of implants into extraction sockets. Int J Oral Maxillofac Implants 1996;11:205.
280. Buchanan LS. The art of endodontics: a rationale for treatment. DentToday 1993;12:30.
281. Carr GB. Advanced techniques and visual enhancement for endodontic surgery. Endod Rep 1992;7:6.
282. Carr GB. Microscopes in endodontics. Calif Dent Assoc J 1992;20:55.
283. Rubinstein R. Horizons in endodontic surgery. Part I: The operating microscope. Oak County (MI) Review 1991;30:7.
284. Rubinstein R. Horizons in endodontic surgery. Part II: The operating microscope. Oak County (MI) Review 1992;30:9.
285. Pecora G, Andreana S. Use of dental operating microscope in endodontic surgery. Oral Surg 1993;75:751.
286. Ruddle CJ. Surgical endodontic retreatment. Calif Dent Assoc J 1991;19:61.
287. Selden HS. The role of the dental operating microscope in endodontics. Pa Dent J 1986;55:36.
288. Bellizzi R, Loushine R. Adjuncts to posterior endodontic surgery. J Endod 1990;16:604.
289. Reuben HL, Apotheker H. Apical surgery with the dental microscope. Oral Surg 1984;57:433.
290. Rubinstein R. Endodontic microsurgery and the surgical operating microscope. Compend Contin Educ Dent 1997;18:659.
291. Rubinstein RA, Kim S. Short-term observation of the results of endodontic surgery with the use of a surgical operating microscope and Super-EBA as root-end filling material. J Endod 1999;25:43.

Chapter 13

OUTCOME OF ENDODONTIC TREATMENT AND RE-TREATMENT

John I. Ingle, James H. Simon, Pierre Machtou, and Patrick Bogaerts

A question that should be asked of any discipline or technique in dentistry is, "What degree of success should be expected?" Success, in turn, should be measured longitudinally in time—long-range success as opposed to short-term success. The beautiful resin restoration turning an ugly yellow in 1 year is not an unqualified success. By the same token, the denture "worn" in the bureau drawer is far from successful, nor is the well-fitting partial denture successful if it leads to clasp caries in 6 months. Moreover, the endodontically treated tooth with a large periradicular lesion that does not show signs of healing 2 years after treatment cannot be considered a success.

To answer the question, "How successful is endodontic therapy?" a study was undertaken at the University of Washington School of Dentistry to evaluate endodontically treated teeth to determine their rate of success. More important to the study, the rate of failure was also established, and the **causes of failure** were carefully examined. Analysis of the failures led to modifications in technique and treatment. Finally, the entire discipline of endodontic therapy was re-examined, and definitive improvements were made as a result. The improvements in treatment are reflected in the improvement in success, which increased to 94.45% from a former success rate of 91.10%, an improvement of 3.35 percentage points. In other words, **nearly 95% of all endodontically treated teeth were successful.**

There was also a hidden agenda to the Washington study—to prove ourselves to a profession that, at that time, was skeptical of root canal therapy. In light of today's knowledge, the project had some design flaws and misinterpretations and was not that well controlled, even though each phase was subjected to statistical analysis. The null hypothesis was ignored in an effort to prove a point: **root canal therapy could be successful if properly done.** On the other hand, the figures of the Washington study compared favorably with other reports of success.[1–13]

A group at Temple University, for example, reported a 95.2% success rate at the end of **1 year** with 458 canals filled by the gutta-percha-euchapercha method.[5] They found that teeth that started with vital inflamed pulps had more success (98.2%) than teeth with nonvital pulps (93.1%). Contrary to other reports, however, they were far less successful with short-filled canals (71.1%) than with flush-filled or overfilled canals (100%). (Reports of 100% success must be questioned.)

South African researchers enjoyed a success rate similar to that of the Temple University group: 89% success at the end of 1 year.[6] Also, as with the Temple group, they were successful 92% of the time in teeth filled to the apex and 91% of the time if the canals were overfilled. Filling short of the apex reduced their success rate to 82%.[6]

The poorest reported rate of success dealt with 845 Dutch military servicemen.[7] After 17 years, 45% of the endodontically treated teeth had failed in nonaviators, whereas only 7% had failed in aviator patients. There is a simple explanation for this wide discrepancy in failure rate. The aviators were usually treated with gutta-percha or silver point fillings, whereas the nonaviators were more frequently treated by "therapy with special chemical compounds." Furthermore, the aviators' teeth were more frequently crowned.[7]

Hession, a highly respected endodontist in Australia, reported the highest rate of success: 98.7% of 151 teeth.[8] Nelson reported lower rates in England: 81.9% of 299 teeth. With re-treatment, however, Nelson salvaged 11 of the treatment failures, raising the success rate to 85.6%.[9] Kerekes and Tronstad, using the standardized technique recommended in this text, had a success rate similar to the Washington study,[10] as did Sjögren and his associates from Sweden.[11] Their remarkable study of 356 endodontic patients, re-examined 8 to 10 years later, reported a 96% success rate if the teeth had vital pulps prior to treatment. The success rate dropped to 86% if the pulps were necrotic and the teeth had periradicular lesions and dropped still lower to **62% if the teeth had been re-treated.** They concluded by stating that "teeth with pulp necrosis and periradicular lesions and those with periradicular lesions undergoing re-treatment constitute major therapeutic problems..." They surmised that bacteria in "sites inaccessible" might be the cause of increased failure.[11]

Worldwide, most controlled studies seem to agree that a lower success rate is associated with overfilled canals, teeth with preexisting periradicular lesions, and teeth not properly restored after root canal therapy.[11–15] A Swedish group reported a high failure rate if canals were not totally obturated.[13] Sjögren et al., quoted above, also noted a direct correlation between success and the point of termination of the root filling.[11] As Figure 13-1 shows, teeth filled within 0 to 2 mm from the apex enjoyed a 94% success rate, which fell to 76% if the teeth were overfilled and fell further to 68% if they were filled more than 2 mm short.

In reported **re-treatment** of initial endodontic failures, success figures have been unacceptably low. Only 50% of the overfilled teeth were acceptable (Figure 13-2). Similarly, a Japanese group reported a much higher failure rate if root fillings were overextended.[14] Surprisingly, a Dutch group enjoyed as high a healing rate whether or not the canals were filled.[16] The Dutch report was only a 2-year study. Unfilled canals had not been followed over a long period of time (such as 10 to 20 years). Most endodontically treated teeth should last as long as other teeth. Vire examined 116 root-filled teeth that were extracted because of failure and found that only 8.6% failed for endodontic reasons compared with 59.4% restorative failures and 32% periodontal failures.[17]

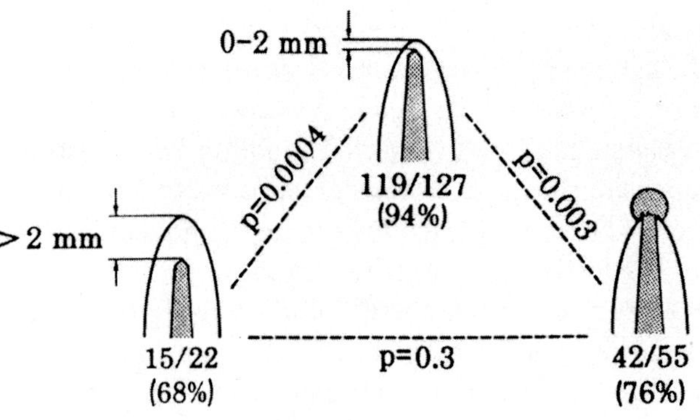

Figure 13-1 Outcome of **treatment** according to the level of the root filling in relation to the root apex in cases with **preoperative pulp necrosis** and **apical periodontitis.** Number of healed lesions/number of preoperative lesions. Reproduced with permission from Sjögren U.[11]

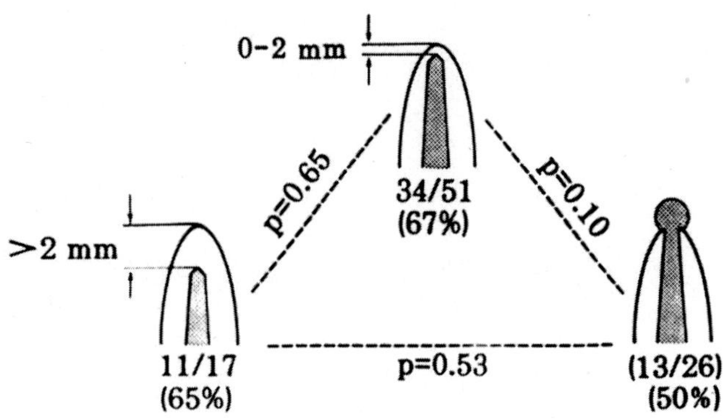

Figure 13-2 Results of **re-treatment** of previously filled roots with **apical periodontitis** with regard to the level of the final root filling in relation to the root apex. Number of healed lesions/number of preoperative lesions. Reproduced with permission from Sjögren U.[11]

The Washington Study

The figures above from the University of Washington are only a few from an exhaustive study encompassing many aspects of endodontic therapy. The modifications in treatment mentioned above were instituted following a pilot study of endodontic success and failure. Even with the limited number of patients in the pilot study, the causes of failure became apparent. Clinical techniques were then changed in an effort to overcome failure. Patients were recalled for follow-up at 6 months, 1 year, 2 years, and 5 years, and the recall radiographs were carefully evaluated for improvement or lack of improvement. Teeth included in the **success** group were those that demonstrated decided periradicular improvement (Figures 13-3 and 13-4) and those with continuing periradicular health (Figure 13-5). The **failures** were made up of those teeth that initially demonstrated periradicular damage and that **had not** improved (Figure 13-6), as well as those that had **deteriorated** since treatment (see Figure 13-6). As soon as a statistically significant group of cases built up in the file, the material was ready to be analyzed.

The 2-year recall series was found to be ideal for this study because a statistically significant sample developed within this group. The 5-year recall sample was also analyzed but in understandably smaller, though significant, numbers. The study did not take into consideration any illnesses or systemic differences between patients.

Two-Year Recall Analysis. Of a total population of 3,678 patients who could have returned for 2 years, 1,229 actually did return, a recall rate of 33.41%—a statistically significant cohort. Before improvements in technique and case selection were instituted, there was

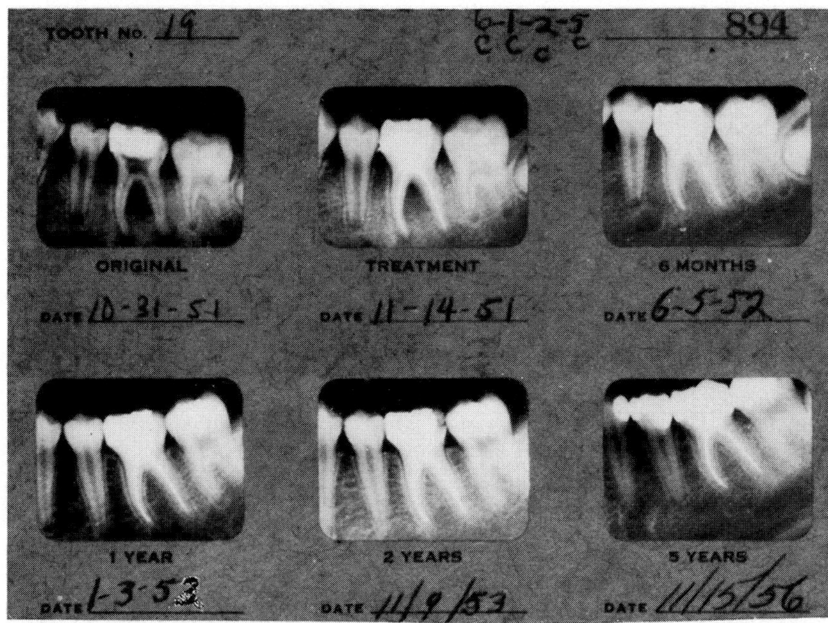

Figure 13-3 Special mount for radiographs taken of each case. Note that recall films are exposed at 6 months, 1 year, 2 years, and 5 years following therapy. Figures at the top of the card indicate that **complete** healing had occurred at 6 months and was maintained for 5 years.

a 91.10% success rate—104 failures of 1,067 cases. After these improvements were instituted, the success rate rose to 94.45%—9 failures of 162 cases.

Five-Year Recall Analysis. From the beginning of the study, enough 5-year recalls had returned to make a statistically valid analysis of these cases. Of the 302 5-year recalls, 281 teeth were successful—a success rate of 93.05%; 21 teeth were considered failures—a failure rate of 6.95%. These figures compare favorably with the 2-year recall analysis.

Two-Year Recall Analysis by Age of Patient. Reference is frequently made to age as a criterion for

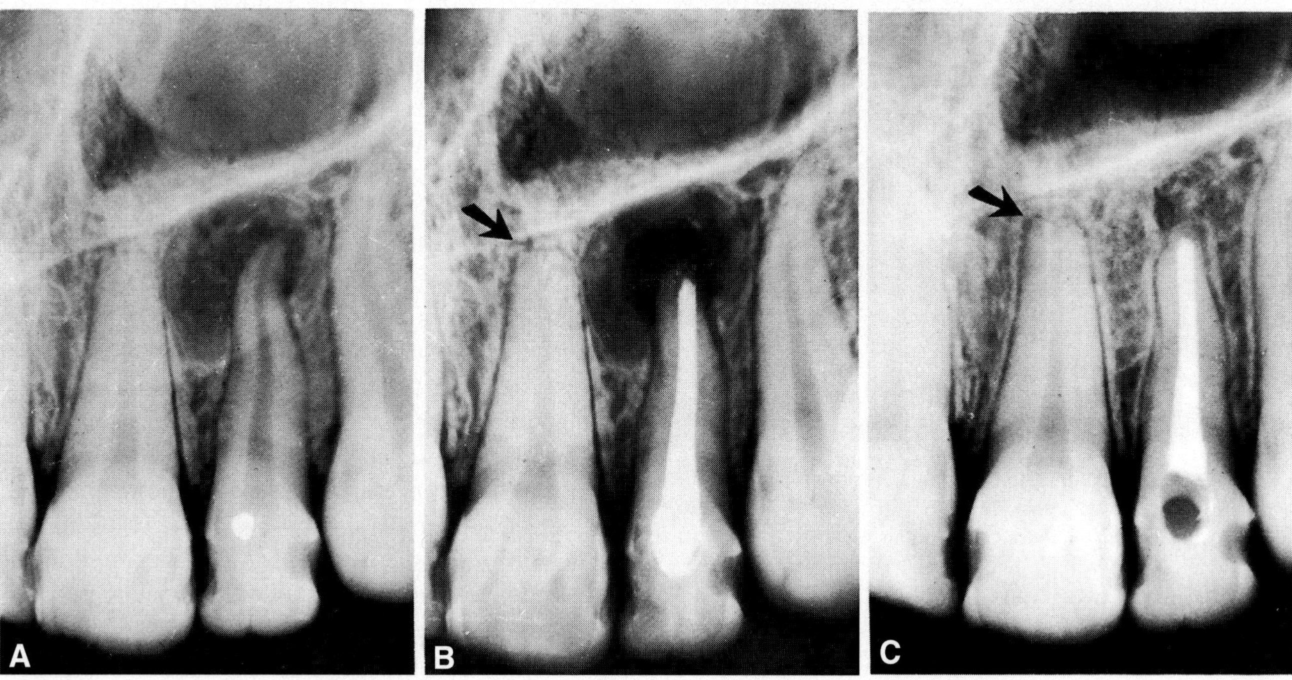

Figure 13-4 A, "Before" radiograph, with large periradicular lesion. B, "Treatment" radiograph immediately following periradicular surgery. Also note the fractured root tip of a central incisor (**arrow**) that tests vital. C, Two-year postoperative radiograph of successfully treated case. Lack of total periradicular repair (**moderate** repair) is related to extensive surface of filling material over which cementum cannot grow. Also note fracture repair (**arrow**) of vital central incisor.

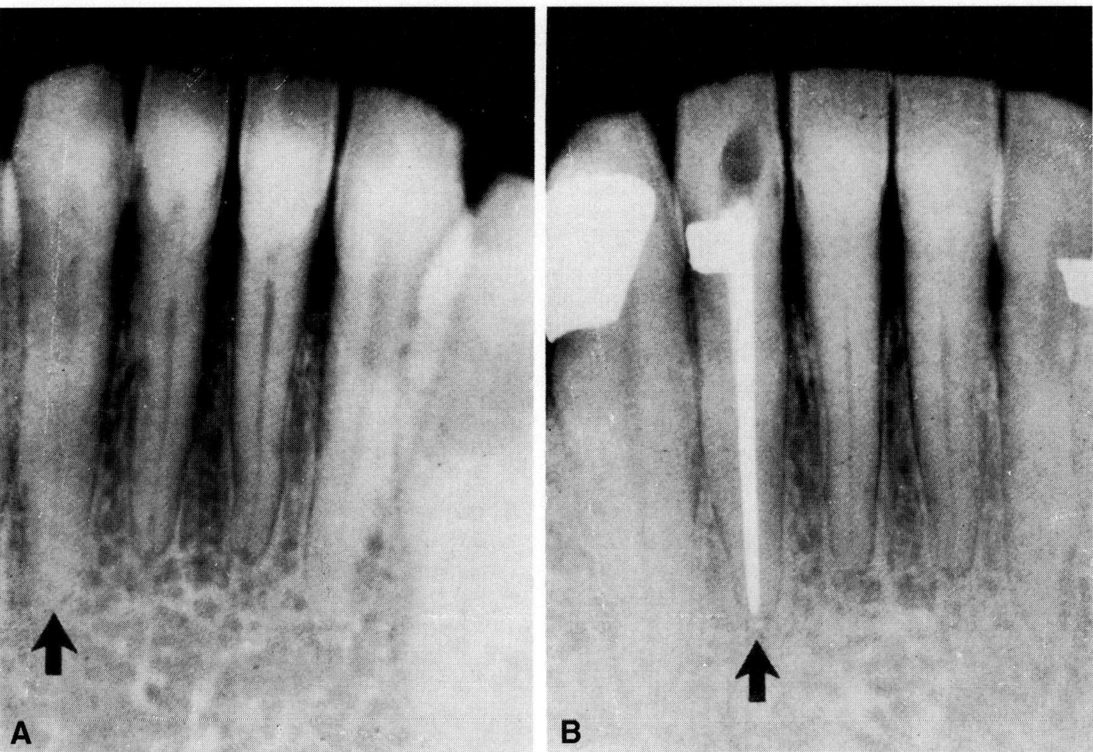

Figure 13-5 A, Pulpless mandibular lateral incisor with no periradicular lesion. **B,** Constant periradicular health is revealed in a 2-year postoperative radiograph, a successful case.

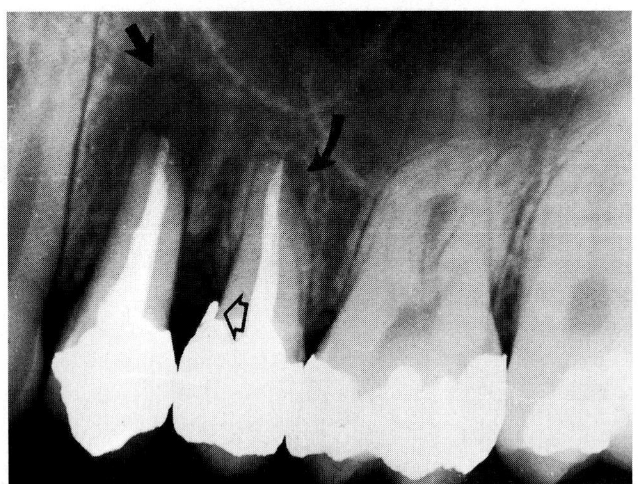

Figure 13-6 Two failure cases demonstrated in a single radiograph. **Curved arrow (right)** points to a lesion that has failed to heal 2 years following endodontic treatment. **Straight arrow (left)** points to a lesion that has grown worse 2 years following therapy. Lack of total obturation of canals is revealed by the fuzzy appearance of root canal fillings. Defective amalgam restoration (**open arrow**) contributes to an interproximal periodontal lesion.

endodontic treatment. The youngest patient treated in the study was 2½ years old; the oldest patient was 92 years old. There was a fairly consistent rate of success and failure according to age as shown by statistical analysis ($\chi^2 = 2.72$; $p > .09$). Age, of course, has a great deal to do with the size and shape of the canal. It was found that older teeth, with more restricted canals, were more successfully obturated than very "young" teeth with large-diameter canals. It also became obvious that the size and shape of the lumen of the canal, as well as the direction of root curvature, play an important part in the successful completion of a root canal filling. Analysis of success, by individual tooth, will demonstrate these points.

Two-Year Recall Analysis by Individual Tooth. No significant difference in failure existed between any of the teeth in either arch ($\chi^2 = 2.45$; $p > .10$). Thus, no particular tooth can be considered a higher endodontic risk, although there was a wide discrepancy between the **mandibular second premolar** with a failure rate of 4.54% and the **mandibular first premolar** with a failure rate of 11.45%. Canal anatomy might account for the greater increase in failure in the first premolar. Pucci and Reig, in their monumental work ***Conductos Radiculares,*** pointed out the great anatomic differences between the two mandibular premolars.[18] Whereas the mandibular second premolar has two canals and two foramina 11.5% of the time, the **mandibular first premolar has branching canals, apical bifurcation, and trifurcation 26.5% of the time.**[18]

Others have found similar discrepancies between mandibular premolars, most recently Trope et al. at the University of Pennsylvania.[19] These researchers confirmed one of Pucci and Reig's findings almost exactly: 23.2% of the **mandibular first premolars** examined had two canals. They also found that 7.8% of second premolars had two canals, a figure differing from Pucci and Reig's 11.5%. This discrepancy could well be explained on an ethnic basis: the researchers at Pennsylvania reporting on a US African American population and Pucci reporting on a Uruguayan population containing some aborigines.

The Pennsylvania study also confirmed the notion that African American patients more frequently have two canals in lower premolars than white patients. In the first premolars, 32.8% had two canals, compared with 13.7% of whites. In the second premolars, 7.8% of African Americans had two canals, compared with 2.8% of whites. Nearly 40% of the African Americans in the study had at least one premolar with two canals and 16% of the time presented **two separate roots** in mandibular first premolars.[19]

Failures in the **maxillary lateral incisor** may also be explained by anatomic differences. Pucci and Reig showed extensive distal curvature of the maxillary lateral incisor root 49.2% of the time.[18] Here again, poor judgment and preparation frequently prevent adequate instrumentation and obturation, with root perforation at the curvature a common occurrence (Figure 13-7). Increased failure rate in the maxillary lateral incisor is also related to continuing root resorption following treatment, a finding peculiar to these teeth.

The overall failure rate, mandible to maxilla, is striking but not statistically significant. Failure in the mandibular arch was encountered 6.65% of the time and 9.03% of the time in the maxilla.

Two-Year Recall Analysis: Nonsurgical versus Surgical Intervention. The degree of success achieved by surgical intervention in treated endodontic cases has long been a contentious point. The Washington study demonstrated that although nonsurgical treatment appears to be slightly more successful than surgical treatment, differences are not statistically significant ($\chi^2 = 3.44$; $p > .05$).

It is tempting to indict case selection as the basis for increased failure of surgical treatment. One of the indications for surgical intervention has been the grossly involved periradicular lesion, where a lower rate of repair might be expected. Although the 10 to 12 mm periradicular lesion appears to heal as readily, if not quite as rapidly, as the 2 mm lesion (Figure 13-8), this may not always be true. Others have shown that larger lesions, or cases with lesions versus those without, are less successful. Nelson reported that the failure rate was three times higher if a periradicular lesion existed before treatment.[9] In another study, the failure rate was the same.[16] The Dutch study, interestingly enough, found that "teeth with periradicular granulomas tend to heal less successfully than teeth showing cysts."[12] Similarly, Japanese researchers reported a wide discrepancy in success between treated teeth that had no periradicular rarefaction (88%) and those with a 5.0 mm or greater rarefaction (38.5%).[14] For those teeth without periradicular lesions, Sjögren et al. reported a 96% success rate, but this rate dropped to 86% if periradicular lesions were present.[11]

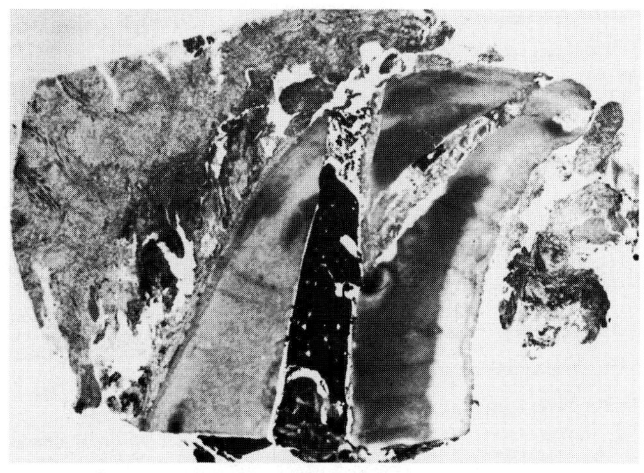

Figure 13-7 Root tip biopsy from the curved apex of a maxillary lateral incisor. Severe inflammatory reaction surrounding the root end is related to perforation as well as failure to débride and obturate the curved portion of the canal. Reproduced with permission from Luebke RG, Glick DH, Ingle JI. Oral Surg 1964;18:97.

Two-Year Recall Analysis of Endodontic Failures. The final and most important portion of the Washington study dealt with 104 failure cases as a group. Careful analysis of these particular cases is most revealing.

Arrangement of Failures by Frequency of Occurrence. As Table 13-1 shows, the most striking finding is the 58.66% of the failures caused by **incomplete obturation** of the canal (Figure 13-9). This is a highly significant figure. This most common cause of failure is almost 50 percentage points ahead of the next greatest cause of failure, **root perforation,** which

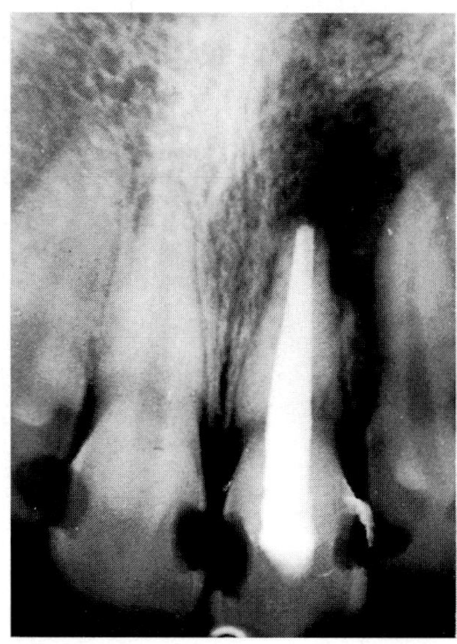

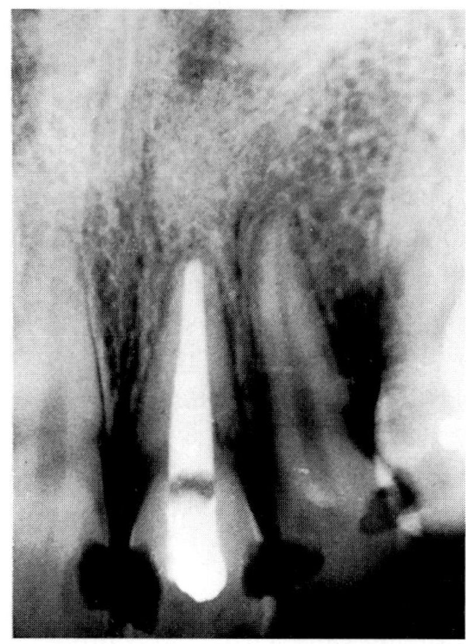

Figure 13-8 Large periradicular lesion (**left**) has healed completely (**right**) within 6 months in a patient 20 years of age.

Table 13-1 Distribution of Failures of Treated Endodontic Cases: Two-Year Recall by Frequency of Occurrence

Causes of Failure	Number of Failures	% Failures
Incomplete obturation	61	58.66
Root perforation	10	9.61
External root resorption	8	7.70
Coexistent periodontal-periradicular lesion	6	5.78
Canal grossly overfilled or overextended	4	3.85
Canal left unfilled	3	2.88
Developing apical cyst	3	2.88
Adjacent pulpless tooth	3	2.88
Silver point inadvertently removed	2	1.92
Broken instrument	1	0.96
Accessory canal unfilled	1	0.96
Constant trauma	1	0.96
Perforation, nasal floor	1	0.96
Total failures	104	100.00

Distribution of 104 endodontic failures 2 years following therapy. When arranged by frequency of occurrence, note that **incomplete obturation** accounts for almost 60% of all failures, followed by **root perforation**, which accounts for nearly 10% of 104 failures. Cause of failure includes infrequently encountered conditions that occur less than 1% of the time.

accounts for 9.61% of the failures. Thus, the two greatest causes of failure stand revealed: **inadequate cleaning and shaping** and **incomplete obturation.** In other words, over two-thirds of all of the endodontic failures in the study were related to inadequate performance of two points of the endodontic triad, "canal instrumentation and canal obturation." This alone would call for improved technique and attention to detail.

Categorical Arrangement of Causes of Failure. The 13 causes of endodontic failure may be arranged in three general categories of causes leading to failure: (1) apical percolation, (2) operative errors, and (3) errors in case selection (Table 13-2). Actually, a clear-cut delineation of the agents of failure is difficult; apical percolation into the canal accounts for almost all of these failures, as Table 13-2 shows.

Apical Percolation. Three of the causes of failure shown in Table 13-2 lead to apical percolation and subsequent diffusion stasis into the canal (Figures 13-10 and 13-11). Factor in the bacteria lurking in the region and these three causes together account for 63.47% of all of the endodontic failures in the study and demonstrate how vital careful therapy is to success. One must also consider the potential of microleakage under and around coronal restorations: bacteria penetrating from the crown to the periapex alongside poorly obturated canals.

Operative Errors. A category made up of errors in coronal cavity preparation and canal preparation accounts for almost 15% of the failures (root perforation, 9.61%; broken instrument, 0.96%; and canal grossly overfilled, 3.85%; total, 14.42% of all of the failures).

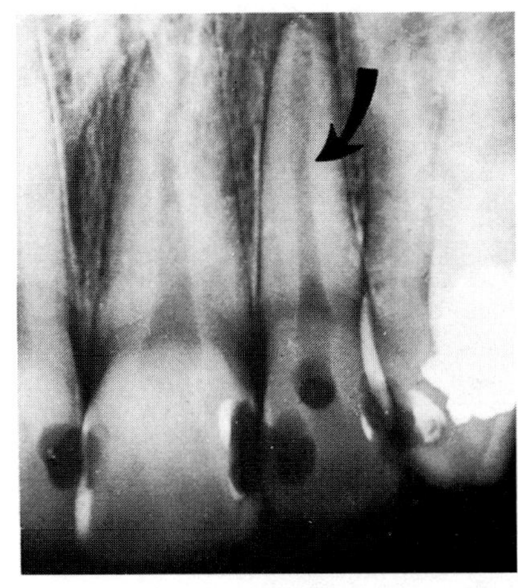

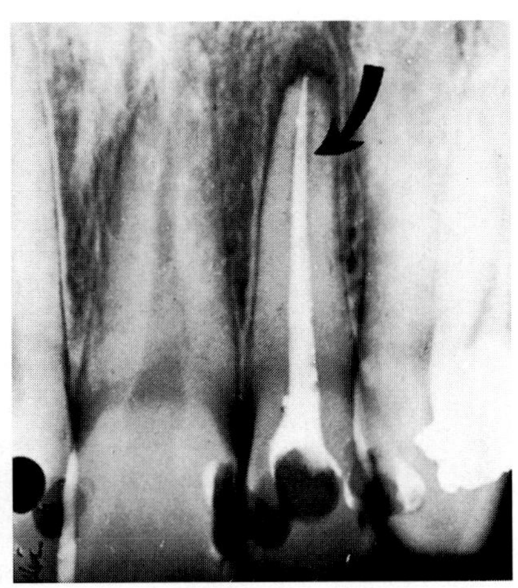

Figure 13-9 **Left,** Careful examination of an initial radiograph reveals internal resorption and widening of the canal apical to the **curved arrow.** **Right,** In a 2-year recall radiograph, periradicular lesion persists owing to failure to totally obliterate the root canal space (**arrow**).

Table 13-2 Distribution of Failures of Treated Endodontic Cases: Two-Year Recall by Category of Cause of Failure

Causes of Failure	Number of Failures	% Failures
Apical percolation—total	**66**	**63.46**
Incomplete obturation	61	58.66
Unfilled canal	3	2.88
Ag point inadvertently removed	2	1.92
Operative error—total	**15**	**14.42**
Root perforation	10	9.61
Canal grossly overfilled or overextended	4	3.85
Broken instrument	1	0.96
Errors in case selection—total	**23**	**22.12**
External root resorption	8	7.70
Coexistent periodontal-periradicular lesion	6	5.78
Developing apical cyst	3	2.88
Adjacent pulpless tooth	3	2.88
Accessory canal unfilled	1	0.96
Constant trauma	1	0.96
Perforation, nasal floor	1	0.96
Total failures	104	100.00

Distribution of 104 endodontic failures 2 years following therapy. Causes of failure may be categorized into three general groupings: **apical percolation,** which accounts for 63.46% of failures; **operative errors,** which account for 14.42% of failures; and **errors in case selection,** which account for 22.12% of the 104 failures.

These operative errors are all related to inadequate coronal cavity preparation, improper use of endodontic instruments and filling materials, and lack of standardization of endodontic equipment and material as it arrives from the manufacturer. The latter problem has now been reduced through instrument standardization.

On the other hand, delicate root canal instruments must not be mistreated by the inexperienced, and one of the common complaints of the neophyte is "instrument breakage." Also, improper use of the instruments causing root perforation and apex perforation accounted for 14 of the 104 failures in the study. Penetrating through the side of a curved root ultimately leads to incomplete instrumentation and incomplete obturation (Figure 13-12).

Opening wide the apical foramen during instrumentation illustrates that this is also a form of perforation and leads to gross overfilling or overextension. Healing is delayed and often incomplete around the grossly overfilled areas that may be caused by foreign-body reaction. Moreover, the perforated apical foramen has destroyed the apical "stop" and does not allow compaction during canal filling. Although the canal may appear overfilled, it is actually incompletely obturated, with resulting percolation and failure (Figure 13-13).

The paucity of failures in this study owing to broken instruments illustrates that this is not as desperate a situation as it is often considered to be. In analyzing the University of Washington caseload, Crump and Natkin found that failure following instrument fragmentation was the same as in other endodontic cases.[20]

Broken instruments, however, are not favored any more than overfilling and underfilling are favored, but, occasionally, both accidents may occur. Surgical treatment is recommended in operable teeth if the instrument is broken off in the apical one-third of the canal

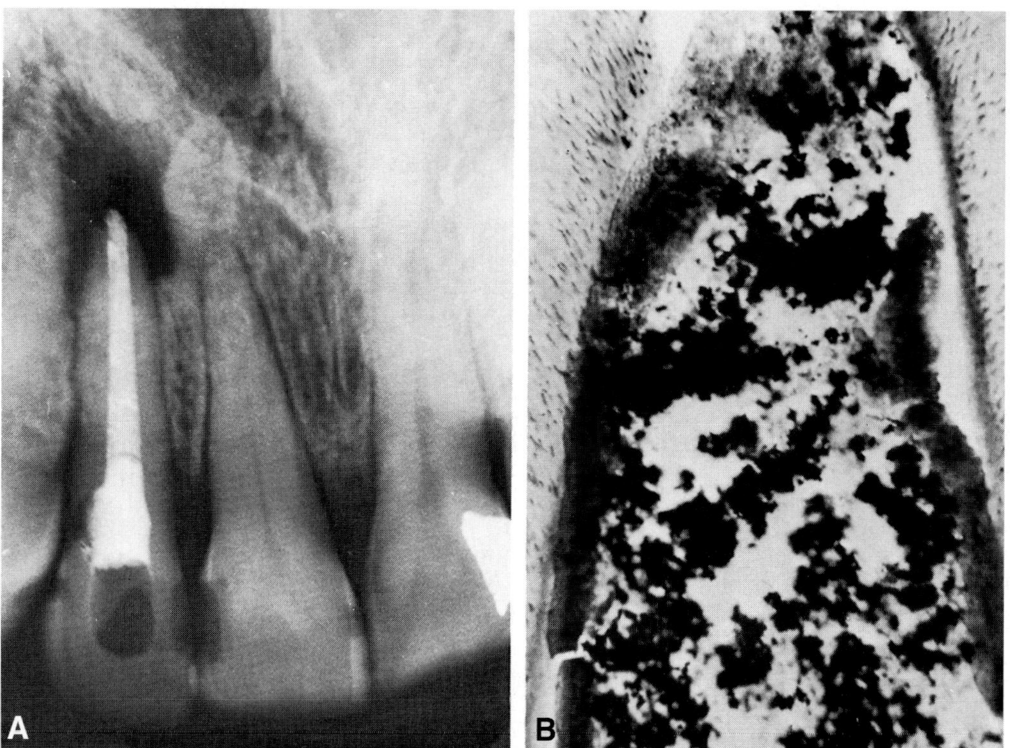

Figure 13-10 **A,** Although the root canal filling appears to be overextended, the fuzzy appearance indicates a lack of density necessary for total obturation. Apical perforation destroyed the apical constriction necessary for compaction of the root canal filling. **B,** Root end biopsy of this failure case shows root canal cement and cellular debris rather than well-condensed gutta-percha filling. Constant percolation into the root canal space provides media for bacterial growth.

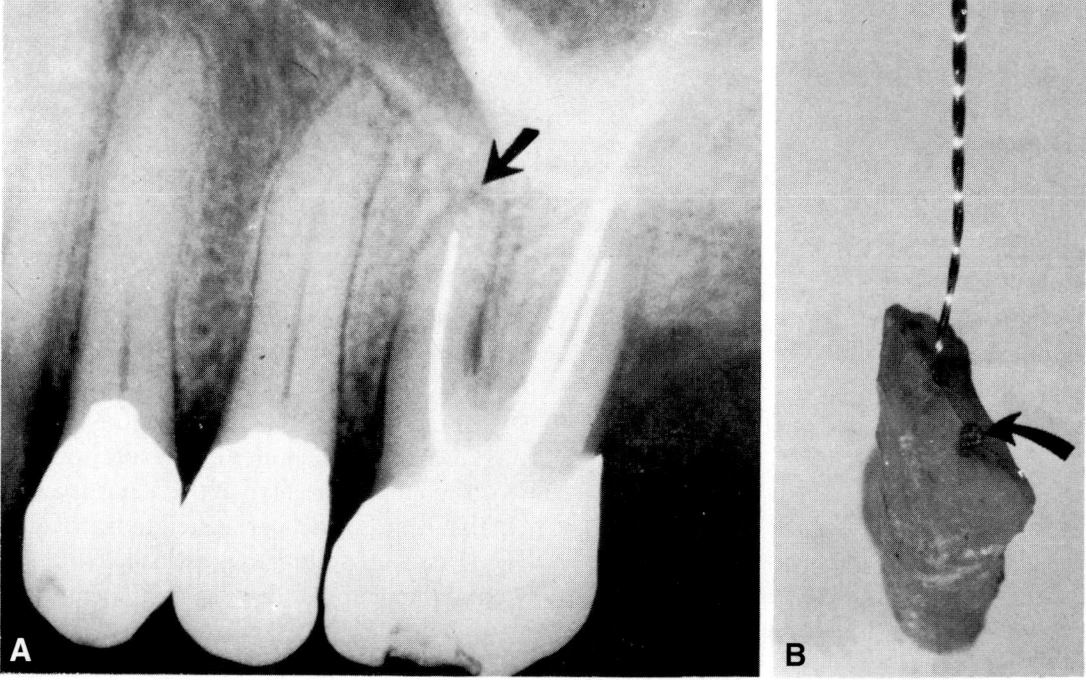

Figure 13-11 **A,** Constantly draining sinus tract opposite the mesiobuccal root of a maxillary first molar (**arrow**) was thought to be related to an advanced periodontal lesion. Total amputation of the mesiobuccal root is indicated. **B,** Amputated root reveals an error in diagnosis. The reamer is in an undetected second canal, whereas the **arrow** points to an obturated primary canal. Secondary canals in mesiobuccal roots of first permanent molars occur about 60% of the time.

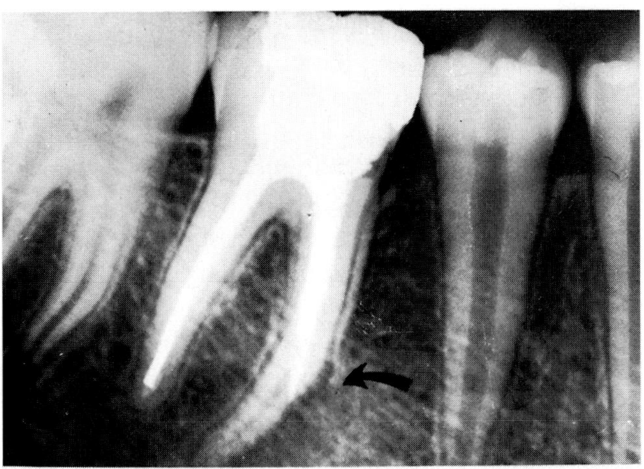

Figure 13-12 Failure owing to root perforation accompanied by incomplete débridement and imperfect obturation. Note the break in the lamina dura opposite the perforation (**arrow**).

and **is loose** in the canal and cannot be removed or bypassed. Surgery may also be the approach if the canal is grossly overfilled with irretrievable gutta-percha and cement. Broken instruments may often be retrieved by "floating" out the piece with an ultrasonically powered instrument. Broken instruments, loose in the canal, have also been seen to "rust out." Failures associated with underfilled canals can usually be remedied by **retreatment** rather than surgery (see Chapter 14).

All of these errors of operation may be prevented by careful cavity preparation and canal obturation. For example, if the operator is unsure of the instrument position in the canal, a radiograph should be taken. Also, more accuracy in fitting the primary or initial filling point will lead to less overfilling. In the final analysis, **operative error** is the simplest cause of failure to control and requires more patience, care, and understanding to overcome.

Errors in Case Selection. Errors in case selection are not as easily overcome as operative errors and may often be listed as the "bad breaks of the game" rather than errors in judgment. Who could predict, for example, that external root resorption would continue, an apical cyst would develop following treatment, an adjacent tooth would become pulpless, or an associated periodontal

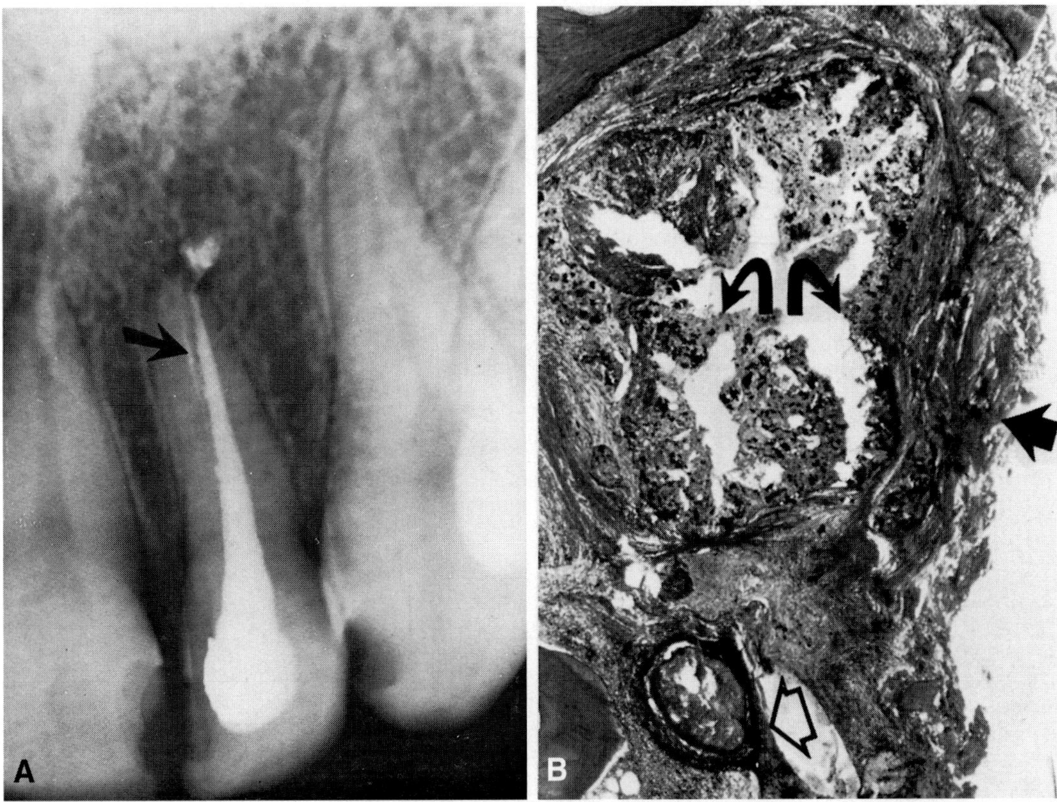

Figure 13-13 A, Although this incisor appears to be grossly overfilled, careful examination (**arrow**) reveals failure to totally obturate the canal. **B**, Tissue reaction to overfilling and underfilling in a single biopsy specimen from this failure case. **Curved arrows** direct attention to a mass of cement forced into periradicular tissue. **Heavy black arrow** (**right**) indicates noninflammatory tissue capsule that has developed as foreign-body reaction. **Open arrow** (**bottom**) points to a violent inflammatory reaction and an abscess related to bacterial products percolating from the unfilled canal.

lesion would lead to failure?[21] These are all factors that led to some of the failures in the Washington study, factors that constitute 22.12% of the total failures. Some could well have been predicted at the time of therapy, but others were entirely unpredictable.

As Table 13-2 shows, there were also minor causes of failure: constant occlusal trauma from bruxism,[22] perforation of the nasal floor, and unfilled accessory or lateral canals. The low incidence of failure associated with unfilled accessory canals came as a surprise considering the degree of emphasis placed by some on the absolute necessity of totally obliterating these lateral canals.

Returning to some of the greater causes of failure, one should note that all eight cases of continuing **root resorption** were in **maxillary lateral incisors.** So one should be wary in evaluating the future of these teeth if they exhibit extensive apical resorption prior to treatment. Most external apical root resorption stops in response to successful root canal treatment!

Endodontic failure associated with **periodontal pockets** is usually the fault of the dentist for not recognizing the pocket's existence. One stumbles ahead with the endodontics before careful probing reveals the presence of an associated pocket and that concurrent periodontal/endodontal therapy will be necessary.[23]

In some cases, concurrent treatment may not solve an unsolvable problem. Witness the destructive and irreparable nature of some *dens invaginatus* or **radicular lingual grooves** extending to the apex[24] (Figure 13-14) or the resorptive invasion from one endodontic lesion causing the necrosis of an adjoining tooth[25] (Figure 13-15).

There are, of course, multiple causes of failure not revealed in the Washington study: retrofilling failures, root tip and foreign bodies left in surgical sites, root fenestration following surgery (Figure 13-16), cracked or split roots, or carious destruction unrelated to the root canal treatment (Figure 13-17). Ultimately, in all of these situations, **bacteria are the final cause of failure.** One must also recognize that one of the most frequent causes of failure of the treated pulpless tooth is fracture of the crown. The **tooth must be carefully protected** by an adequate restoration.

The Washington study has been faulted by some for being only a radiographic study. As Brynolf pointed out in her classic punch biopsy study of root-filled teeth in cadavers, histologic evaluation is a much more accurate method of determining if inflammation remains at the apex than is radiologic evidence.[26] But her research was done on cadavers, proving the impracticality of punch biopsy on live patients. Green and Walton followed up on Brynolf's approach, comparing histologic and radiographic findings on cadavers, and also found that 26% of the teeth with **no radiolucencies** showed chronic inflammation histologically.[27] But that is not to say that these teeth were uncomfortable or contributing to the patient's poor health. How success-

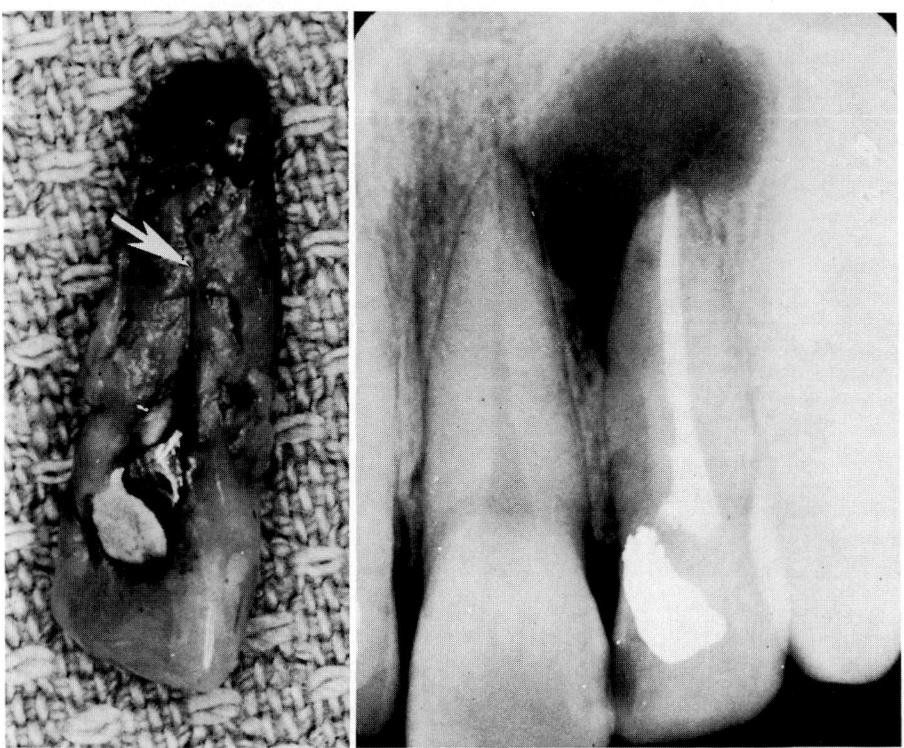

Figure 13-14 Developmental defect, invagination, and radicular lingual groove, resulting in an unattached periodontal ligament tract to the apex. The defect at the cingulum probably communicated with the pulp. Endodontic and periodontic therapy were to no avail. Reproduced with permission from Simon JHS, Glick DH, Frank AL. Oral Surg 1971;37:823.

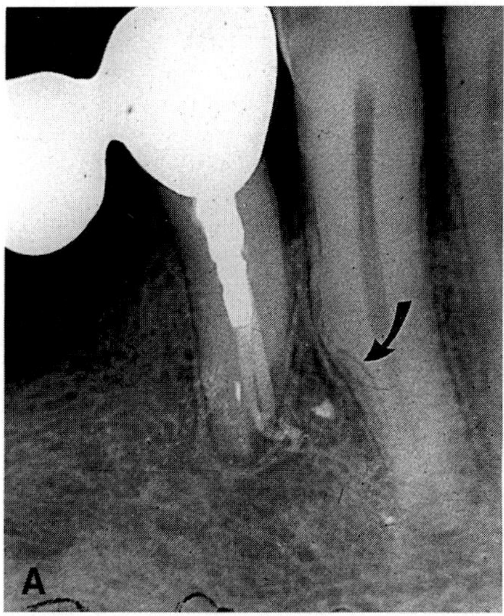

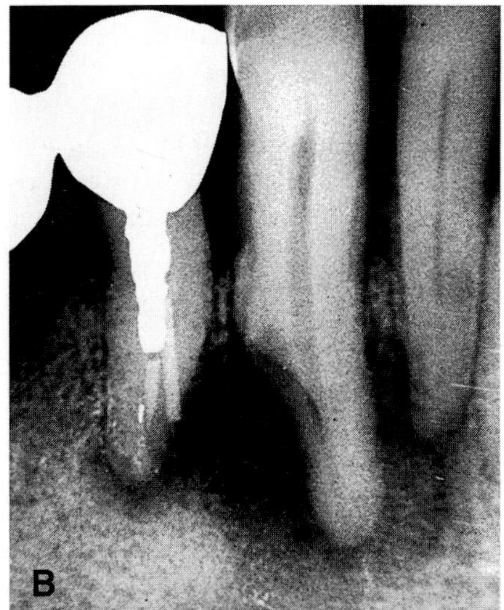

Figure 13-15 **A**, No radiolucency is apparent on a 4-year recall radiograph following root canal filling of a first premolar. Note the anatomic defect on the canine (**arrow**). **B**, Radiograph taken 6 years after the lesion was first noticed. Failed root canal filling in the premolar led to periradicular lesions, inflammatory external resorption of canine, and ultimately necrosis of the canine pulp. Reproduced with permission from Frank AL.[25]

ful is success? Better yet, what are the criteria of success? Comfort and function? Radiographic? Histologic? Since histologic evaluation is impractical, if not illegal, one would have to go with comfort and function and the radiographic findings.

There are well over 50 studies attempting to delineate how successful our treatment procedures are and what the prognosis is for a particular form of treatment.[28] All in all, the studies that have been done suggest the following generalizations:

1. The more extensive and severe the endodontic pathosis, the poorer the prognosis. In other words, the highest percentage of success is with teeth with vital pulps and the worst prognosis is for those with large, long-standing periradicular lesions.
2. The more dental treatment that is done, the poorer the prognosis. In other words, good nonsurgical endodontic treatment has the best prognosis. The worst prognosis lies with teeth that have been **re-treated nonsurgically** and then re-treated **surgically** once or twice more.

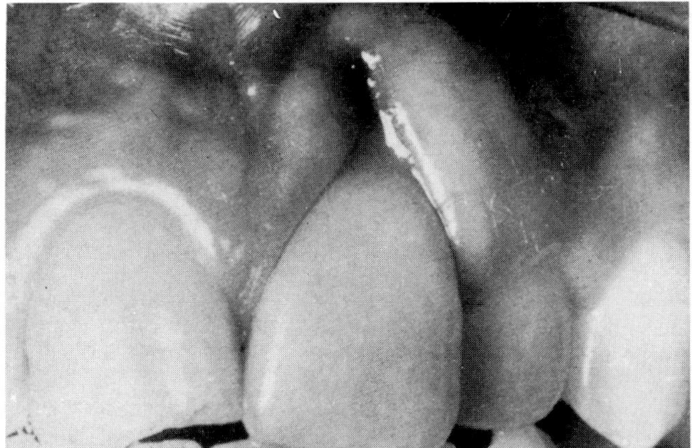

Figure 13-16 Severe bony and soft tissue dehiscence extending to the periapex of a traumatized incisor. Postoperative defects of this type may develop following surgery in an area of osseous fenestration. Reproduced with permission from Luebke RG, Glick DH, Ingle JI. Oral Surg 1964;18:97.

MICROBES

To further elaborate on the role bacteria play in pulpal and periradicular disease, one must turn to the classic research by Kakehashi and his associates at the National Institute of Dental Research.[29] They were able to show, in a gnotobiotic study, that microorganisms alone cause pulpal inflammation and necrosis as well as periradicular infection.[29] It follows that inadequate removal of microbes (ie, bacteria, fungi, and viruses) from the canal leads to continued infection and inflammation[30] and that all of the defects listed in the Washington study are ultimately reduced to bacterial invasion and/or colonization.

But what happens when everything is done right (ie, cleaning, shaping, and obturation), yet failure still occurs?[31–34] Can bacteria still be present after adequate endodontic treatment?

There is strong evidence that bacteria may not be completely eliminated after thorough cleaning, shaping, and disinfection.[35–37] Moreover, when obturation is postponed, bacteria may be able to recolonize in the canal.[38] Furthermore, try as one might, no preparation

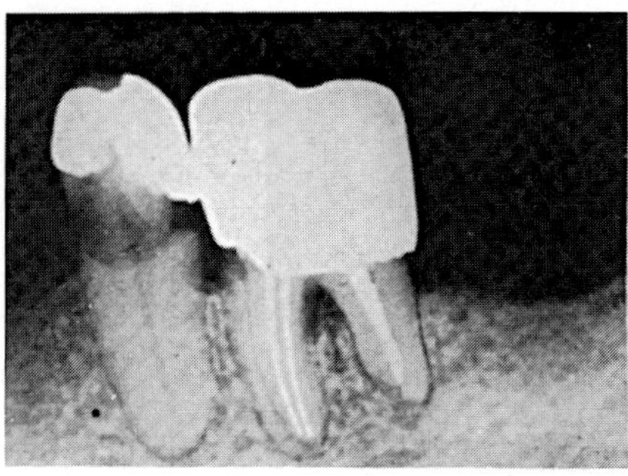

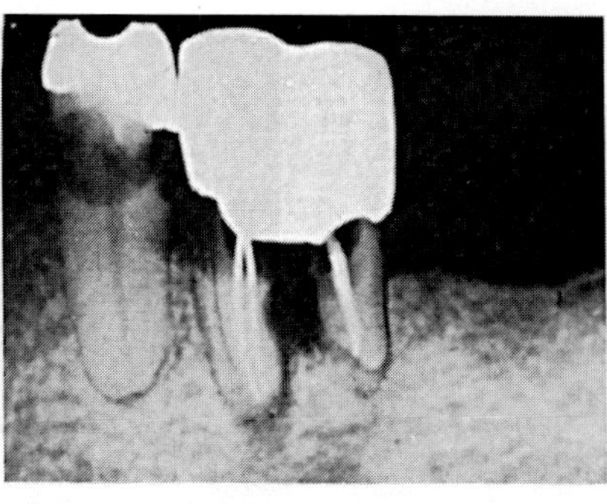

Figure 13-17 Postoperative failure owing to extension of dental caries rather than endodontic therapy *per se*. Loss of these abutment teeth led to full denture in this case.

technique can totally eliminate the intracanal irritants, and a "critical amount" can sustain periradicular inflammation (Figure 13-18).[39,40]

In addition, as stated previously, the obturated canal may be recontaminated from coronal leakage.[41] Indeed, gutta-percha root canal fillings do not resist salivary contamination.[42,43] As Ray and Trope have been able to show, "long term prognosis of treatment seems to correlate directly with the quality of the **coronal seal**."[44]

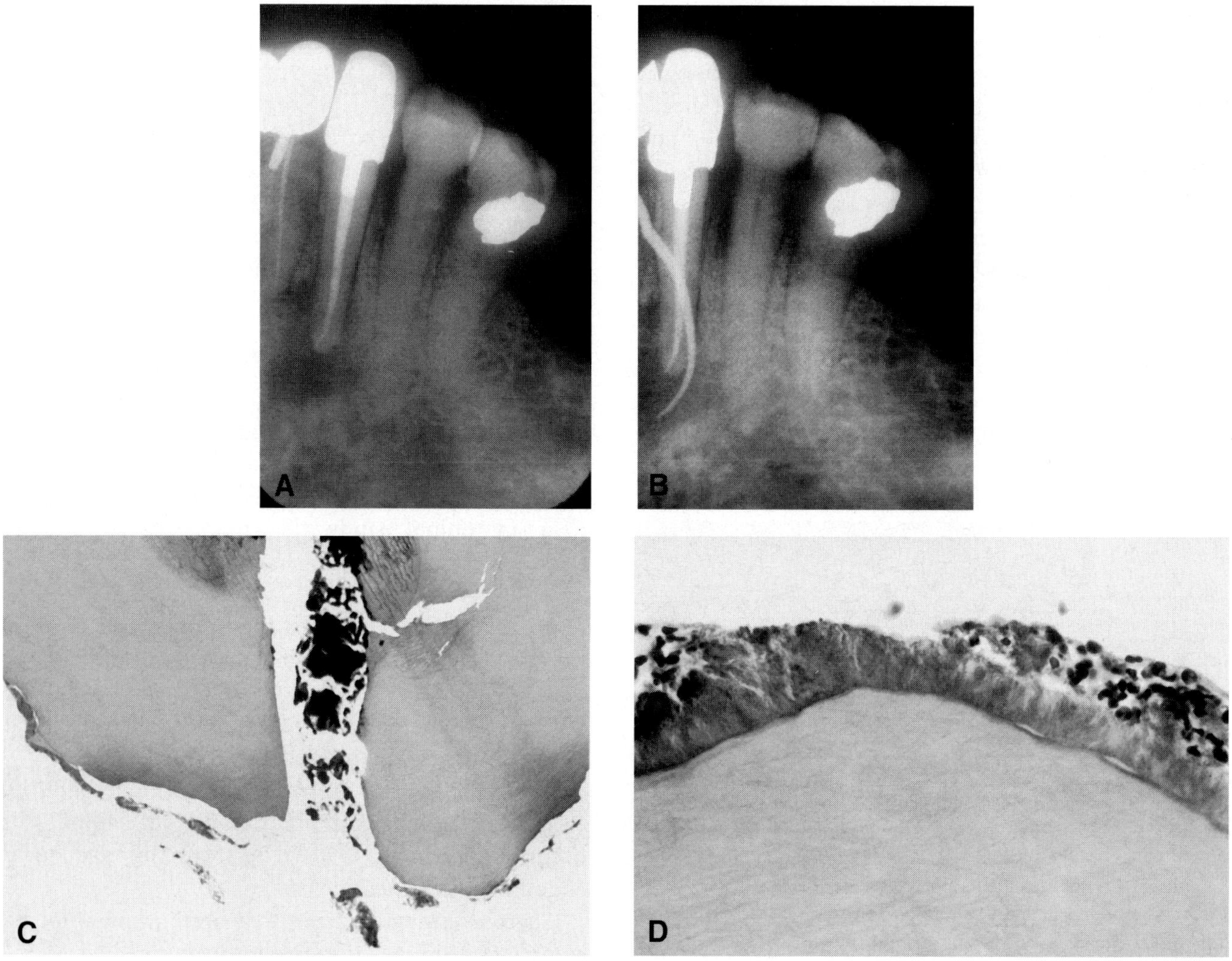

Figure 13-18 A, The radiograph shows a mandibular cuspid that appears well obturated with a well-fitting coronal restoration. B, A sinus tract is traced with a gutta-percha point to the apical lesion that has not responded to treatment. C, Surgical resection of the root end. D, High-power photomicrographs show bacteria containing plaque on the external root surface.

There are also times when an irritant, such as infected dentin chips, is packed at the apex or pushed through the apex, there to serve as a continuing irritant[45,46] that overwhelms the body's defense system. As stated before, the periapical tissue could become colonized by periodontal contamination,[47] the virulence of the bacteria, or extrusion by overaggressive instrument action.[48–50]

In most cases, the host's immune system can overcome these antigens.[51] On the other hand, some bacteria possess mechanisms to resist phagocytosis such as encapsulation or the production of proteases aimed against the immune system.[52,53] Bacteria may also bury themselves in a thick matrix that acts as a sort of apical plaque (see Figure 13-18, D).[54–56]

Many organisms can survive in periradicular lesions: *Actinomyces, Peptostreptococcus,*[57–60] *Propionibacterium,*[61,62] *Prevotella* and *Porphyromonas,* [63–65] *Staphylococcus,*[66,67] and *Pseudomonas aeruginosa.*[35] Barnett, in fact, has stated that *Pseudomonas* **refractory periradicular infection** could be "cured" only by heavy doses of **metronidazole** (Flagyl) following the failure of re-treatment and apicoectomy.[68]

FOREIGN BODIES

In spite of what has been stated above, "foreign-body giant cell reaction" can occur without the presence of bacteria, but no fulminating infection will develop without the bacteria.

A number of foreign bodies have been reported: lentil beans,[69] other vegetables,[70] popcorn kernels[71] (Figure 13-19), paper points, cellulose, and a variety of unidentified materials.[72] Human body defense cells are unable to digest cellulose or cotton pellets.[72,73]

In addition, various lipids, cholesterols, and crystals have also been implicated as periradicular irritants. By their very presence, these intrinsic factors are capable of sustaining an apical lesion despite correct endodontic treatment.[74]

Root canal sealers can also act as a foreign body and thus sustain a lesion, although, over time, extruded sealers (and gutta-percha) may be phagocytized by macrophages.[75]

The cytotoxicity of freshly mixed and unset sealers is well documented.[76] In the long term, however, obturation materials are far less irritating than microbes.[75] It can be concluded that an overfill may cause a delay in healing but will not prevent it.[77]

EPITHELIUM

The role of epithelium must also be taken into account when reviewing failure to heal periapically. If the **resting cells of Malassez** remain in the region, they may respond to the irritants and inflammation and proliferate into a cyst-like attempt to wall off the irritants.[78]

It has been suggested that these latent epithelial cell rests could be activated by the epidermal growth factor present in saliva that contaminates canals left open for drainage.[79,80] In the absence of treatment, or in the presence of persistent bacteria, epithelium continues to proliferate to become a bay (pocket) cyst and eventually a true cyst.[81,82] The distinction between a bay (pocket) cyst (Figure 13-20) and a true cyst is important from a clinical standpoint. Since root canal therapy can directly affect the lumen of the bay (pocket) cyst, the environmental change may bring resolution of the lesion.

There is a controversy over whether cysts heal after nonsurgical endodontic treatment. The **true cyst is independent of the root canal system**, so conventional therapy may have no effect on it. The prevalence of true cysts is less than 10%. [65,66] Most practitioners now realize that true cysts, as well as some bay (pocket) cysts, probably do not heal with nonsurgical therapy. In spite of good cleaning, shaping, and filling, these lesions have to be surgically removed to effect healing.

The dangers delineated above emphasize the point initially stressed: if the case is **carefully selected** before treatment, if the canal is **correctly instrumented** and **obturated,** and if the crown is **properly restored,** the ultimate outcome should be successful.

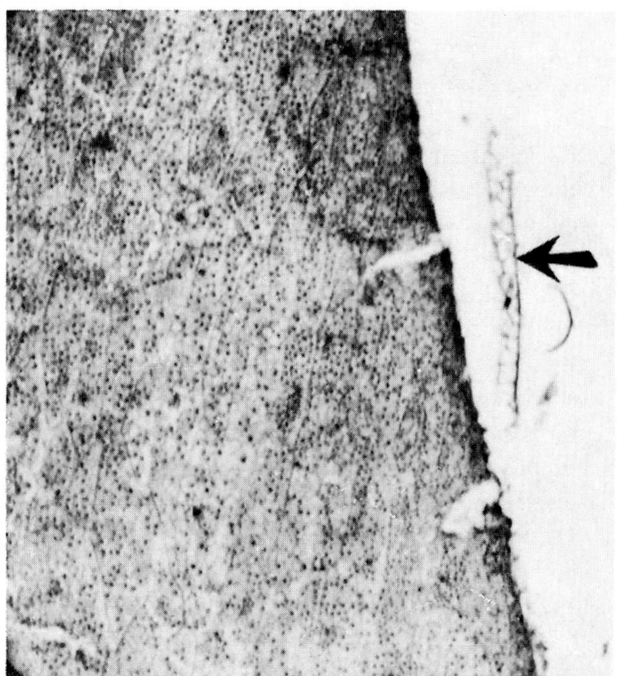

Figure 13-19 Biopsy of what was thought to be a root tip reveals columnar-like cells (**arrow**) of the outer husk of a popcorn kernel that was trapped in a fresh surgical area and served as a severe irritant.

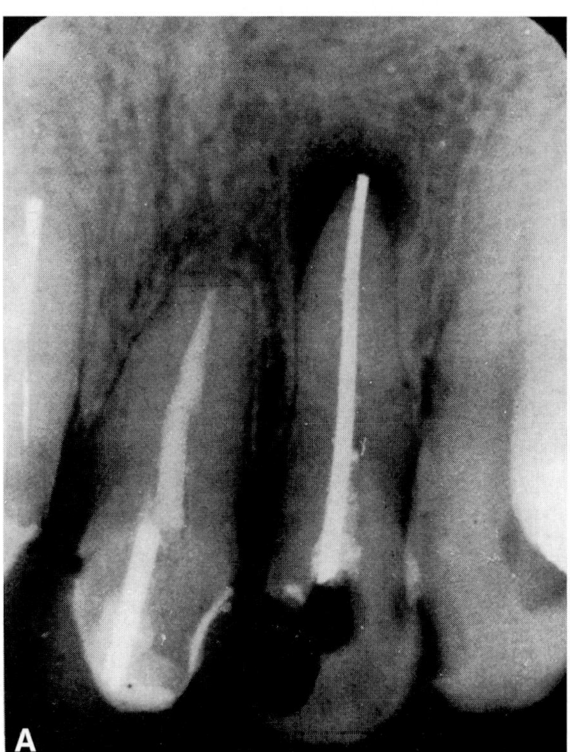

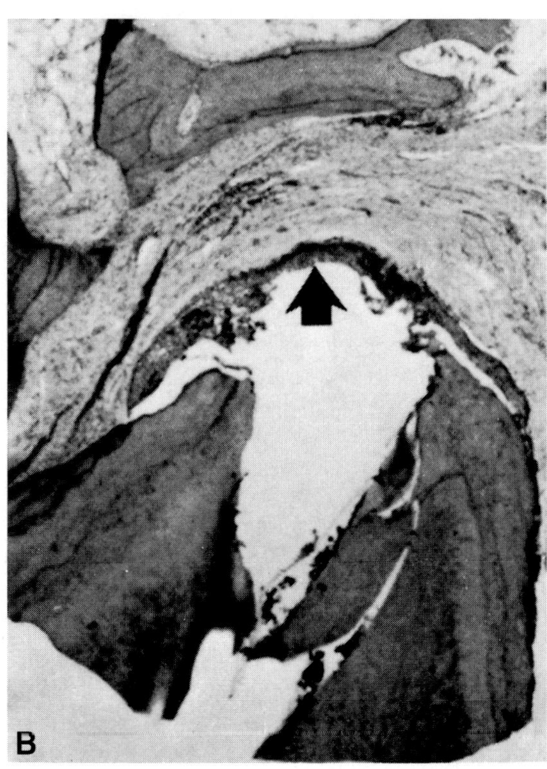

Figure 13-20 **A,** Periradicular lesion persisting 2 years following endodontic therapy appears to be either an apical cyst or chronic apical periodontitis. **B,** Biopsy of the periapex demonstrated the epithelial lining of an apical cyst (**arrow**). Persistence of development of apical cysts led to failure in three cases in study.

Measures to be Employed to Improve Success. One may draw certain conclusions from this study and finally list a number of procedures to improve the rate of success of treated endodontic cases. These are the **Ten Commandments of Endodontics:**

1. **Use great care in case selection.** Be wary of the case that will be an obvious failure, but, at the same time, be daring within the limits of capability.
2. **Use greater care in treatment.** Do not hurry; maintain an organized approach. Be certain of instrument position and procedure before progressing.
3. **Establish adequate cavity preparation** of both the access cavity, which can be improved by modifications of the coronal preparation, and the radicular preparation, which can be improved by more thorough canal débridement—cleaning and shaping.
4. **Determine the exact length of tooth to the foramen** and be certain to operate only to the apical stop, about 0.5 to 1.0 mm from the external orifice of the foramen.
5. **Always use curved, sharp instruments in curved canals,** and especially remember to clean and reshape the curved instrument each time it is used. This applies to stainless steel instruments.
6. **Use great care in fitting the primary filling point.** One must be certain to obliterate the apical portion of the canal. Be more exacting in the total obturation of the entire root canal. **Always** use a root canal sealer cement.
7. **Use periradicular surgery only in those cases for which surgery is definitely indicated.**
8. **Always check the apical density of the completed root canal filling** of the patient undergoing periradicular surgical treatment, and this should be done by using a sharp right-angled explorer. If found wanting, the apical foramen is prepared and retrofilled.
9. **Properly restore each treated pulpless tooth to prevent coronal fracture and microleakage.**
10. **Practice endodontic techniques** until the procedures are as routine as the placement of an amalgam restoration or the extraction of a central incisor. Practice on extracted teeth mounted in acrylic blocks is especially recommended.

Careful attention to details in following the **Ten Commandments of Endodontics** will ensure a degree of success approaching 100%.

PROGNOSIS

All of this having been said, it should be possible to predict the outcome of endodontic treatment. With the benefit of education and experience and some plain luck, one should be able to choose the proper cases for endodontic treatment and reject those that will obviously fail. But it is not quite that simple.

The practicing dentist should not be cited for faulty judgment when even the experts tend to disagree on prognosis. A North Carolina group, for example, found considerable disparity in treatment choice between general practitioners and endodontists who were shown seven controversial cases.[83] In another instance, Holland and his collaborators reviewed 17 prognosis studies dealing with success or failure of teeth with and without periradicular lesions.[84] In the "with lesion" column, successful outcome ranged from a low of 31.8% to a high of 85%. On the other hand, there was general agreement among these 17 experts that a greater success rate may be enjoyed if there is **no initial** periradicular lesion present. This is not to say that teeth with periradicular lesions should be shunned. On the contrary, respectable success rates have been reported by many who have treated teeth with radiolucent lesions.

All in all, one must ultimately develop confidence in one's own abilities. Being able to practice using a variety of techniques and not being "married" to a single approach in every case greatly enhances one's capabilities. This is the basis of good prognosis, the result of skill, knowledge, and self-confidence. On the other hand, if a treated tooth does fail, it may be resurrected by skillful **re-treatment!**

SUCCESSFUL RE-TREATMENT

One must recognize that the patients in the Washington study were all controlled university clinic or specialty practice patients, as were the patients in many of the other success and failure reports, an important consideration in evaluating these outcomes.

In marked contrast, worldwide reports of endodontic success and failure in a cohort of **general practice** patients is an entirely different matter.[44,85–103] To make matters worse, the **periradicular lesions** in these reports were associated with **previously treated endodontic** general practice cases and were much higher (24.5 to 46%) than the periradicular lesions in **non-treated teeth** (1.4 to 10%) (Table 13-3).

There is also a very disappointing finding in a general survey by Buckley and Spångberg at the University of Connecticut; they noted that periradicular lesions are found 5 to 10 times more often in **endodontically** treated teeth than for teeth without root fillings.[101] Mactou pointed out that "the **quality of treatment** plays a decisive role in the successful outcome of endodontic therapy" (Figure 13-21) (personal communication, April 2000).

Fortunately, treated root canals with inadequate results may be **re-treated** to improve the quality of the treatment and heal any apical lesion. (Figure 13-22) Bergenholtz et al., for example, reported on 556 **re-treatment cases** in which 50% completely healed after 2 years, and in an additional 30%, the lesions were significantly reduced in size.[104] In a 2-year follow-up study, Bergenholtz et al. also reported a 94% success rate for re-treatments done for one reason only, to improve root canal filling quality prior to prosthodontic therapy.[105]

Friedman et al. claimed a 100% success rate in **re-treatment** of endodontic cases presenting **without** periradicular lesions, which suggests that if infection is not present, and re-treatment is performed by skilled clinicians, the success rate can be expected to be very high (Table 13-4). On the other hand, if periradicular lesions are present **before re-treatment**, the success rate can be expected to fall to around 70% (Table 13-5).[28]

As many as 22 factors have been listed to affect the prognosis of endodontic re-treatment, the preoperative

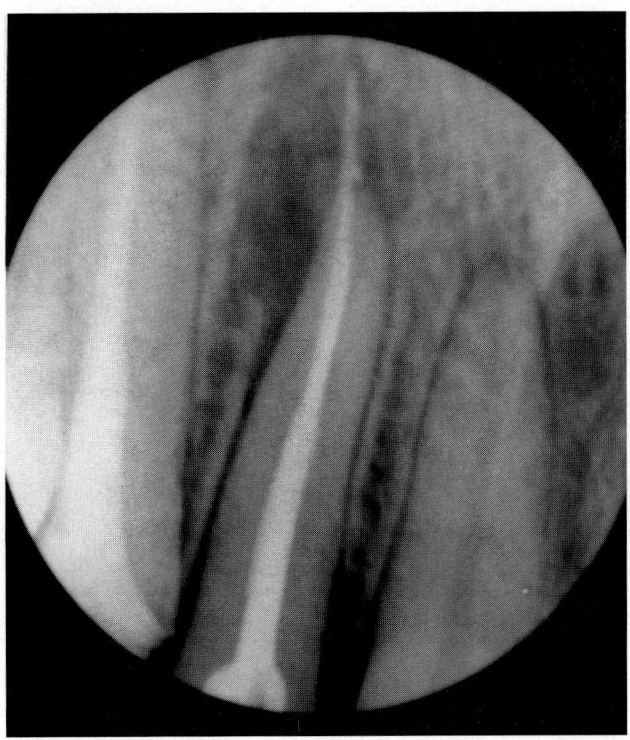

Figure 13-21 Apical perforation through overinstrumentation leads to loss of the apical stop, gross overextension, and failure to compact the canal filling. Notice that instrumentation has resulted in a canal that is short of the apex. (Courtesy of Dr. Pierre Mactou.)

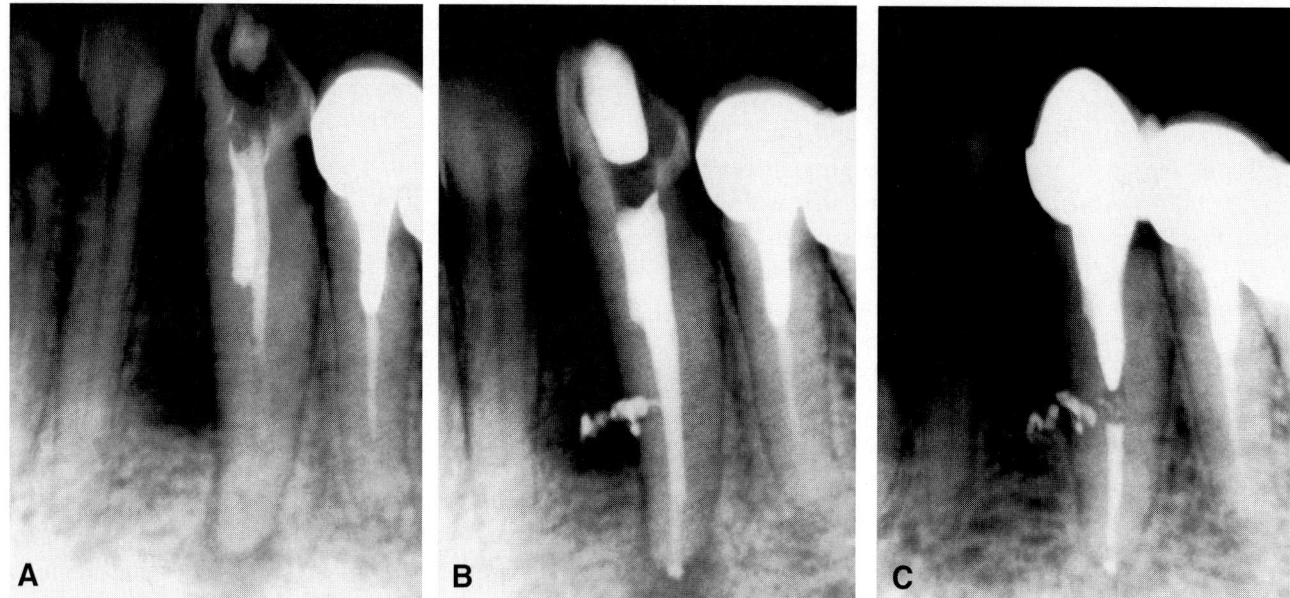

Figure 13-22 **A,** Failure case with apical and lateral periradicular lesions. **B,** Re-treatment eliminates bacterial infection through extensive recleaning, reshaping, and canal medication. Obturation by vertical compaction fills the lateral canal as well. **C,** Complete healing 1 year later. (Courtesy of Dr. Pierre Mactou.)

state of the tooth (as above) obviously being a key factor in outcome.[106] Stabholz et al.[107] and Friedman[108] have noted that causes of endodontic failure fall into three categories: preoperative, intraoperative, and postoperative causes. Of these three, **intraoperative**, that is, iatrogenic, causes are the most prevalent but the most easily controlled.[109] For example, Nair has pointed out that **refractory periradicular infections** are found in acute symptomatic teeth.[110] At the same time, others have noted that these bacteria may have been "planted" there as contaminants during previous endodontic treatment.[110–116] As previously stated, infected dentin chips, extruded from overinstrumentation, may also be the "root" cause of refractory infections.[103] Bergenholtz has stated that"...root filling material [*per se*] was not the immediate cause of the unsuccessful cases, but that

Table 13-3 Cross-sectional Studies on the Presence of Periapical Periodontitis (PAP) in Nontreated and Endodontically Treated Teeth and Quality of Treatment

Lead Author	Country	Teeth with PAP (%)	Endodontically Treated Teeth (%)	Endodontically Treated Teeth with PAP (%)	Technically Inadequate Treatment (%)
Bergenholtz, 1973	Sweden	6	12.7	31	—
Hansen, 1976	Norway	1.5	3.4	46	—
Petersson, 1986	Sweden	6.9	12.4	31	> 60
Allard, 1986	Sweden	10	18	27	69
Eckerbom, 1987	Sweden	5.2	13	26.4	55
Eriksen, 1988	Norway	1.4	3.4	34	59
Odesjo, 1990	Sweden	2.9	8.6	24.5	70
Imfeld, 1991	Switzerland	8	20.3	31	64
De Cleen, 1993	Netherlands	6	2.3	38	50.6
Buckley, 1995	United States	4.1	5.5	31.3	58
Soikkonen, 1995	Finland	4	21	16	75

Table 13-4 Nonsurgical Endodontic Re-treatment Outcome in Pulpless Teeth without Periapical Periodontitis

Authors	Cases	Success (%)
Strindberg, 1956	64	95
Grahnon and Hansson, 1961	323 (roots)	94
Engstrom et al., 1964	68	93
Bergenhotz et al., 1979	322 (roots)	94
Molven and Halse, 1988	76 (roots)	89
Allen et al., 1989	48	96
Sjögren et al., 1990	173 (roots)	98
Friedman et al., 1995	42	100

From Friedman.[28]

Table 13-5 Nonsurgical Endodontic Re-treatment Outcome in Teeth with Periapical Periodontitis

Authors	Cases	Success (%)	Uncertain	Failure (%)
Strindberg, 1956	123	84	—	16
Grahnen and Hansson, 1961	118 (roots)	74	—	26
Engstrom et al., 1964	85	74	—	26
Bergenhotz et al., 1979	234 (roots)	48	30	22
Molven and Halse, 1988	98 (roots)	71	—	29
Sjögren et al., 1990	94 (roots)	62	—	38
Friedman et al., 1995	86	56	34	10
Sundqvist et al., 1998	50	74	—	26

From Friedman.[28]

unsuccessful cases were caused…by a reinfection in the apical areas favored by overinstrumentation"[105] (Figure 13-23).

Mactou has laid out the important factors that must be adhered to if **re-treatment** is to be successful: first of all, **complete re**cleaning and **re**shaping of the canals. This should be carried out in a **step-down** fashion: early coronal enlargement and canal body shaping **prior** to apical preparation (personal communication, April 2000).

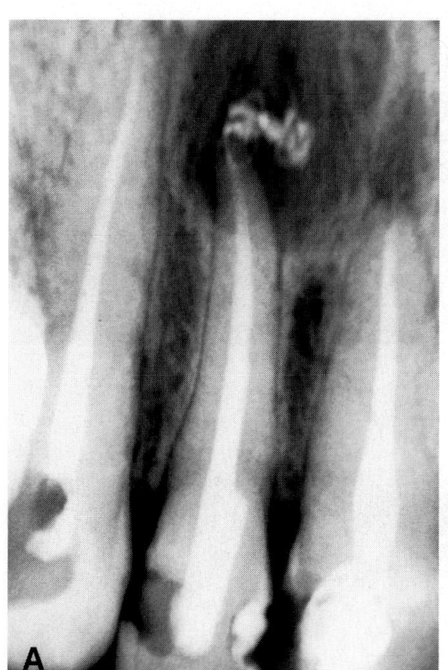

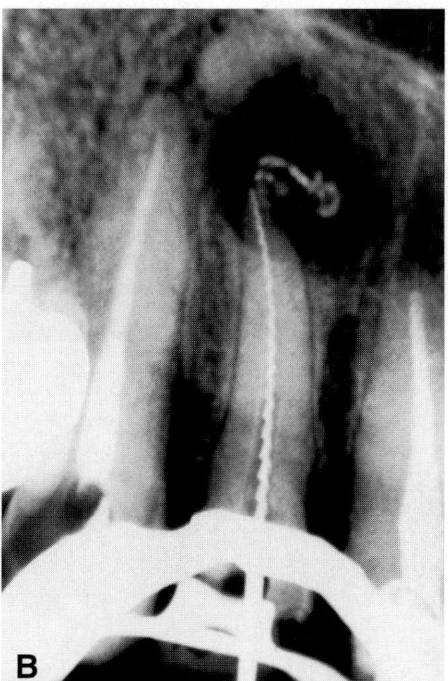

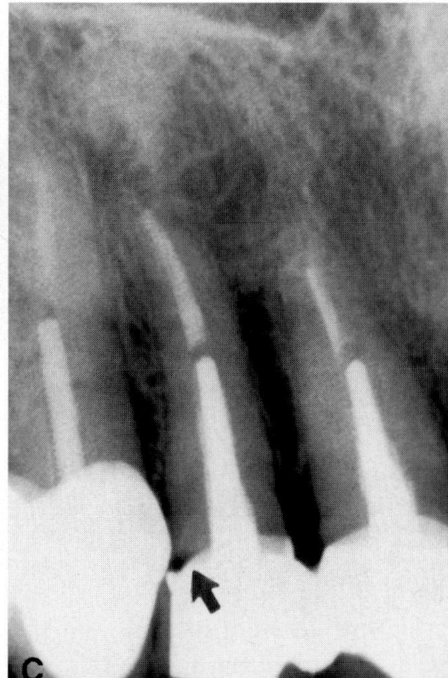

Figure 13-23 **A**, Failed endodontic treatment caused by overinstrumentation and failure to totally obturate the canal. Note the gross overextension of sealer and that the final 6 mm of the canal are sealer only. **B**, Re-treatment by complete recleaning, reshaping, and canal medication before final obturation. **C**, Twelve-year recall shows total healing. Note recurrent decay at the distal margin of the crown (**arrow**) that can lead to microleakage and potential failure. (Courtesy of Dr. Pierre Mactou.)

The canal should be cleaned segment by segment through a coronal reservoir of 2.5% of sodium hypochlorite. Working length at the radiographic terminus is established late in treatment, when the remainder of the canal has already been cleaned and shaped. Maintenance of apical potency and constant recapitulation with fine files avoids canal blockage with dentin debris. It also allows the sodium hypochlorite to reach this area. Great care must be exercised when removing the previous filling material, particularly when solvents such as chloroform are used.

It is very difficult to remove all of the sealer and gutta-percha from the canal walls. Wilcox et al. contended that the last remnants of sealer can be removed only by vigorous reinstrumentation and reshaping of the canal[117,118] but cautioned that overenlargement may result.[119] It would appear that sealer removal is most important since bacteria can easily "hide" under previous sealer.

CANAL MEDICATION

Re-treatment cases are notorious for continued failure! In all probability this is caused by the failure to remove or kill the refractory bacteria responsible for the lesions in the first place. One is warned that these cases are challenging, and this is **probably not the occasion for one-appointment therapy**. Continuing failure is undoubtedly owing to remaining bacteria, and their elimination calls for extra effort. New data regarding failed root canals indicate that these microflora[120–122] **differ** from those of untreated necrotic teeth.

Enterococci, for example, are quite prevalent in **previously root-filled teeth** and are quite difficult to eliminate. *Enterococcus faecalis* is the most frequent strain and, as a monoinfection, is found in 33% of the cases.[123] Entercocci are quite resistant to calcium hydroxide, so Safaui et al. have recommended the addition of iodine potassium iodide in these cases.[124] Heling and Chandler have recommended a mixture of 3% hydrogen peroxide and 1.8% chlorhexidine as an alternative against *E. faecalis.*[125] *Staphylococcus aureus* and *Pseudomonos* are also notorious refractory contaminants and may require a prescription of metronidazole and amoxicillin to rid the periapex of these bacteria.[126–128]

OBTURATION AND RESTORATION

It goes without saying that total obturation is the *sine qua non* of successful re-treatment.

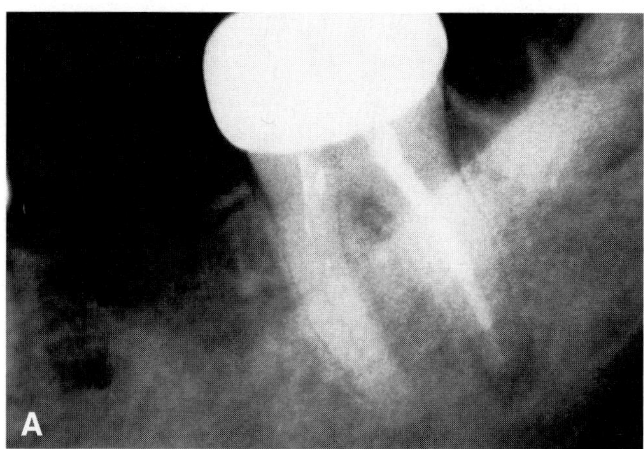

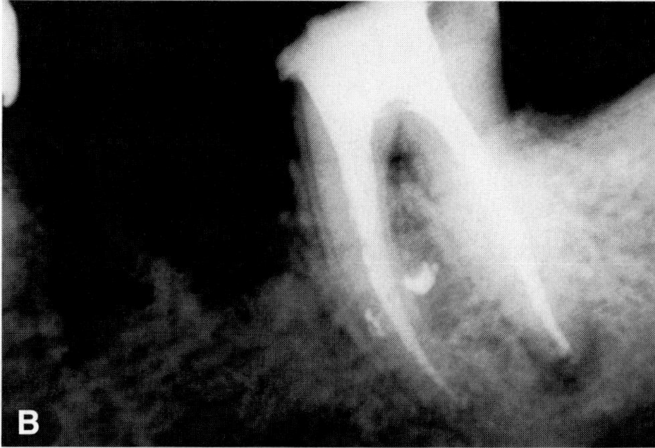

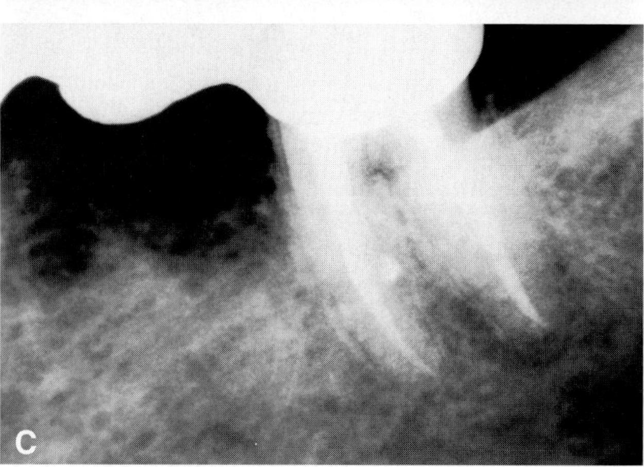

Figure 13-24 A, **Pre**treatment radiograph reveals failed endodontic treatment and a periradicular lesion. B, **Re-treament** by total recleaning, reshaping, and canal medication. Final obturation by vertical compaction fills the lateral canal as well. C, **Six-year** follow-up. (Courtesy of Dr. Pierre Mactou.)

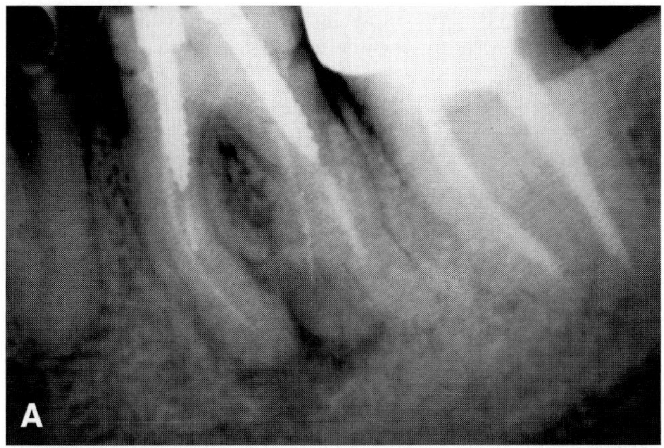

Figure 13-25 A, Pretreatment radiograph reveals failed root canal treatment and the presence of two posts. B, Re-treatment showing complete obturation of the canals including apical branching in the mesial canals. C, One-year follow-up. (Courtesy of Dr. Pierre Mactou.)

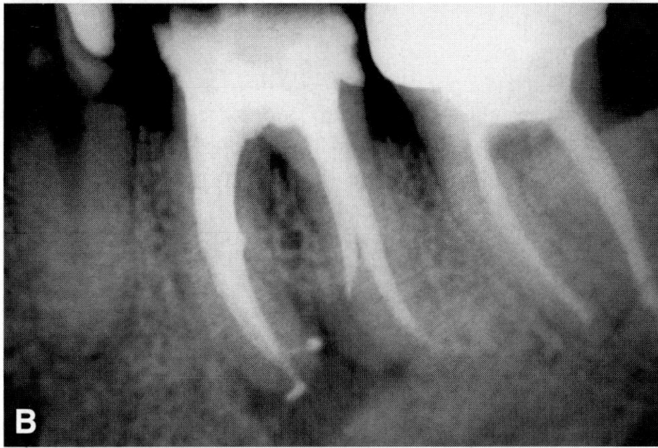

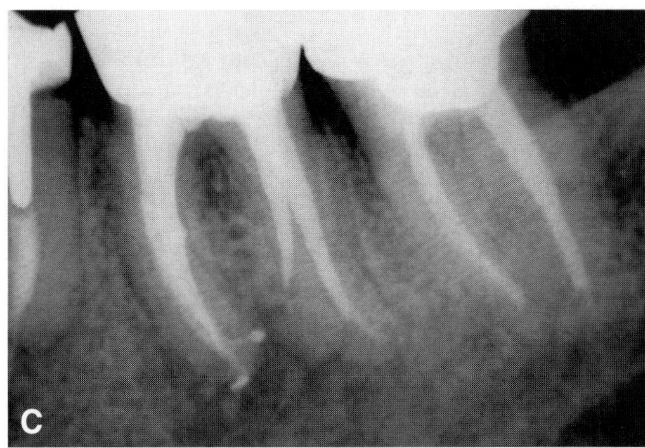

For this, the reader is referred to chapter 11. Furthermore, since many failures are believed to be related to microleakage from around coronal restorations, it is imperative that the re-treated tooth be properly restored, at once, not weeks later (Figure 13-24).

Molven and Halse have said it best: "Success depends on the elimination of root canal infection present when treatment starts, and the prevention of both contamination during treatment and re-infection later. So success rates reflect the standard of the cleaning, shaping and filling of root canals"[129] (Figure 13-25).

REFERENCES

1. Zeldow BJ, Ingle JI. Correlation of the positive culture to prognosis of endodontically treated teeth: a clinical study. J Am Dent Assoc 1963;66:23.
2. Abramson II. A frank appraisal of the present status of the bacterial culture test as a routine endodontic procedure . Presented at the Annual Meeting of the American Association of Endodontists Chicago, February, 1961.
3. Strindberg LL. The dependence of the results of pulp therapy on certain factors. Acta Odontol Scand 1956;Suppl 21 14:175 .
4. Adenubi JO, Rule DC. Success rate for root fillings in young patients. Br Dent J 1976;141:327.
5. Morse DR, et al. A radiographic evaluation of the periradicular status of teeth treated by the gutta-percha-eucapercha endodontic method: a one year follow-up study of 458 root canals, Part III. Oral Surg 1983;56:190.
6. Barbakow FH, et al. Endodontic treatment of teeth with periradicular radiolucent areas in a general dental practice. Oral Surg 1981;51:552.
7. Meeuwissen R, Eschen S. Twenty years of endodontic treatment. JOE 1983;9:390.
8. Hession RW. Long-term evaluation of endodontic treatment: anatomy, instrumentation, obturation—the endodontic practice triad. Int Endodont J 1981;14:179.
9. Nelson IA. Endodontics in general practice—a retrospective survey. Int Endodont J 1982;15:168.
10. Kerekes K, Tronstad L. Long-term results of endodontic treatment performed with a standardized technique. JOE 1979;5:8.
11. Sjögren U, et al. Factors affecting the long-term results of endodontic treatment. JOE 1990;16:498.
12. Mikkonen M, et al. Clinical and radiologic re-examination of apicoectomized teeth. Oral Surg 1983;55:302.
13. Peterson K, et al. Technical quality of root fillings in an adult Swedish population. Endodont Dent Traumatol 1986;2:99.
14. Matsumoto T, et al. Factors affecting successful prognosis of root canal treatment. JOE 1987;13:239.
15. Swartz DB, Skidmore AE, Griffin JA Jr. Twenty years of endodontic success and failure. JOE 1983;9:198.

16. Klevant FJH; Eggink CO. The effect of canal preparation on periradicular disease. Int Endodont J 1983;16:68.
17. Vire DE. Failure of endontically treated teeth: classification and evaluation. JOE 1991;17:338.
18. Pucci FM, Reig R. Conductos radiculares. Vol I. Buenos Aires: Editorial Medico-Quirurgica;1944. p. 219–225.
19. Trope M, Elfenbein L, Tronstad L. Mandibular premolars with more than one root canal in different race groups. JOE 1986;12:343.
20. Crump MC, Natkin E. Relationship of broken root canal instruments to endodontic case prognosis: a clinical investigation. J Am Dent Assoc 1970;80:1341.
21. Ramfjord S. Experimental periodontal reattachment in Rhesus monkeys. J Periodontol 1951;22:73.
22. Ingle JI. Alveolar osteoporosis and pulpal death associated with compulsive bruxism. Oral Surg 1960;13:1371.
23. Simon JH, Glick DH, Frank AL. The relationship of endodontic-periodontic lesions. J Periodontol 1972;43:202.
24. Slowey RR. Radiographic aids in the detection of extra root canals. Oral Surg 1974;37:271.
25. Frank AL. Inflammatory resorption caused by an adjacent necrotic tooth. JOE 1990;7:339.
26. Brynolf I. A histological and roentgenological study of the periapical region of upper incisors. Odont Revy 1967;18:1.
27. Green TL, et al. Radiographic and histologic periapical findings of root canal treated teeth in cadavers. Oral Surg 1997;83:707.
28. Friedman S. Treatment outcome and prognosis of endodontic therapy. In: Ørstavik D, Pitt Ford TR, editors. Essential endodontology. London: Blackwell Scientific; 1998. p. 367–401.
29. Kakehashi S, Stanley HR, Fitzgerald RJ. The effects of surgical exposures of dental pulps in germ-free and conventional rats. Oral Surg 1965;20:340.
30. Moller AJR, et al. Influence on periapical tissues of indigenous oral bacteria and necrotic pulp tissue in monkeys. Scand J Dent Res 1981;89:475.
31. Sjögren U. Success and failure in endodontics [thesis]. Umea (Sweden): Department of Endodontics, Univ Umea.
32. Gutmann JL. Clinical, radiographic, and histologic perspectives on success and failure in endodontics. Dent Clin North Am 1992;36:379.
33. Sundqvist G. Bacteriological studies of necrotic dental pulps [dissertation]. Umea (Sweden): Univ Umea.
34. Lin LM, Skribner JE, Gaengler P. Factors associated with endodontic treatment failures. JOE 1992;18:625.
35. Barnett F, Axelrod P, Tronstad L, et al. Ciprofloxacin treatment of periapical *Pseudomonas aeruginosa* infection. Endod Dent Traumatol 1988;4:132.
36. Bystrom A. Evaluation of endodontic treatment of teeth with apical periodontitis [dissertation]. Umea (Sweden): Univ Umea; 1986.
37. Nair PNR, Sjögren U, Krey G, et al. Intraradicular bacteria and fungi in root filled asymptomatic human teeth with therapy resistant periapical lesions: a long-term light and electron microscopic follow-up study. JOE 1990;16:520.
38. Sundquist G. Ecology of the root canal flora. JOE 1992;18:427.
39. Allard U, Stromberg U, Stromberg T. Endodontic treatment of experimentally induced apical periodontitis in dogs. Endod Dent Traumatol 1987;3:240.
40. Szajkis S, Tagger M. Periapical healing in spite of incomplete root canal debridement and filling. JOE 1983;9:203.
41. Saunders WP, Saunders EM. Coronal leakage as a cause of failure in root-canal therapy: a review. Endod Dent Traumatol 1994;10:105.
42. Khayat A, Lee SJ, Torabinejad M. Human saliva penetration of coronally unsealed obturated root canals. JOE 1993;19:458.
43. Friedman S, Torneck C, et al. *In vivo* model for assessing the functional efficacy of endodontic filling materials and techniques. JOE 1997;23:557.
44. Ray HA, Trope M. Periapical status of endodontically treated teeth in relation to the technical quality of the root filling and the coronal restoration. Int Endod J 1995;28:12.
45. Holland R, de Souza V, Nery MJ, et al. Tissue reaction following apical plugging of the root canal with infected dentin chips: a histologic study in dog's teeth. Oral Surg 1980;49:366.
46. Yusef H. The significance of the presence of foreign material periapically as a cause of failure of root treatment. Oral Surg 1982;54:566.
47. Simon JHS, Glick DH, Frank AL. The relationship of endodontic-periodontic lesions. J Periodontol 1972;43:202.
48. Iwu C, Macfarlane TW, Mackenzie D, Stenhoouse D. The microbiology of periapical granulomas. Oral Surg 1990; 69:502.
49. Wayman B, Murata S, Almeida R, Fowler C. A bacteriological and histological evaluation of 58 periapical lesions. JOE 1992;18:152.
50. Weiger R, Manncke B, Werner H, Lost C. Microbial flora of sinus tracts and root canals of non-vital teeth. Endod Dent Traumatol 1995;11:15.
51. Kettering J, Torabinejad M, Jones S. Specificity of antibodies present in human periapical lesions. JOE 1991;17:213.
52. Haapsalo M. *Bacteroides* spp in dental root canal infections. Endod Dent Traumatol 1989;5:1.
53. Wu M, Henry C, Gutmann J. Bactericidal effects of human neutrophils and sera on selected endodontic pathogenic bacteria in an anaerobic environment. Int Endodont J 1990;23:189.
54. Lomcali G, Sen BH, Cankaya H. Scanning electron microscopic observations of apical root surfaces of teeth with apical periodontitis. Endod Dent Traumatol 1996;12:70.
55. Molven O, Olsen I, Kerekes K. Scanning electron microscopy of bacteria in the apical part of root canals in permanent teeth with periapical lesions. Endod Dent Traumatol 1991;7:226.
56. Tronstad L, Barnett F, Cervone F. Periapical bacterial plaque in teeth refractory to endodontic treatment. Endod Dent Traumatol 1990;6:73.
57. Abou-Rass M, Bogen G. Microorganisms in closed periapical lesions. Int Endod J 1998;31:39.
58. August DS, Levy BAA. Periapical actinomycosis. Oral Surg 1973;36:585.
59. Happonen RP. Periapical actinomycosis: a follow-up study of 16 surgically treated cases. Endod Dent Traumatol 1986;2:205.
60. Sundquist G, Reuterving CO. Isolation of *Actinomyces israelii* from periapical lesions. JOE 1980;6:602.
61. Bystrom A, Happonen RP, Sjögren U, Sundquist G. Healing of periapical lesions of pulpless teeth after endodontic treatment with controlled asepsis. Endod Dent Traumatol 1987;3:58.
62. Sjögren U, Happonen RP, Kahnberg K, Sundquist G. Survival of *Arachnia propionica* in periapical tissue. Int Endod J 1988;21:277.

63. Barnett F, Stevens R, Tronstad L. Demonstration of *Bacteroides intermedius* in periapical tissue using indirect immunofluorescence microscopy. Endod Dent Traumatol 1990;6:153.
64. Haapsalo M, Ranta K, Ranta H. Mixed anaerobic periapical infection with sinus tract. Endod Dent Traumatol 1987;3:83.
65. Van Winkelhoff AJ, Van Steenbergen JM, de Graaff J. *Porphyromonas (Bacteroides) endodontalis*: its role in endodontic infections. JOE 1992;18:431.
66. Reader CM, Boniface M, Bujanda-Wagner S. Refractory endodontic lesion associated with *Staphylococci aureus*. JOE 1994;20:607.
67. Tronstad L, Barnett F, Riso K, Slots J. Extraradicular endodontic infections. Endod Dent Traumatol 1987;3:86.
68. Barnett F. Question and answer session. Palm Springs Seminars, Palm Springs, California, January 18, 1992.
69. Simon JHS, Chimenti R, Mintz G. Clinical significance of the pulse granuloma. JOE 1982;8:116.
70. Yang ZP, Barnett F. Hyaline bodies and giant cells associated with a radicular cyst. Endod Dent Traumatol 1985;1:85.
71. Ingle JI. Endodontics. Baltimore: Williams & Wilkins; 1994.
72. Koppang H, Koppang G, Solheim T, et al. Cellulose fibers from endodontic paper points as an etiologic factor in post-endodontic periapical granulomas and cysts. JOE 1989;15:369.
73. Sedgley CM, Messer HH. Long-term retention of a paper point in the periapical tissues: a case report. Endod Dent Traumatol 1993;9:120.
74. Nair PNR, Sjögren U, Schumacher E, Sundquist G. Radicular cyst affecting a root-filled human tooth: a long-term post-treatment follow-up. Int Endod J 1993;26:225.
75. Brynolf I. A histological and roentgenological study of the periapical region of upper incisors. Odont Revy 1967;18:1.
76. Arenholt-Bindsley D, Hörsted-Bindsley P. A simple model for evaluating relative toxicity of root filling materials in cultures of human oral fibroblasts. Endod Dent Traumatol 1989;5:219.
77. Malooley J, Patterson SS, Kafrawy A. Response of periapical pathosis to endodontic treatment in monkeys. Oral Surg 1979;6:545.
78. Simon JHS. Periapical pathology. In: Cohen S, Burns R, editors. Pathways of the pulp. 6th ed. St. Louis: CV Mosby; 1994. p.337.
79. Torres JOC, Torabinejad M, Matiz RAR, Mantilla EG. Presence of secretory IgA in human periapical lesions. JOE 1994;20:87.
80. Lin LM, Wang SL, Wu-Wang C, et al. Detection of epidermal growth factor receptor in inflammatory periapical lesions. Int Endod J 1996;29:179.
81. Simon JHS. Incidence of periapical cysts in relation to the root canal. JOE 1980;6:845.
82. Nair PNR. New perspectives on radicular cysts: do they heal? Int Endod J 1998;31:155.
83. Smith JW, et al. A survey: controversies in endodontic treatment and retreatment. JOE 1981;7:47.
84. Holland R, Valle GF, Taintor JF, Ingle JI. Influence of bony resorption on endodontic treatment. Oral. Surg 1983;55:191.
85. Bergenholtz G, Malmcrona E, Milthon R. Endodontisk behandling och periapikalstatus. 1—Röntgenologisk undersökning av frekvensen endodontiskt behandlade tänder och frekvensen periapikala destruktioner. Tandlakartidningen 1973;65:64.
86. Bergenholtz G, Malmcrona E, Milthon R. Endodontisk behandling och periapikalstatus. 2—Röntgenologisk bedömning av rotfyllningens kvalitet ställd i relation till förekomst av periapikala destruktioner. Tandlakartidningen 1973;65:269.
87. Hansen BF, Johansen JR. Oral roentgenologic findings in a Norwegian urban population. Oral Surg 1976;41:261.
88. Allard U, Palmqvist S. A radiographic survey of periapical conditions in elderly people in a Swedish county population. Endod Dent Traumatol 1986;2:103.
89. Petersson K, Petersson A, Hakansson J, et al. Endodontic status and suggested treatment in a population requiring substantial dental care. Endod Dent Traumatol 1989;5:153.
90. Petersson K, Lewin B, Olsson B, et al. Technical quality of root fillings in an adult Swedish population. Endod Dent Traumatol 1986;2:99.
91. Petersson K, Hakansson R, Hakansson J, et al. Follow-up study of endodontic status in an adult Swedish population. Endod Dent Traumatol 1991;7:221.
92. Petersson K. Endodontic status of mandibular premolars and molars in Swedish adults. A repeated cross-sectional study in 1974 and in 1985. Endod Dent Traumatol 1993;9:185.
93. Eckerbom M, Andersson E, Magnusson T. Frequency and technical standard of endodontic treatment in a Swedish population. Endod Dent Traumatol 1987;3:245.
94. Eckerbom M, Andersson JE, Magnusson T. A longitudinal study of changes in frequency and technical standard of endodontic treatment in a Swedish population. Endod Dent Traumatol 1989;5:27.
95. Eriksen HM, Bjertness E. Prevalence of apical periodontitis and results of endodontic treatment in an urban adult population in Norway. Endod Dent Traumatol 1988;4:122.
96. Eriksen HM, Bjertness E, Ørstavik D. Prevalence and quality of endodontic treatment in middle-aged adults in Norway. Endod Dent Traumatol 1991;7:1.
97. Eriksen HM, Berset GP, Hansen BF, Bjertness E. Changes in endodontic status 1973–1993 among 35-year-olds in Oslo, Norway. Int Endod J 1995;28:129.
98. Odesjo B, Hellden L, Salonen L, Langeland L. Prevalence of previous endodontic treatment, technical standard and occurrence of periapical lesions in a randomly selected adult general population. Endod Dent Traumatol 1990;6:265.
99. Imfeld TN. Prevalence and quality of endodontic treatment in an elderly urban population of Switzerland. JOE 1991;17:604.
100. De Cleen MJH, Schuurs AHB, Wesselink PR, Wu MK. Periapical status and prevalence of endodontic treatment in an adult Dutch population. Int Endod J 1993;26:112.
101. Buckley M, Spångberg LSW. The prevalence and technical quality of endodontic treatment in an American subpopulation. Oral Surg 1995;79:92.
102. Soikkonen KT. Endodontically treated teeth and periapical findings in the elderly. Int Endod J 1995;28:200.
103. Marques MD, Moreira B, Eriksen HM. Prevalence of apical periodontitis and results of endodontic treatment in an adult Portuguese population. Int Endod J 1998;31:161.
104. Bergenholtz G, Lekholm U, Milthon R, et al. Retreatment of endodontic fillings. Scand J Dent Res 1979;87:217.
105. Bergenholtz G, Lekholm U, Milthon R, Engstrom B. Influence of apical overinstrumentation and overfilling on re-treated root canals. JOE 1979;5:310.
106. Gutmann JL, Pitt-Ford TR. Problems in the assessment of success and failure. In: Gutmann JL, Dumsha TC, Lovdahl PE, Hovland EJ, editors. Problems solving in endodontics. 2nd ed. St. Louis: Mosby-Year Book; 1992; p.1–11.

107. Stabholz A, Friedman I, Tamse A. Endodontic failures and retreatment. In: Cohen S, Burns RC, editors. Pathways of the pulp. 6th ed. St Louis: CV Mosby; 1994. p. 691–728.
108. Friedman S. Retreatment of failures. In: Walton RE, Torabinejad M. Principles and practice of endodontics. 2nd ed. Philadelphia: WB Saunders; 1996. p. 336–53.
109. Morand MA. The true reasons for endodontic failures [abstract]. JDR 1992;71:565.
110. Nair PNR. Light and electron microscope studies on the root canal flora and periapical lesions. JOE 1987;13:29.
111. Iwu C, Macfarlane TW, Mackenzie D, Stenhouse D. The microbiology of periapical granuloma. Oral Surg 1990;69:502.
112. Fukushima H, Yamamoto K, Hirohata K, et al. Localization and identification of root canal bacteria in clinically asymptomatic periapical pathosis. JOE 1990;16:534.
113. Debelian GJ, Olsen I, Tronstad L. Profiling of *Propionibacterium acnes* recovered from root canal and blood during and after endodontic treatment. Endod Dent Traumatol 1992;8:248.
114. Debelian GJ, Olsen I, Tronstad L. Bacteremia in conjunction with endodontic therapy. Endod Dent Traumatol 1995;11:142.
115. Weiger R, Manncke B, Werner H, Lost C. Microbial flora of sinus tracts and root canals of non-vital teeth. Endod Dent Traumatol 1995;11:15.
116. Ruddle CJ. Endodontic canal preparation: breakthrough cleaning and shaping strategies. Dent Today 1994;44, (February).
117. Wilcox LR, Krell KV, Madison S, Rittman B. Endodontic retreatment: evaluation of gutta-percha and sealer removal and canal reinstrumentation. JOE 1987;13:453.
118. Wilcox LR. Endodontic retreatment: ultrasonics and chloroform as the final step in reinstrumentation. JOE 1989;15:125.
119. Wilcox LR, Van Surksum R. Endodontic retreatment in large and small straight canals. JOE 1991;17:119.
120. Molander A, Reit C, Dahlen G, Kvist T. Microbiological examination of root filled teeth with apical periodontitis. Int Endod J 1993.
121. Molander A, Reit C, Dahlen G, Kvist T. Microbiological status of root-filled teeth with apical periodontitis. Int Endod J 1998;31:1.
122. Sundqvist G, Figdor D, Persson S, Sjögren U. Microbiologic analysis of teeth with failed endodontic treatment and the outcome of conservative retreatment. Oral Surg 1998;85:86.
123. Siren EK, Haapasalo MPP, Ranta K, et al. Microbiological findings and clinical treatment procedures in endodontic cases selected for microbiological investigation. Int Endod J 1997;30:91.
124. Safavi KE, Spångberg LSW, Langeland K. Root canal dentinal tubule disinfection. JOE 1990;16:207.
125. Heling I, Chandler NP. Antimicrobial effect of irrigant combinations within dentinal tubules. Int Endod J 1998;31:8.
126. Barnett F, Axelrod P, Tronstad L, et al. Ciprofloxacin treatment of periapical *Pseudomonas aeruginosa* infection. Endod Dent Traumatol 1988;4:132.
127. Ranta K, Haapsolo M, Ranta H. Monoinfection of root canal with *Pseudomonas aeruginosa*. Endod Dent Traumatol 1988;4:269.
128. Sjögren U, Figdor D, Persson S, Sundqvist G. Influence of infection at the time of root filling on the outcome of endodontic treatment of teeth with apical periodontitis. Int Endod J 1997;30:297.
129. Molven O, Halse A. Success rates for gutta-percha and Kloroperka N-O root fillings made by undergraduate students: radiographic findings after 10-17 years. Int Endod J 1988;21:243.

Chapter 14

ENDODONTIC MISHAPS: THEIR DETECTION, CORRECTION, AND PREVENTION

Robert J. Frank

Endodontics is currently in the midst of its own "Industrial Revolution." The technological advances made routinely since the early part of this decade have far exceeded the progress made since the discipline was first recognized as a specialty. The advent of nickel-titanium files, rotary instrumentation, "endosonics," radiovisiography, the endoscope, and the clinical microscope are but a few innovations that have changed the way in which endodontics is practiced. This progress has increased both productivity and quality of care. The public's awareness and interest in preserving their teeth are increasing, and cases that heretofore were not attempted are now being successfully managed. Improved instruments and equipment have contributed to the quality of care. On the other hand, the complexity of the cases being treated by both general dentists and endodontists is increasing, with the result that new problems are being created. "Re-treatodontics" and "disassembly" are new terms that have arisen as the profession attempts to correct these new problems, or **procedural mishaps** as they are called. The purpose of this chapter is to present common mishaps and the treatment approaches for managing them.

Endodontic mishaps or procedural accidents are those unfortunate occurrences that happen during treatment, some owing to inattention to detail, others totally unpredictable. The mishaps listed in Table 14-1 will be described in detail, including how to recognize them, how to correct them, how they affect prognosis, and how to prevent them.

Recognition of a mishap is the first step in its management; it may be by radiographic or clinical observation or as a result of a patient complaint; for example, during treatment, the patient tastes sodium hypochlorite owing to a perforation of the tooth crown allowing the solution to leak into the mouth.

Correction of a mishap may be accomplished in one of several ways depending on the type and extent of procedural accident. Unfortunately, in some instances, the mishap causes such extensive damage to the tooth that it may have to be extracted.

Re-evaluation of the prognosis of a tooth involved in an endodontic mishap is necessary and important. The re-evaluation may affect the entire treatment plan and may involve dentolegal consequences. Dental standard of care requires that **patients be informed about any procedural accident.**

How can mishaps be **prevented?** The literature provides much information that can help prevent acci-

Table 14-1 Endodontic Mishaps

Access related
Treating the wrong tooth
Missed canals
Damage to existing restoration
Access cavity perforations
Crown fractures
Instrumentation related
Ledge formation
Cervical canal perforations
Midroot perforations
Apical perforations
Separated instruments and foreign objects
Canal blockage
Obturation related
Over- or underextended root canal fillings
Nerve paresthesia
Vertical root fractures
Miscellaneous
Post space perforation
Irrigant related
Tissue emphysema
Instrument aspiration and ingestion

dents. It is also true that experience can teach many valuable lessons if one pays attention. Put another way, we learn from our own and others' mistakes, and that can be true of endodontic mishaps as well. So when a file separates in a canal, the floor of the chamber is perforated while searching for canal orifices, or any of several other unfortunate procedural accidents occur, **immediately inform the patient**, correct the mishap, and re-evaluate the prognosis. Examine the various steps that led to the mishap and determine how it could have been avoided. Treatment evaluation can help prevent future occurrences.

Endodontic mishaps sometimes have dentolegal consequences. These can be minimized or avoided by providing patients with adequate information prior to the endodontic procedure. The following suggestions can help in establishing good patient communication:

1. Inform the patient before treatment about the possible risks involved. If the patient has been told that a porcelain crown may chip during treatment, when this occurs it will not be unexpected.
2. When a procedural accident occurs, explain to the patient the nature of the mishap, what can be done to correct it, and what effect the mishap may have on the tooth's prognosis and on the entire treatment plan.
3. If a procedural accident leads to a situation that is beyond the treating dentist's training and ability to handle, he or she should recognize the need to refer the patient to a specialist. It is important to note here that the standard of care in endodontics has only one level; both general dentists and specialists are held to the same standard.

For a more extensive discussion of endodontics and the law and informed consent, see chapter 1.

ACCESS-RELATED MISHAPS

Treating the Wrong Tooth

If there is no question about diagnosis, treating the wrong tooth falls within the category of inattention on the part of the dentist. Obviously, misdiagnosis may happen and should not be automatically considered an endodontic mishap. But if tooth #23 has been diagnosed with a necrotic pulp and the rubber dam is placed on tooth #24 and that tooth opened, that is a mishap.

Recognition that the wrong tooth has been treated is sometimes a result of re-evaluation of a patient who continues to have symptoms after treatment. Other times, the error may be detected after the rubber dam has been removed. In the first instance, the error was probably a misdiagnosis; in the second instance, a tooth adjacent to the one scheduled for treatment was inadvertently opened.

Correction includes appropriate treatment of both teeth: the one incorrectly opened and the one with the original pulpal problem. It is not prudent to hide such an error from the patient. Mistakes happen in all aspects of dental care. When a mistake does happen, the safest approach, even if embarrassing, is to explain to the patient what happened and how the problem may be corrected.

Prevention. Mistakes in diagnosis can be reduced by attention to detail and obtaining as much information as possible before making the diagnosis. In terms of arriving at a correct diagnosis, the baseball rule of "three strikes and y'er out" can be applied to endodontics: before making a definitive diagnosis, obtain at least three good pieces of evidence supporting the diagnosis. For example, a radiograph showing a tooth with an apical lesion may **suggest** pulp necrosis. But to be certain of that diagnosis, it is necessary to have additional information such as a lack of response to electric pulp testing. A draining sinus tract leading to the tooth apex should be proved radiographically with a gutta-percha point inserted in the tract and radiographed. Three such pieces of information make a diagnosis of pulp necrosis reasonable and a treatment plan that includes root canal therapy logical.

If less than three pieces of information are available, a definitive diagnosis may not be possible. The patient, however, may request that something be done because the symptoms are too unpleasant to endure. In such a case, it may be necessary to extirpate the pulp as a **diagnostic procedure** to obtain more information for a **definitive diagnosis.** If the patient agrees and understands that such a diagnostic procedure also requires completion of the root canal therapy even if it turns out that the problem is with another tooth, then it is not unreasonable to proceed. It is, however, usually best, if the diagnosis is tentative, to apply the remedy of "tincture of time" to allow signs and symptoms to become more specific. This may prevent unnecessary procedures or an incorrect diagnosis.

Once a correct diagnosis has been made, the embarrassing situation of opening the wrong tooth can be prevented by marking the tooth to be treated with a pen before isolating it with a rubber dam (Figure 14-1).

Missed Canals

Some root canals are not easily accessible or readily apparent from the chamber; additional canals in the mesial roots of maxillary molars and distal roots of

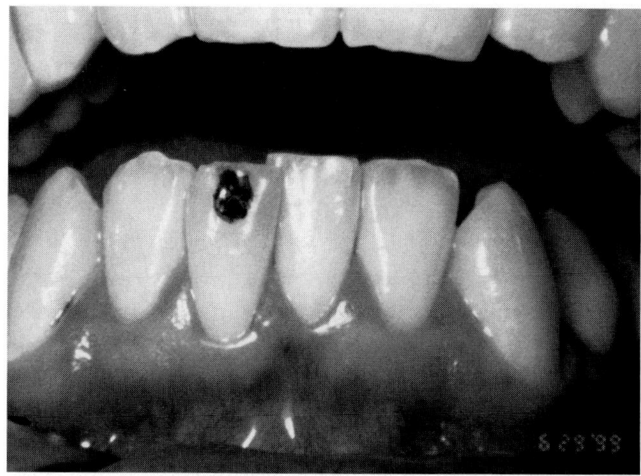

Figure 14-1 Tooth #25 has been marked with a felt tip pen in preparation for placement of the rubber dam. Marking a tooth will prevent placing the rubber dam incorrectly, which could result in treating the wrong tooth.

mandibular molars are good examples of canals often left untreated. Other canals are also missed because of a lack of knowledge about root canal anatomy or failure to adequately search for these additional canals.

Recognition of a missed canal can occur during or after treatment. During treatment, an instrument or filling material may be noticed to be other than exactly centered in the root, indicating that another canal is present (Figure 14-2).

In addition to standard radiographs for the determination of missed canals, computerized digital radiography has increased the chances of locating extra canals by enhancing the density and contrast and magnifying the image.

The advent of high-resolution magnification has also increased the ability to locate canals. Magnifying loupes, the microscope, and the endoscope may be used to clinically determine the presence of additional canals (Figure 14-3) (see chapters 9 and 12).

In some cases, however, recognition may not occur until failure is detected later.

Correction. Re-treatment is appropriate and should be attempted before recommending surgical correction (see chapters 12 and 13).

Prognosis. A missed canal decreases the prognosis and will most likely result in treatment failure. In some teeth with multicanal roots, two canals may have a common apical exit. As long as the apical seal adequately seals both canals, it is possible that the bacterial content in a missed canal may not affect the outcome for some time.

Prevention. Locating all of the canals in a multicanal tooth is the best prevention of treatment failure. **Adequate coronal access** allows the opportunity to find all canal orifices. Additionally, radiographs taken from mesial and/or distal angles will help to determine if the one canal that has been located is centered in the root, recalling that an eccentrically located canal is highly

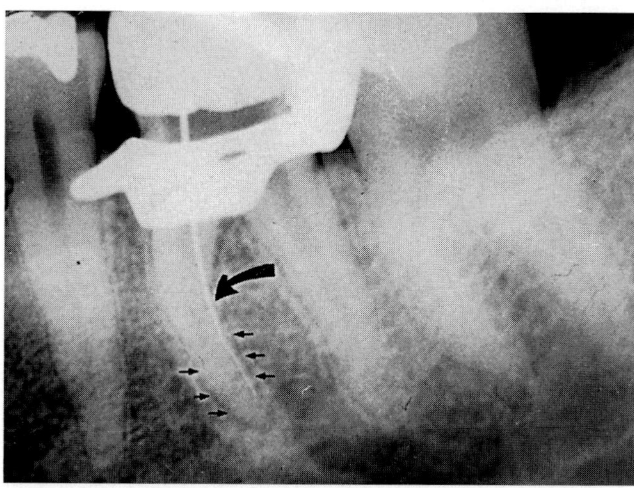

Figure 14-2 Radiograph indicating the presence of a second, or missed, canal. By following the lamina dura of the root (**small arrows**), the eccentric position of the file (**large arrow**), with relation to the outline of the root, **suggests** the presence of a missed canal. In this case, a perforation is confirmed: the file is in the periodontal ligament, and the mesial canals have not been negotiated.

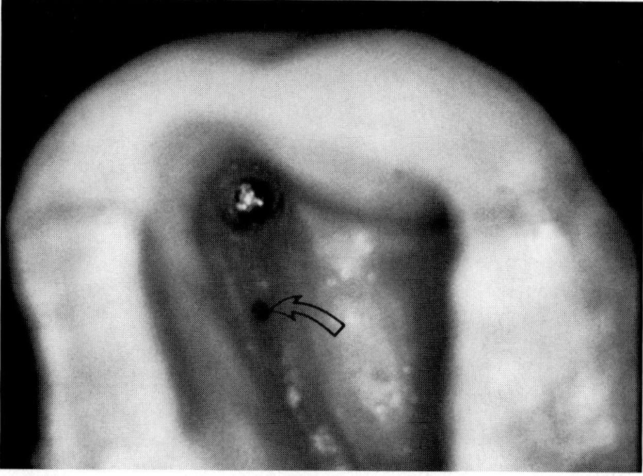

Figure 14-3 Various magnification systems such as the endoscope and the surgical microscope may be used to help detect extra canals. The second mesiobuccal canal (**arrow**) is readily apparent under magnification.

suggestive of the presence of another canal yet to be found (see Figure 14-2). Knowledge of root canal morphology and knowing which teeth have multiple canals is a good foundation. Assuming at the outset that certain teeth have roots with multiple canals and diligently searching for those canals is a prudent preventive procedure.

Damage to Existing Restoration

An existing porcelain crown presents the dentist with its own unique challenges. In preparing an access cavity through a porcelain or porcelain-bonded crown, the porcelain will sometimes chip, even when the most careful approach using water-cooled diamond stones is followed. There is usually no way to predict such an occurrence. Knowing when to exercise caution can, however, reduce unwanted results.

Correction. Minor porcelain chips can at times be repaired by bonding composite resin to the crown. However, the longevity of such repairs is unpredictable.

Prevention. Placing a rubber dam clamp directly on the margin of a porcelain crown is asking for trouble. This may result in damage to the crown margin and/or fracture of the porcelain. Even removal of a **provisionally** cemented new crown prior to endodontic therapy may also pose a problem. These crowns can be difficult to remove, and often a margin will be damaged, or the porcelain may chip.

Justman and Krell described a technique for **removing provisionally cemented crowns** that can help prevent both crazing of the porcelain, damage to the margin, or aspiration of the crown by the patient.[1] They recommended that the rubber dam be attached to the wings of a clamp and the jaws of the clamp placed **coronal** to the margin of the restoration. The rubber dam is released from the wings and positioned with the rubber between the jaws of the retainer and the restoration **to provide a buffer.** The beaks of a Steiglitz forceps can then be placed in the retainer holes, with leverage more safely applied until the restoration is loosened.

An alternative to prevent damage to an existing, **permanently cemented crown** is to remove it before treatment. Preservation of the integrity of the restoration is sometimes possible by using special devices such as the Metalift Crown and Bridge Removal System (Classic Practice Resources, Inc, Baton Rouge, La.). The system allows for removal with little or no damage to the crown. After completion of root canal therapy, the crown can be recemented and the pilot hole repaired. Other techniques such as vibrations have also been used successfully.

Access Cavity Perforations

Undesirable communications between the pulp space and the external tooth surface may occur at any level: in the chamber or along the length of the root canal. They may occur during preparation of the access cavity, root canal space, or post space. In this section, the problem of access cavity perforations will be addressed.

Access preparations are made to allow the locating, cleaning, and shaping of all root canals. In the process of searching for canal orifices, perforations of the crown can occur, either peripherally through the sides of the crown or through the floor of the chamber into the furcation.

Recognition. If the access cavity perforation is **above the periodontal attachment**, the first sign of the presence of an accidental perforation will often be the presence of leakage: either saliva **into** the cavity or sodium hypochlorite **out** into the mouth, at which time the patient will notice the unpleasant taste.

When the crown is perforated **into the periodontal ligament**, bleeding into the access cavity is often the first indication of an accidental perforation. To confirm the suspicion of such an unwanted opening, place a **small** file through the opening and take a radiograph; the film should clearly demonstrate that the file is not in a canal. In some instances, a perforation may initially be thought to be a canal orifice; placing a file into this opening will provide the necessary information to identify this mishap (Figure 14-4).

Correction. Perforations of the coronal walls **above the alveolar crest** can generally be repaired intracoronally without need for surgical intervention

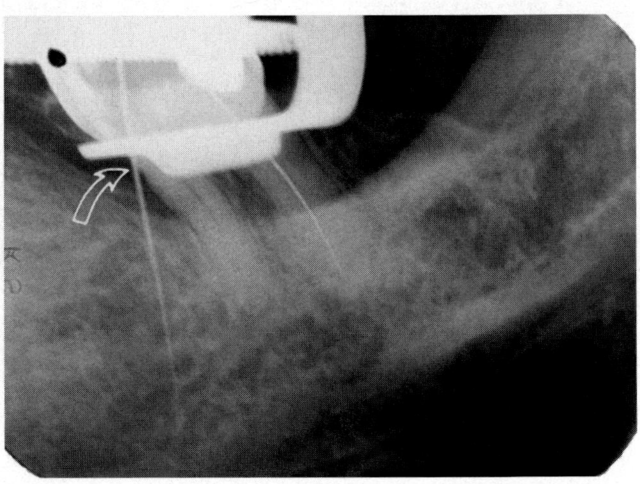

Figure 14-4 Placing a file in a site of suspected perforation (**arrow**) and taking a radiograph will show the position of the file in relation to the root. Note that in this tipped molar, the distal canal has been properly located, but the mesial orifices were missed.

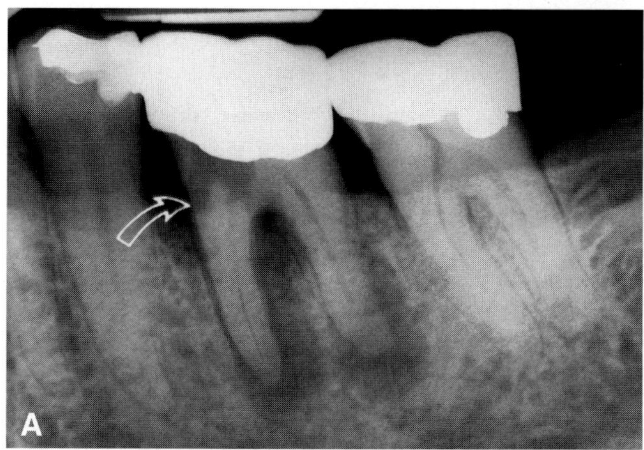

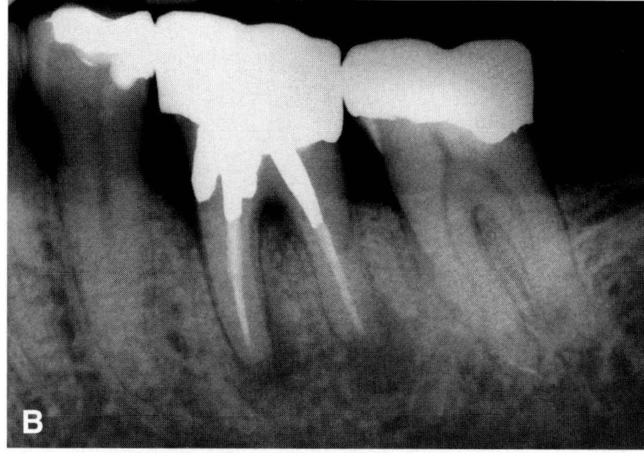

Figure 14-5 Supracrestal perforation repair. **A**, Note the perforation (**arrow**) made in the mesial wall during access preparation. **B**, Repair was done with amalgam; a matrix band was placed to confine the alloy, following which the filling was carved smooth.

(Figure 14-5). Cavit (Premier Dental Products, King of Prussia, Pa.) will usually serve to seal these types of perforations **during endodontic treatment.**

Perforations into the periodontal ligament, whether laterally or into the furcation, should be done as soon as possible to minimize the injury to the tooth's supporting tissues. It is also important that the material used for the repair provides a good seal and does not cause further tissue damage.

Several materials have been recommended for perforation repair: Cavit,[2] amalgam,[3] calcium hydroxide paste,[4] Super EBA,[5] glass ionomer cement,[6] gutta-percha,[7] tricalcium phosphate,[8] or hemostatic agents such as Gelfoam.[9] An *in vitro* dye penetration study creating an artificial floor using either calcium sulfate or hydroxyapatite and then repairing the perforation with Vitrebond (3M, St. Paul, Minn.) was reported by Alhadainy and Abdalla.[10] The results indicated that calcium sulfate and hydroxyapatite, used as barriers, significantly improved the sealing ability of Vitrebond and provided successful barriers against its overextension.

Mittal and coworkers reported their *in vitro* repair of furcation perforations using plaster of Paris with various other materials.[11] Evaluation using dye leakage showed amalgam to have the highest amount of leakage, followed in decreasing order by glass ionomer, composite, IRM, and AH26. An *in vivo* application of this technique is necessary, however, to evaluate periradicular responses to these materials and long-term success.

The concept of using an artificial barrier against which to condense and help confine the repair material has led to the use of absorbable, hemostatic collagen products, such as Collastat OBP (Vitaphore Corp.) and CollaCote (Colla-Tec, Inc, Plainsboro, N.J.).

A material recently approved by the US Food and Drug Administration, mineral trioxide aggregate (MTA) (Pro-Root, Dentsply/Tulsa Dental, Tulsa, Okla.), has shown **convincing** results (Figure 14-6),[12] and several new studies have supported its use for perforation repairs.[12–17]

Hartwell and England reported less than promising results using Teflon and/or decalcified freeze-dried bone to repair furcal perforations in monkeys.[18] No reparative bone formation developed, and epithelial downgrowth from the sulcus separated the connective tissue and bone from cementum. It is apparent that a furcal perforation that is not successfully repaired will soon communicate with the sulcus, resulting in a more serious problem.

Prior to repair of a perforation, it is important to control bleeding, both to evaluate the size and locations of the perforation and to allow placement of the repair material. Calcium hydroxide placed in the area of perforation and left for at least a few days will leave the area dry and allow inspection of perforation. Mineral trioxide aggregate, in contrast to all other repair materials, may be placed in the presence of blood since it requires moisture to cure. It is nevertheless preferable to control bleeding prior to repair so that the location can be more accurately determined.

Prognosis for a perforated tooth must generally be downgraded. How much it is downgraded is a clinical decision based on the circumstances such as the perforation size and the existing periodontal condition. Sinai proposed that the prognosis for a tooth with a perforation depends on the location of the perforation, the length of time the perforation is open to contamination, the ability to seal the perforation, and accessibili-

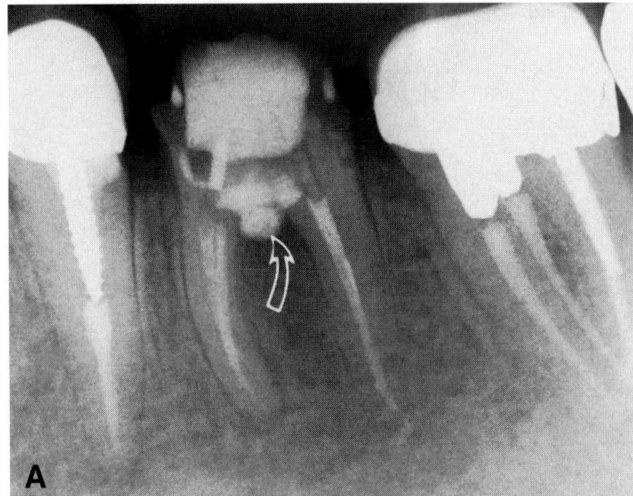

Figure 14-6 Furcation repair using mineral trioxide aggregate (MTA). A, Radiograph shows repair of perforation using MTA (arrow). B, Six months after repair. C, Eighteen months after repair, intact furcation support is evident.

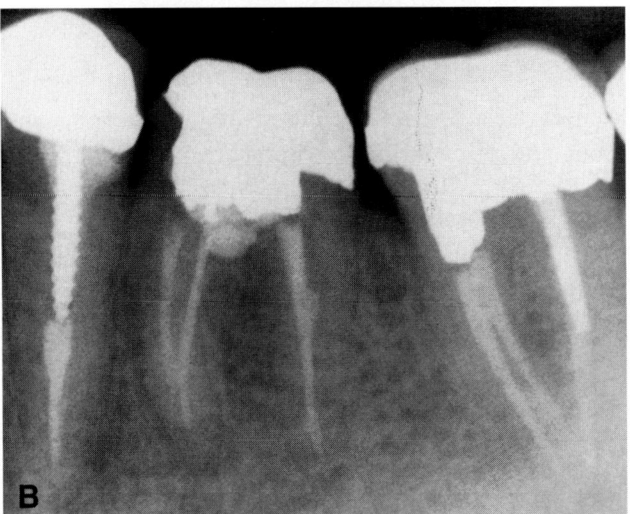

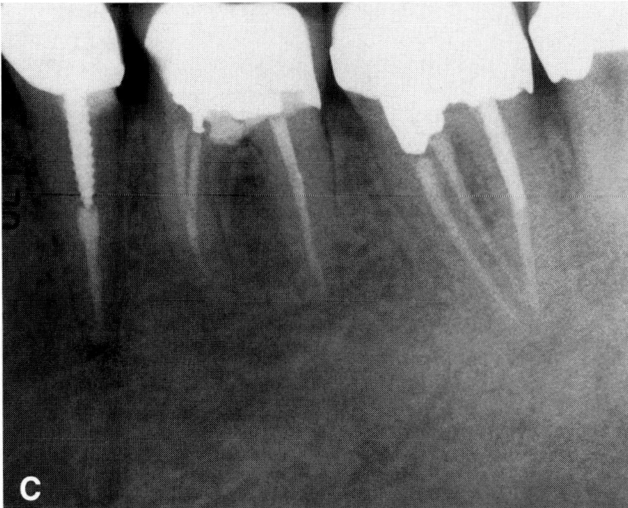

ty to the main canal.[19] The overall success rate for perforation repairs based on 55 cases was reported by Kvinnsland et al. as 92%.[20] Generally, it can be said that the **sooner repair is undertaken**, the better the chance of success. Surgical corrections may be necessary in refractory cases.

Prevention. Thorough examination of diagnostic preoperative radiographs is the paramount step to avoid this mishap. Checking the long axis of the tooth and **aligning the long axis of the access bur with the long axis of the tooth** can prevent unfortunate perforations of a tipped tooth. The presence, location, and degree of calcification of the pulp chamber noted on the preoperative radiograph are also important information to use in planning the access preparation. Perforations can also often be associated with an inadequate access preparation. Prevention of procedural mishaps is best accomplished by close attention to the principles of access cavity preparation: adequate size and correct location, both permitting direct access to the root canals. A thorough knowledge of tooth anatomy, specifically pulpal anatomy, is essential for anyone performing root canal therapy.

Crown Fractures

Crown fractures of teeth undergoing root canal therapy are a complication that can be avoided in many instances. The tooth may have a preexistent infraction that becomes a true fracture when the patient chews on the tooth weakened additionally by an access preparation.

Recognition of such fractures is usually by direct observation. It should be noted that infractions are often recognized first after removal of existing restoration in preparation of the access. When infractions become true fractures, parts of the crown may be mobile.

Treatment. Crown fractures usually have to be treated by extraction unless the fracture is of a "chisel type" in which only the cusp or part of the crown is involved; in such cases, the loose segment can be removed and treatment completed. If the fracture is more extensive, the tooth may not be restorable (Figure 14-7) and needs to be extracted. Crowns with infractions should be supported with circumferential bands or temporary crowns during endodontic treatment.

Prognosis for a tooth with a crown fracture, if it can be treated at all, is likely to be less favorable than for an intact tooth, and the outcome is unpredictable. Crown infractions may spread to the roots, leading to vertical root fractures.

Prevention is simple: reduce the occlusion before working length is established. In addition to preventing this mishap, it also will aid in reducing discomfort following endodontic therapy. As described above, bands and temporary crowns are also valuable.

INSTRUMENTATION-RELATED MISHAPS

Instrumentation-related mishaps can often be associated with excessive and inappropriate dentin removal during the cleaning and shaping phase of endodontics. Most of the procedural mishaps in this section can in some way be related to overinstrumentation. Excessive canal preparation to accommodate large pluggers or spreaders can lead to weakening of the tooth and even fracture of the root tip.[21] Roots that have an hourglass configuration in cross-section (eg, mesial roots of mandibular molars and roots of maxillary premolars) are particularly prone to "canal stripping"—a term used when root perforations result from excessive flaring during canal preparation. Such flaring can also weaken the tooth, with the result that a vertical root fracture occurs during the filling procedure (Figure 14-

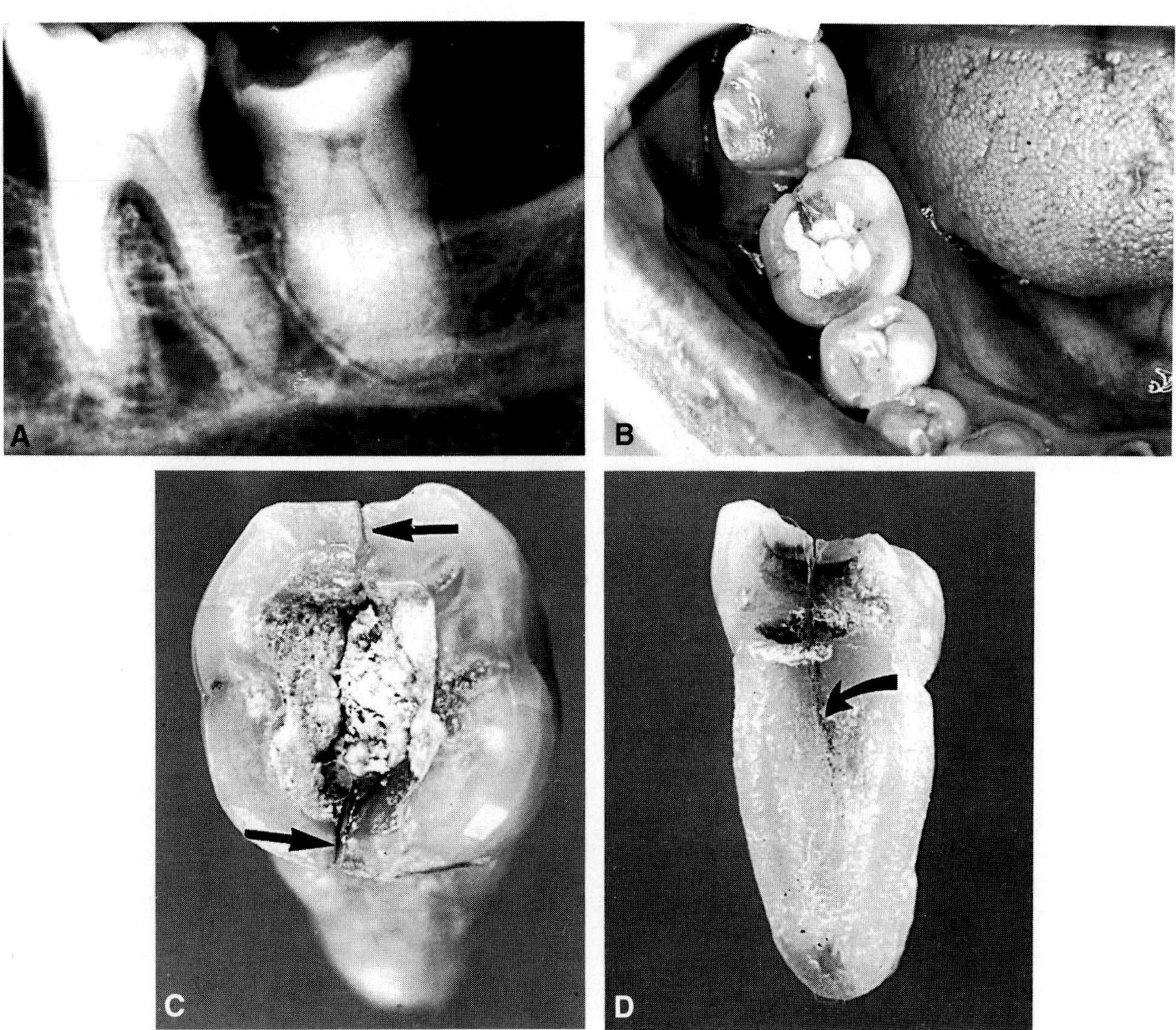

Figure 14-7 Tooth loss resulting from failure to reduce occlusion at onset of endodontic therapy. **A**, Preoperative radiograph. **B**, Occlusal view as the patient presented on the second visit. **C**, Occlusal view of extracted tooth with **arrows** pointing to the mesiodistal fracture line. **D**, **Arrow** indicating that the fracture had extended to the root surface.

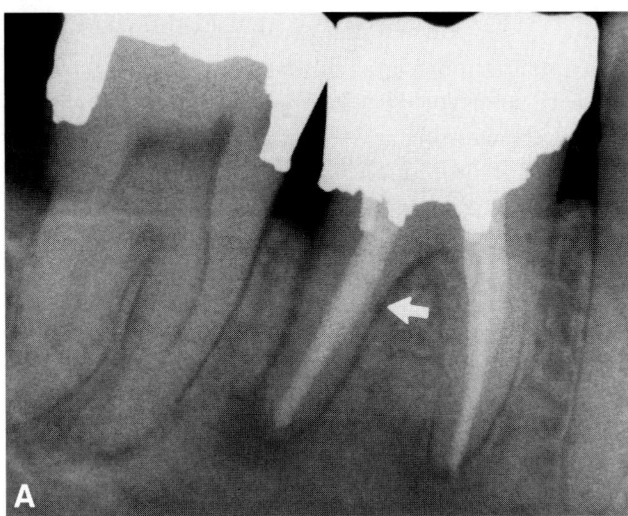

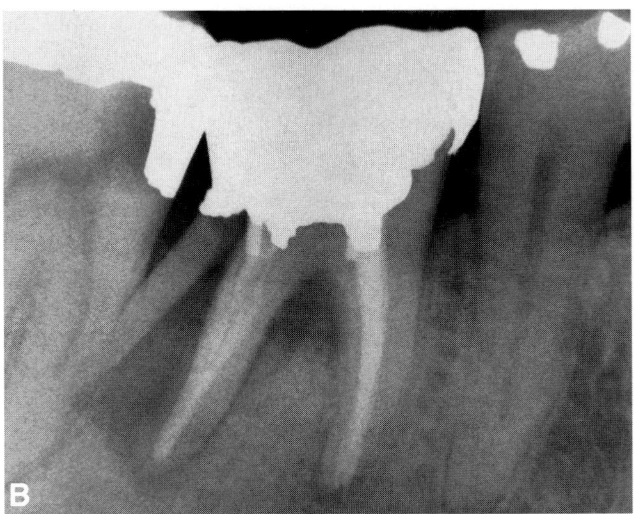

Figure 14-8 Vertical root fracture associated with overzealous canal preparation. **A**, Postoperative radiograph shows distal canals prepared and filled leaving a thin-walled root (**arrow**). **B**, Twelve months later, the patient reported with a vertical root fracture. It should also be noted that the pin placed before root canal therapy may also have contributed to a weakened root.

8). Also related to overinstrumentation are canal ledgings and apical transportations and perforations. Gutmann and Dumsha proposed a range of sizes to be used as a guideline for the apical termination of the canal preparation.[22] For a detailed description of proper instrumentation techniques, refer to chapter 10.

Ledge Formation

Ledges in canals can result from a failure to make access cavities that allow direct access to the apical part of the canals or from using straight or too-large instruments in curved canals (Figure 14-9). The newer instruments with noncutting tips have reduced this problem by allowing the instruments to track the lumen of the canal, as have nickel-titanium files. Occasionally, even skilled and careful clinicians develop canal ledges when treating teeth with unsuspected aberrations in canal anatomy.

One of the anatomic complexities in root canal therapy is the curved root, which is generally evident on radiographs. However, roots that curve toward or away from the central x-ray beam, that is, toward the buccal or lingual, are much more difficult to discover. The frequent finding (55%) of a **buccal curvature** of the palatal root of the maxillary first molar and the **labial or lingual curvature** of the maxillary central incisor and canine are examples of anatomic variations that can complicate root canal treatment (see chapter 10, Plates 4, 6, and 21). Occasionally, the curvature in line with the central beam shows up as a "bull's-eye" or "target" at the apex of the root returning on itself—a subtle and easily missed radiographic characteristic.

Recognition. Ledge formation should be suspected when the root canal instrument can no longer be inserted into the canal to full working length. There may be a loss of normal tactile sensation of the tip of the instrument binding in the lumen. This feeling is supplanted by that of the instrument point hitting against a solid wall: a loose feeling with no tactile sensation of tensional binding (see Figure 14-9, A).

When ledge formation is suspected, a radiograph of the tooth with the instrument in place will provide additional information. The central x-ray beam should be directed through the involved area. If the radiograph shows that the instrument point appears to be directed away from the lumen of the canal, completion of the canal preparation must include an effort to bypass the ledge formation.

Correction. The use of a small file, No. 10 or 15, with a distinct curve at the tip (see Figure 10–49, B), can be used to explore the canal to the apex. The curved tip should be pointed toward the wall opposite the ledge. This is a situation in which the "tear-shaped" silicone instrument stops are valuable. The "tear" is pointed in the same direction as the curve of the instrument. The *vaivén* or "watch-winding" motion often helps advance the instrument. Whenever resistance is met, the file is slightly retracted, rotated, and advanced again until it bypasses the ledge. If the exploring instrument can be introduced to full working length, a radiograph should confirm the return of the

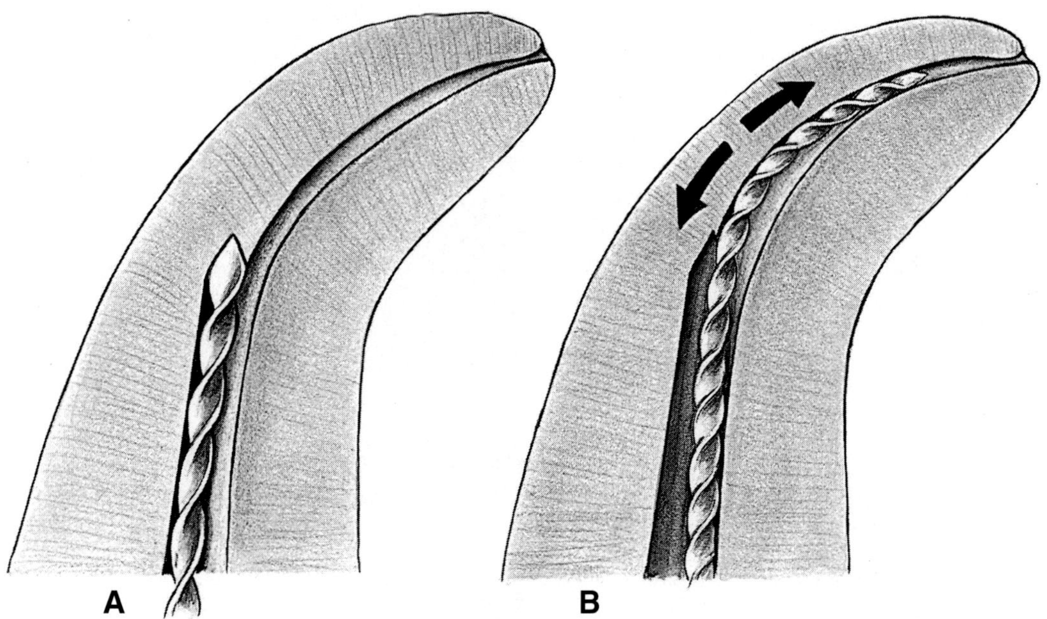

Figure 14-9 Cause and correction of ledge formation in a curved canal. **A,** A large straight instrument used in a curved canal cuts the ledge at the curve. **B,** The ledge may be painstakingly removed with a severely curved file, rasping against the ledge (**arrows**) in the presence of sodium hypochlorite or a lubricant such as Prolube (Dentsply/Tulsa Dental, Tulsa, Okla.). To bypass the ledge, the tip of a correcting file should be severely curved to hug the inside wall of the curve.

file to the apical portion of the canal. Subsequent files should be used in the same manner as the exploring file to maintain the true pathway.

Completion of canal preparation can best be accomplished by following these recommendations: Use a lubricant, irrigate frequently to remove dentin chips, maintain a curve on the file tip, and, using short file strokes, press the instrument against the canal wall where the ledge is located (see Figure 14-9, B). The canal should be constantly irrigated to wash out dentin filings. The tip of the file must be checked repeatedly to be certain that the curve is maintained. If the instrument is allowed to straighten, it will again catch on the ledge, and repeated filing will lead to deepening of the ledge, or worse, a perforation. The possibility of perforation is enhanced by chelation with ethylenediaminetetraacetic acid (EDTA); hence, this medicament should not be used in these situations.

Prevention. The best solution for ledge formation is prevention. Accurate interpretation of diagnostic radiographs should be completed before the first instrument is placed in the canal. Awareness of canal morphology is imperative throughout the instrumentation procedure. Finally, precurving instruments and not "forcing" them is a sure preventive measure. Failing to precurve instruments and forcing large files into curved canals are perhaps the most common causes of this mishap. Using instruments with noncutting tips and nickel-titanium files has been shown to be very beneficial in maintaining root canal curvatures.

Perforations

Accidental canal perforations may be categorized by location. Perforation of the pulp chamber has already been described (access cavity perforations). Radicular perforations can be identified as either cervical, midroot, or apical root perforations.

Perforations in all of these locations may be caused by two errors of commission: (1) creating a ledge in the canal wall during initial instrumentation and perforating through the side of the root at the point of canal obstruction or root curvature and (2) using too large or too long an instrument and either perforating directly through the apical foramen or "wearing" a hole in the lateral surface of the root by overinstrumentation (canal "stripping").

Cervical Canal Perforations

The **cervical portion** of the canal is most often perforated during the process of locating and widening the canal orifice or inappropriate use of Gates-Glidden burs.

Recognition often begins with the sudden appearance of blood, which comes from the periodontal ligament space. Rinsing and blotting (with a cotton pellet) may allow direct visualization of the perforation; magnification with either loupes, an endoscope, or a microscope is very useful in these situations. If direct visualization is not adequate to make a definitive identification of a perforation, it may be necessary to place a small file into the area that has been exposed and take a radiograph of the tooth; the film should clear up any uncertainty. The electronic apex locator has been shown to be very valuable in these situations.[23]

Correction of the perforation may include both internal and external repair. A small area of perforation may be sealed from inside the tooth. If the perforation is large, it may be necessary to seal first from the inside and then surgically expose the external aspect of the tooth and repair the damaged tooth structure; a material that has been recommended for this is Geristore (Den-Mat Corp., Santa Maria, Ca.).[24,25]

Many materials have been used (amalgam, Cavit, glass ionomer), but the most promising material for almost all types of perforations is MTA.[14] It has been shown to provide a very excellent seal of perforated areas, and since it requires moisture for setting, it is very useful in areas of bleeding (Figure 14-10).

Prognosis must be considered to be reduced in these types of perforations, and surgical correction may be necessary if a lesion or symptoms develop.

Prevention may be achieved by reviewing each tooth's morphology prior to entering its pulp space. Additionally, radiographically verifying one's position in the tooth can turn one back on track before it is too late.

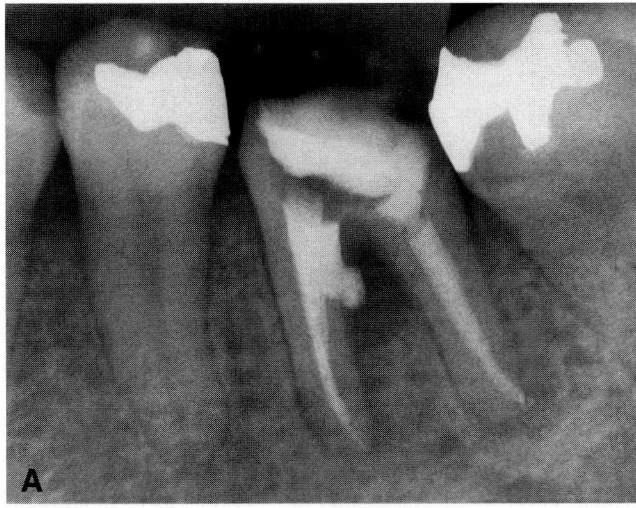

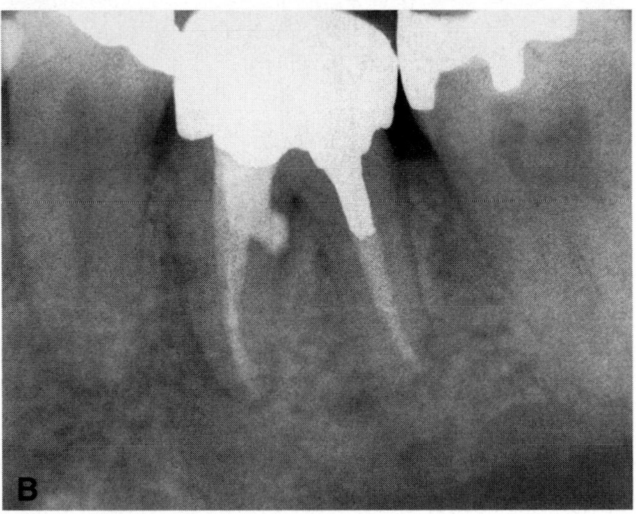

Figure 14-10 Cervical perforation. **A**, Radiograph of a molar with repair of perforation of the mesial root using mineral trioxide aggregate. **B**, Eighteen months re-evaluation shows excellent repair. (Courtesy of Dr. M. Torabinejad, Loma Linda University, California.)

Midroot Perforations

Lateral perforations at midroot level tend to occur mostly in curved canals, either as a result of perforating when a ledge has formed during initial instrumentation or along the inside curvature of the root as the canal is straightened out. The latter is often referred to as canal "stripping" and results in a fairly long perforation that seriously compromises the outcome of treatment.

Recognition. "Stripping" is a lateral perforation caused by overinstrumentation through a thin wall in the root and is most likely to happen on the inside, or concave, wall of a curved canal, such as the **distal wall of the mesial roots** in mandibular first molars (Figure 14-11). Stripping is easily detected by the sudden appearance of hemorrhage in a previously dry canal or by a sudden complaint by the patient. A paper point placed in the canal can confirm the presence and location of the perforation (Figure 14-12).

Correction. Successful repair of a lateral perforation is contingent on the adequacy of the seal established by the repair material. Since the primary concern is to prevent overextension, unless a resorbable material is first introduced against which to condense, the material is often forced out into the ligament space despite gentle placement, and a likely poor seal will result. Using CollaCote and EBA, Castellucci has surmounted this problem (personal communication, April 2000) (Figure 14-13).

Access to midroot perforation is most often difficult, and repair is not predictable. Calcium hydroxide has been used in the hope of stimulating a biologic barrier against which to pack filling material (Figure 14-14), but usually filling material ends up into the perforation area.

Repair of strip perforations has been attempted both nonsurgically and surgically. A majority of the tech-

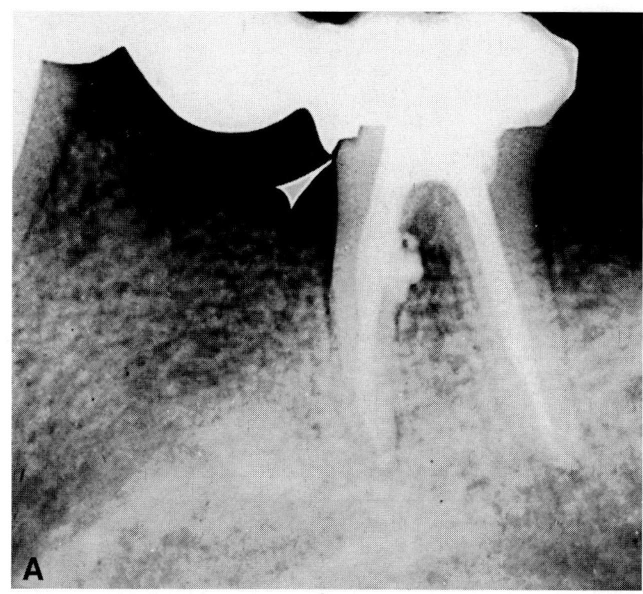

Figure 14-11 A, Lateral perforation by wearing through the thin distal wall of a mesial root. Also note the open margin (**arrow**). B, Schematic cross-section of a curved root depicting thickness of walls, safety zone, and endangered zone. C, Anticurvature filing allows modified access to the apex, avoiding the thin inner wall and flaring toward the thicker wall. (A Courtesy of Dr. J. D. Zidell. B and C reproduced with permission from Abou-Rass M et al.[32])

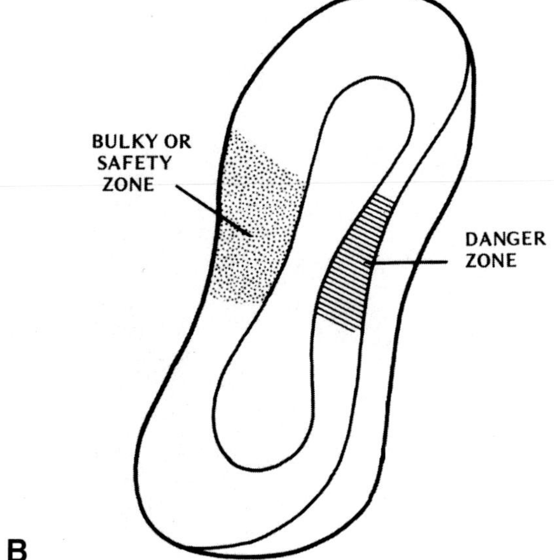

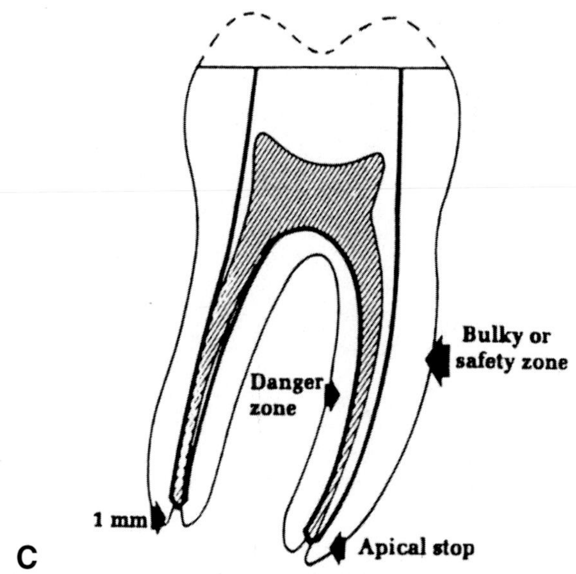

niques, however, propose a two-step method wherein the root canals are first obturated, and then the defect is repaired surgically. Removal of the excess gutta-percha using a hot spatula and cold burnishing the perforation site was reported by Allam.[26] Use of amalgam, gutta-percha, and calcium hydroxide was reported by Biggs et al.,[27] and the results using glass ionomer were reported by Goon and Lundergan.[28] All have reported **limited success**, if any. Based on the impressive results using MTA for perforations other than strip perforations,[12–17] the material might be expected to perform as well for strip perforation repairs also.

Prognosis. Both "stripping" perforation and direct lateral perforation of the root result in a reduction of the prognosis. Loss of tooth structure and integrity of the root wall can lead to subsequent fractures or microleak-

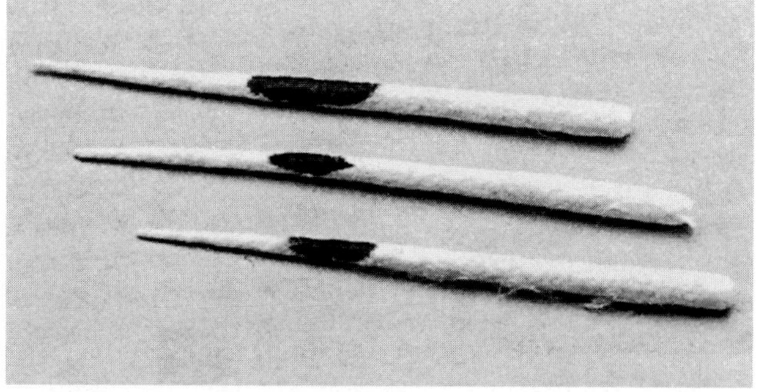

Figure 14-12 Paper points confirming strip perforation. The area of hemorrhage mapped on the point indicates the area where the strip has occurred.

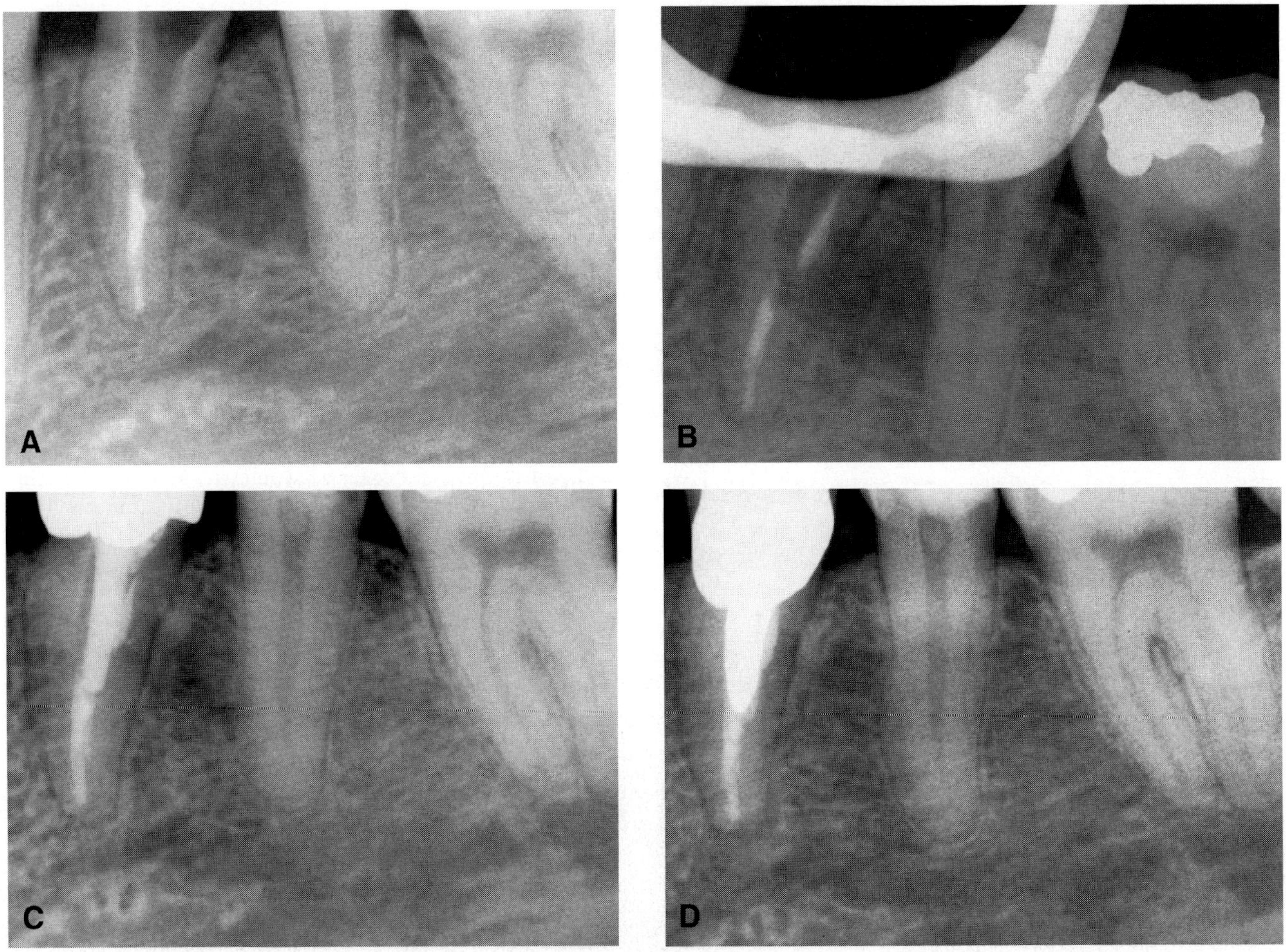

Figure 14-13 Midroot perforation repair. **A**, The lower first premolar has a midroot buccal perforation. The crown and post have been removed and the lesion has been sealed with resorbable collagen. **B**, Using the surgical operating microscope, the perforation has been filled with Super EBA (Harry J. Bosworth Co. Skokie Ill.). **C**, Seven-month recall shows evidence of healing. **D**, Two-year recall with a new restoration in place. (Courtesy of Dr. A. Castellucci, Florence, Italy.)

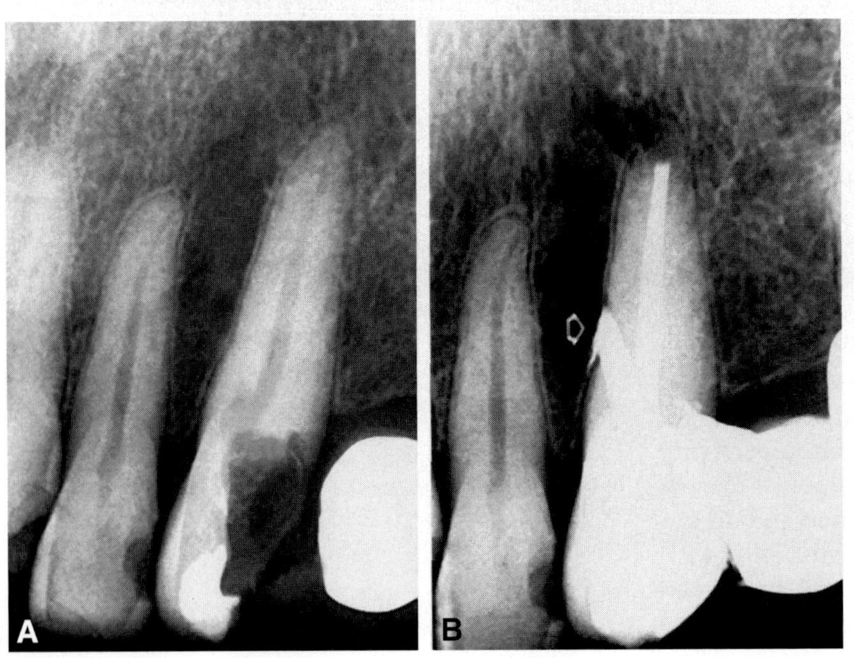

Figure 14-14 Repair of mechanical perforation following calcium hydroxide therapy. **A**, Preoperative radiograph. Gross perforation is caused by a misdirected bur. The main canal was located, cleansed, and shaped in addition to the perforated "canal" prepared with large blunted files. A thick paste of calcium hydroxide was inserted. The patient was reappointed 6 weeks later. **B**, Post-filling radiograph. The gutta-percha point was fitted for each canal and well condensed. Note how a new matrix of healing is demonstrated by the form of sealer and gutta-percha at the site of perforation (**arrow**). Reproduced with permission from Frank AL. Dent Clin North Am 1974;18:465.

age owing to inability to properly seal the perforation. The reduced prognosis must be considered when evaluating the tooth's role in an overall treatment plan.

Prevention. Berutti and Fedou have shown how delicate the tooth structure is in these areas. In lower first molars at 1.5 mm below the bifurcation, they found the dentin of the root to be 1.2 to 1.3 mm thick from the canal to the cementum. The **mesiobuccal canal** is in most danger of being stripped.[29]

There must always have been concern about this mishap. Peeso, writing as early as 1903, spoke of perforated roots, often caused by a rotary instrument, no doubt including the one he designed.[30] Two endodontic groups faced this problem and modified preparations to avoid these "stripping" accidents. Endodontics at the University of Southern California (USC) may have experienced these particular perforations through their advocacy of Peeso power-driven reamers "as an auxiliary aid in enlarging the cervical third" of the preparation.[31] To overcome the problem, they developed a technique they termed **anticurvature filing,**[32] stressing the importance of **maintaining mesial pressure** on the enlarging instruments to avoid the delicate "danger zone" of the distal wall where the root is so thin (see Figure 14-11, C). A similar technique was advocated at Ohio State University.[33] Others reported the same encouraging results.[34,35]

Stripping can be prevented by exercising caution in two areas: careful use of rotary instruments inside the canal and following recommendations for canal preparation in curved roots, as proposed by the USC group.[32]

Apical Perforations

Perforations in the **apical segment** of the root canal may be the result of the file not negotiating a curved canal or not establishing accurate working length and instrumenting beyond the apical confines. Perforation of a curved root is the result of "ledging," "apical transportation," or "apical zipping." The glossary of accepted endodontic terminology defines "transportation" as "removal of canal wall structure on the outside curve in the apical half of the canal due to the tendency of files to restore themselves to their original linear shape during canal preparation." [36] The term "apical zip" is also defined as "an elliptical shape that may be formed in the apical foramen during preparation of a curved canal when a file extends through the apical foramen and subsequently transports that outer wall."[36] Owing to their curvatures, the maxillary lateral incisor, mesiobuccal, and palatal roots of maxillary molars and the mesial root of mandibular molars are most often the sites of these types of perforations.

Recognition. An apical perforation should be suspected if the patient suddenly complains of pain during treatment, if the canal becomes flooded with hemorrhage, or if the tactile resistance of the confines of the canal space is lost. If any of these occur, it is important to confirm one's suspicions radiographically and attempt to correct them before further damage is done. A paper point inserted to the apex will confirm a suspected apical perforation (Figure 14-15).

Correction. Efforts to repair may be to attempt to renegotiate the apical canal segment or to consider the perforation site as the new apical opening and then decide what treatment the untreated apical root segment will require. One is now dealing with two foramina: one natural, the other iatral. Obturation of both of these foramina and of the main body of the canal requires the vertical compacting techniques with heat-softened gutta-percha (Figure 14-16). Often surgery is necessary, particularly if a lesion is present apically.

Apical perforation can also occur in a perfectly straight canal if instrument use exceeds the correct working length. This destroys the Resistance Form of the root canal preparation at the cementodentinal junction, making it difficult to control the apical extensions of the root canal filling.

If the perforation is caused by overinstrumentation, corrective treatment includes re-establishing tooth length **short of the original length** and then enlarging the canal, with larger instruments, to that length. A **careful adaptation of the primary filling point**, often blunted, is imperative. The canal is then cautiously filled to that length cautiously so that the Resistance Form thus created will prevent filling extrusion out the apex.

Creating an **apical barrier** is another technique that can be used to prevent overextensions during root canal filling. Materials used for developing such barriers include dentin chips,[37] calcium hydroxide powder, Proplast (Vitek Inc. Houston Tex.), hydroxyapatite,[38,39] and, more recently, MTA.[14] In deciding which material to use, it is, as with so much in endodontics, more a

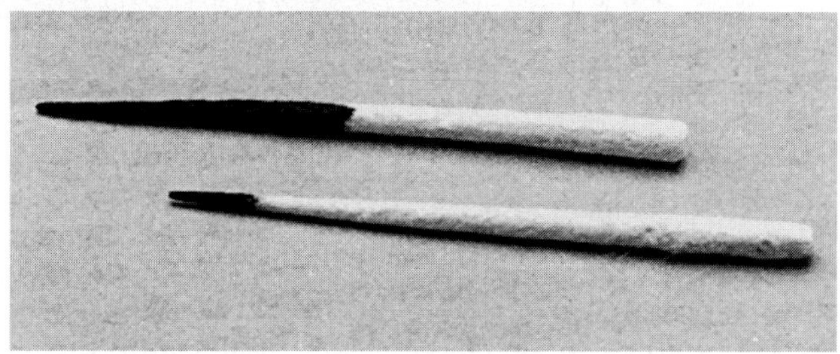

Figure 14-15 Location of hemorrhage at the tip of a paper point suggests apical perforation.

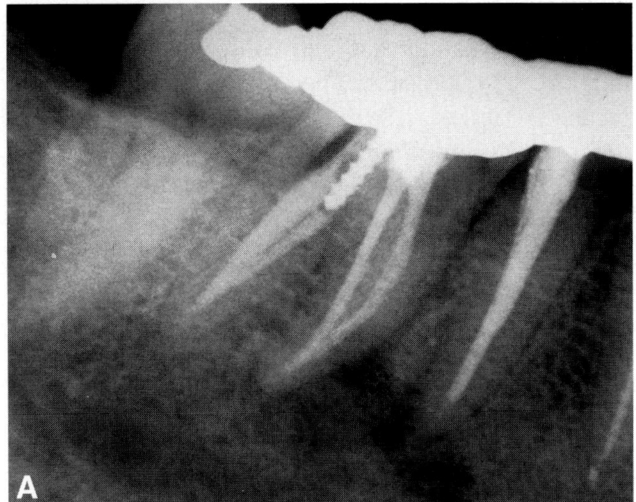

Figure 14-16 **A,** The patient presented with pain and localized swelling buccal to tooth #30. Endodontic treatment had been done 5 years previously. **B,** Mesial canals were re-treated, and the **apical root perforation** was sealed with calcium hydroxide. Later the root canals were obturated with gutta-percha and Roth's sealer. **C,** Two-year post-treatment radiograph. (Courtesy of Dr. Steven Morrow, Loma Linda University, California.)

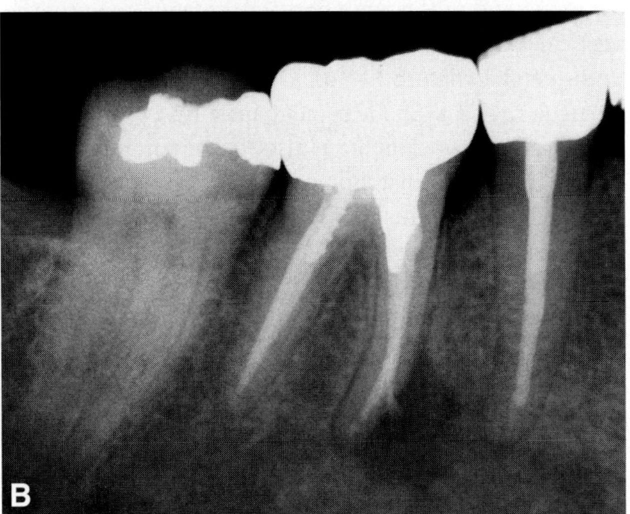

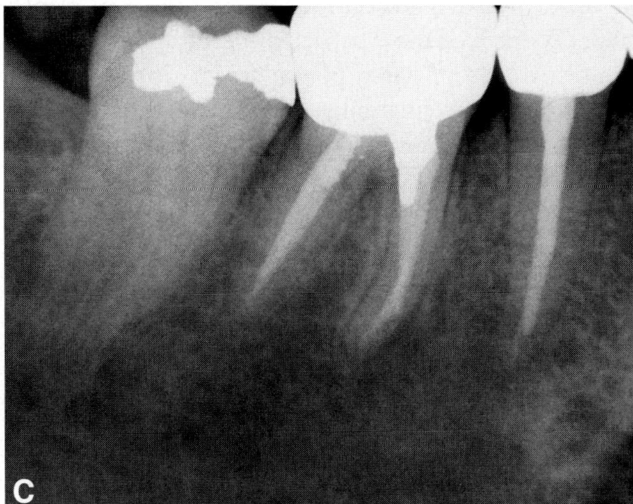

question of what works best in the hands of the individual clinician. The solution is often a compromise but is usually preferable to a surgical correction.

Prognosis. There are probably more apical perforations than perforations in other areas of the pulp space. Fortunately, with successful repair, apical perforations have less adverse effect on prognosis than more coronal perforations.

Prevention. A detailed discussion addressing the prevention of these problems can be found in chapter 10 on instrumentation.

Separated Instruments and Foreign Objects

Many objects have been reported to break or separate and subsequently become lodged in root canals. Glass beads from sterilizers, burs, Gates-Glidden drills, amalgam, lentulo paste fillers, files and reamers, and tips of dental instruments have all found their way into canals, complicating treatment. Chenail and Teplitsky reviewed iatral and patient-placed foreign objects and listed, in addition to the above, nails, pencil lead, toothpicks, tomato seeds, hat pins, needles, pins, and other metal objects and advocated use of orthograde ultrasonics for removal.[40] Most commonly, files and reamers are involved in these types of procedural mishaps. Usually, the instrument is advanced into the canal until it binds, and efforts to remove it then lead to breakage, leaving a segment of it in the canal. Other common errors leading to this mishap are using a "stressed" instrument (Figure 14-17), placing exaggerated bends on instruments to negotiate curved canals, and forcing a file down a canal before the canal has been opened sufficiently with the previous, smaller file and then using it in a reaming motion. The result is fracturing of the instrument.

Rotary instruments such as Gates-Glidden drills, if stressed, will break close to the shank, leaving a piece that can be grasped and easily retrieved. The Stieglitz

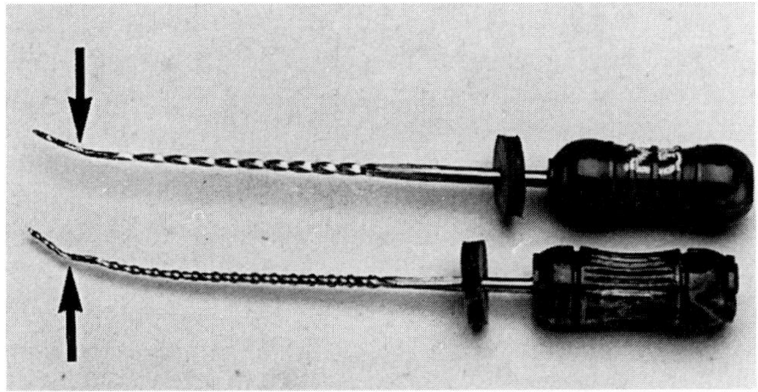

Figure 14-17 Instruments showing stress (**arrows**) from faulty instrumentation techniques. Instruments with these signs of potential fracture should be discarded.

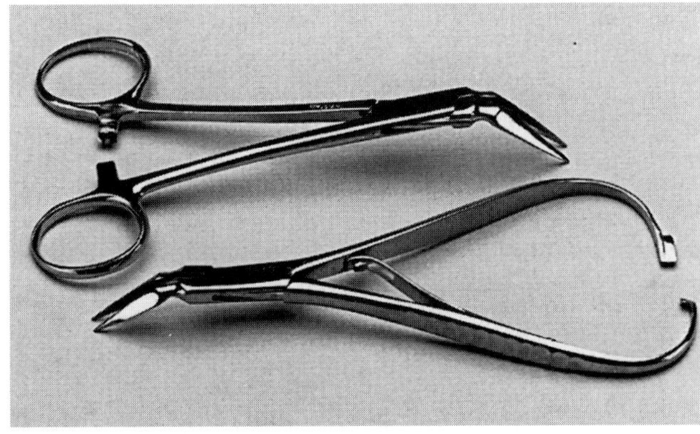

Figure 14-18 Useful armamentaria for retrieving separated instruments from root canals.

forceps (Figure 14-18) are especially useful for this. If the break occurs closer to the bur head, retrieval is much more difficult.

Correction. The optimal correction of instrument fracture or the presence of other foreign objects in a canal is to remove the obstruction. As a general rule, efforts to remove instrument fragments should be made as the initial approach to corrective treatment. **Ultrasonic** fine instruments have proven most effective in loosening and "flushing out" broken fragments. Using microscopy and special fine diamond tips (Figure 14-19), a tunnel can be created around the separated instrument, which can then be vibrated and dislodged (see chapter 10). Martin (personal communication to J Ingle, April 1984) and Japanese researchers[41] have had remarkable success removing broken instruments with ultrasonic devices that loosen the fragments and float them out. Use of ultrasonic devices is advocated in two different case reports wherein a tunnel is created around the separated instrument and a sleeve is positioned in the canal and around the separated instrument. In one study, cyanoacrylate is used to bind and remove the instrument,[42] and in the other, a Hedstrom file is wedged in the sleeve until the instrument is locked between the flutes of the file and the wall of the sleeve.[43] The efficacy of these techniques can be judged only on the basis of the few case reports presented and may be attempted with no predictably favorable result. Recently, Hulsmann reported on the successful use of the Canal Finder System in combination with ultrasonic devices in bypassing and removing fractured instruments.[44] Failing that, one of the following steps may be taken:

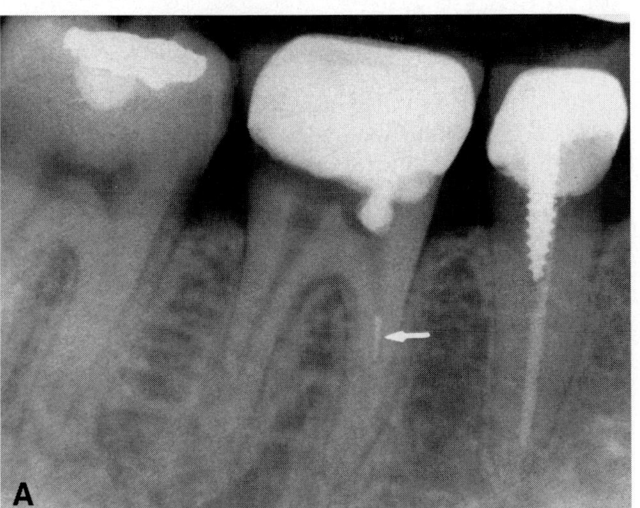

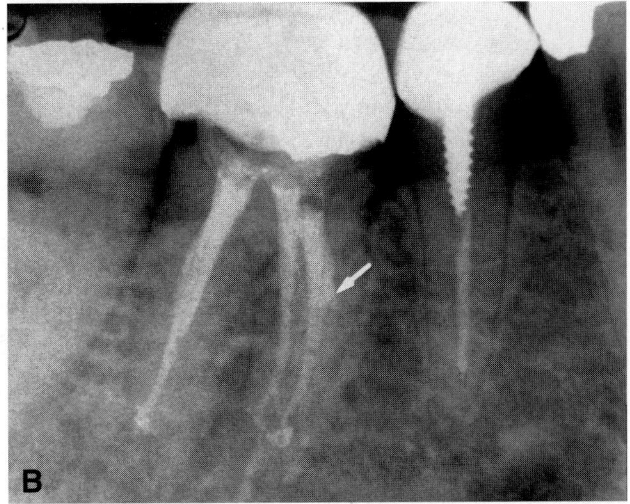

Figure 14-19 A, **Arrow** pointing to a separated rotary instrument in the mesiolingual canal of tooth #30. **B**, Postobturation film with an **arrow** identifying "tunneling" that was created with an ultrasonic instrument to remove the separated instrument. (Courtesy of Dr. Marshall Gomes, Lodi, California.)

1. If the instrument fragment is totally within the root canal system, one may attempt to bypass it with a small file or reamer. Often the instruments that break do so along the walls of the canal, being stuck between irregularities of secondary dentin or calcifications. Broken instruments can often be bypassed if the canals are oval or irregular in shape. Bypassing is made easier with a lubricant. If successful, the canal preparation can be completed and the canal filled regardless of whether the instrument segment is removed during the process of canal preparation. The instrument segment thus becomes part of the filling material. The effort to bypass a broken instrument has its own risk: possible perforation of the canal.
2. If the fragment cannot be bypassed, one can prepare and fill the canal to the level to which instrumentation can be accomplished. As long as the separated instrument fragment is not protruding through the apex, further treatment such as apical surgery may not be necessary. The instrument itself, if embedded in the dentin before fragmentation, may help to seal the canal. Studies by Crump and Natkin[45] and by Fox et al.[46] have shown that success following instrument separation is equal to that of teeth without such mishaps.
3. If the fragment extends past the apex and efforts to remove it nonsurgically are unsuccessful, the corrective treatment will probably include apical surgery. The first step, though, will be to complete cleaning, shaping, and filling the canal, as described above. Following that, apical surgery would include removal of the part of the instrument fragment that extends beyond the apex and retrofilling if indicated (Figure 14-20).

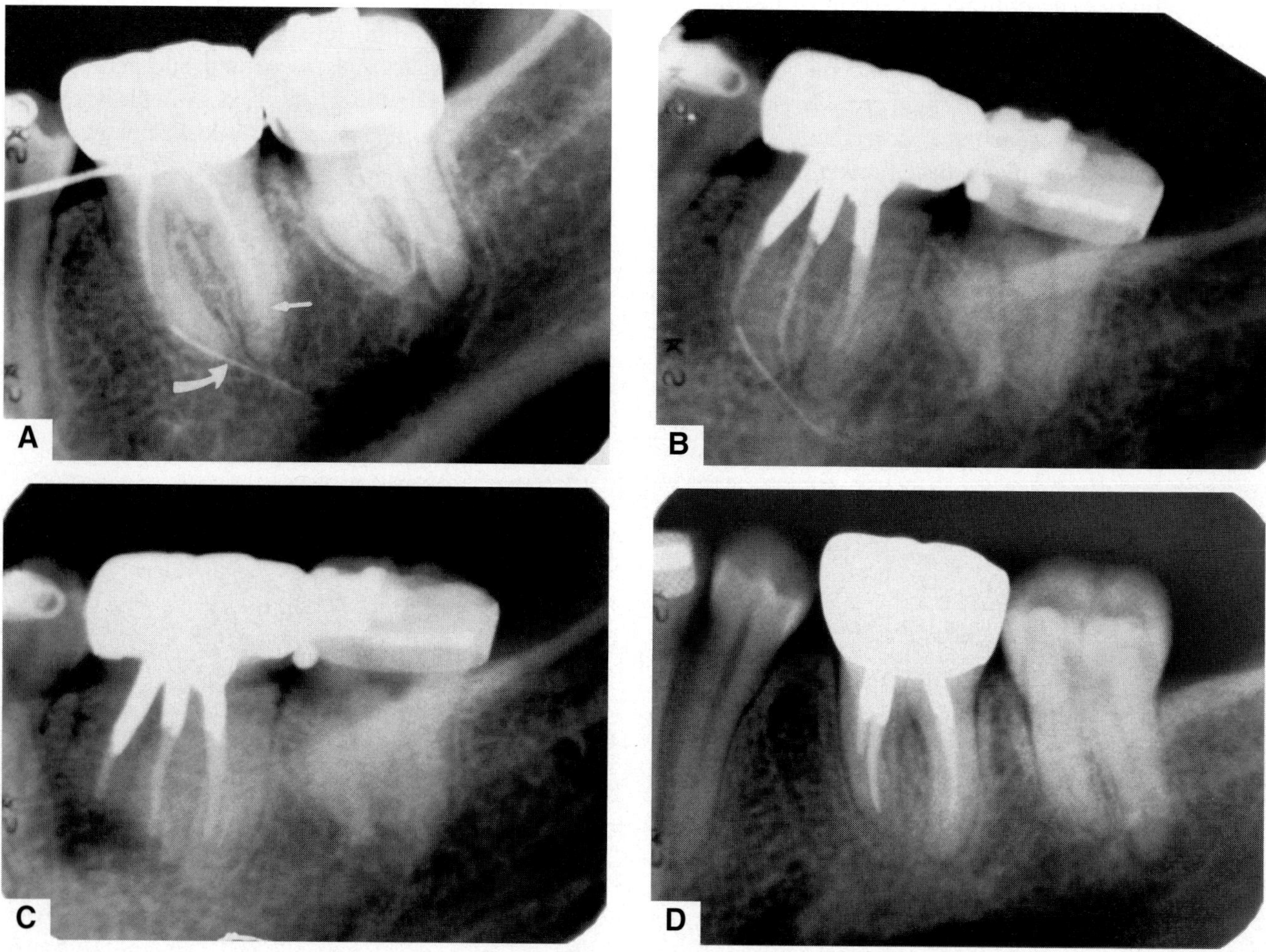

Figure 14-20 Treatment of a broken instrument past the apex. **A,** The patient presented with tooth #19 showing a broken file past the apex of the mesial root (**curved arrow**) and also a small piece of a broken file in one of the distal canals (**small arrow**). The small file fragment is within the root canal system. **B,** The root canals were re-treated; note that neither broken file could be removed. **C,** Film showing the result of apical resection of the mesial root to remove the file fragment extending into the alveolus. No retrofillings were indicated since the canals were adequately obturated. **D,** Twelve-month re-evaluation shows satisfactory healing. (Courtesy of Dr. Donald Peters, Loma Linda University, California.)

Prognosis for a tooth with a separated instrument may not change very much if the instrument can be bypassed. If surgical correction is needed, the prognosis may be reduced, depending on the outcome of corrective treatment. In any event, it is important to tell the patient about the nature of the procedural mishap, what effect it may have on the prognosis, and what corrective measures may be needed.

Prevention of separation mishaps can be partially accomplished by careful handling of instruments. Some instruments, however, will break even with cautious handling and utmost care. As mentioned earlier, a "stressed" instrument is the one most likely to separate in a canal. A stressed instrument, as shown in Figure 14-17, may be recognized by the flutes, which may appear "unwound." When the spacing appears uneven between the cutting edges of a reamer or file, the instrument is stressed and should not be used. Small instruments, such as Nos. 08, 10, 15, and 20, should be examined carefully during use to check for signs of stress. **Instruments No. 08 and 10 should be used only once.** These smaller instruments should not be forced or wedged into a canal; rather, they should be teased gently into place. An instrument that cannot be inserted to the desired depth should be removed and the tip modified slightly by bending before resuming the pathfinding process. The use of a canal lubricant will also help. This process may have to be repeated several times before the path of the canal is negotiated.

Two other important points will aid in prevention of separation: sequential instrumentation, using the "quarter-turn" technique, and increasing file size only after the current working file fits loosely into the canal without binding. The gradual increase in file sizes, even to include the currently available half-sizes, and avoiding the rush to finish will go a long way toward preventing mishaps.

Canal Blockage

When a canal suddenly does not permit a working file to be advanced to the apical stop, a situation sometimes referred to as a "blockout" has occurred. Buchanan pointed out that "...blockage occurs when files compact apical debris into a hardened mass." He further noted that "fibrous blockage occurs when vital pulp tissue is compacted and solidified against the apical constricture."[47] The group at The University of Indiana reported much the same.[48]

Recognition occurs when the confirmed working length is no longer attained. Evaluation radiographically will demonstrate that the file is not near the apical terminus.

Correction is accomplished by means of recapitulation. Starting with the smallest file used, the quarter-turn technique using a chelating agent can be helpful. If the blockout occurs at a curve or bend of the root, gently precurving the instruments to redirect it is also effective. Caution must be employed in attempting to recover from a blockout occurring at a curve or bend. An all too common and unfortunate result is the creation of a ledge and/or lateral perforation. Precurving instruments during the redirection process and radiographic confirmation are essential.

Prognosis depends on the stage of instrumentation completed when the blockout occurs. If the canal has been adequately cleaned, it should have little or no effect. If, however, the blockout occurs before the canal is clean, prognosis will be reduced. Teeth with vital pulps have a better prognosis than those with necrotic pulps.

Accidental blockage of the apical end of the canal should not be confused with the technique for creating an apical stop using dentin chips, as advocated by Marshall[49] (see chapter 11). In that technique, dentin chips are purposely placed **after cleaning and shaping,** and the dentin used is clean. Infected chips and pulpal debris have been shown to deter healing.[50]

Prevention consists of frequent irrigation during canal preparation to remove dentin debris. The use of water-soluble lubricants such as File-Eze or K-Y Jelly is also a preventive measure.

OBTURATION-RELATED MISHAPS

Over- or Underextended Root Canal Fillings

Although controversy still may exist regarding apical termination of the root canal filling, there is general agreement that the ideal location is at or near the dentinocemental junction. A number of studies have supported the apical termination of the filling material just short of the radiographic apex.[51–54]

Root canal filling material is sometimes inadvertently extruded beyond the apical limit of the root canal system, ending up in the periradicular bone, sinus, or mandibular canal or even protruding through the cortical plate. Gross overextensions can lead to symptoms and treatment failure. A frequent cause of this mishap is apical perforation with loss of apical constriction against which gutta-percha is compacted. Treatment failure may be less from irritation of the filling material and more from leakage around a poorly compacted filling. Roane and associates have attempted to minimize apical canal transportation—a frequent cause of overextrusion of root canal filling—by use of the "balanced forced" approach[55,56] (see chapter 10). The results have been promising.

Underextension of root canal filling material may be caused by failure to fit the master gutta-percha point accurately. It can also result from a poorly prepared canal, particularly in the apical part of the canal.

No section addressing overextensions can be considered complete without the inclusion of extruded pastes. Case reports citing materials such as N2,[57] Hydron,[58] AH26,[59] Diaket,[60] and even zinc oxide–eugenol–based sealers[61] have been published. These articles have shown that, in addition to the effects of the material, the sequelae and untoward effects are location related. The risk of this occurrence rises in the root canal wherein the apical stop is inadequately prepared. Rowe stated that, in teeth with apices approximating the inferior alveolar canal, "the most frequent cause of damage is excess filling material which has passed through the apices and either caused pressure on the neurovascular bundle in the inferior dental canal or produced a neurotoxic effect on the nerve trunk"[62] (Figure 14-21). Overextension of materials into the alveolar cancellous bone near other teeth that are not close to a sensory nerve can also be expected to produce mild, to moderate, to severe discomfort until the initial inflammatory response subsides.

Recognition of an inaccurately placed root canal filling usually takes place when a post-treatment radiograph is examined.

Correction of an underextended filling is accomplished by **re-treatment**: removal of the old filling followed by proper preparation and obturation of the canal. Correction of an **overextended filling** is more difficult. An attempt to remove the overextension is sometimes successful if the entire point can be removed with one tug. Many times, however, the point will break off, leaving a fragment loose in the periradicular tissue. Attempts at removing a laterally condensed overextension, by using chloroform and a Hedstroem file, will usually produce the same results as trying to retrieve an overextended thermoplastic filling material; it may be pushed further into the periradicular tissue. If the overextended filling cannot be removed through the canal, it will be necessary to remove the excess surgically if symptoms or radicular lesions develop or increase in size. Root canal filling material such as gutta-percha and many sealers are generally well tolerated by the surrounding tissues, and overextended fillings do not automatically require surgical removal if asymptomatic and not associated with lesions. If symptoms persist from a tooth with an overextended gutta-percha filling, surgical removal of the excess material is usually a relatively minor procedure (Figure 14-22). If the root canal has been adequately cleaned and filled, a retro-filling is not necessary.

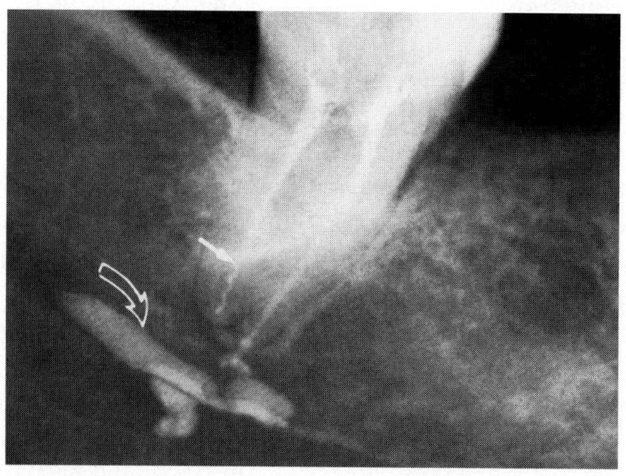

Figure 14-21 Example of the risk in using a paste-type filling material. The root canals in this tooth were filled using a lentulo spiral paste filler; note that part of the instrument is still in a canal (**small arrow**). More serious is the presence of paraformaldehyde paste in the mandibular canal (**open arrow**)—a consequence of spinning the paste into the root canal with the lentulo paste filler.

In re-treatments, the material being removed and the method of removal both affect the potential for overextension and extent of damage to the surrounding tissues. Spångberg studied the effect of various root canal filling materials on HeLa cells and found that amalgam, gutta-percha, and zinc phosphate had the least toxic effect, followed by calcium hydroxide paste, AH26, and Tubliseal (Kerr, Orange, Calif.). Chloropercha, Diaket, and N2 had the strongest toxicity.[63–66]

Prognosis. The effects of over- or underextensions on prognosis vary. Endodontic textbooks recommend that care be used in obtaining good apical seals.[67,68] Consequently, if the overextended filling provides an adequate seal, treatment may still be successful. In cases of underextended fillings, the prognosis depends on the presence or absence of a periradicular lesion and the content of the root canal segment that remains unfilled. If a lesion is present or the apical canals have necrotic or infected material in them, the prognosis diminishes considerably without re-treatment.

Prevention. As with most mishaps, attention to detail is the best form of prevention. Accurate working lengths and care to maintain them will help prevent overextensions. Modifying the obturation technique may also be preventive. In younger patients with wider root canal systems or in teeth with apical resorption, the apical stop may not be adequate to prevent gutta-percha from being extruded. Techniques that create apical barriers with calcium hydroxide, dentin chips, or MTA may be useful in these cases.

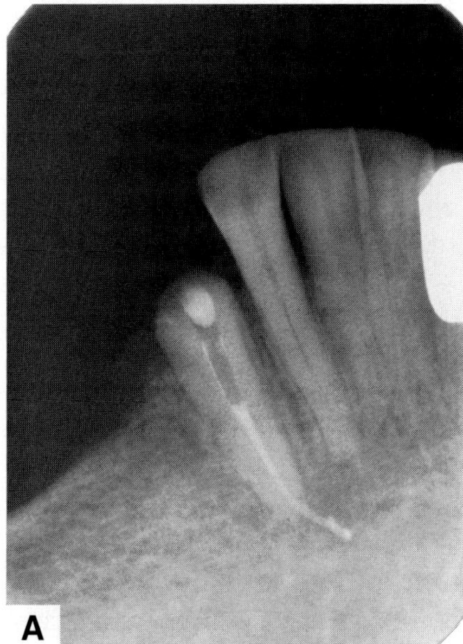

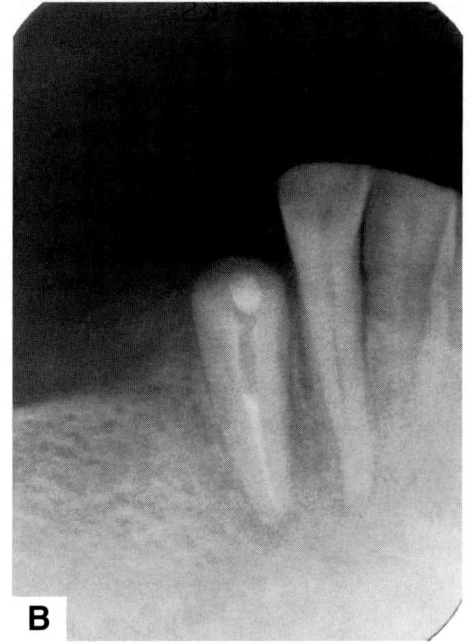

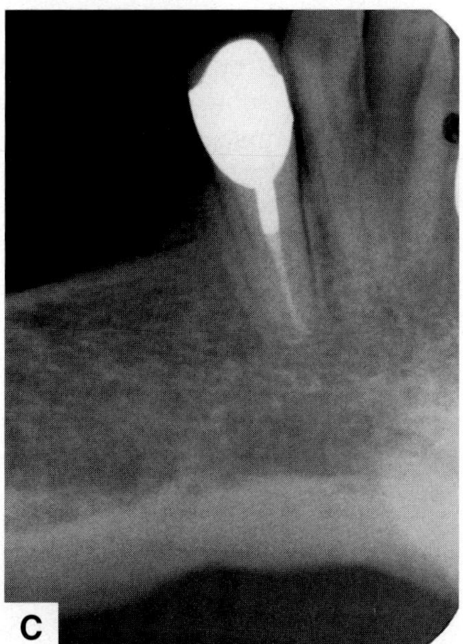

Figure 14-22 Overextended root canal filling. **A**, Radiograph shows overextension of gutta-percha. Symptoms were mild but persistent, so surgical removal of the excess filling material was done. **B**, Radiograph shows the tooth after apical curettage of excess gutta-percha. No retrofilling was needed. **C**, Radiograph shows completed restoration of the tooth 6 months later; the symptoms subsided after the surgical procedure.

Incorporation of two simple steps into one's root canal treatment technique can significantly decrease the chance of aberrant fillings; first, confirmation and adherence to canal working length throughout the instrumentation procedure and, second, taking a radiograph during the initial phases of the obturation to allow for corrective action, if indicated.

Nerve Paresthesia

There have been both local factors and systemic diseases reported as causative agents for paresthesia. Local factors in dental-related paresthesias are not limited to iatral root canal therapy. Patients presenting with this symptom should routinely be screened for an adjacent tooth with necrotic pulp. Cohenca and Rotstein reported a case wherein endodontic therapy completely resolved the patient's paresthesia.[69] The converse of this, however, is unfortunately also possible: the endodontic therapy can cause paresthesia. Overextensions and/or overinstrumentations are the causative factors most often found in paresthesia secondary to orthograde endodontic therapy.

Although it is true that most minor overextensions do not require anything more than periodic observation, nerve paresthesias or dysesthesias subsequent to gross overextensions of root canal–filling materials do occur (see Figure 14-21).[60,62] The nerve damage may be transient or permanent and may be instituted by overinstrumentation, overextensions, or injury to the inferior alveolar nerve, which is also a potential problem in surgical procedures. Finally, the use of formaldehyde-containing pastes has been shown to have a high incidence of nerve toxicity.[70]

Correction of these iatral neuropathies is often through nonintervention and observation. Gatot and Tovi suggested the use of systemic prednisone to shorten the course of the condition, prevent secondary fibrosis, and lessen the severity of sequelae.[71] Surgical decompression has also been reported, often with unpredictable results.[72] Although specifically addressing paresthesia from a surgical procedure, Girard proposed caution in any procedure with the potential of causing nerve damage:

> The most important process the dentist can practice is **prevention**; one should be judicious in his selection of cases. If another treatment for a problem is available, iatral neuropathies can be circumvented by using it. If there is no alternative treatment and neural damage is possible, the patient should be appropriately advised of the problem before surgery. Explicit written consent signed by the patient and witnessed is becoming standard.[73]

Vertical Root Fractures

Vertical root fractures can occur during different phases of treatment: instrumentation, obturation, and post placement. In both lateral and vertical condensation techniques, the risk of fracture is high if too much force is exerted during compaction. Similarly, during post placement, if the post is **forced** apically during seating or cementation, the risk of fracture is high, particularly if the post is tapered.

Recognition is often unmistakable. The sudden crunching sound, similar to that referred to as crepitus in the diseased temporomandibular joint, accompanied with pain reaction on the part of the patient, is a clear indicator that the root has fractured. A suggestive "teardrop" radiolucency may appear in the radiograph of a long-standing vertical root fracture (Figure 14-23) and may be associated with only minor symptoms of soreness in the tooth. To confirm the diagnosis of a vertical fracture, exploratory surgery is a good way to visualize the fracture, but finding a deep periodontal pocket of recent origin in a tooth with a long-present root canal filling is most suggestive of a vertical fracture.

Correction. Unfortunately in most cases of vertical fracture, extraction is the only treatment available at this time. One may speculate that in the future it may be possible to "glue" such fractures. Glass ionomer cement repairs for **furcal perforations** have been reported by Alhadainy and Himel.[74] The bonding ability of glass ionomer cement has led other investigators to use it in attempts to repair vertical root fractures. A 1-year success was reported in a single case.[75] To date, no consistently successful techniques have been reported to correct this problem.

Because this mishap produces irreversible damage to the tooth, it is most important to recognize the causes and adjust the techniques that might cause them.

Prevention involves avoidance of overpreparing canals and the use of a passive, less forceful obturation technique and seating of posts. Helfer et al. found a 9% moisture loss in pulpless teeth compared with vital teeth.[76] As a result of that study, they concluded that endodontically treated teeth are more brittle. Lewinstein and Grajower, however, found no such increased brittleness.[77] Although controversy still exists concerning the brittleness, Tidmarsh remarked that the change in architecture of an endodontically treated tooth required a restoration that will protect the tooth during function.[78] Full cuspal coverage was recommended.

Vertical root fracture can be attributed to overinstrumentation ("overflaring") of the canal, resulting in unnecessary removal of dentin along the canal walls, with subsequent weakening. In Figure 14-8, the result of overpreparation combined with pin placement has created a situation that could well have been prevented with more conservative preparation.

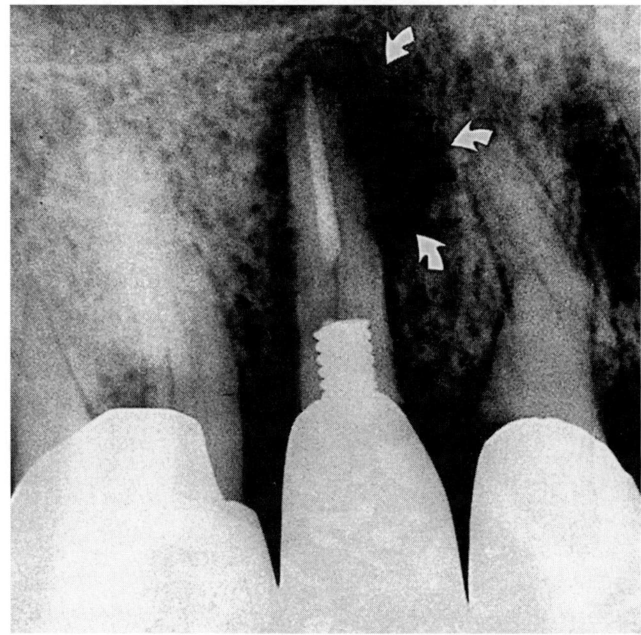

Figure 14-23 Vertical root fracture. **Arrows** surround the typical "halo" radiolucency often seen in vertical root fractures. Note the enormous "screw-type" post.

MISCELLANEOUS

Post Space Perforation

A well-done root canal procedure can be destroyed in a few seconds by a misdirected post space preparation. End-cutting drills such as those used for the Para-post system (Coltene/Whaledent, Mahwah, N.J.) need careful attention to avoid lateral perforation; round burs can also be dangerous if care is not exercised in watching the direction of the bur.

Recognition is similar to that of instrumentation-related lateral root perforations: sudden presence of blood in the canal (post preparation) or radiographic evidence.

Correction consists of sealing the perforation, if possible, as described for other perforations (see Figure 14-14). The use of a resin composite bonded to adjacent root dentin with a dentin bonding agent has been reported for both retro root-filling material[79,80] and as a retro sealing in root perforations associated with improper post placement.[81] A 15% failure rate was reported for perforation repairs located in areas other than the furcation, which had a slightly higher (18%) failure rate.[81]

Prognosis is least affected if the perforation is totally within bone; if it is closer to the gingival sulcus, the risk of periodontal pocket formation is high, but, in any case, the tooth must be considered weakened.

Prevention is associated with a good knowledge of root canal anatomy and planning the post space preparation based on radiographic information regarding the location of the root and its direction in the alveolus. Preparing the space at the time the root canal is obturated reduces the risk of perforating. It is safer to do so with a hot instrument or a file than with a round bur or an end-cutting bur. Gates-Glidden and Peeso drills are not likely to be at risk in causing perforations; however, they can lead to excessive removal of tooth structure and therefore can potentially lead to "stripping" or root fracture.

Irrigant-Related Mishaps

Various irrigants have been used in the chemomechanical preparation of the root canal system. Saline, hydrogen peroxide, alcohol, and sodium hypochlorite are among those most commonly used. Any irrigant, regardless of toxicity, has the potential to cause problems if extruded into periradicular tissues. The fear of toxicity of sodium hypochlorite as an irritant of periradicular tissue has tended to deter its use. In one study, however, no significant inflammatory difference was noted after 7 to 24 days when solutions of sodium hypochlorite ranging from 8.4 to 0.9% were implanted in polyethylene tubes into the backs of guinea pigs.[82]

On the other hand, forcibly injecting sodium hypochlorite, or any irrigating solution, through the canal into the surrounding tissue is another matter entirely. The number of cases reported probably does not truly reflect the incidence of this occurrence. Becker et al. described the damaging effects of an accidental injection of sodium hypochlorite beyond the apex.[83] Bhat reported the same effects with hydrogen peroxide (Figure 14-24).[84] Injection of hydrogen peroxide causes tissue emphysema, which can be managed similarly to that produced by compressed air.

An unfortunate sequence of events is triggered after the solution is injected into the root canal system and forced into the periradicular tissues. With alcohol or sodium hypochlorite, an immediate inflammatory response followed by tissue destruction ensues (Figure 14-25).

Recognition of an irrigant-related mishap will be readily apparent. The patient may immediately complain of severe pain, and swelling can be violent and alarming. Several case reports describing these events have been published.[85–94] The effects on the patient will, of course, depend on the type of solution used, the concentration, and amount of exposure. The initial response stage may be characterized by swelling, pain, interstitial hemorrhage, and ecchymosis.

Treatment. Because of the potential for spread of infection related to tissue destruction, it is advisable to prescribe antibiotics in addition to analgesics for pain. Antihistamines can also be helpful. Ice packs applied initially to the area, followed by warm saline soaks the following day, should be initiated to reduce the swelling.[85] The use of intramuscular steroids, and, in more severe cases, hospitalization and surgical intervention with wound débridement, may be necessary.[86] Monitoring the patient's response is essential until the initial phase of the reaction subsides.

Prognosis is favorable, but immediate treatment, proper management, and close observation are important. The long-term effects of irrigant injection into the tissues have included paresthesia, scarring, and muscle weakness.[90]

Prevention of inadvertent extrusion of irrigants past the apex can be attained by using **passive placement** of a modified needle. No attempt should be made to force the needle apically. The needle **must not be wedged** into the canal, and the solution should be delivered slowly and without pressure. Special endodontic irrigating needles such as the Monoject Endodontic Needle (Sherwood Medical, St. Louis, Mo.) with a

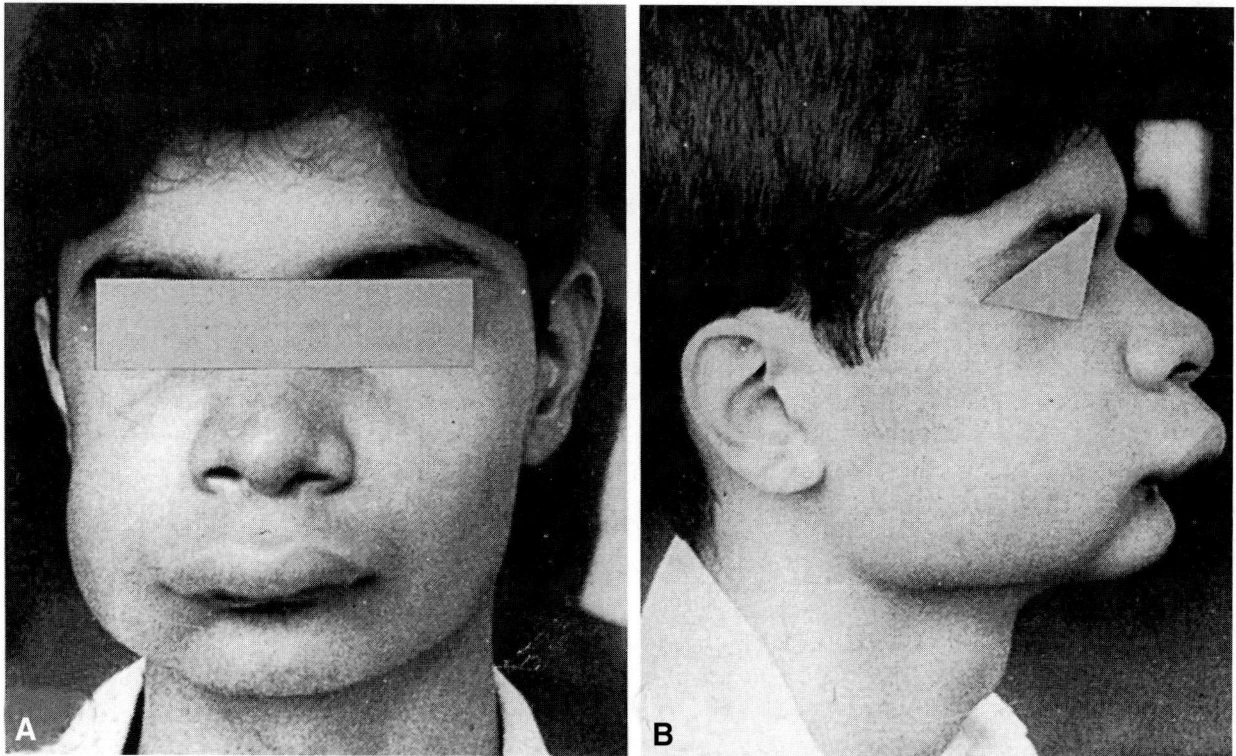

Figure 14-24 A and B, Severe tissue emphysema caused by injecting hydrogen peroxide irrigant into tissues. Reproduced with permission from Bhat KS.[84]

modified tip and side orifice or the blunt-end Prorinse (Dentsply/Tulsa Dental, Tulsa, Okla.) will prevent this mishap.

In the event that sodium hypochlorite is inadvertently injected into the maxillary sinus, immediate lavage of the sinus through the same root canal pathway of at least 30 mL of sterile water or saline should prevent damage of the sinus lining.[92]

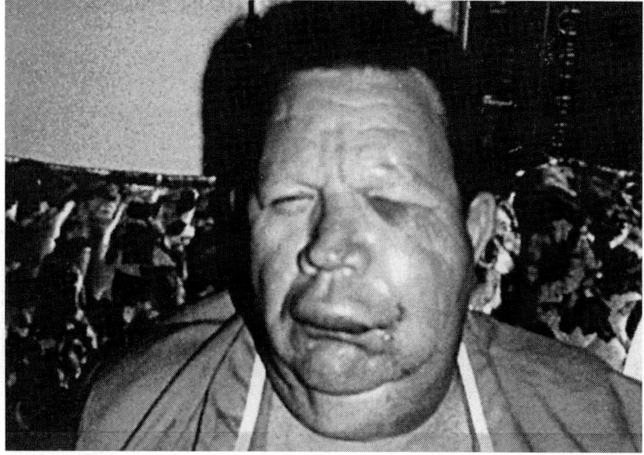

Figure 14-25 Gross swelling caused by inadvertent injection of 5.25% sodium hypochlorite periradicular to a maxillary premolar. Demerol poorly controlled the pain. Swelling, pain, and discoloration disappeared within 10 days. Reproduced with permission from Sabala CL and Powell SE.[85]

Becking reported three cases from Holland, including an accidental injection through a perforation followed by a severe secondary infection. He warned again that the irrigating needle should always be loose in the canal and that excessive pressure should not be exerted on the syringe.[93] A similar case reported from Israel involved massive swelling and secondary infection in spite of postoperative cortisone and antibiotic therapy.[86]

Hypersensitivity to sodium hypochlorite may occur, as has been reported from Tel Aviv. A patient reported a sensitivity to household bleach, and a forearm patch test confirmed it. Wisely, the dentist chose to use a substitute irrigant during endodontic therapy.[94]

Tissue Emphysema

Subcutaneous or periradicular **air emphysema** is, fortunately, relatively uncommon. Tissue space emphysema has been defined as the passage and collection of gas in tissue spaces or fascial planes.[95] It has been reported as an untoward event subsequent to various dental procedures, such as an amalgam restoration,[96] periodontal treatment,[97] endodontic treatment,[98] and exodontia.[99] The common etiologic factor is compressed air being forced into the tissue spaces. Two procedures in endodontics, if carried out improperly, have the potential to cause a problem. First, during canal preparation, a blast of air to dry the canal, and second, during apical surgery, air from a high-speed drill can lead to air emphysema. Any time a stream of air is directed toward exposed soft tissues, the potential for a problem exists.

Recognition. The usual sequence of events is rapid swelling, erythema, and crepitus. Hayduk et al. regard crepitus as pathognomonic of tissue space emphysema and therefore easily distinguished from angioedema.[100] Although pain is not a major complaint, dysphagia[101] and dyspnea[102] have been reported. Unlike irrigant extrusion reactions, tissue space emphysema remains in the subcutaneous connective tissue and usually does not spread to the deep anatomic spaces.[103] Migration of air into the neck region could cause respiratory difficulty, and progression into the mediastinum could cause death.

For obvious reasons, the problem should not be treated lightly. Noble stated,

> There are several diagnostic signs of mediastinal emphysema. First, a sudden swelling of the neck is seen. Second, the patient may have difficulty breathing and his voice will sound brassy. Third, the characteristic crackling can be induced when the swollen regions are palpated. Finally, the mediastinal crunching noise is heard on auscultation, and air spaces are seen in anteroposterior and lateral chest radiographs.[104]

Correction. Treatment recommendations vary from palliative care and observation to immediate medical attention if the airway or mediastinum is compromised. Broad-spectrum antibiotic coverage is indicated in all cases to prevent the risk of secondary infection.[105] The majority of reported cases have followed a benign course followed by total recovery.[106–108]

Preventive measures that should be taken to avoid the risk of this occurrence during endodontic procedures include using paper points to dry root canals. If the air syringe is to be used, Jerome suggested horizontal positioning over the access opening, using the "Venturi effect" to aid in drying the canal.[109] In surgical procedures, once a flap is reflected, apical access can be made with the slow-speed or high-speed handpieces that **do not direct jets** of air into surgery sites.

Instrument Aspiration and Ingestion

Aspiration or ingestion of a foreign object is a complication that can occur during any dental procedure. Endodontic instruments, used in the absence of a rubber dam, can easily be aspirated or swallowed if inadvertently dropped in the mouth. Case reports have been published with reamers or files located in either the food or air passages. The common denominator in all is **failure to use a rubber dam**. The standard of care for endodontic therapy **requires** the use of a rubber dam. **It is not an option to not use it.** The all too familiar scenario is the student, taught the technique in dental school, who abandons its use in private practice, supposedly to save time. Practitioners performing endodontic therapy without the use of a rubber dam are placing themselves in unnecessary legal jeopardy. Thomsen et al. reported an unfortunate result of doing endodontic therapy without the use of a rubber dam (Figure 14-26).[110] The patient developed appendicitis from the ingested file and required surgery. It should be pointed out that all intraoral procedures involve risks: Mejia et al. reported a situation in which a patient swallowed a rubber dam clamp that accidentally was dropped in the mouth. The patient fortunately passed the clamp successfully, but the report illustrated the need for constant care and attention.[111]

Recognition in these cases is perhaps better termed "suspicion" because sometimes aspiration may not be recognizable. If an instrument aspiration or ingestion is apparent, the patient must be taken immediately to a medical emergency facility for examination, which should include radiographs of the chest and abdomen. It is also helpful to bring a sample file along so that the physician, who may be searching for an instrument in the alveolar tree, has a better idea of the size and shape of the instrument.

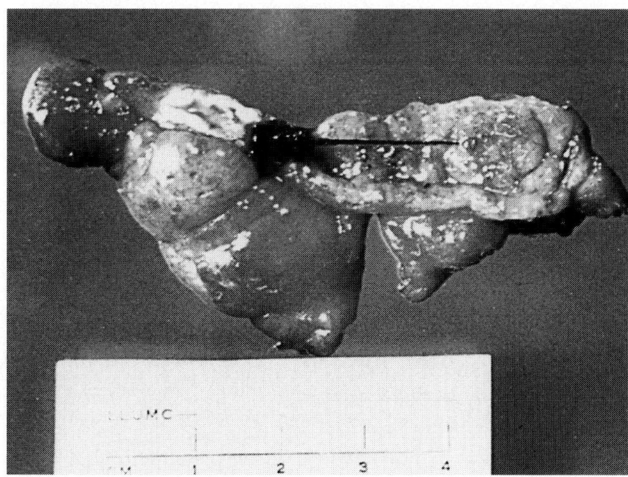

Figure 14-26 Appendix removed from a patient receiving endodontic therapy. Rubber dam placement would have prevented this accident. Reproduced with permission from Thomsen LC.[110]

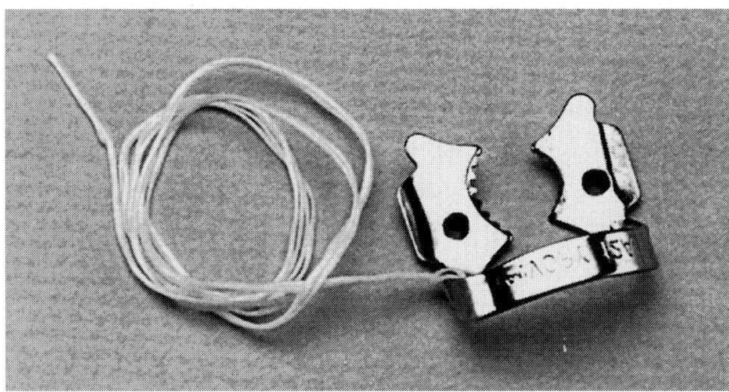

Figure 14-27 Routine placement of floss around the rubber dam retainer will allow retrieval in the event that the patient aspirates it.

Correction in the dental operatory is limited to removal of objects that are readily accessible in the throat. High-volume suction, particularly if fitted with a pharyngeal tip, can be useful in retrieving lost items. Hemostats and cotton pliers can also be used. Once aspiration has taken place, timely transport to a medical emergency facility is essential. The dentist should accompany the patient there.

Prevention can best be accomplished by strict adherence to the use of a rubber dam during all phases of endodontic therapy. If a rubber dam clamp is placed on the tooth to be treated before rubber dam placement, aspiration of a loosened clamp can be avoided by attaching floss to the clamp before placement (Figure 14-27).

REFERENCES

1. Justman BC, Krell KV. A safe technique for removal of provisionally cemented crowns. JOE 1993;19:97.
2. Harris WE. A simplified method of treatment for endodontic perforations. JOE 1976;2:126.
3. El Deeb ME, et al. An evaluation of the use of amalgam, Cavit, and calcium hydroxide in the repair of furcation perforations. JOE 1982;8:459.
4. Martin LR, et al. Management of endodontic perforations. Oral Surg 1982;54:668.
5. Oynick J, Oynick T. Treatment of endodontic perforations. JOE 1985;11:191.
6. Alhadainy HA, Himel VT. Evaluation of the sealing ability of amalgam, Cavit, and glass ionomer cement in the repair of furcation perforations. Oral Surg 1993;75:362.
7. Lantz B, Persson P. Periodontal tissue reactions after root perforations in dog's teeth: a histologic study. Odont Revy 1970;21:51.
8. Himel VT, et al. Evaluation of repair of mechanical perforations of the pulp chamber floor using biodegradable tricalcium phosphate or calcium hydroxide. JOE 1985;11:161.
9. Walia H, et al. Use of a hemostatic agent in the repair of procedural errors. JOE 1988;14:465.
10. Alhadainy HA, Abdalla AI. Artificial floor technique used for the repair of furcation perforations: a microleakage study. JOE 1998;24:33.
11. Mittal M, et al. An evaluation of plaster of Paris barriers used under various materials to repair furcation perforations (in vitro study). JOE 1999;25:385.
12. Lee SJ, Monsef M, Torabinejad M. Sealing ability of mineral trioxide (MT) aggregate for repair of lateral root perforations. JOE 1993;19:541.
13. Schwartz RS, et al. Mineral trioxide aggregate: a new material for endodontics. J Am Dent Assoc 1999;130:967.
14. Torabinejad M, et al. Clinical applications of mineral trioxide aggregate. JOE 1999;25:197.
15. Sluyk SR, et al. Evaluation of setting properties and retention characteristics of mineral trioxide aggregate when used as a furcation perforation repair material. JOE 1998;24:768.
16. Koh ET, et al. Cellular response to mineral trioxide aggregate. JOE 1998;24:543.
17. Nakata TT, et al. Perforation repair comparing mineral trioxide aggregate and amalgam using an anaerobic bacterial leakage model. JOE 1998;24:184.
18. Hartwell GR, England MC. Healing of furcation perforations in primate teeth after repair with decalcified freeze-dried bone: a longitudinal study. JOE 1993;19:357.
19. Sinai IH. Endodontic perforations: their prognosis and treatment. J Am Dent Assoc 1977;95:90.
20. Kvinsland I, et al. A clinical and roentgenological study of 55 cases of root perforation. Int Endod J 1989;22:75.
21. Fava LRG. One appointment root canal treatment: incidence of postoperative pain using a modified double-flared technique. Int Endod J 1991;24:258.
22. Gutmann JL, Dumsha T. In: Cohen S, Burns R, editors. Pathways of the pulp. 4th ed. St. Louis: CV Mosby; 1987. p. 170.
23. Fuss Z, et al. Determination of location of root perforations by electronic apex locators. Oral Surg 1996;82:324.
24. Scherer W, Dragoo MR. New subgingival restorative procedures with Geristore resin ionomer. Pract Periodontics Aesthet Dent 1995;7(1 Suppl):1.
25. Abitbol T, Santi E, Scherer W, Palat M. Using a resin-ionomer in guided tissue regenerative procedures: technique and application-case reports. Periodont Clin Invest 1996;18(1):17.
26. Allam CR. Treatment of stripping perforations. JOE 1996;22:699.
27. Biggs JT, et al. Treatment of iatrogenic root perforations with associated osseous lesions. JOE 1988;14:620.
28. Goon WWY, Lundergan WP. Redemption of a perforated furcation with a multidisciplinary treatment approach. JOE 1995;21:576.
29. Berutti E, Fedoy G. Thickness of the cementum/dentin in mesial roots of mandibular first molars. JOE 1992;18:545.
30. Peeso FA. The treatment of perforated roots. Dent Cosmos 1903;45:277.
31. Abou-Rass M, Jastrab RJ. The use of rotary instruments as auxillary aids to root canal preparation of molars. JOE 1982;8:78.
32. Abou-Rass M, Frank A, Glick DH. Anticurvature filing. J Am Dent Assoc 1980;101:792.
33. Brilliant JD, Christie WH. A taste of endodontics. Acad Gen Dent J 1975;23:29.
34. Kessler JR, et al. Comparison of the relative risk of molar root perforations using various endodontic instrumentation techniques. JOE 1983;9:439.

35. Lim SS, Stock CJR. The risk of perforation in the curved canal; anticurvature filing compared with the step-back technique. Int Endod J 1987;20:33.
36. Contemporary terminology for endodontics. 6th ed. Chicago: American Association of Endodontists; 1998.
37. Oswald RJ, Friedman CE. Periradicular response to dental fillings. Oral Surg 1980;49:344.
38. Eleazer PD, et al. Proplast as an apical barrier in root canal therapy. JOE 1984;10:487.
39. Pitts DL, Jones JE, Oswald RJ. A histological comparison of calcium hydroxide plugs and dentin plugs used for the control of gutta-percha root canal filling material. JOE 1984;10:283.
40. Chenail BL, Teplitsky PE. Orthograde ultrasonic retrieval of root canal obstructions. JOE 1987;13:186.
41. Nagai O, et al. Ultrasonic removal of broken instruments in root canals. Int Endod J 1986;19:298.
42. Gettleman BH, et al. Removal of canal obstructions with the Endo Extractor. JOE 1991;17:608.
43. Suter B. A new method for retrieving silver points and separated instruments from root canals. JOE 1998;24:446.
44. Hulsmann M. Removal of fractured instruments using a combined automated/ultrasonic technique. JOE 1994;20:144.
45. Crump MC, Natkin E. Relationship of broken root canal instruments to endodontic case diagnosis. J Am Dent Assoc 1970;80:1341.
46. Fox J, et al. Filling root canals with files: radiographic evaluation of 304 cases. N Y State Dent J 1972;38:154.
47. Buchanan LS. Working length and apical patency: the control factors. Endod Rep 1987;Fall/Winter:6.
48. Yee RDJ, et al. The effect of canal preparation on the formation and leakage characteristics of the apical dentin plug. JOE 1984;10:308.
49. Marshall FJ. Clinical syllabus. Portland (OR): Oregon Health Sciences University; 1981.
50. Holland R, et al. Tissue reaction following apical plugging of the root canal with infected dentin chips. Oral Surg 1980;49:366.
51. Nygaard-Østby B. The role of the blood clot in endodontic therapy. Acta Odont Scand 1961;19:323.
52. Seltzer S, Bender IB, Turkenkopf S. Factors affecting successful repair after root canal therapy. J Am Dent Assoc 1963;67:651.
53. Heling B, Kischinovsky D. Factors affecting successful endodontic therapy. J Br Endod Soc 1979;12:138.
54. Engström B, Lundberg M. The correlation between positive culture and prognosis of root canal therapy after pulpectomy. Odontol Rev 1965;16:193.
55. Roane JB, Sabala CL, et al. The "balanced force" concept for instrumentation of curved canals. JOE 1985;11:203.
56. Sabala CL, Roane JB, et al. Instrumentation of curved canals using a modified tipped instrument: a comparison study. JOE 1988;14:59.
57. Orlay H. Overfilling in root canal treatment: two incidents with N2. Br Dent J 1966;120:8.
58. Pyner DA. Paresthesia of the inferior alveolar nerve caused by Hydron: a case report. JOE 1980;6:527.
59. Speilman A, et al. Anesthesia following endodontic overfilling with AH26. Oral Surg 1981;52:554.
60. Ørstavik D, et al. Paresthesia following endodontic treatment: survey of the literature and report of a case. Int Endod J 1983;16:167.
61. Brodin P, et al. Neurotoxic effects of root-filling materials on rat phrenic nerve in vitro. J Dent Res 1982;61:1020.
62. Rowe AHR. Damage to the inferior dental nerve during or following endodontic treatment. Br Dent J 1983;153:306.
63. Spångberg L. Biologic effects of root canal filling materials. II. Effect *in vitro* of water-soluble components of root canal filling materials on HeLa cells. Odontol Rev 1969;20:133.
64. Spångberg L. Biological effects of root canal filling materials. IV. Effect *in vitro* of solubilised root canal filling materials on HeLa cells. Odontol Rev 1969;20:289.
65. Spångberg L. Biological effects of root canal filling materials. V. Toxic effect *in vitro* of root canal filling materials on HeLa cells and human fibroblasts. Odontol Rev 1969;20:427.
66. Spangberg L. Biological effects of root canal filling materials. VI. The inhibitory effect of solubilised root canal filling materials on respiration of HeLa cells. Odontol Tidskr 1969;77:121.
67. Grossman LI, Oliet S, Del Rio C. Endodontics. 11th ed. Philadelphia: Lea and Febiger; 1988.
68. Ingle JI, Bakland LK. Endodontics. 4th ed. Philadelphia: Williams and Wilkins; 1995.
69. Cohenca C, Rotstein I. Mental nerve paresthesia associated with a non-vital tooth. Endod Dent Traumatol 1996;12:298.
70. Newton CW, et al. Studies of Sargenti's technique of endodontic treatment: six-month and one-year responses. JOE 1980;6:509.
71. Gatot A, Tovi F. Prednisone treatment for injury and compression of inferior alveolar nerve: report of a case of anesthesia following endodontic overfilling. Oral Surg 1986;62:704.
72. Evans AW. Removal of endodontic paste from the inferior alveolar nerve by sagittal splitting of the mandible. Br Dent J 1988;164:18.
73. Girard K. Considerations in the management of damage to the mandibular nerve. J Am Dent Assoc 1989;98;65.
74. Alhadainy HA, Himel VT. Evaluation of the sealing ability of amalgam, Cavit, and glass ionomer cement in the repair of furcation perforations. Oral Surg 1993;75:362.
75. Trope M, Rosenberg ES. Multidisciplinary approach to the repair of vertically fractured teeth. JOE 1992;18:460.
76. Helfer AR, Melnick S, Schilder H. Determination of the moisture content of vital and pulpless teeth. Oral Surg 1972;34:661.
77. Lewinstein I, Grajower R. Root dentin hardness of endodontically treated teeth. JOE 1981;7:421.
78. Tidmarsh BG. Restoration of endodontically treated teeth. JOE 1976;2:374.
79. Rud J, et al. Root filling with composite and a dentin bonding agent. 1. Endod Dent Traumatol 1991;7:118.
80. Rud J, et al. Root filling with composite and a dentin bonding agent. 2. Endod Dent Traumatol 1991;7:126.
81. Rud J, et al. Retrograde sealing of accidental root perforations with dentin-bonded composite resin. JOE 1998;24:671.
82. Thé SD, et al. Reactions of guinea pig subcutaneous connective tissue following exposure to sodium hypochlorite. Oral Surg 1980;49:160.
83. Becker GL, et al. The sequelae of accidentally injecting sodium hypochlorite beyond the root apex. Oral Surg 1974;38:633.
84. Bhat KS. Tissue emphysema caused by hydrogen peroxide. Oral Surg 1974;38:304.
85. Sabala C, Powell SE. Sodium hypochlorite injection into periradicular tissues. JOE 1989;15:490.
86. Gatot A, et al. Effects of sodium hypochlorite on soft tissues after its inadvertent injection beyond the root apex. JOE 1991;17:573.

87. Herrmann JW, Heicht RC. Complication in therapeutic use of sodium hypochlorite. JOE 1979;5:160.
88. Reeh ES, Messer HH. Long-term paresthesia following inadvertent forcing of sodium hypochlorite through perforation in incisor. Endod Dent Traumatol 1989;5:200.
89. Patterson CJW, McLundie AC. Apical penetration by a root canal irrigant: a case report. Int Endod J 1989;22:197.
90. Joffe E. Complication during root canal therapy following accidental extrusion of sodium hypochlorite through the apical foramen. Gen Dent 1991;39:460.
91. Pashley EL, et al. Cytotoxic effects of sodium hypochlorite on vital tissue. JOE 1985;11:525.
92. Ehrich DG, Brian JD Jr, Walker WA. Sodium hypochlorite accident: inadvertent injections into the maxillary sinus. JOE 1993;19:180.
93. Becking AG. Complications in the use of sodium hypochlorite during endodontic treatment. Oral Surg 1991;71:346.
94. Kaufman AY, Keila S. Hypersensitivity to sodium hypochlorite. JOE 1989;15:224.
95. McGrannahan WW. Tissue space emphysema from an air turbine handpiece. J Am Dent Assoc 1965;71:884.
96. Duncan JM, Ferrillo PJ. Interstitial emphysema after an amalgam restoration. J Am Dent Assoc 1967;74:407.
97. McClendon JL, Hooper WC. Cervicofacial emphysema after air blown into a periodontal pocket. J Am Dent Assoc 1961;63:810.
98. Hirschmann PN, Walker RT. Facial emphysema during endodontic treatment—two case reports. Int Endod J 1983;16:130.
99. Reznik JB, Ardary WC. Cervicofacial subcutaneous air emphysema after dental extraction. J Am Dent Assoc 1990;120:417.
100. Hayduk S, et al. Subcutaneous emphysema after operative dentistry: report of a case. J Am Dent Assoc 1970;80:1362.
101. Lloyd RE. Surgical emphysema as a complication in endodontics. Br Dent J 1975;138:393.
102. Madden PW, Averett JN. Subcutaneous emphysema. Gen Dent 1987;35:474.
103. Horowitz I, et al. Pneumomediastinum and subcutaneous emphysema following surgical extraction of mandibular third molars: three case reports. Oral Surg 1987;63:25.
104. Noble W. Mediastinal emphysema resulting from extraction of an impacted mandibular third molar. J Am Dent Assoc 1972;84:368.
105. Bodal CF, DiFiore PM. Subcutaneous emphysema in dental practice. Gen Dent 1992;40:328.
106. Minton G, Kai TH. Pneumomediastinum pneumothorax, and cervical emphysema following mandibular fractures. Oral Surg 1984;57:490.
107. Munsell WP. Pneumomediastinum. JAMA 1967;202:689.
108. Lee HY, et al. Extensive post traumatic subcutaneous emphysema and pneumomediastinum following a minor facial injury. J Oral Maxillofac Surg 1987;45:812.
109. Jerome CE. Effective methods for drying root canals. Gen Dent 1992;40:400.
110. Thomsen LC, et al. Appendicitis induced by an endodontic file. Gen Dent 1989;37:50.
111. Mejia JL, et al. Accidental swallowing of a dental clamp. JOE 1996;22:619–20.

Chapter 15

ENDODONTIC CONSIDERATIONS IN DENTAL TRAUMA

Leif K. Bakland

The outcome of traumatic events involving teeth depends on three factors: the extent of injury, the quality and timeliness of initial care, and the follow-up evaluation and care.

The extent of injury is influenced by the severity of the traumatic event[1] and the presence or absence of protective gear such as mouthguards, face shields, airbags, and seatbelts.[2] Direction of force against the teeth and supporting structures and the type of impact—blunt or sharp—also can determine how much tissue damage will result. It is well recognized that preventive measures such as tooth and face protection during sporting events and seatbelts and airbags used in cars can significantly reduce the severity of injuries.[2]

The quality and timeliness of initial care contribute to a desirable outcome by promoting healing. A good example is the avulsed tooth: if it is replanted within the first few minutes after avulsion, the prognosis is good, with a high rate of success.[3] It is important to note, however, that the quality of initial care also is important. As Andreasen has pointed out, the initial treatment should not **add** more trauma to already injured tissues.[4] A good example of this principle is with respect to luxated teeth: the repositioning of displaced teeth and adjacent tissues must be done very gently to promote desirable wound healing and long-term favorable outcome.

Follow-up evaluation and care are important components of long-term successful outcomes.[1] A replanted avulsed tooth may show an excellent initial response—healing of the severed periodontal ligament—but if the necrotic pulp is allowed to harbor bacteria, the resultant root resorption will lead to loss of the tooth. Often the long-term outlook for a traumatized tooth is related to the response of the tooth's pulp—thus the importance of endodontic considerations in dental trauma.

This chapter contains information both on the preservation, when indicated, of pulp vitality after a traumatic injury and the appropriate endodontic intervention when pulp necrosis is present or expected.

ETIOLOGY AND INCIDENCE

Sudden impact involving the face or head may result in trauma to the teeth and supporting structures. The most frequent causes are falling while running, followed by traffic accidents, acts of violence, and sports.[5]

Automobile accidents are often very destructive. One estimate suggests that 20 to 60% of all traffic accidents produce some injury to the facial regions. When such injuries involve teeth, avulsions or intrusions are the most common sequelae.[6] Sports activities, both team and individual, can lead to dental injuries, which have been shown to be common in high school athletes who do not use mouthguards.[7]

The incidence of dental trauma continues to be investigated. A large US study indicated that 25% of the population 6 to 50 years of age may have sustained traumatic injuries to the anterior teeth.[8] Surprisingly, some are unaware of their dental injuries, and many choose not to seek dental treatment.

Most dental injuries occur during the first two decades of life. The most accident-prone time period is from ages 8 to 12 years. Frequent dental injuries also occur from ages 2 to 3 years.[5] As might be expected, boys tend to injure their teeth more frequently than girls, by ratios varying from 2:1 to 3:1. One exception is in the preschool age, during which time little gender difference is noted.[5] Maxillary central incisors, followed by maxillary lateral incisors and then the mandibular incisors, are the teeth most frequently involved.[5] The most commonly observed dental trauma involves fracture of enamel, or enamel and dentin, but without pulp involvement.[5]

Finally, it is becoming apparent that dental injuries can result from child abuse or "battered child syndrome." The dentist may be the first health care provider to observe pediatric injuries resulting from abuse. More than half of the reported cases of child abuse include evidence of orofacial trauma. Many of these unfortunate children have intraoral injuries, such as tooth and jaw fractures. It is the responsibility of all professionals to report suspected cases of child abuse or neglect.[9]

The following observations have been recommended as possible indicators of an abused child; none, however, are pathognomonic, and the absence of any of them does not preclude the diagnosis of abuse[10]:

1. There is a delay in seeking medical (dental) help (or help is not sought at all).
2. The story of the "accident" is vague, is lacking in detail, and may vary with each telling and from person to person.
3. The account of the accident is not compatible with the injury observed.
4. The parents' mood is abnormal. Normal parents are full of creative anxiety for the child, whereas abusing parents tend to be more preoccupied with their own problems—for example, how they can return home as soon as possible.
5. The parents' behavior gives cause for concern—for example, they may become hostile and rebut accusations that have not been made.
6. The child's appearance and interaction with the parents are abnormal. The child may look sad, withdrawn, or frightened.
7. The child may say something concerning the injury that is different from the parents' story.

Most hospitals have personnel who can offer advice to health care providers unsure about how to report suspected abuse.

CLASSIFICATION

The purpose of classifying dental injuries is to provide a description of specific conditions, allowing dentists to recognize and treat using recommended treatment remedies. It also allows data collection worldwide to monitor many aspects of dental traumatology: etiology, incidence, and treatment outcome. The currently recommended classification is one based on the World Health Organization classification of diseases and modified by Andreasen and Andreasen.[5] This classification is used by the International Association of Dental Traumatology and is preferred over previous outdated systems.[11] It is also the classification that will be followed in this chapter (Table 15-1).

EXAMINATION

Patients with dental injuries should be examined as soon after the traumatic incident as possible.[12,13] The examination process of trauma patients is similar to the regular examination of all endodontic patients, as described in chapter 6. However, owing to the possibility of concomitant injury to adjacent tissues and the frequent need to provide insurance and/or a legal report, it is prudent to pay particular attention to a careful examination and recording of clinical findings. For that reason, the following sections have been given emphasis.

History

The clinical dental history is primarily the subjective statement by the patient. It includes the chief complaint, history of the present illness (injury), and pertinent medical history.

Chief Complaint

The chief complaint may appear obvious in traumatic injuries. However, the patient should be asked about severe pain and other significant symptoms. A bloody lip appears more dramatic, but a concomitant broken

Table 15-1 Dentofacial Injuries

Soft tissues
Lacerations
Contusions
Abrasions
Tooth fractures
Enamel fractures
Crown fractures—uncomplicated (no pulp exposure)
Crown fractures—complicated (with pulp exposure)
Crown-root fractures
Root fractures
Luxation injuries
Tooth concussion
Subluxation
Extrusive luxation
Lateral luxation
Intrusive luxation
Avulsion
Facial skeletal injuries
Alveolar process—maxilla/mandible
Body of maxillary/mandibular bone
Temporomandibular joint

jaw may produce more pain and must be considered a higher priority. The chief complaint may include several subjective symptoms, and these should be listed in order of importance to the patient. Also note the duration of each symptom.

History of Present Illness (Injury)

Obtain information about the accident in chronologic order and determine what effect it has had on the patient. Note any treatment before this examination and question the patient about previous injuries involving the same area. The information can be gathered by using questions such as the following:

- **When and where did the injury happen?** Record the time and date as closely as the patient can recall. Note the location, for example, playground, car accident, etc. All of this may be highly pertinent if legal or insurance problems later develop.
- **How did the injury happen?** This question can provide important information. A blow to the face by a blunt object, such as a fist, often produces a different injury than if the chin is hit during a car accident or if the patient falls off a bicycle.[14] Further, since children with "battered child syndrome" may be seen, a high degree of suspicion should be maintained in cases with a marked discrepancy between the clinical findings and the history supplied by the parent or guardian.[10,11]
- **Have you had treatment elsewhere before coming here?** Prior treatment affects both the treatment plan and the prognosis. If the tooth was avulsed, was it replanted immediately or how soon after the accident? Was it washed?
- **Have you had similar injuries before?** Repeated injuries to teeth affect the pulps and their ability to recover from trauma. Previous trauma may also explain clinical findings not in harmony with the description of the most recent injury. This is particularly true of abused children.
- **Have you noticed any other symptoms since the injury?** This type of question can provide very useful information about the possible effects of the injury on the nervous system. Signs and symptoms to watch for are dizziness; vomiting; severe headaches; seizures or convulsions; blurred vision; unconsciousness; loss of smell, taste, hearing, sight, or balance; or bleeding from the nose or ears. Affirmative response to any of the above indicates the need for emergency medical evaluation.[12]
- **What specific problems have you had with the traumatized tooth/teeth?** Pain, mobility, and occlusal interference are the most commonly reported symptoms. In addition, the patient should be asked about any symptoms from adjacent soft tissues such as tongue, lips, cheeks, gingiva, and alveolar mucosa.

Medical History

The following aspects of the medical history are emphasized for their importance in trauma cases:

1. **Allergic reactions to medications.** Because both antibiotics and analgesics are frequently prescribed for trauma patients, it is necessary to know if the patient can tolerate the prescribed medication.
2. **Disorders, such as bleeding problems, diabetes, and epilepsy.** These are only some of the many physical and medical conditions that may affect the management of a trauma patient. Because patients with medical problems sometimes neglect to note such a disorder on the questionnaire, the dentist may have to question in more depth. Patients suffering from **grand mal** epilepsy, for example, may have telltale chipped or fractured teeth that were injured during seizures.
3. **Current medications.** To avoid unwanted drug interactions, the dentist must know which drugs the patient is currently taking, including over-the-counter medications.
4. **Tetanus immunization status.** For clean wounds, no booster dose is needed if no more than 10 years have elapsed since the last dose. For contaminated wounds, a booster dose should be given if more than 5 years have elapsed since the last dose.[15]

Clinical Examination

A careful, methodical approach to the clinical examination will reduce the possibility of overlooking or missing important details. The following areas should be examined.

Soft Tissues

Soft tissue trauma, for the most part, is not covered in this chapter, at least not in regard to treatment, such as suturing. It is important, however, to examine all soft tissue injuries because it is not unusual for tooth fragments to be buried in the lips. The radiographic examination should include specific exposures of the lips and cheeks if lacerations and fractured teeth are present (Figure 15-1). In any event, all areas of **soft tissue** injury should be noted, and the lips, cheeks, and tongue adjacent to any fractured teeth should be carefully examined and **palpated.**

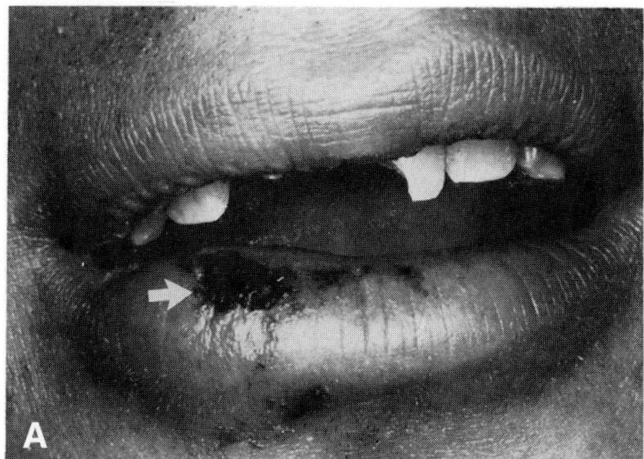

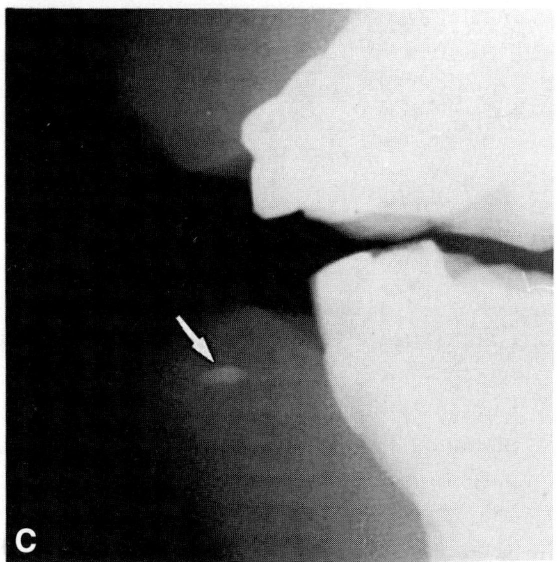

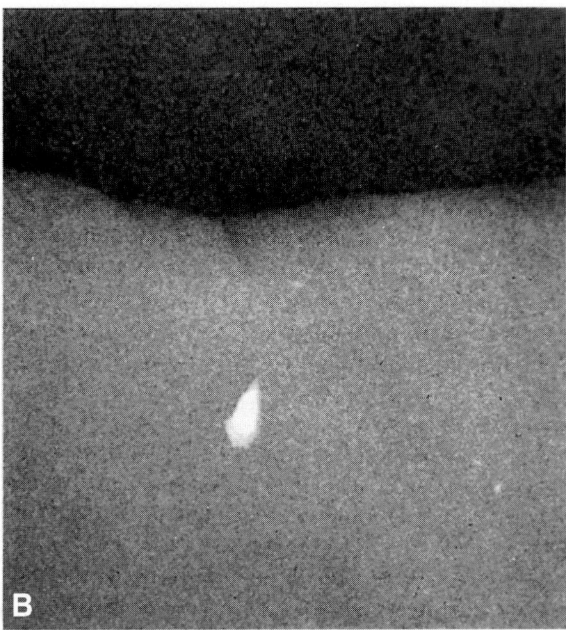

Figure 15-1 **A**, Lacerated lips and cheeks should be radiographed for embedded tooth fragments. **B**, Radiograph placed lingual to the lower lip exposed about one half that used for teeth and shows a hard tissue fragment embedded in the lip. **C**, Lateral film also demonstrates a tooth fragment in the lip (**arrow**).

Facial Bones

The maxilla, mandible, and temporomandibular joint should be examined visually and by palpation, seeking distortions, malalignment, or indications of fractures. Indications of possible fractures should be followed up radiographically. Also note possible tooth dislocation, gross occlusal interference, and development of apical pathosis.

Teeth

The teeth must be examined for fractures, mobility, displacement, injury to periodontal ligament and alveolus, and pulpal trauma. Remember to examine the teeth in the opposite arch also. They, too, may have been involved to some degree.

Tooth Fracture

The crowns of the teeth should be cleaned and examined for extent and type of injury. Crown infractions or enamel cracks can be detected by changing the light beam from side to side, shining a fiber-optic light through the crown, or using disclosing solutions.

If tooth structure has been lost, note the extent of loss: enamel only, enamel and dentin, or enamel and dentin with pulp exposure. Further, indicate the exact location on the crown, such as the "distal-incisal corner" or the "incisal one-third horizontal." Such information can be useful if you are called on later to describe the injury. Photographs are very useful as part of the patient record.[12]

If a crown fracture extends subgingivally, the fractured part often remains attached but loose. Also check for discoloration of the crown or changes in translucency to fiber-optic light. Both may indicate pulp changes.

Mobility

Examine the teeth for mobility in all directions, including axially. If adjacent teeth move along with the tooth being tested, suspect alveolar fracture. Root fractures often result in crown mobility, the degree depending on the proximity of the fracture to the crown. The degree of mobility can be recorded as follows: 0 for no mobility, 1 for slight mobility, 2 for marked mobility, and 3 for mobility and depressibility. Examine for and record the depths of any periodontal pockets.

Displacement

Note any displacement of the teeth that may be intrusive, extrusive, or lateral (either labial or lingual) or complete avulsion. Sometimes the change is minimal, and the patient should be asked about any occlusal interference that developed suddenly. In occlusal changes, consider the possibility of jaw or root fractures or extrusions.

Injury to Periodontal Ligament and Alveolus

The presence and extent of injury to the periodontal ligament and supporting alveolus can be evaluated by tooth percussion. Include all teeth suspected of having been injured and several adjacent and opposing ones. The results may be recorded as "normal response," "slightly sensitive," or "very sensitive" to percussion. Careful tapping with a mirror handle is generally satisfactory. In cases of extensive apical periodontal damage, however, it may be advisable to use no more than a fingertip for percussion. Normal, noninvolved teeth should be included for comparison.

In impact trauma with no fractures or displacement, the percussion test is very important. In some apparently undamaged teeth, the neurovascular bundle, entering the apical canal, may have been damaged, and the possibility of subsequent pulp degeneration exists. Such teeth are often sensitive to percussion.

Pulpal Trauma

The condition of the dental pulp should be evaluated both initially and at various times following the traumatic incident. The response of the pulp to trauma largely determines the treatment of and prognosis for injured teeth. Often the initial treatment may be no treatment but rather monitoring of the pulp response. Pulps may deteriorate and become necrotic months or years after the original trauma, so periodic re-evaluation is important in the management of dental injuries.[1]

Several means of evaluating traumatized pulps are available.[1,12] The electric pulp test (EPT) has been shown as reliable in determining pulpal status, that is, in differentiating between vital and necrotic pulps. The EPT should be used, and the **results recorded**, at the initial visit and at subsequent recall visits. Often, after an impact injury, the pulp does not respond to the EPT for some time. But when the pulp recovers, its sensitivity to the EPT gradually returns. Such recovery can be monitored with the test. Other times, the pulp later becomes necrotic after initially responding positively or even after apparent recovery from the initial injury. The EPT can provide much useful information if its advantages, as well as its limitations, are considered.

Cold stimulus in the form of carbon dioxide or ice is used extensively for pulp testing and is quite reliable. The response, however, is not easily quantified. The usefulness of cold is most applicable in differentiating between reversible and irreversible pulpitis. Hot stimulus has limited use in pulp testing traumatically injured teeth. However, subjective symptoms can be useful, particularly a history of spontaneous pain, indicating irreversibility.

Discoloration, particularly a grayish hue, involving permanent teeth is indicative of pulp necrosis, whereas a yellowish hue means that extensive calcification has occurred. The **latter** is not necessarily associated with irreversible pulpitis or pulp necrosis.[16,17]

Radiographic Examination

Radiography is indispensable in the diagnosis and treatment of dental trauma. Detection of dislocations, root fractures, and jaw fractures can be made by radiographic examination. Extraoral radiography is indicated in jaw and condylar fractures or when one suspects trauma to the succedaneous permanent teeth by intruded primary teeth. Soft tissue radiographic evaluation is indicated when tooth fragments or possible foreign objects may have been displaced into the lips, for example see Figure 15-1. The film should be placed between the lip and the jaw, and short exposure at minimal KVP is advocated.[12]

The size of the pulp chamber and the root canal, the apical root development, and the appearance of the periodontal ligament space may all be evaluated by intraoral radiographs. Such films are of prime importance both immediately after injury and for follow-up evaluation.[18] Changes in the pulp space, both resorptive and calcific, may suggest pulp degeneration and indicate therapeutic intervention (Figure 15-2). Other radiographic views may be indicated in more extensive injuries than those confined to the dentition. Finally, it is also important to carefully file all radiographs for future references and comparisons.

Follow-up Evaluation

Trauma patients should be evaluated often enough, and over a long enough period of time, either to determine that complete recovery has taken place or to

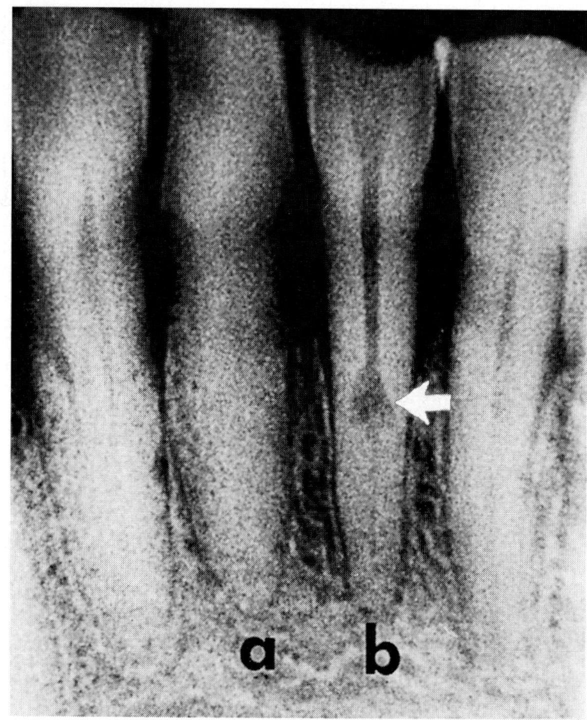

Figure 15-2 Subsequent to trauma one central incisor (a) shows pulpal calcification, whereas the adjacent one (b) undergoes internal resorption (arrow). The latter requires endodontic intervention, whereas pulpal calcification in and of itself does not.

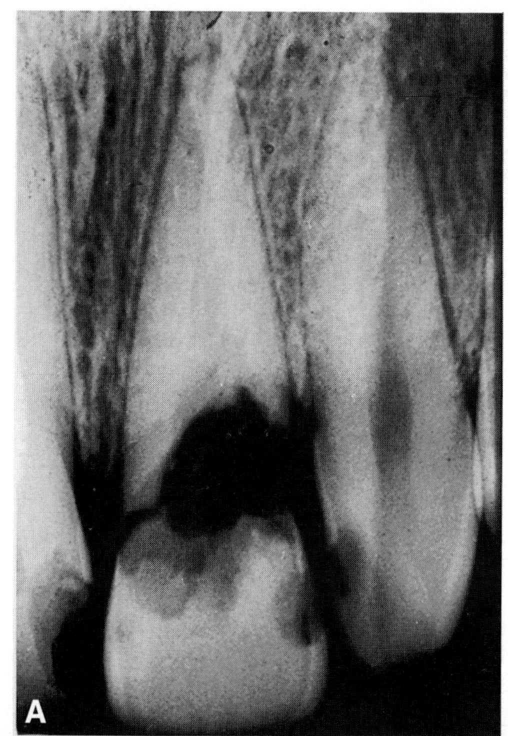

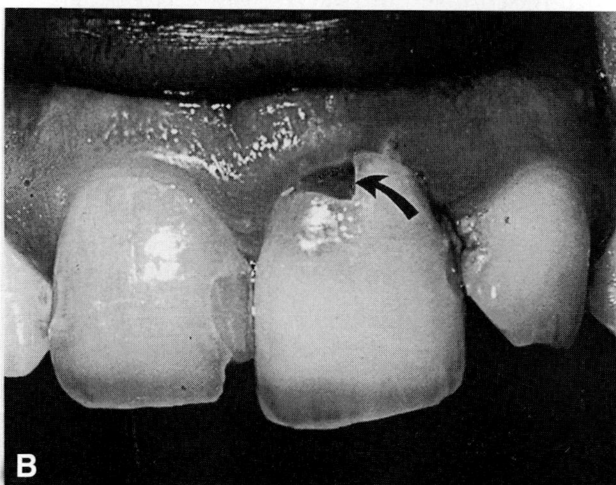

Figure 15-3 Extensive resorption (arrow) following trauma. Such destructive results can often be minimized by timely endodontic intervention.

detect as early as possible pulpal deterioration and root resorption. If pulpal recovery (eg, revascularization) is to be monitored, frequent initial re-evaluations (every 3 to 4 weeks for the first 6 months) and then yearly are recommended.[1,11] Radiographs and pulp testing should be included in the evaluations. If inflammatory resorption or pulp necrosis occurs, endodontic treatment is indicated immediately (Figure 15-3). In permanent teeth, pulp necrosis should be suspected in the presence of a graying crown discoloration, no response to the EPT, and radiographic indication of apical periodontitis. A lack of response to the EPT alone is not sufficient to diagnose pulp necrosis and recommend pulpectomy.[19]

Root canal therapy may be indicated if the pulp lumen diminishes at a rapid pace, as determined by radiographs taken at frequent intervals. No general agreement exists, however, about this indication for treatment.[19]

Examination of Old Injuries

At times, patients request treatment of dental conditions, the etiology of which is uncertain. For instance, an anterior tooth with no restorations and no loss of tooth structure may develop symptoms of pulp necrosis and apical periodontitis (Figure 15-4). Some patients may not remember any traumatic incidents, whereas others may recall specific accidents but only after lengthy efforts at memory recall or after discussions with their families. Some may have received treatment at the time of injury but somewhat later developed new symptoms. In this case, the dental history and chief complaint will be related to the current symptoms.

Information suggesting previous trauma as the etiology would include crown discoloration, gingival dehiscence, reduced pulp canal lumen, root resorption,

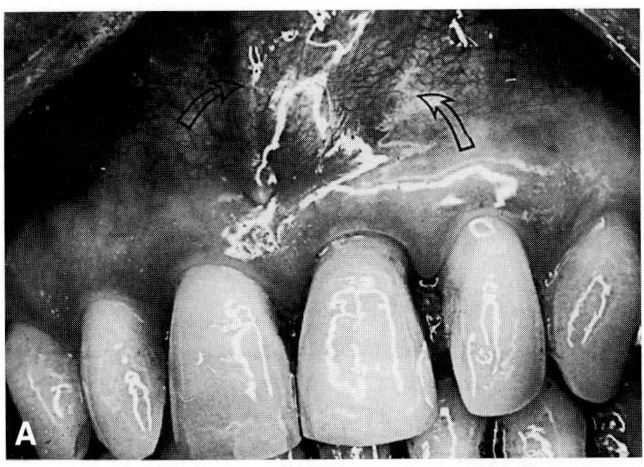

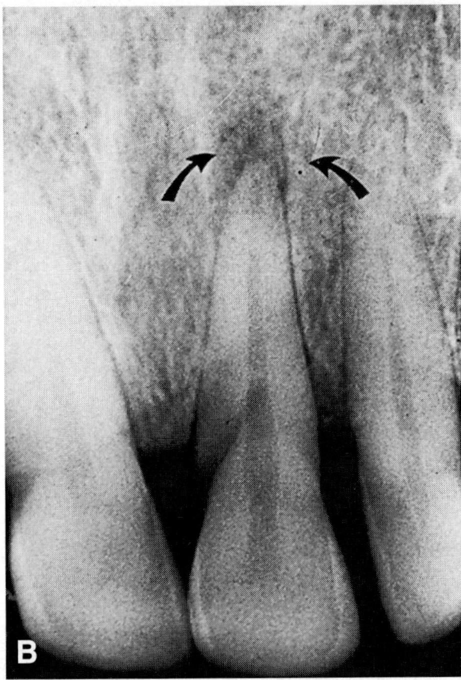

Figure 15-4 Maxillary left central incisor developed an apical abscess 30 years after a traumatic basketball accident. **A**, Note labial swelling (**open arrows**) and **B**, apical radiolucency. Pulp did not respond to an electric pulp test, and the crown was slightly discolored.

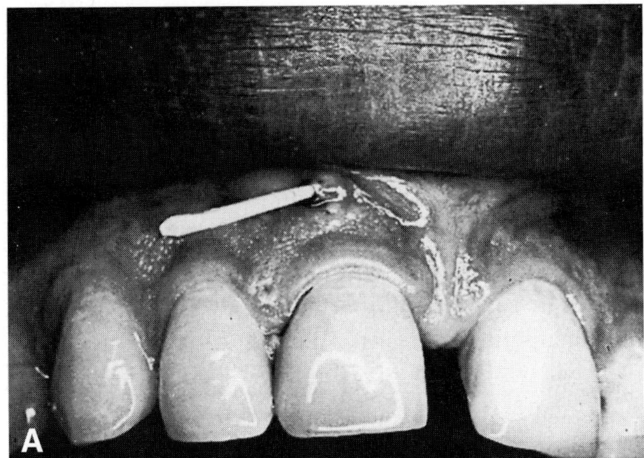

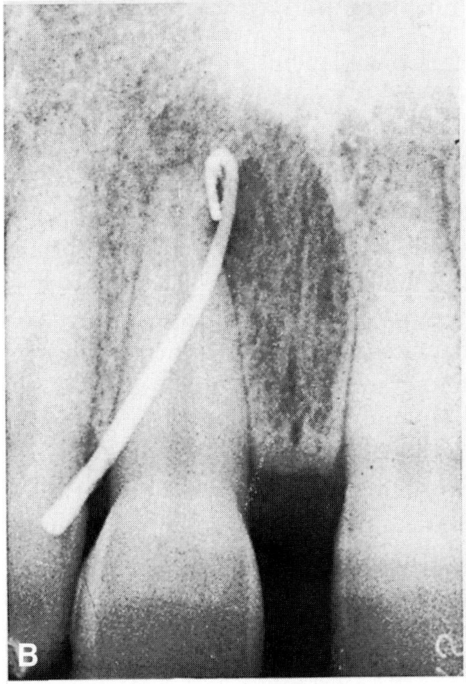

Figure 15-5 **A**, Fistulous tract traced with gutta-percha point from labial orifice to **B**, apical lesion.

and pulp necrosis not related to other obvious causes such as caries and/or tooth infractions. Sinus tracts are sometimes the first indication of a previous injury; these tracts should be traced to identify areas of origin (Figure 15-5).

TRAUMATIC INJURIES

Soft Tissue Injuries

Description. Injuries to oral soft tissues can be lacerations, contusions, or abrasions of the epithelial layer or a combination of injuries.[1] If treatment is indicated, it consists of controlling bleeding, repositioning displaced tissues, and suturing. Oral soft tissues heal rather quickly.

Tooth Fractures

This category of injuries includes all fractures from enamel infractions to complicated crown-root fractures. They are the most commonly reported types of dental injuries, with an incidence of 4 to 5% of the population (United States)[8,20] accounting for over one-third of all dental trauma.[21]

Enamel Fractures

Description. Enamel fractures include chips and cracks confined to the enamel and not crossing the enamel-dentin border. These enamel infractions[22] can be seen by indirect light or transillumination or by the use of dyes. In anterior teeth, the enamel chips often involve either the mesial or distal corners or the central lobe of the incisal edge.[22]

When treatment is indicated, it involves minor smoothing of rough edges or adding some composite resin using the acid-etch technique. One other consideration needs mentioning. Since it is difficult to predict the long-term pulpal response to trauma, pulp vitality tests should be performed both immediately after the injury and again in 6 to 8 weeks.[22] It must be kept in mind that, even with minor traumatic injuries, such as enamel fractures, damage to the apical neurovascular bundle may have occurred (Figure 15-6). The prognosis, however, for teeth with enamel fractures is very good.[22]

Crown Fractures—Uncomplicated (No Pulp Exposure)

Description. Crown fractures involving enamel and dentin without pulp exposure are called uncomplicated crown fractures by Andreasen[5] and Class 2 fractures by Ellis.[23] They may include incisal-proximal corners, incisal edges or lingual "chisel"-type fractures in anterior teeth, and, frequently, cusps in posterior teeth. Cusp fractures in posterior teeth are often related to blows to the face. Because anterior teeth are more often involved in traumatic injuries, the description in this chapter will refer only to these teeth.

Crown fractures that expose dentinal tubules may potentially lead to contamination and inflammation of the pulp. The outcome may be either formation of irritational dentin or pulp necrosis. Which outcome occurs depends on a number of factors: proximity of the fracture to the pulp, surface area of dentin exposed, age of the patient (pulp recession and size of dentinal tubules), concomitant injury to the pulp's blood supply, length of time between trauma and treatment, and possibly the type of initial treatment performed.[1,22]

Incidence. The enamel/dentin type of crown fracture is a very common type of injury; a distinction, however, is not always made between fractures involving only enamel and those involving both enamel and dentin. The two groups together certainly comprise the vast majority of dental injury cases.[8,20,21]

Diagnosis. The diagnosis of crown fracture without pulp involvement is made by clinical examination with a mirror and an explorer. In addition, it is also important to determine the status of the pulp and periradicular tissues by the usual examination procedures.

Treatment. The primary goal of treatment in teeth with crown fractures is to protect the pulp by sealing the dentinal tubules.[24] The most effective method is by direct application of dentin bonding agents and bonded restorations. Placement of unsightly stainless steel or temporary acrylic crowns is now a thing of the past for enamel/dentin fractures.

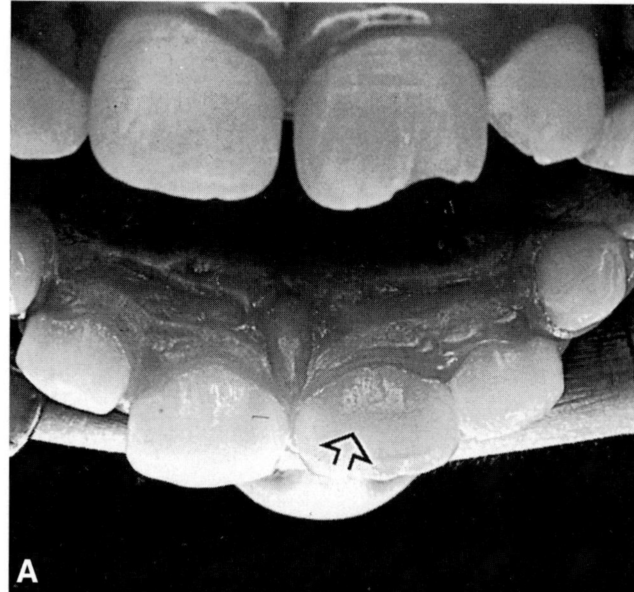

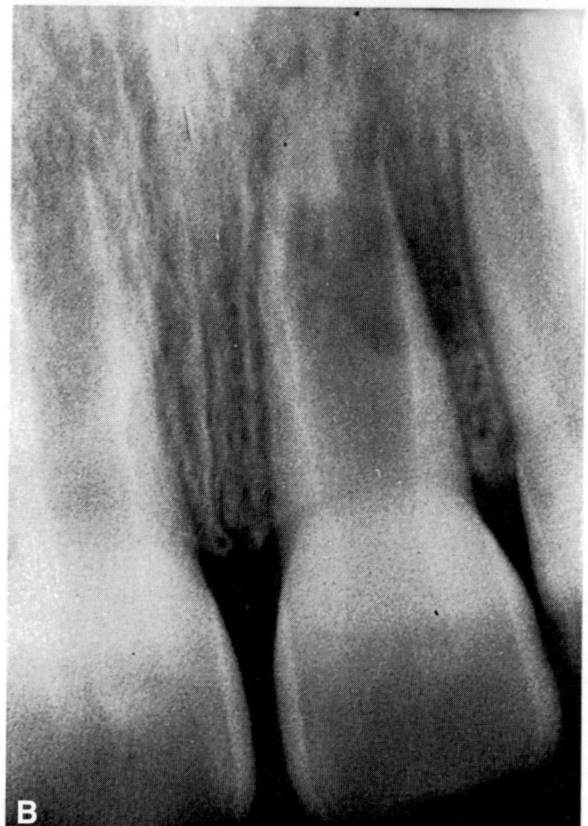

Figure 15-6 Sequelae to injury that initially produced only an enamel fracture, **A**, but includes, in part **B**, pulpal necrosis, arrested root development, and apical periodontitis. Note crown discoloration in A, visible in transmitted light (**arrow**)

If the fractured crown fragment is available, it is often advantageous to use it to restore the tooth. The technique for **reattachment** (Figure 15-7) is as follows[25–27]:

Anesthetize the tooth and place a rubber dam to isolate the tooth. Clean the tooth segment and fractured tooth with pumice and water. Determine the reattachment path of insertion, using a sticky wax handle to hold the coronal fragment. Care should be taken to accurately refit the fragment since it can easily be misaligned anteroposteriorly. Apply a suitable etchant, according to its manufacturer's directions, to both the tooth and the coronal segment extending 2 mm beyond the cavosurface margins. Rinse well. Apply a dentinal primer followed by application of an unfilled resin. Next, dilute a light-cured composite resin with unfilled resin to a creamy consistency and apply it to the tooth and coronal fragment. Carefully re-insert the fragment onto the tooth, taking care that the path of insertion is correct. Remove excess resin and apply the curing light circumferentially. (Alternatively, a dual-cure resin luting agent may be used.) Polish the resin and check the orclusion, which can be adjusted if necessary.

The expected outcome is usually good, although resistance to refracture is about 50% less than an intact tooth's resistance.[25]

Early treatment of crown fractures is desirable. The length of time between injury and treatment has a direct adverse effect on the pulp's ability to survive. The closeness of the fracture to the pulp and the size of the dentinal tubules also have a bearing on the pulp's continued vitality, the latter being significant in young patients.[1,22]

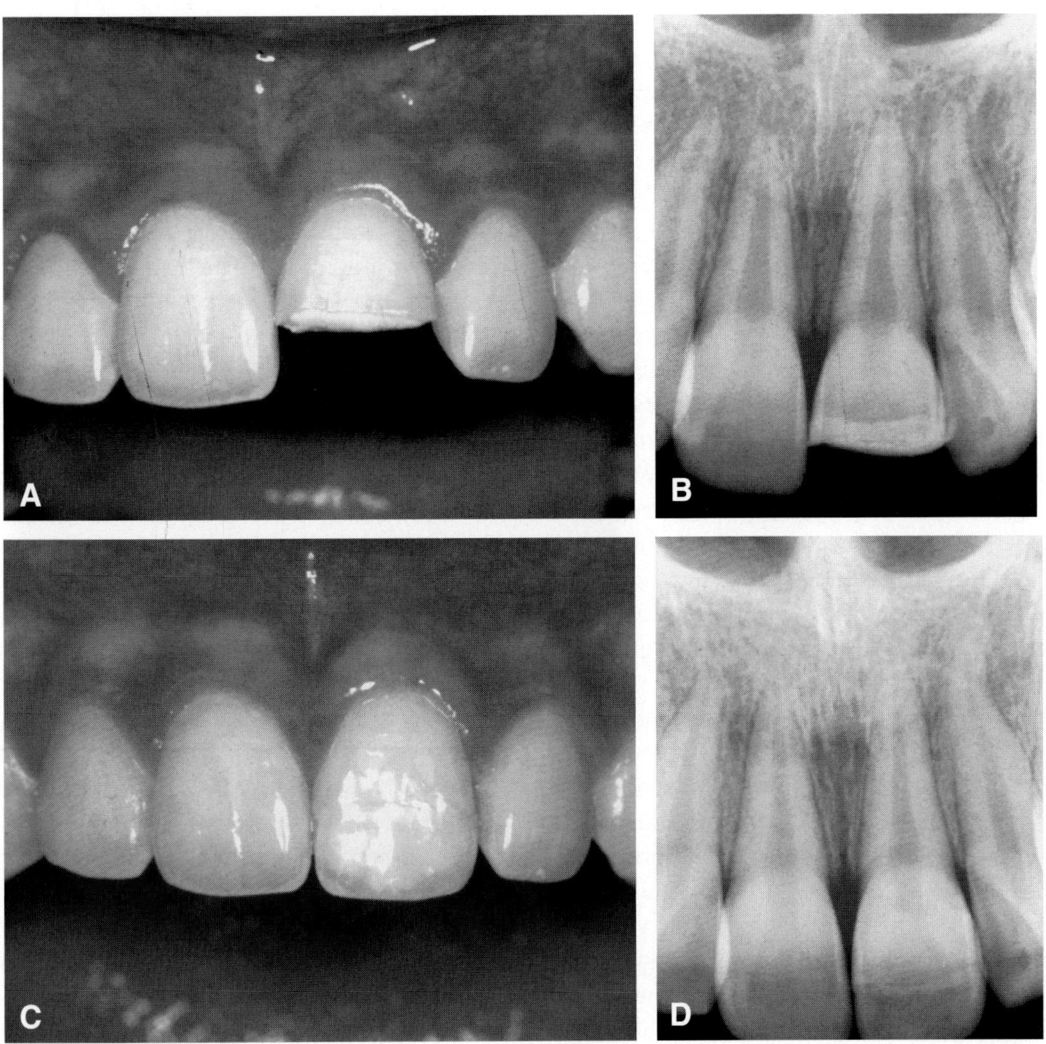

Figure 15-7 A, Uncomplicated fracture, central incisor. The dentin has been temporarily covered with glass ionomer. **B**, Radiograph, showing fracture with incisal glass ionomer. **C**, The incisal tooth fragment, which had been kept in water for several days, has been bonded to the tooth after removal of the glass ionomer. **D**, The tooth as it appears 2½ years after incisal fragment reattachment. (Courtesy of Dr. Mitsuhiro Tsukiboshi.)

Follow-up and Prognosis. As with most traumatic injuries, patients with crown fractures need to be reevaluated periodically to determine pulpal status. Traumatized teeth can develop pulp necrosis some time after the initial injury, and if necrosis occurs, endodontic therapy is indicated.[22]

The prognosis is usually good for teeth with crown fractures in which the pulps are not exposed.[1,22] The unpredictable part is determining the extent of concomitant pulp injury.

Primary Teeth. Crown fractures are rare in the primary dentition, but when they occur, the pulps are exposed more often than in the permanent dentition. When the pulps are **not** exposed, treatment consists of smoothing rough edges or repairing with composite resin by the acid-etch technique.[22]

Crown Fractures—Complicated (With Pulp Exposure)

Description. Crown fractures involving enamel, dentin, and pulp are called complicated crown fractures by Andreasen and Andreasen[22] and Class 3 fractures by Ellis and Davey.[23] The degree of pulp involvement varies from a pinpoint exposure to a total unroofing of the coronal pulp.

The exposure of the pulp in complicated crown fractures makes the treatment more difficult. Bacterial contamination of the pulp precludes healing and repair unless the exposure can be covered to prevent further contamination. The initial reaction is hemorrhage at the site of the pulp wound. Next, a superficial inflammatory response occurs, followed by either a destructive (necrotic) or proliferative ("pulp polyp") reaction.[28]

Incidence. It is fortunate, considering the treatment complications, that crown fractures exposing the pulps are far less common than those not involving the pulp. The incidence, compared with all types of dental injuries, ranges from 2 to 13%.[22]

Diagnosis. The diagnosis of crown fracture with pulp involvement can be made by clinical observation. In addition, it is important to determine the condition of the pulp. If the tooth has been luxated in addition to the crown fracture, pulpal recovery is compromised, and the longer the pulp is exposed before being protected, the poorer the prognosis for pulpal survival.[22]

Treatment. Traditionally, these injuries have often resulted in automatic pulp extirpation, even in young, developing teeth. Such drastic measures are not always necessary; vital pulp therapy preserves the potential for continued root development—an important consideration in a tooth with a thin, weak root structure owing to a lack of complete tooth development.

Treatment planning is influenced by tooth maturity and extent of fracture. Every effort must be made to preserve pulps in immature teeth. Conversely, in mature teeth with extensive loss of tooth structure, pulp extirpation and root canal therapy are prudent before post/core and crown restoration.

Pulp preservation by vital pulp therapy includes pulp capping and pulpotomy. Both procedures permit preservation of pulp tissue for continued root development.

Pulp capping is a time-honored procedure that is sometimes quite successful. However, in recent years, a modified pulpotomy technique ("Cvek type")[29] has shown itself to be more predictable. This pulpotomy technique may be termed "shallow pulpotomy" in contrast to the older method of removing coronal pulp tissue deeply to the cervical, or deeper, level. The "deep pulpotomy" techniques were difficult technically and failed to deliver what vital pulp therapy should: preservation of pulp tissue in the critical cervical area of the tooth, where subsequent fractures can occur in thin, weak walls of pulpless teeth.

The procedure for shallow pulpotomy (also referred to as a partial or "Cvek-type" pulpotomy) can be performed by any well-trained dentist[30,31] (Figures 15-8 and 15-9). After anesthesia and rubber dam isolation, remove granulation tissue from the exposure site using a spoon excavator. This permits evaluation of the size of exposure. Next, with a water-cooled, round diamond stone, remove pulp tissue from the pulp proper, to a depth of 1 to 2 mm. Visualize the removal, layer by layer, rather than a quick cut with the stone. Allow plenty of coolant water spray to irrigate and prevent heat damage to the subjacent pulp tissue.

After preparing the pulp tissue, rinse the wound with saline and allow the bleeding to stop (a cotton pellet moistened with saline can be used to control the bleeding), then wash the wound gently with saline, and it is ready for coverage with a calcium hydroxide material.

Apply the calcium hydroxide over the wound and also cover all exposed adjacent dentin. A hard-setting calcium hydroxide such as Dycal (Dentsply/Caulk, Tulsa, Okla.) is easy to use. Next, an intermediate base of hard-setting zinc phosphate cement or glass ionomer cement is placed before restoring with dentin adhesive and composite resin.

After radiographic evidence of mineralization of the exposed pulpal area, it is recommended that the initial filling and liner be replaced to prevent microleakage. This may occur 6 to 12 months after the initial treatment.[29,30]

An alternative to the use of calcium hydroxide is a new material, mineral trioxide aggregate (MTA)

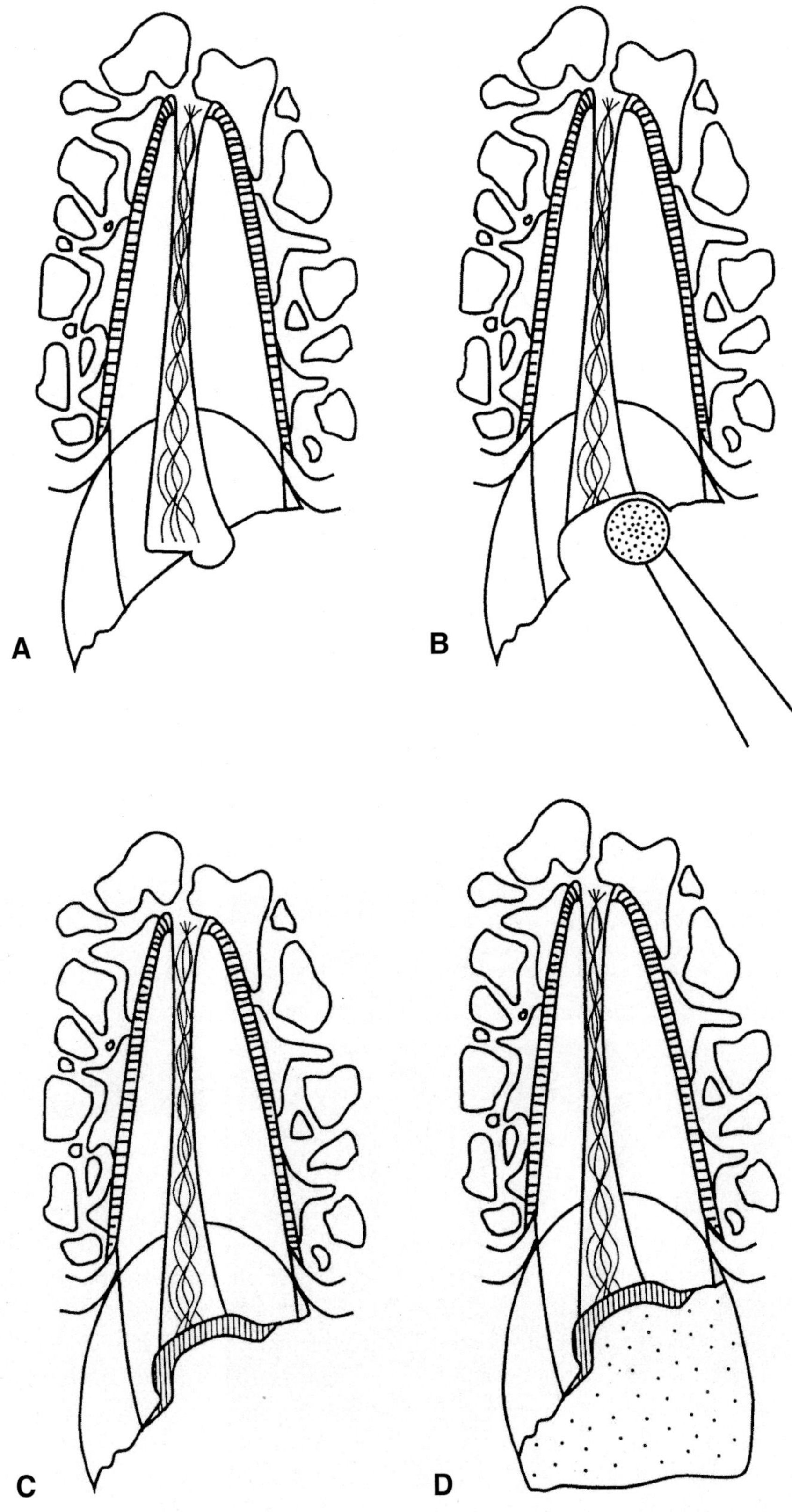

Figure 15-8 Shallow pulpotomy. **A**, Crown fracture exposes pulp. **B**, Remove pulp tissue with a round diamond bur to a depth of about 2 mm; use water spray to cool the diamond. **C**, After bleeding has stopped, wash the pulp wound with saline and apply a calcium hydroxide liner on top of which a base must be placed. The base can be glass ionomer cement. **D**, The lost tooth structure is replaced with acid-etched composite resin.

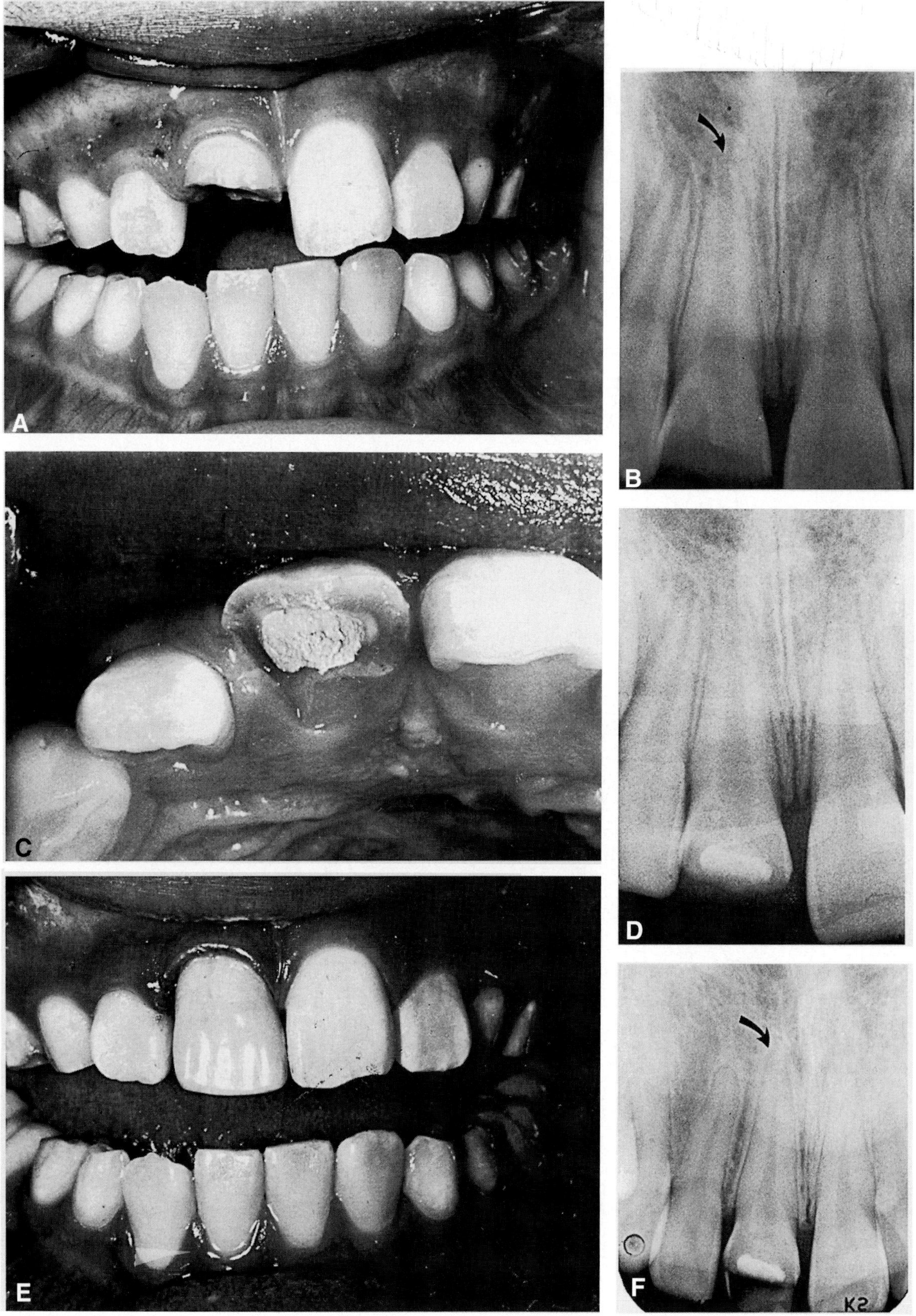

Figure 15-9 **A**, Crown fracture exposing pulp. **B**, Patient's age (10 years) and stage of root development (open apex) indicate need for perserving radicular pulp. **C** and **D**, Pulpotomy and calcium hydroxide to cervical level. **E**, Acid-etched composite restoration. (Restoration by Dr. James Dunn.) **F**, Radiograph taken years after accident. Note continued root development (**arrow**).

(ProRoot MTA, Tulsa Dental/Dentsply, Tulsa, Okla.), which has found many uses in endodontics.[32] It has been shown to be very effective in vital pulp therapy[33–36] (Figure 15-10).

The technique for managing a traumatic pulp exposure using MTA is in many ways similar to that used with calcium hydroxide, with some minor modifications:

1. The tooth must be anesthetized and should be isolated with a rubber dam.
2. The tooth, fractured surface, and wound area should be disinfected using a solution such as sodium hypochlorite.
3. A shallow pulpotomy is done to provide space for the MTA. A round diamond stone is used in a high-speed handpiece with water irrigation to remove exposed pulp tissue to a depth of at least 2 mm into the pulp proper. Bleeding is allowed to stop (which usually takes 2 to 3 minutes) before MTA is placed directly into the pulp wound. The presence of a small amount of blood in the wound area is not a contraindication to placing MTA; in fact, some moisture is required for the proper curing of the material.
4. Since access is not a problem when performing a shallow pulpotomy, the placement of MTA is not as difficult as it often can be when used for other purposes, such as repair of perforations. The mixture of MTA powder and liquid should be of such a consistency that it can be carried from the mixing pad to the pulp wound using a dental instrument such as a spoon excavator. A small amount of MTA should be placed on the wound surface and gently tapped with a moist cotton pellet so that it covers the exposed

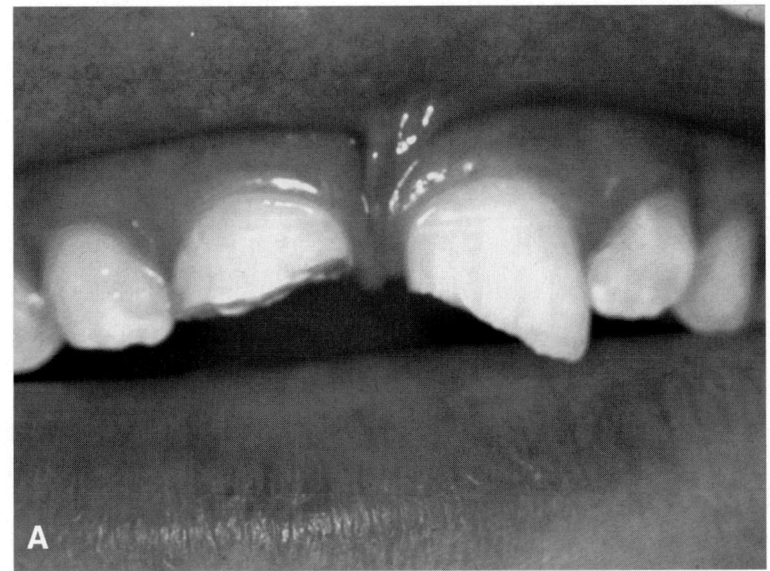

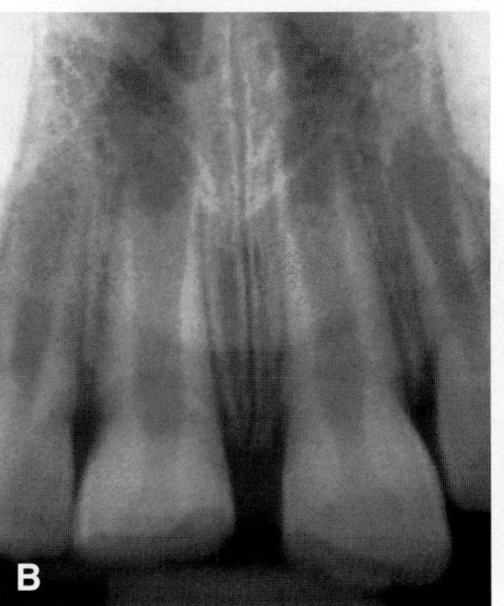

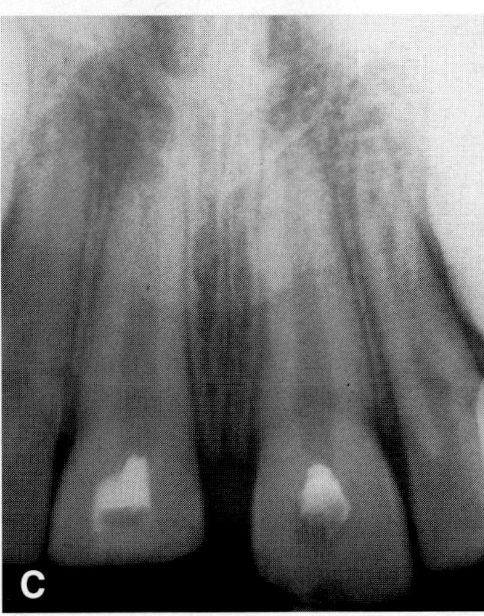

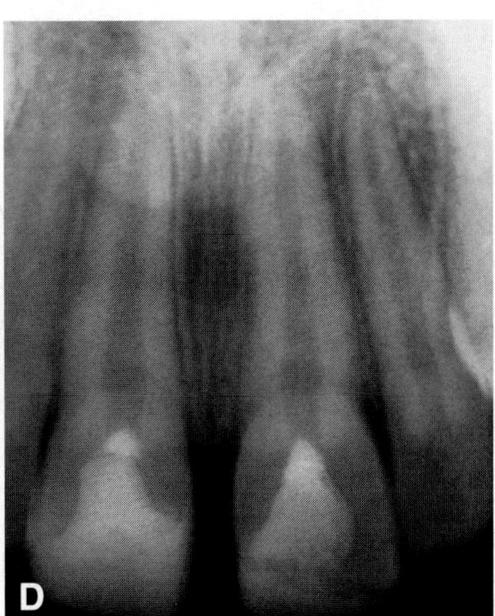

Figure 15-10 **A,** Complicated crown fractures with pulp exposure in both central incisors. **B,** Radiograph shows immature, developing roots with wide open apices. Shallow pulpotomy was done on both teeth, using mineral trioxide aggregate to protect the underlying pulp. **C,** Radiograph taken 2 years later shows excellent continued root formation in both teeth. **D,** Three years after vital pulp therapy.

pulp. Next, the entire access into the pulp should be filled in a similar manner using small amounts of MTA. Any excess moisture should be removed from the surface of the MTA using a dry cotton pellet.
5. The rubber dam can then be removed, and the patient can be dismissed. Leaving the MTA exposed to saliva will allow it to cure. A minimum of 6 hours should be allowed for the material to adequately cure, but clinical experience indicates that waiting at least 24 hours is better. The tooth can then be restored with a definitive restoration.

Previous research[34,35] has shown that the pulp responds favorably to the protection provided by an MTA layer. The reparative dentin is consistently more uniform and thicker under MTA compared with calcium hydroxide. As has been convincingly demonstrated,[37] the pulp can tolerate almost any dental material and produce new dentin as long as it can be protected against microleakage, a function that MTA appears to perform better than any material with which it has been compared.

The differences in the vital pulp therapy technique when MTA is used in place of calcium hydroxide are important to consider. First, it is not important that the pulp wound bleeding be completely stopped prior to placing the MTA; in fact, the presence of a small amount of blood provides necessary moisture for curing of the material and has been shown to work as well as any other fluid.[38] Second, since the MTA needs to cure prior to placement of a definitive restoration, it is necessary to schedule two appointments for this procedure: the first to perform the shallow pulpotomy and place the MTA on the pulp wound and the second to complete the restoration after the material has cured. Future material development may be expected to result in a faster-curing MTA. Third, it is not necessary to reenter the pulpotomy site later to remove the pulp capping material, as has been recommended for calcium hydroxide pulpotomies.[29,30] Mineral trioxide aggregate does not appear to deteriorate and disintegrate with time; thus, space for microleakage does not develop as it does with calcium hydroxide.

In mature, fully developed teeth, particularly those treatment planned for full-crown coverage, conventional root canal therapy is the treatment of choice. It should be pointed out that shallow pulpotomies can be performed in mature teeth, thus preserving pulp tissue and accomplishing repair quite conservatively. But it should probably be reserved for instances of crown fractures in which the fractured segment can be restored with composite resin or when rebonding of the fractures segment is possible.

With respect to the length of time pulp tissue can be exposed and still permit vital pulp therapy to be performed, studies by Heide[28] and Cvek[29] indicate that it may be safe to proceed with shallow pulpotomies up to 1 week post fracture. After that, it is probably questionable in mature, fully formed teeth, although in young, developing teeth with wide-open apices, it is worth attempting to save pulps even when they have been exposed for more than a week. The goal is to promote continued root formation.

Follow-up and Prognosis. A number of studies have evaluated the prognosis of traumatized anterior teeth, including those with crown fractures.[39–43] The teeth need periodic evaluation, radiographically and clinically, to determine pulpal status. Discoloration associated with the interphase between tooth structure and bonded resin material may indicate microleakage, and the restoration should be replaced to prevent bacterial contamination of the exposure site. Acceptable results of evaluation following pulpotomy should be all of the following[42]:

1. No clinical signs or symptoms
2. No evidence of periradicular pathologic changes
3. No evidence of resorption, either internal or external
4. Evidence of continued root formation in developing teeth

Evidence of root canal obliteration by calcified tissue is often taken as a sign of pulp degeneration. Lumen reduction can be seen years after trauma and treatment,[44,45] but such calcification is not necessarily an indication of pulp necrosis.[45] The decision to intervene endodontically in cases of apparent pulp space calcification should be based on evidence of pulp necrosis and not on pulp calcification.

If root canal treatment has been performed, either immediately after the injury or subsequent to pulp capping or pulpotomy, follow-up evaluation of healing should be done, particularly if luxation of the tooth occurred, to monitor for possible root resorption.[1]

Primary Teeth. Crown fractures involving the pulp are not common in the primary dentition.[46] When such injuries occur, pulpotomies or pulpectomies may be considered. Pulp capping is generally not successful in primary teeth, and endodontic treatment is difficult owing to the tortuous and fine canal structure. Patient management is a further complicating factor in treating fractured primary teeth. The result of poor cooperation is often tooth extraction.[47]

Pulpotomy is indicated when the pulp is still healthy and pulpectomy when the pulp is not expected to recover. The procedures are the same as described above for the permanent dentition, except that the root canal filling material should be a resorbable cement such as zinc oxide–eugenol. For additional details, see chapter 17.

Crown-Root Fractures

In these fractures, enamel, dentin, and cementum are involved. If the pulp is also involved, the case is considered more complicated.

Description. Crown-root fractures in anterior teeth are usually caused by direct trauma.[48] This may result in a chisel-type fracture, with the apical extent of the fracture below the lingual gingiva (Figure 15-11). These fragments may be single or multiple, leaving the fragment or fragments loose and attached only by periodontal ligament fibers (Figure 15-12). The pulp may also be involved, depending on the depth of fracture into the dentin, further complicating a difficult traumatic injury.

In posterior teeth, the causes of crown-root fractures have been attributed to indirect trauma including large-size restorations, thermal cycling, high-speed instrumentation, pin placement, and direct trauma, such as accidental blows to the face and jaws. The role of restorative procedures is not well understood, particularly in regard to occlusal restoration size and resultant fractures.[49]

As in anterior teeth, two types of crown-root fractures are recognized in posterior teeth: those with and those without pulpal involvement.

The vertical fracture of endodontically treated teeth is an additional type of crown-root fracture involving both anterior and posterior teeth (Figure 15-13). Most appear to be caused by the endodontic treatment itself or by subsequent inlay or dowel placement[49] (see Chapters 13 and 19).

Incidence. Crown-root fractures per se are not generally recognized as a separate entity, and little information is available about their frequency of occurrence. Andreasen and Andreasen reported a 5% incidence of total dental injuries.[48] However, when one includes the so-called cracked tooth syndrome and vertical fractures of endodontically treated teeth (all are caused by trauma in one form or another), the total incidence may be higher. For additional information, see chapter 13.

Diagnosis. Crown-root fractures result in complaints of pain, particularly when the loose fragment or fragments are manipulated. The fragments are generally easy to move, and bleeding from the periodontal ligament or pulp often fills the fracture line. Because of the mobile parts, percussion is seldom useful in determining apical periodontal involvement. However, that may be done later, after removal of the loose fragments. Unless the pulp is exposed, EPT should be performed on the injured and adjacent teeth.

Radiographs of anterior crown-root fractures are often difficult to interpret. It is very important to take more than one angulation to assess the extent of fractures. Angulations of films should include both additional horizontal and vertical angulations.

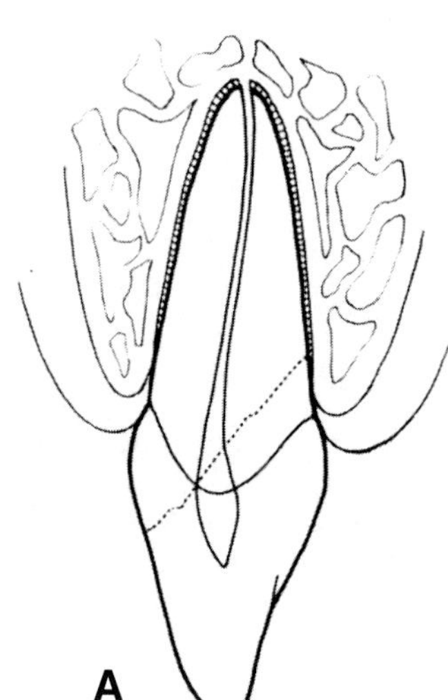

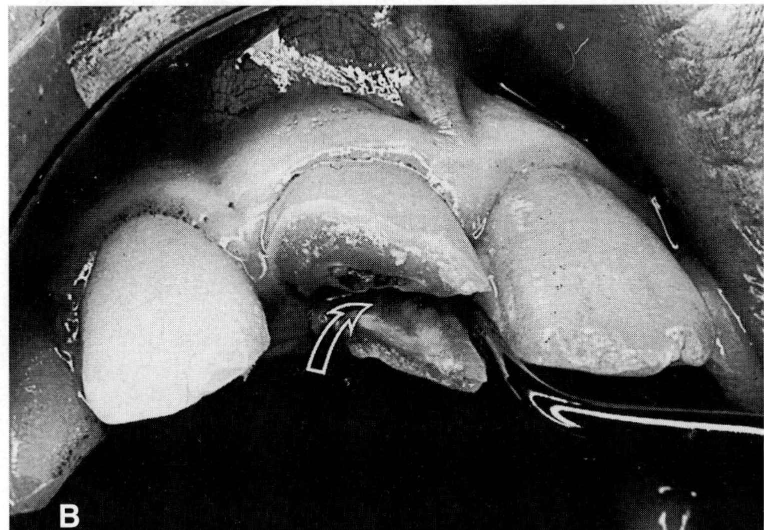

Figure 15-11 **A**, Crown-root fracture of the "chisel type" extending below the alveolar crest palatally. **B**, Such teeth may be orthodontically extruded for restorative reasons.

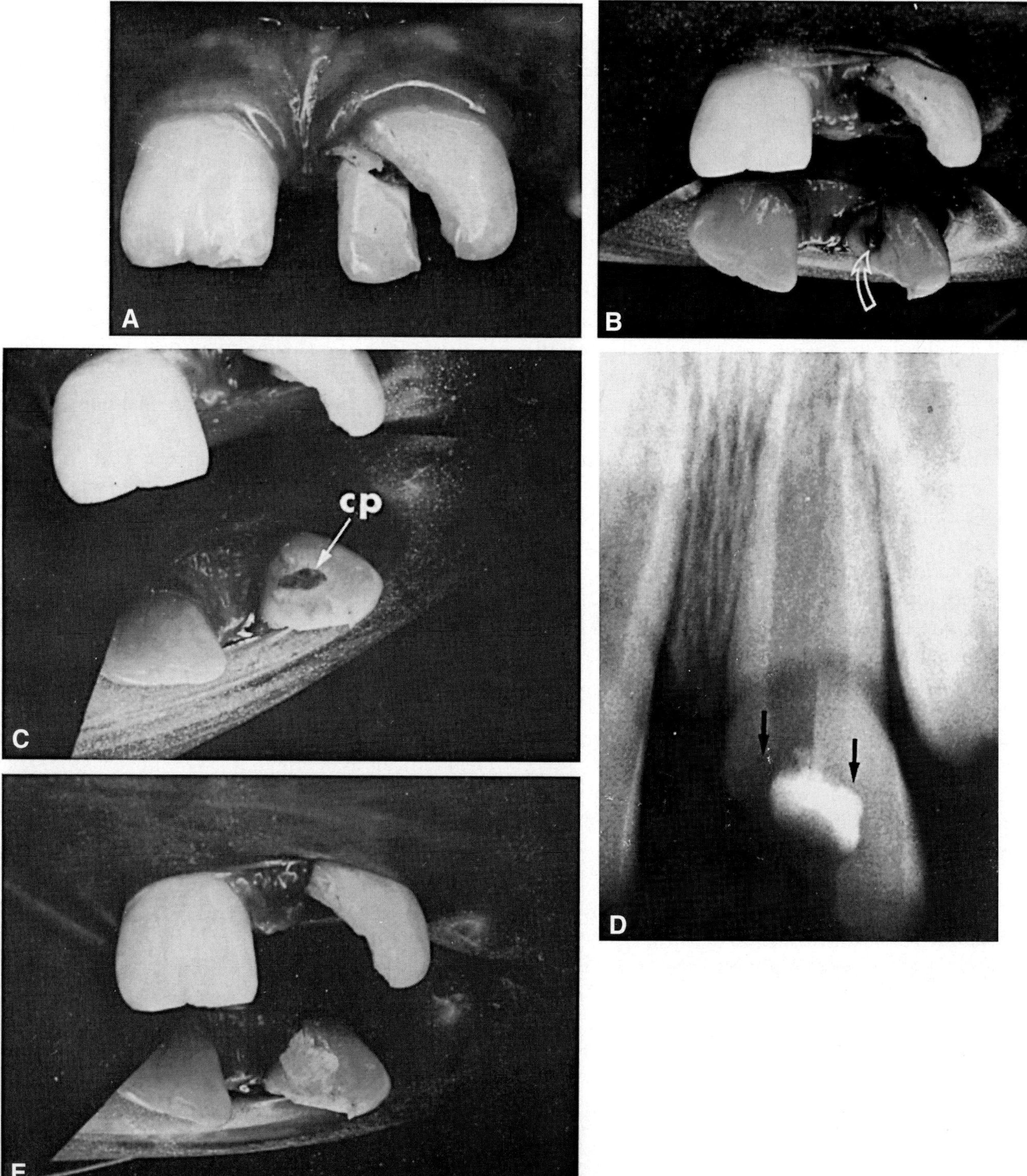

Figure 5-12 Crown-root fracture with pulp exposure. **A,** Note loose mesial crown fragments, which are attached by periodontal ligament fibers. **B,** After anesthesia, loose fragments are removed and rubber dam applied. Note exposure of radicular pulp (arrow). **C,** The remainder of coronal pulp tissue is amputated and the surface of pulp allowed to coagulate. Cotton pellet (CP) aids by controlling initial bleeding. **D,** After surface coagulation, the area is irrigated and calcium hydroxide placed directly over pulp tissue. It helps to prepare a shelf around the pulp orifice to support the base and prevent the cement from being pushed into the underlying pulp tissue (arrows point to shelf in dentin). **E,** After placement of base, acid-etched composite will be used for final restoration.

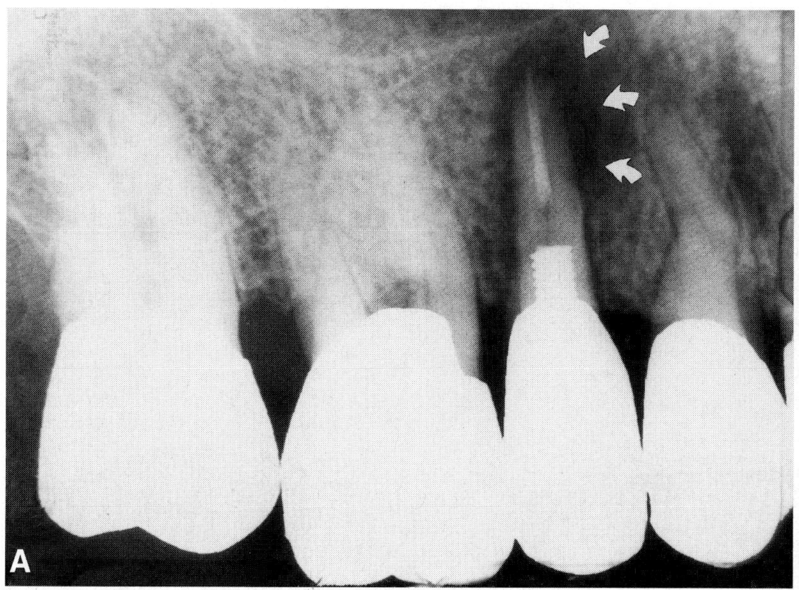

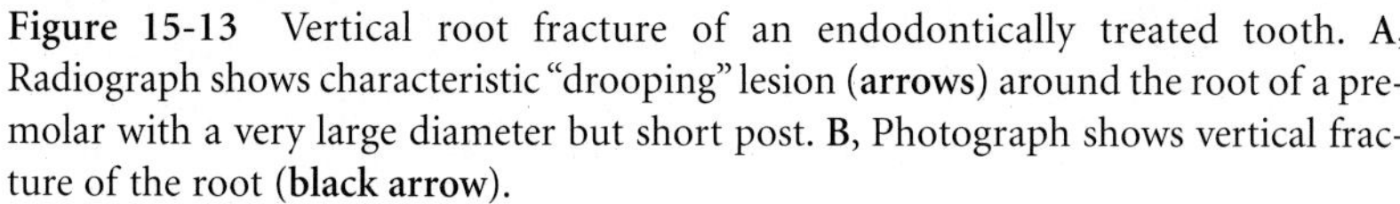

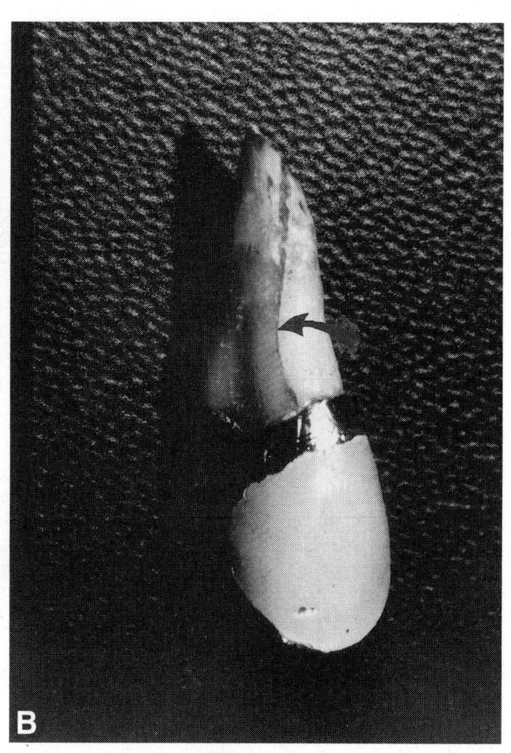

Figure 15-13 Vertical root fracture of an endodontically treated tooth. **A**, Radiograph shows characteristic "drooping" lesion (**arrows**) around the root of a premolar with a very large diameter but short post. **B**, Photograph shows vertical fracture of the root (**black arrow**).

Posterior crown-root fractures may be very difficult to diagnose because they are more inconspicuous. The examination and diagnosis of cracked tooth syndrome are discussed in chapters 6 and 7.

Treatment. There are several treatment options available for crown-root fractures, depending on the extent of the fracture.[1] If the fragment can be reattached by bonding, and no pulp exposure has occurred, that is the most conservative and convenient approach.

If pulp exposure has resulted from the fracture (see Figure 15-12), either a shallow pulpotomy procedure (if the tooth is still developing) or root canal treatment (fully developed teeth) must be done prior to any rebonding or crown restoration.[50]

Crown-root fractures extending well below the alveolar crest may require surgical repositioning of the tissues to expose the level of fracture. Long-term esthetic problems may, however, result from such surgical procedures.[1]

Extrusion—either surgical[51] or orthodontic[52]—can also be done to allow better restoration of the fractured tooth. See Figures 15-14 and 15-15 for illustrations of orthodontic extrusion.

Prognosis and Follow-up. The quality of the restorative procedure is an important factor in determining the long-term success of treating crown-root fractures. Both the loss of significant tooth structure and often the difficulty in restoring normal crown contour contribute to a guarded prognosis.

If the pulp is not initially involved, its continued vitality depends on one's ability to protect it from contamination. If possible, the condition of the pulp should be evaluated for a sufficient period of time to detect necrosis should it occur.

Primary Teeth. Fractures involving crowns and roots of primary teeth occur infrequently, and when they do, extraction is indicated.[48]

Root Fractures

This type of fracture involves the roots only: cementum, dentin, and pulp (Figure 15-16).

Incidence and Description. Intra-alveolar root fractures do not occur frequently compared with other dental injuries and account for probably less than 3% of all dental trauma. These fractures are generally transverse to oblique and may be single or multiple, complete or incomplete.[53] Incompletely formed roots rarely fracture, but when they do, the prognosis is usually very good.[54]

Diagnosis. Root fractures are not always horizontal; in fact, probably more often than not, the angulation of fractures is diagonal (Figure 15-17). This fact probably explains why root fractures are often missed radiographically. With the conventional 90-degree-angulation periradicular x-ray film, if the fracture is diagonal, it is very likely that it will be missed. Only when the x-ray beam can pass directly through the fracture line does it show on the radiograph. It is there-

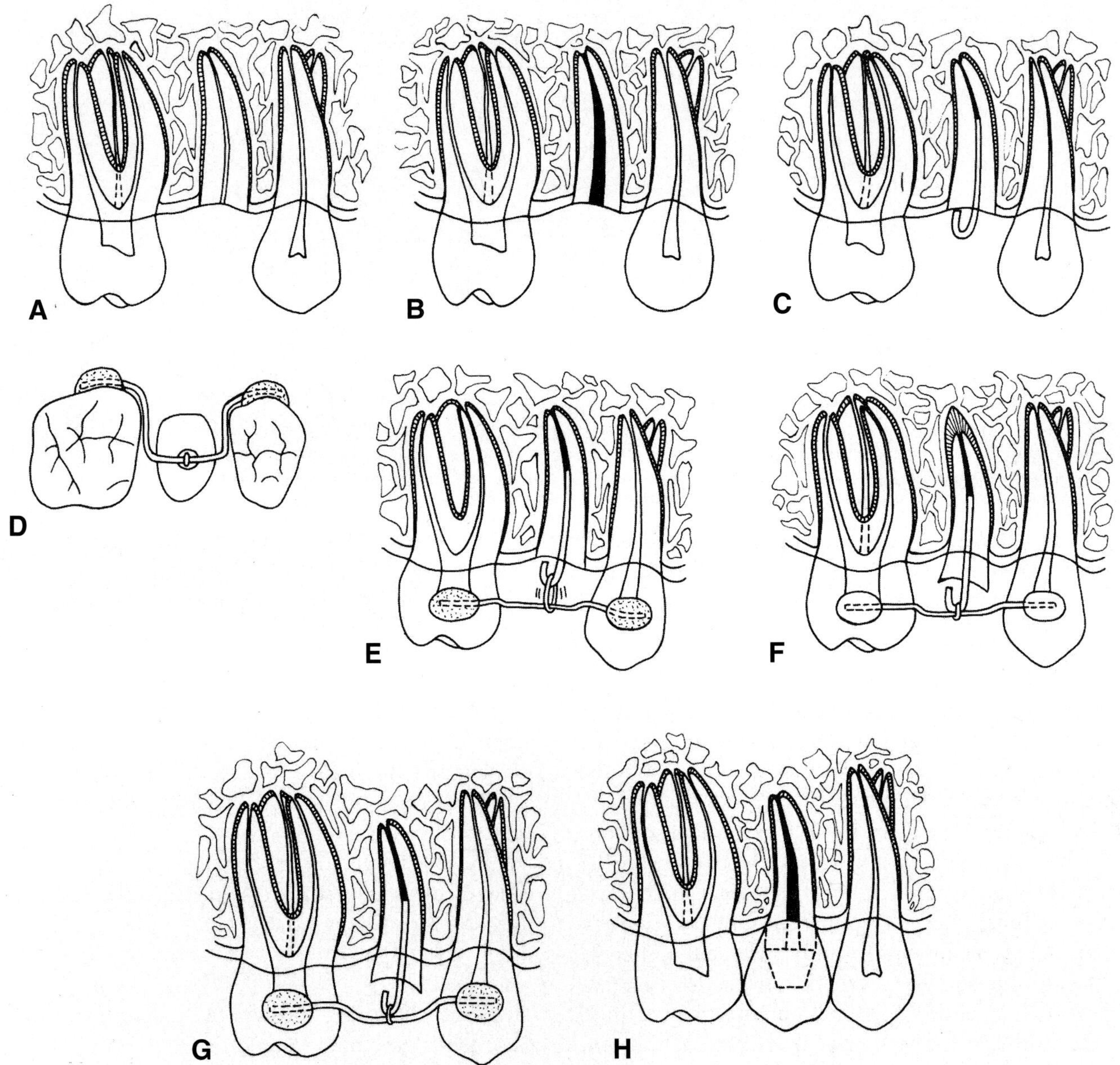

Figure 15-14 Basic technique for root extrusion. **A,** Root fracture at or below crestal bone. **B,** Root canal therapy completed. **C,** Cementation of a post-hook. **D,** Occlusal view; horizontal wire is bent to cross midline of the tooth to be extruded. Wire is embedded with acid-etched composite on adjacent teeth. **E,** Elastic is attached to activate extrusion. **F,** When satisfactory extrusion has been completed, the tooth is stabilized until periodontal and bony repair are complete. **G,** Periodontal and bony repair completed. **H,** Permanent restoration. (See also Figure 15-15.)

fore imperative to take additional film angulations when root fracture is suspected.[53]

One additional film angulation (foreshortened or 45 degrees) will, when combined with the standard 90-degree positioning, reveal most of the traumatic root fractures.[55]

Treatment. If there is no mobility and the tooth is symptomless, the fracture is likely to be in the apical one-third of the root, and no treatment is necessary (Figure 15-18). If the coronal fragment is mobile, treatment is indicated. The initial treatment consists of repositioning the coronal segment (if it is displaced) and then stabilizing the tooth to allow healing of the periodontal ligament supporting the coronal segment[53] (Figure 15-19).

Repositioning can be as simple as pushing the tooth into place with finger pressure, or orthodontic intervention may be required to move the displaced segment

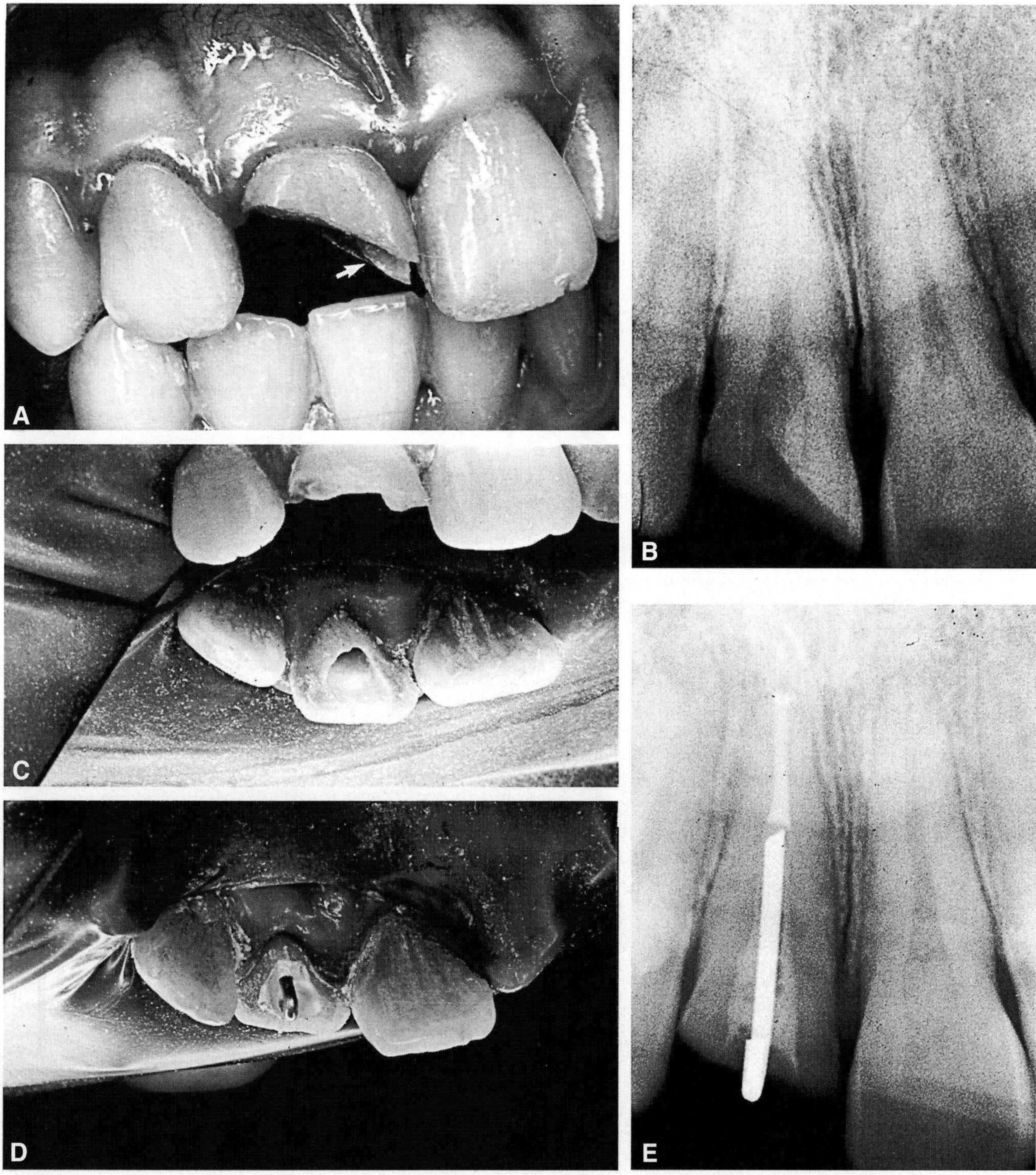

Figure 15-15 A, Crown-root fracture of a right central incisor necessitating orthodontic extrusion owing to palatal extension of fracture. Note that the loose palatal segment (**arrow**) is still present. **B**, Adequate remaining tooth length allows use of the technique. **C**, One-visit root canal therapy performed after removal of loose palatal fragement. **D** and **E**, Extrusion hook cemented in prepared post space.

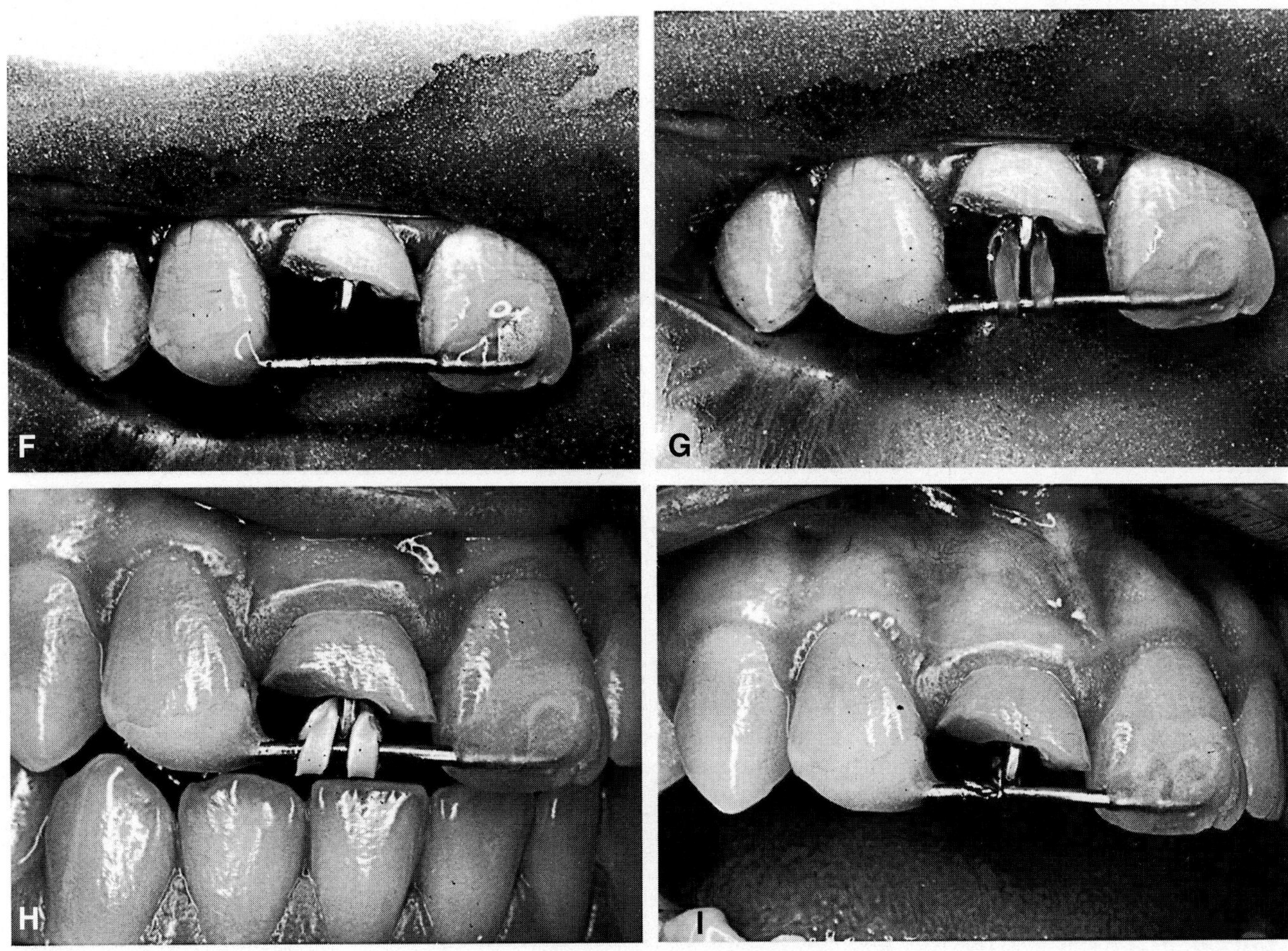

Figure 15-15 (Continued) **F**, Horizontal wire attached to adjacent teeth at desired position by acid-etched composite. **G**, Activation elastic placed over hook and wire. **H**, Two weeks later, the tooth has extruded the desired distance. **I**, It is now stabilized for 8 weeks by use of ligature wire.

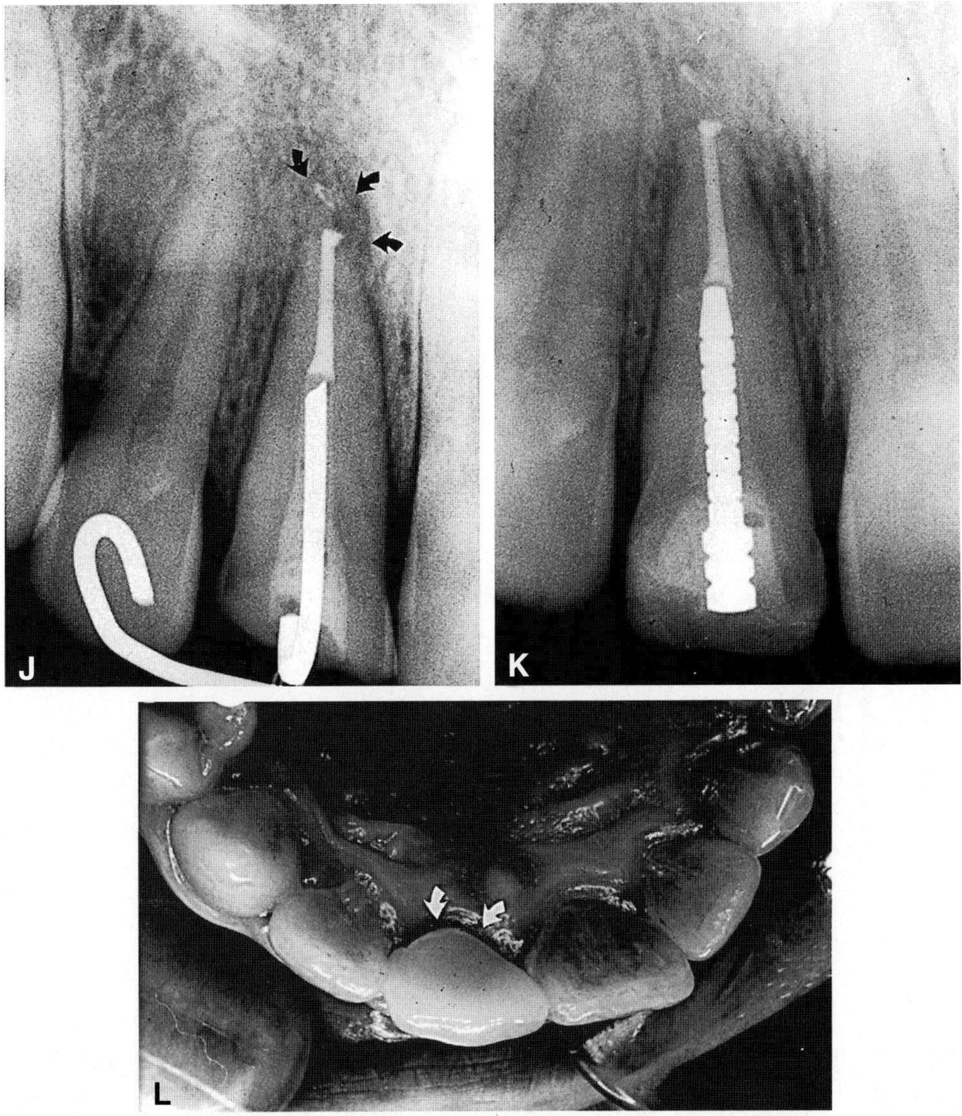

Figure 15-15 (Continued) **J**, Note apical radiolucency (**arrows**) immediately following extrusion and **K**, recalcification after 8 weeks of stabilization. **L**, Palatal tissue shows good adaptation to crown (**arrows**). As a result of extrusion, gingival bevel could be placed on newly exposed tooth structure.

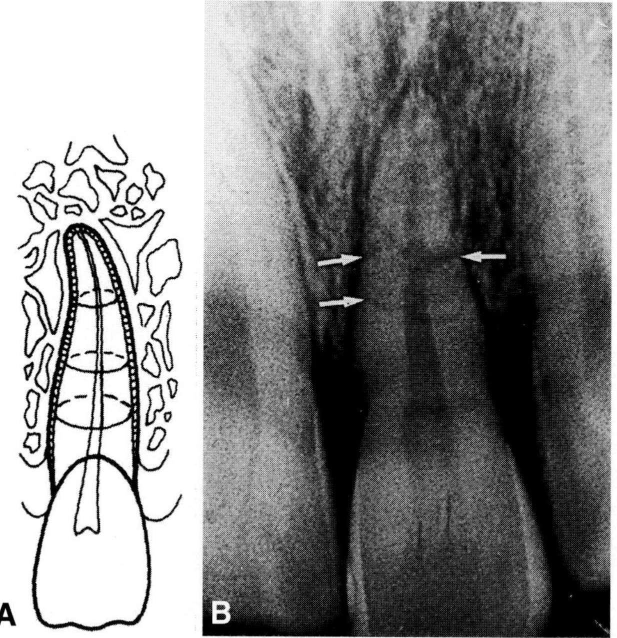

Figure 15-16 A, Root fractures involve cementum, dentin, and pulp and may occur in any part of the root: apical, middle, or coronal thirds. B, Fractures may also be comminuted (arrows).

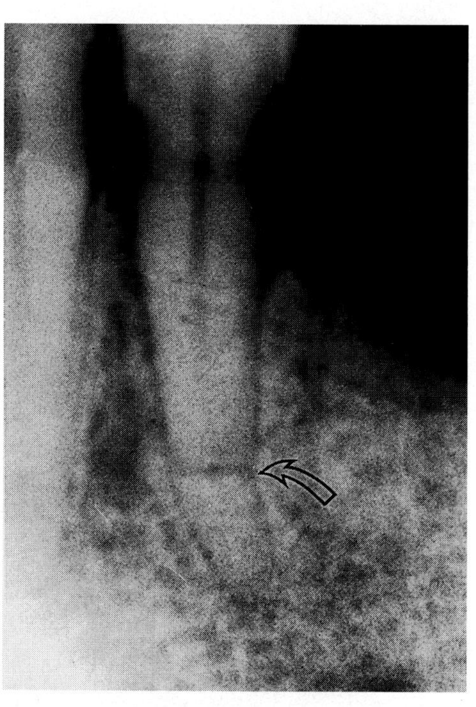

Figure 15-18 Root fracture (arrow) healed spontaneously. The patient was unaware of the fracture.

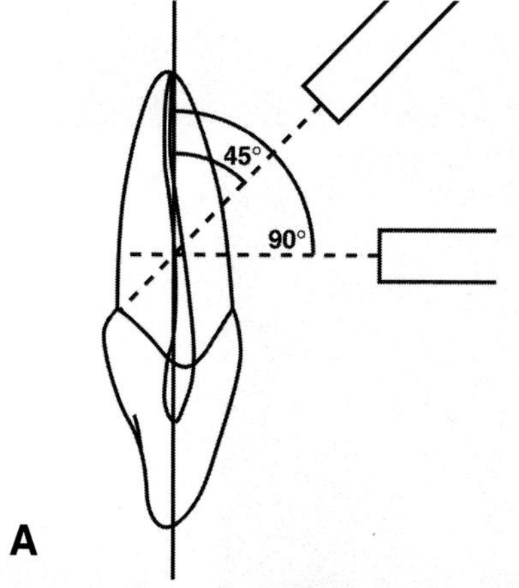

Figure 15-17 A, Graphic illustration showing two angulations (90 and 45 degrees) to better detect root fractures. B, Photograph showing a root fracture (arrow) that could not be detected with a 90-degree angulation C, By changing the angulation to a more foreshortened view (approximately 45 degrees). D, The fracture is easily demonstrated (arrow).

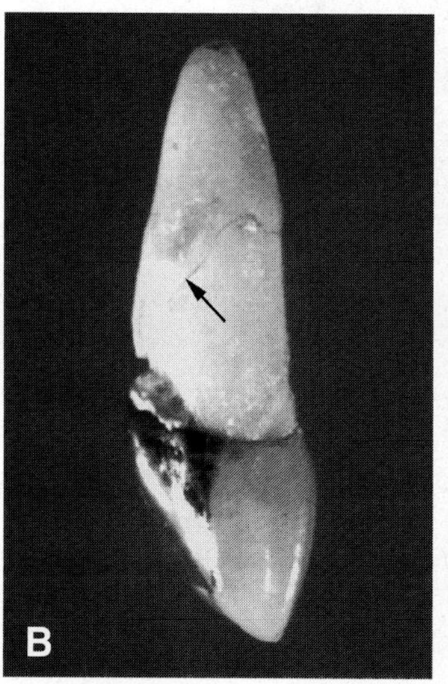

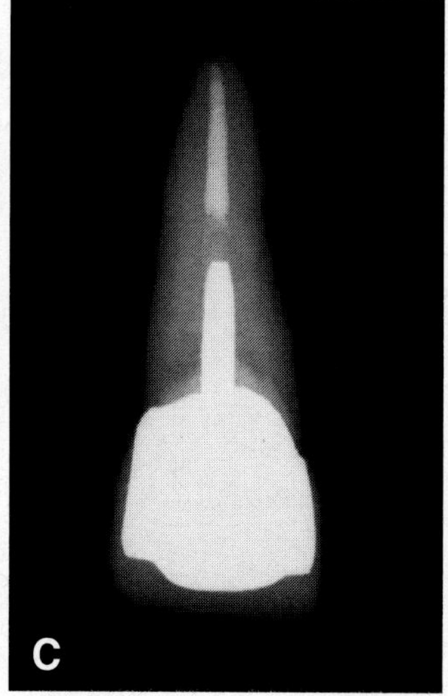

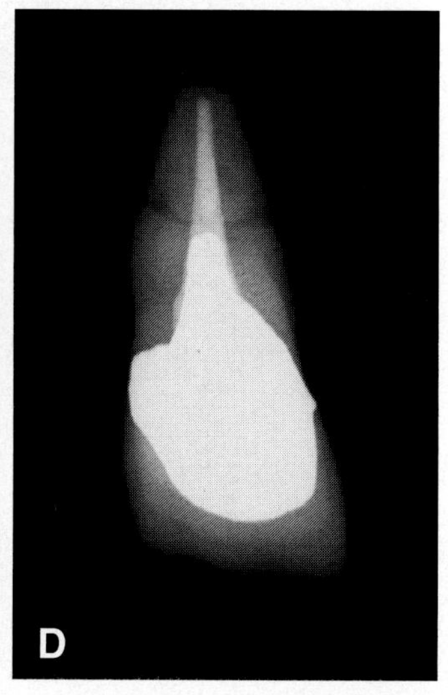

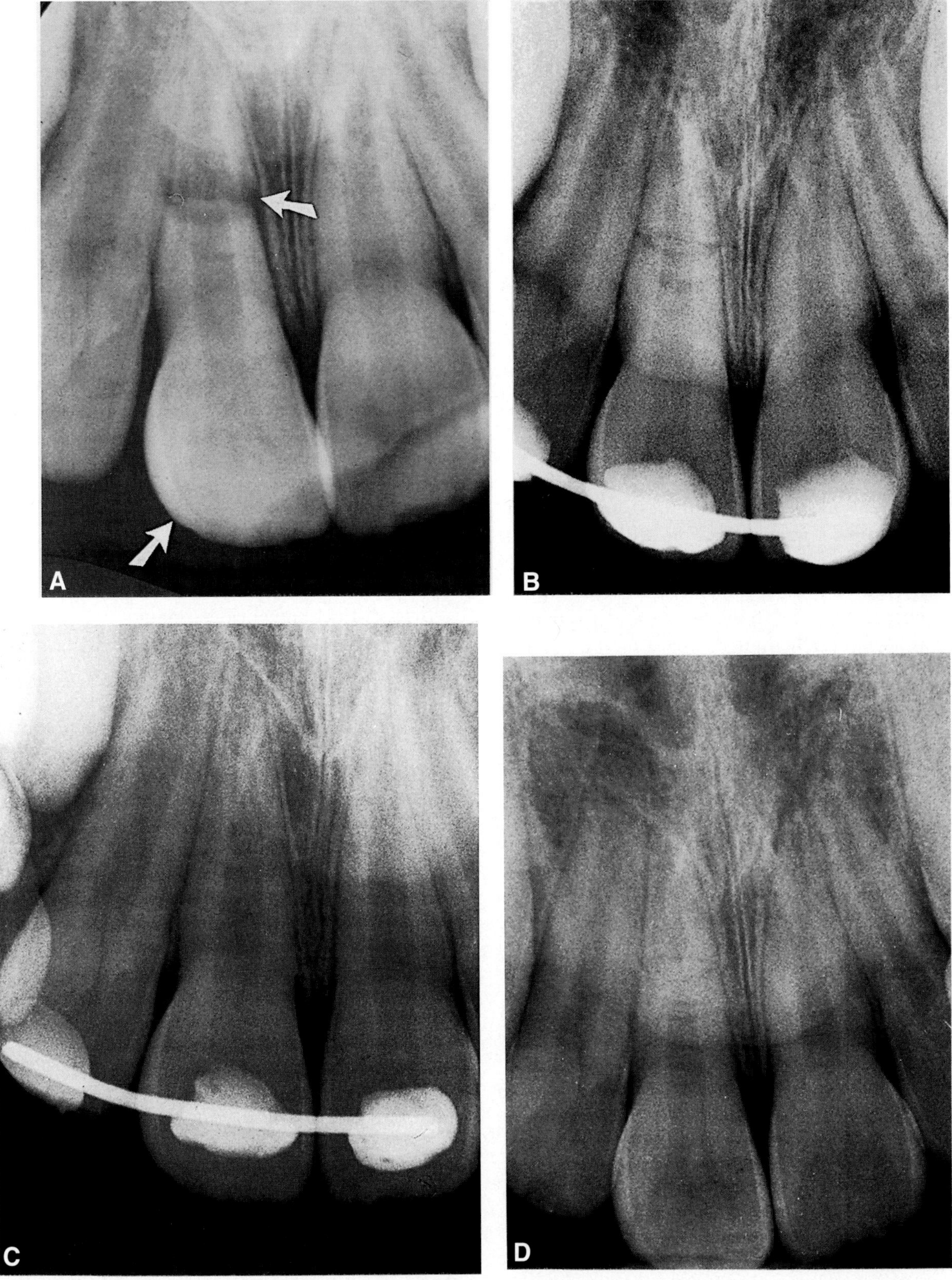

Figure 15-19 Root fracture. **A**, Immediately after the accident. Note displacement of the coronal segment (**arrows**). **B**, The coronal segment has been repositioned and the splint has been attached to stabilize the fractured tooth. **C**, Radiograph taken just before removal of the splint. **D**, Control radiograph taken 1 year after removal of the splint. The tooth is comfortable and responds to the electric pulp test within normal limits. There is no abnormal mobility or discoloration of the tooth. (Courtesy of Dr. Donald Peters.)

into proper alignment. Generally, if considerable time has elapsed between the injury and the treatment appointment, it is more difficult to reposition the coronal segment in line with the apical segment ("reducing the fracture").

Splinting is best accomplished by incorporating a thin orthodontic wire into labially bonded composite resin. The splint should allow for functional movement of the tooth to promote healing, and the length of stabilization time is 4 to 6 weeks.[56]

Following initial treatment by reduction and stabilization, repair by calcific and/or fibrous deposition is very likely. About 80% of properly treated root fractures heal successfully. The prognosis is related to the amount of dislocation, stage of root development, and probably whether treatment was done. Fracture location apparently matters less as long as it is not too close to the alveolar crest.[57]

The amount of dislocation and the degree of mobility of the coronal segment affect the prognosis because the more severe the dislocation (and therefore the mobility), the less likely it is that fracture reduction can be accomplished, and also the more likely it is that the pulp has been severely injured.[58]

The stage of root development matters in root fractures because, with other dental injuries, the more immature the tooth, the better the ability of the pulp to recover from trauma. The rich vascular supply to a young, immature tooth promotes repair.[59]

The conventional wisdom of dentists for years was that root fractures occurring in the coronal half had a poorer prognosis than those taking place more apically. In the important study by Zachrisson and Jacobsen on root fracture outcome, it was surprising to see that location did not influence outcome.[58] Apparently, then, if a tooth can be stabilized long enough for repair to occur, the location of the fracture is immaterial. The only exception naturally would be fractures that occur so close to the crest of the alveolar bone that the support of the tooth is compromised. Also, if communication develops between gingival sulcus and the fracture site, the prognosis has to be considered poor.

Sequelae to root fractures may be divided into four types, as proposed by Andreasen and Hjörting-Hansen[60]:

1. **Healing with calcified tissue.** Radiographically, the fracture line is discernible, but the fragments are in close contact (see Figure 15-19, D).
2. **Healing with interproximal connective tissue.** Radiographically, the fragments appear separated by a narrow radiolucent line, and the fractured edges appear rounded (Figure 15-20).

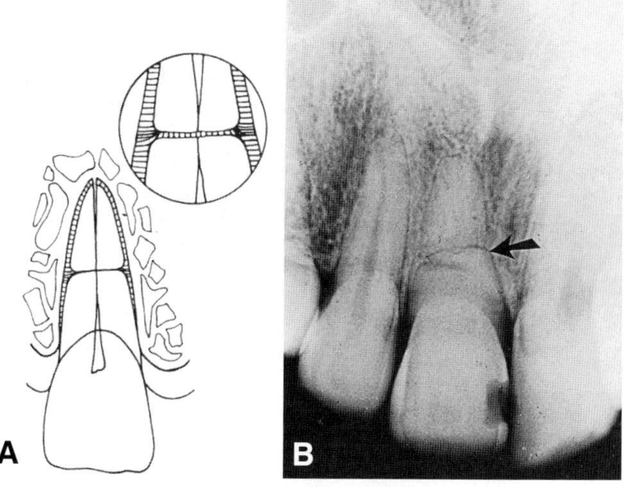

Figure 15-20 A, Root fracture in which healing resulted in connective tissue between the segments. B, Note that the segments appear to be separated by narrow radiolucent lines (**arrows**) and the rounding effect of the fractured edges.

3. **Healing with interproximal bone and connective tissue.** Radiographically, the fragments are separated by a distinct bony bridge (Figure 15-21).
4. **Interproximal inflammatory tissue without healing.** Radiographically, a widening of the fracture line and/or a developing radiolucency corresponding to the fracture line become apparent (Figure 15-22).

The first three types are considered successfully healed injuries; they are asymptomatic, probably respond to electric vitality tests, and may, over time, show only signs of coronal discoloration (yellowing) owing to coronal calcification.[57,58] Fractures that do not heal need additional endodontic treatment. Failing root fractures have characteristic lesions that develop adjacent to the fracture sites, not apically, as in most teeth with necrotic pulps.[60] Further, there is good reason to expect the apical segment of the root-fractured tooth to contain vital, healthy pulp tissue, whereas the coronal pulp is necrotic. The treatment options are therefore many:

1. **Root canal therapy of both segments.** This may be indicated in fracture cases when the segments are not separated, allowing passage of files and filling materials from the coronal segment across the fracture site into the apical segment (Figure 15-23).
2. Root canal treatment of the coronal segment only (Figure 15-24). This is the current recommendation, particularly with the view that the apical segment may contain vital, healthy pulp tissue.[54] A variation to this approach has been recommended by Cvek.[61] He used an apexification procedure in the coronal

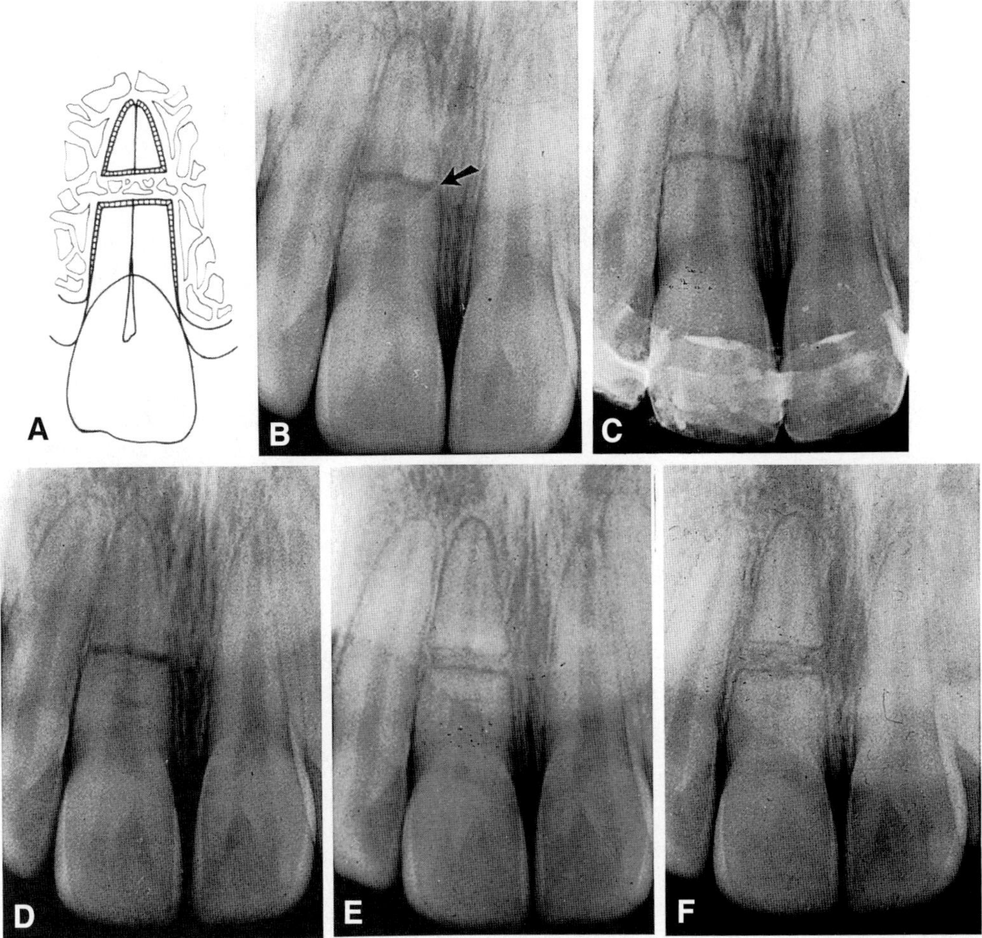

Figures 15-21 A, Healing by interproximal bone. **B**, Root fracture (**arrow**) resulting in total separation of fragments. **C**, Midroot facture stabilized for 3 months. **D**, Note that after removing the splint, the incisal edges are even, yet a space is apparent between the segments. **E**, Eight months later, bone is now apparent between segments. **F**, The interproximal space has enlarged further 2 years after the accident. The tooth is firm and functional. Note calcification of the pulp space. (Courtesy of Dr. Milton Siskin.)

segment, inducing a hard tissue barrier at the exit of the coronal root canal. Although there are no studies at the present time reporting on the use of MTA in root fractures, it would be reasonable to expect that this material could be used instead of calcium hydroxide in root fractures.[9]

3. The use of an intraradicular splint has been recommended by Weine et al.[62] It is similar to the first procedure described; both segments are treated endodontically. Following root canal filling, a post space is prepared in the canal to extend from the coronal segment into the apical one, allowing placement of a rigid-type post (cobalt-chromium alloy [vitallium]) to stabilize the two root segments.
4. Root extrusion is a solution for teeth with root fractures at or near the alveolar crest.[52] This treatment plan must be evaluated carefully because the length of root left after the extrusion must be enough to

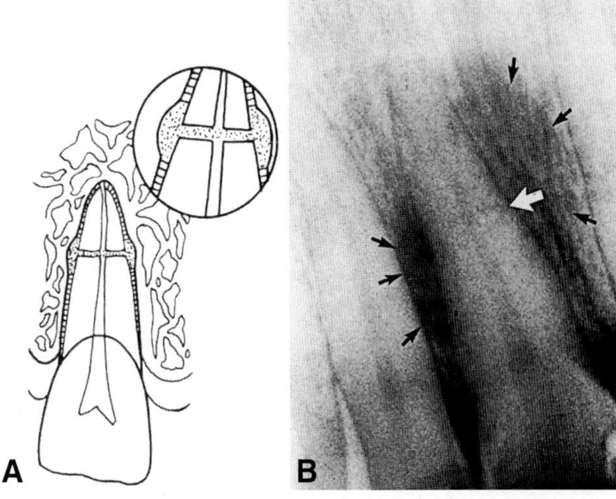

Figure 15-22 A, Root fracture resulting in interproximal inflammatory tissure. **B**, Large periradicular lesion (**small arrows**) adjacent to fracture line (**white arrow**).

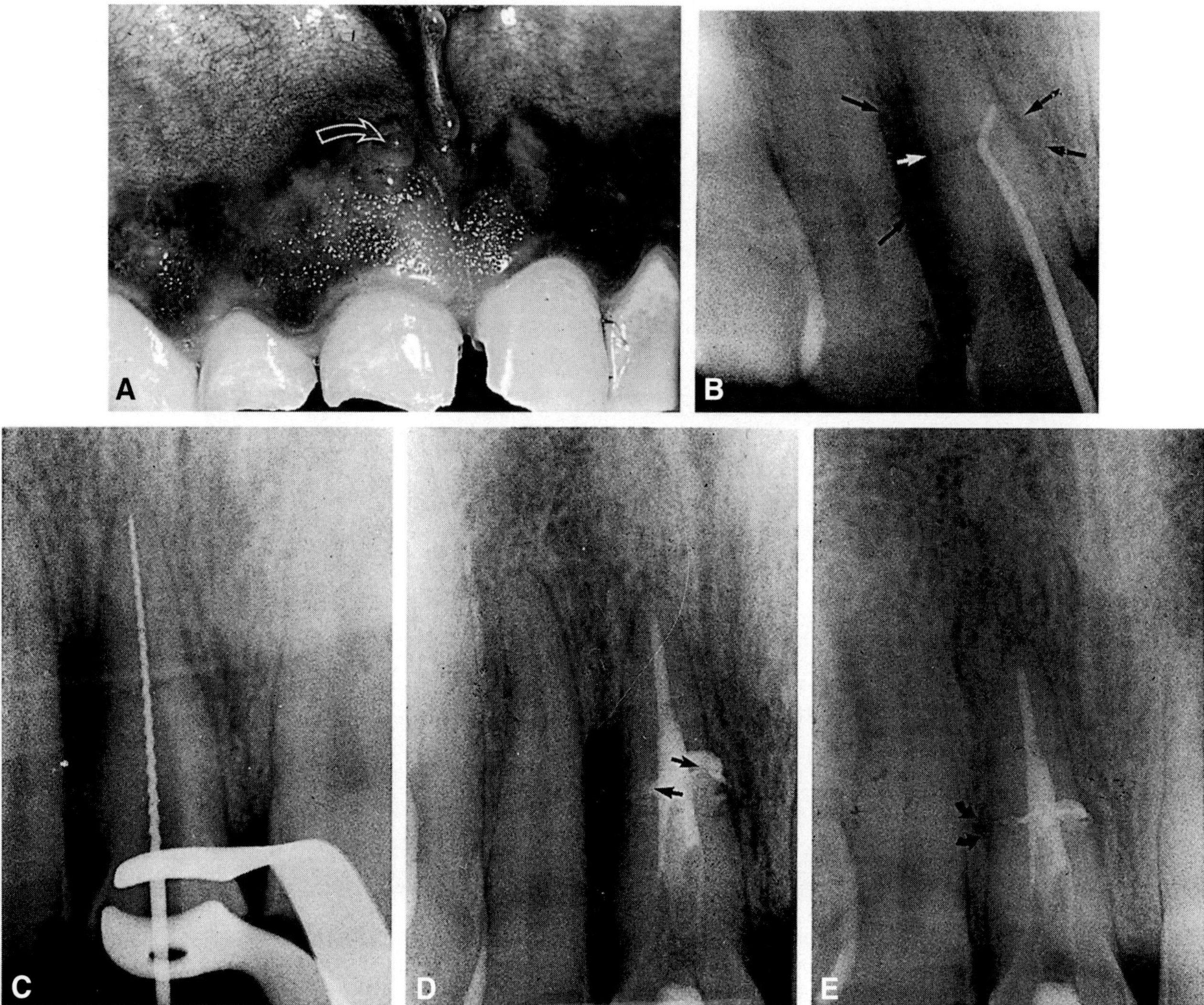

Figure 15-23 Root fracture treated by root canal therapy of both apical and coronal fragments. **A,** Note the fistulous tract. **B,** Tract traced with a gutta-percha point to the root fracture (**white arrow**). Periodontal lesion associated with fracture is evident (**dark arrows**). **C,** Segments aligned properly so that instrumentation is possible. **D,** Sealer extruded into the interproximal area (**arrows**). **E,** Follow-up at 11 months shows resolution of the lesion with a small remaining area expected to heal.

support a new crown. A reasonable guide is to consider a crown-root ratio of 1:1 to have adequate support. See Figures 15-14 and 15-15 for extrusion technique.

Follow-up and Prognosis. It is a commonly held opinion that teeth with root fractures have a poor prognosis, particularly if the fracture is in the middle or coronal third. Whereas it may be true that the prognosis is poor for longitudinal fractures, it appears unfounded for transverse fractures[56] (see Figure 15-19).

A slight discoloration of the crown is a frequent observation in **healed** root-fractured teeth, usually seen as a yellowing effect with reduced transparency.[63] It is associated with pulp obliteration and occasionally a loss of response to the EPT. Endodontic treatment is not indicated unless other evidence, such as root resorption or periradicular radiolucencies, indicates pulp necrosis. Usually, if the pulp space becomes obliterated, no radiolucencies are seen apically or associated with the fracture lines. Endodontic treatment then becomes a decision based on other factors pertinent to each individual case.[57]

Teeth requiring endodontic treatment after root fractures also have a good prognosis with proper treatment unless the fracture is so close to the alveolar ridge that it communicates with the gingival crevice.[57,58] In the latter case, removing the coronal fragment and extruding the root orthodontically may be the treatment of choice.[52]

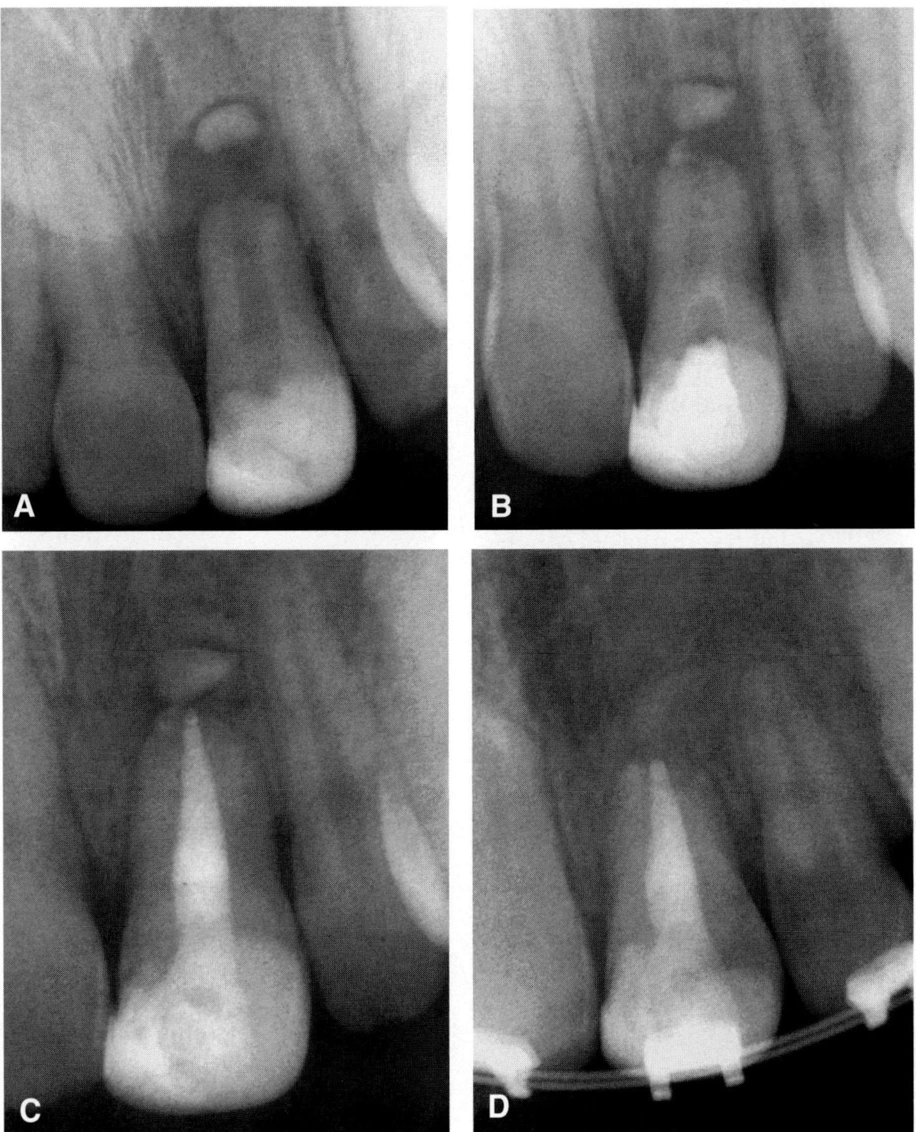

Figure 15-24 A, Radiograph shows a central incisor with an apical root fracture and a crown fracture repaired with composite resin 7 years earlier. The pulp had not survived the original injury, and the patient had an apical abscess. Note the separated apical root segment. B, Radiograph taken 4 months after initial treatment: root canal cleaning and calcium hydroxide medications. C, The tooth immediately after root canal filling. Note that the apical lesion responded favorably to the initial endodontic therapy and the apical root fragment is not involved. D, Twelve months after filling the root canal, the radiograph shows good repair; the apical root fragment can be left in place.

Long-term follow-up with radiographs and clinical tests is indicated in root fractures cases, as with all other types of dental injury. It would appear that few root-fractured teeth need to be extracted. With proper treatment, even those with coronal-third involvement can be expected to survive, although some will require endodontic and possibly orthodontic intervention.

Primary Teeth. Root fractures are infrequent in primary teeth. When they occur, however, the coronal fragment should be extracted. If the removal of the apical segment requires much manipulation, it may be left in its socket. It will resorb during the growth and emergence of the succedaneous tooth. Excessive manipulation may damage the permanent tooth bud.[53]

Luxation Injuries

This category of dental injuries includes impact trauma that ranges from minor crushing of the periodontal ligament and the neurovascular supply to the pulp to more major trauma such as forceful and sometimes total displacement of teeth (avulsion).

Injury to a tooth's supporting structure seldom spares the pulp from trauma. Only in cases of minimal trauma does the pulp have a good chance of recovering. Otherwise, when a tooth is impacted by a blow, the force is very likely to damage the vasculature entering the apical canal opening, with the result that the pulpal blood supply is compromised[64,65] (see chapter 4).

Besides pulpal injuries, impact trauma may also affect the tooth's periodontal support. Loss of attachment, if not restored by subsequent repair, will result in pocket formation and reduction in tooth support. The goal in treatment of luxation injuries is to promote recovery of both pulpal and periodontal health; realistically, except in young, immature teeth, pulpal recovery is not as likely to occur as periodontal repair.[66]

Incidence. Tooth luxation (not including avulsion) is a frequent injury, comprising the largest group of injuries in the classification of dental trauma, ranging from 30 to 44%.[66] These figures are probably on the low side since many instances of mild luxation, such as concussion, go unreported. In severe injuries, luxations may go unnoticed in the face of more obvious injuries. It is important, though, to record findings indicating luxations, even mild ones, because of the high rate of subsequent pulp necrosis, osteitis or apical periodontitis, and root resorption associated with such injuries. Following extrusion-luxation, Dumsha and Hovland reported pulp necrosis in 51 of 52 teeth after a period that ranged from 4 weeks to 18 months.[67]

A frequently overlooked cause of luxation injuries, including avulsions, occurs during intubation in the operating room. Damaged teeth were the most frequent anesthesia-related insurance claim during the time period 1976 to 1983.[68]

Diagnosis. Luxated teeth that have been loosened or slightly displaced are sensitive to biting and chewing. In concussion, this may be the only symptom, and it is noted by percussing the tooth. In more severe injuries, such as subluxation and extrusive luxation, signs and symptoms in addition to percussion sensitivity may be present: sensitivity to pressure and palpation of the alveolus, mobility, dislocation, and possibly bleeding from the periodontal ligament. Radiographs do not always reveal the extent of injuries to the supporting structures but are important nonetheless; it is also important to include additional radiographic angulations. Discoloration of the crown may also be noted and, if present shortly after the injury, is indicative of severe pulp damage. Lateral and intrusive luxations are usually firmly displaced and may not be sensitive to percussion.[66]

Electric pulp testing should be carried out and recorded in cases of luxation, in spite of the fact that an initial "no response" is common. The results of the EPT provide the basis for later evaluation. It is generally found that teeth with an initial normal response but a negative response later have developed either pulp necrosis or calcification. However, without other indications of pulp necrosis, endodontic intervention should not be based solely on a negative response.

Treatment. Initial treatment can be as simple as doing nothing while the patient avoids use of the tooth. In more serious luxations, treatment may range from slight occlusal adjustment to repositioning (reduction) and splinting (stabilization) for 2 to 6 weeks. If symptoms and other conditions (crown fracture with pulp exposure) indicate irreversible pulp involvement, endodontic treatment is indicated immediately after injury. Follow-up evaluation will determine possible later need for root canal therapy.[69–73]

Concussion

This is the mildest form of luxation injury, and it is characterized by sensitivity to percussion only. **No displacement has taken place**, and there is no mobility as a result of the injury. Concussion is probably present in most cases of crown, root, and crown-root fractures.[66]

Treatment for concussion is symptomatic: allow the tooth to rest as much as possible to promote recovery of trauma to periodontal ligament and apical vessels. Monitor pulpal status by EPT and watch clinically for tooth color changes and radiographically for evidence of resorption. The prognosis is good.[66]

Subluxation

When a tooth, as a result of trauma, is sensitive to percussion and has increased mobility, it is classified as subluxated. Electric pulp test results may be either no response or positive; if they are the former, damage to the apical neurovascular bundle is more severe, and pulpal recovery becomes questionable, except in developing teeth.[69–73]

Treatment initially may be none, except to recommend minimal use, or it may be necessary to stabilize the tooth for a short period of time (2 to 3 weeks) to promote periodontal ligament recovery and reduction in mobility[1] (Figure 15-25).

Subluxated teeth need to be evaluated long enough to be certain that the pulps have fully recovered. It may take **2 or more years** before one can make such a final determination. Pulps that do not recover sensitivity to EPT should be assumed to be necrotic even if they are asymptomatic. Definitive treatment for subluxated teeth often includes root canal therapy for fully developed teeth.[71]

Extrusive Luxation

Displacement of a tooth axially in a coronal direction results in a partial avulsion. The tooth is highly mobile

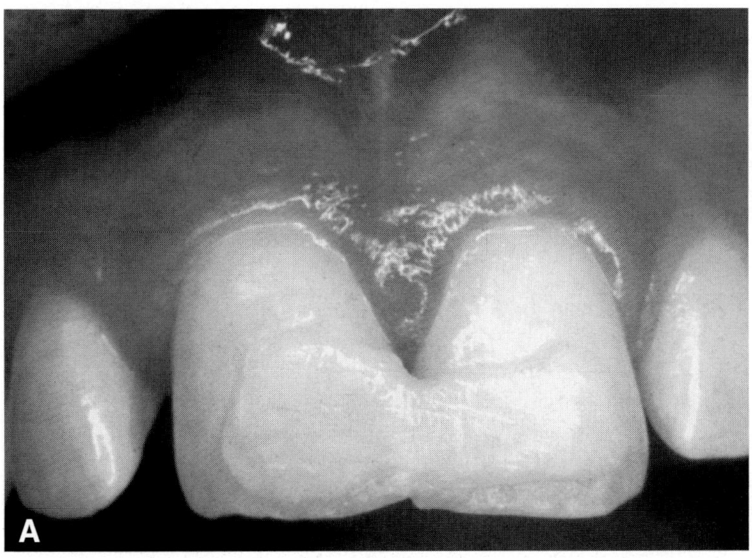

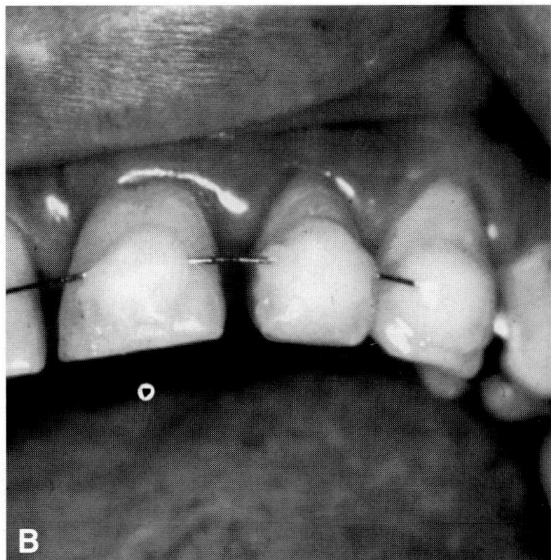

Figure 15-25 Examples of two types of functional splints. **A**, Unfilled resin is bonded to small, etched labial areas. Avoid etching interproximally. **B**, A thin (0.3 mm) orthodontic wire can be bonded to small, etched labial areas with resin.

and is likely to be continually traumatized by contact with opposing teeth, owing to the premature occlusal condition, all of it contributing to patient discomfort and severe tooth mobility[66] (Figure 15-26).

Immediate urgent care consists of repositioning the tooth, usually more easily accomplished than in lateral luxation, and stabilizing it by a functional splint for 4 to 8 weeks (see Figure 15-25). The relatively long stabilization period is to allow realignment of the periodontal ligament fibers supporting the tooth. It is important during this period that gingivitis be prevented. Gingival inflammation will negate any attempt of the tissue to repair itself. During recovery, progress can be monitored by periodontal probing. When reattachment has occurred, probing depth should be similar to pretrauma depth.[1,66]

Definitive treatment for extrusive luxation is likely to include root canal therapy,[71] except in young, developing teeth in which the pulps are more prone to recover.[69] It is important to watch for signs of root resorption if endodontic therapy, for any reason, is not included in the early treatment plan. Root canal therapy should be performed if the pulpal condition at any time is judged to be either irreversible pulpitis or pulp necrosis. It should be done without delay once the decision to do so has been made to reduce the chances of inflammatory root resorption.[1,67]

Lateral Luxation

Traumatic injuries may result in displacement of a tooth labially, lingually, distally, or mesially (Figure 15-27). Such displacement is called lateral luxation, and it is often very painful, particularly when the displacement results in the tooth being moved into a position of premature occlusion. An example of such lateral luxation is when a maxillary incisor is pushed palatally. The crown makes occlusal contact long before centric occlusion. The tooth is painful from the injury alone, and the additional constant trauma of premature contact results in severe pain.

Initial, urgent care for lateral luxation cases includes repositioning the tooth and stabilization if the tooth is mobile after being repositioned. Repositioning a laterally luxated tooth may require pressure application at the apical end of the root in the direction of the root apex's original location or by partially extracting the tooth with forceps prior to repositioning. The splinting, if needed, should be nonrigid and may need to be in place for 3 to 4 weeks, depending on how soon the supporting tissues recover.[1,66]

Definitive treatment for laterally luxated teeth includes root canal therapy (Figure 15-27, D), except in developing teeth, which may revascularize.[69,70] The tooth displacement has probably severed the blood vessels supplying the pulp, resulting in an infarct of the pulp owing to hypoxia. The end result is coagulation necrosis, which, even if asymptomatic, requires root canal therapy. If a decision to delay endodontic treatment is made, it is imperative to monitor the tooth radiographically for possible external, inflammatory root resorption. The prognosis for lateral luxation is good if proper endodontic therapy is performed when indicated.[66]

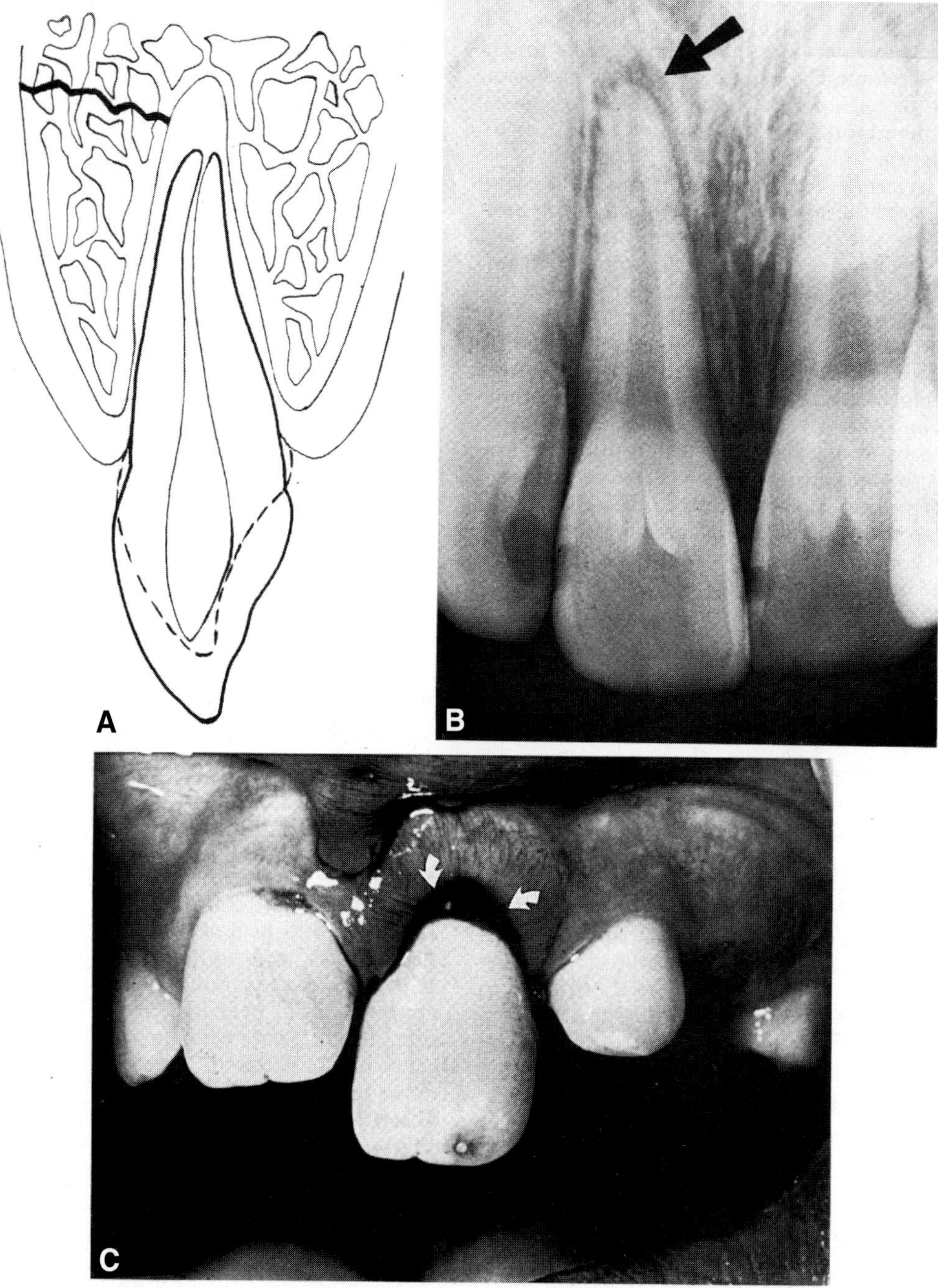

Figure 15-26 A, Tooth extrusion is similar to luxation in that the tooth is displaced, but the direction is axial. It may be accompanied by fracture of the alveolus. B, Note outline of root socket at apex (**arrow**). C, Bleeding is frequently seen from the gingival sulcus (**arrows**).

Intrusive Luxation

A tooth may be pushed into its socket, resulting in a very firm, almost ankylosed tooth (Figure 15-28). Such intrusive luxations require diverse treatment approaches depending on the stage of tooth development: little or no treatment for very immature teeth, **aggressive initial treatment** for more mature teeth.[1,66]

In cases of intrusive luxation of developing, immature teeth, the theory behind not doing anything initially is based on the expectation that a tooth with a wide open apex has the potential to re-erupt spontaneously and establish a normal occlusal alignment within a few weeks or months[74] (Figure 15-29). Monitor the progress of re-eruption, and if the tooth

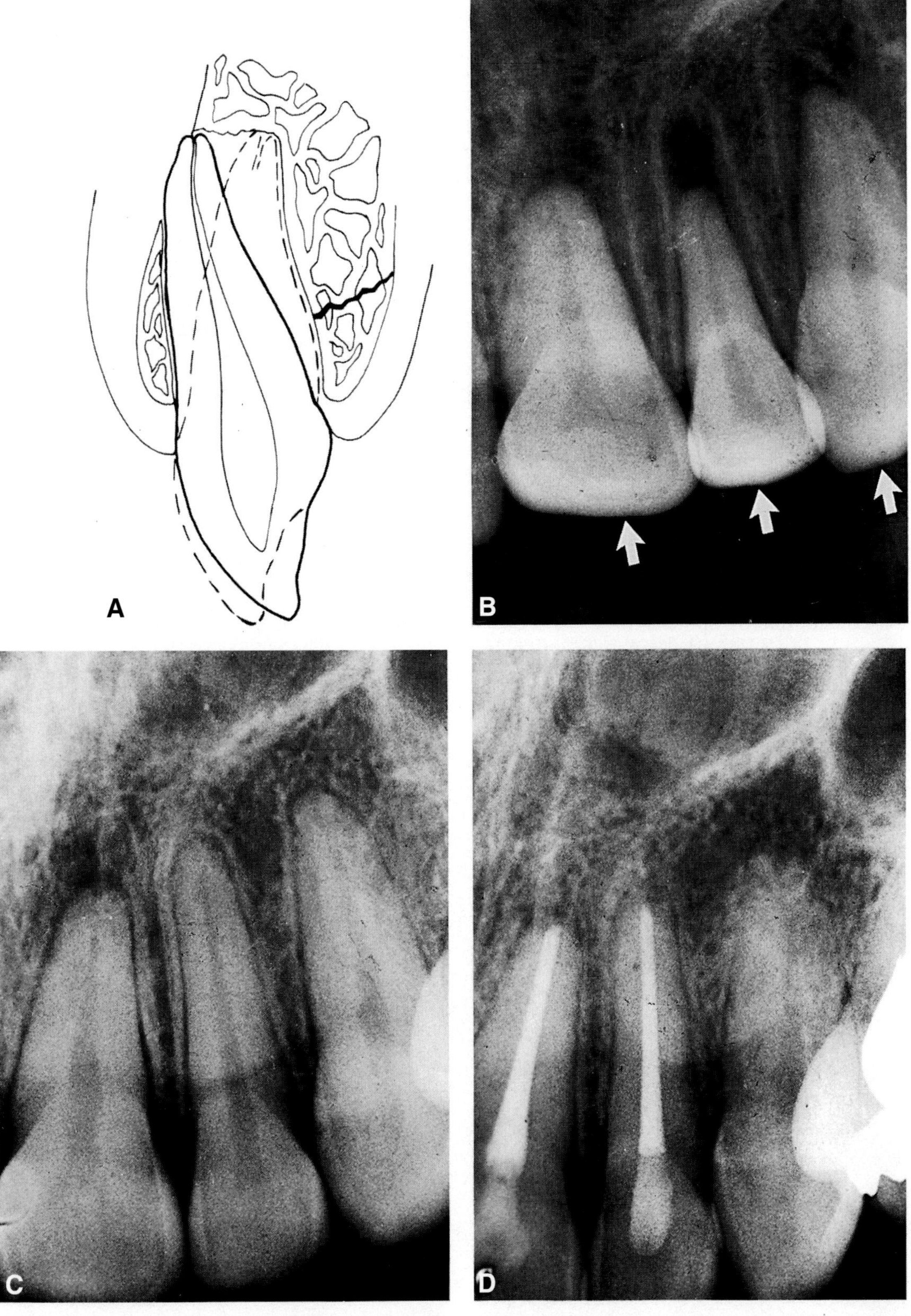

Figure 15-27 **A**, Tooth luxation with loosening and displacement is often accompanied by fracture or comminution of the alveolar socket. **B**, Luxation displacement of left central and lateral incisor and canine (**arrows**). **C**, After repositioning. **D**, The incisor required root canal therapy about 3 months later. Canine retained its pulp vitality. (Courtesy of Dr. Raleigh Cummings.)

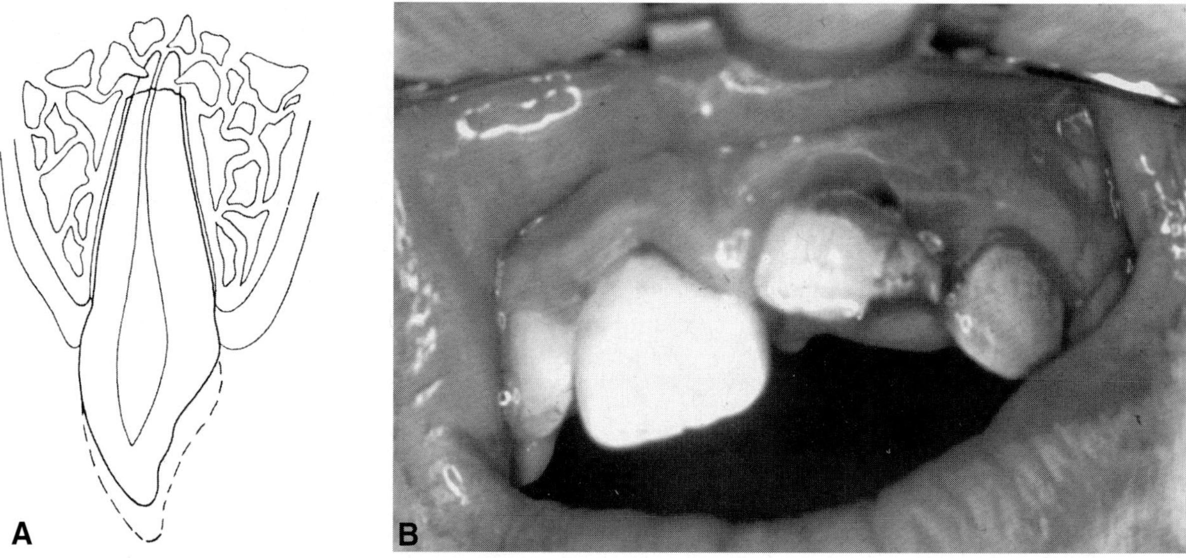

Figure 15-28 A, Graphic illustration of a tooth intruded into the alveolar bone. B, Clinical photograph of intruded incisor. Note bleeding from injured labial gingiva.

does in fact erupt into the normal position, no other treatment is needed. Radiographic control will probably show some bizarre pulpal calcification, but, lacking other evidence of pulpal deterioration, root canal therapy is not likely to be indicated.

Fully developed teeth, however, and those in which the roots are close to being developed should be repositioned either surgically or orthodontically or by a combination of both.[1] If allowed to remain in an intruded position, the tooth is very likely to become ankylosed, and later attempts at extrusion will probably be unsuccessful. The pulp should be prophylactically extirpated as soon as feasible, followed by completion of the root canal treatment after healing of the periodontal ligament (Figure 15-30). The exception to endodontic treatment is when spontaneous eruption takes place in young, developing teeth[1,66] (see Figure 15-29).

Prognosis and Follow-up Evaluation. Complications following luxation injuries are frequent. Pulp necrosis occurs in over half of the cases of lateral luxation, and even in subluxations, pulp death occurs in 12 to 20% of cases.[66] Extension of pulp necrosis to the periradicular tissues may take some time. Often apical periodontitis is not detected for several years post trauma, emphasizing the absolute need for long-term follow-up.[71]

Other complications are crown discoloration and reduction of the pulp lumen by calcification (Figure

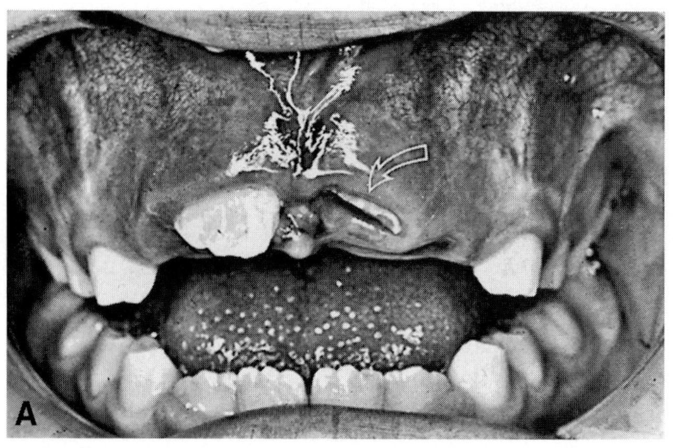

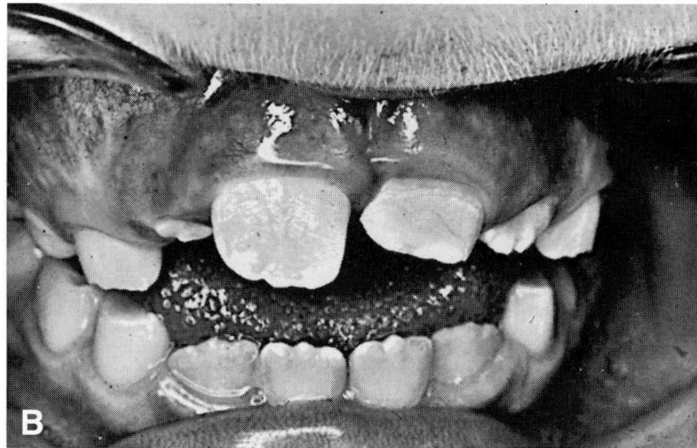

Figure 15-29 A, Intruded immature tooth (arrow). B, Six weeks later. Note re-eruption of the left central incisor, almost catching up with its contralateral mate.

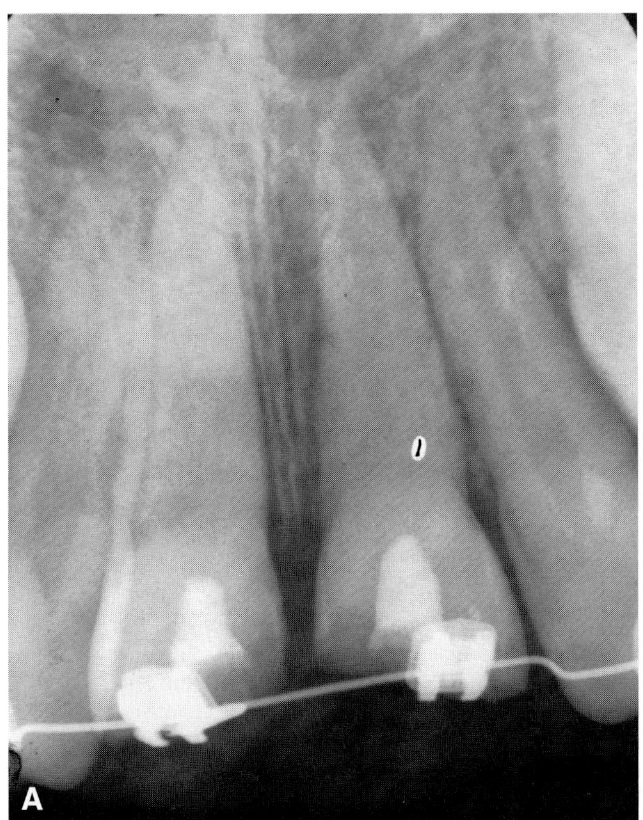

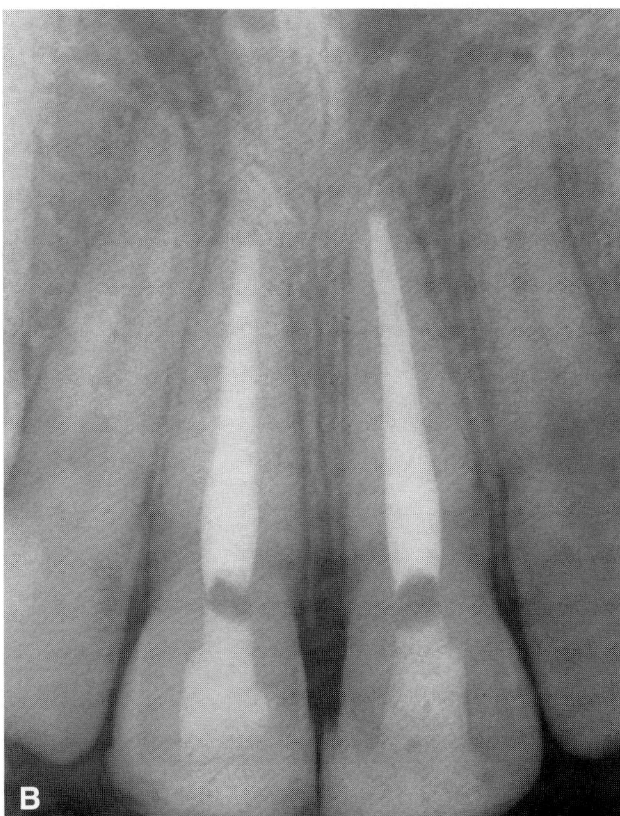

Figure 15-30 Maxillary central incisors were intruded; the crowns fractured also. **A**, The intruded teeth were orthodontically extruded and the pulps were extirpated, followed by placement of calcium hydroxide in the canals. **B**, Radiographs taken after extrusion was accomplished and the root canals were filled. The entire procedure took place over a 2-year period. No evidence of ankylosis is present. (Courtesy of Dr. Arthur LeClaire.)

15-31). A yellow discoloration is indicative of pulp space calcification, whereas a gray color indicates pulp necrosis. Lumen obliteration, as observed radiographically, is a very common occurrence but does not always indicate pulp necrosis and does not alone indicate the need for endodontic therapy even if the pulp does not respond to EPT, as so often happens.[64–67,69,74]

Resorption (external or internal) occurs in 5 to 15% of luxation injuries, usually within the first year and often within the first 2 to 5 months[66] (Figures 15-32 and 15-33). The possibility of resorption shows the need for follow-up. During the first year after trauma, evaluation should be done after 4 to 6 weeks and after 6 months. After that, yearly recalls are indicated.[71]

Treatment for resorption is root canal therapy, which can arrest the resorptive process if it is inflammatory external or internal resorption.[66,75]

If root formation is **incomplete** at the time of trauma, its continuation may be interrupted if the pulp dies. This presents serious treatment problems. Apexification procedures will provide an apical stop for root canal filling (Figures 15-34 and 15-35), but the

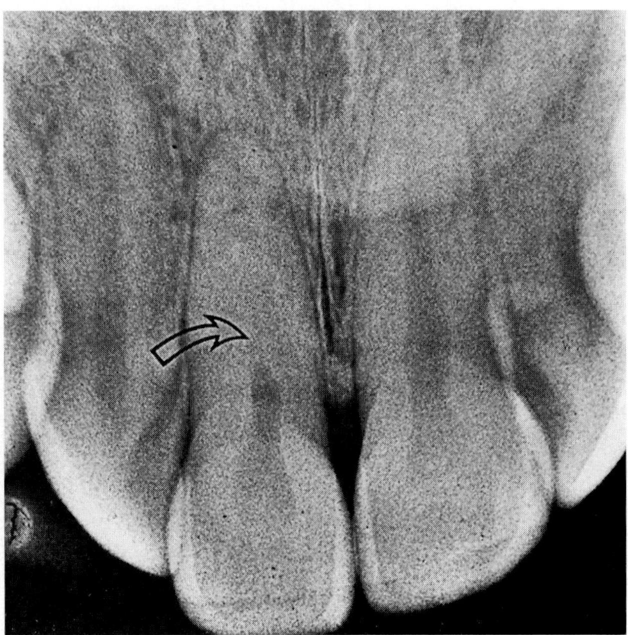

Figure 15-31 Right central incisor had been intruded in an accident when the patient was about 6 years old. The tooth re-erupted, and many years later the tooth is functional, asymptomatic, and responds to electric pulp testing, but shows dystrophic radicular calcification.

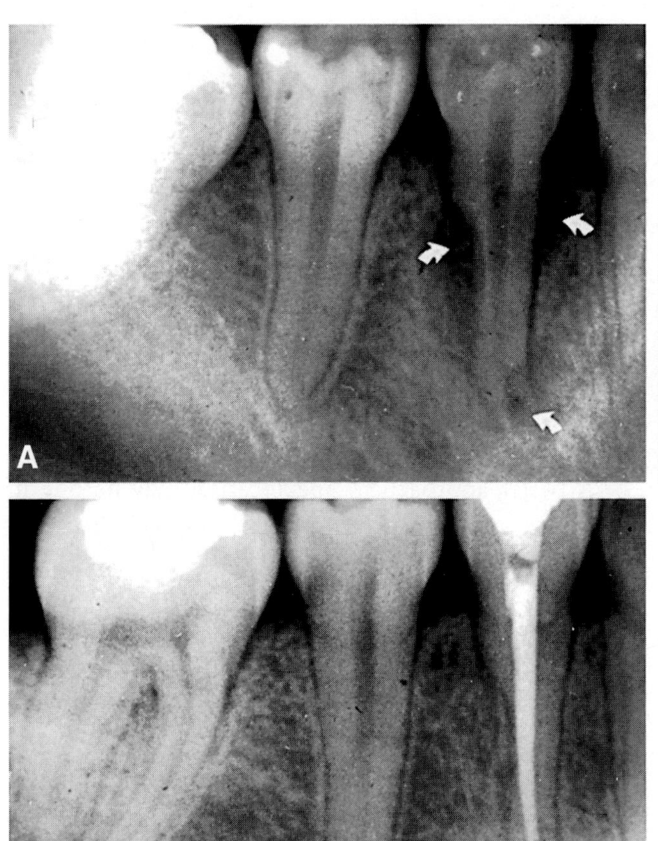

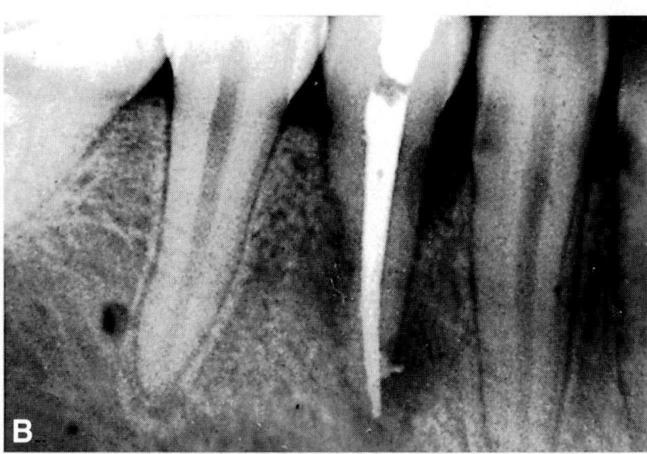

Figure 15-32 External inflammatory resorption. A, Accidentally luxated tooth, radiograph taken 8 weeks after the incident. Note resorption of both dental hard tissues as well as adjacent alveolar bone. B, Immediately after root canal therapy. C, Control radiograph taken 12 months later. Note repair of the alveolus and establishment of a new periodontal ligament space. The root canal procedure arrested the resorptive process. (Courtsey of Dr. Romulo de Leon.)

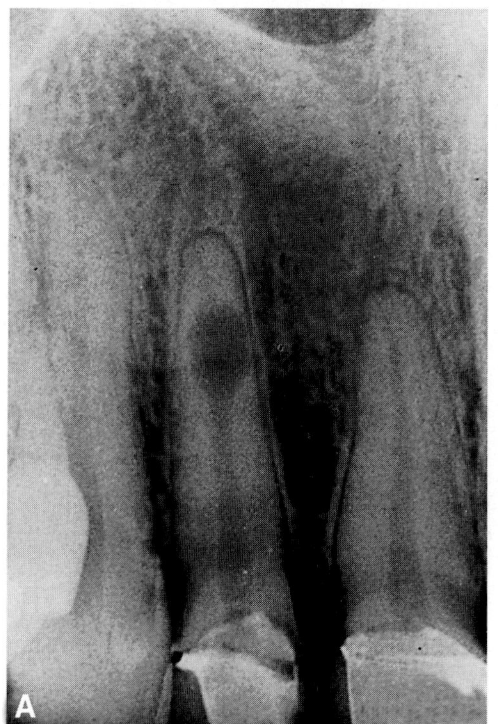

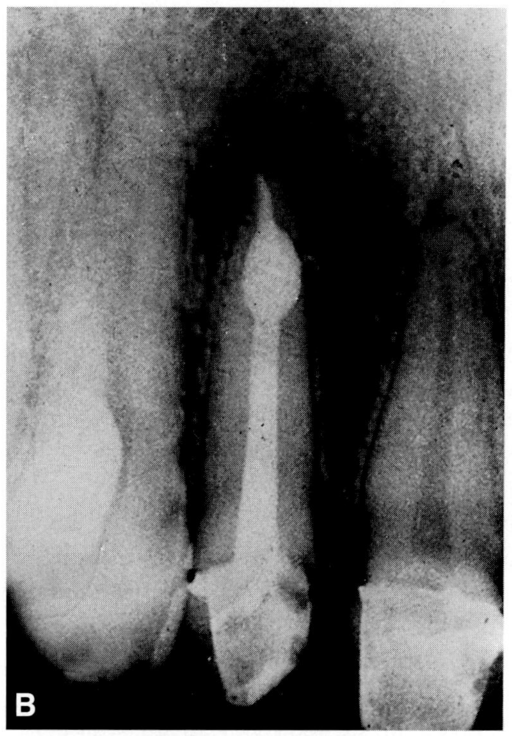

Figure 15-33 A, Internal resorption with a history of trauma. B, Immediately following root canal therapy.

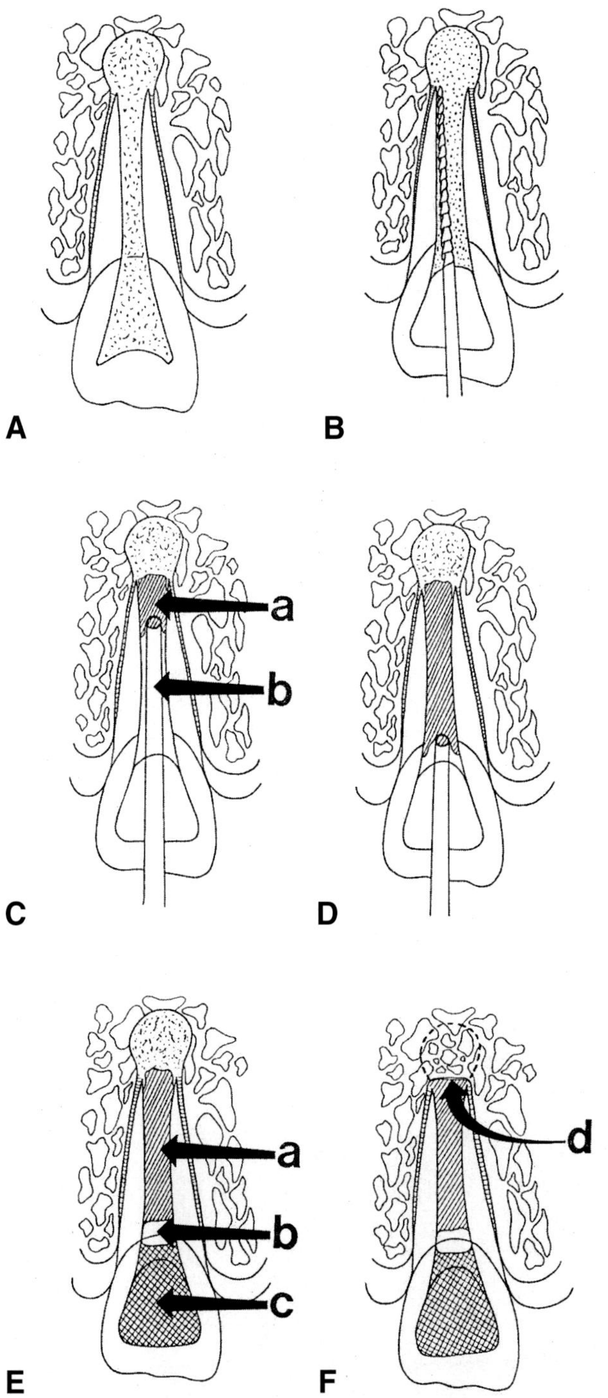

Figure 15-34 Graphic illustration of apexification procedure using calcium hydroxide to induce apical closure. **A**, Tooth with a necrotic pulp and an open, divergent apex. **B**, The thin root canal walls dictate that canal preparation be done very gently with minimal removal of dentin. The canal must be irrigated frequently. **C**, After careful cleansing of the canal, it can be filled with calcium hydroxide (a) to the level of vital tissue. Using a prepared calcium hydroxide paste deposited by a syringe and needle (b) combination facilitates the procedure. **D**, The needle is withdrawn as the material is deposited in the canal. **E**, During the treatment phase, the canal is filled with calcium hydroxide (a), on top of which is placed a cotton pellet (b), followed by a reinforced zinc oxide–eugenol paste or an acid-etched bonded resin. **F**, The goal is to induce an apical hard barrier (d).

teeth are weak and prone to fractures (Figure 15-36). Cvek showed that, after 4 years, fractures ranged from 77% of the most immature teeth to 28% of the most fully developed teeth.[75] Every effort should be made to promote revascularization of pulps in traumatized, developing teeth to allow continued root formation.

It is possible that a reason for the high incidence of cervical root fractures in teeth that have undergone calcium hydroxide apexification—in addition to the thin root walls of developing teeth—may be an adverse effect of calcium hydroxide on dentin, in which the dentin becomes progressively more brittle as it continues to be in contact with calcium hydroxide.[76]

A better approach to apexification may be one in which a combination procedure is done (see Figure 15-36):

1. Use calcium hydroxide for a short period of time—about 2 weeks—to assist in disinfection of the root canal.[77]
2. Place MTA in the apical part of the canal to serve as an apical plug that promotes apical repair.[78]
3. After checking that the MTA has cured, complete the root canal treatment with gutta-percha and a bonded resin restoration extending below the cervical level of the tooth to strengthen the root's resistance to fracture.[79]

Primary Teeth. Injury involving primary teeth results in damage to the supporting structures much more frequently than in crown or root fractures.[80] The initial observation is often a grayish discoloration of the crown, which may change to a yellow color, indicating calcification (Figure 15-37). This is in contrast to permanent teeth, in which a grayish crown discoloration indicates pulp necrosis. In primary teeth, the most frequent sequela to trauma is pulp space obliteration by calcification, although internal and external resorption, apical lesions, and discoloration can occur.[81]

Since the primary crown changes color in most trauma cases, treatment, whether endodontic or exodontic, should be done only in the presence of other clinical or radiographic signs of pulp necrosis. Electric pulp testing of primary teeth is not practical, so one has to rely on other information, such as periradicular osteitis.[81]

If periradicular lesions develop, either endodontic or exodontic treatment is indicated. Although periradicular inflammation of short duration appears to have little or no effect on the succedaneous permanent tooth, lesions present for protracted periods of time do cause defects in the permanent successor[82] (Figures 15-39 and 15-40).

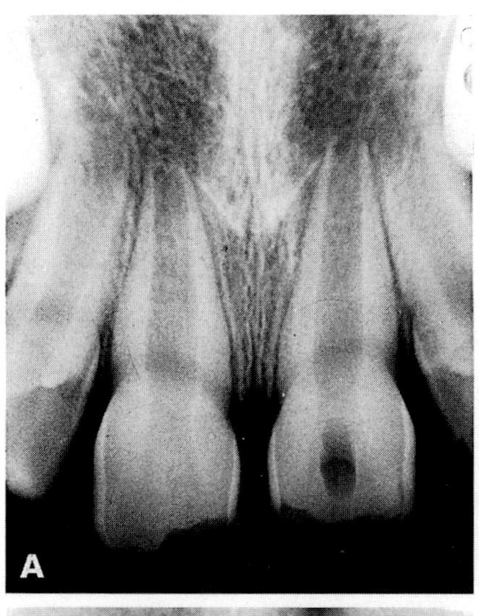

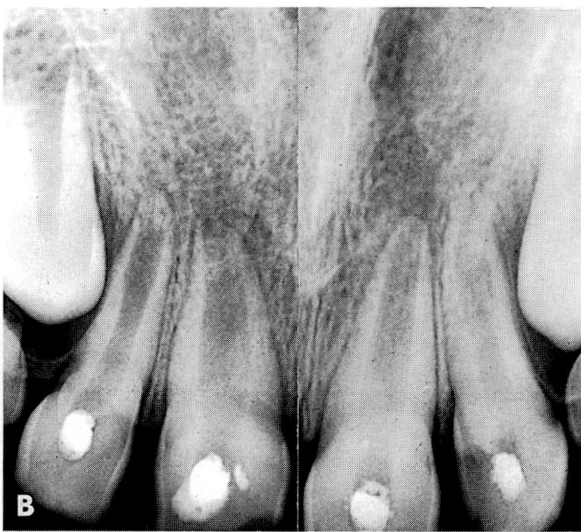

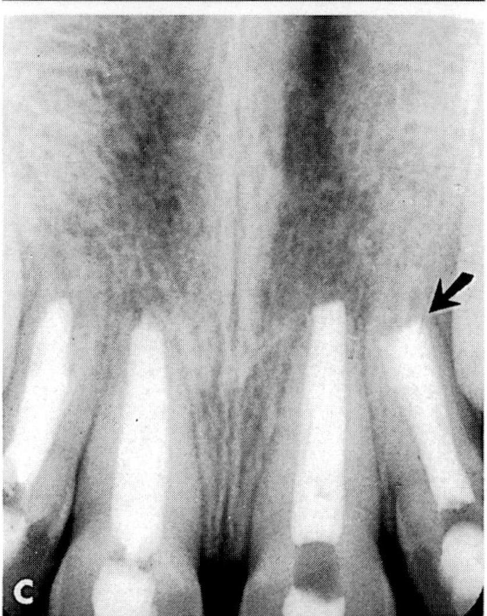

Figure 15-35 Induction of root-end closure with calcium hydroxide paste. **A**, Pulps of all four maxillary incisors have been devitalized by a traumatic accident. The apices are wide open. **B**, Seven months after filling with calcium hydroxide paste, the root apices have closed sufficiently to allow root canal filling. **C**, Root canals filled with gutta-percha. Total apical closure is shown by dense blunted fillings (**arrow**). (Courtesy of Dr. Alfred L. Frank.)

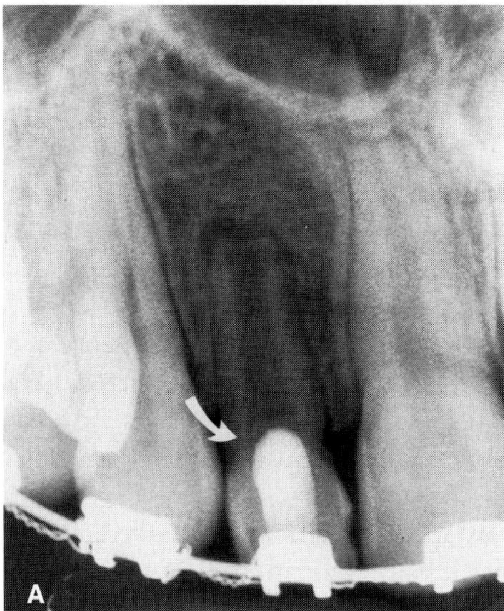

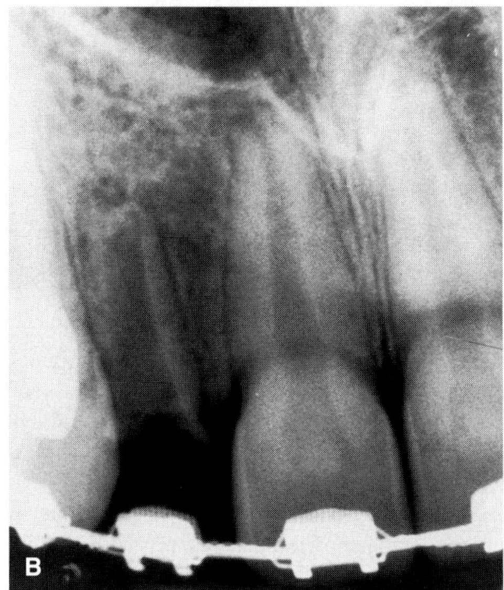

Figure 15-36 Fracture prone tooth. **A**, Owing to pulp necrosis in a developing tooth, apexification was begun with a good initial result; the apex was developing a hard tissue barrier. But the tooth is weak and prone to fracture cervically (**arrow**). **B**, The tooth did fracture as a result of a minor injury to the teeth.

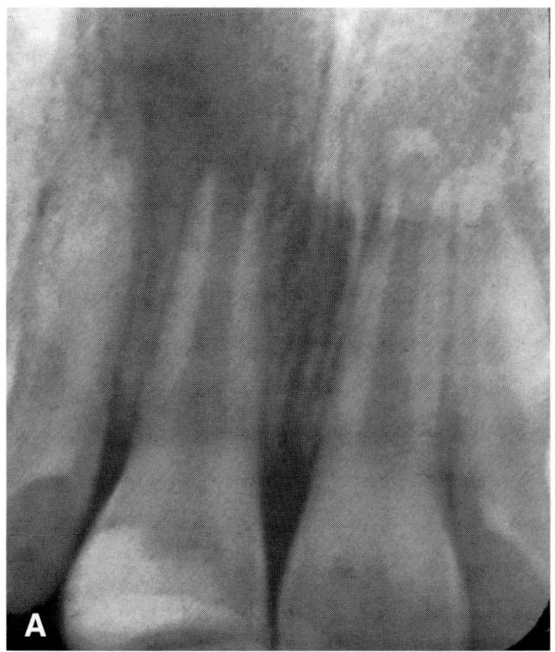

Figure 15-37 The use of mineral trioxide aggregate (MTA) for apexification. **A**, A combination of luxation injury and crown fractures led to pulp necrosis in the central incisors. After pulp extirpation, the canals were medicated with calcium hydroxide for 2 weeks, followed by placement of MTA in the apical portion of the canals. **B**, After the MTA had cured, the coronal portions of the canals were filled with bonded resin and the access cavities were restored with composite. **C**, Two years later, the radiograph shows good periradicular repair and evidence of apical hard tissue. (Courtesy of Dr. Mahmoud Torabinejad.)

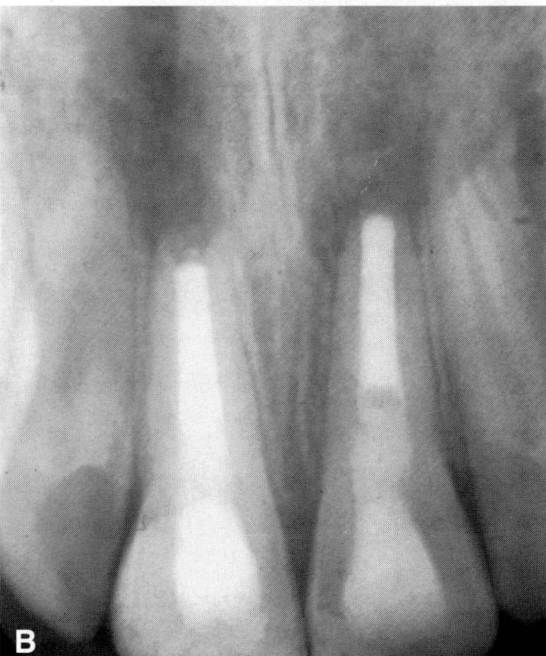

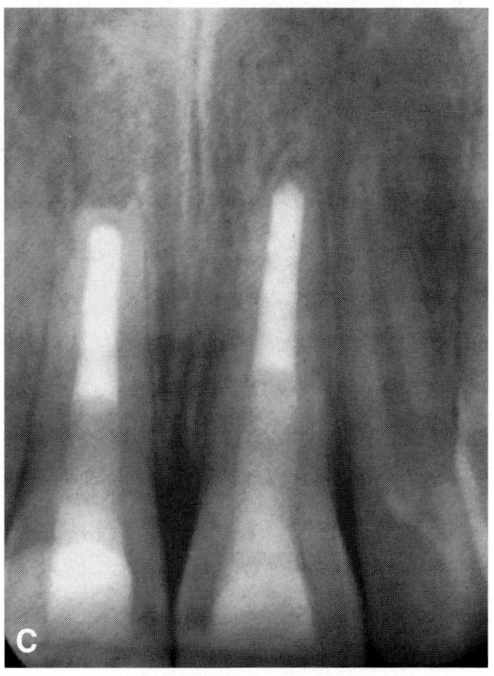

Because little or no hard tissue barrier is present apical to primary teeth, traumatic intrusion of a primary tooth affects the odontogenesis and the eruption of the permanent tooth. On the other hand, the damage is usually minor, and the majority of intruded primary teeth re-erupt within 6 months. Treatment is only symptomatic, but follow-up evaluation is important. If evidence of apical inflammation becomes apparent, endodontic treatment or extraction is indicated to protect the permanent successor.[82–84]

The most common observation of intruded primary teeth is a yellow crown discoloration, indicating pulpal calcification. No treatment is indicated for such teeth unless pulp necrosis and apical periodontitis occur[81] (see Figure 15-38).

Tooth Avulsion

An avulsed tooth is completely displaced out of its socket; this trauma has also been referred to as an exarticulation.[85]

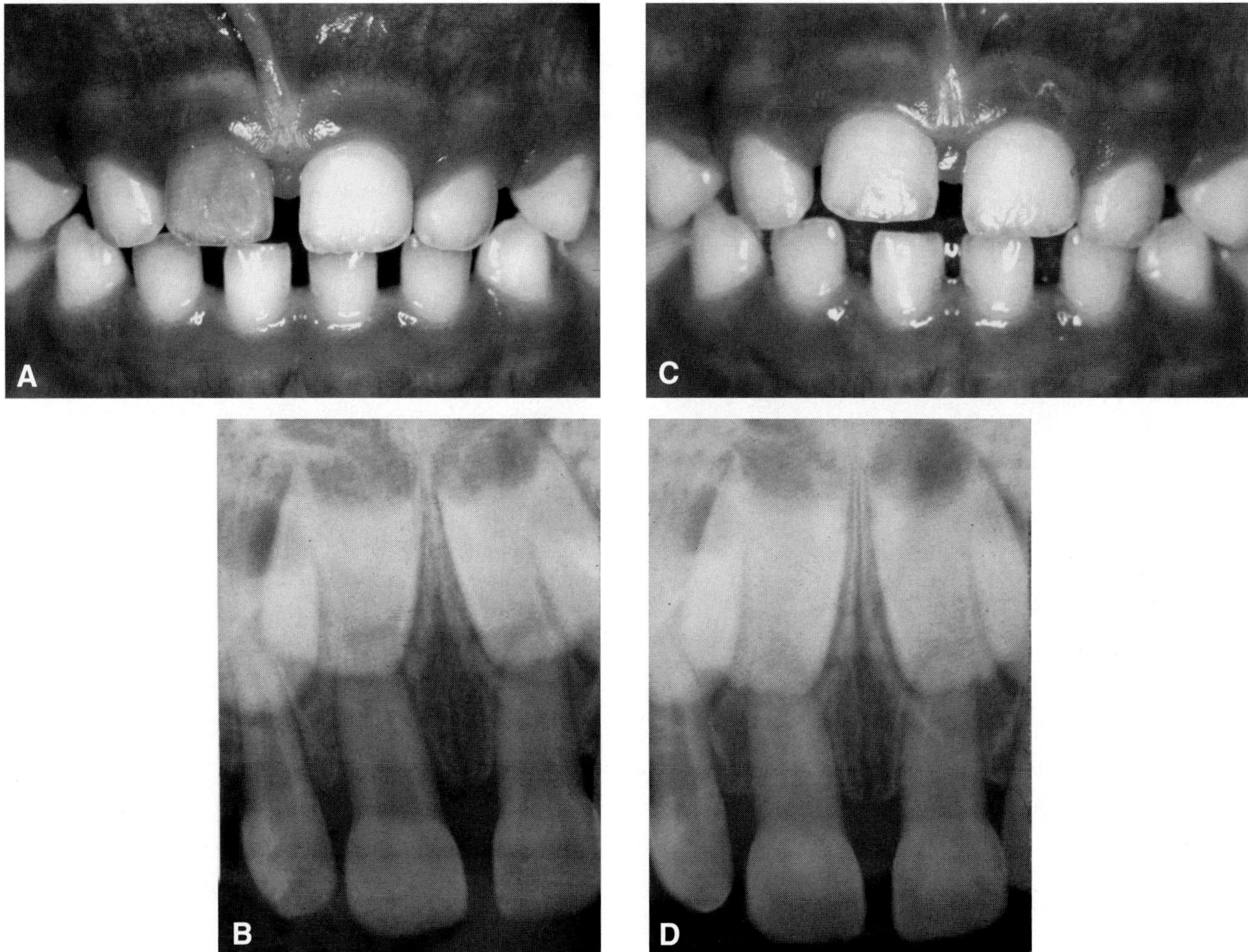

Figure 15-38 Luxation injury to primary tooth. **A**, After injury to the right primary central incisor, the crown showed discoloration, but the tooth was otherwise asymptomatic. **B**, The radiograph shows no displacement of the tooth. **C**, Six months later, the discoloration is no longer present, and **D**, the radiograph shows that the pulp has undergone calcific metamorphosis as a response to the trauma. (Courtesy of Dr. Mitsuhiro Tsukiboshi)

Description and Incidence. Teeth can be avulsed in many trauma situations. Sports and automobile accidents are the most frequent causes. The incidence of avulsion is reported to be less than 3% of all dental injuries.[85]

Tooth avulsion is a true dental emergency since timely attention to replantation could save many teeth.[85] Unfortunately, avulsed teeth are usually lost at the accident scene, and both accident victims and those attending them may neglect to consider the value of finding and saving the teeth. This may gradually change as the public continues to become aware of the possibilities that avulsed teeth can be saved.

Examination. The patient should be carefully examined regardless of whether the tooth has been replanted before coming to the dental office. Radiographs and clinical examination are necessary to help detect possible alveolar fractures. Such fractures of the tooth socket may reduce the prognosis but are not always a contraindication. Examine the tooth carefully for debris or contamination. Record the time of the avulsion. The length of extra-alveolar time determines both treatment procedures and prognosis. If the tooth has been left dry for less than 1 hour or kept in milk for no more than 4 to 6 hours, the protocol for treatment is described as "immediate" replantation; more than 1 hour of dry time is "delayed" replantation.[1,11,85]

Treatment: Immediate Replantation. Treatment success for avulsed teeth can be directly related to the extra-alveolar time before replantation: the sooner an avulsed tooth is replanted, the better the prognosis.[86] With that in mind, dentists and their staff should be prepared to advise parents and others who may call to report a tooth avulsion (Table 15-2).

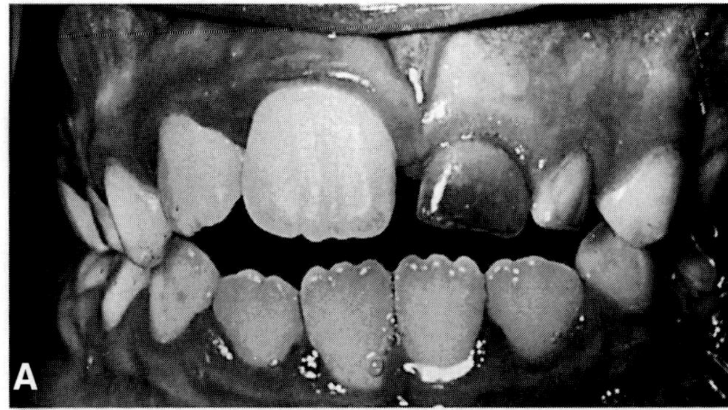

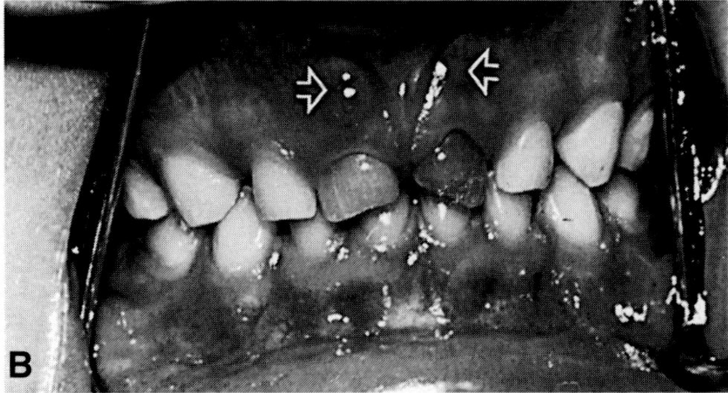

Figure 15-39 Discolored primary teeth indicating pulp trauma. **A**, The left **primary** central and lateral incisors have been retained by ankylosis, whereas the permanent right incisors have already erupted. **B**, Another case; both primary central incisors have necrotic pulps, evidenced by discoloration and labial swelling over apices (**open arrows**).

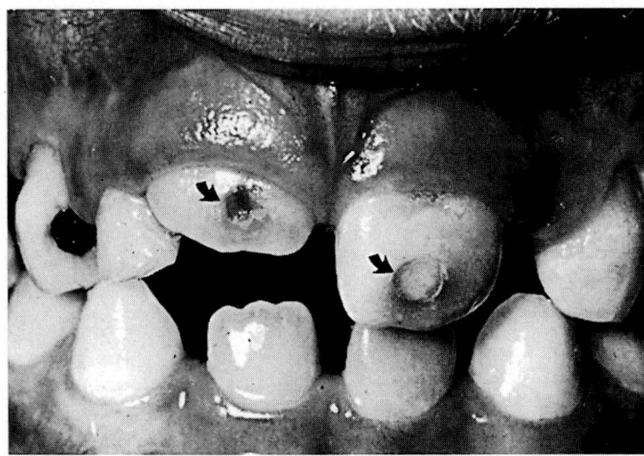

Figure 15-40 Injury to primary teeth led to defects in crowns of succedaneous central incisors.

Table 15-2 Guidelines for Replantation

Ideally, if an avulsed tooth can be replanted at the site of injury, the prognosis is better than waiting until the patient is transported to a treatment facility. The following advice can be given over the telephone to someone able to assist the victim:

1. Rinse the tooth in cold running water. The purpose is to rinse off any obvious debris that may have collected on the root surfaces.
2. Do not scrub the tooth. The less the root surface is touched, the less damage to fibers and cells. Suggest that the person applying these first-aid measures handle the tooth by holding on to the crown of the tooth and not the root.
3. Replace the tooth in the socket. Many individuals, even parents, may be squeamish about this step. A relatively easy way out is for the first-aid person to place the tooth, root tip first, partly into the socket, then let the patient bite down gently on a piece of cloth such as a handkerchief to move the tooth back into its normal, or nearly normal, position.
4. Bring the patient to the dental office right away to complete the treatment of replantation.

Often the person calling is not able to follow instructions to replant the tooth. Rather than waste time trying to explain a procedure to someone who is not prepared to follow the steps described, it is often more practical to urge that the patient and the tooth be brought immediately to the dental office. The manner in which the tooth is transported is important and needs to be explained to the person who accompanies the patient.

The ideal way to transport the tooth is to have it replaced in its socket, even if it will need to be repositioned in the dentist's office.[86] **Hank's Balanced Salt Solution** has been recommended as a transport medium to be kept in places where avulsion may occur.[87] Milk is more readily available and can serve satisfactorily for several hours to maintain cell vitality.[88,89] The least favorable medium is water; however, that is better than allowing the tooth to dry. If no milk is available, or while milk is being obtained, the tooth should be kept in the vestibule of the patient's mouth (or saliva) if possible.[1]

When the patient arrives, place the avulsed tooth in saline while the examination and preparation for replantation take place. Saline will support the survival of periodontal ligament cells on the tooth's root surface and allow the time necessary to prepare for treatment.[90]

Replantation in the office (Figure 15-41) must be preceded by a careful evaluation of the traumatized alveolus and the avulsed tooth. Radiograph the alveolar segment involved and any other oral area that appears also to have been injured. Look for evidence, both clinically and radiographically, of alveolar fracture. Inspect

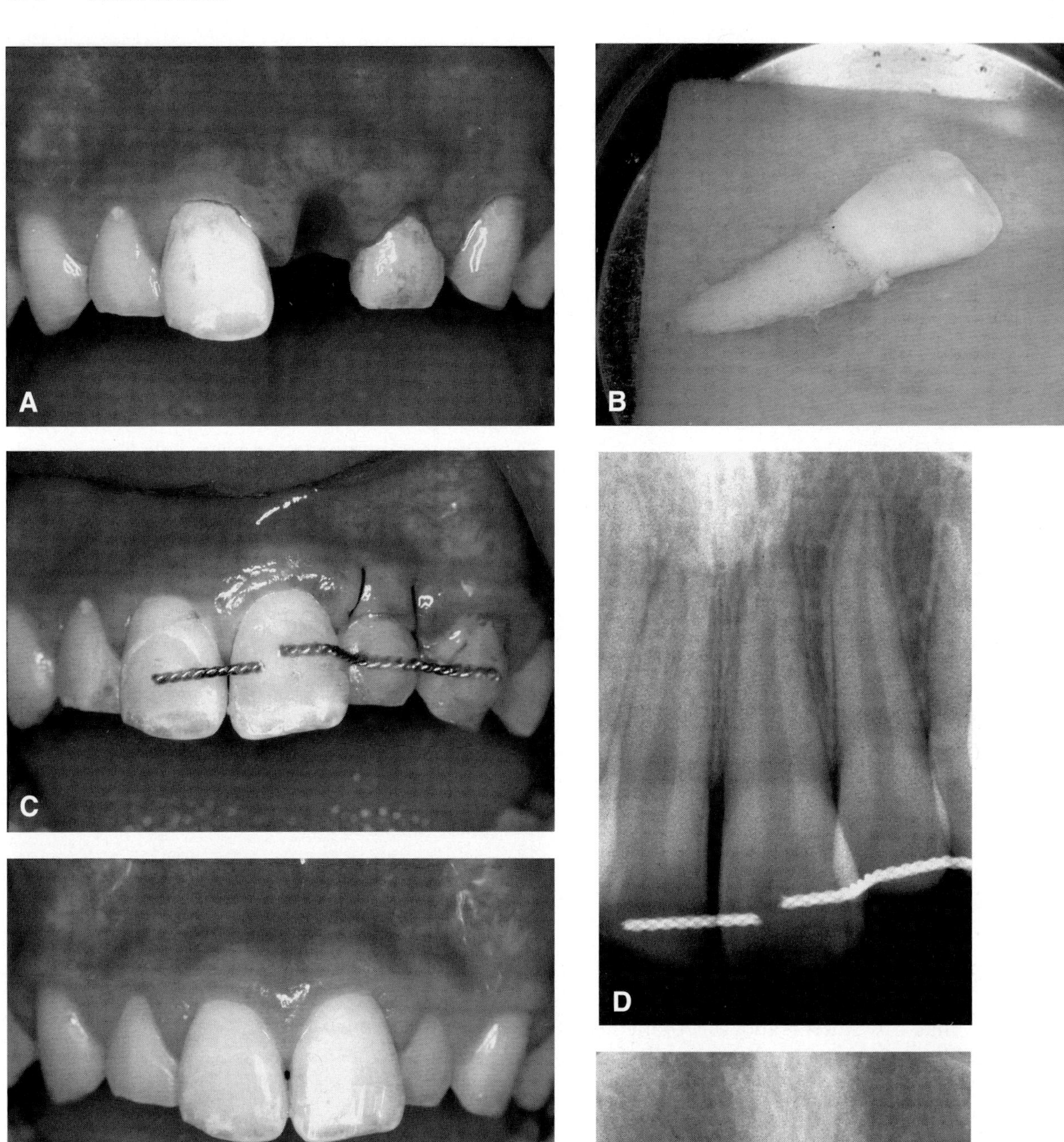

Figure 15-41 Replantation of avulsed tooth; the extra-alveolar time was less than 1 hour. **A** and **B**, The patient brought the tooth in his mouth. In the office, the tooth was placed in saline while the alveolar socket was examined. **C** and **D**, The avulsed tooth was replanted and splinted; the lacerated gingiva labial to the adjacent lateral incisor was sutured. Two weeks later, the splint was removed and endodontic therapy initiated. **E** and **F**, One year later, the tooth is functioning well, the tissues have healed, and, radiographically, the replantation looks satisfactory. (Courtesy of Dr. Mitsuhiro Tsukiboshi.)

the alveolar socket for foreign bodies and debris, **taking care not to scrape the bony walls.** The blood clot in the socket can be gently suctioned and the socket irrigated with saline. Check the avulsed tooth for debris on the root; if such debris cannot be rinsed off with saline or water, gently pick it off with cotton pliers. While inspecting the tooth, it can be held by the crown with a pair of extraction forceps. This permits examination of the tooth without touching the root surface.

After examining the alveolus and the tooth, begin replantation. Gently insert the tooth into the socket; anesthesia will probably not be necessary. The insertion should be slow and gentle so that pressure is minimized. When the tooth is nearly in place, have the patient complete the process by biting on a piece of gauze. Even small children will be able to follow the instruction to bite gently, and it allows them a measure of participation in the treatment.

The following steps in the replantation treatment also apply to situations in which the tooth may have been replanted before the patient's arrival. Check it for alignment with respect to adjacent and opposing teeth. **It is most important that it not be in hyperocclusion.** Such premature contact would delay or prevent recovery.[85]

Next, evaluate the need for stabilization. Splinting may not be necessary if the tooth fits firmly in its socket. If there is mobility, however, it should be stabilized with a functional splint (see Figure 15-25). Use either a thin orthodontic wire (0.3 mm) attached with acid-etched resin to the labial surfaces of the replanted and adjacent teeth or use only an unfilled resin bonded to small etched labial spots. In mixed dentition and cases of missing, nonreplaceable adjacent teeth, other types of splints may be necessary.[1,85,86]

The splint should be left in place only long enough for the initial reattachment of periodontal ligament fibers; in most cases, that can be expected to take place in 1 to 2 weeks, after which the splint should be removed [1,85,86] (Figure 15-42).

Further support of the replantation procedure consists of initial antibiotic coverage, tetanus prevention, and root canal therapy. The latter is ideally performed 10 to 14 days after replantation.

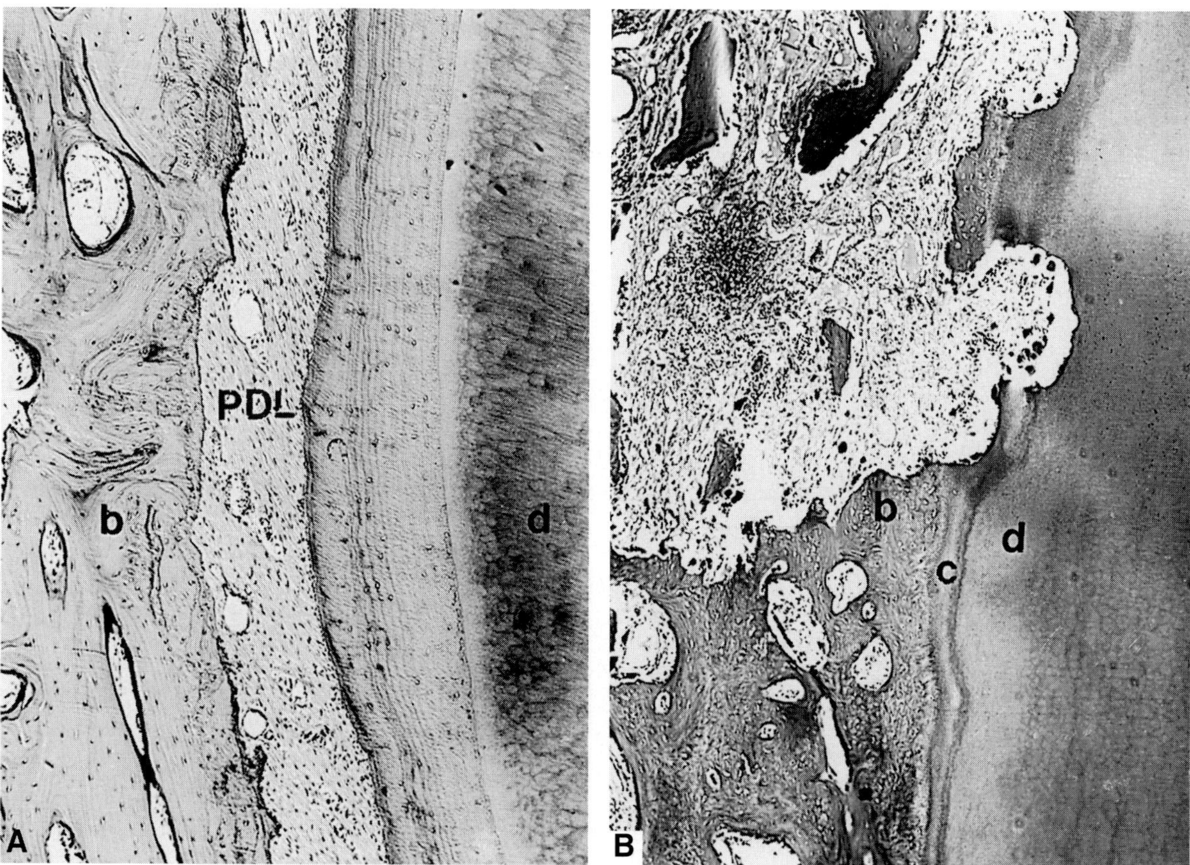

Figure 15-42 A, Replanted tooth **splinted for 7 days.** A normal periodontal ligament (PDL) is evident in this 4-month specimen. B, Replanted tooth **splinted for 30 days.** Replacement and inflammatory resorption covered the apical half of the tooth. b = bone; c = cementum; d = dentin. Reproduced with permission from Nasjleti CE, Castelli, WA, Caffesse RG. Oral. Surg 1982; 53:557.

Antibiotics should be administered from the time of replantation; prescribe a dosage regimen similar to that recommended for a mild to moderate dental infection. Coverage for 5 to 7 days should suffice.[85,91]

If the patient has not had a tetanus vaccination, referral to a hospital or physician is indicated. If the patient has had a vaccination, but more than 5 years have passed since the vaccination or any subsequent booster injections, a booster injection following the replantation is necessary.

The optimal time for root canal therapy in a replanted avulsed tooth is about 10 to 14 days after replantation.[85,89,92] The only exception to the rule of root canal therapy for avulsed teeth is when the tooth is still developing and has a wide open apical foramen[93–95] (Figure 15-43). Such teeth have the potential for pulp revascularization. If the replanted tooth falls into this category, monitor its progress carefully with frequent, periodic radiographs. If the pulp does not revascularize, it will become necrotic and lead to the same postreplantation sequelae that can be expected from any replanted tooth that has not been treated endodontically: inflammatory resorption (Figure 15-44).

Calcium hydroxide has been recommended as an intracanal medication during root canal therapy.[85,96,97] Based on current evidence,[89,92,97–99] it appears reasonable to use calcium hydroxide for canal disinfection (about 2 weeks), and in situations in which resorption has begun, use the calcium hydroxide until resorption has ceased. The completion of the root canal treatment must include a proper root canal filling and a protective coronal restoration.

Treatment: Delayed Replantation. The treatment for teeth with more than 1 hour of extra-alveolar time includes efforts to slow the inevitable replacement resorption:

1. Examine the avulsed tooth for debris. In contrast to avulsed teeth with less than 1 hour extra-alveolar time, those with more than 1 hour are not expected to retain the vitality of periodontal ligament cells and fibers. Therefore, it is best to remove pieces of soft tissue attached to the root surface. This needs to be accomplished without overtly scraping the root surface.[1,11,85]
2. Perform root canal therapy with the tooth in vitro. This can often be best accomplished by holding the tooth by the crown and proceeding with the endodontic treatment through an apical approach. Cut off 2 to 3 mm of the root apex to expose the root canal, extirpate the content of the canal and pulp chamber, and then fill with gutta-percha and sealer. An advantage in doing root canal therapy this way, along with convenience, is that the crown of the tooth can be left intact.

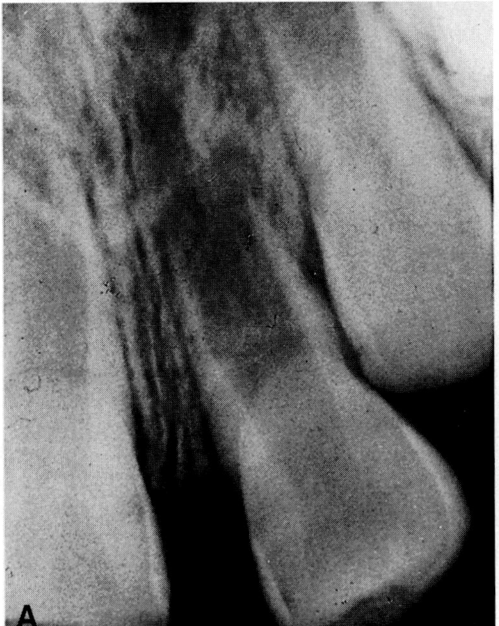

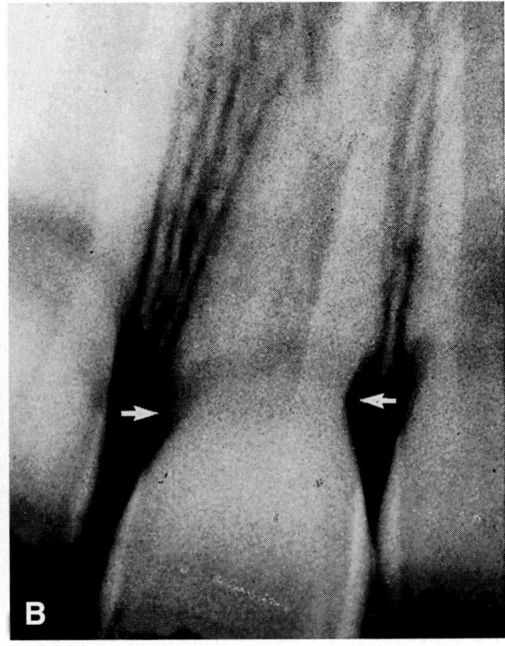

Figure 15-43 An avulsed left central incisor in a 6-year-old boy was replanted immediately. **A**, When re-evaluated after 8 weeks, there was still response to electric pulp testing. **B**, One year after trauma, the tooth was in the normal position and had no discoloration but did not respond to electric pulp testing. The root has continued to develop and the pulp appears to be calcifying. Also note hourglass erosion/resorption cervically (**arrows**). (Courtesy of Dr. Robert Bravin.)

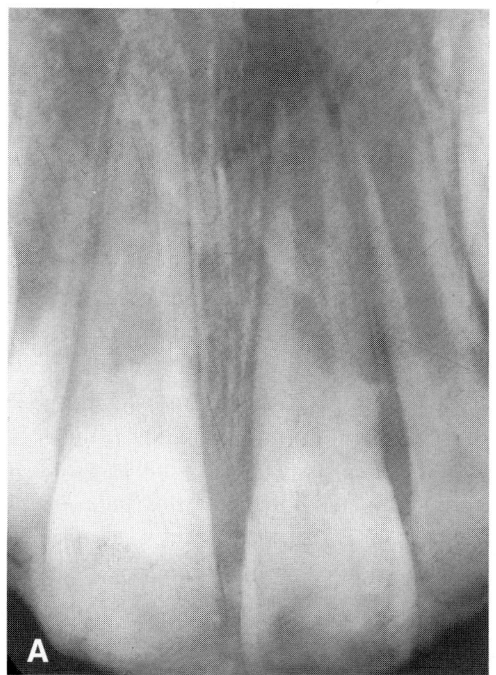

Figure 15-44 Replanted avulsed tooth in which revascularization did not occur. A, Radiograph of a left central incisor taken 2 weeks after replantation. Note the open apex. B, Radiograph taken 4 months later shows aggressive inflammatory resorption. In an effort to try to keep the tooth for some time, the pulp was extirpated, and calcium hydroxide was placed in the canal. C, Six months later, the radiograph shows remarkable response to treatment—an indication of the result that could have been accomplished if endodontic therapy had been initiated much earlier.

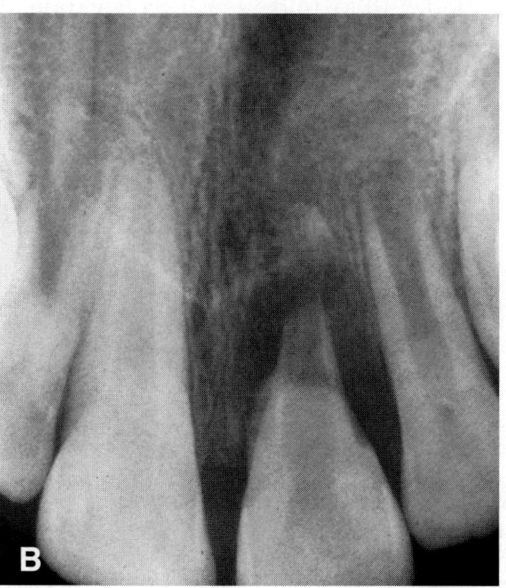

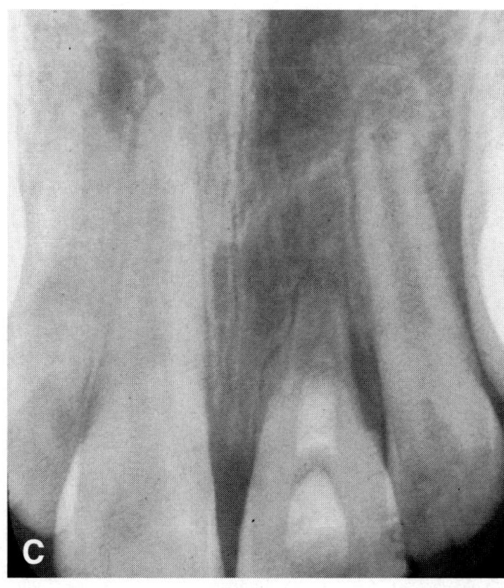

3. Soak the tooth in a 2.4% fluoride solution acidulated at pH 5.5 for 20 minutes or more. The fluoride will slow the resorptive process.[1,85]
4. Prepare the tooth socket by gently curetting the blood clot out of the alveolar socket and then irrigate with saline.[1,85]
5. Rinse the tooth thoroughly in saline and then insert it into the socket and splint for 6 weeks.[1,85]
6. An additional procedure that is showing promise in reducing resportion is to fill the tooth socket with Emdogain (Biora, Inc, Chicago, Illinois) prior to replantation.[100]

Because replanted teeth with more than 1 hour of extra-alveolar time are expected to resorb and ankylose, it is probably reasonable to expect only a limited length of service from such teeth.[101] However, if the resorption is relatively slow, several years of service may result, and this is probably reason enough for performing this relatively simple procedure. It must be noted, however, that in young patients, such ankylosis can result in a lack of alveolar ridge development, so when infraocclusion becomes apparent in a growing child, it may be advisable to remove the crown in a process termed "decoronation" to allow proper ridge development.[102]

Avulsed Teeth with Open Apices. The only exception to the rule that replanted teeth must be treated endodontically is the situation in which a very immature, developing tooth with a wide open apex has been avulsed and replanted (see Figure 15-43). Such teeth have the potential for revascularization and therefore should be monitored after replantation to look for signs of revascularization (ie, continued root formation and absence of resorption and ankylosis).[95,103,104] It has been recommended to soak the avulsed tooth in a solution of doxycycline (1 mg/20 mL saline) prior to replantation.[11,104]

Primary Teeth. Most authors advise against replantation of **primary** teeth unless ideal conditions exist to prevent trauma to the permanent succedaneous tooth.[105]

Prognosis and Follow-up Evaluation. Resorption is the most frequent sequela to luxation injuries; three different types of resorption have been identified: surface, inflammatory, and replacement (ankylotic) resorption[106–108]:

- **Surface resorption**: small superficial cavities in cementum and outermost dentin. This type is not visible on radiographs and is usually repaired by new cementum. It may be transitory or progressive. The former leads to repair, the latter to further resorption (see below). Surface resorption is usually detectable only histologically and probably represents part of the process that takes place both during recovery and as a prelude to more severe resorption.[107]
- **Inflammatory resorption**: radiographically seen as a bowl-shaped resorptive area of the root and associated with adjacent bony radiolucencies. It involves both tooth structure and adjacent bone. Radiographically, there is apparent tooth loss along with adjacent bony destruction. This type of resorption is typical in the apical area involving any tooth with a necrotic pulp; replanted teeth that have not had root canal treatment often show these resorptive lesions laterally as well as apically. Root canal therapy can be expected to arrest inflammatory resorption that involves replanted teeth; the resorption can be prevented by judicious timing of the root canal therapy. Optimally, that is about 10 to 14 days post replantation[1,11,85,86,106] (see Figure 15-44).
- **Replacement resorption**: resorption of the root surface and its substitution by bone, resulting in anky-

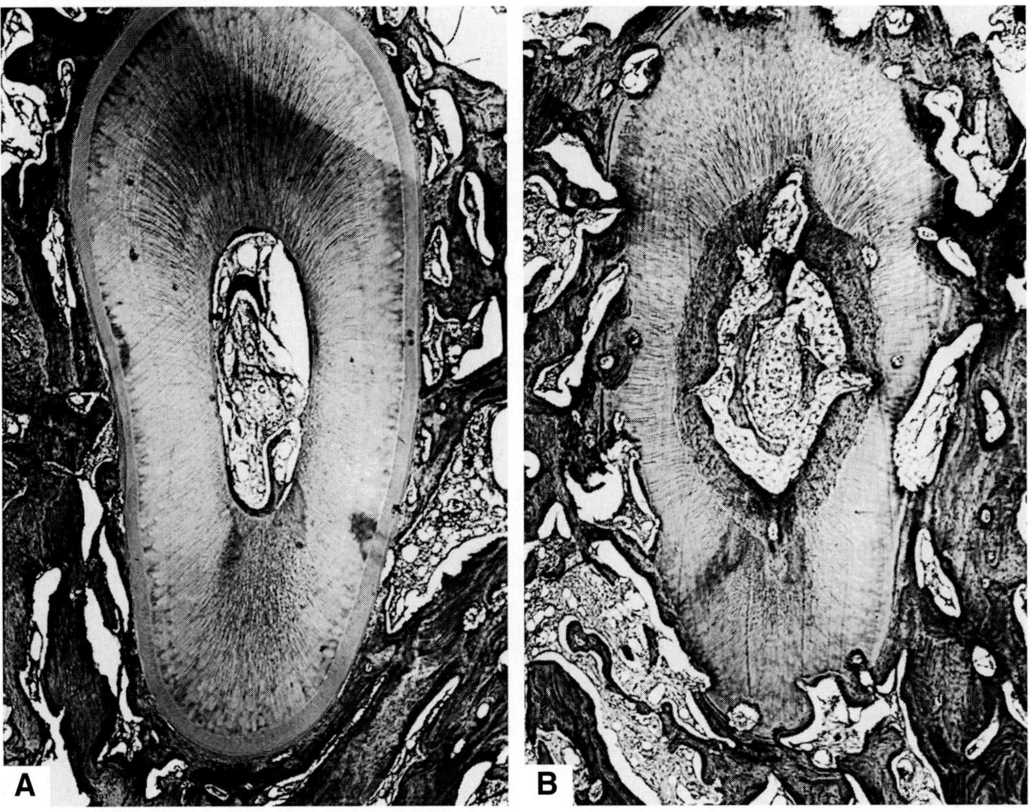

Figure 15-45 A, Reattachment of a replanted tooth treated enzymatically with hydrochloric acid, hyaluronidase, and glutaraldehyde. B, Control tooth, untreated and replanted, with extensive inflammatory and replacement resorption. Reproduced with permission from Nevins AJ, La Porta RF, Borden BG, Lorenzo P. Oral Surg 1980; 50:277.

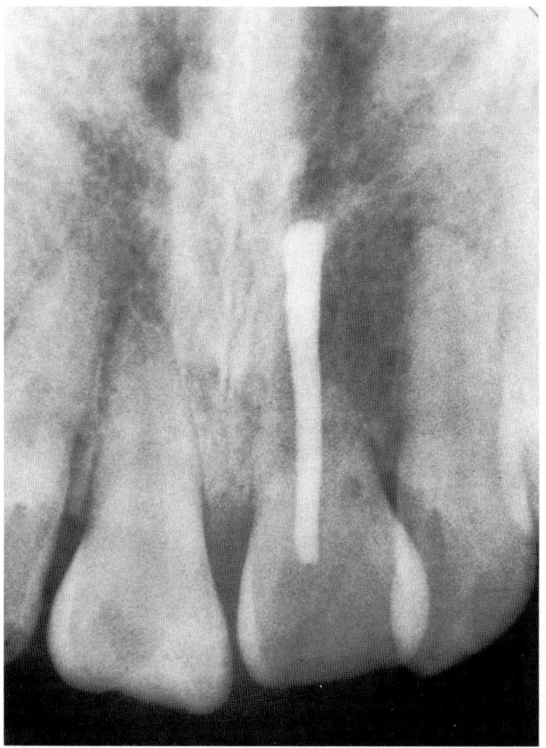

Figure 15-46 Radiograph showing replacement resorption 5 years after replantation of an avulsed tooth with more than 2 hours extra-alveolar time. Note infraocclusion owing to the ankylosis.

losis (Figure 15-45). This is a frequent sequela to replantation. As tooth structure is resorbed, it is replaced with bone that fuses to the tooth structure, thereby producing ankylosis. Root canal therapy has no effect on replacement resorption (Figure 15-46). Replacement resorption can be expected in replanted teeth in which the root surface elements have become necrotic, usually owing to the drying effect of too long extra-alveolar time. Teeth not replanted within 1 hour of avulsion can be expected to fall into this category.[106,107]

Facial Skeletal Injuries

Fractures of the Alveolar Process and the Mandible and Maxilla. These are closed fractures or comminutions (crushing or compression) that involve the socket walls in the case of the alveolar process fractures and may or may not involve the tooth sockets in fractures of the body of the mandible or the maxilla[109] (Figure 15-47).

It was common practice in the past to remove teeth located in a jaw fracture line. Today, however, it is recognized that removal of such teeth does not improve the prognosis for the bone fracture. With the use of antibiotics, fractures involving teeth can be treated conservatively.[109–114]

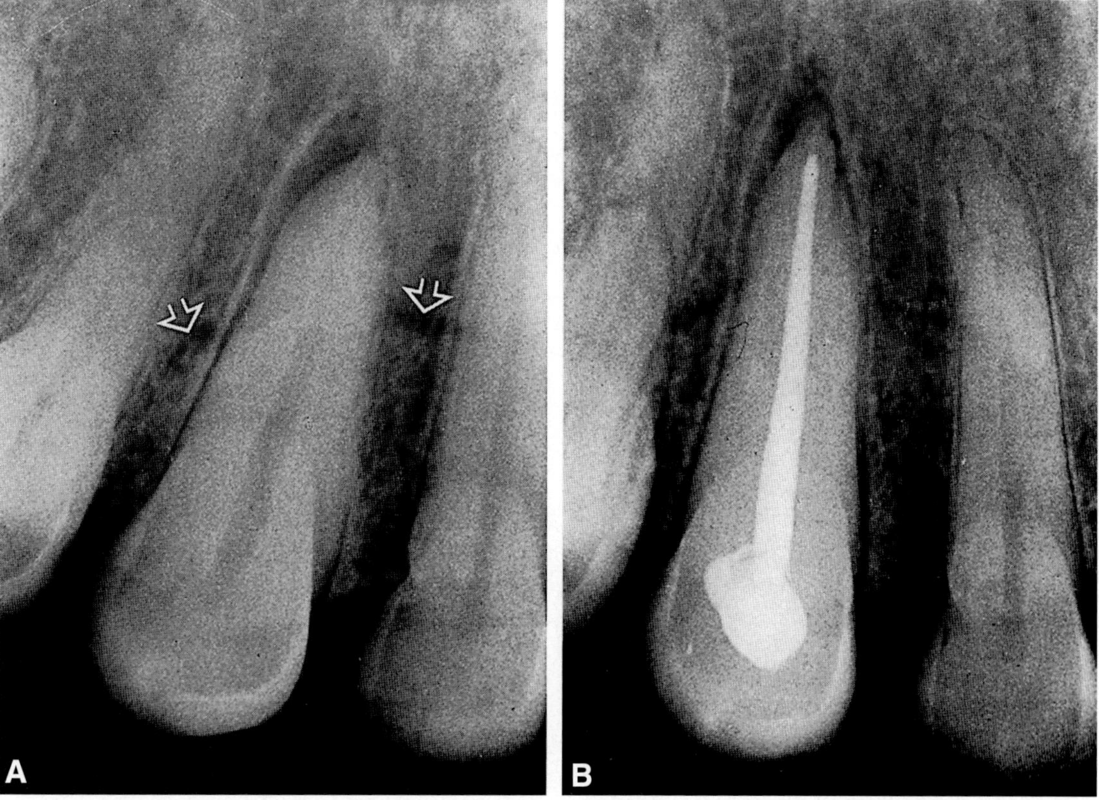

Figure 15-47 A, Alveolar fracture (**arrows**) and displacement of right canine treated by repositioning the tooth. B, A few weeks later symptoms indicative of apical periodontitis developed, and root canal therapy was performed. (Courtesy of Dr. Eugene Kozel.)

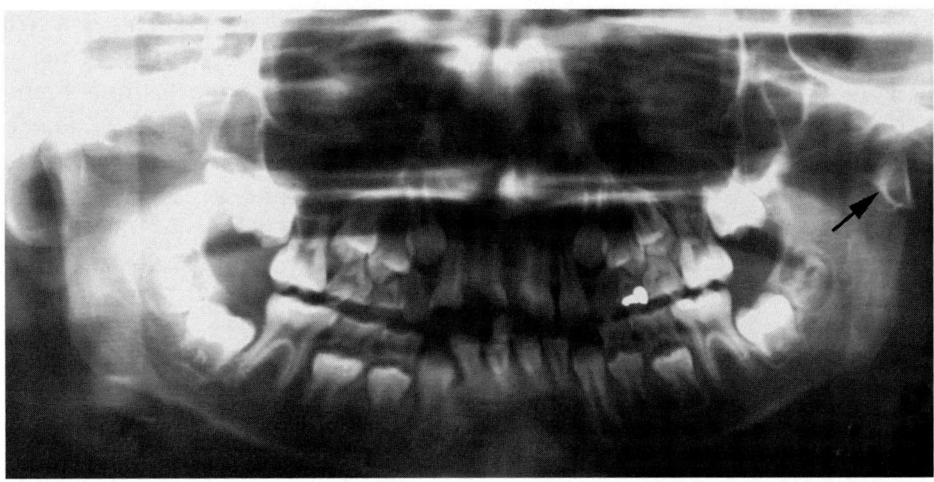

Figure 15-48 Panoramic film of an 8-year-old patient after a bicycle accident. In addition to maxillary anterior crown fractures, the left temporomandibular condyle also fractured.

Examination and Diagnosis. Fist fights and bicycle and traffic accidents account for most cases of jaw fractures. The most frequent locations are in the mandible—the angles near the third molars and the canine areas.[110] Teeth involved in the fracture lines should be pulp tested; a transitory negative response is common, and of the teeth not responding initially, about 25% can be expected to recover.[112] Locating the fracture and identifying the involved teeth are the basic considerations in the examination of this group of injuries.

Treatment. Initial treatment consists of reduction of the fracture and stabilization by splinting for 3 to 4 weeks.[112–114] Analgesic and antibacterial supportive treatment is needed. Stabilization must be carefully done because persistent dislocations increase the chances for pulp necrosis in affected teeth. Stabilization should be carried out as soon as possible.[112] The length of time between trauma and treatment adversely affects the prognosis of involved teeth.[111] Unless concomitant tooth fractures occur, no treatment of the teeth is needed **initially**.

Prognosis and Follow-up. Although teeth involved in jaw fractures need not be extracted and may help stabilization, 25 to 40% develop pulp necrosis and in time develop periradicular lesions.[111,113] For that reason, **follow-up evaluation is important** and should be done at 3-, 6-, and 12-month periods after initial treatment. Yearly examination for several years alerts one to pulp complications necessitating treatment intervention. Although it may not be mandatory to treat all teeth not responding to the EPT, it should be noted that in one report, all five such teeth that were opened were found to have necrotic pulps.[111–113]

Temporomandibular Joint

A blow to the mandible may result in injuries to the temporomandibular joints. In young children, the condylar necks are rather thin and can easily fracture, particularly if the blow causes a retrusive force on the mandible[115] (Figure 15-48).

Clinically, traumatized joints may be painful to palpation; in more severe injuries, mandibular function may be compromised, and the patient may have difficulty moving the lower jaw.[116]

Immediate care of temporomandibular joint injury involves jaw stabilization and symptomatic treatment of joint pain. Careful evaluation, both radiographic and clinical, must be made to determine what, if any, definitive treatment will be necessary. Fractures of the condylar neck with displacement of the condylar head are usually treated by closed reduction in young children. The displaced condyle remodels well to a normal upright position.[117] The main factors to remember about trauma involving the temporomandibular joints are (1) to not overlook the possibility of such fractures, particularly in young children,[115] and (2) that preventive measures—seatbelts and airbags in cars and face and mouth protection in sports—can be very effective in reducing injuries.[2]

REFERENCES

1. Andreasen JO, Andreasen FM, Bakland LK, Flores MT. Traumatic dental injuries—a manual. Copenhagen; Munksgaard; 1999.
2. Padilla R, Dorney B, Balikov S. Prevention of oral injuries. Can Dent Assoc J 1996;24:30.
3. Andreasen JO, et al. Replantation of 400 avulsed permanent incisors. Endod Dent Traumatol 1995;11:51.

4. Andreasen JO. 35 years of dental traumatology. Lecture to the International Association of Dental Traumatology, Melbourne, Australia, March 15, 1999.
5. Andreasen JO, Andreasen FM. Classification, etiology and epidemiology of traumatic dental injuries. In: Andreasen JO, Andreasen FM, editors. Textbook and color atlas of traumatic injuries to the teeth. 3rd ed. Copenhagen: Munksgaard; 1993. p. 151–77.
6. Huelke DF, Compton CP. Facial injuries in automobile crashes. J Oral Maxillofac Surg 1993;41:241.
7. Kvittem B, et al. Incidence of orofacial injuries in high school sports. J Public Health Dent 1998;58:288.
8. Kaste LM, et al. Prevalence of incisors trauma in persons 6 to 50 years of age: United States, 1988–1991. J Dent Res 1996;75:696.
9. Boyd J. Child abuse: P.A.N.D.A. program designed to help dental professionals diagnose and refer abuse victims. Can Dent Assoc 1994; Update 6(8):8.
10. Speight N. Nonaccidental injury. In: Meadow R, editor. The ABC's of child abuse. BMJ 1989.
11. International Association of Dental Traumatology. Guidelines for the evaluation and management of traumatic dental injuries. Dent Traumatol 2001;17:1, 49, 97, 145, 193.
12. Andreasen FM, Andreasen JO. Examination and diagnosis of dental injuries. In: Andreasen JO, Andreasen FM, editors. Textbook and color atlas of traumatic injuries to the teeth. 3rd ed. Copenhagen: Munksgaard; 1993. p. 196–215.
13. Bakland LK, Andreasen JO. Examination of the dentally traumatized patient. Can Dent Assoc J 1996;24:35.
14. Oikarinen K. Pathogenesis and mechanism of traumatic injuries to teeth. Endod Dent Traumatol 1987;3:220.
15. Nelson WE, Vaughan VC III, McKay RJ Jr, Behrman RE. Textbook of pediatrics. Philadelphia: WB Saunders; 1979.
16. Andreasen FM, et al. Relationship between pulp dimensions and development of pulp necrosis after luxation injuries of the permanent dentition. Endod Dent Traumatol 1986;2:90.
17. Crona-Larson G, et al. Effect of luxation injuries on permanent teeth. Endod Dent Traumatol 1991;7:199.
18. Blinkhorn FA, Mackie IC. The value of radiographs in the assessment of previously traumatized anterior teeth. Eur J Paediatr Dent 2000;4:157.
19. Andreasen FM, Vestergaard Pedersen B. Prognosis of luxated permanent teeth—the development of pulp necrosis. Endod Dent Traumatol 1985;1:207.
20. Bader JD, et al. Preliminary estimates of the incidence and consequences of tooth fractures. J Am Dent Assoc 1995;126:1650.
21. Gassner R, et al. Prevalence of dental trauma in 6000 patients with facial injuries. Oral Surg 1999;87:27.
22. Andreasen JO, Andreasen FM. Crown fractures. In: Andreasen JO, Andreasen FM, editors. Textbook and color atlas of traumatic injuries to the teeth. 3rd ed. Copenhagen: Munksgaard; 1993. p. 219–56.
23. Ellis GE, Davey KW. The classification and treatment of injuries to the teeth of children. 5th ed. Chicago: Year Book Medical; 1970.
24. Olgart L, Brännström M, Johnson G. Invasion of bacteria into dentinal tubules. Acta Odontol Scand 1974;32:61.
25. DiAngelis AJ. Bonding of fractured tooth segments: a review of the past 20 years. Can Dent Assoc J 1998;26:753.
26. Worthington RB, et al. Incisal edge reattachment: the effect of preparation utilization and design. Quintessence Int 1999;30:637.
27. Farik B, et al. Drying and rewetting anterior crown fragments prior to bonding. Endod Dent Traumatol 1999;15:113.
28. Heide S. The effect of pulp capping and pulpotomy on hard tissue bridges of contaminated pulps. Int Endod J 1991;24:126.
29. Cvek M. A clinical report on partial pulpotomy and capping with calcium hydroxide in permanent incisors with complicated crown fractures. JOE 1978;4:232.
30. Cvek M, Lundberg M. Histological appearance of pulps after exposure by a crown fracture, partial pulpotomy, and clinical diagnosis of healing. JOE 1983;9:8.
31. Bakland LK, Milledge T, Nation W. Treatment of crown fractures. Can Dent Assoc J 1996;24:45.
32. Torabinejad M, Chivan N. Clinical application of mineral trioxide aggregate. J Endod 1999;2:197.
33. Pitt Ford TR, Torabinejad M, et al. Mineral trioxide aggregate as a pulp capping material. J Am Dent Assoc 1996;127:1491.
34. Junn D. Assessment of dentin bridge formation following pulp capping with mineral trioxide aggregate [thesis]. Loma Linda (CA): Loma Linda University School of Dentistry; 2000.
35. Faraco IM Jr, Holland R. Response of the pulp of dogs to capping with mineral trioxide aggregate or a calcium hydroxide cement. Dent Traumatol 2001;17:163.
36. Bakland LK. Management of traumatically injured pulps in immature teeth using MTA. Can Dent Assoc J 2000;28:855.
37. Cox CF, et al. Biocompatibility of surface-sealed dental materials against exposed pulps. J Prosthet Dent 1987;57:1.
38. Torabinejad M, Hong CU, Pitt Ford TR. Physical properties of a new root end filling material. J Endod 1995;21:349.
39. Andreasen FM, et al. Long-term survival of fragment bonding in the treatment of fractured crowns: a multicenter clinical study. Quintessence Int 1995;26:669.
40. Ravn JJ. Follow-up study of permanent incisors with enamel-dentin fractures after acute trauma. Scand J Dent Res 1981;89:355.
41. Ravn JJ. Follow-up study of permanent incisors with complicated crown fractures after acute trauma. Scand J Dent Res 1982;90:363.
42. Cvek M. A clinical report on partial pulpotomy and capping with calcium hydroxide in permanent incisors with complicated crown fracture. J Endod 1978;4:232.
43. Cvek M. Partial pulpotomy in crown-fractured incisors—results 3 to 15 years after treatment. Acta Stomatol Croat 1993;27:167.
44. Jacobsen I, Kerekes K. Long-term prognosis of traumatized permanent anterior teeth showing calcifying processes in the pulp cavity. Scand J Dent Res 1977;85:588.
45. Lundberg M, Cvek M. A light microscopy study of pulps from traumatized permanent incisors with reduced pulpal lumen. Acta Odontol Scand 1980;38:89.
46. Jacobsen I, Sangnes F. Traumatized primary anterior teeth. Acta Odontol Scand 1978;36:199.
47. Cvek M. Endodontic management of traumatized teeth. In: Andreasen JO, Andreasen FM, editors. Textbook and color atlas of traumatic injuries to the teeth. 3rd ed. Copenhagen: Munksgaard; 1993. p. 517–85.
48. Andreasen FM, Andreasen JO. Crown-root fractures. In: Andreasen JO, Andreasen FM, editors. Textbook and color atlas of traumatic injuries to the teeth. 3rd ed. Copenhagen: Munksgaard; 1993. p. 257–76.

49. Meister F Jr, Lommel TJ, Gerstein H. Diagnosis and possible causes of vertical root fractures. Oral Surg 1980;49:243.
50. Warfvinge J, Kahnberg K-E. Intraalveolar transplantation of teeth. IV. Endodontic considerations. Swed Dent J 1989;13:229.
51. Kahnberg K-E. Surgical extrusion of root-fractured teeth—a follow-up study of two surgical methods. Endod Dent Traumatol 1988;4:85.
52. Malmgren O, Malmgren B, Frykholm A. Rapid orthodontic extrusion of crown root and cervical root fractured teeth. Endod Dent Traumatol 1991;7:49.
53. Andreasen FM, Andreasen JO. Root fractures. In: Andreasen JO, Andreasen FM, editors. Textbook and color atlas of traumatic injuries to the teeth. 3rd ed. Copenhagen: Munksgaard; 1993. p. 279–311.
54. Andreasen FM, et al. Prognosis of root-fractured permanent incisors—prediction of healing modalities. Endod Dent Traumatol 1989;5:11.
55. Bender IB, Freedland JB. Clinical considerations in diagnosis and treatment of intra-alveolar root fracture. J Am Dent Assoc 1983;107:595.
56. Cvek M, Andreasen JO, Borum MK. Healing of 208 intraalveolar root fractures in patients aged 7–17 years. Dent Traumatol 2001;7:53.
57. Jacobsen I, Zachrisson BU. Repair characteristics of root fractures in permanent anterior teeth. Scand J Dent Res 1975;83:355.
58. Zachrisson BU, Jacobsen I. Long-term prognosis of 66 permanent anterior teeth with root fracture. Scand J Dent Res 1975;83:345.
59. Jacobsen I. Root fractures in permanent anterior teeth with incomplete root formation. Scand J Dent Res 1976;84:210.
60. Andreasen JO, Hjörting-Hansen E. Intra-alveolar root fractures: radiographic and histologic study of 50 cases. J Oral Surg 1967;25:414.
61. Cvek M. Treatment of non-vital permanent incisors with calcium hydroxide. IV. Periodontal healing and closure of the root canal in the coronal fragment of teeth with intra alveolar root fracture and vital apical segment. Odont Revy 1974;25:239.
62. Weine FA, Altman A, Healey HJ. Treatment of fractures of the middle third of the root. J Dent Child 1971;38:215.
63. Andreasen FM, Andreasen JO. Resorption and mineralization processes following root fracture of permanent incisors. Endod Dent Traumatol 1988;4:202.
64. Andreasen FM, Vestergaard Pedersen B. Prognosis of luxated permanent teeth—the development of pulp necrosis. Endod Dent Traumatol 1985;1:207.
65. Andreasen FM. Pulpal healing after luxation injuries and root fracture in the permanent dentition. Endod Dent Traumatol 1989;5:111.
66. Andreasen JO, Andreasen FM. Luxation injuries. In: Andreasen JO, Andreasen FM, editors. Textbook and color atlas of traumatic injuries to the teeth. 3rd ed. Copenhagen: Munksgaard; 1993. p. 315–82.
67. Dumsha T, Hovland EJ. Pulpal prognosis following extrusive luxation injuries in permanent teeth with closed apexes. JOE 1982;8:410.
68. Lockhard PB, et al. Dental complications during and after tracheal intubation. J Am Dent Assoc 1986;112:480.
69. Andreasen FM, et al. Relationship between pulp dimensions and development of pulp necrosis after luxation injuries of the permanent dentition. Endod Dent Traumatol 1986;2:90.
70. Andreasen FM. Transient apical breakdown and its relation to color and sensibility changes after luxation injuries to teeth. Endod Dent Traumatol 1986;2:9.
71. Oikarinen K, et al. Late complications of luxation injuries to teeth. Endod Dent Traumatol 1987;3:296.
72. Andreasen FM, et al. Occurrence of pulp canal obliteration after luxation injuries in the permanent dentition. Endod Dent Traumatol 1987;3:103.
73. Crona-Larson G, et al. Effect of luxation injuries on permanent teeth. Endod Dent Traumatol 1991;7:199.
74. Jacobsen I. Clinical follow-up study of permanent incisors with intrusive luxation after acute trauma. J Dent Res 1983;62:4.
75. Cvek M. Prognosis of luxated non-vital maxillary incisors treated with calcium hydroxide and filled with gutta percha. A retrospective clinical study. Endod Dent Traumatol 1992;8:45.
76. Andreasen JO. Controversies and challenges in the managemnent of luxated teeth. Lecture at the American Association of Endodontists Annual Session, 2001.
77. Byström A, Claesson R, Sundqvist G. The antibacterial effect of camphorated paramonochlorphenol, camphorated phenol and calcium hydroxide in the treatment of infected root canals. Endod Dent Traumatol 1985;1:170.
78. Shabahang S, Torabinejad M. Treatment of teeth with open apices using mineral trioxide aggregate. Pract Periodont Aesthet Dent 2000;12:315.
79. Katebzadeh J, et al. Strengthening immature teeth during and after apexification. JOE 1998;24:256.
80. Borum MK, Andreasen JO. Sequelae of trauma to primary maxillary incisors. I. Complications in the primary dentition. Endod Dent Traumatol 1998;14:31.
81. Jacobsen I, Sangnes F. Traumatized primary anterior teeth. Acta Odontol Scand 1978;36:199.
82. Andreasen JO. Injuries to developing teeth. In: Andreasen JO, Andreasen FM, editors. Textbook and color atlas of traumatic injuries to the teeth. 3rd ed. Copenhagen: Munksgaard; 1993. p. 459–91.
83. Ben Bassat Y, Brin I, Fuks A, Zilberman Y. Effect of trauma to the primary incisors on permanent successors in different development stages. Pediatr Dent 1985;7:37.
84. Zilberman Y, Ben Bassat Y, Lustman J. Effect of trauma to primary incisors on root development of their permanent successors. Pediatr Dent 1986;8:289.
85. Andreasen JO, Andreasen FM. Avulsions. In: Andreasen JO, Andreasen FM, editors. Textbook and color atlas of traumatic injuries to the teeth. 3rd ed. Copenhagen: Munksgaard; 1993. p. 282–420.
86. Andreasen JO, et al. Replantation of 400 avulsed permanent incisors. Endod Dent Traumatol 1995;11:51.
87. Krasner P, Person P. Preserving avulsed teeth for replantation. J Am Dent Assoc 1992;123:80.
88. Huang S-C, et al. Effects of long-term exposure of human periodontal ligament cells to milk and other solutions. J Endod 1996;22:30.
89. Barrett EJ, Kenny DJ. Avulsed permanent teeth: a review of the literature and treatment guidelines. Endod Dent Traumatol 1997;13:153.
90. Andreasen JO, Schwartz O. The effect of saline storage before replantation upon dry damage of the periodontal ligament. Endod Dent Traumatol 1986;2:67.
91. Hammarström L, et al. Replantation of teeth and antibiotic treatment. Endod Dent Traumatol 1986;2:51.

92. Trope M. A protocol for treating the avulsed tooth. Can Dent Assoc J 1996;24:43.
93. Andreasen JO. The effect of pulp extirpation or root canal treatment on periodontal healing after replantation of permanent incisors in monkeys. JOE 1981;7:245.
94. Johnson WT, Goodrich JL, James GA. Replantation of avulsed teeth with immature root development. Oral Surg 1985;60:420.
95. Kling M, Cvek M, Mejàre I. Rate and predictability of pulp revascularization in therapeutically reimplanted permanent incisors. Endod Dent Traumatol 1986;2:83.
96. Trope M, et al. Effect of different endodontic treatment protocols on periodontal repair and root resorption of replanted dog teeth. JOE 1992;18:492.
97. Trope M, Moshonov J, Nissan R, et al. Short versus long-term calcium hydroxide treatment of established inflammatory root resorption in replanted dog teeth. Endod Dent Traumatol 1995;11:124.
98. Lengheden A, et al. Effect of immediate calcium hydroxide treatment and permanent root-filling on periodontal healing in contaminated replanted teeth. Scand J Dent Res 1991;99:139.
99. Lengheden A, et al. Effect of delayed calcium hydroxide treatment on periodontal healing in contaminated replanted teeth. Scand J Dent Res 1991;99:147.
100. Filippi A, et al. Treatment of replacement resorption with Emdogain—preliminary results after 10 months. Dent Traumatol 2001;17:134.
101. Andersson L, Blomlöf L, Lindskog S, et al. Tooth ankylosis. Clinical, radiographic, and histological assessments. Int J Oral Surg 1984;13:423.
102. Malmgren B, Cvek M, et al. Surgical treatment of ankylosed and infrapositioned reimplanted incisors in adolescents. Scand J Dent Res 1984;92:391.
103. Cvek M, et al. Pulp revascularization in reimplanted immature monkey incisors—predictability and the effect of antibiotic systemic prophylaxis. Endod Dent Traumatol 1990;6:157.
104. Cvek M, et al. Effect of topical application of doxycycline on pulp revascularization and periodontal healing in reimplanted monkey incisors. Endod Dent Traumatol 1990;6:170.
105. Andreasen JO, Ravn JJ. The effect of traumatic injuries to primary teeth on their permanent successors. II. A clinical and radiographic follow-up study of 213 teeth. Scand J Dent Res 1971;79:284.
106. Hammarström L, Pierce AM, Blomlöf L, et al. Tooth avulsion and replantation—a review. Endod Dent Traumatol 1986;2:1.
107. Andreasen JO, Hjörting-Hansen E. Replantation of teeth. II. Histological study of 22 replanted anterior teeth in humans. Acta Odontol Scand 1966;24:287.
108. Coccia CT. A clinical investigation of root resorption rates in reimplanted young permanent incisors: a five-year study. J Endod 1980;6:413.
109. Andreasen JO. Injuries to the supporting bone. In: Andreasen JO, Andreasen FM, editors. Textbook and color atlas of traumatic injuries to the teeth. 3rd ed. Copenhagen: Munksgaard; 1993. p. 427–53.
110. Andreasen JO. Fractures of the alveolar process of the jaw. A clinical and radiographic follow-up study. Scand J Dent Res 1970;78:263.
111. Roed-Petersen B, Andreasen JO. Prognosis of permanent teeth involved in jaw fractures. Scand J Dent Res 1970;78:343.
112. Kahnberg KE, Ridell A. Prognosis of teeth involved in the line of mandibular fractures. Int J Oral Surg 1979;8:163.
113. Oikarinen K, et al. Prognosis of permanent teeth in the line of mandibular fractures. Endod Dent Traumatol 1990;6:177.
114. Markowitz NR. Evaluations and treatment of mandibular and midface fractures. Can Dent Assoc J 1996;24:53.
115. Ellis E III, Moos KF, El-Attar A. Ten years of mandibular fractures: an analysis of 2,137 cases. Oral Surg 1985;59:120.
116. Bakland LK, Christiansen EL, Strutz JM. Frequency of dental traumatic events in the etiology of temporomandibular disorders. Endod Dent Traumatol 1988;4:182.
117. Boyne PJ. Osseous repair and mandibular growth after subscondylar fractures. J Oral Surg 1967;25:300.

Chapter 16

TOOTH DISCOLORATION AND BLEACHING

Ilan Rotstein

Tooth discoloration usually occurs owing to patient- or dentist-related causes[1,2] (Table 16-1).

PATIENT-RELATED CAUSES

Pulp Necrosis

Bacterial, mechanical, or chemical irritation to the pulp may result in tissue necrosis and release of disintegration by-products that may penetrate tubules and discolor the surrounding dentin. The degree of discoloration is directly related to how long the pulp has been necrotic. The longer the discoloration compounds are present in the pulp chamber, the greater the discoloration. Such discoloration can usually be bleached intracoronally (Figures 16-1 and 16-2).

Intrapulpal Hemorrhage

Intrapulpal hemorrhage and lysis of erythrocytes are a common result of traumatic injury to a tooth. Blood disintegration products, presumably iron sulfides, flow into the tubules and discolor the surrounding dentin. If the pulp becomes necrotic, the discoloration persists and usually becomes more severe with time. If the pulp recovers, the discoloration may be reversed, with the tooth regaining its original shade. The severity of such discoloration is time dependent; intracoronal bleaching is usually quite effective in this type of discoloration.[3–5]

Table 16-1 Causes of Tooth Discoloration

Patient-Related Causes	Dentist-Related causes
Pulp necrosis	Endodontically related
Intrapulpal hemorrhage	Pulp tissue remnants
Dentin hypercalcification	Intracanal medicaments
Age	Obturating materials
Tooth formation defects	Restoration related
Developmental defects	Amalgams
Drug-related defects	Pins and posts
	Composites

Dentin Hypercalcification

Excessive formation of irregular dentin in the pulp chamber and along canal walls may occur following certain traumatic injuries. In such cases, a temporary disruption of blood supply occurs, followed by destruction of odontoblasts. These are replaced by undifferentiated mesenchymal cells that rapidly form irregular dentin on the walls of the pulp lumen. As a result, the translucency of the crowns of such teeth gradually decreases, giving rise to a yellowish or yellow-brown discoloration.

Extracoronal bleaching may be attempted first. However, sometimes root canal therapy is required followed by intracoronal bleaching.

Age

In elderly patients, color changes in the crown occur physiologically, a result of excessive dentin apposition, thinning of the enamel, and optical changes. Food and beverages also have a cumulative discoloration effect. These become more pronounced in the elderly, owing to the inevitable cracking, crazing, and incisal wear of the enamel and underlying dentin. In addition, amalgam and other coronal restorations that degrade over time cause further discoloration. When indicated, bleaching can be successfully done for many types of discolorations in elderly patients.

TOOTH FORMATION DEFECTS

Developmental Defects

Discoloration may result from developmental defects during enamel and dentin formation, either hypocalcific or hypoplastic. Enamel ***hypocalcification*** is a distinct brownish or whitish area, commonly found on

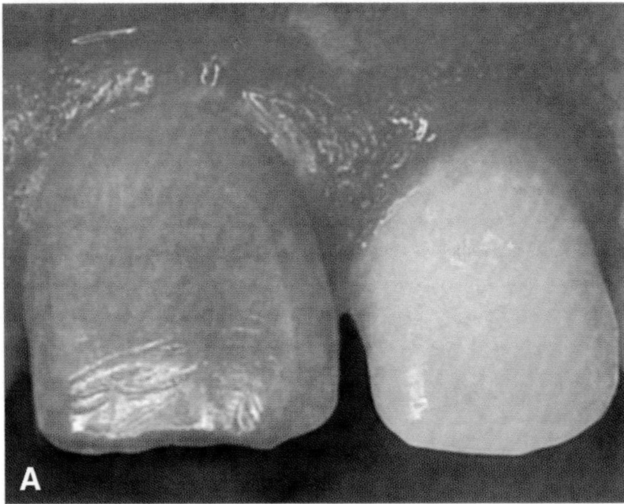

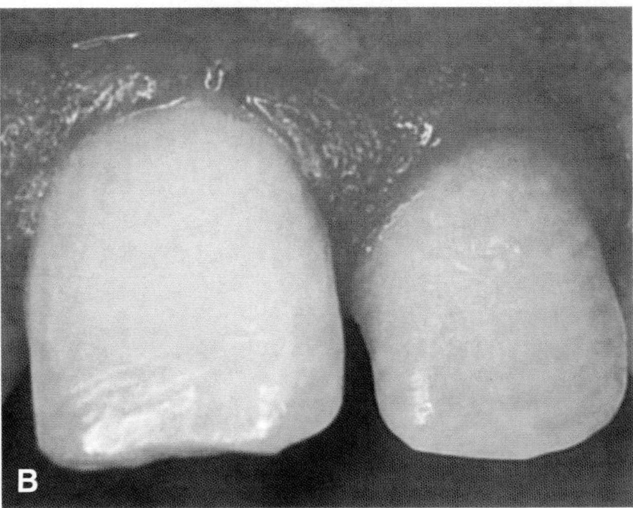

Figure 16-1 A, Post-traumatic discoloration of a maxillary left central incisor. B, A mixture of perborate and distilled water, placed in the chamber 2 times over 3 weeks, achieved the lightening of the tooth to its natural color. Reproduced with permission from Docteur Anne Claisse-Crinquette. L'eclaireissement des dyschromies: une longue histoire. Paris, France, Endo Contact 1999;2:16.

the facial aspect of affected crowns. The enamel is well formed with an intact surface.

Enamel ***hypoplasia*** differs from hypocalcification in that the enamel is defective and porous. This condition may be hereditary, as in amelogenesis imperfecta, or a result of environmental factors such as infections, tumors, or trauma. Presumably, during enamel formation, the matrix is altered and does not mineralize properly. The defective enamel is porous and readily discolored by materials in the oral cavity. In such cases, bleaching effect may not be permanent depending on the severity and extent of hypoplasia and the nature of the discoloration.

Several other systemic conditions may cause tooth discoloration. Erythroblastosis fetalis, for example, may occur in the fetus or newborn because of Rh incompatibility factors, with resulting massive systemic lysis of erythrocytes. Large amounts of hemosiderin pigment are released, which subsequently penetrate and discolor the forming dentin. This condition may also present a variety of systemic complications.[6] However, such discoloration is now uncommon and is not amenable to bleaching. High fever during tooth formation may also result in chronologic hypoplasia, a temporary disruption in enamel formation that gives rise to banding-type surface discoloration. Porphyria, a

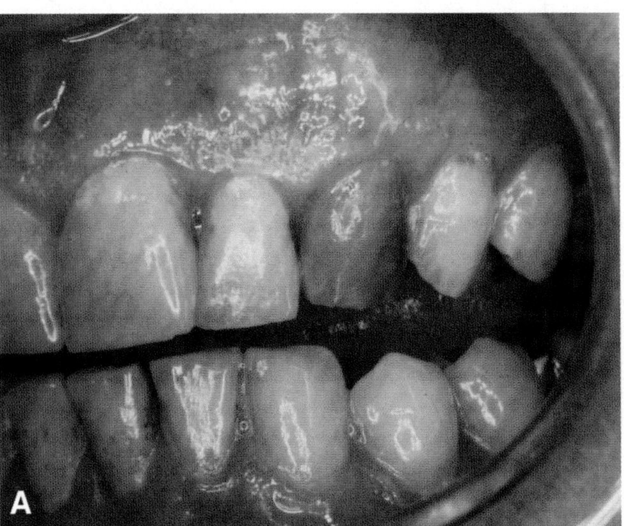

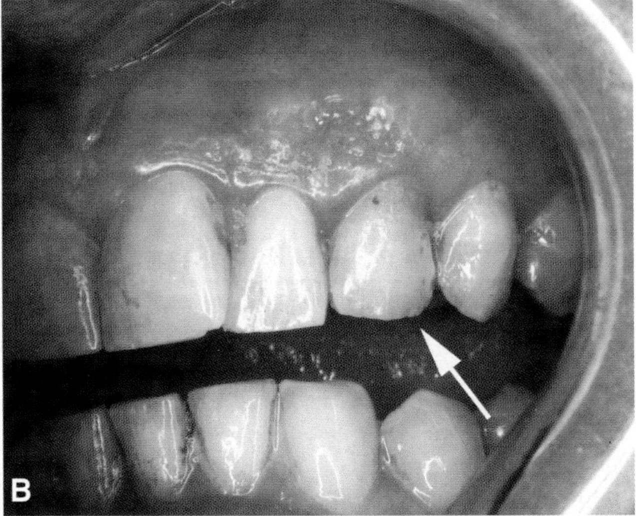

Figure 16-2 Traumatic pulp necrosis and dentin discoloration of a maxillary central incisor. A, Before treatment. B, Esthetic results following one treatment of "walking bleach" with sodium perborate mixed with Superoxol. Reproduced with permission from Nutting EB, Poe GS. Dent Clin North Am 1967;655.

metabolic disease, may also cause red or brownish discoloration of deciduous and permanent teeth. Thalassemia and sickle cell anemia may cause intrinsic blue, brown, or green discolorations. Amelogenesis imperfecta may result in yellow or brown discolorations. Dentinogenesis imperfecta can cause brownish violet, yellowish, or gray discoloration. These conditions are usually not amenable to bleaching and should be corrected by restorative means.

Drug-Related Defects

Administration or ingestion of certain drugs during tooth formation may cause severe discoloration both in enamel and dentin.[7,8]

Tetracycline. This antibiotic was used extensively during the 1950s and 1960s for prophylactic protection and for the treatment of chronic obstructive pulmonary disease, *Mycoplasma*, and rickettsial infections. It was sometimes prescribed for long periods of time, years in some cases, and therefore was a common cause of tooth discoloration in children. Although, today, tetracycline is not usually administrated chronically, dentists still face the residue of damage to the appearance of the teeth of the prior two generations.

Tooth shades can be yellow, yellow-brown, brown, dark gray, or blue, depending on the type of tetracycline, dosage, duration of intake, and patient's age at the time of administration. Discoloration is usually bilateral, affecting multiple teeth in both arches. Deposition of the tetracycline may be continuous or laid down in stripes depending on whether the ingestion was continuous or interrupted (Figure 16-3).

The mechanism of tetracycline discoloration is not fully understood. Tetracycline bound to calcium is thought to be incorporated into the hydroxyapatite crystal of both enamel and dentin. However, most of the tetracycline is found in dentin.

Tetracycline discoloration has been classified into three groups according to severity.[9] First-degree discoloration is light yellow, light brown, or light gray and occurs uniformly throughout the crown, without banding. Second-degree discoloration is more intense and also without banding. Third-degree discoloration is very intense, and the clinical crown exhibits horizontal color banding. This type of discoloration usually predominates in the cervical regions.

Repeated exposure of tetracycline-discolored tooth to ultraviolet radiation can lead to formation of a reddish-purple oxidation by-product that permanently discolors the teeth. In children, the anterior teeth often discolor first, whereas the less exposed posterior teeth are discolored more slowly. In adults, natural photobleaching of the anterior teeth is observed, particularly in individuals whose teeth are excessively exposed to sunlight owing to maxillary lip insufficiency.

Two approaches have been used to treat tetracycline discoloration: (1) bleaching the external enamel surface[9–11] (Figure 16-4) and (2) intracoronal bleaching following intentional root canal therapy[12–14] (Figure 16-5).

Endemic Fluorosis. Ingestion of excessive amounts of fluoride during tooth formation may produce a defect in mineralized structures, particularly in the enamel matrix, causing hypoplasia. The severity and degree of subsequent staining generally depend on the degree of hypoplasia and are directly related to the amount of fluoride ingested during odontogenesis.[15] The teeth are not discolored on eruption, but their surface is porous and will gradually absorb colored chemicals present in the oral cavity.

Discoloration is usually bilateral, affecting multiple teeth in both arches. It presents as various degrees of intermittent white spotting, chalky or opaque areas, yellow or brown discoloration, and, in severe cases, surface pitting of the enamel. Since the discoloration is in the porous enamel, such teeth can be bleached externally.

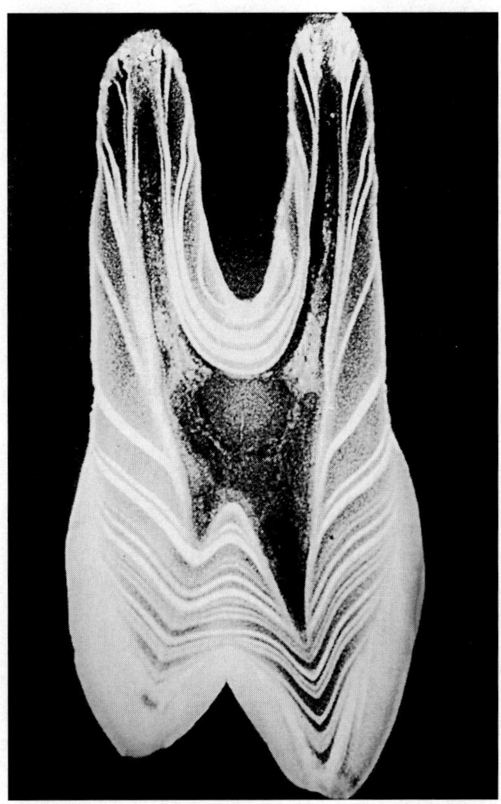

Figure 16-3 Fluorescent photomicrograph of tetracycline-discolored tooth. Tetracycline deposition is seen as stripes caused by start and stop ingestion. (Courtesy of Dr. David L. Myers.)

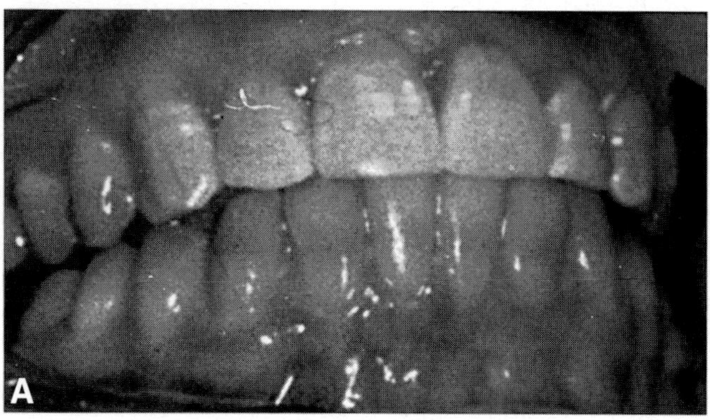

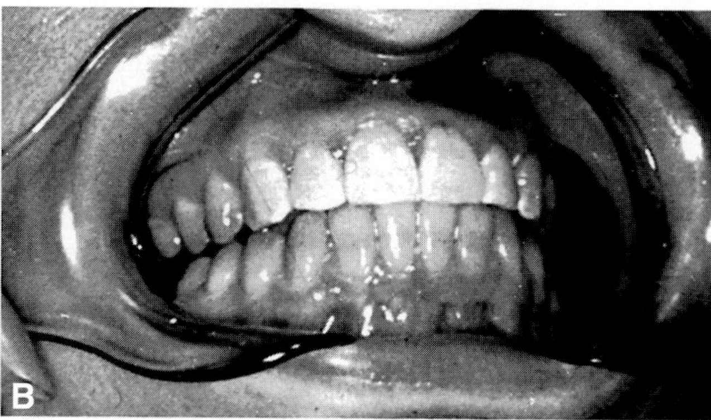

Figure 16-4 Extracoronal bleaching of tetracycline-discolored maxillary incisors. **A**, Before bleaching. **B**, After three sessions of bleaching with *Hi Lite Dual Activated Bleach* as compared to unbleached discolored area of mandibular incisors. (Courtesy of Drs. Fred and Scott Hanosh.)

DENTIST-RELATED CAUSES

Discolorations owing to various dental materials or unsuitable operating techniques do occur; such dentist-related discolorations are usually preventable and should be avoided.

Endodontically Related

Pulp Tissue Remnants. Tissue remaining in the pulp chamber disintegrates gradually and may cause discoloration. Pulp horns must always be included in the access cavity to ensure removal of pulpal remnants and to pre-

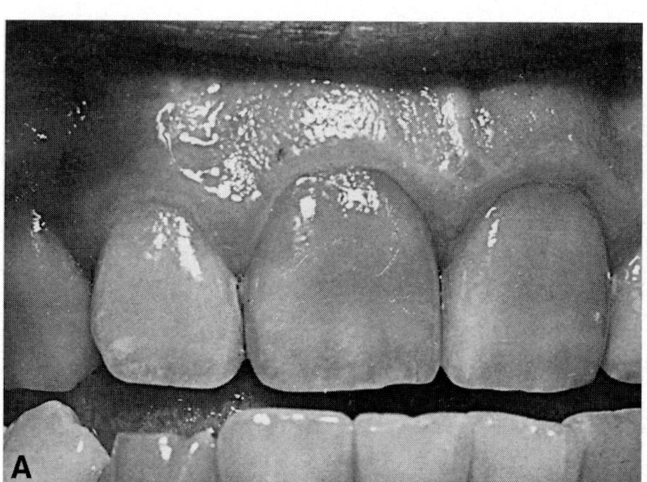

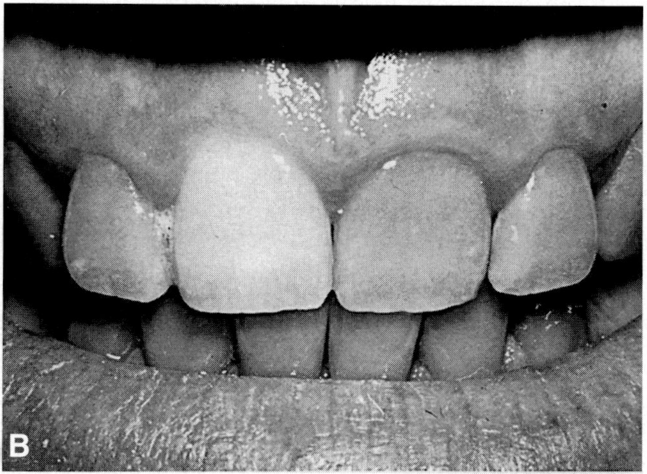

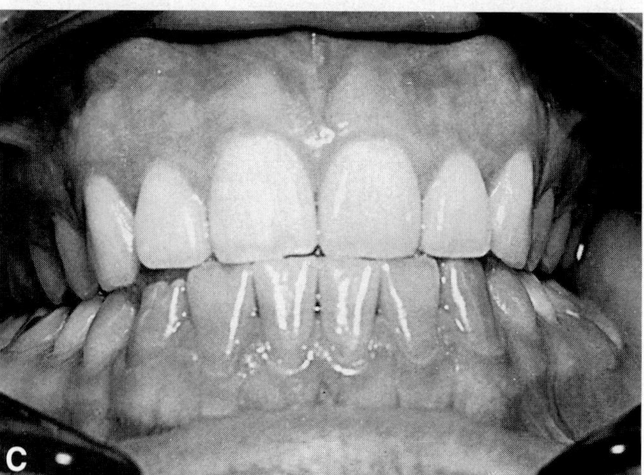

Figure 16-5 Intentional pulp devitalization and root canal obturation followed by intracoronal bleaching of tetracycline-discolored teeth. **A**, All anterior teeth badly discolored from tetracycline ingestion when the patient was 2 to 3 years old. **B**, Trial treatment tooth (central incisor) successfully bleached. **C**, All six maxillary anterior teeth subsequently bleached. Contrast with discolored mandibular incisors is apparent. Reproduced with permission from Abou-Rass M. Alpha Omegan. 1982;75:57.

vent retention of sealer at a later stage. Intracoronal bleaching in these cases is usually successful.

Intracanal Medicaments. Several intracanal medicaments are liable to cause internal staining of the dentin. Phenolics or iodoform-based medicaments sealed in the root canal and chamber are in direct contact with dentin, sometimes for long periods, allowing penetration and oxidization. These compounds have a tendency to discolor the dentin gradually.

Obturating Materials. This is a frequent and severe cause of single tooth discoloration. Incomplete removal of obturating materials and sealer remnants in the pulp chamber, mainly those containing metallic components,[16] often results in dark discoloration. This is easily prevented by removing all materials to a level just below the gingival margin (Figure 16-6).

Intracoronal bleaching is the treatment of choice; prognosis, however, in such cases depends on the type of sealer and duration of discoloration.

Restoration Related

Amalgams. Silver alloys have severe effects on dentin owing to dark-colored metallic components that can turn the dentin dark gray. When used to restore lingual access preparations or a developmental groove in anterior teeth, as well as in premolar teeth, amalgam may discolor the crown. Such discolorations are difficult to bleach and tend to rediscolor with time.

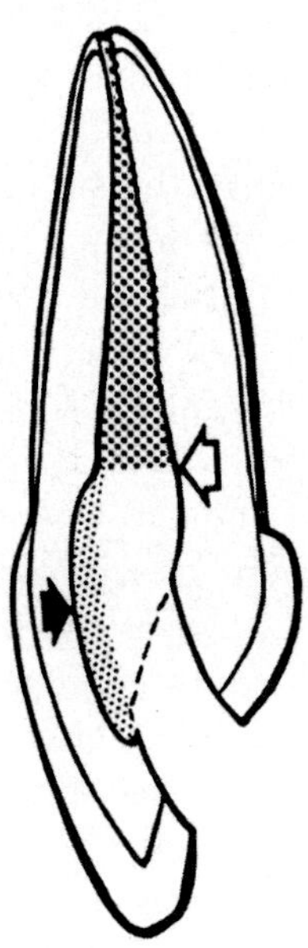

Figure 16-6 Gutta-percha and dentin removal prior to bleaching. **Heavyily dotted area** represents gutta-percha filling, which is removed to a level just below the gingival level (**open arrow**). **Lightly dotted area** represents removal of dentin to eliminate heavy stain concentration and pulp horn material (**black arrow**).

Sometimes the dark appearance of the crown is caused by the amalgam restoration that can be seen through the tooth structure. In such cases, replacing the amalgam with an esthetic restoration usually corrects the problem.

Pins and Posts. Metal pins and prefabricated posts are sometimes used to reinforce a composite restoration in the anterior dentition. Discoloration from inappropriately placed pins and posts is caused by the metal seen through the composite or tooth structure. In such cases, coverage of the pins with a white cement or removal of the metal and replacement of the composite restoration is indicated.

Composites. Microleakage around composite restorations causes staining. Open margins may allow chemicals to enter between the restoration and the tooth structure and discolor the underlying dentin. In addition, composites may become discolored with time, affecting the shade of the crown. These conditions are generally corrected by replacing the old composite restoration with a new, well-sealed one.

BLEACHING MATERIALS

Many different bleaching agents are available today; the ones most commonly used are hydrogen peroxide, sodium perborate, and carbamide peroxide. Hydrogen peroxide and carbamide peroxide are mainly indicated for extracoronal bleaching, whereas sodium perborate is used for intracoronal bleaching.

Hydrogen Peroxide. Various concentrations of this agent are available, but 30 to 35% stabilized aqueous solutions (Superoxol, Perhydrol Merck & Co.; West Point, Pa.) are the most common. Silicone dioxide gel forms containing 35% hydrogen peroxide are also available, some of them activated by a composite curing light (Figure 16-7).

Hydrogen peroxide is caustic and burns tissues on contact, releasing toxic free radicals, perhydroxyl anions, or both. High-concentration solutions of hydrogen peroxide must be handled with care as they are thermodynamically unstable and may explode unless refrigerated and kept in a dark container.

Sodium Perborate. This oxidizing agent is available in a powdered form or as various commercial preparations. When fresh, it contains about 95% perborate, corresponding to 9.9% of the available oxygen. Sodium perborate is stable when dry. In the presence of acid, warm air, or water, however, it decomposes to form sodium metaborate, hydrogen peroxide, and nascent oxygen.

Three types of sodium perborate preparations are available: monohydrate, trihydrate, and tetrahydrate. They differ in oxygen content, which determines their

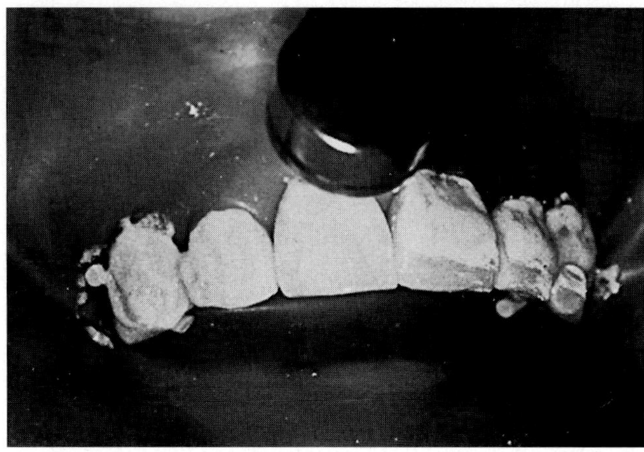

Figure 16-7 Bleaching gel applied to labial surfaces of maxillary teeth and activated by resin curing light. Note the rubber dam carefully protecting gingiva from bleaching agent. (Courtesy of Shofu Dental Corp.;San Marcos, Calif.)

bleaching efficacy.[17] Commonly used sodium perborate preparations are alkaline, and their pH depends on the amount of hydrogen peroxide released and the residual sodium metaborate.[18]

Sodium perborate is more easily controlled and safer than concentrated hydrogen peroxide solutions. Therefore, it should be the material of choice in most intracoronal bleaching procedures (Figure 16-8).

Carbamide Peroxide. This agent, also known as urea hydrogen peroxide, is available in the concentration range of 3 to 45%. However, popular commercial preparations contain about 10% carbamide peroxide, with a mean pH of 5 to 6.5. Solutions of 10% carbamide peroxide break down into urea, ammonia, carbon dioxide, and approximately 3.5% hydrogen peroxide.

Bleaching preparations containing carbamide peroxide usually also include glycerine or propylene glycol, sodium stannate, phosphoric or citric acid, and flavor additives. In some preparations, carbopol, a water-soluble polyacrylic acid polymer, is added as a thickening agent. Carbopol also prolongs the release of active peroxide and improves shelf life.

Carbamide peroxide–based preparations have been associated with various degrees of damage to the teeth and surrounding mucosa.[19–23] They also may adversely affect the bond strength of composite resins and their marginal seal.[24,25] Since long-term studies are not yet available, these materials must be used with caution.

BLEACHING MECHANISM

The mechanism of tooth bleaching is unclear. It differs according to the type of discoloration involved and the chemical and physical conditions at the time of the

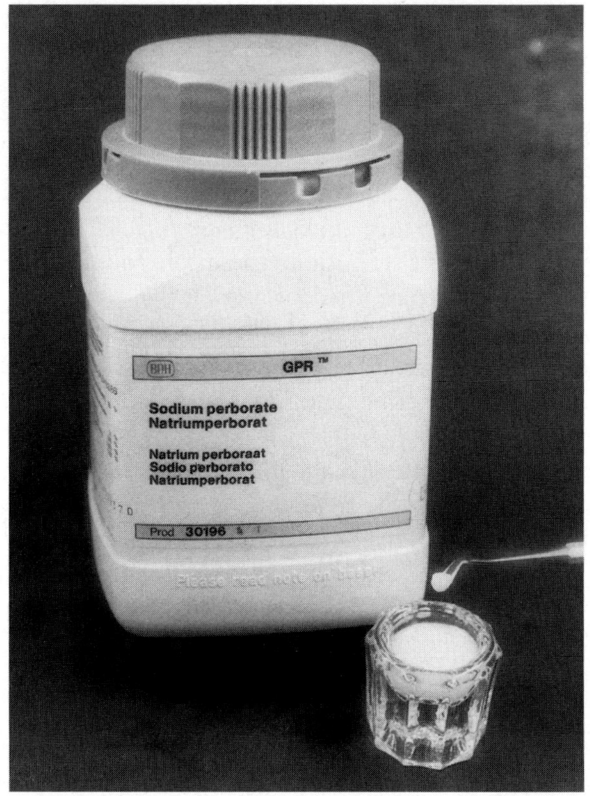

Figure 16-8 Sodium perborate powder and liquid are mixed to a thick consistency of wet sand.

reaction. Bleaching agents, mainly oxidizers, act on the organic structure of the dental hard tissues, slowly degrading them into chemical by-products, such as carbon dioxides, that are lighter in color. Inorganic molecules do not usually break down as well. The oxidation-reduction reaction that occurs during bleaching is known as a redox reaction. Generally, the unstable peroxides convert to unstable free radicals. These free radicals may oxidize (remove electrons from) or reduce (add electrons to) other molecules.

Most bleaching procedures use hydrogen peroxide because it is unstable and decomposes into oxygen and water. The **mouthguard** bleaching technique employs mainly carbamide peroxide as a vehicle for the delivery of lower concentrations of hydrogen peroxide, which require more exposure time. The rate of hydrogen peroxide decomposition during mouthguard bleaching depends on its concentration and the levels of salivary peroxidase. With high levels of hydrogen peroxide, a zero-order reaction occurs, so that the time required to clear the hydrogen peroxide is proportional to its concentration. The longer it takes to clear the hydrogen peroxide, the greater the exposure to reactive oxygen species and their adverse effects.

BLEACHING TECHNIQUES FOR ENDODONTICALLY TREATED TEETH

Intracoronal bleaching of endodontically treated teeth may be successfully carried out many years after root canal therapy and discoloration. A successful outcome depends mainly on the etiology, correct diagnosis, and proper selection of bleaching technique (Table 16-2).

The methods most commonly employed to bleach endodontically treated teeth are the **walking bleach** and the **thermocatalytic** techniques. Walking bleach is preferred since it requires less chair time and is safer and more comfortable for the patient.[26,27]

Walking Bleach

The walking bleach technique should first be attempted in all cases requiring ***intracoronal*** bleaching. It involves the following steps:

1. Familiarize the patient with the possible causes of discoloration, procedure to be followed, expected outcome, and possibility of future **re**discoloration.
2. Radiographically assess the status of the periapical tissues and the quality of the endodontic obturation. Endodontic failure or questionable obturation should **always be re-treated** prior to bleaching.
3. Assess the quality and shade of any restoration present and replace if defective. Tooth discoloration frequently is the result of leaking or discolored restorations. In such cases, cleaning the pulp chamber and replacing the defective restorations will usually suffice.
4. Evaluate tooth color with a shade guide and, if possible, take clinical photographs at the beginning of and throughout the procedure. These provide a point of reference for future comparison.
5. Isolate the tooth with a rubber dam. The dam must fit tightly at the cervical margin of the tooth to prevent possible leakage of the bleaching agent onto the gingival tissue. Interproximal wedges and ligatures may also be used for better isolation. If Superoxol is used, a protective cream, such as Orabase or Vaseline, must be applied to the surrounding gingival tissues prior to dam placement.
6. Remove all restorative material from the access cavity, expose the dentin, and refine the access. Verify that the pulp horns and other areas containing pulp tissue are clean.
7. Remove all materials to a level just below the labial-gingival margin. ***Orange solvent***, chloroform, or xylene on a cotton pellet may be used to dissolve sealer remnants. Etching the dentin with phosphoric acid is unnecessary and may not improve the prognosis.
8. Apply a sufficiently thick layer, at least 2 mm, of a protective white cement barrier, such as polycarboxylate cement, zinc phosphate cement, glass ionomer, ***IRM*** (Dentsply/Caulk; York, Pa.) or ***Cavit*** (Premier Dental Products, King of Prussia, Pa.), to cover the endodontic obturation. The coronal height of the barrier should protect the dentinal tubules and conform to the external epithelial attachment.[28]
9. Prepare the walking bleach paste by mixing sodium perborate and an inert liquid, such as water, saline, or anesthetic solution, to a thick consistency of wet sand (Figure 16-8). Although a sodium perborate and 30% hydrogen peroxide mixture bleaches faster, in most cases, long-term results are similar to those with sodium perborate and water alone and therefore need not be used routinely.[4,5,29] With a plastic instrument, pack the pulp chamber with the paste. Remove excess liquid by tamping with a cotton pellet. This also compresses and pushes the paste into all areas of the pulp chamber.
10. Remove excess bleaching paste from undercuts in the pulp horn and gingival area and apply a thick well-sealed temporary filling (preferably ***IRM***) directly against the paste and into the undercuts. Carefully pack the temporary filling, at least 3 mm thick, to ensure a good seal.
11. Remove the rubber dam and inform the patient that bleaching agents work slowly and significant lightening may not be evident for several days.
12. Evaluate the patient 2 weeks later and, if necessary, repeat the procedure several times.[29] Repeat treatments are similar to the first one.
13. As an optional procedure, if initial bleaching is not satisfactory, strengthen the walking bleach paste by mixing the sodium perborate with gradually increasing concentrations of hydrogen peroxide (3 to 30%) instead of water. The more potent oxidizers may have an enhanced bleaching effect but are not used routinely because of the possibility of permeation into the tubules and damage to the cervical periodontium by these more caustic agents.

Table 16-2 Indications and Contraindications for Bleaching Endodontically Treated Teeth

Indications	Contraindications
Discolorations of pulp chamber	Superficial enamel discolorations
Dentin discolorations	Defective enamel formation
Discolorations not amenable to extracoronal bleaching	Severe dentin loss
	Presence of caries
	Discolored composites

Thermocatalytic

This technique involves placement of the oxidizing chemical, generally 30 to 35% hydrogen peroxide *(Superoxol)*, in the pulp chamber followed by heat application either by electric heating devices or specially designed lamps.

Potential damage by the thermocatalytic approach is external **cervical root resorption** caused by irritation to the cementum and periodontal ligament. This is possibly attributable to the oxidizing agent combined with heating.[30,31] Therefore, application of highly concentrated hydrogen peroxide and heat during intracoronal bleaching is questionable and should not be carried out routinely.

Ultraviolet Photo-Oxidation

This technique applies ultraviolet light to the labial surface of the tooth to be bleached. A 30 to 35% hydrogen peroxide solution is placed in the pulp chamber on a cotton pellet followed by a 2-minute exposure to ultraviolet light. Supposedly, this causes oxygen release, like the thermocatalytic bleaching technique.[32]

Intentional Endodontics and Intracoronal Bleaching

Intrinsic tetracycline and other similar stains are incorporated into tooth structure during tooth formation, mostly into the dentin, and are therefore more difficult to treat from the external enamel surface. Intracoronal bleaching of tetracycline-discolored teeth has been shown clinically[12] and experimentally[13,14] to lead to significant lightening.

The technique involves standard endodontic therapy (pulpectomy, cleaning and shaping, and obturation) followed by an intracoronal walking bleach technique. Preferably, only intact teeth without coronal defects, caries, or restorations should be treated. This prevents the need for any additional restoration, thereby reducing the possibility of coronal fractures and failures. The most discolored tooth should be selected for trial treatment (see Figure 16-5).

The procedure should be carefully explained to the patient, including the possible complications and sequelae. A treatment consent form is necessary! Sacrificing pulp vitality should be considered in terms of the overall psychological and social needs of the individual patient as well as the possible complications of other treatment options. The procedure has been shown to be predictable and without significant clinical complications.[12,33]

Complications and Adverse Effects to Bleaching

External Root Resorption. Clinical reports[34–44] and histologic studies[30,31,45] have shown that intracoronal bleaching may induce external root resorption (Table 16-3 and Figure 16-9). This is probably caused by the oxidizing agent, particulary 30 to 35% hydrogen peroxide. The mechanism of bleaching-induced damage to the periodontium or cementum has not been fully elucidated. Presumably, the irritating chemical diffuses via unprotected dentinal tubules and cementum defects[46,47] and causes necrosis of the cementum, inflammation of the periodontal ligament, and, finally, root resorption. The process may be enhanced if heat is applied[48] or in

Table 16-3 Clinical Reports of External Root Resorption Associated with Hydrogen Peroxide Bleaching

Authors	No. of Cases	Age of Patients	Previous Trauma		Heat Applied		Barrier Used	
			Yes	No	Yes	No	Yes	No
Harrington and Natkin[34]	7	10–29	7	0	7	0	0	7
Lado et al.[35]	1	50	0	1	1	0	0	1
Montgomery[36]	1	21	1	0	?	?	?	?
Shearer[37]	1	?	0	1	1	0	0	1
Cvek and Lindvall[38]	11	11–26	10	1	11	0	0	11
Latcham[39]	1	8	1	0	0	1	0	1
Goon et al.[40]	1	15	?	?	0	1	0	1
Friedman et al.[41]	4	18–24	0	4	3	1	0	4
Gimlin and Schindler[42]	1	13	1	0	1	0	0	1
Al-Nazhan[43]	1	27	0	1	1	0	0	1
Heithersay et al.[44]	4	10–20	4	0	4	0	0	4

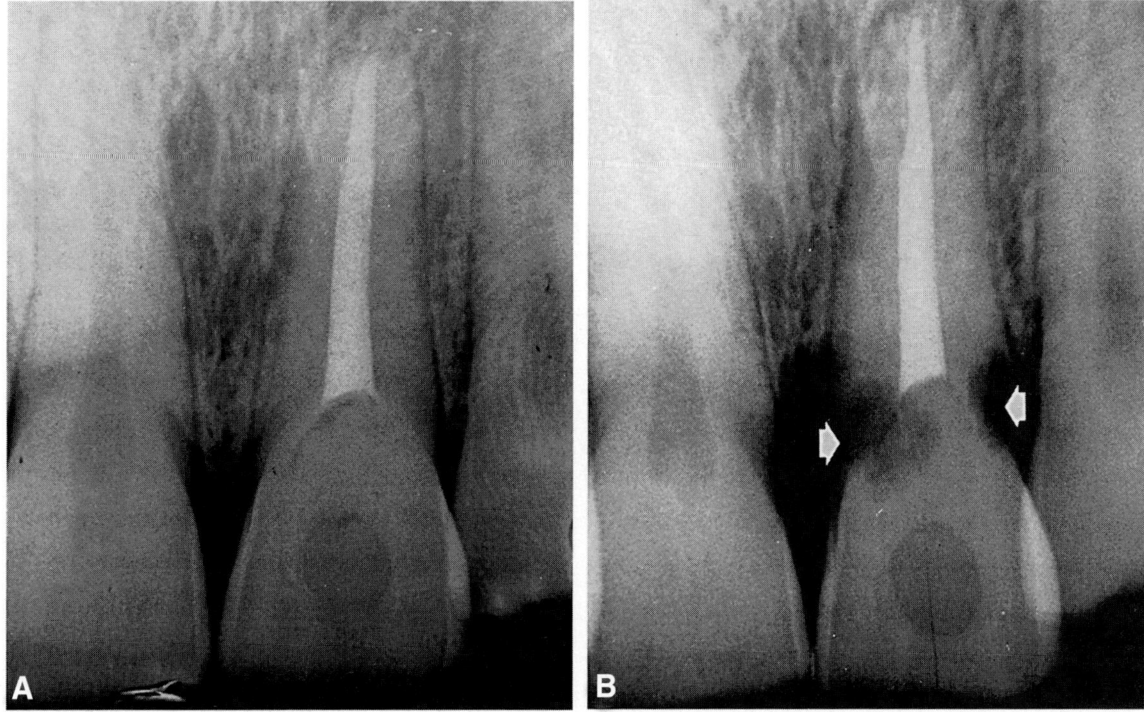

Figure 16-9 Postbleaching external root resorption. **A**, Nine-year recall radiograph of a central incisor devitalized by trauma and treated endodontically shortly thereafter. **B**, Radiograph taken 2 years following bleaching. Superoxol and heat were used first and followed by "walking bleach" with Superoxol and sodium perborate. (Courtesy of Drs. David Steiner and Gerald Harrington.)

the presence of bacteria.[38,49] Previous traumatic injury and age may act as predisposing factors.[34]

Chemical Burns. Thirty percent hydrogen peroxide is caustic and causes chemical burns and sloughing of the gingiva. When using such solutions, the soft tissues should always be protected with *Vaseline* or *Orabase.*

Damage to Restorations. Bleaching with hydrogen peroxide may affect bonding of composite resins to dental hard tissues.[50] Scanning electron microscopy suggests a possible interaction between composite resin and residual peroxide, causing inhibition of polymerization and an increase in resin porosity.[51] This presents a clinical problem when immediate esthetic restoration of the bleached tooth is required. It is therefore recommended that residual hydrogen peroxide be totally eliminated prior to composite placement.

It has been shown that immersion of peroxide-treated dental tissues in water at 37°C for 7 days prevents the reduction in bond strength.[52] In another study, the efficacy of **catalase** in removing residual hydrogen peroxide from the pulp chamber of human teeth, as compared to prolonged rinsing in water, was assessed.[53] Three minutes of catalase treatment effectively removed all of the residual hydrogen peroxide from the pulp chamber.

Suggestions for Safer Bleaching of Endodontically Treated Teeth

- **Isolate the tooth effectively.** Intracoronal bleaching should always be carried out with rubber dam isolation. Interproximal wedges and ligatures may also be used for better protection.
- **Protect the oral mucosa.** Protective creams, such as *Orabase* or *Vaseline*, must be applied to the surrounding oral mucosa to prevent chemical burns by caustic oxidizers. Animal studies suggest that catalase applied to oral tissues prior to hydrogen peroxide treatment totally prevents the associated tissue damage.[54]
- **Verify adequate endodontic obturation.** The quality of root canal obturation should always be assessed clinically and radiographically prior to bleaching. Adequate obturation ensures a better overall prognosis of the treated tooth. It also provides an additional barrier against damage by oxidizers to the periodontal ligament and periapical tissues.
- **Use protective barriers.** This is essential to prevent leakage of bleaching agents that may infiltrate between the gutta-percha and root canal walls, reaching the periodontal ligament via dentinal tubules, lateral canals, or the root apex. In none of the clinical reports of post-bleaching root resorption was a protective barrier used.

Various materials can be used for this purpose. Barrier thickness and its relationship to the cementoenamel junction are most important.[28,55] The ideal barrier should protect the dentinal tubules and conform to the external epithelial attachment (Figure 16-10).

- **Avoid acid etching.** It has been suggested that acid etching of dentin in the chamber to remove the smear layer and open the tubules would allow better penetration of the oxidizer. This procedure has not proven beneficial.[56] The use of caustic chemicals in the pulp chamber is undesirable as periodontal ligament irritation may result.
- **Avoid strong oxidizers.** Procedures and techniques applying strong oxidizers should be avoided if they are not essential for bleaching. Solutions of 30 to 35% hydrogen peroxide, either alone or in combination with other agents, should not be used routinely for intracoronal bleaching.

  Sodium perborate is mild and quite safe, and no additional protection of the soft tissues is usually required. Generally, however, oxidizing agents should not be exposed to more of the pulp space and dentin than absolutely necessary to obtain a satisfactory clinical result.
- **Avoid heat.** Excessive heat may damage the cementum and periodontal ligament as well as dentin and enamel, especially when combined with strong oxidizers.[30,31] Although no direct correlation has been found between heat applications alone and external cervical root resorption, it should be limited during bleaching procedures.
- **Recall periodically.** Bleached teeth should be frequently examined both clinically and radiographically. Root resorption may occasionally be detected as early as 6 months after bleaching. Early detection improves the prognosis since corrective therapy may still be applied.

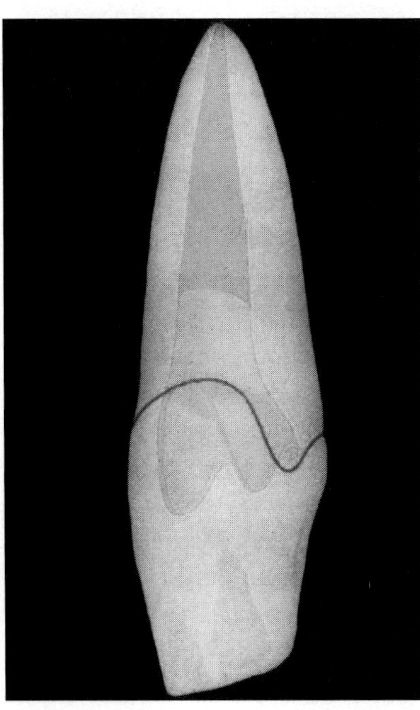

Figure 16-10 Schematic illustration of the intracoronal protective bleach barrier. The shape of the barrier matches the contour of the external epithelial attachment. Reproduced with permission from Steiner DR, and West JD.[28]

Post-Bleaching Tooth Restoration

Proper tooth restoration is essential for long-term sucessful bleaching results. Coronal microleakage of lingual access restorations is a problem,[57] and a leaky restoration may lead to rediscoloration.

There is no ideal method for filling the chamber after tooth bleaching. The pulp chamber and access cavity should be carefully restored with a light-cured acid-etched composite resin, light in shade. The composite material should be placed at a depth that seals the cavity and provides some incisal support. Light curing from the labial surface, rather than the lingual surface, is recommended since this results in shrinkage of the composite resin toward the axial walls, reducing the rate of microleakage.[58]

Placing white cement beneath the composite access restoration is recommended. Filling the chamber completely with composite may cause loss of translucency and difficulty in distinguishing between composite and tooth structure during rebleaching.[59]

As previously stated, residual peroxides from bleaching agents, mainly hydrogen peroxide and carbamide peroxide, may affect the bonding strength of composites.[25,50] Therefore, waiting for a few days after bleaching prior to restoring the tooth with composite resin has been recommended. Catalase treatment at the final visit may enhance the removal of residual peroxides from the access cavity; however, this requires further clinical investigation.[53]

Packing calcium hydroxide paste in the pulp chamber for a few weeks prior to placement of the final restoration, to counteract acidity caused by bleaching agents and to prevent root resorption, has also been suggested; this procedure, however, is unnecessary with walking bleach.[18]

VITAL BLEACHING TECHNIQUES

Many techniques have been advocated for extracoronal bleaching of vital teeth. In these techniques, oxidizers are applied to the external enamel surface of the teeth.

Thermo/Photo Bleaching

This technique basically involves application of 30 to 35% hydrogen peroxide and heat or a combination of heat and light or ultraviolet rays to the enamel surface (Table 16-4). Heat is applied either by electric heating devices or heat lamps. The technique involves the following steps:

1. Familiarize the patient with the probable causes of discoloration, procedure to be followed, expected outcome, and possibility of future rediscoloration.
2. Make radiographs to detect the presence of caries, defective restorations, and proximity to pulp horns. Well-sealed small restorations and minimal amounts of exposed incisal dentin are not usually a contraindication for bleaching.
3. Evaluate tooth color with a shade guide and take clinical photographs before and throughout the procedure.
4. Apply a protective cream to the surrounding gingival tissues and isolate the teeth with a rubber dam and waxed dental floss ligatures. If a heat lamp is used, avoid placing rubber dam metal clamps as they are subjected to heating and may be painful to the patient.
5. **Do not inject a local anesthetic.**
6. Position protective sunglasses over the patient's and the operator's eyes.
7. Clean the enamel surface with pumice and water. Avoid prophylaxis pastes containing glycerine or fluoride.
8. As an optional procedure, acid etch the darkest or most severely stained areas with buffered phosphoric acid for 10 seconds and rinse with water for 60 seconds. A gel form of acid provides optimum control. Enamel etching for extracoronal bleaching is controversial and should not be carried out routinely.
9. Place a small amount of 30 to 35% hydrogen peroxide solution into a dappen dish. Apply the hydrogen peroxide liquid on the labial surface of the teeth using a small cotton pellet or a piece of gauze. A bleaching gel containing hydrogen peroxide may be used instead of the aqueous solution (see Figure 16-4).
10. Apply heat with a heating device or a light source. The temperature should be at a level the patient can comfortably tolerate, usually between 125°F and 140°F (52°C to 60°C). Rewet the enamel surface with hydrogen peroxide as necessary. If the teeth become too sensitive, discontinue the bleaching procedure immediately. Do not exceed 30 minutes of treatment even if the result is not satisfactory.
11. Remove the heat source and allow the teeth to cool down for at least 5 minutes. Then wash with warm water for 1 minute and remove the rubber dam. Do not rinse with cold water since the sudden change in temperature may damage the pulp or can be painful to the patient.
12. Dry the teeth and gently polish them with a composite resin polishing cup. Treat all of the etched and bleached surfaces with a neutral sodium fluoride gel for 3 to 5 minutes.
13. Inform the patient that cold sensitivity is common, especially during the first 24 hours after treatment. Also, instruct the patient to use a fluoride rinse daily for 2 weeks.
14. Re-evaluate the patient approximately 2 weeks later on the effectiveness of bleaching. Take clinical photographs with the same shade guide used in the preoperative photographs for comparison purposes. If necessary, repeat the bleaching procedure.

Table 16-4 Indications and Contraindications for Thermo/Photo Extracoronal Bleaching

Indications	Contraindications
Light enamel discolorations	Severe dark discolorations
Mild tetracycline discolorations	Severe enamel loss
Endemic fluorosis discolorations	Proximity of pulp horns
Age-related discolorations	Hypersensitive teeth
	Presence of caries
	Large/poor coronal restorations

Complications and Adverse Effects. *Postoperative Pain.* A number of short- and long-term symptoms may occur following extracoronal bleaching of vital teeth. A common immediate postoperative problem is pulpalgia characterized by intermittent shooting pain. It may occur during or after the bleaching session and usually persists for between 24 and 48 hours. The intensity of the pulpalgia is related to duration and the temperature of the bleaching procedure. Shorter bleaching periods are therefore recommended. If long-term sensitivity to cold develops, topical fluoride treatments and desensitizing toothpastes should be used to alleviate these symptoms.

Pulpal Damage. Extracoronal bleaching with hydrogen peroxide and heat has been associated with some pulpal damage. Although investigators have not found significant irreversible effects on the pulp,[10,60,61] these procedures must be approached and carried out with caution[62] and not in the presence of caries, areas of exposed dentin, or in close proximity to pulp horns.

Defective restorations must be replaced prior to bleaching. Teeth with large coronal restorations should not be bleached.

Dental Hard Tissue Damage. Hydrogen peroxide has been shown to cause morphologic and structural changes in enamel, dentin, and cementum in vitro.[20–23,63] A reduction in microhardness has been observed.[64] These changes may cause dental hard tissues to be more susceptible to degradation and to secondary caries formation.

Mucosal Damage. Caustic bleaching agents in contact with the oral mucosa may cause peroxide-induced tissue damage.[54] Ulceration and sloughing of the mucosa are caused by oxygen gas bubbles in the tissue. Generally, the mucosa appears white but does not become necrotic or leave scar tissue. The associated burning sensation is extremely uncomfortable for the patient. Treatment is by extensive water rinses until the whiteness is reduced. In more severe cases, a topical anesthetic, limited movements, and good oral hygiene aid healing. Application of protective cream or catalase can prevent most of these complications.

Laser-Activated Bleaching

Recently, a technique has been introduced using lasers for extracoronal bleaching. Two types of lasers can be employed: the argon laser that emits a visible blue light and a carbon-dioxide laser that emits invisible infrared light. These lasers can be targeted to stain molecules and, with the use of a catalyst, rapidly decompose hydrogen peroxide to oxygen and water. The catalyst/peroxide combination may be damaging; therefore, exposed soft tissues, eyes, and clothing should be protected.

Combination of both lasers can effectively reduce intrinsic stains in the dentin. An argon laser can be targeted at stain molecules without overheating the pulp. It is easy to use and is best for removal of initial dark stains, such as those caused by tetracycline. However, visible blue light becomes less effective as the tooth whitens, and there are fewer stain molecules. On the other hand, the carbon-dioxide laser interacts directly with the catalyst/peroxide combination and removes the stain regardless of the tooth color.

Some techniques involve high-concentration hydrogen peroxide formulations as active ingredients (35 to 50%). It was reported that such laser bleaching techniques lightened teeth faster. However, short-term postoperative sensitivity can be profound.

Laser bleaching is a relatively new technique, and there are currently no long-term studies regarding its benefits or adverse effects.[65]

Mouthguard Bleaching

This technique has been widely advocated as a home bleaching technique, with a wide variety of materials, bleaching agents, frequency, and duration of treatment. Numerous products are available, mostly containing either 1.5 to 10% hydrogen peroxide or 10 to 15% carbamide peroxide, that degrade slowly to release hydrogen peroxide. The carbamide peroxide products are more commonly used. Higher concentrations of the active ingredient are also available and may reach up to 50% (Table 16-5).

Treatment techniques may vary according to manufacturers' instructions. The following step-by-step instructions should be used only as a general guideline. The procedure is as follows:

1. Familiarize the patient with the probable causes of discoloration, procedure to be followed, and expected outcome.
2. Carry out prophylaxis and assess tooth color with a shade guide. Take clinical photographs before and throughout the procedure.
3. Make an alginate impression of the arch to be treated. Cast the impression and outline the guard on the model. It should completely cover the teeth, although second molars need not be covered unless required for retention. Place two layers of die relief on the buccal aspects of the cast teeth to form a small reservoir for the bleaching agent. Fabricate a vacuum-form soft plastic matrix, approximately 2 mm thick, trim with crown and bridge scissors to 1 mm past the gingival margins, and adjust with an acrylic trimming bur.
4. Insert the mouthguard to ensure a proper fit. Remove the guard and apply the bleaching agent in the space of each tooth to be bleached. Reinsert the mouthguard over the teeth and remove excess bleaching agent.
5. Familiarize the patient with the use of the bleaching agent and wearing of the guard. The procedure is usually performed 3 to 4 hours a day, and the bleaching agent is replenished every 30 to 60 minutes. Some clinicians recommend wearing the guard during sleep for better long-term esthetic results.
6. Instruct patients to brush and rinse their teeth after meals. The guard should not be worn while eating. Inform the patient about thermal sensitivity and minor irritation of soft tissues and to discontinue use of the guard if uncomfortable.
7. Treatment should be for between 4 and 24 weeks. Recall the patient every 2 weeks to monitor stain lightening. Check for tissue irritation, oral lesions,

Table 16-5 Common Commercial Brands of Home-Use Bleaching Products

Brand	Company	Active Ingredient	Concentrations Available, %
BriteSmile	BriteSmile	10% HP	6, 8, 10
Contrast P.M.	Interdent	10% CP	10, 15, 20
Denta-Lite	Challenge	10% CP	10
Karisma	Confi-Dental	10% CP	10
Natural White	Aesthete	6% HP	6
Nite White	Discus Dental	10% CP	5, 10, 16, 22
Nupro Gold	Dentsply/Ash	10% CP	10
NuSmile	M&M	15% CP	15
Opalescence	Ultradent	10% CP	10, 35
Perfecta	Am Dent Hygienics	11% CP	11, 13, 16
Rembrandt	Den-Mat	10% CP	10, 15, 22
Spring White	Spring Health	10% CP	10
White & Brite	Omnii	10% CP	10, 16
Platinum	Colgate	10% CP	10
Zaris System	3-M	10% CP	10, 16

HP = hydrogen peroxide; CP = carbamide peroxide.

enamel etching, and leaky restorations. If complications occur, stop treatment and re-evaluate the feasibility of continuation at a later date. Note that frequently the incisal edges are bleached more readily than the remainder of the crown (Table 16-6).

The long-term esthetic results of this method are unknown. However, it appears that rediscoloration is not more frequent than with the other techniques. To date, no conclusive experimental or clinical studies on the safety of long-term use of these bleaching agents are available. Therefore, caution should be exercised in their prescription and application.[66] Of major concern is the products marketed to the public over the counter, often without professional control. Their use should be discouraged.

Table 16-6 Indications and Contraindications for Mouthguard Vital Bleaching

Indications	Contraindications
Superficial enamel discolorations	Severe enamel loss
Mild yellow discolorations	Hypersensitive teeth
Brown fluorosis discolorations	Presence of caries
Age-related discolorations	Defective coronal restorations
	Allergy to bleaching gels
	Bruxism

Complications and Adverse Effects. *Systemic Effects.* Controlled mouthguard bleaching procedures are considered relatively safe.[19] However, some concern has been raised over bleaching gels inadvertently swallowed by the patient. Accidental ingestion of large amounts of these gels may be toxic and cause irritation to the gastric and respiratory mucosa.[67] Bleaching gels containing carbopol, which retards the rate of oxygen release from peroxide, are usually more toxic. Therefore, it is advisable to pay specific attention to any adverse systemic effects and to discontinue treatment immediately if they occur.

Dental Hard Tissue Damage. *In vitro* studies indicate morphologic and chemical changes in enamel, dentin, and cementum associated with some agents used for **mouthguard** bleaching.[20–23] Long-term in vivo studies are still required to determine the clinical significance of these changes.

Tooth Sensitivity. Transient tooth sensitivity to cold may occur during or after mouthguard bleaching. In most cases, it is mild and ceases on termination of treatment. Treatment for sensitivity consists of removal of the mouthguard for 2 to 3 days, reduction of wearing time, and re-adjustment of the guard.

Pulpal Damage. Long-term effects of mouthguard bleaching on the pulp are still unknown. To date, no correlation has been found between carbamide peroxide bleaching and permanent pulpal damage.[19] The pulpalgia associated with tooth hypersensitivity is usually transient and uneventful.

Mucosal Damage. Minor irritations or ulcerations of the oral mucosa have been reported to occur during the initial course of treatment. This infrequent occurrence is usually mild and transient. Possible causes are mechanical interference by the mouthguard, chemical irritation by the bleaching active agent, and allergic reaction to gel components. In most cases, readjustment and smoothing the borders of the guard will suffice. However, if tissue irritation persists, treatment should be discontinued.

Damage to Restorations. Some *in vitro* studies suggest that damage of bleaching gels to composite resins might be caused by softening and cracking of the resin matrix.[24,25] It has been suggested that patients are informed that previously placed composites may require replacement following bleaching. Others have reported no significant adverse effects on either surface texture or color of restorations.[19] Generally, however, if composite restorations are present in esthetically critical areas, they may need replacement to improve color matching following successful bleaching.

It has also been reported that both 10% carbamide peroxide and 10% hydrogen peroxide may enhance the liberation of mercury and silver from amalgam restorations and may increase exposure of patients to toxic by-products.[68] Although bleaching gels are mainly applied to the anterior dentition, excessive gel may inadvertently make contact with posterior teeth. Coverage of posterior amalgam restorations with a protective layer of dental varnish prior to gel application may prevent such hazards.

Occlusal Disturbances. Typically, occlusal problems related to the mouthguard may be mechanical or physiologic. From a mechanical point of view, the patient may occlude only on the posterior teeth rather than on all teeth simultaneously. Removing posterior teeth from the guard until all of the teeth are in contact rectifies this problem. From a physiologic point of view, if the patient experiences temporomandibular joint pain, the posterior teeth can be removed from the guard until only the anterior guidance remains. In such cases, wearing time should be reduced.

For further information on extracoronal, home-bleaching methods, the reader is referred to the writings of Haywood and colleagues.[69–74]

REFERENCES

1. Walton RE, Rotstein I. Bleaching discolored teeth: Internal and external. In: Walton RE, Torabinejad M, editors. Principles and practice of endodontics. 2nd ed. Philadelphia: WB Saunders; 1996. p. 385.
2. Rotstein I. Bleaching nonvital and vital discolored teeth. In: Cohen S, Burns RC, editors. Pathways of the pulp. 7th ed St. Louis: CV Mosby; 1998. p. 674.
3. Freccia WF, et al. An in vitro comparison of non-vital bleaching techniques in the discolored tooth. JOE 1982;8:70.
4. Rotstein I, et al. *In vitro* efficacy of sodium perborate preparations used for intracoronal bleaching of discolored non-vital teeth. Endod Dent Traumatol 1991;7:177.
5. Rotstein I, Mor C, Friedman S. Prognosis of intracoronal bleaching with sodium perborate preparations *in vitro*: 1 year study. JOE 1993;19:10.
6. Atasu M, Genc A, Ercalik S. Enamel hypoplasia and essential staining of teeth from erythroblastosis fetalis. J Clin Pediatr Dent 1998;22:249.
7. Lochary ME, Lockhart PB, Williams WT Jr. Doxycycline and staining of permanent teeth. Pediatr Infect Dis J 1998;17:429.
8. Livingston HM, Dellinger TM. Intrinsic staining of teeth secondary to tetracycline. Ann Pharmacother 1998;32:607.
9. Jordan RE, Boskman L. Conservative vital bleaching treatment of discolored dentition. Compend Contin Educ Dent 1984;5:803.
10. Arens DE, Rich JJ, Healey HJ. A practical method of bleaching tetracycline-stained teeth. Oral Surg 1972;34:812.
11. Cohen S, Parkins FM. Bleaching tetracycline-stained vital teeth. Oral Surg 1970;29:465.
12. Abou-Rass M. The elimination of tetracycline discoloration by intentional endodontics and internal bleaching. JOE 1982;8:101.
13. Lake F, O'Dell N, Walton R. The effect of internal bleaching on tetracycline in dentin. JOE 1985;11:415.
14. Walton RE, O'Dell NL, Lake FT. Internal bleaching of tetracycline stained teeth in dogs. JOE 1983;9:416.
15. Driscoll WS, et al. Prevalence of dental caries and dental fluorosis in areas with optimal and above-optimal water fluoride concentrations. J Am Dent Assoc 1983;107:42.
16. Van der Burgt TP, Plasschaert AJM. Bleaching of tooth discoloration caused by endodontic sealers. JOE 1986;12:231.
17. Weiger R, Kuhn A, Löst C. *In vitro* comparison of various types of sodium perborate used for intracoronal bleaching. JOE 1994;20:338.
18. Rotstein I, Friedman S. pH variation among materials used for intracoronal bleaching. JOE 1991;17:376.
19. Haywood VB, Heymann HO. Nightguard vital bleaching: how safe is it? Quintessence Int 1991;22:515.
20. Rotstein I, et al. Histochemical analysis of dental hard tissues following bleaching. JOE 1996;22:23.
21. Seghi RR, Denry I. Effects of external bleaching on indentation and abrasion characteristics of human enamel *in vitro*. J Dent Res 1992;71:1340.
22. Zalkind M, Arwaz JR, Goldman A, Rotstein I. Surface morphology changes in human enamel, dentin and cementum following bleaching: a scanning electron microscopy study. Endod Dent Traumatol 1996;12:82.
23. Bitter NC. A scanning electron microscope study of the long-term effect of bleaching agents on the enamel surface *in vivo*. Gen Dent 1998;46:84.

24. Crim GA. Post-operative bleaching: effect on microleakage. Am J Dent 1992;5:109.
25. Titley KC, Torneck CD, Ruse ND. The effect of carbamide-peroxide gel on the shear bond strength of a microfil resin to bovine enamel. J Dent Res 1992;71:20.
26. Spasser HF. A simple bleaching technique using sodium perborate. N Y State Dent J 1961;27:332.
27. Nutting EB, Poe GS. A new combination for bleaching teeth. J South Calif Dent Assoc 1963;31:289.
28. Steiner DR, West JD. A method to determine the location and shape of an intracoronal bleach barrier. JOE 1994;20:304.
29. Holmstrup G, Palm AM, Lambjerg-Hansen H. Bleaching of discoloured root-filled teeth. Endod Dent Traumatol 1988;4:197.
30. Madison S, Walton RE. Cervical root resorption following bleaching of endodontically treated teeth. JOE 1990; 16:570.
31. Rotstein I, et al. Histological characterization of bleaching-induced external root resorption in dogs. JOE 1991;17:436.
32. Lin LC, Pitts DL, Burgess LW. An investigation into the feasibility of photobleaching tetracycline-stained teeth. JOE 1988;14:293.
33. Anitua E, Zabalegui B, Gil J, Gascon F. Internal bleaching of severe tetracycline discolorations: four-year clinical evaluation. Quintessence Int 1990;21:783.
34. Harrington GW, Natkin E. External resorption associated with bleaching of pulpless teeth. JOE 1979;5:344.
35. Lado EA, Stanley HR, Weisman MI. Cervical resorption in bleached teeth. Oral Surg 1983;55:78.
36. Montgomery S. External cervical resorption after bleaching a pulpless tooth. Oral Surg 1984;57:203.
37. Shearer GJ. External resorption associated with bleaching of a non-vital tooth. Aust Endod Newslett 1984;10:16.
38. Cvek M, Lindvall AM. External root resorption following bleaching of pulpless teeth with oxygen peroxide. Endod Dent Traumatol 1985;1:56.
39. Latcham NL. Postbleaching cervical resorption. JOE 1986;12:262.
40. Goon WWY, Cohen S, Borer RF. External cervical root resorption following bleaching. JOE 1986;12:414.
41. Friedman S, et al. Incidence of external root resorption and esthetic results in 58 bleached pulpless teeth. Endod Dent Traumatol 1988;4:23.
42. Gimlin DR, Schindler WG. The management of postbleaching cervical resorption. JOE 1990;16:292.
43. Al-Nazhan S. External root resorption after bleaching: a case report. Oral Surg 1991;72:607.
44. Heithersay GS, Dahlstrom SW, Marin PD. Incidence of invasive cervical resorption in bleached root-filled teeth. Aust Dent J 1994;39:82.
45. Heller D, Skriber J, Lin LM. Effect of intracoronal bleaching on external cervical root resorption. JOE 1992;18:145.
46. Rotstein I, Torek Y, Misgav R. Effect of cementum defects on radicular penetration of 30% H_2O_2 during intracoronal bleaching. JOE 1991;17:230.
47. Koulaouzidou E, et al. Role of cementoenamel junction on the radicular penetration of 30% hydrogen peroxide during intracoronal bleaching *in vitro*. Endod Dent Traumatol 1996;12:146.
48. Rotstein I, Torek Y, Lewinstein I. Effect of bleaching time and temperature on the radicular penetration of hydrogen peroxide. Endod Dent Traumatol 1991;7:196.
49. Heling I, Parson A, Rotstein I. Effect of bleaching agents on dentin permeability to *Streptococcus faecalis*. JOE 1995;21:540.
50. Titley KC, Torneck CD, Ruse ND, Krmec D. Adhesion of a resin composite to bleached and unbleached human enamel. JOE 1993;19:112.
51. Titley KC, et al. Scanning electron microscopy observations on the penetration and structure of resin tags in bleached and unbleached bovine enamel. JOE 1991;17:71.
52. Torneck CD, Titley KC, Smith DC, Adibfar A. Effect of water leaching on the adhesion of composite resin to bleached and unbleached bovine enamel. JOE 1991;17:156.
53. Rotstein I. Role of catalase in the elimination of residual hydrogen peroxide following tooth bleaching. JOE 1993;19:567.
54. Rotstein I, Wesselink PR, Bab I. Catalase protection against hydrogen peroxide-induced injury in rat oral mucosa. Oral Surg 1993;75:744.
55. Rotstein I, Zyskind D, Lewinstein I, Bamberger N. Effect of different protective base materials on hydrogen peroxide leakage during intracoronal bleaching *in vitro*. JOE 1992;18:114.
56. Casey LJ, Schindler WG, Murata SM, Burgess JO. The use of dentinal etching with endodontic bleaching procedures. JOE 1989;15:535.
57. Wilcox LR, Diaz-Arnold A. Coronal microleakage of permanent lingual access restorations in endodontically treated anterior teeth. JOE 1989;15:584.
58. Lemon R. Bleaching and restoring endodontcally treated teeth. Curr Opin Dent 1991;1:754.
59. Freccia WF, Peters DD, Lorton L. An evaluation of various permanent restorative materials' effect on the shade of bleached teeth. JOE 1982;8:265.
60. Cohen SC. Human pulpal response to bleaching procedures on vital teeth. JOE 1979;5:134.
61. Robertson WD, Melfi RC. Pulpal response to vital bleaching procedures. JOE 1980;6:645.
62. Nathanson D. Vital tooth bleaching: sensitivity and pulpal considerations. J Am Dent Assoc 1998;128 Suppl:41S.
63. Rotstein I, Lehr T, Gedalia I. Effect of bleaching agents on inorganic components of human dentin and cementum. JOE 1992;18:290.
64. Lewinstein I, Hirschfeld Z, Stabholz A, Rotstein I. Effect of hydrogen peroxide and sodium perborate on the microhardness of human enamel and dentin. JOE 1994;20:61.
65. Garber DA. Dentist-monitored bleaching: a discussion of combination and laser bleaching. J Am Dent Assoc 1997;128 Suppl:26S.
66. Li Y. Toxicological considerations of tooth bleaching using peroxide-containing agents. J Am Dent Assoc 1997;128 Suppl:31S.
67. Redmond AF, Cherry DV, Bowers DE Jr. Acute illness and recovery in adult female rats following ingestion of a tooth whitener containing 6% hydrogen peroxide. Am J Dent 1997;10:268.
68. Rotstein I, Mor C, Arwaz JR. Changes in surface levels of mercury, silver, tin and copper of dental amalgam treated with carbamide peroxide and hydrogen peroxide. Oral Surg 1997;83:506.
69. Haywood VB, Heymann HO. Response of normal and tetracycline-stained teeth with pulp-size variation to nightguard vital bleaching. J Esthet Dent 1994;6:109.

70. Haywood VB. Nightguard vital bleaching: current concepts and research. J Am Dent Assoc 1997;128 Suppl:19S.
71. Haywood VB. Bleaching vital teeth: current concepts. Quintessence Int 1997;28:424.
72. Leonard RH, Haywood VB, Phillips C. Risk factors for developing tooth sensitivity and gingival irritation in nightguard vital bleaching. Quintessence Int 1997;28:527.
73. Haywood VB. Extended bleaching of tetracycline stained teeth: a case report. Contemp Esthet Restor Pract 1997;1:14.
74. Haywood VB. Critical appraisal: at home bleaching. J Esthet Dent 1998;10:94.

Chapter 17

PEDIATRIC ENDODONTICS

Clifton O. Dummett Jr and Hugh M. Kopel

Treatment of pulpally inflamed primary and permanent teeth in children presents a unique challenge to the dental clinician. Pulp diagnosis in the child is imprecise as clinical symptoms do not correlate well with histologic pulpal status. Age and behavior can compromise the reliability of pain as an indicator of the extent of pulp inflammation. Furthermore, treatment goals are developmentally oriented and may be relatively short term by comparison to the long-term restorative permanence of adult endodontics. Because of this latter fact, a major focus in pediatric pulp therapy is vital pulp treatment, that capitalizes on the healing potential of the noninflamed remaining portions of the pulp. With instances of irreversibly inflamed and necrotic radicular pulps, conventional concepts of nonvital pulp treatment are indicated. However, they must be modified to accommodate physiologic root resorption in primary teeth and continued root development in young permanent teeth.

Lewis and Law succinctly stated the ultimate objective of pediatric pulp therapy: "The successful treatment of the pulpally involved tooth is to retain that tooth in a healthy condition so it may fulfill its role as a useful component of the primary and young permanent dentition."[1] Premature loss of primary teeth from dental caries and infection may result in the following sequelae:

- Loss of arch length
- Insufficient space for erupting permanent teeth
- Ectopic eruption and impaction of premolars
- Mesial tipping of molar teeth adjacent to primary molar loss
- Extrusion of opposing permanent teeth
- Shift of the midline with a possibility of crossbite occlusion
- Development of certain abnormal tongue positions

It is for this reason that maximum attempts must be made to preserve primary teeth in a healthy state until normal exfoliation occurs. A major contention in contemporary research involving vital pulp treatment is the definition of "healthy pulp status" ascribed to many of the treatment outcomes. This issue will be addressed in more detail later in this chapter.

Vital pulp therapy is based on the premise that pulp tissue has the capacity to heal. In addition to the biologic basis for the healing capacity of the pulp, differences between primary and permanent teeth exist from a morphologic and histologic standpoint. These differences must be addressed by the clinician to successfully treat pulpally inflamed teeth in children.

PULP MORPHOLOGY

Anatomic Differences Between Primary and Permanent Teeth

Anatomic differences between the pulp chambers and root canals of primary teeth and those of young permanent teeth have been described[2] (Figure 17-1): (1) **Pulp chamber** anatomy in primary teeth approximates the surface shape of the crown more closely than in permanent teeth. (2) The pulps of primary teeth are proportionately larger and the pulp horns extend closer to the outer surfaces of the cusps than in permanent teeth. (3) The pulp-protecting dentin thickness between the pulp chamber and the dentinoenamel junction is less than in permanent teeth. These three factors increase the potential for pulp exposure from mechanical preparation, dental caries, and trauma. (4) An increased number of accessory canals and foramina, as well as porosity in pulpal floors of primary teeth, has been noted in comparison with permanent teeth.[3] This is thought to account for the consistent pulp necrosis response of furcation radiolucency in primary teeth versus periapical radiolucency in permanent teeth.[4–6]

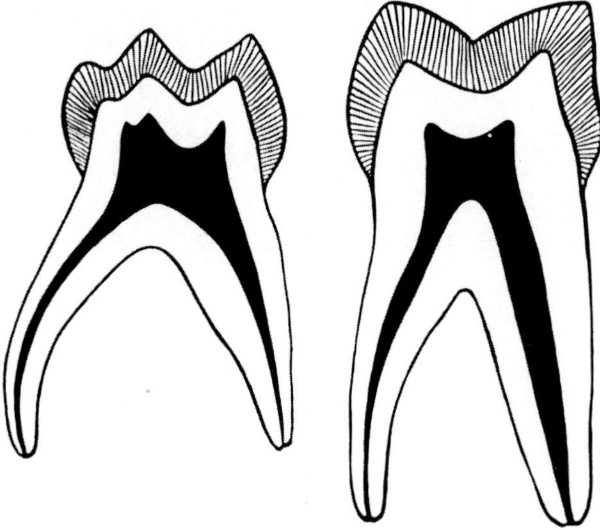

Figure 17-1 Comparative anatomy between primary (**left**) and permanent (**right**) molars. Primary teeth are smaller in all dimensions; their enamel cap is thinner, with less tooth structure protecting the pulp. Primary pulp horns are higher, particularly mesial. The roots of primary molars are longer and more slender, are "pinched in" at the cervical part of the tooth, and flare more toward the apex to accommodate permanent tooth buds. All of these factors tend to increase the incidence of pulp involvement from caries or complicate canal preparation and obturation. Reproduced with permission from Finn SB.[2]

A comparison of **root canals** in primary teeth with those of young permanent teeth reveals the following characteristics: (1) the roots of primary teeth are proportionately longer and more slender; (2) primary root canals are more ribbon-like and have multiple pulp filaments within their more numerous accessory canals; (3) the roots of primary molars flare outward from the cervical part of the tooth to a greater degree than permanent teeth and continue to flare apically to accommodate the underlying succedaneous tooth follicle; (4) the roots of primary anterior teeth are narrower mesiodistally than permanent anterior tooth roots; and (5) in contrast to permanent teeth, the roots of primary teeth undergo physiologic root resorption. These factors make complete extirpation of pulp remnants almost impossible and increase the potential of root perforation during canal instrumentation. As a result, the requirements of primary root canal filling materials must encompass germicidal action, good obturation, and resorptive capability.[3]

Histologic Considerations

Numerous descriptions of pulp histology exist that identify the various cell components of pulp tissue.[7,8] Consistently, the pulp is primarily connective tissue and has considerable healing potential. Features that distinguish pulp tissue from other connective tissue include the presence of odontoblasts, absence of histamine-releasing mast cells, tissue confinement in a hard cavity with little collateral circulation, and vascular access limited to the root apex.[7,8] Pulp healing capability is affected by endogenous factors of coronal cellularity and apical vascularity. Both are increased in primary and young permanent teeth.[8] Pulps become more fibrous, less cellular, and less vascular with age.[8] Exogenous factors affecting pulp healing include bacterial invasion and chemical/thermal insult. Current research in pulp biology and restorative materials strongly substantiates the need for bacterial microleakage control in maximizing pulp survival.[9]

Fox and Heeley concluded that, histologically, no structural differences exist between primary pulp tissue and young permanent pulp tissue with the exception of the presence of a cap-like zone of reticular and collagenous fibers in the primary coronal pulp.[10] However, many clinicians have noted different pulp responses between primary and young permanent teeth to trauma, bacterial invasion, irritation, and medication. Anatomic differences may contribute to these responses. **Primary** roots have an enlarged apical foramen, in contrast to the foramen of permanent roots, which is constricted. The resultant reduced blood supply in mature permanent teeth favors a calcific response and healing by "calcific scarring."[11] This hypothesis is exemplified in older pulps, in which more calcified nodules and ground substance are found than in young pulps. Primary teeth, with their abundant blood supply, demonstrate a more typical **inflammatory response** than that seen in mature permanent teeth.

The exaggerated inflammatory response in primary teeth may account for increased internal and external root resorption from calcium hydroxide pulpotomies. The alkalinity of calcium hydroxide can produce severe pulp inflammation and subsequent metaplasia with resultant internal primary root resorption. It has been shown that the greater the inflammation, the more severe the resorption (Figure 17-2). Although it is suspected that pulps of primary teeth have a different function from those of permanent teeth, no supporting data are available.

Some clinicians believe that primary teeth are less sensitive to pain than permanent teeth, probably because of differences in the number and/or distribution of neural elements. When comparing primary and permanent teeth, Bernick found differences in the final distribution of pulp nerve fibers.[12] In permanent teeth, these fibers terminate mainly among the odontoblasts and even beyond the predentin. In primary teeth, pulp

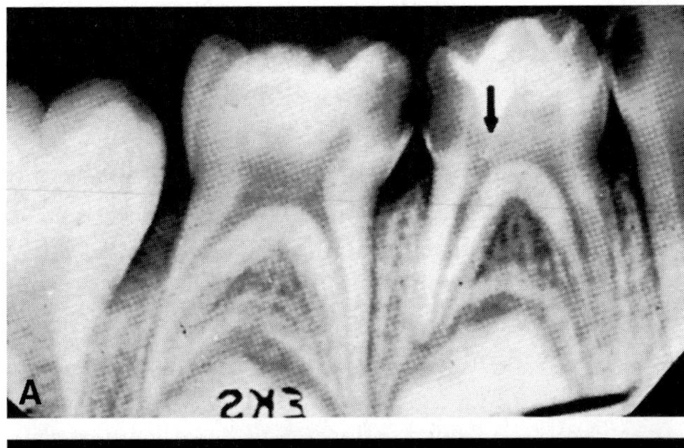

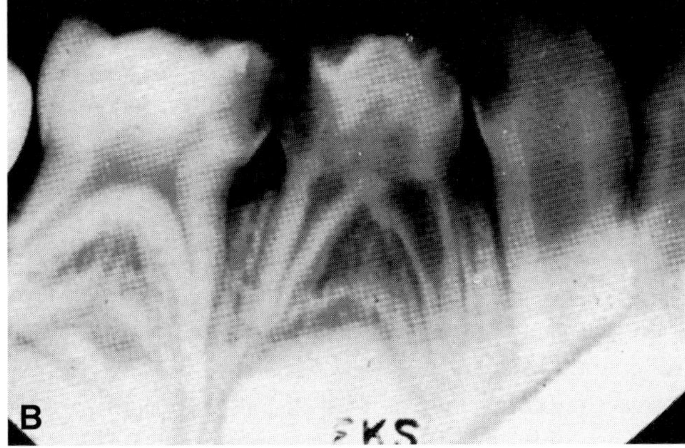

Figure 17-2 Internal resorption triggered by inflammation. **A**, Advanced caries in a 5-year-old child. Note calcification (**arrow**) in the first primary molar (contraindication for pulp therapy). **B**, Same patient 6 months later. Marked internal resorption, forecast in the earlier radiograph, indicates advanced degenerative changes. Reproduced with permission from Law DB, Lewis TM, Davis JM. An atlas of pedodontics. Philadelphia: WB Saunders; 1969.

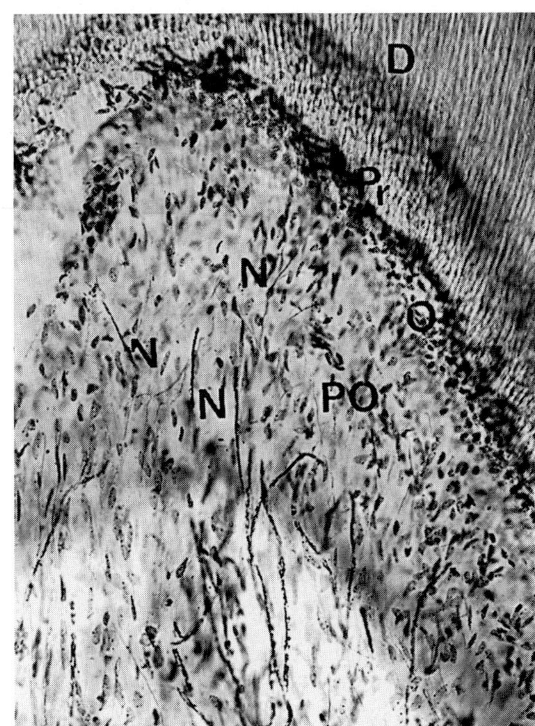

Figure 17-3 Section of pulp from a human **primary** molar. Note that the majority of nerves terminate at the pulp-odontoblastic (PO) border. Only isolated nerve fiber penetrates the P-O border to terminate in the zone of Weil. D = dentin; N = nerve fiber; O = odontoblasts; Pr = predentin; PO = pulp-odontoblast border. Reproduced with permission from Bernick S.[12]

nerve fibers pass to the odontoblastic area, where they terminate as free nerve endings. Bernick postulated that if primary teeth were not so short-lived in the oral cavity, their nerve endings might terminate among the odontoblasts and in the predentin as in permanent teeth[12] (Figure 17-3).

Rapp and associates concurred with Bernick's hypothesis and also stated that the density of the innervation of the primary tooth is not as great as that of the permanent tooth and may be the reason why primary teeth are less sensitive to operative procedures.[13] They agree, however, that as the primary teeth resorb, there is a degeneration of the neural elements as with other pulp cells. **Neural tissue** is the first to degenerate when root resorption begins, just as it **is the last tissue to mature** when the pulp develops.

Primary and permanent teeth also differ in their cellular responses to irritation, trauma, and medication. It has been shown, for example, that the incidence of reparative dentin formation beneath carious lesions is more extensive in primary than in permanent teeth.[14–17] McDonald reported that the localization of infection and inflammation is poorer in the primary pulp than in the pulp of permanent teeth.[18]

MANAGEMENT OF DEEP CARIOUS LESIONS AND PULP INFLAMMATION IN PRIMARY AND YOUNG PERMANENT TEETH

Pulp therapy for primary and young permanent teeth has historically been subject to change and controversy. Pulp medicaments, such as zinc oxide–eugenol (ZOE) cement, calcium hydroxide, and formocresol, have been the basis for much of this controversy. A better understanding of the reactions of the pulp and dentin to these medicaments has developed over time, primarily through improvements in histologic techniques. Anderson and colleagues felt that the pulp and dentin should be considered as one organ.[19] Frankl determined that this pulpodentinal system reaction is proportional to the intensity and duration of the offending agents of caries, trauma, medicaments, or restorative materials.[20]

A correct diagnosis of pulp conditions in primary teeth is important for treatment planning. McDonald and Avery have outlined several diagnostic aids in selecting teeth for vital pulp therapy.[3] Eidelman et al.[21] and Prophet and Miller[22] have emphasized that **no single** diagnostic means can be relied on for determining a diagnosis of pulp conditions. Rayner and Southam have stated that the inflammation response to the effects of dentin caries in the deciduous pulp is more rapid than in the permanent pulp.[23] Yet Taylor concluded that in spite of being inflamed and infected by the carious process, primary molars are still capable of marked defense reactions similar to those observed in permanent teeth.[24]

The goal in managing the deep carious lesion is preservation of pulp vitality before arbitrarily instituting endodontic therapy. A suggested outline for determining the pulpal status of cariously involved teeth in children involves the following:

1. Visual and tactile examination of carious dentin and associated periodontium
2. Radiographic examination of
   a. periradicular and furcation areas
   b. pulp canals
   c. periodontal space
   d. developing succedaneous teeth
3. History of spontaneous unprovoked pain
4. Pain from percussion
5. Pain from mastication
6. Degree of mobility
7. Palpation of surrounding soft tissues
8. Size, appearance, and amount of hemorrhage associated with pulp exposures

Pediatric pulp therapy for primary and young permanent teeth involves the following techniques:

1. Indirect pulp capping
2. Direct pulp capping
3. Coronal pulpotomy
4. Pulpectomy

The **first three methods are vital techniques** that involve conservative management of portions of inflamed pulp tissue with the preservation of the remaining vital pulp. The **pulpectomy procedure is a nonvital technique** and involves the complete extirpation of the irreversibly inflamed and/or necrotic pulp followed by canal obturation with a resorbable medicament in primary teeth and conventional root canal filling in permanent teeth.

INDIRECT PULP CAPPING

Indirect pulp capping is defined as the application of a medicament over a thin layer of remaining carious dentin, after deep excavation, with no exposure of the pulp. In 1961, Damele described the purpose of indirect pulp capping as the use of "reconstructed" dentin to prevent pulp exposure.[25] The treatment objective is to avoid pulp exposure and the necessity of more invasive measures of pulp therapy by stimulating the pulp to generate reparative dentin beneath the carious lesion. This results in the arrest of caries progression and preservation of the vitality of the nonexposed pulp.[26] This technique can be used as a one-sitting procedure or the more classic two-sitting procedure. The latter involves re-entry after a 6 to 8-week interval to remove any remaining carious dentin and place the final restoration[3,27] (Figure 17-4).

DiMaggio found, in a histologic evaluation of teeth selected for indirect treatment, that 75% would have been pulp exposures if all of the caries had initially been removed. Using **clinical** criteria, this same study showed a **failure** rate of only **1%** for **indirect** pulp caps compared with **25% failure** for **direct** caps.[28] A **histologic examination,** however, raised these failure rates to **12%** and **33%**, respectively. Trowbridge and Berger stated that complete removal of softened dentin, with ensuing pulp exposure, may contribute nothing of diagnostic value in estimating the extent of existing pulp disease.[29] In fact, other studies have shown that the true picture of pulp disease cannot be assessed on the basis of such diagnostic criteria as history of pain, response to temperature change, percussion, and electric pulp testing.[30,31]

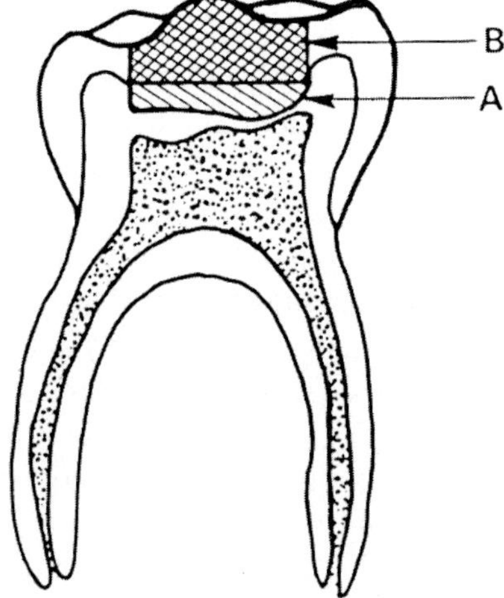

Figure 17-4 Indirect pulp-capping technique. **A**, Medicament, either zinc oxide–eugenol cement, calcium hydroxide, or both, against remaining caries. **B**, Lasting temporary restoration. Following repair, both materials are removed along with softened caries, and final restorations are placed.

Historical Review

The concept of indirect pulp capping was first described by Pierre Fauchard as reported by John Tomes in the mid-18th century, who recommended that all caries should not be removed in deep, sensitive cavities "for fear of exposing the nerve and making the cure worse than the disease."[32] John Tomes, in his mid-19th century textbook, stated, "It is better that a layer of discolored dentin should be allowed to remain for the protection of the pulp rather than run the risk of sacrificing the tooth."[32] Although neither of these dental pioneers referred to any specific medication for the softened dentin, they recognized the healing capacity of the pulp.

In 1891, W. D. Miller discussed various "antiseptics" that should be used for sterilizing dentin.[34] In contrast to these early reports advocating conservative management of deep lesions, G. V. Black felt that in the interest of scientific dental practice, no decayed or softened material should be left in a cavity preparation, whether or not the pulp was exposed.[35]

Rationale

Indirect pulp capping is based on the knowledge that decalcification of the dentin precedes bacterial invasion within the dentin.[36–38] This technique is predicated on removing the outer layers of the carious dentin, that contain the majority of the microorganisms, reducing the continued demineralization of the deeper dentin layers from bacterial toxins, and sealing the lesion to allow the pulp to generate reparative dentin. Fusayama and colleagues demonstrated that in **acute caries**, dentin discoloration occurred far in advance of the microorganisms, and as much as **2 mm of softened or discolored dentin was not infected.**[38] In a later study, Fusayama found that carious dentin actually consists of two distinct layers having different ultramicroscopic and chemical structures.[39] The outer carious layer is irreversibly denatured, infected, and incapable of being remineralized and should be removed. The inner carious layer is **reversibly** denatured, **not infected**, and capable of being remineralized and should be preserved. The two layers can be differentiated clinically by a solution of basic fuchsin.[39]

Whitehead and colleagues compared deep excavations in primary and permanent teeth.[40] After all softened dentin had been removed from the cavity floor, they found that 51.5% of the permanent teeth were free from all signs of organisms, and a further 34% had only 1 to 20 infected dentinal tubules in any one section.[40] Primary teeth, however, showed a much higher percentage of bacteria in the cavity floor after all softened dentin was removed. These results were further supported by Shovelton, who found that although the deepest demineralized layers of dentin were generally free from infection, the possibility of a few dentinal tubules containing organisms did exist, especially in primary teeth.[41] This finding was supported by Seltzer and Bender.[42] Thus, complete clinical removal of carious dentin does not necessarily ensure that all infected tubules have been eradicated. Conversely, the presence of softened dentin does not necessarily indicate infection.

A number of investigators have provided evidence that the pulp can readily cope with minute contamination. Reeves and Stanley[43] and Shovelton[44] showed that when the carious lesion proximity to the pulp was greater than 0.8 mm (including reparative dentin when present), no significant disturbance occurred within the pulp of permanent teeth. Rayner and Southam, in studying carious primary teeth, found the mean depth of pulp inflammatory changes from bacterial dentin penetration to be 0.6 mm in proximity to the pulp, with some changes occurring within a 1.8 mm pulp proximity.[23] Massler considered that pulp reactions under deep carious lesions result from bacterial toxins rather than the bacteria themselves.[45] Massler and Pawlak used the terms "affected" and "infected" to describe pulp reaction to deep carious attack.[46] This histologic study showed that the "affected" pulp, beneath a deep carious lesion with a thin layer of dentin between the pulp and the bacterial front, was often inflamed and painful but contained no demonstrable bacteria. However, when significant numbers of bacteria were found within the "infected" pulp, a microscopic exposure in the carious dentin was seen. Canby and Bernier concluded that the deeper layers of carious dentin tend to impede the bacterial invasion of the pulp because of the acid nature of the affected dentin.[47]

The results of these studies indicate the presence of three dentinal layers in a carious lesion: (1) a necrotic, soft, brown dentin outer layer, teeming with bacteria and not painful to remove; (2) a firmer, discolored dentin layer with fewer bacteria but painful to remove, suggesting the presence of viable odontoblastic extensions from the pulp; and (3) a hard, discolored dentin deep layer with a minimal amount of bacterial invasion that is painful to instrumentation.

Response to Treatment

Sayegh found three distinct types of new dentin in response to **indirect pulp capping**: (1) cellular fibrillar dentin at 2 months post-treatment, (2) presence of globular dentin during the first 3 months, and (3) tubular dentin in a more uniformly mineralized pattern.[17] In this study of 30 primary and permanent teeth, Sayegh concluded that new dentin forms fastest in teeth with the thinnest dentin remaining after cavity preparation. He also found that the longer treatment times enhanced dentin formation.[17]

Diagnosis of the type of caries influences the treatment planning for indirect pulp capping. In the **active** lesion, most of the caries-related organisms are found in the outer layers of decay, whereas the deeper decalcified layers are fairly free of bacteria. In the **arrested** lesion, the surface layers are not always contaminated, especially where the surface is hard and leathery. The deepest layers are quite sclerotic and free of microorganisms.[48] Deep carious dentin is even more resistant to decomposition by acids and proteolysis than is normal dentin. This was especially true in arrested caries.[49,50]

Procedures for Indirect Pulp Capping

Case selection based on clinical and radiographic assessment to substantiate the health of the pulp is critical for success. **Only those teeth free from irreversible signs and symptoms should be considered for indirect pulp capping.** The following measures should be employed for those teeth appropriate for this technique.

Indications. The decision to undertake the indirect pulp capping procedure should be based on the following findings:

1. History
   a. Mild discomfort from chemical and thermal stimuli
   b. Absence of spontaneous pain
2. Clinical examination
   a. Large carious lesion
   b. Absence of lymphadenopathy
   c. Normal appearance of adjacent gingiva
   d. Normal color of tooth
3. Radiographic examination
   a. Large carious lesion in close proximity to the pulp
   b. Normal lamina dura
   c. Normal periodontal ligament space
   d. No interradicular or periapical radiolucency

Contraindications. Findings that contraindicate this procedure are listed below:

1. History
   a. Sharp, penetrating pain that persists after withdrawing stimulus
   b. Prolonged spontaneous pain, particularly at night
2. Clinical examination
   a. Excessive tooth mobility
   b. Parulis in the gingiva approximating the roots of the tooth
   c. Tooth discoloration
   d. Nonresponsiveness to pulp testing techniques
3. Radiographic examination
   a. Large carious lesion with apparent pulp exposure
   b. Interrupted or broken lamina dura
   c. Widened periodontal ligament space
   d. Radiolucency at the root apices or furcation areas

If the indications are appropriate for indirect pulp capping, such treatment may be performed as a two-appointment or a one-appointment procedure.

Two-Appointment Technique (First Sitting).

1. Administer local anesthesia and isolate with a rubber dam.
2. Establish cavity outline with a high-speed handpiece.
3. Remove the majority of soft, necrotic, infected dentin with a large round bur in a **slow-speed** handpiece **without exposing** the pulp.
4. Remove peripheral carious dentin with sharp spoon excavators. Irrigate the cavity and dry with cotton pellets.
5. Cover the remaining affected dentin with a hard-setting calcium hydroxide dressing.
6. Fill or base the remainder of the cavity with a **reinforced** ZOE cement (IRM Dentsply-Caulk; Milford.) or a glass-ionomer cement to achieve a good seal.
7. Do not disturb this sealed cavity for 6 to 8 weeks. It may be necessary to use amalgam, composite resin, or a stainless steel crown as a final restoration to maintain this seal.

Two-Appointment Technique (Second Sitting, 6 to 8 Weeks Later). If the tooth has been asymptomatic, the surrounding soft tissues are free from swelling, and the temporary filling is intact, the second step can be performed:

1. Bitewing radiographs of the treated tooth should be assessed for the presence of reparative dentin.
2. Again use local anesthesia and rubber dam isolation.
3. **Carefully** remove all temporary filling material, especially the calcium hydroxide dressing over the deep portions of the cavity floor.
4. The remaining affected carious dentin should appear dehydrated and "flaky" and should be easily removed. The area around the potential exposure

should appear whitish and may be soft; this is **"predentin." Do not disturb!**

5. The cavity preparation should be irrigated and gently dried.
6. Cover the entire floor with a **hard-setting** calcium hydroxide dressing.
7. A base should be placed with a **reinforced** ZOE or glass ionomer cement, and the tooth should receive a final restoration.

One-Appointment Technique. The value of re-entry and re-excavation has been questioned by some clinicians when viewed in light of numerous studies reporting success rates of indirect pulp capping with calcium hydroxide ranging from 73 to 98% (Table 17-1). On this basis, the need to uncover the residual dentin to remove dehydrated dentin and view the sclerotic changes has been questioned. The second entry subjects the pulp to potential risk of exposure owing to overzealous re-excavation.[7]

Leung et al.[51] and Fairbourn and colleagues[52] have been able to show a significant decrease of bacteria in deep carious lesions after being covered with calcium hydroxide (Dycal, Dentsply-Caulk; Milford.) or a modified ZOE (IRM) for periods ranging from 1 to 15 months. These investigators suggested that re-entry to remove the residual minimal carious dentin after capping with calcium hydroxide may not be necessary if the final restoration maintains a seal and the tooth is asymptomatic.

After cavity preparation, if all carious dentin was removed except the portion that would expose the pulp, re-entry might be unnecessary.[7] Conversely, if the clinician had to leave considerably more carious dentin owing to patient symptoms, re-entry would be advised to confirm reparative dentin and pulp exposure status. If a pulp exposure occurs during re-entry, a more invasive vital pulp therapy technique such as direct pulp capping or pulpotomy would be indicated. Tooth selection for one-appointment indirect pulp capping must be based on clinical judgment and experience with many cases in addition to the previously mentioned criteria.

Evaluation of Therapy. A histologic evaluation of pulp reactions to indirect pulp capping has been reported in a varying number of samples. Law and Lewis reported irritational dentin formation, an active odontoblastic layer, an intact zone of Weil, and a slightly hyperactive pulp with the presence of some inflammatory cells.[53] Held-Wydler demonstrated irritational dentin in 40 of 41 young molars in which the carious dentin was covered with ZOE cement.[54] The pulp tissue was either completely normal or mildly inflamed over a period of

Table 17-1 Studies on Indirect Pulp Capping in Primary and Young Permanent Teeth

Study	Agent	Cases	Observation Period	% of Success
Sowden, 1956	$Ca(OH)_2$	4,000	Up to 7 y	"Very high"
Law and Lewis, 1961	$Ca(OH)_2$	38	Up to 2 y	73.6
Hawes and DiMaggio, 1964	$Ca(OH)_2$	475	Up to 4 y	97
Kerkhove et al., 1964	$Ca(OH)_2$	41	12 mo	95
	ZOE	35	12 mo	95
Held-Wydler, 1964	$Ca(OH)_2$	41	35–630 d	88
King et al., 1965	$Ca(OH)_2$	21	25–206 d	62
	ZOE	22		88
Aponte, 1966	$Ca(OH)_2$	30	6–46 mo	93
Jordan and Suzuki, 1971	$Ca(OH)_2$	243	10–12 wk	98
Nordstrom et al., 1974	$Ca(OH)_2$	64	94 d	84
	SnFl			90
Magnusson, 1977	$Ca(OH)_2$	55		85
Sawusch, 1982	$Ca(OH)_2$	184	13–15 mo	97
Nirschl and Avery, 1983	$Ca(OH)_2$	38	6 mo	94
Coll, 1988	$Ca(OH)_2$	26	20–58 mo	92.3

$Ca(OH)_2$ = calcium hydroxide; ZOE = zinc oxide–eugenol; SnFI = stannous fluoride.

34 to 630 days. In the histologic sections, four layers could be demonstrated (Figure 17-5): (1) carious decalcified dentin, (2) rhythmic layers of irregular reparative dentin, (3) regular tubular dentin, and (4) normal pulp with a slight increase in fibrous elements.

Clinical studies have shown no significant differences in the ultimate success of this technique regardless of whether calcium hydroxide or ZOE cement is used over residual carious dentin.[55–57] However, Torstenson et al. demonstrated slight to moderate inflammation when ZOE was used in deep unlined cavities that were less than 0.5 mm to the pulp itself.[58] Nordstrom and colleagues reported that carious dentin, wiped with a 10% solution of stannous fluoride for 5 minutes and covered with ZOE, can be remineralized.[59] It was further stated that no particular difference was found in failure rates of teeth treated with calcium hydroxide and those treated with stannous fluoride. As so many others have also concluded, the results for primary and young permanent teeth do not differ significantly (see Table 17-1).

King and associates,[60] as well as Aponte et al.[61] and Parikh et al.,[62] determined that the residual layer of carious dentin, left in the indirect pulp-capping technique, can be **sterilized** with either ZOE cement or calcium hydroxide. However, it cannot be presumed that all of the remaining infected or affected dentin becomes **remineralized.** In contrast to ZOE, residual dentin will increase in mineral content when in contact with calcium hydroxide.[63,64]

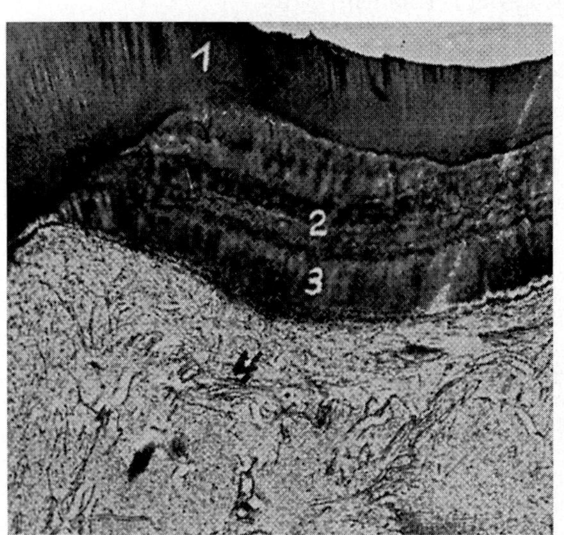

Figure 17-5 Photomicrograph of four layers of healing under indirect pulp capping of a permanent molar of a 14½-year-old child. Zinc oxide–eugenol cement capping after excavation of the necrotic dentin layer only. No pain 480 days later when extracted. 1 = carious decalcified dentin; 2 = rhythmic layers of irregular irritational dentin; 3 = regular tubular dentin; 4 = normal pulp with slight increase in fibrous elements. Reproduced with permission from Held-Wydler E.[54]

Sawusch evaluated calcium hydroxide liners for indirect pulp capping in primary and young permanent teeth. After periods ranging from 13 to 21 months, he concluded that Dycal was a highly effective agent.[65]

Nirschl and Avery reported greater than 90% success rates for both Dycal and LIFE (SybronEndo/Kerr Corp.; Orange, Calif.) calcium hydroxide preparations when used as bases in both primary and permanent teeth for indirect pulp-capping therapy.[66]

Coll et al., in an evaluation of several modes of pulp therapy in primary incisors, stated that the success rates of indirect pulp cappings in primary incisors did not differ from comparable molar rates.[67] They showed a 92.3% success rate for treated incisors after a mean follow-up time of 42 months.

The medicament choice for indirect pulp capping can be based on the clinical history of the carious tooth in question. Some investigators recommend ZOE because of its sealing and obtundant properties, which reduce pulp symptoms. Others recommend calcium hydroxide because of its ability to stimulate a more rapid formation of reparative dentin. Stanley believes that it makes no difference which is used because neither is in direct contact with pulp tissue, and increased dentin thickness was observed to occur beneath deep lesions treated with both agents.[57] However, in case of an undetected microscopic pulp exposure during caries excavation, calcium hydroxide will better stimulate a dentinal bridge.[57,68] Primosch et al. noted that the majority of US pediatric dentistry undergraduate programs used calcium hydroxide as the principal indirect pulp capping medicament in their teaching protocols.[69]

Lado and Stanley demonstrated that light-cured calcium hydroxide compounds were equally effective in inhibiting growth of organisms commonly found at the base of cavity preparations.[70]

A minimum indirect pulp post-treatment time period of 6 to 8 weeks should be allowed to produce adequate remineralization of the cavity floor.[7,17,71] This desirable outcome is essentially dependent on the maintenance of a patent seal against microleakage by the **temporary** and final restorations. In this regard, the newer resin-reinforced glass ionomer cements and dentin bonding agents should be considered.

DIRECT PULP CAPPING

Direct pulp capping involves the placement of a biocompatible agent on **healthy** pulp tissue that has been inadvertently exposed from caries excavation or trau-

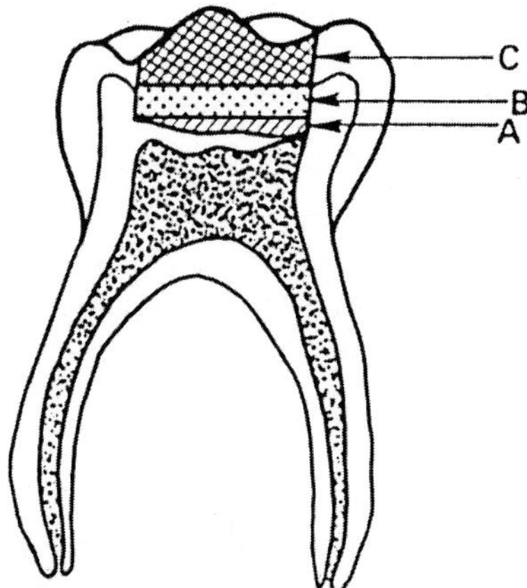

Figure 17-6 Direct pulp-capping technique. A, Capping material covers pulp exposure and the floor of the cavity. B, Protective base of zinc oxide–eugenol cement. C, Amalgam restoration.

matic injury[72] (Figure 17-6). The treatment objective is to seal the pulp against bacterial leakage, encourage the pulp to wall off the exposure site by initiating a dentin bridge, and maintain the vitality of the underlying pulp tissue regions (Figure 17-7).

Case Selection

Success with direct pulp capping is dependent on the coronal and radicular pulp being healthy and free from bacterial invasion.[73,74] The clinician must rely on the physical appearance of the exposed pulp tissue, radiographic assessment, and diagnostic tests to determine pulpal status.

Indications. Tooth selection for direct pulp capping involves the same vital pulp therapy considerations mentioned previously, to rule out signs of irreversible pulp inflammation and degeneration. The classic indication for direct pulp capping has been for "pinpoint" mechanical exposures that are surrounded with sound dentin.[3,7,21–24] The exposed pulp tissue should be bright red in color and have a slight hemorrhage that is easily controlled with dry cotton pellets applied with minimal pressure. Frigoletto noted that **small exposures** and a **good blood supply** have the best healing potential.[75] Although imprecise, the term "pinpoint" conveys the concept of smallness to the exposed tissue, which should have the lowest possibility of bacterial access. An empirical guideline has been to limit the technique to exposure diameters of less than 1 mm. Stanley has

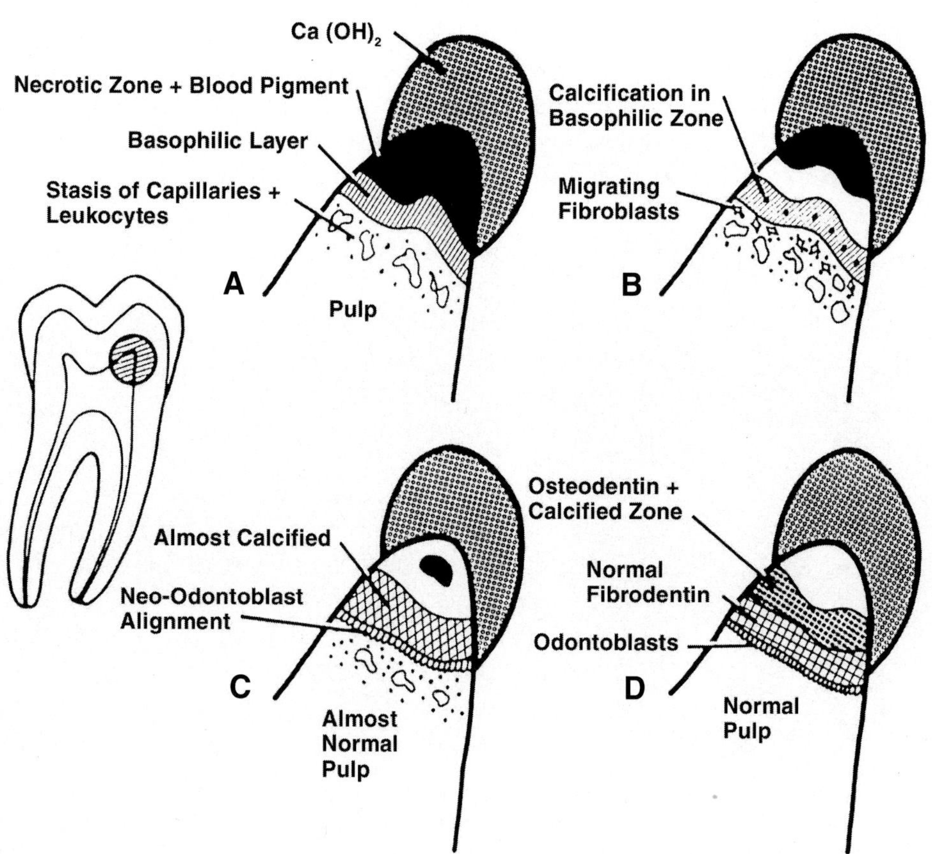

Figure 17-7 Effect of calcium hydroxide and time on the healing of the capped pulp. A, Twenty-four hours after application of calcium hydroxide. B, After 2 or 3 weeks. C, After 4 or 5 weeks. D, After 8 weeks. Reproduced with permission from Vermeersch AG.[107]

determined, however, that the size of the exposure is less significant than the quality of the capping technique in avoiding contamination and mechanical trauma to the exposure site and careful application of the medicament to hemostatically controlled pulp tissue.[74] Equally important is the quality of the temporary or permanent restoration to exclude microleakage.

Contraindications. Contraindications to **direct** pulp-capping therapy include a history of (1) spontaneous and nocturnal toothaches, (2) excessive tooth mobility, (3) thickening of the periodontal ligament, (4) radiographic evidence of furcal or periradicular degeneration, (5) uncontrollable hemorrhage at the time of exposure, and (6) purulent or serous exudate from the exposure.

Clinical Success

The salient features of a clinically successful direct pulp-capping treatment (with or without bridging) are (1) maintenance of pulp vitality, (2) absence of sensitivity or pain, (3) minimal pulp inflammatory responses, and (4) absence of radiographic signs of dystrophic changes.

Permanent Teeth. Several investigators have provided evidence that direct pulp capping cannot be successful in the presence of pulpal inflammation and identify this condition as a contraindication to direct pulp capping.[2] Tronstad and Mjör capped inflamed pulps in monkey teeth with calcium hydroxide or ZOE and found no beneficial healing of the exposed pulp when calcium hydroxide was used.[76] More recently, however, other investigators have shown in animal studies that pulp healing can take place irrespective of the presence of overt inflammation.[77,78] Cotton observed that when there is minimal pulp inflammation, a bridge may form against the capping material, but when inflammation is more severe, the bridge is apt to form at a distance from the exposure.[79]

Dentin bridge formation has been considered to be the sine qua non for success in response to direct pulp-capping procedures.[73,80–82] Weiss and Bjorvatn have demonstrated, however, that a healthy pulp can exist beneath a direct pulp cap even in the absence of a dentinal bridge.[83] Kakehashi et al., in a germ-free animal study, found pulp exposure healing **with bridging** even when left uncovered[84] (Figure 17-8). Seltzer and Bender[42] and Langeland et al.[85] have shown that a dentin bridge is not as complete as it appears, which can ultimately lead to untoward pulp reactions. Cox and Subay found that 89% of bridges formed in response to calcium hydroxide direct pulp caps demonstrated tunnel defects, which allowed access of microleakage products beneath the restoration into the pulp. They found recurrent pulp inflammation beneath 41% of all bridges formed in the sample.[86]

It is generally considered that pulps inadvertently exposed and asymptomatic in the preoperative period are more apt to survive when capped. The prognosis is far less favorable if an attempt is made to cap an inflamed pulp infected from caries or trauma.[87] Also, the wide-open apices and high vascularity of young permanent teeth enhance the successful outcome of direct capping techniques.

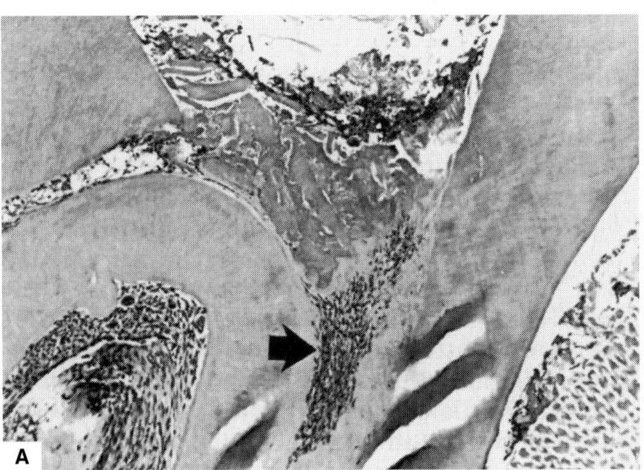

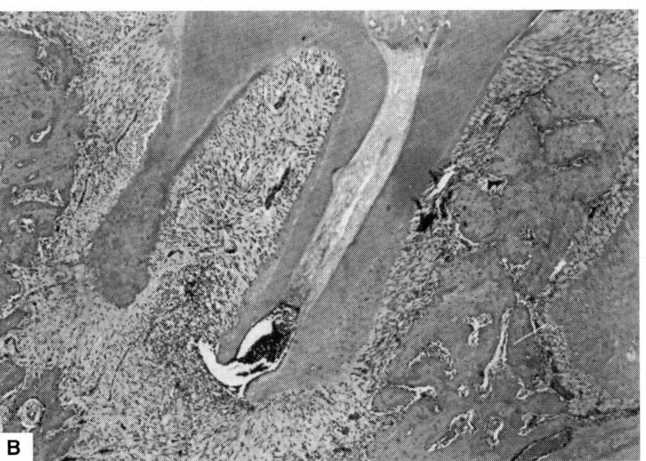

Figure 17-8 Role of bacteria in dentin repair following pulp exposure. **A**, **Germ-free** specimen, obtained 14 days after surgery, with food and debris in occlusal exposure. Nuclear detail of the surviving pulp tissue (**arrow**) can be observed beneath the bridge consisting of dentin fragments united by a new matrix. **B**, Intentional exposure of a first molar in a control rat (with bacteria) 28 days postoperatively. Complete pulp necrosis with apical abscess. **A** reproduced with permission from Kakehashi S et al.[84] **B** reproduced with permission from Clark JW and Stanley HR. Clinical dentistry. Hagerstown (MD): Harper & Row; 1976.

Primary Teeth. Kennedy and Kapala attributed the high cellular content of pulp tissue to be responsible for direct pulp-capping failures in primary teeth.[88] Undifferentiated mesenchymal cells may give rise to **odontoclastic** cells in response to either the caries process or the pulp-capping material, resulting in internal resorption.

Because of the pulp cellular content, increased inflammatory response, and increased incidence of internal resorption, some pediatric dentists feel that the direct capping procedure is contraindicated in primary teeth.[27,89,90] Starkey and others feel that a high degree of success with direct pulp capping in primary teeth can be achieved in carefully selected cases using specific criteria and treatment methods.[91–94]

Treatment Considerations

Débridement. Kalins and Frisbee have shown that necrotic and infected dentin chips are invariably pushed into the exposed pulp during the last stages of caries removal.[95] This debris can impede healing in the area by causing further pulpal inflammation and encapsulation of the dentin chips. Therefore, it is prudent to remove peripheral masses of carious dentin before beginning the excavation where an exposure may occur. When an exposure occurs, the area should be appropriately irrigated with nonirritating solutions such as normal saline to keep the pulp moist.[81]

Hemorrhage and Clotting. Hemorrhage at the exposure site can be controlled with cotton pellet pressure. A blood clot must not be allowed to form after the cessation of hemorrhage from the exposure site as it will impede pulpal healing.[96] The capping material must directly contact pulp tissue to exert a reparative dentin bridge response. Hemolysis of erythrocytes results in an excess of hemosiderin and inflammatory cellular infiltrate, which prolongs pulpal healing.[74]

Exposure Enlargement. There have been recommendations that the exposure site be enlarged by a modification of the direct capping technique known as **pulp curettage** or **partial pulpotomy** prior to the placement of the capping material.[3,93,96,97] Enlarging this opening into the pulp itself serves three purposes: (1) it removes inflamed and/or infected tissue in the exposed area; (2) it facilitates removal of carious and noncarious debris, particularly dentin chips; and (3) it ensures intimate contact of the capping medicament with healthy pulp tissue below the exposure site.

Cvek[98] and Zilberman et al.[99] have described highly favorable results with this partial pulpotomy technique for pulp-exposed, traumatized, anterior teeth and carious molars. After a 24-month waiting period, Mejare and Cvek were able to show a 93.5% success rate of partial pulpotomy in **permanent** posterior teeth with deep carious lesions with exposed pulps.[100] Fuks et al. found similar partial pulpotomy success rates above 90% in permanent incisors with fracture-exposed pulps.[101]

Bacterial Contamination. Watts and Paterson[102] and Cox[103] have both emphasized the fact that **bacterial microleakage** under various restorations causes pulpal damage in deep lesions, not the toxic properties of the cavity liners and/or restorative materials. The success of pulp-capping procedures is dependent on prevention of microleakage by an adequate seal. Cox et al. have shown that pulp healing is more dependent on the capacity of the capping material to prevent bacterial microleakage rather than the specific properties of the material itself.[104]

Medications and Materials. Many medicaments and materials have been suggested to cover pulp exposures and initiate tissue healing and/or hard structure repair. Calcium hydroxide, in one form or another, has been singled out by a myriad of authors as the medicament of choice for pulp exposures.[80,82,105,106] Antibiotics, calcitonin, collagen, corticosteroids, cyanoacrylate, formocresol, and resorbable tricalcium phosphate ceramic have also been investigated, with varying degrees of success. These latter compounds, with the exception of formocresol, have not had sufficient clinical impact to be adopted as the material of choice in direct pulp capping, especially in the pediatric age groups.

Calcium Hydroxide. Calcium hydroxide produces coagulation necrosis at the contact surface of the pulp. The underlying tissue then differentiates into odontoblasts, which elaborate a matrix in about 4 weeks.[107] This results in the formation of a reparative dentin bridge, caused by the irritating quality of the highly alkaline calcium hydroxide, which has a pH of 11 to 12.[108] Stanley has identified that the dentin bridging effects of calcium hydroxide occur only when the agent is in direct contact with healthy pulp tissue.[74] Tamburic et al. summarized the mineralizing effects of calcium hydroxide, which include cellular adenosine triphosphate activation resulting from calcium and hydroxyl ion enhancement of alkalinity in the mineralization process.[109]

Yoshiba et al. provided immunofluorescence evidence of the possible contribution of calcium hydroxide to odontoblastic differentiation. They found increased amounts of fibronectin, an extracellular glycoprotein implicated in cell differentiation, among migrating fibroblasts and newly formed odontoblasts in areas of initial bridge calcification in response to calcium hydroxide. They noted that although calcium hydroxide was not unique in initiating reparative dentinogenesis, it demonstrated the most rapid tubular dentin formation in comparison to calcium phosphate ceramics and tricalcium phosphate.[110]

Calcium hydroxide has significant antibacterial action, which has been identified as an additional benefit in capping procedures.[111,112] Estrela et al. summarized the antibacterial properties of calcium hydroxide, which include hydrolyzing bacterial cell wall lipopolysaccharides, neutralizing bacterial endotoxins, and reducing anaerobic organisms through carbon dioxide absorption.[113]

There is some controversy as to the source of calcium ions necessary for dentinal bridge repair at the exposure site. Sciaky and Pisanti[114] and Attalla and Noujaim[115] demonstrated that calcium ions from the capping material were not involved in the bridge formation. Stark and his colleagues, however, believe that calcium ions from the capping medicament do enter into bridge formation.[116] Holland et al. provided additional evidence to support this concept.[117]

Seltzer and Bender identified the osteogenic potential of calcium hydroxide.[42] It is capable of inducing calcific metamorphosis, resulting in obliteration of the pulp chamber and root canals. This fact has raised concern among clinicians.[42] Lim and Kirk, in an extensive review of direct pulp capping literature, found little support for pulp obliteration and internal resorption being a major complication of pulp capping.[81] Although internal resorption has been documented following calcium hydroxide **pulpotomies** in primary teeth, it does not appear to be a problem in permanent teeth.

Jeppersen, in a long-term study using a creamy mix of calcium hydroxide placed on exposed pulps of primary teeth, reported a 97.6% clinical success and 88.4% histologic success.[93] Although calcium hydroxide pastes have been shown to be effective in promoting dentin bridges, their higher pH, water solubility, and lack of physical barrier strength led manufacturers to introduce modified calcium hydroxide cements that set quickly and **hard** for lining cavities and pulp capping.

Various studies have shown successful results of up to 80% with calcium hydroxide pulp capping of involved primary teeth with or without coronal inflammation.[65,94,96,118] These investigations support the use of hard-set calcium hydroxide cements in place of calcium hydroxide pastes without causing pathologic sequelae, such as internal resorption, associated with pulp-capping failure. For example, the so-called "necrobiotic" and inflammatory zones are minimal, and dentin bridges seem to form directly under these commercial compounds instead of at a distance from the paste forms.[82,118,119] Antibacterial properties and physical strength to support amalgam condensation have been shown for the hard-set calcium hydroxide cements.[51,103,120]

After a clinical investigation of two formulas of a hard, self-setting calcium hydroxide compound (Dycal), Sawusch found calcium hydroxide liners to be effective agents for direct and indirect pulp capping in both primary and young permanent teeth.[65] He also found that **failures in this study tended to be associated with failed restorations and microleakage.** Fuks et al. observed an 81.5% success in young permanent fractured teeth with pinpoint exposures when calcium hydroxide was the capping material of choice.[121]

With the advent of visible light-curing restorative resins, it was inevitable that, in the interest of efficiency and improving the hardness of a cavity lining material, light-cured calcium hydroxide pulp-capping products were introduced. Stanley and Pameijer[122] and Seale and Stanley,[123] in histologic studies, found that a calcium hydroxide product (Prisma VLC Dycal, L. D. Caulk Co.), cured by visible light, maintained all of the characteristics of healing and bridge formation equivalent to the original self-curing Dycal. Lado, in an in vitro study comparing the bacterial inhibition of these new light-cured products to the self-setting calcium hydroxide cements, also found no differences.[112] Howerton and Cox reported the same results as Stanley and Pameijer[122] and Seale and Stanley[123] using light-cured calcium hydroxide in monkeys.[124]

Alternative Agents to Calcium Hydroxide Suggested for Direct Pulp Capping in Primary and Permanent Teeth

Zinc Oxide–Eugenol Cement. Glass and Zander found that ZOE, in direct contact with the pulp tissue, produced chronic inflammation, a lack of calcific barrier, and an end result of necrosis.[80]

Hembree and Andrews, in a literature review of ZOE used as a direct pulp-capping material, could find no positive recommendations.[125] Watts also found mild to moderate inflammation and no calcific bridges in the specimens under his study,[126] and this was confirmed by Holland et al.[127] Weiss and Bjorvatn, on the other hand, noted negligible necrosis of the pulp in direct contact with ZOE but stated that any calcific bridging of an exposure site was probably a layer of dentinal chips.[83] They also found no apparent difference in the pulp reactions of primary and permanent teeth.

In spite of the reported lack of success with ZOE cement, Sveen reported 87% success with the capping of primary teeth with ZOE **in ideal situations** of pulp exposure.[128] He offered no histologic evidence, but Tronstad and Mjör, comparing ZOE with calcium hydroxide, found ZOE more beneficial for inflamed, exposed pulps and felt that the production of a calcific bridge is not necessary if the pulp is free of inflammation following treatment.[76]

Corticosteroids and Antibiotics. Corticosteroids and/or antibiotics were suggested for direct pulp capping in the pretreatment phase and also to be mixed in with calcium hydroxide with the thought of reducing or preventing pulp inflammation. These agents included neomycin and hydrocortisone,[129] Cleocin,[130] cortisone,[131] Ledermix (calcium hydroxide plus prednisolone),[132] penicillin,[133] and Keflin (cephalothin sodium).[134] Although many of these combinations reduced pain for the most part, they were found only to **preserve chronic inflammation** and/or reduce reparative dentin. Also, Watts and Paterson cautioned that anti-inflammatory compounds should not be used in patients at risk from bacteremia.[135] Gardner et al. found, however, that vancomycin, in combination with calcium hydroxide, was somewhat more effective than calcium hydroxide used alone and stimulated a more regular reparative dentin bridge.[136]

Polycarboxylate Cements. These cements have also been suggested as a direct capping material. The material was shown to lack an antibacterial effect and did not stimulate calcific bridging in the pulps of monkey primary and permanent teeth.[134] Negm et al. placed calcium hydroxide and zinc oxide into a 42% aqueous polyacrylic acid and used this combination for direct pulp exposure in patients from 10 to 45 years of age. This mixture showed faster dentin bridging over the exposures in 88 to 91% of the patients when compared to Dycal as the control.[137]

Inert Materials. Inert materials such as **isobutyl cyanoacrylate**[138] and **tricalcium phosphate ceramic**[139] have also been investigated as direct pulp-capping materials. Although pulpal responses in the form of reduced inflammation and unpredictable dentin bridging were found, to date, none of these materials have been promoted to the dental profession as a viable technique. At Istanbul University, dentists capped 44 pulps, half with tricalcium phosphate hydroxyapatite and half with Dycal (calcium hydroxide). At 60 days, none of the hydroxyapatite-capped pulps exhibited hard tissue bridging but instead had mild inflammation. Nearly all of the Dycal-capped pulps, however, were dentin bridged, with little or no inflammation.[140]

Collagen Fibers. Because collagen fibers are known to influence mineralization, Dick and Carmichael placed modified wet collagen sponges with reduced antigenicity in pulp-exposed teeth of young dogs.[141] Although the material was found to be relatively less irritating than calcium hydroxide, and with minimal dentin bridging in 8 weeks, it was concluded that collagen was not as effective in promoting a dentin bridge as was calcium hydroxide. Fuks et al. did find dentin bridges after 2 months in 73% of pulpotomized teeth that had been capped with an enriched collagen solution.[142] They felt that a different mechanism exists for the production of a truer dentin when a collagen solution is used rather than with calcium hydroxide because no coagulation necrosis was seen.

Formocresol. Because of the clinical success of formocresol when used in primary pulp therapy such as pulpotomies and pulpectomies, several investigators have been intrigued by the possibility of its use as a medicament in **direct pulp-capping** therapy. Arnold applied full-strength formocresol for 2 minutes over enlarged pulp exposures in primary teeth and found a 97% clinical "success" **after 6 months.**[97] Ibrahim et al. reported the absence of inflammation along with dentin bridging in 15 experimental teeth when exposures were medicated with formocresol for 5 minutes and capped with a mixture of formocresol and ZOE cement.[143] More recently, Garcia-Godoy obtained a 96% clinical and radiographic success rate in human exposed primary molars when capped with a paste of one-fifth diluted formocresol mixed with a ZOE paste and covered with a reinforced ZOE cement.[144]

Hybridizing Bonding Agents. Recent evidence has shown that elimination of bacterial microleakage is the most significant factor affecting restorative material biocompatibility.[145,146] A major shortcoming of calcium hydroxide preparations is their lack of adhesion to hard tissues and resultant inability to provide an adequate seal against microleakage.[9,147] Furthermore, calcium hydroxide materials have been found to dissolve under restorations where microleakage has occurred, resulting in bacterial access to the pulp.[148] Currently, hybridizing dentinal bonding agents (such as AmalgamBond or C & B MetaBond, Parkell Products, Farmingdale, N.Y.) represent the state of the art in mechanical adhesion to dentin with resultant microleakage control beneath restorations.[9,149,150] Miyakoshi and et al. have shown the effectiveness of **4-META-MMA-TBB adhesives** in obtaining an effective biologic seal.[151] Cox et al. demonstrated that pulps sealed with 4-META "showed reparative dentin deposition without subjacent pulp pathosis."[152,153]

A number of investigators have proposed that sealing vital pulp exposures with **hybridizing dentin bonding agents** may provide a superior outcome to calcium hydroxide direct pulp-capping techniques.[9,154] Because of their superior adhesion to peripheral hard tissues, an effective seal against microleakage can be expected. These proposals have been made in spite of concerns with the effects of acid etchant and resin materials on pulp tissue.

Snuggs et al. demonstrated that pulpal healing occurred, with bridge formation, in exposed primate teeth capped with acidic materials such as silicate cement and zinc phosphate cement. This was contingent on the fact of the biologic surface seal of the overlying restoration remaining intact.[147] Kashiwada and Takagi demonstrated 60 of 64 teeth to be vital and free of any clinical and radiographic signs of pulp degeneration 12 months after pulp capping with a resin bonding agent and composite resin. The pulp tissue was not exposed to acid conditioner during the technique. Selected third molars receiving this treatment were histologically studied and demonstrated dentin bridge formation below the area of exposure.[155]

Heitman and Unterbrink studied a glutaraldehyde-containing dentin bonding agent, in direct pulp-capping exposed pulps, in eight permanent teeth. All exposed pulps were protected with calcium hydroxide during application of the acid conditioner. After rinsing away the calcium hydroxide dressing and conditioner, the bonding agent was applied directly to the exposed pulp tissue and surrounding dentin. All teeth were vital after a 6-month postoperative period.[156] These results have been further substantiated by Cox and White and Bazzuchi et al.[153,157] Kanca reported a 4-year clinical and radiographic success with dentin bonding agent application following etching material applied directly to a fracture-induced exposed pulp and dentin in rebonding a tooth fragment.[158]

Conversely, other investigators provide conflicting evidence that does not support using dentin bonding agents in pulp-capping techniques. Stanley has stated that acid conditioning agents can harm the pulp when placed in direct contact with exposed tissues.[159] In a primate tooth sample with pulp exposures treated with total-etch followed by application of a dentin bonding agent, Pameijer and Stanley found that 45% became nonvital and 25% exhibited bridge formation after 75 days. In the "no etch" calcium hydroxide pulp-capping sample, 7% became nonvital and 82% exhibited bridge formation after the same time period.[160] After 1 year, Araujo et al. experienced a clinical and radiographic success rate of 81% in primary tooth exposures etched and capped with resin adhesives. Histologic assessment of extracted sample teeth in advent of their exfoliation demonstrated inflammatory infiltrate, microabscess formation, and no dentin bridging. Furthermore, bacterial penetration occurred in 50% of the histologically studied teeth. This occurred in spite of the final composite resin restorations being resealed at 6-month intervals from the time of initial placement.[161]

Gwinnett and Tay, using light microscopic and electron microscopic techniques, identified early and intermediate pulp responses to total-etch followed by a resin bonding agent and composite resin restoration in human teeth. Some specimens demonstrated signs of initial repair with dentin bridge formation along the exposed site and reparative dentin adjacent to the exposed site. Other specimens demonstrated persistence of chronic inflammation with a foreign body response in the form of resin globules imbedded within the exposed pulp tissue that were surrounded by pulpal macrophages. This was also accompanied by a mononuclear inflammatory infiltrate and an absence of calcific bridge formation.[162]

Although using dentin bonding agents as a replacement for calcium hydroxide in the direct pulp-capping technique has been advocated,[163] more long-term evidence and histologic evaluation are needed. Until such evidence is available, the clinician would be prudent to employ a combination of calcium hydroxide as a medicament for the exposed pulp followed by a hybridizing resin bonding agent for a successful microbiologic seal.[164,165] This concept is further substantiated by Katoh et al., who reported improved direct pulp-capping results with dentin bonding agents when they were used in conjunction with calcium hydroxide.[166,167]

Cell-Inductive Agents. A number of cell-inductive agents have been proposed as potential direct pulp-capping alternatives to calcium hydroxide. These contemporary substances mimic the reciprocal inductive activities seen in embryologic development and tissue healing that are receiving so much attention at this time.

Mineral trioxide aggregate (MTA) (Dentsply, Tulsa; Tulsa, Okla.) cement was developed at Loma Linda by Torabinejad for the purposes of root-end filling and furcation perforation repair.[168] The material consists of tricalcium silicate, tricalcium aluminate, tricalcium oxide, and silicate oxide. It is a hydrophilic material that has a 3-hour setting time in the presence of moisture. Major MTA advantages include excellent sealing ability, good compressive strength (70 MPa) comparable to IRM, and good biocompatibility. Pitt Ford et al. documented superior bridge formation and preservation of pulp vitality with MTA when compared with calcium hydroxide in a direct pulp-capping technique.[169] They also reported normal cytokine activity in bone and cementum regeneration in response to MTA, which is indicative of its cell-inductive potential.[169]

Calcium phosphate cement has been developed for repairing cranial defects following brain neurosurgery. The components of this material include tetracalcium phosphate and dicalcium phosphate, which react in an aqueous environment to form hydroxyapatite, the mineral component of hard tissues. Chaung et al. histologically compared calcium phosphate cement with calcium hydroxide as a direct pulp-capping agent. Although both materials produced similar results with respect to pulp biocompatibility and hard tissue barrier formation, calcium phosphate cement was suggested as a viable alternative because of (1) its more neutral pH resulting in less localized tissue destruction, (2) its superior compressive strength, and (3) its transformation into hydroxyapatite over time.[170]

Yoshimine et al. demonstrated the potential benefits of direct pulp capping with **tetracalcium phosphate–based cement.** As with calcium phosphate cement, this material has the ability to be gradually converted into hydroxyapatite over time. In contrast to calcium hydroxide, tetracalcium phosphate cement induced bridge formation with no superficial tissue necrosis and significant absence of pulp inflammation.[171]

Summary: Direct Pulp Capping. Adherence to established criteria for case selection is important to achieve success. Although somewhat controversial based on the previously reviewed studies, **direct pulp capping has been found to be less successful in primary teeth** than indirect pulp therapy or coronal pulpotomy. However, **direct pulp capping tends to be more successful in young permanent teeth.**

PULPOTOMY

Pulpotomy is the most widely used technique in vital pulp therapy for primary and young permanent teeth with carious pulp exposures. A pulpotomy is defined as the surgical removal of the entire coronal pulp presumed to be partially or totally inflamed and quite possibly infected, leaving intact the vital radicular pulp within the canals.[2] A germicidal medicament is then placed over the remaining vital radicular pulp stumps at their point of communication with the floor of the coronal pulp chamber. This procedure is done to promote healing and retention of the vital radicular pulp. Dentin bridging may occur as a treatment outcome of this procedure depending on the type of medicament used (Figure 17-9). Additional variables thought to influence treatment outcome include the medication type, concentration, and time of tissue contact.

Indications. According to Dannenberg, pulpotomies are indicated for cariously exposed **primary** teeth when their retention is more advantageous than extraction and replacement with a space maintainer.[172] Pulpotomy candidates should demonstrate clinical and radiographic signs of radicular pulp vitality, absence of pathologic change, restorability, and at least two-thirds remaining root length. Pulpotomized teeth should receive stainless steel crowns as final restorations to avoid potential coronal fracture at the cervical region. Pulpotomy is also recommended for **young permanent teeth** with **incompletely formed apices** and **cariously** exposed pulps that give evidence of extensive coronal tissue inflammation.

Contraindications. According to Mejare, contraindications for pulpotomy in **primary teeth** exist when (1) root resorption exceeds more than one-third of the root length; (2) the tooth crown is nonrestorable; (3) highly viscous, sluggish, or absent hemorrhage is observed at the radicular canal orifices; as well as (4) marked tenderness to percussion; (5) mobility with locally aggravated gingivitis associated with partial or total radicular pulp necrosis exists; and (6) radiolucency exists in the furcal or periradicular areas.[173]

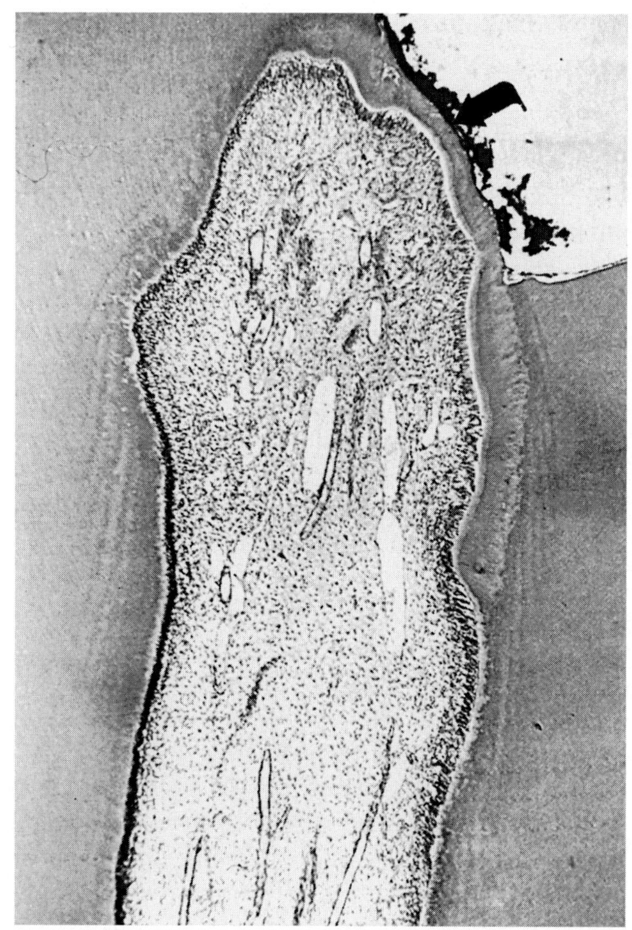

Figure 17-9 Dentin bridge following calcium hydroxide pulpotomy with LIFE. (Courtesy of SybronEndo/Kerr Orange, Ca.)

Persistent toothaches and coronal pus should also be considered contraindications.

Treatment Approaches for Primary Teeth. Ranly, in reviewing the rationale and various medicaments that have guided the historical development of the pulpotomy procedure, provided three categories of treatment approaches. **Devitalization** was the first approach to be used with the intention of "mummifying" the radicular pulp tissue.[174] The term "mummified" has been ascribed to chemically treated pulp tissue that is inert, sterilized, metabolically suppressed, and incapable of autolysis.[174] This approach involved the original two-sitting formocresol pulpotomy, which resulted in complete devitalization of the radicular pulp. Also included were the 5-minute formocresol and 1:5 diluted formocresol techniques, which both result in partial devitalization with persistent chronic inflammation.[174,175]

The **preservation** approach involved medicaments and techniques that provide minimal insult to the orifice tissue and maintain the vitality and normal histologic appearance of the entire radicular pulp. Pharmacotherapeutic agents included in this category are corticosteroids, glutaraldehyde, and ferric sulfate. Nonpharmacotherapeutic techniques in this category include electrosurgical and laser pulpotomies.[174]

The **regeneration** approach includes pulpotomy agents that have cell-inductive capacity to either replace lost cells or induce existent cells to differentiate into hard tissue–forming elements. Historically, calcium hydroxide was the first medicament to be used in a "regenerative" capacity because of its ability to stimulate hard tissue barrier formation. The calcium hydroxide pulpotomy is predicated on the healing of pulp tissue beneath the overlying dentin bridge. Recently, its regenerative capacity has been questioned owing to the fact that calcium hydroxide tissue response is more reactive than inductive. Examples of true cell-inductive agents include transforming growth factor-β (TGF-β) in the form of bone morphogenetic proteins,[176,177] freeze-dried bone,[178] and MTA.[168,169] These materials are more representative of the regeneration category and provide the direction for future research in vital pulp therapy.[174]

Formocresol Pulpotomy

Formocresol was introduced in 1904 by Buckley, who contended that equal parts of formalin and tricresol would react chemically with the intermediate and end products of pulp inflammation to form a "new, colorless, and non-infective compound of a harmless nature."[179] Buckley's formula, formocresol, consists of tricresol, 19% aqueous formaldehyde, glycerine, and water.*

The formocresol pulpotomy technique currently used is a modification of the original method reported by Sweet in 1930.[180] By 1955, Sweet claimed 97% clinical success in 16,651 cases.[181] It should be noted, however, that in this report, about one half of the primary teeth exfoliated early.

Histology. In spite of regional popularity, the multiple-visit pulpotomy did not receive wide acceptance because it was regarded as a nonvital or devitalization method. In addition, histologic studies to support its use were also lacking. It became overshadowed by the so-called "vital" pulpotomy for primary teeth using calcium hydroxide, which at that time was supported by clinical and histologic evidence. Interest in formocresol was renewed, however, with a reported increase in clinical failures and radiographic evidence of internal resorption with calcium hydroxide, even in the presence of dentinal bridging.[188] At the same time, improved clinical and histologic success rates were reported with formocresol.[182]

In spite of histologic studies that showed formalin, creosol, and paraformaldehyde to be connective tissue irritants, it was recognized early that formocresol is an efficient bactericide. It was also found to have the ability to prevent tissue autolysis by the complex chemical binding of formaldehyde with protein. However, this binding reaction may be reversible as the protein molecule does not change in its basic overall structure.[175]

Massler and Mansukhani conducted a detailed histologic investigation of the effect of formocresol on the pulps of 43 human primary and permanent teeth in multiple treatment intervals.[183] Fixation of the tissue directly under the medicament was apparent. After a 7- to 14-day application, the pulps developed three distinctive zones: (1) a broad eosinophilic zone of fixation, (2) a broad pale-staining zone with poor cellular definition, and (3) a zone of inflammation diffusing apically into normal pulp tissue. After 60 days, in a limited number of samples, the remaining tissue was believed to be completely fixed, appearing as a strand of eosinophilic fibrous tissue.[183]

Emmerson et al. also described the action of formocresol on human pulp tissue.[184] They reported

*The formocresol used in this technique may be obtained under the trade name Buckley's Formocresol (Roth, Chicago, IL). Composition: 35% cresol, 19% formalin in a vehicle of glycerine and water at a pH of approximately 5.1. To dilute formocresol to one-fifth strength, thoroughly mix three parts of glycerine with one part of distilled water. Add these four parts to one part of concentrated commercial formocresol compound.

that the effect on the pulp varied with the length of time formocresol was in contact with the tissue. A 5-minute application resulted in surface fixation of normal tissue, whereas an application sealed in for 3 days produced calcific degeneration. They concluded that formocresol pulpotomy in primary pulp therapy may be classified as either vital or nonvital, depending on the duration of the formocresol application.

Formocresol versus Calcium Hydroxide. Doyle et al. compared the formocresol pulpotomy technique with the calcium hydroxide technique in primary canines and found the formocresol technique to be 95% clinically successful at the end of 1 year.[182] Although fixation of pulp tissue and some loss of cellular definition were seen histologically, **healthy, vital tissue existed in the apical third.** The calcium hydroxide technique was considered to be 61% clinically successful, and dentin bridge formation was seen in 50% of the cases examined.

Spedding et al. also studied these two medicaments in monkeys and produced essentially the same results as Doyle and colleagues.[185] Law and Lewis evaluated the clinical effectiveness of the formocresol technique over a 4-year period and reported a 93 to 98% success rate. Their failure rate was greatest between the first and second years.[186]

Formocresol versus Zinc Oxide–Eugenol. Berger compared the pulpotomy effects of using a one-appointment formocresol medication with those of ZOE paste alone on the amputated pulps of cariously exposed human primary molars.[187] Periods of evaluation ranged from 3 to 38 weeks postoperatively. Clinically and radiographically, 97% of the formocresol-treated teeth were judged successful, whereas only 58% of the teeth treated with ZOE were considered successful. Histologically, 82% of the formocresol group was judged successful, compared to **total failure** with ZOE.[187]

An intriguing part of this study was the finding of a total absence of cellular detail in the apical third at 3 weeks, but by 7 weeks, connective tissue of a granular type had ingrown through the apical foramen. In specimens obtained after longer postoperative periods, granulation tissue progressively replaced the necrotic pulp tissue up to the coronal area. Small areas of resorption of the dentinal walls were also being replaced by osteodentin.[187]

Spamer also conducted a histologic study of caries-free human primary canines following a one-appointment formocresol pulpotomy in which the final pulp covering was ZOE.[188] Again, the three typical zones were distinguishable, including the apical one-third tissue, which was normal and free of inflammatory reaction. Initially, Spamer observed an acute inflammatory reaction, succeeded by a chronic inflammatory response, proliferation of odontoblasts, and an increase in collagen fibers. By 6 months, deposition of mature dentin and vital tissue was seen throughout.[188]

Formocresol Pulpotomy Outcomes: Primary Teeth. Rolling and Thylstrup reported a clinical 3-year follow-up study of pulpotomized primary molars using formocresol.[189] Their results showed a progressively decreasing survival rate of 91% at 3 months, 83% at 12 months, 78% at 24 months, and 70% at 36 months after treatment. These investigators concluded that although their rate of success was less than previous studies had shown, the formocresol method must be considered an acceptable clinical procedure compared with other methods. Possibly, bacterial microleakage over the longer time span accounted for their decreasing success rate.

Rolling and coworkers, in later studies, investigated the morphologic and enzyme histochemical reactions of pulpotomies done with formocresol in human primary molars for periods ranging from 3 to 24 months and 3 to 5 years.[190,191] In these studies, a wide range of pulpal reactions occurred, from normal pulps to total chronic inflammation. In most instances, however, the pulp tissue in the apical region was vital with minimal inflammation, which was in agreement with many other studies. It was concluded from both studies that the formocresol method should be regarded as only a means to keep primary teeth with pulp exposures functioning for a relatively short period of time.

Magnusson investigated "therapeutic" (ie, formocresol) pulpotomies and stated that his histologic examinations revealed early "capricious" diffusion of the medicament through the pulp tissue, producing chronic inflammation and no healing in the apical areas along with a small percentage of internal resorption.[192] From a biologic standpoint, Magnusson felt that formocresol was biologically inferior to calcium hydroxide in the pulpotomy technique as the latter manifested true signs of healing but in a low percentage in primary teeth.[192] Ranley and Lazzari concluded, however, that variations in the interpretation of histologic studies with formocresol, on either vital or nonvital tissue, are attributable to the length of exposure of the radicular tissue to the drug, but there is no true "healing."[193]

In general, the results of many histologic studies on the formocresol pulpotomy have shown that several distinct zones are usually present in the pulp following the application of the medicament:

1. Superficial debris along with dentinal chips at the amputation site
2. Eosinophil-stained and compressed tissue
3. A palely stained zone with loss of cellular definition
4. An area of fibrotic and inflammatory activity
5. An area of normal-appearing pulp tissue considered to be vital

Formocresol Addition to Sub-base. Beaver et al. investigated the differences in pulp reactions between a 5-minute application of formocresol using sub-bases of either ZOE cement alone or with the addition of formocresol.[194] There was no appreciable difference in a histologic reaction of the remaining radicular pulp tissue under either of these two types of sub-bases.

An alternative procedure reported clinically and histologically successful is to **incorporate diluted formocresol** into the ZOE dressing and then place it on the pulpal stumps instead of a moistened formocresol cotton pellet.[17,195,196] Ranly and Pope have shown in vitro and in vivo that formocresol can leach out from a ZOE sub-base when the two substances are combined.[197] They have suggested that the initial application of a formocresol-saturated cotton pellet on the pulp might be an unnecessary step.

Formocresol Dilution. Venham suggested that formocresol might be reduced to one-quarter strength in the pulpotomy application.[198] The combined investigations of Straffon and Han[199,200] and Loos et al.[201] on the histologic and biochemical effects of formocresol introduced new thinking in this type of pulp therapy. Straffon and Han concluded from a study of connective tissue in hamster pulps exposed to formocresol that the medicament does not interfere with a prolonged recovery of connective tissue and may even suppress the initial inflammatory reaction. In a later report, they concluded that formocresol at 1:5 strength might be equally effective and possibly a less damaging pulpotomy agent. Loos and colleagues concurred with the previous work in a further study of diluted formocresol.[201] Morawa and colleagues, in a 5-year clinical study of 70 cases, found that the formocresol pulpotomy, using a 1:5 concentration, was as effective as a full concentration and also has the advantage of reduced postoperative complications in the periradicular region. In only five teeth was there limited radicular internal resorption.[202]

Fuks and Bimstein used this one-fifth dilution of formocresol in a clinical and radiographic study of primary teeth over a period of 4 to 36 months.[203] The clinical success rate was reported at 94.3%, and 39% of 41 cases showed a slightly higher rate of premature root resorption. Twenty-nine percent had radiographic evidence of a root canal obliteration process. In a later study with rhesus monkeys, using full-strength formocresol compared with a 20% dilution, these investigators found the same premature root resorption but a milder pulpal inflammatory response with the diluted concentration.[204] Garcia-Godoy, however, did not find any differences histologically between full-strength and a one-fifth dilution of formocresol when applied in several ways over the amputated pulps.[195]

Outcomes. Citing an 80% success rate of primary molars pulpotomized with formocresol, Wright and Widmer also found early root resorption of the pulpotomized molars in comparison to the untreated antimeres.[205] The permanent successors, however, were not found to erupt significantly earlier, as has been previously reported.

The hard tissue deposition or "calcification" of the root canal walls following a formocresol pulpotomy has also been observed radiographically in several other studies.[203,206,207] These findings imply that the use of formocresol does not result in a complete loss of pulp vitality.

More recently, the findings of a retrospective radiographic study of the formocresol pulpotomy technique with a post-treatment time ranging from 24 to 87 months were reported by Hicks et al.[196] In this study, a ZOE paste into which full-strength formocresol was incorporated was placed in the pulp chamber after coronal amputation followed by restoration with a stainless steel crown. Based on radiographic evaluation criteria, which included abscess formation, radiolucencies, pathologic root resorption, calcific metamorphosis, and advanced or delayed exfoliation, the procedure was considered to be successful in 93.8% of the cases. Coll et al. compared the techniques of formocresol pulpotomy versus pulpectomy in primary incisors. They concluded that the pulpotomy was the preferred technique for these teeth.[67]

Formocresol Pulpotomy Technique in Primary Teeth

Correct diagnosis is essential to ensure the clinician that inflammation is limited to the coronal pulp.[208] Biopsy studies of pulp tissue removed from the opening of root canals under pulpotomies have demonstrated the unreliability of clinical assessments in primary teeth.[192] Radiographic examinations are therefore necessary to confirm the need for pulpotomy therapy in primary teeth. It is judicious to take bitewing and periradicular radiographs so that the depth of caries may be observed and the condition of the periradicular tissues determined. Mejare found **only a 55% success rate** in primary molars with either coronal or total **chronic**

pulpitis that were treated by formocresol pulpotomy after 2½ years.[209]

One-Appointment Pulpotomy. *Indications.* This method of treatment should be carried out only on those restorable teeth in which it has been determined that inflammation is confined to the coronal portion of the pulp. When the coronal pulp is amputated, only vital, healthy pulp tissue should remain in the root canals (Figure 17-10).

Contraindications. Teeth with a history of spontaneous pain should not be considered. If profuse hemorrhage occurs on entering the pulp chamber, the one-step pulpotomy is also contraindicated. Other contraindications are pathologic root resorption, roots that are two-thirds resorbed or internal root resorption, interradicular bone loss, presence of a fistula, or presence of pus in the chamber (Figure 17-11).

Procedure.

1. Anesthetize the tooth and tissue.
2. Isolate the tooth to be treated with a rubber dam.
3. Excavate all caries.
4. Remove the dentin roof of the pulp chamber with a high-speed fissure bur (Figure 17-12, A).
5. Remove all coronal pulp tissue with a slow-speed No. 6 or 8 round bur (Figure 17-12, B). Sharp spoon excavators can remove residual tissue remnants.
6. Achieve hemostasis with dry cotton pellets under pressure.
7. Apply **diluted** formocresol to the pulp on a cotton pellet for **3 to 5 minutes**[210] (Figure 17-12, C).

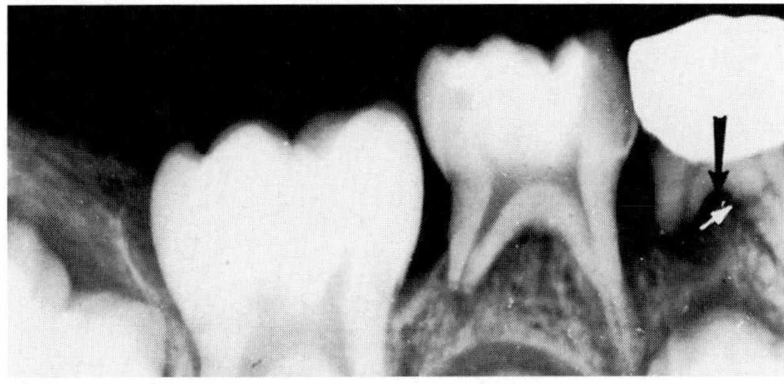

Figure 17-11 Final failure of formocresol pulpotomy, mandibular first primary molar. Root resorption and interradicular bone loss (**arrows**) prior to treatment forecast eventual failure. The tooth was extracted. Reproduced with permission from Law DB, Lewis TM, Davis JM. An atlas of pedodontics. Philadelphia: WB Saunders; 1969.

8. Place a ZOE cement base without incorporation of formocresol (Figure 17-12, D).
9. Restore the tooth with a stainless steel crown.

Two-Appointment Pulpotomy. *Indications.* The two-appointment technique is indicated if there is (1) evidence of sluggish or profuse bleeding at the amputation site, (2) difficult-to-control bleeding, (3) slight purulence in the chamber but **none** at the amputation site, (4) thickening of the periodontal ligament, or (5) a history of spontaneous pain without other contraindications. The two-step pulpotomy can also be used when shorter appointments are necessary to facilitate patient management problems. Miyamoto suggested the two-appointment technique for uncoopera-

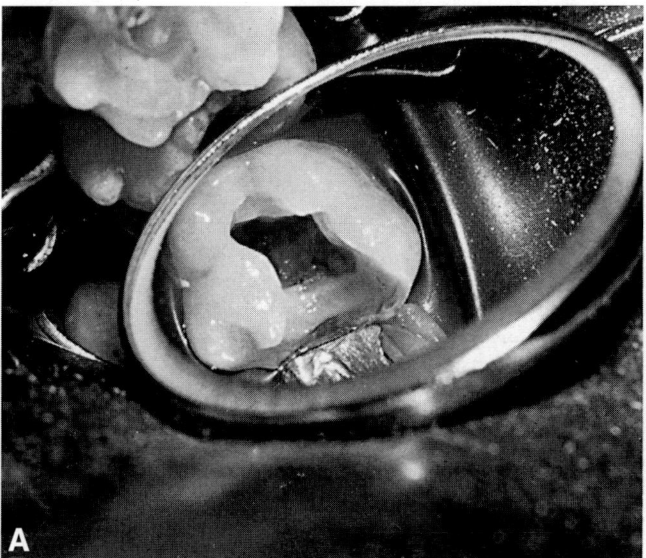

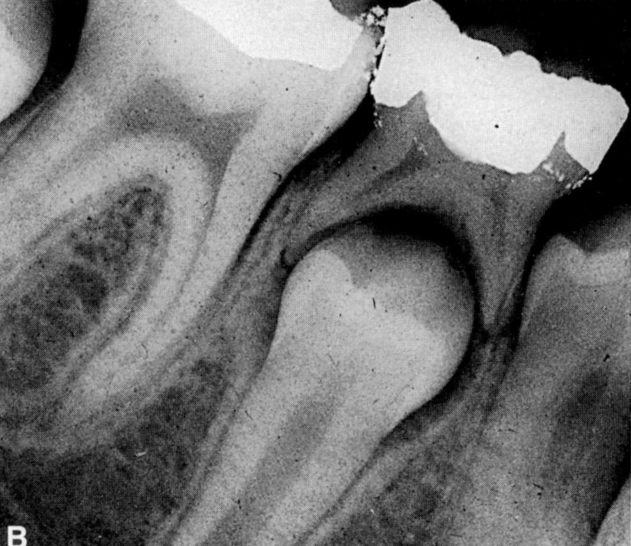

Figure 17-10 One-appointment formocresol pulpotomy. **A**, Root of the pulp chamber and coronal pulp removed. Cotton pellet with formocresol in place for 5 minutes. **B**, Successful formocresol pulpotomy 1 year following treatment. (**A** courtesy of Dr. Constance B. Greeley; **B** courtesy of Dr. Mark Wagner.)

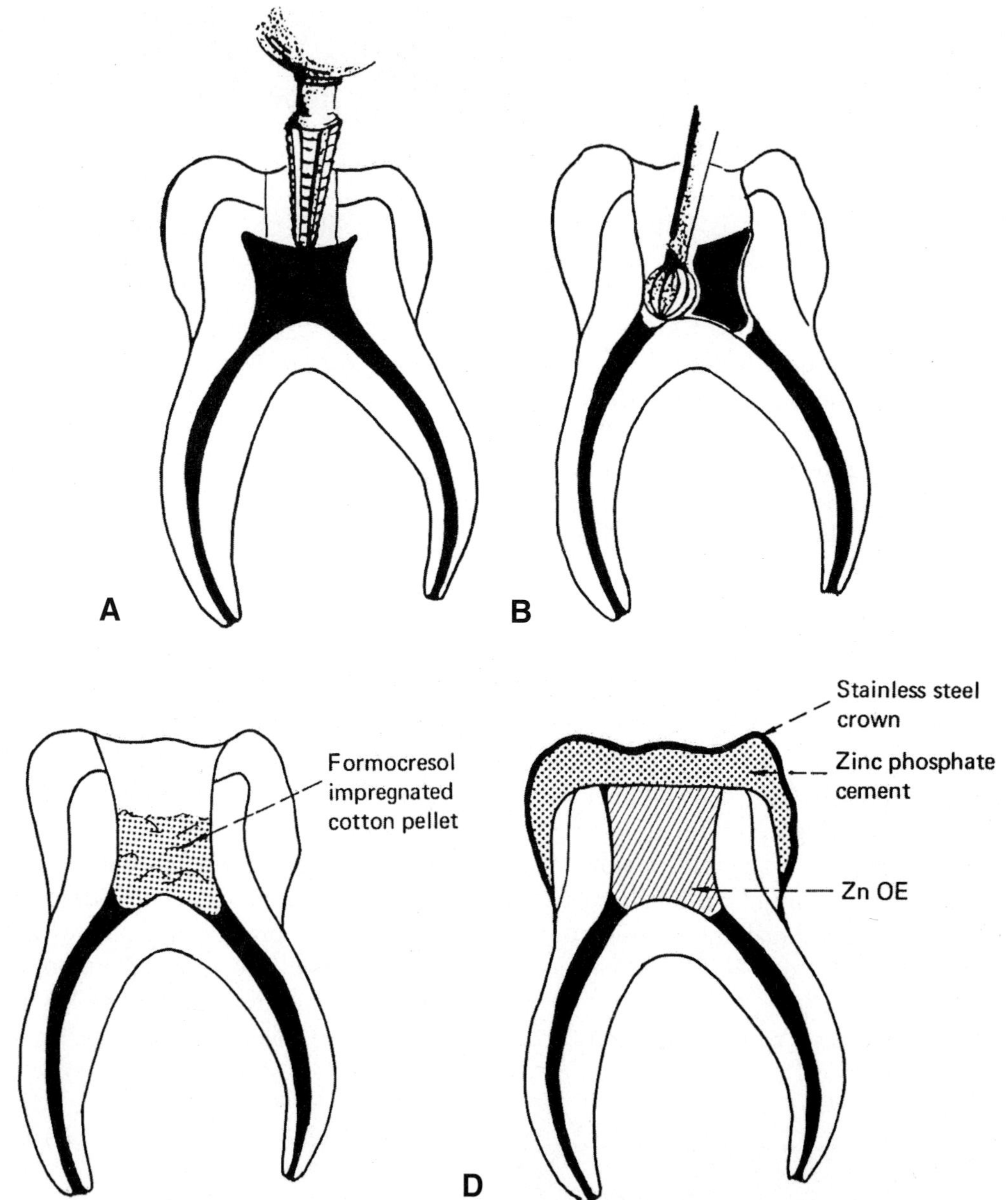

Figure 17-12 Step-by-step technique in one-appointment formocresol pulpotomy. **A**, Exposure of pulp by roof removal. **B**, Coronal pulp amputation with a round bur. Hemostasis with dry cotton or epinephrine. **C**, Application of formocresol for 1 minute. Excess medicament is expressed from cotton before placement. **D**, Following formocresol removal, zinc oxide–eugenol base and stainless steel crown are placed.

tive children to minimize chair time, especially for the initial operative visit.[211]

Contraindications. This technique should not be done for teeth that are (1) nonrestorable, (2) soon to be exfoliated, or (3) necrotic.

Procedure.

1. The steps are the same as for the one-appointment procedure through step 6.
2. A cotton pellet moistened with **diluted** formocresol is sealed into the chamber for 5 to 7 days with a durable temporary cement.
3. At the second visit, the temporary filling and cotton pellet are removed and the chamber is irrigated with hydrogen peroxide.
4. A ZOE cement base is placed.
5. The tooth is restored with a stainless steel crown. As previously stated, Verco and Allen found no difference in the success rate between one-stage and two-stage procedures.[212]

Avram and Pulver surveyed Canadian, American, and selected dental schools throughout the world as well as a limited number of pediatric dental specialists to determine medicament choice and clinician attitude toward pulpotomy therapy prevalent at the time of investigation.[213] The most prevalent medicament used in pediatric dental departments (40.8%) was full-strength formocresol, followed by 36% for the 1:5 dilution. This 1:5 dilution was used by 50% of the pediatric specialists, whereas 42% used-full strength formocresol. Primosch et al. surveyed predoctoral pediatric dentistry programs in 53 US dental schools to determine the prevalence and types of primary tooth pulp therapy techniques taught in those institutions. Formocresol was the most widely taught pulpotomy medicament, with 71.7% of the programs using diluted formocresol and 22.6% full-strength formocresol. Zinc oxide–eugenol was the base material of choice for 92.4% of all programs surveyed. [69]

Clinical experience has shown that pulpotomized **primary** molars are susceptible to cuspal and cervical fracture. For this reason, the restoration of choice is a well-fitted stainless steel crown. Additional advantages of this restoration include elimination of recurrent decay, elimination of intracoronal restoration fracture, and reduction of microleakage. Although composite resin restorations, incorporating the dentin bonding agents, have been proposed for pulpotomized primary molars, more studies are indicated to determine their effectiveness relative to stainless steel crowns.

PULPOTOMY FOR YOUNG PERMANENT TEETH

Treatment of severely decayed and pulpally involved **young permanent teeth** in the child or adolescent creates a dilemma. Complete endodontic therapy and a cast full-crown restoration have been considered to be the ideal treatment. However, this is time consuming and, in many instances, beyond the family financial resources. Most importantly, canal obturation for incompletely formed roots and open apices presents unique problems with conventional endodontic techniques. The relatively thin dentin walls of the large obturated canals place the tooth at greater risk for root fracture over time. In these instances, the treatment objective is to maximize the opportunity for apical development and closure, known as **apexogenesis**, and enhance continual root dentin formation. These objectives can occur only if the radicular pulp is maintained in a healthy state—the intent of the pulpotomy technique. Although **calcium hydroxide** has been the most recommended pulpotomy medicament for pulpally involved vital **young permanent** teeth with incomplete apices, formocresol has also been proposed as an alternative.

Formocresol

The well-documented success with formocresol pulpotomies in primary teeth has led a number of clinicians to extrapolate the use of this medication in young **permanent** teeth with a **vital** or, in some instances, **nonvital** pulp status at the start of operative treatment.

Canosa reported the widespread use of formocresol pulpotomy in Cuba for all restorable molars with **vital** pulps only. Restorable necrotic molars, as well as premolars and anterior teeth, received full root canal therapy. She reported an empirical success rate of 75% with formocresol pulpotomies. Those cases that failed were treated by endodontic cleaning, shaping, and filling (I Canosa, personal communication, March 1994).

Ibrahim et al. studied the use of formocresol as a pulpotomy medication in the permanent teeth of two dogs and a monkey for up to 20 weeks.[214] Radiographically, no evidence of apical pathosis was seen. Histologically, calcification in the canal, continued apical closure, and partial bridging were noted. Areas of inflammation were replaced with connective tissue.

Using formocresol, Trask reported clinical success treating 43 permanent teeth with necrotic pulps in an age range of 7 to 23 years.[215] Eight of these patients were under 10 years of age, when root apices are presumed to be still open. Trask sealed a small formocresol cotton pellet in the pulp chamber by amalgam restoration or stainless steel crown for an observed period of 14 to 33 months. The treated teeth were asymptomatic except in one instance in which the tooth had to be retreated in the same manner. He felt that the permanent tooth formocresol pulpotomy was a better alternative than extraction as conventional endodontics was economically unfeasible in this cohort of patients. He considered it to be a **temporizing** treatment only and not a substitute for complete root canal therapy, which was advocated at a later date.[215]

Myers also conducted a clinical study of formocresol treatment in **pulpless** permanent molars. Sixty-six cases were evaluated clinically for periods of time ranging from 3 to 22 months. Fifty-six of the treated teeth (85%) radiographically demonstrated elimination or marked reduction of initial periradicular rarefaction. Three of the teeth (4.5%) showed no change in appearance, and seven teeth (10.6%) exhibited an increase in periradicular rarefaction. An important finding was the observation that all of the teeth treated with formocresol exhibited continued apexification and increase in root length.[216] Armstrong et al. found the same as well as intracanal "calcification."[217]

Fiskio undertook a 5-year clinical study of 148 permanent teeth, using either a one-step or two-step formocresol pulpotomy.[218] Ninety-one percent required no further treatment. In the remaining 9%, the initial use of formocresol did not prevent endodontic therapy at a later date. The age of the patients at the start of treatment had no significant effect.

Spedding, in discussing the use of formocresol for permanent molars, stated that a "plug" of fixed tissues forms in the root canals that can easily be removed with endodontic instruments.[219] This is in contrast to teeth treated with calcium hydroxide. He concluded, however, that although few failures with formocresol had been reported in permanent teeth, this treatment rationale is empirical, and more definite information about failures is needed.

Rothman observed 165 pulpotomized human permanent teeth for 2 years with a two-treatment formocresol medication.[220] He reported an average success rate of 71% as judged clinically and radiographically. Intracanal calcification was seen in only three teeth.

Fuks et al., in studying radiographs of formocresol pulpotomies in young permanent teeth of monkeys at the end of 1 year, observed a favorable response with both full-strength and diluted medication for continuing root development and closed apices.[204] Histologically, mild internal resorption was seen at a later date. The investigators stated that neither concentration produced ideal results, but a milder degree of inflammation was seen in the diluted group.

Schwartz, surveying a group of Canadian practitioners and faculty on the use of formocresol for pulpotomies in young permanent teeth, found that the respondents felt that the procedure was a compromise and that the teeth should be treated with conventional endodontics at a later date.[221]

Muniz et al. histologically studied 26 young permanent teeth treated with the formocresol technique 5 to 20 months postoperatively.[222] This investigation was based on an earlier study by Muniz in which he found an overall success rate of 92% in both vital and nonvital permanent teeth. He found inflammation and necrosis in the cervical third but fibrosis and osteodentin predominantly in the apical third, a response that seems to indicate stages of biologic scar healing that probably require around 10 to 20 months to be seen.

Akbar investigated the differences in formocresol pulpotomy in permanent teeth with acute and chronic pulpitis over a 5-year period.[223] On the basis of clinical criteria only, he found the treatment to be more successful in the acute pulpitis group (81%) than in the chronic pulpitis group (70%).

In reviewing the literature on apical histologic response to formocresol pulpotomies, Nishino identified a fallacy in extrapolating its success in primary teeth to its use in permanent teeth.[224] A consistent finding in pulpotomized primary teeth has been the ingrowth of connective tissue through the apex in a coronal direction through the pulpal areas of chronically inflamed and fibrosed tissue. He identified that favorable clinical responses could mask the reality of histologic pulpal degeneration. Late symptoms from pulp degeneration in pulpotomized **primary teeth** are eliminated owing to their exfoliation. Young permanent teeth, however, may have a greater potential for developing periradicular infection with this technique owing to the longer time exposure to the inflammatory degenerative process. Conversely, he hypothesized that the formocresol treatment might be effective because the open apical foramen of immature permanent teeth would be conducive to an ingrowth of connective tissue at the apex in the form of proliferating fibroblasts.[224]

Because linear osteodentin calcification may develop as a response to formocresol pulpotomies over time, there has been considerable concern expressed by endodontists of the difficulty in renegotiating treated young permanent canals after the apices have closed.

Calcium Hydroxide

Calcium hydroxide was most favored as a pulpotomy agent in the 1940s and mid-1950s because it was thought to be more biologically acceptable owing to the fact that it promoted reparative dentin bridge formation and pulp vitality was maintained. This rationale was introduced by Teuscher and Zander in 1938, who described it as a "vital" technique.[225] Their histologic studies showed that the pulp tissue adjacent to the calcium hydroxide was first necrotized by the high pH (11 to 12) of the calcium hydroxide. This necrosis was accompanied by acute inflammatory changes in the underlying tissue. After 4 weeks, a new odontoblastic layer and, eventually, a bridge of dentin developed (Figure 17-13). Later investigations showed three identifiable histologic zones under the calcium hydroxide in 4 to 9 days: (1) coagulation necrosis, (2) deep-staining basophilic areas with varied osteodentin, and (3) relatively normal pulp tissue, slightly hyperemic, underlying an odontoblastic layer.

As with direct pulp capping, the presence of a dentinal bridge is not the sole criterion of success. The bridge may be incomplete and may appear histologically as doughnut, dome, or funnel shaped or filled with tissue inclusions.[226,227] It is also possible for the remaining pulp to be walled off by fibrous tissue with no dentin bridge evident radiographically. Initial reports by Berk and Brown indicated a success rate

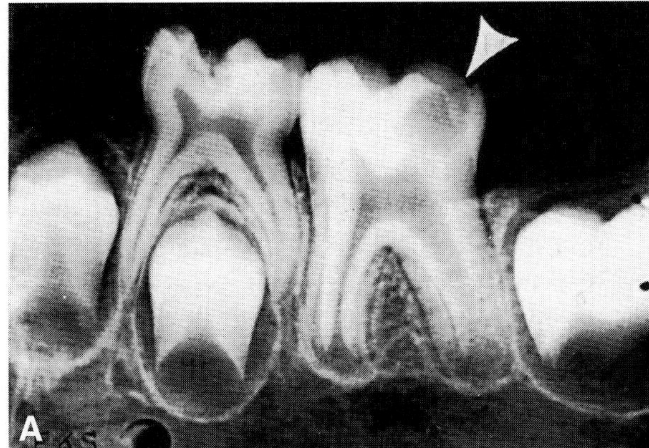

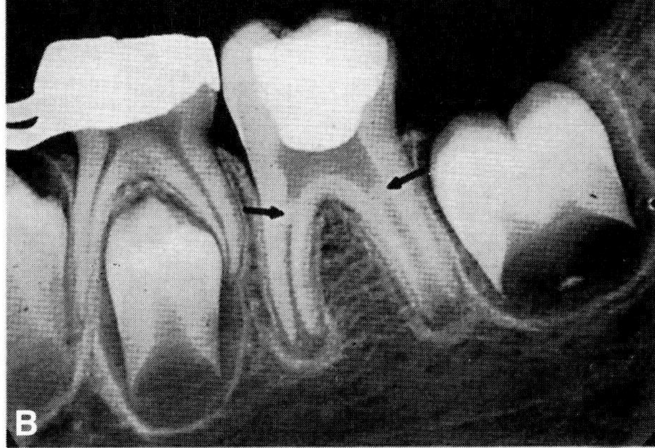

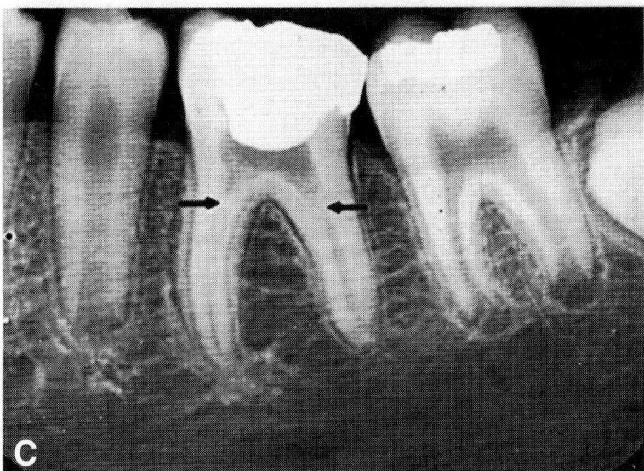

Figure 17-13 Calcium hydroxide pulpotomy, young permanent molar. **A**, Pulp of a first permanent molar exposed by caries (**white arrow**). **B**, Calcified dentin bridges (**arrows**) over vital pulp in canals. Note open apices. **C**, Pulp recession (**arrows**) and continued root development indicative of continuing pulp vitality. Reproduced with permission from McDonald RE. Dentistry for the child and adolescent. 2nd ed. St. Louis: CV Mosby; 1974.

with calcium hydroxide for primary and young permanent teeth in the range of 30 to 90%.[228,229]

Calcium Hydroxide Pulpotomy Outcomes in Primary Teeth

Via, in a 2-year study of calcium hydroxide pulpotomies in primary teeth, had only a 31% success,[230] and Law reported only a 49% success in a 1-year study.[231] In all investigations, failure was the result of chronic pulpal inflammation and internal resorption. Magnusson[192] and Schröder and Granath[232] found similar high failure rates with calcium hydroxide in pulpotomized primary molars.

Internal resorption may result from overstimulation of the primary pulp by the highly alkaline calcium hydroxide. This alkaline-induced overstimulation could cause metaplasia within the pulp tissue, leading to the formation of odontoclasts (Figure 17-14). In addition, undetected microleakage could allow large numbers of bacteria to overwhelm the pulp and nullify the beneficial effects of calcium hydroxide.

Schröder also evaluated the progress of 33 pulpotomized primary molars with calcium hydroxide as a wound dressing.[233] After 2 years, the success rate was 59%, with failures manifested as internal resorption. Histologic study revealed extra pulpal blood clots, over the amputated sites, which Schröder felt interfered with pulpal healing and dentin bridge formation.

In spite of these earlier discouraging reports, Phaneuf et al. demonstrated significant primary tooth pulpotomy success with calcium hydroxide in commercial preparations such as Pulpdent (Pulpdent Corporation

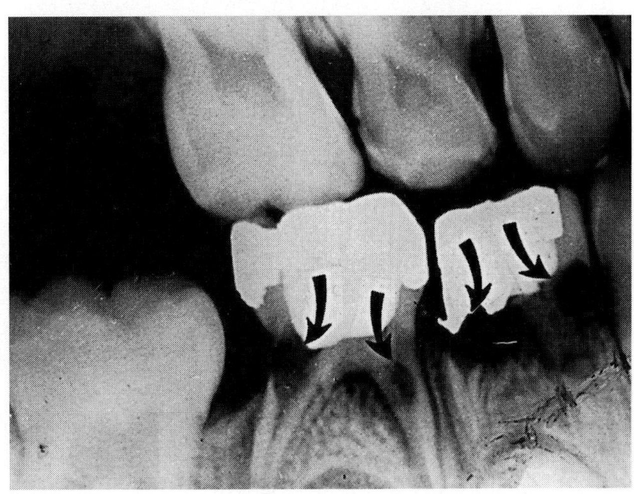

Figure 17-14 Massive internal resorption (**arrows**) of primary mandibular molars after calcium hydroxide pulpotomy.

of America; Watertown, Mass.) and Dycal.[106] The difference in pulp response to these commercial preparations might be attributed to their lower pH values. Calcium hydroxide incorporated in a methylcellulose base, such as Pulpdent, showed earlier and more consistent bridging than did other types of calcium hydroxide preparations. Berk and Krakow[234] and Schröder[233] have extensively studied calcium hydroxide pulpotomies and believe that the state of the pulp, surgical trauma, or amputation treatment may be more important than the calcium hydroxide per se in inducing success. At present, the **calcium hydroxide pulpotomy technique cannot be generally recommended for primary teeth** owing to its low success rate.[89,184,235]

Permanent Tooth Pulpotomy: Indications and Contraindications

Because of improved clinical outcomes, **calcium hydroxide is the recommended pulpotomy agent** for carious and traumatic exposures in **young permanent teeth,** particularly with incomplete apical closure (Figure 17-15). Following the closure of the apex, it is generally recommended that conventional root canal obturation be accomplished to avoid the potential long-term outcome of root canal calcification.[236]

Procedure.

1. Anesthetize the tooth to be treated and isolate under a rubber dam.
2. Excavate all caries and establish a cavity outline.
3. Irrigate the cavity with water and lightly dry with cotton pellets.
4. Remove the roof of the pulp chamber with a high-speed fissure bur.
5. Amputate the coronal pulp with a large low-speed round bur or a high-speed diamond stone with a light touch.[237]
6. Control hemorrhage with a cotton pellet applied with pressure or a damp pellet of hydrogen peroxide.
7. Place a **calcium hydroxide mixture** over the radicular pulp stumps at the canal orifices and dry with a cotton pellet.
8. Place quick-setting ZOE cement or resin-reinforced glass ionomer cement over the calcium hydroxide to seal and fill the chamber.
9. If the crown is severely weakened by decay, a stainless steel crown rather than an amalgam restoration should be used to prevent cusp fractures (Figure 17-16).

ALTERNATIVES TO FORMOCRESOL IN PRIMARY TEETH

Although **diluted formocresol is currently the recommended agent for pulpotomy treatment** for carious pulp exposures in vital **primary teeth,** some concern has been expressed regarding its use as a pulp medication because of its biocompatibility deficiencies. The formaldehyde component of the medicament and its

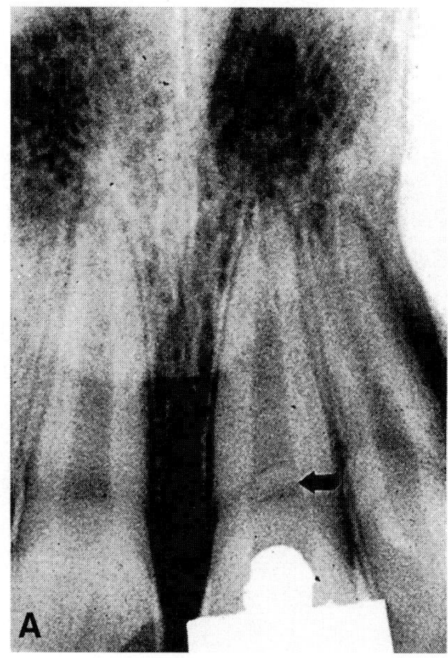

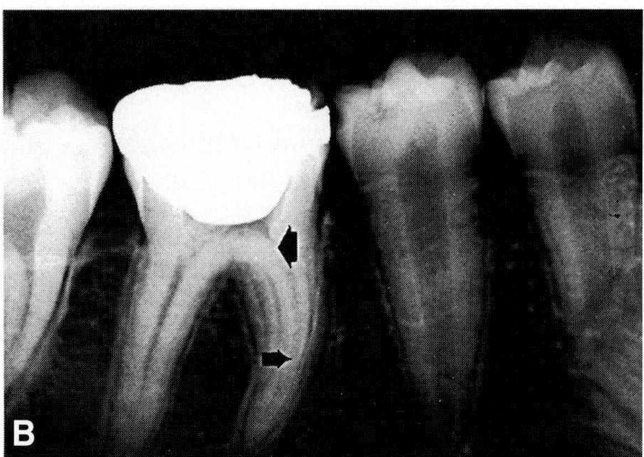

Figure 17-15 Calcium hydroxide pulpotomies in young permanent teeth. **A,** Crown fracture exposure of a central incisor. The apex was open at the time of pulpotomy. Note root growth, apical closure, and the dentin bridges (**arrows**). **B,** Partial root canal calcification (**arrows**) following pulpotomy in a young first permanent molar.

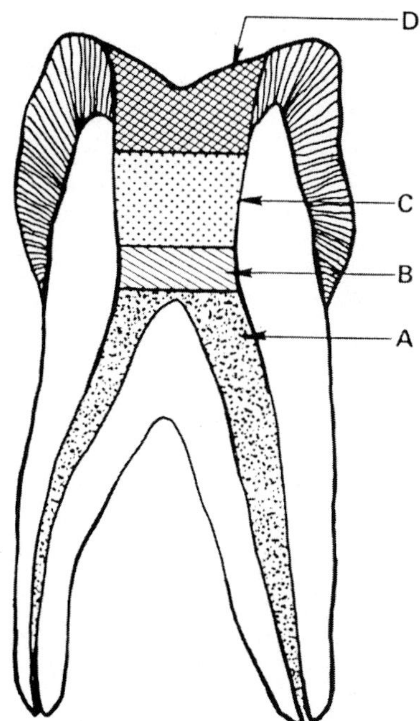

Figure 17-16 Calcium hydroxide pulpotomy in a young permanent molar. The cavity is prepared, caries and the chamber roof are removed, and the pulp is amputated to the canal orifices. Following hemostasis, commercial calcium hydroxide is placed and protected with zinc oxide–eugenol and amalgam filling or a stainless crown. **A**, Vital pulp. **B**, Calcium hydroxide. **C**, Zinc oxide–eugenol quick-set cement. **D**, Amalgam.

close derivatives have been implicated for exerting potentially harmful systemic and local effects.

Formocresol may not be confined solely to the radicular tissue. Various investigations by Pashley et al.[238] and Myers et al.[239] showed systemic uptake and tissue injury of labeled formaldehyde that was later found in dentin, periodontal tissue, bone, plasma, kidneys, and lungs. Ranly and Horn, in studying the ingredients and actions of formocresol, stated that although high levels of formaldehyde or cresol can be mutagenic or carcinogenic and produce histologic failures pulpally, it is not realistic that enough multiple pulpotomies would be performed to bring about a toxic systemic level.[240,241]

Messer et al. reported a significant number of enamel defects in the succedaneous teeth under formocresol pulpotomies.[242] Rollings and Paulsen[243] and Mulder et al.,[244] however, found no difference in the prevalence of enamel defects in permanent teeth in relation to formocresol pulpotomies.

Because of the potential concerns in the use of formaldehyde in dentistry, it has been suggested that research in alternative formulations be conducted for use in pediatric pulpal therapy.[245] In spite of these concerns, formocresol remains as the benchmark medicament to which alternative agents are compared.

Sandler et al. sealed in Cresatin as the medicament in pulpotomy and protected it with a covering of Cavit (Premier Dental Products, Plymouth Meeting, Mass.).[246] Clinically, only one failure occurred in their test group. Histologically, tissue fixation appeared at the amputation site, and the apical-third pulp demonstrated vital tissue in 84% of the 21 cases examined.

Nevins et al. were very successful in producing dentin bridging and canal calcification using collagen-calcium phosphate gel cross-linked with 0.6% glutaraldehyde to increase firmness and fiber stability.[247]

Fuks et al., using native collagen solutions enriched with cell nutrients that promote cell proliferation and healing of incision wounds, showed complete healing of pulpotomized teeth in dogs and monkeys.[142]

Glutaraldehyde

It was suggested by 's-Gravenmade that formaldehyde did not represent the ideal pulp fixative in clinical endodontic therapy. Inflamed tissue that produces toxic by-products should be **fixed** rather than treated with strong disinfectants.[248] He felt that satisfactory fixation with formocresol requires an excessive amount of medication, as well as a longer period of interaction. These requirements may lead to undesirable effects at the periapex.

Also, the reactions of formaldehyde with proteins should be considered less than stable and may be reversible. He felt that a **glutaraldehyde** solution might replace formocresol in endodontic therapy because of its fixative properties and bactericidal effectiveness and result in less destruction of tissue.

Hill et al. compared glutaraldehyde to formocresol in vitro with respect to its antimicrobial and cytotoxic effects. Minimal antimicrobial concentrations were 3.125% for glutaraldehyde and 0.75% for formocresol. More importantly, at these concentrations, glutaraldehyde was found to be less cytotoxic "when used as a pulpotomy agent." Formocresol at its lower concentration, however, was considerably more antimicrobial than glutaraldehyde.[249]

Wernes and 's-Gravenmade, in an in vivo study of permanent and primary dentitions, in which some teeth were vital and others nonvital, found no evidence of periradicular inflammation after the application of glutaraldehyde.[250] Dankert and colleagues found only minimal diffusion through the apices.[251]

The following attributes have been ascribed to **glutaraldehyde** as a more desirable medicament for pulpal therapy when compared to formocresol: (1) it is a bifunctional reagent, which allows it to form strong intra- and intermolecular protein bonds, leading to superior fixation by cross-linkage; (2) its diffusibility is limited; (3) it is an excellent antimicrobial agent; (4) it causes less necrosis of pulpal tissue; and (5) it causes less dystrophic calcification in pulp canals.

In an initial clinical study, Kopel and colleagues used a 2% glutaraldehyde solution as a medicament for pulpotomies in vivo for cariously exposed primary molars.[252] Histologic evaluations were made on extracted teeth at 1 month, 3 months, 6 months, and 1 year. The most striking finding from this study was that, histologically, the remaining root pulp tissue did not resemble pulp tissue subjected to formocresol. There was an initial zone of fixation adjacent to the dressing that did not proceed apically. The tissue adjoining the fixed zone and down to the apex had the cellular detail of normal pulp and was presumably vital (Figure 17-17). It was suggested that **2% glutaraldehyde,** because of its biochemical effects on the pulp, **can be used for pulpotomies in primary teeth.**

Following this initial clinical investigation with glutaraldehyde, many in vitro and in vivo studies began with important implications and findings for its use in pediatric pulp therapy. Dilly and Courts found that glutaraldehyde did not stimulate a significant immune response.[253] Lekka et al. later found that only a minimal amount of glutaraldehyde diffused through the radicular pulp tissue when compared to formocresol.[254]

Clinical studies in primary teeth have been conducted by Garcia-Godoy,[255] Fuks et al.,[256] and Alacam[257] for periods ranging from 12, 19, and 42 months. Respective success rates were found to be 98, 90.4, and 96%. Root canal obliteration and internal resorption were seen in the radiographs in a small percentage of the cases in Fuks et al.'s study. Other studies have investigated various aspects in the use of glutaraldehyde as a pulpotomy medicament such as concentration, pH, time, and method of application as contrasted to the original values when it was first used.[258–260]

After several investigations, Ranly et al. concluded that buffering glutaraldehyde, increasing its concentration, and applying it for longer time periods all enhanced the degree of fixation.[261] They suggested that clinical treatment might involve buffered glutaraldehyde at either 4% for 4 minutes or 8% for 2 minutes. Lloyd et al. felt that the tissue becomes more stable with longer application times of 2% glutaraldehyde.[260]

Although Ranly and coworkers originally suggested that glutaraldehyde might be incorporated in a ZOE base over a pulpotomy,[261] a later clinical study found a 48.6% rate of failure with this procedure.[262]

Hernandez et al. evaluated the clinical and radiographic results of pulpotomies in permanent molars medicated with either formocresol or 2% glutaraldehyde.[263] The observations showed a return to a more normal trabecular bone pattern in perialveolar bone after 2 years with the glutaraldehyde compared to the formocresol treatment.

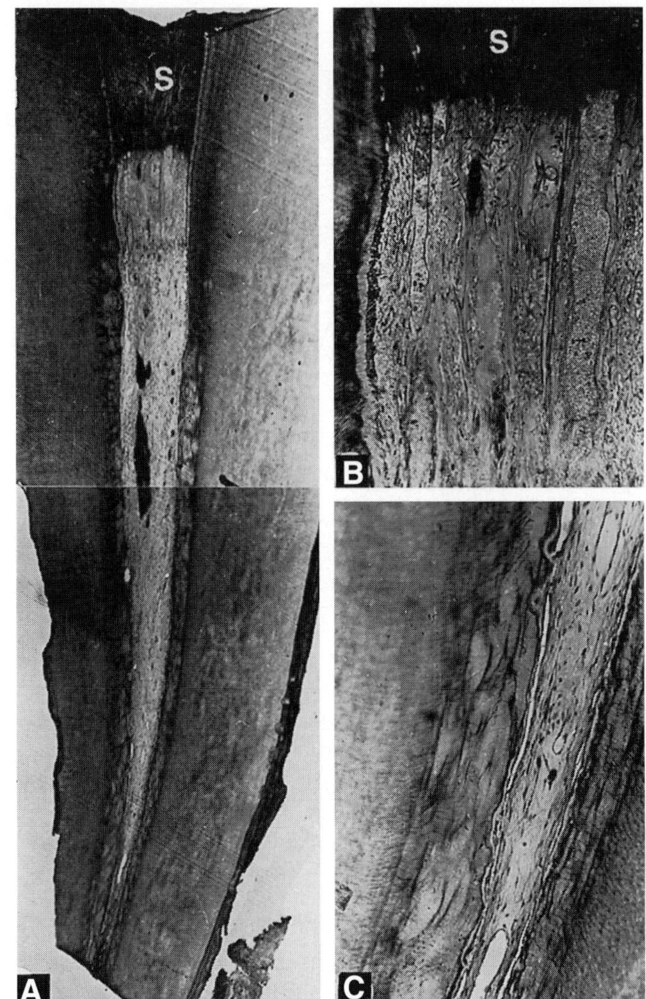

Figure 17-17 Glutaraldehyde pulpotomy. **A,** Section of the root of a primary molar treated with glutaraldehyde 1 month earlier. Note the Schiff-positive homogenous zone (S) in the coronal region. **B,** Pulp tissue adjacent to the coronal region has dilated veins and absence of inflammatory cells. **C,** Tissue in the apical region is also free of inflammatory cells. A wide area of new irritational dentin is evident. At 1 year, the collagen concentration increases with mild inflammation. Reproduced with permission from Kopel HM, et al. The effect of gluteraldehyde on primary pulp tissue following coronal amputation. J Dent Child 1980;47:425.

The same concerns that related to the systemic absorption of formocresol have been expressed with the use of glutaraldehyde in pulp therapy. Myers et al. demonstrated some systemic absorption with ultimate excretion of ^{14}C-glutaraldehyde following a 5-minute application of 2% glutaraldehyde to multiple pulpotomy sites in dogs.[264]

Ranly et al. also investigated the systemic distribution of 4% infused glutaraldehyde pulpotomies in rats and found only an approximate 25% of the applied dose. These investigators concluded that the use of glutaraldehyde as a pulpotomy agent in humans would be free of any significant toxicity.[265]

Astringents

Schröder and Granath documented the fact that pulpal hemorrhage control is critical for pulpotomy success.[232] Kouri et al. compared formocresol pulpotomies in primary teeth using **epinephrine** versus sterile water and cotton pellets for hemorrhage control. After 6-week to 3-month post-treatment periods, histologic and electron microscopic evidence of healing was similar for both groups. Bleeding times for the epinephrine-treated pulps were 50 seconds versus 251 seconds for the sterile water–treated pulps. Less extravasated blood occurred with the epinephrine-treated pulps and was limited to the amputation site. No clinical or radiographic failures occurred for either group.[266]

Helig et al. compared **aluminum chloride** versus sterile water in achieving hemostasis prior to medicament placement in calcium hydroxide pulpotomies for primary teeth in humans. They found a 25% radiographic failure rate in the sterile water group versus no radiographic failures with the aluminum chloride group after 9 months.[267]

Ferric sulfate has received the most recent attention as a formocresol alternative in pulpotomy choices. This material, when in contact with tissue, forms a ferric ion-protein complex that mechanically occludes capillaries at the pulpal amputation site. The subjacent pulp tissue is then allowed to heal. Landau and Johnson found a more favorable pulpal response to a 15.5% ferric sulfate solution than calcium hydroxide in primate pulpotomies after 60 days.[268] Fei et al. found a combined clinical and radiographic success rate of 96.3% for ferric sulfate pulpotomies versus a 77.8% success rate for diluted formocresol pulpotomies in humans after 12 months.[269]

Fuks et al. found a 92.7% success rate with ferric sulfate versus 83.8% with diluted formocresol in primary tooth pulpotomies after a mean post-treatment time of 20.5 months. They noted that these differences were not statistically significant and therefore concluded the success rates to be similar for both groups.[270] Fuks et al. conducted a histologic study of ferric sulfate versus diluted formocresol–treated pulps in primate teeth at 4- and 8-week observation periods. Mild inflammation was evident in 58% of the ferric sulfate group versus 48% of the diluted formocresol group. Severe inflammation was noted in 35% of the ferric sulfate group versus 29% of the diluted formocresol group. Abscess and necrosis were noted in 3% of the ferric sulfate group versus 13% of the diluted formocresol group. They concluded that histologic results were similar for both groups and did not compare favorably with previously reported clinical findings of ferric sulfate potential superiority.[271]

Cell-Inductive Agents

Mineral trioxide aggregate and **calcium phosphate cement** have already been described with respect to their potential cell-inductive properties in the context of direct pulp-capping techniques. Their use in pulpotomy techniques remains to be substantiated from control studies. Mineral trioxide aggregate was identified as a potentially effective pulpotomy agent in a review of this material with case examples by Abedi and Ingle.[272]

Higashi and Okamoto reviewed the use of **calcium phosphate ceramics** and **hydroxyapatite** as potential pulpotomy agents. They studied the particle size effects of hydroxyapatite and β-tricalcium phosphate as variables in pulpotomy success as determined by hard tissue formation. Osteodentin and tubular dentin formation occurred around large particles (300 mu) in contrast to small particles (40 mu), which demonstrated pulp tissue inflammation.[273] Yoshiba et al. provided evidence of α-tricalcium phosphate in combination with calcium hydroxide being successful in bridge formation with less local destruction of pulp tissue than with calcium hydroxide alone.[274]

Bone morphogenetic proteins have been proposed as potential capping agents in direct pulp-capping and pulpotomy techniques. Bone morphogenetic proteins 2 to 8 belong to TGF-β, that are signaling proteins that regulate cell differentiation. Bone morphogenetic proteins 2 and 4 have been implicated in odontoblastic differentiation. Nakashima demonstrated dentin bridging in dog tooth coronal pulp amputation when the remaining tissue was capped with BMP-2 and BMP-4, along with recombinant human dentin matrix. After a 2-month time interval, tubular dentin and osteodentin were found histologically in response to both BMP types.[177]

Fadhavi and Anderson compared **freeze-dried bone**, calcium hydroxide, and ZOE in primate deciduous tooth pulpotomies with respect to histologic inflammation and clinical/radiopathic pathology. After 6-week and 6-month time periods, vital pulps with moderate inflammation were found in 83.3% of the freeze-dried bone group. This was in contrast to the calcium hydroxide group, which demonstrated moderate to severe inflammation in 50% of the cases and signs of partial necrosis in 100%. Dentin bridge formation occurred in 100% of the freeze-dried bone group versus 50% in the calcium hydroxide group. All of the ZOE-treated teeth were necrotic at 6 months. They concluded that freeze-dried bone was superior to calcium hydroxide within the parameters of their study and might have potential as a pulpotomy agent if substantiated by studies in humans.[178]

Nonpharmacotherapeutic Pulpotomy Techniques: Controlled Energy

Controlled energy in the form of electrosurgical and laser heat application to the pulp stumps at the canal orifice site has been proposed as an alternative to the more traditional pharmacotherapeutic techniques, particularly those using formocresol. Ruemping et al. identified electrosurgical pulpotomy advantages that can be applied to the controlled energy category at large and include (1) quick and efficient, (2) self-limiting, (3) good hemostasis, (4) good visibility of the field, (5) no systemic effects, and (6) sterilization at the site of application.[275]

Electrosurgery. Ruemping et al. histologically compared electrosurgery with formocresol in pulpotomy techniques for primate primary and young permanent teeth. They mechanically amputated coronal pulps and then either applied formocresol to the pulp stump or performed momentary electrosurgery, followed by ZOE cement placement.[275] After an 8-week post-treatment period, the histologic appearance for both groups was similar, with no evidence of pulp necrosis or abscess formation. In the electrosurgery group, secondary dentin was deposited along the lateral canal walls, and the apical two-thirds of the pulp revealed a slightly fibrotic to normal appearance.[275] Shaw et al. compared, after 6 months, the histologic effects of electrosurgery with formocresol on the radicular pulp. They found similar success rates of 80% for the formocresol and 84% for the electrosurgical groups according to their histologic criteria. They concluded that neither technique was superior.[276]

Conversely, Shulman et al. histologically compared electrosurgery, formocresol, and electrosurgery plus formocresol in primate pulpotomies.[277] They used ^{14}C-labeled formocresol and performed coronal amputation with electrosurgery subsequent to pulp chamber roof removal. They found more periradicular and furcal pathologic change after 65 days in the electrosurgery group. They also noted that combining the two techniques of electrosurgery and formocresol produced no better results. Both electrosurgical groups were inferior to the formocresol group.[277] Sheller and Morton histologically studied the effects of electrosurgical pulpotomies on the remaining radicular tissue in 11 primary canines at 6-day, 2-week, 8-week, and 13-week post-treatment intervals. Varying degrees of inflammation, edema, and necrosis were seen at all time periods, with the most favorable tissue appearance occurring at the longer intervals. Those teeth judged to be successful demonstrated reparative dentin formation along the lateral aspect of the radicular canal walls but not across the amputation site. They concluded that their results did not support the concept of electrosurgery being less harmful to pulp tissue than conventional pharmacotherapeutic techniques.[278]

A form of electrosurgery, known as **electrofulguration,** has been suggested for pulpotomies in primary teeth.[279] It involves establishing an electrical arc to the targeted tissue without direct contact of the probe, which ideally confines heat to the superficial tissue level. Mack and Dean investigated the electrofulguration pulpotomy technique in 164 primary molars.[279] After a 26-month post-treatment period, they found a 99.4% clinical and radiographic success rate. They felt that this compared favorably with a 93.9% formocresol pulpotomy success rate in a retrospective study by Hicks et al. with a similar protocol.[196,279] Conversely, Fishman et al. compared calcium hydroxide with ZOE when used as a base over electrofulgurated pulp tissue. Although the overall clinical success rate for the entire sample was 77 to 81%, the radiographic success was 57.3% for the electrofulguration plus calcium hydroxide group and 54.6% for the electrofulguration plus ZOE group.[280]

Lasers. Application of laser irradiation in vital pulp therapy has been proposed as another alternative to pharmacotherapeutic techniques. Its advantages and disadvantages are the same as for electrosurgery. Adrian reported that irradiation of the buccal tooth surface with the neodymium: yttrium-aluminum-garnet (Nd:YAG) laser produced less pulp damage than the ruby laser with less histologic evidence of coagulation and focal necrosis.[281] Shoji et al. histologically studied the carbon-dioxide laser in the pulpotomy procedure. They noted that the least amount of pulp tissue injury occurred with defocused irradiation with lower power settings and shorter application. More tissue destruction occurred in the defocused mode with higher irradiation power settings.[282] Kato et al. studied the effects of the Nd:YAG laser on pulpotomized rat molars at low (5 watts) and high (15 watts) power settings. At 2 weeks, histologic evidence showed osteodentin covering the amputated pulps with the low power setting and fibrous dentin formation at the orifice wall of the root canal with the high power setting. Normal root development was observed in all specimens.[283] McGuire et al. compared the Nd:YAG laser with formocresol in permanent tooth pulpotomies in dogs at 6- and 12-week post-treatment periods. No significant differences in radiographic pathology were found between the two groups. Histologically, the frequency of pulpal inflammation was higher for the laser group (29%) at 12 weeks than for the formocresol group (0%). No differences were found with respect to periradicular inflammation and root resorption.[284]

Studies on controlled-energy pulpotomy techniques are equivocal as to their effectiveness in reducing post-treatment inflammation when compared to conventional pharmacotherapeutic techniques. Although clinical reports of success exist, more controlled clinical and histologic investigations are needed to address the variables of power settings, application times, continuous versus pulsed modes of application, and degree of heat dissipation in the radicular pulp and surrounding hard tissues.

NONVITAL PULP THERAPY IN PRIMARY TEETH: PULPECTOMY

The treatment objectives in nonvital pulp therapy for primary teeth are to (1) maintain the tooth free of infection, (2) biomechanically cleanse and obturate the root canals, (3) promote physiologic root resorption, and (4) hold the space for the erupting permanent tooth. The treatment of choice to achieve these objectives is **pulpectomy,** which involves the removal of necrotic pulp tissue followed by filling the root canals with a resorbable cement. Indications for this procedure include teeth with poor chance of **vital** pulp treatment success, strategic importance with respect to space maintenance, absence of severe root resorption, absence of surrounding bone loss from infection, and expectation of restorability.

Most negative attitudes toward primary teeth complete pulpectomy have been based on the difficulty in cleaning and shaping the bizarre and tortuous canal anatomy of these teeth.[285,286] This was especially true for primary molars with their resorbing and open apices.[287,288] Removal of abscessed primary teeth has been suggested because of their potential to create developmental defects in the underlying permanent successors.[289–291] In spite of these objections, successful root canal obturation of irreversibly inflamed and nonvital primary teeth can be successfully accomplished. Modifications of adult endodontic techniques, however, must be implemented because of the aforementioned anatomic differences between primary and permanent teeth.

Marsh and Largent indicated that the goal of the pulpectomy procedure in primary teeth should be to eliminate the bacteria and the contaminated pulp tissue from the canal.[292] In **primary teeth,** more emphasis is placed on **chemical means** in conjunction with limited mechanical débridement to disinfect and remove necrotic pulp remnants from the somewhat inaccessible canals rather than conventional "shaping" of the canals. Complete pulpectomy procedures have been recommended for primary teeth even with evidence of severe chronic inflammation or necrosis in the radicular pulp.[293–295]

Resorbable cements such as ZOE and iodoform-containing pastes have been recommended as canal obturants. **Nonresorbable** materials such as gutta-percha and silver points **are contraindicated** as they will not enhance the primary root physiologic resorptive process (Figure 17-18). Rifkin identified criteria for an ideal pulpectomy obturant that include it being (1) resorbable, (2) antiseptic, (3) noninflammatory and nonirritating to the underlying permanent tooth germ, (4) radiopaque, (5) easily inserted, and (6) easily removed.[296] No currently available obturant meets all of these criteria.

Owing to primary tooth exfoliation, the standard for long-term pulpectomy success is shorter than for adult endodontics. Primary tooth pulpectomies are successful if the root is (1) firmly attached, (2) remains in function without pain or infection until the permanent successor is ready to erupt, (3) undergoes physiologic resorption, and (4) is free from fistulous tracts. Radiographically, success is judged by the absence of furcation or periradicular lesions and the re-establishment of a normal periodontal ligament.

Historical Perspective

Sweet described a four- or five-step technique using formocresol for the treatment of pulpless teeth with and without fistulae.[180] A study of pediatric endodontic procedures was reported by Rabinowitz in which nonvital primary molars were treated with a 2- to 3-day application of formocresol, followed by precipitation of silver nitrate and a sealer of ZOE cement into the canals.[297,298] Although he reported a high success rate, his complicated procedure involved a range of 4 to 17 visits, with an average of 5.5 visits for teeth without periradicular involvement and 7.7 visits for those with periradicular involvement.

Hobson described pulpectomy techniques for necrotic primary teeth in which the canals were not débrided. Beechwood creosote was used as a disinfectant, usually for 2 weeks, followed by filling the pulp

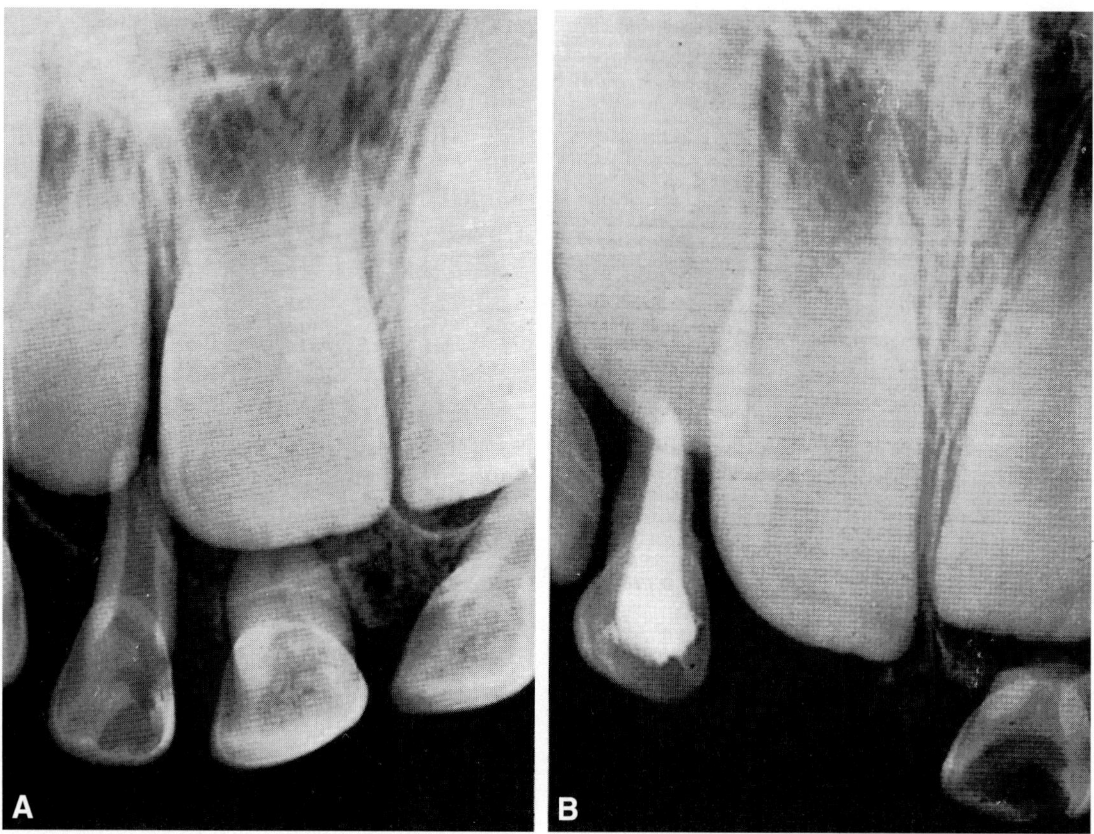

Figure 17-18 Root canal filling of a pulpless, maxillary primary lateral incisor. **A**, Carious exposure and pulp death—a candidate for endodontic therapy. **B**, Six months following successful root canal filling with resorbable zinc oxide–eugenol cement. Care must be taken not to perforate the apex or overfill and injure the developing permanent tooth bud. Reproduced with permission from Law DB, Lewis TM, Davis JM. An atlas of pedodontics. Philadelphia: WB Saunders; 1969.

chamber with a ZOE cement. Treatment proved equally successful for teeth with necrotic pulps or vital infected pulps.[299]

In treating primary molars, Lewis and Law used conventional endodontics in canal preparation where they instrumented, irrigated with sodium hypochlorite, and dried the canals, which were then medicated for 3 to 7 days with either eugenol, camphorated parachlorophenol, or formocresol.[1] On the second visit, the canals were mechanically prepared with files and filled with one of various resorbable mixtures, such as ZOE cement or ZOE mixed with iodoform crystals (see Figure 17-18).

Judd and Kenny advocated a different complete pulpectomy method for deciduous teeth.[300] For vital pulp extirpation, two Hedstroem files, usually size 20, were slid along opposite sides of the canal to entangle pulp tissue. Ideal placement of the files just short of the apex, with two or three rotations, will ensnare the pulp. When withdrawn, the vital pulp will be removed in toto. If the pulp has degenerated, "then the canal should be filed with a single No. 20 to allow access for a red No. 1 Lentulo paste filler."[300] After water irrigation and air drying, canals were obturated with "a thin mix (viscosity similar to toothpaste) of a fine-grained, nonreinforced ZOE cement (ZOE 2200, Dentsply-Caulk; Milford, Dela.) using a Lentulo spiral paste filler."[300]

Gould reported a clinical study of primary teeth in 27 children, age 3½ years to 8½ years, using a one-appointment technique.[301] In 35 "frankly infected" primary molars, a cotton pellet of camphorated parachlorophenol was placed in the chamber for 5 minutes after the canals had been débrided with files over two-thirds of their length. Zinc oxide–eugenol cement was then pressed into the prepared canals. After 26 months of clinical and radiographic observation, 83% were judged to be therapeutically successful on the basis of no lesions being detected.

In asymptomatic necrotic primary teeth, Frigoletto suggested that canals be débrided with a barbed broach, irrigated with sodium hypochlorite, and dried. Canals were then filled with root canal paste using a specially designed pressure syringe.[75] In instances of symptomatic teeth, Cresatin was mixed with the paste.

Starkey has described a **one-appointment** and **multiappointment** method of treating cariously involved primary pulp tissue.[91] The **one-appointment** method is used in cases with **vital** pulp tissue, in which inflammation extends beyond the coronal pulp and no radiographic evidence of periradicular involvement is present. In these cases, Starkey recommended a **partial pulpectomy** to remove the coronal aspects of the radicular pulp, **controlling hemorrhaging** and **filling the canals** and crown with a creamy mix of ZOE cement.

Starkey's **multiappointment** method was advocated for cases with **necrotic pulps** and **periradicular involvement.**[91] At the first appointment, coronal pulp debris is removed, but the canals are not instrumented. A medicament such as formocresol or camphorated monochlorophenol is placed in the pulp chamber and sealed with IRM for 1 week. If the tooth and surrounding gingival tissues are asymptomatic and clinically negative at the second visit, the canals are mechanically cleansed and débrided and then filled with ZOE cement (Figure 17-19). Modifications of these procedures have been described by Cullen,[302] Dugal and Curgon,[303] Goerig and Camp,[304] Kopel,[305] Mathewson and Primosch,[89] and Spedding.[306]

It should be noted that some controversy exists with respect to the relative effectiveness of the one-sitting and two-sitting pulpectomy procedures. Coll et al. reported an 80 to 86% success rate with the one-sitting technique.[307] Primosch et al. noted that 60% of US undergraduate dental programs teach the one-sitting technique versus 26% teaching the two-sitting technique.[69]

Extension of formocresol use to the pulpectomy technique was a logical sequence. Vander Wall et al. have shown formocresol to be more effective than either camphorated parachlorophenol or Cresatin as a root canal medicament for inhibiting bacterial growth.[308] Several studies have evaluated the clinical and radiographic findings of the pulpectomy procedure for nonvital primary molars and primary anteriors using formocresol. Coll et al. evaluated a one-appointment formocresol pulpectomy technique for nonvital primary molars. After a mean observation period of 70 months, 86.1% were judged successful.[307] They also found that successful pulpectomized primary molars were not over-retained and the successor premolars had a very low incidence of hypoplastic defects.[307]

Barr et al., in a radiographic retrospective evaluation of primary molar pulpectomies performed in a private practice with a mean observation period of 40.2 months, found an overall success rate of 85.5%.[309] Noteworthy findings included 88% complete ZOE paste resorption and a 25.8% reduction of preoperative

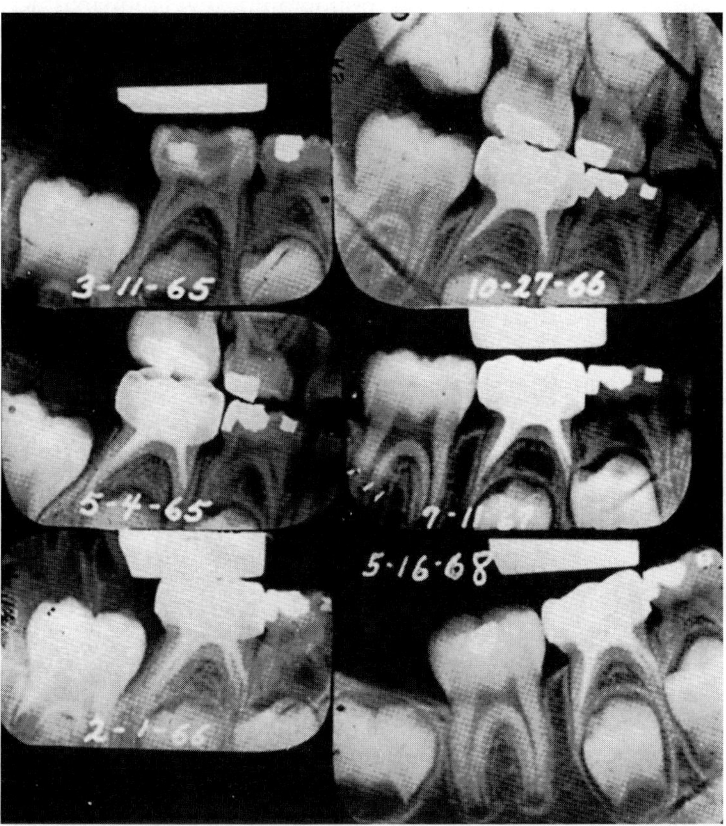

Figure 17-19 Three-year successful root canal filling of mandibular second primary molar. (Courtesy of Dr. Paul E. Starkey.) The canals have been thoroughly filed and irrigated at the first appointment and medicated with formocresol or camphorated parachlorophenol. At the second appointment, the canals were filled with resorbable zinc oxide–eugenol cement. Reproduced with permission from Law DB, Lewis TM, Davis JM. An atlas of pedodontics. Philadelphia: WB Saunders; 1969.

radiolucencies. These clinicians suggested that posterior primary molar pulpectomies have a relatively high success rate in private practice.

Coll et al. and Flaitz et al. also evaluated the results of pulpectomy treatment in primary anterior teeth.[310,311] Using clinical and radiographic evaluations, Coll and colleagues completed 27 pulpectomies in primary incisors and found that their 78% success rate did not differ statistically from comparable primary molar rates after a mean of 45 months.[310] Seventy-three percent were considered to have exfoliated normally. These investigators concluded, however, that documented success rates for indirect pulp capping and pulpotomies in primary anterior teeth were higher than for pulpectomies.

Flaitz et al.'s contrasting study compared 57 **pulpotomies** versus 87 **pulpectomies** in primary anterior teeth followed for a mean of 37 months.[311] Based on the final radiographs in the study, treatment was successful in 68.5% of the pulpotomized group of anterior teeth versus 84% of the pulpectomized group. They concluded overall that pulpectomy was a better treatment option for primary incisors even though they may have shown more radiographic pathosis at the time of the diagnosis.

Yacobi and Kenny have twice monitored their success rates in vital pulpectomy and immediate ZOE (ZOE 2200, L. D. Caulk Co.; Milford, Dela.) filling. At 6 months, their success rate was comparable to the formocresol results of 89% for anterior teeth and 92% for posterior teeth.[312] At 2 years, reporting on 81 patients and 253 teeth, Payne et al., using ZOE, reported a mean success rate of 83% for anterior teeth and 90% for posterior teeth. They conjectured that the discrepancy in rates between anterior and posterior teeth was related to the final restorations—microleakage from composite resin in the anterior regions and stainless crowns in the posterior.[313] They believed this to be a most acceptable alternative method for saving primary teeth while avoiding the compromising effects of the aldehydes.

Alternative Pulpectomy Canal Obturants

Zinc oxide–eugenol cement has been the most frequently used obturant in the pulpectomy technique. Primosch et al. noted that 90% of US pediatric dentistry undergraduate programs teach ZOE as the pulpectomy obturant of choice.[69] Although considered to be resorbable, Coll et al., in a 6-year follow-up of 41 pulpectomized primary molars, found that ZOE particle retention in the gingival sulcus occurred in 8 of 17 patients followed to the time of premolar eruption.[307] Their technique included a 5-minute formocresol-blotted paper point treatment of the canals prior to obturation. As previously mentioned, there has been concern about the use of formocresol in any form in pediatric endodontic therapy. Alternative pulpectomy agents have been proposed to improve on the biocompatibility limitations of ZOE and formocresol.

Hendry et al. compared **calcium hydroxide** with ZOE as a pulpectomy obturant in primary teeth of dogs. At 4 weeks post-treatment, canals treated with calcium hydroxide exhibited less inflammation, less pathologic root resorption, and more hard tissue apposition than ZOE and control-treated teeth.[314]

Barker and Lockett identified the potential benefits of **Kri paste,** an **iodoform compound**, also containing parachlorophenol, camphor, and menthol. The advantages of this material include bactericidal properties and excellent resorbability. Histologically, they found that this material easily resorbed even when extruded beyond the apex of the treated teeth. An ingress of connective tissue was seen in the apical portions of the treated canals.[315] Bactericidal iodoform pastes have been reintroduced as a root canal filling.[245,316,317] Garcia-Godoy obtained a 95.6% success clinically and radiographically with Kri paste during a 24-month period for 43 teeth.[318] It was noted that this paste would resorb within 2 weeks if found in the periradicular or furcation areas.[319] Rifkin reported an 89% clinical and radiographic success rate after 1 year with Kri paste pulpectomies in primary teeth.[296] Holan and Fuks clinically and radiographically compared Kri paste with ZOE in human primary molars after 48 months postoperatively. They found overall success rates of 84% with the Kri paste group versus 65% with the ZOE group. Kri paste was almost twice as successful in primary first molars as ZOE. However, no significant differences between these two agents occurred in primary second molars. Overfills with Kri paste resulted in 79% success versus 41% success with ZOE. They concluded that iodoform-containing paste had a potential advantage over ZOE in the pulpectomy procedure for primary teeth.[319]

Treatment Considerations

The preceding review demonstrates the varied techniques and successes for mastering pulp therapy for nonvital and irreversibly inflamed primary teeth. Before outlining treatment methods, special considerations, indications, and contraindications must be addressed by the clinician.

General Considerations.

1. The patient should be healthy and cooperative. If any systemic disorders are present that would com-

promise a child's responses, the child's physician or medical team should be consulted.

2. Informed consent, with a clear explanation of the procedure to the parents, must be obtained.

Dental Considerations.

1. The tooth must be restorable after the root canal treatment.
2. Chronologic and dental age must be evaluated to rule out teeth with eminent exfoliation.
3. Psychological or cosmetic factors (anterior primary teeth) must be considered, which are often more important to the parent than to the child.
4. The number of teeth to be treated and strategic importance to the developing occlusion must be evaluated.
5. Primary molar root anatomy, along with the proximity of the underlying succedaneous tooth, must be evaluated.

Indications for a Pulpectomy Procedure.

1. Primary teeth with pulpal inflammation extending beyond the coronal pulp but with roots and alveolar bone free of pathologic resorption
2. Primary teeth with necrotic pulps, minimum root resorption, and minimum bony destruction in the bifurcation area
3. Pulpless primary teeth with sinus tracts
4. Pulpless primary teeth without permanent successors
5. Pulpless primary second molars before the eruption of the permanent first molar
6. Pulpless primary teeth in hemophiliacs
7. Pulpless primary anterior teeth when speech, crowded arches, or esthetics are a factor
8. Pulpless primary teeth next to the line of a palatal cleft
9. Pulpless primary molars supporting orthodontic appliances
10. Pulpless primary molars when arch length is deficient
11. Pulpless primary teeth when space maintainers or continued supervision are not feasible (handicapped or isolated children[†])

[†]Owing to the isolation of the children involved in its Bureau of Indian Health Affairs, the US Public Health Service has recommended root canal filling of primary teeth, whenever feasible, rather than space maintainers that require lengthy supervision.[320]

Contraindications.

1. Teeth with nonrestorable crowns
2. Periradicular involvement extending to the permanent tooth bud
3. **Pathologic** resorption of at least one-third of the root with a fistulous sinus tract
4. Excessive internal resorption
5. Extensive pulp floor opening into the bifurcation
6. Young patients with systemic illness such as congenital or rheumatic heart disease, hepatitis, or leukemia and children on long-term corticosteroid therapy or those who are immunocompromised
7. Primary teeth with underlying dentigerous or follicular cysts

Clinical Procedures: Partial Pulpectomy

Partial pulpectomy can be considered an extension of the pulpotomy procedure in that the coronal portion of the radicular pulp is amputated, leaving vital tissue in the canal that is assumed to be healthy. Although discussed in the context of nonvital pulp therapy, technically, it is a vital pulp therapy technique. The decision to implement the partial pulpectomy is made after removing the coronal pulp from the chamber and encountering difficulty with hemorrhage control from the radicular orifice.

Hemorrhage control is achieved with endodontic broaches used to remove one-third to one half of the coronal portion of the **radicular pulp** tissue from the canals. The canals and chamber are irrigated with hydrogen peroxide followed by sodium hypochlorite and then dried with cotton pellets. If hemorrhage is still impossible to control, all remaining radicular pulp tissue is to be removed, and the complete **pulpectomy** procedure must be implemented.

After successful hemorrhage control from the amputated radicular pulp, a formocresol-dampened cotton pellet, squeezed dry, is placed in the pulp chamber for 1 to 5 minutes. The pellet is removed, and a nonreinforced fast-setting ZOE cement is packed with pressure into the chamber and canals. A radiograph is then taken, and if the canals appear to be adequately filled, a stainless steel crown is placed as a permanent restoration (Figure 17-20).

Clinic Procedures: Complete Pulpectomy

The child with a necrotic primary tooth presents a considerable challenge for the clinician. In some instances, the tooth may be totally asymptomatic from a clinical standpoint. In other instances, the tooth may be acutely or chronically abscessed, mobile and painful, with

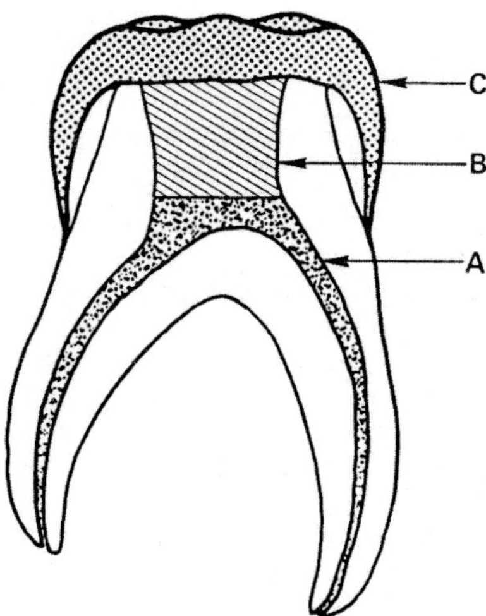

Figure 17-20 Root canal obturation and crown restoration for a pulpless primary molar. At the first appointment, following mechanical and chemical canal débridement, medicament is sealed in place for 1 week. The canal is obturated at the second appointment with resorbable zinc oxide–eugenol cement. **A**, Zinc oxide–eugenol cement root canal filling. **B**, Oxyphosphate of zinc cement. **C**, Stainless steel crown.

swollen periodontal tissues. In the latter case, the child may be apprehensive and irritable, making relief of pain and swelling the highest priority. In cases of nondraining alveolar abscesses and cellulitis from odontogenic origin, **antibiotic therapy** using first- or second-generation **penicillins** should be immediately prescribed for a period of 4 to 7 days. Canal instrumentation can then be implemented.

The complete pulpectomy procedure involves the following considerations. Under local anesthesia, the pulp chamber is carefully opened with a high-speed bur to relieve any pressure from the infected pulp. A low-speed round bur or a spoon excavator may be used to clean out the pulp chamber, which is then irrigated with sodium hypochlorite. In cases of acute inflammation, a camphorated monochlorophenol-dampened cotton pellet is placed in the coronal chamber as an **interim** medicament to chemically sterilize the pulp canals. In cases of **chronic abscess formation**, a formocresol-dampened cotton pellet is generally used as the interim medicament. The chambers are then sealed with a fast-setting ZOE cement, and the tooth may need to be equilibrated to avoid hyperocclusion.

At the end of 1 week, if all acute symptoms including pain and soft tissue swelling have resolved, final canal preparation—careful enlargement and débridement—is completed with **Hedstroem** files. Canal irrigation is accomplished with hydrogen peroxide and sodium hypochlorite. Tooth length should be carefully determined, and instrumentation should not extend beyond the apex. Fine files, in ultrasonic or sonic endodontic handpieces, with copious irrigation can be considered in this protocol.

The ribbon-shaped and tortuous root canals of primary teeth present a time-consuming problem in obtaining adequate obturation. A pressure syringe was developed by Greenberg for filling primary canals.[321] This technique has been described in detail by Spedding[306] and by Krakow et al..[322] The material of choice for filling the root canals of pulpectomized primary teeth is pure ZOE, first mixed as a slurry and carried into the canals using either paper points, a syringe, a "Jiffy tube," or a lentulo spiral root canal filler. Aylard and Johnson showed that the lentulo was the best overall ZOE root canal–filling instrument for curved canals and the pressure syringe technique was best for straight canals.[323] The slurry may be further compressed into the canals by packing the chamber with a stiffer mix of ZOE. After the canals are estimated to be filled to the chamber floor, the chamber itself is filled with a suitable cement such as a reinforced ZOE or a glass ionomer. As previously mentioned, the tooth is prepared for the placement of a stainless steel crown after evaluation of the canal filling by a radiograph.[90]

Mack and Halterman described the rationale and technique for an innovative approach to pulpectomy for **primary anterior teeth** by using a **labial** entry to the canal instead of the traditional lingual opening. This allows greater ease of instrumentation and provides incorporation of the access chamber in the esthetic labial veneer preparation. Bonded composite resin is used to complete the final **esthetic** restoration.[324]

Clinical Variation: Pulpotomy for Nonvital Primary Teeth

Less demanding techniques than the pulpectomy have been reported for treating **irreversibly inflamed** primary teeth, usually involving the formocresol pulpotomy technique. Ripa recommended that, owing to the anatomy of primary tooth canals, it would be much easier to perform complete débridement in nonvital primary molars using a pulpotomy technique, with appropriate medicaments.[325] Although there is evidence to support such a concept, the consensus is that the pulpotomy technique should be confined to teeth meeting the selection criteria for vital pulp therapy.[326]

Velling[327] and Droter[328] reported high degrees of success in nonvital primary molars with a coronal pulpotomy only, using formaldehyde-type medicaments in either one- or two-appointment visits. The final dressing in the coronal pulp chamber was usually a modified ZOE cement. Full described complete success in 20 children with chronically abscessed primary molars and draining fistulae in a two-appointment formocresol technique.[329] All of the draining fistulae were reported to be resolved. As an extension of this technique, Meyer and Sayegh used a combination treatment of formocresol in the pulp chamber and curettage of the bifurcation to achieve an 87% clinical success at 5 years postoperatively.[330]

In a survey of members of the American Academy of Pediatric Dentistry, success rates of 72% were reported in nonvital primary molars that had been treated by cleaning only the coronal chamber and placing formocresol versus instrumenting the canals. Both treatments were concluded by filling the respectively cleansed areas with a resorbable medicated cement and placing a stainless steel crown.[331]

Myers et al., in a recent histologic study of failed pulpotomies in primary molars, stated that the development of a furcation lesion has the potential for cystic transformation and the tooth should be extracted.[332] This conclusion also implies that pulpectomy treatment for nonvital primary molars **with furcation lesions** is contraindicated.

Pulpectomy Outcomes

Negative sequelae from endodontically treated primary teeth in the form of accelerated resorption and exfoliation have been a major concern of many clinicians. Starkey felt that delayed eruption of the permanent successors sometimes followed pulpotomy and pulpectomy treatment of primary molars, with some possible deflection in the eruption path.[333] This sequela was not seen in the studies by Barr et al.[309] and Coll et al..[310] Ankylosis of the primary tooth with a root canal filling has also been noted. Erausquin and Devoto have shown that formaldehyde-containing cements frequently caused partial ankylosis at different levels of the periodontal ligament.[334] Coll and Sadrian, in a retrospective study of pulpectomy outcomes, noted two parameters that were the highest predictors of success. **Pretreatment pathologic root resorption,** when evident, resulted in a 44.4% prevalence of enamel defects in underlying permanent teeth after their eruption. In the absence of pretreatment pathologic root resorption, the pulpectomy success rate was 91.7%. The **quality of canal fill relative to the apex** was another outcome determinant, with 86.5% success rates occurring for canals filled short of the apex, 88.9% success for canals filled to the apex, and 57.7% success for canals filled beyond the apex.[335]

SUMMARY

The rationale for pediatric pulp therapy has developed out of extensive clinical studies and improved histologic techniques. Ongoing research will result in modifications that will enhance treatment outcomes.

A successful pediatric endodontic outcome should be based on (1) re-establishment of healthy periodontal tissues; (2) freedom from pathologic root resorption; (3) maintenance of the primary tooth in an infection-free state to hold space for the eruption of its permanent successor; (4) in the case of young permanent teeth, maintenance of the maximum amount of noninflamed portions of pulp tissue to enhance apexogenesis and root dentin formation. With adherence to sound principles in case selection and techniques, pediatric pulp therapy is a major health benefit to the child. The treatment modalities and medicaments that have been

Table 17-2 Pulp Treatment Summary: Current Recommendations

Indirect pulp cap	Permanent teeth, primary teeth—**calcium hydroxide** glass ionomer cement, resin bonding agent
Direct pulp cap	Permanent teeth—**calcium hydroxide**, mineral trioxide aggregate, resin bonding agent (?)
Direct pulp cap	Primary teeth (mechanical exposures only)—**calcium hydroxide**
Pulpotomy	Primary teeth—**diluted and full-strength formocresol**, glutaraldehyde, ferric sulfate (?), controlled energy techniques (?)
Pulpotomy	Permanent teeth (**apexogenesis)—calcium hydroxide**, formocresol (?), glutaraldehyde(?)
Partial pulpectomy	Primary teeth—**zinc oxide–eugenol**, zinc oxide–eugenol + formocresol
Complete pulpectomy	Permanent teeth (**apexification)—calcium hydroxide**
Complete pulpectomy	Primary teeth—**zinc oxide–eugenol, zinc oxide–eugenol + formocresol**, iodoform-containing pastes (?), calcium hydroxide (?)

discussed are summarized in Table 17-2, highlighting the most substantiated and qualifying those that need further confirmation by additional research. The clinician must realize that these recommendations are not absolute and will continue to be modified.

REFERENCES

1. Lewis TM, Law DC. Pulpal treatment of primary teeth. In: Finn SB, editor. Clinical pedodontics. 4th ed. Philadelphia: WB Saunders; 1973.
2. Finn SB. Morphology of the primary teeth. In: Finn SB, editor. Clinical pedodontics. 4th ed. Philadelphia: WB Saunders; 1973.
3. McDonald RE, Avery DR. Treatment of deep caries, vital pulp exposure and pulpless teeth. In: McDonald RE, Avery DR, editors. Dentistry for the child and adolescent. 6th ed. St. Louis: CV Mosby; 1995. p. 428–54.
4. Moss SJ, Addleston H. Histologic study of the pulpal floor of deciduous molars. J Am Dent Assoc 1965;70:372.
5. Rengelstein D, Slow WK. The prevalence of furcation foramina in primary molars. Pediatr Dent 1989;11:198.
6. Wrbas KT, Kielbassa AM, Hellwig E. Microscopic studies of accessory canals in primary molar furcations. J Dent Child 1997;64:118.
7. Greely CB. Pulp therapy for the primary and young permanent dentition. In: Forrester DJ, Wagner ML, Fleming J, editors. Pediatric dental medicine. Philadelphia: Lea & Febiger; 1981. p. 456–60.
8. Seltzer S, Bender IB. The dental pulp—biologic considerations in dental procedures. 3rd ed. Philadelphia: JB Lippincott; 1984.
9. Cox CF, Suzuki S. Re-evaluating pulp protection: calcium hydroxide liners vs. cohesive hybridization. J Am Dent Assoc 1994;125:823.
10. Fox AG, Heeley JD. Histologic study of human primary teeth. Arch Oral Biol 1980;25:103.
11. Massler M. Preventive endodontics: vital pulp therapy. Dent Clin North Am 1967; p.670.
12. Bernick S. Innervation of the teeth and periodontium. Dent Clin North Am 1959; p.503.
13. Rapp R, et al.. The distribution of nerves in human primary teeth. Anat Rec 1967;159:89.
14. Benzer G, Bevelander S. Morphology and incidence of secondary dentin in human teeth. J Am Dent Assoc 1943;30:1075.
15. Ireland RI. Secondary dentin formation in deciduous teeth. J Am Dent Assoc 1941;28:1626.
16. Corbett MD. The incidence of secondary dentin in carious teeth. Br Dent J 1963;114:142.
17. Sayegh FS. Qualitative and quantitative evaluation of new dentin in pulp capped teeth. J Dent Child 1968;35:7.
18. McDonald RE. Diagnostic aids and vital pulp therapy for deciduous teeth. J Am Dent Assoc 1956;53:14.
19. Anderson AW, Sharav Y, Massler M. Reparative dentin formation and pulp morphology. Oral Surg Oral Patts Oral Med 1948;26:837.
20. Frankl SH. Pulp therapy in pedodontics. Oral Surg 1972;34:192.
21. Eidelman E, et al. Pulp pathology in deciduous teeth: clinical and histological correlations. Isr J Med Sci 1968;4:1244.
22. Prophet AS, Miller J. The effect of caries on the deciduous pulp. Br Dent J 1955;99:105.
23. Rayner JA, Southam II. Pulp changes in deciduous teeth associated with deep carious dentin. J Dent 1970;7:39.
24. Taylor B, et al. Response of the pulp and dentine to dental caries in primary molars. J Int Assoc Dent Child 1971;2:3.
25. Damele J. Clinical evaluation of indirect pulp capping: a progress report. J Dent Res 1961;40:756.
26. Belanger G K. Pulp therapy for young permanent teeth. In: Pinkham JR, Cassamassimo PS, Fields HW, et al., editors. Pediatric dentistry—infancy through adolescence. 2nd ed. Philadelphia: WB Saunders; 1988. p. 483–91.
27. Troutman K, et al. Vital pulp therapy: part 1. In: Stewart RE, et al., editors. Pediatric dentistry. St. Louis: CV Mosby; 1982. p. 916.
28. DiMaggio JJ, et al. Histological evaluation of direct and indirect pulp capping [abstract]. J Dent Res 1963.
29. Trowbridge H, Berger J. The clinical management of deep carious lesions. Calif Dent J 1971;47:26.
30. Ishibaski M. A comparison between results of clinical and histo-pathological diagnosis of disease of deciduous tooth pulp. Dent Abstr 1958;3:547.
31. Reynolds RL. The determination of pulp vitality by means of thermal and electrical stimuli. Oral Surg 1966;22:231.
32. Tomes J. A system of dental surgery. London: I. Churchill; 1859.
34. Miller WD. What antiseptics should be used for sterilizing cavities before filling. Dent Cosmos 1891;33:337.
35. Black GV. A work on operative dentistry. Vol 2. Chicago: Medico-Dental Publishing; 1908.
36. Dorfman A, Stephan RM, Muntz JA. In vitro studies of carious dentin. II. Extent of infection in carious lesions. J Am Dent Assoc 1943;30:1901.
37. MacGregor AB, et al. Experimental studies of dental caries. I. The relationship of bacterial invasions to softening of the dentine. Br Dent J 1956;101:203.
38. Fusayama T, et al. Relationship between hardness, discoloration and microbial invasion in carious dentin. J Dent Res 1966;45:1033.
39. Fusayama T. Two layers of carious dentin: diagnosis and treatment. Oper Dent 1979;4:63.
40. Whitehead FI, et al. The relationship of bacterial invasion of softening of the dentin in permanent and deciduous teeth. Br Dent J 1960;108:261.
41. Shovelton DS. A study of deep carious dentin. Int Dent J 1968;18:392.
42. Seltzer S, Bender IB. The dental pulp. Philadelphia: JB Lippincott; 1965. p. 184–98.
43. Reeves R, Stanley HR. The relationship of bacterial penetration and pulpal pathosis in carious teeth. Oral Surg 1966;22:59.
44. Shovelton DS. Studies of dentin and pulp in deep caries. Int Dent J 1970;20:283.
45. Massler M. Op Cit. Ref no. 11.
46. Massler M, Pawlak J. The affected and infected pulp. Oral Surg 1977;43:929.
47. Canby CP, Bernier JL. Bacteriologic studies of carious dentin. J Am Dent Assoc 1936;23:2083.
48. Kuwabara RK, Massler M. Pulpal reactions to active and arrested carious lesions. J Dent Child 1966;33:190.
49. Bradford EW. The dentin, a barrier to caries. Br Dent J 1960;109:387.

50. Young MA, Massler M. Some physical and chemical characteristics of carious dentin. Br Dent J 1963;115:406.
51. Leung RL, et al. Effect of Dycal on bacteria in deep carious lesions. J Am Dent Assoc 1980;10:193.
52. Fairbourn DR, et al. Effect of improved Dycal and IRM on bacteria in deep carious lesions. J Am Dent Assoc 1980;100:547.
53. Law DB, Lewis TM. The effects of calcium hydroxide on deep carious lesions. Colorado Dent J 1964;42:27.
54. Held-Wydler E. Natural (indirect) pulp capping. J Dent Child 1964;31:107.
55. Kerkhove BC, et al. A clinical and television densitometric evaluation of the indirect pulp capping technique. J Dent Child 1967;34:192.
56. Ehrenreich DV. A comparison of the effects of zinc oxide-eugenol and calcium hydroxide in carious dentin in human primary molars. J Dent Child 1968;35:451.
57. Stanley HR. Pulpal response to dental techniques and materials. Dent Clin North Am 1971;15:115.
58. Torstenson B, et al. Pulp reaction to IRM [abstract]. J Dent Res 1982;61:573.
59. Nordstrom DO, et al. Use of stannous fluoride for indirect pulp capping. J Am Dent Assoc 1974;88:997.
60. King J, et al. Indirect pulp capping: a bacteriologic study of deep carious dentin in human teeth. Oral Surg 1965;20:663.
61. Aponte AJ, Hartsook JT, Crowley MC. Indirect pulp capping verified. J Dent Child 1966;33:164.
62. Parikh SR, Massler M, Bahn A. Microorganisms in active and arrested carious lesions of dentin. N Y State Dent J 1963;29:347.
63. Eidelman E, et al. Remineralization of carious dentin treated with calcium hydroxide. J Dent Child 1965;32:218.
64. Mjör IA, et al. The effect of calcium hydroxide and amalgam on noncarious vital dentin. Arch Oral Biol 1961;3:283.
65. Sawusch RH. Direct and indirect pulp capping with two new products. J Am Dent Assoc 1982;104:459.
66. Nirschl R, Avery D. Evaluation of a new pulp capping agent in indirect pulp therapy. J Dent Child 1983;50:25.
67. Coll JA, et al. An evaluation of pulp therapy in primary incisors. Pediatr Dent 1988;10:178.
68. Schroder A. Indirect capping and the treatment of deep carious lesions. Int Dent J 1968;18:381.
69. Primosch RE, Glomb TA, Jerrell RG. Primary tooth pulp therapy as taught in predoctoral pediatric dental programs in the United States. Pediatr Dent 1997;19:118–22.
70. Lado EA, Stanley HR. An in vitro study of bacterial inhibition by VLC calcium hydroxide pulp cap compounds. Pediatr Dent 1987;9:292.
71. Jordan RE, Suzuki M. Conservative treatment of deep carious lesions. Can Dent Assoc J 1971;37:337.
72. Fuks AB. Pulp therapy for the primary dentition. In: Pinkham JR, Cassamassimo PS, Fields HW, et al., editors. Pediatric dentistry—infancy through adolescence. 2nd ed. WB Saunders; 1988. p. 326–38.
73. Langeland K. Capping exposed pulpal tissue. Dent Clin North Am 1974;2:1.
74. Stanley HR. Criteria for standardizing and increasing credibility of direct pulp capping studies. Am. J Dent 1998;11:S17.
75. Frigoletto RT. Pulp therapy in pedodontics. J Am Dent Assoc 1973;86:1344.
76. Tronstad L, Mjör I.A. Capping of the inflamed pulp. Oral Surg 1972;34:477.
77. Cox CF, Bergenholtz G. Healing sequence in capping inflamed dental pulps of rhesus monkeys. Int Endod J 1986;19:113.
78. Heide S, Kerekes K. Delayed direct pulp capping in permanent incisors of monkeys. Int Endod J 1987;20:65.
79. Cotton WR. Bacterial contamination as a factor in healing of pulp exposures. Oral Surg 1974;38:441.
80. Glass RL, Zander HA. Pulp healing. J Dent Res 1949;28:97.
81. Lim KC, Kirk EE. Direct pulp capping: a review. Endod Dent Traumatol 1987;3:213.
82. Stanley HR, Lundy T. Dycal therapy for pulp exposures. Oral Surg 1972;34:818.
83. Weiss MD, Bjorvatn K. Pulp capping in deciduous and newly erupted permanent teeth of monkeys. Oral Surg 1970;29:769.
84. Kakehashi S, Stanley HR, Fitzgerald R J. The effects of surgical exposures of the dental pulp in germ free and conventional laboratory rats. Oral Surg 1965;20:340.
85. Langeland K, et al. Human pulp changes of iatrogenic origin. Oral Surg 1971;32:943.
86. Cox CF, Subay RK, Ostro E, et al. Tunnel defects in dentin bridges: their formation following direct pulp capping. Oper Dent 1996;21:4.
87. Baume L, Holz J. Long-term clinical assessment of direct pulp capping. Int Dent J 1981;31:251.
88. Kennedy DB, Kapala JT. The dental pulp: biologic considerations of protection and treatment. In: Braham RL, Morris ME, editors. Textbook of pediatric dentistry. 2nd ed. Baltimore: Williams and Wilkins; 1985. p. 492–522.
89. Mathewson RJ, Primosch R. Pulp treatment. In: Fundamentals of pediatric dentistry. 3rd ed. Chicago: Quintessence; 1995. p. 257–84.
90. Camp J. Pulp therapy for primary and young permanent teeth. Dent Clin North Am 1984;28:651.
91. Starkey PE. Treatment of pulpally involved primary molars. In: McDonald RE, et al., editors. Current therapy in dentistry. Vol VII. St. Louis: CV Mosby; 1980.
92. Weine DM. The effect of calcium hydroxide in direct pulp capping in primary teeth [thesis]. Ann Arbor [MA]: Univ. of Michigan School of Dentistry; 1963.
93. Jeppersen K. Direct pulp capping on primary teeth—a long-term investigation. Int Assoc Dent Child 1971;12:10.
94. Jerrell RG, Courts FK, Stanley HR. A comparison of two calcium hydroxide agents in direct pulp capping of primary teeth. J Dent Child 1984;51:34.
95. Kalins V, Frisbee HE. The effect of dentine fragments on the healing of the exposed pulp. Arch Oral Biol 1960;2:96.
96. Schröder U, et al. A one-year follow-up of partial pulpotomy and calcium hydroxide capping in primary molars. Endod Dent Traumatol 1987;3:304.
97. Arnold DS. The use of formocresol as a pulp capping agent in human primary teeth [thesis]. Lincoln, NE: Univ. of Nebraska School of Dentistry; 1970.
98. Cvek M. A clinical report on partial pulpotomy and capping with calcium hydroxide in permanent incisors with complicated crown fracture. J Endod 1978;4:232.
99. Zilberman U, et al. Partial pulpotomy in carious permanent molars. Am J Dent 1989;2:147.
100. Mejare I, Cvek M. Partial pulpotomy in young permanent teeth with deep carious lesions. Endod Dent Traumatol 1993;9:238.
101. Fuks AB, Chosack A, Klein H, Eidelman E. Partial pulpotomy as a treatment alternative for exposed pulps in crown-fractured permanent incisors. Endod Dent Traumatol 1987;3:100.

102. Watts A, Paterson RC. Bacterial contamination as a factor influencing the toxicity of materials to the exposed pulp. Oral Surg 1987;64:466.
103. Cox CF. Pulp capping of dental pulp mechanically exposed to oral microflora: a 1-2 year observation of wound healing in the monkey. J Oral Pathol 1985;14:156.
104. Cox CF, et al. Biocompatibility of surface sealed dental materials against exposed pulps. J Prosthet Dent 1987;57:1.
105. Nyborg H. Capping of the pulp. The processes involved and their outcome. Odontol Tidskr 1958;66:296.
106. Phaneuf RA, Frankl S, Reuben M. A comparative histological evaluation of three calcium hydroxide preparations on human primary dental pulp. J Dent Child 1968;35:61.
107. Vermeersch AC. Pulp conservation. Oper Dent 1977;2:105.
108. Joos RW. Calcium hydroxide as a pulp capping agent. Northwest Dent 1974;53:362.
109. Tamburic SD, Vuleta GM, Ognjanovic JM. In vitro release of calcium and hydroxyl ions from two types of calcium hydroxide preparations. Int Endod J 1993;26:125.
110. Yoshiba K, Yoshiba N, Nakamura H, et al., editors. Immunolocalization of fibronectin during reparative dentinogenesis in human teeth after pulp capping with calcium hydroxide. J Dent Res 1996;75:1590.
111. Fisher FJ. The effect of a calcium hydroxide/water paste on micro-organisms in carious dentine. Br Dent J 1972;143:231.
112. Lado EA. In vitro antimicrobial activity of six pulp capping agents. Oral Surg 1986;61:197.
113. Estrela C, Fabiana CP, Yoto I, Bammann LL. In vitro determination of direct antimicrobial effect of calcium hydroxide. JOE 1998;24:15.
114. Sciaky I, Pisanti S. Localization of calcium placed over amputated pulps in dogs teeth. J Dent Res 1960;39:1128.
115. Attalla MN, Noujaim AA. Role of calcium hydroxide in the formation of reparative dentin. Can Dent Assoc J 1969;35:267.
116. Stark MM, et al. The localization of radioactive $Ca(OH)_2$ (Ca45) over exposed pulps in rhesus monkey teeth: a preliminary report. J Oral Ther Pharmacol 1964;3:290.
117. Holland R, et al. Histochemical analysis of the dog's dental pulp after pulp capping with calcium, barium, and strontium hydroxides. JOE 1982;8:444.
118. Turner C, Courts FJ, Stanley HR. A histological comparison of direct pulp capping agents in primary canines. J Dent Child 1987;54:423.
119. Tronstad L. Reaction of the exposed pulp to Dycal treatment. Oral Surg 1974;38:945.
120. Drahein R, Murrey A. Compressive strength of two calcium hydroxide bases. J Prosthet Dent 1985;54:365.
121. Fuks AB, et al. Clinical and radiographic assessment of direct pulp capping and pulpotomy in young permanent teeth. Pediatr Dent 1982;4:240.
122. Stanley HR, Pameijer CH. Pulp capping with a new visible-light-curing calcium hydroxide composition. Oper Dent 1985;10:156.
123. Seale NS, Stanley HR. Pulpal response to a new visible light cured composite calcium hydroxide pulp capping agent in human premolars. Pediatr Dent 1988;10:239.
124. Howerton B, Cox CF. Pulpal biocompatibility of two photo-cured $Ca(OH)_2$ containing materials [abstract]. JOE 1987;13:129.
125. Hembree JH, Andrews IT. Zinc oxide as a pulp capping agent. Miss Dent J 1974;30:10.
126. Watts A. Zinc oxide as a pulp capping agent [abstract]. J Dent Res 1977;56:D104.
127. Holland R, et al. The influence of the sealing material in the healing process of inflamed pulps capped with calcium hydroxide or zinc oxide-eugenol cement. Acta Odontol Pediatr 1981;2:5.
128. Sveen OB. Pulp capping of primary teeth with zinc oxide-eugenol. Odontol Tidskr 1969;77:427.
129. Brosch JW. Capping pulps with a compound of calcium phosphate, neomycin and hydrocortisone. J Dent Child 1966;33:42.
130. Soldali GD. Pulp capping with antibiotics. Fla Dent J 1975;46:18.
131. Bhaskar SH, et al. Tissue response to cortisone-containing and cortisone-free calcium hydroxide. J Dent Child 1969;36:1.
132. Ulmansky M, Sela J. Response of pulpotomy wounds in normal human teeth to successively applied Ledermix and Calxyl. Arch Oral Biol 1971;16:1393.
133. Haskell EW, et al. Direct pulp capping treatment: a long-term follow-up. J Am Dent Assoc 1978;97:607.
134. McWalter G, et al. Long-term study of pulp capping in monkeys with three agents. J Am Dent Assoc 1976;933:105.
135. Watts A, Paterson RC. The response of the mechanically exposed pulp to prednisolone and triamcinolone acetonide. Int Endod J 1988;21:9.
136. Gardner DE, Mitchell DF, McDonald RE. Treatment of pulps of monkeys with vancomycin and calcium hydroxide. JDR 1971;50:1273.
137. Negm M, et al. Clinical and histologic study of human pulpal response to new cements containing calcium hydroxide. Oral Surg 1980;50:462.
138. Bhaskar SH, et al. Human pulp capping with isobutylcyanoacrylate. J Dent Res 1972;51:50.
139. Heys DR, Cox CF, Avery JK. Histological considerations of direct pulp capping agents. J Dent Res 1981;68:1371.
140. Subay RK, Asci S. Human pulpal response to hydroxyapatite and a calcium hydroxide material as direct capping agents. Oral Surg 1993;76:485.
141. Dick HM, Carmichael DJ. Reconstituted antigen poor collagen preparations as potential pulp capping agents. JOE 1980;6:641.
142. Fuks AB, et al. Enriched collagen solution as a pulp dressing in pulpotomized teeth in monkeys. Pediatr Dent 1984;6:243.
143. Ibrahim SM, Mitchell DF, Healy HG. A histopathologic study of the effects of formocresol in pulp capping of permanent teeth. Egypt Dent J 1970;16:219.
144. Garcia-Godoy F. Direct pulp capping and partial pulpotomy with diluted formocresol in primary molars. Acta Odontol Pediatr 1984;5:57.
145. Bergenholtz G, et al. Bacterial leakage around dental restorations: its effect on the dental pulp. J Oral Pathol 1982;11:439.
146. Cox CF. Evaluation and treatment of bacterial microleakage. Am J Dent 1994;7:293–5.
147. Snuggs HM, Cox CF, Powell CS, White KC. Pulpal healing and dentinal bridge formation in an acidic environment. Quintessence Int 1993;24:501.
148. Barnes IE, Kidd EAM. Disappearing Dycal. Br Dent J 1980;111:147.
149. Cox CF. Effects of adhesive resins and various dental cements on the pulp. Oper Dent 1992;55:165.

150. Kanca J III. Bonding to tooth structure—a rationale for a clinical protocol. J Esthet Dent 1989;1:135–8.
151. Miyakoshi S, et al. Interfacial interaction of 4-META-MMA-TBB resin and the pulp [abstract]. J Dent Res 1993;72:220.
152. Cox CF, et al. Pulp response following in vivo etching and 4-META bonding. J Dent Res 1993;72:213.
153. Cox CF, White KC. Biocompatibility of amalgam on exposed pulps employing a biological seal [abstract]. J Dent Res 1992;71:187.
154. Tsuneda Y, Hayakawa T, Yamamoto H, et al. A histopathological study of direct pulp capping with adhesive resins. Oper Dent 1995;20:223.
155. Kashiwada T, Takagi M. New restoration and direct pulp capping systems using adhesive composite resin. Bull Tokyo Med Dent Univ 1991;38:45.
156. Heitman T, Unterbrink G. Direct pulp capping with a dentinal adhesive resin system—a pilot study. Quintessence Int 1995;26:765.
157. Bazzuchi M, et al. Pulp response to direct capping of adhesive resins and glass ionomer cements [abstract]. J Dent Res 1995;74:555.
158. Kanca J III. Replacement of a fractured incisor fragment over pulpal exposure: a long-term case report. Quintessence Int 1996;27:829.
159. Stanley HR. Pulpal consideration of adhesive materials. Oper Dent 1992;55:151.
160. Pameijer CH, Stanley HR. The disastrous effects of the "total etch" technique in vital pulp capping in primates. Am J Dent 1998;11:S45.
161. Araujo FB, Barata JS, Costa CAS, Garcia-Godoy F. Clinical, radiographical and histological evaluation of direct capping with a resin adhesive in primary teeth [abstract]. J Dent Res 1996;75:280.
162. Gwinnett AJ, Tay FR. Early and intermediate time response of the dental pulp to an acid etch technique in vivo. Am J Dent 1998;11:S35.
163. Kopel HM. The pulp capping procedure in primary teeth "revisited." J Dent Child 1997;64:327.
164. Cox CF, et al. Biocompatibility of various dental materials: pulp healing with a surface seal. Int J Periodont Rest Dent 1996;16:241.
165. Stanley HR, Pameijer CH. Dentistry's friend—calcium hydroxide. Oper Dent 1997; 22:1.
166. Katoh Y, et al. Direct capping effects on exposed pulp of macaca fascicularis [abstract]. J Dent Res 1996;75:34.
167. Katoh Y, Kimura T, Inaba T. Clinical prognosis of pulp tissue direct-capping with adhesive resins [abstract]. J Dent Res 1997;76:162.
168. Torabinejad M, et al. Physical and chemical properties of a new root-end filling material. JOE 1995;21:349.
169. Pitt Ford TR, Torabinejad M, Abedi HR, et al. Using mineral trioxide aggregate as a pulp capping material. J Am Dent Assoc 1996;127:1491.
170. Chaung HM, et al. Comparison of calcium phosphate cement mixture and pure calcium hydroxide as direct pulp-capping agents. J Formos Med Assoc 1996;95:545.
171. Yoshimine Y, Maeda K. Histologic evaluation of tetracalcium phosphate-based cement as a direct pulp-capping agent. Oral Surg Oral Med Oral Pathol Oral Radiol Endod 1995;79:351.
172. Dannenberg JL. Pedodontic endodontics. Dent Clin North Am 1974;18:367.
173. Mejare I. Pulpotomy of primary molars with coronal or total pulpitis using formocresol technique. Scand J Dent Res 1979;87:208.
174. Ranly DM. Pulpotomy therapy in primary teeth: new modalities for old rationales. Pediatr Dent 1994;16:403.
175. Berger JE. A review of the erroneously labeled "mummification" techniques of pulp therapy. Oral Surg 1972;34:131.
176. Urist M. Bone formation by autoinduction. Science 1965;150:893.
177. Nakashima M. Induction of dentin formation on canine amputated pulp by recombinant human bone morphogenetic proteins (BMP)-2 and -4. J Dent Res 1994;73:1515.
178. Fadhavi S, Anderson AW. A comparison of the pulpal response to freeze-dried bone, calcium hydroxide, and zinc oxide-eugenol in primary teeth in two cynomolgus monkeys. Pediatr Dent 1996;18:52.
179. Buckley JP. The chemistry of pulp decomposition with a rational treatment for this condition and its sequelae. J Am Dent Assoc 1904;3:764.
180. Sweet CA. Procedure for treatment of exposed and pulpless deciduous teeth. J Am Dent Assoc 1930;17:1150.
181. Sweet CA. Treatment of vital primary teeth with pulpal involvement—therapeutic pulpotomy. Colorado State Dent Assoc J 1955;33:10.
182. Doyle WA, McDonald RE, Mitchell DF. Formocresol versus calcium hydroxide in pulpotomy. J Dent Child 1962;29:86.
183. Massler M, Mansukhani H. Effects of formocresol on the dental pulp. J Dent Child 1959;26:277.
184. Emmerson CC, Miyamoto O, Sweet CA Sr, Bhatia HD. Pulpal changes following formocresol applications on rat molars and human primary teeth. South Calif Dent Assoc J 1959;27:309.
185. Spedding RH, Mitchell DF, McDonald RE. Formocresol and calcium hydroxide therapy. J Dent Res 1965;44:1023.
186. Law DB, Lewis TM. Formocresol pulpotomy in deciduous teeth. J Am Dent Assoc 1964;69:601.
187. Berger J. Pulp tissue reaction from formocresol and zinc oxide and eugenol. J Dent Child 1965;32:13.
188. Spamer RG. The formocresol pulpotomy: a histological study of a single application of formocresol on the dental pulp of human primary teeth [thesis]. Seattle (WA): Univ. of Washington School of Dentistry; 1965.
189. Rolling I, Thylstrup A. A three-year clinical follow up study of pulpotomized primary molars treated with the formocresol technique. Scand J Dent Res 1975;83:47.
190. Rolling I, Hasselgren G, Tronstad L. Morphologic and enzyme histochemical observations on the pulp of human primary molars 3 to 5 years after formocresol condition. Oral Surg 1976;42:518.
191. Rolling I, Lambjerg-Hansen H. Pulp condition of successfully formocresol-treated primary molars. Scand J Dent Res 1978;86:267.
192. Magnusson BO. Pulpotomy in primary molars: long-term clinical and histological evaluation. Int Dent J 1980;13:143.
193. Ranly DM, Lazzari EP. The formocresol pulpotomy: the past, the present and the future. J Pedod 1978;3:115.
194. Beaver HA, Kopel HM, Sabes WR. The effect of zinc oxide-eugenol cement on a formocresolized pulp. J Dent Child 1966;33:381.
195. Garcia-Godoy F. Penetration and pulpal response by two concentrations of formocresol using two methods of application. J Pedod 1981;5:102.

196. Hicks JH, et al. Formocresol pulpotomies in primary molars: a radiographic study in a pediatric dentistry practice. J. Pedod 1986;10:331.
197. Ranly DM, Pope HO. An in vitro comparison of the release of ^{3}H-formaldehyde and ^{14}C-p-cresol from zinc oxide eugenol cement. Pharm Ther Dent 1979;4:53.
198. Venham LJ. Pulpal responses to variations on the formocresol pulpotomy technique [thesis]. Columbus, OH: Ohio State Univ. College of Dentistry; 1967.
199. Straffon LH, Han SS. The effect of formocresol on hamster connective tissue cells: a histologic and quantitative radioautographic study with proline H3. Arch Oral Biol 1968;13:271.
200. Straffon LH, Han S S. Effects of varying concentrations of formocresol on RNA synthesis of connective tissue in sponge implants. Oral Surg 1970;29:915.
201. Loos PJ, Straffon LH, Han SS. Biological effects of formocresol. J Dent Child 1973;40:193.
202. Morawa AP, et al. Clinical evaluation of pulpotomies using dilute formocresol. J Dent Child 1975;45:28.
203. Fuks A, Bimstein E. Clinical evaluation of diluted formocresol pulpotomies in the primary teeth of school children. Pediatr Dent 1981;3:321.
204. Fuks A, et al. A radiographic and histologic evaluation of the effect of two concentrations of formocresol on pulpotomized primary and young permanent teeth in monkeys. Pediatr Dent 1983;5:9.
205. Wright FA, Widmer RP. Pulpal therapy in primary molar teeth: a retrospective study. J Pedod 1979;3:195.
206. Willard RM. Radiographic changes following formocresol pulpotomies in primary molars. J Dent Child 1976;43:34.
207. Garcia-Godoy F. Radiographic evaluation of root canal "calcification" following formocresol pulpotomy. J Dent Child 1983;50:430.
208. Koch G, Nyborg H. Correlation between clinical and histologic indications for pulpotomy of deciduous teeth. J Int Assoc Dent Child 1970;1:3.
209. Mejare I. Pulpotomy of primary molars with coronal or total pulpitis using formocresol technique. Scand J Dent Res 1979;87:208.
210. Garcia-Godoy F, et al. Pulpal response to different application times of formocresol. J Pedod 1982;6:176.
211. Miyamoto O. Current status of pulpal therapy on primary and young permanent teeth. J Acad Dent Handicapped 1974;1:27.
212. Verco PJ, Allen KR. Formocresol pulpotomies in primary teeth. J Int A Dent Child 1984;15:51.
213. Avram DC, Pulver F. Pulpotomy medicaments for vital primary teeth. J Dent Child 1989;56:426.
214. Ibrahim SM, et al. A histopathological study of the effects of formocresol in pulp capping of permanent teeth. Egypt Dent J 1970;16:219.
215. Trask PA. Formocresol pulpotomy in young permanent teeth. J Am Dent Assoc 1972;85:1316.
216. Myers DA. Effects of formocresol on pulps of cariously exposed permanent molars [thesis]. Memphis, TN: University of Tennessee School of Dentistry; 1972.
217. Armstrong RL, et al. Comparison of Dycal and formocresol pulpotomies in young permanent teeth in monkeys. Oral Surg 1979;48:160.
218. Fiskio HM. Pulpotomies in vital and non-vital permanent teeth. Gen Dent 1974;22:27.
219. Spedding RH. Formocresol pulpotomies for permanent teeth. In: Goldman HM, et al., editors. Current therapy in dentistry. Vol 5. St. Louis: CV Mosby; 1975.
220. Rothman MS. Formocresol pulpotomy: a practical procedure for permanent teeth. Gen Dent 1977;25:29.
221. Schwartz EA. Formocresol vital pulpotomy on permanent dentition. Can Dent Assoc J 1980;46:570.
222. Muniz MA, et al. The formocresol technique in young permanent teeth. Oral Surg 1983;55:611.
223. Akbar A. A five year clinical study of formocresol treatment in 120 cases of pulpotomy in permanent molars. J Pedod 1987;11:242.
224. Nishino PK. Apical histologic response to formocresol pulpotomy. Chron Omaha Dent Soc 1974;37:242.
225. Teuscher GW, Zander HA. A preliminary report on pulpotomy. Northwest Univ Grad Bull 1938;39:4.
226. Ulmansky M, et al. Scanning electron microscopy of calcium hydroxide induced bridges. J Oral Pathol 1972;1:244.
227. Goldberg F, et al. Evaluation of the dentinal bridge after pulpotomy and calcium hydroxide dressing. JOE 1984;10:318.
228. Berk H. Effects of calcium hydroxide methyl-cellulose paste on the dental pulp. J Dent Child 1950;17:65.
229. Brown WE Jr. The vital pulpotomy technique for the management of vital exposed pulps in primary and young permanent teeth. Univ Mich Alumni Bull 1947;48:14.
230. Via WR Jr. Evaluation of deciduous molars treated by pulpotomy and calcium hydroxide. J Am Dent Assoc 1955; 50:34.
231. Law DB. An evaluation of the vital pulpotomy technique. J Dent Child 1956;23:40.
232. Schröder U, Granath LE. On internal dentin resorption in deciduous molars treated by pulpotomy and capped with calcium hydroxide. Odontol Revy 1971;22:179.
233. Schröder U. A 2-year follow-up of primary molars, pulpotomized with a gentle technique and capped with calcium hydroxide. Scand J Dent Res 1978;86:273.
234. Berk H, Krakow A. A comparison of the management of pulpal pathosis in primary and permanent teeth. Oral Surg 1952;34:944.
235. Berson RB, Good D. Pulpotomy and pulpectomy for primary teeth. In: Stewart RL, et al. editors. Pediatric dentistry: scientific foundation and clinical practice. St. Louis: CV Mosby; 1982. p. 917–26.
236. Patterson SS. Pulp calcification due to operative procedures—pulpotomy. Int Dent J 1967;17:490.
237. Bimstein CD, et al. Histologic evaluation of the effect of different cutting techniques on pulpotomized teeth. Am J Dent 1989;2:151.
238. Pashley EL, et al. Systemic distribution of ^{14}C-formaldehyde from formocresol-treated pulpotomy sites. J Dent Res 1980;59:603.
239. Myers DR, et al. Tissue changes induced by the absorption of formocresol from pulpotomy sites in dogs. Pediatr Dent 1983;5:6.
240. Ranly DM. Formocresol toxicity: current knowledge. Acta Odontol Pediatr 1984;5:93.
241. Ranly DM, Horn D. Assessment of the systemic distribution and toxicity of formaldehyde following pulpotomy treatment. Part Two. J Dent Child 1987;54:404.
242. Messer LB, et al. Long-term effects of primary molar pulpotomies on succedaneous bicuspids. J Dent Res 1980;59:116.

243. Rollings I, Paulsen S. Formocresol pulpotomy of primary teeth and occurrence of enamel defects of permanent successors. Acta Odontol Scand 1978;36:243.

244. Mulder GR, et al. Consequences of endodontic treatment of primary teeth. Part II. A clinical investigation into the influence of formocresol pulpotomy on the permanent successor. J Dent Child 1987;54:35.

245. American Academy of Pediatric Dentistry. Use of formocresol in pedodontics: a committee report. Chicago: 1984.

246. Sadler ES, Frankl S, Ruben MP. The histological response of the dental pulp to Cresatin. J Dent Child 1971;38:49.

247. Nevins AJ, et al. Pulpotomy and partial pulpectomy procedures in monkey teeth using cross-linked collagen-calcium phosphate gel. Oral Surg 1980;49:360.

248. 's-Gravenmade E J. Some biochemical considerations in endodontics. JOE 1975;1:233.

249. Hill SD, et al. Comparison of antimicrobial and cytotoxic effects of glutaraldehyde and formocresol. Oral Surg 1991;71:89.

250. Wernes JC, 's-Gravenmade EJ. Glutaraldehyde: a new fixative in endodontics [abstract]. JDR 1973;52:601.

251. Dankert J, et al. Diffusion of formocresol and glutaraldehyde through dentin and cementum. JOE 1976;2:42.

252. Kopel HM, Bernick S, Zachrisson E. The effects of glutaraldehyde on primary pulp tissue following coronal amputation: an in vivo histologic study. J Dent Child 1980;47:425.

253. Dilly G, Courts FJ. Immunological response to four pulpal medicaments. Pediatr Dent 1981;3:179.

254. Lekka M, et al. Comparison between formaldehyde and glutaraldehyde diffusion through root tissues of pulpotomy treated teeth. J Pedod 1984;8:185.

255. Garcia-Godoy F. A 42 month clinical evaluation of glutaraldehyde pulpotomies in primary teeth. J Pedod 1986;10:148.

256. Fuks A, Bernstein E, Klein H. Assessment of a 2% buffered glutaraldehyde solution in pulpotomized primary teeth of children: a preliminary report. J Pedod 1986;10:323.

257. Alacam A. Pulpal tissue changes following pulpotomies with formocresol, glutaraldehyde-calcium hydroxide, glutaraldehyde-zinc oxide eugenol pastes in primary teeth. J Pedod 1989;13:123.

258. Davis M, et al. An alternative to formocresol for vital pulpotomy. J Dent Child 1982;49:176.

259. Fuks AB, et al. Glutaraldehyde as a pulp dressing after pulpotomy in primary teeth of baboon monkeys. Pediatr Dent 1986;8:32.

260. Lloyd JM, et al. The effects of various concentrations and lengths of application of glutaraldehyde on monkey pulp tissue. Pediatr Dent 1988;10:115.

261. Ranly DM, Garcia-Godoy F, et al. Time, concentration and pH parameters for the use of glutaraldehyde as a pulpotomy agent: an in vitro study. Pediatr Dent 1987;9:199.

262. Garcia-Godoy F, Ranly DM. Clinical evaluation of pulpotomies with ZOE as the vehicle for glutaraldehyde. Pediatr Dent 1987;9:144.

263. Hernandez JRP, et al. Evaluaion clinica y radiografica de pulpotomies on formocresol o glutaraldehydo en dientes phmonentes [abstract]. Acta Odontol Pediatr 1987;8:59.

264. Myers DR, et al. Systemic absorption of ^{14}C-glutaraldehyde from glutaraldehyde-treated pulpotomy sites. Pediatr Dent 1986;8:134.

265. Ranly DB, et al. Assessment of the systemic distribution and toxicity of glutaraldehyde as a pulpotomy agent. Pediatr Dent 1989;11:8.

266. Kouri EM, Matthews JL, Taylor PP. Epinephrine in pulpotomy. J Dent Child 1969;36:123

267. Helig J, Yates J, Siskin M, et al. Calcium hydroxide pulpotomy for primary teeth: a clinical study. J Am Dent Assoc 1984;108:775–8.

268. Landau M, Johnson D. Pulpal responses to ferric sulfate in monkeys [abstract]. J Dent Res 1988;67:215.

269. Fei AL, Udin RD, Johnson R. A clinical study of ferric sulfate as a pulpotomy agent in primary teeth. Pediatr Dent 1991;13:327.

270. Fuks AB, Holan G, Davis JM, Eidelman E. Ferric sulfate versus dilute formocresol in pulpotomized primary molars: long-term follow-up. Pediatr Dent 1997;19:327.

271. Fuks AB, Eidelman E, Cleaton-Jones P, Michaeli Y. Pulp response to ferric sulfate, diluted formocresol, and IRM in pulpotomized primary baboon teeth. J Dent Child 1997;64:254–9.

272. Abedi HR, Ingle JI. Mineral trioxide aggregate: a review of a new cement. Calif Dent Assoc J 1995;23:36.

273. Higashi T, Okamoto H. Influence of particle size of calcium phosphate ceramics as a capping agent on the formation of a hard tissue barrier in amputated pulp. J Endod 1996;22:281.

274. Yoshiba K, Yoshiba N, Iwaku M. Histological observations of hard tissue barrier formation in amputated dental pulp capped with alpha-tricalcium phosphate containing calcium hydroxide. Endod Dent Traumatol 1994;10:113.

275. Ruemping DR, et al. Electrosurgical pulpotomy in primates—a comparison with formocresol. Pediatr Dent 1983;5:14.

276. Shaw DW, Sheller B, Barrus BD, Morton TH Jr. Electrosurgical pulpotomy—a 6-month study in primates. JOE 1987;13:500.

277. Shulman ER, et al. Comparison of electrosurgery and formocresol as pulpotomy techniques in monkey primary teeth. Pediatr Dent 1987;9:189.

278. Sheller B, Morton TH. Electrosurgical pulpotomy: a pilot study in humans. JOE 1987;13:69.

279. Mack RB, Dean JA. Electrosurgical pulpotomy: a retrospective human study. J Dent Child 1993;60:107.

280. Fishman SA, Udin RD, Good DL, Rodef F. Success of electrofulguration pulpotomies covered by zinc oxide-eugenol or calcium hydroxide: a clinical study. Pediatr Dent 1996;18:385.

281. Adrian JC. Pulp effect of neodymium laser. Oral Surg Oral Med Oral Pathol Oral Radiol Endod 1977;44:301.

282. Shoji S, Nakamura M, Horiuchi H. Histopathological changes in dental pulps irradiated by CO_2 laser: a preliminary report on laser pulpotomy. JOE 1985;11:379.

283. Kato J, Hashimoto M, Ono H. Pulp reactions after pulpotomy with Nd:YAG laser irradiation [abstract]. J Dent Res 1991;70:384.

284. McGuire S, et al. Comparison of Nd:YAG laser with formocresol in permanent tooth pulpotomies in dogs [abstract]. J Dent Res 1995;74:160.

285. Hibbard ED, Ireland RL. Morphology of the root canals of the primary molar teeth. J Dent Child 1957;24:250.

286. Barker BC, et al. Anatomy of root canals. IV. Deciduous teeth. Austr Dent J 1975;20:101.

287. Hartsook JT. Pulpal therapy in primary and young permanent teeth. Dent Clin North Am 1966; p.385.

288. Hallett GE. Endodontic treatment and conservation of temporary teeth. Int Dent J 1968;18:520.

289. Matsumiya S. Experimental pathological study on the effect of treatment of infected root canals in the deciduous tooth on growth of the permanent tooth germ. Int Dent J 1968;18:546.
290. Valdenhaug J. Periradicular inflammation in primary teeth and its effect on the permanent successors. Int J Oral Surg 1974;3:171.
291. Brook AH, Winter GB. Developmental arrest of permanent tooth germs following pulpal infection of deciduous teeth. Br Dent J 1975;139:9.
292. Marsh SJ, Largent MD. A bacteriological study of the pulp canals of infected primary molars. J Dent Child 1967;34:460.
293. O'Riordan MW, Coll J. Pulpectomy procedure for deciduous teeth with severe pulpal necrosis. J Am Dent Assoc 1979;99:480.
294. Tagger E, Sarnat H. Root canal therapy of infected primary teeth. Acta Odontol Pediatr 1984;5:63.
295. Camp JH. Pedodontic-endodontic treatment. In: Cohen S, Burns RC, editors. Pathways of the pulp. St. Louis: CV Mosby; 1987. p. 685–722.
296. Rifkin A. A simple, effective safe technique for the root canal treatment of abscessed primary teeth. J Dent Child 1980;47:435.
297. Rabinowitz BZ. Pulp management of primary teeth. Oral Surg 1953; 6:542.
298. Rabinowitz BZ. Pulp management of primary teeth. Oral Surg 1953;6:671.
299. Hobson P. Pulp treatment of deciduous teeth. Br Dent J 1970;128:275.
300. Judd P, Kenny D. Non-aldehyde pulpectomy technique for primary teeth. Ontario Dentist 1991;68:25.
301. Gould JM. Root canal therapy for infected primary molar teeth - preliminary report. J Dent Child 1970;34:23.
302. Cullen CL. Endodontic therapy of deciduous teeth. Compend Contin Educ 1983;4:302.
303. Dugal MS, Curgon ME. Restoration of the broken down primary molar: 1. Pulpectomy technique. Dent Update 1989;16:26.
304. Goerig AC, Camp JH. Root canal treatment in primary teeth: a review. Pediatr Dent 1983;5:33.
305. Kopel HM. Root canal therapy for primary teeth. Mich Dent Assoc J 1970;52:28.
306. Spedding R. Endodontic treatment of primary molars. In: Goldman HM, et al., editors. Current therapy in dentistry. St. Louis: CV Mosby; 1977. p. 558–69.
307. Coll JA, Josell S, Casper JS. Evaluation of a one appointment formocresol pulpectomy technique for primary molars. Pediatr Dent 1985;7:123.
308. Vander Wall GL, et al. Endodontic medicaments. Oral Surg 1972;25:238.
309. Barr ES, et al. Radiographic evaluation of primary molar pulpectomies in a pediatric dental practice [abstract]. Pediatr Dent 1986;8:180.
310. Coll JA, et al. An evaluation of pulpal therapy in primary incisors. Pediatr Dent 1988;10:178.
311. Flaitz CM, et al. Radiographic evaluation of pulpal therapy for primary anterior teeth. J Dent Child 1989;56:182.
312. Yacobi R, et al. Evolving primary pulp therapy techniques. J Am Dent Assoc 1991;122:83.
313. Payne RG, Kenny DJ, Johnston DH, Judd PL. Two year outcome study of zinc oxide-eugenol root canal treatment for vital primary teeth. J Can Dent Assoc 1993;59:1.
314. Hendry J, Jeansonne BG, Dummett CO Jr, Burrell W. Comparison of calcium hydroxide and zinc oxide and eugenol pulpectomies in primary teeth of dogs. Oral Surg Oral Med Oral Pathol Oral Radiol Endod 1982;54:445.
315. Barker BC, Lockett BC. Endodontic experiments with resorbable paste. Aust Dent J 1971;16:364.
316. Rifkin A. The root canal treatment of abscessed primary teeth: a 3-4 year follow-up. J Dent Child 1982;49:428.
317. Zilberman UL, Mass E. Endodontic treatment of infected primary teeth using Maisto's paste. J Dent Child 1989;56:117.
318. Garcia-Godoy F. Evaluation of an iodoform paste in root canal therapy for infected primary teeth. J Dent Child 1987;54:30.
319. Holan G, Fuks AB. A comparison of pulpectomies using ZOE and Kri Paste in primary molars: a retrospective study. Pediatr Dent 1993;15:403.
320. Glauser RO. Preventive orthodontics and limited treatment procedures. US Public Health Service, Division of Indian Health; 1967.
321. Greenberg M. Filling root canals of deciduous teeth by an injection technique. Dent Dig 1961;67:574.
322. Krakow A, et al. Advanced endodontics in pedodontics. In: White G, editor. Clinical oral pediatrics. Chicago: Quintessence; 1981. p. 248–64.
323. Aylard S, Johnson R. Assessment of filling techniques for primary teeth. Pediatr Dent 1987;9:195.
324. Mack RB, Halterman CW. Labial pulpectomy access followed by esthetic composite resin restoration for nonvital maxillary deciduous incisors. J Am Dent Assoc 1980;100:374.
325. Ripa LW. Pulp therapy for the primary dentition. II. The treatment of teeth with non-vital or degenerating pulps. Conn State Dent Assoc J 1970;44:210.
326. American Academy of Pediatric Dentistry guidelines for pulp therapy for primary and young permanent teeth. Pediatr Dent 1998;20:43.
327. Velling RJ. A study of the treatment of infected and necrotic primary teeth. J Dent Child 1961;28:213.
328. Droter JA. Pulp therapy in primary teeth. J Dent Child 1967;34:507.
329. Full CA. Pulpotomy treatment of fistulated primary molars. Quintessence Int 1979;10:73.
330. Meyer FW, Sayegh FS. Wound healing following curettement of bifurcation abscesses of human primary molars. Oral Surg 1979;47:267.
331. Parkins FM, et al. Coronal vs. canal therapy for non-vital primary molars: a clinical trial [abstract]. JDR 1977;56:143.
332. Myers DR, et al. Histopathology of radiolucent furcation lesions associated with pulpotomy-treated primary molars. Pediatr Dent 1988;10:291.
333. Starkey P. Treatment of pulpally involved primary molars. In: McDonald RE, et al, editors. Current therapy in dentistry. St. Louis: CV Mosby; 1980. p. 414.
334. Erausquin J, Devoto FC. Alveolodental ankylosis induced by root canal treatment in rat molars. Oral Surg 1970;30:105.
335. Coll JA, Sadrian R. Predicting pulpectomy success and its relationship to exfoliation and succedaneous dentition. Pediatr Dent 1996;18:57.

Chapter 18

PHARMACOLOGY FOR ENDODONTICS

Paul D. Eleazer

Infections concur with many endodontic conditions. Accordingly, it behooves the practitioner to be well prepared to use drugs that help fight infection. Unfortunately, **pain** has also become associated with endodontics, at least in the public's mind. Fortunately, for both pre- and postoperative pain, relief through drugs is readily available. In addition to pain, **anxiety** about endodontic treatment is also rampant. Again, modern antianxiety drugs have been developed, displacing the sedatives, hypnotics, and soporifics often misused to control anxiety in the past. In the present-day pharmacy, drugs are available that work directly against anxiety without many of the side effects, making dental treatment easier for the patient and the practitioner alike, enabling more patients to receive optimal dental care.

The up-to-date dentist, and the endodontist in particular, must be prepared to handle any pharmacologic exigency. One must know not only actions and reactions to drugs but also indications and contraindications, as well as side effects, toxicity, half-life, and any interaction the newly prescribed drug may have with other drugs the patient may be taking.

This chapter is meant to be a specific overview of drugs vital to endodontics. For in-depth details about any of these drugs, the reader is referred to a pharmacology text, the *Physicians' Desk Reference (PDR)*, or the *U.S. Pharmacopeia (USP)*.

INFECTION CONTROL

The overwhelming importance of microorganisms to endodontics was highlighted in 1965 by the classic experiment of Kakehashi et al.[1] They found that exposing the pulps of **germ-free** rats to the oral environment caused **no pulpal destruction** beyond the operative wound. In **control animals,** however, with **normal oral flora**, the same pulpal exposure resulted in pulpal **necrosis** and periradicular **abscess,** just as it does in the endodontic patient.

In the usual scenario, pulpal invasion begins with a mixed infection of aerobes and anaerobes. As the infection continues, oxygen is depleted, and **obligate** anaerobic bacteria and **facultative** bacteria predominate.[2] For many years, endodontists suspected bacteria as the pathogens in necrotic pulps but were not able to prove the point because of inadequate culture methods. After the development of anaerobic culture techniques, however, investigators were able to show nearly 100% infection of necrotic pulps (Table 18-1).[3]

One of the primary goals of endodontic treatment is to eliminate a hospitable place for microorganisms to grow. Débridement of the canal soft tissues and debris should be as thorough as possible. The space should be totally obturated to isolate any remaining tissue from the body and to close off that path for oral bacteria to reach beyond the apex. Sterile technique should be used throughout the procedures to avoid introducing any new microbes into the patient. Attention to proper technique also protects the entire staff from receiving pathogens from the patient.

Periapically, bacteria do not usually hold the advantage, and infection is less likely. Without a doubt, situations occur where chronic infections persist in the periapex following root canal therapy. Tronstad believes that most periapical granulomas are infected.[4] Gatti et al. showed bacterial presence in chronic asymptomatic, enlarging, periapical radiolucent lesions discovered at postendodontic recall.[5]

Table 18-1 Bacterial Pathways to the Pulp

Caries
Periodontal disease
Fractures
Dentinal tubules not covered by cementum
Anachoresis

They used the highly accurate deoxyribonucleic acid (DNA) probe technique. Ratner et al. have shown anaerobes within bone lesions from old extraction sites to be related to trigeminal neuralgia.[6] Others discovered similar-appearing lesions around failing root canals at surgery.[7]

ANTIBIOTICS

Antibacterial agents, commonly called **antibiotics**, are very useful because they kill bacteria without damage to the host. These drugs attack cell structure and metabolic paths unique to bacteria and not shared with human cells. Systemic antibiotics are used frequently in the practice of medicine and dentistry. Some say they are overused. Although this is probably true, it is also difficult to tell when an infection might spread to cause life-threatening problems, such as cavernous sinus thrombosis, Ludwig's angina, danger-space swelling reaching into the mediastinum, brain abscess, or endocarditis, all of which have developed as sequelae of root canal therapy. It is probably wise to use systemic antibiotics when there is a reasonable possibility of microorganisms beyond the root canal. The immunologically compromised patient should also be considered an indication for antibiotic therapy, regardless of the condition of the canal.

This discussion of antibiotics will not include parenteral-use drugs or drugs used rarely in dental patients, which need monitoring by a physician because of potential side effects. The dental practitioner should be acutely aware of signs of infection not responding to oral antibiotic therapy and be speedy in referring such patients to an infection specialist.

CLASSIFICATION

Antibiotics may be classified into two main categories: those that kill bacteria rapidly and those that kill more slowly by retarding bacterial protein synthesis (Table 18-2 and 18-3). Generally speaking, the faster-killing antibacterial agents are more desirable.

Table 18-2 Types of Antibiotics

Types of Antibiotics
Rapid-killing antibiotics
Penicillins and cephalosporins
Metronidazole (Flagyl®)
Fluoroquinolones
Antibiotics that slow protein synthesis
Erythromycins (macrolides)
Clindamycin (Cleocin®)
Tetracyclines

Table 18-3 Common Examples of Oral Penicillins and Cephalosporins

Drugs
Penicillins
Penicillin V 500 mg qid
Ampicillin 500 mg qid
Amoxicillin 500 mg tid/qid
Augmentin 500 mg tid/qid
Cephalosporins
First generation
Cephalexin (Keflex®) 500 mg qid
Cefadroxil (Duricef®) 500 mg qid
Second generation
Cefuroxime (Ceftin®) 250 or 500 mg bid
Cefaclor (Ceclor®) 500 mg tid
Third generation
Cefixime (Suprax®) 400 mg daily

Dosages may vary with the specific situation.

Fast-killing antibacterial agents are often called **bactericidal**, meaning that they are observed to kill quickly in the laboratory. **Penicillins, cephalosporins, and metronidazole** are the bactericidal antibiotics commonly used against endodontic pathogens. The first two kill by integrating into and weakening a newly made cell wall, whereas the latter impedes DNA manufacture. Both require actively growing organisms to be effective, so antibiotics that fight bacteria by slowing their protein synthesis (bacteriostatic antibiotics) are generally not given along with these bactericidal drugs.

Allergies

Serious anaphylactic allergic reactions are rare with **oral** penicillins and cephalosporins, although they are possible. If allergic to one penicillin, the patient should be considered allergic to all penicillins and possibly to cephalosporins as well. Because of a close molecular structure, there is about a 10% cross-reactivity between these groups, that is, 1 in 10 who are allergic to penicillins will be allergic to cephalosporins and vice versa.

Resistance

The main biochemical structural similarity of penicillins and cephalosporins is the β-lactam ring. Some bacteria can produce an enzyme, called β-lactamase or penicillinase, which cleaves this ring, thus disabling the antibiotic. Microbiologists have identified about 30 different types of this enzyme. Some penicillins and cephalosporins have been altered to defeat this bacterial trick with altering a slightly different three-dimensional structure. Potassium clavulanate has been added to **amoxicillin**, for example, to make it stable in the presence of β-lactamase. The combination is called **Augmentin®**.

Bacterial resistance may also be developed by mutation of the DNA molecule or can be acquired from other bacteria by DNA transfer, even from one species of bacteria to another. In addition to enzymatic destruction of antibiotic molecules, as with β-lactamase, bacteria sometimes become resistant by not allowing an antibiotic to pass through the cell wall or cell membrane. Another resistance situation occurs when the bacteria can pump the antibiotic molecule overboard faster than it can enter.

Bacteria generally pass on their resistance genes to their offspring. Fortunately, if not used, this DNA will sometimes not be passed on to future generations. Although recent laboratory research is developing new antibiotics awaiting approval, these new drugs will probably fall prey to new forms of bacterial resistance. It behooves the professions to limit antibiotic therapy to those situations in which the patient will likely benefit from treatment and not expose the "wonder drugs" to bacteria's resistance-making mechanisms.

Replantation of avulsed teeth, on the other hand, calls for **systemic antibiotic therapy** in conjunction with endodontic treatment for best results. Success, as measured by the degree of inflammatory root resorption, was judged to be superior by Hammarstrom and coworkers when permanent incisors of monkeys were replanted under controlled conditions.[8]

Penicillins

Penicillins have a short half-life, limited to about 1 hour. It is important to tell patients the need to be prompt in taking their pills. Because they are excreted unchanged by the kidneys, they are very useful in treating urinary tract infections, where they accumulate in powerful killing levels. In patients with compromised kidney function, reducing the dosage is appropriate. The dentist should discuss with the patient's physician, if the individual patient is undergoing kidney dialysis, and tailor the penicillin or cephalosporin dosage according to the dialysis schedule.

Penicillins are unique in their lack of toxicity. That is, if the patient is not allergic, there is no maximum dose of penicillin and no side effects from overdosage. **Amoxicillin** is generally considered the penicillin of first choice because of its somewhat better absorption from the gut.

Cephalosporins

Cephalosporins have been developed over the last three decades. Because of the β-lactam ring, many consider them a subgroup of the penicillin family. Their improvement has seen three major improvements in their ability to kill stubborn infections, so the drugs are classed as first, second, and third generation. **First-generation cephalosporins** have the most value in dentistry since they kill most oral pathogens and should be considered for use in most infections. Second- and third-generation cephalosporins are used for refractory infections, probably after laboratory results of a culture. Oral cephalosporins lag behind parenteral ones in the development process. One must give consideration to hospitalization and intravenous antibiotic therapy if the seriously ill patient does not respond to oral drug therapy.

Metronidazole

Metronidazole (Flagyl®) is also considered a bactericidal drug because of its fast killing time. It attacks the bacteria's DNA and works against obligate anaerobes but not against facultative bacteria or aerobes. **Metronidazole** is often used in combination with another antibiotic, usually **amoxicillin,** to combat the stomach ulcer–causing *Helicobacter pylori.* This combination of two fast-killing drugs also helps in severe dental infections. Periodontists find metronidazole helpful in destroying deep-pocket anaerobes, bacteria that obviously infect the root canal in many instances. Metronidazole shares properties with disulfiram (Antabuse®), a drug used to help alcoholics avoid alcohol by inducing violent vomiting. So patients taking metronidazole should be cautioned about not using alcohol for the time they are taking the drug plus 1 day following to allow the drug to be eliminated from their system.

The half-life of metronidazole is in the 8- to 10-hour range. Side effects include an unpleasant, metallic taste and brown discoloration of the urine, effects that are dose related.

Fluoroquinolones

Fluoroquinolones interfere with DNA replication, classifying them as bactericidal. However, they are not effective against microbes commonly seen in endodontic infections. Their use in dentistry should probably be limited to cases in which culture and sensitivity results prove their indication.

Macrolides

Erythromycins kill bacteria by slowing the manufacture of bacterial protein but do not alter the rate of human protein synthesis. Because of their large molecule, **erythromycins** are also called macrolides (Table 18-4). These drugs kill about the same bacteria as penicillins, albeit by different means, so they are the drug of choice for patients allergic to penicillins. They are notorious for causing stomach cramps because they increase gut motility, and many patients who are susceptible to this phenomenon report that they are "allergic." True allergy exists, so the doctor must use judgment based on a thorough history before deciding to use this type of drug. The macrolides kill many gram-positive bacteria but have a limited spectrum for gram-negative bacteria. At one time, dentists were particularly fond of using erythromycins because of the lack of risk of life-threatening anaphylactic allergic reaction, but recently discovered serious interactions with other drugs have lessened their popularity. The wider-spectrum new macrolides, **azithromycin** and **clarithromycin,** are more useful for dental infections if the practitioner is cautious of potential drug interactions. The newer macrolides also develop higher tissue concentrations.

These recently discovered problems with other drugs are because they share the same metabolic pathway. The first discovered problem drugs were the large-molecule antihistamines terfenadine (Seldane®) and astemizole (Hismanal®). Seldane is no longer available in the United States because of fatal reactions with other drugs metabolized similarly. Mid-size molecule antihistamines, fexofenadine (Allegra®), loratidine (Claritin®), and cetirizine (Zyrtec), do not seem to be a problem.

Cisapride (Propulsid®), given to increase gut motility and treat esophageal reflux, has been associated with fatal heart arrhythmias when these patients have concurrently taken macrolide antibiotics. The elimination half-life of cisapride is 8 to 10 hours. This serious contraindication should encourage all practitioners to update the patient's medical history frequently.

Another serious potential problem lies with the bronchodilator theophylline, used for asthmatic patients, often at doses near the toxic level, in whom there is real potential for severe complications with the macrolides. Both of these drugs share the same metabolic pathway. Too many molecules of the drug overwhelm the pathway and high systemic levels result, giving rise to toxic manifestations such as cardiac arrhythmias. It should be noted that clarithromycin (Biaxin®) is metabolized by both the liver **and** the kidney, perhaps causing less bottleneck in the liver. Caution is warranted, however, in patients with either kidney or liver compromise because the half-life of the drug is prolonged.

The half-life of most erythromycins is in the range of 1 to 2 hours, whereas the newer ones remain active longer. Clarithromycin's half-life is 6 hours, and azithromycin has a remarkable **40-hour** half-life.

There are a few case reports of severe muscle weakness in patients taking lovastatin (Mevacor®) for cholesterol reduction who have been given a macrolide. Although this relationship is not clearly defined, it would be wise to select another antibiotic when the patient is taking this type of cholesterol-lowering drug (Table 18-5).[9]

Clindamycin

Clindamycin (Cleocin®) is often indicated in endodontic infections. It is rapidly and completely absorbed and has a good spectrum of killing oral pathogens, including many anaerobes. It was, however, the first antibiotic to be associated with causing pseudomembranous colitis, a life-threatening condition in which large patches of gut slough epithelium because of toxins from overgrowth of the nonsusceptible organism *Clostridium difficile.* This serious condition requires hospital management with intravenous fluids and antibiotics specific for the causative *Clostridium.* Patients being treated with clindamycin who experience diarrhea or another gut problem should immediately be referred to their physician for evaluation. Other broad-spectrum antibiotics have been associated with this phenomenon as well.

The average half-life of clindamycin is about 3 hours. Although clindamycin does not cross the blood-brain barrier, it does penetrate into abscesses and other areas of poor circulation rather well.

Tetracyclines

There is one standout among the tetracycline family of antibiotics: **doxycycline** (Vibramycin®). It has a long

Table 18-4 Macrolide Antibiotics

Erythromycin base 250–500 mg qid
Erythromycin stearate 250–500 mg qid
Erythromycin estolate (Ilosone®) 250–500 mg qid
Clarithromycin (Biaxin®) 250–500 mg bid
Azithromycin (Zithromax®) 500 mg bid × 1 d, then one daily

Table 18-5 Other Oral Antibiotics Commonly Used in Dentistry

Metronidazole (Flagyl®) 250–500 mg qid
Clindamycin (Cleocin®) 150–300 mg qid
Doxycycline (Vibramycin®) 100 mg bid

half-life and is least affected by heavy metal ions such as calcium, so the patient does not have to avoid dairy products and antacids. Tetracyclines kill the broadest spectrum of microbes of all antibiotics. They have recently found a place in periodontal infection fighting and should be included in the endodontist's armamentarium since periodontal pathogens frequently invade the root canal and periapical tissues.

Recall that all tetracyclines cause staining of developing teeth as they bind to calcium during formation of teeth and bones. This means that their use should be avoided in children and pregnant women if at all possible.

A rare side effect is phototoxicity, where exposure to the sun causes severe sunburn or rash. Patients should be cautioned to avoid sun exposure while taking tetracyclines unless they are sure that they are not susceptible to this side effect. Half-lives of most tetracyclines are about 10 hours, whereas doxycycline's half-life is 16 hours, allowing twice-daily dosing.

Sulfa Drugs

Sulfa drugs, often combined with trimethoprim to reduce resistance problems, are frequently used for urinary tract infections. Sulfa drugs predate penicillin by a decade but were quickly replaced by the more dramatic bacteria killer. Sulfa drugs cannot kill rapidly because they merely compete with a precursor in the bioformation of folic acid, which many bacteria cannot obtain from other sources and must manufacture for themselves. Their kill speed is dependent on the amount of natural precursors in the environment. In other words, sulfa drugs are the slowest of the slow, the poorest of bacteriostatic antibiotics. Their main plus is that they accumulate in the bladder. They are not generally useful in dentistry.

Caveats

In prescribing antibiotics, it seems warranted to continue therapy for 2 or 3 days after symptoms have resolved. In theory, if viable bacteria are present when antibiotic levels drop below the killing threshold, mutations can occur more readily. Patients are often not conscientious about continuing medications once their symptoms resolve. A reminder telephone call to check on their condition and reinforce the need to finish their prescription is well advised.

Females of childbearing age should be told that perhaps antibiotics will interfere with the effectiveness of oral contraceptives. If they need antibiotics, other means of birth control should be used through the next cycle. Some researchers believe that antibiotic-induced reduction in the gut flora causes malabsorption of the hormones in birth control pills. This side effect remains unproved.

Change in gut flora is definitely associated with increased levels of digitalis preparations, commonly used in heart conditions. Dangerously high levels can occur, and such patients need a consultation with their physician. Diminution of gut bacteria by antibiotics also changes output of vitamin K, needed in blood clotting, so patients on anticoagulant therapy should also be cautioned to consult with their physician.

Endodontists are in a unique position among dentists because of the preponderance of anaerobes in the conditions treated. A good specimen for culturing can often be obtained by needle aspiration from an abscess that has not yet drained. The specimen should be placed in an oxygen-free container available from a local hospital laboratory. A culture can be a big advantage when a patient does not respond to the first antibiotic. The practitioner can telephone the laboratory and quickly learn which drug to use next.

Hospitalization for administration of antibiotics intravenously should be considered when the patient is not responding to oral antibiotics. Many new-generation antibiotics are available only parenterally, and the continuous dosage of intravenous administration gives higher blood levels without the complication of oral-dosing variables such as half-life and patient compliance. The results of culture and sensitivity tests can greatly aid in selection of the appropriate drug when hospitalization is warranted.

Use of corticosteroids to reduce inflammation remains popular among some practitioners. Reducing inflammation relieves symptoms but also reduces the efficiency of white blood cells, which are crucial to infection fighting. Sometimes prophylactic antibiotics are prescribed as a precaution when corticosteroids are used.

Antibiotic Prophylaxis

Dentists should all be aware of the need, before dental treatment, to premedicate with antibiotics patients who have certain heart ailments. Systemic diseases compromising the immune system also call for consideration of prophylactic antibiotics in situations for which they might not otherwise be indicated. The goal of **antibiotic prophylaxis** is to prevent clinical infection by helping destroy small numbers of bacteria present before or introduced during treatment. Oral bacteria released during dental treatment clearly can cause heart and artificial joint infections. Oral streptococci, in particular, have been indicted as causative organisms for seeding heart and implanted joints, causing morbidity or even death.

Oral streptococci are weak pathogens known as "*viridans* strep." They are α-hemolytic, meaning that they cannot totally metabolize blood on a culture plate. They can, however, store energy molecules intra- and extracellularly. These external stores are long-chain polysaccharides, also known as the sticky substance of dental plaque. These long chains become seriously pathogenic when "*viridans*" colonies form on heart valves, trapping blood cells and fibrin and thereby reducing heart efficiency by hindering closure of the valves. Furthermore, portions of the sticky "vegetations," as they are called, break off and lodge in small vessels at distant sites, causing ischemia with possibly disastrous consequences.

For many years, the American Heart Association has made recommendations for antibiotic therapy to kill bacteria released into the bloodstream when certain dental procedures are performed. These recommendations have been updated as new knowledge became available. The most recent was in 1997.[10] Following these suggestions, the American Academy of Orthopaedic Surgeons and the American Dental Association collaborated to make further recommendations for patients with artificial joints.[11]

There was an addendum to these recommendations in late 1997 about patients taking the diet pills commonly known as "fen-phen" because of a propensity of these drugs to **cause heart valve defects.**[12] The drugs fenfluramine (Pondamin®) or dexfenfluramine (Redux®), with or without phentermine (Adipex® or Fastin®), have been associated with an alarming development of permanent, serious heart valve defects, primarily in women. Patients who have taken these diet pills, even for a short time, should be premedicated unless an echocardiogram has proven that their heart is properly functioning. Over-the-counter diet pills have not been associated with any heart problem.

It is important to note that all of these recommendations are guidelines, not mandates, and that modifications may be needed for some situations. Consultation with the patient's physician is always in order if any doubt exists.

Bender et al. pointed out the value of destroying intraoral bacteria with an antiseptic prior to invasive procedures.[13] Heimdahl and coworkers also demonstrated bacteremia from endodontic procedures confined to the canal (Table 18-6).[14]

PAIN CONTROL

There are three categories of pain control medications. **Narcotics** are the most powerful. They have three types of receptors in the brain. **Aspirin** and the **nonsteroidal anti-inflammatory drugs** (NSAIDS) make up the second category. These act at the site of injury to reduce pain-invoking prostaglandins that are made within the damaged cell. Although not classed as a pain reliever, corticosteroids relieve pain by this mechanism as well but have many side effects. Finally, **acetaminophen** (Tylenol®) is the third type. Acetaminophen acts primarily on the brain to relieve pain.

Modern endodontic therapy does not elicit much pain. However, many patients associate it with pain, partly because pain **was** a hallmark of early endodontic treatment and partly because the media often portray endodontics in this light. Just as a placebo will alleviate symptoms if the brain is convinced it will work, the patient who anticipates pain usually needs higher doses or stronger types of drug for relief. For patients anticipating pain, a prescription drug is often the only thing that will be effective (Table 18-7). Surgical pain, postoperative pain, and where the patient has significant preoperative pain usually warrant narcotics.

Narcotics can cause addiction, with characteristics unique from other types of addiction. Both physical and psychological addiction occur. Patients may present a "story" of drug allergies, leaving the practitioner no choice but to prescribe narcotics. Be aware of this type of patient and make certain that there is a real medical need for narcotics; otherwise, you may be feeding someone's addiction or helping a drug pusher obtain his stock.

Narcotics are central nervous system (CNS) depressants and work synergistically with all other CNS depressants. The most commonly available CNS depressant, alcohol, is contraindicated with narcotics. Narcotics reduce reaction times, and narcotized patients must not drive or operate machinery. Usually, narcotics are combined with acetaminophen or aspirin or an NSAID to make them more effective without excessive narcotic side effects.

Propoxyphene was originally introduced as a non-narcotic; however, it is now known as a rather weak narcotic. It works for many patients, perhaps in part because its characteristic, dizziness, makes the patient feel that it must be helping with the pain. Darvon® is available plain or with aspirin; with acetaminophen, it is called Darvocet-N®.

Codeine has been a standard drug in dentistry for many years because it is usually powerful enough to control dental pain. It is irritating to the stomach in high doses, however, so addicts are seldom appeased. Unfortunately, many patients with legitimate pain are troubled with this gastrointestinal upset.

Hydrocodone (Vicodin®), a development of the 1980s, is less irritating to the gut and has become very

Table 18-6 Summary of Guidelines for Antibiotic Prophylaxis for Heart and Artificial Joint Patients

Medical History	
Prophylaxis Needed	**Prophylaxis Not Needed**
Heart patients	
Any artificial valve	Isolated atrial-septal defect
Previous endocarditis	Coronary artery bypass graft
Pulmonary shunt	Surgical repair of septal defect
Most congenital defects	Functional murmur
Rheumatic heart disease	Rheumatic fever without valve damage
Hypertrophic cardiomegaly	Pacemaker
MVP with regurgitation	MVP without regurgitation
"Fen-phen" diet pill history	"Fen-phen" with a normal echocardiogram
Artificial joint patients	
Immunocompromised/immunosuppressed	
Inflammatory arthropathies	
Rheumatoid arthritis	
Systemic lupus erythematosus	
Disease, drug, or radiation immunosuppression	
Other patients	
Insulin-dependent diabetes mellitus	
Artificial joint within past 2 y	
History of failed artificial joint	
Malnutrition	
Hemophilia	
Dental Treatment	
Prophylaxis Needed	**Prophylaxis Not Needed**
Extraction	Restorative treatment even with retraction cord
Periodontal procedures, even probing	Radiographs
Subgingival antibiotic fiber placement	Local anesthesia, except PDL
Prophylaxis	Impressions and partial dentures
Implants	Fluoride treatments
Instrumentation beyond apex	**Endoscope within canal**
Intraligamentary (PDL) injection	Rubber dam
Ortho band placement	Suture removal
	Shedding of primary teeth
Prophylactic Antibiotic Regimen	
Amoxicillin 2000 mg	
Cephalexin (Keflex®) 2000 mg	
Clindamycin (Cleocin®) 600 mg	
Azithromycin (Zithromax®) or clarithromycin (Biaxin®) 500 mg	

All dosages are given 1 hour preoperatively, with **no** following doses, unless otherwise indicated.
Macrolides are **NOT** recommended for prophylaxis of artificial joints
MVP = mitral valve prolapse; fen-phen = fenfluramine-phentermine.

Table 18-7 Pain Control Medications Taken Orally

Narcotics
Propoxyphene: Darvon® (plain or with aspirin), Darvocet-N® (with acetaminophen)
Codeine: Phenaphen®, Empirin® (with aspirin), Tylenol with Codeine®
Hydrocodone: Vicodin®, Lorcet®, Lortab®, Vicoprofen® (with ibuprofen)
Oxycodone: Percodan® (with aspirin), Percocet®, or Tylox® (with acetaminophen)
Meperidine: Demerol®
Morphine: Oramorph®, others
Aspirin and nonsteroidal anti-inflammatory drugs (NSAIDS)
Aspirin
Ibuprofen: Motrin®, Advil®, Nuprin®
Etodolac: Lodine®
Fenoprofen: Nalfon®
Naproxen: Aleve®, Naprosyn®, Anaprox®
Cyclooxygenase 2 inhibitor NSAIDS
Celecoxib: Celebrex®
Rofecoxib: Vioxx®
Acetaminophen
Tylenol®

popular in dentistry. It is less powerful than its cousin **oxycodone**, which is notoriously famous among drug addicts for its euphoria. Percodan® is oxycodone with aspirin, whereas Percocet® and Tylox® are oxycodone with acetaminophen. Occasionally, patients will experience sufficient pain from endodontic procedures to require high-level narcotics, such as oxycodone or **meperidine** (Demerol®). A stronger drug effect carries more frequent side effects, including constipation, euphoria, sedation, impaired coordination, and pupillary constriction. **Morphine** is available orally as Oramorph® and by other trade names. Like most other drugs given orally, because of rapid liver metabolism following oral dosing, a larger dose is required than is typical of the parenteral dose. Morphine pills are available in 10, 15, 30, 60, and 100 mg amounts. The higher levels are reserved for terminal cancer patients. For severe dental pain, such as when the bony cortical plates confine infection pressure, necessitating very strong drug therapy, morphine remains a viable choice for the astute practitioner.

Tramadol (Ultram®) is a new, potent, synthetic pain reliever that has similarities and differences with the classic opiates. Similarly, it binds with the mu opioid receptor, decreases respiration, and increases intracranial pressure. It also causes dizziness, nausea, and constipation and potentiates other CNS depressants. Unlike other opiates, tramadol is not fully reversed by naloxone (Narcan®). Further, it inhibits reuptake of serotonin and norepinephrine, a monoamine; hence, concomitant administration with monoamine oxidase inhibitor drugs is **not recommended**. Tramadol is well absorbed orally, and the usual adult dose is 50 to 100 mg four times a day.

Aspirin has been a standard drug for dental pain for many years and is still useful. It, however, prolongs bleeding, and for this reason is a poor presurgical drug. The anticoagulant effect comes from interference with platelet formation. Aspirin **irreversibly** binds the enzyme cyclooxygenase, key to the pathway from injury-induced arachidonic acid, that is released from the membranes of all cells, leading to production of inflammation and pain-causing prostaglandins. Platelets in circulation do not have enough protein synthesis reserves to replace the bound cyclooxygenase and are thus unable to participate in clotting for the remainder of their cell life—around 11 days. Many patients are on routine, low-dosage aspirin therapy for prophylaxis against stroke or heart attack. Prior to endodontic surgery, consultation with their physician may be in order.

For patients with stomach problems, consider the use of coated aspirin, such as Ecotrin®. The coating will not dissolve until reaching the alkaline conditions of the small intestine. This means that drug action will be delayed for the usual 2-hour stomach transit time. Alternatively, aspirin buffered with chemicals such as magnesium, calcium, or aluminum compounds to decrease stomach complaints (Bufferin®, Ascripton®) can be considered for sensitive patients.

Nonsteroidal anti-inflammatory drugs (Motrin/Advil) do not cause interruption of platelet synthesis for nearly as long because their binding to cyclooxygenase is **reversible**. Bleeding profiles return to normal shortly after NSAIDS are metabolized. Nonsteroidal anti-inflammatory drugs were found to be superior to 60 mg of codeine for pain relief in many pain studies. They have also been injected locally into the jaws, with good result in diminishing postoperative pain associated with pulpectomy.[15]

Both NSAIDS and aspirin cause stomach upset and can be ulcerogenic. The deleterious stomach (and kidney) effects of aspirin and NSAIDS are caused by action on one of the cyclooxygenase enzymes, cyclooxygenase 1 (COX-1), which seems to predominate in the stomach and kidney. Arachidonic acid is released by damaged cell membranes. Two forms of the enzyme cyclooxygenase transform the arachidonic acid into prostaglandins, which have diverse actions. The action we are interested in moderating is the one that produces inflammation and pain, which is catalyzed by the **cyclooxygenase 2 (COX-2) pathway.**

Celecoxib (Celebrex) and **rofecoxib** (Vioxx) have the unique capability of limiting prostaglandin synthesis from the pathways controlled by **COX 2**. This spares the side effects of prostaglandin inhibition of the COX-1 pathway that can harm the gut and/or kidneys.[16] The other NSAIDS have action on both pathways.

These new COX-2 inhibitor NSAIDS were introduced with great promise of exclusive targeting of the pain-inducing prostaglandin production. Unfortunately, clinical use has shown them to have serious gut and kidney side effects in some patients. The incidence of these side effects is lower than with classic NSAIDS. As with all new drugs, the practitioner should carefully weigh the potential benefits with the higher costs always related to development of new drugs, as well as the potential for yet undiscovered side effects.

Acetaminophen (Tylenol) gives patients relief via its action directly on an unknown site in the brain. It was discovered many years ago, and its cousin phenacetin was popularized in the now unavailable "APC" formulation of aspirin, phenacetin, and caffeine. Although it is effective against pain and fever, inflammation remains unchanged by acetaminophen. Some practitioners alternate acetaminophen and aspirin every 2 hours to enhance pain relief. Excedrin®, Goody's Headache Powder®, and other preparations contain aspirin and acetaminophen.

Acetaminophen is metabolized by the liver and should be used cautiously in patients with liver disease or chronic alcohol use. Considerable controversy exists about use of acetaminophen in alcohol abusers with compromised liver function. Most recent evidence suggests that a metabolite is the problem and that abrupt cessation of alcohol intake can lead to higher levels of the toxic metabolite than if some alcohol intake was continued.[17] Obviously, it is best to avoid acetaminophen when liver capability is in question.

On the positive side, acetaminophen does not cause stomach irritation. Also interesting is the fact that research data show that acetaminophen is better for elevation of the threshold for sharp pain, such as with dental treatment, than other types of pain relievers.[18]

ANXIETY REDUCTION

As mentioned earlier, many patients view endodontic therapy as a painful process and avoid treatment, to the detriment of their dental and general health. In a recent study, nearly 30% of laypersons surveyed said that they were nervous about going to the dentist. Over half of this group said that they would go to the dentist more often if given a "**sedative drug.**"[19] It is a common observation in practice that patients arrive fearful. To worsen matters, epinephrine, commonly administered to retain local anesthetic in the area of injection, increases anxiety. Caffeine can also release endogenous catecholamines and aggravate the fear reaction. Perhaps it would be wise to recommend avoiding caffeine and to reduce epinephrine if feasible for anxious patients. Smoking also prolongs caffeine's half-life of 5 to 7 hours.

For many years, anxious patients were treated by verbally belittling their fear or by inappropriate drug therapy. Narcotics and/or barbiturates and other sedatives were used without much success. They were not working on the fear itself. **Benzodiazepines** are now available that act directly on the brain centers that control fear. This class of drug not only relieves anxiety but is also an anticonvulsant, an amnestic, a sedative, and a muscle relaxant.

The first of the benzodiazepines discovered was **diazepam** (Valium®). Its usefulness is limited by its long half-life, approaching 60 hours. One reason for the long life span of the drug is that two of its metabolites are pharmacologically active. By administering one of these metabolites or a similar drug with a shorter half-life, the duration of drug effect is lessened. **Lorazepam** (Ativan®) is an example of using a diazepam metabolite as the administered drug, with its half-life in the 14-hour range. **Triazolam** (Halcion®), a slightly different molecule, has a half-life of approximately 3 hours and is popular for dental procedures.

Any drug administered orally has considerable variation because of the "first-pass effect," as drug-laden blood from the stomach and small intestine goes first to the liver, where significant metabolism immediately reduces the drug level before it reaches its target. Berthold and coworkers showed that slowly dissolving a 0.25 mg tablet of triazolam intraorally gives higher blood plasma levels than swallowing the same amount of drug, probably by allowing absorption through the oral mucosa that does not progress directly to the liver.[20] Ehrich et al. also found oral 0.25 mg triazolam superior to 5.0 mg diazepam for decreasing anxiety, superior amnesia, and better patient perception of drug effectiveness.[21]

Oral drug administration should occur in the office to allow monitoring and should occur about 1 hour prior to treatment. As with all CNS depressants, one must consider lowering the dose when the patient is concurrently taking another CNS depressant. Patients must not be allowed to drive or operate machinery. Anxious patients will gladly make arrangements for a driver to escort them home.

An additional positive effect of the benzodiazepine drugs is their amnesia. Patients frequently think that the treatment took significantly less time than it actually did and also have gaps in their recall of events during the procedure, probably from a direct drug effect on their brain. Obviously, it is necessary to have a second person in the treatment room at all times. Although there are wide safety margins with dose, safety is further enhanced by the recent development of a specific drug antagonist, **flumazenil** (Romazicon®), which is injected parenterally to offset adverse effects.

REFERENCES

1. Kakehashi G, Stanley HR, Fitzgerald R. The effects of surgical exposures of dental pulps in germ-free and conventional laboratory rats. Oral Surg 1965;20:340.
2. Nair PNR. Apical periodontitis: a dynamic encounter between root canal infection and host response. Periodontology 1997;13:121.
3. Kantz WE, Henry CA. Isolation and classification of anaerobic bacteria from intact pulp chambers of non-vital teeth in man. Arch Oral Biol 1974;19:91.
4. Tronstad L.Extraradicular endodontic infections. Endodont Dent Traumatol 1987;3:86.
5. Gatti J, Skobe Z, Dubeck JM, et al. Bacterial DNA in periapical lesions using two surgical techniques [abstract]. J Dent Res 1997;76:58.
6. Ratner EJ, et al. Jawbone cavities and trigeminal and atypical facial neuralgias. Oral Surg 1979;48:3.
7. McMahon RE, Adams W, Spolnick KJ. Diagnostic anesthesia for referred trigeminal pain: part 1. Compend Contin Educ Dent 1992;13:980.
8. Hammarstrom L, Blomlof L, Anderson L, Lindskog S. Replantation of teeth and antibiotic treatment. Endod Dent Traumatol 1996;2:51.
9. Corpier CL, et al. Rhabdomyolysis and renal injury with lovastatin use. JAMA 1988;260:239.
10. Dajani AS, et al. Prevention of bacterial endocarditis. JAMA 1997;277:1794.
11. Advisory statement: antibiotic prophylaxis for dental patients with total joint replacements. J Am Dent Assoc 1997;129:1004.
12. US Department of Health and Human Services Interim Public Health Recommendation. MMWR Morb Mortal Wkly Rep 1997;46:1061–6.
13. Bender IB, Naidorf IJ, Garvey GJ. Bacterial endocarditis: a consideration for the physician and dentist. J Am Dent Assoc 1984;109:415.
14. Heimdahl A, Hall G, Hedberg M, et al. Detection and quantitation by lysis-filtration of bacteremia after different oral surgical procedures. J Clin Microbiol 1990;28:2205.
15. Penniston SG, Hargreaves KM. Evaluation of periapical injection of ketorolac for management of endodontic pain. J Endod 1996;22:55.
16. Pennisi E. Building a better aspirin. Science 1998;280:1191.
17. Slattery JT, Nelson SD, Thummel KE. The complex interaction between ethanol and acetaminophen. Clin Pharmacol Ther 1996;60:241.
18. Carnes PL, Cook B, Eleazer PD, Scheetz JP. Change in pain threshold to sharp pain by meperidine, naproxen, and acetaminophen as determined by electric pulp testing. Anesth Prog 1998;45:139.
19. Dionne RA, et al. Assessing the need for anesthesia and sedation in the general population. J Am Dent Assoc 1998;129:167.
20. Berthold CE, Corey SE, Dionne RA. Triazolam drug levels following sublingually and orally administered premedication [abstract]. J Dent Res 1997;76:114.
21. Ehrich DG, Lundgren JP, Dionne RA, et al. Comparison of triazolam, diazepam, and placebo as outpatient oral premedication for endodontic patients. J Endod 1997;23:181.

Chapter 19

RESTORATION OF ENDODONTICALLY TREATED TEETH

Charles J. Goodacre and Joseph Y. K. Kan

Various methods of restoring pulpless teeth have been reported for more than 200 years. In 1747, Pierre Fauchard described the process by which roots of maxillary anterior teeth were used for the restoration of single teeth and the replacement of multiple teeth (Figure 19-1).[1] Posts were fabricated of gold or silver and held in the root canal space with a heat-softened adhesive called "mastic."[1,2] The longevity of restorations made using this technique was attested to by Fauchard: "Teeth and artificial dentures, fastened with posts and gold wire, hold better than all others. They sometimes last fifteen to twenty years and even more without displacement. Common thread and silk, used ordinarily to attach all kinds of teeth or artificial pieces, do not last long."[1]

In Fauchard's day, replacement crowns were made from bone, ivory, animal teeth, and sound natural tooth crowns. Gradually, the use of these natural substances declined, to be slowly replaced by porcelain. A pivot (what is today termed a post) was used to retain the artificial porcelain crown into a root canal, and the crown-post combination was termed a "pivot crown." Porcelain pivot crowns were described in the early 1800s by a well-known dentist of Paris, Dubois de Chemant.[2] Pivoting (posting) of artificial crowns to natural roots became the most common method of replacing artificial teeth and was reported as the "best that can be employed" by Chapin Harris in *The Dental Art* in 1839.[3]

Early pivot crowns in the United States used seasoned wood (white hickory) pivots.[4] The pivot was adapted to the inside of an all-ceramic crown and also into the root canal space. Moisture would swell the wood and retain the pivot in place.[2] Surprisingly, Prothero reported removing two central incisor crowns with wooden pivots that had been successfully used for 18 years.[2] Subsequently, pivot crowns were fabricated using wood/metal combinations, and then more durable all-metal pivots were used. Metal pivot retention was achieved by various means such as threads,

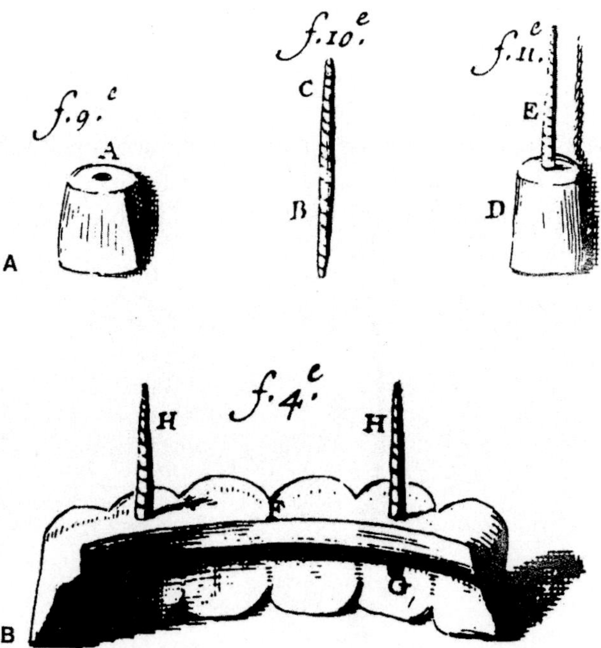

Figure 19-1 Early attempts to restore single or multiple units. **A**, "Pivot tooth" consisting of crown, post, and assembled unit. **B**, Six-unit anterior bridge "pivoted" in lateral incisors with canines cantilevered. Crowns were fashioned from diversity of materials. Human, hippopotamus, sea horse, and ox teeth were used, as well as ivory and oxen leg bones. Posts were usually made from precious metals and fastened to crown and root using a heated sticky "mastic" prepared by gum, lac, turpentine, and white coral powder. (Reproduced with permission from Fauchard P.[1])

*The authors are indebted to Drs. Kenneth C. Trabert, Joseph P. Cooney, Angelo A. Caputo, and Jon P. Standlee of the University of California School of Dentistry, Los Angeles, who contributed so generously the many fine illustrations, photographs, and laboratory findings found in this chapter.

pins, surface roughening, and split designs that provided mechanical spring retention.[2]

Unfortunately, adequate cements were not available to these early practitioners—cements that would have enhanced post retention and decreased abrasion of the root caused by movement of metal posts within the canal. One of the best representations of a pivoted tooth appears in *Dental Physiology and Surgery*, written by Sir John Tomes in 1849 (Figure 19-2).[5] Tomes's post length and diameter conform closely to today's principles in fabricating posts.

Endodontic therapy by these dental pioneers embraced only minimal efforts to clean, shape, and obturate the canal. Frequent use of the wood posts in empty canals led to repeated episodes of swelling and pain. Wood posts, however, did allow the escape of the so-called "morbid humors." A groove in the post or root canal provided a pathway for continual suppuration from the periradicular tissues.[1]

Although many of the restorative techniques used today had their inception in the 1800s and early 1900s, **proper endodontic treatment was neglected until years later.** Today, both the endodontic and prosthodontic aspects of treatment have advanced significantly, new materials and techniques have been developed, and a substantial body of scientific knowledge is available on which to base clinical treatment decisions.

The purpose of this chapter is to answer questions frequently asked when dental treatment involves pulpless teeth and to describe the techniques commonly employed when restoring endodontically treated teeth. Whenever possible, the answers and discussion will be supported by scientific evidence.

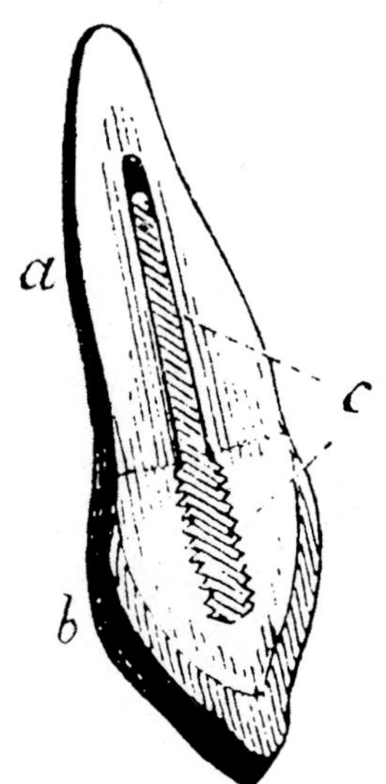

Figure 19-2 Principles used today in selecting post length and diameter were understood and taught by early practitioners during mid-1800s. Reproduced with permission from Tomes J.[5]

SHOULD CROWNS BE PLACED ON ENDODONTICALLY TREATED TEETH?

A retrospective study of 1,273 teeth endodontically treated 1 to 25 years previously compared the clinical success of anterior and posterior teeth.[6] Endodontically treated teeth with restorations that encompassed the tooth (onlays, partial- or complete-coverage metal crowns, and metal ceramic crowns) were compared with endodontically treated teeth with no coronal coverage restorations. It was determined that **coronal coverage crowns did not significantly improve the success of endodontically treated anterior teeth.** This finding supports the use of a conservative restoration such as an etched resin in the access opening of otherwise intact or minimally restored anterior teeth. Crowns are indicated only on endodontically treated anterior teeth when they are structurally weakened by the presence of large and/or multiple coronal restorations or they require significant form/color changes that cannot be effected by bleaching, resin bonding, or porcelain laminate veneers. Scurria et al. collected data from 30 insurance carriers in 45 states regarding the procedures 654 general dentists performed on endodontically treated teeth.[7] The data indicated that 67% of endodontically treated anterior teeth were restored without a crown, supporting the concept that many anterior teeth are being satisfactorily restored without the use of a crown.

When endodontically treated **posterior teeth** (with and without coronal coverage restorations) were compared, **a significant increase in the clinical success** was noted when **cuspal coverage crowns** were placed on maxillary and mandibular molars and premolars.[6] Therefore, restorations that encompass the cusps should be used on posterior teeth that have interdigitation with opposing teeth and thereby receive occlusal forces that push the cusps apart. The previously discussed insurance data indicated that 37 to 40% of posterior pulpless teeth were restored by practitioners without a crown, a method of treatment not supported by the long-term clinical prognosis of posterior endodontically treated teeth that do not have cusp-encompassing crowns.[7] There are, however, certain posterior teeth (not as high as 40%) that do not have substantive occlusal interdigitation or have an occlusal form that precludes interdigitation of a nature that attempts to separate the cusps (such as **mandibular first premolars** with small, poorly developed lingual cusps). When these teeth are intact or minimally restored, they would be reasonable candidates for restoration of only the access opening without use of a coronal coverage crown.

Multiple clinical studies of fixed partial dentures, many with long spans and cantilevers, have determined that endodontically treated abutments failed more often than abutment teeth with vital pulps owing to tooth fracture,[8–12] supporting the greater fragility of endodontically treated teeth and the need to design restorations that reduce the potential for both crown and root fractures when extensive fixed prosthodontic treatment is required.

Gutmann reviewed the literature and presented an overview of several articles that identify what happens when teeth are endodontically treated.[13] These articles provide background information important to an understanding of why **coronal coverage crowns help prevent fractures of posterior teeth.** Endodontically treated dog teeth were found to have 9% less moisture than vital teeth.[14] Also, with aging, greater amounts of peritubular dentin are formed, which decreases the amount of organic materials that may contain moisture. It has been shown that endodontic procedures reduce tooth stiffness by 5%, attributed primarily to the access opening.[15]

Tidmarsh described the structure of an intact tooth that permits deformation when loaded occlusally and elastic recovery after removal of the load.[16] The direct relationship between tooth structure removed during tooth preparation and tooth deformation under load of mastication has been described.[17] Dentin from endodontically treated teeth has been shown to exhibit significantly lower shear strength and toughness than vital dentin.[18] Rivera et al. stated that the effort required to fracture dentin may be less when teeth are endodontically treated because of potentially weaker collagen intermolecular cross-links.[19]

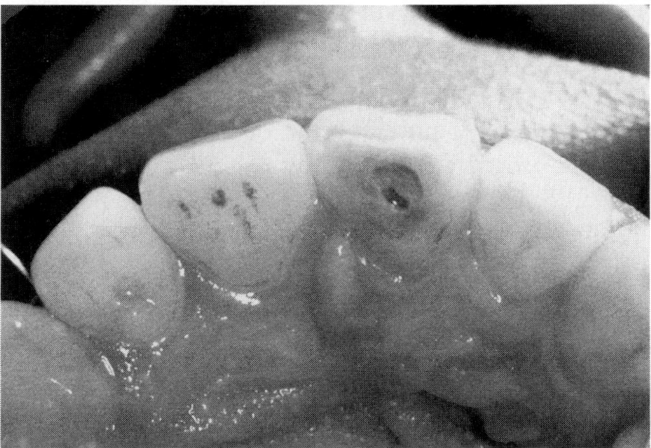

Figure 19-3 Incisal view of an intact central incisor that required endodontic treatment owing to trauma. Placement of a bonded resin restoration in the access opening is the only treatment required since crowns do not enhance the longevity of anterior endodontically treated teeth. A crown would only be used when esthetic and functional needs cannot be achieved through more conservative treatments.

Conclusions

Restorations that encompass the cusps of endodontically treated posterior teeth have been found to increase the clinical longevity of these teeth. Therefore, **crowns should be placed on endodontically treated posterior teeth that have occlusal interdigitation with opposing teeth** of the nature that places expansive forces on the cusps. Since **crowns do not enhance the clinical success of anterior endodontically treated teeth**, their use on relatively sound teeth should be limited to situations in which esthetic and functional requirements cannot be adequately achieved by other, more conservative restorations (Figure 19-3).

WITH PULPLESS TEETH, DO POSTS IMPROVE LONG-TERM CLINICAL PROGNOSIS OR ENHANCE STRENGTH?

Laboratory Data

Virtually all laboratory studies have shown that placement of a post and core either fails to increase the fracture resistance of extracted endodontically treated teeth or decreases the fracture resistance of the tooth when a force is applied via a mechanical testing machine.[20–25] Lovdahl and Nicholls found that endodontically treated maxillary central incisors were stronger when the natural crown was intact, except for the access opening, than when they were restored with cast posts and cores or pin-retained amalgams.[20] Lu found that posts placed in intact endodontically treated central incisors did not lead to an increase in the force required to fracture the tooth or in the position and angulation of the fracture line.[21] McDonald et al. found no difference in the impact fracture resistance of mandibular incisors with or without posts.[22] Eshelman and Sayegh[25a] reported similar results when posts were placed in extracted dog lateral incisors. Guzy and Nicholls determined that there was no significant reinforcement achieved by cementing a post into an endodontically treated tooth that was intact except for the access opening.[23] Leary et al. measured the root deflection of endodontically treated teeth before and after posts of various lengths were cemented into prepared root canals.[24] They found no significant differences in strength between the teeth with or without a post. Trope et al. determined that preparing a post space weakened endodontically treated teeth compared with ones in which only an access opening was made but no post space.[25]

A potential situation in which a post and core could strengthen a tooth was identified by Hunter et al. using photoelastic stress analysis.[26] They determined that removal of internal tooth structure during endodontic therapy is accompanied by a proportional increase in stress. They also determined that minimal root canal enlargement for a post does not substantially weaken a tooth, but when excessive root canal enlargement has occurred, a post strengthens the tooth. Therefore, **if the walls of a root canal are thin** owing to removal of internal root caries or overinstrumentation during post preparation, then **a post may strengthen the tooth**.

Two-dimensional finite element analysis was used in one study to determine the effect of posts on dentin stress in pulpless teeth.[27] When loaded vertically along the long axis, a post reduced maximal dentin stress by as much as 20%. However, only a small (3 to 8%) decrease in dentin stress was found when a tooth with a post was subjected to masticatory and traumatic loadings at 45 degrees to the incisal edge. The authors proposed that the reinforcement effect of posts is doubtful for anterior teeth because they are subjected to angular forces.

Clinical Data

Sorenson and Martinoff clinically evaluated endodontically treated teeth with and without posts and cores.[28] Some of the teeth were restored with single crowns, whereas others served as either fixed or removable partial-denture abutments. Posts and cores significantly decreased the clinical success rate of teeth with single crowns and improved the clinical success of removable partial-denture abutment teeth but had little influence on the clinical success of fixed partial-denture abutments. Eckerbom et al. examined the radiographs of 200 consecutive patients and radiographically re-examined the same patients 5 to 7 years later to determine the prevalence of apical periodontitis.[29] Of the 636 endodontically treated teeth evaluated, 378 had posts and 258 did not have posts. At both examinations, **apical periodontitis was significantly more common in teeth with posts** than in endodontically treated teeth without posts.

Morfis evaluated the incidence of vertical root fracture in 460 endodontically treated teeth, 266 with posts.[30] There were 17 teeth with root fracture after a time period of at least 3 years. Nine of the 17 fractured teeth had posts, and 8 root fractures were in teeth without posts. Morfis concluded that the endodontic technique can cause vertical root fracture.[30] **None of the clinical data provide definitive support for the concept that posts and cores strengthen endodontically treated teeth or improve their long-term prognosis.**

Purpose of Posts

Since clinical and laboratory data indicate that teeth are not strengthened by posts, **their purpose is for retention** of a core that will provide appropriate support for the definitive crown or prosthesis. Unfortunately, this primary purpose has not been completely recognized. Hussey and Killough noted that 24% of general dental practitioners felt that a post strengthens teeth.[31] A 1994 survey (with responses from 1,066 practitioners and educators) revealed some interesting but erroneous facts.[32] Ten percent of the dentist respondents felt that each endodontically treated tooth should receive a post. Sixty-two percent of dentists over age 50 believed that a post reinforces the tooth, whereas only 41% of the dentists under age 41 believed in that concept. Thirty-nine percent of part-time faculty, 41% of full-time faculty, and 56% of nonfaculty practitioners felt that posts reinforce teeth.[32]

Conclusions

Both laboratory and clinical data fail to provide definitive support for the concept that posts strengthen endodontically treated teeth. Therefore, **the purpose of a post is to provide retention for a core.**

WHAT IS THE CLINICAL FAILURE RATE OF POSTS AND CORES?

Several studies provide clinical data regarding the number of posts and cores that failed over certain time periods (Table 19-1).[33–42] When this number is divided by the total number of posts and cores placed, the absolute failure rate is determined. A 9% overall average for absolute failure was calculated by averaging the absolute failure percentages from eight studies (an average study length of 6 years). In these studies, the absolute percent of failure ranged from 7 to 14%.

A review of more specific details from the eight studies provides insight into the length of each study and the number of posts and cores evaluated. The findings of a 5-year retrospective study of 52 posts and cores indicated that there were 6 failures and a 12% absolute failure rate.[33] Another study found that 17 of 154 posts failed after 3 years, for an 11% absolute failure rate.[34] An absolute failure rate of 9% was found in three studies.[35–37] A study of 138 posts in service for 10 years or more reported a 7% absolute post and core failure rate after 10 years or more (9 of 138 posts failed).[38] An 8% absolute failure rate (39 of 516 posts and cores) was published when 516 posts and cores placed by senior dental students were retrospectively evaluated,[39] whereas another study recorded a 14% failure rate (8 failures in 56

Table 19-1 Clinical Failure Rate of Posts and Cores

Lead Author	Study Length	% Clinical Failure
Turner, 1982*[33]	5 y	12 (6 of 52)
Sorenson, 1984[35]	1–25 y	9 (36 of 420)
Bergman, 1989*[36]	5 y	9 (9 of 96)
Weine, 1991*[38]	10 y or more	7 (9 of 138)
Hatzikyriakos, 1992*[34]	3 y	11 (17 of 154)
Mentink, 1993*[39]	1–10 y (4.8 mean)	8 (39 of 516)
Wallerstedt, 1984*[40]	4–0 y (7.8 mean)	14 (8 of 56)
Torbjörner, 1995[37]	1–69 mo	9 (72 of 788)
Mean values†	**6 yr 9 (196 of 2,220)**	

*Studies used to calculate mean study length.
†Calculation made by averaging numeric data from all studies.

posts and cores) from posts and cores placed by dental students.[40]

Kaplan-Meier survival statistics (percent survival over certain time periods) were presented or could be calculated from the data in seven studies (Table 19-2).[41] The survival rates ranged from a high of 99% after 10 years or more of follow-up to a 78% survival rate after a mean time of 5.2 years. The percent failure per year has also been calculated and ranged from 1.56%/year[36] to 4.3%/year.[42]

Conclusions

Posts and cores had an average absolute rate of failure of 9% (7 to 14% range) when the data from eight studies were combined (average study length of 6 years).

Table 19-2 Kaplain-Meier Survival Data (%) of Posts and Cores

Lead Author	Study Length	% Survival
Roberts, 1970[42]	5.2 y mean	78
Wallerstedt, 1984[40]	4–10 y range	83
Sorenson, 1985[28]	1–25 y range	90
Weine, 1991[38]	>10 y	99
Hatzikyriakos, 1992[34]	3 y	92
Mentink, 1993[39]	10 y	82
Creugers, 1993[41] (meta-analysis)	6 y	81 (threaded posts), 91 (cast posts)

WHAT ARE THE MOST COMMON TYPES OF POST AND CORE FAILURES?

Seven studies indicate that **post loosening is the most common cause of post and core failure** (Figure 19-4).[33,34,36,37,39,43,44] Turner reported on 100 failures of post-retained crowns and indicated that post loosening was the most common type of failure.[43] Of the 100 failures, 59 were caused by post loosening. The next most common occurrences were 42 apical abscesses followed by 19 carious lesions. There were 10 root fractures and 6 post fractures. In another article by Turner, he reported the findings of a 5-year retrospective study of 52 post-retained crowns.[33] Six posts had come loose, which was the most common failure. Lewis and Smith presented data regarding 67 post and core failures after 4 years.[44] Forty-seven of the failures (70%) resulted from posts loosening, 8 from root fractures, 7 from caries, and 4 from bent or fractured posts. Bergman et al. found 8 failures in 96 posts after 5 years.[36] Six posts had come loose, and 2 roots fractured. Hatzikyriakos et al. reported on 154 posts and cores after 3 years.[34] Five posts had come loose, 5 crowns had come loose, 4 roots fractured, and caries caused 3 failures. Mentink et al. identified 30 post loosenings and 9 tooth fractures when evaluating 516 posts and cores over a 1- to 10-year time period (4.8 years mean study length).[39] Torbjörner et al. reported on the frequency of 3 technical failures (loss of retention, root fracture, and post fracture).[37] They did not report biologic failures. Loss of retention was the most frequent post failure, accounting for 45 of the 72 post and core failures (62.5%). Root fracture was the second most common failure cause, followed by post fracture (Figure 19-5).

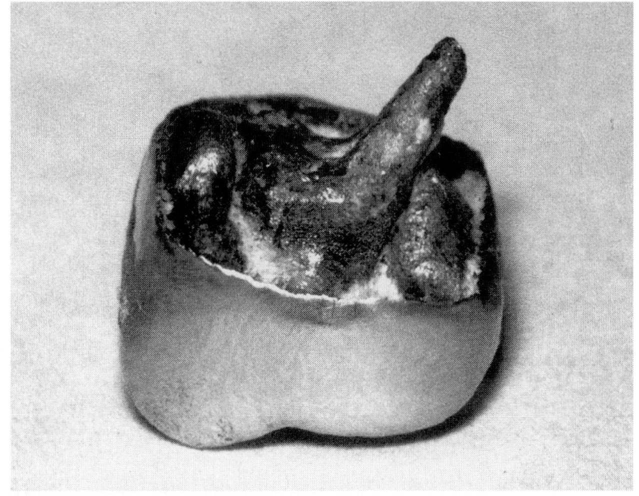

Figure 19-4 Mandibular molar crown that failed because the post loosened from the distal root.

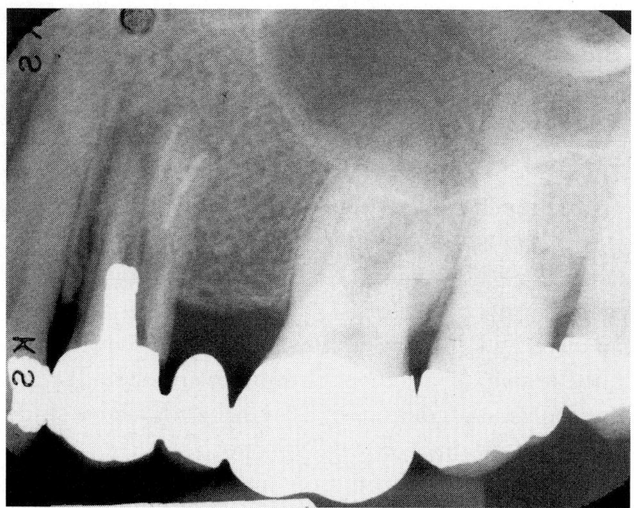

Figure 19-5 Radiograph of a fractured maxillary first premolar caused by a post with an excessive diameter and insufficient length, two problems frequently seen in conjunction with fractured roots.

In two studies, factors other than loss of retention were listed as the most common cause of failure.[35,38] Sorenson and Martinoff evaluated 420 posts and cores and recorded 36 failures.[35] Of the 36 failures, 8 were related to restorable tooth fractures, 12 to nonrestorable tooth fractures, and 13 to loss of retention and 3 were caused by root perforations. Weine et al. found 9 failures in 138 posts and cores after 10 years or more.[38] Three failures were caused by restorative procedures, 2 by endodontic treatment, 2 by periodontal problems, and 2 by root fracture. No posts failed owing to loss of retention.

Four studies provided data on the incidence of tooth fracture but did not provide information regarding post loosening. Linde reported that 3 of 42 teeth fractured,[45] Ross found no fractures with 86 posts,[46] Morfis found that 10 of 266 teeth fractured,[30] and Wallerstedt et al. identified 2 fractures with 56 posts.[40]

Loss of retention and tooth fracture are the two most common causes of failure (in that order of occurrence) when these studies are collectively analyzed by averaging the numeric data from all of the studies. Five percent of the posts placed (105 of 2,178 posts) experienced loss of retention (Table 19-3). Three percent of the posts placed (66 of 2,628 posts) failed via tooth fracture (Table 19-4).

Conclusions

Loss of retention and tooth fracture are the two most common causes of post and core failure.

WHICH POST DESIGN PRODUCES THE GREATEST RETENTION?

Laboratory Data

There have been many laboratory studies comparing the retention of various post designs. Threaded posts provide the greatest retention, followed by cemented, parallel-sided posts. Tapered cemented posts are the least retentive. Cemented, parallel-sided posts with ser-

Table 19-3 Clinical Loss of Retention Associated with Posts and Cores

Lead Author	Study Length	% of Posts Placed That Loosened	Post Form	% of Failures Owing To Loosening
Turner, 1982[33]	5 y	9 (6 of 66)	Appeared to be tapered	*
Turner, 1982[33]	1–5 y or more	*	Tapered	59 (59 of 100)
Sorenson, 1984[35]	1–25 y	3 (13 of 420)	Tapered and parallel	36 (13 of 36)
Lewis, 1988[44]	4 y	*	Threaded, tapered, and parallel	70 (47 of 67)
Bergman, 1989	5 y	6 (6 of 96)	Tapered	67 (6 of 9)
Weine, 1991[38]	10 or more	0 (0 of 138)	Tapered	0 (0 of 9)
Hatzikyriakos, 1992[34]	3 y	3 (5 of 154)	Threaded, parallel, and tapered	29 (5 of 17)
Mentink, 1993[39]	1–10 y (4.8 mean)	6 (30 of 516)	Tapered	77 (30 of 39)
Torbjörner, 1995[37]	4–5 y	6 (45 of 788)	Tapered and parallel	63 (45 of 72)
Mean values†		**5 (105 of 2,178)**		**59 (205 post loosenings of 349 total failures)**

*Data not available in publication.
†Calculation made by averaging numeric data from all studies.

Table 19-4 Clinical Tooth Fractures Associated with Posts and Cores

Lead Author	Study Length	% of Teeth Restored with Posts That Fractured	Post Form(s) Studied	% of Failures Owing To Fracture	
Turner, 1982[33]	5 y	0 (0 of 66)	Appear to be tapered	*	
Turner, 1982[33]	1–5 y or more	*	Tapered, parallel, and threaded	10	(10 of 100)
Sorenson, 1984[35]	1–25 y	3 (12 of 420)	Tapered and parallel	33	(12 of 36)
Linde, 1984[45]	2–10 y (5 y, 8 mo) mean	7 (3 of 42)	Threaded	38	(3 of 8)
Lewis, 1988[44]	4 y	*	Threaded, tapered, and parallel	12	(8 of 67)
Bergman, 1989[36]	5 y	3 (3 of 96)	Tapered	33	(3 of 9)
Ross, 1980[46]	5 y or more	0 (0 of 86)	Tapered, parallel, and threaded	0	(0 of 86)
Morfis, 1990[30]	3 y at least	4 (10 of 266)	Threaded and parallel	*	
Weine, 1991[38]	10 y or more	1 (2 of 138)	Tapered	50	(2 of 4)
Hatzikyriakos, 1992[34]	3 y	3 (4 of 154)	Threaded, parallel, and tapered	3	(4 of 17)
Mentink, 1993[39]	1–10 y (4.8 mean)	2 (9 of 516)	Tapered	23	(9 of 39)
Wallerstedt, 1984[40]	7.8 y	4 (2 of 56)	Threaded	25	(2 of 8)
Torbjörner, 1995[37]	1–6 y	3 (21 of 788), 3% mean	Parallel and tapered	29	(21 of 72)
Mean values†		**3 (66 of 2,628)**		**17**	**(74 tooth fractures of 446 total failures)**

*Data not available in publication.
†Calculation made by averaging numeric data from all studies.

rations are more retentive than cemented, smooth-sided parallel posts.

Clinical Data

There is clinical support for these laboratory studies. Torbjörner et al. reported significantly greater loss of retention with tapered posts (7%) compared with parallel posts (4%).[37] Sorenson and Martinoff determined that 4% of tapered posts failed by loss of retention, whereas 1% of parallel posts failed in that manner.[35] Turner indicated that tapered posts loosened clinically more frequently than parallel-sided posts.[43] Lewis and Smith also found a higher loss of retention with smooth-walled tapered posts than parallel posts.[44] Bergman et al.[36] and Mentink et al.[39] evaluated only tapered posts, and both studies reported that 6% of tapered posts failed via loss of retention, values higher than those recorded by Torbjörner et al.[37] and Sorenson and Martinoff[35] for parallel posts.

Contrasting results were reported by Weine et al.[38] They found no clinical failures from loss of retention with cast tapered posts. Hatzikyriakos et al. studied tapered threaded posts, parallel cemented posts, and tapered cemented posts.[34] The only posts that loosened from the root were parallel cemented posts.

Conclusions

Tapered posts are the least retentive and threaded posts the most retentive in laboratory studies. Most of the clinical data support the laboratory findings.

IS THERE A RELATIONSHIP BETWEEN POST FORM AND THE POTENTIAL FOR ROOT FRACTURE?

Laboratory Data

Using photoelastic stress analysis, Henry determined that threaded posts produced undesirable levels of stress.[47] Another study used strain gauges attached to the root and compared four parallel-sided threaded posts with one parallel-sided nonthreaded post.[48] Two of the threaded posts produced the highest strains, whereas two other threaded posts caused strains comparable to the nonthreaded post. Standlee et al., using photoelastic methods, indicated that tapered, threaded posts were the worst stress producers.[49] When three types of threaded posts were compared in extracted teeth, Deutsch et al. found that **tapered, threaded posts increased root fracture by 20 times that of the parallel threaded posts.**[50]

Laboratory testing of **split-threaded posts** has provided varying results, but more research groups have concluded that they **do not reduce the stress associated with threaded posts.** Thorsteinsson et al. determined that split-threaded posts did not reduce stress concentration during loading.[51] In another study, split, threaded posts were found to produce installation stresses comparable to other threaded posts.[52] Greater stress concentrations than some other threaded posts were reported under simulated functional loading.[53–55] Rolf et al. found that a split, threaded post produced comparable stress to one type of threaded post and less stress than a third threaded post design.[56] Ross et al. determined that a split-threaded post produced less root strain than two other threaded posts and comparable strain to a third threaded post and a nonthreaded post.[48] Another research group concluded that the split, threaded design reduced the stresses caused during cementation compared with a rigid, threaded post design.[57]

Multiple photoelastic stress studies concluded that **posts designed for cementation produced less stress than threaded posts.**[47,49,56]

When parallel-sided cemented posts have been compared with tapered cemented posts, photoelastic stress testing results have generally favored parallel-sided posts. Using this methodology, Henry found that parallel-sided posts distribute stress more evenly to the root.[47] Finite-element analysis studies produced similar results.[58,59] Two additional photoelastic studies concluded that parallel posts concentrate stress apically and tapered posts concentrate stress at the post-core junction.[51,54] Also, using photoelastic testing, Assif et al. found that tapered posts showed equal stress distribution between the cementoenamel junction and the apex compared with parallel posts, which concentrated the stress apically.[60]

When fracture patterns in extracted teeth were used to compare parallel and tapered posts, the evidence favoring parallel posts is less favorable. Sorenson and Engelman determined that tapered posts caused more extensive fractures than parallel-sided posts, but the load required to create fracture was significantly higher with tapered posts.[61] Lu, also using extracted teeth, found no difference in the fracture location between prefabricated parallel posts and cast posts and cores.[21] Assif et al. tested the resistance of extracted teeth to fracture when the teeth were restored with either parallel or tapered posts and complete crowns.[62] No significant differences were noted, and post design did not influence fracture resistance.

In analyzing the stress distribution of posts, it was noted that tapered posts generate the least cementation stress and should be considered for teeth that have thin root walls, are nearly perforated, or have perforation repairs.[54]

Clinical Data

There are several clinical studies that provide data related to the incidence of root fracture associated with different post forms. Some of these studies provide a comparison of multiple post forms, whereas other studies evaluated only one type of post. Combining all of the root fracture data for each post form from both types of studies reveals some interesting trends (Table 19-5). Five studies present data regarding root fractures and threaded posts,[30,35,40,45,46] four regarding fracture associated with parallel-sided cemented posts,[30,35,37,46] and seven related to tapered, cemented posts.[30,35–39,46] If the total number of threaded posts evaluated in the five studies is divided into the total number of fractures found with threaded posts, a percent value can be determined that represents the average incidence of tooth fracture associated with threaded posts in the five studies. The same data can be calculated for parallel cemented and tapered cemented posts, permitting a comparison of the root fracture incidences associated with these three post forms.

Combining the five studies that reported data relative to **threaded posts** produced a mean **fracture rate of 7%** (11 fractures from 169 posts). The four clinical studies that contain fracture data from **parallel-sided cemented posts** produced a mean **fracture incidence of 1%** (9 fractures from 687 posts). From the seven studies reporting root fracture with **tapered posts**, there is a mean **fracture rate of 3%** (50 root fractures from 1,553 posts). These combined study data support the previously cited photoelastic laboratory stress tests, indicating that the greatest incidence of root fractures occurred with threaded posts and that the lowest percentage of root fracture was associated with parallel cemented posts. In a meta-analysis of selected clinical studies, Creugers et al. calculated a 91% tooth survival rate for cemented **cast posts** and cores and an 81% survival rate for **threaded posts** with resin cores.[41]

Although the combined data from all of the studies for each type of post revealed certain trends, analysis of

Table 19-5 Post Form and Tooth Fracture

Clinical Data (% of Post and Cores Studied That Failed via Tooth Fracture)		
Threaded Posts (Lead Author)	Parallel-Sided Posts (Lead Author)	Tapered Posts (Lead Author)
40 (2 of 5) (Sorenson[35])	0 (0 of 170) (Sorenson[35])	7 (18 of 245) (Sorenson[35])
0 (0 of 10) (Ross[46])	2 (5 of 332) (Torbjöner[37])	4 (16 of 456) (Torbjöner[37])
4 (2 of 56) (Wallerstedt[40])	0 (0 of 39) (Ross[46])	1 (2 of 138) (Weine[38])
7 (3 of 42) (Linde[45])	3 (4 of 146) (Morfis[30])	2 (9 of 516) (Mentink[39])
7 (4 of 56) (Morfis[30])		3 (3 of 96) (Bergman[36])
		0 (0 of 38) (Ross[46])
		3 (2 of 64) (Morfis[30])
7% Mean* (11 of 169)	**1% Mean* (9 of 687)**	**3% Mean* (50 of 1,553)**

*Calculation made by averaging numeric data from all studies.

individual studies (where multiple post forms were compared in the same study) produced less conclusive results. One study of threaded and cemented posts determined that teeth with threaded posts were lost more frequently than teeth with cast posts.[29] In three other clinical comparisons of threaded and cemented posts, no tooth fracture differences were noted between threaded and cemented posts.[30,34,46] In addition to the comparisons of threaded and cemented posts, four clinical studies provide data comparing the tooth fracture incidences associated with parallel-sided and tapered posts. In comparing parallel and tapered posts by reviewing dental charting records, a higher failure rate was reported with tapered posts than parallel posts in two studies,[35,37] and the failures were judged to be more severe with tapered posts. Two other clinical studies determined that there were no differences between tapered and parallel-sided posts.[34,46] Hatzikyriakos et al. found no significant differences between 47 parallel cemented posts and 44 tapered cemented posts after 3 years of service.[34] Ross evaluated 86 teeth with posts and cores that had been restored at least 5 years previously.[46] No fracture differences were found between 38 tapered cemented posts and 39 parallel cemented posts.

Unfortunately, the total number of clinical studies that compared multiple post forms in the same study is limited. Also, several factors may have affected the findings of available studies. Two of the articles that contained a comparison of multiple post forms covered sufficiently long time periods (10 to 25 years) that the tapered cemented posts may have been in place for much longer time periods than the parallel-sided cemented posts (owing to the later introduction of parallel posts into the dental market).[35,37] The mean time since placement for each post form was not identified in these studies. Also, both of these studies were based on reviews of patient records (rather than clinical examinations) and depended on the accuracy of dental charts in determining if and when posts failed, as well as the cause of the failure. Another factor that affected the results of many of the referenced clinical studies was the length of the posts. For instance, in Sorenson and Martinoff's study, 44% of the tapered cemented posts had a length that was half (or less than half) the incisocervical/occlusocervical dimension of the crown whereas only 4% of the parallel cemented posts were that short.[35] Since short posts have been associated with higher root stresses in laboratory studies, the difference in post length may have affected their findings in which tooth fractures occurred with 18 of 245 tapered posts compared with no fractures with 170 parallel posts.

Conclusions

When evaluating the relationship between post form and root fracture, **laboratory tests** generally indicate that all types of **threaded posts produce the greatest potential for root fracture**. When comparing tapered and parallel cemented posts using photoelastic stress analysis, the results generally favor the parallel cemented posts. However, the evidence is mixed when the comparison between tapered and parallel posts is based on fracture patterns in extracted teeth created by applying a force via a mechanical testing machine.

When evaluating the combined data from multiple **clinical studies, threaded posts generally produced the highest root fracture incidence** (7%) compared with tapered cemented posts (3%) and parallel cemented posts (1%). Analysis of individual clinical studies as opposed to the combined data produces less conclusive results. Additional comparative clinical studies would be beneficial, including designs that have not yet been evaluated in comparative studies.

WHAT IS THE PROPER LENGTH FOR A POST?

A wide range of recommendations have been made regarding post length, which includes the following: (1) the post length should equal the incisocervical or occlusocervical dimension of the crown[63–70]; (2) the post should be longer than the crown[71]; (3) the post should be one and one-third the crown length[72]; (4) the post should be half the root length[73,74]; (5) the post should be two-thirds the root length[75–79]; (6) the post should be four-fifths the root length[80]; (7) the post should be terminated halfway between the crestal bone and root apex[81–83]; and (8) the post should be as long as possible without disturbing the apical seal.[47] A review of scientific data provides the basis for differentiating between these varied guidelines.

Although short posts have never been advocated, they have frequently been observed during radiographic examinations (Figure 19-6). Grieve and McAndrew found that only 34% of 327 posts were as long as the incisocervical length of the crown.[84] In a clinical study of 200 endodontically treated teeth, Ross determined that only 14% of posts were two-thirds or more of the root length and 49% of the posts were one-third or less of the root length.[46] A radiographic study of 217 posts determined that only 5% of the posts were two-thirds to three-quarters the root length.[85] In a retrospective clinical study of 52 posts, Turner radiographically compared the length of the post with the maximum length available if 3 mm of gutta-percha were retained.[33] Posts that came loose used only 59% of the ideal length, and only 37% of the posts were longer than the proposed minimum length. Nine millimeters were proposed as the ideal length.

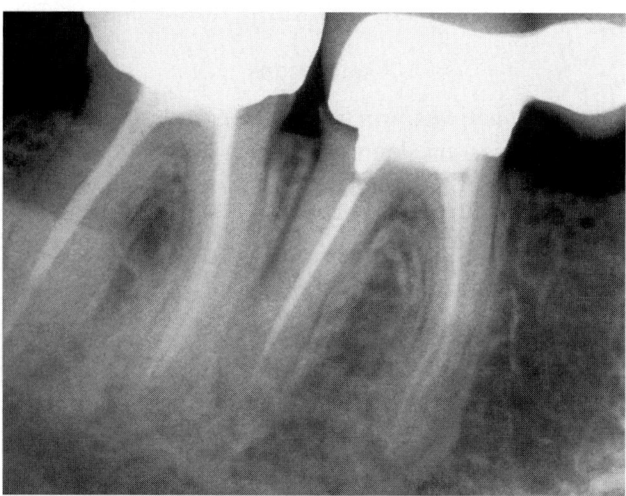

Figure 19-6 Radiograph showing a very short post in the distal root of the first molar that has loosened and caused prosthesis failure.

Sorensen and Martinoff determined that clinical success was markedly improved when the post was equal to or greater than the crown length.[35] Johnson and Sakumura determined that posts that were three-quarters or more of the root length were up to 30% more retentive than posts half of the root length or equal to the crown length.[86] Leary et al. indicated that posts with a length at least three-quarters of the root offered the greatest rigidity and least root bending.[87]

These data indicate that post length would appropriately be three-quarters that of root length. However, some interesting results occur when post length guidelines of two-thirds to three-quarters the root length are applied to teeth with average, long, and short root lengths. It was determined that a post approaching this recommended length range is not possible without compromising the apical seal by retaining less than 5 mm of gutta-percha.[88] When post length was half that of the root, the apical seal was rarely compromised on average-length roots. However, when posts were two-thirds the root length, many of the average- and short-length roots would have less than the optimal gutta-percha seal. Shillingburg et al. also indicated that making the post length equal the clinical crown length can cause the post to encroach on the 4.0 mm "safety zone" required for an apical seal.[89]

Abou-Rass et al. proposed a post length guideline for maxillary and mandibular molars based on the incidence of lateral root perforations occurring when post preparations were made in 150 extracted teeth.[90] They determined that molar posts should not be extended more than 7 mm apical to the root canal orifice.

When teeth have diminished bone support, stresses increase dramatically and are concentrated in the dentin near the post apex.[91] A recent finite-element model study established a relationship between post length and alveolar bone level.[92] To minimize stress in the dentin and in the post, the post should extend more than 4 mm apical to the bone.

Conclusions

Reasonable clinical guidelines for length include the following: (1) Make the post approximately **three-quarters the length of the root when treating long-rooted teeth;** (2) when average root length is encountered, then post length is dictated by **retaining 5 mm of apical gutta-percha** and extending the post to the gutta-percha (Figure

19-7); (3) whenever possible, posts should **extend at least 4 mm apical to the bone crest** to decrease dentin stress; and (4) molar posts should **not be extended more than 7 mm** into the root canal apical to the base of the pulp chamber (Figure 19-8).

HOW MUCH GUTTA-PERCHA SHOULD BE RETAINED TO PRESERVE THE APICAL SEAL?

It has been determined that when 4 mm of gutta-percha are retained, only 1 of 89 specimens showed leakage, whereas 32 of 88 specimens (36%) leaked when only 2 mm of gutta-percha were retained.[93] Two studies found no leakage at 4 mm, whereas another study found that 1 of 8 specimens leaked at 4 mm.[94,95] Portell et al. found that most specimens with only 3 mm of apical gutta-percha had some leakage.[96] When the leakage associated with 3, 5, and 7 mm of gutta-percha was compared, Mattison et al. found significant leakage differences between each of the dimensions.[97] They proposed that at least 5 mm of gutta-percha are required for an adequate apical seal. Nixon et al. compared the sealing capabilities of 3, 4, 5, 6, and 7 mm of apical gutta-percha using dye penetration.[98] The greatest leakage occurred when only 3 mm were retained, and it was significantly different from the other groups. They also noted that a significant decrease in leakage occurred when 6 mm of gutta-percha remained. Kvist et al. examined radiographs from 852 clinical endodontic treatments.[99] Posts were present in 424 of the teeth. Roots with posts in which the remaining root filling material was shorter than 3 mm showed a significantly higher frequency of periapical radiolucencies.

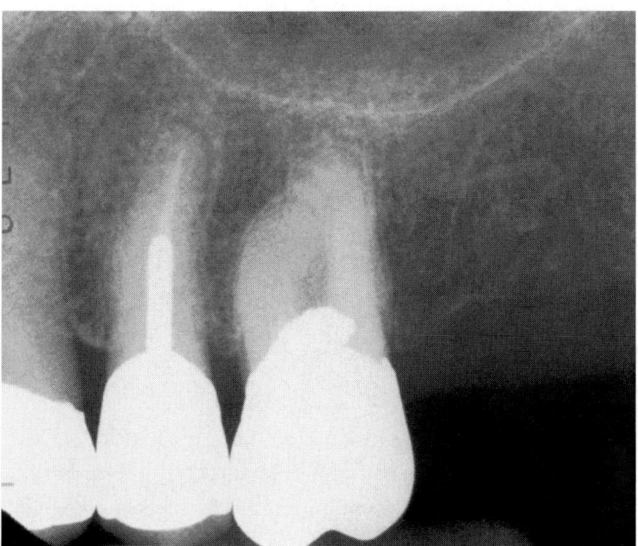

Figure 19-7 Five millimeters of gutta-percha were retained in the maxillary premolar and the post extended to that point.

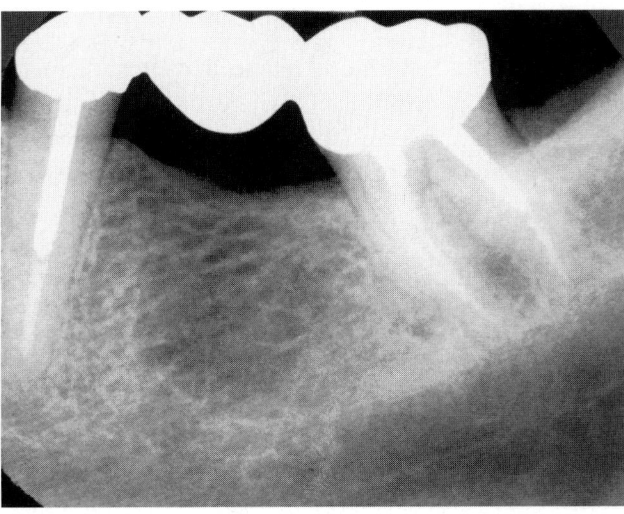

Figure 19-8 Distal post in the mandibular molar was extended to a maximal length of 7 mm.

Conclusions

Since there is greater leakage when only 2 to 3 mm of gutta-percha are present, 4 to 5 mm should be retained apically to ensure an adequate seal. Although studies indicate that 4 mm produce an adequate seal, stopping precisely at 4 mm is difficult, and radiographic angulation errors could lead to retention of less than 4 mm. **Therefore, 5 mm of gutta-percha should be retained apically** (see Figure 19-7).

DOES POST DIAMETER AFFECT RETENTION AND THE POTENTIAL FOR TOOTH FRACTURE?

Studies relating post diameter to post retention have failed to establish a definitive relationship. Two studies determined that there was an increase in post retention as the diameter increased,[89,100] whereas three studies found no significant retention changes with diameter variations.[101–103] Krupp et al. indicated that post length was the most important factor affecting retention and post diameter was a secondary factor.[104]

A more definitive relationship has been established between post diameter and stress in the tooth. **As the post diameter increased**, Mattison found that **stress increased in the tooth.**[105] Trabert et al. measured the impact resistance of extracted maxillary central incisors as post diameter increased and found that increasing post diameter decreased the tooth's resistance to fracture.[106] Deutsch et al. determined that there was a sixfold increase in the potential for root fracture with every millimeter the tooth's diameter was decreased.[50] However, two finite-element studies failed to find higher tooth stresses with larger-diameter posts.[58,59]

Conclusions

Laboratory studies relating retention to post diameter have produced mixed results, whereas a more definitive relationship has been established between root fracture and large-diameter posts (Figure 19-9).

WHAT IS THE RELATIONSHIP BETWEEN POST DIAMETER AND THE POTENTIAL FOR ROOT PERFORATIONS?

In a literature review of guidelines associated with post diameter, Lloyd and Palik indicated that there are three distinct philosophies of post space preparation.[107] One group advocated the narrowest diameter for fabrication of a certain post length (the conservationists). Another group proposed a space with a diameter that does not exceed one-third the root diameter (the proportionists). The third group advised leaving at least 1 mm of sound dentin surrounding the entire post (the preservationists).

Based on the proportional concept of one-third the root diameter, three articles measured the root diameters of extracted teeth and proposed post diameters that would not exceed that proportion.[89,90,108] Tilk et al. examined 1,500 roots.[108] They measured the narrowest mesiodistal dimension at the apical, middle, and cervical one-thirds of the teeth except the palatal root of the maxillary first molar, which was measured faciolingually. Based on a 95% confidence level that post width would not exceed one-third the apical width of the root, they proposed the following post widths (Table 19-6): small teeth such as mandibular incisors, about 0.6 to 0.7 mm; large-diameter roots such as maxillary central incisors and the palatal root of the maxillary first molar, about 1.0 mm; and for the remaining teeth, about 0.8 to 0.9 mm.

Shillingburg et al. measured 700 root dimensions to determine the post diameters that would minimize the risk of perforation.[89] Also based on not exceeding one-third the mesiodistal root width, they recommended the following post diameters (see Table 19-6): mandibular incisors, 0.7 mm; maxillary central incisors or other large roots, 1.7 mm, which was the maximal recommended dimension; post tip diameter, at least 1.5 mm less than root diameter at that point; and post diameter at the middle of the root length, 2.0 mm less than the root diameter.

Post spaces were prepared in 150 extracted maxillary and mandibular molars using different instrument diameters, and the resulting incidences of perforations were recorded.[90] The authors determined that the **mesial roots of mandibular molars and the buccal roots of maxillary molars should not be used for posts** owing to the higher risk of perforation on the furcation side of the root. For the principal roots (mandibular distal and maxillary palatal), they determined that posts should not be extended more than 7 mm into the root canal (apical to the pulp chamber) owing to the risk of perforation. Regarding instrument size, they concluded that post preparations can be safely completed using a No. 2 Peeso instrument, but perforations are more likely when the larger No. 3 and 4 Peeso (Dentsply/Maillefer North America; Tulsa, Okla.; Moyco/Union Broach; York, Pa.) instruments were used.

Raiden et al. evaluated several instrument diameters (0.7, 0.9, 1.1, 1.3, 1.5, and 1.7 mm) to determine which

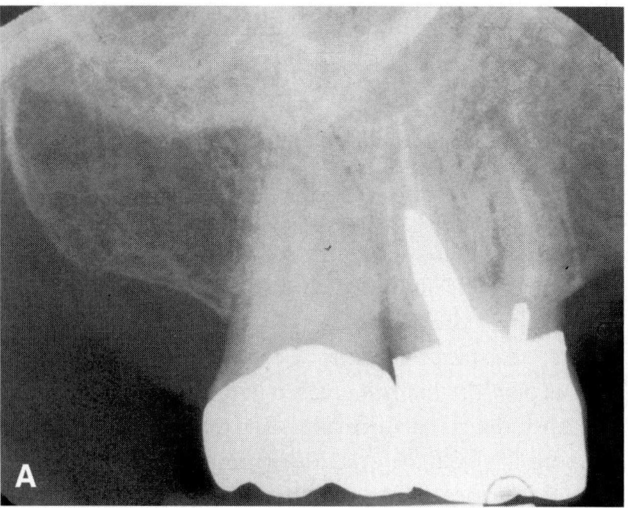

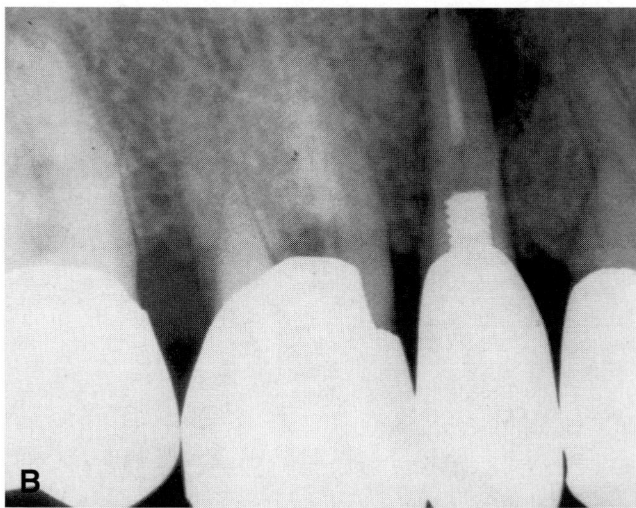

Figure 19-9 Excessive post diameters. **A,** A large-diameter post placed in the palatal root of the maxillary molar. **B,** A large-diameter threaded post caused fracture of the maxillary second premolar. The radiographic appearance of the bone is typical of a fractured root—a teardrop-shaped lesion with a diffuse border.

Table 19-6 Post Space Preparation Widths (in mm)

	Maxillary			Mandibular	
	Tilk et al.[108]	Shillingburg et al.[89]		Tilk et al.[108]	Shillingburg et al.[89]
Central incisor	1.1	1.7		0.7	0.7
Lateral incisor	0.9	1.3		0.7	0.7
Canine	1.0	1.5		0.9	1.3
First premolar					
(B)	0.9	0.9			
(L)	0.9	0.9			
Second premolar	0.9	1.1		0.9	1.3
First molar					
(MB)	0.9	1.1	(MB)	0.9	1.1
(DB)	0.8	1.1	(ML)	0.8	0.9
(L)	1.0	1.3	(D)	0.9	1.1
Second molar					
(MB)	—	1.1	(MB)	—	0.9
(DB)	—	0.9	(ML)	—	0.9
(L)	—	1.3	(D)	—	1.1

one(s) would preserve at least 1 mm of root wall thickness following post preparation in maxillary first premolars.[109] They determined that instrument diameter must be small (0.7 mm or less) for maxillary first premolars with single canals because the mesial and distal developmental root depressions restrict the amount of available tooth structure in the centrally located single root canal. However, when there are dual canals, the instrument can be as large as 1.1 mm because the canals are located buccally and lingually into thicker areas of the roots.

Conclusions

Instruments used to prepare posts should be related in size to root dimensions to avoid excessive post diameters that lead to root perforation (Figure 19-10). Safe instrument diameters to use are 0.6 to 0.7 mm for small teeth such as mandibular incisors and 1 to 1.2 mm for large-diameter roots such as the maxillary central incisor. Molar posts longer than 7 mm have an increased chance of perforations and therefore should be avoided even when using instruments of an appropriate diameter.

CAN GUTTA-PERCHA BE REMOVED IMMEDIATELY AFTER ENDODONTIC TREATMENT AND A POST SPACE PREPARED?

Several studies indicate that there is no difference in the leakage of the root canal filling material when the post space is prepared immediately after completing endodontic therapy.[94,110–112] Bourgeois and Lemon found no difference between immediate preparation of a post space and preparation 1 week later when 4 mm of gutta-percha were retained.[110] Zmener found no difference in dye penetration between gutta-percha removal after 5 minutes and 48 hours.[111] Two sealers were tested, and 4 mm of gutta-percha were retained apically. When lateral condensation of gutta-percha was used, Madison and Zakariasen found no difference in the dye penetration between immediate removal and 48-hour removal.[94] Using the chlorpercha filling technique,

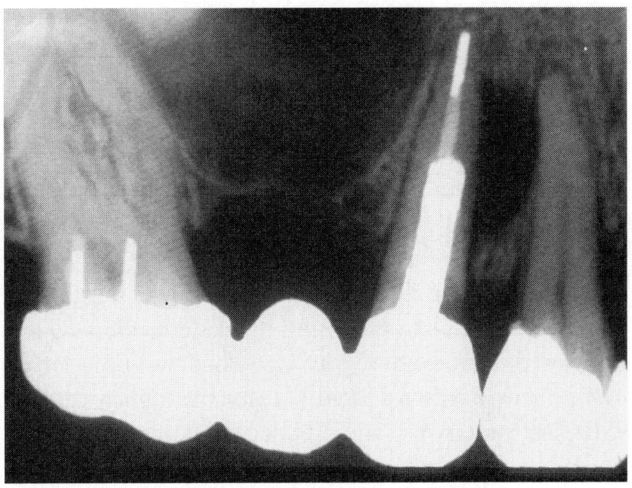

Figure 19-10 The excessive post diameter in the maxillary second premolar created a perforation in the mesial root concavity. Note the distinct border and round form of the radiolucent lesion, characteristics indicative of a root perforation.

Schnell found no difference between immediate removal of gutta-percha and no removal of gutta-percha.[112] By contrast, Dickey et al. found significantly greater leakage with immediate gutta-percha removal.[113]

Kwan and Harrington tested the effect of immediate gutta-percha removal using both warm and rotary instruments.[114] There was no significant difference between the controls and immediate removal using warm pluggers and files. Compared to the controls, there was significantly less leakage with immediate removal of gutta-percha when using Gates-Glidden (Dentsply/Maillefer North America; Tulsa, Okla.; Moyco/Union Broach; York, Pa.) drills.

Karapanou et al. compared immediate and delayed removal of two sealers (a zinc oxide–eugenol sealer and a resin sealer).[115] No difference between immediate and delayed removal was noted with the resin sealer, but delayed removal of the zinc oxide–eugenol sealer produced significantly greater leakage.

Portell et al. found that delayed gutta-percha removal (after 2 weeks) caused significantly more leakage than immediate removal when only 3 mm of gutta-percha were retained apically.[96] Fan et al. found more leakage from delayed removal of gutta-percha.[116]

Conclusions

Adequately condensed gutta-percha can be safely removed immediately after endodontic treatment.

WHAT INSTRUMENTS REMOVE GUTTA-PERCHA WITHOUT DISTURBING THE APICAL SEAL?

Multiple studies have determined that there is no difference in leakage between removing gutta-percha with hot instruments and removing it with rotary instruments.[93,97,117] Suchina and Ludington[117] and Mattison et al.[97] found no difference between hot instrument removal and removal with Gates-Glidden burs. Camp and Todd found no difference between Peeso reamers, Gates-Glidden burs, and hot instruments.[93] Hiltner et al. compared warm plugger removal with two types of rotary instruments (GPX burs; Brassler, Savannah, Georgia, and Peeso reamers).[118] There were no significant differences in dye leakage between any of the groups. Contrasting results were found by Haddix et al.[119] They measured significantly less leakage when the gutta-percha was removed with a heated plugger than when either a GPX instrument or Gates-Glidden drills were used.

Conclusions

Both rotary instruments and hot hand instruments can safely be used to remove adequately condensed gutta-percha when 5 mm are retained apically.

CAN A PORTION OF A SILVER POINT BE REMOVED AND STILL MAINTAIN THE APICAL SEAL?

In one study, all of the specimens leaked when 1 mm of a 5-mm-long silver point was removed using a round bur.[111] Neagley found that removal of the filling material coronal to the silver point with a Peeso reamer caused no leakage.[95] However, when all of the filling material and 1 mm of the silver point were removed, complete dye penetration occurred in eight of nine specimens.

Conclusions

The removal of a portion of a silver point during post preparation causes apical leakage.

DOES THE USE OF A CERVICAL FERRULE (CIRCUMFERENTIAL BAND OF METAL) THAT ENGAGES TOOTH STRUCTURE HELP PREVENT TOOTH FRACTURE?

Survey data indicate the percentage of respondents who felt that a ferrule increased a tooth's resistance to fracture.[32] Fifty-six percent of general dentists, 67% of prosthodontists, and 73% of board-certified prosthodontists felt that core ferrules increased a tooth's fracture resistance. To investigate this concept, several research studies have been performed. Some of the studies indicate that ferrules are beneficial, whereas others found no increase in fracture resistance.

The results appear indecisive until three differences between study designs are analyzed. First, some of the studies tested ferrules that were part of a cast metal core (core ferrules),[120–124] whereas other studies evaluated the effectiveness of ferrules created by the overlying crown engaging tooth structure.[125–128] One study evaluated both core and crown ferrules.[129] Second, there were differences in the form of the ferrule and therefore the manner by which the metal engaged tooth structure (beveled sloping surface versus extension over relatively parallel prepared tooth structure). Third, there were variations in the amount of tooth structure encompassed by the ferrules. Table 19-7 provides a comparison of the studies and the effectiveness of the various core and crown ferrules.

The data generally indicate that ferrules formed as part of the core are less effective than ferrules created when the overlying crown engages tooth structure. In four of the six core ferrule studies, they were found to be ineffective.[121,122,124,129] Also, in one of the two studies in which the core ferrule was effective, the ferrule form was a 2 mm parallel extension of the core over tooth structure[120] as opposed to a bevel. In the other

Table 19-7 Core Ferrules

Study	Ferrule Form	Was Ferrule Effective?	Materials/Type of Test
Barkhordar, 1989	2 mm parallel extension of core over the tooth	Yes	Extracted teeth/angular lingual force applied to p and c (no overlying crown)
Sorensen, 1990	1 mm wide 60-degree bevel at the tooth-core junction	No	Extracted teeth/angular lingual force applied to p and c (with overlying crown)
Tjan, 1985	60-degree bevel at the tooth-core junction	No	Extracted teeth/angular lingual force applied to p and c (no overlying crown)
Loney, 1990	1.5 mm parallel extension of core over the tooth	No	Photoelastic teeth/angular lingual force applied to p and c (no overlying crown)
Hemmings, 1991	45-degree bevel	Yes	Extracted teeth/torsional force applied to p and c (no overlying crown)
Saupe, 1996	2 mm parallel extension of core over *thin* dentin wall (0.5–0.75 mm thick)	No	Extracted teeth/angular lingual force applied to p and c (no overlying crown)
Sorensen, 1990	130-degree sloping finish line	No	Extracted teeth/p and c with crown
	1–2 mm of tooth grasped by crown	Yes	Extracted teeth/p and c with crown
Libman, 1995	0.5–1 mm of prepared tooth grasped by crown	No	Extracted teeth/p and c with crown/cyclic loading
	1.5–2 mm of prepared tooth grasped by crown	Yes	Extracted teeth/p and c with crown/cyclic loading
Milot, 1992	1 mm wide 60-degree bevel grasped by crown	Yes	Plastic analogies of teeth/p and c with crowns
Isidor, 1999	1.25 mm of prepared tooth grasped by crown	Yes	Bovine teeth/cyclic angular load/p and c with crown
	2.5 mm of prepared tooth grasped by crown	Yes, but more effective than 1.25 mm	Bovine teeth/cyclic angular load/p & c with crown
Hoag, 1982	1–2 mm of prepared tooth grasped by crown	Yes	Extracted teeth/p and c with crown

p and c = post and core.

study in which core ferrules were found to be effective,[123] a torsional force was used as opposed to an angular lingual force.

In the crown ferrule studies, most of the ferrules effectively increased a tooth's resistance to fracture. Only when the crown ferrule was of minimal dimension[125] or a sloping form[129] was it found to be ineffective. In support of these studies, Rosen and Partida-Rivera found that a 2 mm cast gold collar (not part of the post and core) was very effective in preventing root fracture when a tapered screw post was intentionally threaded into roots so as to induce fracture.[130] Assif et al. found no difference in the tooth fracture patterns of parallel posts, tapered posts, and parallel posts with a tapered end when they were covered by a crown that grasped 2 mm of tooth structure.[62]

The data also support the concept that ferrules that grasp larger amounts of tooth structure are more effective than those that engage only a small amount of tooth structure. In both the core and crown ferrule studies, the tooth's resistance to fracture was increased when a substantive amount of tooth structure was engaged (2 mm in the core ferrule studies and 1 to 2 mm in the crown ferrule studies). Libman and Nicholls found the 0.5 to 1.0 mm crown ferrule to be ineffective,[125] whereas a 1.5 to 2.0 mm crown ferrule was effective. Isidor et al. determined that increasing crown ferrule length significantly increased the number of cyclic cycles required to cause specimen failure.[127] They compared no ferrule with 1.25 and 2.55 mm crown ferrules and concluded that **ferrule length was more important than post length** in increasing a tooth's resistance to fracture under cyclic loading.

The form of the prepared ferrule also appears to affect a tooth's fracture resistance in the previously cited studies. Only one beveled/sloping ferrule was effective in enhancing a tooth's fracture resistance, and that was when a torsional force was applied to the tooth.

Conclusions

Differences of opinion exist regarding the effectiveness of ferrules in preventing tooth fracture. Ferrules have been tested when they are part of the core and also when the ferrule is created by the overlying crown-engaging tooth structure. Most of the data indicate that **a ferrule created by the crown**-encompassing tooth structure **is more effective** than a ferrule that is part of the post and core (Figure 19-11). Ferrule effectiveness is enhanced by grasping larger amounts of tooth structure. The amount of tooth structure engaged by the overlying crown appears to be more important than the length of the post in increasing a tooth's resistance to fracture. **Ferrules are more effective** when the crown encompasses relatively **parallel prepared tooth structure** than when it engages beveled/sloping tooth surfaces.

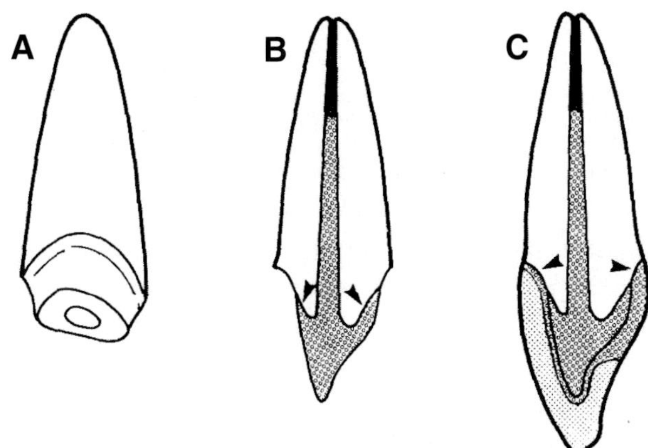

Figure 19-11 Types of ferrules. **A**, Tooth prepared for a post and core. **B**, A post and core has been cemented into the tooth. The **arrows** note how the core has created a ferrule around the tooth (core ferrule). **C**, A metal ceramic crown has been cemented over the core. The **arrows** show how the crown encompasses the tooth cervically, establishing a crown ferrule.

POST AND CORE PLACEMENT TECHNIQUES

Pretreatment Data Review

When it has been determined that a post and core is required to properly retain a definitive single crown or fixed partial denture, the following characteristics should be determined prior to beginning the clinical procedures associated with fabrication of a post and core:

1. Post length
2. Post diameter
3. Anatomic/structural limitations
4. Type of post and core that will be used (prefabricated post and restorative material core or anatomically customized cast post and core)
5. Root selection in multirooted teeth
6. Type of definitive restoration being placed and its effect on core form and tooth reduction depths.

Post Length

Since 5 mm of gutta-percha should be retained apically to ensure a good seal (as measured radiographically), posts should be extended to that length in all teeth except molars. With molars, posts should be placed in the primary roots (palatal root of maxillary molars and distal roots of mandibular molars) and should not be extended more than 7 mm apical to the origin of the root canal in the base of the pulp chamber. Extension beyond this length can lead to root perforation or only very thin areas of remaining tooth structure.

Post Diameter

A frequently used and clinically appropriate guideline for **post diameter is to not exceed one-third the root diameter.** It has been determined that when a root canal is prepared for a post and the diameter is increased beyond one-third of the root diameter, the tooth becomes exponentially weaker. Each millimeter of increase (beyond one-third the root diameter) causes a sixfold increase in the potential for root fracture.[50] Based on measuring the root dimensions of 1,500 teeth (125 of each tooth) and using the guideline that the post should be one-third the root diameter, optimal post diameter measurements have been determined to be about 0.6 mm for mandibular incisors and 1.0 mm for maxillary central incisors, maxillary and mandibular canines, and the palatal root of the maxillary first molar.[108] The recommended post diameter for the other teeth was 0.8 mm.[108] Another study of 700 teeth recommended that post diameter should range from 0.7 mm for mandibular incisors to a maximum of 1.7 mm for maxillary central incisors.[89]

Anatomic/Structural Limitations

The practitioner who completed the endodontic treatment is ideally suited to identify characteristics of the pulp chamber, the anatomy of the root canal(s), and completed endodontic filling that should be reviewed before placing a post and core. These characteristics include the presence and extent of dentinal craze lines, identification of teeth for which further root preparation (beyond that needed to complete endodontic instrumentation) will result in less than 1 mm of remaining dentin or a post diameter greater than one-third the root diameter area, information regarding areas in which the remaining tooth structure is thin, and the point at which significant root curvature begins.

Craze Lines

Craze lines in dentin are areas of weakness where further crack propagation may result in root fracture and tooth loss. The patient should be informed of their presence with appropriate chart documentation of crack location. It is prudent to avoid post placement, if possible, in favor of a restorative material core. If a **post** is required, it should **passively fit** the canal, and the definitive restoration should entirely encompass the cracked area, whenever possible, by forming a ferrule.

Dentin Thickness After Endodontic Treatment

Following normal and appropriate endodontic instrumentation, teeth can possess less than 1 mm of dentin, indicating that there should be no further root preparation for the post. When these teeth are encountered, it is best to fabricate a post that fits into the existing morphologic form and diameter rather than additionally preparing the root to accept a prefabricated type of post. This characteristic is one of the primary indications for use of a **custom cast post and core.** One study determined that canines (maxillary and mandibular), maxillary central and lateral incisors, and the palatal root of maxillary first molars possessed more than 1 mm of dentin after endodontic cleaning and shaping.[131] All other teeth had roots with less than 1 mm of remaining dentin following endodontic treatment. With the goal of preserving 1 mm of remaining dentin lateral to posts, it has been determined that single-canal maxillary first premolars should have posts that are 0.7 mm in diameter or less.[109] Mandibular premolars with oval- or ribbon-shaped canals should not be subjected to any preparation of the root canal for a post since this will result in less than 1 mm of dentin.[132] Preparation of the mesial root canals in mandibular molars and the buccal root canals in maxillary molars can result in perforation or only thin areas of remaining dentin. Based on measurements of residual dentin thickness, it is recommended that posts not be placed in these roots if possible.

Root Curvature

When root curvature is present, post length must be limited to preserve remaining dentin, thereby helping to prevent root fracture or perforation. Root curvature occurs most frequently in the apical 5 mm of the root. Therefore, if 5 mm of gutta-percha are retained apically, curved portions of the root are usually avoided. As discussed previously under post length, molar posts should not exceed 7 mm in the primary roots because of the potential for perforation owing to root curvature and the presence of developmental root depressions. Molar roots are frequently curved, and the post should terminate at the point where substantive curvature begins.

Type of Post and Core

Posts or dowels can be generally classified as cement/bonded posts or threaded posts. Cemented posts depend on their close proximity to prepared dentin walls and the cementing medium. Examples are custom-cast posts and cores (Figure 19-12) and a variety of prefabricated designs (Figure 19-13). The prefabricated designs include parallel-sided metal posts, such as the Para-Post (Coltene/Whaledent, Mahwah, New Jersey) (Figure 19-14) or different types of threaded posts. Threaded posts depend primarily on engaging the tooth—either through threads formed in the dentin as the post is screwed into the root or through threads previously "tapped" into the dentin (eg, the Kurer post; Marie Reiko, Inc, Reno, Nevada). Examples of threaded posts include the Kurer post (Figure 19-15), the Dentatus (Dentatus USA, New York, New York) post, and the Flexi-Post (Essential Dental, South Hackensack, New Jersey) (Figure 19-16).

Recently, posts made of carbon fiber (C-Post, Aesthetic Post, and Light Post, Bisco, Inc, Schaumburg, Illinois), ceramic materials (Cerapost, Brasseler, Savannah, Georgia; Cosmopost, Ivoclar-Vivadent, Amherst, New York), and fiber-reinforced polymers (Ribbond, Ribbond, Inc, Seattle, Washington; Fibrekor Post System, Jeneric/Pentron, Wallingsford, Connecticut) have been introduced. Carbon fiber posts are made of unidirectional carbon fibers embedded in an epoxy matrix.[133–138] Esthetic versions of this post have a quartz exterior that makes the post tooth colored. Ceramic posts are made from zirconium dioxide.[139–142] Fiber-reinforced posts are made of a woven polyethylene fiber ribbon that is coated with a dentin bonding agent and packed into the canal, where it is then light polymerized in position.[143]

Research indicates that carbon fiber posts possess adequate rigidity,[134] are not prone to produce tooth fracture,[135,136,138] and have been shown to be clinically successful.[137] It is reported that carbon fiber posts can

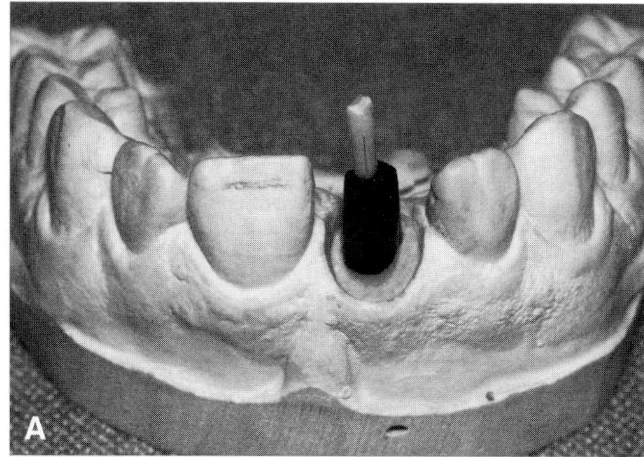

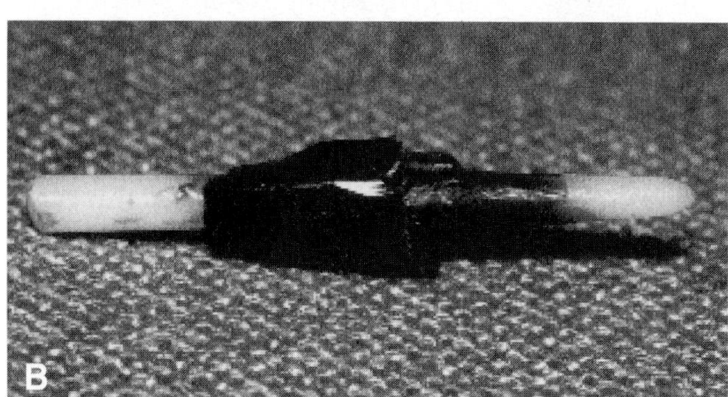

Figure 19-12 Custom-cast post and core. **A**, Wax pattern form around plastic post on a cast. **B**, Pattern removed from the cast. **C**, Casting has been finished and seated on the cast.

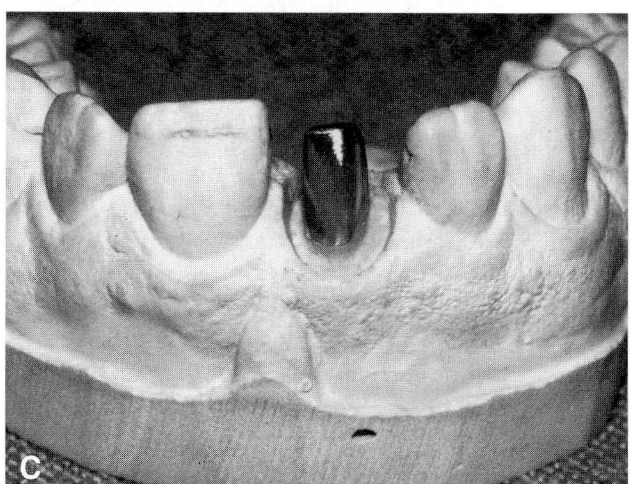

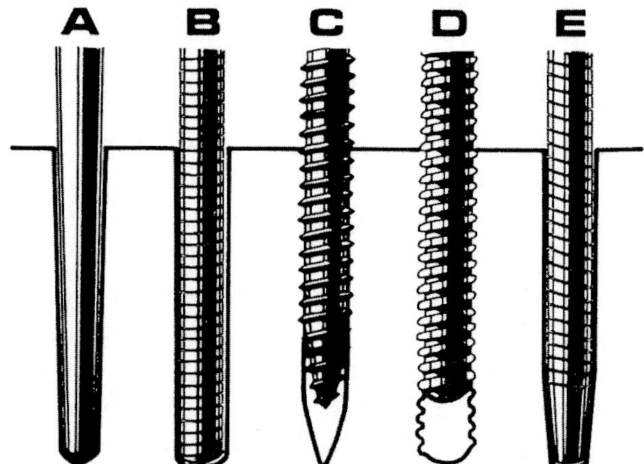

Figure 19-13 Prefabricated post designs. **A**, Tapered, smooth. **B**, Parallel, serrated. **C**, Tapered, self-threading. **D**, Parallel, threaded. Note that the post fits into pretapped threads in the dentin. **E**, Parallel, serrated, tapered end.

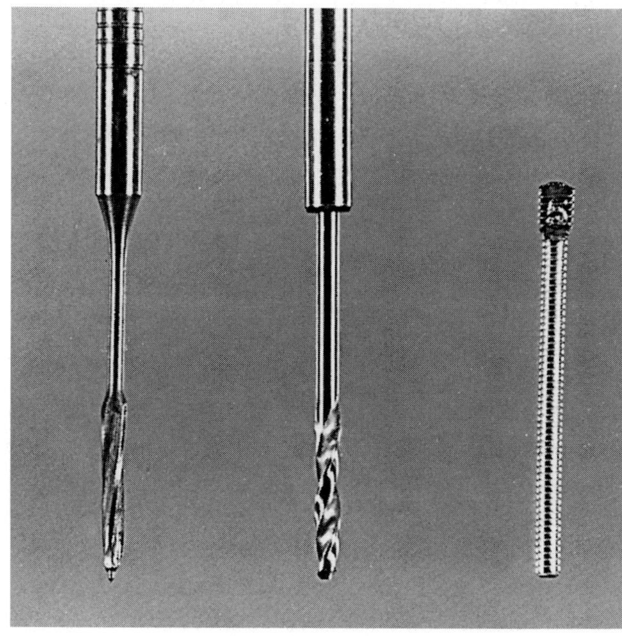

Figure 19-14 Whaledent, parallel-sided, vented, serrated post (**right**). The canal is enlarged with a Peeso reamer (**left**) and the final channel preparation is made with a matched twist drill (**center**).

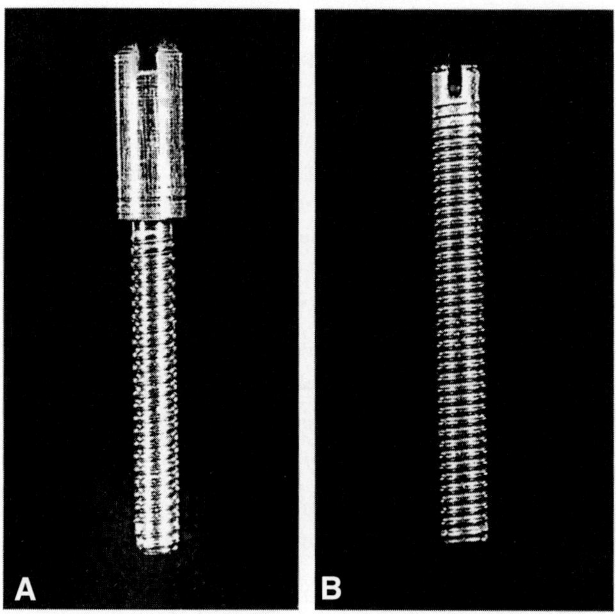

Figure 19-15 Kurer posts. A, Standard anchor. B, Crown saver.

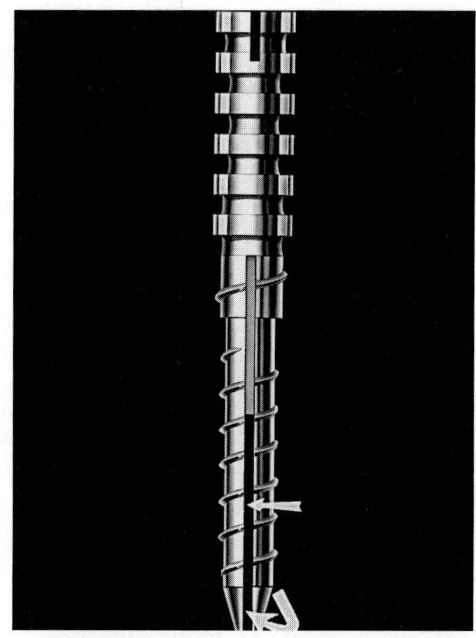

Figure 19-16 Flexi-post. Note the "split" in the apical portion of the post that permits some flexion to occur during placement.

be removed from the tooth. Ceramic posts have very high flexual strengths and are very hard.[139,141] When polyethylene fiber-reinforced posts were compared with metal posts in the laboratory, the fiber-reinforced posts reduced the incidence of vertical root fracture.[143]

The authors prefer to use posts designed for cementation whenever possible. However, when post retention is a critical success factor and available root length is limited, threaded designs are appropriate and necessary.

For teeth with large and/or round roots with substantial remaining root thickness after endodontic treatment is completed, either a prefabricated post or custom cast post can be used. If root preparation required to accommodate a prefabricated (round) post form will reduce dentin thickness to less than a millimeter, then a custom-cast post becomes the safest type of post.

Root Selection for Multirooted Teeth

When posts and cores are needed in molars, posts are best placed in roots that have the greatest dentin thickness and the smallest developmental root depressions. The most appropriate roots (the primary roots) in maxillary molars are the palatal roots, and in mandibular molars, they are the distal roots. The buccal roots of maxillary molars and the mesial root of mandibular molars should be avoided if at all possible. If these roots must be used in addition to the primary roots, then the post length should be short (3 to 4 mm) and a small-diameter instrument should be used (no larger than a No. 2 Peeso instrument, which is 1.0 mm in diameter). When 7 mm long posts were placed in the mesial root of mandibular molars, 20 of the 75 tested teeth had only a thin layer of remaining dentin or were perforated.[90]

Type of Definitive Restoration

It is important to know the type of single crown or retainer (all-metal, all-ceramic, metal ceramic) that will be used as the definitive restoration for each endodontically treated tooth that requires a post and core. This knowledge permits the tooth to be reduced in accordance with the reduction depths and form recommended for each type of crown/retainer.

TECHNICAL PROCEDURES

Coronal Tooth Preparation

Post and core fabrication can often best be done after the coronal tooth preparation has been completed (Figure 19-17). The amount of tooth structure that needs to be removed is related to the type of crown to be used, and that, in turn, determines the extent of core fabrication. For instance, if some of the remaining tooth structure is very thin after the coronal preparations, it is better to remove that part of dentin and replace it as part of the core.

Pulp Chamber Preparation

The pulp chamber should be cleaned of any filling material prior to post space preparation (Figure 19-18). If a

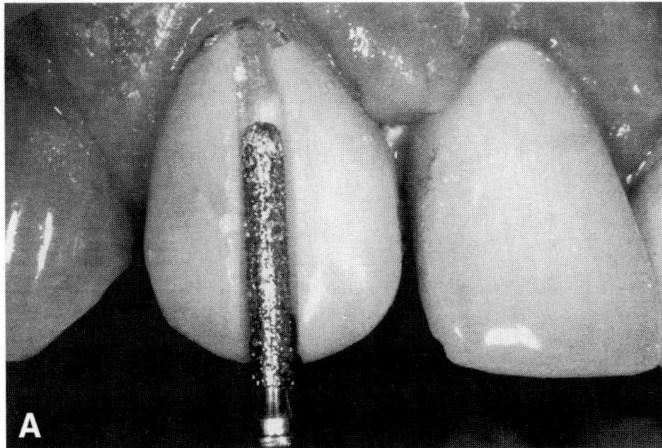

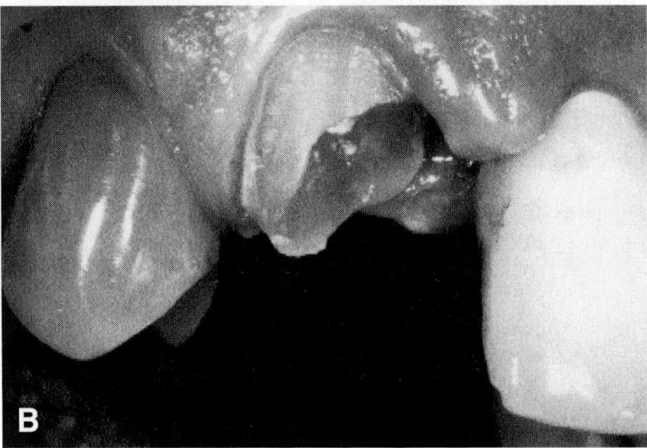

Figure 19-17 Coronal tooth preparation. **A**, Existing crown being removed on an endodontically treated tooth. **B**, Initial reduction of the tooth has been completed to permit assessment of the integrity of the remaining coronal tooth structure.

prefabricated post is to be used, undercuts and irregularities in the pulp chamber will help retain the core material. If a custom-cast post is indicated, the undercuts in the chamber should be blocked out with filling material or eliminated by removing tooth structure.

Root Canal Preparation

The best time to prepare the post space is at the time the root canal treatment is completed. If the post space needs to be prepared later, the gutta-percha can be removed using either a warm endodontic plugger or an endodontic file or a slow-speed rotary instrument such as a Gates-Glidden drill (Figure 19-19) or a Peeso drill (Figure 19-20). It is always prudent to isolate the tooth with a rubber dam during these procedures. The root canal filling material should be removed incrementally until the desired post space depth is achieved (Figure 19-21). A periodontal probe is well suited for measuring preparation depth.

Prefabricated Cemented or Bonded Post/Restorative Material Core (see Figures 19-22, 19-23, 19-24)

1. The root canal filling material is removed using a warm endodontic plugger or a small-diameter rotary instrument until the desired post depth is achieved (Figure 19-24, A).
2. The canal is enlarged in size using the rotary instrument that corresponds to the final dimension of the selected post. Selected post dimensions should correspond to those previously recommended post diameters for specific teeth (Figure 19-24, B). The post should fit passively into the post space without substantial movement (Figure 19-24, C).
3. At least the apical half of the post should fit closely to the preparation. The coronal half of the post may not fit as well because of root canal flaring. However, this lack of adaptation can be corrected when the core material is placed around the cemented post.
4. If the root canal cannot be prepared to conform to the round shape of the post and have adequate

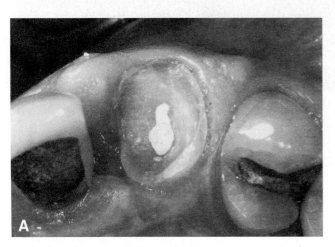

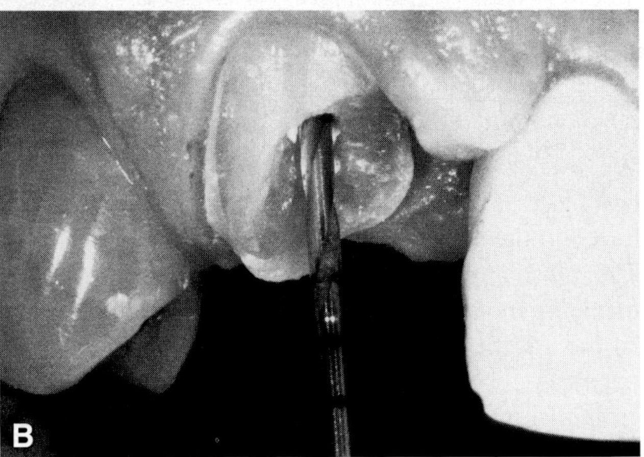

Figure 19-18 Pulp chamber preparation. **A**, Incisal view showing presence of provisional material sealing the coronal access. **B**, Rotary instrument being used to remove provisional material.

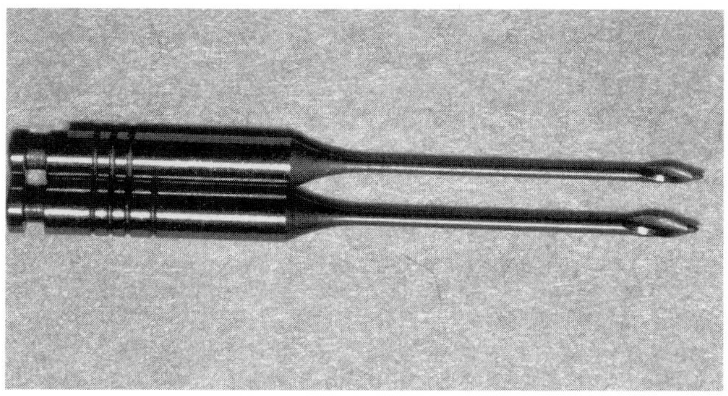

Figure 19-19 Two different diameters of Gates-Glidden drills.

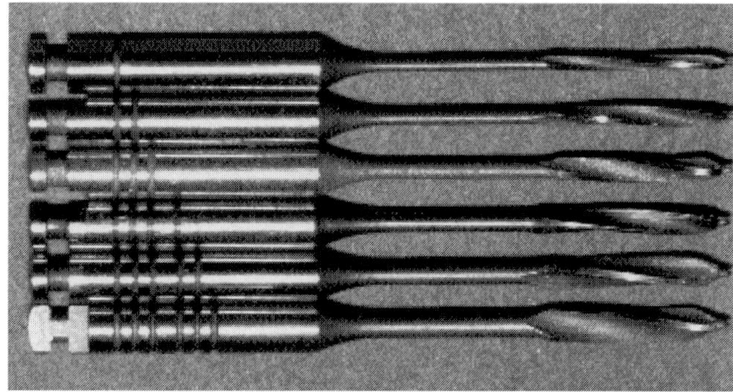

Figure 19-20 Set of six Peeso reamers.

approximation to the root canal walls, then a custom-cast post may be preferable.

5. Care must be taken not to remove more dentin at the apical extent of the post space than is necessary.
6. Radiographic confirmation is important to ensure proper seating and length of the post.
7. The incisal/occlusal end of the post is shortened (Figure 19-24, D) so that it does not interfere with the opposing occlusion, but it must provide support and retention for the restorative core material (2 to 3 mm).
8. When metal posts are used, they can be bent coronally, if necessary, to align them within the core material (Figure 19-25). Post bending is done outside the mouth with orthodontic pliers.
9. The post is cemented into the root canal using **resin bonding procedures** (Figure 19-24, E).
10. If there is little or no remaining coronal tooth structure to provide resistance to core rotation, an auxiliary threaded pin (TMS pins, minimum or regular; Coltene/Whaledent; Mahwah, N.J.) should be placed into the remaining tooth structure (Figure 19-24, F).

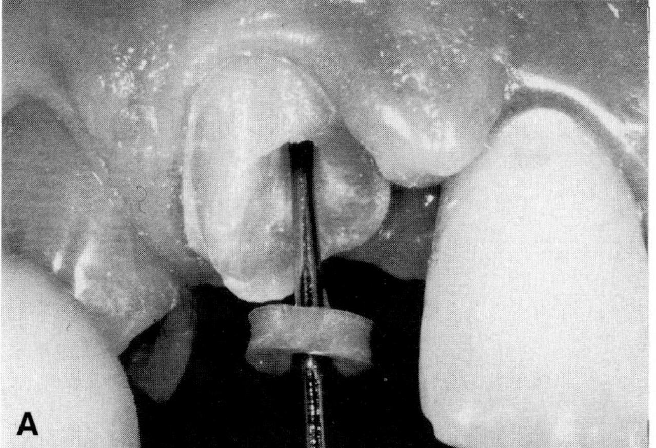

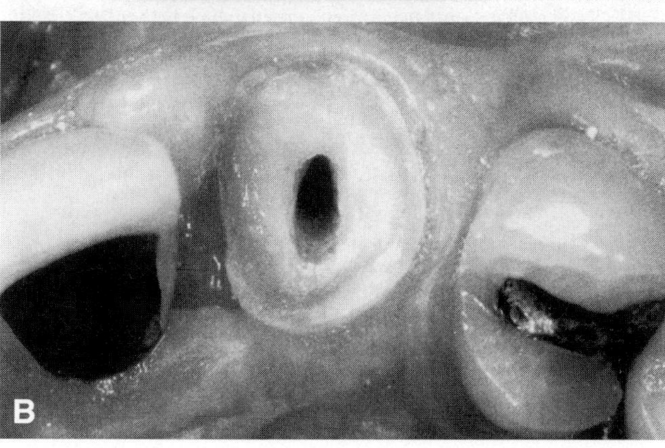

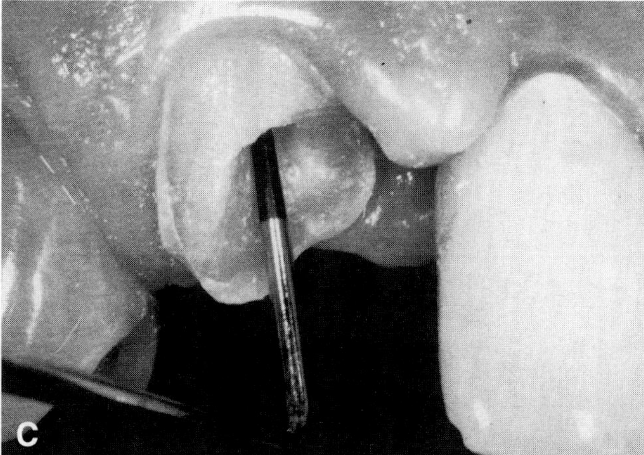

Figure 19-21 Root canal preparation. **A,** Rotary instrument being used to prepare post space in a root canal. Note the rubber ring around the instrument to identify the appropriate apical extension of the post preparation. **B,** Post space preparation completed. **C,** Periodontal probe being used to measure post space depth.

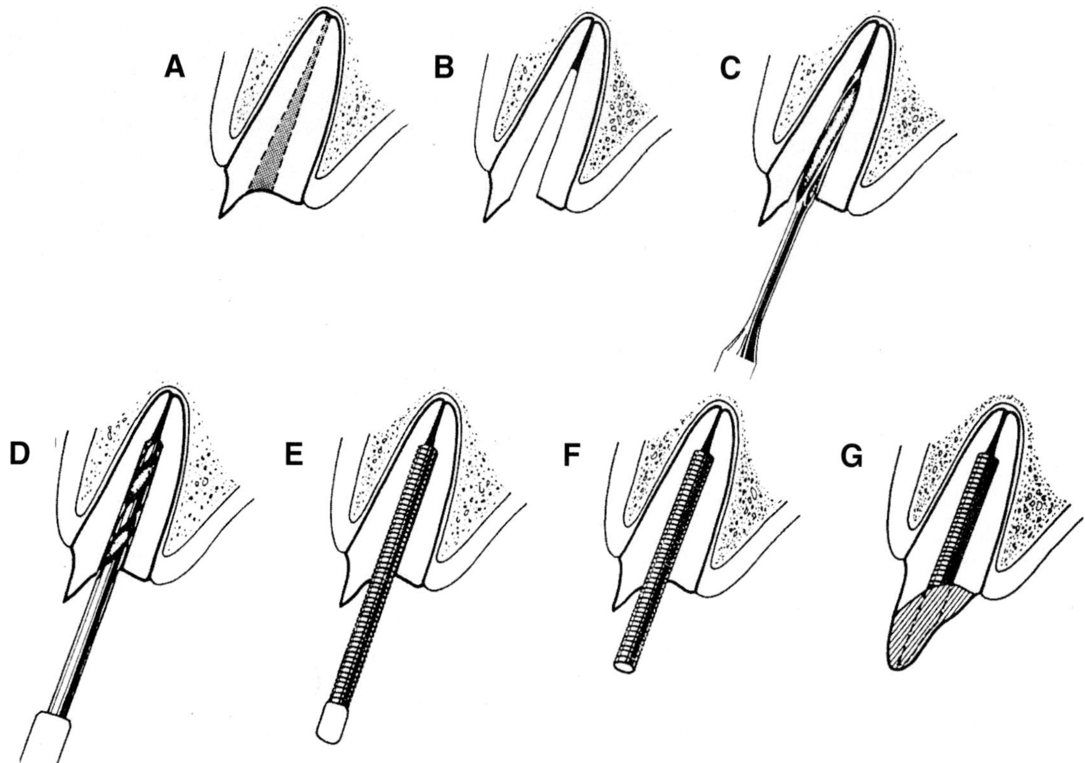

Figure 19-22 Placement of parallel-walled Para-Post and composite resin core in an anterior tooth. **A,** Endodontic treatment completed and initial crown preparation formed on remaining coronal tooth structure. **B,** Gutta-percha removed. **C,** Post space being formed using a Peeso instrument. **D,** Post space being refined using a Para-Post drill. **E,** Trial placement of the post to verify adequate approximation to post space without binding. **F,** The post has been shortened so that it does not interfere with occlusal closure and there will be space for fabrication of the crown. The post was cemented after shortening. **G,** The tooth has been etched and a bonded composite resin core formed and then shaped using rotary instruments.

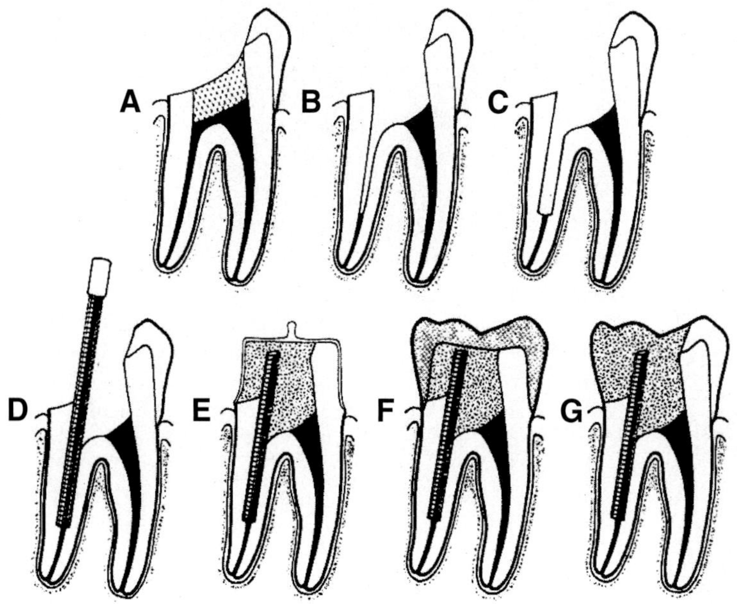

Figure 19-23 Placement of Para-Post and restorative material core in a molar. **A,** Endodontic treatment completed. **B,** Provisional restorative material in the pulp chamber has been removed and gutta-percha removed from the distal root. **C,** Post space formed with a drill. **D,** Trial placement of the post. **E,** The post has been shortened and cemented. A restorative material core has been formed. **F,** The core has been prepared, an impression made, and the definitive crown cemented. **G,** If there will be an extended time delay between placement of the core and preparation of the tooth for a crown, the core can be built to full tooth contour to serve as the interim restoration.

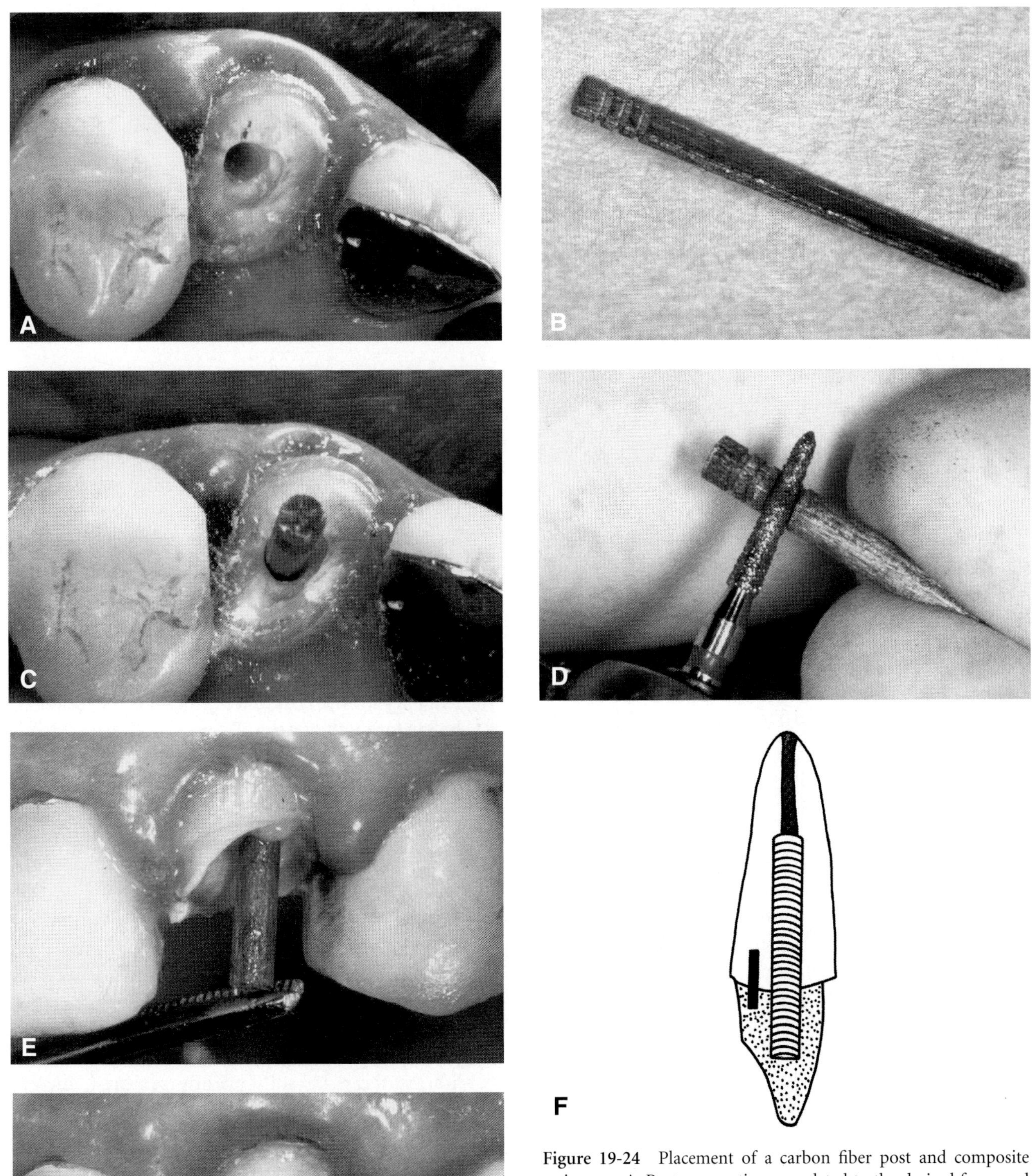

Figure 19-24 Placement of a carbon fiber post and composite resin core. **A**, Post preparation completed to the desired form and depth. Note the antirotation notch prepared into the dentin. **B**, Carbon fiber post. **C**, Post placed into the canal to verify adequate adaptation and passivity. **D**, Post being shortened using a diamond instrument so that there is adequate occlusal clearance. **E**, The post has been bonded into the root canal. **F**, Diagram showing placement of a threaded pin because there was a lack of coronal tooth structure to augment core retention. **G**, The composite resin core has been bonded to the dentin. The tooth preparation can now be completed by decreasing the total occlusal convergence, refining the finish line, and smoothing the surfaces.

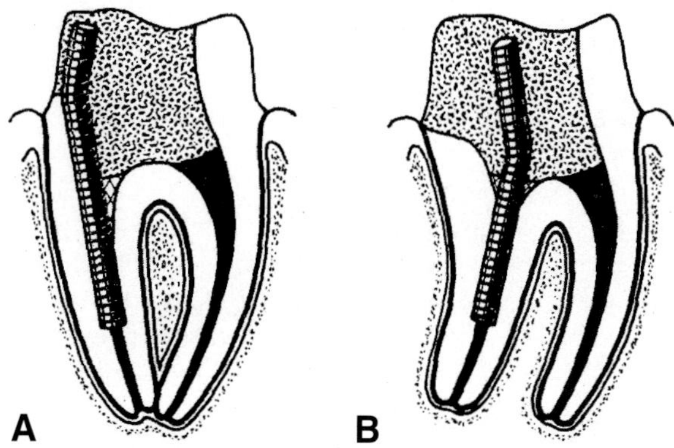

Figure 19-25 Coronal portion of posts are bent prior to cementation to place them more strategically within core. A, For containment inside preparation contour. B, For a more central location in core material.

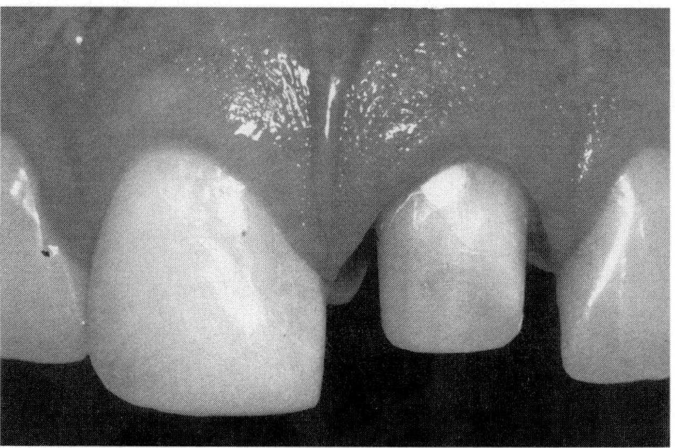

Figure 19-26 Definitive tooth preparations. Composite resin core and remaining coronal tooth structure of a maxillary central incisor have been prepared for a definitive all-ceramic crown.

11. Restorative material is then condensed around the post or bonded to the post and remaining tooth structure. A slight excess of material is placed, and this is removed during crown preparation (Figure 19-24, G).
12. The definitive tooth preparation is then completed (Figure 19-26), and an impression is made for the crown.

Prefabricated Threaded Post/ Restorative Material Core

1. The root canal filling material is removed as described.
2. The canal is sequentially enlarged using the manufacturer's provided rotary instruments until the desired diameter is achieved.
3. The Kurer post system uses a root facer to prepare a flat area on the coronal surface of the root against which the incorporated metal core can seat (Figure 19-27). Other threaded posts (such as the Flexi-post) use a restorative material for the core (Figure 19-28) and therefore do not need such an instrument.
4. Either the root is threaded using a hand tap (Kurer) or the post is threaded into the canal (Flexi-post).
5. The core is formed by either reshaping the attached metal core (Kurer) or building a restorative material core to the desired dimensions and then preparing it for the definitive crown.

Custom-Cast Post and Core

This procedure for making a custom-cast post and core is illustrated in Figure 19-29:

1. The root canal filling material is removed as described. It is not necessary or desirable to make the post space round.
2. Since most custom-cast posts and cores will possess a slightly tapered form, a flat area should be prepared in the remaining coronal tooth structure if there is not one already present in existing morphology. This flat area (formed perpendicular to the long axis of the post) will serve as a positive stop during cementation of the post and during subsequent application of occlusal forces, thereby helping to minimize any tendency for the post to wedge against the tooth.
3. The custom-cast post and core can either be made indirectly on a cast obtained from an impression or fabricated from a pattern made directly on the tooth. The indirect process is often the technique of choice for teeth with difficult or limited access.

Direct Procedure

1. Select a plastic post that fits within the confines of the post preparation without binding (Figure 19-30, A). Leave the post sufficiently long that it can be easily grasped.
2. Lightly lubricate the canal (using a water-soluble lubricant such as die lubricant helps ensure that all lubricant can be subsequently removed, thereby not interfering with cement retention).
3. Place notches on the side of a plastic post pattern if the post is smooth and seat it to the depth of the prepared canal.
4. Use the bead-brush technique to apply resin to the prepared canal and the body of the plastic post. Seat the post into the full depth of the canal.
5. **Do not allow** the resin to completely harden within the canal. Remove and reseat the post and attached resin several times while the resin is still in its rubbery stage so that the pattern does not inadvertently become locked into the canal (Figure 19-30, B).

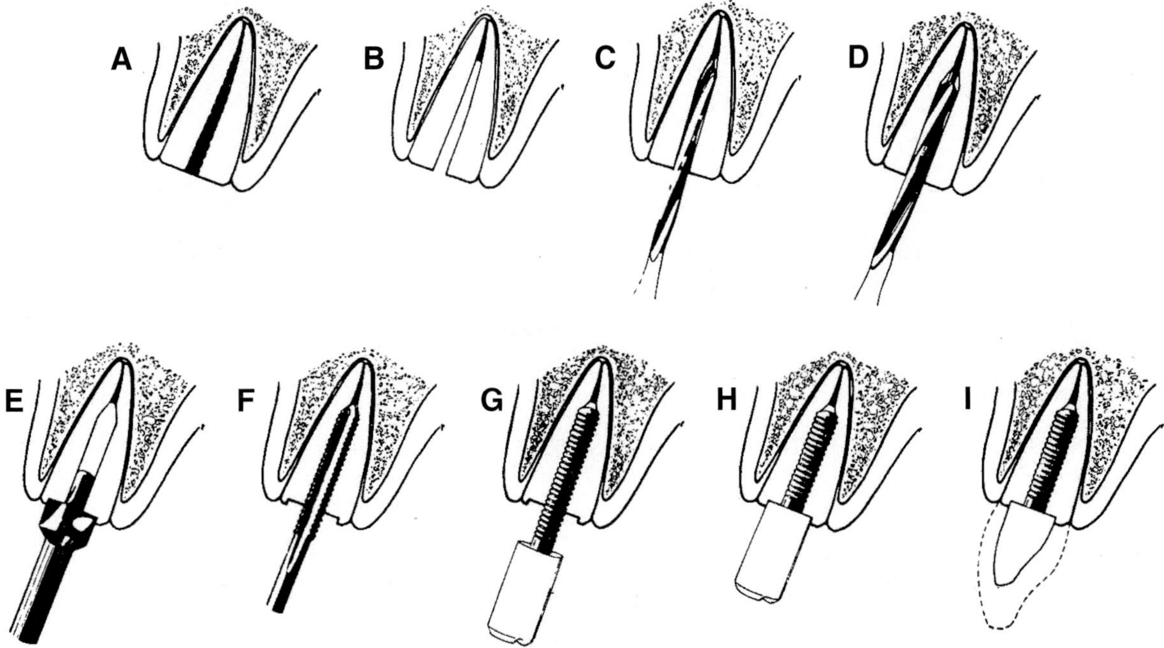

Figure 19-27 Placement of a prefabricated, threaded Kurer post. A, Completed endodontic therapy. B, Gutta-percha removed. C, Initial preparation of the root canal. D, Final diameter established, which also determines the size of the tap and the post that will be used. E, Preparing countersink using a Root Facer instrument (Kurer, Kerr Corporation, Orange. California). F, Hand tap being used to create threads in the root. G, Trail placement of a post to determine how much of the post must be shortened. H, Shortened post in place. I, The prefabricated metal core has been prepared to a form that represents the shape of a prepared tooth and will provide appropriate space for fabrication of a crown.

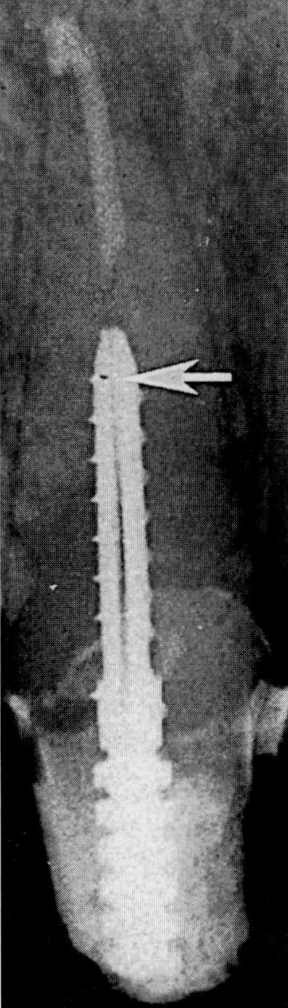

Figure 19-28 Flexi-post has been placed into the root and a composite resin material built around the post.

6. Remove the polymerized pattern and inspect the resin for integrity and lack of voids. Reseat the post and test for adaptation and passivity.
7. Add additional coronal resin to form the desired dimensions of the core (Figure 19-30, C). Remove and reseat the pattern as previously described to prevent it from becoming locked into the coronal tooth structure (Figure 19-30, D). A slight excess of core resin is added (Figure 19-30, E) so that the hardened core can be prepared with a high-speed diamond and water spray to the desired form (Figure 19-30, F).
8. The core is then removed, invested, and cast.
9. The post and core are trial placed, adjusted, and then cemented. The definitive tooth preparation can then be completed.
10. A pattern can also be developed using wax rather than resin.

Indirect Procedure

1. Nonaqueous elastomeric impression materials make accurate impressions of the prepared root canal, but some method of supporting the impression material prevents distortion/displacement of the set material during removal from the mouth and pouring of the cast.

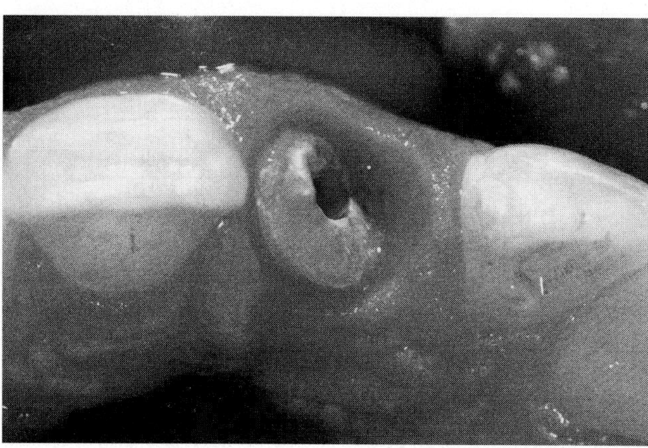

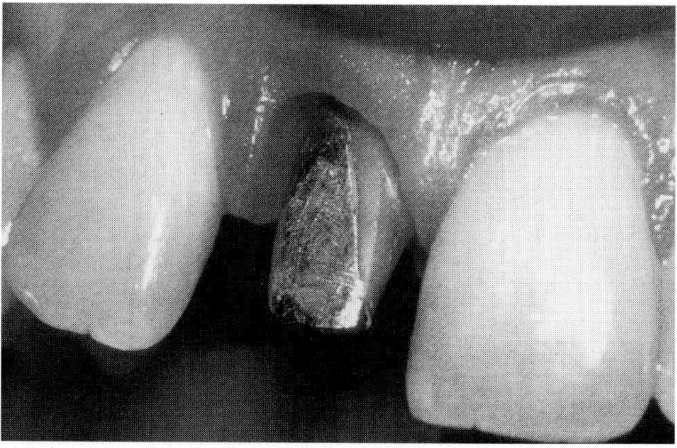

Figure 19-29 Custom-cast post and core. **A**, Traumatically fractured central incisor after endodontic treatment and post space preparation. **B**, Cast post and core seated in the tooth.

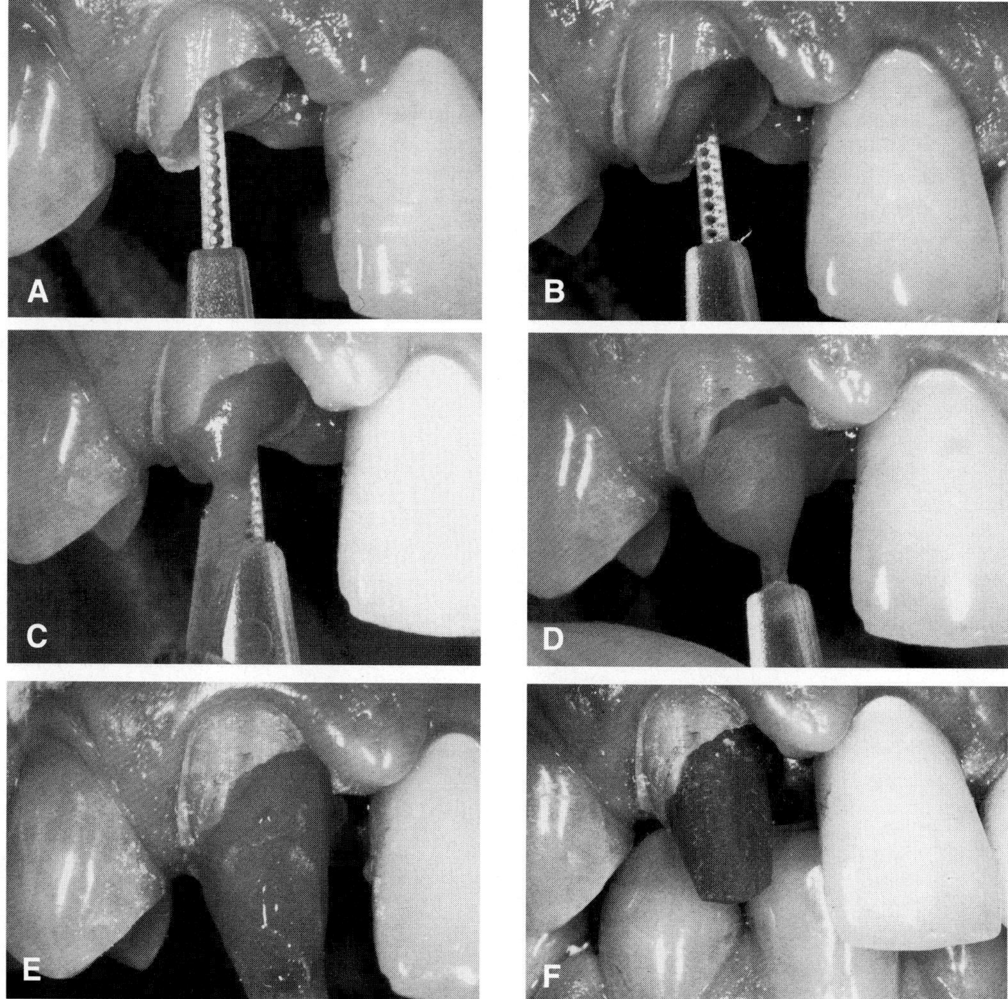

Figure 19-30 Fabrication of a direct pattern for a custom-cast post and core. **A**, Plastic post selected that fits passively into the prepared post space. **B**, Resin has been placed into the prepared root canal and the plastic post seated to the depth of the canal. Note that the plastic post is being removed before the resin completely hardens to ensure that the resin post does not become locked into the prepared post space. **C**, Additional unfilled resin is being applied using a bead-brush technique to build a core. **D**, The core buildup is being removed before it completely hardens to again prevent the resin from becoming locked into position. **E**, Excess core material has been applied. **F**, Initial preparation of the resin core has been completed. The pattern can now be removed and cast and the final tooth preparation completed after the post and core are cemented.

2. Several methods of support are available. A metal wire that returns to its original shape when slightly distorted is desirable. Safety pins (Figure 19-31, A) and orthodontic wire have been used for this purpose. Metal wire such as a paper clip can be bent on impression removal and be permanently distorted. Plastic posts are also used to support the impression material (Figure 19-32, C). They can be flexed in slightly curved canals or if they contact coronal tooth structure. Subsequent removal of the post after the impression material sets allows straightening of the plastic post to occur, resulting in distortion. Only use plastic posts when they are **totally passive and do not bind** on any tooth structure.
3. When a safety pin or orthodontic wire is selected as the means of supporting the impression material, the coronal portion of the wire should be bent over to form a handle and to help retain it in the impression material (Figure 19-31, B).
4. Notch the wire and coat it with adhesive (see Figure 19-31, B).
5. Fill the prepared canal with impression material using a slowly rotating lentulo spiral instrument (Dentsply Maillefer North America, Tulsa, Ok) (Figure 19-31, C) accompanied by an up and down motion (Figure 19-31, D).
6. Alternately, an anesthetic needle can be placed to the depth of the post space (to serve as an air escape channel) and impression material syringed down the canal (Figure 19-32, A and B).
7. Seat the wire or plastic post through the impression material to the full depth of the canal (Figure 19-31, E), syringe additional impression material around the supporting device as well as the prepared tooth (Figure 19-31, F), and seat the impression tray (Figure 19-31, G).
8. Remove the impression (Figure 19-31, H), evaluate it, and pour a cast.
9. Make an interocclusal record and obtain an opposing cast and appropriately sized plastic post to be used in forming a wax pattern (Figure 19-33, A).
10. Lightly lubricate the canal of the working cast with die lubricant (Figure 19-33, B).
11. Place notches on the side of a plastic post that seats to the full depth of the canal preparation.
12. Apply a very thin layer of sticky wax to the plastic post and then add soft inlay wax in small increments, fully seating the plastic post after each increment of wax is added (see Figure 19-33, B).
13. Ensure that the pattern is well adapted but passive (Figure 19-33, C).
14. After the post pattern has been fabricated, the wax core is added (Figure 19-33, D) and shaped, and then the pattern is cast in metal (see Figure 19-33, E).
15. The cast post and core are then cemented in the tooth and the definitive tooth preparation completed (Figure 19-33, F).

PREPARATION FOR OVERDENTURES

An overdenture is a complete denture supported by retained teeth and the residual alveolar ridge.[144] Because the retained teeth are shortened, contoured, and altered to be covered, they need to be endodontically treated (Figure 19-34).

In 1969, Lord and Teel coined the term "overdenture" and described the combined endodontic-periodontic-prosthodontic technique applied thereto.[145] As early as 1916, however, Prothero had referred to the use of root support, stating, "Oftentimes two or three widely separated roots or teeth can be utilized for supporting a denture."[2] It should also be noted that much earlier, in 1789, George Washington's first lower denture, constructed of ivory by John Greenwood, was in part supported by a left mandibular premolar.[146]

Retaining roots in the alveolar process is based on the proven observation that as long as the root remains, the bone surrounding it remains (Figure 19-35). This overcomes the age-old prosthetic problem of ridge resorption. Ideally, then, retaining four teeth, two molars and two canines—one each at the four divergent points of an arch—should provide good balance and long "life" to a full overdenture (Figure 19-36). Unfortunately, patients requiring prostheses seldom present just these ideal conditions, and the dentist must make do with the best that can be devised from the dentition remaining. One situation to be **warned against**, however, is the **diagonal cross-arch arrangement** —a molar abutment on one side, for example, and a canine on the opposite side. The rocking and torquing action set up by this arrangement leads to problems and loss of one or both abutments. The molar abutment alone is preferable to the diagonal cross-arch situation.

If the selected abutment teeth are reduced to a short rounded or **bullet shape**—literally "tucking" the abutments inside the denture base—the crown-root ratio of the tooth is vastly improved, especially when periodontally involved teeth have lost some alveolar support. As shortened teeth, however, they can serve quite well as abutments for full overdentures.

Indications and Advantages

The indications for overdentures include the psychic support some patients receive from **not** being totally

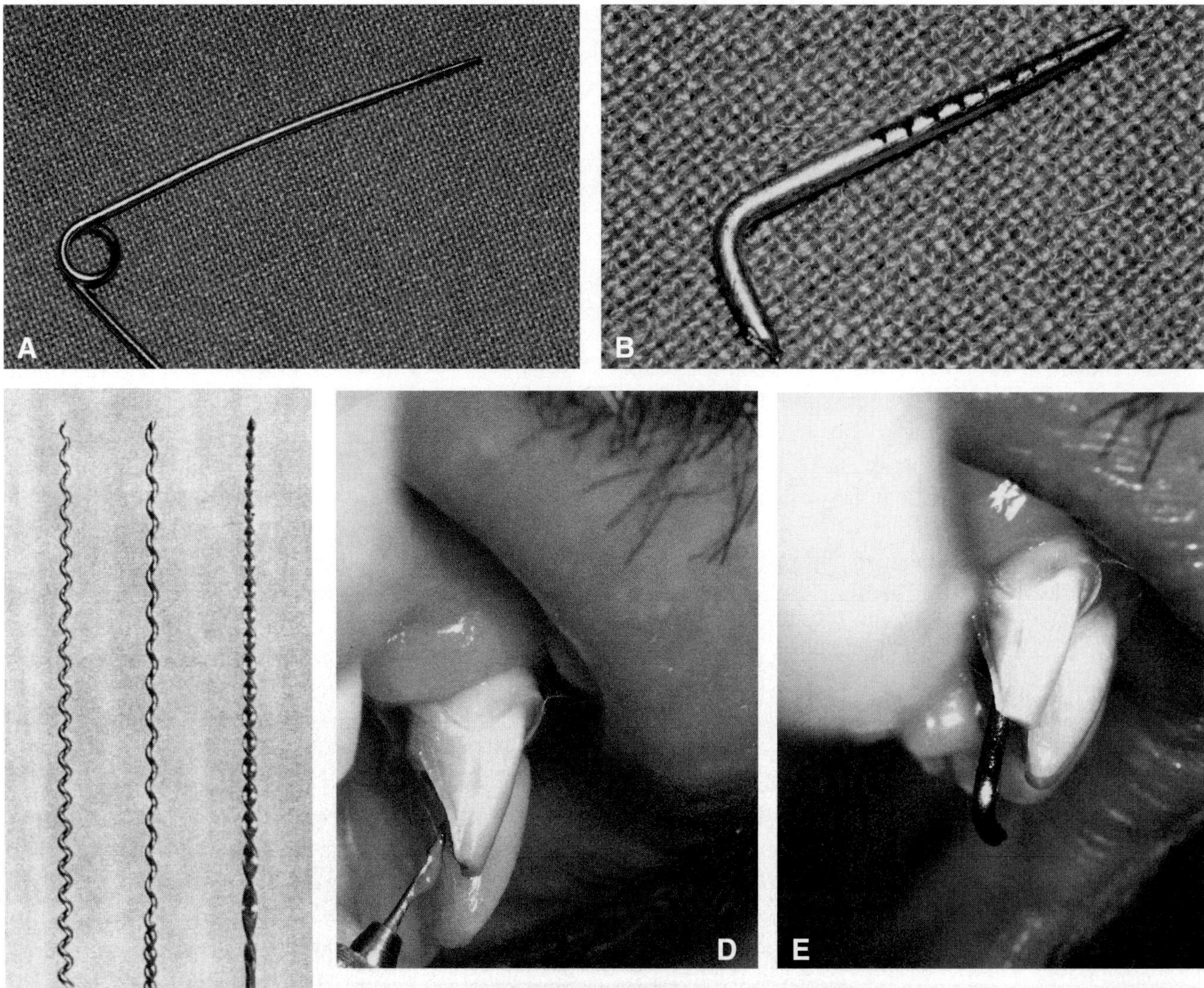

Figure 19-31 Post and core impression using safety pin wire and a spiral instrument for placing impression material. **A,** A safety pin that will be sectioned. **B,** The safety pin has been sectioned and bent so that the point extends to the depth of the post preparation and the bent portion projects above the tooth. The bent portion serves as a handle and also as a means of helping retain the wire in the impression material. Note that notches have been ground into the wire to facilitate retention of the impression material. The wire will now be coated with impression material adhesive. **C,** A lentulo spiral instrument that will be used to "spin" impression material to the apical portion of the post preparation. The corkscrew form of the instrument, when slowly rotating toward the root apex in a slow-speed handpiece, spirals the impression material to the depth of the prepared post space. **D,** A small portion of mixed impression material is picked up with the spiral instrument and placed into the prepared post space. The spiral instrument is being slowed rotated by the handpiece and moved up and down in the canal to place the impression into all aspects of the prepared post space. **E,** A section of the safety pin has been fully seated into the prepared post space.

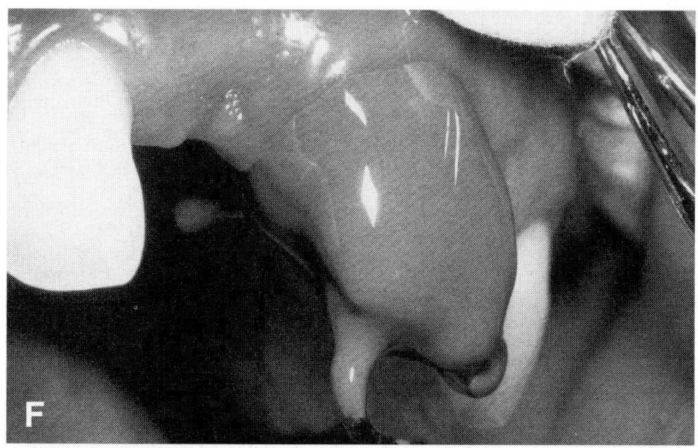

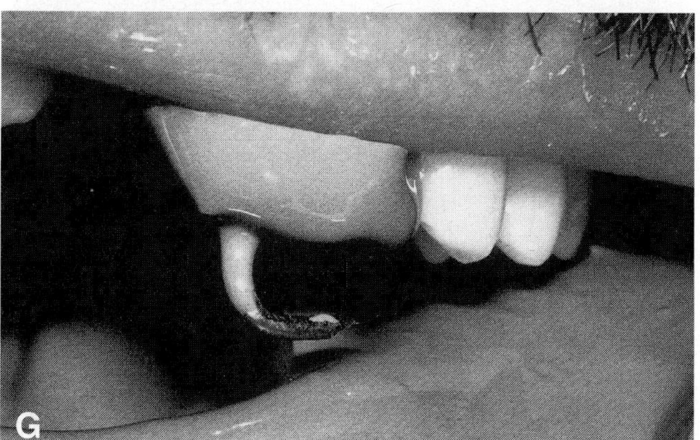

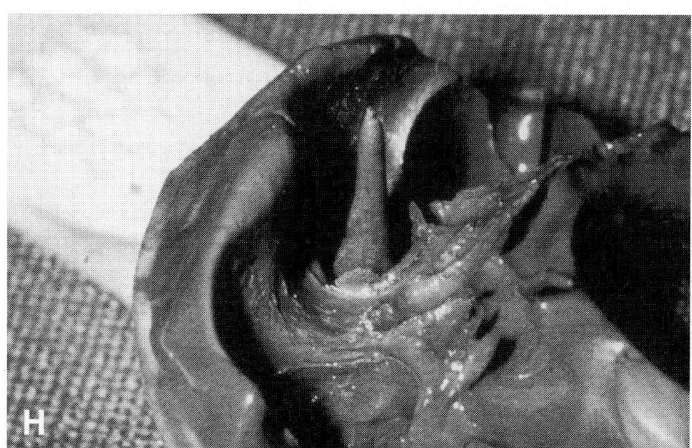

Figure 19-31 (*Continued*) **F**, Additional impression material has been syringed over the prepared tooth. **G**, Impression tray being seated. **H**, Completed impression.

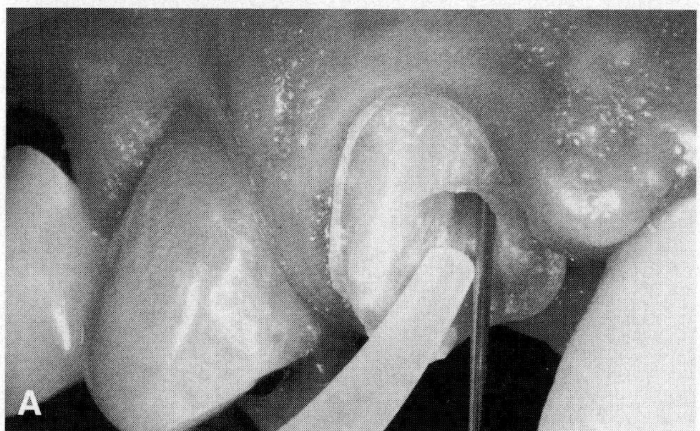

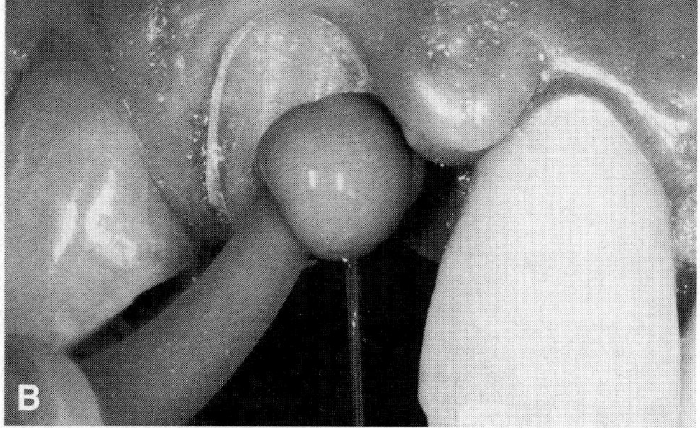

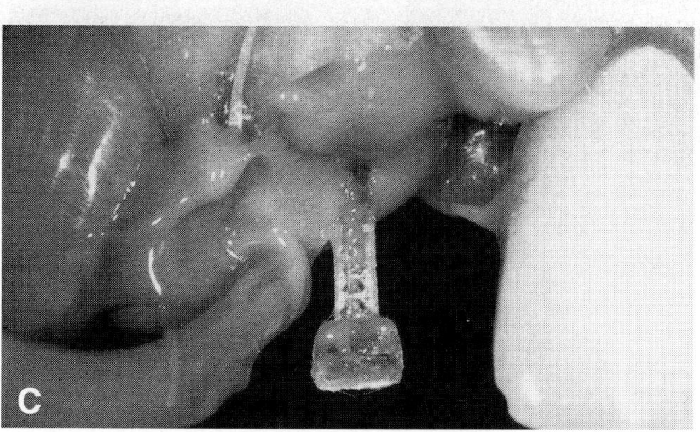

Figure 19-32 Post and core impression using an anesthetic needle, impression syringe, and poly (vinyl siloxane) impression material. **A**, An anesthetic needle seated to the base of a prepared post space and an impression syringe tip in position. **B**, Impression material being syringed down the prepared canal. **C**, A plastic post that fits passively into the canal is fully seated through impression material.

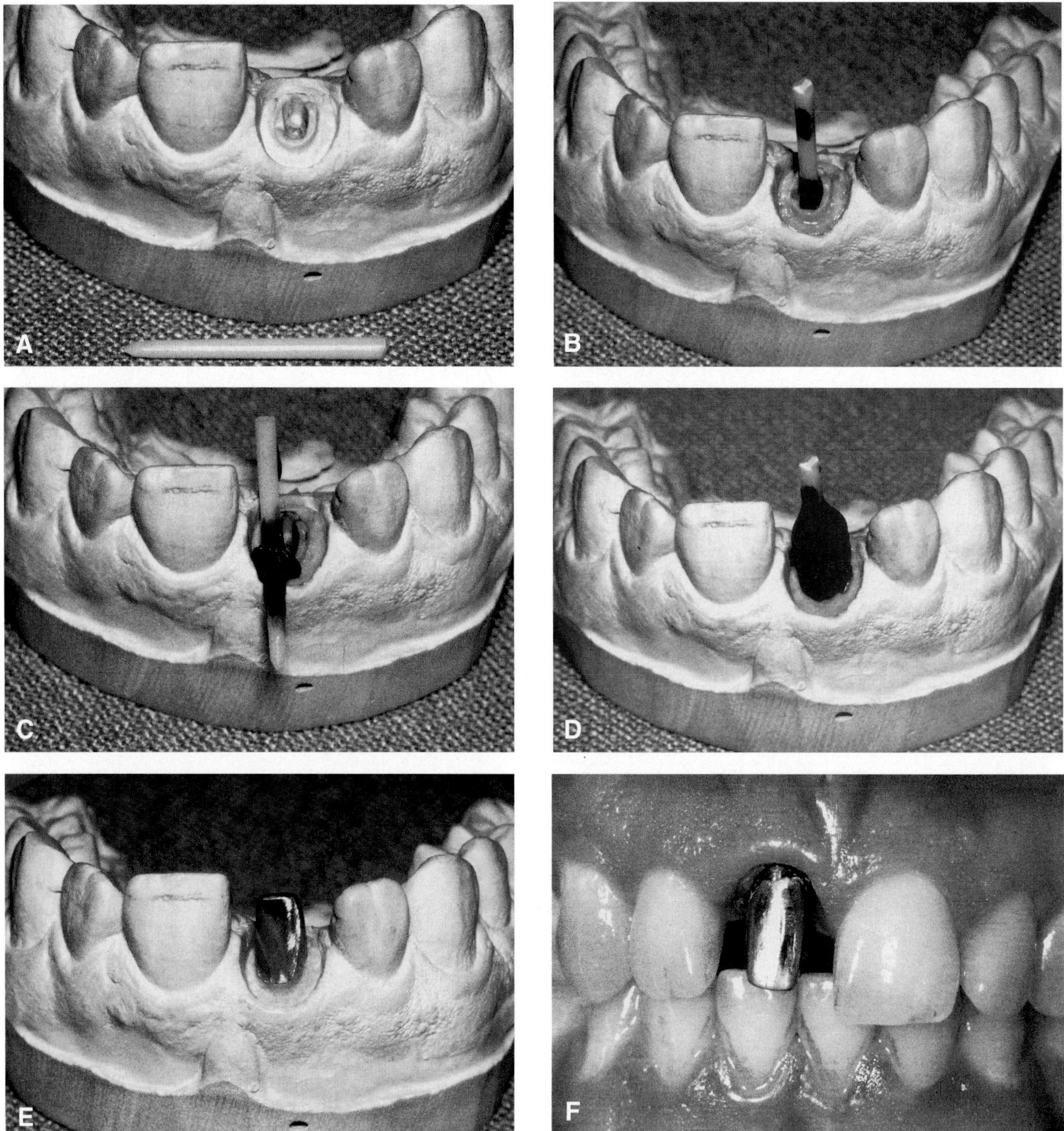

Figure 19-33 Indirect post fabrication on a working cast. **A,** Working cast with plastic post around which a wax pattern will be formed. The apical portion of the post has good approximation to the cast but is passive. **B,** The cast has been lubricated, a thin layer of wax applied to the plastic post, and the post fully seated into the cast while the wax is soft. **C,** A plastic post removed from the cast so that the wax adaptation can be evaluated. **D,** Wax added to the adapted post to form a core. The core will now be carved to the final form and then invested and cast. **E,** Casting seated on the working cast. The cast can be hand articulated with the opposing cast to establish the required occlusal clearance. **F,** Cast post and core cemented and preparation completed.

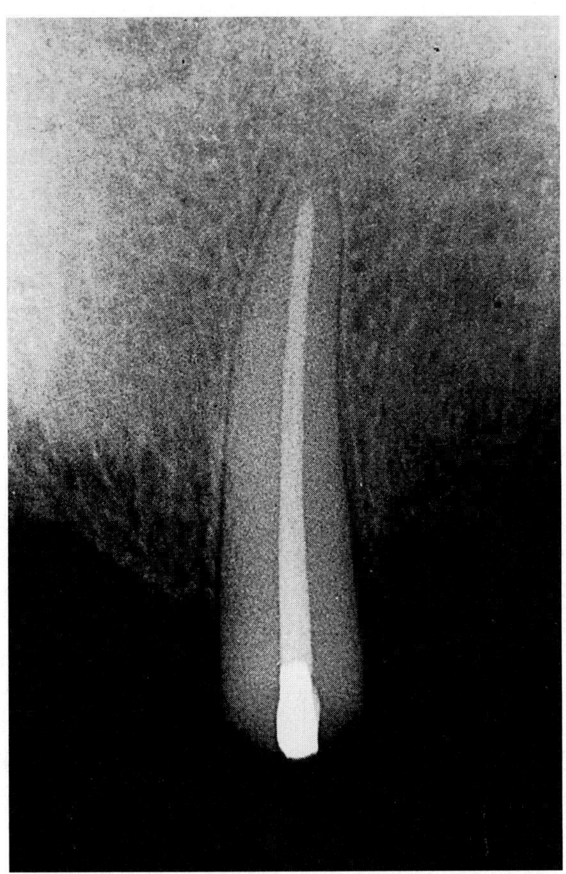

Figure 19-34 Overdenture abutment, well obturated and restored with amalgam. Note excellent bony support. (Courtesy of Dr. David H. Wands.)

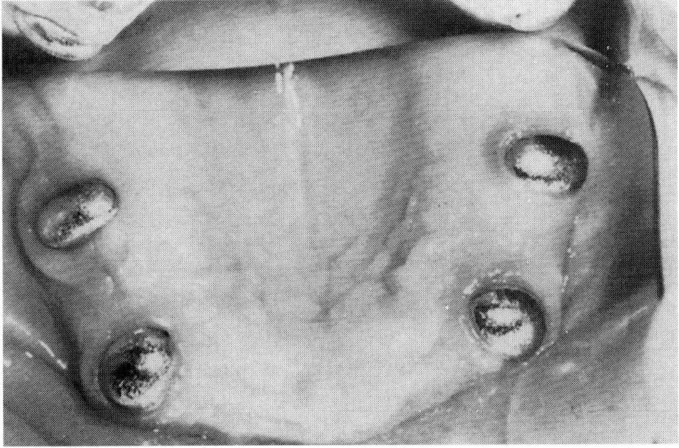

Figure 19-36 Mirror view of four retained abutments providing ideal support for an overdenture. Reproduced with permission from Brewer AA and Morrow RM.[149]

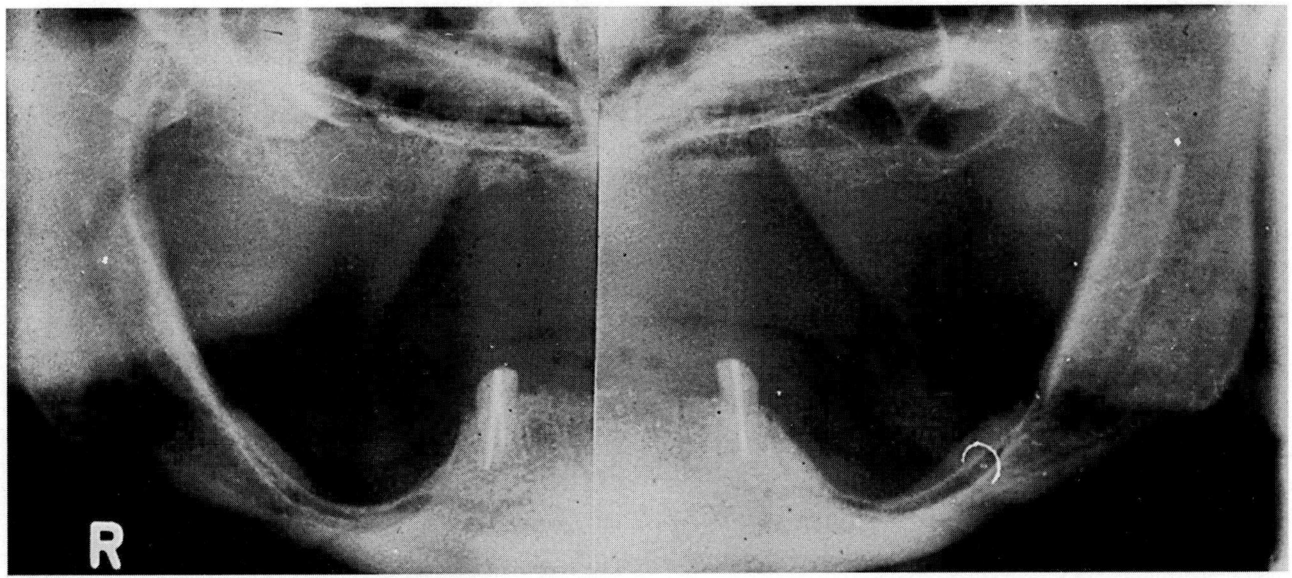

Figure 19-35 Dramatic demonstration of alveloar bone remaining around retained canines but badly resorbed under full upper and osterior lower partial dentures. Reproduced with permission from Lord JL and Teel S.[144]

edentulous. Even more important is the preservation of the alveolar ridge and the shielding of the ridge from stress provided by firm abutment teeth. One should also be aware that vertical dimension is better preserved if ridge height is maintained. A bonus to all of these advantages is the support, stability, and retention derived from firm abutments.

Contraindications

Overdentures are contraindicated when remaining alveolar support is so lacking that no tooth can be retained for very long. Overdentures are also contraindicated if the remaining natural teeth are adequate to restore the mouth with fixed or removable partial dentures.

Abutment Tooth Selection

A healthy abutment tooth for an overdenture must have minimal mobility, a manageable sulcus depth, and an adequate band of attached gingiva.[145] If these prerequisites are lacking, the pocket depth can be reduced and the attached gingiva developed by proper periodontal procedures.

Abutment Tooth Location

The ideal teeth to retain are those located where occlusal forces wreak greatest destruction on the ridges. Opposite a natural dentition, the canine teeth are ideal to retain. In edentulous patients, the anterior portion of the arches is particularly susceptible to resorption, so canines and premolars are again the first choice to be saved, with incisors the second choice. It is especially important to save mandibular teeth because of difficulties encountered in retaining lower dentures. Even saving a single tooth, a molar in particular, may contribute greatly to long-term denture success.

Technique

After the selection of the proper abutment teeth, the key to successful overdenture construction is simplicity of technique. If an immediate denture is to be placed, the endodontic therapy, extractions, and periodontal treatment may all be done at the denture placement appointment. The teeth to receive root canal fillings are anesthetized, and a rubber dam is placed. The crowns of these teeth are then amputated 3 to 4 mm above the gingival level. The length of the remaining tooth is established radiographically, and the pulps are removed. The canals are then properly cleaned, shaped, and obturated with gutta-percha by means of the filling technique appropriate to the canal anatomy. The coronal 3 to 5 mm of the gutta-percha filling are then removed, the preparation is undercut, and a well-condensed amalgam filling is placed to cap the canal obturation. At this time as well, the abutments should be properly shaped to rise 2 to 3 mm above the tissue and to be rounded or bullet shaped with a slope back from the labial surface to accommodate the denture tooth to be set above it. They should then be highly polished (Figure 19-37). The abutments must not be too short or the tissue will grow over them as a "lawn grows over a sidewalk,"[144] nor should they be too long, compromising the denture contour and placing greater stress on the supporting teeth (Figure 19-38).

The denture is relieved over the abutment until it fits securely on the tissue without **touching the abutment teeth**. It is then related to the abutment teeth with a small amount of self-curing acrylic. This proper relationship of denture to tissue and tooth is important for denture stability and to keep the stresses on the teeth within physiologic limits.

This entire operation is neither complex nor time consuming. Removing the crown from the tooth greatly simplifies and speeds the endodontic therapy. Some candidates for overdenture abutment teeth may not need root canal therapy. The pulpless teeth may already have been successfully treated. Other teeth may be so abraded that the pulp has receded to a level where the tooth only needs shortening, proper contouring, and polishing (Figure 19-39).

If the abutment teeth are involved periodontally or are not surrounded by a good collar of attached gingiva, periodontal therapy will be needed to correct these aberrations.

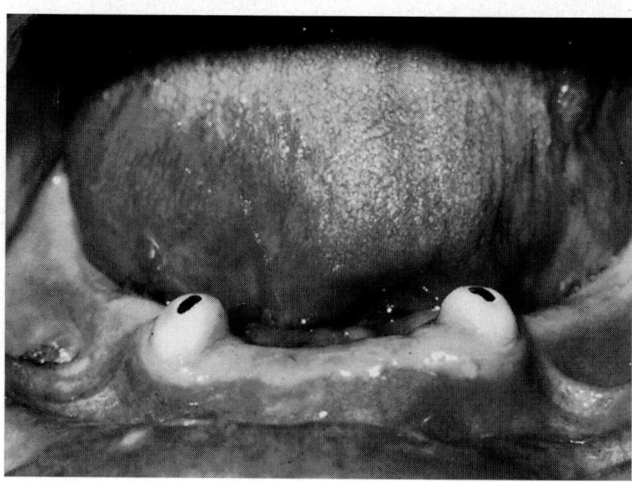

Figure 19-37 Mandibular canines that have served as overdenture abutments for years. Reproduced with permission from Fenton A, Brewer A. Dent Clin North Am 1973;17:723.

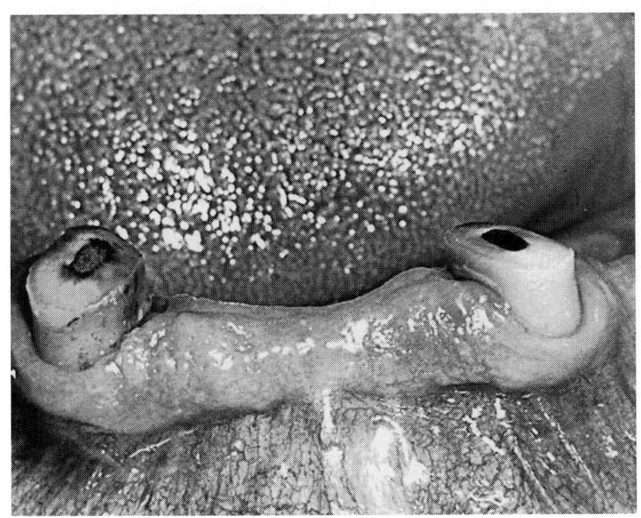

Figure 19-38 Improperly contoured overdenture abutments. Square edge invites grip by overdenture and torquing action. Prominent buccal contour and extra height comprised the contour of the overdenture. (Courtesy of Dr. David H. Wands.)

Problems

A number of problems have arisen with overdentures, most of them related to poor patient selection and lack of patient cooperation.

The most serious problems are associated with dental caries and periodontal disease. One must remember that, throughout their lives, candidates for complete dentures have usually been neglectful of their teeth and supporting structures and have a history of extensive dental disease. That is why they have reached this sad point (Figure 19-40). In recommending overdentures, the dentist takes an obvious chance that the patient's habits will change and that he will become motivated and adept at oral hygiene to retain the vestiges of this dentition. That some do not should come as no surprise (Figure 19-41). The importance of good home care must be emphasized to the overdenture patient.

Other challenges related to the use of endodontically treated teeth include wear of the dentin and the need for retention.

Possible Solutions to the Problems

Quite naturally, the prime solution to the caries-periodontal problem is better patient cooperation in home care. A special 0.4% stannous fluoride gel has been introduced to be placed in the "well" in the base plate to remineralize the dentin.[147,148] This, of course, will do nothing for periodontal disease, which can be controlled only by plaque removal and by proper and equal force placed on the abutments. More frequent denture relines may also be required.

Coverage of the dentin surfaces is recommended for those situations wherein severe abrasion of the tooth has occurred (Figures 19-42 and 19-43). Bruxism would be the principal etiologic factor. Even gold may eventually be worn through,[149] but it takes a much longer time.

A possible solution to inadequate denture retention or to the rotational problem centering around the single anterior abutment tooth may be with mechanical attachments. There are a number on the market, and

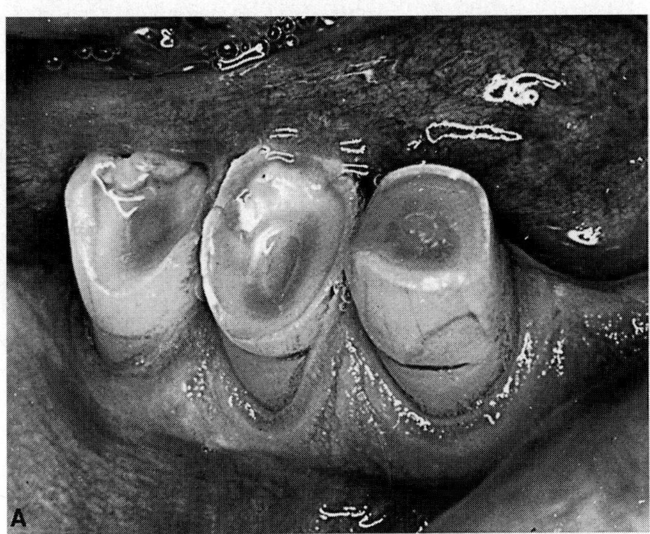

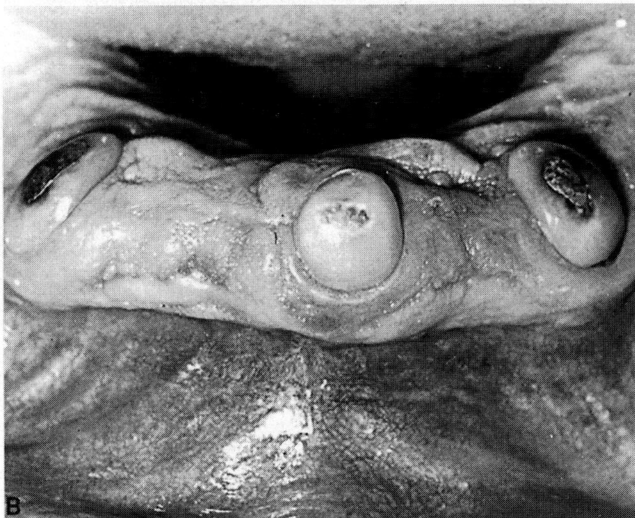

Figure 19-39 **A,** Vital teeth with severe abrasion and receded pulps—ideal overdenture abutments. **B,** Incisor overdenture abutment not requiring therapy owing to pulp recession. The calcified pulp area should be carefully explored for the pulp horn. (Courtesy of Dr. David H. Wands.)

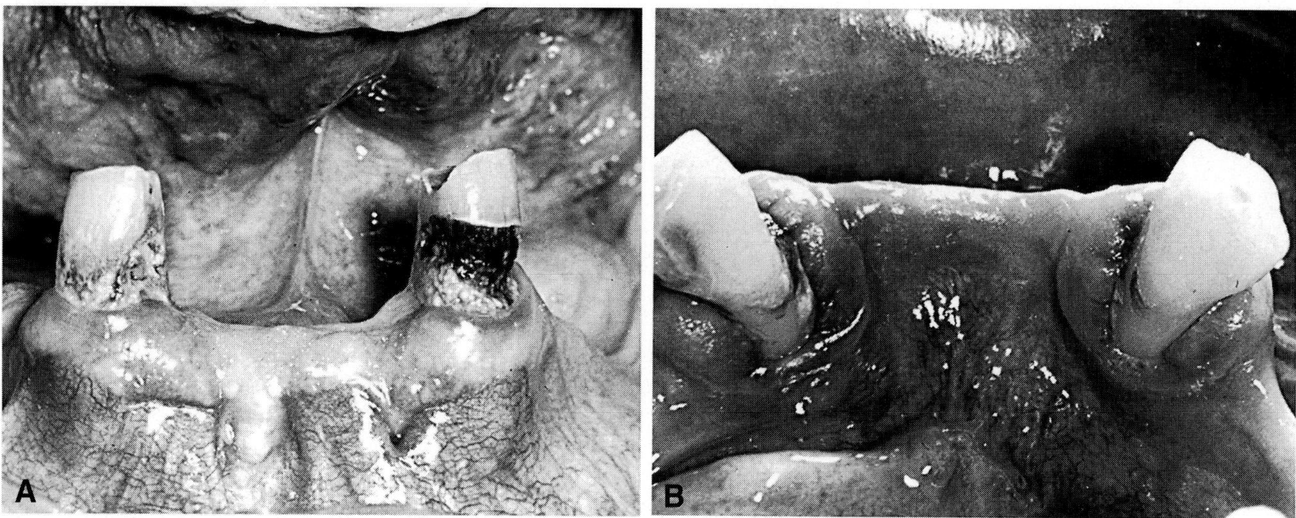

Figure 19-40 **A,** Rather typical neglect by many denture patients. Caries and periodontal disease forecast probable lack of future patient cooperation. **B,** Mirrow view of lingual gingiva of two possible overdenture abutments. Because it is virtually impossible to develop attached gingiva in the lingual area, use of these teeth as abutments is **contraindicated.** (Courtesy of Dr. David H. Wands.)

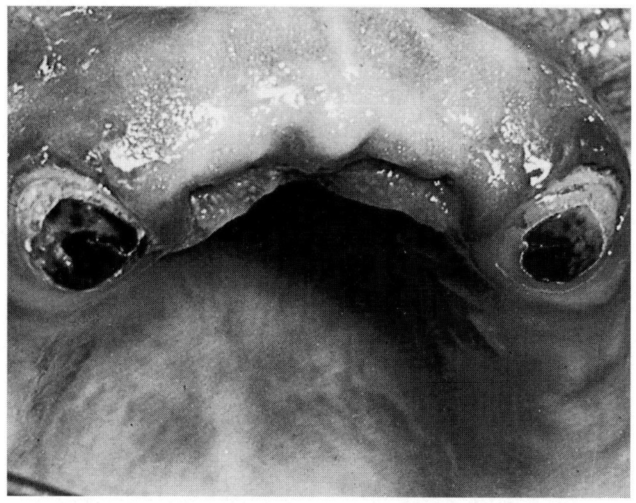

Figure 19-41 Two-year recall reveals advanced caries and periodontal disease of abutments. The patient did not remove the denture for days at a time. (Courtesy of Dr. David H. Wands.)

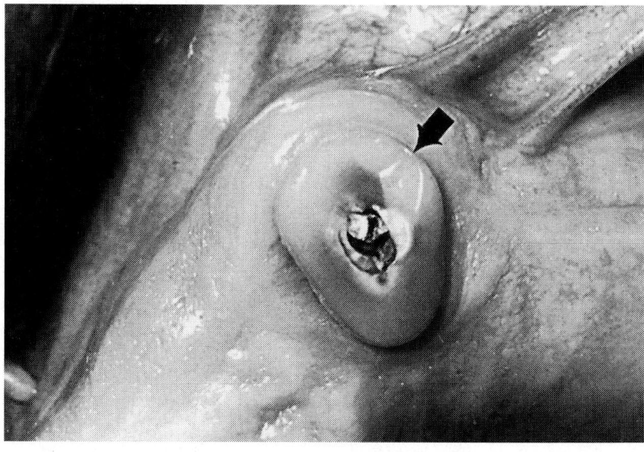

Figure 19-42 Severe abrasion (**arrow**) caused by bruxism. For long-term overdenture success, such an abutment needs post and coping. Reproduced with permission from Robbins JW. J Am Dent Assoc 1980;100:858.

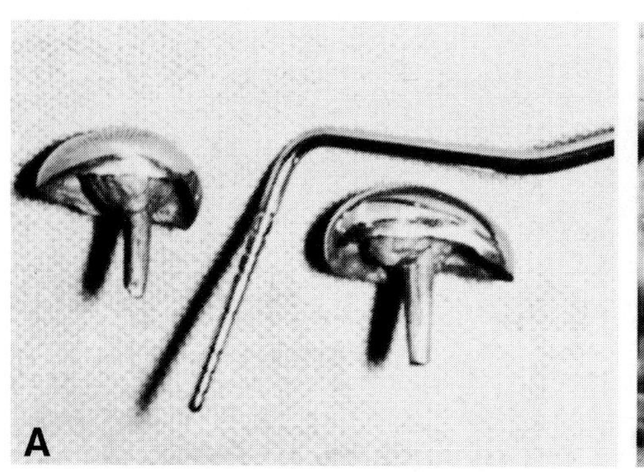

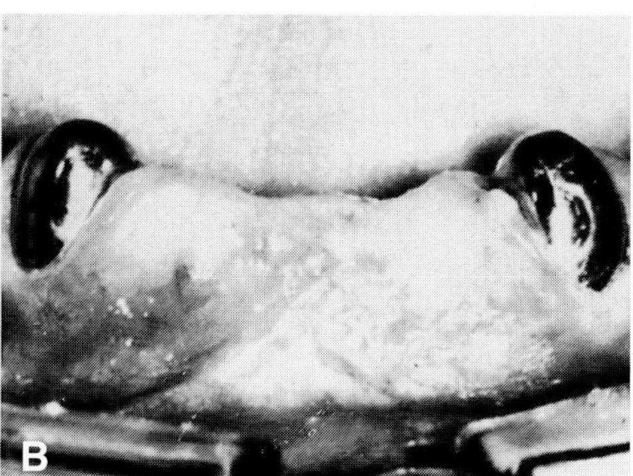

Figure 19-43 **A,** Cast post and copings, properly contoured and polished to restore abutment teeth. **B,** Two-year recall shows a healthy response to this ideal, albeit expensive, restorative method. Reproduced with permission from Lord JL and Teel S.[145]

they include ball and socket type of attachments, o-rings, and magnets.

REFERENCES

1. Fauchard P. The surgeon dentist. 2nd ed. Vol II. Birmingham (AL): Classics of Dentistry Library; 1980.
2. Prothero JH. Prosthetic dentistry. 2nd ed. Chicago: Medico-Dental Publishing; 1916.
3. Harris CA. The dental art. Baltimore: Armstrong and Berry; 1839.
4. Richardson J. A practical treatise on mechanical dentistry. Philadelphia: Lindsay and Blakiston; 1880.
5. Tomes J. Dental physiology and surgery. London: John W. Parker, West Strand; 1848.
6. Sorensen JA, Martinoff JT. Intracoronal reinforcement and coronal coverage: a study of endodontically treated teeth. J Prosthet Dent 1984;51:780.
7. Scurria MS, Shugars DA, Hayden WJ, Felton DA. General dentists' patterns of restoring endodontically treated teeth. J Am Dent Assoc 1995;126:775.
8. Reuter JE, Brose MO. Failures in full crown retained dental bridges. Br Dent J 1984;157:61.
9. Randow K, Glantz PO, Zöger B. Technical failures and some related clinical complications in extensive fixed prosthodontics. Acta Odontol Scand 1986;44:241.
10. Karlsson S. A clinical evaluation of fixed bridges, 10 years following insertion. J Oral Rehabil 1986;13:423.
11. Palmqvist S, Swartz B. Artificial crowns and fixed partial dentures 18 to 23 years after placement. Int J Prosthodont 1993;6:279.
12. Sundh B, Ödman P. A study of fixed prosthodontics performed at a university clinic 18 years after insertion. Int J Prosthodont 1997;10:513.
13. Gutmann JL. The dentin-root complex: anatomic and biologic considerations in restoring endodontically treated teeth. J Prosthet Dent 1992;67:458.
14. Helfer AR, Schilder H. Determination of the moisture content of vital and pulpless teeth. Oral Surg Oral Med Oral Pathol 1972;34:661.
15. Reeh ES, Messer HH, Douglas WH. Reduction in tooth stiffness as a result of endodontic and restorative procedures. J Endod 1989;15:512.
16. Tidmarsh BG. Restoration of endodontically treated posterior teeth. J Endod 1976;2:374.
17. Grimaldi J. Measurement of the lateral deformation of the tooth crown under axial compressive cuspal loading [thesis]. Dunedin (New Zealand): Univ. of Otago; 1971.
18. Carter JM, Sorensen SE, Johnson RR, et al. Punch shear testing of extracted vital and endodontically treated teeth. J Biomech 1983;16:841.
19. Rivera E, Yamauchi G, Chandler G, Bergenholtz G. Dentin collagen cross-links of root-filled and normal teeth. J Endod 1988;14:195.
20. Lovdahl PE, Nicholls JI. Pin-retained amalgam cores vs. cast-gold dowel-cores. J Prosthet Dent 1977;38:507.
21. Lu YC. A comparative study of fracture resistance of pulpless teeth. Chin Dent J 1987;6:26.
22. McDonald AV, King PA, Setchell DJ. An in vitro study to compare impact fracture resistance of intact root-treated teeth. Int Dent J 1990;23:304.
23. Guzy GE, Nicholls JI. In vitro comparison of intact endodontically treated teeth with and without endo-post reinforcement. J Prosthet Dent 1979;42:39.
24. Leary JM, Aquilino SA, Svare CW. An evaluation of post length within the eleastic limits of dentin. J Prosthet Dent 1987;57:277.
25. Trope M, Maltz DO, Tronstad L. Resistance to fracture of restored endodontically treated teeth. Endod Dent Traumatol 1985;1:108.

25a. Eshelman EG Jr, Sayegh FS. Dowel materials and root fracture. J Prosthet Dent 1983;50:342.

26. Hunter AJ, Feiglin B, Williams JF. Effects of post placement on endodontically treated teeth. J Prosthet Dent 1989;62:166.
27. Ko CC, Chu CS, Chung KH, Lee MC. Effects of posts on dentin stress distribution in pulpless teeth. J Prosthet Dent 1992;68:421.
28. Sorensen JA, Martinoff JT. Endodontically treated teeth as abutments. J Prosthet Dent 1985;53:631.
29. Eckerbom M, Magnusson T, Martinsson T. Prevalence of apical periodontitis, crowned teeth and teeth with posts in a Swedish population. Endodont Dent Traumatol 1991;7:214.
30. Morfis AS. Vertical root fractures. Oral Surg Oral Med Oral Pathol 1990;69:631.
31. Hussey DL, Killough SA. A survey of general dental practitioners' approach to the restoration of root-filled teeth. Int Endod J 1995;28:91.
32. Morgano SM, Hashem AF, Fotoohi K, Rose L. A nationwide survey of contemporary philosophies and techniques of restoring endodontically treated teeth. J Prosthet Dent 1994;72:259.
33. Turner CH. The utilization of roots to carry post-retained crowns. J Oral Rehabil 1982;9:193.
34. Hatzikyriakos AH, Reisis GI, Tsingos N. A 3-year postoperative clinical evaluation of posts and cores beneath existing crowns. J Prosthet Dent 1992;67:454.
35. Sorensen JA, Martinoff JF. Clinically significant factors in dowel design. J Prosthet Dent 1984;52:28.
36. Bergman B, Lundquist P, Sjögren U, Sundquist G. Restorative and endodontic results after treatment with cast posts and cores. J Prosthet Dent 1989;61:10.
37. Torbjörner A, Karlsson S, Ödman PA. Survival rate and failure characteristics for two post designs. J Prosthet Dent 1995;73:439.
38. Weine FS, Wax AH, Wenckus CS. Restrospective study of tapered, smooth post systems in place for ten years or more. J Endod 1991;17:293.
39. Mentink AGB, Meeuwissen R, Käyser AF, Mulder J. Survival rate and failure characteristics of the all metal post and core restoration. J Oral Rehabil 1993;20:455.
40. Wallerstedt D, Eliasson S, Sundström F. A follow-up study of screwpost-retained amalgam crowns. Swed Dent J 1984;8:165.
41. Creugers NHJ, Mentink AGB, Käyser AF. An analysis of durability data on post and core restorations. J Dent 1993;21:281.
42. Roberts DH. The failure of retainers in bridge prostheses. Br Dent J 1970;128:117.
43. Turner CH. Post-retained crown failure: a survey. Dent Update 1982;9:221.
44. Lewis R, Smith BGN. A clinical survey of failed post retained crowns. Br Dent J 1988;165:95.

45. Linde LÅ. The use of composites as core material in root-filled teeth. Swed Dent J 1984;8:209.
46. Ross IF. Fracture susceptibility of endodontically treated teeth. J Endod 1980;6:560.
47. Henry PJ. Photoelastic analysis of post core restorations. Aus Dent J 1977;22:157.
48. Ross RS, Nicholls JI, Harrington GW. A comparison of strains generated during placement of five endodontic posts. J Endod 1991;17:450.
49. Standlee JP, Caputo AA, Holcomb JP. The dentatus screw: comparative stress analysis with other endodontic dowel designs. J Oral Rehabil 1982;9:23.
50. Deutsch AS, Musikant BL, Cavallari J, et al. Root fracture during insertion of prefabricated posts related to root size. J Prosthet Dent 1985;53:786.
51. Thorsteinsson TS, Yaman P, Craig RG. Stress analyses of four prefabricated posts. J Prosthet Dent 1992;67:30.
52. Standlee JP, Caputo AA. The retentive and stress distributing properties of split threaded endodontic dowels. J Prosthet Dent 1992;68:436.
53. Standlee JP, Caputo AA, Holcomb J, Trabert KC. The retentive and stress-distributing properties of a threaded endodontic dowel. J Prosthet Dent 1980;44:398.
54. Standlee JP, Caputo AA, Collard EW, Pollack MH. Analysis of stress distribution by endodontic posts. Oral Surg 1972;33:952.
55. Caputo AA, Hokama SN. Stress and retention properties of a new threaded endodontic post. Quintessence Int 1987;18:431.
56. Rolf KC, Parker MW, Pelleu GB. Stress analysis of five prefabricated endodontic dowel designs: A photoelastic study. Oper Dent 1992;17:86.
57. Cohen BI, Musikant BL, Deutsch AS. Comparison of the photoelastic stress for a split-shank threaded post versus a threaded post. J Prosthodont 1994;3:53.
58. Davy DT, Dilley GL, Krejci RF. Determination of stress patterns in root-filled teeth incorporating various dowel designs. J Dent Res 1981;60:1301.
59. Peters MCRB, Poort HW, Farah JW, Craig RG. Stress analysis of a tooth restored with a post and core. J Dent Res 1983;62:760.
60. Assif D, Oren E, Marshak BL, Aviv I. Photoelastic analysis of stress transfer by endodontically treated teeth to the supporting structure using different restorative techniques. J Prosthet Dent 1989;61:535.
61. Sorensen JA, Engelman MJ. Effect of post adaptation on fracture resistance of endodontically treated teeth. J Prosthet Dent 1990;64:419.
62. Assif D, Bitenski A, Pilo R, Oren E. Effect of post design on resistance to fracture of endodontically treated teeth with complete crowns. J Prosthet Dent 1993;69:36.
63. Harper RH, Lund MR. Treatment of the pulpless tooth during post and core construction. Oper Dent 1976;1:55.
64. Mondelli J, Piccino AC, Berbert A. An acrylic resin pattern for a cast dowel and core. J Prosthet Dent 1971;25:413.
65. Pickard HM. Variants of the post crown. Br Dent J 1964;117:517.
66. Blaukopf ER. Direct acrylic davis crown technic. J Am Dent Assoc 1944;31:1270.
67. Sheets CE. Dowel and core foundations. J Prosthet Dent 1970;23:58.
68. Goldrich N. Construction of posts for teeth with existing restorations. J Prosthet Dent 1970;23:173.
69. Rosen H. Operative procedures on mutilated endodontically treated teeth. J Prosthet Dent 1961;11:973.
70. Rosenberg PA, Antonoff SJ. Gold posts. Common problems in preparation and technique for fabrication. N Y State Dent J 1971;37:601.
71. Silverstein WH. Reinforcement of weakened pulpless teeth. J Prosthet Dent 1964;14:372.
72. Dooley BS. Preparation and construction of post retention crowns for anterior teeth. Aust Dent J 1967;12:544.
73. Baraban DJ. The restoration of pulpless teeth. Dent Clin North Am 1967;11:633–53.
74. Jacoby WE. Practical technique for the fabrication of a direct pattern for a post core restoration. J Prosthet Dent 1976;35:357.
75. Dewhirst RB, Fish DW, Schillingburg HT. Dowel core fabrication. J South Calif Dent Assoc 1969;37:444.
76. Hamilton AI. Porcelain dowel crowns. J Prosthet Dent 1959;9:639.
77. Larato DC. Single unit cast post crown for pulpless anterior tooth roots. J Prosthet Dent 1966;16:145.
78. Christy JM, Pipko DJ. Fabrication of a dual post veneer crown. J Am Dent Assoc 1967;75:1419.
79. Bartlett SO. Construction of detached core crowns for pulpless teeth in only two sittings. J Am Dent Assoc 1968;77:843.
80. Burnell SC. Improved cast dowel and base for restoring endodontically treated teeth. J Am Dent Assoc 1964;68:39.
81. Perel ML, Muroff FI. Clinical criteria for posts and cores. J Prosthet Dent 1972;28:405.
82. Stern N, Hirschfeld Z. Principles of preparing endodontically treated teeth for dowel and core restorations. J Prosthet Dent 1973;30:162.
83. Hirschfeld Z, Stern N. Post and core—the biomechanical aspect. Aus Dent J 1972;17:467.
84. Grieve AR, McAndrew R. A radiographic study of post-retained crowns in patients attending a dental hospital. Br Dent J 1993;174:197.
85. Martin N, Jedynakiewicz N. A radiographic survey of endodontic post lengths [abstract]. J Dent Res 1989;68:919.
86. Johnson JK, Sakumura JS. Dowel form and tensile force. J Prosthet Dent 1978;40:645.
87. Leary JM, Aquilino SA, Svare CW. An evaluation of post length within the elastic limits of dentin. J Prosthet Dent 1987;57:277.
88. Zillich RM, Corcoran JF. Average maximum post lengths in endodontically treated teeth. J Prosthet Dent 1984;52:489.
89. Shillingburg HT, Kessler JC, Wilson EL. Root dimensions and dowel size. Calif Dent Assoc J 1982;10:43.
90. Abou-Rass M, Jann JM, Jobe D, Tsutsui F. Preparation of space for posting: effect on thickness of canal walls and incidence of perforation in molars. J Am Dent Assoc 1982;104:834.
91. Reinhardt RA, Krejci RF, Pao Y, Stannard JG. Dentin stresses in post-reconstructed teeth with diminishing bone support. J Dent Res 1983;62:1002.
92. Buranadham S, Aquilino SA, Stanford CM. Relation between dowel extension and bone level in anterior teeth [abstract]. J Dent Res 1999;78:222.
93. Camp LR, Todd MJ. The effect of dowel preparation on the apical seal of three common obturation techniques. J Prosthet Dent 1983;50:664.

94. Madison S, Zakariasen KL. Linear and volumetric analysis of apical leakage in teeth prepared for posts. J Endod 1984;10:422.
95. Neagley RL. The effect of dowel preparation on the apical seal of endodontically treated teeth. Oral Surg Oral Med Oral Pathol 1969;28:739.
96. Portell FR, Bernier WE, Lorton L, Peters DD. The effect of immediate versus delayed dowel space preparation on the integrity of the apical seal. J Endod 1982;8:154.
97. Mattison GD, Delivanis PD, Thacker RW, Hassell KJ. Effect of post preparation on the apical seal. J Prosthet Dent 1984;51:785.
98. Nixon C, Vertucci FJ, Swindle R. The effect of post space preparation on the apical seal of root canal obturated teeth. Todays FDA 1991;3:1–6C.
99. Kvist T, Rydin E, Reit C. The relative frequency of periapical lesions in teeth with root canal-retained posts. J Endod 1989;15:578.
100. Turner CH, Willoughby AFW. The retention of vented-cast dental posts. J Dent 1985;13:267.
101. Standlee JP, Caputo AA, Hanson EC. Retention of endodontic dowels: effects of cement, dowel length, diameter, and design. J Prosthet Dent 1978;39:401.
102. Kurer HG, Combe EC, Grant AA. Factors influencing the retention of dowels. J Prosthet Dent 1977;38:515.
103. Hanson EC, Caputo AA. Cementing mediums and retentive characteristics of dowels. J Prosthet Dent 1974;32:551.
104. Krupp JD, Caputo AA, Trabert KC, Standlee JP. Dowel retention with glass-ionomer cement. J Prosthet Dent 1979;41:163.
105. Mattison GD. Photoelastic stress analysis of cast-gold endodontic posts. J Prosthet Dent 1982;48:407.
106. Trabert KC, Caputo AA, Abou-Rass M. Tooth fracture—a comparison of endodontic and restorative treatments. J Endod 1978;4:341.
107. Lloyd PM, Palik JF. The philosophies of dowel diameter preparation: a literature review. J Prosthet Dent 1993;69:32.
108. Tilk MA, Lommel TJ, Gerstein H. A study of mandibular and maxillary root widths to determine dowel size. J Endod 1979;5:79.
109. Raiden G, Costa L, Koss S, Hernández J, Aceñolaza V. Residual thickness of root in first maxillary premolars with post space preparation. J Endod 1999;25:502.
110. Bourgeois RS, Lemon RR, Dowel space preparation and apical leakage. J Endod 1981;7:66.
111. Zmener O. Effect of dowel preparation on the apical seal of endodontically treated teeth. J Endod 1980;6:687.
112. Schnell FJ. Effect of immediate dowel space preparation on the apical seal of endodontically filled teeth. Oral Surg 1978;45:470.
113. Dickey DJ, Harris GZ, Lemon RR, Leubke RG. Effect of post space preparation on apical seal using solvent techniques and peeso reamers. J Endod 1982;8:351.
114. Kwan EH, Harrington GW. The effect of immediate post preparation on apical seal. J Endod 1981;7:325.
115. Karapanou V, Vera J, Cabrera P, et al. Effect of immediate and delayed post preparation on apical dye leakage using two different sealers. J Endod 1996;22:583.
116. Fan B, Wu MK, Wesselink PR. Coronal leakage along apical root fillings after immediate and delayed post space preparation. Endod Dent Traumatol 1999;15:124.
117. Suchina JA, Ludington JR. Dowel space preparation and the apical seal. J Endod 1985;11:11.
118. Hiltner RS, Kulild JC, Weller RN. Effect of mechanical versus thermal removal of gutta-percha on the quality of the apical seal following post space preparation. J Endod 1992;18:451.
119. Haddix JE, Mattison GD, Shulman CA, Pink FE. Post preparation techniques and their effect on the apical seal. J Prosthet Dent 1990;64:515.
120. Barkhordar RA, Radke R, Abbasi J. Effect of metal collars on resistance of endodontically treated teeth to root fracture. J Prosthet Dent 1989;61:676.
121. Tjan AHL, Whang SB. Resistant to root fracture of dowel channels with various thicknesses of buccal dentin walls. J Prosthet Dent 1985;53:496.
122. Loney RW, Kotowicz WE, McDowell GC. Three-dimensional photoelastic stress analysis of the ferrule effect in cast post and cores. J Prosthet Dent 1990;63:506.
123. Hemmings KW, King PA, Setchell DJ. Resistance to torsional forces of various post and core designs. J Prosthet Dent 1991;66:325.
124. Saupe WA, Gluskin AH, Radke RA Jr. A comparative study of fracture resistance between morphologic dowel and cores and a resin-reinforced dowel system in the intraradicular restoration of structurally compromised roots. Quintessence Int 1996;27:483.
125. Libman WJ, Nicholls JI. Load fatigue of teeth restored with cast posts and cores and complete crowns. Int J Prosthodont 1995;8:155.
126. Milot P, Stein RS. Root fracture in endodontically treated teeth related to post selection and crown design. J Prosthet Dent 1992;68:428.
127. Isidor F, Brøndum K, Ravnholt G. The influence of post length and crown ferrule length on the resistance to cyclic loading of bovine teeth with prefabricated titanium posts. Int J Prosthodont 1999;12:78.
128. Hoag EP, Dwyer TG. A comparative evaluation of three post and core techniques. J Prosthet Dent 1982;47:177.
129. Sorensen JA, Engelman MJ. Ferrule design and fracture resistance of endodontically treated teeth. J Prosthet Dent 1990;63:529.
130. Rosen H, Partida-Rivera M. Iatrogenic fracture of roots reinforced with a cervical collar. Oper Dent 1986;11:46.
131. Ouzounian ZS, Schilder H. Remaining dentin thickness after endodontic cleaning and shaping before post space preparation. Oral Health 1991;81:13.
132. Pilo R, Tamse A. Residual dentin thickness in mandibular premolars prepared with Gates Glidden and ParaPost drills. J Prosthet Dent 2000;83:617.
133. Isidor F, Ödman P, Brøndum K. Intermittent loading of teeth restored using prefabricated carbon fiber posts. Int J Prosthodont 1996;9:131.
134. Purton DG, Payne JA. Comparison of carbon fiber and stainless steel root canal posts. Quintessence Int 1996;27:93.
135. Sidoli GE, King PA, Stechell DJ. An in vitro evaluation of a carbon fiber-based post and core system. J Prosthet Dent 1997;78:5.
136. Dean JP, Jeansonne BG, Sarkar N. In vitro evaluation of a carbon fiber post. J Endod 1998;24:807.
137. Fredriksson M, Astbäck J, Pamenius M, Arvidson K. A retrospective study of 236 patients with teeth restored by carbon fiber-reinforced epoxy resin posts. J Prosthet Dent 1998;80:151.

138. Martinez-Insua A, da-Silva L, Rilo B, Santana U. Comparison of the fracture resistances of pulpless teeth restored with a cast post and core or carbon-fiber post with a composite core. J Prosthet Dent 1998;80:527.
139. Asmussen E, Peutzfeldt A, Heitmann T. Stiffness, elastic limit, and strength of newer types of endodontic posts. J Dent 1999;27:275.
140. Kakehashi Y, Luthy H, Naef R, et al. A new all-ceramic post and core system: clinical, technical, and in vitro results. Int J Periodont Restor Dent 1998;18:586.
141. Rosentritt M, Furer C, Behr M, et al. Comparison of in vitro fracture strength of metallic and tooth-coloured posts and cores. J Oral Rehabil 2000;27:595.
142. Koutayas SO, Kern M. All-ceramic posts and cores: the state of the art. Quintessence Int 1999;30:383.
143. Sirimai S, Riis DN, Morgano SM. An in vitro study of the fracture resistance and the incidence of vertical root fracture of pulpless teeth restored with six post-and-core systems. J Prosthet Dent 1999;81:262.
144. Lord JL, Teel S. The overdenture: patient selection, use of copings, and follow-up evaluation. J Prosthet Dent 1974;32:41.
145. Lord JL, Teel S. The overdenture. Dent Clin North Am 1969;13:871.
146. Sognnaes RF. America's most famous teeth. Smithsonian 1973;3:47.
147. Shannon IL. Chemical preventive dentistry for overdenture patients. In: Brewer AA, Morrow RM, editors. Overdentures. 2nd ed. St. Louis: CV Mosby; 1980. p. 322–40.
148. Key MC. Topical fluoride treatment of overdenture abutments. Gen Dent 1980;28:58.
149. Brewer AA, Morrow RM. Overdenture problems. In: Brewer AA, Morrow RM, editors. Overdentures. 2nd ed. St. Louis: CV Mosby; 1980. p. 345.

INDEX

Page numbers followed by "f" indicate figures; page numbers followed by "t" indicate tables.